471.47

05/18/12: 799.18

MILADY STANDARD

AUTHORS FOR
2012 EDITION:
Catherine M. Frangie
Alisha Rimando Botero
Colleen Hennessey
Dr. Mark Lees
Bonnie Sanford
Frank Shipman
Victoria Wurdinger

EDITORIAL CONTRIBUTORS
FOR 2012 EDITION:
John Halal
Randy Ferman
Jim McConnell
Janet McCormick
Vicki Peters
Douglas Schoon

COSMETOLOGY

CENGAGE Learning™
Australia Brazil Japan Korea Mexico Singapore Spain United Kingdom United States

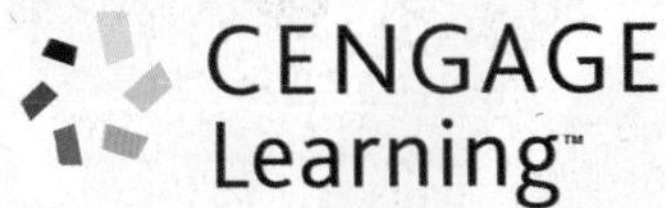

Milady Standard Cosmetology
Author: Milady

President, Milady: Dawn Gerrain
Senior Product Manager: Philip Mandl
Editorial Assistant: Maria K. Hebert
Director of Beauty Industry Relations: Sandra Bruce
Executive Marketing Manager: Gerard McAvey
Production Director: Wendy Troeger
Senior Content Project Manager: Angela Sheehan
Senior Content Project Manager: Nina Tucciarelli
Design Director: Bruce Bond
Art Director: Benj Gleeksman
Senior Art Director: Joy Kocsis
Cover and title page photo: © Adrianna Williams/Corbis

© 2012, 2008, 2004, 2000, 1996, 1991, 1985, 1981, 1972, 1967, 1965, 1959, 1954, 1938 Milady®, a part of Cengage Learning

ALL RIGHTS RESERVED. No part of this work covered by the copyright herein may be reproduced, transmitted, stored, or used in any form or by any means graphic, electronic, or mechanical, including but not limited to photocopying, recording, scanning, digitizing, taping, Web distribution, information networks, or information storage and retrieval systems, except as permitted under Section 107 or 108 of the 1976 United States Copyright Act, without the prior written permission of the publisher.

For product information and technology assistance, contact us at
Professional & Career Group Customer Support, 1-800-648-7450

For permission to use material from this text or product, submit all requests online at **cengage.com/permissions.**
Further permissions questions can be e-mailed to
permissionrequest@cengage.com.

Library of Congress Control Number: 2007941007

Hardcover
ISBN-13: 978-1-4390-5930-2
ISBN-10: 1-4390-5930-6

Softcover
ISBN-13: 978-1-4390-5929-6
ISBN-10: 1-4390-5929-2

Milady
5 Maxwell Drive
Clifton Park, NY 12065-2919
USA

Cengage Learning products are represented in Canada by Nelson Education, Ltd.

For your lifelong learning solutions, visit **milady.cengage.com.**

Visit our corporate Web site at **cengage.com**.

Notice to the Reader

Publisher does not warrant or guarantee any of the products described herein or perform any independent analysis in connection with any of the product information contained herein. Publisher does not assume, and expressly disclaims, any obligation to obtain and include information other than that provided to it by the manufacturer. The reader is expressly warned to consider and adopt all safety precautions that might be indicated by the activities described herein and to avoid all potential hazards. By following the instructions contained herein, the reader willingly assumes all risks in connection with such instructions. The publisher makes no representations or warranties of any kind, including but not limited to, the warranties of fitness for particular purpose or merchantability, nor are any such representations implied with respect to the material set forth herein, and the publisher takes no responsibility with respect to such material. The publisher shall not be liable for any special, consequential, or exemplary damages resulting, in whole or part, from the readers' use of, or reliance upon, this material.

Printed in the United States of America
1 2 3 4 5 XXX 15 14 13 12 11

MILADY STANDARD

AUTHORS FOR
2012 EDITION:
Catherine M. Frangie
Alisha Rimando Botero
Colleen Hennessey
Dr. Mark Lees
Bonnie Sanford
Frank Shipman
Victoria Wurdinger

EDITORIAL CONTRIBUTORS
FOR 2012 EDITION:
John Halal
Randy Ferman
Jim McConnell
Janet McCormick
Vicki Peters
Douglas Schoon

COSMETOLOGY

CENGAGE Learning™

Australia Brazil Japan Korea Mexico Singapore Spain United Kingdom United States

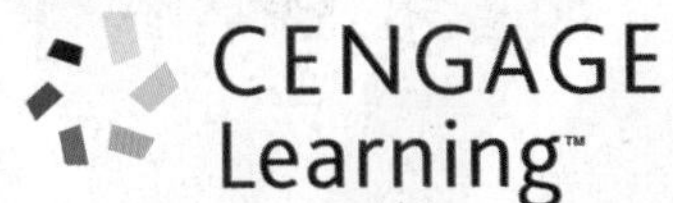

Milady Standard Cosmetology
Author: Milady

President, Milady: Dawn Gerrain
Senior Product Manager: Philip Mandl
Editorial Assistant: Maria K. Hebert
Director of Beauty Industry Relations: Sandra Bruce
Executive Marketing Manager: Gerard McAvey
Production Director: Wendy Troeger
Senior Content Project Manager: Angela Sheehan
Senior Content Project Manager: Nina Tucciarelli
Design Director: Bruce Bond
Art Director: Benj Gleeksman
Senior Art Director: Joy Kocsis
Cover and title page photo: © Adrianna Williams/Corbis

© 2012, 2008, 2004, 2000, 1996, 1991, 1985, 1981, 1972, 1967, 1965, 1959, 1954, 1938 Milady®, a part of Cengage Learning

ALL RIGHTS RESERVED. No part of this work covered by the copyright herein may be reproduced, transmitted, stored, or used in any form or by any means graphic, electronic, or mechanical, including but not limited to photocopying, recording, scanning, digitizing, taping, Web distribution, information networks, or information storage and retrieval systems, except as permitted under Section 107 or 108 of the 1976 United States Copyright Act, without the prior written permission of the publisher.

For product information and technology assistance, contact us at
Professional & Career Group Customer Support, 1-800-648-7450
For permission to use material from this text or product,
submit all requests online at **cengage.com/permissions.**
Further permissions questions can be e-mailed to
permissionrequest@cengage.com.

Library of Congress Control Number: 2007941007

Hardcover
ISBN-13: 978-1-4390-5930-2
ISBN-10: 1-4390-5930-6

Softcover
ISBN-13: 978-1-4390-5929-6
ISBN-10: 1-4390-5929-2

Milady
5 Maxwell Drive
Clifton Park, NY 12065-2919
USA

Cengage Learning products are represented in Canada by Nelson Education, Ltd.

For your lifelong learning solutions, visit **milady.cengage.com.**

Visit our corporate Web site at **cengage.com**.

Notice to the Reader
Publisher does not warrant or guarantee any of the products described herein or perform any independent analysis in connection with any of the product information contained herein. Publisher does not assume, and expressly disclaims, any obligation to obtain and include information other than that provided to it by the manufacturer. The reader is expressly warned to consider and adopt all safety precautions that might be indicated by the activities described herein and to avoid all potential hazards. By following the instructions contained herein, the reader willingly assumes all risks in connection with such instructions. The publisher makes no representations or warranties of any kind, including but not limited to, the warranties of fitness for particular purpose or merchantability, nor are any such representations implied with respect to the material set forth herein, and the publisher takes no responsibility with respect to such material. The publisher shall not be liable for any special, consequential, or exemplary damages resulting, in whole or part, from the readers' use of, or reliance upon, this material.

Printed in the United States of America
1 2 3 4 5 XXX 15 14 13 12 11

Contents in Brief

Table of Contents

Procedures at a Glance

Preface

Milady Standard Cosmetology

Congratulations! You are about to begin a journey that can take you in many directions and that holds the potential to make you a confident, successful professional in cosmetology. As a cosmetologist, you will become a trusted professional, the person your clients rely on to provide ongoing services that enable them to look and feel their best. You will become as personally involved in your clients' lives as their physicians or dentists, and with study and practice, you will have the opportunity to showcase your artistic and creative ideas for the entire world to see!

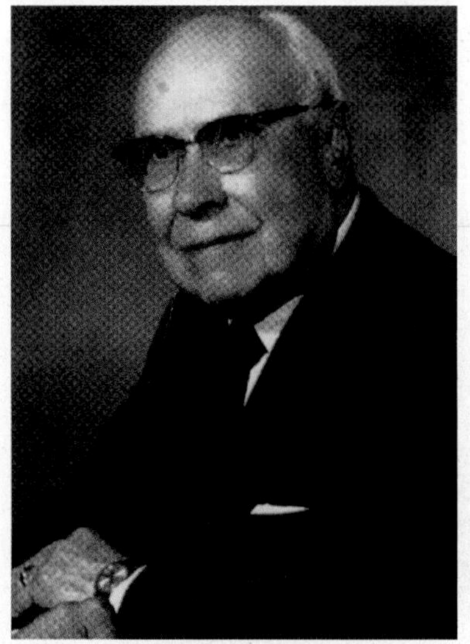

© Milady, a part of Cengage Learning.

Mr. Nicholas F. Cimaglia, Founder of Milady Publishing Company.

You and your school have chosen the perfect course of study to accomplish all of this and more. *Milady Standard Cosmetology* was the creation of Nicholas F. Cimaglia, founder of Milady Publishing Company, in 1927. The very first edition of *Milady Standard Cosmetology* was published in 1938, and since that time, it has consistently been the most-used cosmetology textbook in the world. Many of the world's most famous, sought-after, successful, and artistic professional cosmetologists have studied this very book!

Milady employs experts from all aspects of the beauty profession—hair care, skin care, nail care, massage, makeup, infection control, and business development—to write for and consult on every textbook published. Since the field of cosmetology is always changing, progressing, and discovering new technologies, services, and styles, Milady keeps a close eye on its texts and is committed to investing the time, energy, resources, and efforts to revising its educational offerings to provide the beauty industry with the most up-to-date and all-encompassing tools available.

So you see, by studying the *Milady Standard Cosmetology*, you have not simply opened the cover of a textbook, you've been adopted by a family of the most well-known and highly respected professional cosmetology educators in the world!

Foreword

A Little Advice from Successful Professionals

You have one decision to make today: Are you going to be your very best self or just get by? That's it. After all, 90 percent of success is showing up, mentally—*and* physically. Are you committed to putting a laser focus on learning?

Education makes your life better, happier, richer. Specialized learning builds confidence, leads to a specific career, and opens dozens of unexpected doors. And if you listen to those who have already traversed the path before you, cosmetology training will provide you with the foundation for an exciting, artistic, limitless career that can fulfill what celebrity stylist Ted Gibson calls "Your Big, BIG dream."

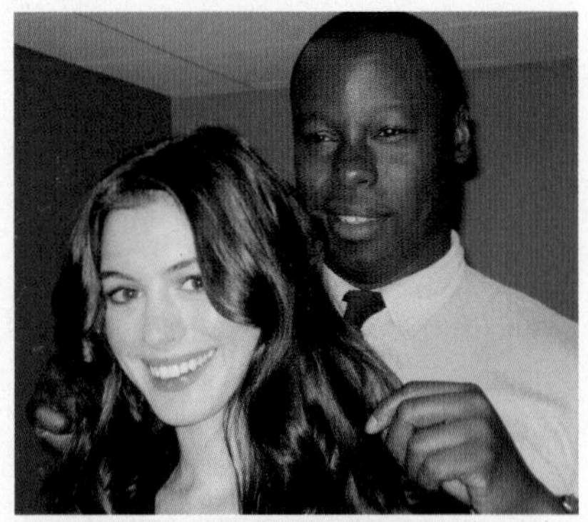

"All my training was the best, because now I can say I am a beauty school graduate and very proud of it. I feel fortunate to have found what makes my heart sing."—Ted Gibson

Ted Gibson styling actress Anne Hathaway. Photo courtesy of Ted Gibson Celebrity Hair Stylist and Owner of the Ted Gibson Salon, NYC.

The 2010 host of TLC's *What Not To Wear* and owner of namesake salons in NYC and Washington, D.C., Gibson says that a solid, basic education is vital because what you learn in beauty school will carry you through your career:

> *"Your cosmetology education gives you the opportunity to do so many things, from working behind the chair to styling celebrities to doing platform work, TV, and movies," says Gibson. "I love this business!"*

The Road to Success

Before you compose your own song of success, take stock of what it will take: hard work, dedication, and plenty of practice. If you've been styling friends' hair since you were ten, you may think you know a lot already, but that's a trap.

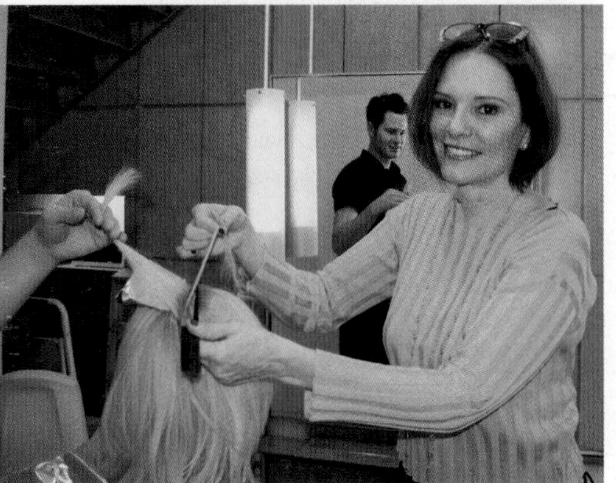

"Being a hairdresser is like being an athlete. Work hard, focus, and ask for more responsibility. If you do, you'll get the honor of being included with successful people." —Beth Minardi

Photo courtesy of Beth Minardi, President Minardi Salon.

Beth Minardi didn't become the country's most accomplished haircolor educator or premiere Manhattan salon owner by happenstance. When she recognized that haircolor was uniquely challenging, she did what all super-successful hairdressers do—she took a chance in order to learn all she could. Armed with a B.A. in Education and Theatre and a cosmetology license, she applied for a job with Clairol. Of her four weeks in training, the first was spent on semipermanent color, the second on the lift and deposit shades, the third on bleaching and toning, and the fourth on special effects.

> *"After each week, you were tested, and if you failed any test, you were fired," recalls Minardi. "It made me realize that there is no fashion without foundation, no creativity without the basics."*

While Minardi credits her mentors for understanding that being a great colorist meant mastering theory and all color products, she stresses that success also requires commitment and a healthy body and mind: "When you go to work, it's show time; there's no room for gossip, personal problems or partying."

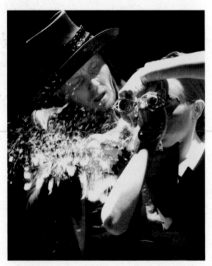

"Developing a great habit of going to school every day will benefit your career as a salon professional. Motivation doesn't change things; good habits do."—Robert Cromeans

Robert Cromeans. Photo courtesy of John Paul Mitchell Systems.

As for creative ideas, the old adage is true: they originate from more perspiration than inspiration. Robert Cromeans, Global Artistic Director for Paul Mitchell and a Paul Mitchell The School owner, is known for cutting hair with a fork, using electric clippers to create a bob, and even using a staple gun. Here's what he says about creative genius:

> *"The truth of the matter is that without the foundation of haircutting under my belt, I would never have been able to create these techniques. It is pivotal to know and understand the rules before you can break them."*

Where Milady Comes In

As you show up each day, ready to be at your mental and physical best, you will have the support of the hundreds of professionals who contributed to the creation of this revised edition of *Milady Standard*

Cosmetology. Milady was part of Cromeans' cosmetology curriculum, as well as Minardi's and Gibson's. Gibson says he still refers to Milady textbooks regularly. In other words, successful stylists never stop learning.

At the Eric Fisher Academy in Wichita, KS, salon and school owner Eric Fisher, who has won numerous artistic and business awards, chose this very textbook for his students because he considers it the most comprehensive one available.

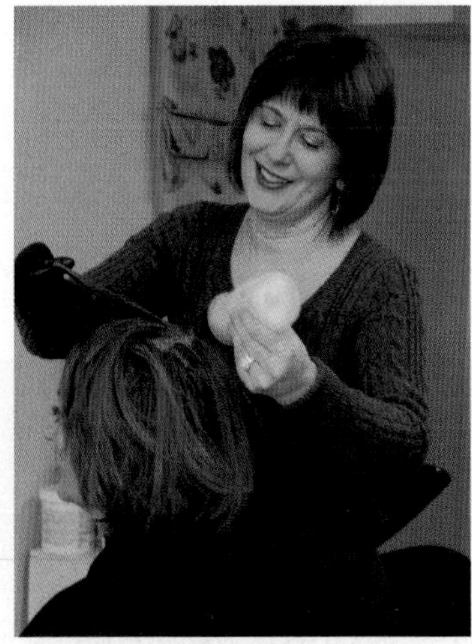

Photo courtesy of Aviva Maller Photography.

"Don't be afraid to admit you have to learn more. Remember, knowledge is power." —Colleen Hennessey

Technical and Artistic Fundamentals

Look through the Table of Contents, and you'll see everything from cutting, coloring, perming, and relaxing to the body's structures, infection control, makeup application, and braiding. Within each chapter, learning objectives are clearly established, terms are simply defined, and review questions help you recall all you've learned.

"Sometimes, you don't even know that you have stumbled upon an aspect of the profession that you will love for the rest of your career," comments Colleen Hennessey, a colorist, salon owner, and P&G School Manager Consultant. "That's why it is important to learn all that you can. Without being exposed to all cosmetology has to offer, you can't make sound choices about the direction you want to take."

Even if you think you already know which area of cosmetology interests you most, developing skills in many disciplines is important because—combined—they provide the solid foundation that can take you anywhere.

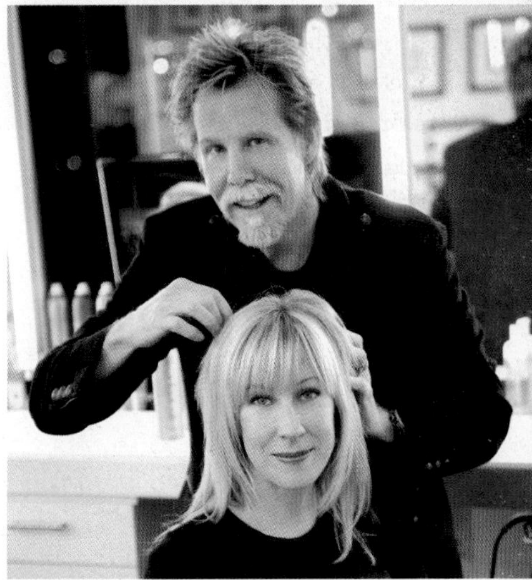

Photo courtesy of Eric Fisher Academy-Salons.

"If you practice anything for one hour every day for 365 days, you can be a national expert. You need the attitude that goes with it, which means embracing the positive. Smile often. Make others feel welcome and important." —Eric Fisher

"When I went to school, I learned roller placement, how to accommodate the hair's movement, and how to work with bone structure," recalls Fisher. "I'm grateful for those basics because they eventually allowed me to travel the world, own a successful business, do hair for video shoots, and more. It's like basketball: you can run, pass, and alley-oop, but the game is won at the free throw line. Fundamentals—strong foundations—build houses that can survive any threat from inside or out."

At Fisher's Academy, the motto is *student for life*, and it works well. His students have gone on to work at top New York City salons, travel the world, and even win the student category at the North American Hairdressing Awards (something Fisher himself won in other categories).

"Every day in school, think about the kind of person you want to be," advises Fisher. "You don't have to be a superstar to achieve greatness—repetition and practice lead to success. Offer to help others just for the opportunity to learn. You have to do more than you get paid for, before you can get paid for more than you do."

Strong Interpersonal Skills

With focus, foundation, repetition, and practice, anyone can master the technical aspects of this wonderful profession. But hairdressing

is also an emotional field, one that requires you to be a *people person.* What that really means is that you must have a positive attitude and be able to listen, read others, and speak their language.

That's why this textbook includes details on conducting a great consultation, working with difficult clients and co-workers, and other life skills that you'll begin to hone during the clinic phase of your training. Throughout the chapters, activities and real-life examples help you develop the good work habits and interpersonal skills that accomplished professionals say are a must.

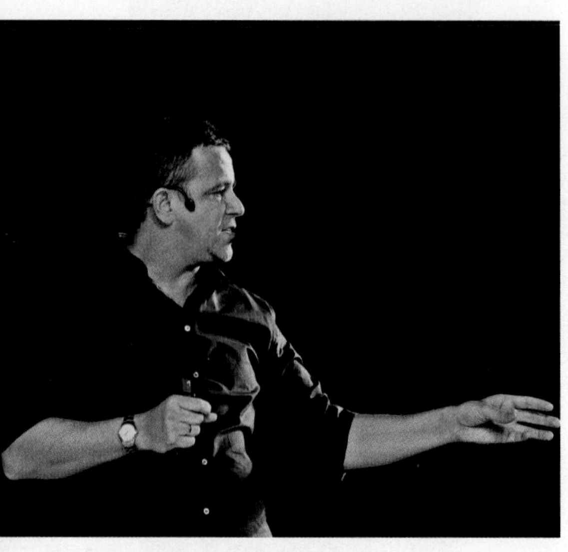

"I believe anyone who shows professionalism, discipline, and commitment over many years of hard work can do what I do." —Nick Arrojo

Photo courtesy of Jammi York/Arrojo.

"Success as a hairdresser is about more than cutting and coloring skills," notes Nick Arrojo, who educates on platform for Wella, oversees his New York City-based Arrojo Studio and Arrojo Education, and preceded Gibson as the hair guru of TLC's What Not To Wear. "You have to be a great communicator. You need to know the challenges of different hair types, the importance of cleanliness, both of yourself and your environment, and you must be able to retail."

"The so-called non-artistic parts of the profession are actually arts in themselves, because you're learning how to communicate with a person who has different tastes and desires than you do," says Minardi. "Your body language, facial expression, and carriage are all part of being successful. After awhile, applying color is the easier part; it takes longer to do the rest well."

Cromeans adds that developing great habits will help you through both the artistic and interpersonal aspects of hairdressing.

"Focus equally on your technical skills and on your dialogue, chair-side manner, and ability to celebrate each (client)," he says.

Business Basics and Beyond

When it comes down to it, cosmetology comprises three tiers. First, it's an *artistically expressive* field. Second, it relies on *human dynamics and personal interaction*, so that one individual can make another look and feel fabulous. Third, cosmetology is a *business.*

The final chapters of this book, which you will study near the end of your schooling, detail the employment search, the job interview, and business basics, from salon design to personnel management. You'll want to refer to these chapters often as you enter the working world and progress toward achieving your *big* dream.

"Your passion for the art may drive your fire, but to succeed, you also need business discipline," says Fisher. "Each stylist should know his or her average service and retail ticket, retention and prebooking rates, and future goals for next week and next month."

"Being a strong business person is the best way to give your creativity the freedom to flourish," stresses Arrojo. "You must have enough money to pay the bills. Keep learning, stay focused, and continue doing the right things every day. There's no race to the finish line. Technique, creativity, confidence, and communication can all be taught, but only with time can you gain experience. With experience, opportunities follow."

Opportunities for Life

Many professionals say that as they grew into their careers, they found themselves wishing they had paid more attention in school. They also say that they are grateful for everything they learned, even things they hadn't thought useful at the time. Hairdressers are no different.

Whether you want to be a Hollywood stylist, a corporate educator, the owner of a spa, or the world's greatest braider, learning all you can now and finding a great mentor will help you achieve your goal.

"Don't get ahead of yourself and think you're a superstar," cautions Hennessey. "Have a good work ethic. Be a team player. Continue your education. And be willing to put in long hours on your feet."

Arrojo stresses that winners are always on time, respect their peers, and accept criticism as a positive learning experience. Cromeans advises forming good habits and being prepared every day to go for it: "You have to be present to win."

"There are no shortcuts to fame," says Minardi. "Your head, heart, and hands are what will make you a success."

If you're ready to apply all three, take a big step toward your future, and turn the page!

The Industry Standard

This edition of *Milady Standard Cosmetology* is jam-packed with new and compelling information and photography that will enable you to not only pass your licensing exams, but also to ensure your success once you are on the job.

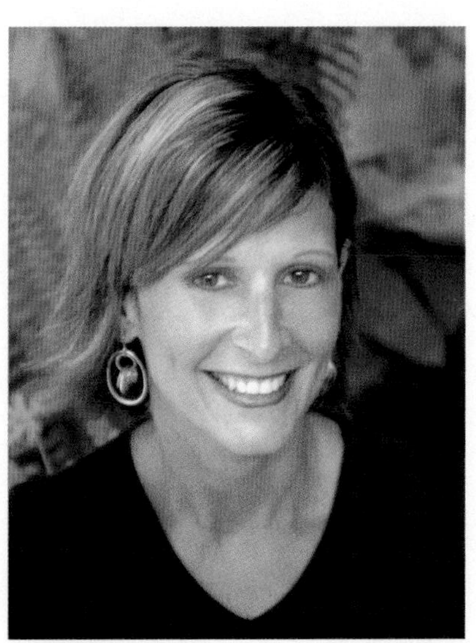

Dawn Gerrain
President
Milady

© Milady, a part of Cengage Learning.

Before beginning this revision, Milady surveyed hundreds of educators and professionals, held focus groups, and received in-depth comments from dozens of reviewers to learn what needed to be changed, added, or deleted from the previous edition. We then consulted with educational experts to learn the best way to present the material, so that all types of learners could understand and remember it. Next we went to several experts in various cosmetology-related fields to write or revise the chapters. Milady then held a seventeen-day photo shoot to update the technical art for chapter and procedural steps. Finally, we sent the finished manuscripts to yet more subject experts to ensure the accuracy and thoroughness of the material. What you hold in your hands is the result. Enjoy it, and best of luck as you start your career in the beauty industry.

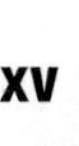

New to this Edition

In response to the suggestions of the cosmetology educators and professionals who reviewed the *Milady Standard Cosmetology* and to those submitted by students who use this text, this edition includes many new features and learning tools.

Alignment

Milady has carefully aligned all of its core textbooks. This means that information appearing in more than one text—whether it be cosmetology, nail technology, or esthetics—now matches from one book to another.

Design

Milady has also dramatically changed the design of the textbook—it now has a very exciting fashion magazine feel—to reflect the innovative and unique energy and artistry found in the beauty business.

Photography and Art

You'll also notice that there are more than 750 new, four-color photographs and illustrations throughout the book, appearing in both chapter content and step-by-step procedures. In addition, all of the new procedure photographs were taken using live models, instead of mannequins.

Pre- and Post-Service Procedures

To drive home the point that pre-service cleaning, disinfecting, and preparing for the client are important, you will find that a unique *Pre-Service Procedure* has been created to specifically address the individual needs of each Part—hair care, skin care, and nail care. Additionally, a *Post-Service Procedure* has been created to address cleaning, disinfecting, and organizing after servicing a client. Both the *Pre-Service* and *Post-Service Procedures* appear in every part of the text for you to quickly and easily refer to and follow.

Why Study This?

Milady knows, understands, and appreciates how excited students are to delve into the newest and most exciting haircutting, styling, and coloring trends, and we recognize that students can sometimes feel restless spending time learning the basics of the profession. To help you understand why you are learning each chapter's material and to help you see the role it will play in your future career as a cosmetologist, Milady has added this new section to each chapter. The section includes three or four bullet points that tell you why the material is important and how you will use the material in your professional career.

Left-Handed Instruction

This new edition includes left-handed procedures in the haircutting, hairstyling, and haircoloring chapters with full color photography. For the first time in a textbook students will see professionals using their left hand to hold and manipulate hair and tools.

All About Shears

One of the most important and costly tools a cosmetologist will buy is a pair—or several pairs—of haircutting shears, so Milady has dedicated an entire section of the haircutting chapter to never-before-available information on how to purchase, use, and maintain your shears. The section is complete with photos of the kinds of shears available and the proper way to care for them.

New Organization of Chapters

The information in this text, along with your teachers' instruction, will enable you to develop the abilities you need to build a loyal and satisfied clientele. To help you locate information more easily, the chapters are grouped into six main parts.

Part 1: Orientation

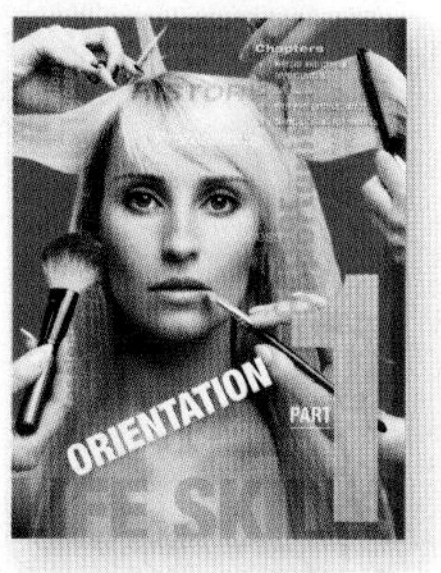

Orientation consists of four chapters that cover the field of cosmetology and the personal skills you will need to become successful. Chapter 1, "History and Career Opportunities," outlines how the profession of cosmetology came into being and where it can take you. In Chapter 2, "Life Skills," the ability to set goals and maintain a good attitude is emphasized, along with the psychology of success. Chapter 3, "Your Professional Image," stresses the importance of inward beauty and health as well as outward appearance, and Chapter 4, "Communicating for Success," describes the important process of building client relationships based on trust and effective communication.

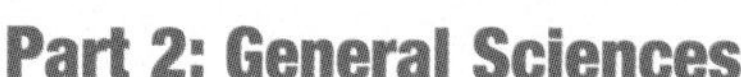

Part 2: General Sciences

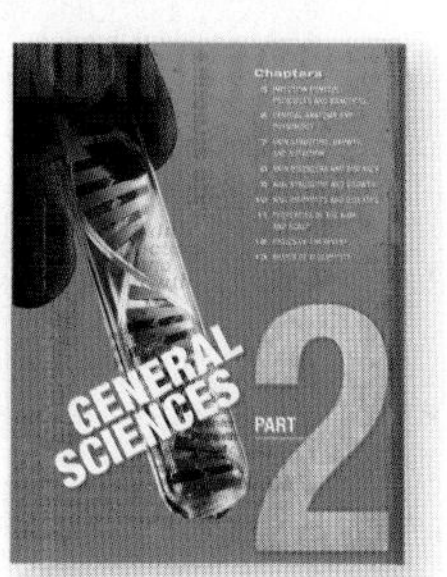

General Sciences includes important information you need to know in order to keep yourself and your clients safe and healthy. Chapter 5, "Infection Control: Principles and Practices," offers the most current, vital facts about hepatitis, HIV, and other infectious viruses and bacteria and tells how to prevent their spread in the salon. The remaining chapters in Part 2—"General Anatomy and Physiology," "Skin Structure, Growth, and Nutrition," "Skin Disorders and Diseases," "Nail Structure and Growth," "Nail Disorders and Diseases," "Properties of the Hair and Scalp," "Basics of Chemistry," and "Basics of Electricity"—provide essential information that will affect how you interact with clients and how you use service products and tools.

Also, you'll notice that the "Skin Disorders and Diseases" and "Nail Disorders and Diseases" chapters were moved from their previous

© Milady, a part of Cengage Learning.

locations to this section, where all of the other science chapters are located—by request of instructors and students.

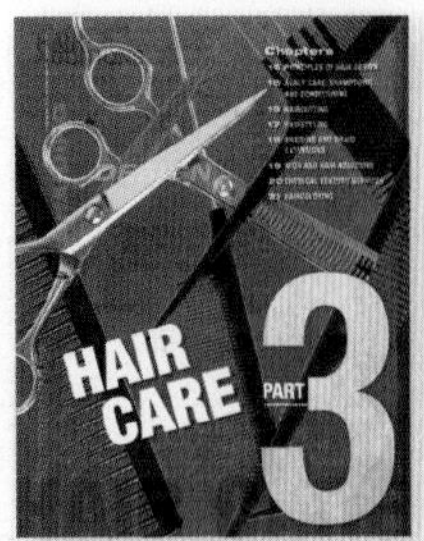

Part 3: Hair Care

Hair Care offers information on every aspect of hair. "Principles of Hair Design" explores the ways hair can be sculpted to enhance a client's facial shape. The foundation of every hair service is covered in "Scalp Care, Shampooing, and Conditioning," followed by an updated "Haircutting" chapter, complete with step-by-step procedures for core cuts with fantastic new glamour shots to show the finished look. Step-by-step procedures are also found in "Hairstyling," which includes information on new tools and techniques. Another revised chapter, "Braiding and Braid Extensions," is followed by "Wigs and Hair Additions," and both "Chemical Texture Services" and "Haircoloring" reflect the most recent advances in these areas.

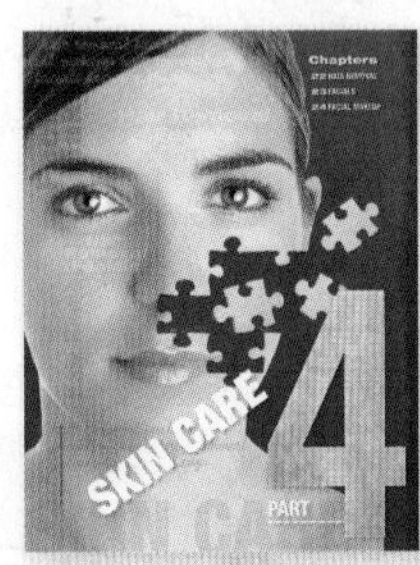

Part 4: Skin Care

Skin Care focuses on another area in which new advances have altered the way students must be trained. This part begins with a chapter on "Hair Removal," which covers waxing, tweezing, and other popular methods of removing unwanted hair from the face and body. Next, the basics of skin care is covered in "Facials" and makeup application in "Facial Makeup." These two chapters offer the critical information you'll need for these increasingly requested services in the expanding field of esthetics. Procedures are included for many of the services offered in salons and day spas.

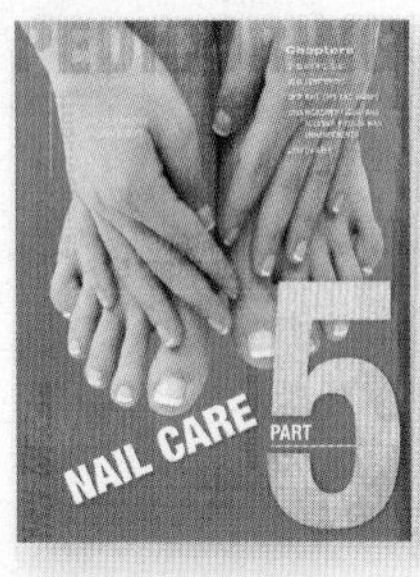

Part 5: Nail Care

Nail Care contains completely revised chapters that are also perfectly aligned with *Milady Standard Nail Technology* ,6e. These chapters include "Manicuring," "Pedicuring," "Nail Tips and Wraps," "Monomer Liquid and Polymer Powder Nail Enhancements," and an expanded "UV Gels" chapter.

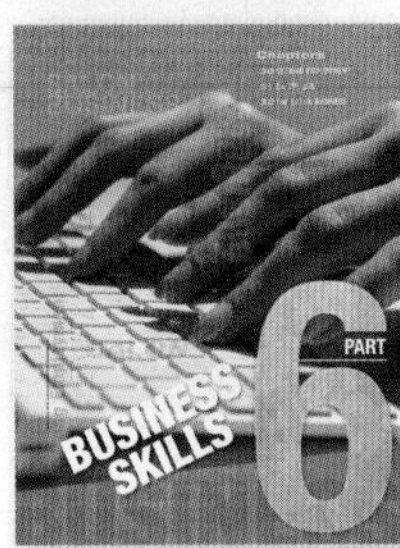

Part 6: Business Skills

Business Skills opens with the updated chapter "Seeking Employment." This chapter prepares students for licensure exams and job interviews, and it explains how to create a resume and a portfolio. What you will be expected to know and do as a newly licensed cosmetologist is described in "On the Job." It offers tips on how to make the most of your first job—including the importance of learning all you can. The final chapter, "The Salon Business," exposes students to the numerous types of salons and salon ownerships available to them.

© Milady, a part of Cengage Learning.

Additional Features of This Edition

As part of this edition, many features are available to help you master key concepts and techniques.

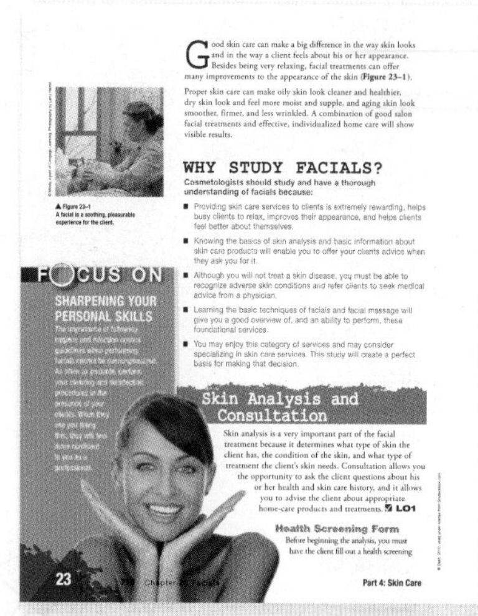

FOCUS ON

Throughout the text, short paragraphs in the outer column draw attention to various skills and concepts that will help you reach your goal. The **Focus On** pieces target sharpening technical and personal skills, ticket upgrading, client consultation, and building your client base. These topics are key to your success as a student and as a professional.

did you know?

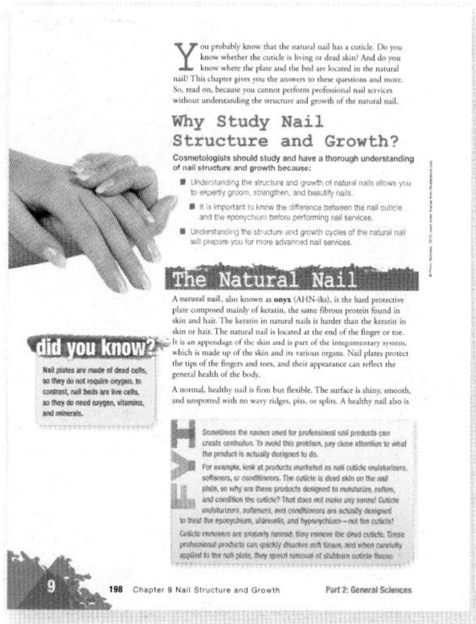

This feature provides interesting information that will enhance your understanding of the material in the text and call attention to a special point.

FYI

FYI's offer important, interesting information related to the content. Often **FYI** boxes direct you to a Web site or other resource for further information.

ACTivity

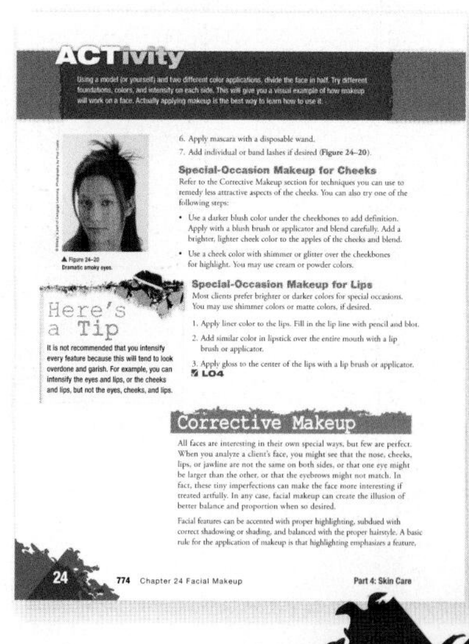

The Activity boxes describe hands-on classroom exercises that will help you understand the concepts explained in the text.

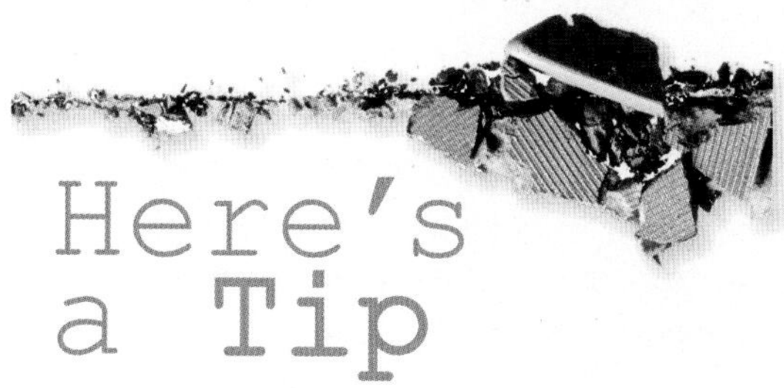

These helpful tips draw attention to situations that might arise and provide quick ways of doing things. Look for these tips throughout the text.

© Milady, a part of Cengage Learning.

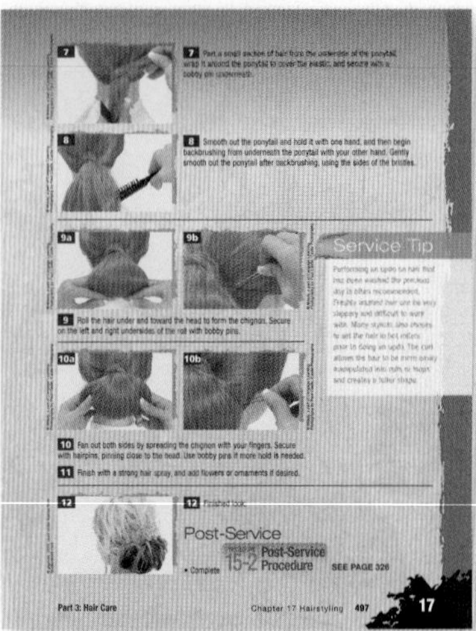

Service Tip

Service Tips draw attention to situations that might arise while performing a service and provide quick ways of doing things. Look for these tips in the procedures.

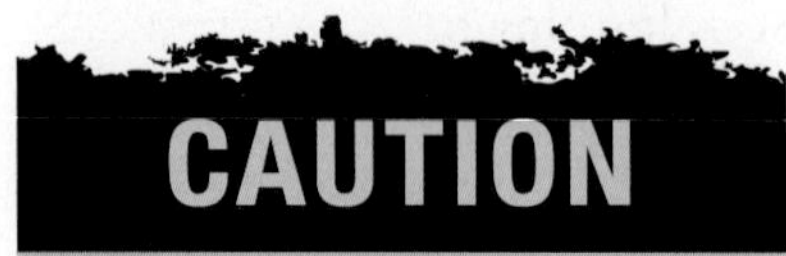

Some information is so critical for your safety and the safety of your clients that it deserves special attention. The text directs you to this information in the **Caution** boxes.

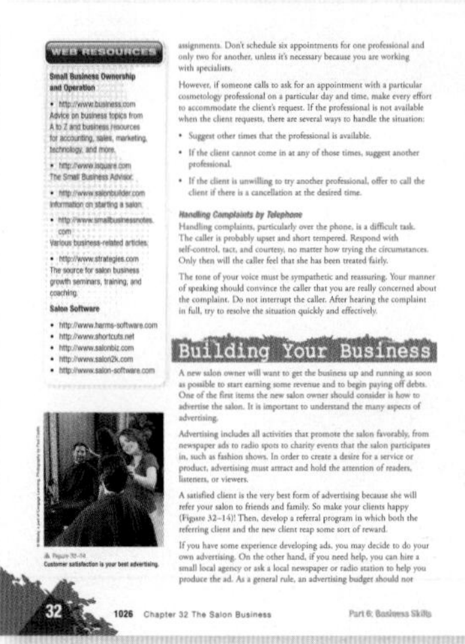

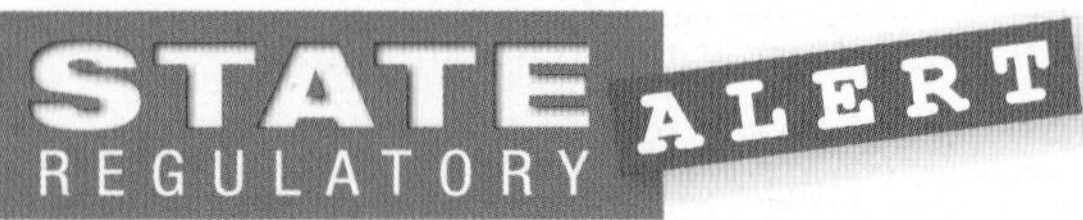

This feature alerts you to check the laws in your region for procedures and practices that are regulated differently from state to state. It is important, while you are studying, to contact state boards and provincial regulatory agencies to learn what is allowed and not allowed. Your instructor will provide you with contact information.

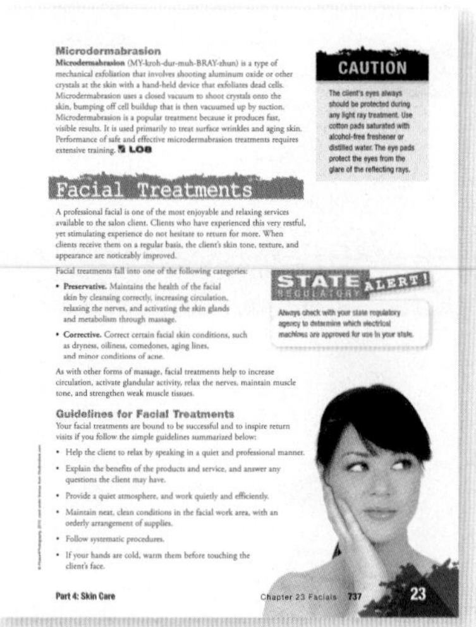

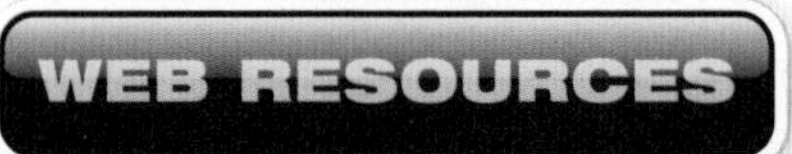

The **Web Resources** provide you with Web addresses where you can find more information on a topic and references to additional sites for more information.

© Milady, a part of Cengage Learning.

Educational Chapter Formatting

Each chapter of *Milady Standard Cosmetology* includes specialized formatting and strategies for the presentation of material to enhance your experience while working with the chapter and to facilitate the learning process.

Learning Objectives

At the beginning of each chapter is a list of learning objectives that tell you what important information you will be expected to know after studying the chapter. Throughout the chapter you will see a special icon that indicates you have finished reading the material that corresponds to one of these Learning Objectives. ☑ **LO1**

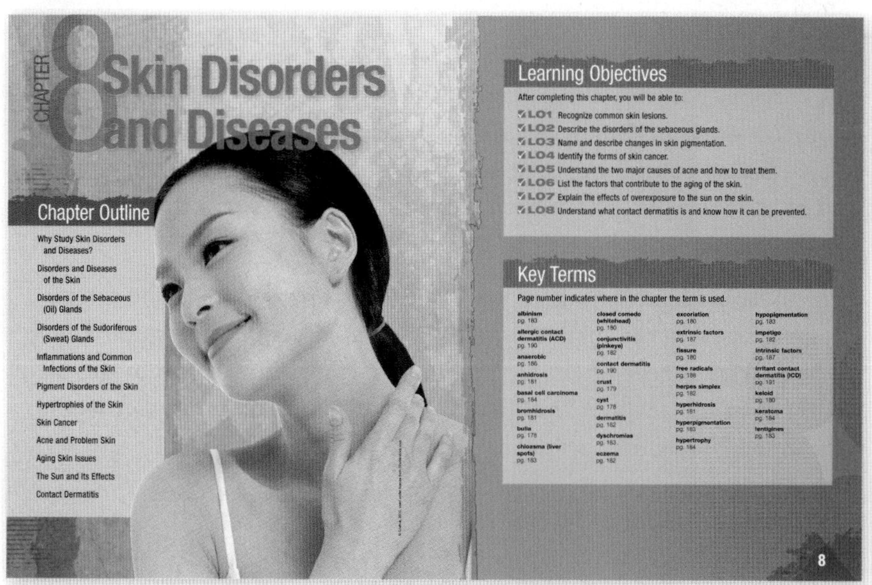

CHAPTER 8 Skin Disorders and Diseases

Chapter Outline

Why Study Skin Disorders and Diseases?
Disorders and Diseases of the Skin
Disorders of the Sebaceous (Oil) Glands
Disorders of the Sudoriferous (Sweat) Glands
Inflammations and Common Infections of the Skin
Pigment Disorders of the Skin
Hypertrophies of the Skin
Skin Cancer
Acne and Problem Skin
Aging Skin Issues
The Sun and Its Effects
Contact Dermatitis

Learning Objectives

After completing this chapter, you will be able to:

LO1 Recognize common skin lesions.
LO2 Describe the disorders of the sebaceous glands.
LO3 Name and describe changes in skin pigmentation.
LO4 Identify the forms of skin cancer.
LO5 Understand the two major causes of acne and how to treat them.
LO6 List the factors that contribute to the aging of the skin.
LO7 Explain the effects of overexposure to the sun on the skin.
LO8 Understand what contact dermatitis is and know how it can be prevented.

Key Terms

Page number indicates where in the chapter the term is used.

albinism pg. 183
allergic contact dermatitis (ACD) pg. 190
anaerobic pg. 186
anhidrosis pg. 181
basal cell carcinoma pg. 184
bromhidrosis pg. 181
bulla pg. 178
chloasma (liver spots) pg. 183
closed comedo (whitehead) pg. 180
conjunctivitis (pinkeye) pg. 182
contact dermatitis pg. 190
crust pg. 179
cyst pg. 178
dermatitis pg. 182
dyschromias pg. 183
eczema pg. 182
excoriation pg. 180
extrinsic factors pg. 187
fissure pg. 180
free radicals pg. 188
herpes simplex pg. 182
hyperhidrosis pg. 181
hyperpigmentation pg. 183
hypertrophy pg. 184
hypopigmentation pg. 183
impetigo pg. 182
intrinsic factors pg. 187
irritant contact dermatitis (ICD) pg. 191
keloid pg. 180
keratoma pg. 184
lentigines pg. 183

8

Key Terms

The words you will need to know in a chapter are given at the beginning of the chapter, in a list of **Key Terms**. When the word is discussed for the first time within the chapter, it appears in boldface type. If the word is difficult to pronounce, a phonetic pronunciation appears after it in parentheses.

Procedures

All step-by-step procedures offer clear, easy-to-understand directions and multiple photographs for learning the techniques. At the beginning of each procedure, you will find a list of the needed implements and materials, along with any preparation that must be completed before the procedure begins. At the end of each procedure, you will find photographs showing the finished result.

© Milady, a part of Cengage Learning.

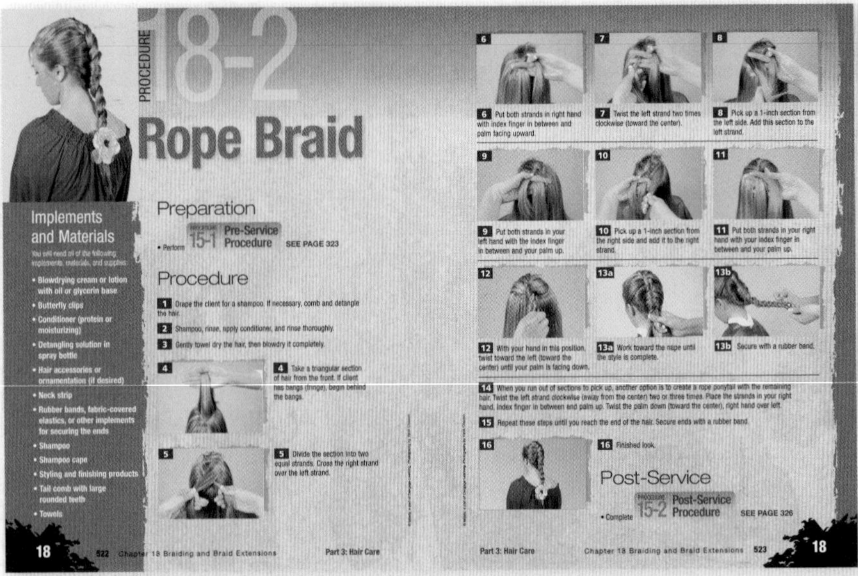

PROCEDURE 18-2

Rope Braid

Implements and Materials

You will need all of the following implements, materials, and supplies:

- Blowdrying cream or lotion with oil or glycerin base
- Butterfly clips
- Conditioner (protein or moisturizing)
- Detangling solution in spray bottle
- Hair accessories or ornamentation (if desired)
- Neck strip
- Rubber bands, fabric-covered elastics, or other implements for securing the ends
- Shampoo
- Shampoo cape
- Styling and finishing products
- Tail comb with large rounded teeth
- Towels

Preparation

- Perform PROCEDURE 15-1 Pre-Service Procedure SEE PAGE 323

Procedure

1. Drape the client for a shampoo. If necessary, comb and detangle the hair.
2. Shampoo, rinse, apply conditioner, and rinse thoroughly.
3. Gently towel dry the hair, then blowdry it completely.
4. Take a triangular section of hair from the front. If client has bangs (fringe), begin behind the bangs.
5. Divide the section into two equal strands. Cross the right strand over the left strand.
6. Put both strands in right hand with index finger in between and palm facing upward.
7. Twist the left strand two times clockwise (toward the center).
8. Pick up a 1-inch section from the left side. Add this section to the left strand.
9. Put both strands in your left hand with the index finger in between and your palm up.
10. Pick up a 1-inch section from the right side and add it to the right strand.
11. Put both strands in your right hand with your index finger in between and your palm up.
12. With your hand in this position, twist toward the left (toward the center) until your palm is facing down.

13a. Work toward the nape until the style is complete.

13b. Secure with a rubber band.

14. When you run out of sections to pick up, another option is to create a rope ponytail with the remaining hair. Twist the left strand clockwise (away from the center) two or three times. Place the strands in your right hand, index finger in between and palm up. Twist the palm down (toward the center), right hand over left.
15. Repeat these steps until you reach the end of the hair. Secure ends with a rubber band.
16. Finished look.

Post-Service

- Complete PROCEDURE 15-2 Post-Service Procedure SEE PAGE 326

18 522 Chapter 18 Braiding and Braid Extensions Part 3: Hair Care

Part 3: Hair Care Chapter 18 Braiding and Braid Extensions 523 18

In previous editions, the procedures interrupted the flow of the main content, often making it necessary for readers to flip through many pages before continuing their study. In order to avoid this interruption, all of the procedures have been moved to a special **Procedures** section at the end of each chapter.

For those students who may wish to review a procedure at the time it is mentioned in the main content, Milady has added Procedural Icons. These icons appear where each procedure is mentioned within the main content of the chapter, and they direct you to the page number where the entire procedure appears.

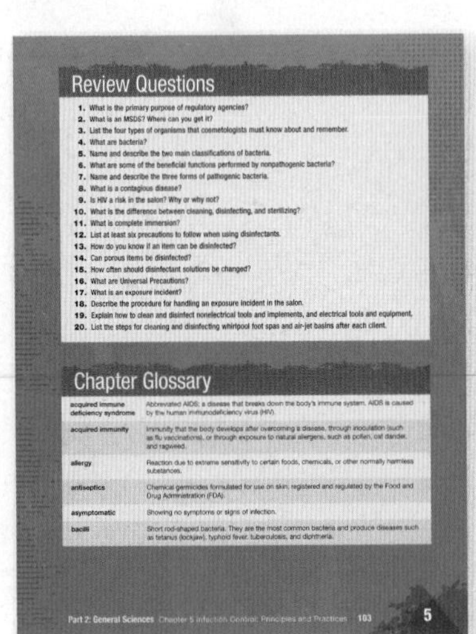

Review Questions

1. What is the primary purpose of regulatory agencies?
2. What is an MSDS? Where can you get it?
3. List the four types of organisms that cosmetologists must know about and remember.
4. What are bacteria?
5. Name and describe the two main classifications of bacteria.
6. What are some of the beneficial functions performed by nonpathogenic bacteria?
7. Name and describe the three forms of pathogenic bacteria.
8. What is a contagious disease?
9. Is HIV a risk in the salon? Why or why not?
10. What is the difference between cleaning, disinfecting, and sterilizing?
11. What is complete immersion?
12. List at least six precautions to follow when using disinfectants.
13. How do you know if an item can be disinfected?
14. Can porous items be disinfected?
15. How often should disinfectant solutions be changed?
16. What are Universal Precautions?
17. What is an exposure incident?
18. Describe the procedure for handling an exposure incident in the salon.
19. Explain how to clean and disinfect nonelectrical tools and implements, and electrical tools and equipment.
20. List the steps for cleaning and disinfecting whirlpool foot spas and air-jet basins after each client.

Chapter Glossary

acquired immune deficiency syndrome	Abbreviated AIDS; a disease that breaks down the body's immune system. AIDS is caused by the human immunodeficiency virus (HIV).
acquired immunity	Immunity that the body develops after overcoming a disease, through inoculation (such as flu vaccinations), or through exposure to natural allergens, such as pollen, cat dander, and ragweed.
allergy	Reaction due to extreme sensitivity to certain foods, chemicals, or other normally harmless substances.
antiseptics	Chemical germicides formulated for use on skin; registered and regulated by the Food and Drug Administration (FDA).
asymptomatic	Showing no symptoms or signs of infection.
bacilli	Short rod-shaped bacteria. They are the most common bacteria and produce diseases such as tetanus (lockjaw), typhoid fever, tuberculosis, and diphtheria.

Part 2: General Sciences Chapter 5 Infection Control: Principles and Practices 103 5

Review Questions

Each chapter ends with questions designed to test your understanding of the chapter's information. Your instructor may ask you to write the answers to these questions as an assignment or to answer them orally in class. If you have trouble answering a chapter review question, go back to the chapter to review the material and then try again. The answers to the **Review Questions** are in your instructor's *Course Management Guide.*

Chapter Glossary

All key terms and their definitions are included in the **Chapter Glossary** at the end of each chapter, as well as in the **Glossary/Index** at the end of the text.

© Milady, a part of Cengage Learning.

Extensive Learning and Teaching Package

While *Milady Standard Cosmetology* is the center of the curriculum, students and educators have a wide range of supplements from which to choose. All supplements have been revised and updated to complement the new edition of the textbook.

STUDENT SUPPLEMENTS	
SUPPLEMENT TITLE	SUPPLEMENT DESCRIPTION
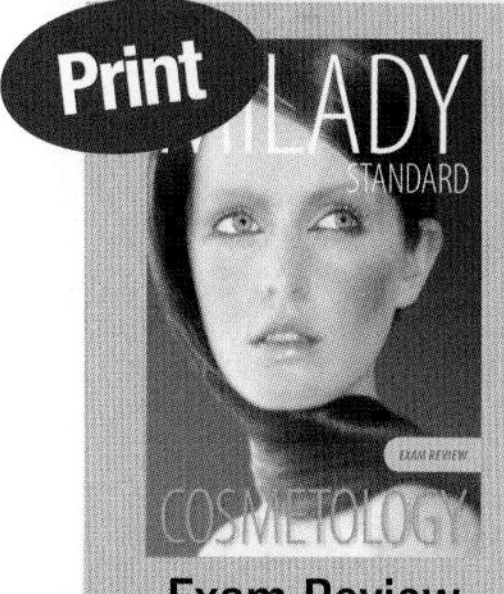 Exam Review	• Contains chapter-by-chapter questions in multiple-choice, true/false, and matching formats to help prepare for the written portion of licensure exams. • Revised to meet the most stringent test-development guidelines. • Questions are for study purposes only and are not the exact questions that will be seen on licensure exams.
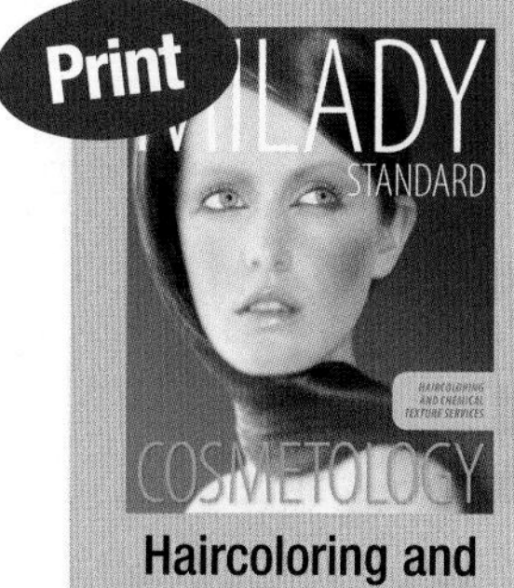 Haircoloring and Chemical Texture Services	• Full-color, spiral-bound guide • Showcases additional advanced procedures for changing hair texture (10 examples) and hair color (15 examples) with step-by-step accuracy.
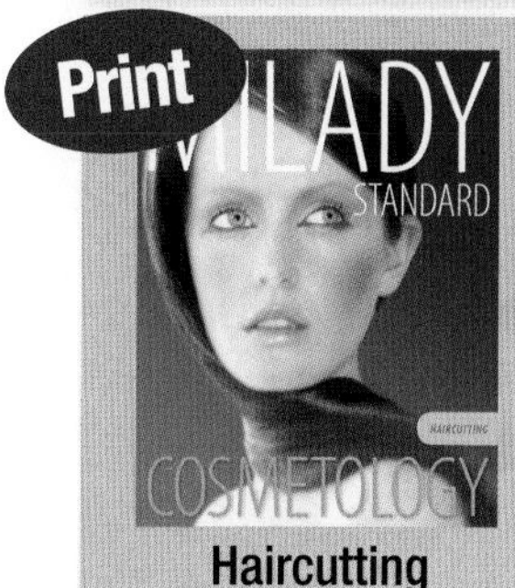 Haircutting	• Full-color, spiral-bound guide • Showcases cuts and styles that build upon content in Milady Standard Cosmetology for both women (15 cuts) and men (10 cuts) with step-by-step accuracy.

STUDENT SUPPLEMENTS

SUPPLEMENT TITLE	SUPPLEMENT DESCRIPTION
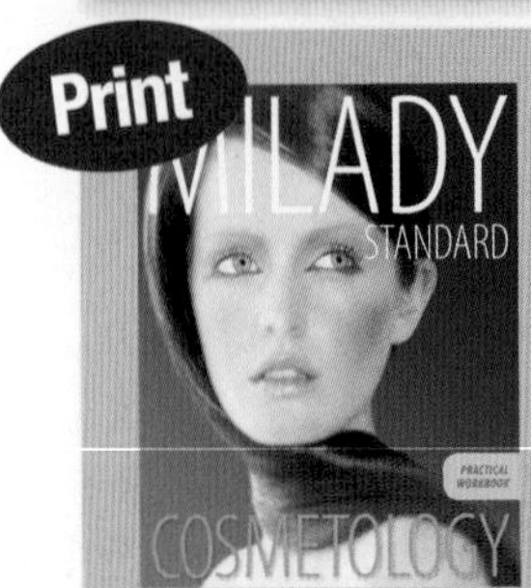 Practical Workbook	• Helps with mastering the techniques, procedures, and product usage needed for licensure as covered in the textbook. • Provides fill-in-the-blank, matching, multiple-choice, and labeling exercises that reinforce practical applications.
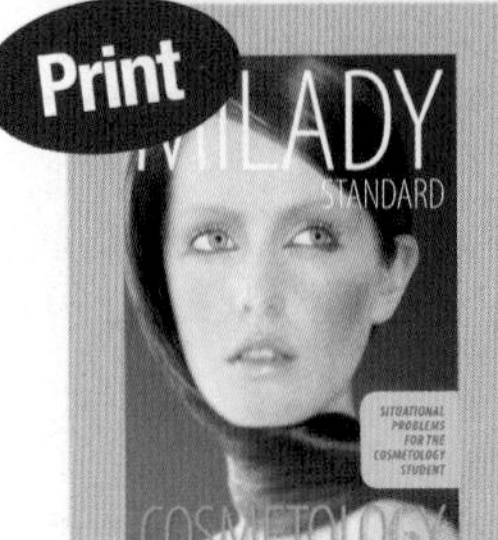 Situational Problems for the Cosmetology Student	• Tests the knowledge of how information that is learned can be applied in real-life situations. • Stories and scenarios closely reflect situations that are likely to arise when working in a salon. • Helps to demonstrate how to use the information learned by calling on the concepts discussed in the classroom and applying them to real-life situations.
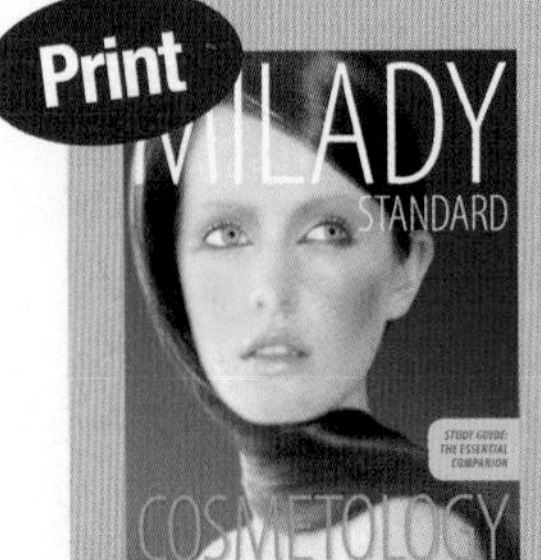 Study Guide: The Essential Companion	The study guide is designed to emphasize active, conceptual learning, and to consolidate understanding of the material in Milady Standard Cosmetology. • Provides six easy-to-follow features for each chapter, presenting the key content in a different manner to help with overall comprehension. • Chapter features: Essential Objectives, Essential Subjects, Essential Concepts, Essential Review, Essential Discoveries, Accomplishments, Rubrics incorporated throughout provide self-assessments to assist in overall learning. • Attractive full-color design provides an engaging experience in order to learn the important theory and practical aspects necessary for licensure and professional success.
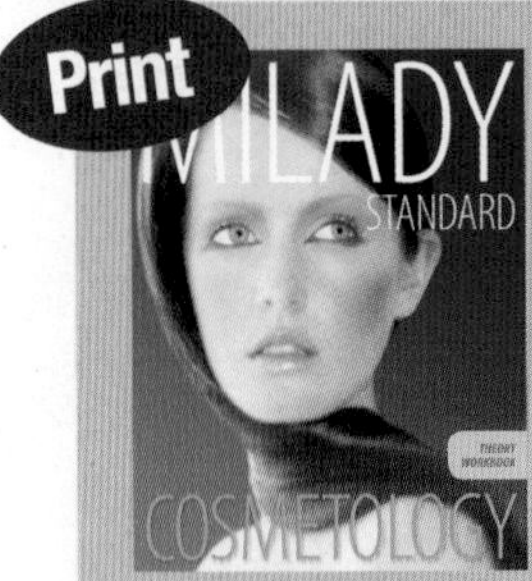 Theory Workbook	• Designed to reinforce classroom and textbook learning. • Contains chapter-by-chapter exercises on theory subjects. • Includes fill-in-the-blank, multiple-choice, matching, and labeling exercises, all coordinated with material from the main text. • Final Review Examinations at the end of the workbook assist with test preparation.

STUDENT SUPPLEMENTS

SUPPLEMENT TITLE	SUPPLEMENT DESCRIPTION
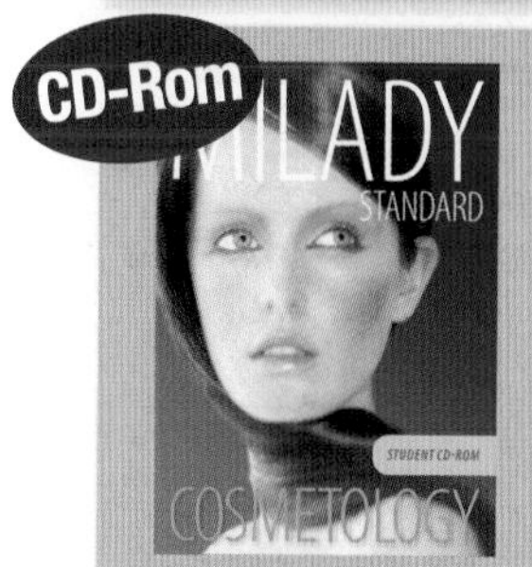 Student CD-Rom	• Interactive resource designed to reinforce classroom learning, stimulate the imagination, and aid in preparation for board exams. • Includes: • Over 100 video clips that demonstrate procedures and theoretical concepts • Chapter quizzes that provide 10 questions at a time but draw from a quiz bank of more than 1,200 questions • An 'arcade' with 4 different types of games • An audio glossary that pronounces each term and provides the definition • Content follows and enhances Milady Standard Cosmetology.
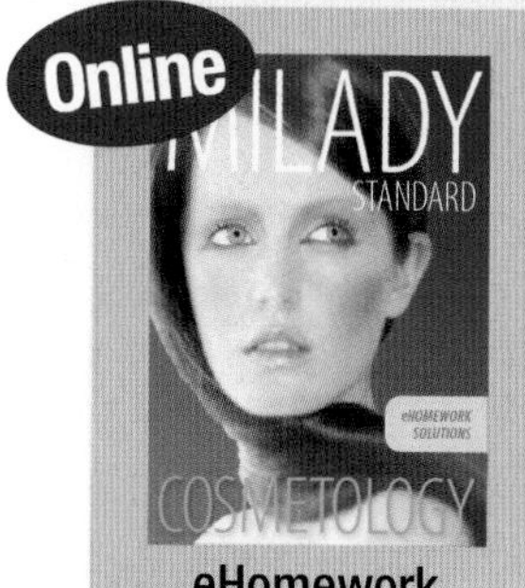 eHomework Solutions	• Content-rich, web-based learning aid that presents information in a new and different way. • 24x7 access • Provides tools and content that allow for more effective management of time, progress checks, exam preparation, and organization of notes. • Designed for integration of additional technology into programs that accommodate the ever-changing learning styles. • Student Features include: Chapter Learning Objectives, Study Sheets, Online Chapter Quizzes, Flash Cards, Discussion Topics, Web Links, FAQs, Glossary, Video, Games
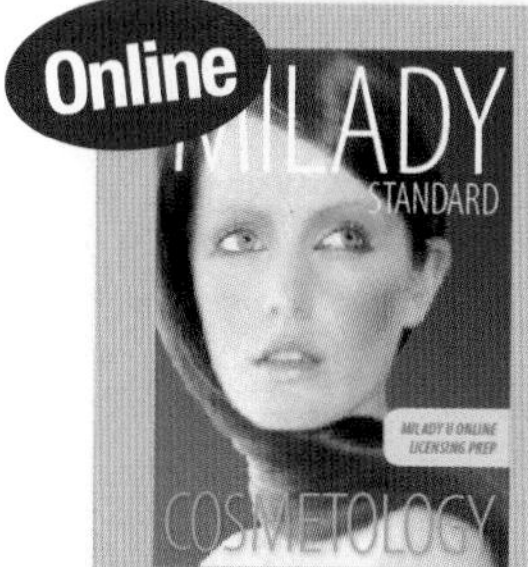 Milady U Online Licensing Prep	• Provides an alternative way to study for licensure exams, whether taken on a computer or on paper. • Offers familiarity with a computerized test environment during licensure exam preparation. • Features include: • 24x7 availability and students have the flexibility to study from any computer • Chapter tests, quizzes and comprehensive exams that draw from more than 1,200 multiple-choice questions • All questions are available in both English and Spanish • Immediate results with rationales to assist with knowledge acquisition • Robust reports that help students determine areas of study they need to focus on **www.miladyonline.cengage.com**

STUDENT SUPPLEMENTS

SUPPLEMENT TITLE	SUPPLEMENT DESCRIPTION

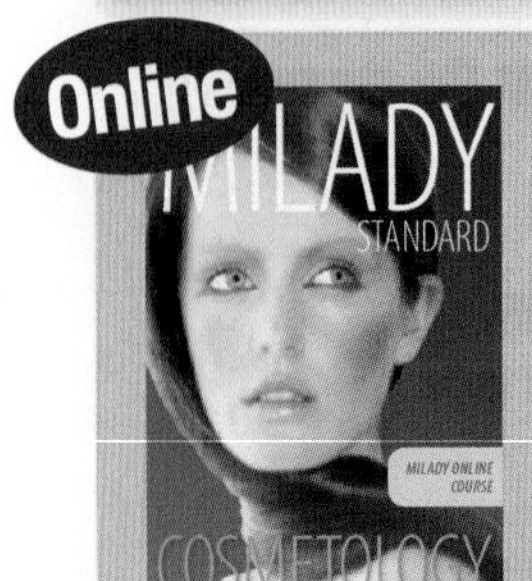 Milady Online Course	Designed to be used in conjunction with Milady Standard Cosmetology textbook and the practical portion of a cosmetology program.
	• Focuses on delivering the theory portions of the cosmetology curriculum in an online format.
	• Extremely interactive which will engage all types of learners
	• Features include:
	  • Interactive lectures with audio
	  • Video
	  • Interactive learning reinforcement activities including situational problems
	  • Games
	  • Automatically graded quizzes and tests
	  • Audio Flashcards with glossary terms and definitions

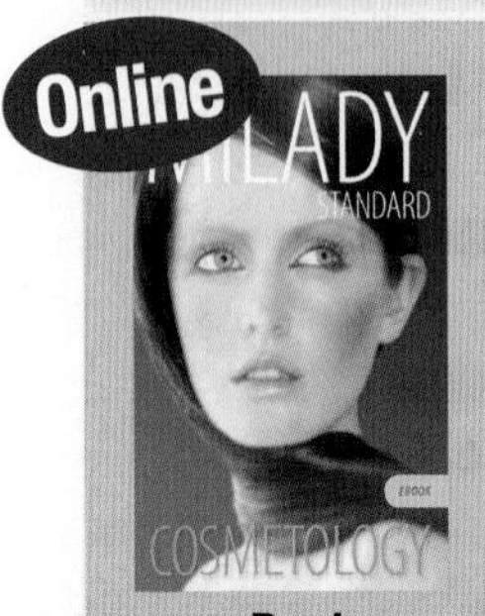 eBook	• Electronic version of Milady Standard Cosmetology for instant online access • Requires an internet connection. • Enables highlighting, note-taking, and bookmarking. • Has search capabilities. • Contains an audio glossary. • Ability to print pages one at a time while connected to the internet

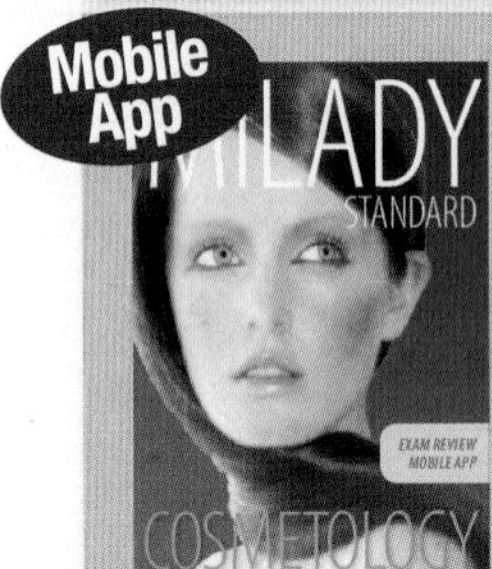 Exam Review Mobile App	• An 'on-the-go' tool designed to help prepare for the written portion of licensure exams.
	• Available for iPhone, iPod Touch, and iPad devices.
	• Features include:
	  • "Question of the Day"
	  • Randomized multiple choice questions for each chapter
	  • Immediate feedback with rationales
	  • Progress reporting for all chapter tests

Educator Supplements

Milady proudly offers a full range of innovative resources created especially for cosmetology educators to make classroom preparation and presentation simple, effective and enjoyable.

SUPPLEMENT TITLE
Milady Standard Cosmetology Course Management Guide Print Binder
Milady Standard Cosmetology Course Management Guide CD
Milady Standard Cosmetology DVD Series
Milady Standard Cosmetology Instructor Support Slides CD
Milady Standard Cosmetology Student CD School/Network Version
Milady Standard Cosmetology Interactive Games CD
Milady Standard Cosmetology Haircutting DVD Series
Milady Standard Cosmetology Haircutting Instructor Resource CD
Milady Standard Cosmetology Haircoloring and Chemical Texture Services DVD Series
Milady Standard Cosmetology Haircoloring and Chemical Texture Services Instructor Resource CD

Thank you for choosing Milady as your Total Learning Solutions Provider. For additional information on the above resources or to place an order please contact your Milady Sales Representative or visit us online at www.milady.cengage.com

Contributing Authors

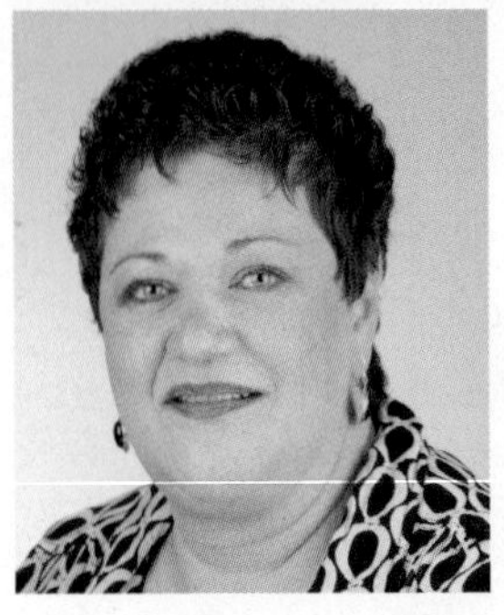

Catherine Frangie

Catherine M. Frangie began her career in 1982 as a licensed cosmetologist, salon owner, and beauty school instructor. Since then, Catherine has held prominent positions in the professional beauty industry, including Marketing, Communications, and Education Vice President; Communications Director; Trade Magazine Editor/Publisher; and Textbook Editor and Author.

Catherine has been a guest lecturer at conferences and trade shows, including the International Beauty Show in NYC. She has authored more than 125 feature-length magazine articles and several books on beauty trends, fashion, and the business of the professional salon. Catherine holds degrees in communications, and marketing.

In 2001, Catherine founded Frangie Consulting, LLC, a marketing, communications, and publishing firm which offers strategies for managing business objectives, creating high-performing teams, and successfully achieving goals. Her experiences and successes have given her a well-deserved reputation as an industry expert in marketing and branding, communications and education. Frangie Consulting earned seven ABBIE Awards—including two Gold ABBIEs—for marketing campaigns, new product launches, and outstanding professional educational programs.

Catherine has been involved with Milady for more than twenty years, and since 2004 has acted as the revision author/editor for its three core textbooks—*Milady Standard Cosmetology, Milady Standard Nail Technology*, and *Milady Standard Esthetics Fundamentals.*

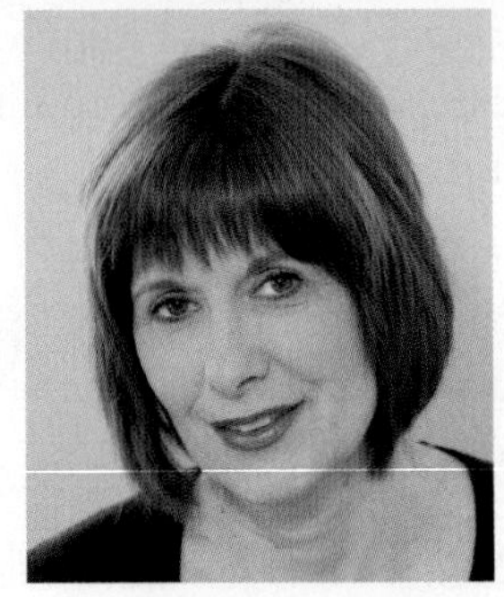

Photo courtesy of Cathy Frangie.

Photo courtesy of Colleen Hennessey.

Colleen Hennessey

Recognized nationally as a Master Haircolorist, Platform Artist, and Technical Educator, Colleen Hennessey brings many years of hands-on coloring experience to the industry. She spent eight years at the renowned Adam Broderick Salon and Spa as a Master Colorist and Director of Salon Education.

Colleen's rare skills as an educator make her a sought-after resource throughout the profession. For eight years she served as Senior Technical Editor of *Haircolor and Design Magazine*, where she wrote an editorial article entitled "The Haircolor Department."

Beauty schools' students also benefit from Colleen's expert knowledge and teaching ability. Colleen is the subject matter expert chosen to write the Haircolor chapter for *Milady Standard Cosmetology.* In addition to her writing projects, she works as a School Manager representing the Procter & Gamble School Partnership Program to help schools keep abreast of all new product introductions and education.

An artist of many talents, Colleen is an established platform artist, performing throughout the United States and attracting crowds at mega trade shows, including Hair Color USA in Long Beach, International Beauty Show in New York City, Haircolor USA, Matrix Logics Tour, and the Midwest Show. Her easy color techniques are popular with stylists, as are her classes in effective client-communication skills, both of which have enabled her and the stylists she works with to build salon haircolor sales.

Formally Clairol Professional's exclusive color designer and Senior Manager of Clairol Professional's Education Department, Colleen has brought techniques and color-correction advice direct to salon mailboxes through Clairol Professional's Creative Connection, an educational membership program free to all licensed cosmetologists. Her color work has also been featured in *Color & Style, Matrix News, Modern Salon*, and *Passion* magazines, as well as Milady educational publications.

Wherever Colleen teaches—on platform, in salons, in textbooks, or in magazines—she communicates her love of haircolor by teaching others the precise, technical, artistic, and communication skills that have earned her the prestigious title of Master Colorist.

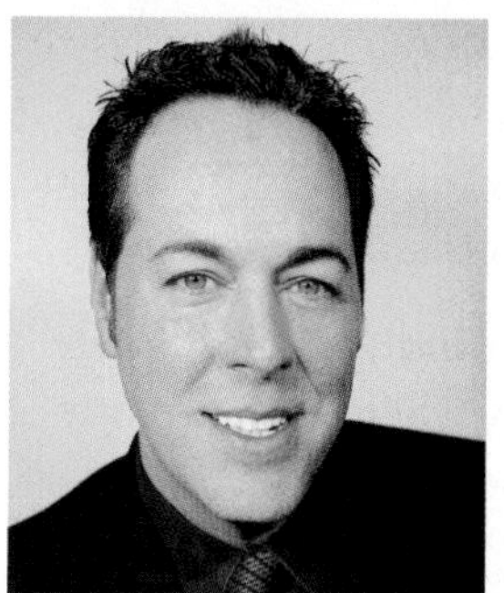

Photo courtesy of Mark Lees.

Dr. Mark Lees

Dr. Mark Lees is one of the country's most noted skin care specialists and an award-winning speaker and product developer. He has been actively practicing clinical skin care for over twenty years at his multi-award winning CIDESCO accredited Florida salon, which has been awarded many honors by the readers of the *Pensacola News-Journal*, including Best Facial, Best Massage, and Best Pampering Place.

His professional awards are numerous and include Esthetician of the Year from *American Salon Magazine*, the Les Nouvelles Esthétiques Crystal Award, the Dermascope Legends Award, the Rocco Bellino Award for outstanding education from the Chicago Cosmetology Association, and Best Educational Skin Care Classroom from the Long Beach International Beauty Expo. Dr. Lees has also been inducted into the National Cosmetology Association's Hall of Renown.

Dr. Lees has been interviewed and quoted by NBC News, The Associated Press, The Discovery Channel, *Glamour, Self, Teen, Shape*, and many other publications.

Dr. Lees is cofounder of both the Skin Care Study Center in Los Angeles and the Institute of Advanced Clinical Esthetics in Seattle, special science-based advanced training programs for clinical estheticians.

Dr. Lees is former Chairman of EstheticsAmerica, the esthetics education division of the National Cosmetology Association (NCA), and has served as a CIDESCO International Examiner. He has also served on the national Board of Directors of the NCA.

Dr. Lees is former Chairman of the Board of the Esthetics Manufacturers and Distributors Alliance, is a member of the Society of Cosmetic Chemists, and is author of the popular book *Skin Care: Beyond the Basics*, now in its third edition, and the recently released *The Skin Care Answer Book.*

Dr. Lees holds a Ph.D. in Health Sciences, a Master of Science in Health, and a CIDESCO International Diploma. He is licensed to practice in both Florida and Washington State. His line of products for problem, sensitive, and sun-damaged skin is available at finer salons and clinics throughout the United States.

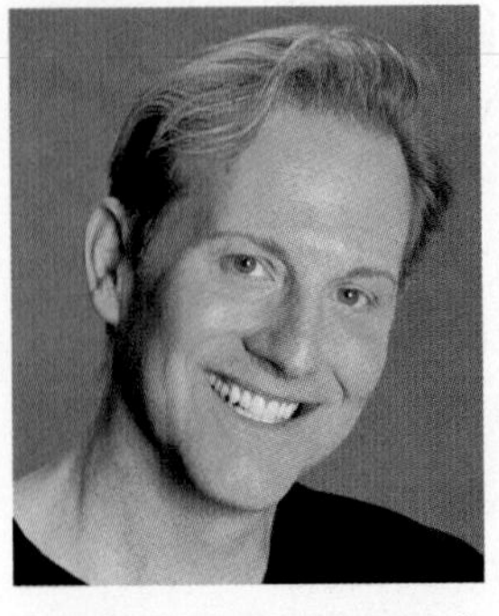

Frank Shipman

Frank Shipman has been making hair look great for more than two decades. As the owner of the nationally recognized Technicolor/TC Salon Spas, Frank is proud to have the privilege of working behind the chair. He also continues to be a beauty educator, writer, and speaker, bringing his own unique perspective to the industry.

In 2005, Frank received the prestigious Diamond Award from the magazine *Day Spa* to add to his many professional awards and honors.

Frank has a graduate degree in art from Boston University and has had his art exhibited nationally and internationally. Today he no longer creates precious objects but instead creates experiences. Frank is happy to be in a profession that allows him to state, "What I do is make people feel good."

Photo courtesy of Frank Shipman.

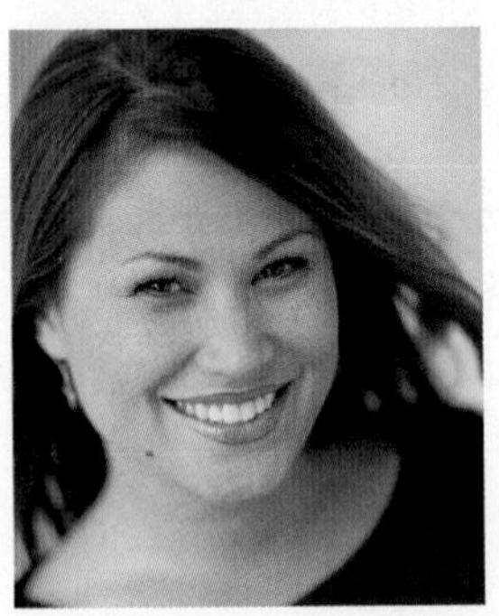

Alisha Rimando Botero

Alisha is recognized as one of the nail industry's leading experts in training and education. In her first two years as an educator, Alisha taught classes in over 100 beauty schools and vo-techs across the US. As she expanded internationally, her focus turned to Asia, where she dedicated eight years to implementing artistic training programs and marketing strategies that resulted in the opening of over 100 nail salons and seven schools in Japan, growing that market to become the industry leader in nail art techniques.

In her fourteen years of experience, her work has been described as "groundbreaking." She has been a platform artist and motivational speaker for more than 1,500 promotional and educational events and has competed in over 100 nail competitions around the globe, winning a World Championship in 2005. She has been featured in multiple training videos and more than 150 beauty and trade publications and blog spots worldwide, such as *Teen Vogue, Bridal Guide, Self, Fitness,* and *Seventeen Magazine,* as well as numerous industry trade magazines like *Nails, Nailpro, Scratch* (UK), and *Stylish Nail* (Japan).

Through the years, Alisha has garnered the attention of large industry manufacturers, small business entrepreneurs, salon franchises, and nail and beauty associations. She has worked with Research and Development chemists to develop artificial nail enhancement products, nanotechnology skin care and cuticle treatments, polish collections, and natural nail treatments. One of her innovative product lines was awarded an industry ABBIE for best packaging, and several others have been recognized with readers' choice awards for best products. Recently, Alisha has added reflexology to her growing list of competencies, ever striving to advance a more holistic approach to natural nail products and services.

Alisha's love and passion for her industry and family have led her to New York State, where she currently resides with her husband and son.

Photo courtesy of Alisha Rimando.

Bonnie Sanford

Bonnie Sanford is a beauty industry consultant, editor, and writer who specializes in marketing, communications, and public relations. She has worked in the professional beauty industry for over fourteen years, beginning as the Managing Editor of a national trade publication. Bonnie moved from the publishing field to the professional products industry, first as the Director of Communications and Creative Services for a leading international hair care company, then as a consultant to various hair care and skin care companies.

Bonnie was a contributing writer for the sixth edition of *Milady Standard Nail Technology Student CD-ROM*. She is honored to continue her work with Milady as a contributing author for *Milady Standard Cosmetology*.

Victoria Wurdinger

Victoria Wurdinger is an award-winning writer and researcher who specializes in beauty, business, and wellness. Her "State of the Professional Haircare Market," originally appearing in *DCI* and later in *Modern Salon* magazine, became the essential annual report on the salon industry for both venture capitalists and industry insiders. As a columnist, she has written about new technology, and her articles on the health-care concerns of small businesses brought notice from as far away as Germany.

Victoria's work has appeared in dozens of publications, among them *Art Business News, Beauty Digest, Beauty Store Business, British Hairdressers Journal, Celebrity Hairstyles, Color and Style, Drug Store News, Day Spa, DCI, Longevity, Modern Salon,* Germany's *Top Hair, Launchpad,* and *Salon Today.* Her travels to salons have taken her from Miami to Moscow and New York to Paris.

Additionally, Victoria has developed educational programs and promotional materials for several major beauty care manufacturers, including ARTec, Clairol, Mizani, Redken, Rusk, and Tocco Magico. As a commercial writer, she was selected to write the packaging and promotional copy for Joan Rivers' infomercial-sold skin care line, *Fundamentals.*

Victoria has authored several books, including *Competition Hairdesign, The Photo Session Handbook, 101 Quick Fixes for Bad Hair Days, The Eric Fisher Salon Training Notebook*, and *Multicultural Markets.* For the latter, she conducted extensive historical research, sometimes working with Spanish translators to explore early methods of hairstyling in the Latino community. *Multicultural Markets* contains the never-before-published history of ethnic beauty culture in the United States.

She has won several American Society of Business Press Editors awards, as well as an international award for her coverage of the British Hair Fashion industry. Most recently, she has provided content for various Web sites. Her own is http://www.victoriawurdinger.com.

Contributing Authors for Previous Editions of *Milady Standard Cosmetology*

Arlene Alpert
Margrit Altenburg
Diane Carol Bailey
Letha Barnes
Lisha Barnes
Deborah Beatty
Mary Brunetti
Jane Crawford
Robert Cromeans
Alyssa Evirs
Catherine M. Frangie
John Halal
Colleen Hennessey
Mary Beth Janssen
Nancy King
Dr. Mark Lees
Toni Love
Vivienne Mackinder
Carey Nash
Ruth Roche
Teresa Sammarco
Sue Sansom
Douglas Schoon
Sue Ellen Schultes
Frank Shipman
Jeryl Spear

Editorial Contributors for the 2012 Edition

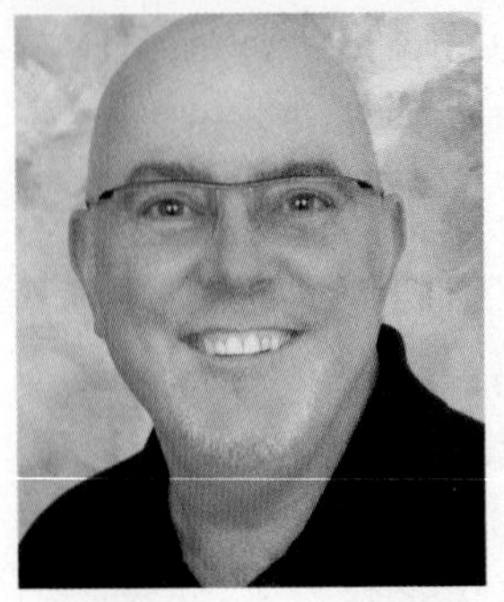

Randy Ferman

Randy Ferman, CEO and Founder of the Shark Fin Shear Co., has a history of introducing new products that revolutionize the way stylists do business. His mission has been to improve stylists' quality of life through innovation and product advancement. Randy Ferman's genuine concern and instinctive ability has resulted in innovative and technologically advanced products for the professional beauty industry.

After teaching at cosmetology schools in the Northeast, Randy Ferman learned that students and instructors were quick to cite the need for a more advanced shear. With traditional shears, the handle openings were too large, causing users' fingers to slide through. This resulted in loss of control and a misalignment of the fingers. Randy Ferman dedicated more than five years to creating a more ergonomically correct shear that enhances both comfort and precision. This unique patented design can help to prevent and may even eliminate conditions such as carpal tunnel syndrome, nerve damage, tendonitis, wrist and arm pain, and shoulder and neck pain.

In 2001, Randy Ferman created a remarkable product for the shear segment of the beauty industry, now called the Shark Fin® Shear. This line of revolutionary shears for stylists has a patented handle design that comes with the SHEAR-FIT® scissor fitting system for a more ergonomically correct fit for the hand. This patented scissor fitting system offers interchangeable ring guards that provide a customized fit for the user's exact ring finger and thumb diameter, providing more control and comfort. Shark Fin® shears are patented throughout the United States, Canada, and Europe, and other patents are pending worldwide. Randy Ferman continues to introduce innovative and exciting products for the hair care industry and holds many patents worldwide.

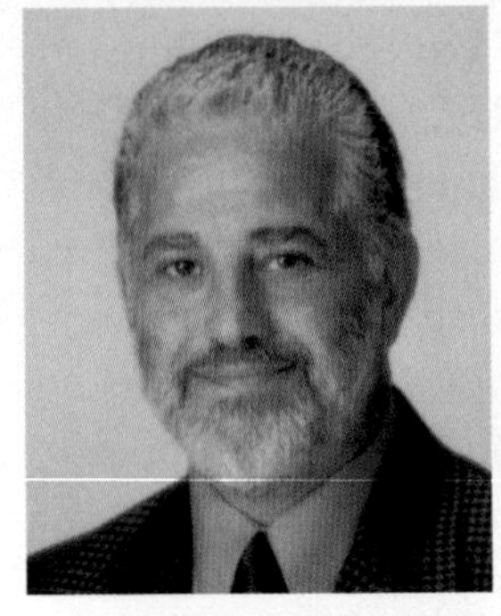

John Halal

John Halal began his career in the beauty industry as a hairstylist over forty years ago. Halal is a former salon owner, a licensed cosmetology instructor, and since 1992, founder and president of Honors Beauty College, Inc.

Halal is an affiliate member of the Society of Cosmetic Chemists (SCC). He is a past President of both the American Association of Cosmetology Schools (AACS) and the Indiana Cosmetology Educators Association (ICEA).

Halal is the author of *Hair Structure and Chemistry Simplified* and *Milady Hair Care and Product Ingredient Dictionary*. He is also a contributing author of the *Milady Standard Cosmetology* and several other Milady publications.

Halal obtained his Associate's Degree, with highest distinction, from Indiana University and is a member of The Golden Key National Honor Society and Alpha Sigma Lambda.

He has authored numerous articles on a wide variety of topics and has been published in several professional trade magazines. He often travels as a guest speaker, addressing both professional and consumer groups.

"I love the beauty industry more than ever," he states proudly. The secret, according to Halal is to "never stop learning."

Photo courtesy of Randy Fermin.

Photo courtesy of John Halal.

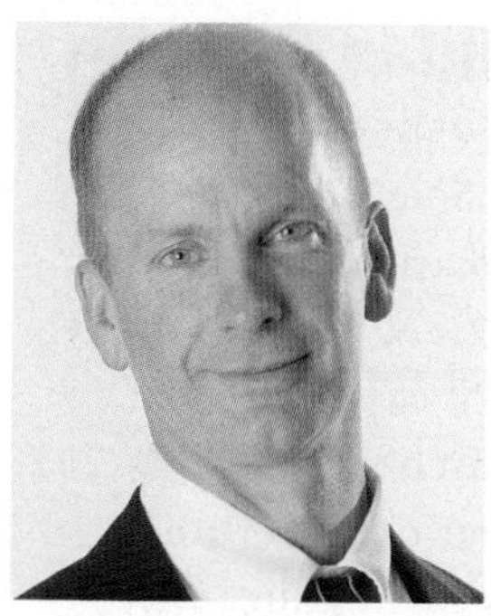

Photo courtesy of Jim McConnell.

Jim McConnell

Jim McConnell received his B.S. in Chemistry from the University of Oregon in 1986. He has been a chemist in the field of polymers since 1988. After graduating from the University of Oregon, Jim worked as a catalytic chemist in the petroleum industry and as a urethane and epoxy chemist in the wood products, concrete coating, and steel coating industries for twelve years. During this time, he was on the board for various committees for the Steel Structures Painting Council (SSPC) and National Association of Corrosion Engineers (NACE).

He and his wife, Lezlie, began McConnell Labs, Inc., in 1998 to make Light Elegance Nail Products for their salon in Eugene, Oregon. After making Light Elegance for use in their own salon, they began selling the UV gel products internationally. Jim contributed to numerous nail technology magazines around the world to answer questions, provide chemistry information, and explain UV light technology prior to starting McConnell Labs with his wife.

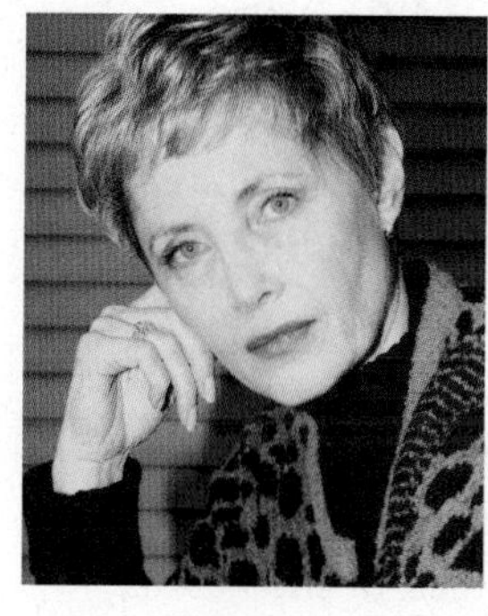

Photo courtesy of Janet McCormick.

Janet McCormick

Janet McCormick is a licensed and experienced esthetician and manicurist, a sought-after trainer, a former spa director, and salon owner. She has been writing for over twenty years, producing hundreds of highly respected articles in beauty industry trade magazines, three books, and chapters covering two specialties for the industry's leading textbooks.

Ms. McCormick is co-owner of the Just For Toenails Nail System, a gel system sold only to podiatrists. She is also co-owner of the Medinail Learning Center, which educates nail professionals and prepares them to work in medical facilities. The Center offers two certification programs: the Advanced Nail Technician certification program for salon-based nail technicians and the Medical Nail Technician certification for technicians who work in podiatry offices. She is also owner of Spa Techniques, a consulting and training firm, and she writes under that banner.

Vicki Peters

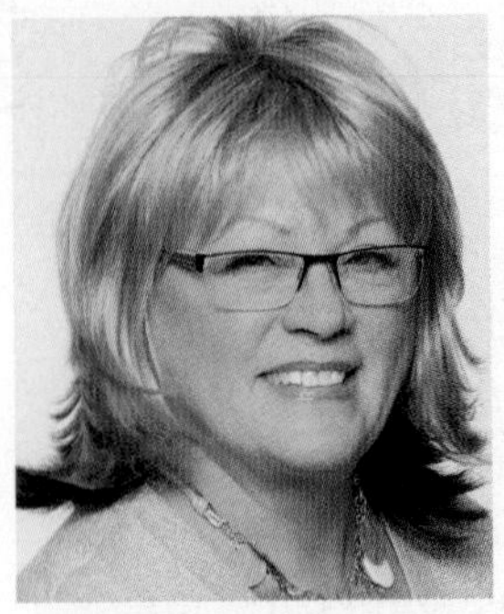

As a nail technician, Vicki Peters has wowed the industry with her championship nails. As a cover artist and author, her work has been published worldwide, more than any other tech in the history of the nail business. As an educator, she has trained techs from Russia, Germany, Japan, Ireland, the United Kingdom, Canada, Mexico, Africa, Australia, and the United States. As an industry leader, she has mentored thousands of nail professionals. As a world-master nail technician, Peters, with her own line of products, promises to lead the industry to new heights.

Vicki Peters is a twenty-eight-year veteran nail technician, former competition champion, competition judge and director, technical educator, and featured business speaker. She is also author of the *Nails Q&A Book, Drilltalk, The Competitive Edge,* and *Novartis' Nail Healthy Guide*. Her nail artistry has been on the covers of *TV Guide, Day Spa, Nails, Nailpro, Nailpro Europe*, and numerous fashion magazines. Her expertise in the nail business ranges from salon work and hands-on technical experience to Research and Development, education, and lecturing worldwide.

Douglas Schoon

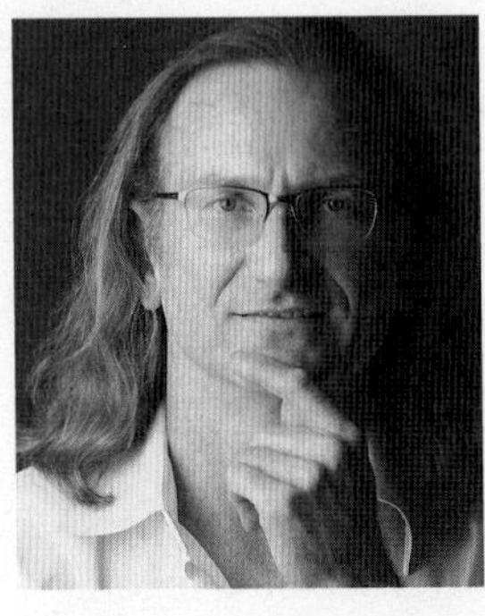

Doug Schoon is the Chief Scientific Advisor for Creative Nail Design (CND). With over thirty years of experience as a research scientist, international lecturer, author, and educator, he has become a recognized authority in the professional beauty industry. Schoon led CND's Research and Development program for nineteen years. Now, as president of his own consulting firm, Schoon Scientific, he continues focusing on assisting CND with scientific, technical, and regulatory issues that help shape the industry. He works as a strong advocate for salon safety and represents the professional nail industry on scientific and technical issues in the U.S., Europe, Canada, Australia, and Japan.

Schoon is the author of several books, video and audio training programs, and dozens of magazine articles about salon chemicals, chemical safety, and disinfection. As a writer and speaker, Schoon is applauded for his ability to make complex chemical theories and concepts seem simple and easy to understand. Schoon's latest book, *Nail Structure & Product Chemistry*, Second Edition, Milady, a part of Cengage Learning, is also considered an excellent resource for nail professionals. Currently, Schoon is a co-chair of the Nail Manufacturers Council (NMC) of the Professional Beauty Association (PBA).

Photo courtesy of Vicki Peters.

Photo courtesy of Doug Schoon.

Acknowledgments

Milady recognizes, with gratitude and respect, the many professionals who have offered their time to contribute to this edition of *Milady Standard Cosmetology* and wishes to extend enormous thanks to the following people who have played an invalueable role in the creation of this edition:

- ***Milady would like to offer our special thanks to the Continental School of Beauty Culture of Rochester, Batavia, Buffalo, West Seneca, Olean, and Syracuse, NY, who, along with their school owners, directors, instructors, and students, welcomed the Milady team to their schools in order to conduct this edition's massive photo shoot and who were wholeheartedly kind, accommodating, and hospitable to all of our crew!***
- Maria Moffre-Lynch, cosmetologist, cosmetology instructor, and consultant, for her invaluable assistance throughout the revision process and for sharing her hairdressing skills and keen eye during the *Milady Standard Cosmetology* photo shoot.
- Yanik Chauvin, professional photographer, whose artistic vision and photographic expertise helped bring many of these pages to life.
- Krissy Ferro, professional makeup artist and founder of Ferro Cosmetics, for her artfully inspired makeup applications and for generously providing much of the makeup product, tools, and supplies used and pictured throughout this edition.
- Colleen Hennessey, for her on-camera haircoloring work, her writing and authoring abilities, and her passion about haircolor education.
- Frank Shipman, for his on-camera haircutting and styling work, his innovative approach, and his love for the beauty industry.
- Tom Carson, professional photographer, for his wonderful finished haircut and styling photos, which truly enhance these pages and are sure to inspire readers.
- Dino Petrocelli, professional photographer, for his photographic expertise for many of the photos in the nail technology chapters.
- Latoyia Anderson, owner of The Hair Extension Room, Rochester, NY, for her enthusiastic and creative braiding styles that are featured in this edition.
- Debbie Harris, professional stylist, Rochester, NY, for her beautiful finger-wave styling.
- Jesse Hajduk, cosmetologist, Averill Park, NY, for her off-camera assistance and on-camera modeling.
- Shear Ego International School of Hair Design, Rochester, NY, for allowing Milady to hold casting calls at their school.

Product Suppliers

- **The Andis Company** for generously providing clippers and trimmers used and pictured throughout this edition.
- **The Burmax Company** for providing many of the tools, implements, and supplies used and pictured throughout this edition.
- **Hairlines Inc. Distributors** for generously providing wet products, flat irons, curling irons, scissors, carving combs, and brushes used and pictured throughout this edition.
- **The Procter & Gamble Co.,** parent company of *Clairol Professional,* for generously providing the haircolor products, swatch books, and other educational materials used and pictured throughout this edition.
- **The Shark Fin Shear Company** and *Randy Ferman* for generously providing the shears and cutting implements used and pictured throughout this edition.
- **Zotos International, Inc.,** for generously providing hair care, texture products, and educational material used and pictured throughout this edition.

Interior Photo Shoot Models

Latoyia Anderson, Nicole Bleier, John Bradley, Charla Buckner, Monique Campbell, Cheryl Carapezza, Sandy Charette, Melissa Christensen, Jennifer East, Latrice Ellis, Emma Eskander, Tracy Eskander, Cassidy Ewing, Krissy Ferro, Maureen Fink, Roberta Alessandra Finn, Yesenia Fonseca, Victoria Gerstner, Jessie Hajduk, Laura Hand, Debbie Harris, Michael Harvey, Maria K. Hebert, Colleen Hennessey, Shadia Jaber, Shantelle Luety, Tracy Lupinetti, Philip Mandl, Orlando Martinez, Kari Maytum, Katie Meynis, Alexandra Mitchell, Bonnie M. Mitchell, Kristin Mitchell, Maria Moffre-Lynch, Jamie Mookel, Renee Moonan, Carrie Morris, Thanh-Van Nguyen, Jaionna Overton, Trina Palmo, Kristie Peraza, Alanna Perna, Courtney Perrotta, Samantha Perry, Matthew Poissant, Joseph Rojo, Dezmarie Ruiz, Yvette Seils, Frank Shipman, Caitlin Siebert, Amanda Spenziero, Crystal Stephan, Ashley Stewart, Lynn A. Strzelecki, Rosemary Suong, Natalie Tchurekow, Nina Vieira, Betty Vieira, Tiffany Vogt, Tiffany Wade, Lisa Wallace

Reviewers of Milady Standard Cosmetology 2012 Edition

Francis Archer, The Nail Clinic School of Manicuring, SC

Brenda Baker, Euphoria/Lincoln College of Technology, FL

RaNae Barker, Southern Oklahoma Technology Center, OK

Jane Barrett, Chisholm Institute, Victoria, Australia

Yota Batsaras, Sephora USA, CA

Laurie Biagi, Skyline Community College, CA

Melinda Borrego, Mindyfingers, CT

Gina Boyce, Gegi Designs, MO

Peggy Braswell, Swainsboro Technical College, GA

Toni Campbell, Sullivan South High School, TN

Phyllis Causey, Hair By Phyllis, TX

Robin Cochran, Gadsden State Community College, AL

Kimberly Cutter, Savannah Technical College, GA

Corrinne Edwards, CTN Systems, MD

Ami Enzweiler, Salon 4 U, OH

Cortney Forster, The Beauty Bar, MI

Laureen Gillis, Kent Career Technical Center, MI

Shari Golightly, Entanglements Inc. Training Center, CO

Keri Gray, State College of Beauty Culture, WI

Kristy Henderson, East Central Technical College, GA

Mary Jean Hernandez, Southeastern Trade Schools, Inc., GA

Jean Hoffer, Capital Region Career and Technical School, NY

Florence Hogan, Bella Vita Spa, MI

MaryAnn Hough, State of Connecticut Unified Vocational School District #1, CT

Patricia Jones, Southern Union State Community College, AL

Dr. Carolyn Kraskey, Central Beauty School, MN

Susan Kolar, David Pressley Professional School of Cosmetology and Transitions-Mott Community College, MI

Fredrick Laurino, House of Heavilin of Kansas Inc., KS

Danielle Lawson, Kenneth Shuler School of Cosmetology, SC

Helen LeDonne, Santa Monica College, CA

Dawn Mango, John Paulos Extreme Beauty School, NY

Laura Manicho, OPI National School Division, OH

Maria Moffre, Orlo School of Hair Design and Cosmetology, NY

Kirby Morris, Wyoming Board of Cosmetology, WY

Alan Murphy, King Research, WI

Ernestine Peete, Tennessee Technology Center at Memphis, TN

Sandra Peoples, Pickens Technical College, CO

Beth Phillips, Heritage College, MO

Robert Powers, Pinellas Technical Education Center, FL

Debbie Eckstine-Weidner, DeRielle Cosmetology Academy, PA

LuAnne Rickey, The Lab – A Paul Mitchell Partner School, NJ

Conrad Sanchez, Central New Mexico Community College, NM

Denise Sauls, Lurleen B. Wallace Community College, AL

Penny Sawyer, Rapid Response Monitoring, NY

Jennifer Schrodt, University of Nebraska, NE

Kimberly Schroeder, Avalon School of Cosmetology, MN

Vickie Servais, New Horizons Regional Education Center, VA

Donna Simmons, Tulsa Tech, OK

Foy Smith, Beech High School and Looks By Foy, TN

Lisa Sparhawk, Self-Employed Private Educator, NY

Kay Stannard, Four County Career Center, OH

Madeline Udod, Brookhaven Technical Center (Eastern Suffolk BOCES), NY

Rebecca Udwary, San Francisco Institute of Esthetics and Cosmetology, CA

Michael Vanacore, Learning Institute for Beauty Sciences, NY

Therese Vogel, Tiffin Academy of Hair Design, OH

Kenneth Young, Hotheads Hair Design, OK

Tamara Yusupoff, Bellus Academy, The Academy of Beauty and Spa, CA

Ida Scarpelli-Zanon, Northern Gateway Division Onoway High School, AB, Canada

Special Thanks to Milady's Infection Control Advisory Panel for Reviewing & Contributing to Chapter 5, Infection Control: Principles and Practices

- Barbara Acello, M.S., R.N., Denton, TX
- Gerri Cevetillo-Tuccillo, General Manager, Dentronix Inc./Ultronics Inc., OH
- Mike Kennamer, Ed.D., Director of Workforce Development & Skills Training, Northeast Alabama Community College
- Janet McCormick, M.S., Cidesco, FL
- Leslie Roste, R.N., National Director of Education & Market Development, King Research/Barbicide, WI
- Robert T. Spalding, Jr., DPM, TN
- David Vidra, CLPN, WCC, MA, President Health Educators, Inc., OH

PART 1 ORIENTATION

Chapters

CHAPTER 1

History and Career Opportunities

Chapter Outline

© Vladimir Wrangel, 2010; used under license from Shutterstock.com.

Learning Objectives

After completing this chapter, you will be able to:

✓ **LO1** Explain the origins of appearance enhancement.

✓ **LO2** Name the advancements made in cosmetology during the nineteenth, twentieth, and early twenty-first centuries.

✓ **LO3** List several career opportunities available to a licensed beauty practitioner.

Key Terms

Page number indicates where in the chapter the term is used.

Cosmetology
pg. 4

Cosmetology (kahz-muh-TAHL-uh-jee) is a term used to encompass a broad range of specialty areas, including hairstyling, nail technology, and esthetics. Cosmetology is defined as the art and science of beautifying and improving the skin, nails, and hair and includes the study of cosmetics and their application. The term comes from the Greek word *kosmetikos*, meaning skilled in the use of cosmetics. Archaeological studies reveal that haircutting and hairstyling were practiced in some form as early as the Ice Age.

The simple but effective cosmetic implements used at the dawn of history were shaped from sharpened flints, oyster shells, or bone. Animal sinew or strips of hide were used to tie the hair back or as adornment. Ancient people around the world used coloring matter on their hair, skin, and nails, and they practiced tattooing. Pigments were made from berries, tree bark, minerals, insects, nuts, herbs, leaves, and other materials. Many of these colorants are still used today.

© Robyn Mackenzie, 2010; used under license from Shutterstock.com.

Why Study Cosmetology History and Career Opportunities?

Cosmetologists should study and have a thorough understanding of the history of cosmetology and the career opportunities available because:

- Many very old methods have evolved into techniques still used today. Studying the origin of these techniques can be useful in fully understanding how to use them today.
- Knowing the history of your profession can help you predict and understand upcoming trends.
- By learning about many possible career paths, you'll see the wide range of opportunities open to cosmotologists.

Brief History of Cosmetology

The Egyptians

The Egyptians were the first to cultivate beauty in an extravagant fashion. They used cosmetics as part of their personal beautification habits, religious ceremonies, and preparation of the deceased for burial.

As early as 3000 BC, Egyptians used minerals, insects, and berries to create makeup for their eyes, lips, and skin. Henna was used to stain their hair and nails a rich, warm red. They were also the first civilization to infuse essential oils from the leaves, bark, and blossoms of plants for use as perfumes and for purification purposes. Queen Nefertiti (circa 1400 BC) stained her nails red by dipping her fingertips in henna, wore lavish makeup designs, and used custom-blended essential oils as signature scents. Queen Cleopatra (circa 50 BC) took this dedication to beauty to an entirely new level by erecting a personal cosmetics factory next to the Dead Sea.

Ancient Egyptians are also credited with creating kohl makeup—originally made from a mixture of ground galena (a black mineral), sulfur, and animal fat—to heavily line the eyes, alleviate eye inflammation, and protect the eyes from the glare of the sun.

In both ancient Egypt and Rome, military commanders stained their nails and lips in matching colors before important battles (**Figure 1–1**).

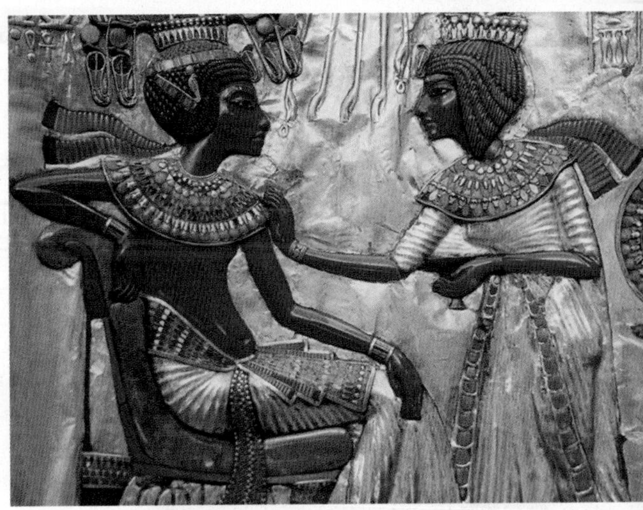

© Corbis

▲ Figure 1–1
The Egyptians wore elaborate hairstyles and cosmetics.

The Chinese

History also shows that during the Shang Dynasty (circa 1600 BC), Chinese aristocrats rubbed a tinted mixture of gum arabic, gelatin, beeswax, and egg whites onto their nails to color them crimson or ebony. Throughout the Chou Dynasty (circa 1100 BC), gold and silver were the royal colors. During this early period in Chinese history, nail tinting was so closely tied to social status that commoners caught wearing a royal nail color faced a punishment of death.

The Greeks

During the golden age of Greece (circa 500 BC), hairstyling became a highly developed art. The ancient Greeks made lavish use of perfumes and cosmetics in their religious rites, in grooming, and for medicinal purposes. They built elaborate baths and developed excellent methods of dressing the hair and caring for the skin and nails. Greek women applied preparations of white lead onto their faces, kohl around their eyes, and vermillion upon their cheeks and lips. Vermillion is a brilliant red pigment, made by grinding cinnabar (a mineral that is the chief source of mercury) to a fine powder. It was mixed with ointment or dusted on the skin in the same way cosmetics are applied today (**Figure 1–2**).

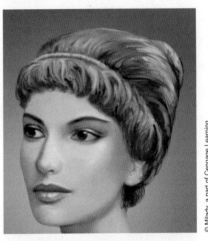

© Milady, a part of Cengage Learning.

▲ Figure 1–2
The Greeks advanced grooming and skin care.

The Romans

Roman women lavishly used fragrances and cosmetics. Facials made of milk and bread or fine wine were popular. Other facials were made of corn with flour and milk, or from flour and fresh butter. A mixture of chalk and white lead was used as a facial cosmetic. Women used hair color to indicate their class in society. Noblewomen tinted their hair red, middle-class women colored their hair blond, and poor women dyed their hair black (**Figure 1–3**).

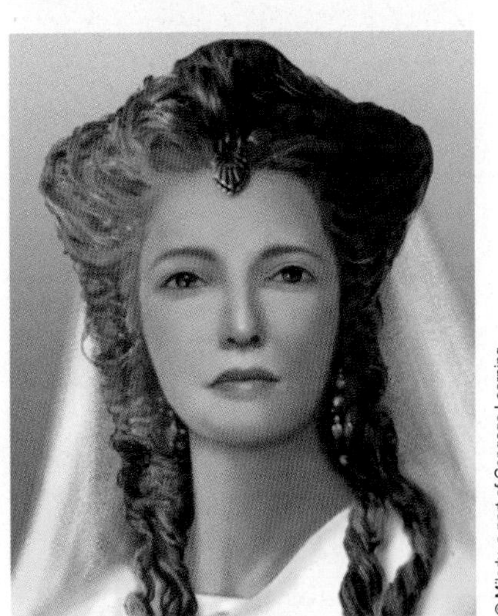

© Milady, a part of Cengage Learning.

▲ Figure 1–3
The Romans applied various preparations to the skin.

The Middle Ages

The Middle Ages is the period of European history between classical antiquity and the Renaissance, beginning with the downfall of Rome, circa AD 476, and lasting until about 1450. Beauty culture is evidenced by tapestries, sculptures, and other artifacts from this period. All of these show towering headdresses, intricate hairstyles, and the use of cosmetics on skin and hair. Women wore colored makeup on their cheeks and lips, but not on their eyes. Around AD 1000, a Persian physician and

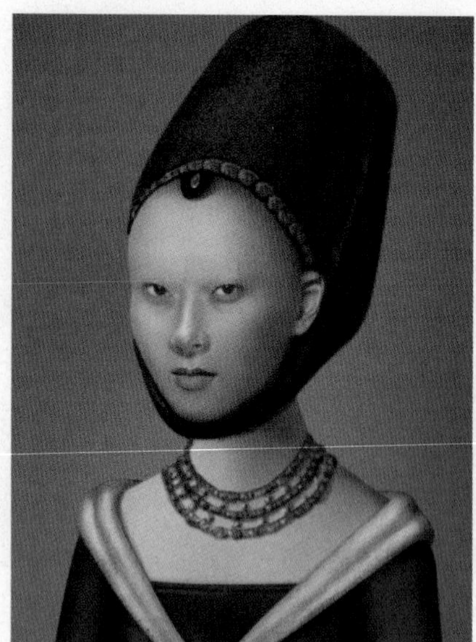

▲ **Figure 1–4**
During the Renaissance, shaving or tweezing of the eyebrows and hairline to show a greater expanse of the forehead was thought to make women appear more intelligent.

alchemist named Avicenna refined the process of steam distillation. This ushered in the modern era of steam-distilled essential oils that we use today.

The Renaissance

This is the period in history during which Western civilization made the transition from medieval to modern history. Paintings and written records tell us a great deal about the grooming practices of the time. One of the most unusual practices was the shaving of the eyebrows and the hairline to show a greater expanse of forehead. A brow-less forehead was thought to give women a look of greater intelligence. During this period, both men and women took great pride in their physical appearance and wore elaborate, elegant clothing. Fragrances and cosmetics were used, although highly colored preparations of the lips, cheeks, and eyes were discouraged (**Figure 1–4**).

The Victorian Age

The reign of Queen Victoria of England, between 1837 and 1901, was known as the Victorian Age. Fashions in dress and personal grooming were drastically influenced by the social mores of this austere and restrictive period in history. To preserve the health and beauty of the skin, women used beauty masks and packs made from honey, eggs, milk, oatmeal, fruits, vegetables, and other natural ingredients. Victorian women are said to have pinched their cheeks and bitten their lips to induce natural color rather than use cosmetics, such as rouge or lip color (**Figure 1–5**). ☑ **LO1**

The Twentieth Century

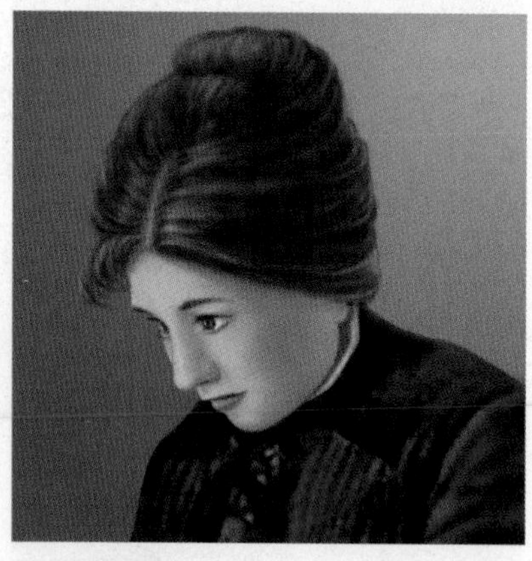

▲ **Figure 1–5**
During the Victorian period, makeup and showy clothing were discouraged except in the theater.

In the early twentieth century, the invention of motion pictures coincided with an abrupt shift in American attitudes. As viewers saw pictures of celebrities with flawless complexions, beautiful hairstyles, and manicured nails, standards of feminine beauty began to change. This era also signaled the spread of industrialization, which brought a new prosperity to the United States. Beauty applications began to follow the trends set by celebrities and society figures (**Figure 1–6**).

1901-1910

In 1904, Max Faktor emigrated from Lodz, Poland, to the United States. By 1908, he had Americanized his name to Max Factor and moved to Los Angeles, where he began making and selling makeup. His makeup was popular with movie stars because it wouldn't cake or crack, even under hot studio lights.

On October 8, 1906, Charles Nessler invented a heavily wired machine that supplied electrical current to metal rods around which hair strands were wrapped. These heavy units were heated during the waving process. They were kept away from the scalp by a complex system of counterbalancing weights that were suspended from an overhead chandelier mounted on a stand. Two methods were used to wind hair

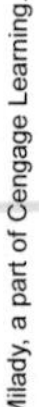
© Milady, a part of Cengage Learning.

strands around the metal units. Long hair was wound from the scalp to the ends in a technique called spiral wrapping. After World War I, when women cut their hair into the short bobbed style, the croquignole (KROH-ken-yohl) wrapping technique was introduced. In this method, shorter hair was wound from the ends toward the scalp. The hair was then styled into deep waves with loose end-curls.

One of the most notable success stories of the cosmetology industry is that of Sarah Breedlove. She was the daughter of former slaves and was orphaned at age seven when she went to work in the cotton fields of the Mississippi delta. In 1906, Sarah married her third husband, C. J. Walker, and became known as Madame C. J. Walker. Sarah suffered from a scalp condition and began to lose her hair, which caused her to experiment with store-bought products and homemade remedies. She began to sell her scalp conditioning and healing treatment called "Madam Walker's Wonderful Hair Grower." She devised sophisticated sales and marketing strategies and traveled extensively to give product demonstrations. In 1910, she moved her company to Indianapolis where she built a factory, hair salon, and training school. As she developed new products, her empire grew. She devoted much time and money to a variety of causes in Indianapolis, including the National Association for the Advancement of Colored People (NAACP) and the Young Men's Christian Association (YMCA). In 1917, she organized a convention for her Madam C. J. Walker Hair Culturists Union of America. This was one of the first national meetings for businesswomen ever held. By the time of her death, she had established herself as a pioneer in the modern African-American hair care and cosmetics industry.

In 1872, Marcel Grateau (AKA Francois Marcel) invented the first curling iron—tongs heated by a gas burner. Later, around 1923, he created an electric version. Because he introduced several electric versions, the actual date of the invention remains in dispute. Grateau went on to develop a permanent wave machine, barbers clippers, a safety razor, and other devices.

1920s

The cosmetics industry grew rapidly during the 1920s. Advertising expenditures in radio alone went from $390,000 in 1927 to $3.2 million in 1930. At first, many women's magazines deemed cosmetics improper and refused to print cosmetic advertisements, but by the end of the 1920s, cosmetics provided one of their largest sources of advertising revenue.

1930s

In 1931, the preheat-perm method was introduced. First, hair was wrapped using the croquignole method. Then, clamps that had been preheated by a separate electrical unit were placed over the wound curls. An alternative to the machine perm was introduced in 1932

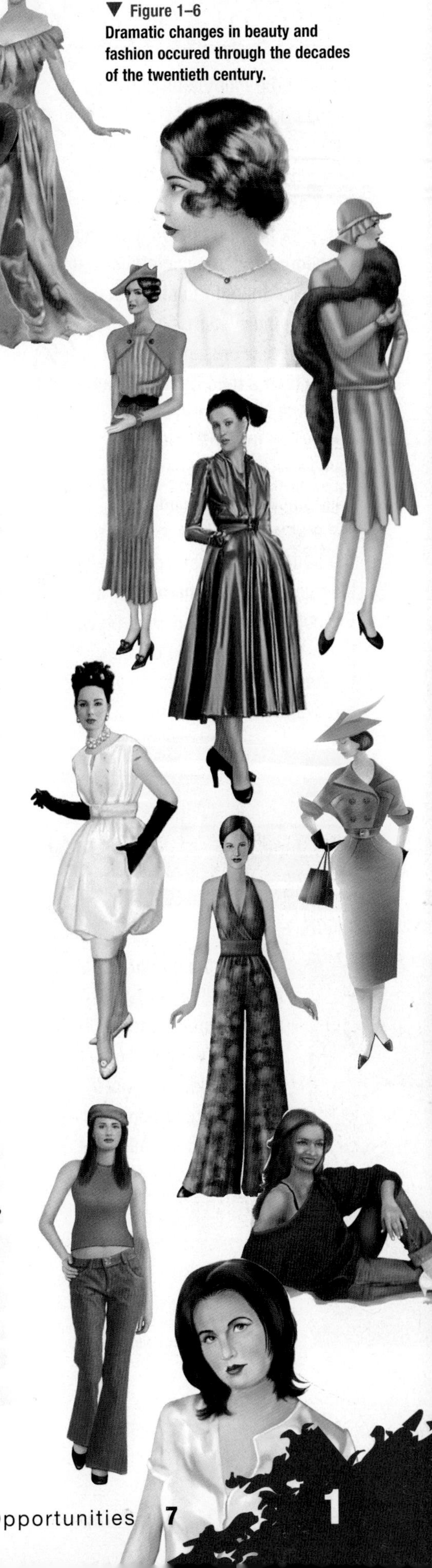

▼ **Figure 1–6**
Dramatic changes in beauty and fashion occured through the decades of the twentieth century.

© Milady, a part of Cengage Learning.

did you know?

Up until the nineteenth century, many barbers also performed minor surgeries and practiced dentistry. In fact, the barber pole, a symbol of the barber–surgeon, has its roots in a medical procedure called bloodletting that was once thought to strengthen the immune system. The pole is believed to represent the staff that patients held tightly to make the veins in their arms stand out during the procedure. The bottom cap represents the basin used to catch the blood. The red and white stripes represent the bandages that stopped the bleeding and were then hung on the pole to dry. As the wind blew, these bandages would become twisted around the pole, forming a red-and-white pattern.

The modern barber pole, then, was originally the symbol of the barber–surgeon, and is believed to represent the bandages (white), blood (red), and veins (blue) involved in bloodletting (Figure 1–7).

Up until the end of the nineteenth century, even in the United States, both men and women wore wigs. Today wigs are making a resurgence as a fashion item, riding the popularity wave of hair extensions.

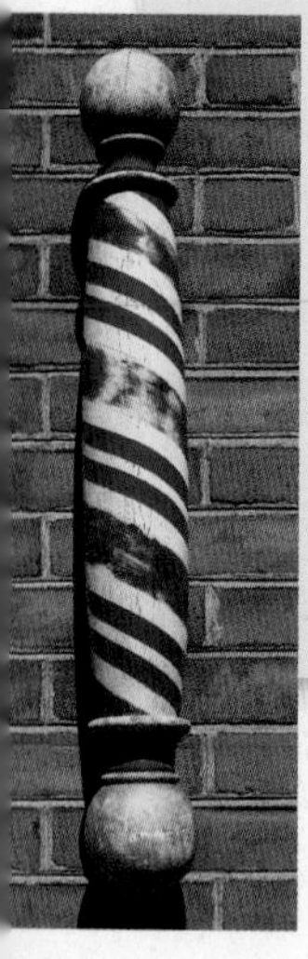

▶ **Figure 1–7**
A traditional barber pole.

© Corbis.

when chemists Ralph L. Evans and Everett G. McDonough pioneered a method that used heat generated by chemical reaction: small flexible pads containing a chemical mixture were wound around hair strands. When the pads were moistened with water, a chemical heat was released that created long-lasting curls. Thus the first machineless permanent wave was born. Salon clients were no longer subjected to the dangers and discomforts of the Nessler machine.

In 1932, nearly 4,000 years after the first recorded nail-color craze, Charles Revson of Revlon fame marketed the first nail polish—as opposed to a nail stain—using formulas that were borrowed from the automobile paint industry. This milestone marked a dramatic shift in nail cosmetics as women finally had an array of nail lacquers available to them. The early screen sirens Jean Harlow and Gloria Swanson glamorized this hip new nail fashion in silent pictures and early talkies by appearing in films wearing matching polish on their fingers and toes.

Also in 1932, Lawrence Gelb, a New York Chemist, introduced the first permanent haircolor product and founded a company called Clairol. In 1935, Max Factor created pancake makeup to make actors' skin look natural on color film. In 1938, Arnold F. Willatt invented the cold wave that used no machines or heat. The cold wave is considered to be the precursor to the modern perm.

1940s

In 1941, scientists developed another method of permanent waving that used waving lotion. Because this perm did not use heat, it was also called a cold wave. Cold waves replaced virtually all predecessors and competitors. In fact, the terms *cold waving* and *permanent waving* became practically synonymous. Modern versions of cold waves, usually referred to as alkaline perms, are very popular today. The term *texture services* is used today to refer to the variety of permanent waving and straightening services available for various hair types and conditions.

1951–2000

The second half of the twentieth century saw the introduction of tube mascara, improved hair care and nail products, and the boom and then death of the weekly salon appointment. In the late 1960s, Vidal Sassoon turned the hairstyling world on its ear with his revolutionary geometric cuts. The 1970s saw a new era in highlighting when French hairdressers introduced the art of hair weaving using aluminum foil. In the 1980s, makeup went full circle, from barely there to heavily made-up "cat-eyes" and the heavy use of eye shadows and blush. In the 1990s, haircolor became gentler, allowing all ethnicities to enjoy being blonds, brunettes, or redheads. In 1998, Creative Nail Design introduced the first spa pedicure system to the professional beauty industry.

The Twenty-First Century

Today, hairstylists have far gentler, no-fade haircolor. Estheticians can noticeably rejuvenate the skin, as well as keep disorders such as sunspots and mild acne at bay. The beauty industry has also entered the age of specialization. Now cosmetologists frequently specialize either in haircolor or in haircutting; estheticians specialize in esthetic or medical-aesthetic services; and nail technicians either offer a full array of services or specialize in artificial nail enhancements, natural nail care, or even pedicures.

Since the late 1980s, the salon industry has evolved to include day spas, a name that was first coined by beauty legend Noel DeCaprio. Day spas now represent an excellent employment opportunity for beauty practitioners (**Figure 1–8**).

Men-only specialty spas and barber spas have also grown in popularity. These spas provide exciting new opportunities for men's hair, nail, and skin-care specialists. **Figure 1–9** on page 10 is a timeline of significant events in the cosmetology industry. ✔ **LO2**

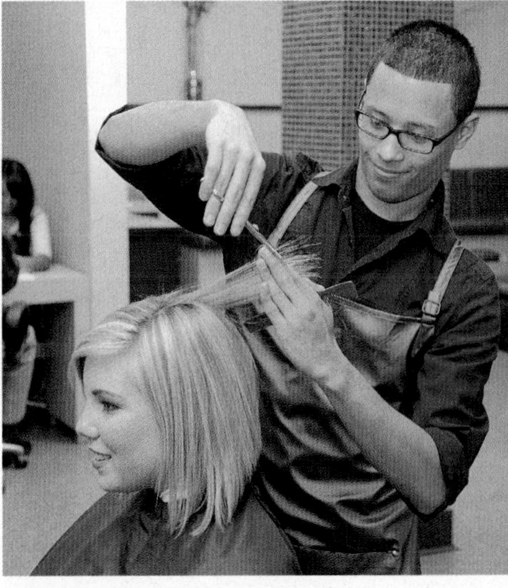

▲ **Figure 1–8**
Day spas are increasing in number and popularity.

Career Paths for Cosmetologists

Once you have completed your schooling and are licensed, you will be amazed at how many career opportunities will open up to you. The possibilities can be endless for a hard-working professional cosmetologist who approaches her or his career with a strong sense of personal integrity. Within the industry there are numerous specialties, such as the following:

- **Haircolor specialist.** Once you have received additional training and experience in haircolor, you may be responsible for training others in your salon to perform color services or work for a product manufacturer, where you will be expected to train other professionals how best to perform color services according to the company's guidelines and product instructions (**Figure 1–10**).
- **Texture specialist.** Once you have received additional training and experience in texture services you may be responsible for training others to perform texture services in the salon, or work for a manufacturer where you will be expected to train others on how best to perform texture services according to your company's guidelines and product instructions. A subspecialty, curly hair specialist, focuses on maintaining natural curl.
- **Cutting specialist.** This position requires a dedicated interest in learning various cutting styles and techniques. After perfecting your own skills and developing your own method of cutting (everyone develops his or her own cutting technique), you may want to study with other reputable haircutters to learn and adopt their systems and techniques. This training will allow you to perform top-quality haircutting in your own salon, as well as to coach those around you, helping them to hone their skills (**Figure 1–11**).

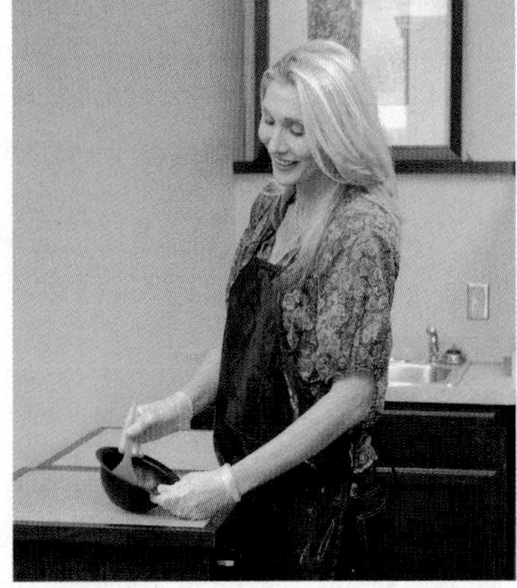

▲ **Figure 1–10**
Haircolor specialists are in great demand.

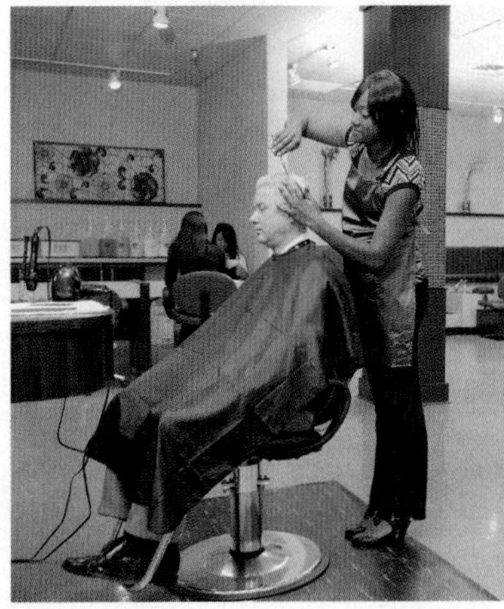

▲ **Figure 1–11**
Cutting hair in a salon is one of the many choices open to you.

© Milady, a part of Cengage Learning. Photography by Yanik Chauvin.

Figure 1–9

A Timeline of Milestones in the Professional Beauty Industry.

3000 BC 2500 2000 1500 1100 BC

3000 BC Egyptians used minerals, insects, and berries to create makeup for their eyes, lips, and skin. Henna was used to stain their hair and nails a rich, warm red. They also infused essential oils from the leaves, bark, and blossoms of plants for use as perfumes and purification purposes.

1600 BC Chinese aristocrats rubbed a tinted mixture of gum arabic, gelatin, beeswax, and egg whites onto their nails to color them crimson or ebony.

1400 BC Queen Nefertiti stained her nails red by dipping her fingertips in henna, wore lavish makeup designs, and used custom-blended essential oils as signature scents.

1100 BC Throughout the Chinese Chou Dynasty, gold and silver were the royal colors. Nail tinting was so closely tied to social status that commoners caught wearing a royal nail color faced a punishment of death.

© Vladimir Wrangel, 2010; used under license from Shutterstock.com.

1900 1905 1910 1915

1872 Marcel Grateau (AKA Francois Marcel) invented the first curling iron—gas burner-heated tongs. About 1923, he created an electric version.

1900s Motion picture viewers saw pictures of celebrities with flawless complexions, beautiful hairstyles, and manicured nails, and standards of feminine beauty began to change.

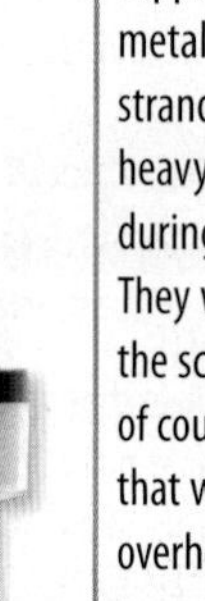

1906 Charles Nessler invented a heavily wired machine that supplied electrical current to metal rods around which hair strands were wrapped. These heavy units were heated during the waving process. They were kept away from the scalp by a complex system of counterbalancing weights that were suspended from an overhead chandelier mounted on a stand.

1908 Max Factor began making and selling makeup to movie stars that wouldn't cake or crack, even under hot studio lights.

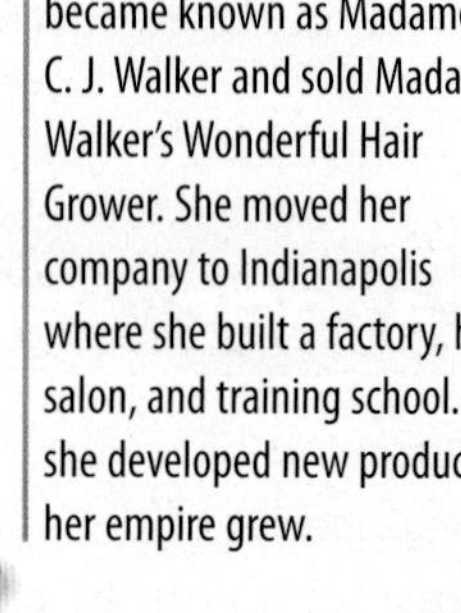

1910 Sarah Breedlove became known as Madame C. J. Walker and sold Madam Walker's Wonderful Hair Grower. She moved her company to Indianapolis where she built a factory, hair salon, and training school. As she developed new products, her empire grew.

© Milady, a part of Cengage Learning.

1940 1950 1960

1935 Max Factor created pancake makeup to make actors' skin look natural on color film.

1938 Arnold F. Willatt invented the cold wave that used no machines or heat. The cold wave is considered to be the precursor to the modern perm.

1941 Scientists developed another method of permanent waving that used waving lotion. Because this perm did not use heat, it was also called a cold wave. Cold waves replaced virtually all predecessors and competitors, and the terms *cold waving* and *permanent waving* became practically synonymous.

1960s Vidal Sassoon turned the hairstyling world on its ear with his revolutionary geometric cuts.

© Milady, a part of Cengage Learning.
© Zastol`skiy Victor Leonidovich, 2010; used under license from Shutterstock.com.

2000 2001 2002 2003 2004 2005

2000 According to a Vance Research Services' study of 1,500 salon owners, 30 percent of salons used a computer for business while at work and 44 percent used it for business at home. Sixty-five percent of respondents had home Internet access, while just 17 percent had it in their salons.

2003 Sebastian International introduces the first consumer-oriented DVD to the professional salon industry, in order to speak directly to the consumer.

2005 Most salons have their own websites and use e-mail to communicate. Point-of-sale software and computerized appointment scheduling are in widespread use.

© Borodaev, 2010; used under license from Shutterstock.com.

500 BC 50 AD 1000 1500 1850

500 BC During the golden age of Greece, hairstyling became a highly developed art. The ancient Greeks made lavish use of perfumes and cosmetics in their religious rites and personal grooming. Greek women applied preparations of white lead onto their faces, kohl around their eyes, and vermillion upon their cheeks and lips.

50 BC Queen Cleopatra took dedication to beauty to an entirely new level by erecting a personal cosmetics factory next to the Dead Sea.

AD 1000 Persian physician and alchemist, Avicenna, refined the process of steam distillation. This ushered in the modern era of steam-distilled essential oils that we use today.

1837–1901 To preserve the health and beauty of the skin, women used beauty masks and packs made from honey, eggs, milk, oatmeal, fruits, vegetables, and other natural ingredients.

© Natalia Lisovskaya, 2010; used under license from Shutterstock.com.

1920 1925 1930

1917 Madame Walker organized a convention for her Madam C. J. Walker Hair Culturists Union of America. This was one of the first national meetings for businesswomen ever held.

1920s The cosmetics industry grew rapidly. Advertising expenditures in radio alone went from $390,000 in 1927 to $3.2 million in 1930.

1931 The preheat perm method was introduced. Hair was wrapped using the croquignole method. Clamps, preheated by a separate electrical unit, were then placed over the wound curls.

1932 Chemists Ralph L. Evans and Everett G. McDonough pioneered a method that used heat generated by chemical reaction: small flexible pads containing a chemical mixture were wound around hair strands. When the pads were moistened with water, a chemical heat was released that created long-lasting curls. Thus the first machineless permanent wave was born. Salon clients were no longer subjected to the dangers and discomforts of the Nessler machine.

Also that year, Charles Revson of Revlon fame marketed the first nail polish—as opposed to a nail stain—using formulas that were borrowed from the automobile paint industry. Lawrence Gelb, a New York Chemist, introduced the first permanent haircolor product and founded a company called Clairol.

© Milady, a part of Cengage Learning.

1970 1980 1990

1970s French hairdressers introduced the art of hair weaving using aluminum foil.

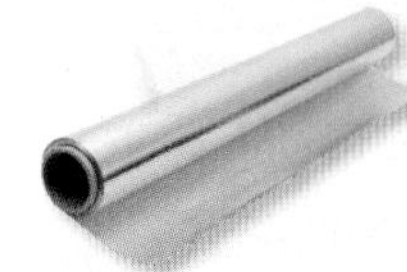

1980s Makeup went full circle, from barely there to heavily made-up "cat-eyes" and the heavy use of eye shadows and blush. Also, the salon industry evolved to include day spas, a name that was first coined by beauty legend Noel DeCaprio.

1990s Haircolor became gentler, allowing all ethnicities to enjoy being blonds, brunettes, or redheads.

1998 Creative Nail Design introduced the first spa pedicure system to the professional beauty industry.

1999 Spas hit their stride as big business. According to the International Spa Association (ISPA), consumers spent $14.2 billion in about 15,000 destination and day spas.

© Bogdan Ionescu, 2010; used under license from Shutterstock.com.
© Milady, a part of Cengage Learning.

2006 2007 2008 2009 2010

2006 Brazilian straightening treatments are introduced in the U.S.

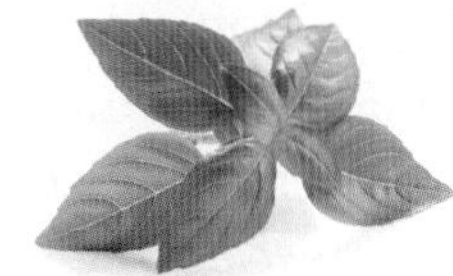

2007 Haircolor becomes the largest hair care category in terms of in-salon, back bar, and take-home color refresher product sales. The green movement takes off in salons, with many positioning themselves as eco salons and spas striving for sustainability. In April, the first American television reality-competition show for salons, Shear Genius, debuts.

2008 There is an explosion in salons using social networking sites to do business. Twitter, which was introduced in March, 2006, becomes the next big thing in social networking with clients.

2009 Many beauty manufacturers have Mobile versions of their Websites. Access to instant online technical education and color formulas becomes common.

© Robyn Mackenzie, 2010; used under license from Shutterstock.com.

did you know?

Although cosmetologists who work in salons and spas do not have to join a union to be considered for work or to be entitled to certain benefits of employment, to work on films, television shows, and theater you may need to join a union.

The unions have different names, one of the largest is the Makeup and Hairstylists Union, also known as the International Alliance of Theatrical Stage Employees, Moving Picture Technicians, Artist and Allied Crafts of the United States and Canada, AFL-CIO, CLC (IA).

You may also need to join the Makeup and Hairstylists Guild, or the Actor's union.

- **Salon trainer.** Many companies, such as manufacturers and salon chains, hire experienced salon professionals and train them to train others. This kind of training can take many forms, from technical training to management and interpersonal relationship training. A salon trainer can work with small salons, as well as large organizations and trade associations, to help develop the beauty industry's most valuable resource—salon staff and personnel.
- **Distributor sales consultant.** The salon industry depends heavily on its relationships with product distributors in order to stay abreast of what is occurring in the marketplace. Distributor sales consultants (DSCs) provide information about new products, new trends, and new techniques. This specialty provides an excellent opportunity for highly skilled and trained cosmetology professionals. The DSC is the salon and its staff's link with the rest of the industry, and this relationship represents the most efficient method that outside companies use to reach the salon stylist.
- **Manufacturer educator.** Most manufacturers hire their own educators to train stylists and salon staff to understand and use the company's hair care, haircolor, and chemical-service products. Mastery of the company's product lines is a must for manufacturer educators. An accomplished educator who is a good public speaker can advance to field educator, regional educator, or even platform educator, appearing on stage at shows in the U.S. and around the world.
- **Cosmetology instructor.** Have you ever wondered how your instructor decided to start teaching? Many instructors had fantastic careers in salons before dedicating themselves to teaching new professionals the tricks of the trade. If this career path interests you, spend some time with your school's instructors and ask them why they went into education. Educating new cosmetologists can be very trying, but it can also be very rewarding.
- **Film or theatrical hairstylist and editorial stylist.** Working behind the scenes at magazine and Internet photo shoots or backstage on movies and TV sets all starts with volunteering to assist. Even someone right out of school can volunteer by calling agencies, networking with photographers, or asking other hairdressers who work behind the scenes for advice. The days are long—up to eighteen hours on soap opera sets—but once you clock the specific number of hours required by your state of residence, you can join the local union, which opens many doors. All you need are persistence, networking skills, reliability, team spirit, and attention to detail.

© FXQuadr, 2010; used under license from Shutterstock.com.

ACTivity

You may think you already know which area of cosmetology interests you most. But as you learn more, that can change. To help you determine the best area of speciality, interview a salon owner or a specialist in your area. Ask the following questions:

- Why did you choose the specialty you did?
- What special skills are required?
- What type of training was required to become a specialist?
- How long did it take you to get really proficient?
- What's the most exciting thing about your specialization?

To find someone to interview, ask your instructors for ideas, visit local salons, go to trade shows, or search the Internet for specialists in your area—or anywhere! Many salon owners, colorists, texture specialists, business experts, and educators can be found through social networks like Facebook, Myspace, LinkedIn, and many others.

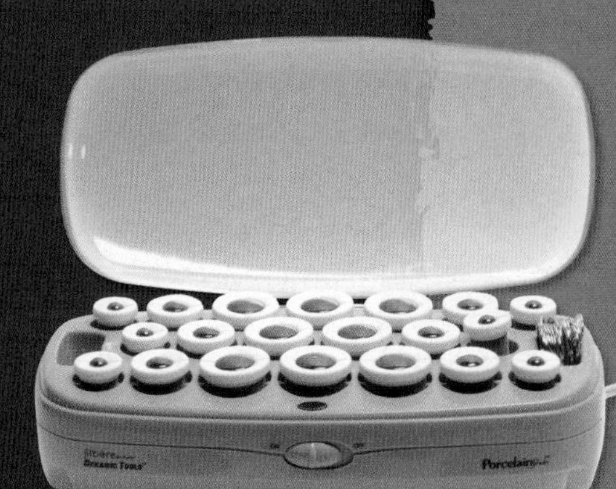
© Milady, a part of Cengage Learning.

This field requires constant continuing education, particularly in working with wigs, hairpieces, and makeup. ✓ **LO3**

These are but a few of the many career paths awaiting you on the road to a lifelong career in cosmetology. The wonderful thing about the professional beauty industry is that there are truly no limits to what you can do if you have a sincere interest in learning and giving back to your industry. Keep developing your skills in the specialities that interest you, and you'll soon be building and enjoying an extremely creative and unique career.

Salon Management

If business is your calling, you will find that management opportunities in the salon and spa industry are quite diverse. They include being an inventory manager, department head, educator, special events manager (promotions), assistant manager, and general manager. With experience, you can also add salon owner to this list of career possibilities. To ensure your success, it is wise to enroll in business classes to learn more about managing products, departments, and—above all—people.

Salon manager is a potential career path for a cosmetologist, but it requires a very different skill set. As a result, some managers of large operations are not cosmetologists. Salon managers must have an aptitude for math and accounting and be able to read documents such as profit and loss statements. They should understand marketing, including the roles of advertising, public relations and promotions, and what makes these programs successful. Much of management involves the business side of the salon—making it profitable—while keeping clients and employees

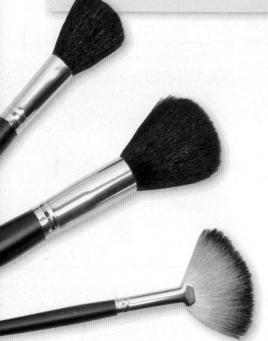

FYI

The field of cosmetology has broadened to encompass areas of specialization, including esthetics and nail technology. As the cosmetology industry continues to grow, opportunities for professionals increase.

According to a study by the National Accrediting Commission of Cosmetology Arts and Sciences (NACCAS), salons employed around 1,683,000 professionals in 2007, and 53 percent of salons had job openings. Nearly three-quarters of salon owners with positions to fill could not find qualified applicants, even though about 38 percent of the jobs were for inexperienced professionals with less than a year on the job.

While many factors, including the national economy, affect the industry, the salon business usually withstands recessions much better than other industries. To make each day in school positively impact your future, focus on your studies, read trade publications cover-to-cover, become a member of relevant trade associations, and attend workshops outside of school. Remember, your license will unlock countless doors, but it is your personal dedication and passion that ultimately determines how successful you become.

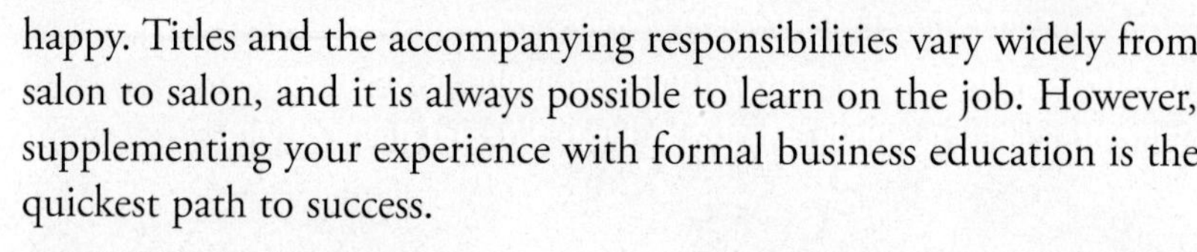

happy. Titles and the accompanying responsibilities vary widely from salon to salon, and it is always possible to learn on the job. However, supplementing your experience with formal business education is the quickest path to success.

Beyond choosing a specialty, you must decide on the type of facility where you will work. Many options are available:

- Specialty salons
- Full-service salons (offering hair, skin, and nail services)
- Photo, video, or film sets (preparing models and actors for camera appearances)
- Day spas (offering services that emphasize both beauty and wellness) (**Figure 1–12**)

© Milady, a part of Cengage Learning.

To learn more about the various types of salon business models, see Chapter 32, The Salon Business. There you will find a wealth of choices, including national and regional chains and low- and high-end salon opportunities.

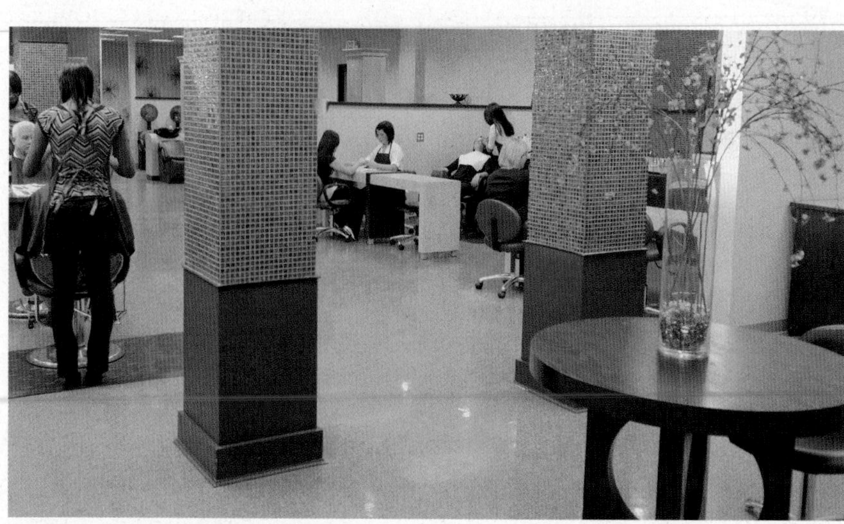

© Milady, a part of Cengage Learning. Photography by Yanik Chauvin.

▶ **Figure 1–12**
A day spa may offer nail, hair, body, and skin services.

Review Questions

1. What are the origins of appearance enhancement?
2. What are some of the advancements made in cosmetology during the nineteenth, twentieth, and early twenty-first centuries?
3. What are some of the career opportunities available to licensed beauty practitioners?

Chapter Glossary

cosmetology	The art and science of beautifying and improving the skin, nails, and hair and includes the study of cosmetics and their application.

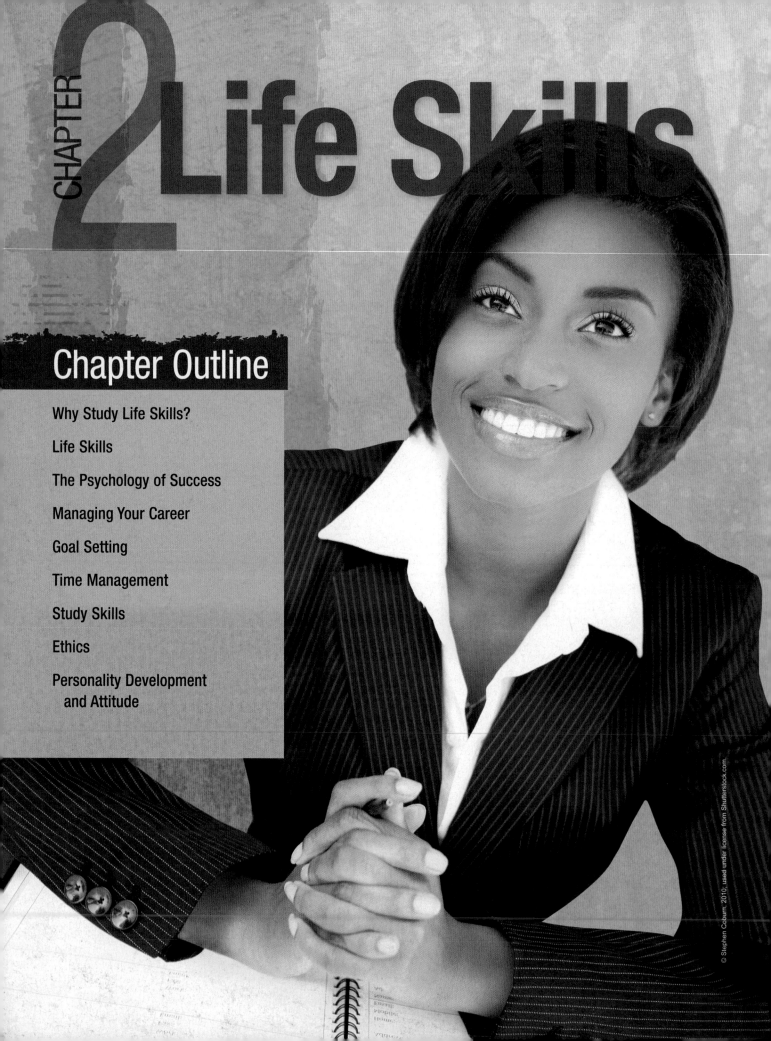

CHAPTER 2 Life Skills

Chapter Outline

- Why Study Life Skills?
- Life Skills
- The Psychology of Success
- Managing Your Career
- Goal Setting
- Time Management
- Study Skills
- Ethics
- Personality Development and Attitude

© Stephen Coburn, 2010, used under license from Shutterstock.com.

Learning Objectives

After completing this chapter, you will be able to:

- ✓ **LO1** List the principles that contribute to personal and professional success.
- ✓ **LO2** Create a mission statement.
- ✓ **LO3** Explain how to set long-term and short-term goals.
- ✓ **LO4** Discuss the most effective ways to manage time.
- ✓ **LO5** Describe good study habits.
- ✓ **LO6** Define ethics.
- ✓ **LO7** List the characteristics of a healthy, positive attitude.

Key Terms

Page number indicates where in the chapter the term is used.

ethics
pg. 29

game plan
pg. 20

goal setting
pg. 24

mission statement
pg. 22

perfectionism
pg. 20

prioritize
pg. 26

procrastination
pg. 20

School has one set of challenges, and staying on course for your entire career has another set of challenges. Life skills are particularly important in the field of cosmetology because the hard-and-fast rules that apply to more structured industries are frequently absent in the salon. By its nature, the salon is a creative workplace where you are expected to exercise your artistic talent. The salon is also a highly social atmosphere that requires strong self-discipline and excellent people skills. Besides making a solid connection with each client, you must always stay focused on the task at hand. You must display competence and enthusiasm every time you take care of a client's needs—no matter how you feel, or how many hours you have been at work. Your livelihood and your personal feelings of success depend on how well you maintain this attitude.

WHY STUDY LIFE SKILLS?

Cosmetologists should study and have a thorough understanding of life skills because:

- Practicing good life skills will lead to a more satisfying and productive career in the beauty industry.
- Hair stylists work with many different types of clients and having good life skills can help you keep those interactions positive, in any situation.
- The ability to deal with difficult clients, coworkers, and even friends comes from having well-developed life skills.
- Having good life skills builds high self-esteem, which in turn helps you achieve your goals.

Life Skills

Some of the most important life skills for you to remember and practice in the salon (and outside it) include:

- Being genuinely caring and helpful to others.
- Making good friends.
- Feeling good about yourself.
- Having a sense of humor to take you through difficult situations.
- Maintaining a cooperative attitude.
- Approaching all of your work with a strong sense of responsibility.
- Being consistent in your work.
- Successfully adapting to different situations.

© Elena Elisseeva, 2010; used under license from Shutterstock.com.

- Sticking to a goal and seeing a job through to completion.
- Mastering techniques that will help you become more organized.
- Developing a deep reservoir of common sense.

The Psychology of Success

Are you passionate about studying? Do you see yourself sustaining this passion one year, five years, or even ten years from now? While cosmetology school is definitely challenging, school becomes much easier when you put that extra amount of effort, enthusiasm, and excitement into your studies. If your talent is not fueled by the passion necessary to sustain you over the course of your career, you can have all the talent in the world and still not be successful (**Figure 2–1**).

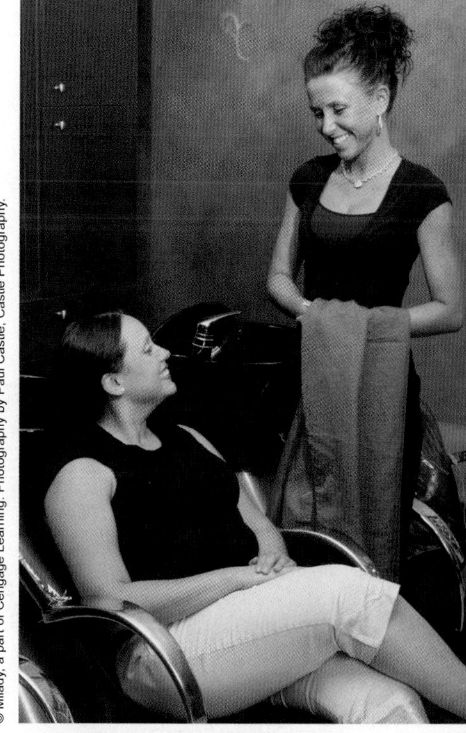
© Milady, a part of Cengage Learning. Photography by Paul Castle, Castle Photography.

▲ **Figure 2–1**
Loving your work is critical to your success.

Guidelines for Success

Defining success is a very personal thing. There are some basic principles, however, that form the foundation of all personal and business success. You can begin your path to success right now by examining and putting these principles into practice:

- **Build self-esteem.** Self-esteem is based on inner strength and begins with trusting your ability to achieve your goals. It is essential that you develop high self-esteem while you are still a student.
- **Visualize success.** Imagine yourself working in your dream salon, competently handling clients, and feeling at ease and happy with your situation. The more you practice visualization, the more easily you will turn your vision into reality.
- **Build on your strengths.** Practice doing whatever helps you maintain a positive self-image. If you are good at doing something (e.g., playing the guitar, running, cooking, gardening, or singing), the time you invest in this activity will allow you to feel good about yourself (**Figure 2–2**). Remember that there may be things you are good at that you may not realize. You may be a good listener, for instance, or a caring and considerate friend.
- **Be kind to yourself.** Stop self-critical or negative thoughts that can work against you. If you make a mistake, tell yourself that it is okay and you will do better next time.
- **Define success for yourself.** Do not depend on other people's definition of success. Instead, become a success in your own eyes. What is right for your sister or a friend, for instance, may not be right for you.
- **Practice new behaviors.** Because creating success is a skill, you can develop it by practicing positive new behaviors, such as speaking with confidence, standing tall, staying true to yourself, or even remembering to use good grammar.

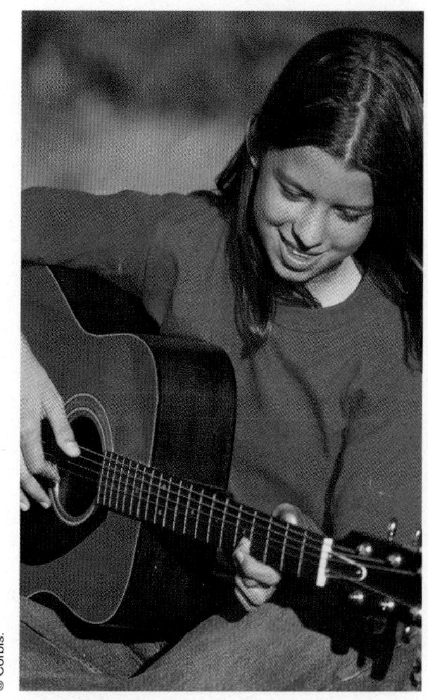
© Corbis.

▲ **Figure 2–2**
Spend time on the things you do well.

- **Keep your personal life separate from your work.** Talking about your personal life and that of others at work is counterproductive and can cause the whole salon to suffer.
- **Keep your energy up.** Successful cosmetologists do not run themselves ragged, nor do they eat, sleep, and drink beauty. They take care of their personal needs by spending time with family and friends, having hobbies, enjoying recreational activities, and living a full life.

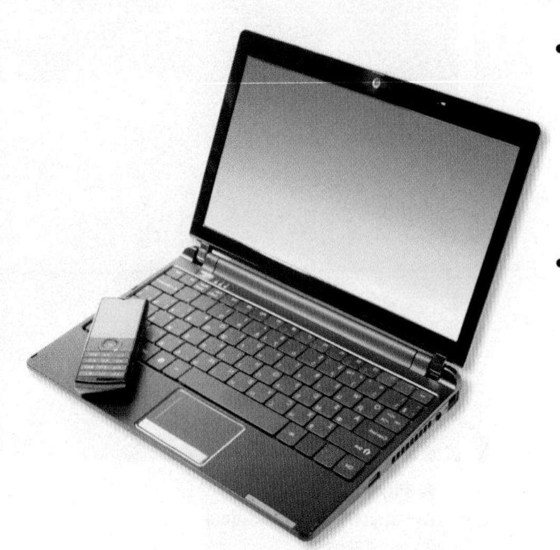

© Borodaev, 2010; used under license from Shutterstock.com.

- **Respect others.** Make a point of relating to everyone you know with a conscious feeling of respect. Exercise good manners with others by using words like *please*, *thank you*, and *excuse me*. Do not interrupt people when they are speaking, and practice being a good listener.
- **Stay productive.** There are three bad habits that can keep you from maintaining peak performance: (1) procrastination, (2) perfectionism, and (3) lack of a game plan. You will see an almost instant improvement in your productivity when you eliminate these troublesome tendencies.

  1. **Procrastination** is putting off until tomorrow what you can do today. This destructive, yet common, habit is a characteristic of poor study habits. (I'll study tomorrow instead of today.) It may also be a symptom of taking on too much, which, in turn, is a symptom of faulty organization.
  2. **Perfectionism** is an unhealthy compulsion to do things perfectly. Success is not defined as doing everything perfectly. In fact, someone who never makes a mistake may not be taking risks necessary for growth and improvement. A better definition of success is not giving up, even when things get really tough.
  3. **Lacking a game plan.** Having a **game plan** is the conscious act of planning your life, instead of just letting things happen. While an overall game plan is usually organized into large blocks of time (five or ten years), it is just as important to set daily, monthly, and yearly goals. Where do you want to be in your career five years from now? What do you have to do this week, this month, and this year to move closer to that goal?

Rules for Success

To be successful, you must take ownership of your education. While your instructors can create motivational circumstances and an environment to assist you in the learning process, the ultimate responsibility for learning is yours. To realize the greatest benefits from your education, commit yourself to the following rules that will take you a long way down the road of success:

- Attend all classes.
- Arrive for class early.

- Have all necessary materials ready.
- Listen attentively to your instructor.
- Highlight important points.
- Take notes for later review.
- Pay close attention during summary and review sessions.
- When something is not clear, ask. If it is still not clear, ask again.

Even after you complete school, you should regularly seek continuing education opportunities. Never stop learning. The cosmetology industry is constantly changing. There are always new trends, techniques, products, and information. Throughout your career you should read industry magazines and books, and you should attend trade shows and advanced educational classes.

Motivation and Self-Management

Motivation propels you to do something. Self-management involves knowing what you want to achieve and keeping yourself on track so that you do eventually achieve your goal. When you are hungry, for example, you are motivated to eat. But it is self-management that helps you to decide how you will get food. A motivated student finds it much easier to learn. The best motivation for learning comes from an inner desire to grow your skills as a professional—a lifelong pursuit that is motivated by the ever-changing world of professional beauty.

If you are personally drawn to cosmetology, then you are likely to be interested in the material you study in school. If your motivation comes from some external source—for instance, your parents, friends, or a vocational counselor—you might have a difficult time finishing school and jump-starting your beauty career. To achieve success, you need more than an external push; you must feel a sense of personal excitement and a good reason for staying the course. You are the one in charge of managing your own life and learning. To do this successfully, you need good self-management skills.

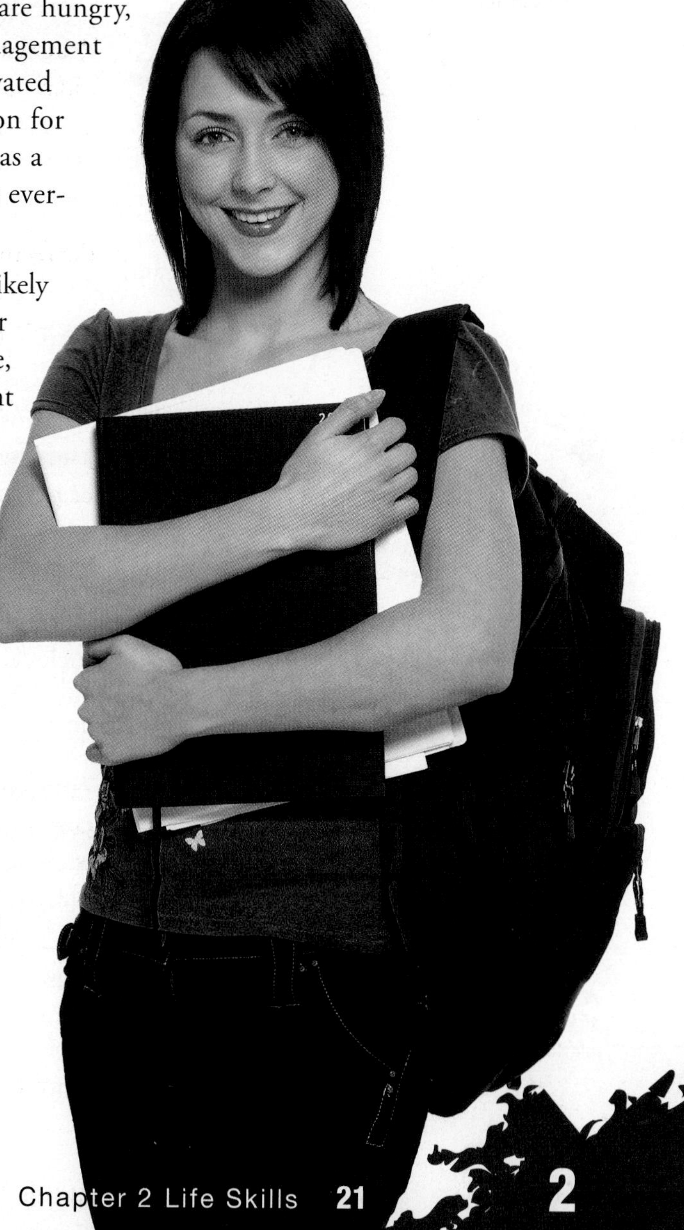

© Dean Mitchell, 2010; used under license from Shutterstock.com.

Your Creative Capability

One self-management skill you can draw on is creativity. Creativity means having a talent such as painting, acting, cutting hair, applying makeup, or doing artificial nails. Creativity is also an unlimited inner resource of ideas and solutions. To enhance your creativity, keep these guidelines in mind:

- **Do not be self-critical.** Criticism blocks the creative mind from exploring ideas and discovering solutions to challenges.

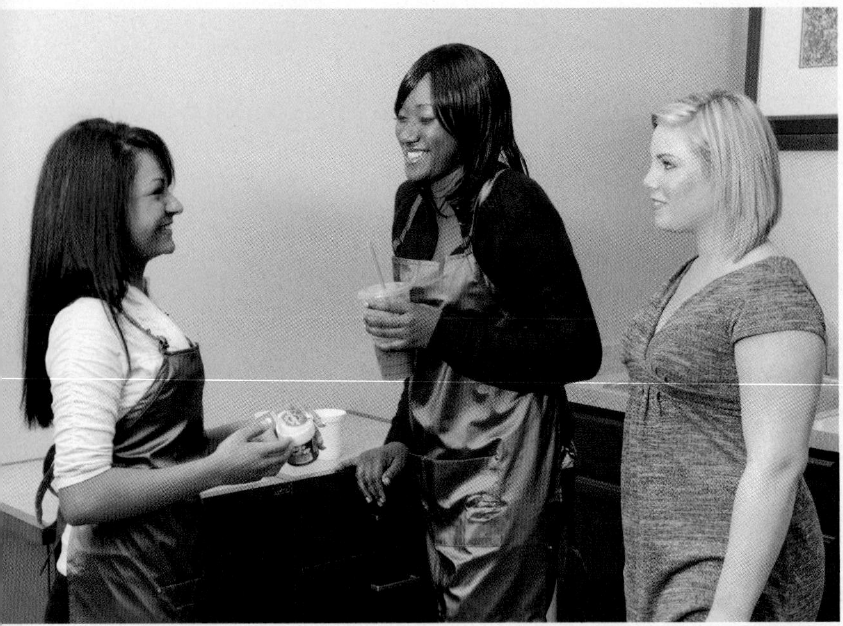

© Milady, a part of Cengage Learning. Photography by Yanik Chauvin.

▲ Figure 2–3
Build strong relationships for support.

- **Do not look to others for motivation.** Tapping into your own energy and creativity will be the best way to manage your success.
- **Change your vocabulary.** Build a positive vocabulary by using active problem-solving words like *explore*, *analyze*, *determine*, and other words of this nature.
- **Do not try to go it alone.** In today's hectic and pressured world, many talented people find that they are more creative in an environment where people work together and share ideas. This is where the value of a strong salon team comes into play (**Figure 2–3**). ☑ **LO1**

Managing Your Career

As you navigate your beauty career, you will come up against difficulties—shallow spots, rocks, swift currents, and even an occasional iceberg—no matter how creative, talented, or motivated you are. Knowing how to manage your career will make all the difference in staying afloat.

Design a Mission Statement

Every successful business has a business plan. An essential part of business plans is the **mission statement**, which establishes values the institution lives by as well as target goals (**Figure 2–4**). If you are going to succeed in life, you will need a well thought-out sense of purpose and a plan that supports that purpose. In other words, like a successful business, you will need a mission statement.

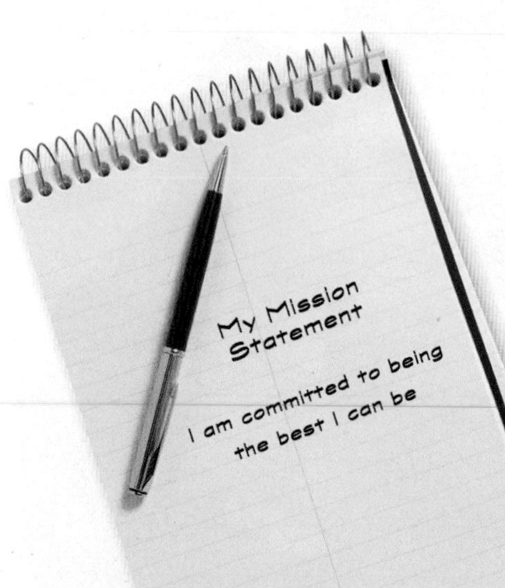

My Mission Statement
I am committed to being the best I can be

© Photodisc.

▲ Figure 2–4
An example of a personal mission statement.

In order to know where you want to go and what your mission statement will include, you will need to know what interests you most and which of these interests you wish to pursue. To help you, take the Interests Self-Test (**Figure 2–5**) before working on your mission statement.

Try to prepare a mission statement in one or two sentences that communicates who you are and what you want for your life. One example of a simple, yet thoughtful, mission statement is: "I am dedicated to pursuing a successful career with dignity, honesty, and integrity." Your career will be directed by the mission statement you make now. Your mission statement will point you in the right direction and help you feel secure when things temporarily go off course. For reinforcement, keep a copy of your mission statement where you can see it, and read it frequently. ☑ **LO2**

The Interests Self-Test

Your personality is tied to your interests. You've already learned about cosmetology specialties. Why not start thinking about which specialty interests you the most? This quick quiz gives you an idea of where your future might lie, based on your personal preferences.

1. Which subject interests you most?

A. Chemistry
B. Geometry
C. Accounting

2. Which of the following would you rather do?

A. Analyze a problem
B. Solve a problem
C. Read about a problem

3. When you look at a painting, what do you notice first?

A. Color
B. Shape
C. Details

4. When it comes to coworkers, would you prefer to:

A. Work with one other person on a specific problem
B. Work with a team to get lots of ideas
C. Work alone or tell them what to do

5. When it comes to salon clients, do you think they:

A. Know exactly what they want, and that's good
B. Are open to new ideas and suggestions, which is fun
C. Probably want a good value

Instructions: Add up the number of As, Bs and Cs. Then check below to see what might be of most interest to you.

Mostly As. Hair color, which involves chemistry, detail work, and solving specific problems might be a good choice for you. Of course, color can be creative, too, but you need strong fundamentals and a mind for detail to reach the top. Additionally, clients frequently bring in a photo of a specific hair color, and you must know how to get from point A (their natural color) to point B (their desired color).

Mostly Bs. Hair cutting involves an understanding of geometry, lines, and shapes. Clients may want a certain look but they can't always have it if their hair type doesn't allow it. That's why the ability to gather ideas and make suggestions is important. At the advanced level, there are several different cutting methods to try out.

Mostly Cs. Business demands an attention to details, the ability to crunch numbers, and an understanding of client's desires and consumer trends. While you sometimes work alone, you also have to be able to manage other people, which is an additional consideration. If you like taking responsibility for yourself and others, you might consider focusing on the business of salons.

Figure 2–5
The Interests Self-Test.

© Milady, a part of Cengage Learning.

Goal Setting

Some people never have a fixed goal in mind. They go through life one day at a time without really deciding what they want, where they can find it, or how they are going to live their lives once they get it. They drift from one activity to the next aimlessly. Does this describe you? Or do you have direction, drive, desire, and a dream? If so, do you have a reasonable idea of how to go about meeting your goal(s)?

> **FYI**
>
> **Real-Life Goal Setting:** Many salon managers help you set goals, based on the salon's criteria. One common goal is for stylists to sell retail products to a specific number or percentage of clients or in an amount equal to a percentage of billed services. For example, stylists might be required to retail at least 30 percent of gross.
>
> Another common salon goal is that stylists should be booked a certain amount of the time and maintain a specific client-retention rate. Usually, you cannot raise your prices unless you are booked 80 to 90 percent of the time and retain about 70 percent of your clients.
>
> Goals that salons set are almost always tied to your income. In turn, goals that stylists set for themselves are often based on what they want to earn. Salon managers will help you break down financial goals into attainable, daily goals. For example, if you want to gross $10,000 more a year, you need to earn an additional $27.39 per day. Of course, you don't work seven days a week. A more realistic number is based on working five days a week, fifty-two weeks out of the year. You need to gross $38.46 more per day, and fortunately there are many different ways to do it in the salon business. You can sell retail to half your clients; you can up-sell color services and back-bar treatments; or you can get more clients.

Goal setting is the identification of long- and short-term goals that help you decide what you want out of your life. When you know what you want, you can draw a circle around your destination and chart the best course to get you there. By mapping out your goals, you will see where you need to focus your attention and what you need to learn in order to fulfill your dreams.

How Goal Setting Works

There are two types of goals: short term and long term. An example of a short-term goal is to get through a competency exam successfully. Another short-term goal would be graduating from cosmetology school. Short-term goals are usually considered to be those you wish to accomplish in a year or less.

Long-term goals are measured in larger sections of time such as five years, ten years, or even longer. An example of a long-term goal is becoming a salon owner in five years.

Once you have organized your thinking around your goals, write them down in short-term and long-term columns and divide each set of goals into workable segments. In this way, your goals will not seem out of sight or overwhelming. For example, one of your long-term goals should be to get your license to practice cosmetology. At first, getting this license might seem to require an overwhelming amount of time and effort. However, when you separate this goal into short-term goals (such as going to class on time, completing homework assignments, and mastering techniques), you see that each step on the way to the long-term goal can be accomplished without too much difficulty or stress.

The important thing to remember about goal setting is to have a plan and to re-examine it often in order to make sure that you are staying on track. Even people who have fame, fortune, and wide-spread respect continue to set goals for themselves. While they may adjust their goals and action plans as they go along, successful people know that goals move them toward additional successes (**Figure 2–6 and Figure 2–7**). ☑ **LO3**

HOW TO SET AND TRACK SHORT-TERM GOALS

NUMBER	GOAL SETTING CHECKLIST	COMPLETION DATE	DONE
1.	Read Chapter 2. Action Steps: Read first part at lunch; finish it after dinner.	6/09/2012	❑
2.	Practice speaking to clients in a pleasing voice. Action Steps: Do with family tonight.	6/10/2012	❑
3.	Create my own mission statement. Action Steps: Review sample in Chapter Two; write my own.	6/15/2012	❑
4.	Start learning trends. Action Steps: Search online, read trade and beauty magazines. Make a 5-word "trend list."	6/20/2012	❑
5.	Prepare to pass the Chapter 2 exam. Action Steps: Review what I read, ask instructor any questions, have study session with 2 friends.	7/10/2012	❑
6.	Practice being on time! Action Steps: Set alarm for 15 minutes earlier. Give self $1 every time I get to class 10 minutes early.	Start 6/20 5 days in a row by 7/20	
7.	Build my vocabulary. Action Steps: Buy book or find Website. Learn 1 new word a day.	Daily	

▲ **Figure 2–6**
A sample of how to set and track short-term goals.

MY GOALS

NUMBER	GOAL SETTING CHECKLIST	COMPLETION DATE	DONE
1.			
2.			
3.			
4.			
5.			
6.			
7.			

© Milady, a part of Cengage Learning.

▲ **Figure 2–7**
Photocopy this template and fill in your own goals!

ACTivity

It is estimated that as much as four hours in the average person's day are spent checking e-mail, looking at Websites, and watching videos. The average teenager sends nearly 80 text messages a day! To find out if you are managing your time well, try this exercise:

- Write down the time in the morning when you first go online, check e-mail, or send a text message.
- Do what you normally do online, then note the time you finish these activities.
- Throughout the day try to estimate (and add to your list) how much additional time you spend on these activities.
- Add up the total time at the end of your day.

Are you surprised? Time-management experts recommend that you work for the first forty-five minutes or hour of the day, avoiding e-mailing, Web browsing, and texting during this time. Instead, use this time to plan your day, review reading materials for school, or do other work. This first hour of the day is often the best time to accomplish something concrete because it is quiet and often interruption-free. Starting your day by being productive helps you develop good time-management skills for life.

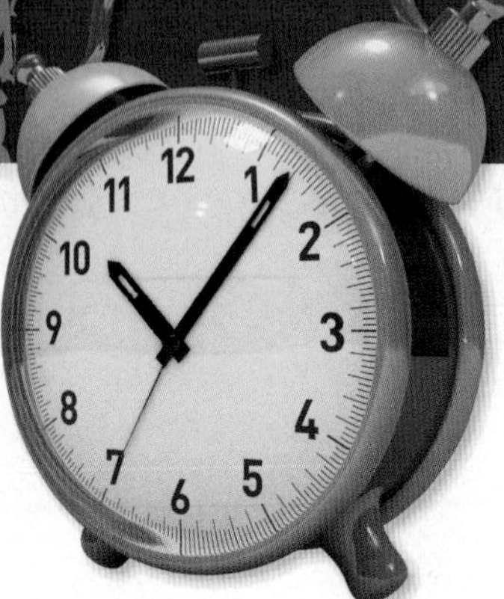

© Zaptik, 2010; used under license from Shutterstock.com.

Time Management

One thing that all time-management experts agree on is that each of us has an *inner organizer*. When we pay attention to our natural rhythms, we can learn how to manage our time efficiently, allowing us to reach our goals faster and with less frustration. Here are some of the most effective ways to manage time:

- Learn to **prioritize** by ordering tasks on your to-do list from most important to least important.
- When designing your own time management system, make sure it will work for you. For example, if you are a person who needs a fair amount of flexibility, schedule in some blocks of unstructured time.
- Never take on more than you can handle. Learn to say "no" firmly but kindly, and mean it. You will find it easier to complete your tasks if you limit your activities and do not spread yourself too thin.
- Learn problem-solving techniques that will save you time and needless frustration.
- Give yourself some down time whenever you are frustrated, overwhelmed, worried, or feeling guilty. You lose valuable time and energy when you are in a negative state of mind. Unfortunately, there may be situations—such as when you are in the classroom—in which you cannot get up and walk away. To handle these difficult times,

try practicing the technique of deep breathing. Just fill your lungs as much as you can and exhale slowly. After about five to ten breaths, you will usually find that you have calmed down and your inner balance has been restored.

- Carry a notepad, an organizer, or your electronic notepad with you at all times. You never know when a good idea might strike or when you will need to add a task to your schedule. Write these things down before they slip your mind!
- Make daily, weekly, and monthly schedules that show exam times, study sessions, and any other regular commitments. Plan your leisure time around these commitments, rather than the other way around (**Figure 2–8**).
- Identify times during the day when you are typically energetic and times when you typically want or need to relax. Plan your schedule accordingly.
- Reward yourself with a special treat or activity for work well done and time managed efficiently.
- Do not neglect physical activity. Remember that exercise and recreation stimulate clear thinking and efficient planning.
- Schedule at least one block of free time each day. This will be your hedge against events that come up unexpectedly, such as car trouble, baby-sitting problems, helping a friend in need, or any other unforeseen circumstance.
- Understand the value of to-do lists for the day and the week. These lists help you prioritize tasks and activities, a key element to organizing your time efficiently (**Figure 2–9**).
- Make time management a habit. ☑ **LO4**

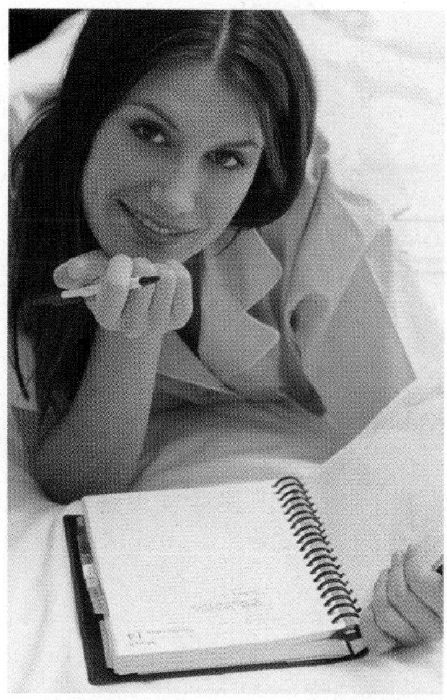

© Corbis.

▲ **Figure 2–8**
Keep a schedule for yourself and refer to it frequently.

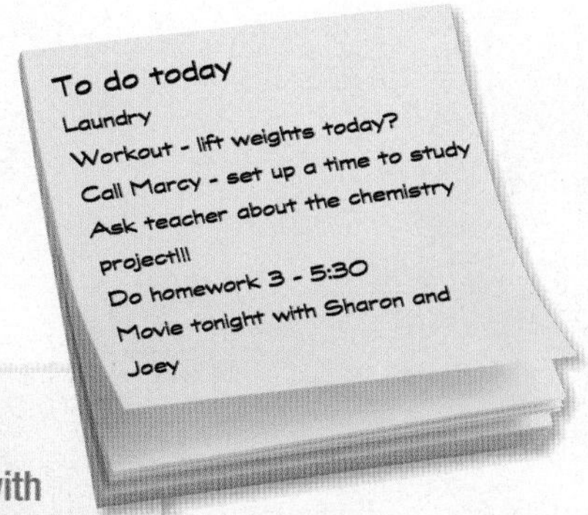

To do today
Laundry
Workout - lift weights today?
Call Marcy - set up a time to study
Ask teacher about the chemistry project!!!
Do homework 3 - 5:30
Movie tonight with Sharon and Joey

© Photodisc.

▲ **Figure 2–9**
An example of a to-do list.

FYI

Real-Life Time Management: In the salon, the most important aspect of time management is staying on schedule with your bookings so that you can greet each client at the scheduled appointment time. This means completing the service during the time allotted. Some salons book haircuts on the hour; others book them in intervals of forty-five minutes. Accomplished stylists do a cut in half an hour, but they usually schedule clients for longer so they can upsell more services if the opportunity presents itself.

Making sure that you arrive on time, start your first client as soon as he or she arrives, and stay on schedule will take you a long way toward success as a stylist. The front desk and salon manager can be a tremendous help if you find yourself falling behind or if you have the opportunity to add-on a color service and need help fitting it into your day. With experience, you'll learn to accommodate late clients and add-on services like a pro.

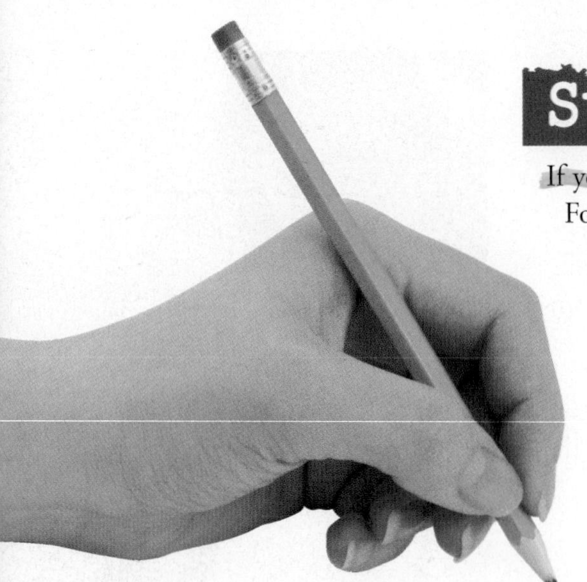

Study Skills

If you find studying overwhelming, focus on small tasks one at a time. For example, instead of trying to study for three hours at a stretch and suffering a personal defeat when you fold after forty minutes, set the bar lower by studying in smaller chunks of time. If your mind tends to wander in class, try writing down key words or phrases as your instructor discusses them. Any time you lose your focus, do not hesitate to stay after class and ask questions based on your notes.

Another way to get a better handle on studying is to find other students who are helpful and supportive. The more you discuss new material with others, the more comfortable you and they will become with the material. In the end, everyone will be more successful. If possible, study together (**Figure 2–10**).

© Tatiana Popova, 2010; used under license from Shutterstock.com.

Establishing Good Study Habits

Part of developing consistently good study habits is knowing where, when, and how to study.

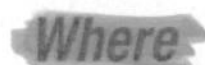

Where

- Establish a comfortable, quiet spot where you can study without interruptions.

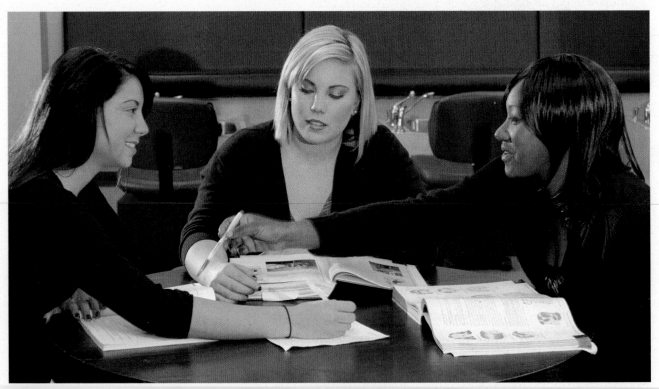

© Milady, a part of Cengage Learning. Photography by Yanik Chauvin.

▲ **Figure 2–10**
Studying with a friend can be effective and fun.

- Have everything you need—books, pens, paper, proper lighting, and so on—before you begin studying.
- Remain as alert as possible by sitting upright. Reclining will make you sleepy!

When

- Start out by estimating how much study time you need.
- Study when you feel most energetic and motivated.
- Practice effective time management by studying during blocks of time that would otherwise be wasted—such as while you are waiting in the doctor's office, taking a bus across town,and so forth.

How

- Study just one section of a chapter at a time, instead of reading the entire chapter at once.
- Make note of key words and phrases as you go along.
- Test yourself on each section to ensure that you understand and remember the key points of each chapter.

Remember that every effort you make to follow through on your education is an investment in your future. The progress you make with your learning will increase your confidence and self-esteem across the board. In fact, when you have mastered a range of information and techniques, your self-esteem will soar right along with your grades. ✓ **LO5**

FOCUS ON

THE GOAL

Determine whether your goal-setting plan is an effective one by asking yourself these key questions:

- Are there specific skills I will need to learn in order to meet my goals?
- Is the information I need to reach my goals readily available?
- Am I willing to seek out a mentor or a coach to enhance my learning?
- What is the best method or approach that will allow me to accomplish my goals?
- Am I open to finding better ways of putting my plan into practice?

Ethics

Ethics are the moral principles by which we live and work. In the salon setting, ethical standards should guide your conduct with clients and fellow employees. When your actions are respectful, courteous, and helpful, you are behaving in an ethical manner.

There are five professional behaviors that will show you are an ethical person. You can practice ethics in the salon every day by:

- Providing skilled and competent services.
- Being honest, courteous, and sincere.
- Avoiding sharing clients' private matters with others—even your closest friends.
- Participating in continuing education and staying on track with new information, techniques, and skills.
- Giving clients accurate information about treatments and products. ✓ **LO6**

FOCUS ON

PROFESSIONAL ETHICS

Ethical people often embody the following qualities:

- **Self-care.** Many service providers suffer from stress and eventually burnout because they focus too much of their energy and time on other people and too little on themselves. If you are to be truly helpful to others, it is essential to take care of yourself. Try The Self-Care Test to assess how you are doing (**Figure 2–11**).
- **Integrity.** Maintain your integrity by matching your behavior and actions to your values. For example, if you believe it is unethical to increase your sales by recommending products that clients don't really need, then do not engage in that behavior. On the other hand, if you feel that a client would benefit from certain products and additional services, it would be unethical not to give the client that information.
- **Discretion.** Do not share your personal issues with clients. Likewise, never breach confidentiality by repeating personal information that clients have shared with you.
- **Communication.** Your responsibility to behave ethically extends to your communications with customers and coworkers. In other words, you should always be honest.

The Self-Care Test

Some people know intuitively when they need to stop, take a break, or even take a day off. Other people forget when to eat. You can judge how well you take care of yourself by noting how you feel physically, emotionally, and mentally. Here are some questions to ask yourself to see how you rate on the self-care scale.

1. Do you wait until you are exhausted before you stop working?
2. Do you forget to eat nutritious food and substitute junk food on the fly?
3. Do you say you will exercise and then put off starting a program?
4. Do you have poor sleep habits?
5. Are you constantly nagging yourself about not being good enough?
6. Are your relationships with people filled with conflict?
7. When you think about the future are you unclear about the direction you will take?
8. Do you spend most of your spare time watching TV?
9. Have you been told you are too stressed and yet you ignore these concerns?
10. Do you waste time and then get angry with yourself?

Score 5 points for each yes. A score of 0-15 says that you take pretty good care of yourself, but you would be wise to examine those questions you answered yes to. A score of 15-30 indicates that you need to rethink your priorities. A score of 30-50 is a strong statement that you are neglecting yourself and may be headed for high stress and burnout. Reviewing the suggestions in these chapters will help you get back on track.

© Milady, a part of Cengage Learning.

▲ **Figure 2–11**
The Self-Care Test.

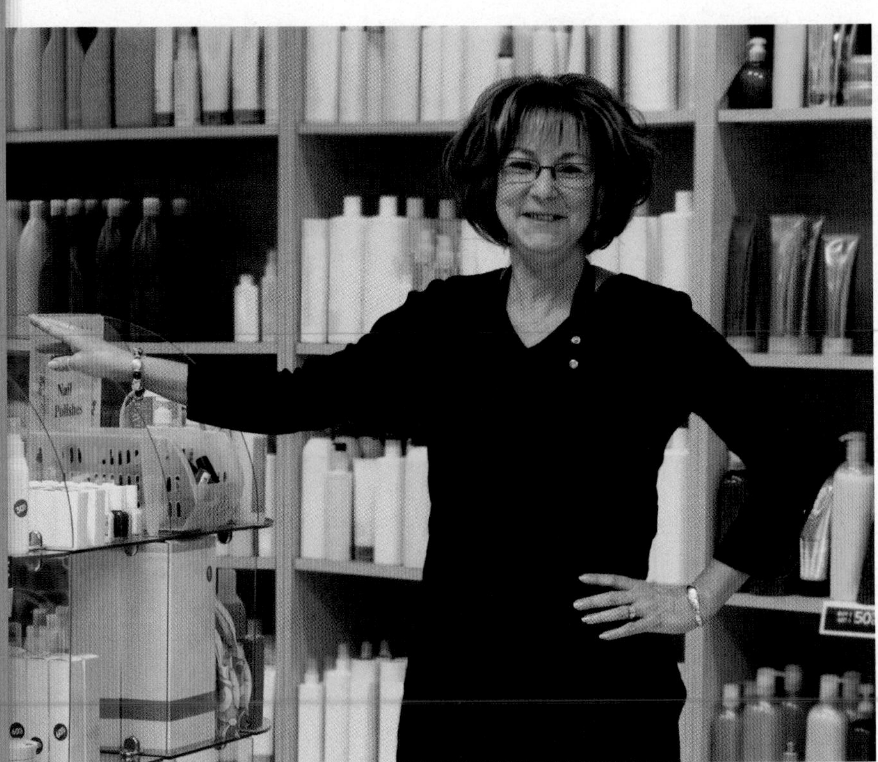

© Melissa Carrol, 2010; used under license from iStockphoto.com.

Personality Development and Attitude

Some occupations require less interaction with people than others. For example, computer programmers do not usually interact with all different sorts of people every day. Cosmetologists, however, deal with people from all walks of life—every day, all day. It is useful, therefore, to have some sense of how different personality traits and attitudes can affect your success.

© Sakala, 2010; used under license from Shutterstock.com.

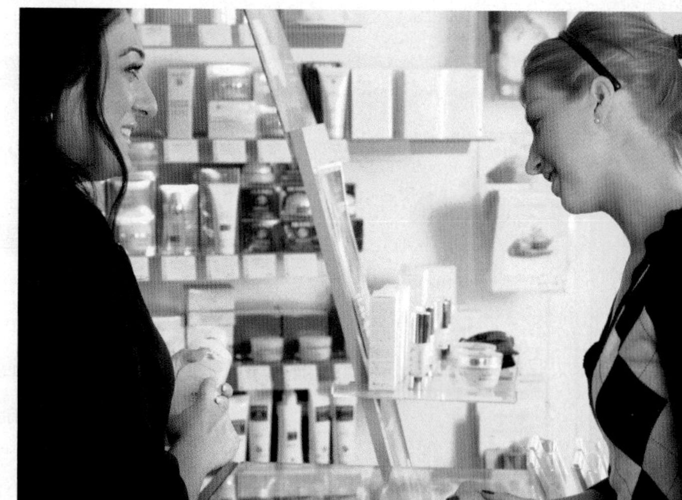

Refer regularly to the following characteristics of a healthy, positive attitude to ensure that they match your self-description.

- **Diplomacy.** Being assertive is a good thing because it helps people understand your position. However, it is a short step from assertive to aggressive or even bullying. Take your attitude temperature to see how well you practice the art of diplomacy. Diplomacy—also known as *tact*—is the ability to deliver truthful, even sometimes critical or difficult, messages in a kind way.
- **Pleasing tone of voice.** The tone of your voice is an inborn personality trait, but if your natural voice is harsh or if you tend to mumble, you can consciously improve by speaking more softly or more clearly. Also, if you have a positive attitude, this will shine through in a pleasant delivery, even if your tone of voice is not ideal.

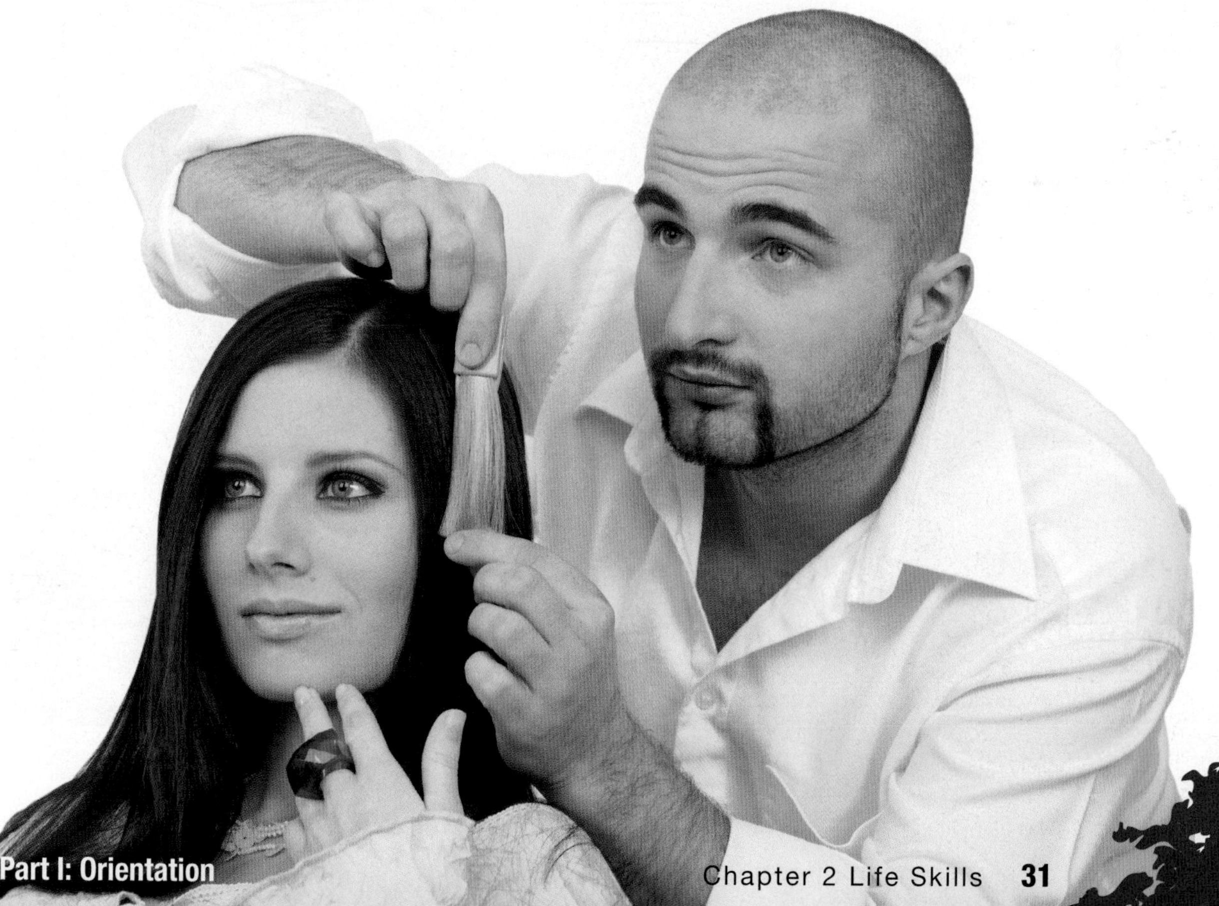

© CandyBox Photography, 2010; used under license from iStockphoto.com.

FOCUS ON

THE WHOLE PERSON

An individual's personality is the sum total of her or his inborn characteristics, attitudes, and behavioral traits. While you may not be able to alter most of your inborn characteristics, you certainly can work on your attitude. Attitude improvement is a process that continues throughout life. In both your business and personal life, a pleasing attitude gains more associates, clients, and friends. You will know you have a pleasing attitude when you are able to see the good in difficult situations. People enjoy the company of individuals who can put a positive "spin" on things.

- **Emotional stability.** Our emotions are important, but they do require some control. Some people express themselves excessively or inappropriately. When they are happy, they get almost frantic; when they are angry, they fly into a rage. Learning how to handle a confrontation and how to share your feelings without going overboard are important indicators of maturity and important demonstrations of emotional stability.
- **Sensitivity.** Sensitivity is a combination of understanding, empathy, and acceptance. Being sensitive means being compassionate and responsive to other people.
- **Values and goals.** Neither values nor goals are inborn characteristics; we acquire them as we move through life. Values and goals guide our behavior and give us direction.
- **Receptivity.** To be receptive means to be interested in other people, and to be responsive to their opinions, feelings, and ideas. Receptivity involves taking the time to really listen, instead of just pretending to do so (**Figure 2–12**).
- **Effective communication skills.** Effective communicators usually have warm, caring personalities. They usually have an easy time talking about themselves and listening to what others have to say. When they want something, they can ask for it clearly and directly, and they pay attention when somebody else is speaking to them.

☑ **LO7**

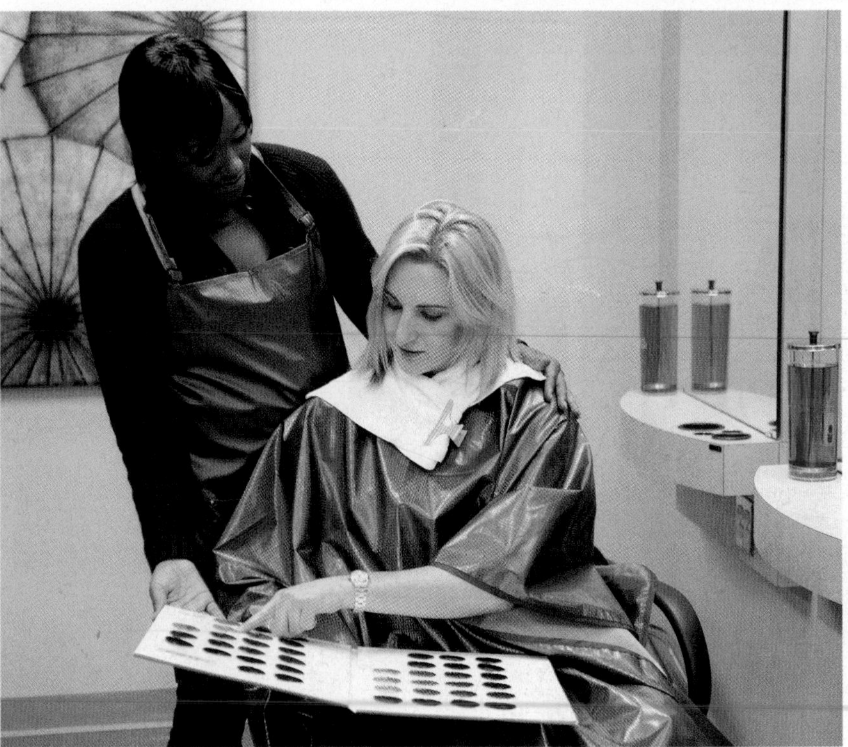

▶ **Figure 2–12 Being receptive is an important personal skill.**

© Milady, a part of Cengage Learning. Photography by Yanik Chauvin.

Review Questions

1. What principles contribute to personal and professional success?
2. How do you create a mission statement? (Give an example.)
3. How do you go about setting long- and short-term goals?
4. What are some of the most effective ways to manage time?
5. How do you describe good study habits?
6. What is the definition of the word ethics?
7. What are the characteristics of a healthy, positive attitude?

Chapter Glossary

ethics	The moral principles by which we live and work.
game plan	The conscious act of planning your life, instead of just letting things happen.
goal setting	The identification of long-term and short-term goals that helps you decide what you want out of life.
mission statement	A statement that establishes the values that an individual or institution lives by, as well as future goals.
perfectionism	An unhealthy compulsion to do things perfectly.
prioritize	To make a list of tasks that needs to be done in the order of most-to-least important.
procrastination	Putting off until tomorrow what you can do today.

CHAPTER 3

Your Professional Image

Chapter Outline

© Diego Cervo, 2010; used under license from Shutterstock.com.

Learning Objectives

After completing this chapter, you will be able to:

- ✓ **LO1** Understand the importance of professional hygiene.
- ✓ **LO2** Explain the concept of dressing for success.
- ✓ **LO3** Demonstrate an understanding of ergonomic principles and ergonomically correct postures and movement.

Key Terms

Page number indicates where in the chapter the term is used.

ergonomics
pg. 41

personal hygiene
pg. 37

physical presentation
pg. 40

professional image
pg. 38

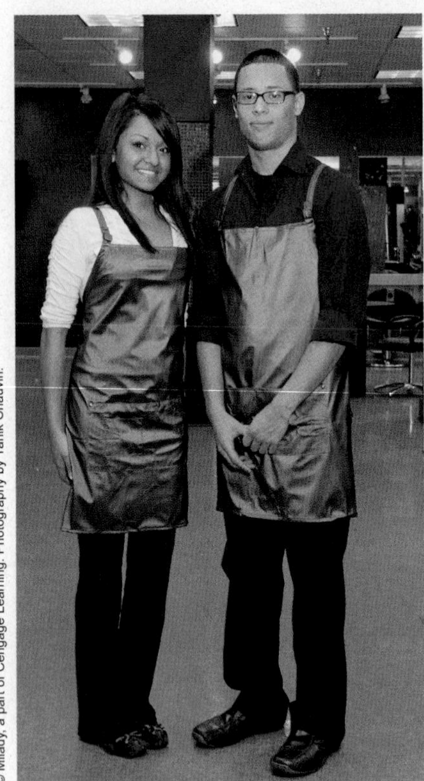
© Milady, a part of Cengage Learning. Photography by Yanik Chauvin.

▲ Figure 3–1
Project a professional image.

First impressions matter a lot, and because you are in the image business, how you look and present yourself has a bigger than usual impact on your success. If you are talking about style, then you need to look stylish; if you are advising your clients about makeup, your makeup must be current and beautifully applied. If you are recommending hand care services, your hands and nails should be well groomed. When your appearance and the way that you conduct yourself are in harmony with the beauty business, your chances of being successful increase dramatically!

Of course your personality and abilities also come into play, but how you look is the first and most important clue that leads potential clients to decide that you can make them look great. Add your behavior, the attitude you project, the way you interact with others, your communication skills, and how you physically hold yourself, and you create a complete, professional image (**Figure 3–1**). Ideally, you should present a great total package.

Why Study the Importance of Your Professional Image?

Cosmetologists should study and have a thorough understanding of the importance of their professional image because:

- Clients rely on beauty professionals to look good, well-cared for, and contemporary. They develop confidence that a professional who has a pleasant professional image can be trusted to perform their beauty services.
- Finding a salon and salon environment with a compatible idea of professional image and behavior is vitally important to working and flourishing in your career.
- Behaving professionally includes having a genuine interest in your own day-to-day activities, as well as being concerned about and for others, and knowing how to interact with managers, coworkers, and clients appropriately.
- Understanding ergonomics can help keep you healthy and gainfully employed.

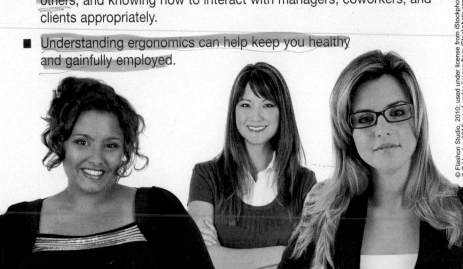

© Flashon Studio, 2010; used under license from iStockphoto.com.
© SJ Locke, 2010; used under license from iStockphoto.com.
© Hugo Silveirinha Felix, 2010; used under license from Shutterstock.com.

Beauty and Wellness

© Djapeman, 2010; used under license from Shutterstock.com.

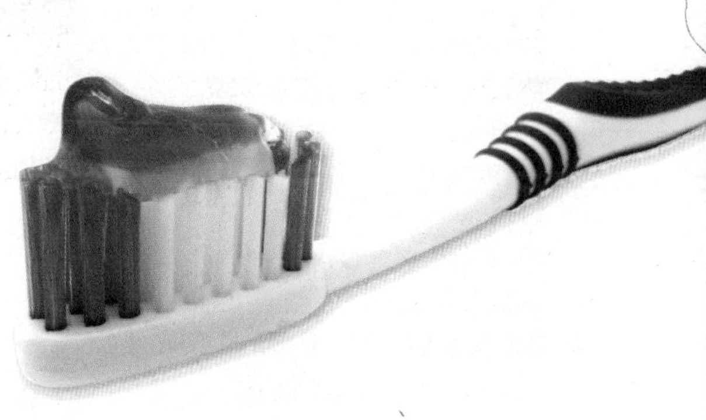

Being well groomed begins with looking and smelling fresh. This is especially important in the beauty business where practitioners are frequently only inches away from their clients during services.

Personal Hygiene

It is a given that you should shower or bathe every day, use deodorant before going to work, and generally be neat and clean. Beyond that, though, there are special considerations when working in a salon.

One weak moment of drinking coffee right before performing a service, for instance, or wearing something that needs laundering because you did not plan ahead, could spell disaster. Rather than telling you that you smell offensive, most clients will simply not return for another service. Equally distressing, they will typically tell three of their friends about the bad experience they had while sitting in your chair.

Personal hygiene is the daily maintenance of cleanliness by practicing good healthful habits (**Figure 3–2**). Working as a stylist behind the chair, or doing makeup, nail care, or skin care means that you'll be physically close to clients, which requires extra attention to your hygiene habits.

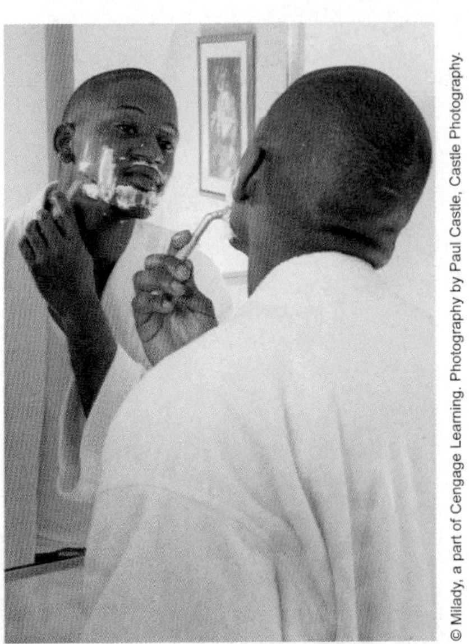

© Milady, a part of Cengage Learning. Photography by Paul Castle, Castle Photography.

▲ **Figure 3–2**
Practice meticulous personal hygiene every day.

One of the best ways to ensure that you always smell fresh and clean is to create a hygiene pack to use at work. This pack should include the following items:

- Toothbrush and toothpaste
- Mouthwash
- Sanitizing hand wipes or liquid to clean your hands between clients (when soap and water are not available)
- Dental floss
- Deodorant or antiperspirant

Your hygiene pack will be useful in maintaining the following good personal hygiene habits:

- Wash your hands throughout the day as required, including at the beginning of each service.
- Use deodorant or antiperspirant.
- Brush and floss your teeth, and use mouthwash or breath mints throughout the day as needed.
- Do self-checks periodically to ensure that you smell and look fresh.
- If you smoke cigarettes, *do not* smoke during work hours. Many clients find the lingering smell offensive. If you smoke during your lunch break, brush your teeth, use mouthwash, and wash your hands afterward! ☑ **LO1**

CAUTION

Many salons have a no-fragrance policy for staff members during work hours because a significant number of people are sensitive or allergic to a variety of chemicals, including perfume oils. Whether or not your salon has a no-fragrance policy, perfume should be saved for after work.

Appearances Count

In the line of work that you have chosen, having well-groomed hair, skin, and nails advertises your commitment to professional beauty. Make sure that you:

- Put thought into your appearance every day.
- Keep your haircut and color fresh.
- Take care of your skin and use a sun block.
- Determine the best length and grooming for your nails, and maintain their appearance.
- Change your style frequently, or as often as you feel comfortable, to keep up with trends. You don't have to be super-trendy, but even a stylist with a classic look or image should get subtle, seasonal updates, such as longer bangs or warmer hair color.

Personal Grooming

Many salon owners and managers view appearance, personality, and poise as being just as important as technical knowledge and skills. One of the most vital aspects of good personal grooming is the careful maintenance of your wardrobe. First and foremost, your clothes must be clean—not simply free of the dirt that you can see, but stain free, a feat that is sometimes difficult to achieve in a salon environment. Because you are constantly coming into contact with products and chemicals that can stain fabric, you should invest in an apron or smock to wear while handling such materials. Be mindful about spills and drips when using chemicals, and avoid leaning on counters in the work area—particularly in the dispensary.

Some salons require employees to wear aprons at all times, while others have dress-code rules, such as anything you wear must be a combination of black and white. These requirements are your first clue as to the culture of a particular salon, and how its stylists dress for success. However, whenever mixing chemicals, using haircolor or performing other services, it is always more professional to wear a smock or apron, and it will protect your clothing.

Dress for Success

What you wear outside of work is your choice. But while you're at work, your wardrobe selection should express a professional image that is consistent with the image of the salon (**Figure 3–3**). Your **professional image** is the impression you project through both your outward appearance and your conduct in the workplace. Common sense should rule when it comes to

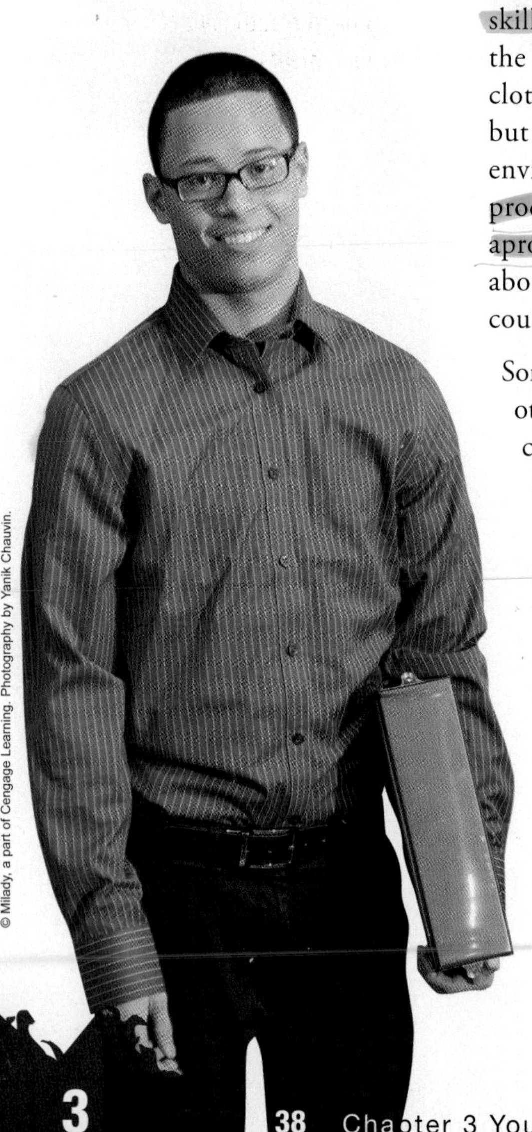

© Milady, a part of Cengage Learning. Photography by Yanik Chauvin.

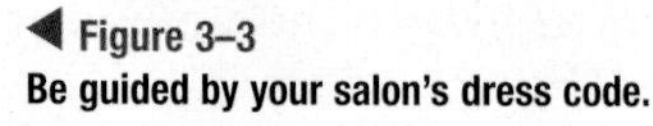

Figure 3–3
Be guided by your salon's dress code.

choosing clothes to wear at work. When shopping for work clothes, you should always visualize how you would look in them while performing professional client services. Is the image you will present one that is acceptable to your clients?

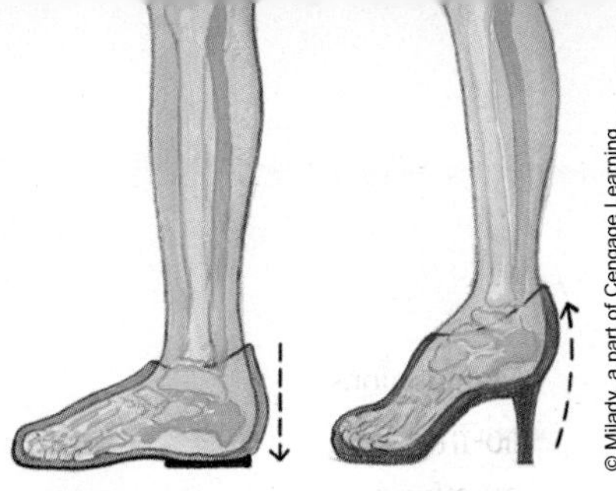
© Milady, a part of Cengage Learning.

▲ Figure 3–4
Working in high heels can throw off the body's balance.

To some degree, your clothing should reflect the fashions of the season. Depending on where you work, you may be encouraged to wear stylish torn jeans and faded tees, or they may be expressly forbidden. Just remember, the best way to ensure that you are dressed for success is to "tune in" to your salon's culture and clientele, so that you can make the best clothing choices.

While you should always follow your salon's dress code, here are some guidelines as to what's appropriate almost anywhere:

- Wear clothing that is clean, fresh, and in step with fashion.
- Choose clothing that is functional and comfortable, as well as stylish.
- Accessorize your outfits, but make sure that your jewelry does not clank and jingle while you work because this can irritate fellow professionals and clients.

Wear shoes that are comfortable, have a low heel, and good arch support. Ill-fitting shoes or high heels are not the best choices to wear when you have to stand all day (**Figure 3–4**). ☑ **LO2**

CAUTION

Not only can wearing inappropriate shoes at work be uncomfortable, it could be dangerous. Flip-flops and open-toed shoes, for example, are not safe to wear around electricity and sharp implements.

Wearing Makeup in the Salon

Makeup is an exciting category for beauty professionals. It helps promote your professional image and represents profitable sales for salons. You should always use makeup to accentuate your best features. With that said, it is important to always wear makeup at work. A freshly scrubbed face may look great for a leisurely day at the beach, but it does nothing to promote your image as a beauty professional. Unless you are working in a trendy urban salon, things like heavily blackened eyes and black nail polish are best left for after work. As with clothing, let the salon's image be your guide in makeup application (**Figure 3-5**).

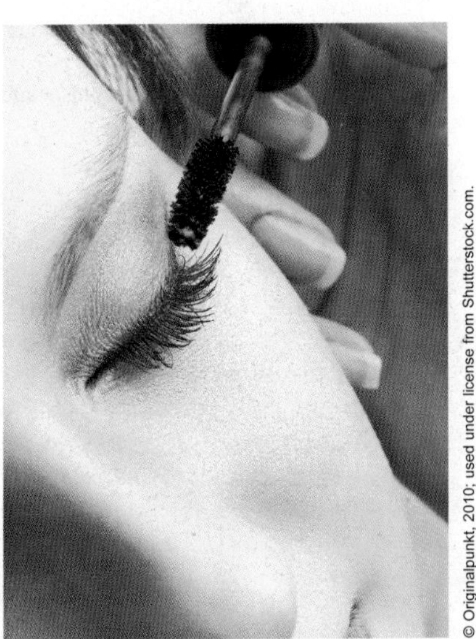
© Originalpunkt, 2010; used under license from Shutterstock.com.

▲ Figure 3–5
Expertly applied makeup is part of having a professional image.

Behaving Professionally

Beyond hygiene, grooming, and clothing, professional image and appearance are affected by your behavior, etiquette, and interactions with others. Keeping a positive attitude at work helps you behave appropriately and project a positive image. Ask yourself how an employee appears to you if he or she is rude to customers, shouts at colleagues, or crudely asks, "Yeah?" to find out what a customer wants.

Politeness is the hallmark of professionalism, even under pressure, and cooperating with colleagues is a great way to learn. If you are rude to your colleagues, you may lose important opportunities. If, on the other hand, when you cheerfully offer to assist a senior stylist with a service, you'll gain a mentor who will be willing to help you out. Specific communication skills will be discussed in Chapter 4, Communicating for Success. For now, keep in mind that all on-the-job behavior is part of your professional image and that it is just as important to be polite to colleagues as clients.

Your Physical Presentation

Your **physical presentation** involves your posture, as well as the way you walk and move. Good posture conveys an image of confidence. From a health standpoint, it can also prevent fatigue and many other physical problems. Sitting improperly can put a great deal of stress on your neck, shoulders, back, and legs. Having good posture, on the other hand, allows you to get through your day feeling good and doing your best work.

Posture

Some guidelines for achieving and maintaining good work posture include the following:

- Keep your neck elongated and balanced directly above the shoulders.
- Lift your upper body so that your chest is out and up (do not slouch).
- Hold your shoulders level and relaxed, not scrunched up.
- Sit with your back straight.
- Pull your abdomen in so that it is flat (**Figure 3–6**).

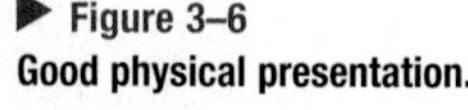

Figure 3–6
Good physical presentation.

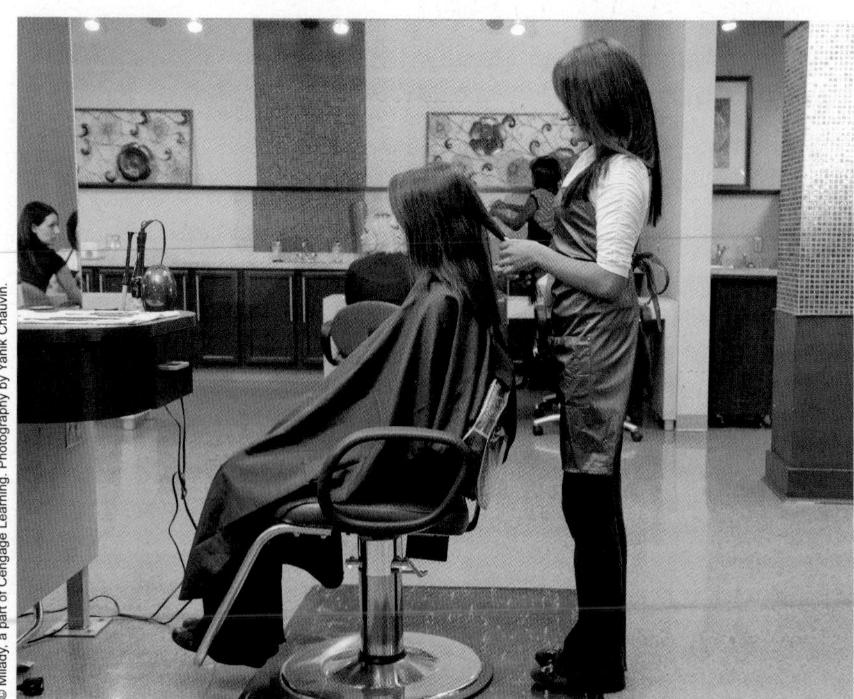

© Milady, a part of Cengage Learning. Photography by Yanik Chauvin.

Ergonomics and Your Body

You can move because your muscles and bones work together as a "musculoskeletal system," allowing you to walk, raise your arms, and use your fingers. **Ergonomics** is the science of designing the workplace as well as its equipment and tools to make specific body movements more comfortable, efficient, and safe. Ergonomics fits the job to the person, rather than the other way around.

For example, a hydraulic chair can be raised or lowered to accommodate stylists of different heights, allowing each to service clients without bending over too far. Certain shears are designed to eliminate hand fatigue when cutting hair because repetitive movements are of particular concern.

Ergonomics is tied to your personal presentation; when you sit or stand up straight, you look more professional. Ergonomics is also important to your ability to work and your body's wellness. Remember, beauty and wellness go hand-in-hand, and wellness starts with self care.

Each year, hundreds of cosmetology professionals report musculoskeletal disorders, including carpal tunnel syndrome (a wrist injury) and back injuries. Beauty professionals may have to stand or sit all day and perform repetitive movements, so they are susceptible to problems of the hands, wrists, shoulders, neck, back, feet, and legs.

Prevention is the key to avoiding these problems. An awareness of your body posture and movements, coupled with good work habits and proper tools and equipment, will enhance your health and comfort (**Figure 3–7**).

Repetitive motions have a cumulative effect on the muscles and joints. To avoid problems, monitor yourself as you work to see if you are falling into these bad habits:

- Gripping or squeezing implements too tightly.
- Bending your wrist up or down repeatedly when using the tools of your profession.
- Holding your arms too far away from your body as you work.
- Holding your elbows at more than a 60-degree angle away from your body for extended periods of time. (Your elbows should be close to your body when cutting.)
- Bending forward and/or twisting your body to get closer to your client.

To avoid ergonomic-related injuries, follow these guidelines: (**Figure 3–8**).

- Keep your wrists in a straight or neutral position as much as possible (**Figure 3–9**).

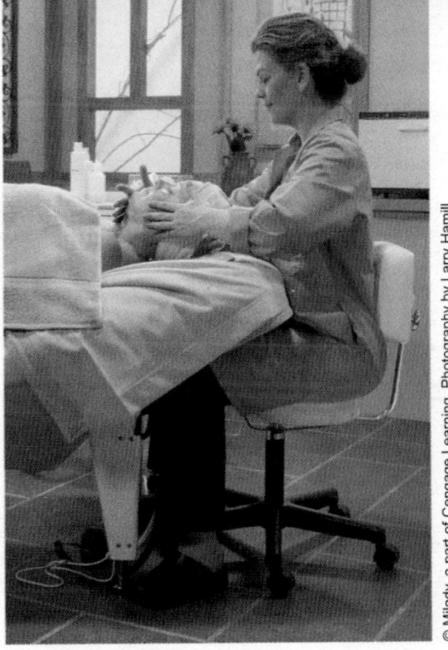
© Milady, a part of Cengage Learning. Photography by Larry Hamill.

▲ **Figure 3–7**
Proper position in relation to the client on the facial bed.

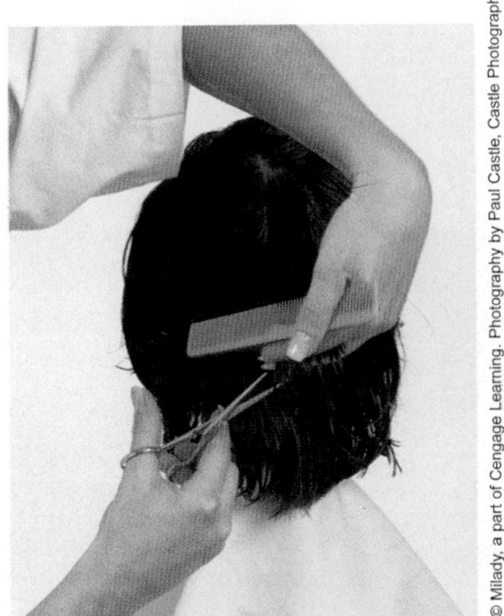
© Milady, a part of Cengage Learning. Photography by Paul Castle, Castle Photography.

▲ **Figure 3–8**
Improper haircutting position.

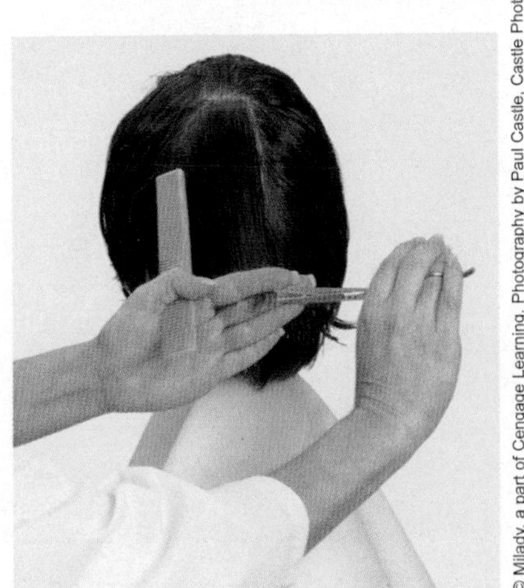
© Milady, a part of Cengage Learning. Photography by Paul Castle, Castle Photography.

▲ **Figure 3–9**
Correct wrist and hand position for haircutting.

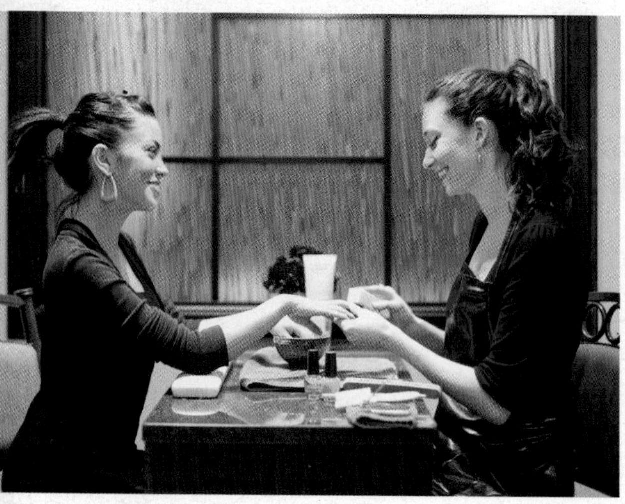
© Milady, a part of Cengage Learning. Photography by Dino Petrocelli.

▲ Figure 3–10
Follow proper ergonomic techniques when giving nail services.

- When giving a manicure, do not reach across the table; have the client extend her hand across the table to you (**Figure 3–10**).
- Use ergonomically designed implements.
- Keep your back and neck straight.
- Stand on an anti-fatigue mat.
- When cutting hair, sit if you can. When standing to cut, position your legs hip-width apart, bend your knees slightly, and align your trunk with your abdomen. ☑ **LO3**

Counter the negative impact of repetitive motions or long periods spent in one position by stretching and walking around at intervals. Always put your well-being first, and you'll enjoy a long and healthy career.

ACTivity

Practice these quick exercises, which will help you relieve stress from repetitive movements or from standing or sitting in one position for too long:

For Wrists

1. Stand up straight.
2. Raise both of your arms straight out.
3. Bend your wrists so your fingers point upward and hold for five seconds.
4. Hold your wrists steady and turn your hands, so your fingers face the floor and hold for five seconds.
5. Repeat the cycle five times.

For Fingers

1. Get a ball the size of a tennis ball or a tension ball.
2. Grip it tightly for a count of five. Release.
3. Repeat five times.

For Shoulders

1. Stand up straight and shrug your shoulders upward.
2. Roll your shoulders back and hold for a count of five.
3. Reverse direction and roll your shoulders forward for a count of five.
4. Repeat five times.

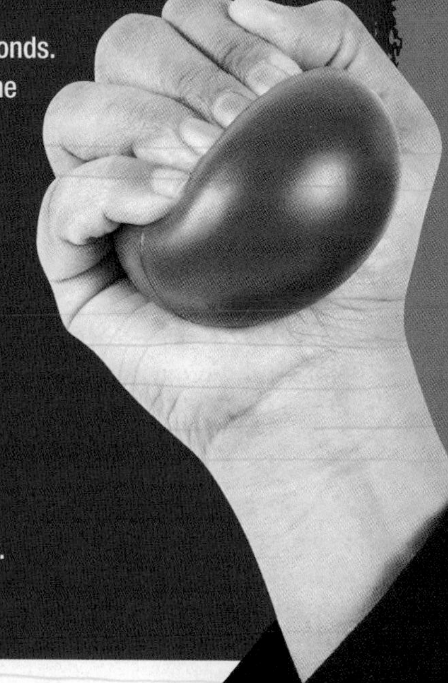
© Vishwanath Bhat, 2010; used under license from iStockphoto.com.

Review Questions

1. What are four good personal hygiene habits?
2. What is the best way to ensure you are dressed for success?
3. What are four ways you can avoid ergonomic-related injuries?

Chapter Glossary

ergonomics	The science of designing the workplace as well as its equipment and tools to make specific body movements more comfortable, efficient, and safe.
personal hygiene	Daily maintenance of cleanliness by practicing good healthful habits.
physical presentation	Your posture, as well as the way you walk and move.
professional image	The impression you project through both your outward appearance and your conduct in the workplace.

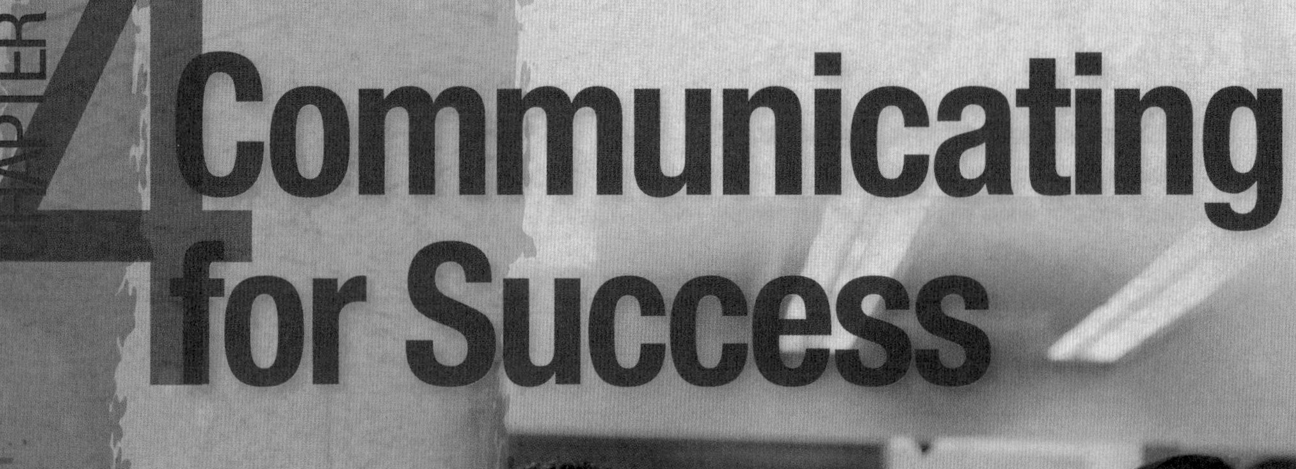

CHAPTER 4 Communicating for Success

Chapter Outline

© Milady, a part of Cengage Learning. Photography by Dino Petrocelli.

Learning Objectives

After completing this chapter, you will be able to:

- ✓ **LO1** List the golden rules of human relations.
- ✓ **LO2** Explain the definition of effective communication.
- ✓ **LO3** Conduct a successful client consultation/needs assessment.
- ✓ **LO4** Handle an unhappy client.
- ✓ **LO5** Build open lines of communication with coworkers.

Key Terms

Page number indicates where in the chapter the term is used.

client consultation (needs assessment)
pg. 52

effective communication
pg. 49

reflective listening
pg. 55

Do you have outstanding technical skills? Are you ready to unleash your artistic talents? If so, then you are on your way to becoming successful in your chosen career path. It is important to realize, though, that technical and artistic skills can only take you so far. In order to have a thriving clientele, you must also master the art of communication (**Figure 4–1**). Effective human relations and communication skills build lasting client relationships, accelerate professional growth, and help prevent misunderstandings in the workplace.

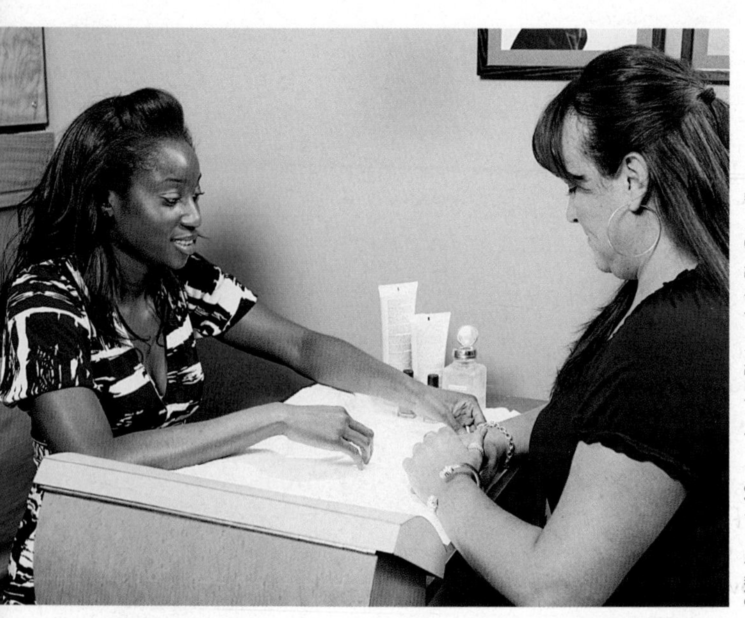

© Milady, a part of Cengage Learning. Photography by Dino Petrocelli.

▲ **Figure 4–1**
Communication is part of building lasting cosmetologist–client relationships.

Why Study Communicating for Success?

Cosmetologists should study and have a thorough understanding of communicating for success because:

- Communicating effectively—with a purpose—is the basis of all long-lasting relationships with clients and coworkers.
- Professionals need to build strong relationships based on trust, clarity, and loyalty in order to have a successful career, and you must be able to verbalize your thoughts and ideas with clients, colleagues, and supervisors.
- The close-knit salon environment will present complex and sometimes difficult interpersonal issues, and you will need effective ways to communicate, in order to navigate them successfully.
- Practicing and perfecting professional communication ensures that clients will enjoy their experience with you, and will encourage their continued patronage.
- The ability to control communication and effectively express ideas in a professional manner is a necessary skill for success in any career. This is particularly true in one as personal as cosmetology.

Human Relations

No matter where you work, you will find some people harder to get along with than others. It is not always possible to understand what people need, even if you know them well. Though you think you understand what people want, you cannot always satisfy their wishes. This can lead to misunderstandings.

The ability to understand people is the key to operating effectively in many professions. It is especially important in cosmetology, where customer service is central to success. Most of your interactions will depend on your ability to communicate successfully with a wide range of people: supervisors, coworkers, clients, and various vendors who come into the salon to sell products. When you understand the motives and needs of others, you will be in a better position to do your job professionally.

People all have the same basic needs, and the best way to understand others is to begin with a clear understanding of yourself. When you know and understand your own motivations, it is easier to appreciate others and to help them meet their goals. When people treat us with respect and listen to us, we feel good about them and about ourselves. By treating others with respect, you create an environment in which customers and staff develop confidence in you. Mutual respect—which transforms a good stylist into a trusted adviser and colleague—follows naturally.

Here is a brief look at the basics of human relations, along with some practical tips for dealing with situations that you are likely to encounter:

- Human beings are social animals. We like to interact with other people. As human beings, we enjoy giving our opinion and take pleasure in having people help us. Also, we feel pride when we use our abilities to help others.
- A fundamental factor in human relations involves a person's sense of security. When people feel secure, they are happy, calm, and confident. When people feel secure, they can be a joy to be around. On the other hand, when people feel insecure, they can become worried, anxious, and overwhelmed.
- No matter how secure you are as an individual and a professional stylist, there will be times when you encounter people and situations that are difficult to handle. Some people create conflict wherever they go. Try to remember that these people are feeling insecure; if they weren't, they wouldn't be acting that way.

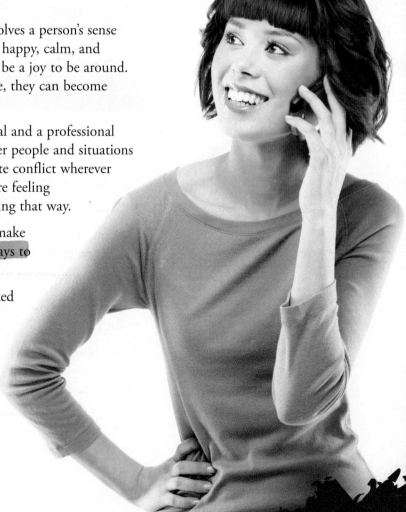

© Chris Gramly, 2010; used under license from iStockphoto.com.

To become skilled in human relations, learn to make the best of any situation. Here are some good ways to handle the ups and downs of human relations:

- **Respond instead of reacting.** A man was asked why he did not get angry when a driver cut him off. "Why should I let someone else dictate my emotions?" he replied. A wise fellow, don't you think? He might have even saved his own life by not reacting with "an eye for an eye" mentality.

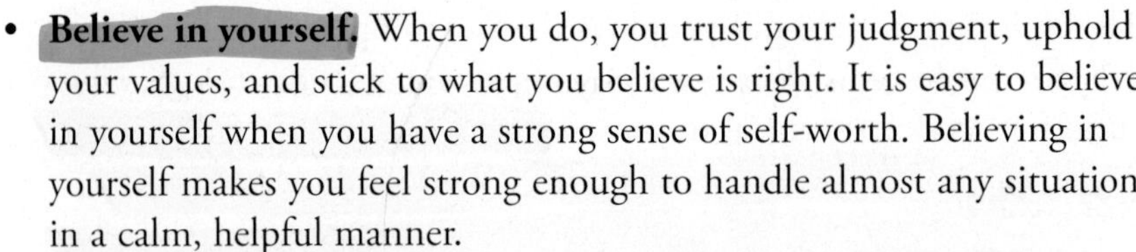

- **Believe in yourself.** When you do, you trust your judgment, uphold your values, and stick to what you believe is right. It is easy to believe in yourself when you have a strong sense of self-worth. Believing in yourself makes you feel strong enough to handle almost any situation in a calm, helpful manner.
- **Talk less, listen more.** There is an old saying that we were given two ears and one mouth for a reason. Listen more than you talk. When you are a good listener, you are fully attentive to what other people are saying.
- **Be attentive.** Each client is different. Some are clear about what they want, some are demanding, and still others may be hesitant. If you have an aggressive client, ask your manager for advice. You will likely be advised that what usually calms difficult clients down is agreeing with them. Follow up by asking what you can do to make the service more satisfactory (**Figure 4–2**).
- **Take your own temperature.** If you are tired or upset, your interactions with clients may be affected. An important part of succeeding in a service profession is taking care of yourself and your own personal conflicts first so that you can take the best possible care of your clients.

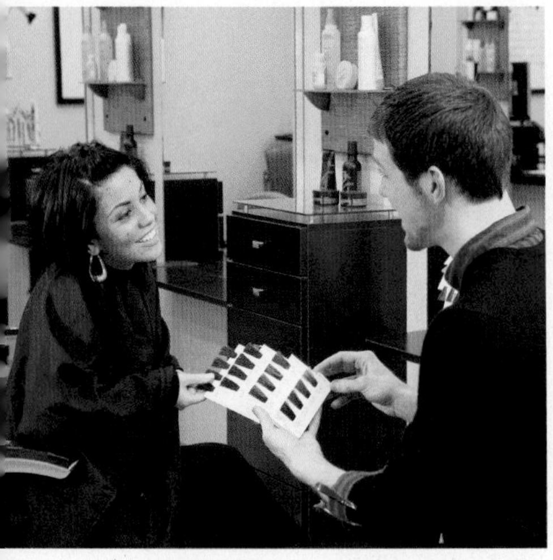

© Milady, a part of Cengage Learning. Photography by Dino Petrocelli.

▲ **Figure 4–2**
Be attentive to your client's needs.

Human relations can be rewarding or demoralizing. The result you achieve will depend on how much you are willing to give and how well you have prepared yourself for that day's services.

The Golden Rules of Human Relations

Keep the following golden rules of human relations in mind, and you will deal with difficult situations more successfully:

- Communicate from your heart; problem-solve from your head.
- A smile is worth a million times more than a sneer.
- It is easy to make an enemy; it is harder to keep a friend.
- See what happens when you ask for help instead of just reacting.
- Show people you care by listening to them and trying to understand their point of view.
- Compliment people even if they are challenging or unpleasant.
- For every service you do for others, do not forget to do something for yourself.
- Laugh often.
- Show patience with other people's flaws.

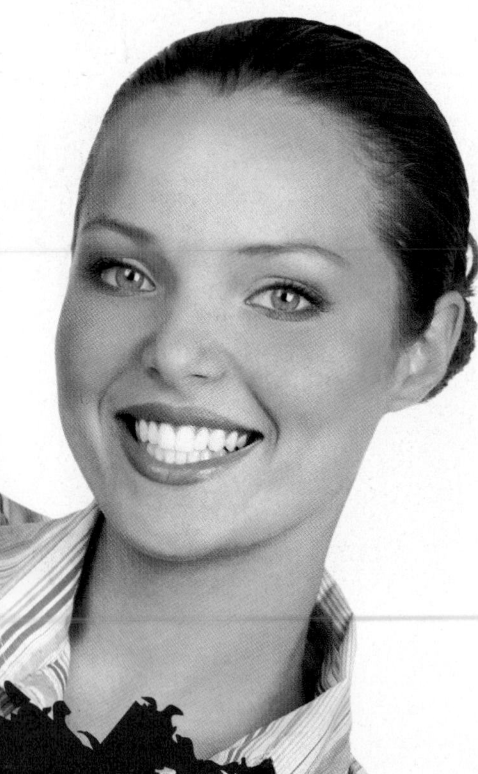

© Kurhan, 2010; used under license from Shutterstock.com.

- Build shared goals; be a team player and a partner to your clients.
- Always remember that listening is the best relationship builder.

☑ **LO1**

Communication Basics

Effective communication is the act of successfully sharing information between two people (or groups of people) so that the information is successfully understood. You can communicate through words, voice inflections, facial expressions, body language, or visual tools (e.g., a portfolio of your work). When you and your client are both communicating clearly about an upcoming service, your chances of pleasing that client soar. ☑ **LO2**

Meeting and Greeting New Clients

One of the most important encounters you will have is the first time you meet a client. Be polite, genuinely friendly, and inviting in every way you communicate with the client. You should keep in mind that your clients are coming to you for services and paying for your expertise with their hard-earned money (**Figure 4–3**). This means you need to court them every time they come to see you; if not, you may lose them to another stylist or salon.

To earn a client's trust and loyalty, you should:

- Always approach the client with a smile on your face. If you are having a difficult day, keep it to yourself. The time you spend with your client is for his or her needs, not yours.
- Always introduce yourself. Names are a powerful communication tool and should be used.
- Set aside a few minutes to take new clients on a quick tour of the salon.
- Introduce clients to people they may have interactions with while in the salon, including potential providers for other services, such as skin care or nail services.
- Be yourself. Do not try to fool clients by representing yourself as someone or something you are not.

▼ **Figure 4–3**
Welcome your client to the salon.

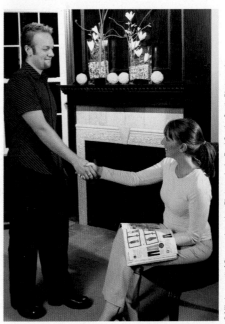

© Milady, a part of Cengage Learning. Photography by Paul Castle, Castle Photography.

Intake Form

Prior to sitting at your station, every new client should fill out an intake form—also called a client questionnaire or consultation card. This form can prove to be an extremely useful communication and business tool (**Figure 4–4**).

Client Intake Form

Dear Client,

Our sincerest hope is to provide you with the best hair care services you've ever received! We not only want you to be happy with today's visit, we also want to build a long-lasting relationship with you.
In order for us to do so, we would like to learn more about you, your hair care needs, and your preferences. Please take a moment now to answer the questions below as completely and as accurately as possible.

Thank you, and we look forward to building a relationship!

Name:______________________________

Address:______________________________

Phone Number: (day)__________ (evening)__________ (cell)__________

E-mail address:__________

Sex: _____ Male _____ Female Age:_____

How did you hear about our salon?______________________________

If you were referred, who referred you?______________________________

Please answer the following questions in the space provided. Thanks!

1. Approximately when was your last salon visit?______________________________
2. In the past year have you had any of the following services either in or out of a salon?
   - ____ Haircut
   - ____ Haircolor
   - ____ Permanent Wave or Texturizing Treatment
   - ____ Chemical Relaxing or Straightening Treatment
   - ____ Highlighting or Lowlighting
   - ____ Full head lightening
   - ____ Manicure
   - ____ Artificial nail services (please describe)
   - ____ Pedicure
   - ____ Facial/Skin Treatment
   - ____ Other (please list any other services you've enjoyed at a salon that may not be listed here).
3. What are your expectations for your hair service(s) today?
4. Are you now, or have you ever been, allergic to any of the products, treatments, or chemicals you've received during any salon service—hair, nails, or skin? (Please explain)

   ____
5. Are you currently taking any medications? (Please list)

   ____
6. Please list all of the products that you use on your hair on a regular basis.

   ____

   ____
7. What tools do you use at home to style your hair?
8. What is the one thing that you want your stylist to know about you/your hair?
9. Are you interested in receiving a skin care, nail care or makeup consultation?
10. Would you like to be contacted via email aboout upcoming promotions and special events?

    Yes_____ No_____

© Milady, a part of Cengage Learning.

▲ **Figure 4–4**
The client intake form gives you an opportunity to build an excellent relationship with your clients.

Continued

NOTE: If this card were used in a cosmetology school setting, it would include a release form at the bottom such as the one below.

Statement of Release: I hereby understand that supervised cosmetology students render these services for the sole purpose of practice and learning, and that by signing this form, I recognize and agree not to hold the school, its employees or the student liable for my satisfaction or the service outcome.

Client signature ______________________________ Date ____________________

Service Notes

Today's Date:

Today's Services:

Notes:

Today's Date:

Today's Services:

Notes:

Today's Date:

Today's Services:

Notes:

Today's Date:

Today's Services:

Notes:

Today's Date:

Today's Services:

Notes:

© Milady, a part of Cengage Learning.

▲ **Figure 4–4**
(Continued)

Some salon intake forms ask for a lot of detailed information; others do not. In cosmetology school, the consultation form may be accompanied by a release statement in which the client acknowledges that the service is being provided by a student who is under instruction. This helps protect the school and the student from legal action.

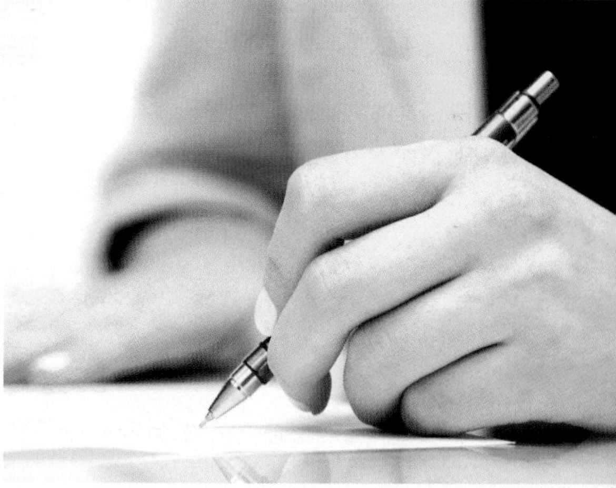

© Wrangler, 2010; used under license from Shutterstock.com.

How to Use the Client Intake Form

The client intake form can be used from the moment a new client calls the salon to make an appointment. When scheduling the appointment, let the client know that you and the salon will require some information before you can begin the service, and that it is important for her to arrive fifteen minutes ahead of her appointment time to fill out a brief form. Also, allow time in your schedule to do a five to fifteen minute client consultation.

FOCUS ON

UNDERSTANDING THE TOTAL LOOK CONCEPT

While the enhancement of your client's image should always be your primary concern, it is important to remember that nails, skin, and hair are reflective of an entire lifestyle. How can you help a client make choices that reflect a personal sense of style? Start by doing a little research. Look for books or articles that describe different fashion styles and become familiar with them. This exercise is useful for developing a profile of the broad fashion categories that you can refer to when consulting with clients.

For example, a person may be categorized as having a classic style if simple and sophisticated clothing, monochromatic colors, and no bright patterns are preferred. A person who prefers classic styling in her clothing would likely want a simple, elegant, and sophisticated look with respect to her nails, makeup, and hair.

Someone who prefers a more dramatic look, on the other hand, will choose nail designs, hairstyles, clothing, and accessories that demand greater attention and allow for more options. These clients are likely to be more willing to try a variety of new products and spend more time having additional services (Figures 4–5 and 4–6).

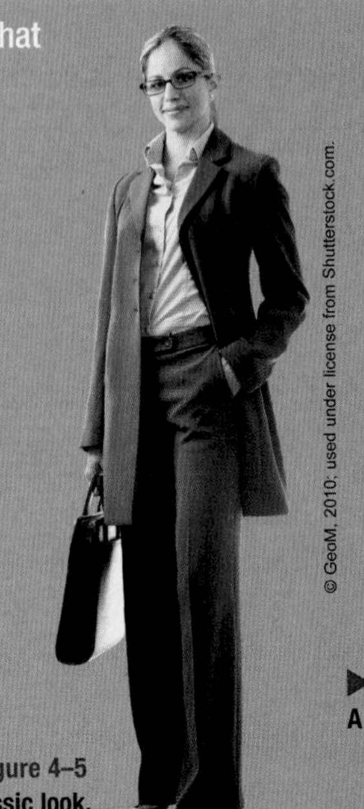

© GeoM, 2010; used under license from Shutterstock.com.

▶ Figure 4–5
A classic look.

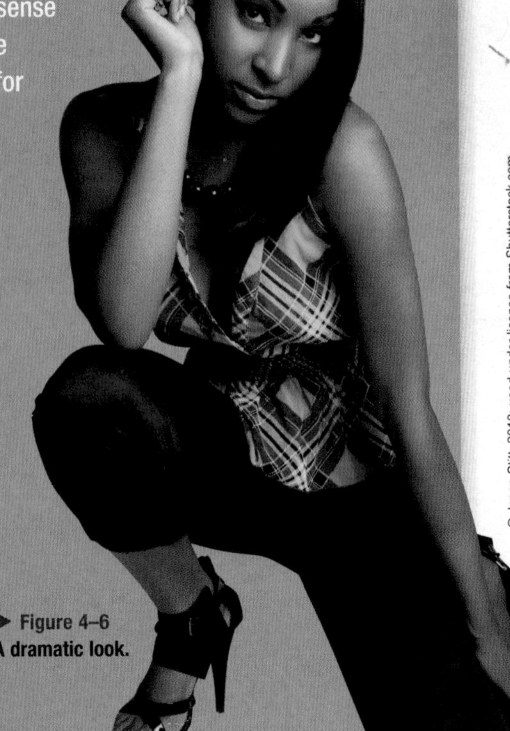

© Jason Stitt, 2010; used under license from Shutterstock.com.

▶ Figure 4–6
A dramatic look.

The Client Consultation / Needs Assessment

The **client consultation**, also known as **needs assessment**, is the verbal communication with a client that determines the client's needs and how to achieve the desired results. The consultation is one of the most important parts of any service and should always be done before starting the actual service. A consultation should be performed, to some degree, as part of every single service and salon visit. The consultation keeps communication on point. Effective client consultations keep your clientele looking current, stylish, and satisfied with your services. A happy client means repeat business for both the salon and you.

Preparing for the Client Consultation / Needs Assessment)

For the client consultation to be effective, it is important that you be well prepared to make the most of this dialogue. To facilitate the process, have certain important items on hand. These include styling books and hair swatches. To properly prepare for a consultation you should:

- Have a variety of styling books that your clients can look through. There should be at least one that depicts short hair, one for medium-length hair, and one with longer styles. You should also have—readily available—an assortment of photos representing all hair color options.
- Have a portfolio of your work on hand. To create one, keep a camera at your station (a disposable or digital camera is fine) and, with the client's permission, take photos after the service.
- When you show the photos, explain why you performed the various services the way you did. This will help new clients understand why certain things can or cannot be achieved, and it will reassure them of your expertise, skill, and knowledge (**Figure 4–7**).

A swatch book or swatch ring is a great tool for discussing hair color options. These are provided by the companies that manufacture haircolor. They are usually packaged in a book, in a ring, or laid out on a paper chart. Swatches are bundles of hair, dyed to match a particular haircolor shade offered by the manufacturer. Usually made from a synthetic material, swatches are very durable and easy to use in consultations. If the swatch is long enough, it can be held up to the client's face or integrated into her own hair to see how it looks.

Many times, you will find yourself consulting with a client who asks for a specific cut or color that she may have heard about from a friend or seen on a celebrity. You know that not every technique or color will work for everyone. In this situation, take the client through the process step-by-step, diplomatically explaining why a specific cut has to be adjusted for her hair type, or why a certain color is either right or wrong for her hair color, skin type, desired maintenance, budget, or lifestyle.

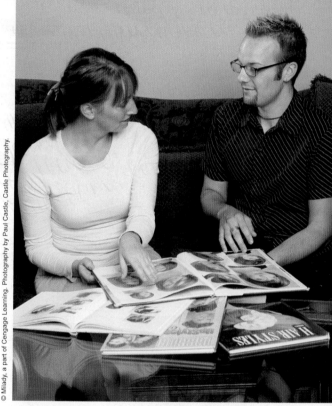

© Milady, a part of Cengage Learning. Photography by Paul Castle, Castle Photography.

▲ **Figure 4–7**
Use a photo collection to help confirm your client's choice.

The Consultation Area

Presentation counts for a lot in a business that is concerned with style and appearance. Once you have brought the client to your station to begin the consultation process, make sure she is comfortable. The two of you are about to begin an important conversation that will clue you in to her needs and preferences. It is your responsibility to find out what the client's needs are and to make recommendations that meet those needs. To do so effectively, you will need a freshly cleaned and uncluttered workspace.

Read the intake form carefully, referring to it often during the consultation process. Throughout the consultation, make notes on the intake form. After the service, record any formulations or products that you used. Include any specific techniques you followed, or goals you are working toward, so that you can remember them for future visits.

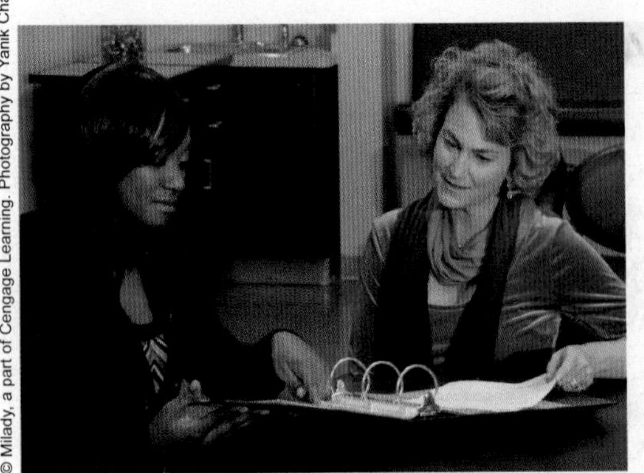

© Milady, a part of Cengage Learning. Photography by Yanik Chauvin.

10-Step Consultation Method

Every consultation should be structured so that you cover all the key points which lead to a successful conclusion. While this may seem like a lot of information to memorize, it will become second nature as you become more experienced. To ensure that you cover all the bases, keep a list of the following 10 key points at your station. Modify the list as needed for each actual service:

1. **Review the intake form.** Feel free to make comments that break the ice and initiate conversation with the client.
2. **Assess the client's current style.** Is it soft and unstructured? Carefully styled? Classic? Avant-garde? Is it in sync with her style of clothing and personal image?
3. **Determine the client's preferences.** Ask your client what they like most and least about their current cut and style. Ask her when was the last time she really loved or liked her hair and other areas of concern (skin, nails, body care). Next ask what she likes least and what challenges she is having. If she could change something what would it be? Is her style too conservative? Does she love the fact that she only has to spend ten minutes a day styling her hair?
4. **Analyze the client's hair.** Assess your client's hair, including its thickness, texture, manageability, and condition. Is her hair particularly thin on top or at the temples? Check for strong hair growth patterns, including unruly cowlicks. Ask your client what at-home products they are using and if they are effective for them. Make notes on the intake form.
5. **Review the client's lifestyle.** Ask your client the following questions about her career and lifestyle:

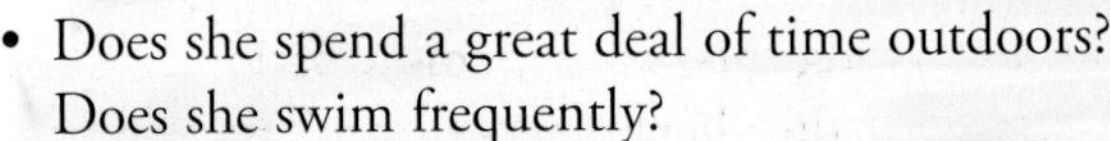

   - Does she spend a great deal of time outdoors? Does she swim frequently?
   - Is she a businesswoman? An artist? A stay-at-home mom?
   - Does she wish to project a strong or specific personal style?
   - What are her styling abilities? How often does she shampoo her hair?
   - How much time does she want to spend on her hair each day?

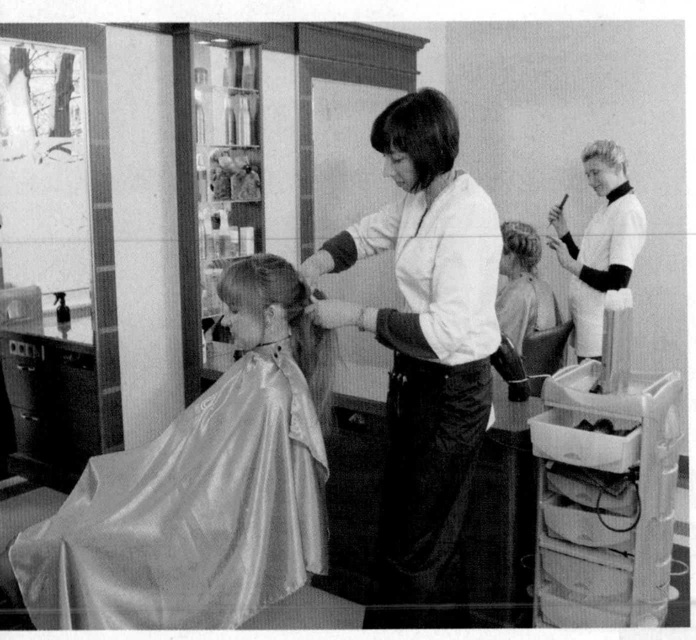

© Iv Mirin, 2010; used under license from Shutterstock.com.

6. **Show and tell.** Encourage your client to flip through your style books and point out styles, or even parts of styles, that she likes and to tell you why she likes them. Does she consistently point out thick, full hairstyles, for instance, when her own hair is quite fineor thin? Is her hair curly, yet she consistently chooses straight styles that would require a chemical straightening service to achieve?

ACTivity

When is the last time you went to a salon for a service yourself? Putting yourself in the client's shoes will help you improve your communication skills in every way. First, recall your most recent salon visit. Now, write down the following information:

- Your first impression of your stylist.
- His or her best verbal and non verbal communications.
- Any questions you asked your stylist and his or her reply.
- Questions you wanted to ask but did not, and why.
- What you would change, knowing what you know now about how to communicate with clients? Would you have asked more questions to make certain you got what you wanted? Would you have avoided a certain subject?
- Do you think you communicated exactly what you wanted? What questions did you ask that your clients may not know to ask, since they are not stylists?

In addition, listen to how she describes hair length. If she says she wants her hair short, for instance, does she mean shoulder length? Above her ears? One-inch long all over her head? When her bangs are dry, does she want them to still touch her eyebrows? In order to make sure you understand what she is saying, repeat what she tells you, using specific terms like *chin-length* or *resting on the shoulders*—as opposed to vague terms like *short* or *long*—and reinforce your words both with pictures and by pointing to where the hair would fall. Listening to the client and then repeating, in your own words, what you think the client is telling you is known as **reflective listening**. It is important to focus on the client and not interrupt while he or she is speaking. After the client is finished, restate and confirm what was said. Following this, ask for confirmation to make certain you understand what the client wants or needs.

7. **Suggest options.** Once you have enough information, ask the client if you may make some recommendations. Before giving any suggestions, wait for her to give you permission to do so. Once she has, base your recommendations on the client's needs and desires. Narrow your selections based on the following criteria:

   - *Lifestyle*. The styles you choose must fit the client's styling parameters (time and ability), meet your client's needs for business and casual looks, and provide options within these looks.
   - *Hair type*. Base your recommendations on whether your client has thick, medium, or thin hair density; fine, medium, or coarse hair texture; straight, wavy, curly, or extremely curly wave patterns.
   - *Face shape*. Point out hairstyles that would look good with her face shape. Is her face narrow across the temple area? If so, you should suggest styles that add a little fullness in this area.

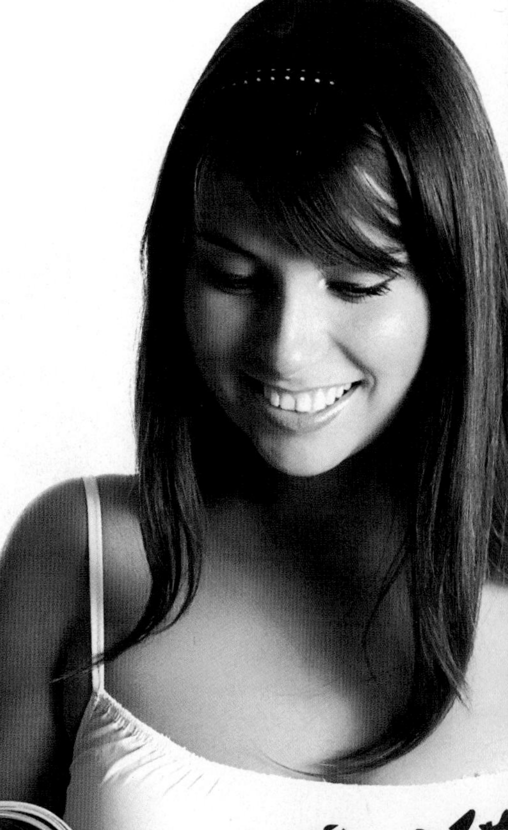

© Raisa Kanareva, 2010; used under license from Shutterstock.com.

FOCUS ON

RETAILING

The best way to make retailing recommendations is to use this three-step plan to discuss the *What, Why,* and *How* of the recommendation:

1. Once you have chosen a product for the client, explain "This is WHAT I recommend…"
2. Next, explain WHY you recommend it for her hair type, to solve some problem or challenge she is having.
3. Finally, describe HOW she should use the product at home.

Educating the client using these three steps helps her to better understand your recommendations and makes selling the home care products much easier.

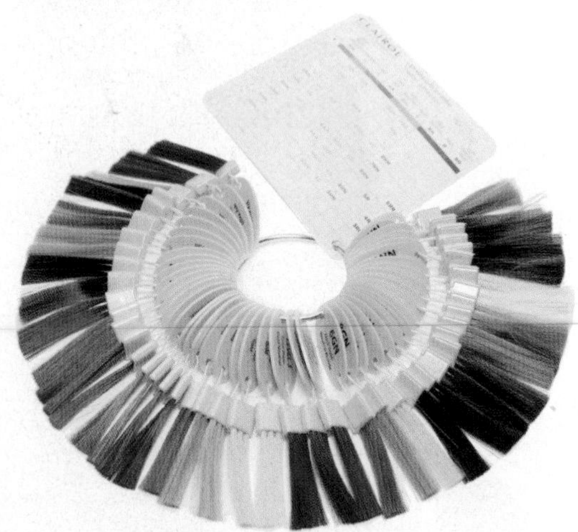

When you make suggestions, qualify them by referencing the above parameters. For example: "I think this hairstyle would work well with the texture of your hair." Tactfully discuss any unreasonable expectations (based on the client's hair and personal needs) that the client expresses. If her hair is damaged, address intensive hair treatments, better home-care products, lifestyle changes, and the need to trim damaged ends.

Never hesitate to suggest additional services (be sure to offer two or more services) that will complete the look or improve it in some way. In addition to color, this could be a texture service for added movement or body, a straightening service to tame her curls, a makeup lesson to complement your client's new style, and so on.

8. **Make color recommendations.** Unless a client absolutely does not want to talk about color, these recommendations should be part of every consultation service. Almost everyone can use a glossing treatment, have her hair color enriched, or add some highlights or low lights to make her hair (and your work) even more attractive.

   Ask if she has colored her hair in the past. If she already has haircolor, find out how long it has been since it was last applied. Has she had color challenges in the past? Does she color her hair at home? Would she like to make a subtle or dramatic hair color change?

   When talking about color, be very careful to make sure you and the client are speaking the same language. Hairstylists are accustomed to the technical side of color and tend to use terms like *multidimensional highlighting*, or *no-ammonia, semi permanent tint*. This can be very confusing and misleading to clients. Use pictures as much as possible. The term *blond* to a stylist might be platinum blond, while *blond* to a client may mean a few fine streaks of medium-blond around the hair line. Let photos be your guide.

9. **Discuss upkeep and maintenance.** Counsel every client on the salon maintenance, lifestyle limitations (blond hair and chlorine, for instance, are not a good match), and at-home maintenance that she will need to commit to in order to look her best. Let the client know that throughout the service you will be educating her on various products that you would recommend for her home use and that at the end of the service she will have an opportunity to choose those home care products that she needs.

10. **Review the consultation.** Reiterate everything that you have agreed upon by using a phrase like, "What I heard you say is . . . " Make sure to speak in measured, precise terms and use visual tools to demonstrate the intended end result. This is the most critical step of the consultation process because it determines the ultimate service(s). Always take your time and be thorough. Pause for your client's confirmation or ask her if you have understood everything correctly. Once you are sure that you both have the same understanding of

© Milady, a part of Cengage Learning.

her needs, ask if she is ready to start the service as you have both outlined. Once your client has agreed, you can proceed with the service. ☑ **LO3**

Concluding the Service

Once the service is finished and the client lets you know they are satisfied, take a few minutes to record the results. Note anything you did that you might want to do again, as well as anything that does not bear repeating. Also, make note of the final results and any retail products that the client purchased. Be sure to date your notes and file them in the proper place.

Special Issues in Communication

Although you may do everything in your power to communicate effectively, you will sometimes encounter situations that are beyond your control. Your reactions to situations and your ability to communicate in the face of challenges are critical to being successful in a people profession.

Handling Tardy Clients

Tardy clients are a fact of life in every service industry. Because beauty professionals depend on appointments and scheduling to maximize working hours, a client who is overly late for an appointment, or one who is habitually late, causes problems. One tardy client can set back your appointment calendar and make you late for every other service that day. The pressure involved in making up for lost time takes its toll. Beyond being rushed and feeling harried, you risk inconveniencing the rest of your clients who are prompt for their appointments. No one benefits—not you, not the salon, and certainly not your clients—when scheduling conflicts arise that are caused by tardy clients.

Here are a few guidelines for handling late clients:

- Know and abide by the salon's appointment policy. Many salons set a limit on the amount of time they allow a client to be late before requiring them to reschedule. Generally, if clients are more than fifteen minutes late, they should be asked to reschedule. Most clients will accept responsibility and be understanding about the rule, but you may come across a few clients who insist on being serviced immediately. Explain to them that you have other appointments and are responsible to those clients as well. Also explain that rushing through the service would be unacceptable to both of you.
- If your tardy client arrives and you have the time to take her without jeopardizing other appointments, let your client know why you are taking her even though she is late. You can deliver this information diplomatically and still remain pleasant and upbeat.

did you know?

When referring to patrons, some salons use the word *client*, while others use *guest*. Spas are more likely to use *guest* because of the amount of time the client spends on the premises and the fact that spa patrons often have lunch during their visits. Some salons have adapted this practice; others feel it personalizes the relationship too much. Medical spas have returned to using *client* because many of these spas are bound by medical privacy laws when it comes to record-keeping. Additionally, *guest* is never used in the professional medical field. Go with the culture of the business in which you're working, and you won't go wrong.

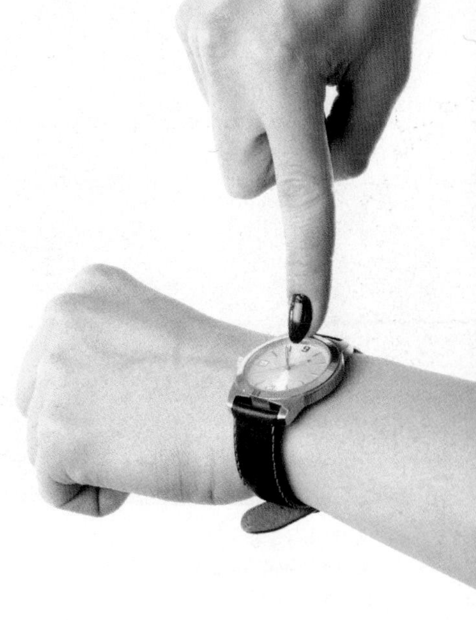

© Totobazilio, 2010; used under license from Shutterstock.com.

- As you get to know your clients, you will learn who is habitually late. You may want to schedule such clients for the last appointment of the day or ask them to arrive earlier than their actual appointment time.
- If you are running very late, have the receptionist call your clients and let them know. The receptionist can give them the opportunity to reschedule or to come a little later than their scheduled time.

Handling Scheduling Mix-Ups

We are all human, and we all make mistakes. Chances are you have gone to an appointment only to discover that you are in the wrong place at the wrong time. The way you are treated at that moment determines whether you patronize that business again. When you, as a professional, are involved with a scheduling mix-up, always remember to be polite. Never argue about who is correct.

Once you have the chance to consult your appointment book, you can say, "Oh, Mrs. Montez, I have you in my appointment book for ten o'clock, and unfortunately I already have clients scheduled for eleven and twelve o'clock. I'm so sorry about the mix-up. Can I reschedule you for tomorrow at ten o'clock?" Even though the client may be fuming, you need to stay detached. Move the conversation away from who is at fault, and squarely into resolving the confusion. Make another appointment for the client and be sure the salon has her telephone number so that the appointment can be confirmed (**Figure 4–8**).

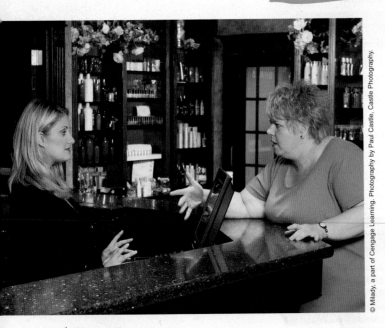
© Milady, a part of Cengage Learning. Photography by Paul Castle, Castle Photography.

▲ Figure 4–8
Accommodate an unhappy client promptly and calmly.

Handling Unhappy Clients

No matter how hard you try to provide excellent service to your clients, once in a while you will encounter a client who is dissatisfied. Remember the ultimate goal: make the client happy enough to pay for the service and return to the salon in the future.

Here are some guidelines:

- Try to find out why the client is unhappy. Ask for specifics.
- If it is possible to change what she dislikes, do so immediately. If that is not possible, look at your schedule book to see how soon you can fit her in to make the adjustment. You may need to enlist the help of the receptionist if you have to reschedule other appointments.
- If the problem cannot be fixed; honestly and tactfully explain why. The client may not be happy but will usually appreciate your honesty. Sometimes you can offer other options that minimize the client's disappointment.
- Never argue with the client or try to force your opinion on her.

ACTivity

At some point in your career you will have a client who is unhappy about something, either related to service or scheduling. The best way to prepare for this scenario is to practice. Role-play with a classmate, taking turns being the client and the stylist.

As you play the role of client:

- Act out different personalities: first shy, then aggressive.
- Act out a problem that was your (the client's) fault. Then evaluate your classmate's (the stylist's) reaction.
- Continue the conversation until you are satisfied.

As you play the role of stylist:

- Pay attention to the tone and level of your voice.
- Make certain you understand the problem.
- Avoid being defensive.
- Offer more than one solution.
- Determine when you should involve a manager.

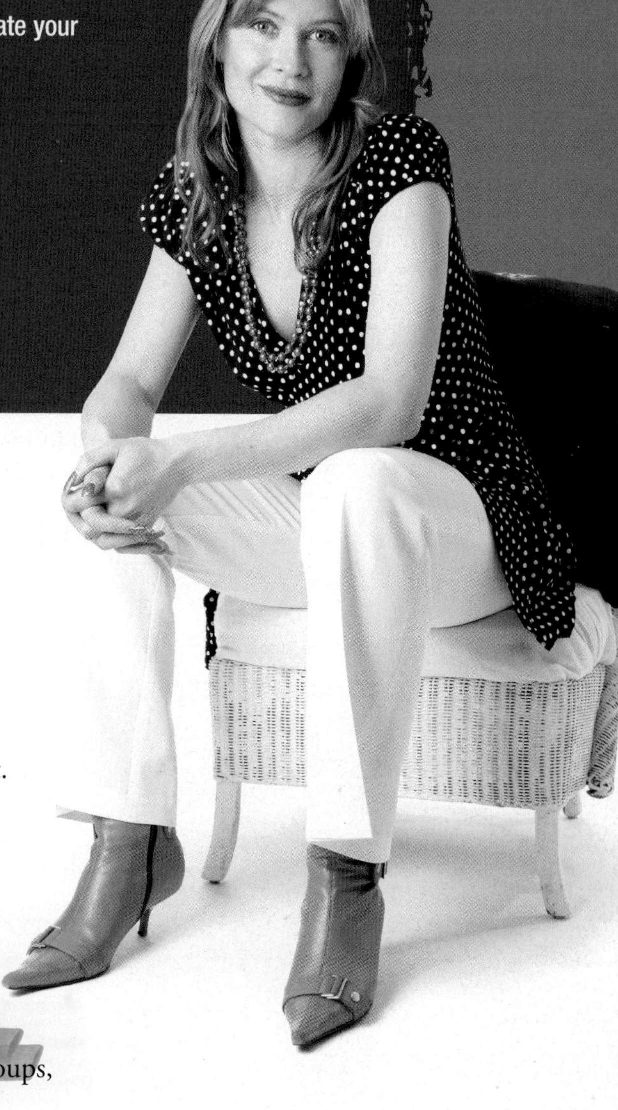

© C Wells Photographic, 2010; used under license from Shutterstock.com.

- Do not hesitate to ask for help from a more experienced stylist or your salon manager. If, after you have tried everything, you are unable to satisfy the client, defer to your manager's advice on how to proceed.
- Confer with your salon manager after the experience. A good manager will not hold the event against you but will view it instead as an inevitable fact of life from which you can learn. Follow your manager's advice and move on to your next client. ☑ **LO4**

Handling Differences

As a stylist, you'll find the clients you are most likely to attract are similar to yourself in age, style, and taste. On the other hand, you will also service clients who are very different from you; this is a positive element in your career as a stylist. Without both older and younger clients, and ones from different social groups, you won't be able to build a solid client base for future business.

When working with clients who come from a different generation, the basic rules of professionalism should guide you. Older clients, in particular, do not like gum chewing, slang, or the use of *yeah* instead of *yes*. They like to hear *please* and *thank you*. They prefer to keep the topics of conversation professional. Some like to be addressed by the honorific, such as "Mrs. Smith," rather than by their first names. When you meet an older client for the first time, ask how he or she would like to be addressed. Some clients are sensitive to verbiage about aging. When delivering skin care services, do not refer to aging skin; instead, talk about dryness and solutions to remedy the condition.

FOCUS ON

TALKING POINTS

Let's imagine a long-time client reveals to you, one day, that she and her husband are going through a messy divorce. You care for her and want to be understanding as she reveals increasingly personal details. Other practitioners and their clients are soon listening to every word of this conversation. You want to be helpful and supportive, but this is not the right time or place. What can you do? Decide which of these solutions you might use:

- Tell her you understand that the situation is very difficult, but that while she is in the salon, you want to do everything in your power to give her a break from it. Let her know gently that while she is in your care, you should both concentrate on her enjoyment of the services and not on the things that are stressing her.
- Change the subject. What topic could you shift to that seems the most natural?
- Find a reason to excuse yourself. When you return, change the subject.
- Acknowledge her by saying, "I'm sorry to hear that." Suggest a mini relaxation service the salon is promoting.

Younger clients may not be up on proper etiquette, but many keep up with the latest celebrity styles, so you need to do the same. If these clients are your peers, relate to their image needs but don't act too much like a peer; it is always better to maintain a professional demeanor.

When it comes to slang, the same word can have a different meaning across cultures, which is why it is always best to avoid using slang terms. If the word is fashion-related and your client uses it, you can too, indicating that you understand and are aware of current trends. Never use cultural slang words or regionalisms you do not fully understand. When in doubt say, "I have never heard that expression before. What, exactly, do you mean?"

Getting Too Personal

Sometimes when a client forms a bond of trust with her stylist, the client can have a hard time differentiating between a professional relationship and a personal one. This will be her problem. Be sure you do not make it your problem. Your job is to handle your client relationships tactfully and sensitively, with professionalism and respect. Do not engage in an attempt to fulfill the role of counselor, career guide, parental sounding board, or motivational coach for any of your clients.

If your client gets too far off topic, use neutral subjects to bring her back to a conversation about her beauty needs. If she tells you about a personal problem, simply listen and tell her you are sorry. Then ask, "What can we do to make your visit better today?"

If your client is gossiping, change the subject as soon as you can. Try something like, "I just noticed your ends are drier than I thought. We'll do a deep-conditioning treatment after your color." Then describe the treatment and home care.

Books, movies, and celebrities can all be used to move into conversations about a particular look or style. As a rule, avoid discussing religion and politics. When you cannot find a way to move the conversation back to something hair- or beauty-related, simply listen; then change the subject. In a worst-case scenario, apologize and excuse yourself, either verbally or physically, to check her client records, to ask another stylist an important question, or to see if a certain conditioner is in stock. When you return your attention to the client, move the conversation back to beauty.

In-Salon Communication

Behaving in a professional manner is the first step in making meaningful in-salon communication a reality. The salon community is a close-knit one in which people spend long hours working side by side. For this reason, it is important to maintain boundaries. Remember, the salon is your place of business and, as such, must be treated respectfully and carefully.

Communicating with Coworkers

In a work environment, you will not have the opportunity to handpick your colleagues. There will always be people you like or relate to better than others. Keep these points in mind as you interact and communicate with coworkers:

- **Treat everyone with respect.** Regardless of whether you like someone, your colleagues are professionals who deserve respect.
- **Remain objective.** Different types of personalities working together over long and intense hours can breed some degree of dissension and disagreement. Make every effort to remain objective. Resist being pulled into spats and cliques.
- **Be honest and sensitive.** Many people use the excuse of being honest as a license to say anything to anyone. While honesty is always the best policy, using unkind words or actions at work is never a good idea. Be sensitive, and think before you speak.
- **Remain neutral.** There may come a time when you are called on to pick a side. Do whatever you can in order to avoid taking sides in a dispute.
- **Avoid gossip.** Gossiping never resolves a problem; it only makes it worse. Participating in gossip can be just as damaging to you as it is to the object of your gossip.
- **Seek help from someone you respect.** If you find yourself at odds with a coworker, seek out someone who is not involved and can be objective, such as the manager. Ask for advice about how to proceed, and then really listen.
- **Do not take things personally.** How many times have you had a bad day, or been thinking about something totally unrelated to work, when a colleague asks you what is wrong, or if you are mad at her? Just because someone is behaving in a certain manner, and you happen to be there, does not mean their behavior involves you. If you are confused or concerned by someone's actions, find a private place and an appropriate time to ask her if something is wrong.
- **Keep your private life private.** There is a time and a place for everything, but the salon is never the place to discuss your personal life and relationships. ☑ **LO5**

Communicating with Managers

Another important relationship for you is the one you will build with your manager. The salon manager is usually the person with the most responsibility regarding the salon's overall operation. The manager's job is a demanding one. Often, in addition to running a hectic salon, he or she also has a personal clientele.

FOCUS ON

YOUR COMMUNICATION SKILLS

If you feel uncertain about how to communicate with salon owners, managers, and clients from a different generation, observe and listen to your peers. Visit colleagues in various professional settings. Stop by a high-end clothing store, and listen to the salesperson. Ask questions at these businesses yourself, and listen closely to the responses. Find someone whose communication skills you admire, and emulate that style. Practice using *yes*, *no*, *please*, *thank you*, and *excuse me* in daily conversation. (Avoid using *yeah*, *nope*, and *thanks*.) Use a dictionary to increase your vocabulary. You can even record yourself (audio or video) and assess your own communication style. The more confident you become when communicating with people from different walks of life and people with different types of jobs, the better.

© Radu Razvan, 2010; used under license from Shutterstock.com.

Your manager is probably the one who hired you and who is responsible for your training. Therefore, your manager has a vested interest in your success. As a salon employee, you might perceive the manager as a powerful figure of authority, but it is important to remember that your manager is a human being. The best thing you can do to support your manager and the salon is to try to understand the decisions and rules that the salon manager makes, whether you agree with them or not.

Here are some guidelines for interacting and communicating with your salon manager:

- **Be a problem solver.** When you need to speak with your manager about some issue or problem, think of possible solutions beforehand. This will indicate that you are working in the salon's best interest and trying to be an asset in the salon's success.
- **Get your facts straight.** Make sure that all your facts and information are accurate before you speak to your salon manager. This way you avoid wasting your manager's time trying to solve a problem that might not really exist.
- **Be open and honest.** When you find yourself in a situation you do not understand or do not have the experience to deal with, tell your salon manager immediately and be willing to listen and learn.
- **Do not gossip or complain about colleagues.** Going to your manager with gossip or to tattle on a coworker could very well lead your manager to consider you a troublemaker. If you are having a legitimate problem with someone and have tried everything you can to handle the problem with your own resources, only then is it appropriate to go to your manager.
- **Check your attitude.** The salon environment, although fun and friendly, can also be stressful, so take a moment between clients to ask yourself how you are feeling. Do you need an attitude adjustment? Be honest with yourself.
- **Be open to constructive criticism.** It is never easy to hear that you need improvement in any area, but keep in mind that part of your manager's job is to

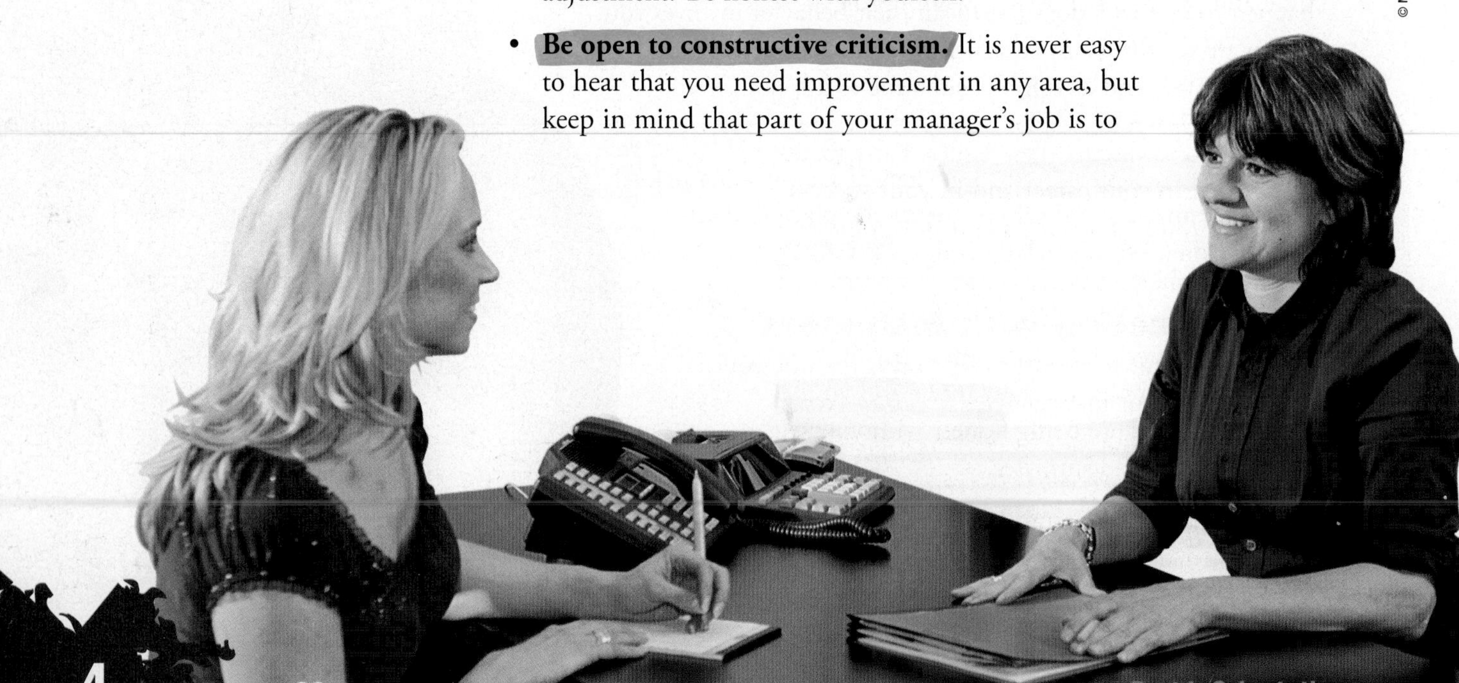

© Milady, a part of Cengage Learning. Photography by Dino Petrocelli.

help you achieve your professional goals and ensure the salon's success. It is her job to evaluate your skills and offer suggestions on how to improve and expand them. Keep an open mind and do not take her criticism personally.

Communicating During an Employee Evaluation

Salons that are well run make it a priority to conduct frequent and thorough employee evaluations. Sometime during the course of your first few days of work, your salon manager will tell you when to expect your first employee evaluation. If she does not mention it, you might ask her about it and request a copy of the form she will use or for a list of the criteria on which you will be evaluated. The following are some points to keep in mind as you begin your tenure in the salon.

- Take some time to look over the employee evaluation document. Be mindful that the behaviors and activities most important to the salon are likely to be the ones on which you will be evaluated. You can begin to review and rate yourself in the weeks and months ahead, so you can assess your progress and performance.
- Remember, the criteria on the evaluation are there for the purpose of helping you become a better stylist and to ensure the salon's success. Make the decision to approach the evaluation positively.
- As the time for the evaluation draws near, try filling out the form yourself. In other words, perform a self-evaluation, even if the salon has not asked you to do so. Be objective, and carefully think out your comments.
- Before your evaluation meeting, write down any thoughts or questions so you can share them with your manager. Do not be shy. If you want to know when you can take on more services, when your pay scale might be increased, or when you might be considered for promotion, this meeting is the appropriate time and place to ask. Many beauty professionals never take advantage of this crucial communication opportunity to discuss their future advancement because they are too nervous, intimidated, or unprepared to discuss these issues. Participate proactively in your career and in your success by communicating your desires and interests.
- When you meet with your manager, show her your self-evaluation and tell her you are serious about your improvement and growth. Your manager will appreciate your input and your initiative. If you are being honest with yourself, there should be no surprises.
- At the end of the meeting, thank your manager for taking the time to do the evaluation and for the feedback and guidance they gave you (**Figure 4–9**).

▼ **Figure 4–9**
Your employee evaluation is a good time to discuss your progress with your manager.

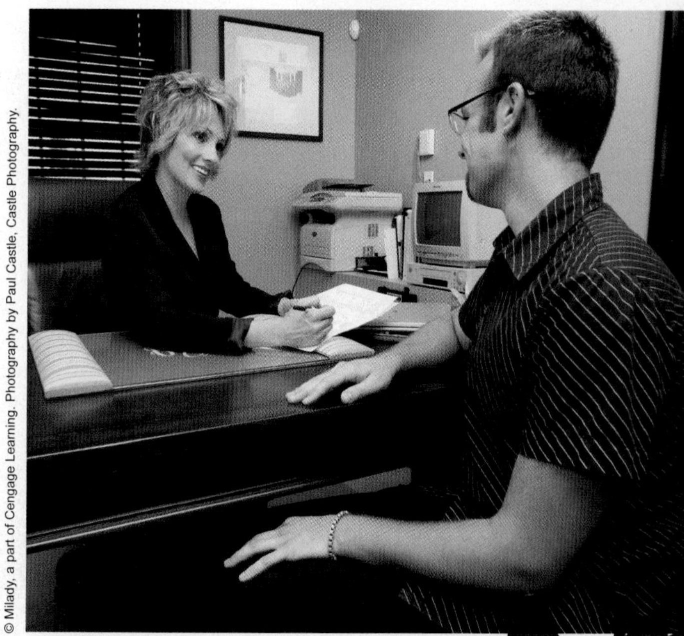

© Milady, a part of Cengage Learning. Photography by Paul Castle, Castle Photography.

Review Questions

1. What are the golden rules of human relations?
2. What is the definition of effective communication?
3. What are the elements of the 10-Step Consultation Method?
4. What are four examples of how a salon professional should handle an unhappy client?
5. List at least five things to remember when communicating with your coworkers.

Chapter Glossary

client consultation	Also known as *needs assessment*; the verbal communication with a client that determines what the client's needs are and how to achieve the desired results.
effective communication	The act of sharing information between two people (or groups of people) so that the information is successfully understood.
reflective listening	Listening to the client and then repeating, in your own words, what you think the client is telling you.

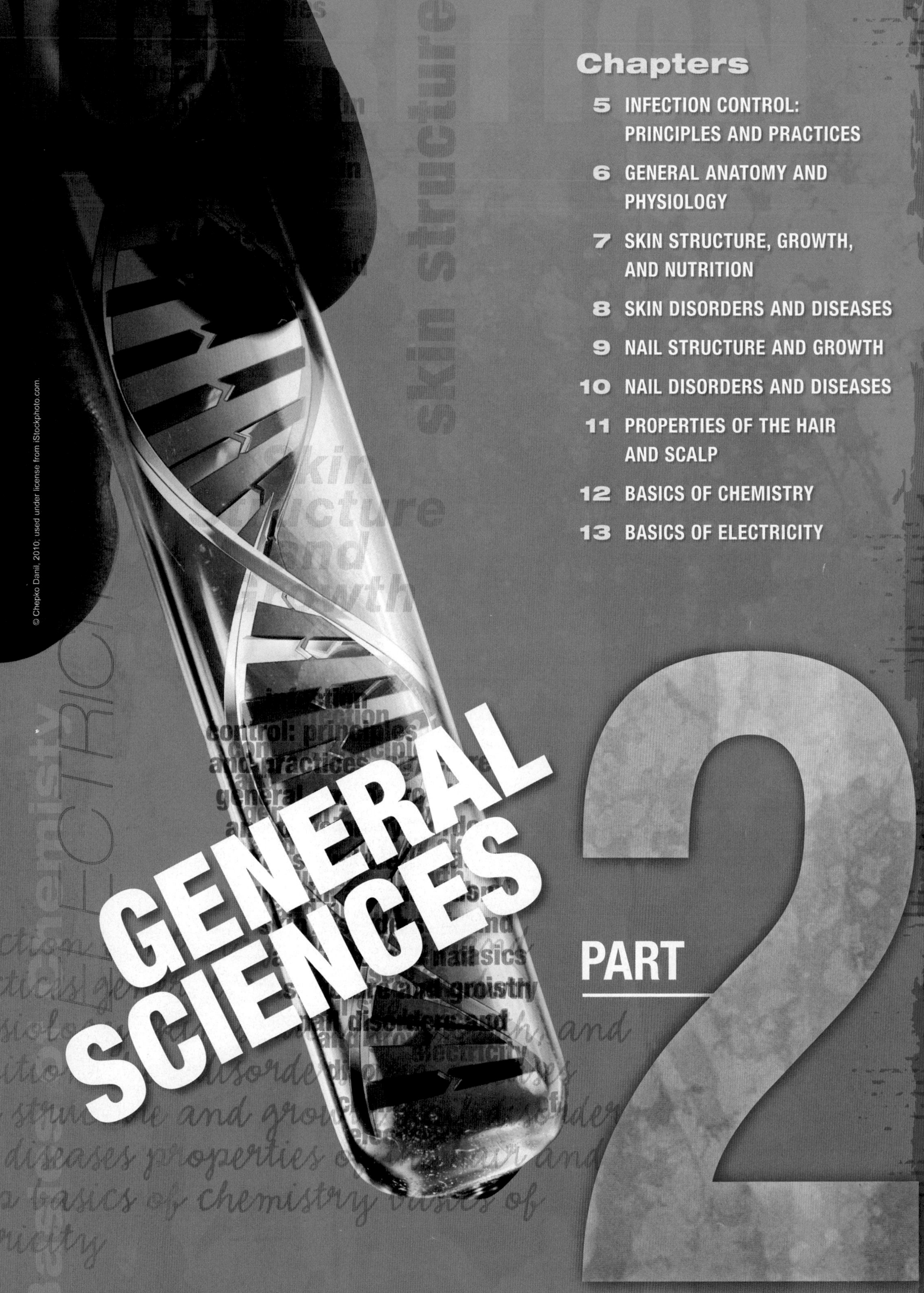
Chapters
5 INFECTION CONTROL: PRINCIPLES AND PRACTICES
6 GENERAL ANATOMY AND PHYSIOLOGY
7 SKIN STRUCTURE, GROWTH, AND NUTRITION
8 SKIN DISORDERS AND DISEASES
9 NAIL STRUCTURE AND GROWTH
10 NAIL DISORDERS AND DISEASES
11 PROPERTIES OF THE HAIR AND SCALP
12 BASICS OF CHEMISTRY
13 BASICS OF ELECTRICITY
GENERAL SCIENCES
PART 2
© Chepko Danil, 2010; used under license from iStockphoto.com.

CHAPTER 5

Infection Control: Principles and Practices

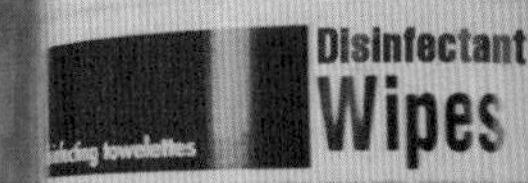

Chapter Outline

Why Study Infection Control?

Regulation

Principles of Infection

Principles of Prevention

Universal Precautions

The Professional Salon Image

Procedures

© Photo courtesy of King Research, Inc.

Learning Objectives

After completing this chapter, you will be able to:

- ✓ **LO1** Understand state laws and rules and the differences between them.
- ✓ **LO2** List the types and classifications of bacteria.
- ✓ **LO3** Define hepatitis and Human Immunodeficiency Virus (HIV) and explain how they are transmitted.
- ✓ **LO4** Explain the differences between cleaning, disinfecting, and sterilizing.
- ✓ **LO5** List the types of disinfectants and how they are used.
- ✓ **LO6** Discuss Universal Precautions.
- ✓ **LO7** List your responsibilities as a salon professional.
- ✓ **LO8** Describe how to safely clean and disinfect salon tools and implements.

Key Terms

Page number indicates where in the chapter the term is used.

acquired immune deficiency syndrome (AIDS)
pg. 80

acquired immunity
pg. 82

allergy
pg. 83

antiseptics
pg. 92

asymptomatic
pg. 93

bacilli
pg. 74

bacteria
pg. 74

bactericidal
pg. 73

binary fission
pg. 76

bioburden
pg. 85

bloodborne pathogens
pg. 79

chelating soaps (chelating detergents)
pg. 90

clean (cleaning)
pg. 73

cocci
pg. 74

contagious disease (communicable disease)
pg. 77

contamination
pg. 78

decontamination
pg. 82

diagnosis
pg. 78

diplococci
pg. 74

direct transmission
pg. 75

disease
pg. 70

disinfectants
pg. 70

disinfection
pg. 73

efficacy
pg. 85

exposure incident
pg. 93

flagella
pg. 76

fungi
pg. 80

fungicidal
pg. 73

hepatitis
pg. 79

hospital disinfectants
pg. 70

human immunodeficiency virus (HIV)
pg. 80

human papilloma virus (HPV, plantar warts)
pg. 79

immunity
pg. 82

indirect transmission
pg. 75

infection
pg. 72

Key Terms

Page number indicates where in the chapter the term is used.

infection control
pg. 72

infectious
pg. 71

infectious disease
pg. 73

inflammation
pg. 76

local infection
pg. 77

Material Safety Data Sheet (MSDS)
pg. 70

methicillin-resistant staphylococcus aureus (MRSA)
pg. 77

microorganism
pg. 74

mildew
pg. 80

motility
pg. 75

multiuse (reusable)
pg. 89

mycobacterium fortuitum
pg. 71

natural immunity
pg. 82

nonpathogenic
pg. 74

nonporous
pg. 70

occupational disease
pg. 78

parasites
pg. 81

parasitic disease
pg. 78

pathogenic
pg. 74

pathogenic disease
pg. 78

phenolic disinfectants
pg. 87

porous
pg. 89

pus
pg. 76

quaternary ammonium compounds (quats)
pg. 87

sanitation (sanitizing)
pg. 68

scabies
pg. 81

single-use (disposable)
pg. 89

sodium hypochlorite
pg. 87

spirilla
pg. 75

staphylococci
pg. 74

sterilization
pg. 84

streptococci
pg. 74

systemic disease
pg. 78

tinea barbae (barber's itch)
pg. 80

tinea capitis
pg. 81

tinea pedis
pg. 81

toxins
pg. 75

tuberculocidal disinfectants
pg. 70

tuberculosis
pg. 70

Universal Precautions
pg. 92

virucidal
pg. 73

virus
pg. 79

Publisher's Note: In previous editions of this chapter the term sanitation, also known as *sanitizing*, was used interchangeably to mean *clean* or *cleaning*. You will also find that many commercially-available products used in the cleaning and disinfecting process continue to use the words sanitize and sanitizing. However, the publisher's goal is to clearly define these terms below and within the glossary because:

- There is much confusion about and misuse of the terms cleaning, sanitizing, disinfecting, and sterilizing within the beauty industry. In an effort to do what we can to clarify these critical terms, Milady opted to consistently use cleaning, instead of using cleaning in one sentence and sanitizing in another sentence.
- Professionals in the health care and scientific communities (of disease prevention and epidemiology) and associations, such as The Association for Professionals in Infection Control and Epidemiology, generally do not use the terms interchangeably either. Instead, it is more common for infection control professionals to use the term cleaning. Infection control professionals consider sanitation a layperson's term or a product marketing term (as in hand sanitizers).

The term clean is defined: A mechanical process (scrubbing) using soap and water or detergent and water to remove all visible dirt, debris, and many disease-causing germs. Cleaning also removes invisible debris that interferes with disinfection. Cleaning is what cosmetologists are required to do before disinfecting.

The term sanitize is defined: A chemical process for reducing the number of disease-causing germs on cleaned surfaces to a safe level.

The term disinfection is defined: A chemical process that uses specific products to destroy harmful organisms (except bacterial spores) on environmental surfaces.

Consider this scenario: You are a new employee of a salon that offers hair and nail services. At the end of the day, the salon manager asks you to help clean and disinfect the counters, workstations, tools, implements, and pedicure equipment. Your manager also tells you to enter the cleaning and disinfection information in the salon's logbook. You know how important it is to follow the proper cleaning and disinfection procedures in the salon. This chapter will give you the principles and practices you need to complete those tasks.

Why Study Infection Control: Principles and Practices?

Cosmetologists should study and have a thorough understanding of infection control principles and practices because:

- To be a knowledgeable, successful, and responsible professional in the field of cosmetology, you are required to understand the types of infections you may encounter in the salon.
- Understanding the basics of cleaning and disinfecting and following federal and state rules will safeguard you and your clients and ensure that you have a long and successful career as a cosmetologist.
- Understanding the chemistry of the cleaning and disinfecting products that you use and how to use them will help keep you, your clients, and your salon environment safe.

Regulation

Many different federal and state agencies regulate the practice of cosmetology. Federal agencies set guidelines for the manufacturing, sale, and use of equipment and chemical ingredients. These guidelines also monitor safety in the workplace and place limits on the types of services you can perform in the salon. State agencies regulate licensing, enforcement, and your conduct when you are working in the salon.

Federal Agencies

Occupational Safety and Health Administration (OSHA)

The Occupational Safety and Health Administration (OSHA) was created as part of the U.S. Department of Labor to regulate and enforce safety and health standards to protect employees in the workplace. Regulating employee exposure to potentially toxic substances and informing employees about the possible hazards of materials used in the workplace are key points of the Occupational Safety and Health Act of 1970. This regulation created the Hazard Communication Standard (HCS), which requires that chemical manufacturers and importers assess and communicate the potential hazards associated with their products. The Material Safety Data Sheet (MSDS) is a result of the HCS.

© Photo Courtesy of King Research, Inc.

WEB RESOURCES

You can find an EPA-approved list of hospital and tuberculocidal disinfectants by going to the EPA's Web site at http://www.epa.gov and entering a search on the homepage for EPA-registered disinfectants.

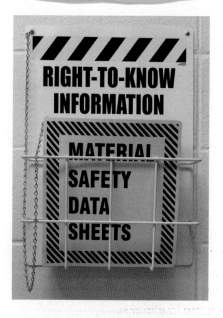

© Travis Klein, 2010; used under license from Shutterstock.com.

The standards set by OSHA are important to the cosmetology industry because of the products used in salons. OSHA standards address issues relating to the handling, mixing, storing, and disposing of products; general safety in the workplace; and your right to know about any potentially hazardous ingredients contained in the products you use and how to avoid these hazards.

Material Safety Data Sheet (MSDS)

Both federal and state laws require that manufacturers supply a **Material Safety Data Sheet (MSDS)** for all products sold. The MSDS contains information compiled by the manufacturer about product safety, including the names of hazardous ingredients, safe handling and use procedures, precautions to reduce the risk of accidental harm or overexposure, and flammability warnings. The MSDS also provides useful disposal guidelines and medical and first aid information. When necessary, the MSDS can be sent to a medical facility, so that a doctor can better assess and treat the patient. OSHA and state regulatory agencies require that MSDSs be kept available in the salon for all products. Both OSHA and state board inspectors can issue fines for salons not having MSDSs available during regular business hours.

Federal and state laws require salons to obtain MSDSs from the product manufacturers and/or distributors for each professional product that is used. MSDSs often can be downloaded from the product manufacturer's or the distributor's Web site. Not having MSDSs available poses a health risk to anyone exposed to hazardous materials and violates federal and state regulations. All employees must read the information included on each MSDS and verify that they have read it by adding their signatures to a sign-off sheet for the product. These sign-off sheets must be available to state and federal inspectors upon request.

did you know?

The term *Hospital Grade* is not a term used by the EPA. The EPA does not grade disinfectants; a product is either approved by the EPA as a hospital disinfectant or it is not.

Environmental Protection Agency (EPA)

The Environmental Protection Agency (EPA) registers all types of disinfectants sold and used in the United States. **Disinfectants** (dis-in-FEK-tents) are chemical products that destroy all bacteria, fungi, and viruses (but not spores) on surfaces. The two types that are used in salons are hospital disinfectants and tuberculocidal disinfectants.

- **Hospital disinfectants** (HOS-pih-tal dis-in-FEK-tents) are effective for cleaning blood and body fluids. They can be used on any nonporous surface in the salon. **Nonporous** (nahn-POHW-rus) means that an item is made or constructed of a material that has no pores or openings and cannot absorb liquids. Hospital disinfectants control the spread of **disease** (dih-ZEEZ), an abnormal condition of all or part of the body, or its systems or organs, that makes the body incapable of carrying on normal function.
- **Tuberculocidal disinfectants** (tuh-bur-kyoo-LOH-sy-dahl dis-in-FEK-tents) are proven to kill the bacteria that cause **tuberculosis**

(tuh-bur-kyoo-LOH-sus), a disease caused by bacteria that are transmitted through coughing or sneezing. These bacteria are capable of forming spores so they are difficult to kill. Tuberculocidal disinfectants are one kind of hospital disinfectant. The fact that tuberculocidal disinfectants are more powerful does not mean that you should automatically reach for them. Some of these products can be harmful to salon tools and equipment, and they require special methods of disposal. Check the rules in your state to be sure that the product you choose complies with state requirements.

It is against federal law to use any disinfecting product contrary to its labeling. Before a manufacturer can sell a product for disinfecting surfaces, tools, implements, or equipment, it must obtain an EPA-registration number that certifies that the disinfectant may be used in the manner prescribed by the manufacturer's label. For example, pedicure tub disinfectants must be approved for that specific use or the manufacturer will be breaking federal law by marketing them for disinfecting pedicure tubs. This also means that if you do not follow the label instructions for mixing, contact time, and the type of

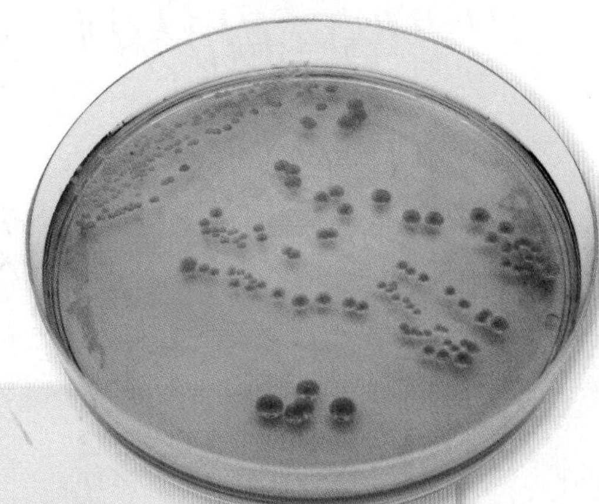

© Guntars Grebezs, 2010; used under license from iStockphoto.com.

did you know?

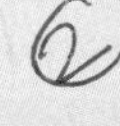

Cosmetologists can put themselves and their clients at risk unless stringent infection control guidelines are performed every day. A case in point was the spread of a bacterium called **Mycobacterium fortuitum** (MY-koh-bak-TIR-ee-um for-TOO-i-tum), a microscopic germ that normally exists in tap water in small numbers. Until an incident occurred, health officials considered the germ to be completely harmless and not **infectious** (in-FEK-shus), caused by or capable of being transmitted by infection.

In 2000, over 100 clients from one California salon developed serious skin infections on their legs after getting pedicures. The infection caused ugly sores that lingered for months, required the use of strong antibiotics, and permanently scarred some of the clients' legs. The source of the infection was traced to the salon's whirlpool foot spas. Salon staff did not clean and disinfect the foot spas properly, resulting in a build-up of hair and debris in the foot spas that created the perfect breeding ground for bacteria.

The outbreak was a catalyst for change in the cosmetology industry. As a result, the state of California issued specific requirements for pedicure equipment in the hope of preventing future outbreaks. In spite of their efforts, there have been other outbreaks affecting hundreds of clients in California and other states. In Texas, family members of a paraplegic woman who died after receiving a pedicure sued a salon. They charged that the woman, who had no feeling in her feet, died because of an improperly disinfected implement that caused an infection on her foot that spread throughout her body and resulted in a fatal heart attack.

While many of the stories in the news have been about diseases caused by manicures or pedicures, not all incidents are related to the nail industry. Take the case of a barber who unintentionally transmitted an infectious disease through a shaving razor. The barber used a disinfectant on the razor, but it was not the proper disinfectant. Several of his clients contracted hepatitis B because the wrong disinfectant was used. This incident demonstrates how important it is for cosmetologists to use the proper disinfectants on tools, such as razors, scissors, and clippers. When in doubt about the disinfectant you should use, consult federal and state regulations.

Media scrutiny has made clients more aware of the infection control practices of salons, and the cosmetology industry has become more enlightened about the importance of cleaning and disinfection practices.

surface the disinfecting product can be used on, you are not complying with federal law. If there is a lawsuit, you can be held responsible.

State Regulatory Agencies

State regulatory agencies exist to protect salon professionals and to protect consumers' health, safety, and welfare while they receive salon services. State regulatory agencies include licensing agencies, state boards of cosmetology, commissions, and health departments. Regulatory agencies require that everyone working in a salon or spa follow specific procedures. Enforcement of the rules through inspections and investigations of consumer complaints is also part of an agency's responsibility. An agency can issue penalties against both the salon owner and the cosmetologist's license. Penalties vary and include warnings, fines, probation, and suspension or revocation of licenses. It is vital that you understand and follow the laws and rules of your state at all times. Your salon's reputation, your license, and everyone's safety depend on it.

FYI

Remember: Salon professionals are not allowed to treat or recommend treatments for infections, diseases, or abnormal conditions. Clients with such problems should be referred to their physicians.

Laws and Rules—What is the Difference?

Laws are written by both federal and state legislatures that determine the scope of practice (what each license allows the holder to do) and that establish guidelines for regulatory agencies to make rules. Laws are also called statutes.

Rules and regulations are more specific than laws. Rules are written by the regulatory agency or the state board, and they determine how the law must be applied. Rules establish specific standards of conduct and can be changed or updated frequently. Cosmetologists must be aware of any changes or updates to the rules and regulations, and they must comply with them. ☑ **LO1**

© MARIA TOUTOUDAKI, 2010; used under license from iStockphoto.com.

Principles of Infection

Being a salon professional is fun and rewarding, but it is also a great responsibility. One careless action could cause injury or **infection** (in-FEK-shun), the invasion of body tissues by disease-causing pathogens. If your actions result in an injury or infection, you could lose your license or ruin the salon's reputation. Fortunately, preventing the spread of infections is easy when you know proper procedures and follow them at all times. Prevention begins and ends with *you* (**Figure 5–1**).

Infection Control

Infection control are the methods used to eliminate or reduce the transmission of infectious organisms. Cosmetologists must understand and remember the following four types of potentially harmful organisms:

- Bacteria
- Fungi
- Viruses
- Parasites

© Milady, a part of Cengage Learning. Photography by Tom Stock.

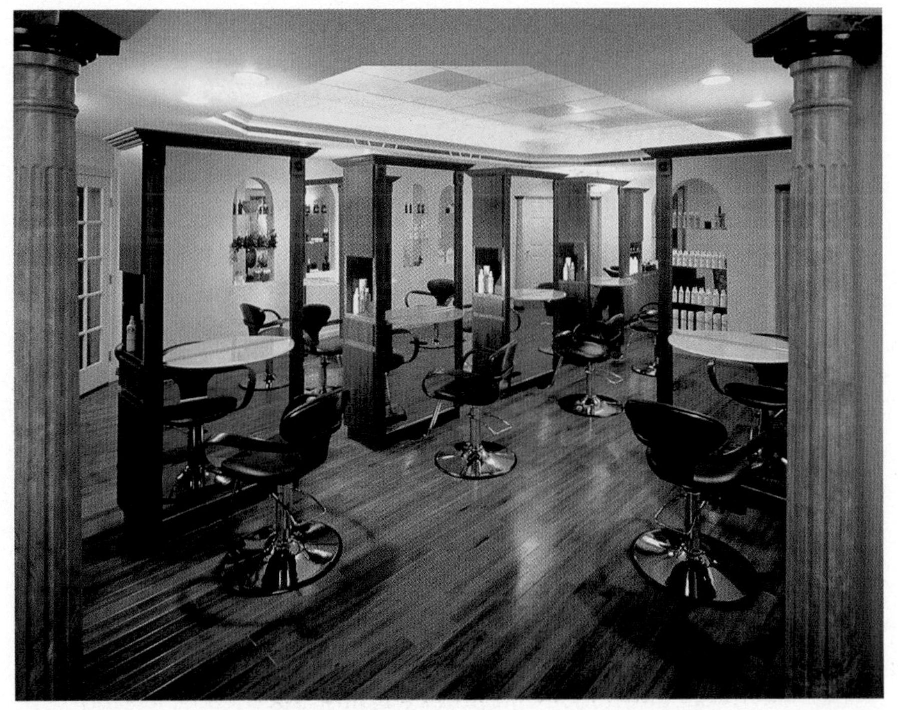

Figure 5–1
A sparkling clean salon gains your clients' confidence.

Under certain conditions, many of these organisms can cause infectious disease. An **infectious disease** (in-FEK-shus dih-ZEEZ) is caused by pathogenic (harmful) organisms that enter the body. An infectious disease may or may not be spread from one person to another person.

In this chapter, you will learn how to properly clean and disinfect the tools and equipment you use in the salon so they are safe for you and your clients. To **clean** (cleaning) is a mechanical process (scrubbing) using soap and water or detergent and water to remove all visible dirt, debris, and many disease-causing germs from tools, implements, and equipment. The process of **disinfection** (dis-in-FEK-shun) destroys most, but not necessarily all, harmful organisms on environmental surfaces. Disinfection is not effective against bacterial spores.

© Milady, a part of Cengage Learning.

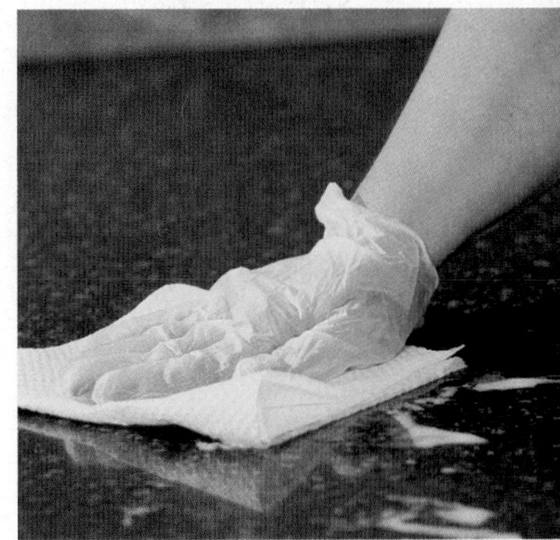

Cleaning and disinfecting procedures are designed to prevent the spread of infection and disease. Disinfectants used in salons must be **bactericidal** (back-teer-uh-SYD-ul), capable of destroying bacteria; **virucidal** (vy-ru-SYD-ul), capable of destroying viruses; and **fungicidal** (fun-jih-SYD-ul), capable of destroying fungi. Be sure to mix and use these disinfectants according to the instructions on the labels so they are safe and effective.

Contaminated salon tools and equipment can spread infections from client to client if the proper disinfection steps are not taken after every service. You have a professional and legal obligation to protect clients from harm by using proper infection control procedures. If clients are infected or harmed because you perform infection control procedures incorrectly, you may be found legally responsible for their injuries or infections.

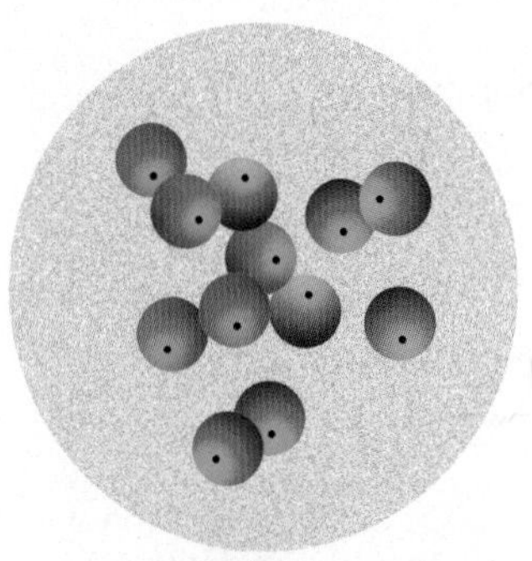

▲ Figure 5–2
Cocci.

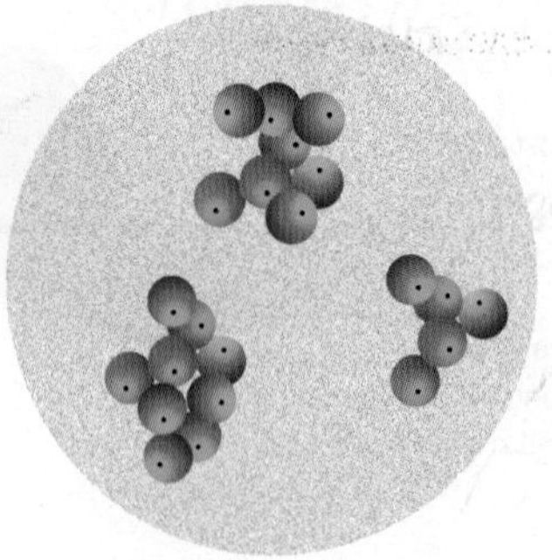

▲ Figure 5–3
Staphylococci.

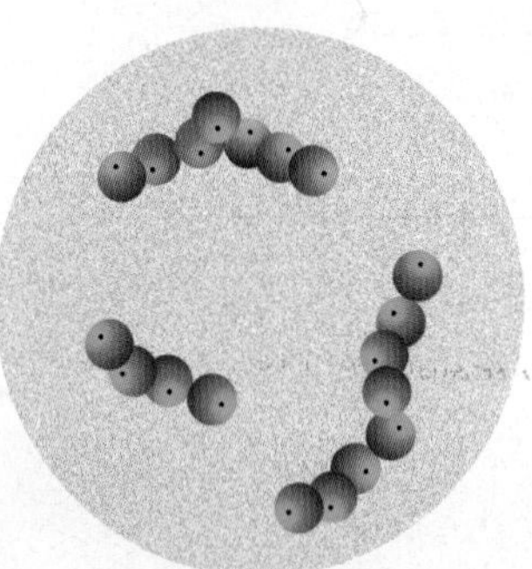

▲ Figure 5–4
Streptococci.

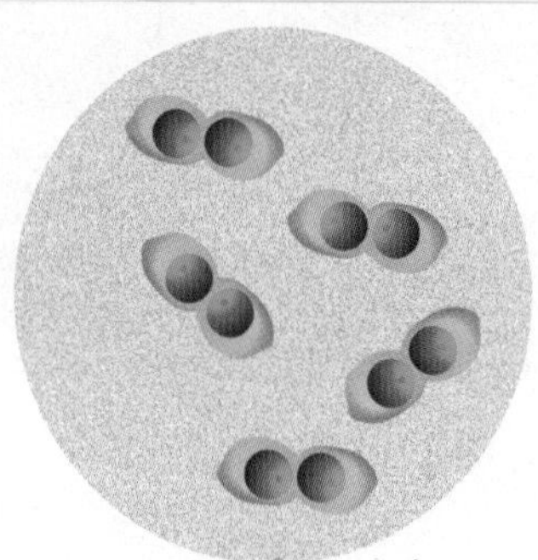

▲ Figure 5–5
Diplococci.

Bacteria

Bacteria (bak-TEER-ee-ah) (singular: bacterium, back-TEER-ee-um) are one-celled microorganisms that have both plant and animal characteristics. A **microorganism** (my-kroh-OR-gah-niz-um) is any organism of microscopic or submicroscopic size. Some bacteria are harmful and some are harmless. Bacteria can exist almost anywhere: on skin, in water, in the air, in decayed matter, on environmental surfaces, in body secretions, on clothing, or under the free edge of nails. Bacteria are so small they can only be seen with a microscope.

Types of Bacteria

There are thousands of different kinds of bacteria that fall into two primary types: pathogenic and nonpathogenic. Most bacteria are **nonpathogenic** (non-path-uh-JEN-ik); in other words, they are harmless organisms that may perform useful functions. They are safe to come in contact with since they do not cause disease or harm. For example, nonpathogenic bacteria are used to make yogurt, cheese, and some medicines. In the human body, nonpathogenic bacteria help the body break down food and protect against infection. They also stimulate the immune system.

Pathogenic (path-uh-JEN-ik) bacteria are harmful microorganisms that can cause disease or infection in humans when they invade the body. Salons and schools must maintain strict standards for cleaning and disinfecting at all times to prevent the spread of pathogenic microorganisms. It is crucial that cosmetologists learn proper infection control practices while in school to ensure that you understand the importance of following them throughout your career. **Table 5–1**, Causes of Disease, presents terms and definitions related to pathogens.

Classifications of Pathogenic Bacteria

Bacteria have three distinct shapes that help to identify them. Pathogenic bacteria are classified as described below.

- **Cocci** (KOK-sy) are round-shaped bacteria that appear singly (alone) or in groups (**Figure 5–2**):
  - **Staphylococci** (staf-uh-loh-KOK-sy) are pus-forming bacteria that grow in clusters like bunches of grapes. They cause abscesses, pustules, and boils (**Figure 5–3**). Some types of staphylococci (or staph as many call it) may not cause infections in healthy humans.
  - **Streptococci** (strep-toh-KOK-sy) are pus-forming bacteria arranged in curved lines resembling a string of beads. They cause infections such as strep throat and blood poisoning (**Figure 5–4**).
  - **Diplococci** (dip-lo-KOK-sy) are spherical bacteria that grow in pairs and cause diseases such as pneumonia (**Figure 5–5**).
- **Bacilli** (bah-SIL-ee) are short rod-shaped bacteria. They are the most common bacteria and produce diseases such as tetanus (lockjaw),

© Milady, a part of Cengage Learning.

CAUSES OF DISEASE

TERM	DEFINITION
BACTERIA	One-celled microorganisms having both plant and animal characteristics. Some are harmful and some are harmless.
DIRECT TRANSMISSION	Transmission of blood or body fluids through touching (including shaking hands), kissing, coughing, sneezing, and talking.
INDIRECT TRANSMISSION	Transmission of blood or body fluids through contact with an intermediate contaminated object, such as a razor, extractor, nipper, or an environmental surface.
INFECTION	Invasion of body tissues by disease-causing pathogens.
GERMS	Nonscientific synonym for disease-producing organisms.
MICROORGANISM	Any organism of microscopic to submicroscopic size.
PARASITES	Organisms that grow, feed, and shelter on or in another organism (referred to as the host), while contributing nothing to the survival of that organism. Parasites must have a host to survive.
TOXINS	Various poisonous substances produced by some microorganisms (bacteria and viruses).
VIRUS	A parasitic submicroscopic particle that infects and resides in cells of biological organisms. A virus is capable of replication only through taking over the host cell's reproductive function.

© Milady, a part of Cengage Learning.

Table 5–1 **Causes of Disease.**

typhoid fever, tuberculosis, and diphtheria (**Figure 5–6**).

- **Spirilla** (spy-RIL-ah) are spiral or corkscrew-shaped bacteria. They are subdivided into subgroups, such as treponema papillida, which causes syphilis, a sexually transmitted disease (STD), and borrelia burgdorferi, which causes Lyme disease (**Figure 5–7**).

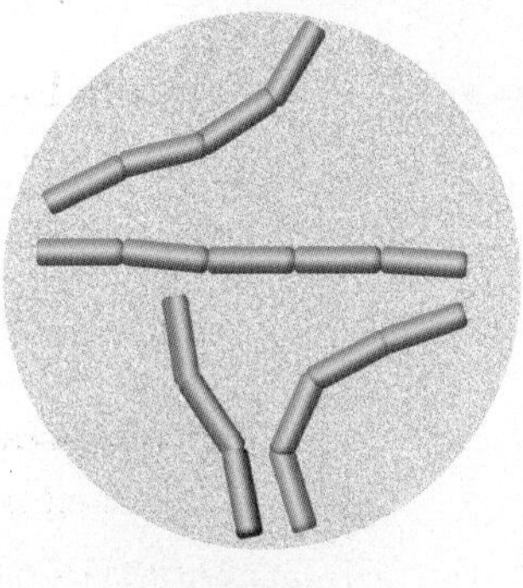

▲ Figure 5–6
Bacilli.

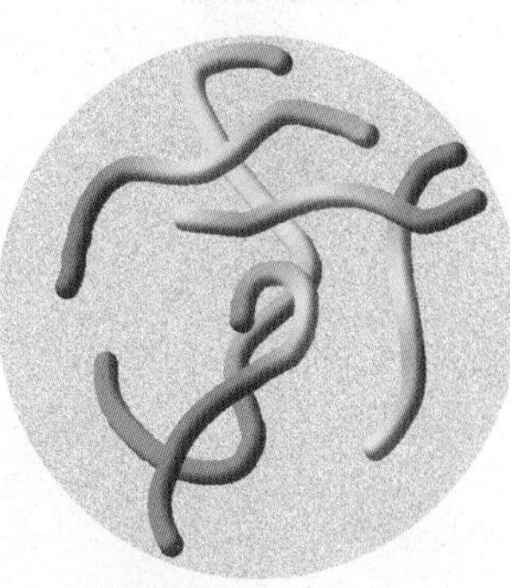

▲ Figure 5–7
Spirilla.

© Milady, a part of Cengage Learning.

Movement of Bacteria

Different bacteria move in different ways. Cocci rarely show active **motility** (MOH-til-eh-tee), which means self-movement. Cocci are transmitted in the air, in dust, or within the substance in which they settle. Bacilli and spirilla are both capable of movement and use slender, hair-like extensions called **flagella** (fluh-JEL-uh) for locomotion (moving about). You may also hear people refer to **cilia** (SIL-ee-uh) as hair-like extensions on cells. Cilia are shorter than flagella, however. Both flagella and cilia move cells, but they have a different motion. Flagella move in a snake-like motion while cilia move in a rowing-like motion.

Bacterial Growth and Reproduction

When seen under a microscope, bacteria look like tiny bags. They generally consist of an outer cell wall that contains liquid called protoplasm. Bacterial cells manufacture their own food through what they absorb from the surrounding environment. They give off waste products, grow, and reproduce. The life cycle of bacteria consists of two distinct phases: the active stage and the inactive or spore-forming stage.

Active stage. During the active stage, bacteria grow and reproduce. Bacteria multiply best in warm, dark, damp, or dirty places. When conditions are favorable, bacteria grow and reproduce. When they reach their largest size, they divide into two new cells. This division is called **binary fission** (BY-nayr-ee FISH-un). The cells that are formed are called daughter cells and are produced every twenty to sixty minutes, depending on the bacteria. The infectious pathogen staphylococcus aureus undergoes cell division every twenty-seven to thirty minutes. When conditions become unfavorable and difficult for them to thrive, bacteria either die or become inactive.

Inactive or spore-forming stage. Certain bacteria, such as the anthrax and tetanus bacilli, coat themselves with wax-like outer shells. These bacteria are able to withstand long periods of famine, dryness, and unsuitable temperatures. In this stage, spores can be blown about and are not harmed by disinfectants, heat, or cold. When favorable conditions are restored, the spores change into the active form and begin to grow and reproduce.

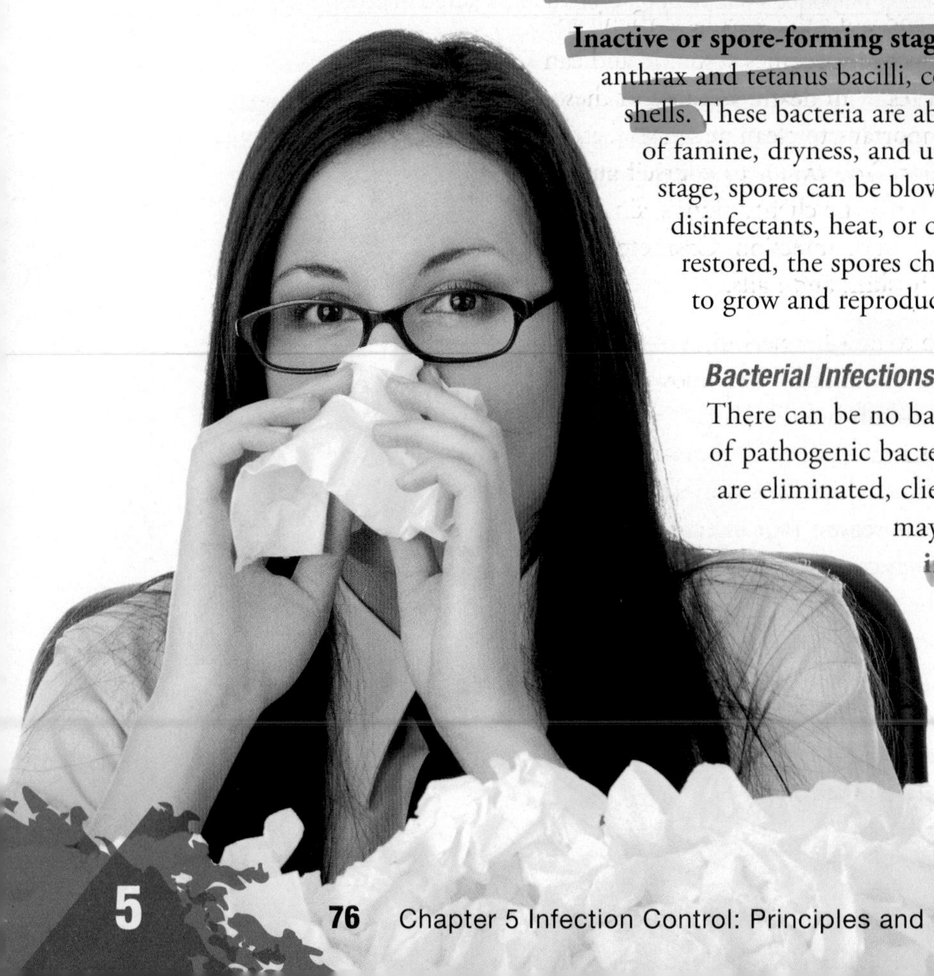

Bacterial Infections

There can be no bacterial infection without the presence of pathogenic bacteria. Therefore, if pathogenic bacteria are eliminated, clients cannot become infected. You may have a client who has tissue **inflammation** (in-fluh-MAY-shun), a condition in which the body reacts to injury, irritation, or infection. An inflammation is characterized by redness, heat, pain, and swelling. **Pus** is a fluid created by

© Piotr Marcinski, 2010; used under license from Shutterstock.com.

infection. It contains white blood cells, bacteria, and dead cells. The presence of pus is a sign of a bacterial infection. A **local infection**, such as a pimple or abscess, is confined to a particular part of the body and appears as a lesion containing pus. Staphylococci are among the most common bacteria that affect humans and are normally carried by about a third of the population. Staph bacteria can be picked up on doorknobs, countertops, and other surfaces, but in the salon they are more frequently spread through skin-to-skin contact (such as shaking hands) or through the use of unclean tools or implements. If these bacteria get into the wrong place, they can be very dangerous. Although lawsuits are rare considering the number of services performed in a salon, every year many salons are sued for allegedly causing staph infections.

© Viorika Prikhodko, 2010; used under license from iStockphoto.com.

Staph is responsible for food poisoning and a wide range of diseases, including toxic shock syndrome. Some types of infectious staph bacteria are highly resistant to conventional treatments such as antibiotics. An example is the staph infection called **methicillin-resistant staphylococcus aureus (MRSA)** (METH-eh-sill-en-ree-ZIST-ent staf-uh-loh-KOK-us OR-ee-us). Historically, MRSA occurred most frequently among persons with weakened immune systems or among people who had undergone medical procedures. Today, it has become more common in otherwise healthy people. Clients who appear completely healthy may bring this organism into the salon where it can infect others. Some people carry the bacteria and are not even aware of their infection, but the people they infect may show more obvious symptoms. MRSA initially appears as a skin infection, such as pimples, rashes, and boils that can be difficult to cure. Without proper treatment, the infection becomes systemic and can have devastating consequences that can result in death. Because of these highly resistant bacterial strains, it is important to clean and disinfect all tools and implements used in the salon. You owe it to yourself and your clients! Also, do not perform services if the client's skin, scalp, neck, hands, or feet show visible signs of abrasion or infection. Cosmetologists are only allowed to work on healthy hair, skin, and nails.

When a disease spreads from one person to another person, it is said to be a **contagious disease** (kon-TAY-jus dih-ZEEZ), also known as **communicable disease** (kuh-MYOO-nih-kuh-bul dih-ZEEZ). Some of the more common contagious diseases that prevent a salon professional from servicing a client are the common cold, ringworm, conjunctivitis (pinkeye), viral infections, and natural nail, toe, or foot infections. The most common way these infections spread is through dirty hands, especially under the fingernails and in the webs between the fingers. Be sure to always wash your hands after using the restroom and before eating. Contagious diseases can also be spread by contaminated implements, cuts, infected nails, open sores, pus, mouth and nose discharges, shared drinking cups, telephone receivers, and towels. Uncovered coughing or sneezing and spitting in public also spread germs. ☑ **LO2**

TERMS RELATED TO DISEASE

TERM	DEFINITION
ALLERGY	Reaction due to extreme sensitivity to certain foods, chemicals, or other normally harmless substances.
CONTAGIOUS DISEASE	Also known as *communicable disease*; disease that is spread from one person to another person. Some of the more contagious diseases are the common cold, ringworm, conjunctivitis (pinkeye), viral infections, and natural nail or toe and foot infections.
CONTAMINATION	The presence, or the reasonably anticipated presence, of blood or other potentially infectious materials on an item's surface or visible debris or residues such as dust, hair, and skin.
DECONTAMINATION	The removal of blood or other potentially infectious materials on an item's surface and the removal of visible debris or residue such as dust, hair, and skin.
DIAGNOSIS	Determination of the nature of a disease from its symptoms and/or diagnostic tests. Federal regulations prohibit salon professionals from performing a diagnosis.
DISEASE	An abnormal condition of all or part of the body, or its systems or organs, that makes the body incapable of carrying on normal function.
EXPOSURE INCIDENT	Contact with nonintact (broken) skin, blood, body fluid, or other potentially infectious materials that is the result of the performance of an employee's duties.
INFECTIOUS DISEASE	Disease caused by pathogenic (harmful) microorganisms that enter the body. An infectious disease may or may not be spread from one person to another person.
INFLAMMATION	Condition in which the body reacts to injury, irritation, or infection. An inflammation is characterized by redness, heat, pain, and swelling.
OCCUPATIONAL DISEASE	Illnesses resulting from conditions associated with employment, such as prolonged and repeated overexposure to certain products or ingredients.
PARASITIC DISEASE	Disease caused by parasites, such as lice and mites.
PATHOGENIC DISEASE	Disease produced by organisms, including bacteria, viruses, fungi, and parasites.
SYSTEMIC DISEASE	Disease that affects the body as a whole, often due to under-functioning or over-functioning internal glands or organs. This disease is carried through the blood stream or the lymphatic system.

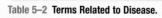

© Milady, a part of Cengage Learning.

Table 5–2 **Terms Related to Disease.**

Table 5–2, Terms Related to Disease, lists terms and definitions that are important for a general understanding of disease.

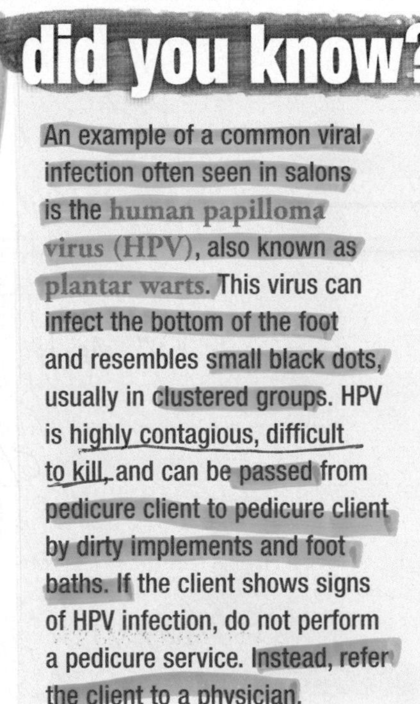

did you know?

An example of a common viral infection often seen in salons is the **human papilloma virus (HPV)**, also known as **plantar warts.** This virus can infect the bottom of the foot and resembles small black dots, usually in clustered groups. HPV is highly contagious, difficult to kill, and can be passed from pedicure client to pedicure client by dirty implements and foot baths. If the client shows signs of HPV infection, do not perform a pedicure service. Instead, refer the client to a physician.

Viruses

A **virus** (VY-rus) (plural: viruses) is a parasitic submicroscopic particle that infects and resides in the cells of a biological organism. A virus is capable of replication only through taking over the host cell's reproductive function. Viruses are so small that they can only be seen under the most sophisticated and powerful microscopes. They cause common colds and other respiratory and gastrointestinal (digestive tract) infections. Other viruses that plague humans are measles, mumps, chicken pox, smallpox, rabies, yellow fever, hepatitis, polio, influenza, and HIV, which causes AIDS.

One difference between viruses and bacteria is that a virus can live and reproduce only by taking over other cells and becoming part of them, while bacteria can live and reproduce on their own. Also, bacterial infections can usually be treated with specific antibiotics, but viruses are not affected by antibiotics. In fact, viruses are hard to kill without harming the body's own cells in the process. Vaccinations prevent viruses from growing in the body. There are many vaccines available for viruses, but not all viruses have vaccines. There is a vaccine available for hepatitis B, however, and you should strongly consider receiving this vaccine. Health authorities recommend that service providers in industries with direct contact to the public—including cosmetologists, teachers, florists, and bank tellers—ask their doctor about getting vaccinated for hepatitis B.

Bloodborne Pathogens

Disease-causing microorganisms that are carried in the body by blood or body fluids, such as hepatitis and HIV, are called **bloodborne pathogens**. In the salon, the spread of bloodborne pathogens is possible through haircutting, chemical burns, shaving, nipping, clipping, facial treatments, waxing, tweezing, or whenever the skin is broken. Use great care to avoid cutting or damaging clients' skin during any type of service.

Cutting living skin is considered outside the scope of the cosmetologist's licensed and approved practices. Federal law allows only qualified medical professionals to cut living skin, since this is considered a medical procedure. This means that cosmetologists are not allowed to trim or cut the skin around the nail plate. Cutting hardened tissue and removing a callus are both considered medical procedures. Even if the client insists, cosmetologists may not intentionally cut any living skin for any reason.

Hepatitis

Hepatitis (hep-uh-TY-tus), is a bloodborne virus that causes disease and can damage the liver. In general, it is difficult to contract hepatitis. However, hepatitis is easier to contract than HIV because hepatitis can be present in all body fluids of those who are infected. In

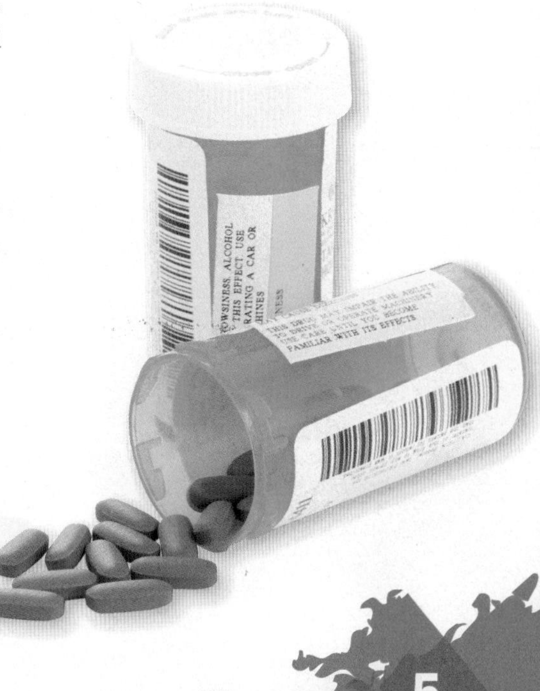

© Kratka Photography, 2010; used under license from Shutterstock.com.

addition, unlike HIV, hepatitis can live on a surface outside the body for long periods of time. For this reason, it is vital that all surfaces that contact a client are thoroughly cleaned and disinfected.

There are three types of hepatitis that are of concern in the salon: hepatitis A, hepatitis B, and hepatitis C. Hepatitis B is the most difficult to kill on a surface, so check the label of the disinfectant you use to be sure that the product is effective against hepatitis B. Hepatitis B and C are spread from person to person through blood and, less often, through other body fluids, such as semen and vaginal secretions.

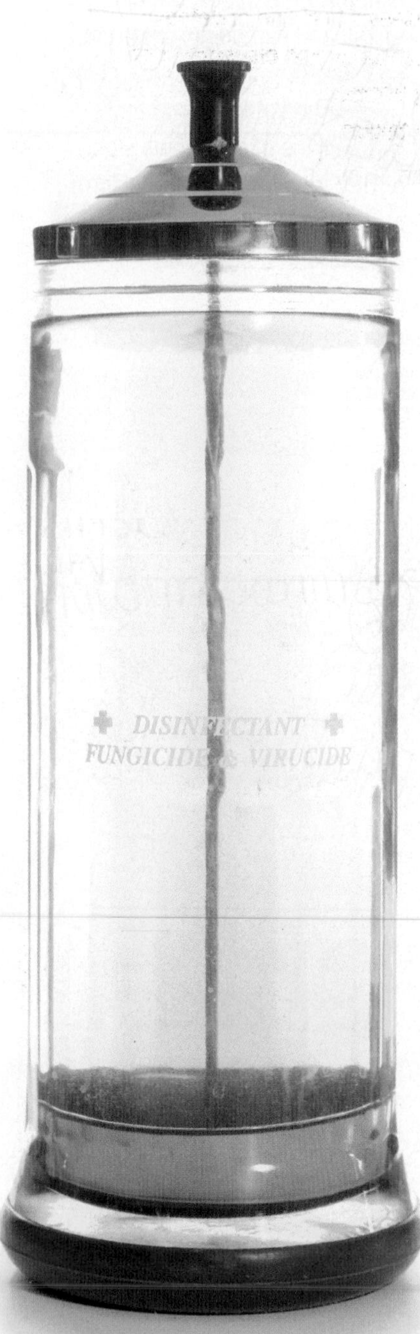

HIV/AIDS

Human immunodeficiency virus (HIV) (HYOO-mun ih-MYOO-noh-di-FISH-en-see VY-rus), abbreviated HIV, is the virus that causes **acquired immune deficiency syndrome (AIDS)** (uh-KWY-erd ih-MYOON di-FISH-en-see sin-drohm), abbreviated AIDS. AIDS is a disease that breaks down the body's immune system. HIV is spread from person to person through blood and, less often, through other body fluids, such as semen and vaginal secretions. A person can be infected with HIV for many years without having symptoms, but testing can determine whether a person is infected within six months after exposure to the virus. Sometimes, people who are HIV-positive have never been tested and do not know they have the potential to infect other people.

The HIV virus is spread mainly through the sharing of needles by intravenous (IV) drug users and by unprotected sexual contact. Less commonly, HIV is spread through accidents with needles in healthcare settings. The virus is less likely to enter the bloodstream through cuts and sores. It is not spread by holding hands, hugging, kissing, sharing food, or using household items such as the telephone or toilet seats. There are no documented cases that indicate the virus can be spread by food handlers, insects, or casual contact during hair, skin, nail, and pedicure salon services.

If you accidentally cut a client who is HIV-positive, the tool will be contaminated. You cannot continue to use the implement without cleaning and disinfecting it. Continuing to use a contaminated implement without cleaning and disinfecting it puts you and others in the salon at risk of infection. ☑ **LO3**

Fungi

Fungi (FUN-jI) (singular: fungus, FUN-gus) are microscopic plant parasites that include molds, mildews, and yeasts. They can produce contagious diseases, such as ringworm. **Mildew** (MIL-doo), another fungus, affects plants or grows on inanimate objects but does not cause human infections in the salon.

The most frequently encountered fungal infection resulting from hair services is **tinea barbae** (TIN-ee-uh BAR-bee), also known as **barber's itch**. Tinea barbae is a superficial fungal infection that commonly affects the skin. It is primarily limited to the bearded areas of the face

© Milady, a part of Cengage Learning.

and neck or around the scalp. This infection occurs almost exclusively in older adolescent and adult males. A person with tinea barbae may have deep, inflamed or noninflamed patches of skin on the face or the nape of the neck. Tinea barbae is similar to **tinea capitis** (TIN-ee-uh KAP-ih-tis), a fungal infection of the scalp characterized by red papules, or spots, at the opening of hair follicles. For more information on tinea capitis, see Chapter 11, Properties of the Hair and Scalp.

FYI

Pathogenic bacteria, viruses, or fungi can enter the body through:

- broken or inflamed skin, such as a cut or a scratch. They also can enter through a bruise or a rash. Intact skin is an effective barrier to infection.
- the mouth (contaminated water, food, or fingers).
- the nose (inhaling different types of dust or droplets from a cough or sneeze).
- the eyes or ears (less likely, but possible).
- unprotected sex.

The body prevents and controls infections with:

- healthy, unbroken skin—the body's first line of defense.
- body secretions, such as perspiration and digestive juices.
- white blood cells that destroy bacteria.
- antitoxins that counteract the toxins.

Hair stylists must clean and disinfect clipper blades to avoid spreading scalp and skin infections. The risk of spreading skin and scalp infections can be reduced by first removing all visible hair and debris from clippers. This can be done effectively and quickly by using compressed air. Then the nonelectrical parts can be cleaned and disinfected properly. Always refer to the manufacturer's directions for proper cleaning and disinfecting methods and recommendations.

Nail infections can be spread by using dirty implements or by not properly preparing the surface of the natural nail before enhancement products are applied. Nail infections can occur on both hands and feet. Fungal infections are much more common on the feet than on the hands, but bacterial infections commonly occur on both hands and feet. The most frequently encountered infection on the foot resulting from nail services is **tinea pedis** (TIN-ee-uh PED-us), a ringworm fungus of the foot. Both bacterial and fungal infections can be spread to an infected client's other nails or to other salon clients unless everything that touches clients is either properly cleaned and disinfected before reuse or is thrown away after use (**Figure 5–8**).

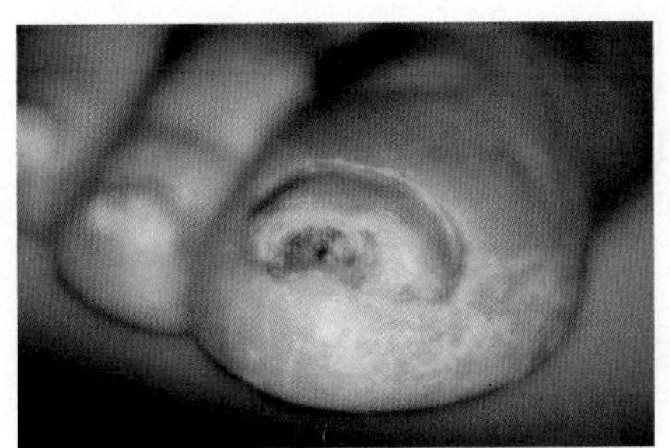

Courtesy of Godfrey F. Mix, DPM Sacramento, CA.

▲ Figure 5–8
Nail fungus.

Parasites

Parasites are organisms that grow, feed, and shelter on or in another organism (referred to as a host), while contributing nothing to the survival of that organism. They must have a host to survive. Parasites can live on or inside of humans and animals. They also can be found in food, on plants and trees, and in water. Humans can acquire internal parasites by eating fish or meat that has not been properly cooked. External parasites that affect humans on or in the skin include ticks, fleas, and mites.

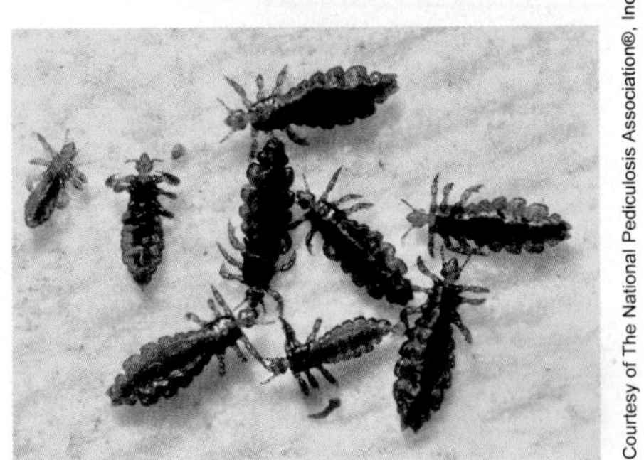

Courtesy of The National Pediculosis Association®, Inc.

▲ Figure 5–9
Head lice.

Head lice are a type of parasite responsible for contagious diseases and conditions (**Figure 5–9**). One condition caused by an infestation of head lice is called **pediculosis capitis** (puh-dik-yuh-LOH-sis KAP-ih-tus). **Scabies** (SKAY-beez) is also a contagious skin disease and is caused

did you know?

In most states cosmetology professionals are not allowed to use needles, lancets, and probes that penetrate the skin, nor are they allowed to offer any invasive services, such as callous removal. You should check your state's regulations about using any implement that may penetrate the skin. If you are allowed to use these implements in your state, be sure to receive the proper training before using them in the salon.

by the itch mite, which burrows under the skin. Contagious diseases and conditions caused by parasites should only be treated by a doctor. Contaminated countertops, tools, and equipment should be thoroughly cleaned and then disinfected with an EPA-registered disinfectant for the time recommended by the manufacturer or with a bleach solution for ten minutes.

Immunity

Immunity is the ability of the body to destroy and resist infection. Immunity against disease can be either natural or acquired and is a sign of good health. **Natural immunity** is partly inherited and partly developed through healthy living. **Acquired immunity** is immunity that the body develops after overcoming a disease, through inoculation (such as flu vaccinations), or through exposure to natural allergens, such as pollen, cat dander, and ragweed.

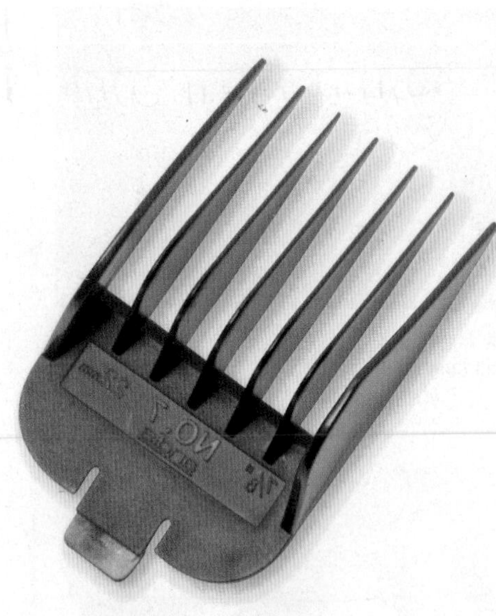

Principles of Prevention

Proper decontamination can prevent the spread of disease caused by exposure to potentially infectious materials on an item's surface. Decontamination also will prevent exposure to blood and visible debris or residue such as dust, hair, and skin.

Decontamination (dee-kuhn-tam-ih-NAY-shun) is the removal of blood or other potentially infectious materials on an item's surface and the removal of visible debris or residue such as dust, hair, and skin. There are two methods of decontamination.

- **Decontamination Method 1:** Cleaning and then disinfecting with an appropriate EPA-registered disinfectant.
- **Decontamination Method 2:** Cleaning and then sterilizing.

Many state regulatory agencies believe there is a lower risk of infection in salons than in medical facilities, where sterilizing is a major concern. Therefore, most salons are only concerned with Decontamination Method 1: cleaning and disinfecting. Some states have upgraded their infection control standards in salons that perform nail services to Decontamination Method 2: cleaning and sterilizing. When done properly, Decontamination Method 2 results in the destruction of all microbes through heat and pressure in an autoclave.

© Milady, a part of Cengage Learning.

Decontamination Method 1

Decontamination Method 1 has two steps: cleaning and disinfecting. Remember that when you clean, you must remove all visible dirt and debris from tools, implements, and equipment by washing with liquid soap and warm water and by using a clean and disinfected nail brush to scrub any grooved or hinged portions of the item.

A surface is properly cleaned when the number of contaminants on the surface is greatly reduced. In turn, this reduces the risk of infection. The vast majority of contaminants and pathogens can be removed from the surfaces of tools and implements through proper cleaning. This is why cleaning is an important part of disinfecting tools and equipment. A surface must be properly cleaned before it can be properly disinfected. Using a disinfectant without cleaning first is like using mouthwash without brushing your teeth—it just does not work properly!

© yummy, 2010; used under license from Shutterstock.com.

Cleaned surfaces can still harbor small amounts of pathogens, but the presence of fewer pathogens means infections are less likely to be spread. Putting antiseptics on your skin or washing your hands with soap and water will drastically lower the number of pathogens on your hands. However, it does not clean them properly. The proper cleaning of the hands requires rubbing hands together and using liquid soap, warm running water, a nail brush, and a clean towel. (See Procedure 5–3, Proper Hand Washing, later in this chapter.) Do not underestimate the importance of proper cleaning and hand washing. They are the most powerful and important ways to prevent the spread of infection.

There are three ways to clean your tools or implements:

- Washing with soap and warm water, then scrubbing them with a clean and properly disinfected nail brush.
- Using an ultrasonic unit.
- Using a cleaning solvent (e.g., on metal bits for electric files).

The second step of Decontamination Method 1 is disinfection. Remember that disinfection is the process that eliminates most, but not necessarily all, microorganisms on nonliving surfaces. This process is not effective against bacterial spores. In the salon setting, disinfection is extremely effective in controlling microorganisms on surfaces such as shears, nippers, and other multiuse tools and equipment (multiuse and single-use tools are discussed later in this chapter). Any disinfectant used in the salon should carry an EPA-registration number and the label should clearly state the specific organisms the solution is effective in killing when used according to the label instructions.

Remember that disinfectants are products that destroy all bacteria, fungi, and viruses (but not spores) on surfaces. Disinfectants are not for use on human skin, hair, or nails. Never use disinfectants as hand cleaners since this can cause skin irritation and **allergy** (AL-ur-jee), a reaction due to extreme sensitivity to certain foods, chemicals, or other normally harmless substances. All disinfectants clearly state on the label that you should avoid skin contact. This means avoid contact with your skin as well as the client's. Do not put your fingers directly into any disinfecting solution.

FYI

Benefits of Sterilizing

Not every tool or implement can be sterilized. Therefore, most state regulatory agencies do not require salons to sterilize tools and implements. However, Texas is one exception. The Texas Department of Licensing and Regulation requires sterilization of nonporous manicure and pedicure tools and implements before each service. Other states may follow. Check with your state regulatory agency to determine whether sterilization of tools and implements is required in your state.

The benefits of sterilization are:

- Sterilization is the most reliable means of infection control.
- Sterilized tools and implements in sealed bags assure clients that you are using fresh instruments during the service. The bag should be opened just before the service to show clients that the tools and implements have been sterilized and that the salon cares about the safety of their clients.

CAUTION

Read labels carefully! Manufacturers take great care to develop safe and highly effective products. However, when used improperly, many otherwise safe products can be dangerous. If you do not follow proper guidelines and instructions, any professional salon product can be dangerous. As with all products, disinfectants must be used exactly as the label instructs.

CAUTION

Disinfectants must be registered with the EPA. Look for an EPA-registration number on the label.

CAUTION

Improper mixing of disinfectants—to be weaker or more concentrated than the manufacturer's instructions—can dramatically reduce their effectiveness. Always add the disinfectant concentrate to the water when mixing and always follow the manufacturer's instructions for proper dilution.

Safety glasses and gloves should be worn to avoid accidental contact with eyes and skin.

Disinfectants are pesticides and can be harmful if absorbed through the skin. If you mix a disinfectant in a container that is not labeled by the manufacturer, the container must be properly labeled with the contents and the date it was mixed. All concentrated disinfectants must be diluted exactly as instructed by the manufacturer on the container's label.

Decontamination Method 2

Decontamination Method 2 also has two steps: cleaning and sterilizing. The word *sterilize* is often used incorrectly. **Sterilization** is the process that completely destroys all microbial life, including spores.

The most effective methods of sterilization use high-pressure steam equipment called autoclaves. Simply exposing instruments to steam is not enough. To be effective against disease-causing pathogens, the steam must be pressurized in an autoclave so that the steam penetrates the spore coats of the spore-forming bacteria. Dry heat forms of sterilization are less efficient and require longer times at higher temperatures. Dry heat sterilization is not recommended for use in salons.

Most people without medical training do not understand how to use an autoclave. For example, dirty implements cannot be properly sterilized without first being properly cleaned. Autoclaves need regular maintenance and testing to ensure they are in good working order. Color indicator strips on autoclave bags can provide false readings so they should never be used solely to determine whether instruments have been sterilized. These strips are only an indication, not verification that the autoclave is working.

The Centers for Disease Control and Prevention (CDC) requires that autoclaves be tested weekly to ensure they are properly sterilizing implements. The accepted method is called a spore test. Sealed packages containing test organisms are subjected to a typical sterilization cycle and then sent to a contract laboratory that specializes in autoclave performance testing. You can find laboratories to perform this type of test by simply doing an Internet search for autoclave spore testing. Other regular maintenance is also required to ensure the autoclave reaches the correct temperature and pressure. Keep in mind that an autoclave that does not reach the intended temperature for killing microorganisms may create a warm, moist place where pathogenic organisms can grow and thrive.

Salons should always follow the autoclave manufacturer's recommended schedule for cleaning, changing the water, service visits, replacement parts, and any required maintenance. Be sure to keep a logbook of all usage, testing, and maintenance for the state board to inspect. Showing your logbook to clients can provide them with peace of mind and confidence in your ability to protect them from infection. ☑ LO4

Choosing a Disinfectant

You must read and follow the manufacturer's instructions whenever you are using a disinfectant. Mixing ratios (dilution) and contact time are very important. Not all disinfectants have the same concentration, so be sure to mix the correct proportions according to the instructions on the label. If the label does not have the word *concentrate* on it, the product is already mixed. It must be used directly from the container and must not be diluted. All EPA-registered disinfectants, even those sprayed on large surfaces, will specify a contact time in their directions for use. Contact time is the amount of time the surface must stay moist with disinfectant in order for the disinfectant to be effective.

Disinfectants must have **efficacy** (ef-ih-KUH-see) claims on the label. Efficacy is the ability to produce an effect. As applied to disinfectant claims, efficacy means the effectiveness with which a disinfecting solution kills organisms when used according to the label instructions.

Professionals have many disinfectants available to them and should choose the one best suited for their specialty. The ideal disinfectant would:

- Maintain efficacy in the presence of **bioburden**, the number of viable organisms in or on an object or surface or the organic material on the surface of an object before decontamination or sterilization.
- Require that it be changed after a longer length of time (at least a week or more, not daily).
- Be inexpensive.
- Be nontoxic and nonirritating.
- Include strips for checking effectiveness.
- Be readily available from multiple manufacturers.
- Be EPA approved.
- Be environmentally friendly (can be disposed down the salon drain).
- Have no odor.
- Be noncorrosive.

Salons and cosmetologists must be aware of the types of disinfectants that are on the market and any new products that become available.

Salons pose a lower infection risk when compared to hospitals. For this reason, hospitals must meet much stricter infection control standards. They often use disinfectants that are too dangerous for the salon environment. Even though salons pose a lower risk of spreading certain types of infections, it is still very important to clean and then disinfect

did you know?

The EPA has recently approved a new disinfectant that can be used in the salon and is available in a spray and an immersion form, as well as wipes.

- **Accelerated hydrogen peroxide (AHP).** This disinfectant is based on stabilized hydrogen peroxide. AHP disinfectant needs to be changed only every 14 days and is nontoxic to the skin and the environment. There is an AHP formula that is available for disinfecting pedicure tubs.

Read the labels of all types of disinfectants closely. Choose the one that is most appropriate for its intended use and is the safest for you and your clients.

CAUTION

Bleach is not a magic potion! All disinfectants, including bleach, are inactivated (made less effective) in the presence of many substances, including oils, lotions, creams, hair, skin, nail dust, and nail filings. If bleach is used to disinfect equipment, it is critical to use a detergent first to thoroughly clean the equipment and remove all debris. Never mix detergents with the bleach.

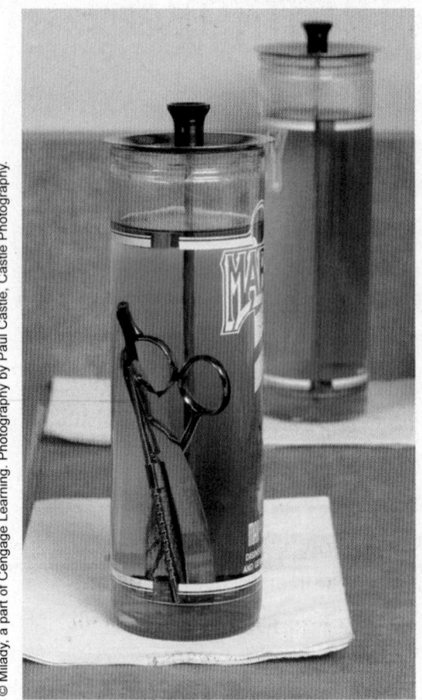

© Milady, a part of Cengage Learning. Photography by Paul Castle, Castle Photography.

▲ **Figure 5–10**
Completely immerse tools in disinfectant.

all tools, implements, surfaces, and equipment correctly. When salon implements accidentally contact blood, body fluids, or unhealthy conditions, they should be properly cleaned and then completely immersed in an EPA-registered hospital disinfectant solution that shows effectiveness against HIV, hepatitis, and tuberculosis. They also can be immersed in a 10 percent bleach solution. Always wear gloves and follow the proper Universal Precautions protocol for cleaning up after an exposure incident (described later in this chapter).

Proper Use of Disinfectants

Implements must be thoroughly cleaned of all visible matter or residue before being placed in disinfectant solution. This is because residue will interfere with the disinfectant and prevent proper disinfection. Properly cleaned implements and tools, free from all visible debris, must be completely immersed in disinfectant solution. Complete immersion means there is enough liquid in the container to cover all surfaces of the item being disinfected, including the handles, for ten minutes or for the time recommended by the manufacturer (**Figure 5–10**).

Disinfectant Tips

- Use only on precleaned, hard, nonporous surfaces—not on single-use abrasive files or buffers.
- Always wear gloves and safety glasses when handling disinfectant solutions.
- Always dilute products according to the instructions on the product label.
- An item must remain submerged in the disinfectant for ten minutes unless the product label specifies differently.
  - To disinfect large surfaces such as tabletops, carefully apply the disinfectant onto the precleaned surface and allow it to remain wet for ten minutes, unless the product label specifies differently.
  - If the product label states, "Complete Immersion," the entire implement must be completely immersed in the solution.
  - Change the disinfectant according to the instructions on the label. If the liquid is not changed as instructed, it will no longer be effective and may begin to promote the growth of microbes.
- Proper disinfection of a whirlpool pedicure spa requires that the disinfecting solution circulate for ten minutes, unless the product label specifies otherwise.

did you know?

Not all household bleaches are effective as disinfectants. To be effective, the bleach must have an EPA-registration number and contain at least 5 percent sodium hypochlorite and be diluted properly to a 10 percent solution—9 parts water to 1 part bleach.

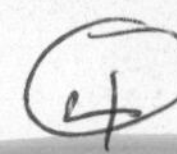

Types of Disinfectants

Disinfectants are not all the same. Some are appropriate for use in the salon and some are not. Some disinfectants should be used on tools and implements that are immersed and some should be used on nonporous surfaces. You should be aware of the different types of disinfectants and the ones that are recommended for salon use.

Disinfectants Appropriate for Salon Use

Quaternary ammonium compounds (KWAT-ur-nayr-ree uh-MOH-neeum KAHM-powndz), also known as **quats** (KWATZ), are disinfectants that are very effective when used properly in the salon. The most advanced type of these formulations is called multiple quats. Multiple quats contain sophisticated blends of quats that work together to dramatically increase the effectiveness of these disinfectants. Quat solutions usually disinfect implements in ten minutes. These formulas may contain anti-rust ingredients, so leaving tools in the solution for prolonged periods can cause dulling or damage. They should be removed from the solution after the specified period, rinsed (if required), dried, and stored in a clean, covered container.

Phenolic disinfectants (fi-NOH-lik dis-in-FEK-tents) are powerful tuberculocidal disinfectants. They are a form of formaldehyde, have a very high pH, and can damage the skin and eyes. Phenolic disinfectants can be harmful to the environment if put down the drain. They have been used reliably over the years to disinfect salon tools; however, they do have drawbacks. Phenol can damage plastic and rubber and can cause certain metals to rust. Phenolic disinfectants should never be used to disinfect pedicure tubs or equipment. Extra care should be taken to avoid skin contact with phenolic disinfectants. Phenolics are known carcinogens.

Bleach

Household bleach, 5.25 percent **sodium hypochlorite** (SOH-dee-um hy-puh-KLOR-ite), is an effective disinfectant and has been used extensively as a disinfectant in the salon. Using too much bleach can damage some metals and plastics, so be sure to read the label for safe use. Bleach can be corrosive to metals and plastics and can cause skin irritation and eye damage.

To mix a bleach solution, always follow the manufacturer's directions. Store the bleach solution away from heat and light. A fresh bleach solution should be mixed every twenty-four hours or when the solution has been contaminated. After mixing the bleach solution, date the container to ensure that the solution is not saved from one day to the next. Bleach can be irritating to the lungs, so be careful about inhaling the fumes.

CAUTION

Some disinfectants are not appropriate for salon use. The following disinfectants should not be used in the salon:

- **Fumigants**
  Years ago, formalin tablets, or paraformaldehyde, were used as fumigants (a gaseous substance capable of destroying pathogenic bacteria) in dry-cabinet sanitizers. This was before EPA-registered disinfectants came on the market and before it was known that paraformaldehyde slowly releases low concentrations of formaldehyde gas. The release of this gas can cause eye, nose, and lung irritation or allergic inhalation sensitivity in individuals who repeatedly breathe these gases. Although the level of formaldehyde gas produced does not cause more serious health problems, these fumigants are no longer used in the salon.
- **Glutaraldehyde**
  Glutaraldehyde is a powerful chemical used to sterilize surgical instruments in hospitals. It produces fumes that are irritating to the lungs, eyes, and skin. While other professions use glutaraldehyde, it is not safe for salon use.

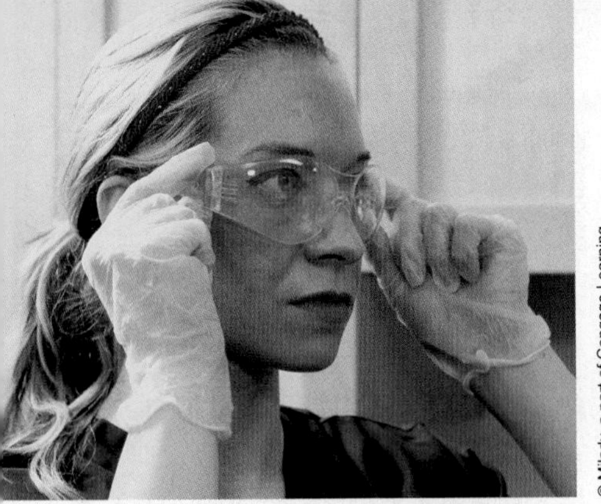

© Milady, a part of Cengage Learning. Photography by Dino Petrocelli.

▲ **Figure 5–11**
Wear gloves and safety glasses while handling disinfectants.

Disinfectant Safety

Disinfectants are pesticides (a type of poison) and can cause serious skin and eye damage. Some disinfectants appear clear while others, especially phenolic disinfectants, are a little cloudy. Always use caution when handling disinfectants, and follow the safety tips below.

Safety Tips for Disinfectants

Always

- Keep an MSDS on hand for the disinfectant(s) you use.
- Wear gloves and safety glasses when mixing disinfectants (**Figure 5–11**).
- Avoid skin and eye contact.
- Add disinfectant to water when diluting (rather than adding water to a disinfectant) to prevent foaming, which can result in an incorrect mixing ratio.
- Use tongs, gloves, or a draining basket to remove implements from disinfectants.
- Keep disinfectants out of reach of children.
- Carefully measure and use disinfectant products according to label instructions.
- Follow the manufacturer's instructions for mixing, using, and disposing of disinfectants.
- Carefully follow the manufacturer's directions for when to replace the disinfectant solution in order to ensure the healthiest conditions for you and your client. Replace the disinfectant solution every day—more often if the solution becomes soiled or contaminated.

CAUTION

Porous or absorbent items must be disposed of properly if the skin is accidentally cut during the service or if they come into contact with unhealthy skin or nails. Remember: When in doubt, throw it out!

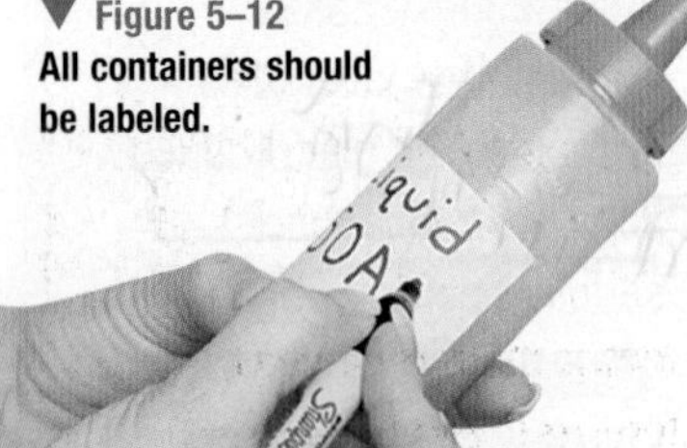

© Milady, a part of Cengage Learning. Photography by Paul Castle, Castle Photography.

▼ **Figure 5–12**
All containers should be labeled.

Never

- Let quats, phenols, bleach, or any other disinfectant come in contact with your skin. If you do get disinfectants on your skin, immediately wash the area with liquid soap and warm water. Then rinse the area and dry the area thoroughly.
- Place any disinfectant or other product in an unmarked container. All containers should be labeled (**Figure 5–12**).

Jars or containers used to disinfect implements are often incorrectly called wet sanitizers. The purpose of disinfectant containers is to disinfect, not to clean. Disinfectant containers must be covered, but not airtight. Remember to clean the container every day and to wear gloves when you do. Always follow the manufacturer's label instructions for disinfecting products. ☑ **LO5**

FYI

Another word that is used (most often in marketing and sales copy) to describe multiuse items is *disinfectable*, which means these items can be disinfected and used again.

Disinfect or Dispose?

How can you tell which items in the salon can be disinfected and reused? There are two types of items used in salons: multiuse (reusable) items, and single-use (disposable) items.

Multiuse, also known as **reusable**, items can be cleaned, disinfected, and used on more than one person even if the item is accidentally exposed to blood or body fluid. These items must have a hard, nonporous surface. Examples of multiuse items are nippers, shears, combs, metal pushers, some nail files, rollers, and permanent wave rods.

Single-use, also known as **disposable**, items cannot be used more than once. These items cannot be properly cleaned so that all visible residue is removed—such as pumice stones used for pedicures—or they are damaged or contaminated by cleaning and disinfecting. Examples of single-use items are wooden sticks, cotton balls, sponges, gauze, tissues, paper towels, and some nail files and buffers. Single-use items must be thrown out after each use.

Porous means that an item is made or constructed of a material that has pores or openings. These items are absorbent. Some porous items can be safely cleaned, disinfected, and used again. Examples of porous items are towels, chamois, linens, and some nail files and buffers.

If a porous item contacts broken skin, blood, body fluid, or any unhealthy skin or nails, it must be discarded immediately. Do not try to disinfect the item. If you are not sure whether an item can be safely cleaned, disinfected, and used again, throw it out.

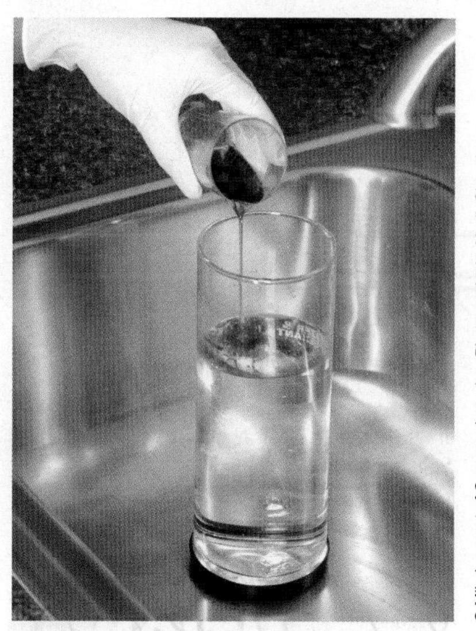

© Milady, a part of Cengage Learning. Photography by Yanik Chauvin.

▲ Figure 5–13
Carefully pour disinfectant into the water when preparing disinfectant solution.

CAUTION

Ultraviolet (UV) sanitizers are useful storage containers, but they do not disinfect or sterilize.

Keep a Logbook

Salons should always follow manufacturers' recommended schedules for cleaning and disinfecting tools and implements, disinfecting foot spas and basins, scheduling regular service visits for equipment, and replacing parts when needed. Although your state may not require you to keep a logbook of all equipment usage, cleaning, disinfecting, testing, and maintenance, it may be advisable to keep one. Showing your logbook to clients provides them with peace of mind and confidence in your ability to protect them from infection and disease.

CAUTION

Electric sterilizers, bead sterilizers, and baby sterilizers cannot be used to disinfect or sterilize implements. These devices can spread potentially infectious diseases and should never be used in salons. Also, UV light units will not disinfect or sterilize implements. State rules require that you use liquid disinfecting solutions! Autoclaves are effective sterilizers. If you decide to use an autoclave, be sure that you know how to operate it properly.

Disinfecting Nonelectrical Tools and Implements

State rules require that all multiuse tools and implements must be cleaned and disinfected before and after every service—even when they are used on the same person. Mix all disinfectants according to the manufacturer's directions, always adding the disinfectant to the water, not the water to the disinfectant (**Figure 5–13**).

PROCEDURE 5-1 Disinfecting Nonelectrical Tools and Implements SEE PAGE 96

Disinfecting Electrical Tools and Equipment

Hair clippers, electrotherapy tools, nail drills, and other types of electrical equipment have contact points that cannot be immersed in liquid. These items should be cleaned and disinfected using an EPA-

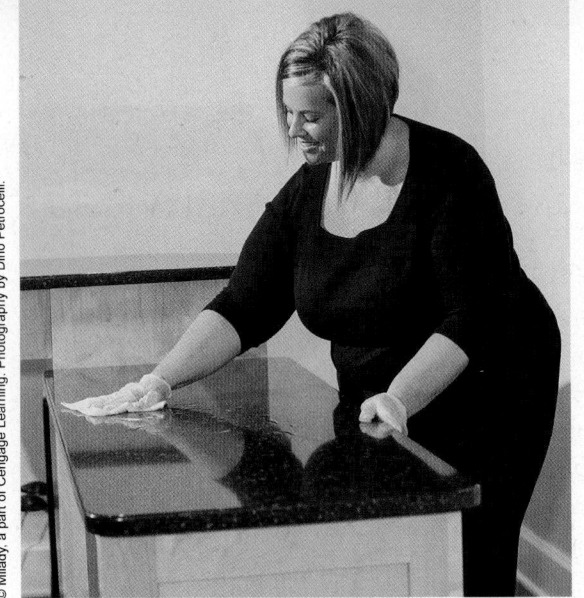

© Milady, a part of Cengage Learning. Photography by Dino Petrocelli.

▲ Figure 5–14
Clean and disinfect manicure tables regularly.

CAUTION

Products and equipment that have the word *sanitizer* on the label are merely cleaners. They do not disinfect. Items must be properly cleaned and disinfected after every use before using them on another client.

CAUTION

Some states require that all procedures for cleaning and disinfecting tools, implements, and equipment must be recorded in a salon logbook. Check with your state's regulatory agency to determine whether you are required to do so. It is a good practice to complete a logbook, even if not required, as it shows clients you are serious about protecting their health.

registered disinfectant designed for use on these devices. Follow the procedures recommended by the disinfectant manufacturer for preparing the solution and follow the item's manufacturer directions for cleaning and disinfecting the device.

Disinfecting Work Surfaces

Before beginning every client service, all work surfaces must be cleaned and disinfected. Be sure to clean and disinfect tables, styling stations, shampoo sinks, chairs, arm rests and any other surface that a customer's skin may have touched (**Figure 5–14**). Clean doorknobs and handles daily to reduce transferring germs to your hands.

Cleaning Towels, Linens, and Capes

Clean towels, linens, and capes must be used for each client. After a towel, linen, or cape has been used on a client, it must not be used again until it has been properly laundered. To clean towels, linens, and capes, launder according to the directions on the item's label. Be sure that towels, linens, and capes are thoroughly dried. Items that are not dry may grow mildew and bacteria. Store soiled linens and towels in covered or closed containers, away from clean linens and towels, even if your state regulatory agency does not require that you do so. Whenever possible, use disposable towels, especially in restrooms. Do not allow capes that are used for cutting, shampooing, and chemical services to touch the client's skin. Use disposable neck strips or towels. If a cape accidentally touches skin, do not use the cape again until it has been laundered.

Disinfecting Foot Spas and Pedicure Equipment

All equipment that contains water for pedicures (including whirlpool spas, pipe-less units, foot baths, basins, tubs, sinks, and bowls) must be cleaned and disinfected after every pedicure, and the information must be entered into a logbook. Inspectors may issue fines if there is no logbook. Some state regulatory agencies allow single-use tub liners in pedicure equipment. Check with your state agency. If single-use liners are allowed in your state, be sure that you clean and disinfect all surfaces of the equipment that are not covered by the liner after every client.

Soaps and Detergents

Chelating soaps (CHE-layt-ing SOHPS), also known as **chelating detergents**, work to break down stubborn films and remove the residue of pedicure products such as scrubs, salts, and masks. The chelating agents in these soaps work in all types of water, are low-sudsing, and are specially formulated to work in areas with hard tap water. Hard tap water reduces the effectiveness of cleaners and disinfectants. If your area has hard water, ask your local distributor for pedicure soaps that are effective in hard water. This information will be stated on the product's label.

Additives, Powders, and Tablets

There is no additive, powder, or tablet that eliminates the need for you to clean and disinfect. Products of this type cannot be used instead of EPA-registered liquid disinfectant solutions. You cannot replace proper cleaning and disinfection with a shortcut. Water sanitizers do not properly clean or disinfect equipment. They are designed for Jacuzzis and hydrotherapy tubs where no oils, lotions, or other enhancements are used. Therefore, water sanitizers do not work well in a salon environment. Never rely solely on water sanitizers to protect your clients from infection. Products that contain Chloramine T, for example, are not effective disinfectants for equipment. These products only treat the water and have limited value in the salon. They do not replace proper cleaning and disinfection. Remember: There are no shortcuts!

PROCEDURE 5-2 Disinfecting Foot Spas or Basins SEE PAGE 97

Dispensary

The dispensary must be kept clean and orderly, with the contents of all containers clearly marked. Always store products according to the manufacturer's instructions and away from heat and out of direct sunlight. Keep the MSDSs for all products used in the salon in a convenient, central location for the employees.

Handling Single-Use Supplies

All single-use supplies, such as wooden sticks, cotton, gauze, wipes, porous nail files and buffers, and paper towels should be thrown away after one use. Anything exposed to blood, including skin care treatment debris, must be double-bagged and marked with a biohazard sticker, separated from other waste, and disposed of according to OSHA standards.

Hand Washing

Properly washing your hands is one of the most important actions you can take to prevent spreading germs from one person to another. Proper hand washing removes germs from the folds and grooves of the skin and from under the free edge of the nail plate by lifting and rinsing germs and contaminants from the surface.

CAUTION

Most pedicure spas hold 5 gallons of water; check with the manufacturer and be sure that you use the correct amount of disinfectant. Also be sure that you are using a disinfectant that is appropriate for the pedicure spa.

Remember:

1 gallon = 128 ounces
5 gallons = 640 ounces

If you are working with a pedicure spa that holds 5 gallons of water, you will have to measure the correct amount of water needed to cover the jets and then add the correct amount of disinfectant.

CAUTION

Never place a client's feet in water that contains a disinfectant.

CAUTION

Follow this rule for all tools and supplies: If you *cannot* disinfect your tools or supplies, you *must* discard them.

© Milady, a part of Cengage Learning.

© Milady, a part of Cengage Learning.

CAUTION

When washing hands, use liquid soaps in pump containers. Bar soaps can grow bacteria.

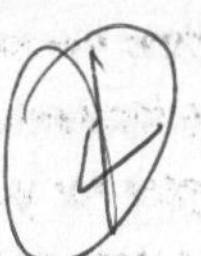

You should wash your hands thoroughly before and after each service. Follow the hand washing procedure in this chapter. And, if you perform nail services, your client should first wash his or her hands using a clean and disinfected nail brush before the service begins.

Antimicrobial and antibacterial soaps can dry the skin, and medical studies suggest that they are no more effective than regular soaps or detergents. Therefore, it is recommended that you minimize the use of antimicrobial and antibacterial soaps. Repeated hand washing can also dry the skin, so using a moisturizing hand lotion after washing is a good practice. Be sure the hand lotion is in a pump container, not a jar.

Avoid using very hot water to wash your hands because this is another practice that can damage the skin. Remember: You must wash your hands thoroughly before and after each service, so do all you can to reduce any irritation that may occur.

CAUTION

Taking the time to conduct a thorough hair and scalp analysis will enable you to determine whether a client has any open wounds or abrasions. If the client does have an open wound or abrasion, do not perform services of any kind for the client.

PROCEDURE 5-3 **Proper Hand Washing** SEE PAGE 102

Waterless Hand Sanitizers

Antiseptics (ant-ih-SEP-tiks) are chemical germicides formulated for use on skin and are registered and regulated by the Food and Drug Administration (FDA). Antiseptics can contain either alcohol or benzalkonium chloride (ben-ZAHL-khon-ee-um KLOHR-yd), which is less drying to the skin than alcohol. Neither type of antiseptic can clean the hands of dirt and debris; this can only be accomplished with liquid soap, a soft-bristle brush, and water. Use hand sanitizers only after properly cleaning your hands. Never use an antiseptic to disinfect instruments or other surfaces. They are ineffective for that purpose.

Universal Precautions

Universal Precautions are guidelines published by OSHA that require the employer and employee to assume that all human blood and body fluids are infectious for bloodborne pathogens. Because it may not be possible to identify clients with infectious diseases, strict

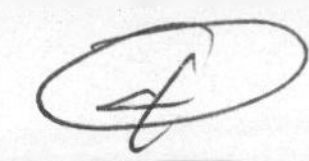

infection control practices should be used with all clients. In most instances, clients who are infected with the hepatitis B virus or other bloodborne pathogens are **asymptomatic**, which means that they show no symptoms or signs of infection. Bloodborne pathogens are more difficult to kill than germs that live outside the body.

OSHA sets safety standards and precautions that protect employees in situations when they could be exposed to bloodborne pathogens. Precautions include proper hand washing, wearing gloves, and properly handling and disposing of sharp instruments and any other items that may have been contaminated by blood or other body fluids. It is important that specific procedures are followed if blood or body fluid is present.

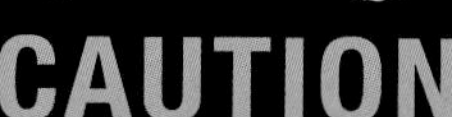

CAUTION

Since cosmetologists work with an array of sharp implements and tools, cutting yourself is a very real possibility. If you do suffer a cut and blood is present, you must follow the steps for an exposure incident outlined in this chapter for your safety and the safety of your client.

An Exposure Incident: Contact with Blood or Body Fluid

You should never perform a service on any client who comes into the salon with an open wound or an abrasion. Sometimes accidents happen while a service is being performed in the salon, however.

An **exposure incident** is contact with nonintact (broken) skin, blood, body fluid, or other potentially infectious materials that is the result of the performance of an employee's duties. Should the client suffer a cut or abrasion that bleeds during a service, follow these steps for the client's safety, as well as your own:

1. Stop the service.
2. Put on gloves to protect yourself from contact with the client's blood.
3. Stop the bleeding by applying pressure to the area with a clean cotton ball or piece of gauze.
4. When bleeding has stopped, clean the injured area with an antiseptic wipe. Every salon must have a first aid kit.
5. Bandage the cut with an adhesive bandage.
6. Clean and disinfect your workstation or styling station, using an EPA-registered disinfectant designed for cleaning blood and body fluids.
7. Discard all single-use contaminated objects such as wipes or cotton balls by double-bagging (place the waste in a plastic bag and then in a trash bag). Place a biohazard sticker (red or orange) on the bag, and deposit the bag into a container for contaminated waste. Deposit sharp disposables in a sharps box (**Figure 5–15**).
8. Before removing your gloves, make sure that all multiuse tools and implements that have come into contact with blood or other body fluids are thoroughly cleaned and completely immersed in an EPA-registered disinfectant solution designed for cleaning blood and body fluids or 10 percent bleach solution for at least ten minutes or for the time recommended by the manufacturer

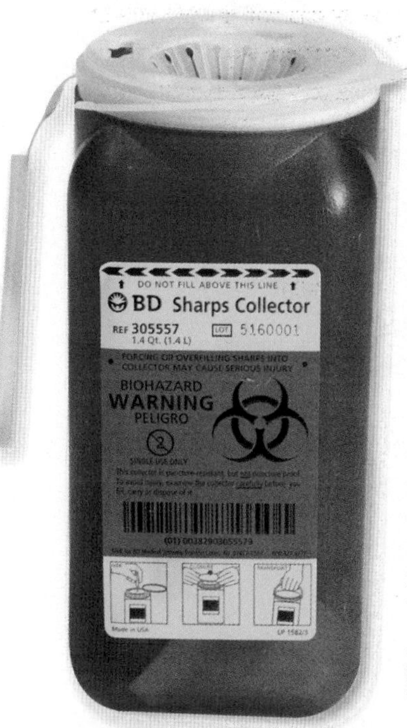

© Milady, a part of Cengage Learning. Photography by Paul Castle. Castle Photography.

▲ **Figure 5–15**
Always use a sharps box to dispose of sharp, disposable implements.

did you know?

You should never attempt to clean or disinfect any used tool or implement at your workstation. Proper cleaning and disinfecting should only be accomplished in a specified area of the salon and requires the use of clean, warm running water, a scrub brush, and liquid soap for cleaning and disinfectant solution for disinfecting. Tools and implements must also be completely rinsed after being disinfected and then dried and kept in a dry, covered container until use.

of the product. Be sure that you do not touch other work surfaces in the salon, such as faucets and counters. If you do, these areas must also be properly cleaned and disinfected. Remember: Blood may carry pathogens, so you should never touch an open sore or a wound.

9. Remove your gloves and seal them in the double bag along with the other contaminated items for disposal. Thoroughly wash your hands and clean under the free edge of your nails with soap and warm water before returning to the service.
10. Recommend that the client see a physician if any signs of redness, swelling, pain, or irritation develop. ☑ LO6

Professional Salon Image

Infection control practices should be a part of the normal routine for you and your coworkers so that the salon and staff project a steadfast professional image. The following are some simple guidelines that will keep the salon looking its best.

- Keep floors and workstations dust-free. Sweep hair off the floor after every client. Mop floors and vacuum carpets every day.
- Control dust, hair, and other debris.
- Keep trash in a covered waste receptacle to reduce chemical odors and fires.
- Clean fans, ventilation systems, and humidifiers at least once each week.
- Keep all work areas well-lit.
- Clean and disinfect restroom surfaces, including door handles.
- Provide toilet tissue, paper towels, liquid soap, properly disinfected soft-bristle nail brushes, and a container for used brushes in the restroom.
- Do not allow the salon to be used for cooking or living purposes.
- Never place food in the same refrigerator used to store salon products.
- Prohibit eating, drinking, and smoking in areas where services are performed or where product mixing occurs (e.g., back bar area). Consider having a smoke-free salon. Even when you do not smoke in the service areas, the odor can flow into those areas.
- Empty waste receptacles regularly throughout the day. A metal waste receptacle with a self-closing lid works best.
- Make sure all containers are properly marked and properly stored.

- Never place any tools or implements in your mouth or pockets.
- Properly clean and disinfect all multiuse tools before reusing them.
- Store clean and disinfected tools in a clean, covered container. Clean drawers may be used for storage if only clean items are stored in the drawers. Always isolate used implements away from disinfected implements.
- Avoid touching your face, mouth, or eye areas during services.
- Clean and disinfect all work surfaces after every client.
- Have clean, disposable paper towels for each client.
- Always properly wash your hands before and after each service.
- Use clean linens and disposable towels on clients. Keep soiled linens separate from clean linens. Use single-use neck strips or clean towels to avoid skin contact with shampoo capes and cutting or chemical protection gowns. If a cape touched the client's skin, do not reuse that cape until it is properly laundered.
- Never provide a nail service to clients who have not properly washed their hands and carefully scrubbed under the free edge of their nails with a disinfected nail brush.
- Use effective exhaust systems in the salon. This will help ensure proper air quality in the salon.

Your Professional Responsibility

You have many responsibilities as a salon professional, but none is more important than protecting your clients' health and safety. Never take shortcuts for cleaning and disinfecting. You cannot afford to skip steps or save money when it comes to safety.

- It is your professional and legal responsibility to follow state and federal laws and rules.
- Keep your license current and notify the licensing agency if you move or change your name.
- Check your state's Web site weekly for any changes or updates to rules and regulations. ✔ LO7

© Stephen Coburn, 2010; used under license from Shutterstock.com.

PROCEDURE 5-1

Disinfecting Nonelectrical Tools and Implements

Nonelectrical tools and implements include items such as combs, brushes, clips, hairpins, metal pushers, makeup brushes, tweezers, and nail clippers.

1 It is important to wear safety glasses and gloves while disinfecting nonelectrical tools and implements to protect your eyes from unintentional splashes of disinfectant and to prevent possible contamination of the implements by your hands and to protect your hands from the powerful chemicals in the disinfectant solution.

2 Rinse all implements with warm running water, and then thoroughly clean them with soap, a nail brush, and warm water. Brush grooved items, if necessary, and open hinged implements to scrub the revealed area.

3 Rinse away all traces of soap with warm running water. The presence of soap in most disinfectants will cause them to become inactive. Soap is most easily rinsed off in warm, not hot, water. Hotter water is not more effective. Dry implements thoroughly with a clean or disposable towel, or allow them to air dry on a clean towel. Your implements are now properly cleaned and ready to be disinfected.

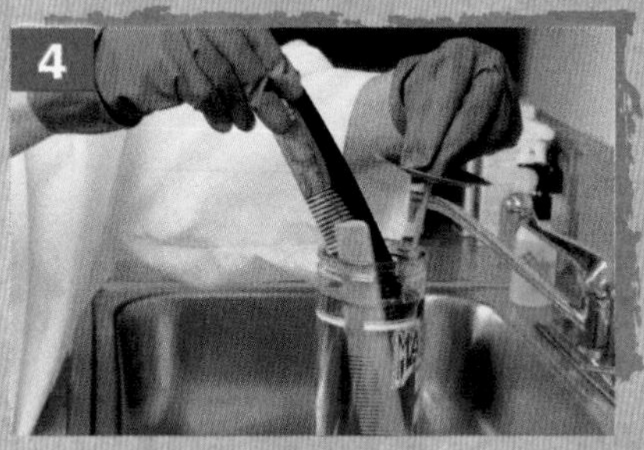

4 It is extremely important that your implements be completely clean before you place them in the disinfectant solution. If implements are not clean, your disinfectant may become contaminated and ineffective. Immerse cleaned implements in an appropriate disinfection container holding an EPA-registered disinfectant for the required time (at least ten minutes or according to the manufacturer's instructions). Remember to open hinged implements before immersing them in the disinfectant. If the disinfection solution is visibly dirty, or if the solution has been contaminated, it must be replaced.

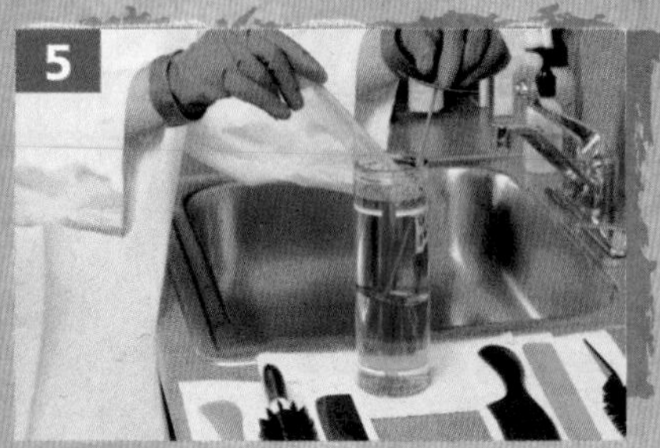

5 After the required disinfection time has passed, remove tools and implements from the disinfection solution with tongs or gloved hands, rinse the tools and implements well in warm running water, and pat them dry.

6 Store disinfected tools and implements in a clean, covered container until needed.

7 Remove gloves and thoroughly wash your hands with warm running water and liquid soap. Rinse and dry hands with a clean fabric or disposable towel. ☑ LO8

© Milady, a part of Cengage Learning. Photography by Paul Castle, Castle Photography.

PROCEDURE 5-2

Disinfecting Foot Spas or Basins

Whirlpool Foot Spas and Air-Jet Basins

After every client:

1. Put on gloves. Drain all water from the basin.

2. Scrub all visible residue from the inside walls of the basin with a clean, disinfected brush and liquid soap and clean, warm water. Use a clean, disinfected brush with a handle. Brushes must be cleaned and disinfected after each use.

3. Rinse the basin with clean, warm water and drain.

4. Refill the basin with enough clean, warm water to cover the jets and circulate the correct amount (as indicated in the mixing instructions on the label) of the EPA-registered disinfectant specified by the manufacturer through the basin for ten minutes or for the time recommended by the manufacturer.

5. Drain, rinse with clean, warm water, and wipe the basin dry with a clean paper towel.

At the end of every day:

1. Put on gloves. Remove the screen and any other removable parts. (You may need a screwdriver.)

2. Clean the screen and other removable parts and the areas behind them with a clean, disinfected brush and liquid soap and clean, warm water to remove all visible residue. Replace properly cleaned screen and other removable parts.

3. Fill the basin with clean, warm water and a chelating detergent (cleansers designed for use in hard water). Circulate the chelating detergent through the system for ten minutes or for the time recommended by the manufacturer. If excessive foaming occurs, discontinue circulation, and let the basin soak for the remainder of the time, as instructed.

PROCEDURE

5-2 Disinfecting Foot Spas or Basins continued

4 Drain the soapy solution, and rinse the basin with clean, warm water.

5 Refill the basin with clean, warm water and circulate the correct amount (as indicated in the mixing instructions on the label) of the EPA-registered disinfectant through the basin for ten minutes or for the time recommended by the manufacturer.

6 Drain, rinse with clean, warm water, and wipe the basin dry with a clean paper towel.

7 Allow the basin to dry completely.

At least once each week:

1 Put on gloves. Drain all water from the basin.

2 Remove the screen and any other removable parts. (You may need a screwdriver.)

3 Clean the screen and other removable parts and the areas behind them with a clean, disinfected brush and liquid soap and clean, warm water to remove all visible residue. Replace properly cleaned screen and other removable parts.

4 Scrub all visible residue from the inside walls of the basin with a brush and liquid soap and clean, warm water. Use a clean, disinfected brush with a handle. Brushes must be cleaned and disinfected after each use.

5 Refill the basin with clean, warm water and circulate the correct amount (as indicated in the mixing instructions on the label) of the EPA-registered disinfectant through the basin for ten minutes or for the time recommended by the manufacturer.

6 Do not drain the disinfectant solution. Instead, turn the unit off and leave the disinfecting solution in the unit overnight.

7 In the morning, put on gloves, then drain and rinse the basin with clean, warm water.

8 Refill the basin with clean, warm water and flush the system.

9 Drain, rinse with clean, warm water, and wipe the basin dry with a clean paper towel.

Disinfecting Pipe-less Foot Spas

For units with footplates, impellers, impeller assemblies, and propellers.

After every client:

1 Put on gloves. Drain all water from the basin.

2 Remove impeller, footplate, and any other removable parts according to the manufacturer's instructions.

3 Thoroughly scrub impeller, footplate, and other parts and the areas behind each with a liquid soap, clean, disinfected brush and clean, warm water to remove all visible residue. Reinsert impeller, footplate, and other parts.

4 Refill the basin with clean, warm water and circulate the correct amount (as indicated in the mixing instructions on the label) of the EPA-registered disinfectant through the basin for ten minutes or for the time recommended by the manufacturer.

5 Drain, rinse with clean, warm water, and wipe the basin dry with a clean paper towel.

At the end of every day:

1 Put on gloves. Fill the basin with clean, warm water and chelating detergent, and circulate the chelating detergent through the system for ten minutes or for the time recommended by the manufacturer. If excessive foaming occurs, discontinue circulation and let soak for the remainder of the time recommended by the manufacturer.

2 Drain the soapy solution and rinse the basin with clean, warm water.

3 Refill the basin with clean, warm water and circulate the correct amount (as indicated in mixing instructions on the label) of the EPA-registered disinfectant through the basin for ten minutes or for the time recommended by the manufacturer.

4 Drain, rinse with clean, warm water, and wipe the basin dry with a clean paper towel.

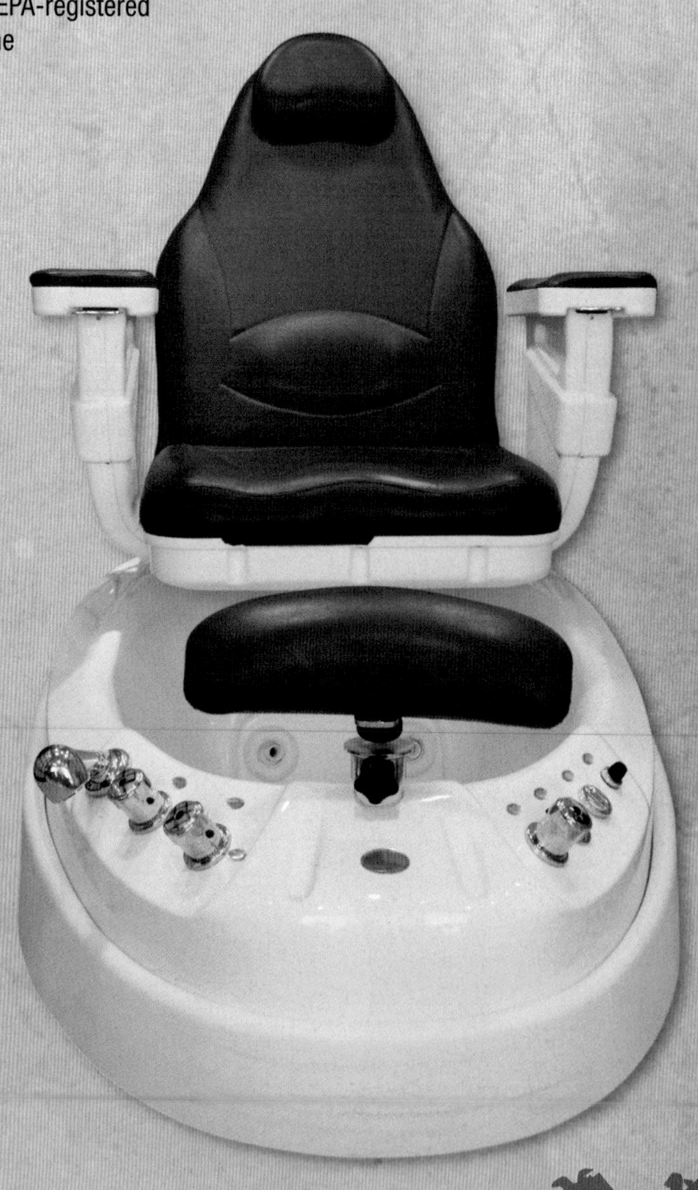

© Dave Wetzel, 2010; used under license from Shutterstock.com.

5-2 Disinfecting Foot Spas or Basins continued

At least once each week:

1 Put on gloves. Drain all water from the basin.

2 Remove impeller, footplate, and any other removable parts according to the manufacturer's instructions.

3 Thoroughly scrub impeller, footplate, and other parts and the areas behind each with a liquid soap and clean, warm water to remove all visible residue. Reinsert impeller, footplate, and other parts.

4 Refill the basin with clean, warm water and circulate the correct amount (as indicated in mixing instructions on the label) of the EPA-registered disinfectant through the basin for ten minutes or for the time recommended by the manufacturer.

5 Do not drain the disinfectant solution. Instead, turn the unit off and leave the disinfecting solution in the unit overnight.

6 In the morning, put on gloves, then drain and rinse the basin with clean, warm water.

7 Refill the basin with clean, warm water and flush the system.

8 Drain, rinse with clean, warm water, and wipe the basin dry with a clean paper towel.

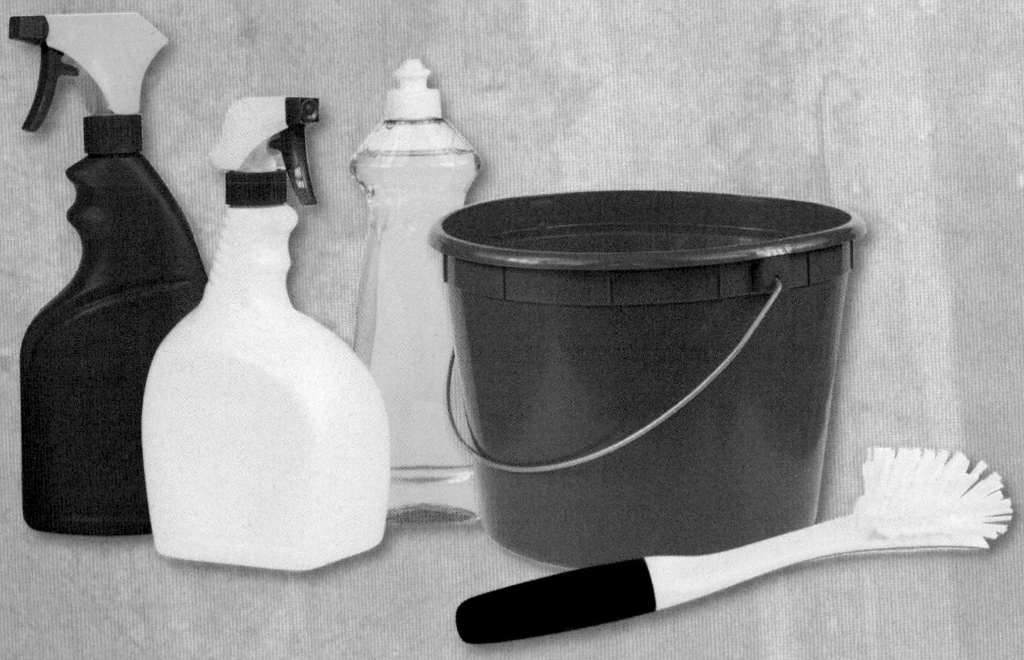

© Natallia Bokach, 2010; used under license from iStockphoto.com.

Disinfecting Nonwhirlpool Foot Basins or Tubs

This includes basins, tubs, footbaths, sinks, and bowls—all nonelectrical equipment that holds water for a client's feet during a pedicure service.

After every client:

1. Put on gloves. Drain all water from the foot basin or tub.

2. Clean all inside surfaces of the foot basin or tub to remove all visible residue with a clean, disinfected brush and liquid soap and clean, warm water.

3. Rinse the basin or tub with clean, warm water and drain.

4. Refill the basin with clean, warm water and the correct amount (as indicated in mixing instructions on the label) of the EPA-registered disinfectant. Leave this disinfecting solution in the basin for ten minutes or for the time recommended by the manufacturer.

5. Drain, rinse with clean, warm water, and wipe the basin dry with a clean paper towel.

At the end of every day:

1. Put on gloves. Drain all water from the foot basin or tub.

2. Clean all inside surfaces of the foot basin or tub to remove all visible residue with a clean, disinfected brush and liquid soap and clean, warm water.

3. Fill the basin or tub with clean, warm water and the correct amount (as indicated in mixing instructions on the label) of the EPA-registered disinfectant. Leave this disinfecting solution in the basin for ten minutes or for the time recommended by the manufacturer.

4. Drain, rinse with clean water, and wipe the basin dry with a clean paper towel.

PROCEDURE 5-3

Proper Hand Washing

Hand washing is one of the most important procedures in your infection control efforts and is required in every state before any service.

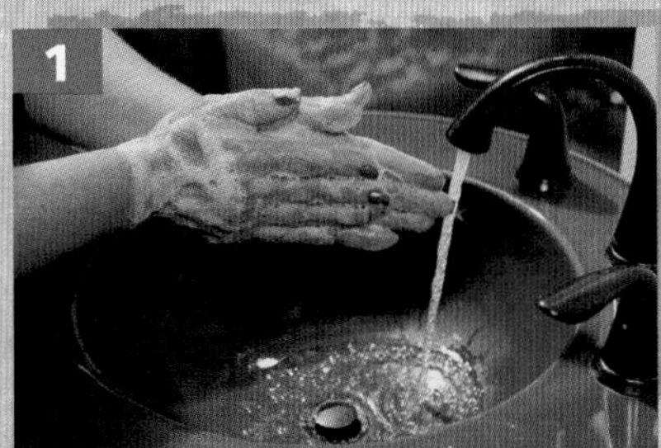

1 Turn on the warm water, wet your hands, and then pump soap from a pump container onto the palm of your hand. Rub your hands together, all over and vigorously, until a lather forms. Continue for a minimum of twenty seconds.

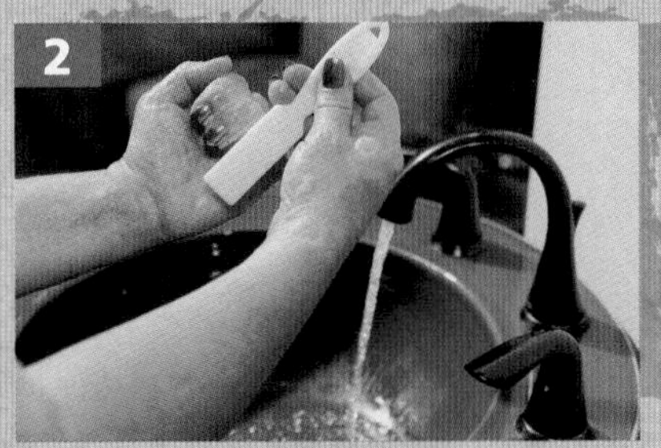

2 Choose a clean, disinfected nail brush. Wet the nail brush, pump soap on it, and brush your nails horizontally back and forth under the free edges. Change the direction of the brush to vertical and move the brush up and down along the nail folds of the fingernails. The process for brushing both hands should take about sixty seconds to finish. Rinse hands in running warm water.

FYI

Dirty nail brushes should be stored together in a closed container until you are ready to clean and disinfect them. Then nail brushes should be properly cleaned, rinsed, dried, and immersed for the required disinfection time, in a disinfectant that does not harm plastics. After they have been disinfected, rinse the brushes in clean, warm water, dry them, and place them in a clean storage location.

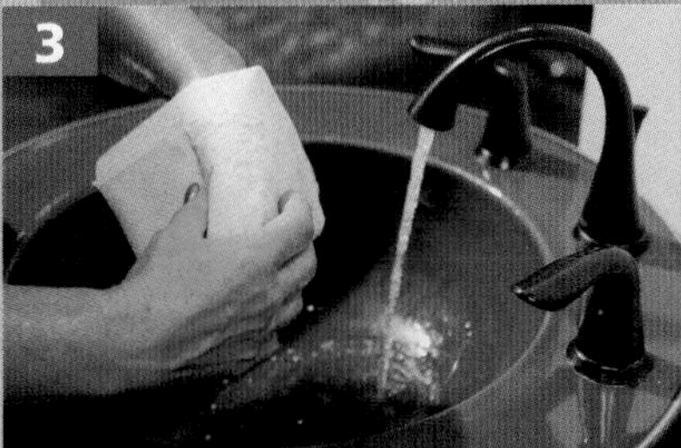

3 Use a clean cloth or paper towel, according to the salon policies, for drying your hands.

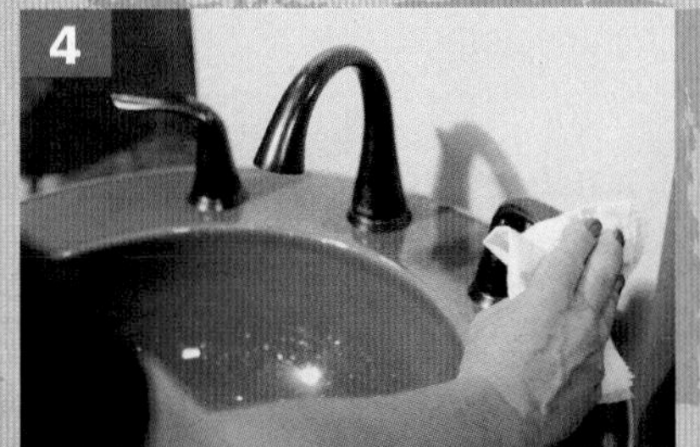

4 After drying your hands, turn off the water with the towel and dispose of the towel.

© Milady, a part of Cengage Learning. Photography by Dino Petrocelli.

Review Questions

1. What is the primary purpose of regulatory agencies?
2. What is an MSDS? Where can you get it?
3. List the four types of organisms that cosmetologists must know about and remember.
4. What are bacteria?
5. Name and describe the two main classifications of bacteria.
6. What are some of the beneficial functions performed by nonpathogenic bacteria?
7. Name and describe the three forms of pathogenic bacteria.
8. What is a contagious disease?
9. Is HIV a risk in the salon? Why or why not?
10. What is the difference between cleaning, disinfecting, and sterilizing?
11. What is complete immersion?
12. List at least six precautions to follow when using disinfectants.
13. How do you know if an item can be disinfected?
14. Can porous items be disinfected?
15. How often should disinfectant solutions be changed?
16. What are Universal Precautions?
17. What is an exposure incident?
18. Describe the procedure for handling an exposure incident in the salon.
19. Explain how to clean and disinfect nonelectrical tools and implements, and electrical tools and equipment.
20. List the steps for cleaning and disinfecting whirlpool foot spas and air-jet basins after each client.

Chapter Glossary

acquired immune deficiency syndrome	Abbreviated AIDS; a disease that breaks down the body's immune system. AIDS is caused by the human immunodeficiency virus (HIV).
acquired immunity	Immunity that the body develops after overcoming a disease, through inoculation (such as flu vaccinations), or through exposure to natural allergens, such as pollen, cat dander, and ragweed.
allergy	Reaction due to extreme sensitivity to certain foods, chemicals, or other normally harmless substances.
antiseptics	Chemical germicides formulated for use on skin; registered and regulated by the Food and Drug Administration (FDA).
asymptomatic	Showing no symptoms or signs of infection.
bacilli	Short rod-shaped bacteria. They are the most common bacteria and produce diseases such as tetanus (lockjaw), typhoid fever, tuberculosis, and diphtheria.

Chapter Glossary

bacteria (singular: bacterium)	One-celled microorganisms that have both plant and animal characteristics. Some are harmful; some are harmless.
bactericidal	Capable of destroying bacteria.
binary fission	The division of bacteria cells into two new cells called daughter cells.
bioburden	The number of viable organisms in or on an object or surface or the organic material on a surface or object before decontamination or sterilization.
bloodborne pathogens	Disease-causing microorganisms carried in the body by blood or body fluids, such as hepatitis and HIV.
chelating soaps	Also known as *chelating detergents*; detergents that break down stubborn films and remove the residue of pedicure products such as scrubs, salts, and masks.
clean (cleaning)	A mechanical process (scrubbing) using soap and water or detergent and water to remove all visible dirt, debris, and many disease-causing germs. Cleaning also removes invisible debris that interferes with disinfection. Cleaning is what cosmetologists are required to do before disinfecting.
cocci	Round-shaped bacteria that appear singly (alone) or in groups. The three types of cocci are staphylococci, streptococci, and diplococci.
contagious disease	Also known as *communicable disease*; disease that is spread from one person to another person. Some of the more contagious diseases are the common cold, ringworm, conjunctivitis (pinkeye), viral infections, and natural nail or toe and foot infections.
contamination	The presence, or the reasonably anticipated presence, of blood or other potentially infectious materials on an item's surface or visible debris or residues such as dust, hair, and skin.
decontamination	The removal of blood or other potentially infectious materials on an item's surface and the removal of visible debris or residue such as dust, hair, and skin.
diagnosis	Determination of the nature of a disease from its symptoms and/or diagnostic tests. Federal regulations prohibit salon professionals from performing a diagnosis.
diplococci	Spherical bacteria that grow in pairs and cause diseases such as pneumonia.
direct transmission	Transmission of blood or body fluids through touching (including shaking hands), kissing, coughing, sneezing, and talking.
disease	An abnormal condition of all or part of the body, or its systems or organs, that makes the body incapable of carrying on normal function.
disinfectants	Chemical products that destroy all bacteria, fungi, and viruses (but not spores) on surfaces.
disinfection (disinfecting)	A chemical process that uses specific products to destroy harmful organisms (except bacterial spores) on environmental surfaces.
efficacy	The ability to produce an effect.
exposure incident	Contact with nonintact (broken) skin, blood, body fluid or other potentially infectious materials that is the result of the performance of an employee's duties.

Chapter Glossary

flagella	Slender, hairlike extensions used by bacilli and spirilla for locomotion (moving about). May also be referred to as cilia.
fungi (singular: fungus)	Microscopic plant parasites, which include molds, mildews, and yeasts; can produce contagious diseases such as ringworm.
fungicidal	Capable of destroying fungi.
hepatitis	A bloodborne virus that causes disease and can damage the liver.
hospital disinfectants	Disinfectants that are effective for cleaning blood and body fluids.
human immunodeficiency virus	Abbreviated HIV; virus that causes aquired immune deficiency syndrome (AIDS).
human papilloma virus	Abbreviated HPV and also known as *plantar warts*; a virus that can infect the bottom of the foot and resembles small black dots, usually in clustered groups.
immunity	The ability of the body to destroy and resist infection. Immunity against disease can be either natural or acquired and is a sign of good health.
indirect transmission	Transmission of blood or body fluids through contact with an intermediate contaminated object such as a razor, extractor, nipper, or an environmental surface.
infection	The invasion of body tissues by disease-causing pathogens.
infection control	Are the methods used to eliminate or reduce the transmission of infectious organisms.
infectious	Caused by or capable of being transmitted by infection.
infectious disease	Disease caused by pathogenic (harmful) microorganisms that enter the body. An infectious disease may or may not be spread from one person to another person.
inflammation	A condition in which the body reacts to injury, irritation, or infection; characterized by redness, heat, pain, and swelling.
local infection	An infection, such as a pimple or abscess, that is confined to a particular part of the body and appears as a lesion containing pus.
Material Safety Data Sheet	Abbreviated MSDS; information compiled by the manufacturer about product safety, including the names of hazardous ingredients, safe handling and use procedures, precautions to reduce the risk of accidental harm or overexposure, and flammability warnings.
methicillin-resistant staphylococcus aureus	Abbreviated MRSA; a type of infectious bacteria that is highly resistant to conventional treatments such as antibiotics.
microorganism	Any organism of microscopic or submicroscopic size.
mildew	A type of fungus that affects plants or grows on inanimate objects, but does not cause human infections in the salon.
motility	Self-movement.

Chapter Glossary

multiuse	Also known as *reusable*; items that can be cleaned, disinfected, and used on more than one person, even if the item is accidentally exposed to blood or body fluid.
mycobacterium fortuitum	A microscopic germ that normally exists in tap water in small numbers.
natural immunity	Immunity that is partly inherited and partly developed through healthy living.
nonpathogenic	Harmless microorganisms that may perform useful functions and are safe to come in contact with since they do not cause disease or harm.
nonporous	An item that is made or constructed of a material that has no pores or openings and cannot absorb liquids.
occupational disease	Illness resulting from conditions associated with employment, such as prolonged and repeated overexposure to certain products or ingredients.
parasites	Organisms that grow, feed, and shelter on or in another organism (referred to as the host), while contributing nothing to the survival of that organism. Parasites must have a host to survive.
parasitic disease	Disease caused by parasites, such as lice and mites.
pathogenic	Harmful microorganisms that can cause disease or infection in humans when they invade the body.
pathogenic disease	Disease produced by organisms, including bacteria, viruses, fungi, and parasites.
phenolic disinfectants	Powerful tuberculocidal disinfectants. They are a form of formaldehyde, have a very high pH, and can damage the skin and eyes.
porous	Made or constructed of a material that has pores or openings. Porous items are absorbent.
pus	A fluid created by infection.
quaternary ammonium compounds	Also known as *quats*; disinfectants that are very effective when used properly in the salon.
sanitation	Also known as *sanitizing*; a chemical process for reducing the number of disease-causing germs on cleaned surfaces to a safe level.
scabies	A contagious skin disease that is caused by the itch mite, which burrows under the skin.
single-use	Also known as *disposable*; items that cannot be used more than once. These items cannot be properly cleaned so that all visible residue is removed—such as pumice stones used for pedicures—or they are damaged or contaminated by cleaning and disinfecting.

Chapter Glossary

sodium hypochlorite	Common household bleach; an effective disinfectant for the salon.
spirilla	Spiral or corkscrew-shaped bacteria that cause diseases such as syphilis and Lyme disease.
staphylococci	Pus-forming bacteria that grow in clusters like a bunch of grapes. They cause abscesses, pustules, and boils.
sterilization	The process that completely destroys all microbial life, including spores.
streptococci	Pus-forming bacteria arranged in curved lines resembling a string of beads. They cause infections such as strep throat and blood poisoning.
systemic disease	Disease that affects the body as a whole, often due to under-functioning or over-functioning of internal glands or organs. This disease is carried through the blood stream or the lymphatic system.
tinea barbae	Also known as *barber's itch*; a superficial fungal infection that commonly affects the skin. It is primarily limited to the bearded areas of the face and neck or around the scalp.
tinea capitis	A fungal infection of the scalp characterized by red papules, or spots, at the opening of the hair follicles.
tinea pedis	A ringworm fungus of the foot.
toxins	Various poisonous substances produced by some microorganisms (bacteria and viruses).
tuberculocidal disinfectants	Disinfectants that kill the bacteria that causes tuberculosis.
tuberculosis	A disease caused by bacteria that are transmitted through coughing or sneezing.
Universal Precautions	A set of guidelines published by OSHA that require the employer and the employee to assume that all human blood and body fluids are infectious for bloodborne pathogens.
virucidal	Capable of destroying viruses.
virus (plural: viruses)	A parasitic submicroscopic particle that infects and resides in cells of biological organisms. A virus is capable of replication only through taking over the host cell's reproductive function.

CHAPTER 6

General Anatomy and Physiology

Chapter Outline

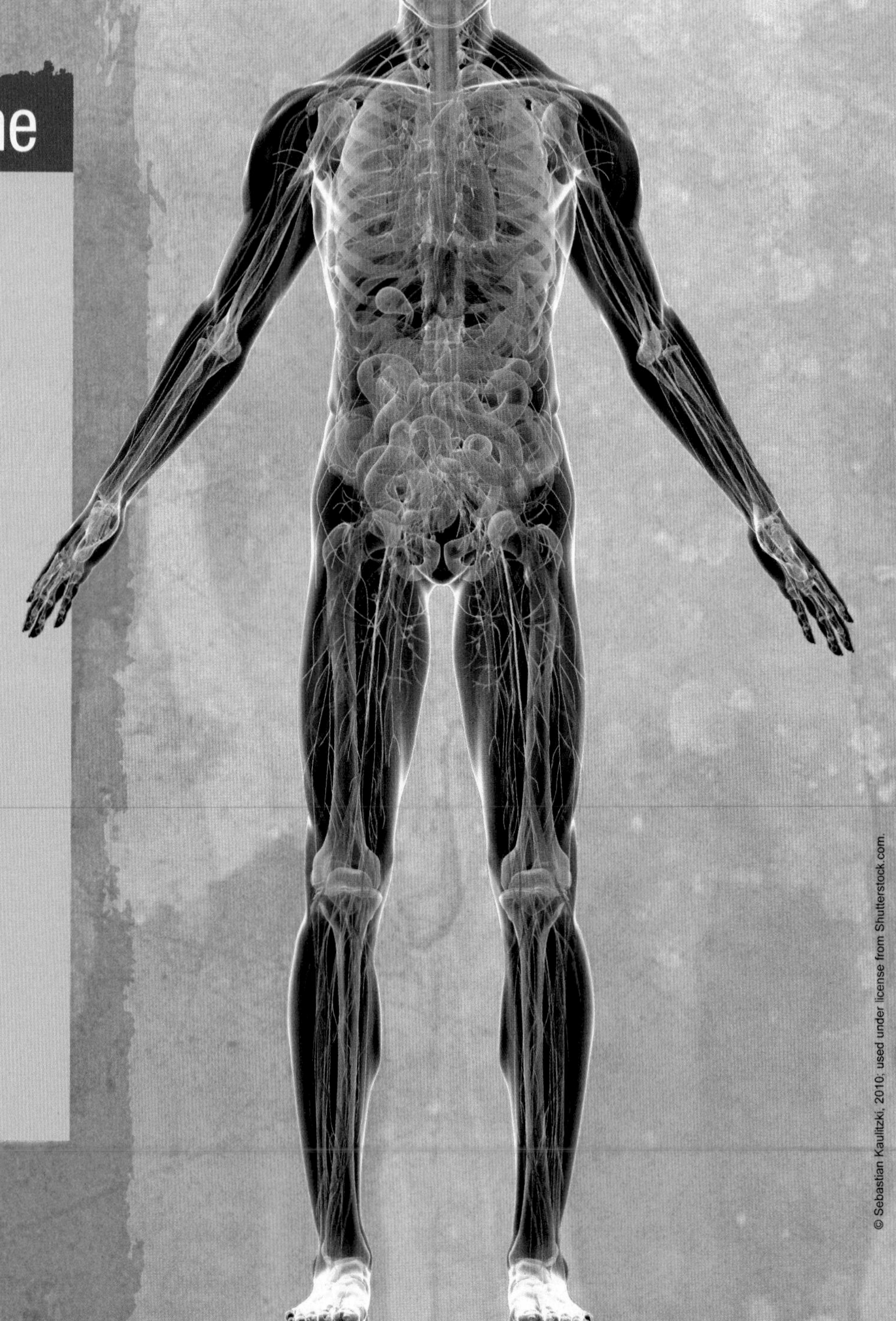

© Sebastian Kaulitzki, 2010; used under license from Shutterstock.com.

Learning Objectives

After completing this chapter, you will be able to:

- ✓ **LO1** Define and explain the importance of anatomy, physiology, and histology to the cosmetology profession.
- ✓ **LO2** Describe cells, their structure, and their reproduction.
- ✓ **LO3** Define tissue and identify the types of tissues found in the body.
- ✓ **LO4** Name the 9 major body organs and the 11 main body systems and explain their basic functions.

Key Terms

Page number indicates where in the chapter the term is used.

abductor digiti minimi
pg. 126

abductor hallucis
pg. 126

abductors
pg. 125

adductors
pg. 125

adipose tissue
pg. 114

adrenal glands
pg. 138

anabolism
pg. 114

anatomy
pg. 112

angular artery
pg. 135

anterior auricular artery
pg. 135

anterior tibial artery
pg. 136

aorta
pg. 133

arteries
pg. 133

arterioles
pg. 133

atrium
pg. 131

auricularis anterior
pg. 121

auricularis posterior
pg. 121

auricularis superior
pg. 121

auriculotemporal nerve
pg. 128

autonomic nervous system (ANS)
pg. 126

axon
pg. 127

axon terminal
pg. 127

belly
pg. 120

bicep
pg. 124

blood
pg. 133

blood vessels
pg. 133

body systems (systems)
pg. 114

brain
pg. 127

buccal nerve
pg. 129

buccinator muscle
pg. 123

capillaries
pg. 133

cardiac muscle
pg. 120

carpus (wrist)
pg. 119

catabolism
pg. 114

cell membrane
pg. 113

cells
pg. 113

central nervous system (CNS)
pg. 126

centrioles
pg. 113

cervical cutaneous nerve
pg. 129

cervical nerves
pg. 129

cervical vertebrae
pg. 118

circulatory system (cardiovascular system, vascular system)
pg. 131

clavicle (collarbone)
pg. 118

common carotid arteries
pg. 134

common peroneal nerve
pg. 130

connective tissue
pg. 114

corrugator muscle
pg. 122

cranium
pg. 116

cytoplasm
pg. 113

deep peroneal nerve (anterior tibial nerve)
pg. 130

deltoid
pg. 124

dendrites
pg. 127

depressor labii inferioris muscle (quadratus labii inferioris muscle)
pg. 123

diaphragm
pg. 140

digestive enzymes
pg. 139

digestive system (gastrointestinal system)
pg. 138

digital nerve
pg. 129

Key Terms

Page number indicates where in the chapter the term is used.

dorsal nerve (dorsal cutaneous nerve)
pg. 130

dorsalis pedis artery
pg. 136

eleventh cranial nerve (accessory nerve)
pg. 129

endocrine glands (ductless glands)
pg. 137

endocrine system
pg. 137

epicranial aponeurosis
pg. 121

epicranius (occipito-frontalis)
pg. 121

epithelial tissue
pg. 114

ethmoid bone
pg. 117

excretory system
pg. 139

exhalation
pg. 140

exocrine glands (duct glands)
pg. 138

extensor digitorum longus
pg. 125

extensor hallucis longus
pg. 125

extensors
pg. 124

external carotid artery
pg. 134

external jugular vein
pg. 136

eyes
pg. 115

facial artery (external maxillary artery)
pg. 135

facial skeleton
pg. 117

femur
pg. 119

fibula
pg. 119

fifth cranial nerve (trifacial nerve, trigeminal nerve)
pg. 128

flexor digiti minimi
pg. 126

flexor digitorum brevis
pg. 126

flexor
pg. 125

frontal artery
pg. 135

frontal bone
pg. 117

frontalis
pg. 121

gastrocnemius
pg. 125

glands
pg. 137

greater auricular nerve
pg. 129

greater occipital nerve
pg. 129

heart
pg. 131

hemoglobin
pg. 133

histology (microscopic anatomy)
pg. 112

hormones
pg. 138

humerus
pg. 118

hyoid bone
pg. 118

inferior labial artery
pg. 135

infraorbital artery
pg. 134

infraorbital nerve
pg. 128

infratrochlear nerve
pg. 128

inhalation
pg. 140

insertion
pg. 121

integumentary system
pg. 140

internal carotid artery
pg. 134

internal jugular vein
pg. 136

interstitial fluid
pg. 137

intestines
pg. 115

joint
pg. 116

kidneys
pg. 115

lacrimal bones
pg. 118

latissimus dorsi
pg. 123

levator anguli oris muscle (caninus muscle)
pg. 123

levator labii superioris muscle (quadratus labii superioris muscle)
pg. 123

liver
pg. 115

lungs
pg. 140

lymph
pg. 137

lymph capillaries
pg. 137

lymph nodes
pg. 137

lymphatic/immune system
pg. 137

mandible
pg. 118

mandibular nerve
pg. 128

marginal mandibular nerve
pg. 129

masseter
pg. 122

maxillae
pg. 118

maxillary nerve
pg. 128

median nerve
pg. 130

mental nerve
pg. 128

mentalis muscle
pg. 123

metabolism
pg. 114

metacarpus
pg. 119

metatarsal
pg. 119

middle temporal artery
pg. 135

mitosis
pg. 113

mitral valve (bicuspid valve)
pg. 132

motor nerves (efferent nerves)
pg. 127

muscle tissue
pg. 114

muscular system
pg. 120

myology
pg. 120

nasal bones
pg. 117

nasal nerve
pg. 128

nerve tissue
pg. 114

nerves
pg. 127

nervous system
pg. 126

neurology
pg. 126

neuron (nerve cell)
pg. 127

nonstriated muscles (smooth muscles)
pg. 120

nucleus
pg. 113

occipital artery
pg. 135

occipital bone
pg. 117

occipitalis
pg. 121

-ology
pg. 112

ophthalmic nerve
pg. 128

Key Terms

Page number indicates where in the chapter the term is used.

orbicularis oculi muscle
pg. 122

orbicularis oris muscle
pg. 123

organs
pg. 114

origin
pg. 120

os
pg. 115

osteology
pg. 115

ovaries
pg. 138

pancreas
pg. 138

parathyroid glands
pg. 138

parietal artery
pg. 135

parietal bones
pg. 117

patella (accessory bone, kneecap)
pg. 119

pectoralis major
pg. 124

pectoralis minor
pg. 124

pericardium
pg. 131

peripheral nervous system (PNS)
pg. 126

peroneus brevis
pg. 125

peroneus longus
pg. 125

phalanges (digits)
pg. 119

physiology
pg. 112

pineal gland
pg. 138

pituitary gland
pg. 138

plasma
pg. 134

platelets
pg. 134

platysma muscle
pg. 122

popliteal artery
pg. 136

posterior auricular artery
pg. 136

posterior auricular nerve
pg. 129

posterior tibial artery
pg. 136

procerus muscle
pg. 122

pronator
pg. 125

protoplasm
pg. 113

pulmonary circulation
pg. 131

radial artery
pg. 136

radial nerve
pg. 130

radius
pg. 119

red blood cells
pg. 133

reflex
pg. 127

reproductive system
pg. 141

respiration
pg. 140

respiratory system
pg. 140

ribs
pg. 118

risorius muscle
pg. 123

saphenous nerve
pg. 130

scapula (shoulder blade)
pg. 118

sciatic nerve
pg. 130

sensory nerves (afferent nerves)
pg. 127

serratus anterior
pg. 124

seventh cranial nerve (facial nerve)
pg. 129

skeletal system
pg. 115

skin
pg. 115

skull
pg. 116

smaller occipital nerve (lesser occipital nerve)
pg. 129

soleus
pg. 125

sphenoid bone
pg. 117

spinal cord
pg. 127

sternocleidomas-toideus
pg. 122

sternum (breastbone)
pg. 118

stomach
pg. 115

striated muscles (skeletal muscles)
pg. 120

submental artery
pg. 135

superficial peroneal nerve (musculo-cutaneous nerve)
pg. 130

superficial temporal artery
pg. 135

superior labial artery
pg. 135

supinator
pg. 125

supraorbital artery
pg. 134

supraorbital nerve
pg. 128

supratrochlear nerve
pg. 129

sural nerve
pg. 130

systemic circulation (general circulation)
pg. 131

talus (ankle bone)
pg. 119

tarsal
pg. 119

temporal bones
pg. 117

temporal nerve
pg. 129

temporalis
pg. 122

testes
pg. 138

thorax (chest, pulmonary trunk)
pg. 118

thyroid gland
pg. 138

tibia
pg. 119

tibial nerve
pg. 130

tibialis anterior
pg. 125

tissue
pg. 114

transverse facial artery
pg. 135

trapezius
pg. 124

triangularis muscle
pg. 123

tricep
pg. 124

tricuspid valve
pg. 132

ulna
pg. 119

ulnar artery
pg. 136

ulnar nerve
pg. 130

valves
pg. 131

veins
pg. 133

ventricle
pg. 131

venules
pg. 133

white blood cells (white corpuscles, leukocytes)
pg. 134

zygomatic bones (malar bones, cheekbones)
pg. 118

zygomatic nerve
pg. 129

zygomaticus major muscles
pg. 123

zygomaticus minor muscles
pg. 123

Cosmetologists are licensed to touch and perform services on clients in ways that are not permitted in many other occupations. This is a very important responsibility, and, as a cosmetologist, you should consider it an honor to be able to aid others in achieving a greater sense of well-being. How can you do this? You can begin by having a solid understanding of the anatomy and physiology of the human body.

WHY STUDY ANATOMY AND PHYSIOLOGY?

Cosmetologists should study and have a thorough understanding of anatomy and physiology because:

- Understanding how the human body functions as an integrated whole is a key component in understanding how a client's hair, skin, and nails may react to various treatments and services.
- You will need to be able to recognize the difference between what is considered normal and what is considered abnormal for the body in order to determine whether specific treatments and services are appropriate.
- Understanding the bone and muscle structure of the human body will help you use the proper application of services and products for scalp manipulations and facials.

Anatomy, Physiology, and You

While you should have an overall knowledge of human anatomy, cosmetology is primarily limited to the skin, muscles, nerves, circulatory system, and bones of the head, face, neck, shoulders, arms, hands, lower legs, and feet. Understanding the anatomy of these areas will help you develop techniques that can be used during scalp massage, facials, manicures, pedicures, and as part of a ritual at the shampoo station. In addition, knowing the bones of the skull and facial structure is important to designing flattering hairstyles that gracefully drape the head and for skillfully applying cosmetics.

Anatomy (ah-NAT-ah-mee) is the study of the human body structures that can be seen with the naked eye and how the body parts are organized; it is the science of the structure of organisms or of their parts.

Physiology (fiz-ih-OL-oh-jee) is the study of the functions and activities performed by the body's structures. The ending **-ology** means *study of.*

Histology (his-TAHL-uh-jee), also known as **microscopic anatomy** (mi-kroh-SKAHP-ik ah-NAT-ah-mee), is the study of tiny structures found in living tissues. ☑ LO1

© Supri Suharjoto, 2010; used under license from Shutterstock.com.

Cells

Cells are the basic units of all living things, from bacteria to plants to animals, including human beings. Without cells, life does not exist. As a basic functional unit, the cell is responsible for carrying on all life processes. There are trillions of cells in the human body, and they vary widely in size, shape, and purpose.

▼ **Figure 6–1**
Basic structure of the cell.

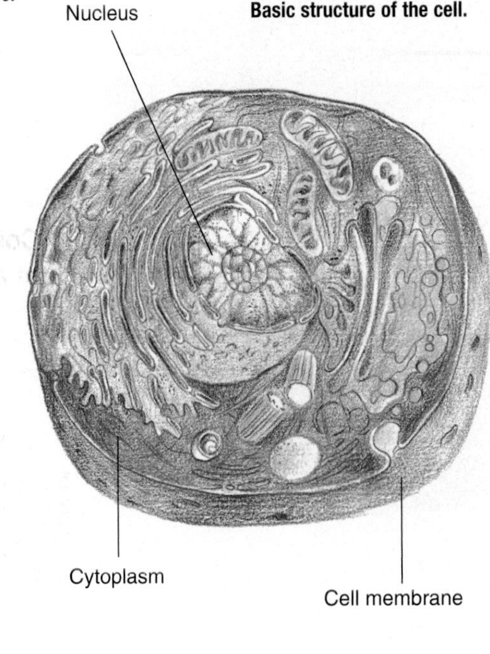

Basic Structure of the Cell

The cells of all living things are composed of a substance called **protoplasm** (PROH-toh-plaz-um), a colorless jelly-like substance found inside cells in which food elements such as proteins, fats, carbohydrates, mineral salts, and water are present. You can visualize the protoplasm of a cell as being similar to raw egg white. In addition to protoplasm, most cells also include a nucleus, cytoplasm, and the cell membrane (**Figure 6–1**).

The **nucleus** (NOO-klee-us) is the dense, active protoplasm found in the center of the cell; it plays an important part in cell reproduction and metabolism. You can visualize the nucleus as the yolk in the middle of a raw egg.

The **cytoplasm** (sy-toh-PLAZ-um) is the protoplasm of a cell, except for the protoplasm in the nucleus, that surrounds the nucleus; it is the watery fluid that cells need for growth, reproduction, and self-repair.

The **cell membrane** (SELL MEM-brayn) is the cell part that encloses the protoplasm and permits soluble substances to enter and leave the cell.

Cell Reproduction and Division

Cells have the ability to reproduce, thus providing new cells for the growth and replacement of worn or injured ones. **Mitosis** (my-TOH-sis) is the usual process of cell reproduction of human tissues that occurs when the cell divides into two identical cells called daughter cells. Two small structures near the nucleus called **centrioles** (SEN-tree-olz) move to each side during the mitosis process to help divide the cell. As long as conditions are favorable, the cell will grow and reproduce. Favorable conditions include an adequate supply of food, oxygen, and water; suitable temperatures; and the ability to eliminate waste products. If conditions become unfavorable, the cell will become impaired or may die. Unfavorable conditions include toxins (poisons), disease, and injury (**Figure 6–2**). ☑ **LO2**

▼ **Figure 6–2**
Phases of mitosis.

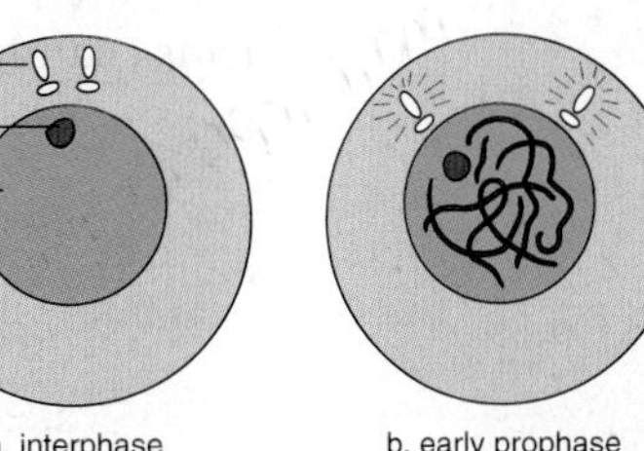

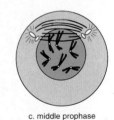

a. interphase

b. early prophase

c. middle prophase

d. late prophase

e. metaphase

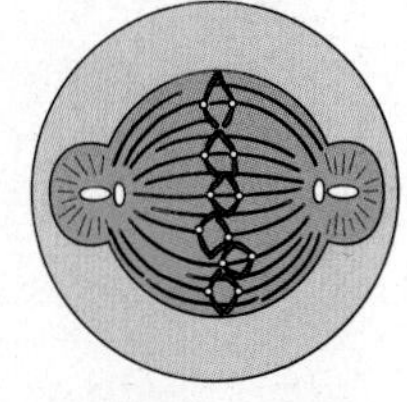

f. early anaphase

g. late anaphase

h. telophase

i. interphase

© Milady, a part of Cengage Learning.

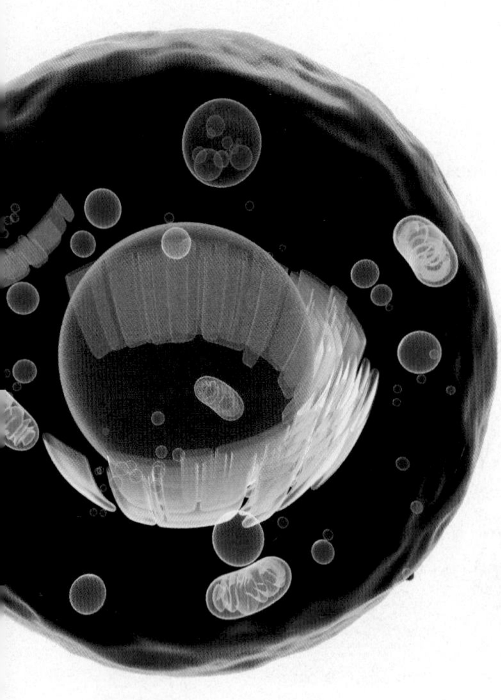

Cell Metabolism

Metabolism (muh-TAB-uh-liz-um) is a chemical process that takes place in living organisms, through which the cells are nourished and carry out their activities. Metabolism has two phases.

- **Anabolism** (uh-NAB-uh-liz-um) is constructive metabolism, the process of building up larger molecules from smaller ones. During this process, the body stores water, food, and oxygen for the times when these substances will be needed for cell growth, reproduction, or repair.
- **Catabolism** (kuh-TAB-uh-liz-um) is the phase of metabolism that involves the breaking down of complex compounds within the cells into smaller ones. This process releases energy that has been stored.

Anabolism and catabolism are carried out simultaneously and continuously within the cells as part of their normal processes.

© Sebastian Kaulitzki; 2010; used under license from Shutterstock.com.

Tissues

Tissue (TISH-oo) is a collection of similar cells that perform a particular function. Each kind of tissue has a specific function and can be recognized by its characteristic appearance. Body tissues are composed of large amounts of water, along with various other substances. There are four types of tissue in the body:

- **Connective tissue** is fibrous tissue that binds together, protects, and supports the various parts of the body. Examples of connective tissue are bone, cartilage, ligaments, tendons, blood, lymph, and **adipose tissue** (ADD-ih-pohz TISH-oo), a technical term for fat. Adipose tissue gives smoothness and contour to the body.
- **Epithelial tissue** (ep-ih-THEE-lee-ul TISH-oo) is a protective covering on body surfaces, such as skin, mucous membranes, the tissue inside the mouth, the lining of the heart, digestive and respiratory organs, and the glands.
- **Muscle tissue** contracts and moves various parts of the body.
- **Nerve tissue** carries messages to and from the brain and controls and coordinates all bodily functions. Nerve tissue is composed of special cells known as neurons that make up the nerves, brain, and spinal cord. ☑ **LO3**

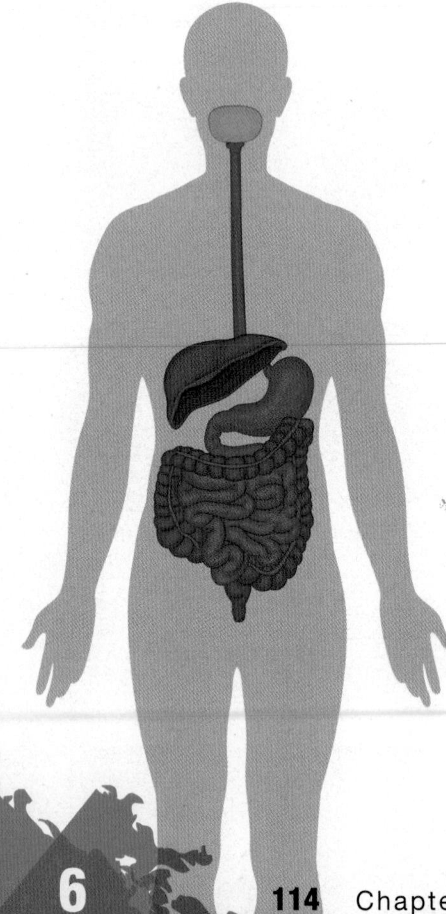

© Matthew Cole, 2010; used under license from Shutterstock.com.

Organs and Body Systems

Organs are structures composed of specialized tissues designed to perform specific functions in plants and animals. **Body systems**, also known as **systems**, are groups of body organs acting together to perform one or more functions. Table 6–1, Nine Major Body Organs

NINE MAJOR BODY ORGANS AND THEIR FUNCTIONS	
ORGAN	**FUNCTION**
BRAIN	Controls the body.
EYES	Control the body's vision.
HEART	Circulates the blood.
KIDNEYS	Excrete water and waste products.
LUNGS	Supply oxygen to the blood.
LIVER	Removes waste created by digestion.
SKIN	Covers the body and is the external protective coating.
STOMACH	Digests food, along with the intestines.
INTESTINES	Digest food, along with the stomach.

© Milady, a part of Cengage Learning.

Table 6–1 **Nine Major Body Organs and Their Functions.**

and Their Functions, and **Table 6–2** (see next page), Eleven Main Body Systems and Their Functions, list some of the most important organs of the body and the main body systems and their functions. ☑ **LO4**

The Skeletal System

The **skeletal system** forms the physical foundation of the body and is composed of 206 bones that vary in size and shape and are connected by movable and immovable joints. **Osteology** (ahs-tee-AHL-oh-jee) is the study of the anatomy, structure, and function of the bones. **Os** (AHS) means *bone*. It is used as a prefix in many medical terms, such as osteoarthritis, a joint disease.

Except for the tissue that forms the major part of the teeth, bone is the hardest tissue in the body. It is composed of connective tissue consisting of about one-third organic matter, such as cells and blood, and two-thirds minerals, mainly calcium carbonate and calcium phosphate.

The primary functions of the skeletal system are to:

- Give shape and support to the body.
- Protect various internal structures and organs.
- Serve as attachments for muscles and act as levers to produce body movement.

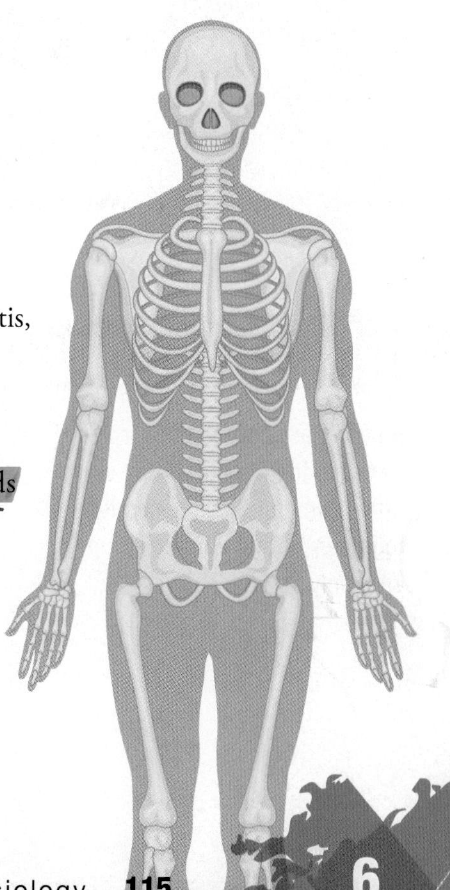

© Matthew Cole, 2010; used under license from Shutterstock.com.

ELEVEN MAIN BODY SYSTEMS AND THEIR FUNCTIONS

SYSTEM	FUNCTION
CIRCULATORY	Controls the steady circulation of the blood through the body by means of the heart and blood vessels.
DIGESTIVE	Breaks down foods into nutrients and wastes; consists of mouth, stomach, intestines, salivary and gastric glands, and other organs.
ENDOCRINE	Affects the growth, development, sexual functions, and health of the entire body; consists of specialized glands.
EXCRETORY	Purifies the body by eliminating waste matter; consists of kidneys, liver, skin, large intestine, and lungs.
INTEGUMENTARY	Serves as a protective covering and helps regulate the body's temperature; consists of skin and its accessory organs, such as oil and sweat glands, sensory receptors, hair, and nails.
LYMPHATIC/IMMUNE	Protects the body from disease by developing immunities and destroying disease-causing toxins and bacteria.
MUSCULAR	Covers, shapes, and holds the skeletal system in place; the muscular system contracts and moves various parts of the body.
NERVOUS	Controls and coordinates all other systems of the body and makes them work harmoniously and efficiently; composed of the brain, spinal cord, and nerves.
REPRODUCTIVE	Produces offspring and passes on the genetic code from one generation to another.
RESPIRATORY	Enables breathing, supplying the body with oxygen, and eliminating carbon dioxide as a waste product; consists of the lungs and air passages.
SKELETAL	Forms the physical foundation of the body; composed of 206 bones that vary in size and shape and are connected by movable and immovable joints.

© Milady, a part of Cengage Learning.

Table 6–2 **Eleven Main Body Systems and Their Functions.**

- Help produce both white and red blood cells (one of the functions of bone marrow).
- Store most of the body's calcium supply, as well as phosphorus, magnesium, and sodium.

did you know?

Humans are born with over 300 bones in their bodies. Then as we grow, some of these bones fuse together, so that adults end up with only 206 bones.

A **joint** is the connection between two or more bones of the skeleton. There are two types of joints: movable, such as elbows, knees, and hips; and immovable, such as the joints found in the pelvis and skull, which allow little or no movement.

Bones of the Skull

The **skull** is the skeleton of the head and is divided into two parts:

- **Cranium** (KRAY-nee-um). An oval, bony case that protects the brain.

- **Facial skeleton**. The framework of the face that is composed of 14 bones (**Figure 6–3**).

Bones of the Cranium

The following are the cranium's eight bones:

- **Occipital bone** (ahk-SIP-ih-tul BOHN). Hindmost bone of the skull, below the parietal bones; forms the back of the skull above the nape.
- **Parietal bones** (puh-RY-uh-tul BOHNS). Bones that form the sides and top of the cranium. There are two parietal bones.
- **Frontal bone** (FRUNT-ul BOHN). Bone that forms the forehead.
- **Temporal bones** (TEM-puh-rul BOHNS). Bones that form the sides of the head in the ear region. There are two temporal bones.
- **Ethmoid bone** (ETH-moyd BOHN). Light spongy bone between the eye sockets; forms part of the nasal cavities.
- **Sphenoid bone** (SFEEN-oyd BOHN). Bone that joins all of the bones of the cranium together.

The ethmoid and sphenoid bones are not affected when performing services or giving a massage.

Bones of the Face

Of the 14 bones of the face, the bones directly involved in facial massage are the following:

- **Nasal bones** (NAY-zul BOHNS). Bones that form the bridge of the nose. There are two nasal bones.

did you know?

People often complain of joint pain; however, the pain is usually caused by inflammation of the tissue surrounding the joint and not by the joint itself.

You have over 230 moveable and semi-moveable joints in your body.

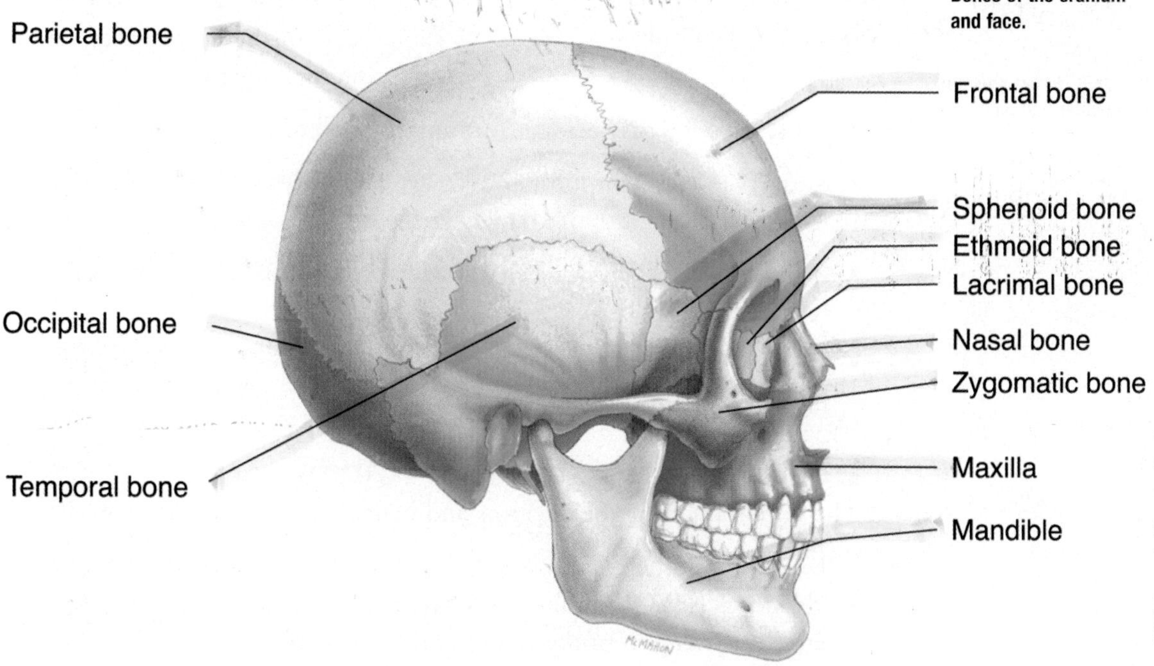

▼ **Figure 6–3** **Bones of the cranium and face.**

© Milady, a part of Cengage Learning.

did you know?

Painful inflammation involving the carpus area can be caused by repetitive motions, such as flexing your wrist excessively or locking it in a bent position. Keeping the wrist straight can help prevent these injuries.

- **Lacrimal bones** (LAK-ruh-mul BOHNS). Small, thin bones located at the front inner wall of the orbits (eye sockets). There are two lacrimal bones.
- **Zygomatic bones** (zy-goh-MAT-ik BOHNS), also known as **malar bones** or **cheekbones**. Bones that form the prominence of the cheeks. There are two zygomatic bones.
- **Maxillae** (mak-SIL-ee) (singular: maxilla, mak-SIL-uh). Bones of the upper jaw. There are two maxillae.
- **Mandible** (MAN-duh-bul). Lower jawbone; largest and strongest bone of the face.

Bones of the Neck

The main bones of the neck are the following:

- **Hyoid bone** (HY-oyd BOHN). U-shaped bone at the base of the tongue that supports the tongue and its muscles.
- **Cervical vertebrae** (SUR-vih-kul VURT-uh-bray). The seven bones of the top part of the vertebral column, located in the neck region (**Figure 6–4**).

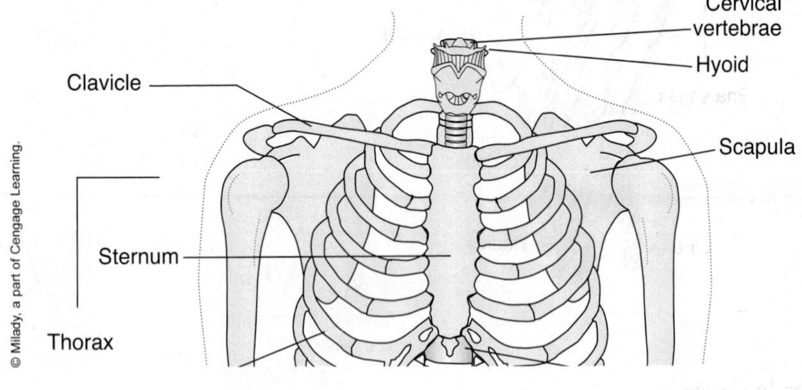

© Milady, a part of Cengage Learning.

▲ Figure 6–4
Bones of the neck, shoulder, and back.

Bones of the Chest, Shoulder, and Back

The bones of the trunk or torso are the following:

- **Thorax** (THOR-aks), also known as **chest** or **pulmonary trunk**. Consists of the sternum, ribs, and thoracic vertebrae. It is an elastic, bony cage that serves as a protective framework for the heart, lungs, and other internal organs.
- **Ribs**. Twelve pairs of bones forming the wall of the thorax.
- **Scapula** (SKAP-yuh-luh), also known as **shoulder blade**. Large, flat, triangular bone of the shoulder. There are two scapulas.
- **Sternum** (STUR-num), also known as **breastbone**. Flat bone that forms the ventral (front) support of the ribs.
- **Clavicle** (KLAV-ih-kul), also known as **collarbone**. Bone that joins the sternum and scapula.

Bones of the Arms and Hands

The important bones of the arms and hands that you should know include the following:

- **Humerus** (HYOO-muh-rus). Uppermost and largest bone in the arm, extending from the elbow to the shoulder.

- **Ulna** (UL-nuh). Inner and larger bone in the forearm (lower arm), attached to the wrist and located on the side of the little finger.
- **Radius** (RAY-dee-us). Smaller bone in the forearm (lower arm) on the same side as the thumb (**Figure 6–5**).
- **Carpus** (KAR-pus), also known as **wrist**. Flexible joint composed of a group of eight small, irregular bones (carpals) held together by ligaments.
- **Metacarpus** (met-uh-KAR-pus). Bones of the palm of the hand; parts of the hand containing five bones between the carpus and phalanges.
- **Phalanges** (fuh-LAN-jeez) (singular: phalanx, FAY-langks) also known as **digits**. Bones of the fingers or toes (**Figure 6–6**).

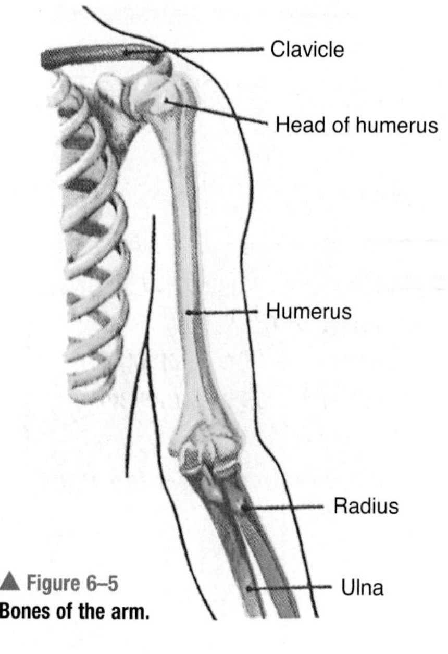

▲ **Figure 6–5**
Bones of the arm.

Bones of the Leg, Ankle, and Foot

The four bones of the leg are the following:

- **Femur** (FEE-mur). Heavy, long bone that forms the leg above the knee.
- **Tibia** (TIB-ee-ah). Larger of the two bones that form the leg below the knee. The tibia may be visualized as a bump on the big-toe side of the ankle.
- **Fibula** (FIB-ya-lah). Smaller of the two bones that form the leg below the knee. The fibula may be visualized as a bump on the little-toe side of the ankle.
- **Patella** (pah-TEL-lah), also known as **accessory bone** or **kneecap**. Forms the kneecap joint (**Figure 6–7**).

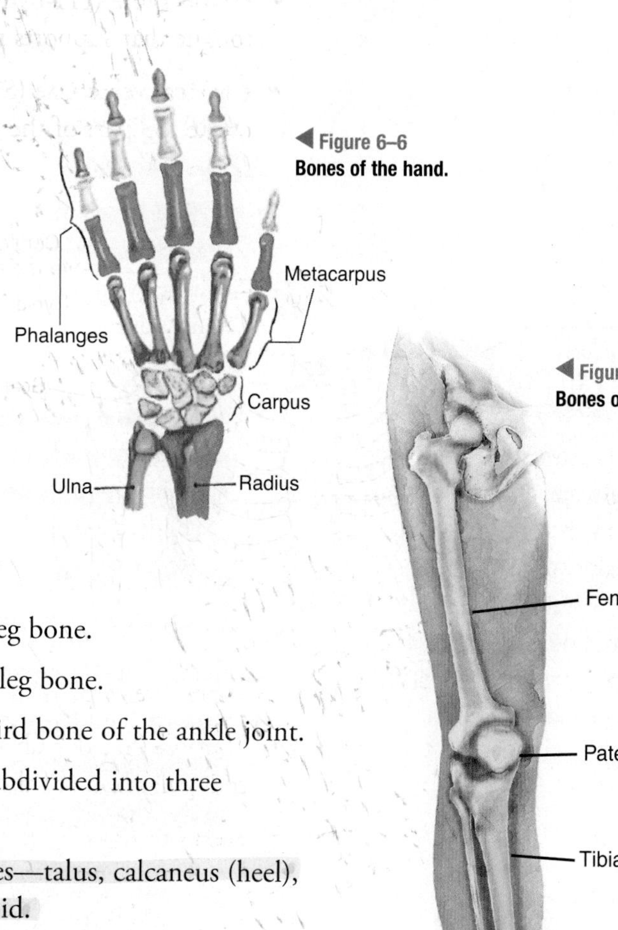

◀ **Figure 6–6**
Bones of the hand.

◀ **Figure 6–7**
Bones of the leg.

The ankle joint is composed of three bones:

- Tibia. Bone that comes down from the lower leg bone.
- Fibula. Bone that comes down from the lower leg bone.
- **Talus** (TA-lus), also known as **ankle bone**. Third bone of the ankle joint.

The foot is made up of 26 bones. These can be subdivided into three general categories:

- **Tarsal** (TAHR-sul). There are seven tarsal bones—talus, calcaneus (heel), navicular, three cuneiform bones, and the cuboid.
- **Metatarsal** (met-ah-TAHR-sul). Long and slender bones, similar to the metacarpal bones of the hand. There are five metatarsal bones.
- Phalanges. Fourteen bones that compose the toes. Toe phalanges are similar to the finger phalanges. There are three phalanges in each toe, except for the big toe, which has only two (**Figure 6–8**).

© Milady, a part of Cengage Learning.

* Read

The Muscular System

The **muscular system** is the body system that covers, shapes, and holds the skeletal system in place; the muscular system contracts and moves various parts of the body.

Cosmetologists must be concerned with the voluntary muscles that control movements of the arms, hands, lower legs, and feet. It is important to know where these muscles are located and what they control. These muscles can become fatigued from excessive work or injury and your clients will benefit greatly from the massaging techniques you incorporate into your services.

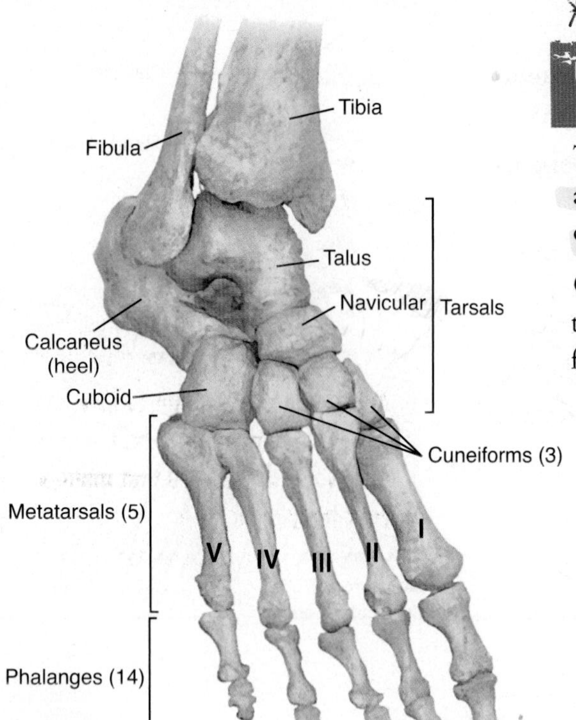

▲ **Figure 6–8**
Bones of the ankle and foot.

Myology (my-AHL-uh-jee) is the study of the nature, structure, function, and diseases of the muscles. The human body has over 630 muscles, which are responsible for approximately 40 percent of the body's weight. Muscles are fibrous tissues that have the ability to stretch and contract according to demands of the body's movements. There are three types of muscle tissue.

- **Striated muscles** (STRY-ayt-ed MUS-uls), also known as **skeletal muscles**. Muscles that are attached to the bones and are voluntary or are consciously controlled. Striated muscles assist in maintaining the body's posture and protect some internal organs (**Figure 6–9**).
- **Nonstriated muscles** (nahn-STRY-ayt-ed MUS-uls), also known as **smooth muscles**. Muscles that are involuntary and function automatically, without conscious will. These muscles are found in the internal organs of the body, such as the digestive or respiratory systems (**Figure 6–10**).
- **Cardiac muscle**. Involuntary muscle that is the heart. This type of muscle is not found in any other part of the body (**Figure 6–11**).

did you know?

Fingernails provide protection for the delicate tips of the phalanges in the hand. If a phalange is accidentally broken, the finger loses much of its fine dexterity, and it becomes more difficult to pick up very small objects such as sewing needles or coins.

A muscle has three parts:

- **Origin**. The part of the muscle that does not move and is attached closest to the skeleton.
- **Belly**. The middle part of the muscle.

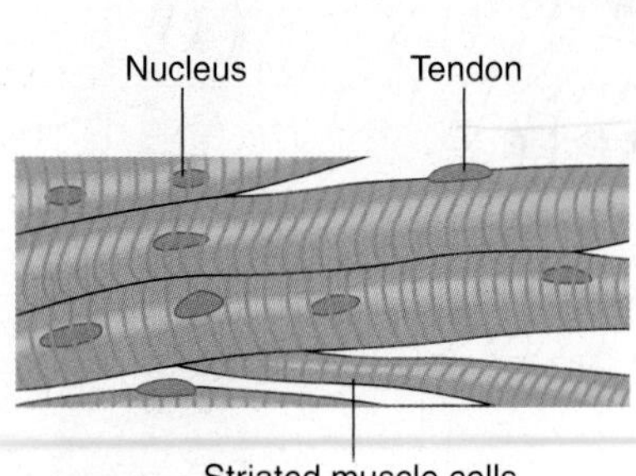

▲ **Figure 6–9**
Striated muscle cells.

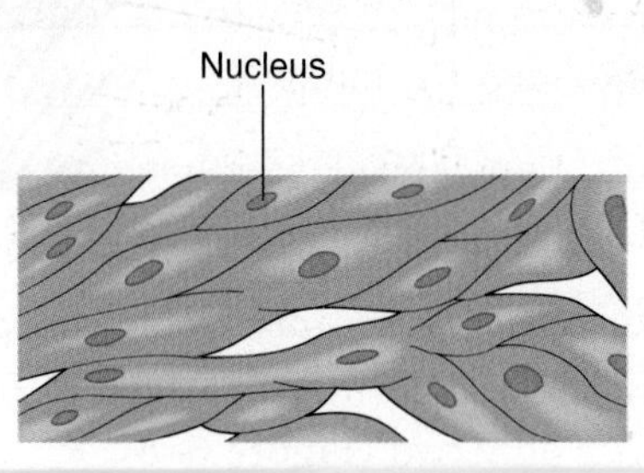

▲ **Figure 6–10**
Nonstriated muscle cells.

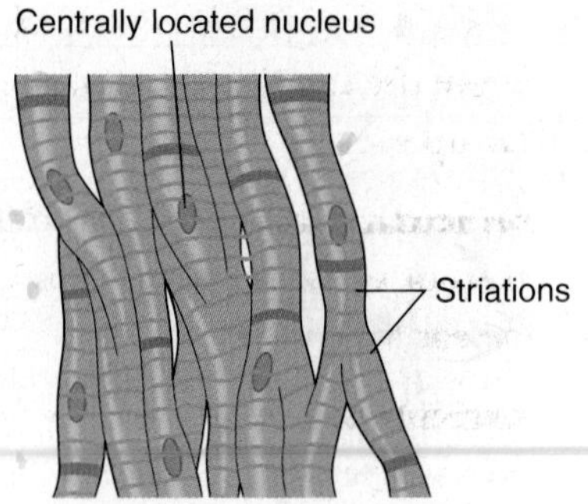

▲ **Figure 6–11**
Cardiac muscle cells.

© Milady, a part of Cengage Learning.

*Read

- **Insertion**. The part of the muscle that moves and is farthest from the skeleton.

Pressure in massage is usually directed from the insertion to the origin.

Muscular tissue can be stimulated by:

- Massage (hand, electric vibrator, or water jets).
- Electrical therapy current. (See Chapter 13, Basics of Electricity, for additional information on types of electrical therapy current.)
- Infrared light.
- Dry heat (heating lamps or heating caps).
- Moist heat (steamers or moderately warm steam towels).
- Nerve impulses (through the nervous system).
- Chemicals (certain acids and salts).

did you know?

About 40 to 50 percent of body weight is in muscles. And there are over 630 muscles that make your body move.

Muscles of the Scalp

The four muscles of the scalp are the following:

- **Epicranius** (ep-ih-KRAY-nee-us), also known as **occipitofrontalis** (ahk-SIP-ih-toh frun-TAY-lus). Broad muscle that covers the top of the skull and consists of the occipitalis and frontalis.
- **Occipitalis** (ahk-SIP-i-tahl-is). Back (posterior) portion of the epicranius; the muscle that draws the scalp backward.
- **Frontalis** (frun-TAY-lus). Front (anterior) portion of the epicranius; the muscle of the scalp that raises the eyebrows, draws the scalp forward, and causes wrinkles across the forehead.
- **Epicranial aponeurosis** (ep-ih-KRAY-nee-al ap-uh-noo-ROH-sus). Tendon that connects the occipitalis and frontalis muscles (**Figure 6–12**).

Muscles of the Ear

The three muscles of the ear are the following:

- **Auricularis superior** (aw-rik-yuh-LAIR-is soo-PEER-ee-ur). Muscle above the ear that draws the ear upward.
- **Auricularis anterior.** Muscle in front of the ear that draws the ear forward.
- **Auricularis posterior.** Muscle behind the ear that draws the ear backward.

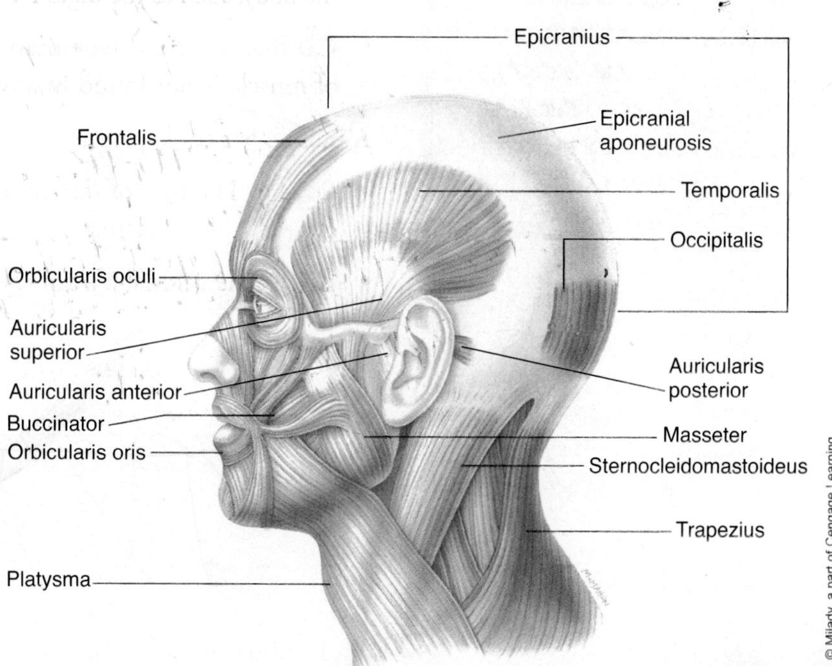

▼ **Figure 6–12**
Muscles of the head, face, and neck.

© Milady, a part of Cengage Learning.

*GO over it.

Although these ear muscles have minimal movement in most humans, some people can contract them and wiggle their ears!

Muscles of Mastication (Chewing)

The main muscles of mastication, also known as the *chewing muscles*, are the following:

- **Masseter** (muh-SEE-tur).
- **Temporalis** (tem-poh-RAY-lis).

These muscles coordinate to open and close the mouth and bring the jaw forward or backward, assisted by the pterygoid (THER-ih-goyd) muscles.

Muscles of the Neck

The muscles of the neck include the following:

- **Platysma muscle** (plah-TIZ-muh MUS-ul). Broad muscle extending from the chest and shoulder muscles to the side of the chin; responsible for lowering the lower jaw and lip.
- **Sternocleidomastoideus** (STUR-noh-KLEE-ih-doh-mas-TOYD-ee-us). Muscle of the neck that lowers and rotates the head.

Muscles of the Eyebrow

The eyebrow muscles include the following:

- **Orbicularis oculi muscle** (or-bik-yuh-LAIR-is AHK-yuh-lye MUS-ul). Ring muscle of the eye socket; enables you to close your eyes.
- **Corrugator muscle** (KOR-oo-gay-tohr MUS-ul). Muscle located beneath the frontalis and orbicularis oculi muscle that draws the eyebrow down and wrinkles the forehead vertically (**Figure 6–13**).

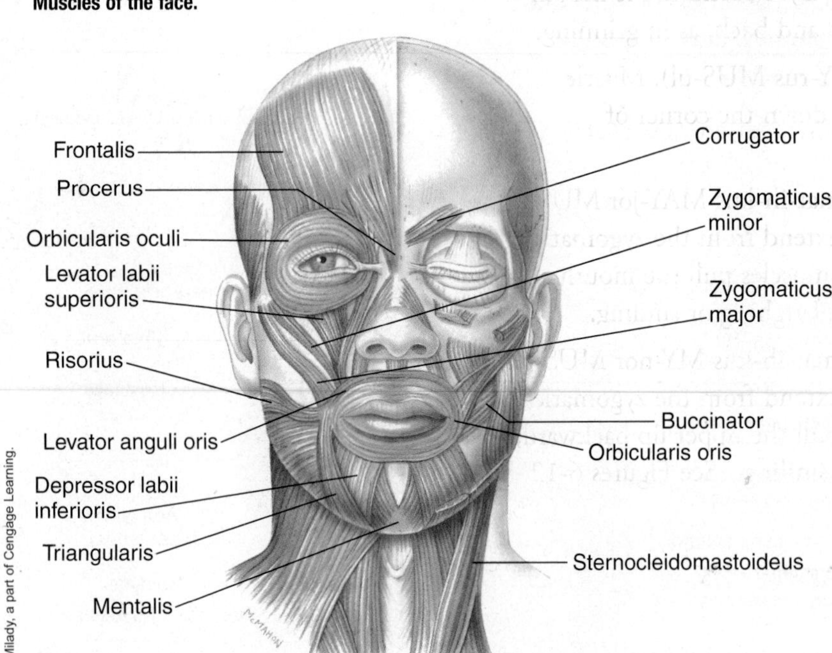

▼ **Figure 6–13**
Muscles of the face.

Muscles of the Nose

The muscle of the nose that you should remember is the following:

- **Procerus muscle** (proh-SEE-rus MUS-ul). Covers the bridge of the nose, lowers the eyebrows, and causes wrinkles across the bridge of the nose.

There are other nasal muscles that contract and expand the openings of the nostrils, but they are not of major concern to cosmetologists.

* Go over it.

Muscles of the Mouth

The important muscles of the mouth are the following:

- **Buccinator muscle** (BUK-sih-nay-tur MUS-ul). Thin, flat muscle of the cheek between the upper and lower jaw that compresses the cheeks and expels air between the lips.
- **Depressor labii inferioris muscle** (dee-PRES-ur LAY-bee-eye in-FEER-ee-or-us MUS-ul), also known as **quadratus labii inferioris muscle** (kwah-DRAY-tus LAY-bee-eye in-feer-ee-OR-is MUS-ul). Muscle surrounding the lower lip; lowers the lower lip and draws it to one side, as in expressing sarcasm.
- **Levator anguli oris muscle** (lih-VAYT-ur ANG-yoo-ly OH-ris MUS-ul), also known as **caninus muscle** (kay-NY-nus MUS-ul). Muscle that raises the angle of the mouth and draws it inward.
- **Levator labii superioris muscle** (lih-VAYT-ur LAY-bee-eye soo-peer-ee-OR-is MUS-ul), also known as **quadratus labii superioris muscle** (kwah-DRA-tus LAY-bee-eye soo-peer-ee-OR-is MUS-ul). Muscle surrounding the upper lip; elevates the upper lip and dilates the nostrils, as in expressing distaste.
- **Mentalis muscle** (men-TAY-lis MUS-ul). Muscle that elevates the lower lip and raises and wrinkles the skin of the chin.
- **Orbicularis oris muscle** (or-bik-yuh-LAIR-is OH-ris MUS-ul). Flat band of muscle around the upper and lower lips that compresses, contracts, puckers, and wrinkles the lips.
- **Risorius muscle** (rih-ZOR-ee-us MUS-ul). Muscle of the mouth that draws the corner of the mouth out and back, as in grinning.
- **Triangularis muscle** (try-ang-gyuh-LAY-rus MUS-ul). Muscle extending alongside the chin that pulls down the corner of the mouth.
- **Zygomaticus major muscles** (zy-goh-mat-ih-kus MAY-jor MUS-ul). Muscles on both sides of the face that extend from the zygomatic bone to the angle of the mouth. These muscles pull the mouth upward and backward, as when you are laughing or smiling.
- **Zygomaticus minor muscles** (zy-goh-mat-ih-kus MY-nor MUS-ul). Muscles on both sides of the face that extend from the zygomatic bone to the upper lips. These muscles pull the upper lip backward, upward, and outward, as when you are smiling. (See Figures 6-12 and 6-13.)

did you know?

You have over 30 muscles in your face that control your expressions.

Muscles that Attach the Arms to the Body

The muscles that attach the arms to the body are the following:

- **Latissimus dorsi** (lah-TIS-ih-mus DOR-see). Large, flat, triangular muscle covering the lower back. It helps extend the arm away from the body and rotate the shoulder.

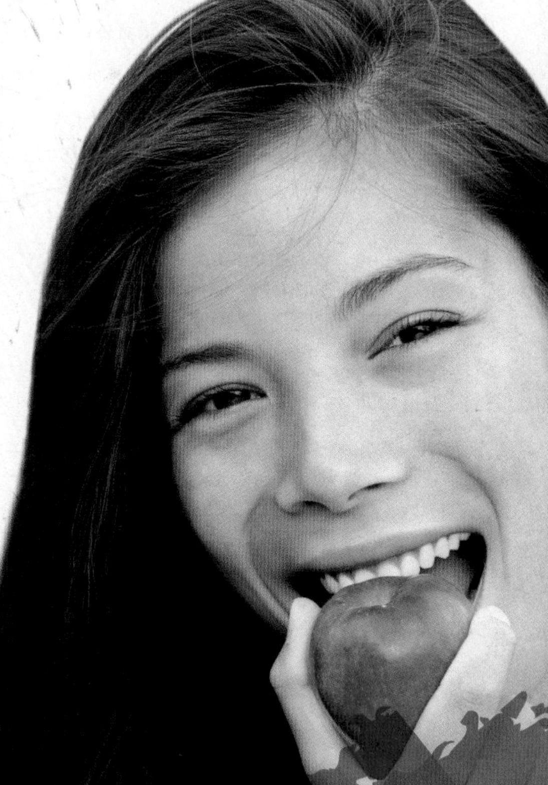

© Maridav, 2010; used under license from Shutterstock.com.

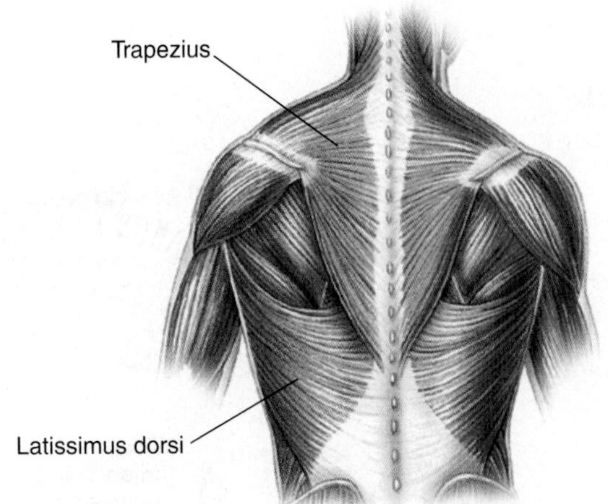

▲ **Figure 6–14**
Muscles of the back that attach the arms to the body.

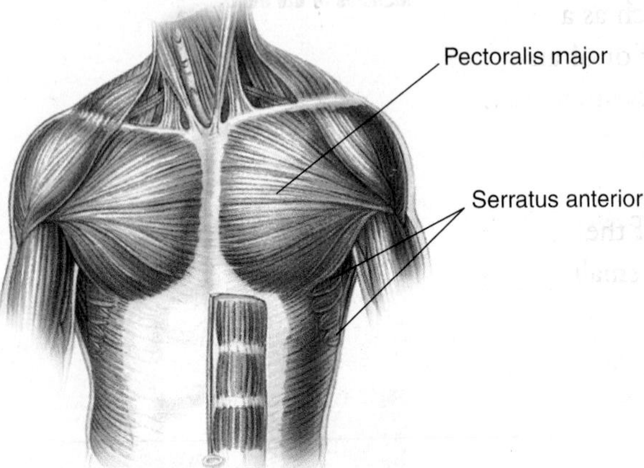

▲ **Figure 6–15**
Muscles of the chest that attach the arms to the body.

- **Pectoralis major** (pek-tor-AL-is MAY-jor) and **pectoralis minor**, located under the pectoralis major (not shown in Figure 6-15). Muscles of the chest that assist the swinging movements of the arm.
- **Serratus anterior** (ser-RAT-us an-TEER-ee-or). Muscle of the chest that assists in breathing and in raising the arm.
- **Trapezius** (trah-PEE-zee-us). Muscle that covers the back of the neck and the upper and middle region of the back; rotates and controls swinging movements of the arm (**Figures 6–14** and **6–15**).

Muscles of the Shoulder and Arm

There are three principal muscles of the shoulders and upper arms (**Figure 6–16**):

- **Bicep** (BY-sep). Muscle that produces the contour of the front and inner side of the upper arm; lifts the forearm and flexes the elbow.
- **Deltoid** (DEL-toyd). Large, triangular muscle covering the shoulder joint that allows the arm to extend outward and to the side of the body.
- **Tricep** (TRY-sep). Large muscle that covers the entire back of the upper arm and extends the forearm.

The forearm is made up of a series of muscles and strong tendons (**Figure 6–16**). As a cosmetologist, you will be concerned with the following muscles of the forearm:

- **Extensors** (ik-STEN-surs). Muscles that straighten the wrist, hand, and fingers to form a straight line.

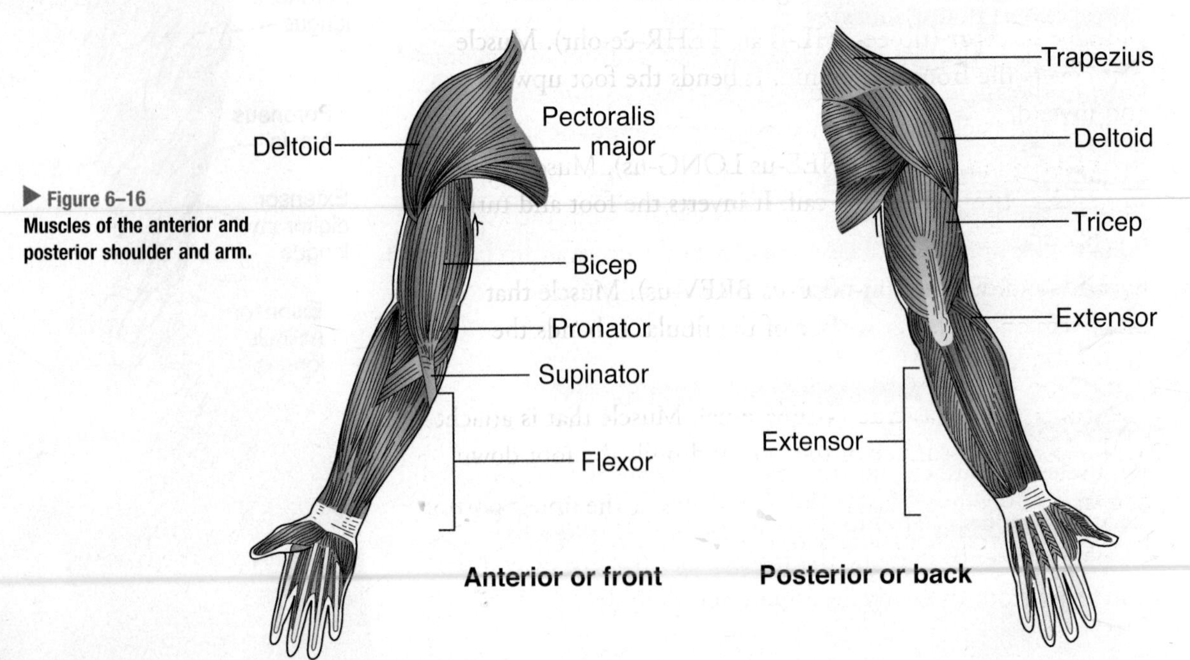

▶ **Figure 6–16**
Muscles of the anterior and posterior shoulder and arm.

© Milady, a part of Cengage Learning.

- **Flexor** (FLEK-sur). Extensor muscle of the wrist involved in flexing the wrist.
- **Pronator** (proh-NAY-tohr). Muscle that turns the hand inward so that the palm faces downward.
- **Supinator** (SOO-puh-nayt-ur). Muscle of the forearm that rotates the radius outward and the palm upward.

Muscles of the Hand

The hand is one of the most complex parts of the body, with many small muscles that overlap from joint to joint and provide the flexibility and strength to open and close the hand and fingers. Important muscles to know include the following:

- **Abductors** (ab-DUK-turz). Muscles that draw a body part, such as a finger, arm, or toe, away from the midline of the body or of an extremity. In the hand, abductors separate the fingers.
- **Adductors** (ah-DUK-turz). Muscles that draw a body part, such as a finger, arm, or toe, inward toward the median axis of the body or of an extremity. In the hand, adductors draw the fingers together (**Figure 6–17**).

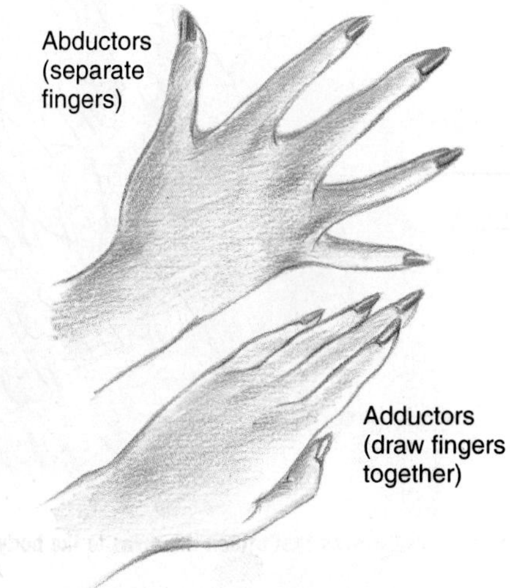

▲ **Figure 6–17**
Muscles of the hand.

Muscles of the Lower Leg and Foot

As a cosmetologist, you will use your knowledge of the muscles of the lower leg and foot during a pedicure. The muscles of the foot are small and provide proper support and cushioning for the foot and leg.

The muscles of the lower leg include the following:

- **Extensor digitorum longus** (eck-STEN-sur dij-it-TOHR-um LONG-us). Muscle that bends the foot up and extends the toes.
- **Extensor hallucis longus** (eck-STEN-sur ha-LU-sis LONG-us). Muscle that extends the big toe and flexes the foot.
- **Tibialis anterior** (tib-ee-AHL-is an-TEHR-ee-ohr). Muscle that covers the front of the shin. It bends the foot upward and inward.
- **Peroneus longus** (per-oh-NEE-us LONG-us). Muscle that covers the outer side of the calf. It inverts the foot and turns it outward.
- **Peroneus brevis** (per-oh-NEE-us BREV-us). Muscle that originates on the lower surface of the fibula. It bends the foot down and out.
- **Gastrocnemius** (gas-truc-NEEM-e-us). Muscle that is attached to the lower rear surface of the heel and pulls the foot down.
- **Soleus** (SO-lee-us). Muscle that originates at the upper portion of the fibula and bends the foot down (**Figure 6-18**).

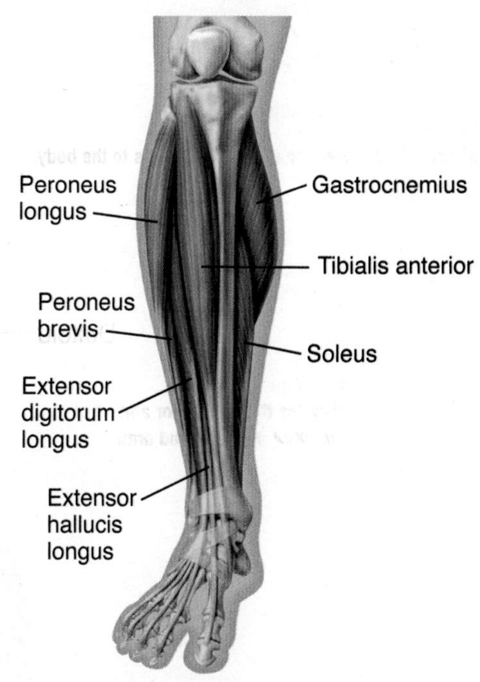

▲ **Figure 6–18**
Muscles of the lower leg.

© Milady, a part of Cengage Learning.

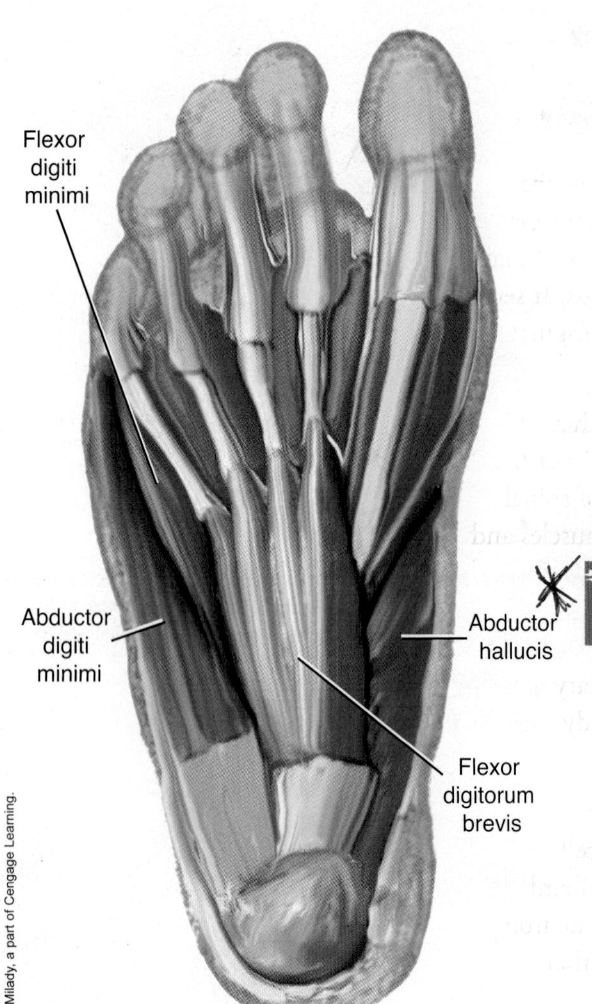

▲ **Figure 6–19**
Muscles of the foot (bottom).

The muscles of the feet include the following:

- **Flexor digiti minimi** (FLEK-sur dij-it-ty MIN-eh-mee). Muscle that moves the little toe.
- **Flexor digitorum brevis** (FLEK-sur dij-ut-TOHR-um BREV-us). Muscle that moves the toes and helps maintain balance while walking and standing.
- **Abductor hallucis** (ab-DUK-tohr ha-LU-sis). Muscle that moves the toes and helps maintain balance while walking and standing.
- **Abductor digiti minimi** (ab-DUK-tohr dij-it-ty MIN-eh-mee). Muscle that separates the toes (**Figure 6–19**).

The Nervous System

The **nervous system** is an exceptionally well-organized body system, composed of the brain, spinal cord, and nerves, that is responsible for controlling and coordinating all other systems of the body and makes them work harmoniously and efficiently. Every square inch of the human body is supplied with fine fibers known as nerves. There are over 100 billion nerve cells, known as neurons, in the body. The scientific study of the structure, function, and pathology of the nervous system is known as **neurology** (nuh-RAHL-uh-jee).

An understanding of how nerves work will help you perform services in a more proficient manner when administering shampoos and massage techniques. It will also help you understand the effects that these treatments have on the body as a whole.

Divisions of the Nervous System

The nervous system is divided into three main subdivisions.

- The **central nervous system (CNS)** consists of the brain, spinal cord, spinal nerves, and cranial nerves. It controls consciousness and many mental activities, voluntary functions of the five senses (seeing, hearing, feeling, smelling, and tasting), and voluntary muscle actions, including all body movements and facial expressions.
- The **peripheral nervous system (PNS)** (puh-RIF-uh-rul NURV-vus SIS-tum) is a system of nerves that connects the peripheral (outer) parts of the body to the central nervous system; it has both sensory and motor nerves. Its function is to carry impulses, or messages, to and from the central nervous system.
- The **autonomic nervous system (ANS)** (aw-toh-NAHM-ik NURV-us SIS-tum) is the part of the nervous system that controls the

involuntary muscles; it regulates the action of the smooth muscles, glands, blood vessels, heart, and breathing (**Figure 6–20**).

The Brain and Spinal Cord

The **brain** is the part of the central nervous system contained in the cranium. It is the largest and most complex nerve tissue and controls sensation, muscles, activity of glands, and the power to think, sense, and feel. On average, the brain weighs a little less than three pounds. It sends and receives messages through 12 pairs of cranial nerves that originate in the brain and reach various parts of the head, face, and neck.

The **spinal cord** is the portion of the central nervous system that originates in the brain and extends down to the lower extremity of the trunk. It is protected by the spinal column. Thirty-one pairs of spinal nerves extending from the spinal cord are distributed to the muscles and skin of the trunk and limbs.

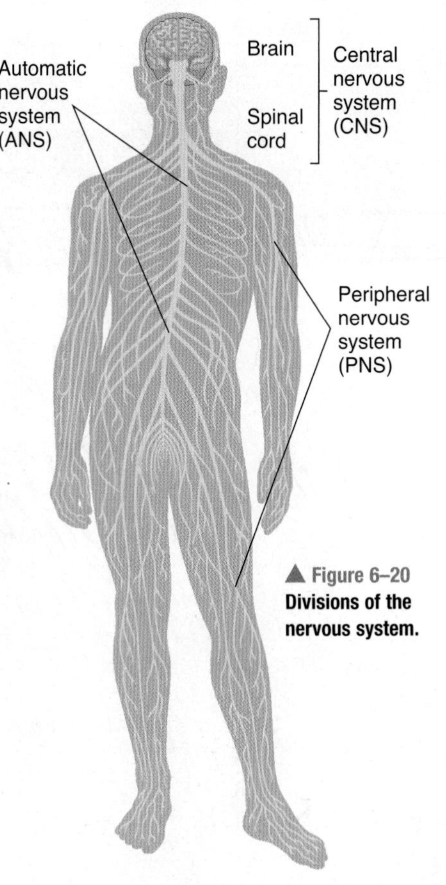

▲ **Figure 6–20** **Divisions of the nervous system.**

Nerve Cell Structure and Function

A **neuron** (NOO-rahn), also known as **nerve cell**, is the primary structural unit of the nervous system, consisting of the cell body, nucleus, dendrites, and the axon.

Dendrites (DEN-dryts) are tree-like branchings of nerve fibers extending from the nerve cell that carry impulses toward the cell and receive impulses from other neurons. The **axon** (AK-sahn) and **axon terminal** (not shown in Figure 6-21) are extensions of a neuron through which impulses are sent away from the cell body to other neurons, glands, or muscles (**Figure 6–21**).

Nerves are whitish cords made up of bundles of nerve fibers held together by connective tissue, through which impulses are transmitted. Nerves have their origin in the brain and spinal cord and send their branches to all parts of the body.

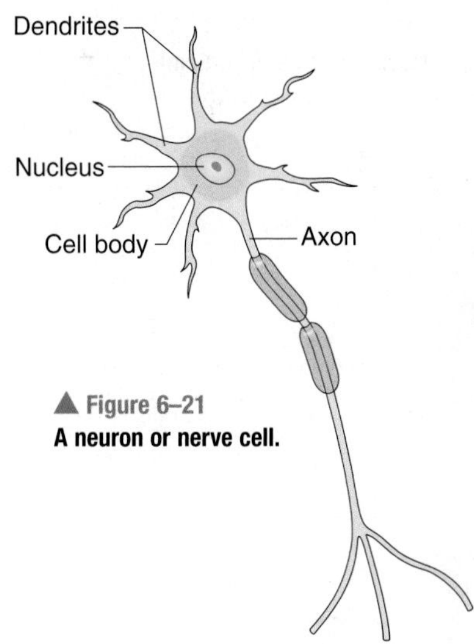

▲ **Figure 6–21** **A neuron or nerve cell.**

Types of Nerves

There are two types of nerves:

- **Sensory nerves**, also known as **afferent nerves** (AAF-eer-ent NURVS), carry impulses or messages from the sense organs to the brain, where sensations such as touch, cold, heat, sight, hearing, taste, smell, pain, and pressure are experienced. Sensory nerve endings called receptors are located close to the surface of the skin. Impulses pass from the sensory nerves to the brain and back through the motor nerves to the muscles; the muscles move as a result of the completed circuit.
- **Motor nerves**, also known as **efferent nerves** (EF-uh-rent NURVS), carry impulses from the brain to the muscles or glands. These transmitted impulses produce movement.

A **reflex** (REE-fleks) is an automatic reaction to a stimulus that involves the movement of an impulse from a sensory receptor along the sensory nerve to the spinal cord. A responsive impulse is sent along a motor

© Milady, a part of Cengage Learning.

ACTivity

There are sensory nerve endings all over the body. Try gently pinching a small piece of the skin on your arm. You feel a slight pressure, right? That is the sensory nerve endings sending a message from your arm to your brain that something is happening to the arm.

neuron to a muscle, causing a reaction (for example, the quick removal of your hand from a hot object). Reflexes do not have to be learned; they are automatic.

Nerves of the Head, Face, and Neck

The largest of the cranial nerves is the **fifth cranial nerve**, also known as **trifacial nerve** (try-FAY-shul NURV) or **trigeminal nerve** (try-JEM-un-ul NURV). It is the chief sensory nerve of the face and serves as the motor nerve of the muscles that control chewing. It consists of three branches:

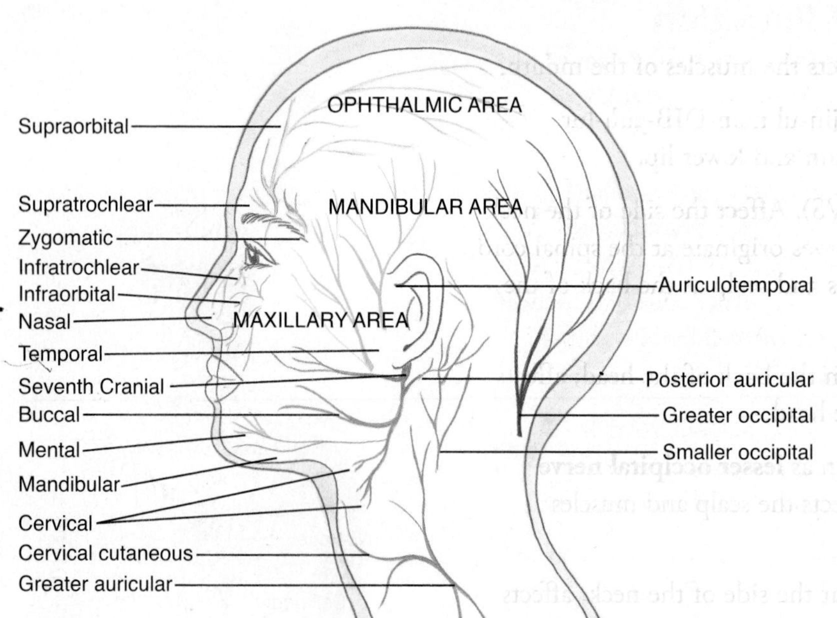

© Milady, a part of Cengage Learning.

▲ **Figure 6–22**
Nerves of the head, face, and neck.

- **Ophthalmic nerve** (ahf-THAL-mik NURV). Supplies impulses to the skin of the forehead, upper eyelids, and interior portion of the scalp, orbit, eyeball, and nasal passage.
- **Mandibular nerve** (man-DIB-yuh-lur NURV). Affects the muscles of the chin, lower lip, and external ear.
- **Maxillary nerve** (MAK-suh-lair-ee NURV). Supplies impulses to the upper part of the face (**Figure 6–22**).

The following are the branches of the fifth cranial nerve that are affected by massage:

- **Auriculotemporal nerve** (aw-RIK-yuh-loh-TEM-puh-rul NURV). Affects the external ear and skin above the temple, up to the top of the skull.
- **Infraorbital nerve** (in-fruh-OR-bih-tul NURV). Affects the skin of the lower eyelid, side of the nose, upper lip, and mouth.
- **Infratrochlear nerve** (in-frah-TRAHK-lee-ur NURV). Affects the membrane and skin of the nose.
- **Mental nerve** (MEN-tul NURV). Affects the skin of the lower lip and chin.
- **Nasal nerve** (NAY-zul NURV). Affects the point and lower side of the nose.
- **Supraorbital nerve** (soo-pruh-OR-bih-tul NURV). Affects the skin of the forehead, scalp, eyebrow, and upper eyelid.

- **Supratrochlear nerve** (soo-pruh-TRAHK-lee-ur NURV). Affects the skin between the eyes and upper side of the nose.
- **Zygomatic nerve** (zy-goh-MAT-ik NURV). Affects the muscles of the upper part of the cheek.

The **seventh cranial nerve**, also known as **facial nerve**, is the chief motor nerve of the face. Its divisions and their branches supply and control all the muscles of facial expression. It emerges near the lower part of the ear and extends to the muscles of the neck. The following are the most important branches of the facial nerve:

- **Posterior auricular nerve** (poh-STEER-ee-ur aw-RIK-yuh-lur NURV). Affects the muscles behind the ear at the base of the skull.
- **Temporal nerve**. Affects the muscles of the temple, side of the forehead, eyebrow, eyelid, and upper part of the cheek.
- Zygomatic nerve (upper and lower). Affects the muscles of the upper part of the cheek.
- **Buccal nerve** (BUK-ul NURV). Affects the muscles of the mouth.
- **Marginal mandibular nerve** (MAR-jin-ul man-DIB-yuh-lur NURV). Affects the muscles of the chin and lower lip.
- **Cervical nerves** (SUR-vih-kul NURVS). Affect the side of the neck and the platysma muscle. Cervical nerves originate at the spinal cord, and their branches supply the muscles and scalp at the back of the head and neck as follows:
  - **Greater occipital nerve**. Located in the back of the head; affects the scalp as far up as the top of the head.
  - **Smaller occipital nerve**, also known as **lesser occipital nerve**. Located at the base of the skull; affects the scalp and muscles behind the ear.
  - **Greater auricular nerve**. Located at the side of the neck; affects the face, ears, neck, and parotid gland.
  - **Cervical cutaneous nerve** (SUR-vih-kul kyoo-TAY-nee-us NURV). Located at the side of the neck; affects the front and sides of the neck as far down as the breastbone.

The **eleventh cranial nerve**, also known as **accessory nerve**, is a motor nerve that controls the motion of the neck and shoulder muscles. This nerve is important to cosmetologists because it is affected during facials, primarily when you are giving a massage to your client.

Nerves of the Arm and Hand

The principal nerves supplying the superficial parts of the arm and hand are the following:

- **Digital nerve** (DIJ-ut-tul NURV). Sensory-motor nerve that, with its branches, supplies impulses to the fingers.

did you know?

If you did not have a central nervous system, you could not taste, smell, see, hear, think, breathe, move, run, sleep, remember, sing, laugh, or write, to name just a few things.

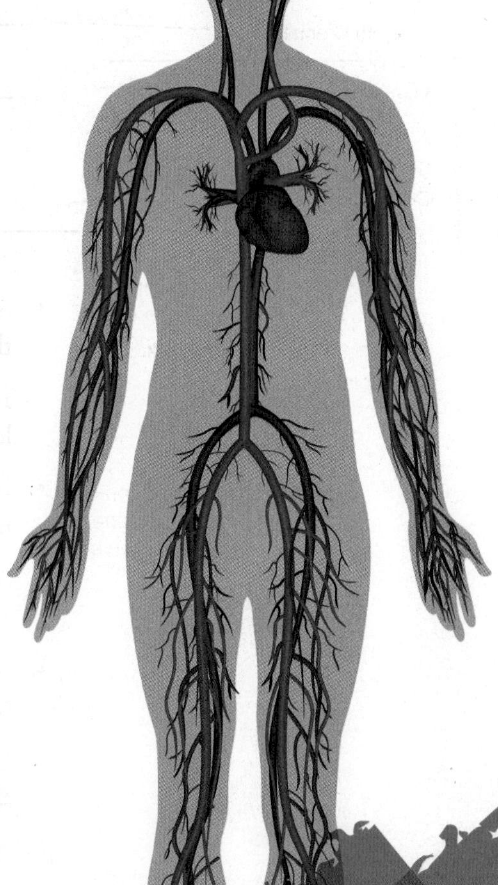

© Matthew Cole, 2010; used under license from Shutterstock.com.

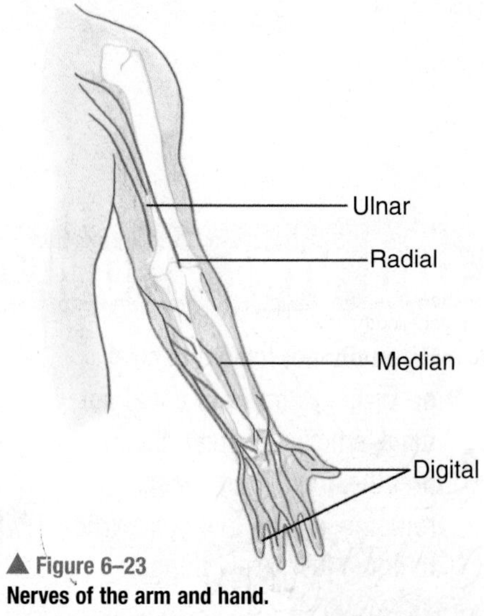

▲ Figure 6–23
Nerves of the arm and hand.

- **Radial nerve** (RAY-dee-ul NURV). Sensory-motor nerve that, with its branches, supplies the thumb side of the arm and back of the hand.
- **Median nerve** (MEE-dee-un NURV). Sensory-motor nerve that is smaller than the ulnar and radial nerves and that, with its branches, supplies the arm and hand.
- **Ulnar nerve** (UL-nur NURV). Sensory-motor nerve that, with its branches, affects the little-finger side of the arm and palm of the hand (**Figure 6–23**).

did you know?

The ulnar nerve runs along the bottom of the elbow. This explains why leaning on the elbows for long periods can cause the little fingers to go numb. This is due to localized inflammation (irritation and swelling) around the nerve.

Nerves of the Lower Leg and Foot

The nerves of the lower leg and foot are the following:

- **Tibial nerve** (TIB-ee-al NURV). Division of the sciatic nerve that passes behind the knee. It subdivides and supplies impulses to the knee, the muscles of the calf, the skin of the leg, and the sole, heel, and underside of the toes. The **sciatic nerve** (sy-AT-ik NURV) is the largest and longest nerve in the body.
- **Common peroneal nerve** (KAHM-un per-oh-NEE-al NURV). Division of the sciatic nerve that extends from behind the knee to wind around the head of the fibula to the front of the leg, where it divides into two branches.
    - **Deep peroneal nerve**, also known as **anterior tibial nerve**. Extends down the front of the leg, behind the muscles. It supplies impulses to these muscles and also to the muscles and skin on the top of the foot and adjacent sides of the first and second toes (not shown in Figure 6-24).
    - **Superficial peroneal nerve**, also known as **musculocutaneous nerve** (MUS-kyoo-loh-kyoo-TAY-nee-us NURV). Extends down the leg, just under the skin, supplying impulses to the muscles and the skin of the leg, as well as to the skin and toes on the top of the foot, where it becomes the **dorsal nerve** (DOOR-sal NURV), also known as **dorsal cutaneous nerve**. The dorsal nerve extends up from the toes and foot, just under the skin, supplying impulses to the toes and foot, as well as the muscles and skin of the leg.
- **Saphenous nerve** (sa-FEEN-us NURV). Supplies impulses to the skin of the inner side of the leg and foot. The saphenous nerve begins in the thigh.
- **Sural nerve** (SUR-ul NURV). Supplies impulses to the skin on the outer side and back of the foot and leg (**Figure 6–24**).

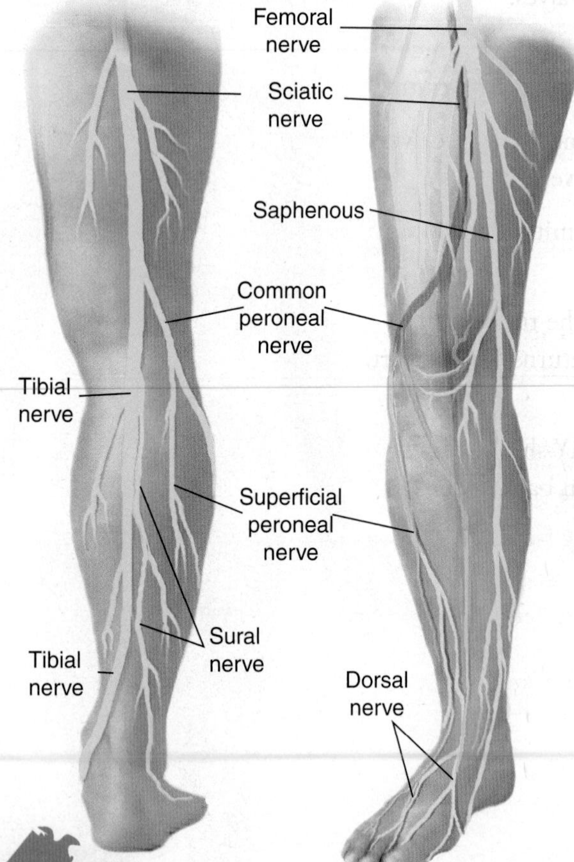

◀ Figure 6–24
Nerves of the lower leg and foot.

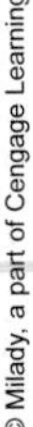
© Milady, a part of Cengage Learning.

The Circulatory System

The **circulatory system**, also known as **cardiovascular system** (KAHRD-ee-oh-VAS-kyoo-lur SIS-tum) or **vascular system**, controls the steady circulation of the blood through the body by means of the heart and blood vessels. The circulatory system consists of the heart, arteries, veins, and capillaries that distribute blood throughout the body.

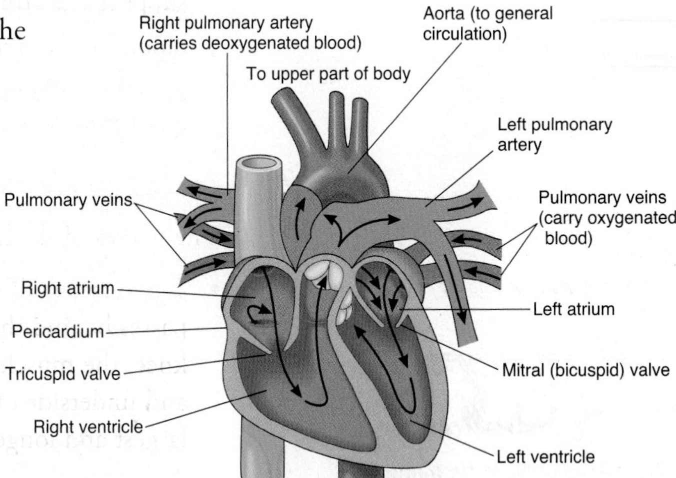

© Milady, a part of Cengage Learning.

The Heart

The **heart** is a muscular, cone-shaped organ that keeps the blood moving within the circulatory system. It is often referred to as the body's pump. The heart is enclosed by a double-layered membranous sac known as the **pericardium** (payr-ih-KAR-dee-um), which is made of epithelial tissue.

The heart is approximately the size of a closed fist, weighs about nine ounces, and is located in the chest cavity. The heartbeat is regulated by the vagus (tenth cranial) nerve and other nerves in the autonomic nervous system. A normal adult heart beats about 60 to 80 times per minute, but it can beat as high as 100 times per minute.

The interior of the heart contains four chambers and four valves.

The **atrium** (AY-tree-um) is an upper, thin-walled chamber through which blood is pumped to the ventricles. There is a right atrium and a left atrium.

The **ventricle** (VEN-truh-kul) is a lower, thick-walled chamber that receives blood from the atrium. There is a right ventricle and a left ventricle.

Valves are structures that temporarily close a passage or permit blood flow in only one direction.

The blood is in constant and continuous circulation from the time that it leaves the heart, is distributed throughout the body, then returns to the heart. Two systems attend to this circulation:

- **Pulmonary circulation** (PUL-muh-nayr-ee sur-kyoo-LAY-shun). Sends the blood from the heart to the lungs to be purified, then back to the heart again.
- **Systemic circulation** (sis-TEM-ik sur-kyoo-LAY-shun), also known as **general circulation**. Carries the blood from the heart throughout the body and back to the heart.

The following is a brief explanation of how the pulmonary circulation system and the systemic circulation system work:

1. Deoxygenated (oxygen-poor) blood flows from the body into the right atrium.

2. From the right atrium, it flows through the **tricuspid valve** (try-KUS-pid VALV), a valve between the right atrium and right ventricle of the heart, into the right ventricle.
3. The right ventricle pumps the blood to the pulmonary arteries, which move the deoxygenated blood to the lungs. When the blood reaches the lungs, it releases the waste gas (carbon dioxide) and receives oxygen. The blood is then considered to be oxygen rich.
4. The oxygen-rich blood returns to the heart through the pulmonary veins and enters the left atrium.
5. From the left atrium, the blood flows through the **mitral valve** (MYE-tral VALV), also known as **bicuspid valve** (by-KUS-pid VALV), the valve between the left atrium and the left ventricle of the heart, into the left ventricle.
6. The blood then leaves the left ventricle and travels throughout the body (**Figure 6–25**).

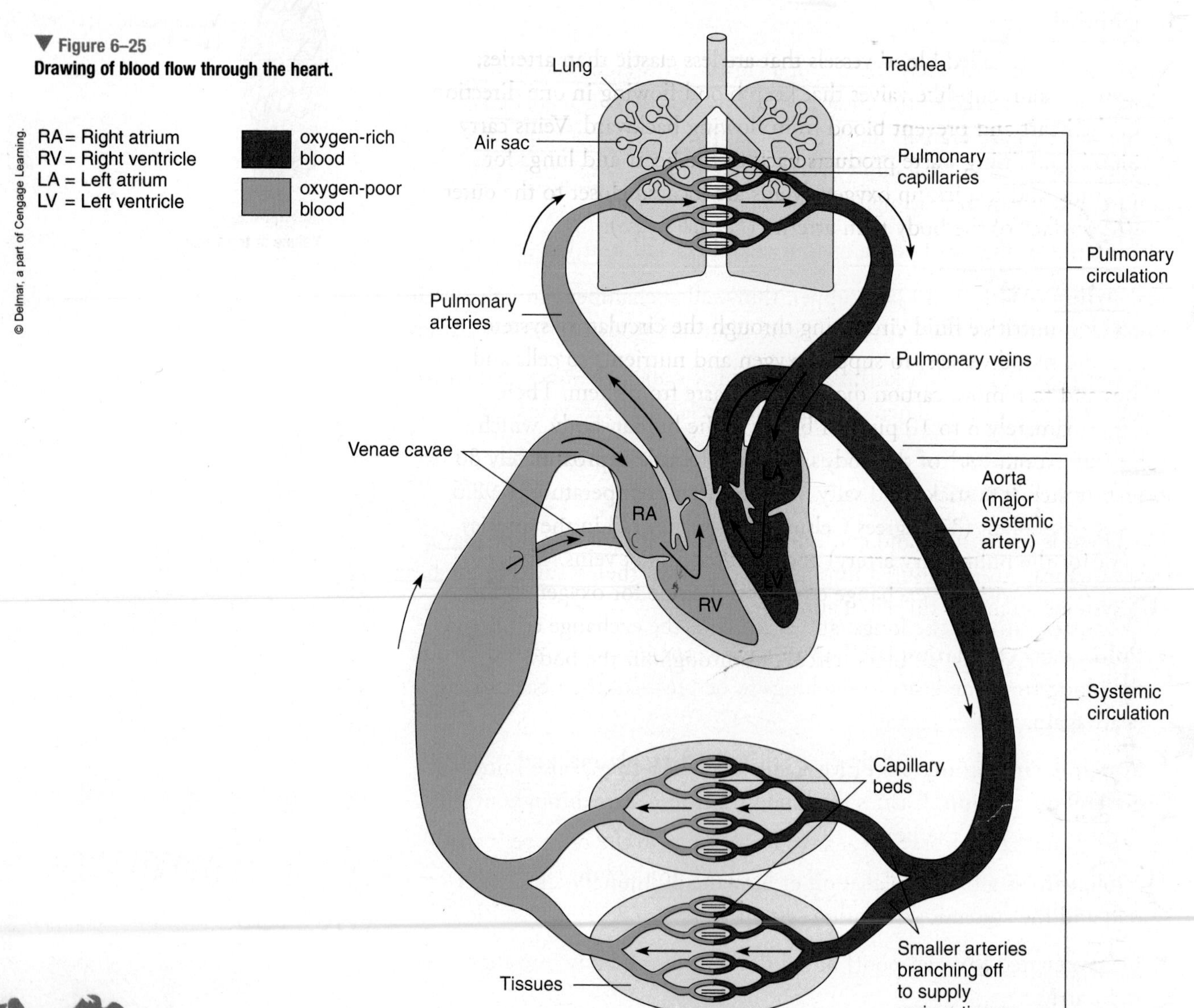

▼ **Figure 6–25**
Drawing of blood flow through the heart.

© Delmar, a part of Cengage Learning.

Blood Vessels

The **blood vessels** are tube-like structures that include the arteries, arterioles, capillaries, venules, and veins. The function of these vessels is to transport blood to and from the heart and then to various tissues of the body. The types of blood vessels found in the body are:

- **Arteries** (AR-tuh-rees). Thick-walled, muscular, flexible tubes that carry oxygenated blood away from the heart to the arterioles. The largest artery in the body is the **aorta** (ay-ORT-uh).
- **Arterioles** (ar-TEER-ee-ohls). Small arteries that deliver blood to capillaries.
- **Capillaries**. Tiny, thin-walled blood vessels that connect the smaller arteries to venules. Capillaries bring nutrients to the cells and carry away waste materials.
- **Venules** (VEEN-yools). Small vessels that connect the capillaries to the veins. They collect blood from the capillaries and drain it into the veins.
- **Veins**. Thin-walled blood vessels that are less elastic than arteries; veins contain cup-like valves that keep blood flowing in one direction to the heart and prevent blood from flowing backward. Veins carry blood containing waste products back to the heart and lungs for cleaning and to pick up oxygen. Veins are located closer to the outer skin surface of the body than arteries (**Figure 6–26**).

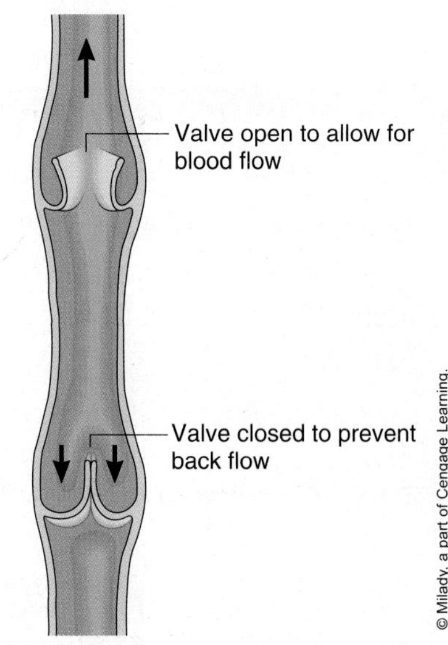

© Milady, a part of Cengage Learning.

▲ **Figure 6–26**
Valves in the veins.

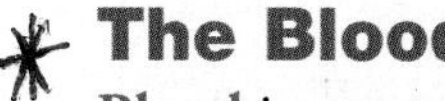

The Blood

Blood is a nutritive fluid circulating through the circulatory system (heart and blood vessels) to supply oxygen and nutrients to cells and tissues and to remove carbon dioxide and waste from them. There are approximately 8 to 10 pints of blood in the human body, which contribute about 1⁄20th of the body's weight. Blood is approximately 80 percent water. It is sticky and salty, with a normal temperature of 98.6 degrees Fahrenheit (37 degrees Celsius). It is bright red in the arteries (except for the pulmonary artery) and dark red in the veins. The color change occurs with the exchange of carbon dioxide for oxygen as the blood passes through the lungs, and again with the exchange of oxygen for carbon dioxide as the blood circulates throughout the body.

Composition of the Blood

Blood is composed of red and white cells, platelets, plasma, and hemoglobin.

- **Red blood cells**. Carry oxygen from the lungs to the body cells and transport carbon dioxide from the cells back to the lungs. Red blood cells contain **hemoglobin** (HEE-muh-gloh-bun), a complex iron protein that binds to oxygen. Hemoglobin gives blood color.

- **White blood cells**, also known as **white corpuscles** (WHYT KOR-pus-uls) or **leukocytes** (LOO-koh-syts). Perform the function of destroying disease-causing toxins and bacteria.
- **Platelets** (PLAYT-lets). Contribute to the blood-clotting process, which stops bleeding. Platelets are much smaller than red blood cells.
- **Plasma** (PLAZ-muh). Fluid part of the blood in which the red and white blood cells and platelets flow. Plasma is about 90 percent water and contains proteins and sugars. The main function of plasma is to carry food and other useful substances to the cells and to take carbon dioxide away from the cells.

did you know?

An adult heart beats about 30 million times a year and pumps nearly 4,000 gallons of blood every day.

Chief Functions of the Blood

Blood performs the following critical functions:

- Carries water, oxygen, and food to all cells and tissues of the body.
- Carries away carbon dioxide and waste products to be eliminated through the lungs, skin, kidneys, and large intestines.
- Helps to equalize the body's temperature, thus protecting the body from extreme heat and cold.
- Works with the immune system to protect the body from harmful toxins and bacteria.
- Seals leaks found in injured blood vessels by forming clots, thus preventing further blood loss.

Arteries of the Head, Face, and Neck

The **common carotid arteries** (KAHM-un kuh-RAHT-ud ART-uh-rees) are the main arteries that supply blood to the head, face, and neck. They are located on both sides of the neck, and each artery is divided into an internal and external branch.

did you know?

Adults have over 60,000 miles of blood vessels in their bodies. If you tied all of your blood vessels together, they would go around the Earth about two and one-half times!

The **internal carotid artery** supplies blood to the brain, eyes, eyelids, forehead, nose, and internal ear. The **external carotid artery** supplies blood to the anterior (front) parts of the scalp, ear, face, neck, and sides of the head (**Figure 6–27**).

Two branches of the internal carotid artery that are important to know are the following:

- **Supraorbital artery** (soo-pruh-OR-bih-tul). Supplies blood to the upper eyelid and forehead.
- **Infraorbital artery** (in-frah-OR-bih-tul). Supplies blood to the muscles of the eye.

There are four branches of the external carotid artery—the facial artery, the superficial temporal artery, the occipital artery, and the posterior auricular artery.

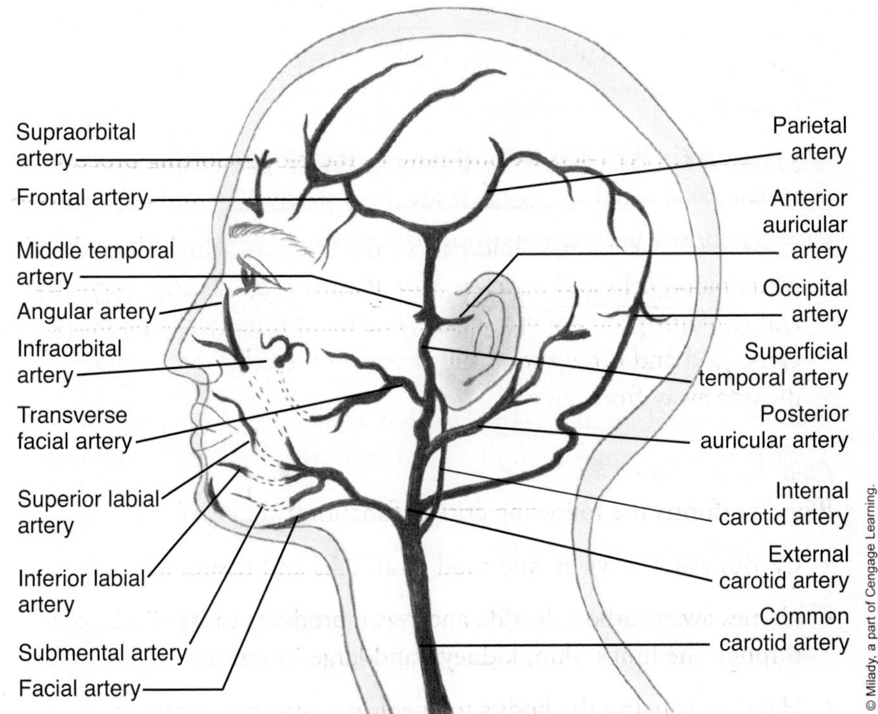

◀ **Figure 6–27**
Arteries of the head, face, and neck.

Read

✱ The **facial artery**, also known as the **external maxillary artery** (eks-TUR-nul MAK-sah-lair-ee ART-uh-ree). Supplies blood to the lower region of the face, mouth, and nose. Some of the important facial artery branches include:

- **Submental artery** (sub-MEN-tul ART-uh-ree). Supplies blood to the chin and lower lip.
- **Inferior labial artery** (in-FEER-ee-ur LAY-bee-ul ART-ur-ee). Supplies blood to the lower lip.
- **Angular artery** (ANG-gyoo-lur ART-ur-ee). Supplies blood to the side of the nose.
- **Superior labial artery**. Supplies blood to the upper lip and region of the nose.

The **superficial temporal artery** is a continuation of the external carotid artery and supplies blood to the muscles of the front, side, and top of the head. Some of the important superficial temporal artery branches include:

- **Frontal artery**. Supplies blood to the forehead and upper eyelids.
- **Parietal artery**. Supplies blood to the side and crown of the head.
- **Transverse facial artery** (tranz-VURS FAY-shul ART-ur-ee). Supplies blood to the skin and masseter muscle.
- **Middle temporal artery**. Supplies blood to the temples.
- **Anterior auricular artery**. Supplies blood to the front part of the ear.

The **occipital artery** supplies blood to the skin and muscles of the scalp and back of the head up to the crown.

The **posterior auricular artery** supplies blood to the scalp, the area behind and above the ear, and the skin behind the ear.

Veins of the Head, Face, and Neck

The blood returning to the heart from the head, face, and neck flows on each side of the neck in two principal veins:

- The **internal jugular vein** (in-TUR-nul JUG-yuh-lur VAYN) is located at the side of the neck to collect blood from the brain and parts of the face and neck.
- The **external jugular vein** is located at the side of the neck and carries blood returning to the heart from the head, face, and neck.

The most important veins of the face and neck are parallel to the arteries and take the same names as the arteries.

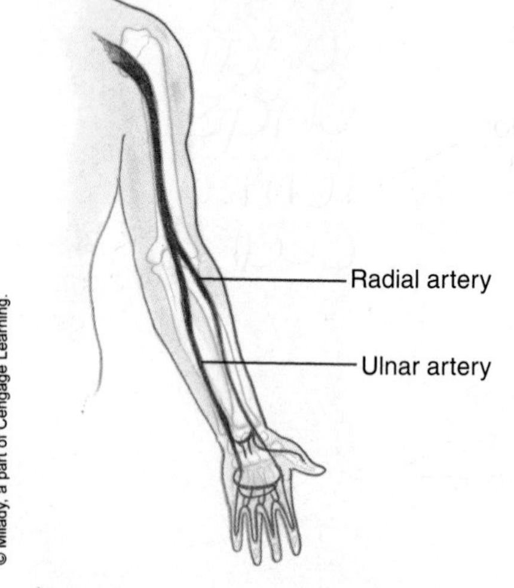

© Milady, a part of Cengage Learning.

▲ **Figure 6–28**
Arteries of the arm and hand.

Blood Supply to the Arm and Hand

The ulnar and radial arteries are the main blood supply of the arms and hands.

The **ulnar artery** and its numerous branches supply blood to the little-finger side of the arm and palm of the hand.

The **radial artery** and its branches supply blood to the thumb side of the arm and the back of the hand; the radial artery also supplies blood to the muscles of the skin, hands, fingers, wrist, elbow, and forearm.

While the arteries are found deep in the tissues, the veins lie nearer to the surface of the arms and hands (**Figure 6–28**).

Blood Supply to the Lower Leg and Foot

The major arteries that supply blood to the lower leg and foot are the popliteal artery and its branches and the dorsalis pedis artery.

The **popliteal artery** (pop-lih-TEE-ul ART-uh-ree), which supplies blood to the foot, divides into two separate arteries known as the anterior tibial artery and the posterior tibial artery.

- **Anterior tibial artery** (an-TEER-ee-ur TIB-ee-al ART-uh-ree). Supplies blood to the lower leg muscles and to the muscles and skin on the top of the foot and adjacent sides of the first and second toes. This artery continues to the foot, where it becomes the dorsalis pedis artery.
- **Posterior tibial artery** (poh-STEER-ee-ur TIB-ee-al ART-uh-ree). Supplies blood to the ankle and the back of the lower leg.

The **dorsalis pedis artery** (DOR-sul-is PEED-us ART-uh-ree) supplies blood to the foot.

As in the arms and hand, the important veins of the lower leg and foot are almost parallel with the arteries and take the same names (**Figure 6–29**).

The Lymphatic/Immune System

The **lymphatic/immune system** (lim-FAT-ik ih-MYOON SIS-tum) is made up of lymph, lymph nodes, the thymus gland, the spleen, and lymph vessels. The lymphatic/immune system carries waste and impurities away from the cells and protects the body from disease by developing immunities and destroying disease-causing microorganisms. **Lymph** (LIMF) is a clear fluid that circulates in the lymph spaces (lymphatics) of the body. Lymph helps carry wastes and impurities away from the cells before it is routed back to the circulatory system. The lymphatic/immune system drains the tissue spaces of excess **interstitial fluid** (in-tur-STISH-al FLOO-id), which is blood plasma found in the spaces between tissue cells. The lymphatic/immune system is closely connected to the cardiovascular system. They both transport streams of fluids, like rivers throughout the body. The difference is that the lymphatic/immune system transports lymph, which eventually returns to the blood where it originated.

Lymphatic vessels start as tubes that are closed at one end. They can occur individually or in clusters that are called **lymph capillaries**, blind-end tubes that are the origin of lymphatic vessels. The lymph capillaries are distributed throughout most of the body (except the nervous system). **Lymph nodes** are gland-like structures found inside lymphatic vessels. Lymph nodes filter the lymphatic vessels, which helps fight infection.

The primary functions of the lymphatic/immune system are to:

- Carry nourishment from the blood to the body cells.
- Act as a defense against toxins and bacteria.
- Remove waste material from the body cells to the blood.
- Provide a suitable fluid environment for the cells.

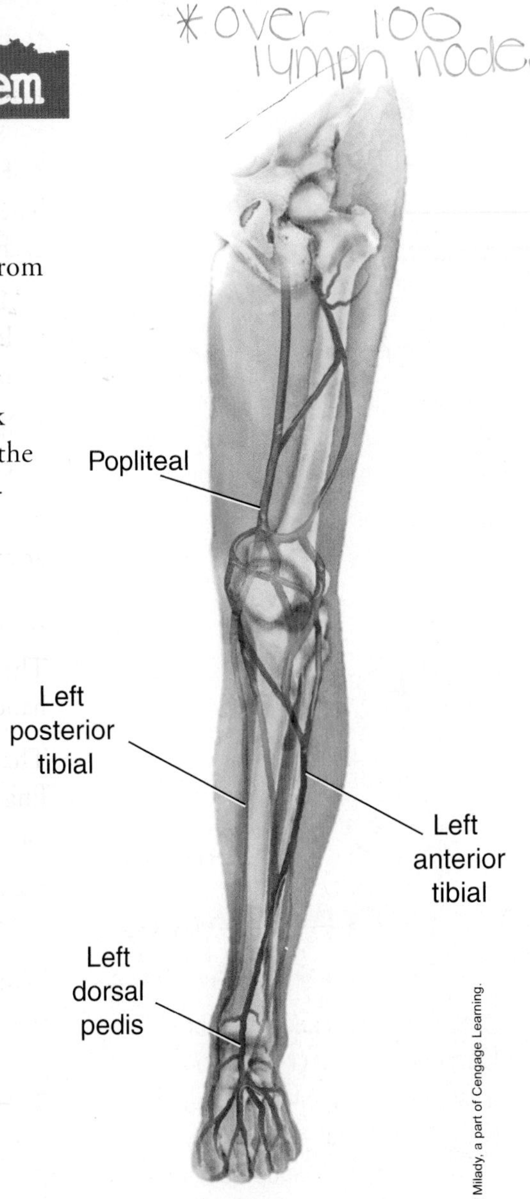

Popliteal
Left posterior tibial
Left anterior tibial
Left dorsal pedis

© Milady, a part of Cengage Learning.

▲ **Figure 6–29**
Arteries of the lower leg and foot (left leg view).

The Endocrine System

The **endocrine system** (EN-duh-krin SIS-tum) is a group of specialized glands that affect the growth, development, sexual functions, and health of the entire body. **Glands** are secretory organs that remove and release certain elements from the blood to convert them into new compounds.

There are two main types of glands:

- **Endocrine glands**, also known as **ductless glands**, such as the thyroid and pituitary glands, release hormonal secretions directly into the bloodstream.

- **Exocrine glands** (EK-suh-krin GLANDZ), also known as **duct glands**, such as sweat and oil glands of the skin, produce a substance that travels through small, tube-like ducts.
- **Hormones** (HOR-mohnz) are secretions, such as insulin, adrenaline, and estrogen, that stimulate functional activity or other secretions in the body. Hormones influence the welfare of the entire body.

did you know?

Hormones are actually chemicals. There are over 30 hormones telling your body what it should do every day.

The endocrine glands and their functions are as follows:

- **Pineal gland** (PY-nee-ul GLAND). Plays a major role in sexual development, sleep, and metabolism.
- **Pituitary gland** (puh-TOO-uh-tair-ee GLAND). Most complex organ of the endocrine system. This gland affects almost every physiologic process of the body: growth, blood pressure, contractions during childbirth, breast-milk production, sexual organ functions in both women and men, thyroid gland function, and the conversion of food into energy (metabolism).
- **Thyroid gland** (THY-royd GLAND). Controls how quickly the body burns energy (metabolism), makes proteins, and how sensitive the body should be to other hormones.
- **Parathyroid glands** (payr-uh-THY-royd GLANDZ). Regulate blood calcium and phosphorus levels so that the nervous and muscular systems can function properly.
- **Pancreas** (PANG-kree-us). Secretes enzyme-producing cells that are responsible for digesting carbohydrates, proteins, and fats. The islet of Langerhans cells within the pancreas control insulin and glucagon production.
- **Adrenal glands** (uh-DREEN-ul GLANDZ). Secrete about 30 steroid hormones and control metabolic processes of the body, including the fight-or-flight response.
- **Ovaries** (OH-vah-reez) (singular: ovary). Female sexual glands; function in reproduction, as well as determining female sexual characteristics (**Figure 6–30**).
- **Testes** (TES-teez) (singular: testicle). Male sexual glands; function in reproduction, as well as determining male sexual characteristics (**Figure 6–30**).

did you know?

The endocrine glands and the hormones they secrete have a tremendous influence on your body. They affect sleep, digestion, growth, sexual development, and many other important functions. You can see that endocrine glands are as important to us as our brain.

The Digestive System

The **digestive system** (dy-JES-tiv SIS-tum), also known as **gastrointestinal system** (gas-troh-in-TES-tun-ul SIS-tum), is responsible for breaking down foods into nutrients and waste. The digestive system consists of the mouth, stomach, intestines, salivary and gastric glands, and other organs.

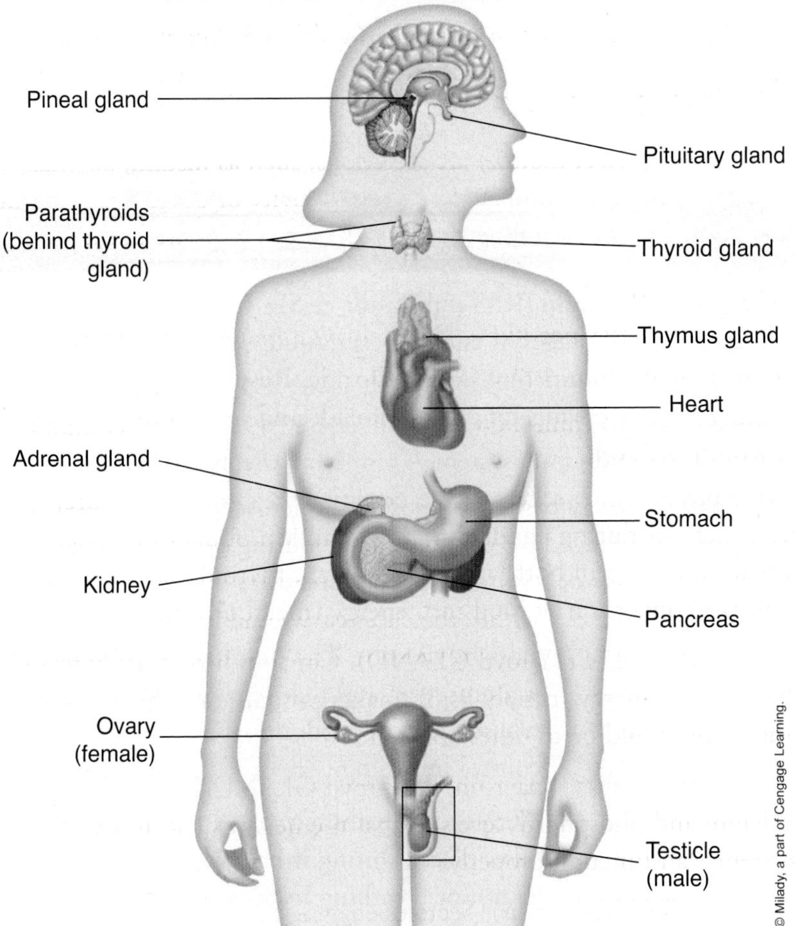

Figure 6–30
Endocrine glands and other body organs.

did you know?

The average adult has about 25 feet of intestines. In your lifetime, your digestive system handles about 50 tons of food.

Digestive enzymes (dy-JES-tiv EN-zymz) are chemicals that change certain types of food into a soluble (capable of being dissolved) form that can be used by the body. The food, in soluble form, is transported by the bloodstream and used by the body's cells and tissues. The entire food digestion process takes about nine hours to complete.

did you know?

Your kidneys make sure that your blood is not too thick or too thin and is not overloaded with wastes made by other parts of your body. About 440 gallons of blood flow through your kidneys every day.

The Excretory System

The **excretory system** (EK-skre-tor-ee SIS-tum) is a group of organs, including the kidneys, liver, skin, large intestine, and lungs, that are responsible for purifying the body by eliminating waste matter. The metabolism of body cells forms toxic substances that, if retained, could poison the body.

Each of the following organs plays a crucial function in the excretory system:

- The kidneys excrete urine (water and waste products).
- The liver discharges toxins produced during digestion.
- The skin eliminates waste through perspiration.

- The large intestine eliminates decomposed and undigested food.
- The lungs exhale carbon dioxide.

did you know?

Your lungs contain almost 1,500 miles of airways that enable you to breathe. Every minute you breathe in about 13 pints of air.

The Respiratory System

The **respiratory system** (RES-puh-ra-tor-ee SIS-tum) consists of the lungs and air passages; it enables respiration, supplying the body with oxygen and eliminating carbon dioxide. **Respiration**, the act of breathing, is the exchange of carbon dioxide and oxygen in the lungs and within each cell.

The **lungs** are spongy tissues composed of microscopic cells in which inhaled air is exchanged for carbon dioxide during one breathing cycle. They are the organs of respiration. The respiratory system is located within the chest cavity and is protected on both sides by the ribs. The **diaphragm** (DY-uh-fram) is a muscular wall that separates the thorax (chest) from the abdominal region and helps control breathing.

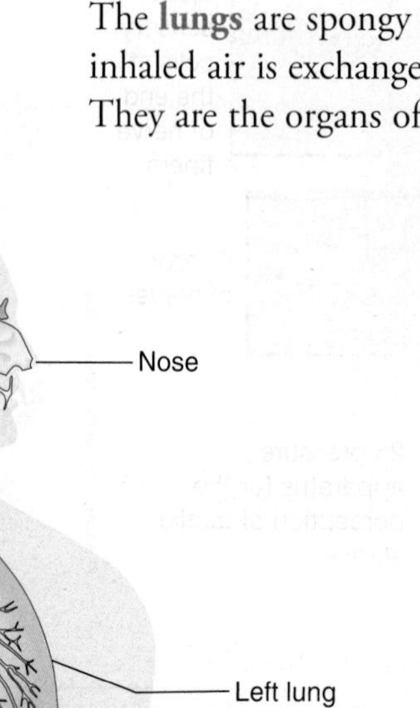

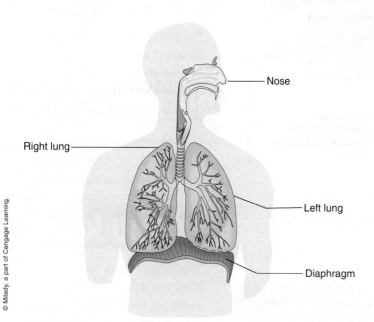

© Milady, a part of Cengage Learning.

▲ **Figure 6–31**
The respiratory system.

With each breathing cycle, an exchange of gases takes place. During **inhalation** (in-huh-LAY-shun), or breathing in through the nose or mouth, oxygen is passed into the blood. During **exhalation** (eks-huh-LAY-shun), or breathing outward, carbon dioxide (collected from the blood) is expelled from the lungs.

Oxygen is more essential than either food or water. People may survive for more than sixty days without food and several days without water. If they are deprived of oxygen, they will die within a few minutes (**Figure 6–31**).

The Integumentary System

The **integumentary system** (in-TEG-yuh-ment-uh-ree SIS-tum) consists of the skin and its accessory organs, such as the oil and sweat glands, sensory receptors, hair, and nails. It is a very complex system that serves as a protective covering and helps regulate the body's temperature (**Figure 6–32**).

The word *integument* means a natural covering. So you can think of the skin as a protective overcoat for your body against the outside elements that you encounter every day, such as germs, chemicals, and sun exposure. Skin is also water-resistant.

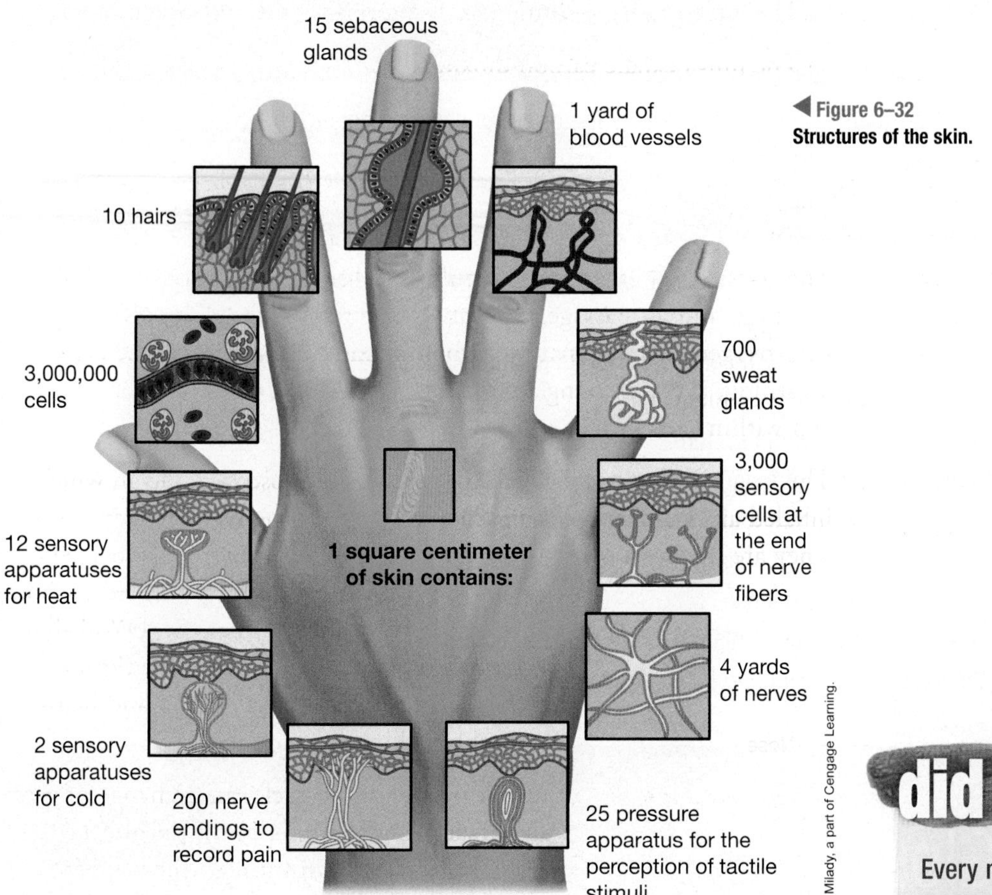

◀ **Figure 6–32**
Structures of the skin.

Skin structure and growth are discussed in detail in Chapter 7, Skin Structure, Growth, and Nutrition.

did you know?

Every minute you shed about 30,000 to 40,000 dead skin cells from your body. That can total up to about 40 pounds of skin in your lifetime!

The Reproductive System

The **reproductive system** (ree-proh-DUK-tiv SIS-tum) includes the ovaries, uterine tubes, uterus, and vagina in the female and the testes, prostate gland, penis, and urethra in the male. This system performs the function of producing offspring and passing on the genetic code from one generation to another.

The reproductive system produces hormones—primarily estrogen in females and primarily testosterone in males. These hormones affect and change the skin in several ways. Acne, loss of scalp hair, facial hair growth and color, and darker skin pigmentations are some of the results of changing or fluctuating hormones. Fortunately, cosmetologists have access to many products and treatments that can address unwanted changes of this nature and help clients feel more comfortable and confident about themselves. This is one more example of how important your role is in your clients' lives.

Review Questions

1. Why is the study of anatomy, physiology, and histology important to cosmetologists?
2. Define anatomy, physiology, and histology.
3. Name and describe the basic structures of a cell.
4. Explain cell metabolism and its purpose.
5. List and describe the functions of the four types of tissue found in the human body.
6. What are organs?
7. List and describe the functions of the 9 major organs found in the body.
8. Name the 11 main body systems and their functions.
9. List the primary functions of the skeletal system.
10. Name and describe the three types of muscular tissue found in the body.
11. Name and describe the types of nerves found in the body and how they react.
12. Name and briefly describe the types of blood vessels found in the body.
13. List and describe the composition of blood.
14. Name and discuss the two main types of glands found in the human body.
15. List the organs of the excretory system and their functions.

Chapter Glossary

abductor digiti minimi	Muscle that separates the fingers and the toes.
abductor hallucis	Muscle that moves the toes and helps maintain balance while walking and standing.
abductors	Muscles that draw a body part, such as a finger, arm, or toe, away from the midline of the body or of an extremity.
adductors	Muscles that draw a body part, such as a finger, arm, or toe, inward toward the median axis of the body or of an extremity.
adipose tissue	Technical term for fat; gives smoothness and contour to the body.
adrenal glands	Glands of the endocrine system that secrete about 30 steroid hormones and control metabolic processes of the body, including the fight-or-flight response.
anabolism	Constructive metabolism, the process of building up larger molecules from smaller ones.
anatomy	Study of human body structures that can be seen with the naked eye and how the body parts are organized; the science of the structure of organisms or of their parts.
angular artery	Branch of the facial artery that supplies blood to the side of the nose.
anterior auricular artery	Branch of the superficial temporal artery that supplies blood to the front part of the ear.
anterior tibial artery	One of the popliteal arteries (the other is the posterior tibial artery) that supplies blood to the lower leg muscles and to the muscles and skin on the top of the foot and adjacent sides of the first and second toes. This artery continues to the foot where it becomes the dorsalis pedis artery.

Chapter Glossary

aorta	The largest artery in the body.
arteries	Thick-walled, muscular, flexible tubes that carry oxygenated blood away from the heart to the arterioles.
arterioles	Small arteries that deliver blood to capillaries.
atrium	Upper, thin-walled chamber of the heart through which blood is pumped to the ventricles. There is a right atrium and a left atrium.
auricularis anterior	Muscle in front of the ear that draws the ear forward.
auricularis posterior	Muscle behind the ear that draws the ear backward.
auricularis superior	Muscle above the ear that draws the ear upward.
auriculotemporal nerve	Branch of the fifth cranial nerve that affects the external ear and skin above the temple, up to the top of the skull.
autonomic nervous system	Abbreviated ANS; the part of the nervous system that controls the involuntary muscles; regulates the action of the smooth muscles, glands, blood vessels, heart, and breathing.
axon	The extension of a neuron through which impulses are sent away from the body to other neurons, glands, or muscles.
axon terminal	The extension of a neuron through which impulses are sent away from the body to other neurons, glands, or muscles.
belly	Middle part of the muscle.
bicep	Muscle that produces the contour of the front and inner side of the upper arm; lifts the forearm and flexes the elbow.
blood	Nutritive fluid circulating through the circulatory system (heart and blood vessels) to supply oxygen and nutrients to cells and tissues and to remove carbon dioxide and waste from them.
blood vessels	Tube-like structures that include arteries, arterioles, capillaries, venules, and veins.
body systems	Also known as *systems*; groups of body organs acting together to perform one or more functions. The human body is composed of 11 major systems.
brain	Part of the central nervous system contained in the cranium; largest and most complex nerve tissue and controls sensation, muscles, activity of glands, and the power to think, sense, and feel.
buccal nerve	Branch of the seventh cranial nerve that affects the muscles of the mouth.
buccinator muscle	Thin, flat muscle of the cheek between the upper and lower jaw that compresses the cheeks and expels air between the lips.
capillaries	Tiny, thin-walled blood vessels that connect the smaller arteries to the venules. Capillaries bring nutrients to the cells and carry away waste materials.
cardiac muscle	The involuntary muscle that is the heart. This type of muscle is not found in any other part of the body.
carpus	Also known as *wrist*; flexible joint composed of a group of eight small, irregular bones (carpals) held together by ligaments.

Chapter Glossary

catabolism	The phase of metabolism that involves the breaking down of complex compounds within the cells into smaller ones. This process releases energy that has been stored.
cell membrane	Cell part that encloses the protoplasm and permits soluble substances to enter and leave the cell.
cells	Basic units of all living things, from bacteria to plants to animals, including human beings.
central nervous system	Abbreviated CNS; consists of the brain, spinal cord, spinal nerves, and cranial nerves.
centrioles	Structures in a cell near the nucleus that move to each side during the mitosis process to help divide the cell.
cervical cutaneous nerve	Cervical nerve located at the side of the neck; affects the front and sides of the neck as far down as the breastbone.
cervical nerves	Branches of the seventh cranial nerve; originate at the spinal cord and affect the side of the neck and the platysma muscle.
cervical vertebrae	The seven bones of the top part of the vertebral column, located in the neck region.
circulatory system	Also known as *cardiovascular system* or *vascular system*; body system that controls the steady circulation of the blood through the body by means of the heart and blood vessels.
clavicle	Also known as *collarbone*; bone that joins the sternum and scapula.
common carotid arteries	Main arteries that supply blood to the head, face, and neck.
common peroneal nerve	A division of the sciatic nerve that extends from behind the knee to wind around the head of the fibula to the front of the leg where it divides into two branches.
connective tissue	Fibrous tissue that binds together, protects, and supports the various parts of the body. Examples of connective tissue are bone, cartilage, ligaments, tendons, blood, lymph, and fat (see adipose tissue).
corrugator muscle	Muscle located beneath the frontalis and orbicularis oculi muscles that draws the eyebrow down and wrinkles the forehead vertically.
cranium	An oval, bony case that protects the brain.
cytoplasm	The protoplasm of a cell, except for the protoplasm in the nucleus, that surrounds the nucleus; the watery fluid that cells need for growth, reproduction, and self-repair.
deep peroneal nerve	Also known as *anterior tibial nerve*; extends down the front of the leg, behind the muscles. It supplies impulses to these muscles and also to the muscles and skin on the top of the foot and adjacent sides of the first and second toes.
deltoid	Large, triangular muscle covering the shoulder joint that allows the arm to extend outward and to the side of the body.
dendrites	Tree-like branching of nerve fibers extending from the nerve cell; carry impulses toward the cell and receive impulses from other neurons.
depressor labii inferioris muscle	Also known as *quadratus labii inferioris muscle*; muscle surrounding the lower lip; lowers the lower lip and draws it to one side, as in expressing sarcasm.
diaphragm	Muscular wall that separates the thorax from the abdominal region and helps control breathing.

Chapter Glossary

digestive enzymes	Chemicals that change certain types of food into a soluble (capable of being dissolved) form that can be used by the body.
digestive system	Also known as *gastrointestinal system*; body system that is responsible for breaking down foods into nutrients and wastes; consists of the mouth, stomach, intestines, salivary and gastric glands, and other organs.
digital nerve	Sensory-motor nerve that, with its branches, supplies impulses to the fingers.
dorsal nerve	Also known as *dorsal cutaneous nerve*; a nerve that extends up from the toes and foot, just under the skin, supplying impulses to toes and foot, as well as the muscles and skin of the leg, where it is becomes the superficial peroneal nerve.
dorsalis pedis artery	Artery that supplies blood to the foot.
eleventh cranial nerve	Also known as *accessory nerve*; a motor nerve that controls the motion of the neck and shoulder muscles.
endocrine glands	Also known as *ductless glands*; glands such as the thyroid and pituitary gland that release hormonal secretions directly into the bloodstream.
endocrine system	Body system consisting of a group of specialized glands that affect the growth, development, sexual functions, and health of the entire body.
epicranial aponeurosis	Tendon that connects the occipitalis and frontalis muscles.
epicranius	Also known as *occipitofrontalis*; the broad muscle that covers the top of the skull and consists of the occipitalis and frontalis.
epithelial tissue	Protective covering on body surfaces, such as skin, mucous membranes, the tissue inside the mouth, the lining of the heart, digestive and respiratory organs, and the glands.
ethmoid bone	Light spongy bone between the eye sockets; forms part of the nasal cavities.
excretory system	Body system that consists of a group of organs, including the kidneys, liver, skin, large intestine, and lungs, that are responsible for purifying the body by eliminating waste matter.
exhalation	Breathing outward; expelling carbon dioxide (collected from the blood) from the lungs.
exocrine glands	Also known as *duct glands*; produce a substance that travels through small tube-like ducts; sweat glands and oil glands of the skin belong to this group.
extensor digitorum longus	Muscle that bends the foot up and extends the toes.
extensor hallucis longus	Muscle that extends the big toe and flexes the foot.
extensors	Muscles that straighten the wrist, hand, and fingers to form a straight line.
external carotid artery	Artery that supplies blood to the anterior (front) parts of the scalp, ear, face, neck, and sides of the head.
external jugular vein	Vein located at the side of the neck that carries blood returning to the heart from the head, face, and neck.
eyes	Body organs that control the body's vision.
facial artery	Also known as *external maxillary artery*; branch of the external carotid artery that supplies blood to the lower region of the face, mouth, and nose.

Chapter Glossary

facial skeleton	Framework of the face composed of 14 bones.
femur	Heavy, long bone that forms the leg above the knee.
fibula	Smaller of the two bones that form the leg below the knee. The fibula may be visualized as a bump on the little-toe side of the ankle.
fifth cranial nerve	Also known as *trifacial nerve* or *trigeminal nerve*; the chief sensory nerve of the face that serves as the motor nerve of the muscles that control chewing.
flexor digiti minimi	Muscle that moves the little toe.
flexor digitorum brevis	Muscle that moves the toes and helps maintain balance while walking and standing.
flexor	Extensor muscle of the wrist involved in flexing the wrist.
frontal artery	Branch of the superficial temporal artery that supplies blood to the forehead and upper eyelids.
frontal bone	Bone that forms the forehead.
frontalis	Front (anterior) portion of the epicranius; muscle of the scalp that raises the eyebrows, draws the scalp forward, and causes wrinkles across the forehead.
gastrocnemius	Muscle attached to the lower rear surface of the heel and pulls the foot down.
glands	Organs that remove and release certain elements from the blood to convert them into new compounds.
greater auricular nerve	Cervical nerve that is located at the side of the neck; affects the face, ears, neck, and parotid gland.
greater occipital nerve	Cervical nerve that is located in the back of the head; affects the scalp as far up as the top of the head.
heart	Muscular, cone-shaped organ that keeps the blood moving within the circulatory system.
hemoglobin	Complex iron protein in red blood cells that binds to oxygen; gives blood color.
histology	Also known as *microscopic anatomy*; the study of tiny structures found in living tissues.
hormones	Secretions, such as insulin, adrenaline, and estrogen, that stimulate functional activity or other secretions in the body. Hormones influence the welfare of the entire body.
humerus	Uppermost and largest bone in the arm, extending from the elbow to the shoulder.
hyoid bone	U-shaped bone at the base of the tongue that supports the tongue and its muscles.
inferior labial artery	Branch of the facial artery that supplies blood to the lower lip.
infraorbital artery	Branch of the internal carotid artery that supplies blood to the muscles of the eye.
infraorbital nerve	Branch of the fifth cranial nerve that affects the skin of the lower eyelid, side of the nose, upper lip, and mouth.
infratrochlear nerve	Branch of the fifth cranial nerve that affects the membrane and skin of the nose.
inhalation	Breathing in through the nose or mouth.

Chapter Glossary

insertion	The movable part of the muscle that is farthest from the skeleton.
integumentary system	Body system that consists of skin and its accessory organs, such as the oil and sweat glands, sensory receptors, hair, and nails; serves as a protective covering and helps regulate the body's temperature.
internal carotid artery	Artery that supplies blood to the brain, eyes, eyelids, forehead, nose, and internal ear.
internal jugular vein	Vein located at the side of the neck to collect blood from the brain and parts of the face and neck.
interstitial fluid	Blood plasma found in the spaces between tissue cells.
intestines	Body organ that digests food, along with the stomach.
joint	Connection between two or more bones of the skeleton.
kidneys	Body organs that excrete water and waste products.
lacrimal bones	Small, thin bones located at the front inner wall of the orbits (eye sockets).
latissimus dorsi	Large, flat, triangular muscle covering the lower back.
levator anguli oris muscle	Also known as *caninus muscle*; muscle that raises the angle of the mouth and draws it inward.
levator labii superioris muscle	Also known as *quadratus labii superioris muscle*; muscle surrounding the upper lip; elevates the upper lip and dilates the nostrils, as in expressing distaste.
liver	Body organ that removes waste created by digestion.
lungs	Spongy tissues composed of microscopic cells in which inhaled air is exchanged for carbon dioxide during one breathing cycle; organs of respiration.
lymph	Clear fluid that circulates in the lymph spaces (lymphatics) of the body. Lymph helps carry wastes and impurities away from the cells before it is routed back to the circulatory system.
lymph capillaries	Blind-end tubes that are the origin of lymphatic vessels.
lymph nodes	Gland-like structures found inside lymphatic vessels; filter the lymphatic vessels and help fight infection.
lymphatic/immune system	Body system that consists of lymph, lymph nodes, the thymus gland, the spleen, and lymph vessels. It carries waste and impurities away from the cells and protects the body from disease by developing immunities and destroying disease-causing microorganisms.
mandible	Lower jawbone; largest and strongest bone of the face.
mandibular nerve	Branch of the fifth cranial nerve that affects the muscles of the chin, lower lip, and external ear.
marginal mandibular nerve	Branch of the seventh cranial nerve that affects the muscles of the chin and lower lip.
masseter	Muscles that coordinate with the temporalis and pterygoid muscles to open and close the mouth and bring the jaw forward; sometimes referred to as chewing muscles.
maxillae (singular: maxilla)	Bones of the upper jaw.

Chapter Glossary

maxillary nerve	Branch of the fifth cranial nerve that supplies impulses to the upper part of the face.
median nerve	Sensory-motor nerve that is smaller than the ulner and radial nerves and that, with its branches, supplies the arm and hand.
mental nerve	Branch of the fifth cranial nerve that affects the skin of the lower lip and chin.
mentalis muscle	Muscle that elevates the lower lip and raises and wrinkles the skin of the chin.
metabolism	Chemical process that takes place in living organisms, through which the cells are nourished and carry out their activities; metabolism has two phases: anabolism and catabolism.
metacarpus	Bones of the palm of the hand; parts of the hand containing five bones between the carpus and phalanges.
metatarsal	One of three subdivisions of the foot; long and slender bones, similar to the metacarpal bones of the hand. The other two subdivisions are the tarsal and phalanges.
middle temporal artery	Branch of the superficial temporal artery that supplies blood to the temples.
mitosis	Usual process of cell reproduction of human tissues that occurs when the cell divides into two identical cells called daughter cells.
mitral valve	Also known as *bicuspid valve*; the valve between the left atrium and the left ventricle of the heart.
motor nerves	Also known as *efferent nerves*; carry impulses from the brain to the muscles or glands.
muscle tissue	Tissue that contracts and moves various parts of the body.
muscular system	Body system that covers, shapes, and holds the skeleton system in place; muscular system contracts and moves various parts of the body.
myology	Study of the nature, structure, function, and diseases of the muscles.
nasal bones	Bones that form the bridge of the nose.
nasal nerve	Branch of the fifth cranial nerve that affects the point and lower side of the nose.
nerve tissue	Tissue that carries messages to and from the brain and controls and coordinates all bodily functions.
nerves	Whitish cords made up of bundles of nerve fibers held together by connective tissue, through which impulses are transmitted.
nervous system	Body system that consists of the brain, spinal cord, and nerves; controls and coordinates all other systems of the body and makes them work harmoniously and efficiently.
neurology	Scientific study of the structure, function, and pathology of the nervous system.
neuron	Also known as *nerve cell*; primary structural unit of the nervous system, consists of the cell body, nucleus, dendrites, and axon.
nonstriated muscles	Also known as *smooth muscles*; these muscles are involuntary and function automatically, without conscious will.

Chapter Glossary

nucleus	Dense, active protoplasm found in the center of the cell; plays an important part in cell reproduction and metabolism.
occipital artery	Branch of the external carotid artery that supplies blood to the skin and muscles of the scalp and back of the head up to the crown.
occipital bone	Hindmost bone of the skull, below the parietal bones; forms the back of the skull above the nape.
occipitalis	Back (posterior) portion of the epicranius; muscle that draws the scalp backward.
-ology	Word ending meaning *study of*.
ophthalmic nerve	Branch of the fifth cranial nerve that supplies impulses to the skin of the forehead, upper eyelids, and interior portion of the scalp, orbit, eyeball, and nasal passage.
orbicularis oculi muscle	Ring muscle of the eye socket; enables you to close your eyes.
orbicularis oris muscle	Flat band of muscle around the upper and lower lips that compresses, contracts, puckers, and wrinkles the lips.
organs	Structures composed of specialized tissues designed to perform specific functions in plants and animals.
origin	Part of the muscle that does not move; attached closest to the skeleton.
os	Bone.
osteology	The study of anatomy, structure, and function of the bones.
ovaries (singular: ovary)	Female sexual glands of the endocrine system that function in reproduction, as well as determining female sexual characteristics.
pancreas	Gland of the endocrine system that secretes enzyme-producing cells that are responsible for digesting carbohydrates, proteins, and fats.
parathyroid glands	Glands of the endocrine system that regulate blood calcium and phosphorus levels so that the nervous and muscular systems can function properly.
parietal artery	Branch of the superficial temporal artery that supplies blood to the side and crown of the head.
parietal bones	Bones that form the sides and top of the cranium.
patella	Also known as *accessory bone* or *kneecap*; forms the kneecap joint.
pectoralis major	Muscles of the chest that assist the swinging movements of the arm.
pectoralis minor	Muscles of the chest that assist the swinging movements of the arm.
pericardium	Double-layered membranous sac enclosing the heart; made of epithelial tissue.
peripheral nervous system	Abbreviated PNS; system of nerves that connects the peripheral (outer) parts of the body to the central nervous system; it has both sensory and motor nerves.
peroneus brevis	Muscle that originates on the lower surface of the fibula; bends the foot down and out.

Chapter Glossary

peroneus longus	Muscle that covers the outer side of the calf; inverts the foot and turns it outward.
phalanges (singular: phalanx)	Also known as *digits*; bones of the fingers or toes; one of the three subdivisions of the foot. The other two subdivisions are the tarsal and metatarsal.
physiology	Study of the functions and activities performed by the body's structures.
pineal gland	Endocrine system gland that plays a major role in sexual development, sleep, and metabolism.
pituitary gland	The most complex organ of the endocrine system. It affects almost every physiologic process of the body: growth, blood pressure, contractions during childbirth, breast-milk production, sexual organ functions in both women and men, thyroid gland function, and the conversion of food into energy (metabolism).
plasma	Fluid part of the blood in which the red and white blood cells and platelets flow.
platelets	Contribute to the blood-clotting process, which stops bleeding; platelets are much smaller than red blood cells.
platysma muscle	Broad muscle extending from the chest and shoulder muscles to the side of the chin; responsible for lowering the lower jaw and lip.
popliteal artery	Artery that supplies blood to the foot; divides into two separate arteries known as the anterior tibial artery and the posterior tibial artery.
posterior auricular artery	Branch of the external carotid artery that supplies blood to the scalp, the area behind and above the ear, and the skin behind the ear.
posterior auricular nerve	Branch of the seventh cranial nerve that affects the muscles behind the ear at the base of the skull.
posterior tibial artery	One of the popliteal arteries (the other is the anterior tibial artery) that supplies blood to the ankle and the back of the lower leg.
procerus muscle	Muscle that covers the bridge of the nose, lowers the eyebrows, and causes wrinkles across the bridge of the nose.
pronator	Muscle that turn tshe hand inward so that the palm faces downward.
protoplasm	Colorless jelly-like substance found inside cells in which food elements such as protein, fats, carbohydrates, mineral salts, and water are present.
pulmonary circulation	The system that sends the blood from the heart to the lungs to be purified, then back to the heart again.
radial artery	Artery, along with numerous branches, that supplies blood to the thumb side of the arm and the back of the hand; supplies blood to the muscles of the skin, hands, fingers, wrist, elbow, and forearm.
radial nerve	Sensory-motor nerve that, with its branches, supplies the thumb side of the arm and back of the hand.
radius	Smaller bone in the forearm (lower arm) on the same side as the thumb.
red blood cells	Blood cells that carry oxygen from the lungs to the body cells and transport carbon dioxide from the cells back to the lungs.

Chapter Glossary

reflex	Automatic reaction to a stimulus that involves the movement of an impulse from a sensory receptor along the sensory nerve to the spinal cord.
reproductive system	Body system that includes the ovaries, uterine tubes, uterus, and vagina in the female and the testes, prostate gland, penis, and urethea in the male. This system performs the function of producing offspring and passing on the genetic code from one generation to another.
respiration	Act of breathing; the exchange of carbon dioxide and oxygen in the lungs and within each cell.
respiratory system	Body system consisting of the lungs and air passages; enables respiration (breathing), supplying the body with oxygen and eliminating carbon dioxide.
ribs	Twelve pairs of bones forming the wall of the thorax.
risorius muscle	Muscle of the mouth that draws the corner of the mouth out and back, as in grinning.
saphenous nerve	Nerve of the leg that supplies impulses to the skin of the inner side of the leg and foot.
scapula	Also known as *shoulder blade*; large, flat, triangular bone of the shoulder. There are two scapulas.
sciatic nerve	Largest and longest nerve in the body.
sensory nerves	Also known as *afferent nerves*; carry impulses or messages from the sense organs to the brain, where sensations of touch, cold, heat, sight, hearing, taste, smell, pain, and pressure are experienced.
serratus anterior	Muscle of the chest that assists in breathing and in raising the arm.
seventh cranial nerve	Also known as *facial nerve*; chief motor nerve of the face. Its divisions and their branches supply and control all the muscles of facial expression.
skeletal system	Forms the physical foundation of the body, composed of 206 bones that vary in size and shape and are connected by movable and immovable joints.
skin	Body organ that covers the body and is the external protective coating.
skull	Skeleton of the head; divided into two parts: cranium and facial skeleton.
smaller occipital nerve	Also known as *lesser occipital nerve*; cervical nerve located at the base of the skull, affects the scalp and muscles behind the ear.
soleus	Muscle that originates at the upper portion of the fibula and bends the foot down.
sphenoid bone	Bone that joins all of the bones of the cranium together.
spinal cord	Portion of the central nervous system that originates in the brain and extends down to the lower extremity of the trunk. It is protected by the spinal column.
sternocleido–mastoideus	Muscle of the neck that lowers and rotates the head.
sternum	Also known as *breastbone*; flat bone that forms the ventral (front) support of the ribs.
stomach	Body organ that digests food, along with the intestines.
striated muscles	Also known as *skeletal muscles*; muscles that are attached to the bones and that are voluntary or are consciously controlled.

Chapter Glossary

submental artery	Branch of the facial artery that supplies blood to the chin and lower lip.
superficial peroneal nerve	Also known as *musculocutaneous nerve*; extends down the leg, just under the skin, supplying impulses to the muscles and the skin of the leg, as well as to the skin and toes on the top of the foot, where it becomes the dorsal nerve.
superficial temporal artery	A continuation of the external carotid nerve artery; supplies blood to the muscles of the front, side, and top of the head.
superior labial artery	Branch of the facial artery that supplies blood to the upper lip and region of the nose.
supinator	Muscle of the forearm that rotates the radius outward and the palm upward.
supraorbital artery	Branch of the internal carotid artery that supplies blood to the upper eyelid and forehead.
supraorbital nerve	Branch of the fifth cranial nerve that affects the skin of the forehead, scalp, eyebrow, and upper eyelid.
supratrochlear nerve	Branch of the fifth cranial nerve that affects the skin between the eyes and upper side of the nose.
sural nerve	Nerve of the lower left leg that supplies impulses to the skin on the outer side and back of the foot and leg.
systemic circulation	Also known as *general circulation*; system that carries the blood from the heart throughout the body and back to the heart.
talus	Also known as *ankle bone*; one of three bones that comprise the ankle joint. The other two bones are the tibia and fibula.
tarsal	One of three subdivisions of the foot. There are seven bones—talus, calcaneus, navicular, three cuneiform bones, and the cuboid. The other two subdivisions are the metatarsal and the phalanges.
temporal bones	Bones that form the sides of the head in the ear region.
temporal nerve	Branch of the seventh cranial nerve that affects the muscles of the temple, side of the forehead, eyebrow, eyelid, and upper part of the cheek.
temporalis	Muscles that coordinate with the masseter and the pterygoid muscles to open and close the mouth and bring the jaw forward; sometimes referred to as chewing muscles.
testes (singular: testicle)	Male sexual glands of the endocrine system that function in reproduction, as well as determining male sexual characteristics.
thorax	Also known as *chest* or *pulmonary trunk*; consists of the sternum, ribs, and thoracic vertebrae; elastic, bony cage that serves as a protective framework for the heart, lungs, and other internal organs.
thyroid gland	Gland of the endocrine system that controls how quickly the body burns energy (metabolism), makes proteins, and how sensitive the body should be to other hormones.
tibia	Larger of the two bones that form the leg below the knee. The tibia may be visualized as a bump on the big-toe side of the ankle.

Chapter Glossary

tibial nerve	A division of the sciatic nerve that passes behind the knee. It subdivides and supplies impulses to the knee, the muscles of the calf, the skin of the leg, and the sole, heel, and underside of the toes.
tibialis anterior	Muscle that covers the front of the shin; bends the foot upward and inward.
tissue	Collection of similar cells that perform a particular function.
transverse facial artery	Branch of the superficial temporal artery that supplies blood to the skin and masseter muscle.
trapezius	Muscle that covers the back of the neck and upper and middle region of the back; rotates and controls swinging movements of the arm.
triangularis muscle	Muscle extending alongside the chin that pulls down the corner of the mouth.
tricep	Large muscle that covers the entire back of the upper arm and extends the forearm.
tricuspid valve	Valve between the right atrium and right ventricle of the heart.
ulna	Inner and larger bone in the forearm (lower arm), attached to the wrist and located on the side of the little finger.
ulnar artery	Artery, along with numerous branches, that supplies blood to the little-finger side of the arm and palm of the hand.
ulnar nerve	Sensory-motor nerve that, with its branches, affects the little-finger side of the arm and palm of the hand.
valves	Structures of the heart that temporarily close a passage or permit blood flow in only one direction.
veins	Thin-walled blood vessels that are less elastic than arteries; veins contain cup-like valves that keep blood flowing in one direction to the heart and prevent blood from flowing backward.
ventricle	A lower, thick-walled chamber of the heart that receives blood pumped from the atrium. There is a right venticle and a left ventricle.
venules	Small vessels that connect the capillaries to the veins. They collect blood from the capillaries and drain it into veins.
white blood cells	Also known as *white corpuscles* or *leukocytes*; blood cells that perform the function of destroying disease-causing bacteria.
zygomatic bones	Also known as *malar bones* or *cheekbones*; bones that form the prominence of the cheeks.
zygomatic nerve	Branch of the fifth and seventh cranial nerves that affects the muscles of the upper part of the cheek.
zygomaticus major muscles	Muscles on both sides of the face that extend from the zygomatic bone to the angle of the mouth. These muscles pull the mouth backward, upward, and outward, as when you are laughing or smiling.
zygomaticus minor muscles	Muscles on both sides of the face that extend from the zygomatic bone to the upper lips. These muscles pull the upper lip backward, upward, and outward, as when you are smiling.

CHAPTER 7

Skin Structure, Growth, and Nutrition

Chapter Outline

© Oleksii Abramov, 2010, used under license from Shutterstock.com.

Learning Objectives

After completing this chapter, you will be able to:

- ✓ **LO1** Describe the structure and composition of the skin.
- ✓ **LO2** List the functions of the skin.
- ✓ **LO3** List the classes of nutrients essential for good health.
- ✓ **LO4** List the food groups and dietary guidelines recommended by the U.S. Department of Agriculture (USDA).
- ✓ **LO5** List and describe the vitamins that can help the skin.

Key Terms

Page number indicates where in the chapter the term is used.

acne (acne vulgaris) pg. 163

arrector pili muscles pg. 158

callus pg. 157

collagen pg. 161

comedo (blackhead) pg. 163

dermal papillae pg. 159

dermatologist pg. 156

dermatology pg. 156

dermis (derma, corium, cutis, true skin) pg. 158

elastin pg. 161

epidermal–dermal junction pg. 159

epidermis pg. 157

esthetician pg. 156

eumelanin pg. 161

keratin pg. 157

melanin pg. 160

melanocytes pg. 158

motor nerve fibers pg. 160

papillary layer pg. 159

papule (pimple) pg. 163

pheomelanin pg. 161

Propionibacterium acnes (P. acnes) pg. 163

pustule pg. 163

reticular layer pg. 159

sebaceous glands (oil glands) pg. 163

sebum pg. 163

secretory coil pg. 162

secretory nerve fibers pg. 160

sensory nerve fibers pg. 160

stratum corneum (horny layer) pg. 157

stratum germinativum (basal cell layer) pg. 158

stratum granulosum (granular layer) pg. 157

stratum lucidum pg. 157

stratum spinosum pg. 158

subcutaneous tissue (adipose tissue, subcutis tissue) pg. 159

sudoriferous glands (sweat glands) pg. 162

tactile corpuscles pg. 159

vitamin A pg. 166

vitamin C pg. 167

vitamin D pg. 167

vitamin E pg. 167

Clear, glowing skin is one of today's most important hallmarks of beauty. No matter how advanced the latest skin care technology may be, you still have to learn how to care for your client's skin and know what you should do to keep it healthy. That means you must study the structure of the skin, how skin grows, and why it is important to maintain a healthy diet.

Why Study Skin Structure, Growth, and Nutrition?

Cosmetologists should study and have a thorough understanding of skin structure, growth, and nutrition because:

- Knowing the skin's underlying structure and basic needs is crucial in order to provide excellent skin care for clients.
- You will need to recognize adverse conditions, including skin diseases, inflamed skin, and infectious skin disorders so that you can refer clients to medical professionals for treatment when necessary.
- Twenty-first century skin care has entered the realm of high technology so you must learn about and understand the latest developments in ingredients and state-of-the-art delivery systems in order to help protect, nourish, and preserve the health and beauty of your clients' skin.

Anatomy of the Skin

The medical branch of science that deals with the study of skin—its nature, structure, functions, diseases, and treatment—is called **dermatology** (dur-muh-TAHL-uh-jee). A **dermatologist** (dur-muh-TAHL-uh-jist) is a physician who specializes in diseases and disorders of the skin, hair, and nails. Dermatologists attend four years of college, four years of medical school, and about four years of specialty training in dermatology. Because some skin symptoms may be a sign of internal disease, many dermatologists have additional training in internal medicine.

Cosmetologists may be allowed to clean skin, preserve the health of skin, and beautify the skin, depending on the laws and regulations of their state. In some states, a cosmetologist must become an esthetician in order to perform services on the skin. An **esthetician** specializes in the cleansing, beautification, and preservation of the health of skin on the entire body, including the face and neck.

© Lena Clara/fstop, 2010; used under license from CorbisImages.com.

Cosmetologists are not allowed to diagnose, prescribe, or provide any type of treatment for abnormal conditions, illnesses, or diseases. Cosmetologists refer clients with medical issues to dermatologists more than to any other type of physician.

The skin is the largest organ of the body. If the skin of an average adult were stretched out, it would cover over 3,000 square inches and weigh about 6 to 9 pounds. Our skin protects the network of muscles, bones, nerves, blood vessels, and everything else inside our bodies. It is the only natural barrier between our bodies and the environment.

Healthy skin should be free of any visible signs of disease, infection, or injury. It is slightly moist, soft, and flexible. Ideally, healthy skin has a smooth, fine-grained texture (feel and appearance). The surface of healthy skin is slightly acidic, and its immune responses react quickly to organisms that touch or try to enter it. Appendages of the skin include hair, nails, and sudoriferous (sweat) and sebaceous (oil) glands.

Continued, repeated pressure on any part of the skin, especially the hands and feet, can cause it to thicken and develop into a **callus** (KAL-us), which is an important and needed protective layer that prevents damage to the underlying skin.

The skin of the scalp is constructed similarly to the skin elsewhere on the human body, but the scalp has larger and deeper hair follicles to accommodate the longer hair of the head.

The skin is composed of two main divisions: the epidermis and the dermis (**Figure 7–1**).

The **epidermis** (ep-uh-DUR-mis) is the outermost and thinnest layer of the skin. It contains no blood vessels, but has many small nerve endings. The epidermis is made up of five layers.

- The **stratum corneum** (STRAT-um KOR-nee-um), also known as **horny layer** (HOR-nee LAY-ur), is the outer layer of the epidermis. The stratum corneum is the layer we see when we look at the skin and is the layer cared for by salon products and services. Its scale-like cells are continually being shed and replaced by cells coming to the surface from underneath. These cells are made up of **keratin** (KAIR-uh-tin), a fibrous protein that is also the principal component of hair and nails. The cells combine with lipids (fats) produced by the skin to help make the stratum corneum a protective, water-resistant layer.
- The **stratum lucidum** (STRAT-um LOO-sih-dum) is the clear, transparent layer under the stratum corneum; it consists of small cells through which light can pass.
- The **stratum granulosum** (STRAT-um gran-yoo-LOH-sum), also known as **granular layer** (GRAN-yuh-lur LAY-ur), is the layer of the epidermis that is composed of cells that look like granules and are filled with keratin. The cells die as they are pushed to the surface to replace dead cells that are shed from the stratum corneum.

did you know?

A callus is nature's way of protecting the skin from damage and infection. Complete removal of a callus is a medical procedure that should not be performed in the salon.

did you know?

The skin located under our eyes and around the eyelids is the thinnest skin of the body. The skin on the palms of our hands and soles of our feet is the thickest skin.

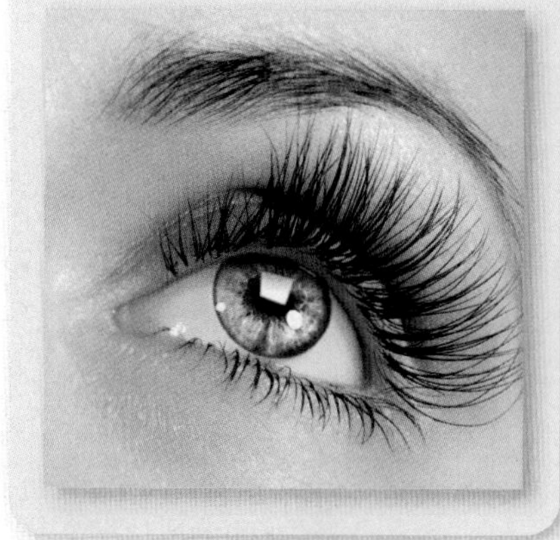

© Ivanova Inga, 2010; used under license from Shutterstock.com.

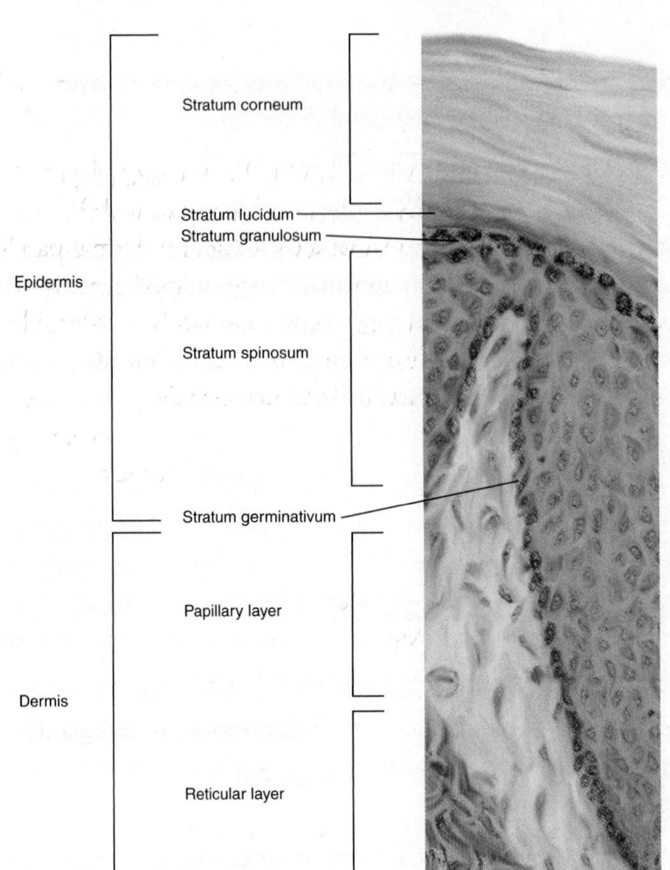

▶ **Figure 7–1**
Layers of the skin.

© Milady, a part of Cengage Learning.

did you know?

The epidermis is only 0.04 millimeter (mm) to 1.5 mm thick. One millimeter is .039 of an inch.

- The **stratum spinosum** (STRAT-um spy-NOH-sum), is the spiny layer just above the stratum germinativum. The spiny layer is where the process of skin cell shedding begins.
- The **stratum germinativum** (STRAT-um jer-mih-nah-TIV-um), also known as **basal cell layer** (CEL LAY-ur), is the deepest layer of the epidermis. This is the live layer of the epidermis that produces new epidermal skin cells and is responsible for the growth of the epidermis. It is composed of several layers of differently shaped cells. The stratum germinativum also contains special cells called **melanocytes** (muh-LAN-uh-syts), which produce the dark skin pigment called melanin. Melanin protects the sensitive cells in the dermis (which is located below the epidermis) from the destructive effects of excessive ultraviolet (UV) light from the sun or from ultraviolet lamps. Melanin is discussed in greater detail later in this chapter.

The **dermis** (DUR-mis), also known as **derma** (DUR-muh), **corium** (KOH-ree-um), **cutis** (KYOO-tis), or **true skin**, is the underlying or inner layer of the skin. The dermis extends to form the subcutaneous tissue. The highly sensitive dermis layer of connective tissue is about 25 times thicker than the epidermis. Within its structure, there are numerous blood vessels, lymph vessels, nerves, sudoriferous (sweat) glands, sebaceous (oil) glands, and hair follicles, as well as arrector pili muscles. **Arrector pili muscles** (ah-REK-tohr PY-leh MUS-uls) are the small, involuntary muscles in the base of the hair that cause goose flesh—or *goose bumps*, as many people call them—and papillae. The dermis is comprised of two layers: the papillary (superficial layer) and the reticular (deeper layer).

- The **papillary layer** (PAP-uh-lair-ee LAY-ur) is the outer layer of the dermis, directly beneath the epidermis. Here you will find the **dermal papillae** (DUR-mul puh-PIL-eye) (singular: dermal papilla; DUR-mul puh-PIL-uh), which are small, cone-shaped elevations at the base of the hair follicles. Some papillae contain looped capillaries, and others contain small epidermal structures called **tactile corpuscles** (TAK-tile KOR-pusuls), with nerve endings that are sensitive to touch and pressure. This layer also contains melanocytes, the pigment-producing cells. The top of the papillary layer where it joins the epidermis is called the **epidermal–dermal junction** (ep-ih-DUR-mul-DUR-mul JUNK-shun).
- The **reticular layer** (ruh-TIK-yuh-lur LAY-ur) is the deeper layer of the dermis that supplies the skin with all of its oxygen and nutrients. It contains the following structures within its network:
    - Fat cells
    - Blood vessels
    - Lymph vessels
    - Sebaceous (oil) glands
    - Sudoriferous (sweat) glands
    - Hair follicles
    - Arrector pili muscles
    - Nerve endings

Subcutaneous tissue (sub-kyoo-TAY-nee-us TISH-oo), also known as **adipose tissue** (AD-uh-pohs TISH-oo) or **subcutis tissue** (sub-KYOO-tis TISH-oo), is the fatty tissue found below the dermis. It gives smoothness and contour to the body, contains fats for use as energy, and also acts as a protective cushion for the skin. Subcutaneous tissue varies in thickness according to the age, gender, and general health of the individual (**Figure 7–2**).

did you know?

Goose bumps often appear on your skin when you are cold or scared. You most likely will see them on the areas of your skin that have little hair.

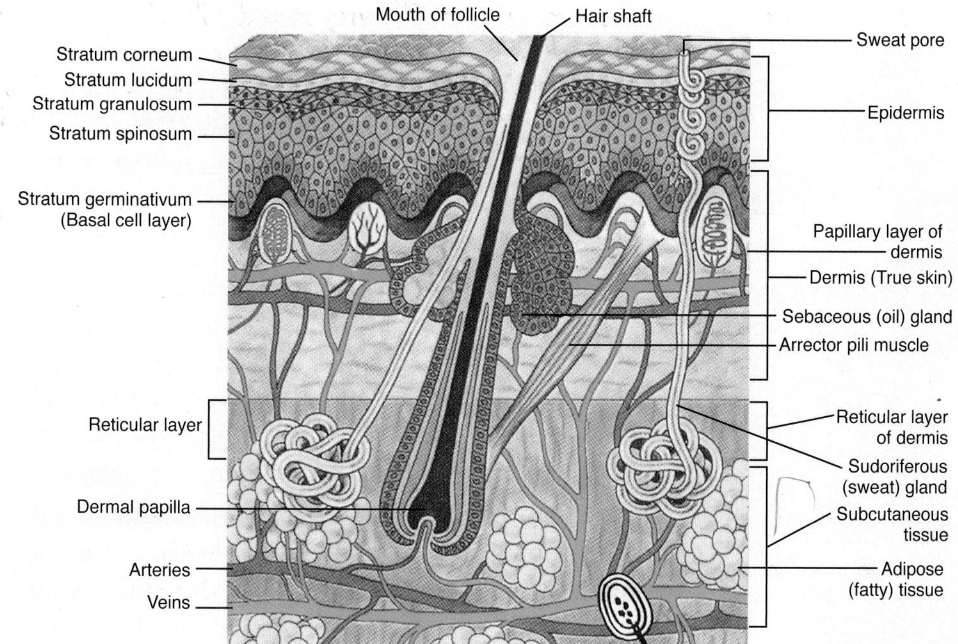

Figure 7–2 Structures of the skin.

© Milady, a part of Cengage Learning.

How the Skin is Nourished

Blood supplies nutrients and oxygen to the skin. Nutrients are molecules from food, such as protein, carbohydrates, and fats. These nutrients are necessary for cell life, repair, and growth. The skin cannot be nourished properly from the outside in with cosmetic products; it must have nourishment from foods that we eat.

Lymph, the clear fluids of the body that bathe the skin cells, remove toxins and cellular waste, and have immune functions that help protect the skin and body against disease. Networks of arteries and lymph vessels in the subcutaneous tissue send their smaller branches to hair papillae, hair follicles, and skin glands.

© ranplett, 2010; used under license from iStockphoto.com.

Nerves of the Skin

The skin contains the surface endings of the following nerve fibers:

- **Motor nerve fibers** (MOH-tur NURV FY-burs) are distributed to the arrector pili muscles attached to the hair follicles. Motor nerves carry impulses from the brain to the muscles.
- **Sensory nerve fibers** (SEN-soh-ree NURV FY-burs) react to heat, cold, touch, pressure, and pain. These sensory receptors send messages to the brain.
- **Secretory nerve fibers** (seh-KREE-toh-ree NURV FY-burs) are distributed to the sudoriferous (sweat) and sebaceous (oil) glands of the skin. Secretory nerves, which are part of the autonomic nervous system, regulate the excretion of perspiration from the sudoriferous glands and control the flow of sebum (a fatty or oily secretion of the sebaceous glands) to the surface of the skin.

Sense of Touch

The papillary layer of the dermis houses the nerve endings that provide the body with the sense of touch, pain, heat, cold, and pressure. Nerve endings are most abundant in the fingertips. Complex sensations, such as vibrations, seem to depend on the sensitivity of a combination of these nerve endings.

Skin Color

The color of the skin—whether fair, medium, or dark—depends primarily on **melanin** (MEL-ah-nin), the tiny grains of pigment (coloring matter) that are produced by melanocytes and then deposited into cells in the stratum germinativum layer of the epidermis and the papillary layers of the dermis. The color of the skin is

© Andre Blais, 2010; used under license from Shutterstock.com.

a hereditary trait and varies among races and nationalities. Genes determine the amount and type of pigment produced in an individual.

The body produces two types of melanin: **pheomelanin** (fee-oh-MEL-uh-nin), which is red to yellow in color, and **eumelanin** (yoo-MEL-uh-nin), which is dark brown to black. People with light-colored skin mostly produce pheomelanin, while those with dark-colored skin mostly produce eumelanin. The size of melanin granules varies from one individual to another.

Melanin helps protect sensitive cells from the sun's UV light, but it does not provide enough protection to prevent skin damage. Daily use of a sunscreen with a sun protection factor (SPF) of 15 or higher can help the melanin protect the skin from burning, skin cancer, and premature aging (**Figure 7–3**).

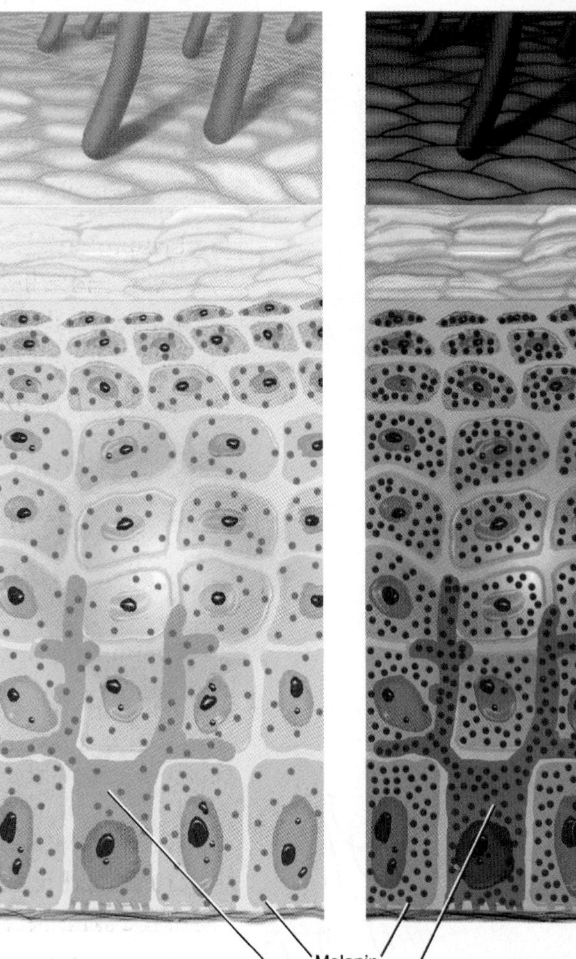

▼ **Figure 7–3**
Melanocytes in the epidermis produce melanin.

Strength and Flexibility of the Skin

The skin gets its strength, form, and flexibility from two specific structures found within the dermis: collagen and elastin. These two structures are composed of flexible protein fibers, and they make up 70 percent of the dermis.

Collagen (KAHL-uh-jen) is a fibrous protein that gives the skin form and strength. This fiber makes up a large percentage of the dermis and provides structural support by holding together all the structures found in this layer. When collagen fibers are healthy, they allow the skin to stretch and contract as needed. If collagen fibers become weakened due to age, lack of moisture, environmental damage such as UV light, or frequent changes in weight, the skin will begin to lose its tone and suppleness. Wrinkles and sagging are often the result of collagen fibers losing their strength.

Elastin (ee-LAS-tin) is a protein base similar to collagen that forms elastic tissue. Elastin is interwoven with the collagen fibers. Elastin fiber gives the skin its flexibility and elasticity. It helps the skin regain its shape, even after being repeatedly stretched or expanded. Elastin can be weakened by the same factors that weaken collagen.

did you know?

The word *collagen* comes from the Greek words *kolla,* meaning glue, and *gennan*, meaning to produce.

Both types of fibers are important to the overall health and appearance of the skin. As we age, gravity causes these fibers to weaken. In the end, a loss of elasticity results in sagging skin.

A majority of scientists now believe that most signs of skin aging are caused by sun exposure over a lifetime. Using high-SPF sunscreen,

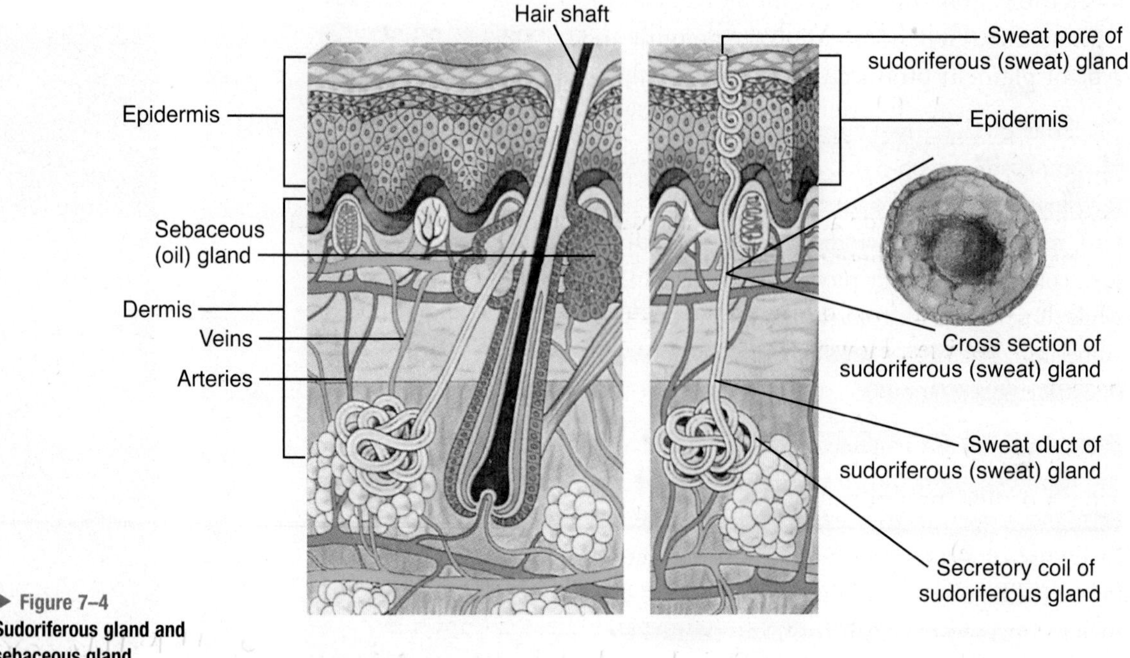

© Milady, a part of Cengage Learning.

▶ **Figure 7–4**
Sudoriferous gland and sebaceous gland.

maintaining a moisturizing skin-care regimen, and keeping skin free of disease will slow the weakening of collagen and elastin fibers and help skin look young longer.

Glands of the Skin

The skin contains two types of duct glands that extract materials from the blood to form new substances. These are sudoriferous glands and sebaceous glands. (See **Figure 7–4.**)

did you know?

Our bodies stop producing elastin around the age of 12 or 13. So what happens when the body stops producing elastin? The skin begins to age.

Sudoriferous (Sweat) Glands

Sudoriferous glands (sood-uh-RIF-uhrus GLANZ), also known as **sweat glands**, excrete perspiration and detoxify the body by excreting excess salt and unwanted chemicals. They consist of a **secretory coil** (seh-KREET-toh-ree KOYL), the coiled base of the sudoriferous gland, and a tube-like sweat duct that ends at the surface of the skin to form the sweat pore. Practically all parts of the body are supplied with sudoriferous glands, which are more numerous on the palms of the hands, the soles of the feet, the forehead, and the underarm (armpit).

The sudoriferous glands regulate body temperature and help eliminate waste products from the body. The evaporation of sweat cools the skin's surface. The activity of sudoriferous glands is greatly increased by heat, exercise, emotions, and certain drugs.

The excretion of sweat is controlled by the nervous system. Normally, 1 to 2 pints of salt-containing liquids are eliminated daily through sweat pores in the skin.

Sebaceous (Oil) Glands

Sebaceous glands (sih-BAY-shus GLANZ), also known as **oil glands**, are connected to the hair follicles. They consist of little sacs with ducts that open into the follicles. These glands secrete **sebum** (SEE-bum), a fatty or oily substance that lubricates the skin and preserves the softness of the hair. With the exception of the palms of the hands and the soles of the feet, these glands are found in all parts of the body, particularly in the face and scalp, where they are larger.

Ordinarily, sebum flows through the oil ducts leading to the mouths of the hair follicles. However, when the sebum hardens and the duct becomes clogged, a pore impaction called a **comedo** (KAHM-uh-doe) (plural: comedones; KAHM-uh-dohnz), also known as **blackhead**, a hair follicle filled with keratin and sebum, is formed. This can lead to acne, a papule, or a pustule.

Acne (AK-nee), also known as **acne vulgaris** (AK-nee vull-GAIR-us), is a skin disorder characterized by chronic inflammation of the sebaceous glands from retained secretions and bacteria known as **Propionibacterium acnes** (pro-PEE-ah-nee-back-tear-ee-um AK-nes), abbreviated P. acnes, the technical term for acne bacteria. A **papule** (PAP-yool), also known as **pimple**, is a small elevation on the skin that contains no fluid but may develop pus. A **pustule** (PUS-chool) is a raised, inflamed papule with a white or yellow center containing pus in the top of the lesion referred to as the head of the pimple. ☑ **LO1**

did you know?

Touch is one of the first senses to develop in the human body.

Functions of the Skin

The six principal functions of the skin are protection, sensation, heat regulation, excretion, secretion, and absorption.

- **Protection** The skin protects the body from injury and bacterial invasion. The outermost layer of the epidermis is rendered water-resistant by a thin layer of sebum and fatty lipids. The fatty lipids exist between the cells and are produced through the cell renewal process. This outermost layer is resistant to wide variations in temperature, minor injuries, chemically active substances, and many forms of bacteria.

- **Sensation** By stimulating different sensory nerve endings, the skin responds to heat, cold, touch, pressure, and pain. When the nerve endings are stimulated, a message is sent to the brain. You respond by saying "Ouch" if you feel pain, by scratching if you have an itch, or by pulling

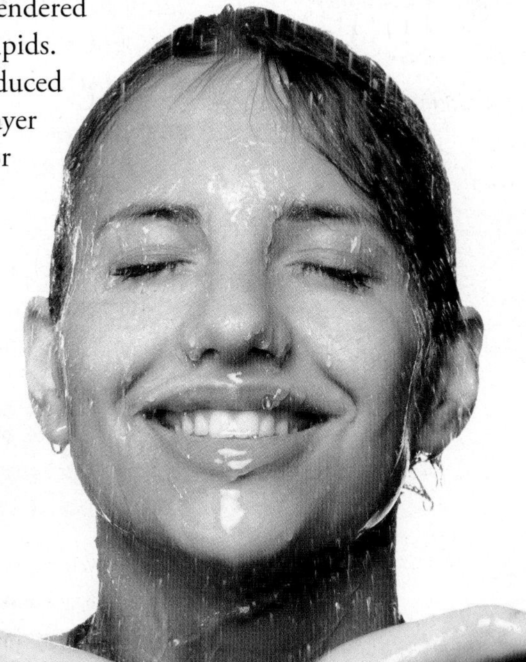

© Raisa Kanareva, 2010; used under license from Shutterstock.com.

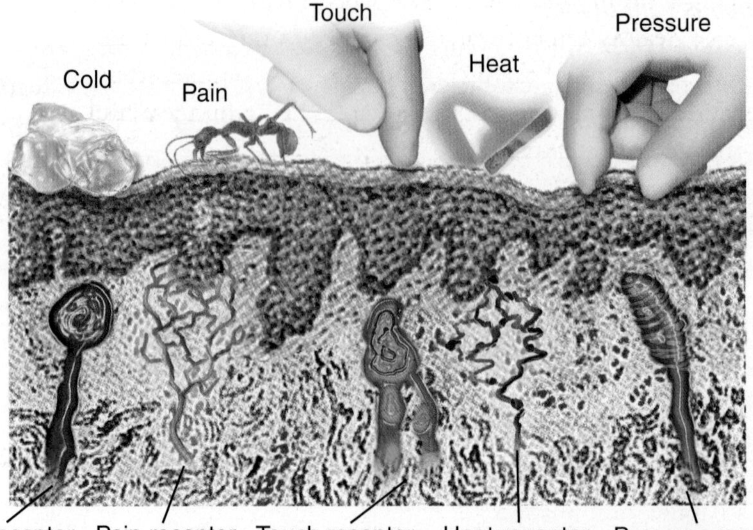

▶ **Figure 7–5**
Sensory nerve endings in the skin.

© Milady, a part of Cengage Learning.

away if you touch something hot. Some sensory nerve endings are located near hair follicles (**Figure 7–5**).

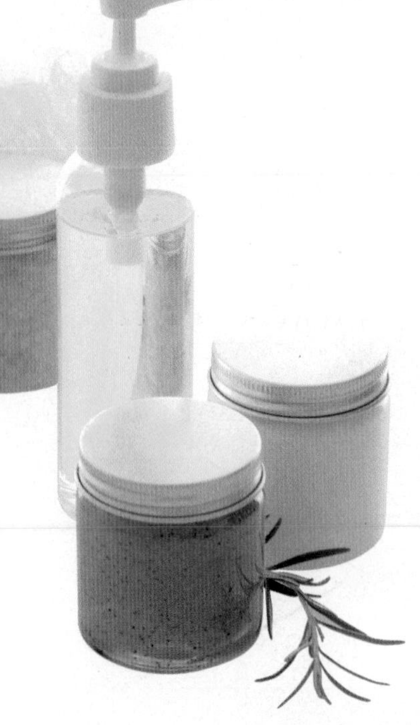

© Khomulo Anna, 2010; used under license from Shutterstock.com.

- **Heat regulation** The skin protects the body from the environment. A healthy body maintains a constant internal temperature of about 98.6 degrees Fahrenheit (37 degrees Celsius). As changes occur in the outside temperature, the blood and sudoriferous glands of the skin make necessary adjustments to allow the body to be cooled by the evaporation of sweat.
- **Excretion** Perspiration from the sudoriferous glands is excreted through the skin. Water lost through perspiration takes salt and other chemicals with it.
- **Secretion** Sebum is secreted by the sebaceous glands. This oil lubricates the skin, keeping it soft and pliable. Oil also keeps hair soft. Emotional stress and hormone imbalances can increase the flow of sebum.
- **Absorption** Some ingredients can be absorbed by the outer layers of the skin, but very few ingredients can penetrate the epidermis. Small amounts of fatty materials, such as those used in many advanced skin care formulations, may be absorbed between the cells and through the hair follicles and sebaceous gland openings. However, cosmetic products are not formulated to penetrate the epidermis. ☑ **LO2**

Nutrition and Maintaining Skin Health

For your own benefit, as well as for the benefit of your clients, you should have a basic understanding of how to maintain healthy skin by making the right nutritional choices. You have heard people say, "You are what you eat." Mainly, that is very true. To keep the body healthy, people must ensure that what they eat helps regulate hydration (keeping a healthy level of water in the body), oil production, and overall function of the cells. Skin disorders, fatigue, stress, depression, and some diseases can be caused by an unhealthful diet or improper hydration.

> **FYI**
> If you want more information about nutrition, you can go to the USDA's Web site at http://www.usda.gov or the U.S. Department of Health and Human Services' Web site at http://www.hhs.gov and enter a search for the word *nutrition*.

Essential Nutrients

There are six classes of nutrients that the body needs:

- Carbohydrates
- Fats
- Proteins
- Vitamins
- Minerals
- Water

These essential nutrients are obtained through eating and drinking. The body cannot make nutrients in sufficient amounts to sustain itself properly. ☑ **LO3**

The United States Department of Agriculture (USDA) developed a food pyramid to help people determine the amounts of food they need to eat from the five basic food groups. Those food groups are:

- Grains
- Vegetables
- Fruits
- Milk
- Meat, poultry, fish, and beans

Eating the recommended amounts of foods from the five basic groups is the best way to support and maintain the health of the skin. See the recommended daily food amounts in **Figure 7–6**.

In addition to following the recommendations included in the daily food pyramid, the USDA and the United States Department of Health and Human Services have established the dietary guidelines below to assist people with a balanced diet.

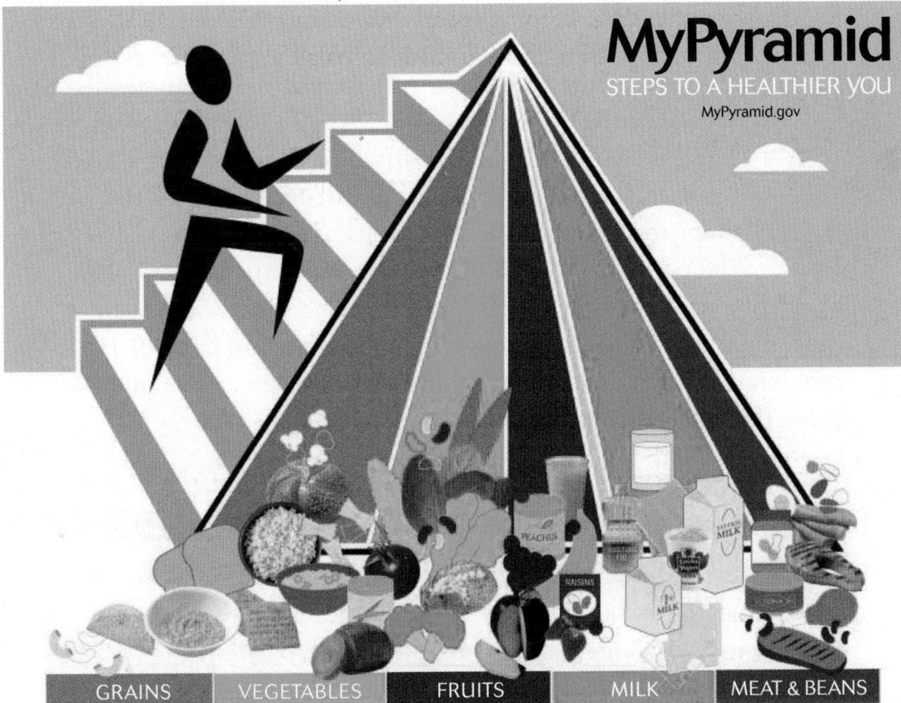

◀ **Figure 7–6**
Daily food pyramid recommended by the USDA.

Courtesy of U.S. Dept. of Agriculture.

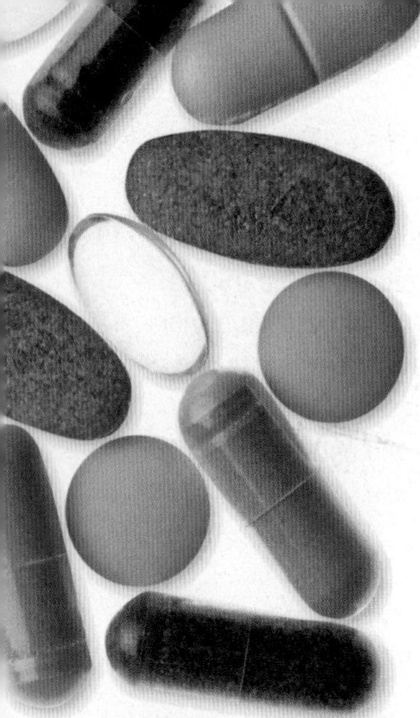

- Eat a variety of foods.
- Select a diet that is high in fresh fruits, vegetables, and grain products and low in fats, saturated fat, and cholesterol.
- Eat moderate amounts of salt and sugar, including the sodium and modified sugars that are in prepared food products.
- Drink an appropriate amount of water. (See the formula in the FYI sidebar to determine the appropriate amount of water based on your body weight.)
- Keep consumption of alcoholic beverages to a minimum.
- Balance your diet with the right amount of physical activity.
- Maintain or improve your weight. ☑ **LO4**

© ZanyZeus, 2010; used under license from Shutterstock.com.

FYI

Do you want to know how much water you should drink every day? Here is an easy formula that will tell you the number of ounces of water you should be drinking each day:

Divide your body weight by two. The result is the number of ounces of water that you should drink every day. Example: 160 pounds ÷ 2 = 80 ounces of water.

Keep in mind that the average water bottle that most people carry with them holds just a bit over 16 ounces (1 pint). Therefore, a person who weighs 160 pounds should drink at least 5 bottles of water. (80 ounces ÷ 16 ounces = 5 bottles.)

People who are very active should drink even more water.

One of the best ways to follow a healthy diet is to read food labels. Food labels can help you select healthy foods. Food labels also contain nutrition facts about serving size, number of servings per container, calorie information, and the quantities of nutrients per serving. If you have any questions or concerns about the ingredients or nutritional value of a food product, contact the manufacturer by telephone or through a Web site to obtain supplemental information.

Vitamins and Dietary Supplements

Vitamins play an important role in the skin's health, often aiding in healing and softening the skin and in fighting diseases. Vitamins such as A, C, D, and E have been shown to have positive effects on the skin's health when taken by mouth. If a person's daily food consumption is lacking in nutrients, vitamin and mineral supplements purchased through a health food store, vitamin store, or pharmacy can help provide some of the nutrients needed. Be sure to read the recommended daily allowance (RDA) for each vitamin and mineral supplement. These recommendations are listed on the supplement labels. Again, if you have any questions or concerns about the supplements, especially if the level of any nutrient is over 100 percent of the RDA, contact the manufacturer either by telephone or through a Web site. Remember that vitamins are nutritional supplements, not cosmetic ingredients. In fact, the law prohibits manufactures from claiming that any skin care product or cosmetic has nutritional value.

The following vitamins can help the skin in significant ways:

- **Vitamin A** supports the overall health of the skin and aids in the health, function, and repair of skin cells. It has been shown to improve the skin's elasticity and thickness.
- **Vitamin C** is an important substance needed for the proper repair of the skin and tissues. This vitamin aids in and accelerates

the skin's healing processes. Vitamin C also is vitally important in fighting the aging process and promotes the production of collagen in the skin's dermal tissues, keeping the skin healthy and firm.

- **Vitamin D** enables the body to properly absorb and use calcium, the element needed for proper bone development and maintenance. Vitamin D also promotes rapid healing of the skin.
- **Vitamin E** helps protect the skin from the harmful effects of the sun's UV light. Some people claim that vitamin E helps to heal damage to the skin's tissues when taken by mouth.

Because the nutrients the body needs for proper functioning and survival must come primarily from what we eat and drink, you should not depend on supplements to make up for poor nutrition. If your daily food consumption is lacking in nutrients, you should strive to improve your diet rather than relying on vitamins and mineral supplements to provide nourishment.

Clients may occasionally ask you about nutrition and their skin. **Table 7–1**, RDA Chart for Vitamins and Minerals: Natural Sources, Functions, and Deficiency Symptoms on the pages that follow, is a good reference for selecting foods that promote a healthy body and healthy skin. If clients ask you detailed questions about nutrition, you should tell them to seek the advice of a physician or a nutritionist. ☑ **LO5**

did you know?

Research suggests that many problems may be caused by insufficient water intake. Here are a few:

- Even mild dehydration will slow metabolism by as much as 3 percent.
- Cracked skin on the feet and lips are often warning signs of dehydration.
- Lack of water is the principal cause of daytime fatigue.
- A 2 percent drop in body water can trigger fuzzy short-term memory, trouble with basic computations, and may cause difficulty focusing on a computer screen or printed page.

Pass the water, please!

Water and the Skin

There is one item that no person can live without: water. To function properly, the body relies heavily on the benefits of water. This is especially true when it comes to the skin. Water composes 50 percent to 70 percent of body weight. The amount of water needed by an individual varies, depending on body weight and the level of daily physical activity (**Figure 7–7**).

Drinking pure water is essential to the health of the skin and body because it sustains the health of the cells, assists with the elimination of toxins and waste, helps regulate the body's temperature, and aids in proper digestion. All these functions, when performing properly, help keep the skin healthy, vital, and attractive.

▼ **Figure 7–7**
Water is essential for healthy skin.

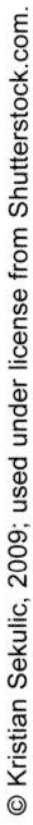

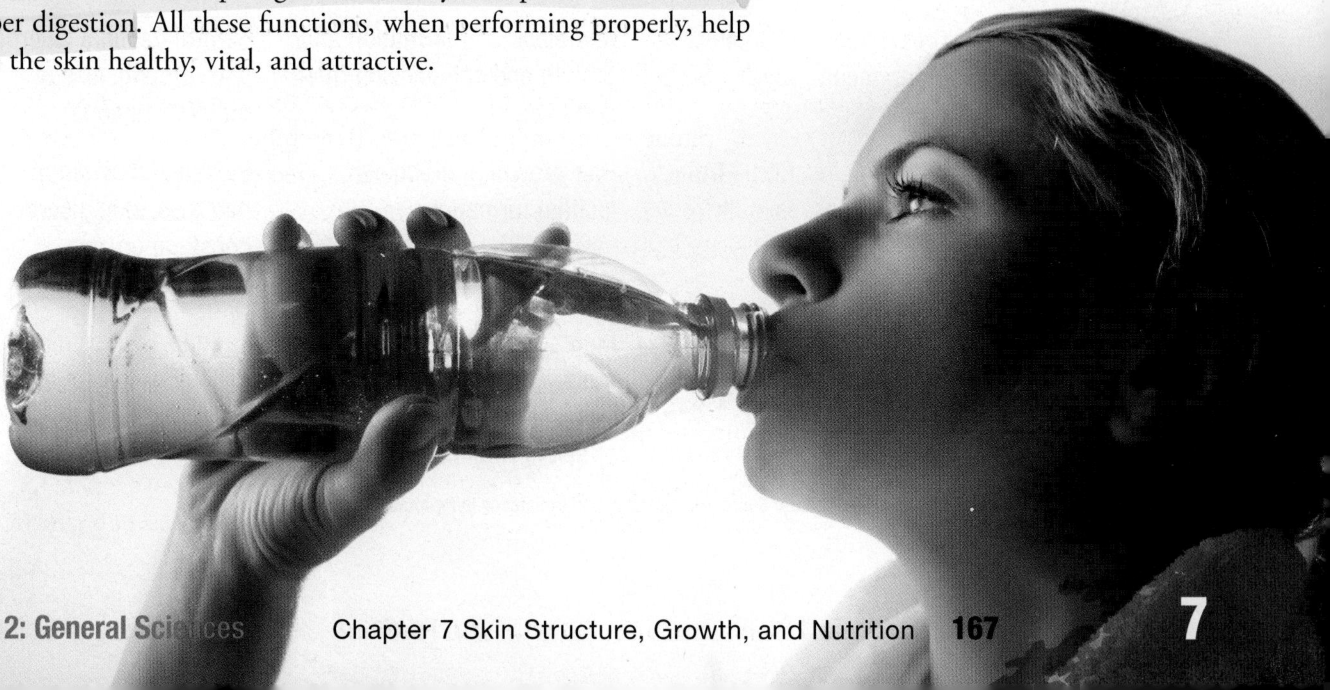

RDA CHART FOR VITAMINS AND MINERALS: NATURAL SOURCES, FUNCTIONS, AND DEFICIENCY SYMPTOMS

VITAMIN/ MINERAL RDA	NATURAL SOURCES	FUNCTIONS	DEFICIENCY SYMPTOMS
A 5,000 IU	Yellow and green fruits and vegetables, carrots, dairy products, fish liver oil, yellow fruits	Growth and repair of body tissues, bone formation, vision	Night blindness, dry scaly skin, loss of smell and appetite, fatigue, bone deterioration
B-1 Thiamine 1.5 mg	Grains, nuts, wheat germ, fish, poultry, legumes, meat	Metabolism, appetite maintenance, nerve function, healthy mental state, muscle tone	Nerve disorders, cramps, fatigue, loss of appetite, loss of memory, heart irregularity
B-2 Riboflavin 1.7 mg	Whole grains, green leafy vegetables, liver, fish, eggs	Metabolism; healthy hair, skin, and nails; cell respiration; formation of antibodies and red blood cells	Cracks and lesions in corners of mouth, digestive disturbances
B-6 Pyridoxine 2 mg	Whole grains, green leafy vegetables, yeast, bananas, organ meats	Metabolism; formation of antibodies; sodium and potassium balance	Dermatitis, blood disorders, nervousness, weakness, skin cracks, loss of memory
B-7 Biotin 300 mcg	Legumes, eggs, grains, yeast	Metabolism, formation of fatty acids	Dry, dull skin, depression, muscle pain, fatigue, loss of appetite
B-12 Cobalamine 6 mcg	Eggs, milk/milk products, fish, organ meats	Metabolism, healthy nervous system, blood cell formation	Nervousness, neuritis, fatigue
Choline (no RDA)	Lecithin, fish, wheat germ, egg yolk, soybeans	Nerve metabolism and transmission; regulation of liver, kidneys, gall bladder	Hypertension, stomach ulcers, liver and kidney conditions
Folic acid Folacin 400 mcg	Green leafy vegetables, organ meats, yeast, milk products	Red blood cell formation and growth and cell division (RNA and DNA)	Gastrointestinal disorders, poor growth, loss of memory, anemia
Inositol (no RDA)	Whole grains, citrus fruits, yeast, molasses, milk	Hair growth, metabolism, lecithin formation	Elevated cholesterol, hair loss, skin disorders, constipation, eye abnormalities
B complex Niacin 20 mg	Meat, poultry, fish, milk products, peanuts	Metabolism; healthy skin, tongue, and digestive system; blood circulation; synthesis of sex hormones	Fatigue, indigestion, irritability, loss of appetite, skin conditions

© Milady, a part of Cengage Learning.

Table 7–1 **RDA Chart for Vitamins and Minerals: Natural Sources, Functions, and Deficiency Symptoms.**

(Continues)

VITAMIN/ MINERAL RDA	NATURAL SOURCES	FUNCTIONS	DEFICIENCY SYMPTOMS
B complex PABA (no RDA)	Yeast, wheat germ, molasses	Metabolism, red blood cell formation, intestines, color of hair, sunscreen	Digestive disorders, fatigue, depression, constipation
B-15 Pantothenic acid 10 mg	Whole grains, pumpkin seeds, sesame seeds	Metabolism, stimulation of nerve and glandular systems, cell respiration	Heart disease, glandular disorders, nerve disorders, poor circulation
C Ascorbic acid 60 mg	Citrus fruits, vegetables, tomatoes, potatoes	Healing, collagen maintenance, resistance to disease	Gum bleeding, bruising, slow healing of wounds, nosebleeds, poor digestion
D 400 IU	Egg yolks, organ meats, fish, fortified milk	Healthy bone formation, circulatory function, nervous system function	Rickets, osteoporosis, poor bone growth, nervous system irritability
E 30 IU	Green vegetables, wheat germ, organ meats, eggs, vegetable oils	Formation of red blood cells, inhibition of blood coagulation, cellular respiration	Muscular atrophy, abnormal fat deposits in muscles, gastrointestinal conditions, heart disease, impotency
F (no RDA)	Wheat germ, seeds, vegetable oils	Respiration of body organs, lubrication of cells, blood coagulation, glandular activity	Brittle nails and hair, dry dandruff, diarrhea, varicose veins, underweight, acne, gallstones
K (no RDA)	Green leafy vegetables, milk, kelp, safflower oil	Blood clotting; proper liver function, longevity	Hemorrhage
P Bioflavonoids (no RDA)	Fruits	Construction of healthy connective tissue; utilization of vitamin C	Tendency to bleed easily, gum bleeding, bruising
Calcium 1000–1400 mg	Dairy products, bone meal	Resilient bones, teeth, and muscle tissue; regulation of heartbeat; blood clotting	Soft, brittle bones; osteoporosis; heart palpitations
Chromium (no RDA)	Corn oil, yeast, clams, whole grains	Utilization of glucose, energy, effective use of insulin	Atherosclerosis, diabetic sugar intolerance
Copper 2 mg	Whole grains, green leafy vegetables, seafood, almonds	Healthy red blood cells, bone growth and formation, elastin formation (when joined with vitamin C)	Skin lesions, general weakness, labored respiration

© Milady, a part of Cengage Learning.

Table 7–1 **RDA Chart for Vitamins and Minerals: Natural Sources, Functions, and Deficiency Symptoms.**

(Continued)

VITAMIN/ MINERAL RDA	NATURAL SOURCES	FUNCTIONS	DEFICIENCY SYMPTOMS
Iodine .15 mg	Iodized table salt, shellfish	Metabolism control	Dry skin and hair, obesity, nervousness, goiters
Iron 18 mg	Meats, fish, green leafy vegetables	Hemoglobin formation, blood quality, resistance to stress and disease	Anemia, constipation, breathing difficulties
Magnesium 400 mg	Nuts, green vegetables, whole grains	Metabolism	Nervousness, agitation, disorientation, blood clots
Manganese 2 mg	Egg yolks, legumes, whole grains	Carbohydrate and fat production, sex hormone production, bone development	Dizziness, loss of muscle coordination
Phosphorus 800 mg	Proteins, grains	Bone development; utilization of protein, fat, and carbohydrates	Soft bones, rickets, loss of appetite, irregular breathing
Potassium 2000 mg	Grains, vegetables, bananas, fruits, legumes	Fluid balance; control of heart muscle, nervous system, kidneys	Irregular heartbeat, muscle cramps (legs), dry skin, general weakness
Sodium 500 mg	Table salt, shellfish, meat, poultry	Maintenance of circulatory, lymphatic, and nervous systems; regulation of body fluid	Muscle weakness, muscle atrophy, nausea, dehydration
Sulphur (no RDA)	Fish, eggs, nuts, cabbage, meat	Formation of collagen, body tissues, and keratin	N/A
Zinc 15 mg	Whole grains, wheat bran	Healthy digestion and metabolism, reproductive system, healing	Stunted growth, delayed sexual maturity, prolonged wound healing
Selenium 055 mcg	Whole grains, liver, meat, fish	Immune system strength	Heart damage, chronic illness
Fluoride	Fluoridated water, toothpaste	Bone formation, tooth formation	Increased tooth decay

© Milady, a part of Cengage Learning.

Table 7–1 **RDA Chart for Vitamins and Minerals: Natural Sources, Functions, and Deficiency Symptoms.**

Review Questions

1. Define dermatology.
2. Briefly describe healthy skin.
3. Name the two main divisions of the skin and the layers within each division.
4. List the three types of nerve fibers found in the skin.
5. Can the skin be nourished with cosmetic products?
6. What are collagen and elastin?
7. Explain how collagen and elastin can be weakened.
8. Name the two types of glands contained within the skin and describe their functions.
9. What are the six important functions of the skin?
10. What are the six classes of nutrients that the body needs and how are they obtained?
11. What are the five basic food groups?
12. Name four vitamins that can help the skin and describe how they help.
13. What is the one essential item that no person can live without? Why is it essential to the skin and body?

Chapter Glossary

acne	Also known as *acne vulgaris*; skin disorder characterized by chronic inflammation of the sebaceous glands from retained secretions and Propionibacterium acnes (P. acnes) bacteria.
arrector pili muscles	Small, involuntary muscles in the base of the hair follicle that cause goose flesh, sometimes called *goose bumps*, and papillae.
callus	Thickening of the skin caused by continued, repeated pressure on any part of the skin, especially the hands and feet.
collagen	Fibrous protein that gives the skin form and strength.
comedo (plural: comedones)	Also known as *blackhead*; hair follicle filled with keratin and sebum.
dermal papillae (singular: dermal papilla)	Small, cone-shaped elevations at the base of the hair follicles that fit into the hair bulb.
dermatologist	Physician who specializes in diseases and disorders of the skin, hair, and nails.
dermatology	Medical branch of science that deals with the study of skin and its nature, structure, functions, diseases, and treatment.
dermis	Also known as *derma*, *corium*, *cutis*, or *true skin*; underlying or inner layer of the skin.
elastin	Protein base similar to collagen that forms elastic tissue.

Chapter Glossary

epidermal–dermal junction	The top of the papillary layer where it joins the epidermis.
epidermis	Outermost and thinnest layer of the skin; it is made up of five layers: stratum corneum, stratum lucidum, stratum granulosum, stratum spinosum, and stratum germinativum.
esthetician	A specialist in the cleansing, beautification, and preservation of the health of skin on the entire body, including the face and neck.
eumelanin	A type of melanin that is dark brown to black in color. People with dark-colored skin mostly produce eumelanin. There are two types of melanin; the other type is pheomelanin.
keratin	Fibrous protein of cells that is also the principal component of hair and nails.
melanin	Tiny grains of pigment (coloring matter) that are produced by melanocytes and deposited into cells in the stratum germinativum layer of the epidermis and in the papillary layers of the dermis. There are two types of melanin: pheomelanin, which is red to yellow in color, and eumelanin, which is dark brown to black.
melanocytes	Cells that produce the dark skin pigment called melanin.
motor nerve fibers	Fibers of the motor nerves that are distributed to the arrector pili muscles attached to hair follicles. Motor nerves carry impulses from the brain to the muscles.
papillary layer	Outer layer of the dermis, directly beneath the epidermis.
papule	Also known as *pimple*; small elevation on the skin that contains no fluid but may develop pus.
pheomelanin	A type of melanin that is red to yellow in color. People with light-colored skin mostly produce pheomelanin. There are two types of melanin; the other type is eumelanin.
Propionibacterium acnes	Abbreviated P. acnes; technical term for acne bacteria.
pustule	Raised, inflamed papule with a white or yellow center containing pus in the top of the lesion referred to as the head of the pimple.
reticular layer	Deeper layer of the dermis that supplies the skin with oxygen and nutrients; contains fat cells, blood vessels, sudoriferous (sweat) glands, hair follicles, lymph vessels, arrector pili muscles, sebaceous (oil) glands, and nerve endings.
sebaceous glands	Also known as *oil glands*; glands connected to hair follicles. Sebum is the fatty or oily secretion of the sebaceous glands.
sebum	A fatty or oily secretion that lubricates the skin and preserves the softness of the hair.
secretory coil	Coiled base of the sudoriferous (sweat) gland.
secretory nerve fibers	Fibers of the secretory nerve that are distributed to the sudoriferous glands and sebaceous glands. Secretory nerves, which are part of the autonomic nervous system (ANS), regulate the excretion of perspiration from the sweat glands and control the flow of sebum to the surface of the skin.
sensory nerve fibers	Fibers of the sensory nerves that react to heat, cold, touch, pressure, and pain. Sensory receptors that send messages to the brain.

Chapter Glossary

stratum corneum	Also known as *horny layer*; outer layer of the epidermis.
stratum germinativum	Also known as *basal cell layer*; deepest, live layer of the epidermis that produces new epidermal skin cells and is responsible for growth.
stratum granulosum	Also known as *granular layer*; layer of the epidermis composed of cells that look like granules and are filled with keratin; replaces cells shed from the stratum corneum.
stratum lucidum	Clear, transparent layer of the epidermis under the stratum corneum.
stratum spinosum	The spiny layer just above the stratum germinativum layer.
subcutaneous tissue	Also known as *adipose* or *subcutis tissue*; fatty tissue found below the dermis that gives smoothness and contour to the body, contains fat for use as energy, and also acts as a protective cushion for the outer skin.
sudoriferous glands	Also known as *sweat glands*; excrete perspiration and detoxify the body by excreting excess salt and unwanted chemicals.
tactile corpuscles	Small epidermal structures with nerve endings that are sensitive to touch and pressure.
vitamin A	Supports the overall health of the skin; aids in the health, function, and repair of skin cells; has been shown to improve the skin's elasticity and thickness.
vitamin C	An important substance needed for proper repair of the skin and tissues; promotes the production of collagen in the skin's dermal tissues; aids in and promotes the skin's healing process.
vitamin D	Enables the body to properly absorb and use calcium, the element needed for proper bone development and maintenance. Vitamin D also promotes rapid healing of the skin.
vitamin E	Helps protect the skin from the harmful effects of the sun's UV light.

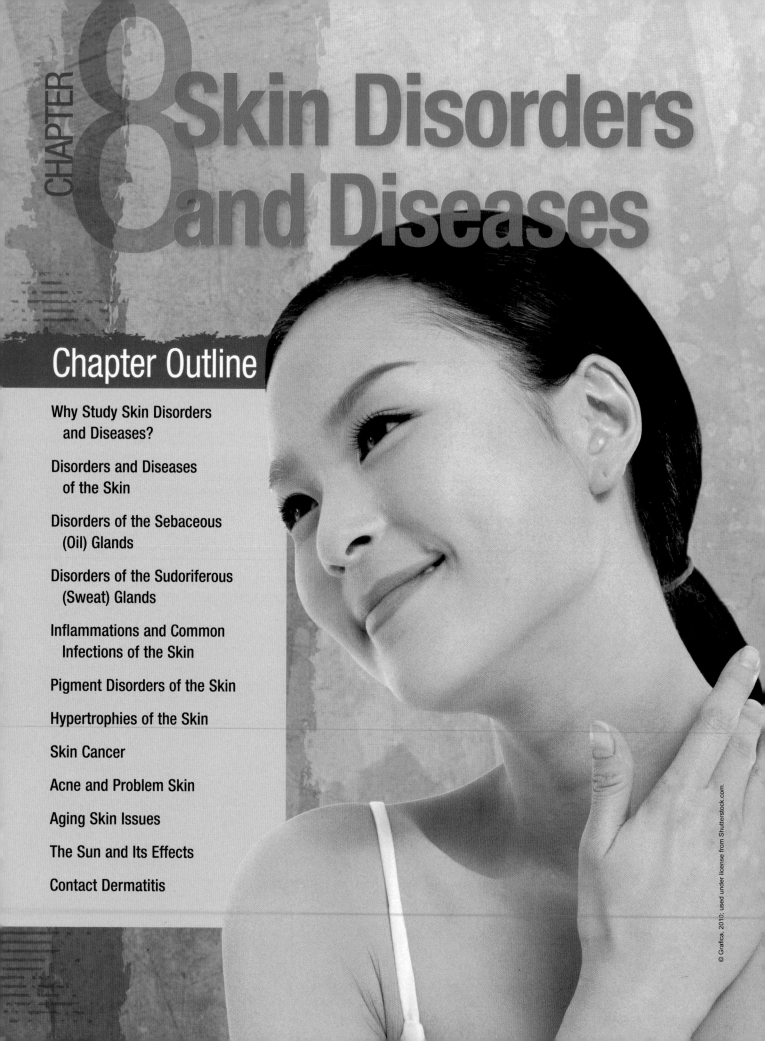

CHAPTER 8

Skin Disorders and Diseases

Chapter Outline

© Grafica, 2010, used under license from Shutterstock.com.

Learning Objectives

After completing this chapter, you will be able to:

✓ **LO1** Recognize common skin lesions.

✓ **LO2** Describe the disorders of the sebaceous glands.

✓ **LO3** Name and describe changes in skin pigmentation.

✓ **LO4** Identify the forms of skin cancer.

✓ **LO5** Understand the two major causes of acne and how to treat them.

✓ **LO6** List the factors that contribute to the aging of the skin.

✓ **LO7** Explain the effects of overexposure to the sun on the skin.

✓ **LO8** Understand what contact dermatitis is and know how it can be prevented.

Key Terms

Page number indicates where in the chapter the term is used.

albinism
pg. 183

allergic contact dermatitis (ACD)
pg. 190

anaerobic
pg. 186

anhidrosis
pg. 181

basal cell carcinoma
pg. 184

bromhidrosis
pg. 181

bulla
pg. 178

chloasma (liver spots)
pg. 183

closed comedo (whitehead)
pg. 180

conjunctivitis (pinkeye)
pg. 182

contact dermatitis
pg. 190

crust
pg. 179

cyst
pg. 178

dermatitis
pg. 182

dyschromias
pg. 183

eczema
pg. 182

excoriation
pg. 180

extrinsic factors
pg. 187

fissure
pg. 180

free radicals
pg. 188

herpes simplex
pg. 182

hyperhidrosis
pg. 181

hyperpigmentation
pg. 183

hypertrophy
pg. 184

hypopigmentation
pg. 183

impetigo
pg. 182

intrinsic factors
pg. 187

irritant contact dermatitis (ICD)
pg. 191

keloid
pg. 180

keratoma
pg. 184

lentigines
pg. 183

Key Terms

Page number indicates where in the chapter the term is used.

lesion
pg. 178

leukoderma
pg. 183

macule
pg. 178

malignant melanoma
pg. 184

milia
pg. 180

miliaria rubra (prickly heat)
pg. 181

mole
pg. 184

nevus (birthmark)
pg. 183

nodule
pg. 178

noncomedogenic
pg. 187

primary lesions
pg. 178

psoriasis
pg. 182

retention hyperkeratosis
pg. 186

rosacea
pg. 181

scale
pg. 180

scar (cicatrix)
pg. 180

sebaceous cyst
pg. 181

seborrheic dermatitis
pg. 181

secondary skin lesions
pg. 179

sensitization
pg. 190

skin tag
pg. 184

squamous cell carcinoma
pg. 184

stain
pg. 183

tan
pg. 183

telangiectasis
pg. 181

tubercle
pg. 179

tumor
pg. 179

ulcer
pg. 180

verruca (wart)
pg. 184

vesicle
pg. 179

vitiligo
pg. 183

wheal
pg. 179

Are you interested in skin care? Have you always thought that it would be interesting to understand the way that the skin functions and how it can be improved and beautified? If so, then skin care is a possible area of specialty for you!

Skin care specialists are in high demand in many salons and spas and earn excellent salaries. Some stylists find caring for the skin less arduous and physically demanding than styling hair and choose to balance their day by scheduling services in both areas. Whatever your reason, skin care is an area of rapid change and growth and a topic on most clients' minds. Knowing the basics of skin care and how the skin functions will allow you to advise clients on their skin care regimens when they seek your professional opinion.

WHY STUDY SKIN DISORDERS AND DISEASES?

Cosmetologists should study and have a thorough understanding of skin disorders and diseases for the following reasons:

- In order to provide even the most basic of skin care services, you must understand the underlying structure of the skin and common skin problems.
- You must be able to recognize adverse conditions, including inflamed skin conditions, skin diseases, and infectious skin disorders, and you must know which of these conditions are treatable by the cosmetologist and which need to be referred to a medical doctor.
- Knowing about and being able to offer skin care treatments adds another dimension of service for your clients.

Disorders and Diseases of the Skin

Like any other organ of the body, the skin is susceptible to a variety of diseases, disorders, and ailments. In your work as a practitioner, you will often see skin and scalp disorders, so you must be prepared to recognize certain common skin conditions and know which you can help to treat and which must be referred to a physician. Occasionally, you may be asked to apply or use on a client a scalp treatment prescribed by a physician. These must be applied in accordance with a physician's directions.

A dermatologist is a physician who specializes in diseases and disorders of the skin, hair, and nails. Dermatologists attend four years of college, four years of medical school, and then about four

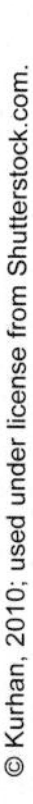
© Kurhan, 2010; used under license from Shutterstock.com.

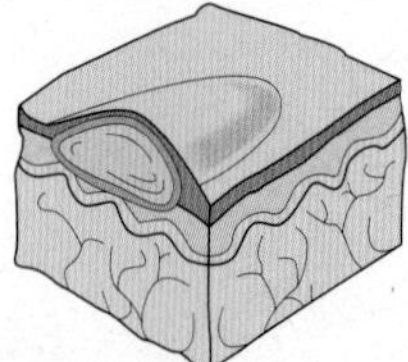

Vesicle:
Accumulation of fluid between the upper layers of the skin; elevated mass containing serous fluid; less than 0.5 cm
Example:
Herpes simplex, herpes zoster, chickenpox

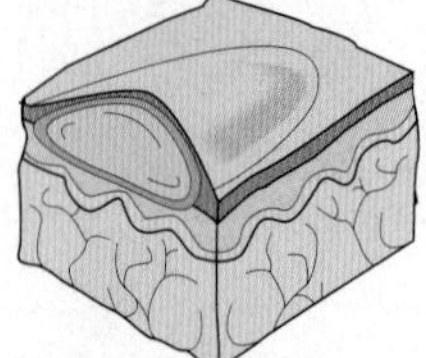

Bulla (plural: bullae):
Same as a vesicle only greater than 0.5 cm
Example:
Contact dermatitis, large second-degree burns, bulbous impetigo, pemphigus

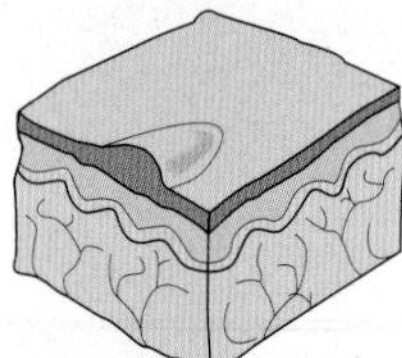

Papule:
Solid, elevated lesion less than 0.5 cm in diameter
Example:
Warts, elevated nevi

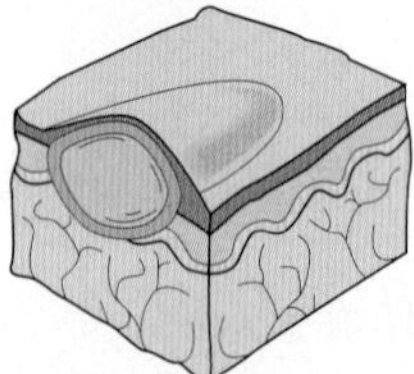

Tubercle:
Solid and elevated; however, it extends deeper than papules into the dermis or subcutaneous tissues, 0.5-2 cm
Example:
Lipoma, erythema, nodosum, cyst

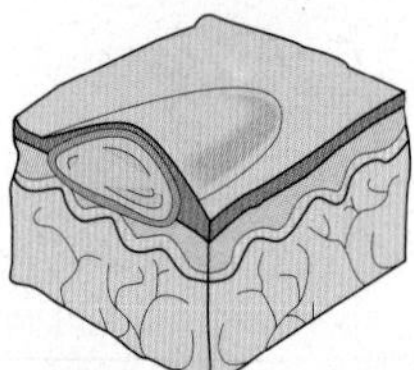

Pustule:
Vesicles or bullae that become filled with pus, usually described as less than 0.5 cm in diameter
Example:
Acne, impetigo, furuncles, carbuncles, folliculitis

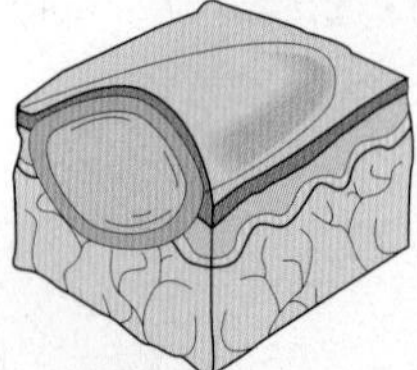

Tumor:
The same as a nodule only greater than 2 cm
Example:
Carcinoma (such as advanced breast carcinoma); not basal cell or squamous cell of the skin

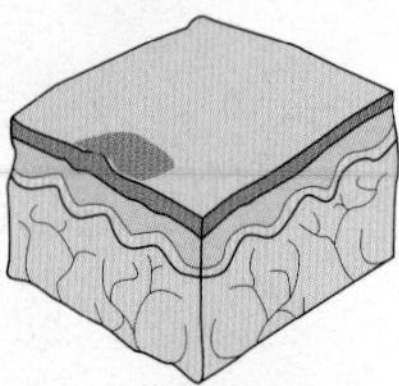

Macule (plural: maculae):
Localized changes in skin color of less than 1 cm in diameter
Example:
Freckle

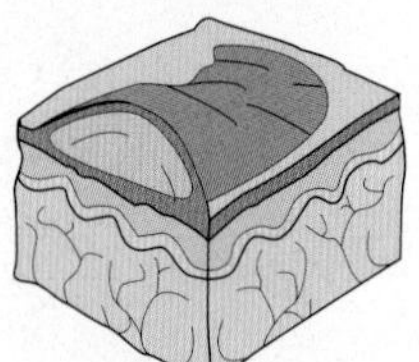

Wheal:
Localized edema in the epidermis causing irregular elevation that may be red or pale
Example:
Insect bite or a hive

▲ Figure 8–1
Primary skin lesions. These illustrations show the size, elevation or depression, and layers of the skin that are affected in each type of lesion.

© Milady, a part of Cengage Learning.

years of specialty training in dermatology. Many have additional training in internal medicine, because some skin symptoms may be reflective of internal disease. Cosmetologists refer clients with medical issues to dermatologists more than any other type of physician.

It is very important that a salon not serve a client who is suffering from an inflamed skin disorder, infectious or not, without a physician's note permitting the client to receive services. The cosmetologist should be able to recognize these conditions and sensitively suggest that proper measures be taken to prevent more serious consequences.

Numerous important terms relating to skin, scalp, and hair disorders that you should be familiar with are described in subsequent sections.

Lesions of the Skin

A **lesion** (LEE-zhun) is a mark on the skin that may indicate an injury or damage that changes the structure of tissues or organs. A lesion can be as simple as a freckle or as dangerous as a skin cancer. Lesions can indicate skin disorders or diseases and sometimes may indicate other internal diseases. Being familiar with the principal skin lesions will help you be able to distinguish between conditions that may and may not be treated in a salon or spa (**Figure 8–1**).

Primary Lesions of the Skin

The terms for different lesions listed below often indicate differences in the area of the skin layers affected and the size of the lesion.

Primary lesions are lesions that are a different color than the color of the skin and/or lesions that are raised above the surface of the skin. Requires medical referral.

Bulla (BULL-uh), (plural: bullae, BULL-ay), is a large blister containing a watery fluid; similar to a vesicle but larger (**Figure 8–2**). Requires medical referral.

Cyst (SIST) is a closed, abnormally developed sac that contains fluid, pus, semifluid, or morbid matter, above or below the skin. Cysts are frequently seen in severe acne cases. Requires medical referral.

Macule (MAK-yool), (plural: maculae, MAK-yuh-ly), is any flat spot or discoloration on the skin, such as a freckle or a red spot, left after a pimple has healed.

Nodule (NOD-yool) is a solid bump larger than .4 inches (1 centimeter) that can be easily felt. Requires medical referral.

Papule is a small elevation on the skin that contains no fluid but may develop pus. Papules are frequently seen in acne.

Pustule is a raised, inflamed, papule with a white or yellow center containing pus in the top of the lesion referred to as the head of the pimple (**Figure 8–3**).

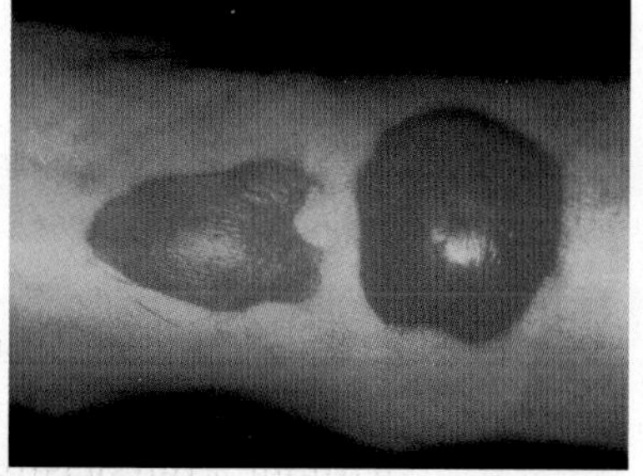

Reprinted with permission from the American Academy of Dermatology. All rights reserved.

▲ Figure 8–2
Bullae.

Reprinted with permission from the American Academy of Dermatology. All rights reserved.

▲ Figure 8–3
Papules and pustules.

Tubercle (TOO-bur-kul) is an abnormal, rounded, solid lump above, within, or under the skin; larger than a papule. Requires medical referral.

Tumor (TOO-mur) is an abnormal mass varying in size, shape, and color. Tumors are sometimes associated with cancer, but the term *tumor* can mean any sort of abnormal mass. Requires medical referral.

Vesicle (VES-ih-kel) is a small blister or sac containing clear fluid, lying within or just beneath the epidermis. Poison ivy and poison oak, for example, produce vesicles (**Figure 8–4**). Requires medical referral.

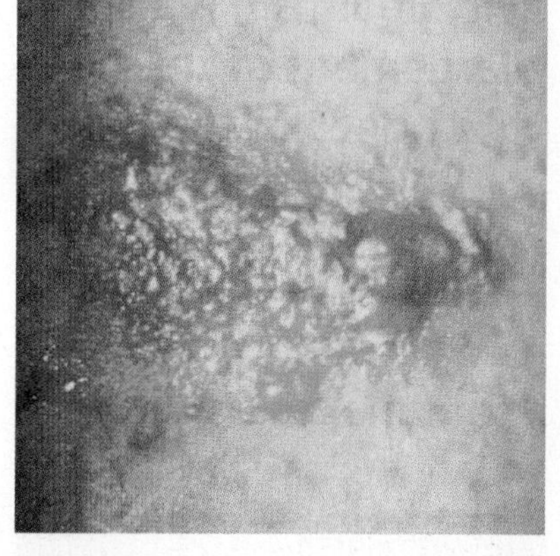

Timothy Berger, MD, Associate Clinical Professor, University of California, San Francisco.

▲ Figure 8–4
Poison oak vesicles.

Wheal (WHEEL) is an itchy, swollen lesion that lasts only a few hours; caused by a blow or scratch, the bite of an insect, urticaria (skin allergy), or the sting of a nettle. Examples include hives and mosquito bites.

Secondary Lesions

Secondary skin lesions are characterized by piles of material on the skin surface, such as a crust or scab, or by depressions in the skin surface, such as an ulcer (**Figure 8–5**).

Crust is dead cells that form over a wound or blemish while it is healing; an accumulation of sebum and pus, sometimes mixed with epidermal material. An example is the scab on a sore.

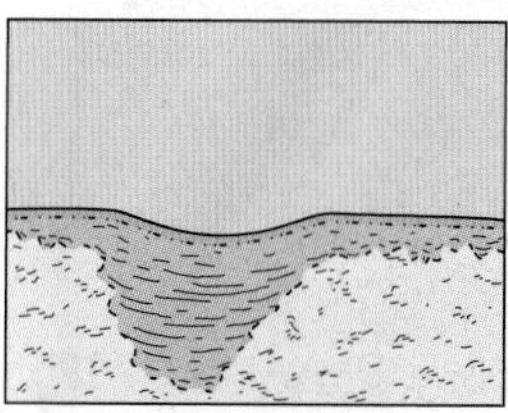

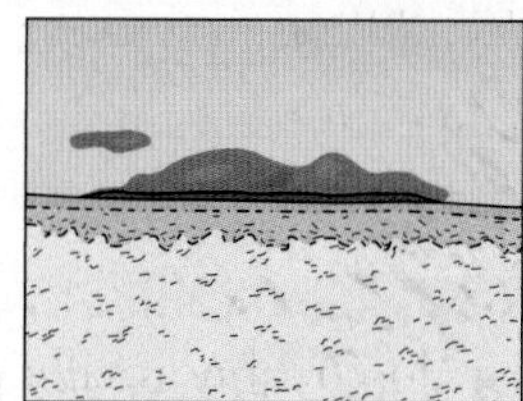

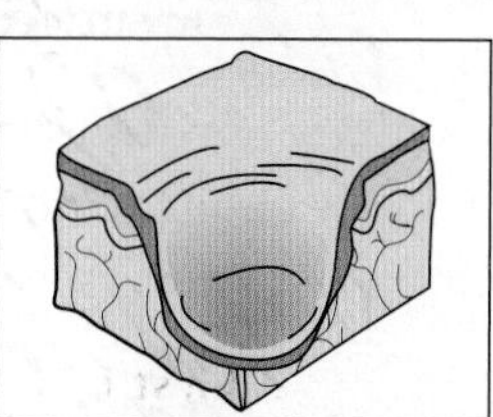

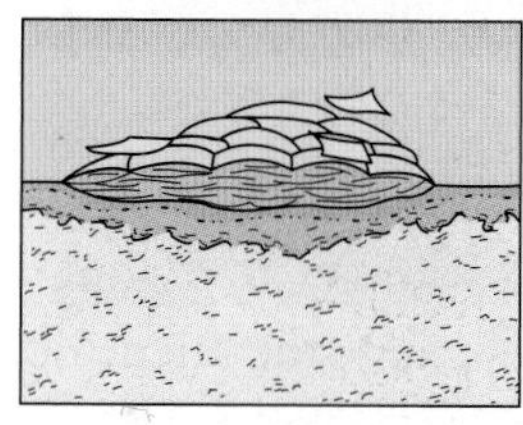

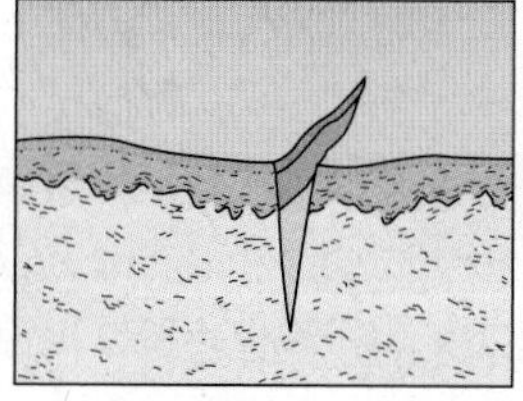

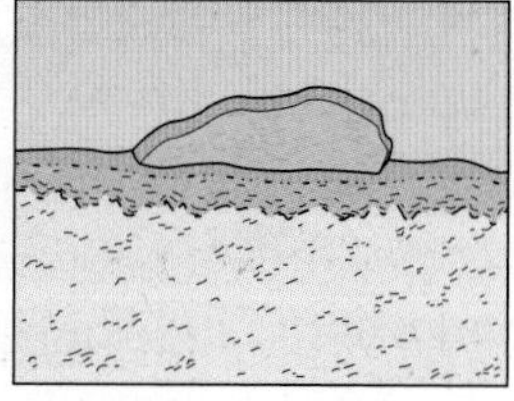

© Milady, a part of Cengage Learning.

◀ Figure 8–5
Secondary skin lesions.

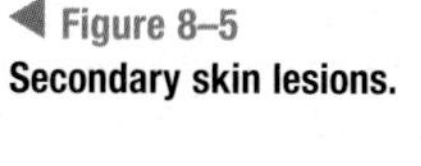

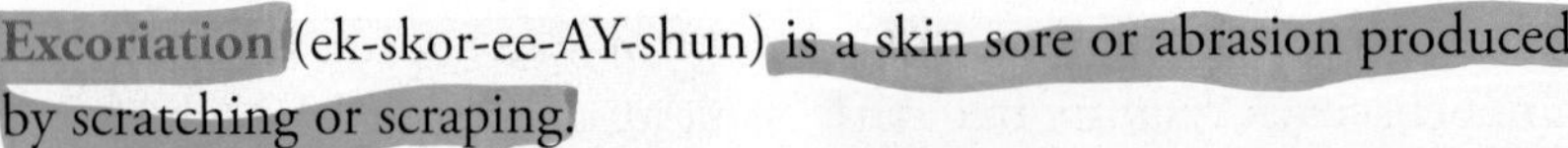

Excoriation (ek-skor-ee-AY-shun) is a skin sore or abrasion produced by scratching or scraping.

Fissure (FISH-ur) is a crack in the skin that penetrates the dermis. Examples are severely cracked and/or chapped hands or lips.

Keloid (KEE-loyd) is a thick scar resulting from excessive growth of fibrous tissue (**Figure 8–6**).

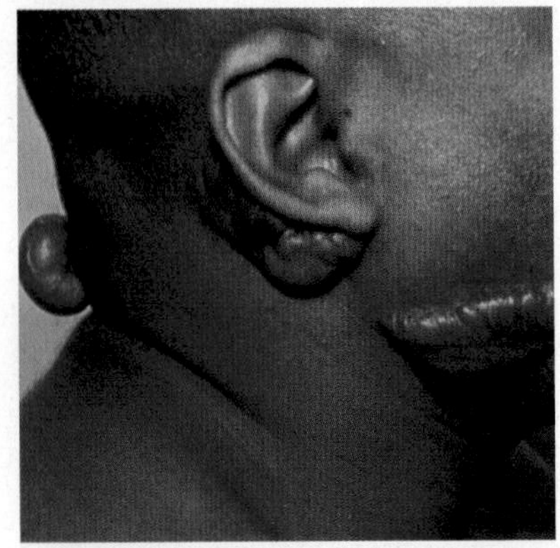

▲ Figure 8–6
Keloids.

Scale is any thin dry or oily plate of epidermal flakes. An example is abnormal or excessive dandruff.

Scar, also known as **cicatrix** (SIK-uh-triks), is a lightly raised mark on the skin formed after an injury or lesion of the skin has healed.

Ulcer (UL-sur) is an open lesion on the skin or mucous membrane of the body, accompanied by loss of skin depth and possibly weeping of fluids or pus. Requires medical referral. ☑ **LO1**

Disorders of the Sebaceous (Oil) Glands

There are several common disorders of the sebaceous (oil) glands that the cosmetologist should be able to understand and identify.

An open comedo, also known as a blackhead, is a hair follicle filled with keratin and sebum. Comedones appear most frequently on the face, especially in the T-zone, the center of the face (**Figure 8–7**). When the sebum of the comedo is exposed to the environment, it oxidizes and turns black. When the follicle is closed and not exposed to the environment, the sebum remains a white or cream color and is a **closed comedo**, also known as **whitehead**, and appears as a small bump just under the skin surface.

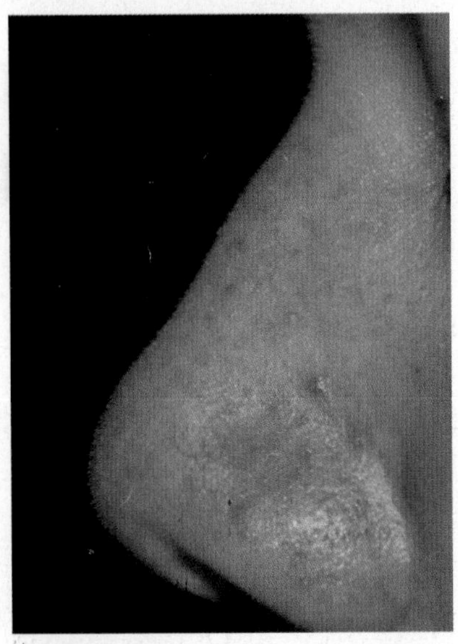

▲ Figure 8–7
Comedones.

Comedones can be removed by trained beauty professionals as long as proper procedures are employed and the procedure is performed in a sanitary environment using extraction implements that have been properly cleaned and disinfected.

Milia (MIL-ee-uh) are benign, keratin-filled cysts that appear just under the epidermis and have no visible opening. They resemble small sesame seeds and are almost always perfectly round. They are commonly associated with newborn babies but can appear on the skin of people of all ages. They are usually found around the eyes, cheeks, and forehead, and they appear as small, whitish masses (**Figure 8–8**). Depending on the state, milia can be treated in the salon or spa.

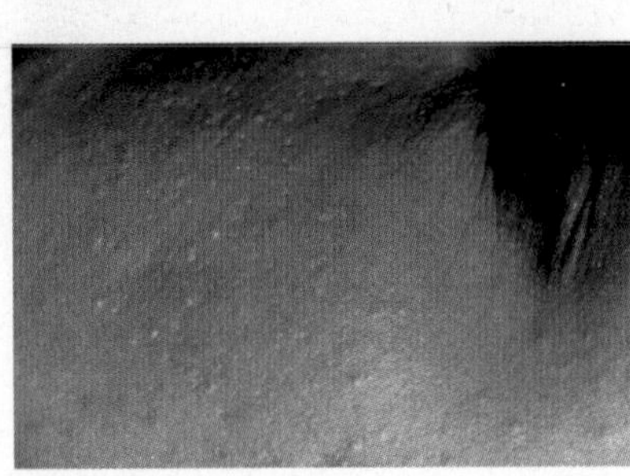

▲ Figure 8–8
Milia.

Acne, also known as acne vulgaris, is a skin disorder characterized by chronic inflammation of the sebaceous glands from retained secretions and bacteria known as propionibacterium acnes (P. acnes), the scientific term for acne bacteria. Acne will be discussed in further detail later in this chapter (**Figure 8–9**).

Reprinted with permission from the American Academy of Dermatology. All rights reserved.

Sebaceous cyst is a large protruding pocket-like lesion filled with sebum. Sebaceous cysts are frequently seen on the scalp and the back. They should be removed surgically by a dermatologist.

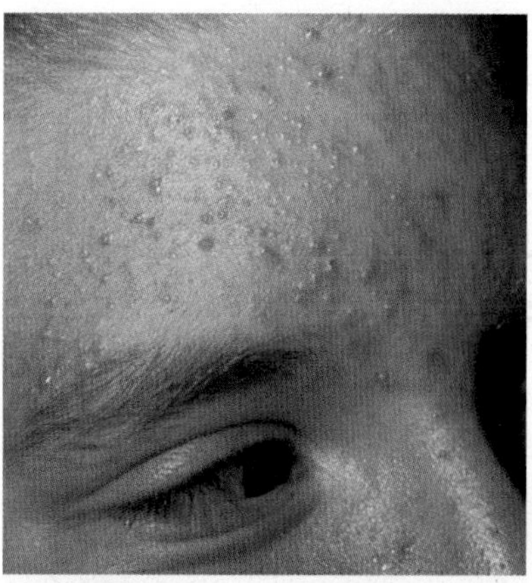

Larry Hamill.

▲ Figure 8–9
Acne.

Seborrheic dermatitis (seb-oh-REE-ick derm-ah-TIE-tus) is a skin condition caused by an inflammation of the sebaceous glands. It is often characterized by redness, dry or oily scaling, crusting, and/or itchiness (**Figure 8–10**). The red, flaky skin often appears in the eyebrows and beard, in the scalp and hairline, at the middle of the forehead, and along the sides of the nose. Mild flares of seborrheic dermatitis are sometimes treated with cortisone creams. Seborrheic dermatitis is a medical condition, but it can be helped in the salon with the application of non-fatty skin care products designed for sensitive skin. Severe cases should be referred to a dermatologist, who will often prescribe topical antifungal medications.

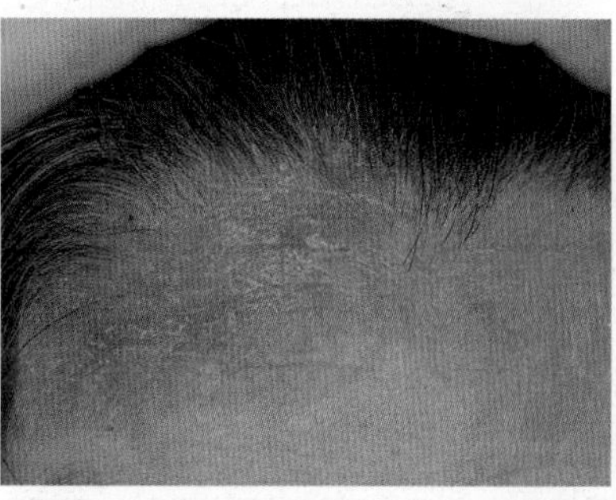

Courtesy of www.dermnet.com.

▲ Figure 8–10
Seborrheic dermatitis.

Rosacea (roh-ZAY-shuh), formerly called *acne rosacea*, is a chronic condition that appears primarily on the cheeks and nose. It is characterized by flushing (redness), **telangiectasis** (tee-lang-jek-tay-shuhz) (distended or dilated surface blood vessels), and, in some cases, the formation of papules and pustules. The cause of rosacea is unknown, but the condition is thought to be genetic. Certain factors are known to aggravate the condition in some individuals. These include exposure to heat, sun, and very cold weather; ingestion of spicy foods, caffeine, and alcohol; and stress. Rosacea can be treated and kept under control by using medication prescribed by a dermatologist, using proper skin care products designed for especially sensitive skin, and avoiding the aggravating flare factors listed above (**Figure 8–11**). ☑ **LO2**

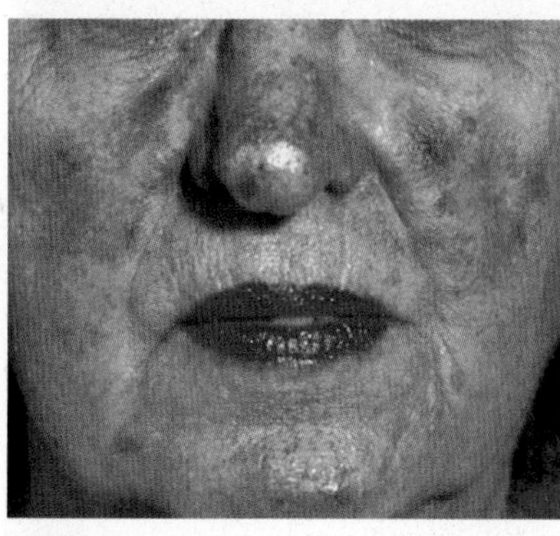

Reprinted with permission from the American Academy of Dermatology. All rights reserved.

▲ Figure 8–11
Rosacea.

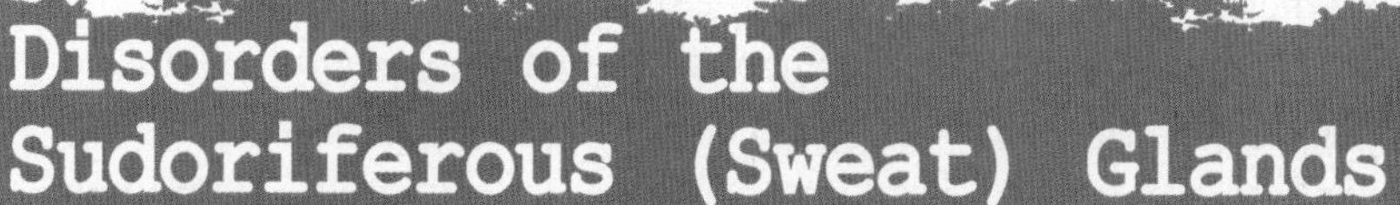

Disorders of the Sudoriferous (Sweat) Glands

Anhidrosis (an-hih-DROH-sis) is a deficiency in perspiration, often a result of fever or certain skin diseases. Requires medical referral.

Bromhidrosis (broh-mih-DROH-sis) is foul-smelling perspiration, usually noticeable in the armpits or on the feet, that is caused by bacteria. Severe cases require medical referral.

Hyperhidrosis (hy-per-hy-DROH-sis) is excessive sweating, caused by heat or general body weakness. Requires medical referral.

Miliaria rubra (mil-ee-AIR-ee-ah ROOB-rah), also known as **prickly heat**, is an acute inflammatory disorder of the sweat glands, characterized by the eruption of small red vesicles and accompanied by burning, itching skin. It is caused by exposure to excessive heat and usually clears in a short time without treatment.

*Read & Summarize!

Inflammations and Common Infections of the Skin

Conjunctivitis (kuhn-juhngk-tuh-VAHY-tis), also known as **pinkeye**, is a common bacterial infection of the eyes. It is extremely contagious, and clients who have conjunctivitis or obviously irritated eyes should be politely rescheduled and referred to a physician immediately. Any product or implements touching infected eyes must be thrown away.

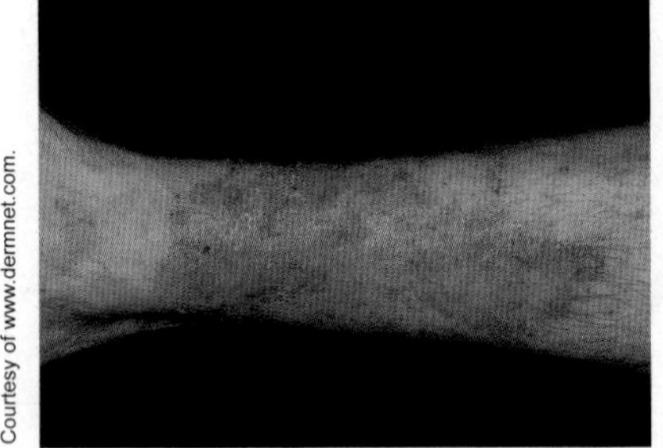

Courtesy of www.dermnet.com.

▲ Figure 8–12
Eczema.

Dermatitis (dur-muh-TY-tis) is a term broadly used to describe any inflammatory condition of the skin.

Eczema (EG-zuh-muh) is an inflammatory, uncomfortable, and often chronic disease of the skin, characterized by moderate to severe inflammation, scaling, and sometimes severe itching. There are several different types of eczema. The most common type is atopic eczema, which is an inherited genetic disorder. All cases of eczema should be referred to a physician for treatment, which is often topical cortisone. Eczema is not contagious (**Figure 8–12**).

Herpes simplex (HER-peez SIM-pleks) is a recurring viral infection that often presents as a fever blister or cold sore. It is characterized by the eruption of a single vesicle or group of vesicles on a red swollen base. The blisters usually appear on the lips, nostrils, or other part of the face, and the sores can last up to three weeks. Herpes simplex is contagious (**Figure 8–13**) and requires medical referral. Drugs are now available to control the symptoms, but the virus always remains in the body of infected persons.

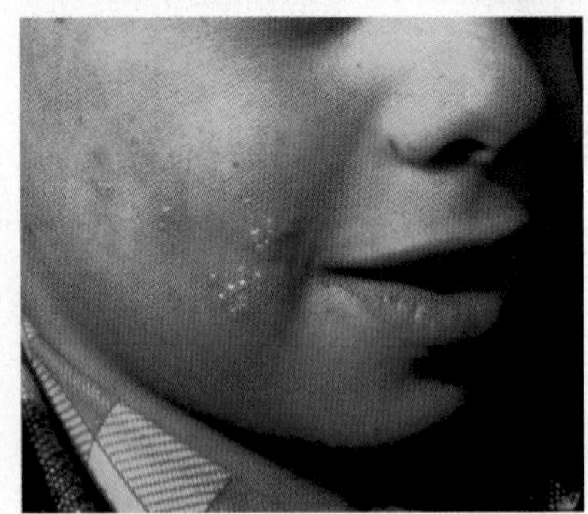

Reprinted with permission from the American Academy of Dermatology. All rights reserved.

▲ Figure 8–13
Herpes simplex.

Impetigo (im-pet-EYE-go) is a contagious bacterial skin infection characterized by weeping lesions. Impetigo normally occurs on the face (especially the chin area) and is most frequently seen in children. Clients with any type of weeping open facial lesions should be politely rescheduled and referred to a physician immediately.

Psoriasis (suh-RY-uh-sis) is a skin disease characterized by red patches covered with silver-white scales and is usually found on the scalp, elbows, knees, chest, and lower back. Psoriasis is caused by the skin cells turning over faster than normal. It rarely occurs on the face. When the condition is irritated, bleeding points can occur. Psoriasis is not contagious (**Figure 8–14**), but it requires medical referral. It is treatable, but it is not curable.

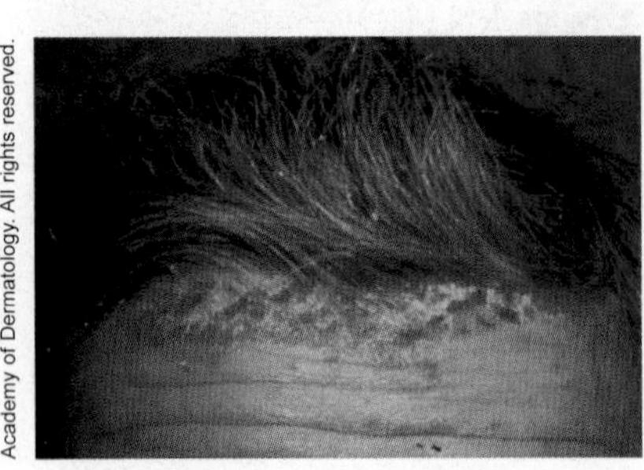

Reprinted with permission from the American Academy of Dermatology. All rights reserved.

▲ Figure 8–14
Psoriasis.

Pigment Disorders of the Skin

Pigment can be affected by internal factors such as heredity or hormonal fluctuations, or by outside factors such as prolonged exposure to the sun. Abnormal colorations, known as **dyschromias** (dis-chrome-ee-uhs), accompany skin disorders and many systemic disorders. A change in pigmentation can also be observed when certain drugs are being taken internally. The following terms relate to changes in the pigmentation of the skin:

Hyperpigmentation (hy-pur-pig-men-TAY-shun) means darker than normal pigmentation, appearing as dark splotches. **Hypopigmentation** (hy-poh-pig-men-TAY-shun) is the absence of pigment, resulting in light or white splotches.

Albinism (AL-bi-niz-em) is congenital hypopigmentation, or absence of melanin pigment in the body, including the skin, hair, and eyes. Hair is silky white. The skin is pinkish white and will not tan. The eyes are pink, and the skin is sensitive to light and ages early.

Chloasma (kloh-AZ-mah), also known as **liver spots**, is a condition characterized by hyperpigmentation on the skin in spots that are not elevated. This is just a commonly-used term; the spots have nothing to do with the liver. They are generally caused by cumulative sun exposure. They can be helped by exfoliation treatments or can be treated by a dermatologist.

Lentigines (len-TIJ-e-neez) (singular: lentigo, len-TY-goh) is the technical term for freckles, small yellow-colored to brown-colored spots on skin exposed to sunlight and air.

Leukoderma (loo-koh-DUR-muh) is a skin disorder characterized by light abnormal patches (hypopigmentation); it is caused by a burn or congenital disease that destroys the pigment-producing cells. Examples are vitiligo and albinism.

Nevus (NEE-vus), also known as **birthmark**, is a small or large malformation of the skin due to abnormal pigmentation or dilated capillaries.

Stain is an abnormal brown-colored or wine-colored skin discoloration with a circular or irregular shape (**Figure 8–15**). Its permanent color is due to the presence of darker pigment. Stains can be present at birth, or they can appear during aging, after certain diseases, or after the disappearance of moles, freckles, and liver spots. The cause is often unknown.

Tan is the change in pigmentation of skin caused by exposure to the sun or ultraviolet light.

Vitiligo (vi-til-EYE-goh) is a hereditary condition that causes hypopigmented spots and splotches on the skin that may be related to thyroid conditions (**Figure 8–16**). Skin with vitiligo must be protected from overexposure to the sun. LO3

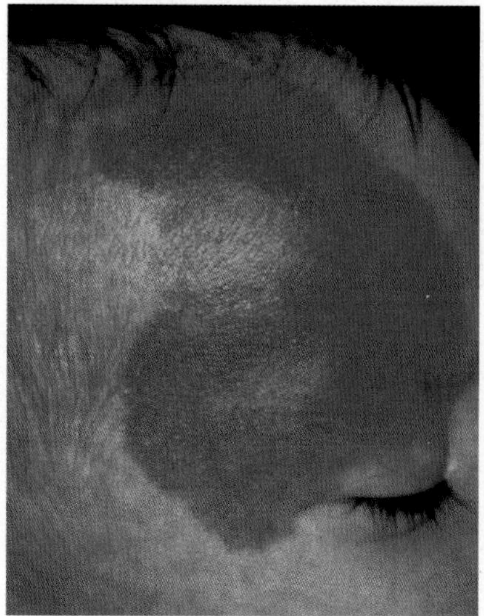

Reprinted with permission from the American Academy of Dermatology. All rights reserved.

▲ Figure 8–15
Port wine stain.

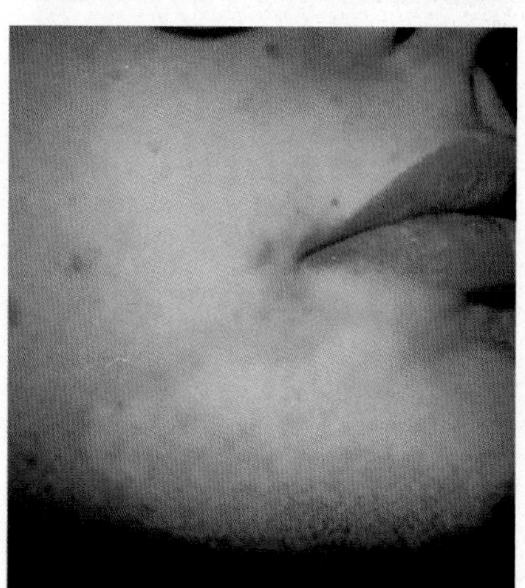

Courtesy of www.dermnet.com.

▲ Figure 8–16
Vitiligo.

CAUTION

Do not treat moles or remove hair from moles. Removing a hair from a mole could irritate or cause a structural change to it. Only a physician should remove a hair from a mole.

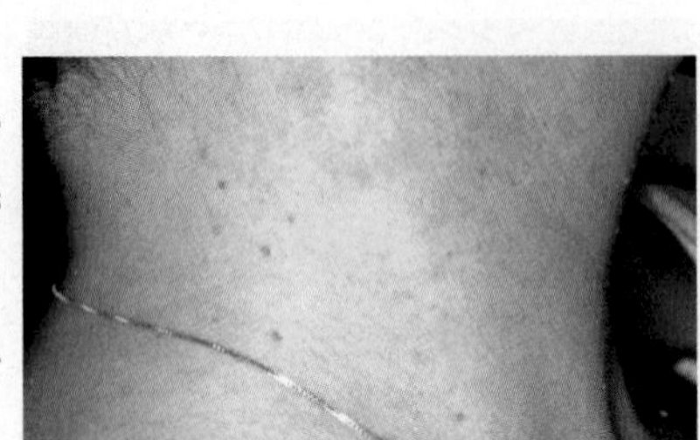

Reprinted with permission from the American Academy of Dermatology. All rights reserved.

▲ Figure 8–17
Skin tags.

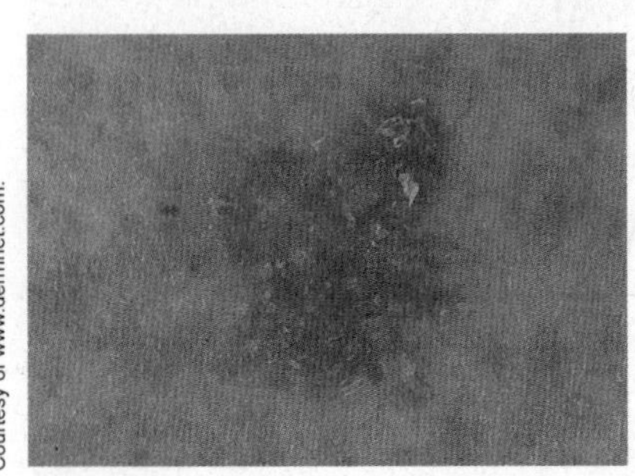

Courtesy of www.dermnet.com.

▲ Figure 8–18
Basal cell carcinoma.

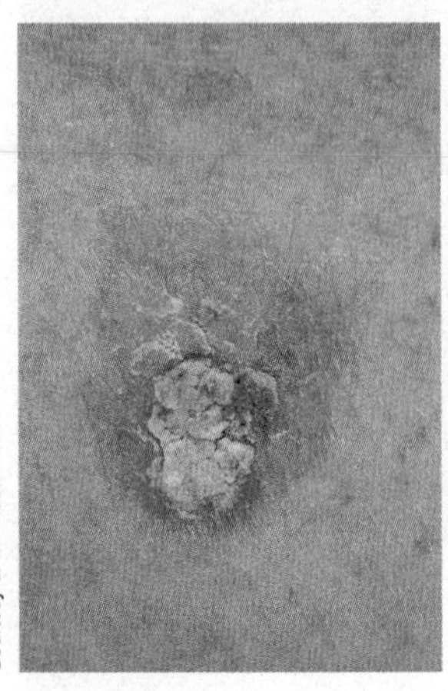

Courtesy of www.dermnet.com.

▲ Figure 8–19
Squamous cell carcinoma.

Hypertrophies of the Skin

A **hypertrophy** (hy-PUR-truh-fee) of the skin is an abnormal growth of the skin. Many hypertrophies are benign, which means they are harmless.

A **keratoma** (kair-uh-TOH-muh) is an acquired, superficial, thickened patch of epidermis. A callus is a keratoma that is caused by continued, repeated pressure or friction on any part of the skin, especially the hands and feet. If the thickening grows inward, it is called a corn.

A **mole** is a small brownish spot or blemish on the skin, ranging in color from pale tan to brown or bluish black. Some moles are small and flat, resembling freckles; others are raised and darker in color. Large dark hairs often occur in moles. Any change in a mole requires medical attention.

A **skin tag** is a small brown-colored or flesh-colored outgrowth of the skin (**Figure 8–17**). Skin tags occur most frequently on the neck of an older person. They can be easily removed by a dermatologist.

A **verruca** (vuh-ROO-kuh), also known as **wart**, is a hypertrophy of the papillae and epidermis. It is caused by a virus and is infectious. Verruca can spread from one location to another, particularly along a scratch in the skin. Requires medical referral.

Skin Cancer

Skin cancer—primarily caused from overexposure to the sun—comes in three distinct forms that vary in severity. Each is named for the type of cells that it affects.

Basal cell carcinoma (BAY-zul SEL kar-sin-OH-muh) is the most common and the least severe type of skin cancer; it is often characterized by light or pearly nodules (**Figure 8–18**). **Squamous** (SKWAY-mus) **cell carcinoma** is more serious than basal cell carcinoma, and often is characterized by scaly red papules or nodules (**Figure 8–19**). The third and most serious form of skin cancer is **malignant melanoma** (muh-LIG-nent mel-uh-NOH-muh), which is often characterized by black or dark brown patches on the skin that may appear uneven in texture, jagged, or raised (**Figure 8–20**). Malignant melanoma is the least common—but also the most dangerous—type of skin cancer.

Clients should be advised to regularly see a dermatologist for checkups of the skin, especially if any changes in coloration, size, or shape of a mole are detected, if the skin bleeds unexpectedly, or a lesion or scrape does not heal quickly.

Home self-examinations can also be an effective way to check for signs of potential skin cancer between scheduled doctor visits. When performing a self-care exam, clients should be advised to check for any changes in existing moles and pay attention to any new visible growths on the skin.

If detected early, anyone with these three forms of skin cancer has a good chance for survival. Cosmetologists serve a unique role by being able to recognize the appearance of serious skin disorders and referring the client to a dermatologist for diagnosis and treatment.

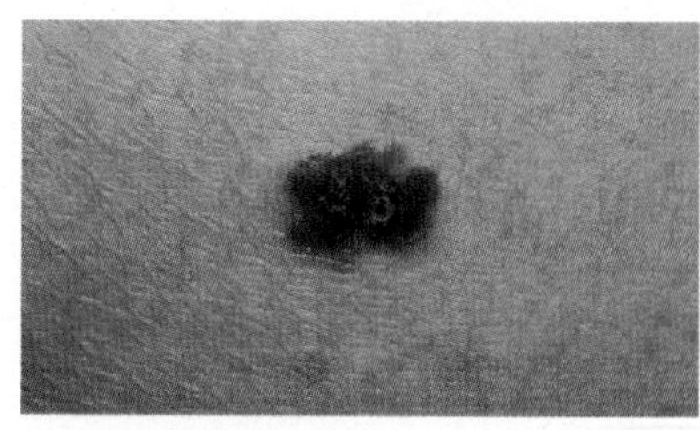

Reprinted with permission from the American Academy of Dermatology. All rights reserved.

▲ Figure 8–20
Malignant melanoma.

FYI

According to the American Cancer Society, professionals should use the ABCDE Cancer Checklist to spot signs of change in existing moles (Figure 8–21 a-f):

- A is for **ASYMMETRY:** the two sides of the lesion are not identical.
- B is for **BORDER:** the border is irregular on these lesions.
- C is for **COLOR:** melanomas are usually dark and have more than one color or colors that fade into one another.
- D is for **DIAMETER:** the lesion in a melanoma is usually at least the size of pencil eraser.
- E is for **EVOLVING:** melanoma as a lesion often changes appearance.

For more information, contact the American Cancer Society at http://www.cancer.org or (800) ACS-2345.

☑ LO4

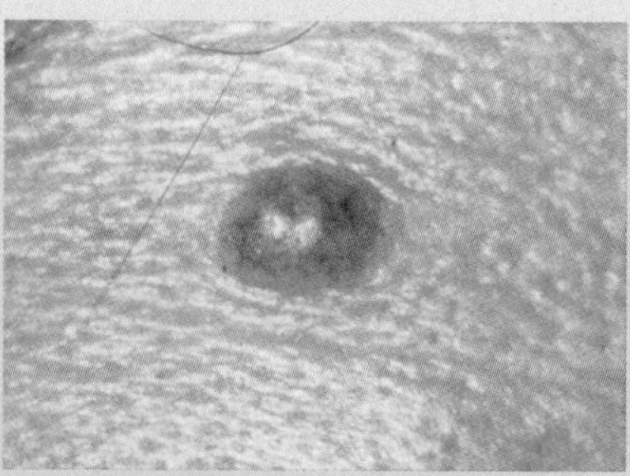

▲ Figure 8–21a
Normal mole with normal symmetry. Both sides of the mole are the same.

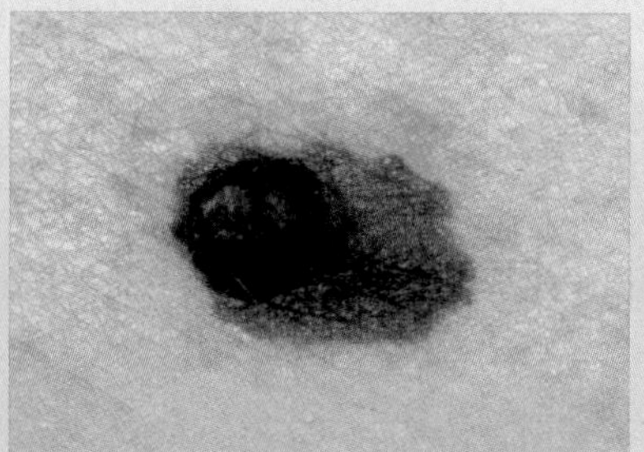

▲ Figure 8–21b
A is for asymmetry. Abnormal mole has uneven symmetry. Two sides of the mole are not the same.

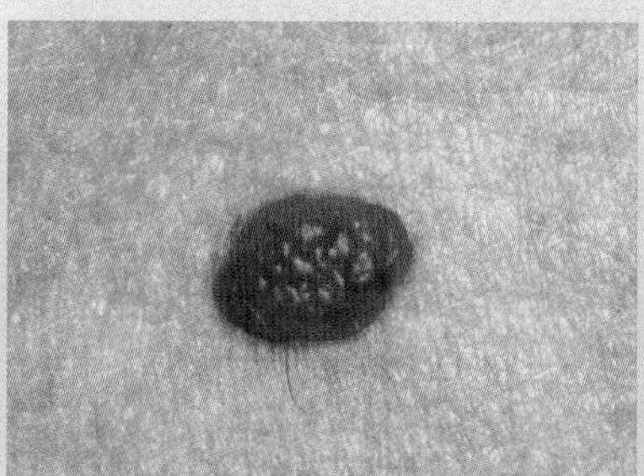

▲ Figure 8–21c
Normal mole with regular even borders.

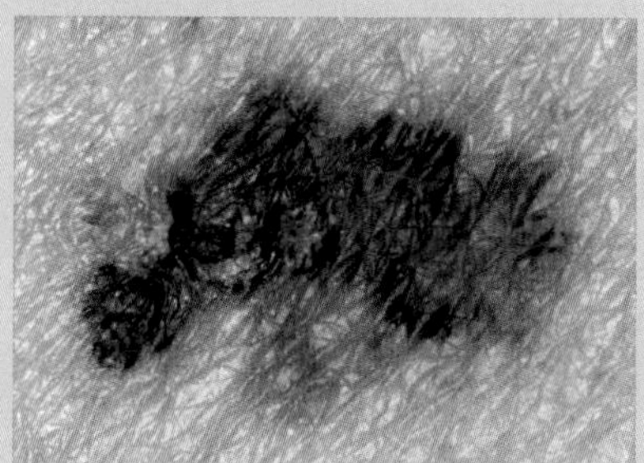

▲ Figure 8–21d
B is for border. Abnormal mole has uneven or jagged borders.

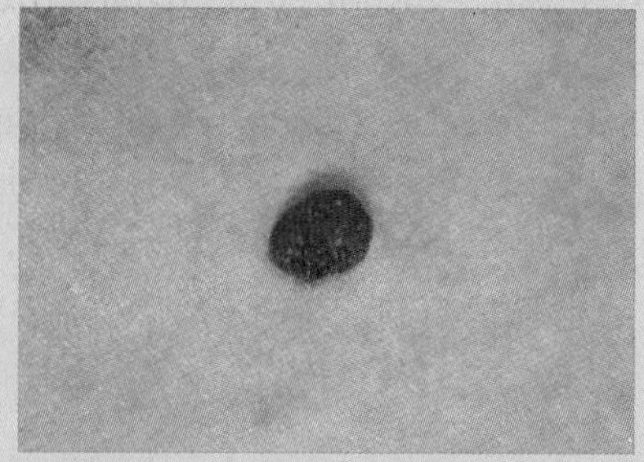

▲ Figure 8–21e
Normal mole with even color.

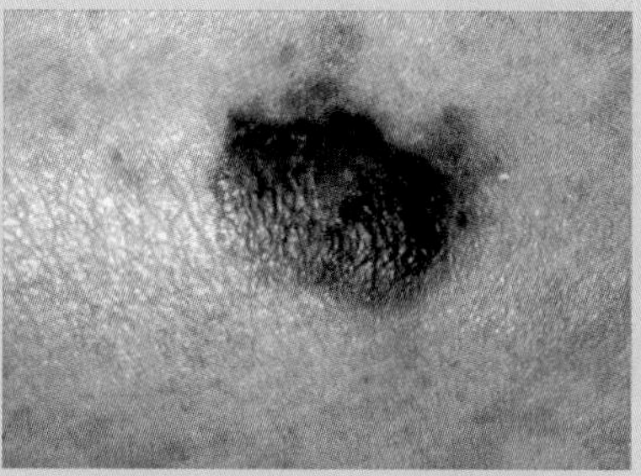

▲ Figure 8–21f
C is for color. Abnormal mole, with more than one dark color.

Courtesy of The Skin Cancer Foundation, http://www.skincancer.org

Acne and Problem Skin

Common skin problems that affect clients' appearance, such as acne, can become a source of great concern. Most people have acne or another skin issue at some time in their lives. Acne is both a skin disorder and an esthetic problem, and it is a major concern to anyone who suffers from it. Frequently misunderstood to be a teenage skin disorder, it can affect people at almost any age. Women often do not have acne problems until they reach their 20s or 30s or beyond. Because it affects the appearance, it is of interest to cosmetologists and estheticians, who are in a position to help their clients with treatment for minor cases or to provide dermatological referral for more severe acne.

Acne is a disorder affected by two major factors: heredity and hormones. People with acne inherit the tendency to retain cells that gather on the walls of the follicle, eventually clumping and obstructing the follicle. **Retention hyperkeratosis** (hy-pur-kair-uh-TOH-sis) is the hereditary tendency for acne-prone skin to retain dead cells in the follicle, forming an obstruction that clogs follicles and exacerbates inflammatory acne lesions such as papules and pustules.

The oiliness of the skin is also hereditary. Overproduction of sebum by the sebaceous gland contributes to the development of acne by coating the dead cell buildup in the follicle with sebum, which hardens due to oxidation. This conglomeration of dead cells and solidified sebum obstruct the follicle.

Propionibacterium acnes are **anaerobic** (ann-air-ROH-bic), which means that these bacteria cannot survive in the presence of oxygen. When the follicles are obstructed, oxygen is blocked from the bottom of the follicles, allowing acne bacteria to multiply.

The main food source for acne bacteria is fatty acids, which are easily obtained from the abundance of sebum in the follicle. These bacteria flourish in this ideal environment, which is void of oxygen and with plenty of food (sebum) for the bacteria. The bacteria multiply, causing inflammation and swelling in the follicle, and eventually rupture the follicle wall. When the wall of the follicle ruptures, the immune system is alerted, causing blood to rush to the ruptured follicle, carrying white blood cells to fight the bacteria. Blood will surround and engulf the follicle, which is what causes the redness in pimples.

An acne papule is an inflammatory acne lesion resulting from this wall rupture and infusion of blood. A pustule forms from the papule when enough white blood cells accumulate to form pus, which is primarily composed of dead white blood cells.

did you know?

Skin cancer is preventable and early detection is possible, if you know what to look for. Be aware of the following as you service your clients:

- Any unusual lesions on the skin or on the scalp or change in an existing lesion or mole.
- Melanomas. These are sometimes found on the scalp and are often first detected by cosmetologists!
- A new lesion or discoloration on the skin or scalp.
- Client complaints about sores that do not heal or unexpected skin bleeding.
- Recurrent scaly areas that may be rough to the touch, especially in sun-exposed areas such as the face, arms, or hands.

If you become aware of any of these conditions, suggest that your client consult a physician.

Acne Treatment

Minor forms of acne can be treated without medical referral. The basics of acne treatment involve:

- The use of cleansers formulated for oily skin. These foamy, rinse-off products remove excess oil from the oily and acne-prone skin. Toners designed for oily skin help to further remove excess sebum.
- Follicle exfoliants are leave-on products that help to remove cell buildup from the follicles, allowing oxygen to penetrate the follicles, killing bacteria. Commonly used ingredients in these products are alpha hydroxy acid, salicylic acid, and benzoyl peroxide. Benzoyl peroxide can be especially effective since it helps to shed cellular debris and also kills the acne bacteria.
- Avoidance of fatty skin care and cosmetic products is important because products that contain large amounts of fatty materials and oils can cause follicles to clog from the outside. Make sure all makeup and skin care products used on acne-prone skin are **noncomedogenic** (non-com-EE-doh-JENN-ic), which means the product has been designed and proven not to clog the follicles.
- Do not use harsh products or over clean acne-prone skin as this can cause inflammation that can worsen the condition.
- Mild and moderate cases of acne are often treated by trained salon and spa professionals who have received specialized education in acne treatment. ✓ **LO5**

Aging Skin Issues

Aging of the skin is a concern of almost every client over thirty years of age. There are two types of factors that influence aging of the skin: intrinsic factors and extrinsic factors.

Intrinsic factors (in-TRIN-zic FAK-torz) are skin-aging factors over which we have little control:

- Genetic aging is how our parents' skin aged, their skin coloring and resistance to sun damage.
- Gravity is the constant pulling downward on our skin and bodies.
- Facial expressions are the repeated movements of the face that result in the formation of expression lines, such as crow's-feet lines that form around the eyes, nasolabial folds that form from the corners of the nose to the corners of the mouth, and scowl lines that form between the eyes.

Extrinsic factors (ex-TRIN-zic FAK-torz) are primarily environmental factors that contribute to aging and the appearance of aging. Many scientists and dermatologists believe that these extrinsic factors are responsible for up to 85 percent of skin aging. Extrinsic factors include:

- Exposure to the sun. Tanning and sun bathing are no-nos, but the cumulative sun that we get in little doses every day is the real

© Kurhan, 2010; used under license from Shutterstock.com.

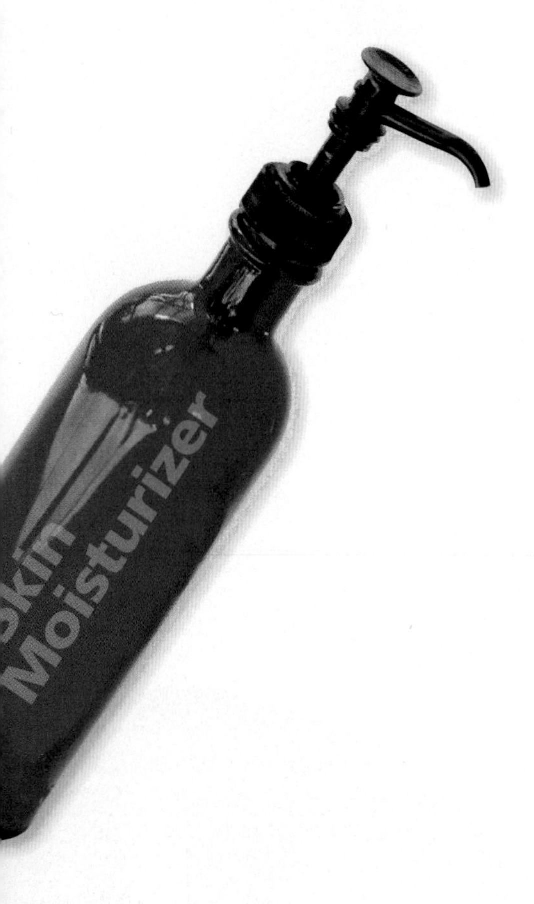

damage-causing sun for most people. Sun is by far the number one cause of the appearance of premature aging. The key to preventing this prominent skin-aging factor is to use a broad-spectrum sunscreen every single day, and the easiest way to do this is to find a daily-use moisturizer with built-in sunscreen. As a cosmetologist, you can help your clients find the best sunscreen and moisturizer to use every day.

- Smoking is bad for the body and the skin. It produces tremendous numbers of **free radicals**, unstable molecules that cause biochemical aging. These molecules, over time, can have a devastating effect on the body, especially wrinkling and sagging of the skin. Smoking causes oxygen deprivation of the skin and body, and it affects blood flow so the skin does not get adequate blood nutrients. Lack of blood flow also causes the accumulation of cellular waste, often called toxins.
- Overuse of alcoholic beverages also has an overall effect on the body and the skin. Alcohol abuse causes the body to repair itself poorly and interferes with proper nutrition distribution for the skin and body's tissues. Alcohol can also dehydrate the skin by drawing essential water out of the tissues, which causes the skin to appear dull and dry.

  Both smoking and overuse of alcoholic beverages contribute to the aging process on their own, but the combination of the two can be devastating to the tissues. The constant dilation and contraction that occur on the tiny capillaries and blood vessels, as well as the constant deprivation of oxygen and water to the tissues, quickly make the skin appear lifeless and dull. It is very difficult for the skin to adjust and repair itself. The damage done by these lifestyle habits is typically hard to reverse or diminish.
- The use of illegal drugs affects the skin as much as smoking does. Some drugs have been shown to interfere with the body's intake of oxygen, thus affecting healthy cell growth. Certain drugs can even aggravate serious skin conditions, such as acne. Others can cause dryness and allergic reactions on the skin's surface.
- Cumulative stress may significantly contribute to aging. Scientists are now learning that stress causes biochemical changes that can lead to the tissue damage that we call aging. Exercise, relaxation techniques, and a healthy state of mind can reduce stress levels, as can relaxing treatments like facials, aromatherapy, and massage.
- Poor nutrition deprives the skin of the proteins, fats, carbohydrates, vitamins, and minerals that are required to maintain, protect, and repair the skin, keeping it looking young and beautiful.
- Exposure to pollution produces free radicals and interferes with proper oxygen consumption. This affects the lungs and other internal organs, as well as the skin. The best defense against pollutants is the simplest one: follow a good daily skin care routine. Routine

© Denise Kappa, 2010; used under license from Shutterstock.com.

washing and mild exfoliating (removing dead surface skin cells) help to remove the buildup of pollutants that have settled on the skin's surface throughout the day. The application of daily moisturizers, protective lotions, and even foundation products all help to protect the skin from airborne pollutants.

The appearance of aging skin can be greatly improved by practicing a good skin care program, especially at home. A professionally designed program for aging skin based on the client's needs, skin type, and condition severity involves a good hydrating sunscreen, an alpha or beta hydroxy acid exfoliating product, and products using state-of-the-art aging skin treatment ingredients such as peptides and topical antioxidants. ✓ **LO6**

The Sun and Its Effects

The sun and its ultraviolet (UV) light have the greatest impact of all extrinsic factors on how skin ages. Approximately 80 to 85 percent of the symptoms of aging skin are caused by the rays of the sun. As we age, the collagen and elastin fibers of the skin naturally weaken. This weakening happens at a much faster rate when the skin is frequently exposed to UV light without proper protection.

UVA rays, also known as *aging rays*, are deep-penetrating rays that can even go through a glass window. These rays weaken the collagen and elastin fibers, causing wrinkling and sagging of the tissues.

UVB rays, also known as *burning rays*, cause sunburns, tanning of the skin, and the majority of skin cancers. These are shorter rays that stop penetration at the base of the epidermis.

Here are some facts to pass on to your clients to educate them about sun safety and aging sun damage prevention:

- The number one way to prevent premature skin aging is to avoid deliberate sun exposure and to use a broad spectrum sunscreen, which is one that filters both UVA and UVB rays and has an SPF (Sun Protection Factor) of at least 15, on a daily basis.
- Avoid prolonged exposure to the sun during peak hours, when UV exposure is highest. This is usually between ten AM and three PM.
- Sunscreen should be applied at least thirty minutes before sun exposure to allow time for absorption. Many people make the mistake of applying sunscreen after they have been exposed to the heat and sun for thirty minutes or more. The already inflamed skin is more

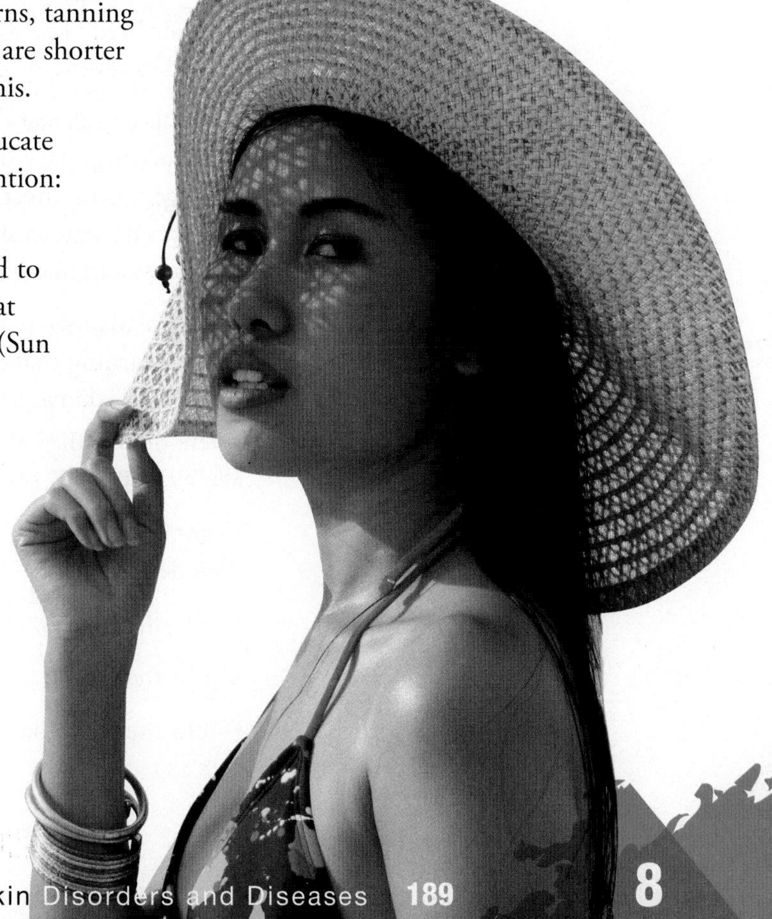

© Gina Smith, 2010; used under license from Shutterstock.com.

likely to react to the sunscreen chemicals when the sunscreen is applied after sun exposure.

- Apply sunscreen liberally after swimming and after activities that result in heavy perspiration. If the skin is exposed to hours of sun, such as during a boat trip or day at the beach, sunscreen should be applied periodically throughout the day as a precaution.
- Avoid exposing children younger than six months of age to the sun.
- People who are prone to burning frequently and easily should wear a hat and protective clothing when participating in outdoor activities, in addition to using sunscreen. Redheads and blue-eyed blonds are particularly susceptible to sun damage. ☑ LO7

© Audrey M. Vasey, 2010; used under license from Shutterstock.com.

Contact Dermatitis

Contact dermatitis is the most common work-related skin disorder for all cosmetology professionals. **Contact dermatitis** is an inflammation of the skin caused by having contact with certain chemicals or substances. Many of these substances are commonly used in cosmetology. There are two types of contact dermatitis: Allergic Contact Dermatitis and Irritant Contact Dermatitis.

Allergic Contact Dermatitis

Allergic contact dermatitis, abbreviated ACD, occurs when the person (cosmetologist or client) develops an allergy to an ingredient or a chemical, usually caused by repeated skin contact with the chemical. **Sensitization** is an allergic reaction created by repeated exposure to a chemical or a substance. Monomer liquids, haircolor, and chemical texture solutions are all capable of causing allergic reactions with repeated exposures.

Once an allergy has been established, all services must be discontinued until the allergic symptoms clear. The person affected by the allergy (cosmetologist or client) must stop using that particular product. In severe or chronic cases, affected people should see a dermatologist for allergy testing.

Common places for allergic contact dermatitis are listed below and include:

- On the fingers, palms, or on the back of the hand.
- On the face, especially the cheeks.
- On the scalp, hairline, forehead, or neckline.

If you examine the area where the problem occurs, you can usually determine the cause. For example, haircolorists often strand test color with their bare fingers and hands, so it is no surprise when they find contact dermatitis on their fingers and hands.

Irritant Contact Dermatitis

Irritant contact dermatitis, abbreviated ICD, occurs when irritating substances temporarily damage the epidermis. Unlike allergic contact dermatitis, irritant contact dermatitis is not usually chronic if precautions are taken.

Corrosive substances or exfoliating agents are examples of products with irritant potential. Contact with irritant chemicals can cause damage to the epidermis because the irritant can enter the skin surface and cause possible inflammation, redness, swelling, itching, and burning. Repeated exposure can worsen the condition.

The way to prevent both types of occupational contact dermatitis is to use gloves or utensils when working with irritating chemicals. Cosmetologists should use gloves or utensils when applying chemicals such as haircolor, straighteners, or permanent wave solutions. Nail technicians should use gloves or utensils when applying nail products such as monomer liquids and polymer powders. Estheticians should use gloves or utensils when applying exfoliants such as peeling products and drying agents. All of these chemicals can irritate the skin of the hands and arms if precautions are not taken to avoid contact.

Frequent hand washing can result in dry hands, with cracks in the skin that can cause more irritation and that can allow penetration of irritant chemicals. Hand washing is important to prevent the spread of disease, but it should be followed by the frequent use of protective hand creams to keep the hands in good condition. ✓ **LO8**

Protect Yourself

Taking the time to keep your implements, tools, equipment, and surfaces clean and disinfected is an important step in protecting yourself and avoiding a skin problem. Practice these suggestions with great diligence:

- Take extreme care to keep brush handles, containers, and table tops clean and free from product, dust, and residue. Repeatedly handling these items will cause overexposure if the items are not kept clean.
- Wear protective gloves whenever using products known to cause irritant or allergic contact dermatitis.
- Keep your hands clean and moisturized. Keeping the skin of the hands in excellent condition will help prevent irritant reactions.

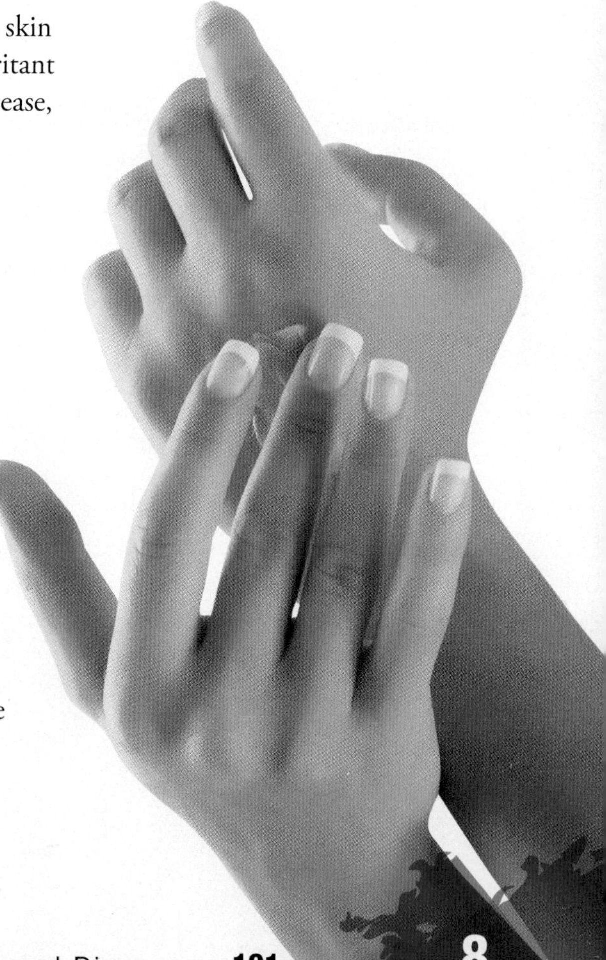

© Liv Friis-Larsen, 2010; used under license from Shutterstock.com.

Review Questions

1. What is a skin lesion?
2. Name and describe at least five disorders of the sebaceous glands.
3. Name and describe at least five changes in skin pigmentation.
4. What are the three forms of skin cancer?
5. What are the two major causes of acne and how should they be effectively treated?
6. List the factors that contribute to the aging of the skin.
7. Explain the skin effects of overexposure to the sun.
8. What is contact dermatitis and how can it be prevented?

Chapter Glossary

albinism	Congenital hypopigmentation, or absence of melanin pigment of the body, including the skin, hair, and eyes.
allergic contact dermatitis	Abbreviated ACD; an allergy to an ingredient or a chemical, usually caused by repeated skin contact withthe chemical.
anaerobic	Cannot survive in the presence of oxygen.
anhidrosis	Deficiency in perspiration, often a result of fever or certain skin diseases.
basal cell carcinoma	Most common and least severe type of skin cancer; often characterized by light or pearly nodules.
bromhidrosis	Foul-smelling perspiration, usually noticeable in the armpits or on the feet, that is caused by bacteria.
bulla (plural: bullae)	Large blister containing a watery fluid; similar to a vesicle but larger.
chloasma	Also known as *liver spots*; condition characterized by hyperpigmentation on the skin in spots that are not elevated.
closed comedo	Also known as *whitehead*; hair follicle is closed and not exposed to the environment; sebum remains a white or cream color and comedone appears as small bump just under the skin surface.
conjunctivitis	Also known as *pinkeye*; common bacterial infection of the eyes; extremely contagious.
contact dermatitis	An inflammation of the skin caused by having contact with certain chemicals or substances; many of these substances are used in cosmetology.

Chapter Glossary

crust	Dead cells that form over a wound or blemish while it is healing; an accumulation of sebum and pus, sometimes mixed with epidermal material.
cyst	Closed, abnormally developed sac that contains fluid, pus, semifluid, or morbid matter above or below the skin.
dermatitis	Inflammatory condition of the skin.
dyschromias	Abnormal colorations of the skin that accompany many skin disorders and systemic disorders.
eczema	An inflammatory, uncomfortable, and often chronic disease of the skin, characterized by moderate to severe inflammation, scaling, and sometimes severe itching.
excoriation	Skin sore or abrasion produced by scratching or scraping.
extrinsic factors	Primarily environmental factors that contribute to aging and the appearance of aging.
fissure	A crack in the skin that penetrates the dermis. Examples are severely cracked and/or chapped hands or lips.
free radicals	Unstable molecules that cause biochemical aging, especially wrinkling and sagging of the skin.
herpes simplex	Recurring viral infection that often presents as a fever blister or cold sore.
hyperhidrosis	Excessive sweating, caused by heat or general body weakness.
hyperpigmentation	Darker than normal pigmentation, appearing as dark splotches.
hypertrophy	Abnormal growth of the skin.
hypopigmentation	Absence of pigment, resulting in light or white splotches.
impetigo	Contagious bacterial skin infection characterized by weeping lesions.
intrinsic factors	Skin-aging factors over which we have little control.
irritant contact dermatitis	Abbreviated ICD; occurs when irritating substances temporarily damage the epidermis.
keloid	Thick scar resulting from excessive growth of fibrous tissue.
keratoma	Acquired, superficial, thickened patch of epidermis. A callus is a keratoma caused by continued, repeated pressure or friction on any part of the skin, especially the hands and feet.
lentigines (singular: lentigo)	Technical term for freckles; small yellow-colored to brown-colored spots on skin exposed to sunlight and air.
lesion	Mark on the skin; may indicate an injury or damage that changes the structure of tissues or organs.

Chapter Glossary

leukoderma	Skin disorder characterized by light abnormal patches (hypopigmentation); caused by a burn or congenital disease that destroys the pigment-producing cells.
macule (plural: maculae)	Flat spot or discoloration on the skin, such as a freckle or a red spot left after a pimple has healed.
malignant melanoma	Most serious form of skin cancer; often characterized by black or dark brown patches on the skin that may appear uneven in texture, jagged, or raised.
milia	Benign, keratin-filled cysts that can appear just under the epidermis and have no visible opening.
miliaria rubra	Also known as *prickly heat*; an acute inflammatory disorder of the sweat glands, characterized by the eruption of small red vesicles and accompanied by burning, itching skin.
mole	Small, brownish spot or blemish on the skin, ranging in color from pale tan to brown or bluish black.
nevus	Also known as *birthmark*; small or large malformation of the skin due to abnormal pigmentation or dilated capillaries.
nodule	A solid bump larger than .4 inches (1 centimeter) that can be easily felt.
noncomedogenic	Product that has been designed and proven not to clog the follicles.
primary lesions	Lesions that are a different color than the color of the skin, and/or lesions that are raised above the surface of the skin.
psoriasis	Skin disease characterized by red patches covered with silver-white scales; usually found on the scalp, elbows, knees, chest, and lower back.
retention hyperkeratosis	The hereditary tendency for acne-prone skin to retain dead cells in the follicle, forming an obstruction that clogs follicles and exacerbates inflammatory acne lesions such as papules and pustules.
rosacea	Chronic condition that appears primarily on the cheeks and nose, and is characterized by flushing (redness), telangiectasis (distended or dialted surface blood vessels), and, in some cases, the formation of papules and pustules.
scale	Any thin dry or oily plate of epidermal flakes. An example is abnormal or excessive dandruff.
scar	Also known as *cicatrix*; a lightly raised mark on the skin formed after an injury or lesion of the skin has healed.

Chapter Glossary

sebaceous cyst	A large protruding pocket-like lesion filled with sebum. Sebaceous cysts are frequently seen on the scalp and the back. They should be removed surgically by a dermatologist.
seborrheic dermatitis	Skin condition caused by an inflammation of the sebaceous glands. It is often characterized by redness, dry or oily scaling, crusting, and/or itchiness.
secondary skin lesions	Characterized by piles of material on the skin surface, such as a crust or scab, or depressions in the skin surface, such as an ulcer.
sensitization	Allergic reaction created by repeated exposure to a chemical or a substance.
skin tag	A small brown-colored or flesh-colored outgrowth of the skin.
squamous cell carcinoma	Type of skin cancer more serious than basal cell carcinoma; often characterized by scaly red papules or nodules.
stain	Abnormal brown-colored or wine-colored skin discoloration with a circular and/or irregular shape.
tan	Change in pigmentation of skin caused by exposure to the sun or ultraviolet light.
telangiectasis	Distended or dilated surface blood vessels.
tubercle	Abnormal, rounded, solid lump above, within, or under the skin; larger than a papule.
tumor	An abnormal mass varying in size, shape, and color.
ulcer	Open lesion on the skin or mucous membrane of the body, accompanied by pus and loss of skin depth and possibly weeping fluids or pus.
verruca	Also known as *wart*; hypertrophy of the papillae and epidermis.
vesicle	Small blister or sac containing clear fluid, lying within or just beneath the epidermis.
vitiligo	Hereditary condition that causes hypopigmented spots and splotches on the skin; may be related to thyroid conditions.
wheal	Itchy, swollen lesion that lasts only a few hours; caused by a blow or scratch, the bite of an insect, urticaria (skin allergy), or the sting of a nettle. Examples include hives and mosquito bites.

CHAPTER 9

Nail Structure and Growth

Chapter Outline

© Ivanova Inga, 2010; used under license from Shutterstock.com.

Learning Objectives

After completing this chapter, you should be able to:

✓ **LO1** Describe the structure and composition of nails.

✓ **LO2** Discuss how nails grow.

Key Terms

Page number indicates where in the chapter the term is used.

bed epithelium
pg. 199

eponychium
pg. 200

free edge
pg. 199

hyponychium
pg. 200

ligament
pg. 200

lunula
pg. 200

matrix
pg. 199

nail bed
pg. 199

nail cuticle
pg. 200

nail folds
pg. 200

nail grooves
pg. 200

nail plate
pg. 199

natural nail (onyx)
pg. 198

natural nail unit
pg. 199

sidewall (lateral nail fold)
pg. 201

You probably know that the natural nail has a cuticle. Do you know whether the cuticle is living or dead skin? And do you know where the plate and the bed are located in the natural nail? This chapter gives you the answers to these questions and more. So, read on, because you cannot perform professional nail services without understanding the structure and growth of the natural nail.

Why Study Nail Structure and Growth?

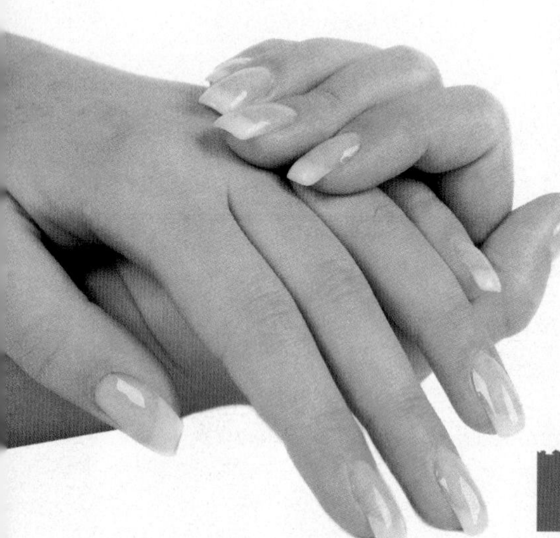

© Perov Stanislav 2010; used under license from Shutterstock.com.

Cosmetologists should study and have a thorough understanding of nail structure and growth because:

- Understanding the structure and growth of natural nails allows you to expertly groom, strengthen, and beautify nails.
- It is important to know the difference between the nail cuticle and the eponychium before performing nail services.
- Understanding the structure and growth cycles of the natural nail will prepare you for more advanced nail services.

The Natural Nail

A **natural nail**, also known as **onyx** (AHN-iks), is the hard protective plate composed mainly of keratin, the same fibrous protein found in skin and hair. The keratin in natural nails is harder than the keratin in skin or hair. The natural nail is located at the end of the finger or toe. It is an appendage of the skin and is part of the integumentary system, which is made up of the skin and its various organs. Nail plates protect the tips of the fingers and toes, and their appearance can reflect the general health of the body.

A normal, healthy nail is firm but flexible. The surface is shiny, smooth, and unspotted with no wavy ridges, pits, or splits. A healthy nail also is

did you know?

Nail plates are made of dead cells, so they do not require oxygen. In contrast, nail beds are live cells, so they do need oxygen, vitamins, and minerals.

FYI

Sometimes the names used for professional nail products can create confusion. To avoid this problem, pay close attention to what the product is actually designed to do.

For example, look at products marketed as nail cuticle moisturizers, softeners, or conditioners. The cuticle is dead skin on the nail plate, so why are these products designed to moisturize, soften, and condition the cuticle? That does not make any sense! Cuticle moisturizers, softeners, and conditioners are actually designed to treat the eponychium, sidewalls, and hyponychium—not the cuticle!

Cuticle removers are properly named; they remove the dead cuticle. These professional products can quickly dissolve soft tissue, and when carefully applied to the nail plate, they speed removal of stubborn cuticle tissue.

whitish and translucent in appearance, with the pinkish color of the nail bed showing through. In some races, the nail bed may have more yellow tones. The water content of the nail varies according to the relative humidity of the surrounding environment; in a humid environment, nails contain more water. A healthy nail may look dry and hard, but its water content is actually between 15 and 25 percent. The water content directly affects the nail's flexibility. The lower the water content, the more rigid the nail becomes. Coating the plate with an oil-based nail conditioner or nail polish improves flexibility by reducing water loss. These products also prevent excessive water absorption.

did you know?

The nail bed does not have sudoiferous (sweat) glands, so the nail cannot perspire. It is the skin around the nail that perspires.

Nail Anatomy

The **natural nail unit** is composed of several major parts, including the nail plate, nail bed, matrix, nail cuticle, eponychium, hyponychium, specialized ligaments, and nail folds.

Nail Plate

The **nail plate** is a hardened keratin plate that sits on and covers the nail bed. It is the most visible and functional part of the nail unit. The nail plate is relatively porous and will allow water to pass through it much more easily than through normal skin of an equal thickness. As it grows, the nail plate slowly slides across the nail bed. The nail plate is formed by the matrix cells. The sole job of the matrix cells is to create nail plate cells. The nail plate may appear to be one solid piece, but is actually constructed of about 100 layers of nail cells. The **free edge** is the part of the nail plate that extends over the tip of the finger or toe.

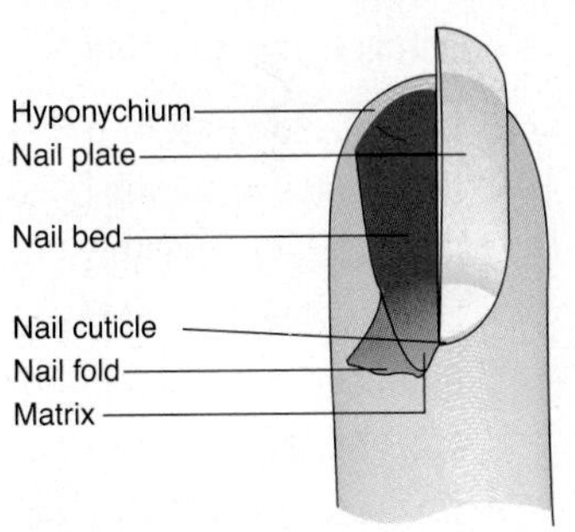

▲ Figure 9–1
Structure of the natural nail.

Nail Bed

The **nail bed** is the portion of living skin that supports the nail plate as it grows toward the free edge. Because it is richly supplied with blood vessels, the nail bed has a pinkish appearance from the lunula to the area just before the free edge of the nail. The nail bed contains many nerves, and is attached to the nail plate by a thin layer of tissue called the **bed epithelium** (BED ep-ih-THEE-lee-um). The bed epithelium helps guide the nail plate along the nail bed as it grows (**Figure 9–1** and **Figure 9–2**).

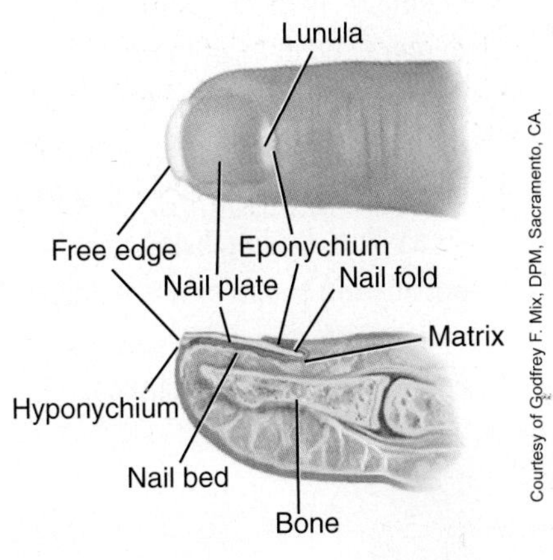

▲ Figure 9–2
Cross-section of the nail.

Matrix

The **matrix** (MAY-trikz) is the area where the nail plate cells are formed; this area is composed of matrix cells that produce the nail plate cells. The matrix contains nerves, lymph, and blood vessels to nourish the matrix cells. As long as it is nourished and healthy, the matrix will continue to create new nail plate cells.

The matrix extends from under the nail fold at the base of the nail plate. The visible part of the matrix that extends from underneath

FYI

Many people cannot tell the difference between the nail cuticle and the eponychium, but it is easy when you use this simple checklist.

- Is the tissue adhering directly to the natural nail plate but easily removed with gentle scraping?
- Is the tissue very thin and colorless but easily visible under close inspection?
- Is the tissue nonliving and not directly attached to living skin?

If you answered "Yes" to any of the questions above, then this tissue is called the cuticle.

- Is the tissue part of the skin that grows up to the base of the natural nail plate?
- Is the tissue part of the skin that covers the nail matrix and lunula?
- If you cut deeply into this tissue, will it bleed?

If you answered "Yes" to any of the questions above, this tissue is called the *eponychium.*

Cosmetologists are permitted to gently push back the eponychium, but are prohibited from cutting or trimming any part of the eponychium, since it is living skin. Cutting living skin is outside the scope of cosmetology and not allowed under any conditions or circumstances.

the living skin is called the **lunula** (LOO-nuh-luh). It is the whitish, half-moon shape at the base of the nail. The whitish color is caused by the reflection of light off the surface of the matrix. The lighter color of the lunula shows the true color of the matrix. Every nail has a lunula, but some lunulas are short and remain hidden under the eponychium.

Growth and appearance of the nails can be affected if an individual is in poor health, if a nail disorder or disease is present, or if there has been an injury to the matrix.

Cuticle

The **nail cuticle** (NAYL KYOO-tih-kul) is the dead, colorless tissue attached to the natural nail plate. The cuticle comes from the underside of the skin that lies above the natural nail plate. This tissue is incredibly sticky and difficult to remove from the nail plate. Its job is to seal the space between the natural nail plate and living skin. This prevents entry of foreign material and microorganisms and helps avoid injury and infection.

Eponychium

The **eponychium** (ep-oh-NIK-eeum) is the living skin at the base of the natural nail plate that covers the matrix area. The eponychium is often confused with the nail cuticle. They are *not* the same. The cuticle is the *dead tissue* adhered to the nail plate; the eponychium is *living tissue* that grows up to the nail plate. The cuticle comes from the underside of this area, where it completely detaches from the eponychium and strongly attaches to the new growth of nail plate. It pulls free to form a seal between the natural nail plate and the eponychium. Cosmetologists are prohibited from cutting the eponychium, even when a client requests it during a service.

Hyponychium

The **hyponychium** (hy-poh-NIK-eeum) is the slightly thickened layer of skin that lies between the fingertip and the free edge of the natural nail plate. It forms a protective barrier that prevents microorganisms from invading and infecting the nail bed.

Specialized Ligaments

A **ligament** (LIG-uh-munt) is a tough band of fibrous tissue that connects bones or holds an organ in place. Specialized ligaments attach the nail bed and matrix bed to the underlying bone. These ligaments are located at the base of the matrix and around the wedges of the nail bed.

Nail Folds

The **nail folds** are folds of normal skin that surround the nail plate. These folds form the **nail grooves,** which are the slits or furrows

© Mark Poprocki, 2010; used under license from Shutterstock.com.

ACTivity

Use a small magnifying glass to examine the hands of at least 10 friends or classmates. Look at the nail cuticle and eponychium on each finger. Observe how the thin cuticle tissue attaches to and rides on top of the nail plate as the cuticle emerges from under the eponychium at the base of the nail plate. Next, examine the eponychium to see how it differs in appearance from the cuticle. Identify which tissue can be removed and which tissue should never be cut.

on the sidewall. The **sidewall**, also known as **lateral nail fold** (LAT-ur-ul NAYL FOHLD), is the fold of skin overlapping the side of the nail. ☑ **LO1**

Nail Growth

In Chapter 7, Skin Structure, Growth, and Nutrition, you learned that nutrition, exercise, and a person's general health can affect the health of the skin. These factors affect the growth and health of the nail plate as well.

A normal nail grows forward from the matrix and extends over the tip of the finger. Normal, healthy nails can grow in a variety of shapes, depending on the shape of the matrix. The length, width, and curvature of the matrix determine the thickness, width, and curvature of the natural nail plate. For example, a longer matrix produces a thicker nail plate, and a highly curved matrix creates a highly curved free edge. No product or procedure can make the nail plate grow thicker because a thicker nail plate would require a larger matrix. Toenails are also thicker and harder than fingernails because the toenail matrix is longer than the fingernail matrix (**Figure 9–3**).

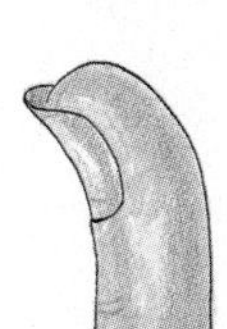
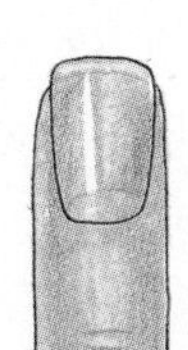
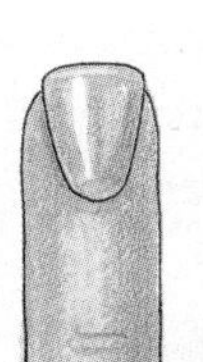
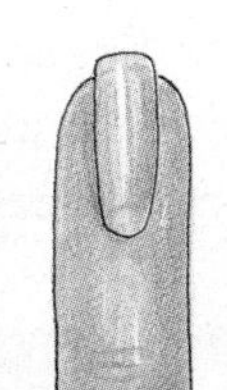
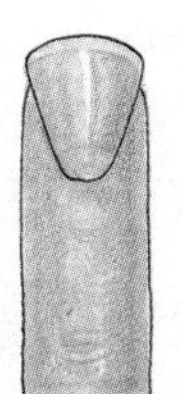
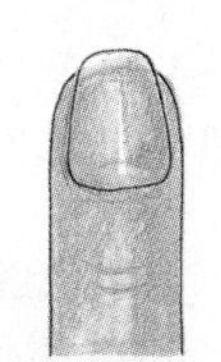
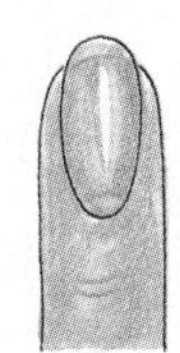
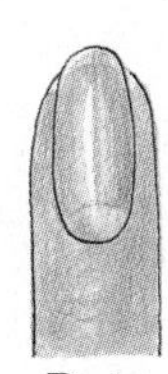
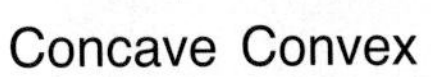
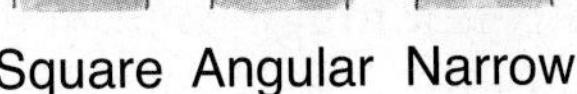
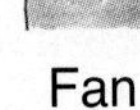
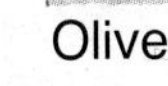

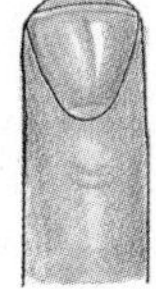
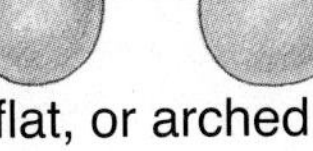
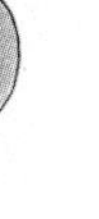
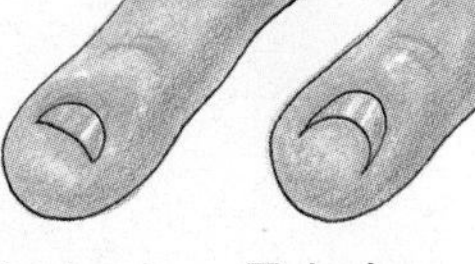
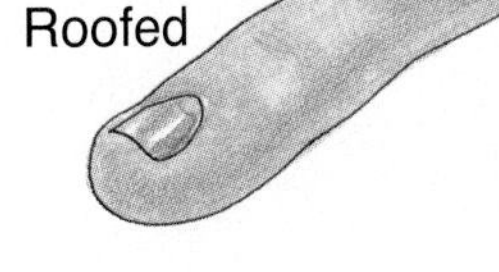

◀ **Figure 9–3 Various shapes of nails.**

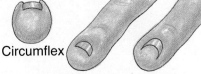

© Milady, a part of Cengage Learning.

did you know?

Typing on a keyboard or lightly touching natural nails on piano keys stimulates the nails and makes them grow.

The average rate of nail growth in the normal adult is about 1/10 of an inch (3.7 mm) per month, but many factors affect this growth rate. Age, for example, affects nail growth. Compared with the nails of an average adult, children's nails grow more rapidly, and elderly adults' nails grow more slowly. Seasons also affect nail growth rate; nails grow faster in the summer than they do in the winter. Pregnancy dramatically affects nail growth because of hormonal changes in the body. Nail growth rates increase dramatically during the last trimester of pregnancy and decrease quickly after delivery, returning to normal as hormone levels return to normal. (In spite of a popular myth, nail growth rates accelerate during pregnancy whether or not a woman takes prenatal vitamins.) A nail's position on the body affects its growth rate. Nail growth rate is fastest on the nail of the middle finger and slowest on the thumb, and toenails grow more slowly than fingernails.

Nail Malformation

If disease, injury, or infection occurs in the matrix, the shape or thickness of the nail plate can change. In fact, these conditions are generally the only reasons that a person will shed a nail. Healthy nails are not shed automatically or periodically in the way that healthy hair is shed. Often after a disease, injury, or infection that has affected the nail's growth, the natural nail will return to its healthy growth as long as the matrix is healthy and undamaged. Ordinarily, replacement of a natural fingernail takes about four to six months. Toenails take about nine months to one year to be fully replaced. ☑ LO2

Know Your Nails

Many cosmetologists are interested in nails because of the creative opportunities they present. As with every other area of cosmetology, this creativity must be grounded in a full awareness of the structure and physiology of the nails and the surrounding tissue.

Working on strong, healthy nails can be a pleasure. Remember that as a licensed cosmetologist, you are allowed to work only on healthy nails and skin with no visible signs of disease or infection.

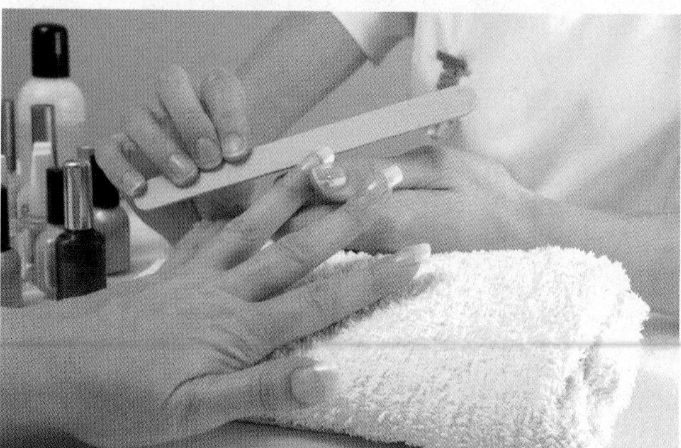

© Christopher Elwell, 2010; used under license from Shutterstock.com.

Review Questions

1. What is the technical term for the natural nail?
2. What protein is in the natural nail?
3. Describe the appearance of a normal, healthy nail.
4. Name the major parts of the natural nail unit.
5. Explain the difference between the nail plate and the nail bed.
6. What part of the natural nail unit contains the nerves, lymph, and blood vessels?
7. What is the difference between the nail cuticle and the eponychium?
8. Why are cosmetologists prohibited from cutting the skin around the base of the nail plate, even when a client requests it during a service?
9. What are three factors that can affect growth of the natural nail?

Chapter Glossary

bed epithelium	Thin layer of tissue that attaches the nail plate and the nail bed.
eponychium	Living skin at the base of the natural nail plate that covers the matrix area.
free edge	Part of the nail plate that extends over the tip of the finger or toe.
hyponychium	Slightly thickened layer of skin that lies between the fingertip and free edge of the natural nail plate.
ligament	Tough band of fibrous tissue that connects bones or holds an organ in place.
lunula	Visible part of the matrix that extends from underneath the living skin; it is the whitish, half-moon shape at the base of the nail.
matrix	Area where the nail plate cells are formed; this area is composed of matrix cells that produce the nail plate.
nail bed	Portion of the living skin that supports the nail plate as it grows toward the free edge.
nail cuticle	Dead, colorless tissue attached to the natural nail plate.
nail folds	Folds of normal skin that surround the natural nail plate.
nail grooves	Slits or furrows on the sides of the sidewall.
nail plate	Hardened keratin plate that sits on and covers the natural nail bed. It is the most visible and functional part of the natural nail unit.
natural nail	Also known as *onyx*; the hard protective plate is composed mainly of keratin, the same fibrous protein found in skin and hair. The keratin in natural nails is harder than the keratin in skin or hair.
natural nail unit	Composed of several major parts of the fingernail including the nail plate, nail bed, matrix, cuticle, eponychium, hyponychium, specialized ligaments, and nail fold. Together, all of these parts form the nail unit.
sidewall	Also known as *lateral nail fold*; the fold of skin overlapping the side of the nail.

CHAPTER 10

Nail Disorders and Diseases

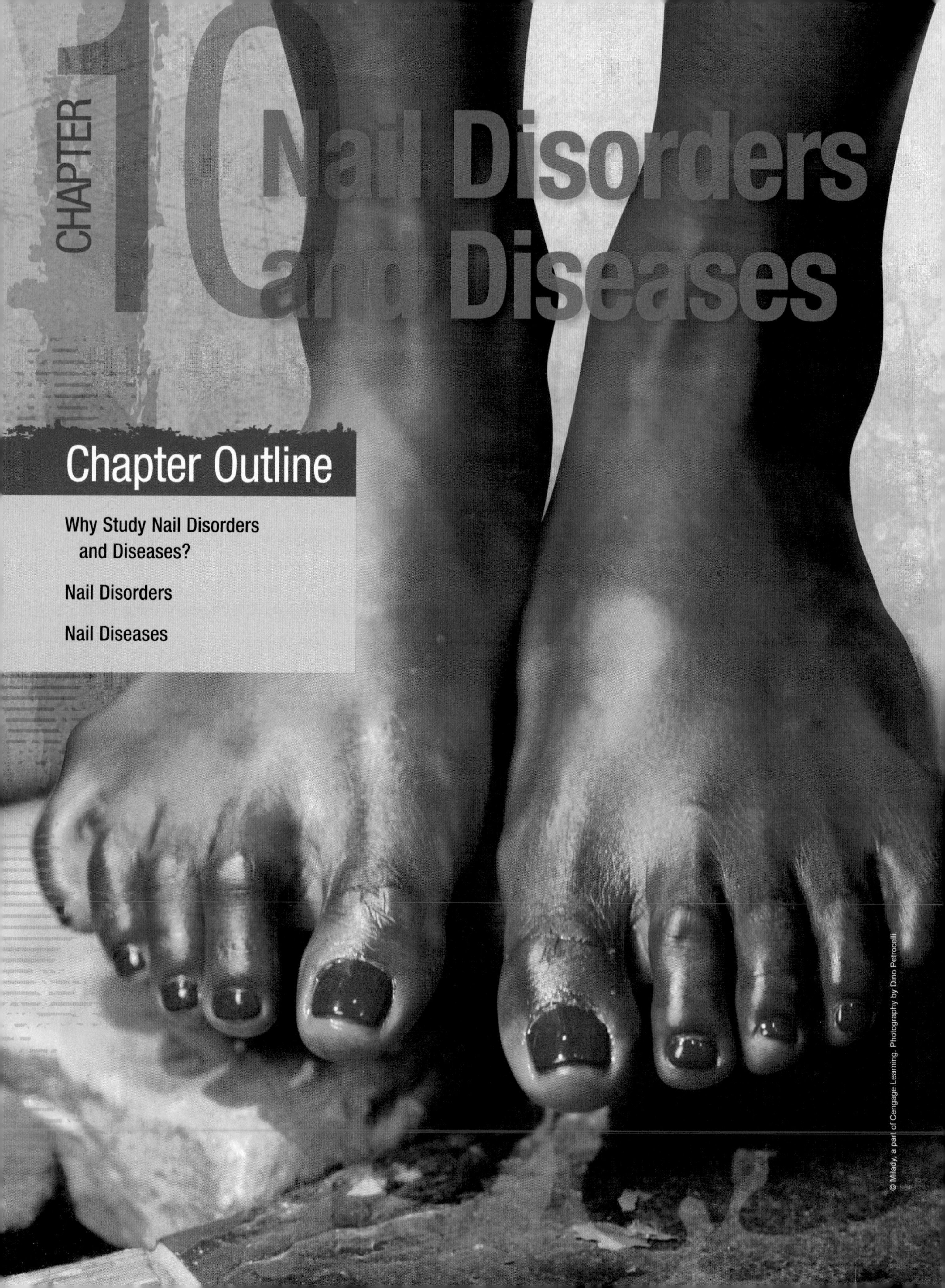

Chapter Outline

© Milady, a part of Cengage Learning. Photography by Dino Petrocelli.

Learning Objectives

After completing this chapter, you will be able to:

- ✓ **LO1** List and describe the various disorders and irregularities of nails.
- ✓ **LO2** Recognize diseases of the nails that should not be treated in the salon.

Key Terms

Page number indicates where in the chapter the term is used.

Beau's lines
pg. 207

bruised nails
pg. 207

discolored nails
pg. 208

eggshell nails
pg. 207

hangnail (agnail)
pg. 207

leukonychia spots (white spots)
pg. 208

melanonychia
pg. 208

nail disorder
pg. 206

nail psoriasis
pg. 214

nail pterygium
pg. 209

onychia
pg. 213

onychocryptosis (ingrown nails)
pg. 213

onycholysis
pg. 213

onychomadesis
pg. 214

onychomycosis
pg. 215

onychophagy (bitten nails)
pg. 208

onychorrhexis
pg. 208

onychosis
pg. 213

paronychia
pg. 214

pincer nail (trumpet nail)
pg. 209

plicatured nail (folded nail)
pg. 209

pseudomonas aeruginosa
pg. 210

pyogenic granuloma
pg. 215

ridges
pg. 209

splinter hemorrhages
pg. 209

tinea pedis
pg. 215

To give clients professional and responsible service and care, you need to learn about the structure and growth of the nail, as you did in Chapter 9, Nail Structure and Growth. Now, you must learn about the disorders and diseases of nails so that you will know when it is safe to work on a client. Nails are an interesting and surprising part of the human body. They are small mirrors of the general health of the entire body. Certain health conditions may first be revealed by a change in the nails, a visible disorder, or poor nail growth. Some conditions are easily treated in the salon—hangnails, for instance, or bruised nail beds that need camouflage—but some are infectious and cannot be treated by salon professionals. Carefully studying this chapter will vastly improve your knowledge and expertise in caring for nails.

Why Study Nail Disorders and Diseases?

Cosmetologists should study and have a thorough understanding of nail disorders and diseases because:

- You must be able to identify any condition on a client's nails that should not be treated in the salon and which may be treated in the salon.
- You must be able to identify infectious conditions that may be present so that you can take the appropriate steps to protect yourself and your clients from the spread of disease.
- You may be in a position to recognize conditions that may signal mild to serious health problems that warrant the attention of a doctor.

Nail Disorders

As you now know, a normal, healthy nail is firm but flexible. The surface is shiny, smooth, and unspotted with no wavy ridges, pits, or splits. A healthy nail also is whitish and translucent in appearance, with the pinkish color of the nail bed showing through. In some races, the nail bed may have more yellow tones. A **nail disorder** is a condition caused by injury or disease of the nail unit. Most, if not all, of your clients have experienced a common nail disorder at some time in their lives. A cosmetologist should recognize normal and abnormal nail conditions, understand what to do, and be able to help a client with a nail disorder in one of two ways:

- You can tell clients that they may have a disorder and refer them to a physician, if required.
- You can cosmetically improve certain nail plate conditions if the problem is cosmetic and not a medical condition or disorder.

©MikLav, 2010; used under license from Shutterstock.com.

It is your professional responsibility and a requirement of your license to know which option to choose. A client whose nail or skin is infected, inflamed, broken, or swollen should not receive services. Instead, the client should be referred to a physician to determine the type of treatment that is required.

did you know?

Clients cannot sign a waiver or verbally give a cosmetologist permission to disobey state or federal rules and regulations.

Bruised nails are a condition in which a blood clot forms under the nail plate, causing a dark purplish spot. These discolorations are usually due to small injuries to the nail bed. The dried blood absorbs into the nail bed epithelium tissue on the underside of the nail plate and grows out with it. Treat this injured nail gently and advise your clients to be more careful with their nails if they want to avoid this problem in the future. Advise them to treat their nails like jewels and not tools! This condition can usually be covered with nail polish or camouflaged with an opaque nail enhancement.

Eggshell nails are noticeably thin, white nail plates that are more flexible than normal. Eggshell nails are normally weaker and can curve over the free edge (**Figures 10–1a** and **10–1b**). The condition is usually caused by improper diet, hereditary factors, internal disease, or medication. Be very careful when manicuring these nails because they are fragile and can break easily. Use the fine side of an abrasive board (240 grit or higher) to file them gently, but only if needed. It is best not to file a nail plate of this type. A thin protective overlay of enhancement product can be helpful, but do not extend these nails beyond the free edge.

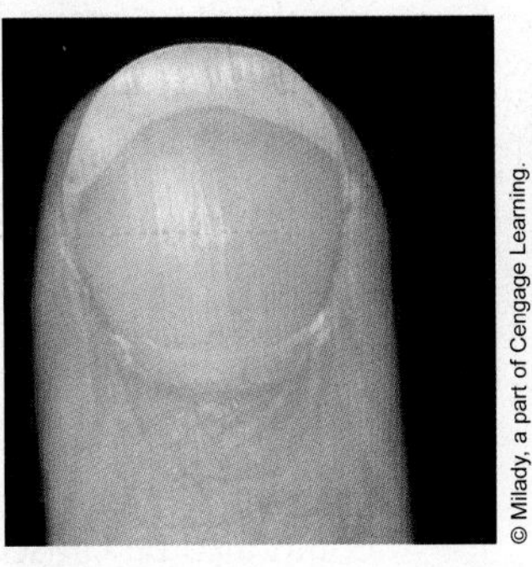

© Milady, a part of Cengage Learning.

▲ Figure 10–1a
Eggshell nail, front view.

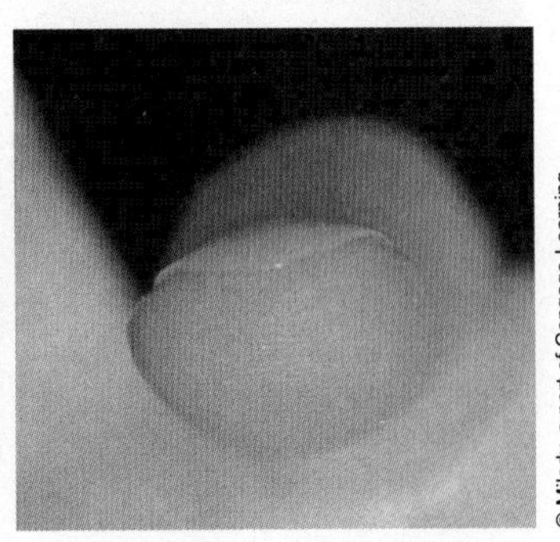

© Milady, a part of Cengage Learning.

▲ Figure 10–1b
Eggshell nail, end view.

Beau's lines are visible depressions running across the width of the natural nail plate (**Figure 10–2**). They usually result from major illness or injury that has traumatized the body, such as pneumonia, adverse drug reaction, surgery, heart failure, massive injury, or a long-lasting high fever. Beau's lines occur because the matrix slows down in producing nail cells for an extended period of time, say a week or a month. This causes the nail plate to grow thinner for a period of time. The nail plate thickness usually returns to normal after the illness or condition is resolved.

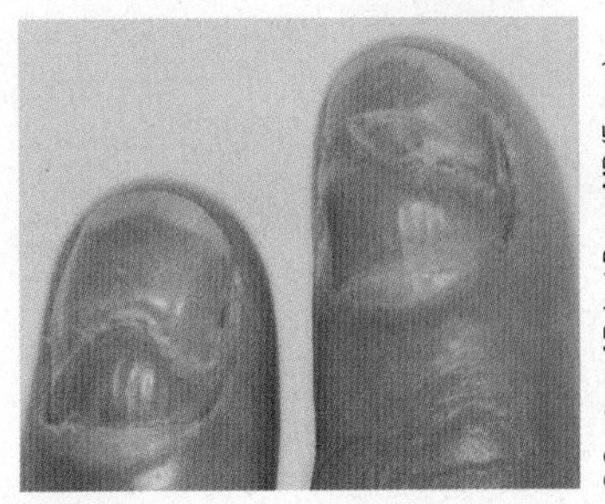

© Courtesy of Robert Baron, MD (France).

▲ Figure 10–2
Beau's lines.

Hangnail, also known as **agnail**, is a condition in which the living skin around the nail plate splits and tears (**Figure 10–3**). Dry skin or small cuts can result in hangnails. If there is no sign of infection or an open wound, advise the client that proper nail care, such as hot oil manicures, will aid in correcting the condition. Also, never cut the living skin around the natural nail plate, even if it is dry and rough looking. Other than to carefully remove the thin layer of dead cuticle tissue on the nail plate, you should not cut skin anywhere on the hands or feet. Hangnails can be carefully trimmed, as long as the living skin is not cut or torn in the process. It is against state board regulations to intentionally cut or tear the client's skin and can lead to serious infections for which you and the salon may be legally liable. If not properly cared

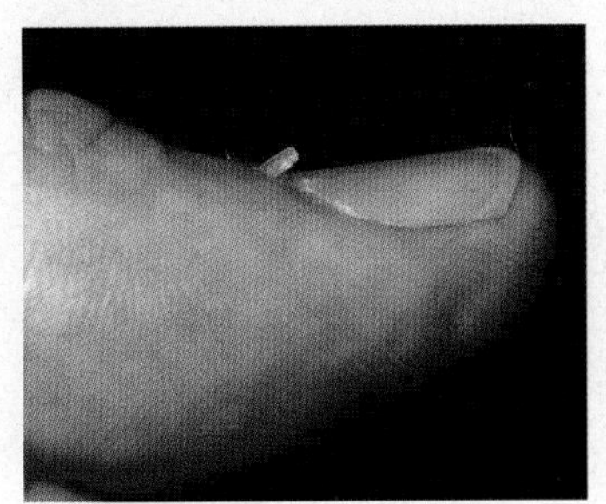

© Milady, a part of Cengage Learning.

▲ Figure 10–3
Hangnail.

for, a hangnail can become infected. Clients with symptoms of infections in their fingers should be referred to a physician. Signs of infection are redness, pain, swelling, or pus.

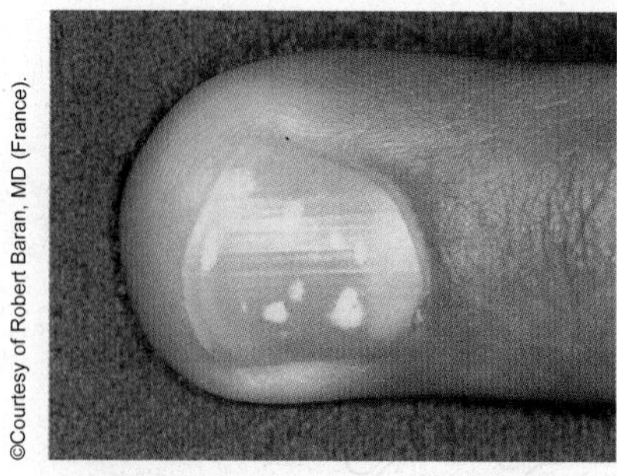

©Courtesy of Robert Baran, MD (France).

▲ Figure 10–4
Leukonychia spots.

Leukonychia spots (loo-koh-NIK-ee-ah SPATS), also known as **white spots**, are whitish discolorations of the nails, usually caused by minor injury to the nail matrix. They are not a symptom of any vitamin or mineral deficiency. It is a myth that these result from calcium or zinc deficiency. They appear frequently in the nails but do not indicate disease. As the nail continues to grow, the white spots eventually disappear (Figure 10–4).

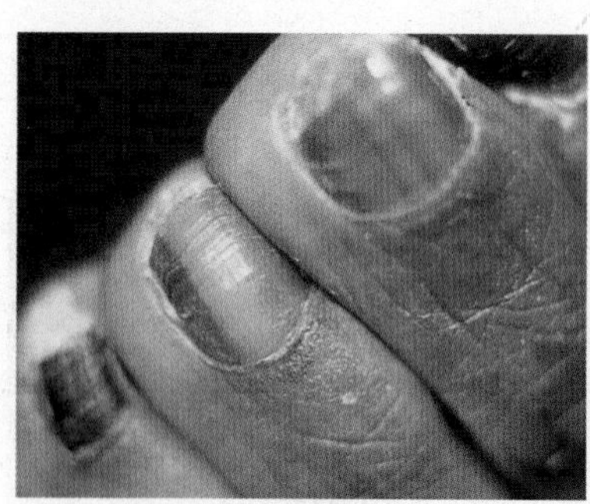

© Courtesy of Godfrey F. Mix, DPM, Sacramento, CA.

▲ Figure 10–5
Melanonychia.

Melanonychia (mel-uh-nuh-NIK-ee-uh) is darkening of the fingernails or toenails. It may be seen as a black band within the nail plate, extending from the base to the free edge. In some cases, it may affect the entire nail plate. A localized area of increased pigment cells (melanocytes), usually within the matrix, is responsible for this condition. As matrix cells form the nail plate, melanin is laid down within the plate by the melanocytes. This is a fairly common occurrence and considered normal in people of color, but could be indicative of a disease condition in Caucasians (Figure 10–5).

Discolored nails are nails that turn a variety of colors, which may indicate surface staining, a systemic disorder, or poor blood circulation. Although quite common, a discolored nail may be caused by several factors, such as: surface stains from nail polish, foods, dyes, or smoking. A discolored nail could also be caused by an internal discoloration of the nail plate due to biological, medical, or even pharmaceutical reasons.

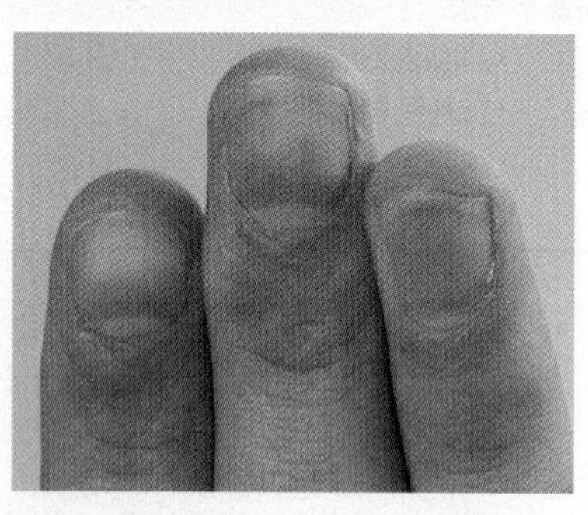

© Milady, a part of Cengage Learning. Photography by Paul Castle, Castle Photography.

▲ Figure 10–6
Bitten nails.

Onychophagy (ahn-ih-koh-FAY-jee), also known as **bitten nails**, is the result of a habit of chewing the nail or the hardened, damaged skin surrounding the nail plate (Figure 10–6). Advise clients that frequent manicures and care of the hardened eponychium can often help them overcome this habit, at the same time improving the health and appearance of the hands. Sometimes, the application of nail enhancements can beautify deformed nails and discourage the client from biting the nails. However, the bitten, damaged skin should not be treated by a cosmetologist. If the skin is broken or infected, no services can be provided until the area is healed.

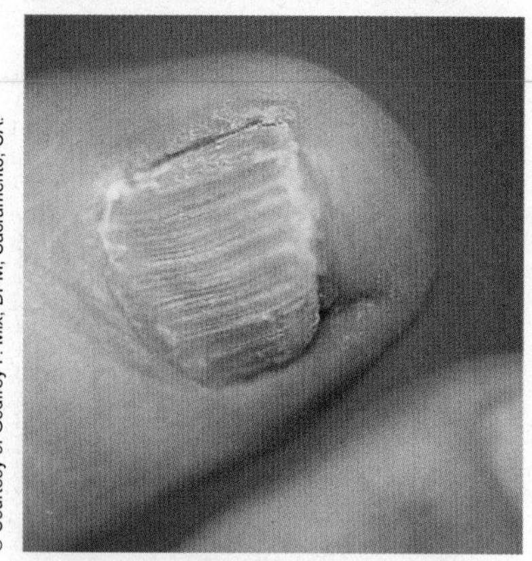

© Courtesy of Godfrey F. Mix, DPM, Sacramento, CA.

▲ Figure 10–7
Onychorrhexis.

Onychorrhexis (ahn-ih-koh-REK-sis) refers to split or brittle nails that have a series of lengthwise ridges giving a rough appearance to the surface of the nail plate. This condition is usually caused by injury to the matrix, excessive use of cuticle removers, harsh cleaning agents, aggressive filing techniques, or heredity. Nail services can be performed only if the nail is not split, exposing the nail bed. Nail enhancement product should never be applied if the nail bed is exposed. This condition may be corrected by softening the nails with a conditioning treatment and discontinuing the use of harsh detergents, cleaners, or improper filing (Figure 10–7). These nail plates often lack sufficient moisture, so twice-daily treatments with a high quality, penetrating nail oil can be very beneficial. Nail hardeners should always be avoided on brittle nails, since these products will increase brittleness.

Plicatured nail (plik-a-CHOORD NAYL), also known as **folded nail**, is a type of highly curved nail plate usually caused by injury to the matrix, but it may be inherited. This condition often leads to ingrown nails (**Figure 10–8**).

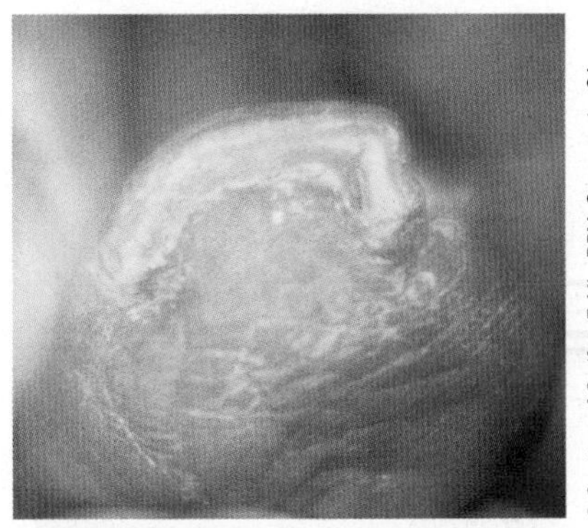

© Courtesy of Godfrey F. Mix, DPM, Sacramento, CA.

▲ **Figure 10–8**
Plicatured nail.

Nail pterygium (teh-RIJ-ee-um) is an abnormal condition that occurs when the skin is stretched by the nail plate. This disorder is usually caused by serious injury, such as burns, or an adverse skin reaction to chemical nail enhancement products (**Figure 10–9**). The terms *cuticle* and *pterygium* do not designate the same thing, and they should never be used interchangeably. Nail pterygium is abnormal and is caused by damage to the eponychium or hyponychium.

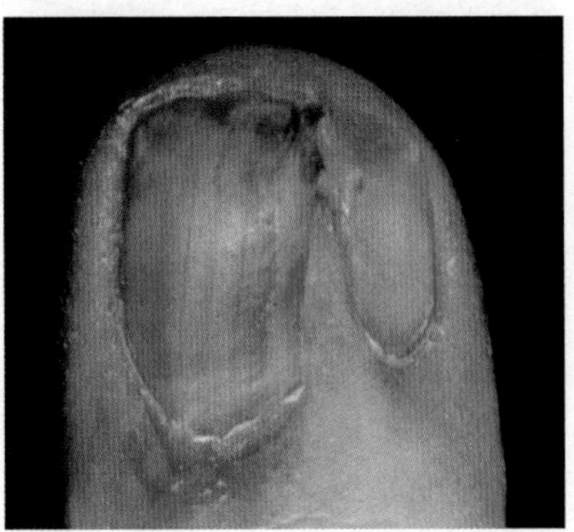

© Courtesy of Godfrey F. Mix, DPM, Sacramento, CA.

▲ **Figure 10–9**
Nail pterygium.

Do not treat nail pterygium and never push the extension of skin back with an instrument. Doing so will cause more injury to the tissues and will make the condition worse. The gentle massage of conditioning oils or creams into the affected area may be beneficial. If this condition becomes irritated, painful, or shows signs of infection, recommend that the client see a physician for examination and proper treatment.

Ridges are vertical lines running down the length of the natural nail plate that are caused by uneven growth of the nails, usually the result of normal aging. Older clients are more likely to have these ridges, and unless the ridges become very deep and weaken the nail plate, they are perfectly normal. When manicuring a client with this condition, carefully buff the nail plate to minimize the appearance of these ridges. This helps to remove or minimize the ridges, but great care must be taken not to overly thin the nail plate, which could lead to nail plate weakness and additional damage. Ridge filler is less damaging to the natural nail plate and can be used with colored polish to give a smooth appearance while keeping the nail plate strong and healthy.

Splinter hemorrhages are caused by physical trauma or injury to the nail bed that damages the capillaries and allows small amounts of blood flow. As a result, the blood stains the bed epithelium tissue that forms rails to guide the nail plate along the nail bed during growth. This blood oxidizes and turns brown or black, giving the appearance of a small splinter underneath the nail plate. Splinter hemorrhages will always be positioned lengthwise in the direction of growth (pointing toward the front and back of the nail plate) because this is how the bed epithelium rails grow. Splinter hemorrhages are normal and usually associated with some type of hard impact or other physical trauma to the fingernail or toenail.

Increased Curvature Nails

Nail plates with a deep or sharp curvature at the free edge have this shape because of the matrix; the greater the curvature of the matrix, the greater the curvature of the free edge. Increased curvature can range from mild to severe pinching of the soft tissue at the free edge. In some cases, the free edge pinches the sidewalls into a deep curve. This is known as **pincer nail**, also known as **trumpet nail**. The nail can also curl in on itself (**Figure 10–10**), may be deformed only on

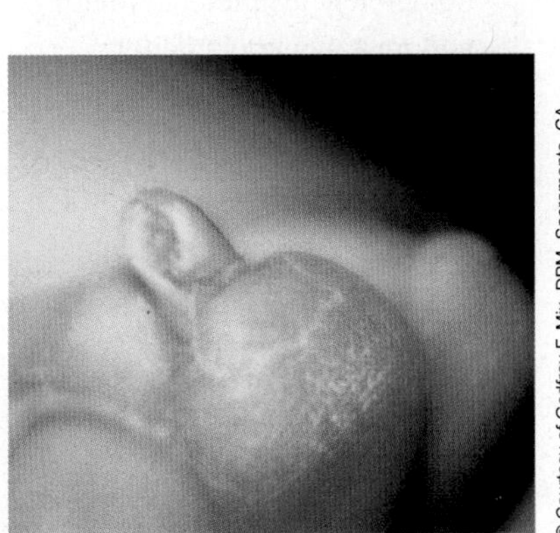

© Courtesy of Godfrey F. Mix, DPM, Sacramento, CA.

▲ **Figure 10–10**
Pincer or trumpet nail.

one sidewall, or the edges of the nail plate may curl around to form the shape of a trumpet or sharp cone at the free edge. In each of these cases, the natural nail plate should be carefully trimmed and filed. Extreme or unusual cases should be referred to a qualified medical doctor or podiatrist. A brief summary of nail disorders is found in **Table 10–1**.

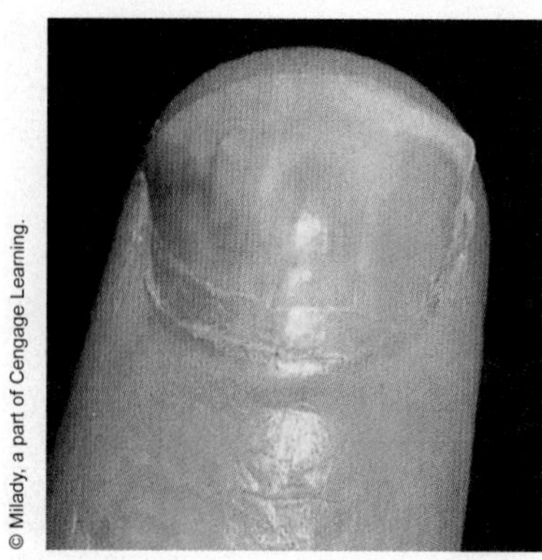
© Milady, a part of Cengage Learning.

▲ **Figure 10–11**
Pseudomonas aeruginosa.

Nail Infections

As you learned in Chapter 5, Infection Control: Principles and Practices, fungi are parasites that may cause infections of the feet and hands. Nail fungi are of concern to the salon because they are contagious and can be transmitted through contaminated implements. Fungi can spread from nail to nail on the client's feet, but it is much less likely that these pathogens will cause fingernail infections. Fungi infections prefer to grow in conditions where the skin is warm, moist, and dark, that is, on feet inside shoes. It is extremely unlikely that a cosmetologist could become infected from a client, but it is possible to transmit fungal infections from one client's foot or toe to another client.

With proper cleaning and disinfection practices the transmission of fungal infections can be easily avoided. Clients with suspected nail fungal infection must be referred to a physician.

CAUTION

Nail infection caused by bacteria and fungi can be avoided by following state board guidelines for proper cleaning and disinfection. Do not omit any of the cleaning and disinfection procedures when performing a nail enhancement service. Do not perform nail services for clients who are suspected of having an infection of any kind on their nails. If you repeatedly encounter nail infections on your clients' nails, you should reexamine your cleaning, disinfection, preparation, and application techniques. Completely disinfect all metal and reusable implements, throw away single-use nail files, wash linens or replace with disposable towels, and thoroughly clean and disinfect the table surface before and after the procedure (Figure 10–12).

It Is Not a Mold!

In the past, discolorations of the nail plate (especially those between the plate and nail enhancements) were incorrectly referred to as *molds*. This term should not be used when referring to infections of the fingernails or toenails. The discoloration is usually a bacterial infection such as **Pseudomonas aeruginosa**, one of several common bacteria that can cause a nail infection, or Staphylococcus aureus. These naturally occurring skin bacteria can grow rapidly to cause an infection if conditions are correct for growth (**Figure 10–11**). Bacterial infections are more likely the cause of infection on the hands, but also can be found on the feet. Bacteria do not need the same growing conditions as fungal organisms, and can thrive on fingernails just as easily as they can on the feet. Infection can be caused by the use of implements that are contaminated with large numbers of these bacteria. These infections are not a result of moisture trapped between the natural nail and nail enhancements. This is a myth! Water does not cause infections. Infections are caused by large numbers of bacteria or fungal organisms on a surface. This is why proper cleaning and preparation of the natural nail plate, as well as cleaning and disinfection of implements, are so important. If these pathogens are not present, infections cannot occur. A typical

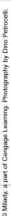

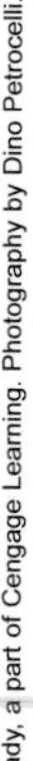
© Milady, a part of Cengage Learning. Photography by Dino Petrocelli.

▶ **Figure 10–12**
Always practice strict rules regarding cleaning and disinfecting when working with nails.

OVERVIEW OF NAIL DISORDERS

DISORDER	SIGNS OR SYMPTOMS
BEAU'S LINES	Visible depressions running across the width of the natural nail plate; usually a result of major illness or injury that has traumatized the body
BRUISED NAILS	Dark purplish spots, usually due to physical injury
DISCOLORED NAILS	Nails turn a variety of colors; may indicate surface staining, a systemic disorder, or poor blood circulation
EGGSHELL NAILS	Noticeably thin, white plate, more flexible than normal and can curve over the free edge; usually caused by improper diet, hereditary factors, internal disease, or medication
HANGNAIL	Living skin around the nail plate (often the eponychium) becomes split or torn
LEUKONYCHIA SPOTS	Also known as *white spots*; whitish discolorations of the nail; usually caused by minor injury to the nail matrix; not related to the body's health or vitamin deficiencies
MELANONYCHIA	Darkening of the fingernails or toenails; may be seen as a black band within the nail plate, extending from the base to the free edge
NAIL PSORIASIS	Nail surface pitting, roughness, onycholysis, and bed discolorations
NAIL PTERYGIUM	Abnormal stretching of skin around the nail plate; usually caused by serious injury, such as burns, or an adverse skin reaction to chemical nail enhancement products or an allergic skin reaction
ONYCHOPHAGY	Also known as *bitten nails*; chewed nails or chewed hardened skin surrounding the nail plate
ONYCHORRHEXIS	Split or brittle nails that have a series of lengthwise ridges giving a rough appearance to the surface of the nail plate
PINCER NAIL	Also known as *trumpet nail*; increased crosswise curvature throughout the nail plate caused by an increased curvature of the matrix; the edges of the nail plate may curl around to form the shape of a trumpet or sharp cone at the free edge
PLICATURED NAIL	Also known as f*olded nail*; a type of highly curved nail plate, usually caused by injury to the matrix, but it may be inherited
RIDGES	Vertical lines running the length of the natural nail plate that are caused by uneven growth of the nails, usually the result of normal aging
SPLINTER HEMORRHAGES	Physical trauma or injury to the nail bed that damages the capillaries and allows small amount of blood flow

© Milady, a part of Cengage Learning.

Table 10–1 **Overview of Nail Disorders.**

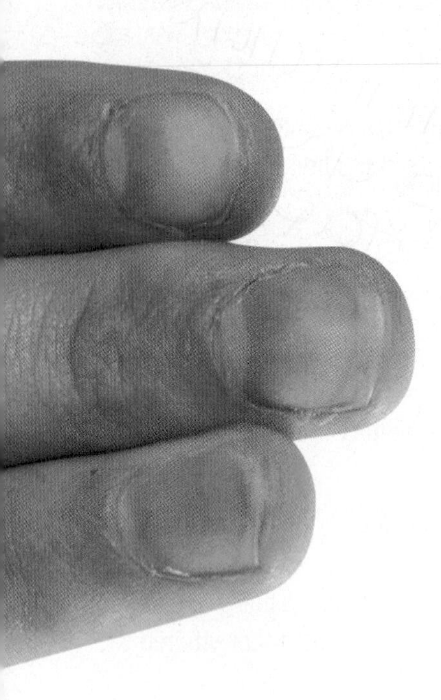

© Milady, a part of Cengage Learning. Photography by Paul Castle, Castle Photography.

bacterial infection on the nail plate can be identified in the early stages as a yellow-green spot that becomes darker in its advanced stages. The color usually changes from yellow to green to brown to black. Clients with these symptoms should be immediately referred to a physician for treatment. It is illegal for a cosmetologist to diagnose or treat a nail infection. Do not remove the nail enhancement unless directed to do so by the client's treating physician.

You should never provide any type of nail services to clients with a nail bacterial or fungal infection. ☑ **LO1**

Nail Diseases

There are several nail diseases that you may come across. A brief overview of nail diseases is found in **Table 10–2**. Any nail disease that shows signs of infection or inflammation (redness, pain, swelling, or pus) should not be diagnosed or treated in the salon. Medical examination is required for all nail diseases and any treatments will be determined by the physician.

A person's occupation can cause a variety of nail infections. For instance, infections develop more readily in people who regularly place their hands in harsh cleaning solutions. Natural oils are removed from the

OVERVIEW OF NAIL DISEASES

DISEASE	SIGNS OR SYMPTOMS
ONYCHIA	Inflammation of the nail matrix, followed by shedding of the nail
ONYCHOLYSIS	Lifting of the nail plate from the nail bed, without shedding, usually beginning at the free edge and continuing toward the luna area
ONYCHOMADESIS	Separation and falling off of a nail plate from the nail bed; can affect fingernails and toenails
NAIL PSORIASIS	Tiny pits or severe roughness on the surface of the nail plate
ONYCHOMYCOSIS	Fungal infection of the natural nail plate
PARONYCHIA	Bacterial inflammation of the tissues around the nail plate causing pus, swelling, and redness, usually in the skin fold adjacent to the nail plate
PYOGENIC GRANULOMA	Severe inflammation of the nail in which a lump of red tissue grows up from the nail bed to the nail plate
TINEA PEDIS	Red, itchy rash on the skin on the bottom of feet and/or between the toes, usually between the fourth or fifth toe

© Milady, a part of Cengage Learning.

Table 10–2 **Overview of Nail Diseases.**

ACTivity

Go to a library or use the Internet to research the term *scope of practice* for medical doctors, dermatologists, and podiatrists. You should be familiar with what these professionals do, as well as the strict limitations placed on cosmetologists' *scope of practice* so that you'll better understand what you cannot do.

skin by frequent exposure to soaps, solvents, and many other types of substances. A cosmetologist's hands are exposed daily to professional products. These products should be used according to manufacturer's instructions to ensure that they are being used correctly and safely. If those instructions or warnings tell you to avoid skin contact, you should take heed and follow such advice. If the manufacturer recommends that you wear gloves, make sure that you do so to protect your skin. Contact the product manufacturer if you are not sure how to use the product safely and obtain the Material Safety Data Sheet (MSDS).

Product manufacturers can always provide you with additional information and guidance. Call them whenever you have any questions related to safe handling and proper use.

Onychosis (ahn-ih-KOH-sis) is any deformity or disease of the natural nail.

Onychia (uh-NIK-ee-uh) is an inflammation of the nail matrix followed by shedding of the natural nail plate. Any break in the skin surrounding the nail plate can allow pathogens to infect the matrix. Be careful to avoid injuring sensitive tissue, and make sure that all implements are properly cleaned and disinfected. Improperly cleaned and disinfected nail implements can cause this and other diseases if an accidental injury occurs.

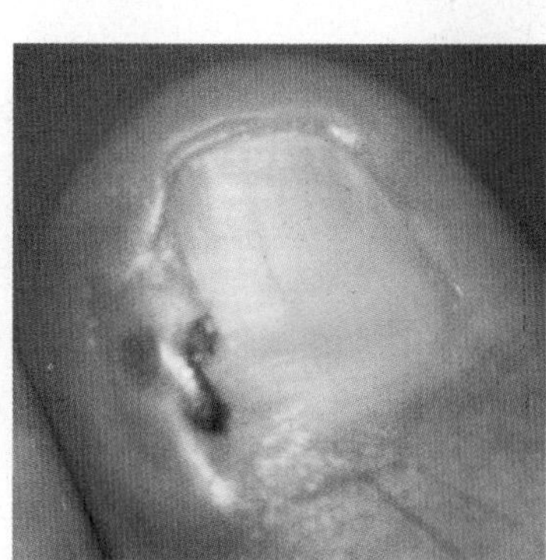

© Courtesy of Godfrey F. Mix, DPM, Sacramento, CA.

▲ Figure 10–13
Onychocryptosis.

Onychocryptosis (ahn-ih-koh-krip-TOH-sis), also known as **ingrown nails**, can affect either the fingers or toes (**Figure 10–13**). In this condition, the nail grows into the sides of the living tissue around the nail. The movements of walking can press the soft tissues up against the nail plate, contributing to the problem. If the tissue around the nail plate is not infected, or if the nail is not imbedded in the flesh, you can carefully trim the corner of the nail in a curved shape to relieve the pressure on the nail groove. However, if there is any redness, pain, swelling, or irritation, you may not provide any services. Cosmetologists are not allowed to service ingrown nails. Refer the client to a physician.

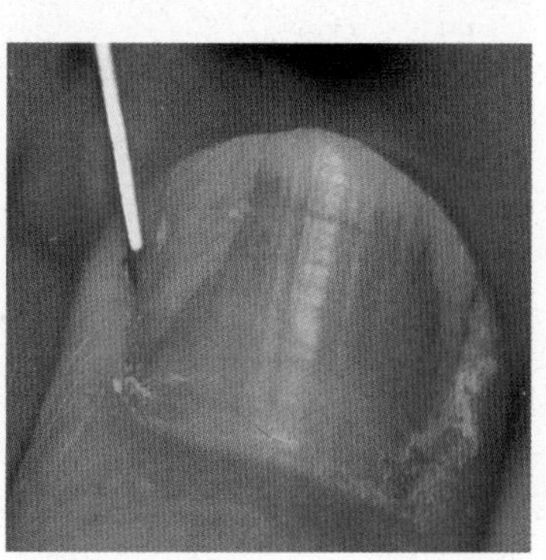

© Courtesy of Robert Baron, MD (France).

▲ Figure 10–14
Onycholysis.

Onycholysis (ahn-ih-KAHL-ih-sis) is the lifting of the nail plate from the bed without shedding, usually beginning at the free edge and continuing toward the lunula area (**Figure 10–14**). This is usually the result of physical injury, trauma, or allergic reaction of the nail bed, and less often related to a health disorder. It often occurs on natural nails when they are filed too aggressively, on nail enhancements when they are improperly removed, or on toenails when clients wear shoes without sufficient room for the toes. If there is no indication of an infection or open sores, a basic manicure or pedicure may be given. The nail plate should be short to avoid further injury, and the area underneath the nail plate should be kept clean and dry. If the trauma that caused the onycholysis is removed, the area will begin to slowly heal itself. Eventually, the nail plate will grow off the free edge and the hyponychium will reform the seal that provides a natural barrier against infection (**Figure 10–15**).

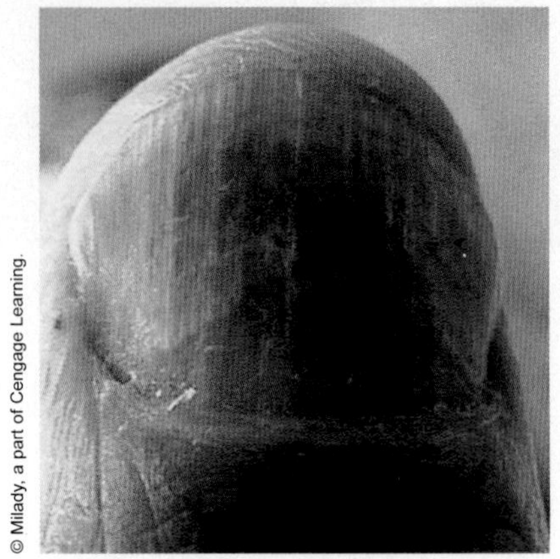
© Milady, a part of Cengage Learning.

▲ Figure 10–15
Onycholysis caused by trauma.

Onychomadesis (ahn-ih-koh-muh-DEE-sis) is the separation and falling off of a nail plate from the nail bed. It can affect fingernails and toenails (**Figure 10–16**). In most cases, the cause can be traced to a localized infection, injuries to the matrix, or a severe systemic illness. Drastic medical procedures, such as chemotherapy, may also be the cause.

Whatever the reason, once the problem is resolved, a new nail plate will eventually grow again. If onychomadesis is present, do not apply enhancements to the nail plate. If there is no indication of an infection or open sores, a basic manicure or pedicure service may be given.

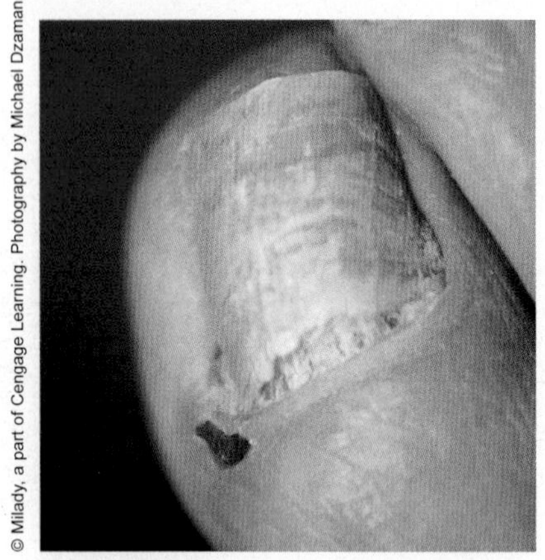
© Milady, a part of Cengage Learning. Photography by Michael Dzaman.

▲ Figure 10–16
Onychomadesis.

Nail psoriasis (NAYL suh-RY-uh-sis) is a noninfectious condition that affects the surface of the natural nail plate causing tiny pits or severe roughness on the surface of the nail plate. Sometimes these pits occur randomly, and sometimes they appear in evenly spaced rows. Nail psoriasis can also cause the surface of the plate to look like it has been filed with a coarse abrasive, can cause a ragged free edge, or can cause both (**Figure 10–17**). People with skin psoriasis often experience this nail disorder. Neither skin nor nail psoriasis are infectious diseases. Nail psoriasis can also affect the nail bed, causing it to develop yellowish to reddish spots underneath the nail plate, called *salmon patches*. Onycholysis is also much more prevalent in people with nail psoriasis. When all of these symptoms are present on the nail unit at the same time, nail psoriasis becomes a likely cause of the client's problem nails, and they should be referred to a physician for diagnoses and treatment, if needed.

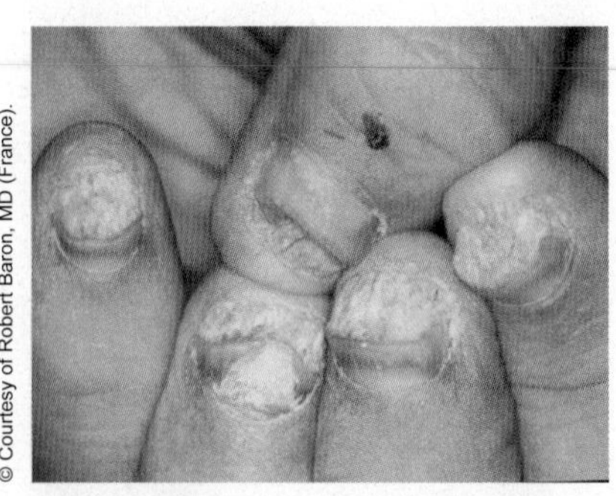
© Courtesy of Robert Baron, MD (France).

▲ Figure 10–17
Nail psoriasis.

Paronychia (payr-uh-NIK-ee-uh) is a bacterial inflammation of the tissues surrounding the nail (**Figure 10–18**). Redness, pus, and swelling are usually seen in the skin fold adjacent to the nail plate.

Individuals who work with their hands in water, such as dishwashers and bartenders, or who must wash their hands continually, such as health-care workers and food processors, are more susceptible because their hands are often very dry or chapped from excessive exposure to water, detergents, and harsh soaps. This makes them much more likely to develop infections.

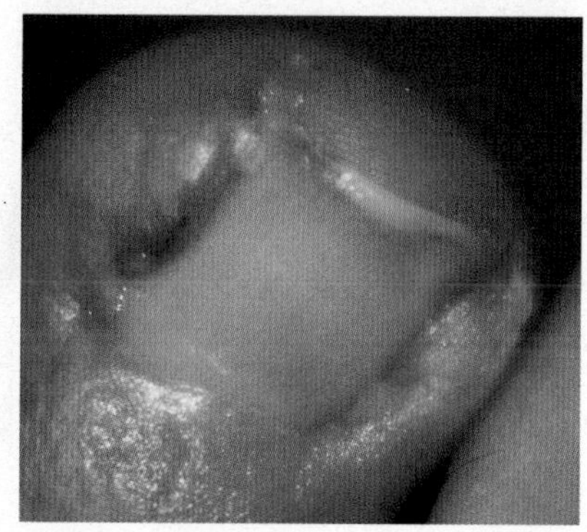
© Milady, a part of Cengage Learning.

▲ Figure 10–18
Chronic paronychia.

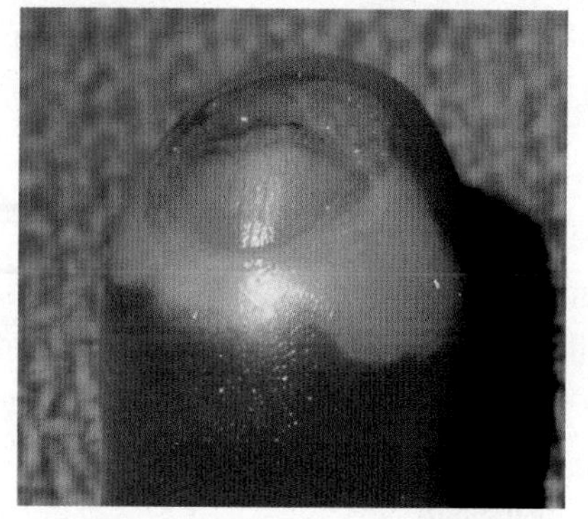
© Milady, a part of Cengage Learning.

▲ Figure 10–19
Paronychia.

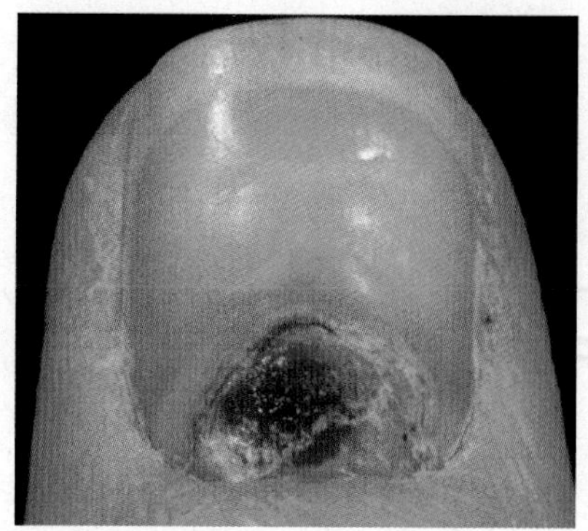
© Milady, a part of Cengage Learning.

▲ Figure 10–20
Pyogenic granuloma.

Toenails, because they spend a lot of time in a warm, moist environment, are often more susceptible to paronychia infections as well (**Figure 10–19**). Use moisturizing hand lotions to keep skin healthy, and keep feet clean and dry.

Pyogenic granuloma (py-oh-JEN-ik gran-yoo-LOH-muh) is a severe inflammation of the nail in which a lump of red tissue grows up from the nail bed to the nail plate (**Figure 10–20**).

Tinea pedis (TIN-ee-uh PED-us) is the medical term for fungal infections of the feet. These infections can occur on the bottoms of the feet and often appear as a red itchy rash in the spaces between the toes, most often between the fourth and fifth toe. There is sometimes a small degree of scaling of the skin. Clients with this condition should be advised to wash their feet every day and dry them completely. This will make it difficult for the infection to live or grow. Advise clients to wear cotton socks and change them at least twice per day. They should also avoid wearing the same pair of shoes each day, since shoes can take up to twenty-four hours to completely dry. Over-the-counter antifungal powders can help keep feet dry and may help speed healing (**Figure 10–21**).

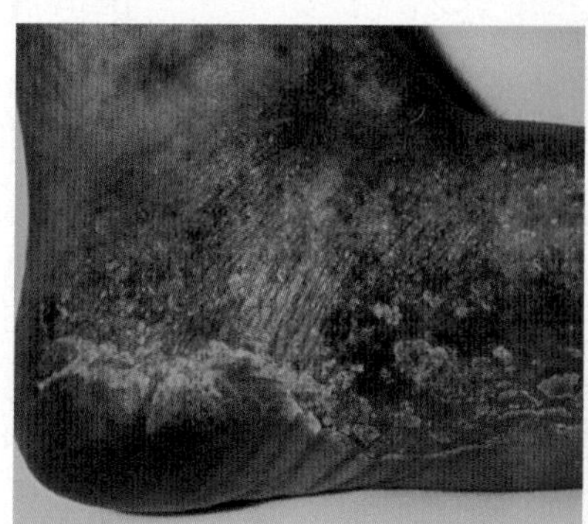
© Reprinted with permission from the American Academy of Dermatology. All rights reserved.

▲ Figure 10–21
Tinea pedis.

Onychomycosis (ahn-ih-koh-my-KOH-sis) is a fungal infection of the natural nail plate (**Figure 10–22**). A common form is whitish patches that can be scraped off the surface of the nail. Another common form of this infection shows long whitish or pale yellowish streaks within the nail plate. A third common form causes the free edge of the nail to crumble and may even affect the entire plate. These types of infection often invade the free edge of the nail and spread toward the matrix. ☑ **LO2**

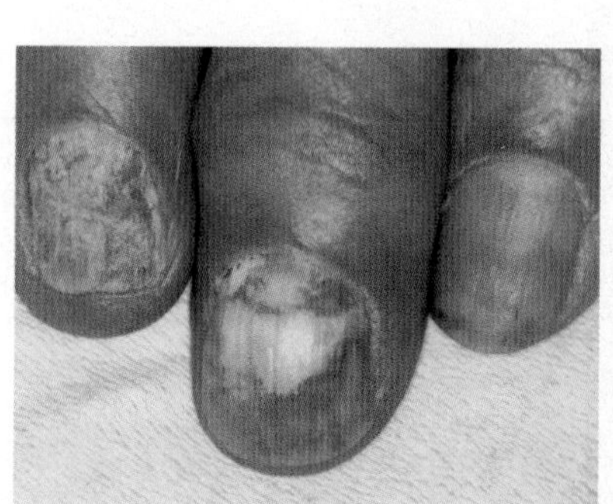
© Courtesy of Robert Baron, MD (France).

▲ Figure 10–22
Onychomycosis.

did you know?

To learn more about the natural nail and understand more about infections, diseases, and disorders, be sure to read *Nail Structure and Product Chemistry*, second edition, by Douglas Schoon. (Published by Milady, a part of Cengage Learning.)

Review Questions

1. In what situation should a nail service not be performed?
2. Name at least eight nail disorders and describe their appearance.
3. What conditions do fungal organisms favor for growth?
4. If a client develops a nail infection, can a cosmetologist offer treatment advice for these conditions? Why?
5. What is the most effective way to avoid transferring infections among your clients?
6. What is pseudomonas aeruginosa? Why is it important to learn about it?
7. Name two common causes of onycholysis.
8. Should a cosmetologist treat an ingrown toenail if there is no sign of pus or discharge? Why?

Chapter Glossary

Beau's lines	Visible depressions running across the width of the natural nail plate; usually a result of major illness or injury that has traumatized the body.
bruised nails	Condition in which a blood clot forms under the nail plate, causing a dark purplish spot. These discolorations are usually due to small injuries to the nail bed.
discolored nails	Nails turn a variety of colors; may indicate surface staining, a systemic disorder, or poor blood circulation.
eggshell nails	Noticeably thin, white nail plates that are more flexible than normal and can curve over the free edge.
hangnail	Also known as *agnail*; a condition in which the living tissue surrounding the nail plate splits or tears.
leukonychia spots	Also known as *white spots*; whitish discolorations of the nails, usually caused by injury to the matrix area; not related to the body's health or vitamin deficiencies.
melanonychia	Darkening of the fingernails or toenails; may be seen as a black band within the nail plate, extending from the base to the free edge.
nail disorder	Condition caused by an injury or disease of the nail unit.
nail psoriasis	A noninfectious condition that affects the surface of the natural nail plate causing tiny pits or severe roughness on the surface of the nail plate.
nail pterygium	Abnormal condition that occurs when the skin is stretched by the nail plate; usually caused by serious injury, such as burns, or an adverse skin reaction to chemical nail enhancement products.
onychia	Inflammation of the nail matrix, followed by shedding of the natural nail.
onychocryptosis	Also know as *ingrown nails*; nail grows into the sides of the tissue around the nail.
onycholysis	Lifting of the nail plate from the nail bed without shedding, usually beginning at the free edge and continuing toward the lunula area.
onychomadesis	The separation and falling off of a nail plate from the nail bed; affects fingernails and toenails.

Chapter Glossary

onychomycosis	Fungal infection of the natural nail plate.
onychophagy	Also known as *bitten nails*; result of a habit of chewing the nail or chewing the hardened skin surrounding the nail plate.
onychorrhexis	Split or brittle nails that have a series of lengthwise ridges giving a rough appearance to the surface of the nail plate.
onychosis	Any deformity or disease of the natural nails.
paronychia	Bacterial inflammation of the tissues surrounding the nail causing pus, swelling, and redness, usually in the skin fold adjacent to the nail plate.
pincer nail	Also known as *trumpet nail*; increased crosswise curvature throughout the nail plate caused by an increased curvature of the matrix. The edges of the nail plate may curl around to form the shape of a trumpet or sharp cone at the free edge.
plicatured nail	Also known as *folded nail*; a type of highly curved nail usually caused by injury to the matrix, but may be inherited.
Pseudomonas aeruginosa	One of several common bacteria that can cause nail infection.
pyogenic granuloma	Severe inflammation of the nail in which a lump of red tissue grows up from the nail bed to the nail plate.
ridges	Vertical lines running through the length of the natural nail plate that are caused by uneven growth of the nails, usually the result of normal aging.
splinter hemorrhages	Hemorrhages caused by trauma or injury to the nail bed that damage the capillaries and allow small amounts of blood flow.
tinea pedis	Medical term for fungal infections of the feet; red, itchy rash of the skin on the bottom of the feet and/or in between the toes, usually found between the fourth and fifth toe.

CHAPTER 11

Properties of the Hair and Scalp

Chapter Outline

Why Study Properties of the Hair and Scalp?

Structure of the Hair

Chemical Composition of Hair

Hair Growth

Hair Loss

Disorders of the Hair

Disorders of the Scalp

Hair and Scalp Analysis

© Yojik, 2010; used under license from Dreamstime.com

Learning Objectives

After completing this chapter, you will be able to:

- ✓ **LO1** Name and describe the structures of the hair root.
- ✓ **LO2** List and describe the three main layers of the hair shaft.
- ✓ **LO3** Describe the three types of side bonds in the cortex.
- ✓ **LO4** Describe the hair growth cycles.
- ✓ **LO5** Discuss the types of hair loss and their causes.
- ✓ **LO6** Describe the options for hair loss treatment.
- ✓ **LO7** Recognize hair and scalp disorders commonly seen in the salon and school and know which ones can be treated by cosmetologists.
- ✓ **LO8** List and describe the factors that should be considered in a hair and scalp analysis.

Key Terms

Page number indicates where in the chapter the term is used.

alopecia pg. 230

alopecia areata pg. 231

alopecia totalis pg. 231

alopecia universalis pg. 231

amino acids pg. 223

anagen phase (growth phase) pg. 227

androgenic alopecia (androgenetic alopecia) pg. 230

canities pg. 232

carbuncle pg. 236

catagen phase pg. 228

COHNS elements pg. 223

cortex pg. 222

cowlick pg. 240

cysteine pg. 224

cystine pg. 225

disulfide bond pg. 224

fragilitas crinium pg. 233

furuncle pg. 236

hair bulb pg. 221

hair cuticle pg. 221

hair density pg. 238

hair elasticity pg. 239

hair follicle pg. 221

hair porosity pg. 238

hair root pg. 220

hair shaft pg. 220

hair stream pg. 240

hair texture pg. 237

helix pg. 223

hydrogen bond pg. 223

hydrophilic pg. 238

hydrophobic pg. 238

hypertrichosis (hirsuties) pg. 232

keratinization pg. 222

lanthionine bonds pg. 225

malassezia pg. 234

medulla pg. 222

monilethrix pg. 233

pediculosis capitis pg. 235

peptide bond (end bond) pg. 223

pityriasis pg. 234

pityriasis capitis simplex pg. 234

pityriasis steatoides pg. 234

polypeptide chain pg. 223

postpartum alopecia pg. 231

proteins pg. 223

ringed hair pg. 232

salt bond pg. 224

scutula pg. 235

side bonds pg. 223

telogen phase (resting phase) pg. 228

terminal hair pg. 227

tinea pg. 235

tinea favosa (tinea favus) pg. 235

trichology pg. 220

trichoptilosis pg. 233

trichorrhexis nodosa pg. 233

vellus hair (lanugo hair) pg. 227

wave pattern pg. 225

whorl pg. 240

From Lady Godiva's infamous horseback ride to the sought-after celebrity styles that make headlines every day, hair has been one of humanity's most enduring obsessions. The term *crowning glory* aptly describes the importance placed on hair, how good we feel when our hair looks great, and just how distressing a bad hair day really can be. This is why hairstylists play such an important role in many people's lives. All professional hair services must be based on a thorough understanding of the growth, structure, and composition of hair.

Why Study Properties of the Hair and Scalp?

Cosmetologists should study and have a thorough understanding of the properties of the hair and scalp because:

- You need to know how and why hair grows and how and why it falls out in order to be able to differentiate between normal and abnormal hair loss.
- Knowing what creates natural color and texture is a vital part of being able to offer a variety of chemical services to clients.
- Spotting an unhealthy scalp condition that could be harboring a communicable disease or even be causing permanent hair loss is a way to aid your client in caring for their scalp and hair's well-being.

Structure of the Hair

The scientific study of hair and its diseases and care is called **trichology** (trih-KAHL-uh-jee), which comes from the Greek words *trichos* (hair) and *ology* (the study of). The hair, skin, nails, and glands are part of the integumentary system. Although we no longer need hair for warmth and protection, hair still has an enormous impact on our psychology.

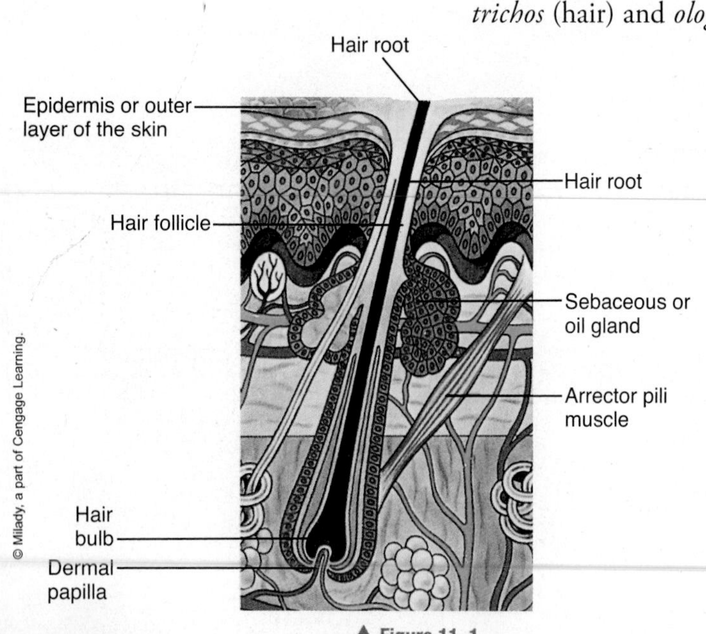

© Milady, a part of Cengage Learning.

▲ **Figure 11–1**
Structures of the hair.

A mature strand of human hair is divided into two parts: the hair root and the hair shaft. The **hair root** is the part of the hair located below the surface of the epidermis (outer layer of the skin). The **hair shaft** is the portion of the hair that projects above the epidermis (**Figure 11–1**).

Structures of the Hair Root

The five main structures of the hair root include the hair follicle, hair bulb, dermal papilla, arrector pili muscle, and sebaceous (oil) glands.

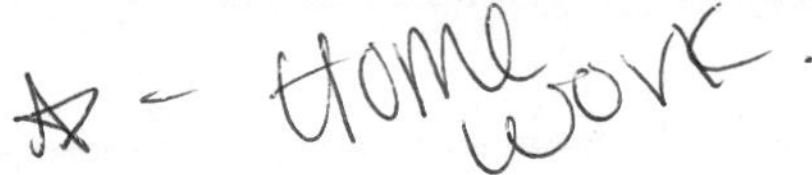

- The **hair follicle** (HAYR FAWL-ih-kul) is the tube-like depression or pocket in the skin or scalp that contains the hair root. Hair follicles are distributed all over the body, with the exception of the palms of the hands and the soles of the feet. The follicle extends downward from the epidermis into the dermis (the inner layer of skin), where it surrounds the dermal papilla. Sometimes more than one hair will grow from a single follicle.
- The **hair bulb** (HAYR BULB) is the lowest part of a hair strand. It is the thickened, club-shaped structure that forms the lower part of the hair root. The lower part of the hair bulb fits over and covers the dermal papilla.
- The dermal papilla (plural: dermal papillae) is a small, cone-shaped elevation located at the base of the hair follicle that fits into the hair bulb. The dermal papilla contains the blood and nerve supply that provides the nutrients needed for hair growth. Some people refer to the dermal papilla as the mother of the hair because it contains the blood and nerve supply that provides the nutrients needed for hair growth.
- The arrector pili muscle is the small, involuntary muscle in the base of the hair follicle. Strong emotions or a cold sensation cause it to contract, which makes the hair stand up straight and results in what we call *goose bumps*.
- Sebaceous glands are the oil glands in the skin that are connected to the hair follicles. The sebaceous glands secrete a fatty or an oily substance called sebum. Sebum lubricates the skin. ☑ **LO1**

did you know?

Have you heard the expression "You are what you eat"? Although a healthy diet does not always guarantee a healthy hair and scalp, it is mainly true that what you eat will affect your hair and scalp. The body can produce 11 of the 20 amino acids that make up hair, but your daily diet must include the remaining 9 essential amino acids that the hair and scalp need. This is why crash dieting and anorexia can cause hair loss, lackluster hair, and unhealthy scalp conditions. Proteins in meat, fish, eggs, and dairy products are good sources of these amino acids, as are food combinations such as peanut butter and bread, rice and beans, and beans and corn.

Structures of the Hair Shaft

The three main layers of the hair shaft are the hair cuticle, cortex, and medulla (**Figure 11–2**).

- The **hair cuticle** (HAYR KYOO-ti-kul) is the outermost layer of the hair. It consists of a single overlapping layer of transparent, scale-like cells that look like shingles on a roof. The cuticle layer provides a barrier that protects the inner structure of the hair as it lies tightly against the cortex. It is responsible for creating the shine and the smooth, silky feel of healthy hair.

To feel the cuticle, pinch a single healthy strand of hair between your thumb and forefinger. Starting near the scalp, pull upward on the strand. The strand should feel sleek and smooth. Next, hold the end of the hair strand with one hand, and then pinch the strand with the thumb and forefingers of your other hand. Move your fingers down the hair shaft. In this direction, the hair feels rougher because

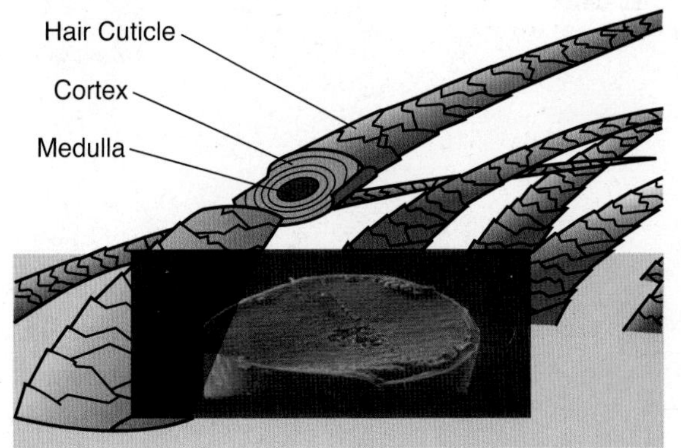

© Milady, a part of Cengage Learning.

▲ **Figure 11–2**
Cross-section of hair cuticle.

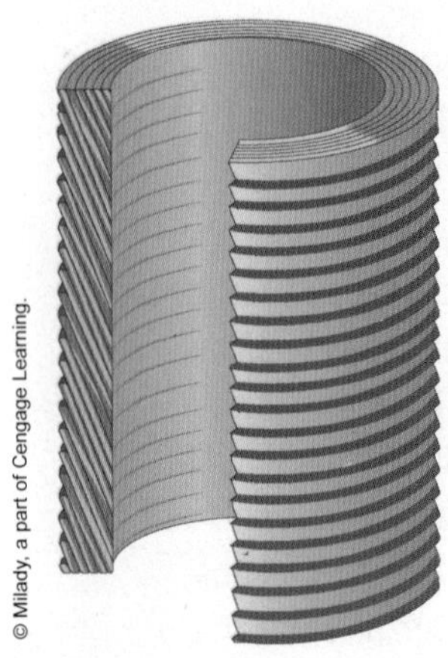

© Milady, a part of Cengage Learning.

▲ **Figure 11–3**
Hair cuticle layer.

you are going against the natural growth of the cuticle layer. A healthy, compact cuticle layer is the hair's primary defense against damage. A lengthwise cross-section of hair shows that although the hair cuticle scales overlap, each individual cuticle scale is attached to the cortex (**Figure 11–3**). These overlapping scales make up the cuticle layer. Swelling the hair by applying substances such as haircolor raises the cuticle layer and opens the space between the scales, which allows liquids to penetrate into the cortex.

A healthy hair cuticle layer protects the hair from penetration and prevents damage to hair fibers. Oxidation haircolors, permanent waving solutions, and chemical hair relaxers must have an alkaline pH to penetrate the cuticle layer, because a high pH swells the cuticle and causes it to lift and expose the cortex.

- The **cortex** (KOR-teks) is the middle layer of the hair. It is a fibrous protein core formed by elongated cells containing melanin pigment. About 90 percent of the total weight of hair comes from the cortex. The elasticity of the hair and its natural color are the result of the unique protein structures located within the cortex. The changes involved in oxidation haircoloring, wet setting, thermal styling, permanent waving, and chemical hair relaxing take place within the cortex (**Figure 11–4**).

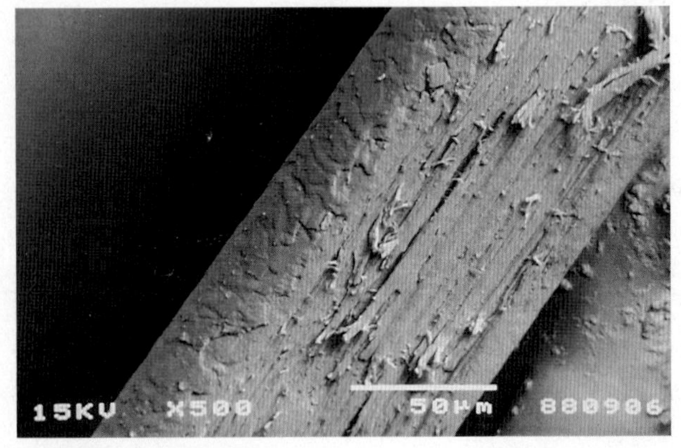

Courtesy of P&G Beauty from John Grey's, The World of Hair Care.

▲ **Figure 11–4**
Hair shaft with part of the hair cuticle stripped off, exposing the cortex.

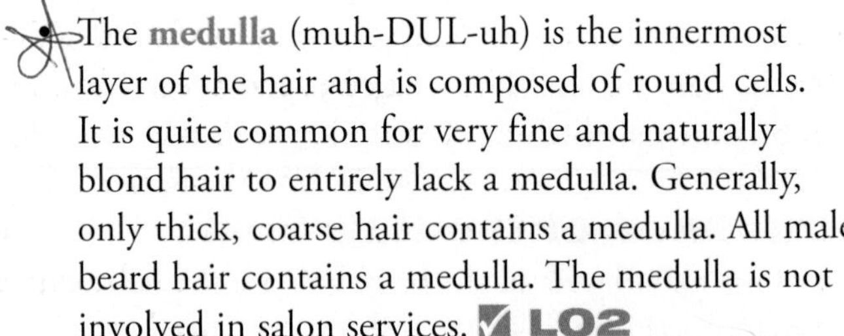

- The **medulla** (muh-DUL-uh) is the innermost layer of the hair and is composed of round cells. It is quite common for very fine and naturally blond hair to entirely lack a medulla. Generally, only thick, coarse hair contains a medulla. All male beard hair contains a medulla. The medulla is not involved in salon services. ☑ **LO2**

Chemical Composition of Hair

Hair is composed of protein that grows from cells originating within the hair follicle. This is where the hair begins. As soon as these living cells form, they begin their journey upward through the hair follicle. They mature in a process called **keratinization** (kair-uh-ti-ni-ZAY-shun). As these newly formed cells mature, they fill up with a fibrous protein called keratin. After they have filled with keratin, the cells move upward, lose their nucleus, and die. By the time the hair shaft emerges from the scalp, the cells of the hair are completely keratinized and are no longer living. The hair shaft that emerges is a nonliving fiber composed of keratinized protein.

Hair is approximately 90 percent protein. The protein is made up of long chains of amino acids, which, in turn, are made up of elements.

THE COHNS ELEMENTS	
ELEMENT	PERCENTAGE IN NORMAL HAIR
CARBON	51%
OXYGEN	21%
HYDROGEN	6%
NITROGEN	17%
SULFUR	5%

Table 11–1 **The COHNS Elements.**

The major elements that make up human hair are carbon, oxygen, hydrogen, nitrogen, and sulfur and are often referred to as the **COHNS elements** (KOH-nz EL-uh-ments). These five elements are also found in skin and nails. **Table 11–1** shows the percentages of each element in a typical strand of hair.

Proteins are made of long chains of **amino acids** (uh-MEE-noh AS-udz), units that are joined together end to end like pop beads. The strong, chemical bond that joins amino acids is a **peptide bond** (PEP-tyd BAHND), also known as **end bond**. A long chain of amino acids linked by peptide bonds is called a **polypeptide chain** (pahl-ee-PEP-tyd CHAYN). **Proteins** (PROH-teenz) are long, coiled complex polypeptides made of amino acids. The spiral shape of a coiled protein is called a **helix** (HEE-licks), which is created when the polypeptide chains intertwine with each other (**Figure 11–5**).

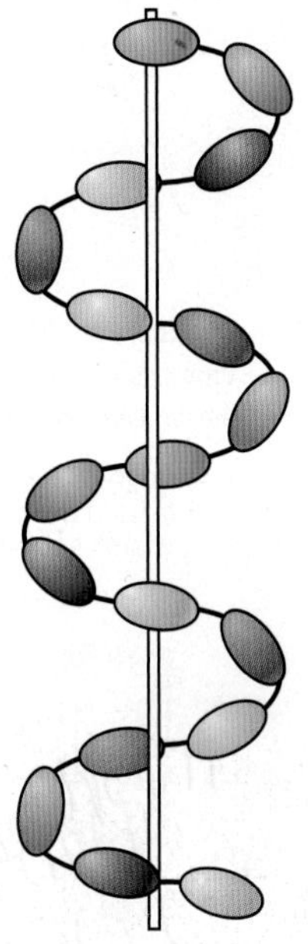

▲ Figure 11–5
Polypeptide chains intertwine in a spiral shape called a helix.

Side Bonds of the Cortex

The cortex is made up of millions of polypeptide chains. Polypeptide chains are cross-linked like the rungs on a ladder by three different types of **side bonds** that link the polypeptide chains together and are responsible for the extreme strength and elasticity of human hair. They are essential to services such as wet setting, thermal styling, permanent waving, and chemical hair relaxing (see Chapter 20, Chemical Texture Services). The three types of side bonds are hydrogen, salt, and disulfide bonds (**Figure 11–6**).

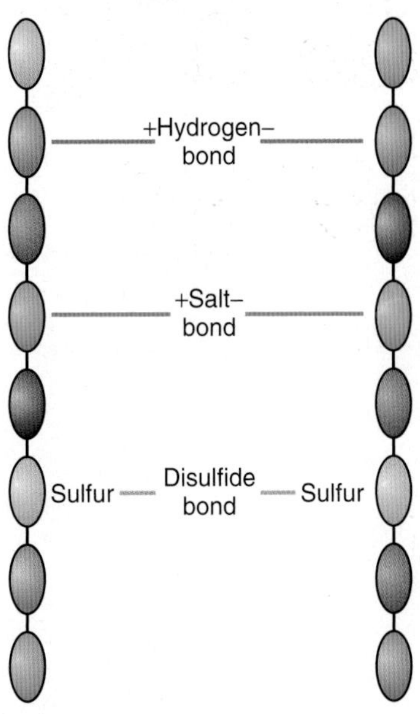

▲ Figure 11–6
Side bonds between polypeptide chains.

© Milady, a part of Cengage Learning.

- A **hydrogen bond** is a weak, physical, cross-link side bond that is easily broken by water or heat. Although individual hydrogen bonds are very weak, there are so many of them that they account for about one-third of the hair's overall strength. Hydrogen bonds are broken by wetting the hair with water (**Figure 11–7**). That allows the hair to be stretched and wrapped around rollers. The hydrogen bonds reform when the hair dries.

- A **salt bond** is also a weak, physical, cross-link side bond between adjacent polypeptide chains. Salt bonds depend on pH, so they are easily broken by strong alkaline or acidic solutions (**Figure 11–8**). Even though they are weak bonds, there are so many of them that they account for about one-third of the hair's overall strength.
- A **disulfide bond** (dy-SUL-fyd BAHND) is a strong, chemical, side bond that is very different from the physical side bond of a hydrogen bond or salt bond. The disulfide bond joins the sulfur atoms of two neighboring **cysteine** (SIS-ti-een) amino acids to create one

▼ **Figure 11–7**
Changes in hair cortex during wet setting.

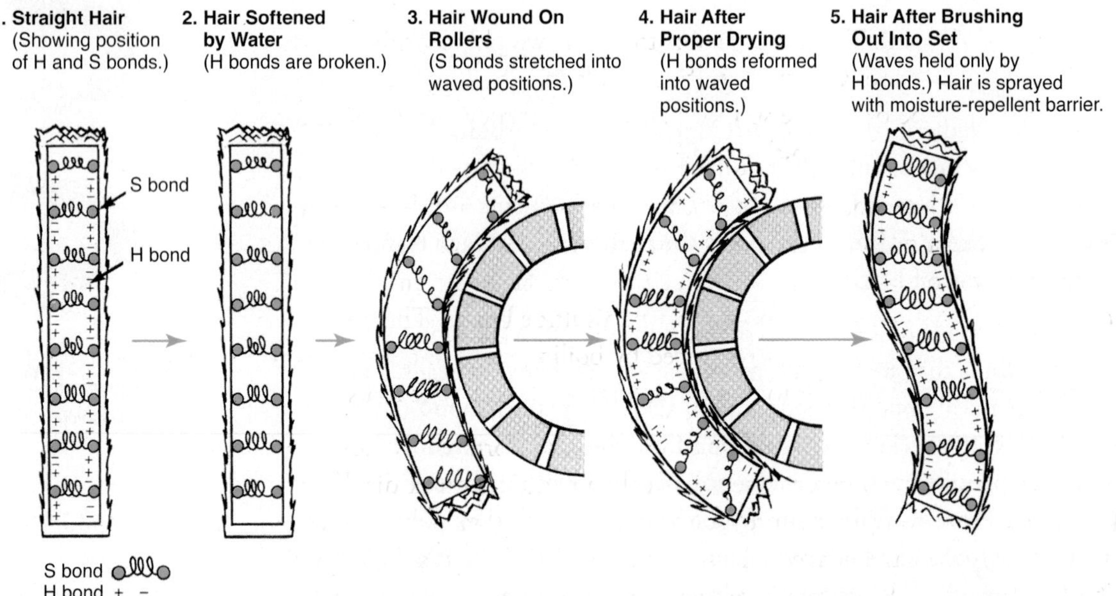
1. Straight Hair
(Showing position of H and S bonds.)
2. Hair Softened by Water
(H bonds are broken.)
3. Hair Wound On Rollers
(S bonds stretched into waved positions.)
4. Hair After Proper Drying
(H bonds reformed into waved positions.)
5. Hair After Brushing Out Into Set
(Waves held only by H bonds.) Hair is sprayed with moisture-repellent barrier.
S bond
H bond
S bond
H bond + –

▼ **Figure 11–8**
Changes in hair cortex during permanent waving.

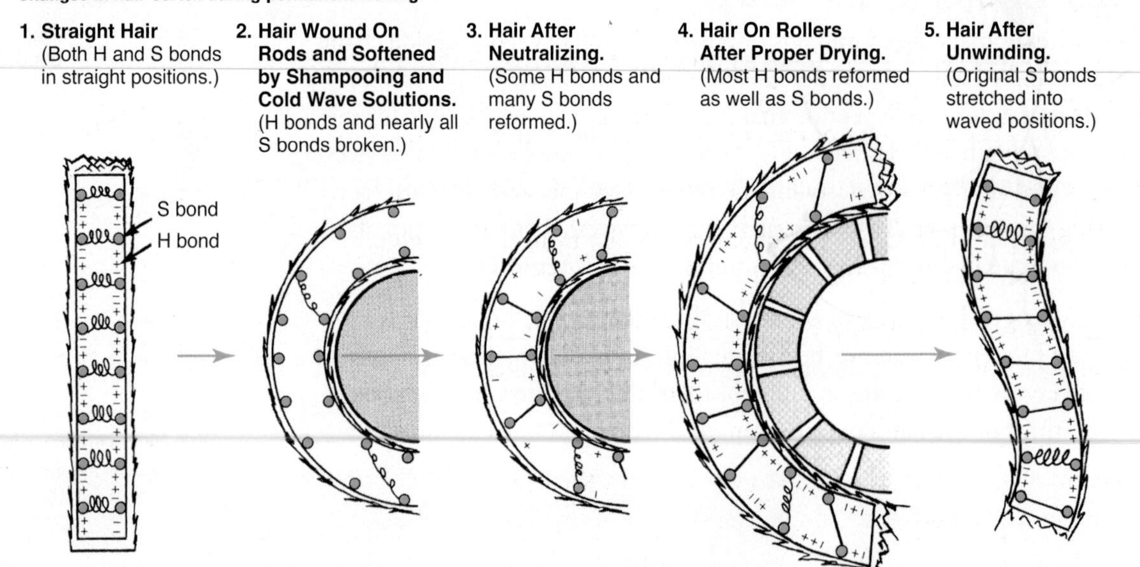
1. Straight Hair
(Both H and S bonds in straight positions.)
2. Hair Wound On Rods and Softened by Shampooing and Cold Wave Solutions.
(H bonds and nearly all S bonds broken.)
3. Hair After Neutralizing.
(Some H bonds and many S bonds reformed.)
4. Hair On Rollers After Proper Drying.
(Most H bonds reformed as well as S bonds.)
5. Hair After Unwinding.
(Original S bonds stretched into waved positions.)
S bond
H bond

© Milady, a part of Cengage Learning.

BONDS OF THE HAIR				
BOND	**TYPE**	**STRENGTH**	**BROKEN BY**	**REFORMED BY**
HYDROGEN	side bond	weak, physical	water or heat	drying or cooling
SALT	side bond	weak, physical	changes in pH	normalizing pH
DISULFIDE	side bond	strong, chemical	1. thio perms and thio relaxers 2. hydroxide relaxers 3. extreme heat	1. oxidation with neutralizer 2. converted to lanthionine bonds
PEPTIDE	end bond	strong, chemical	chemical depilatories	not reformed; hair dissolves

Table 11–2 **Bonds of the Hair.**

cystine (SIS-teen). The **cystine** joins together two polypeptide strands. Although there are far fewer disulfide bonds than hydrogen or salt bonds, disulfide bonds are so much stronger that they also account for about one-third of the hair's overall strength.

Disulfide bonds are not broken by water. They are broken by permanent waves and chemical hair relaxers that alter the shape of hair (**Table 11–2**). Additionally, normal amounts of heat, such as the heat used in conventional thermal styling, do not break disulfide bonds. The bonds can be broken by extreme heat produced by boiling water and some high-temperature thermal styling tools such as straightening or flat irons.

Thio permanent waves break disulfide bonds and reform the bonds with thio neutralizers. Hydroxide chemical hair relaxers break disulfide bonds and then convert them to **lanthionine bonds** (lan-THY-oh-neen BAHNDZ) when the relaxer is rinsed from the hair. The disulfide bonds that are treated with hydroxide relaxers are broken permanently and can never be reformed (see Chapter 20, Chemical Texture Services). ☑ **LO3**

Hair Pigment

All natural hair color is the result of the pigment located within the cortex. Melanin are the tiny grains of pigment in the cortex that give natural color to the hair. The two types of melanin are eumelanin and pheomelanin.

- Eumelanin provides natural dark brown to black color to hair.
- Pheomelanin provides natural colors ranging from red and ginger to yellow and blond tones.

All natural hair color is the result of the ratio of eumelanin to pheomelanin, along with the total number and size of pigment granules.

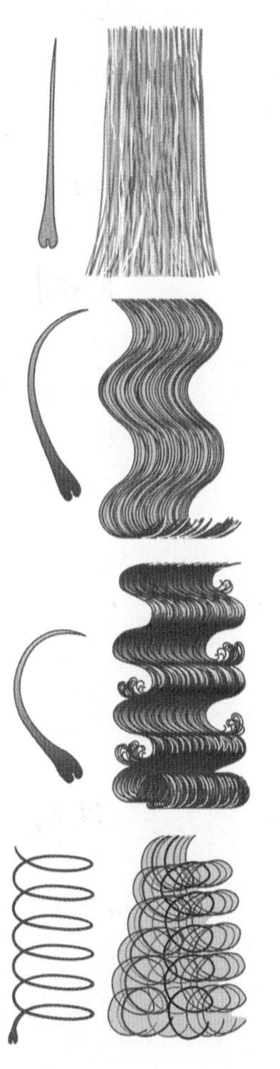

▲ Figure 11–9
Straight, wavy, curly, and extremely curly hair strands.

Wave Pattern

The **wave pattern** of hair refers to the shape of the hair strand. It is described as straight, wavy, curly, or extremely curly (**Figure 11–9**).

© Milady, a part of Cengage Learning.

did you know?

The term hair color (two words) refers to the color of hair created by nature. Haircolor (one word) is the term used in the beauty industry to refer to artificial haircoloring products. Gray hair is caused by the absence of melanin. Gray hair grows from the hair bulb in exactly the same way that pigmented hair grows. It has the same structure, but without the melanin pigment.

Natural wave patterns are the result of genetics. Although there are many exceptions, as a general rule, Asians and Native Americans tend to have extremely straight hair, Caucasians tend to have straight, wavy, or curly hair, and African Americans tend to have extremely curly hair. But straight, wavy, curly, and extremely curly hair occur in all races—anyone of any race, or mixed race, can have hair with varying degrees of curl from straight to extremely curly. The wave pattern may also vary from strand to strand on the same person's head. It is not uncommon for an individual to have different amounts of curl in different areas of the head. Individuals with curly hair often have straighter hair in the crown and tighter curl in other areas.

Several theories attempt to explain the cause of natural curly hair, but there is no single, definite answer that explains why some hair grows straight and other hair grows curly. The most popular theory claims that the shape of the hair's cross-section determines the amount of curl. This theory claims that hair with a round cross-section is straight, hair with an oval to flattened oval cross-section is wavy or curly, and hair with a flattened to flattened oval cross-section is extremely curly (**Table 11–3**).

Another theory that attempts to explain varying degrees of curl is that, in curly hair, one side of the hair strand grows faster than the other side. Since the side that grows faster will be slightly longer than the slower-growing side, tension within the strand causes the long side to curl around the short side. Hair that grows uniformly on both sides does not create tension and results in straight hair. However, this theory is still unproven.

It is true that cross-sections of straight hair tend to be round and curly hair tends to be more oval, but modern microscopes have shown that a cross-section of hair can be almost any shape. So the shape of the cross-section does not always relate to the amount of curl.

Extremely Curly Hair

Extremely curly hair grows in long twisted spirals. Cross-sections appear flattened and vary in shape and thickness along their length. Compared to straight or wavy hair, which tends to possess a fairly regular and uniform diameter along a single strand, extremely curly hair is fairly irregular, showing varying diameters along a single strand. Some extremely curly hair has a natural tendency to form a coil like

WAVE PATTERN AND CROSS-SECTIONS

WAVE PATTERN	SHAPE OF CROSS-SECTION
STRAIGHT HAIR	round cross-section
WAVY OR CURLY	oval to flattened oval cross-section
EXTREMELY CURLY HAIR	flattened cross-section

© Milady, a part of Cengage Learning.

Table 11–3 Wave Pattern and Cross-Sections.

a telephone cord. Coiled hair usually has a fine texture, with many individual strands winding together to form the coiled locks. Extremely curly hair often has low elasticity, breaks easily, and has a tendency to knot, especially on the ends. Gentle scalp manipulations, conditioning shampoo, and a detangling rinse help minimize tangles.

Hair Growth

The two main types of hair found on the body are vellus hair and terminal hair (**Figure 11–10**).

Vellus hair (VEL-us HAYR), also known as **lanugo hair** (luh-NOO-goh HAYR), is short, fine, unpigmented, and downy hair that appears on the body. Vellus hair almost never has a medulla. It is commonly found on infants and can be present on children until puberty. On adults, vellus hair is usually found in places that are normally considered hairless (forehead, eyelids, and bald scalp), as well as nearly all other areas of the body, except the palms of the hands and the soles of the feet. Women normally retain 55 percent more vellus hair than men. Vellus hair helps with the evaporation of perspiration.

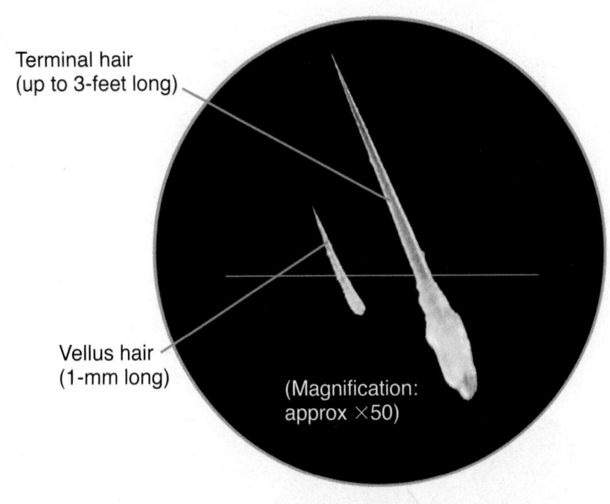

▲ **Figure 11–10**
Vellus hair and terminal hair.

Terminal hair (TUR-mih-nul HAYR) is the long, coarse, pigmented hair found on the scalp, legs, arms, and bodies of males and females. Terminal hair is coarser than vellus hair, and, with the exception of gray hair, it is pigmented. It usually has a medulla.

Hormonal changes during puberty cause some areas of fine vellus hair to be replaced with thicker terminal hair. All hair follicles are capable of producing either vellus or terminal hair, depending on genetics, age, and hormones.

Growth Cycles of Hair

Hair growth occurs in cycles. Each complete cycle has three phases that are repeated over and over again throughout life. The three phases are anagen, catagen, and telogen (**Figure 11–11**).

1. During the **anagen phase** (AN-uh-jen FAYZ), also known as **growth phase**, new hair is produced. New cells are actively manufactured in the hair follicle. During this phase, hair cells are produced faster than any other normal cell in the human body. The average growth of healthy scalp hair is about ½ (0.5) inch (1.25 centimeters) per month. The rate of growth varies on different parts of the body, between sexes, and with age. Scalp hair grows faster on women than on men. Scalp hair grows rapidly between the ages of 15 and 30, but slows down sharply after the age of 50.

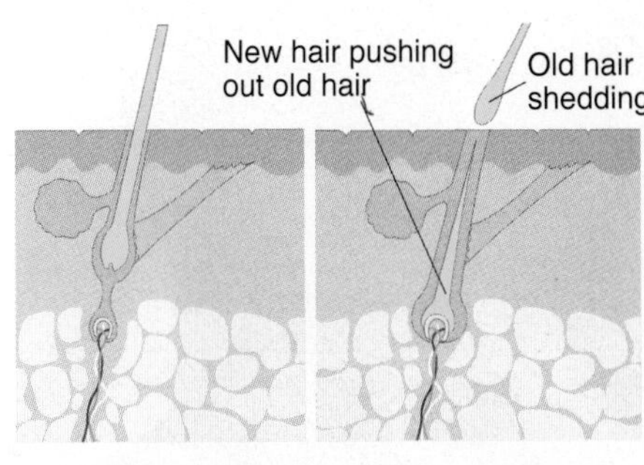

▲ **Figure 11–11**
Cycles of hair growth.

Courtesy of Pfizer Inc.

About 90 percent of scalp hair is growing in the anagen phase at any time. The anagen phase generally lasts from three to five years, but in some cases, it can last as long as 10 years. The longer the anagen cycle is, the longer the hair is able to grow. This is why some people can only grow their hair down to their shoulders, while others can grow it down to the floor!

2. The **catagen phase** (KAT-uh-jen FAYZ) is the brief transition period between the growth and resting phases of a hair follicle. It signals the end of the anagen phase. During the catagen phase, the follicle canal shrinks and detaches from the dermal papilla. The hair bulb disappears and the shrunken root end forms a rounded club. Less than one percent of scalp hair is in the catagen phase at any time. The catagen phase is very short, lasting from one to two weeks.

3. The **telogen phase** (TEL-uh-jen FAYZ), also known as **resting phase,** is the final phase in the hair cycle and lasts until the fully grown hair is shed. The hair is either shed during the telogen phase or remains in place until the next anagen phase, when the new hair growing in pushes it out. About 10 percent of scalp hair is in the telogen phase at any one time.

   The telogen phase lasts for approximately three to six months. As soon as the telogen phase ends, the hair returns to the anagen phase and begins the entire cycle again. On average, the entire growth cycle repeats itself once every four to five years. ☑ **LO4**

Hair Growth Patterns

It is important when shaping and styling hair to consider the hair's growth patterns. Hair follicles usually do not grow out of the head at a perpendicular, 90-degree angle or in a straight direction out from the head. When they do, these growth patterns result in hair streams, whorls, and cowlicks.

Hair growth patterns will be more fully discussed later in this chapter in the Hair Analysis section.

The Truth about Hair Growth

As a stylist, you may hear opinions about hair growth from your clients or from other stylists. Here are some myths and facts about hair growth:

Myth. Shaving, clipping, and cutting the hair on the head makes it grow back faster, darker, and coarser.

Fact. Shaving or cutting the hair on the head has no effect on hair growth. When hair is blunt cut to the same length, it grows back more evenly. Although it may seem to grow back faster, darker, and coarser, shaving or cutting hair on the head has no effect on hair growth.

Myth. Scalp massage increases hair growth.

© Valua Vitaly, 2010; used under license from Shutterstock.com.

© Veronika Vasilyuk, 2010; used under license from iStockphoto.com.

Fact. Scalp massages are very stimulating to the scalp and can increase blood circulation, relax the nerves in the scalp, and tighten the scalp muscles. However, it has not been scientifically proven that any type of stimulation or scalp massage increases hair growth. Minoxidil and finasteride are the only treatments that have been scientifically proven to increase hair growth and are approved for that purpose by the Food and Drug Administration (FDA). Products that claim to increase hair growth are regulated as drugs and are not cosmetics.

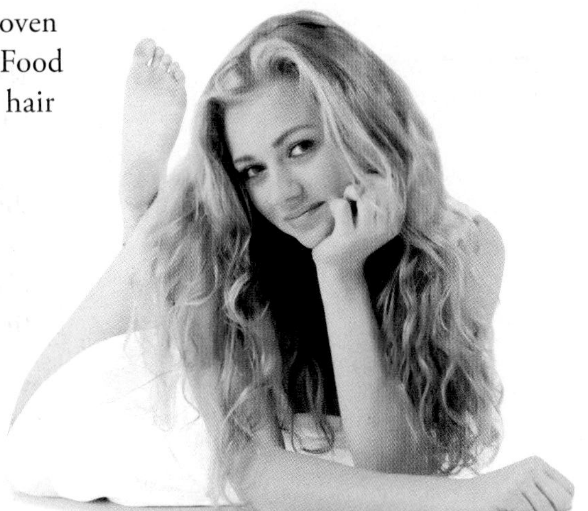

Myth. Gray hair is coarser and more resistant than pigmented hair.

Fact. Other than the lack of pigment, gray hair is exactly the same as pigmented hair. Although gray hair may be resistant, it is not resistant simply because it is gray. Pigmented hair on the same person's head is just as resistant as the gray hair. Gray hair is simply more noticeable than pigmented hair.

Myth. The amount of natural curl is always determined by racial background.

Fact. Anyone of any race, or mixed race, can have hair from straight to extremely curly. It is also true that within races, individuals have hair with varying degrees of curl in different areas of the head.

Myth. Hair with a round cross-section is straight, hair with an oval cross-section is wavy, and hair with a flattened cross-section is curly.

Fact. In general, cross-sections of straight hair are often round, cross-sections of wavy and curly hair tend to be more oval to flattened oval, and cross-sections of extremely curly hair have a flattened cross-section. However, cross-sections of hair can be almost any shape, and the shape of the cross-section does not always relate to the amount of curl or the shape of the follicle.

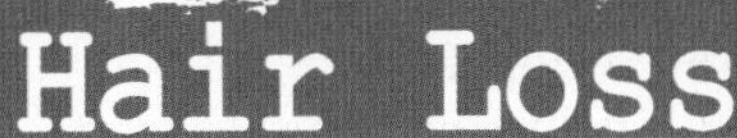

Hair Loss

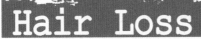

Under normal circumstances, we all lose some hair every day. Normal daily hair loss is the natural result of the anagen, catagen, and telogen phases of the hair's growth cycle that were explained earlier in this chapter.

The growth cycle provides for the continuous growth, fall, and replacement of individual hair strands. A hair that is shed in the telogen phase is replaced by a new hair, in that same follicle, in the next anagen phase. This natural shedding of hair accounts for normal daily hair loss. Although estimates of the rate of hair loss have long been quoted at 100 to 150 hairs per day, recent measurements indicate that the average rate of hair loss is closer to 35 to 40 hairs per day.

The Emotional Impact of Hair Loss

Although the medical community does not always recognize hair loss as a medical condition, the anguish felt by many of those who suffer from abnormal hair loss is very real and all too often overlooked. Results from a study that investigated perceptions of bald and balding men showed that compared to men who had hair, bald men were perceived as:

- less physically attractive (by both sexes).
- less assertive.
- less successful.
- less personally likable.
- older (by about five years).

A study of how bald men perceive themselves showed that greater hair loss had a more significant impact than moderate hair loss. Men with more severe hair loss:

- experience significantly more negative social and emotional effects.
- are more preoccupied with their baldness.
- make some effort to conceal or compensate for their hair loss.

Abnormal hair loss is not as common in women as it is in men, but it can be very traumatic and devastating for women who experience it because, as studies indicate, women have a greater emotional investment in their appearance. Many women with abnormal hair loss feel anxious, helpless, and less attractive. They may think that they are the only ones who have the problem. They also tend to worry that their hair loss is a symptom of a serious illness and sometimes try to disguise it from everyone, even their doctors, which is usually a mistake.

Over 63 million people in the United States suffer from abnormal hair loss. As a professional hairstylist, it is likely that you will be the first person that a hair loss sufferer will confide in, so it is important that you have a basic understanding of the different types of hair loss and the products and services that are available.

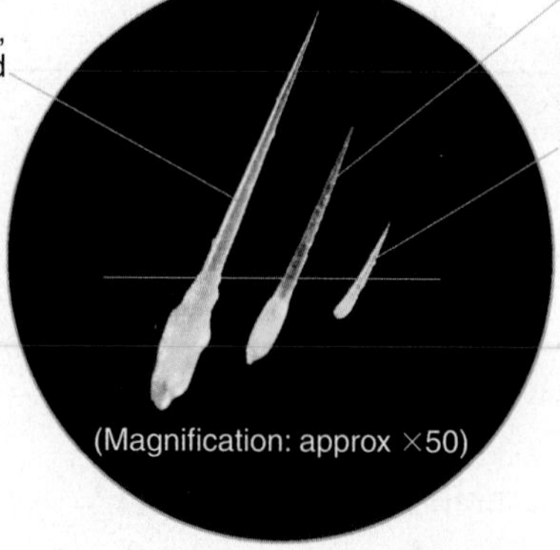

Courtesy of Pfizer Inc.

▲ **Figure 11–12**
Miniaturization of the hair follicle.

Types of Abnormal Hair Loss

Abnormal hair loss is called **alopecia** (al-oh-PEE-shah). The three most common types of abnormal hair loss are androgenic alopecia, alopecia areata, and postpartum alopecia.

Androgenic alopecia (an-druh-JEN-ik al-oh-PEE-shah), also known as **androgenetic alopecia** (an-druh-je-NETik al-oh-PEE-shah), is hair loss that is characterized by miniaturization of terminal hair that is converted into vellus hair. It is usually the result of genetics, age, or hormonal changes that cause terminal hair to miniaturize (**Figure 11–12**).

Androgenic alopecia can begin as early as the teens and is frequently seen by the age of 40. By age 35, almost 40 percent of both men and women show some degree of hair loss.

In men, androgenic alopecia is known as male pattern baldness and usually progresses to the familiar horseshoe-shaped fringe of hair. In women it shows up as generalized thinning over the entire crown area. Androgenic alopecia affects millions of men and women in the United States.

Alopecia areata (al-oh-PEE-shah air-ee-AH-tah) is an autoimmune disorder that causes the affected hair follicles to be mistakenly attacked by a person's own immune system. White blood cells stop the hair growth during the anagen phase. It is a highly unpredictable skin disease that affects an estimated 5 million people in the United States alone. This hair disorder usually begins with one or more small, round, smooth bald patches on the scalp and can progress to total scalp hair loss, known as **alopecia totalis** (al-oh-PEE-shah toh-TAHL-us), or complete body hair loss, called **alopecia universalis** (al-oh-PEE-shah yoo-nih-vur-SAA-lis).

Alopecia areata occurs in males and females of all ages, races, and ethnic backgrounds and most often begins in childhood. The scalp usually shows no obvious signs of inflammation, skin disorder, or disease (Figure 11–13).

Postpartum alopecia (POHST-pahr-tum al-oh-PEE-shah) is temporary hair loss experienced at the end of a pregnancy. For some women, pregnancy seems to disrupt the normal growth cycle of hair. There is very little normal hair loss during pregnancy, but then there is sudden and excessive shedding from three to nine months after delivery. Although this is usually very traumatic to the new mother, the growth cycle generally returns to normal within one year after the baby is delivered. ☑ LO5

FYI

The mission of the National Alopecia Areata Foundation (NAAF) is to support research to find a cure or acceptable treatment for alopecia areata, to support those with the disease, and to educate the public.

The NAAF can be contacted at 14 Mitchell Boulevard, San Rafael, CA 94903, telephone: (415) 472-3780, fax: (415) 472-5343, e-mail: info@NAAF.org, or on the Web at http://www.alopeciaareata.com.

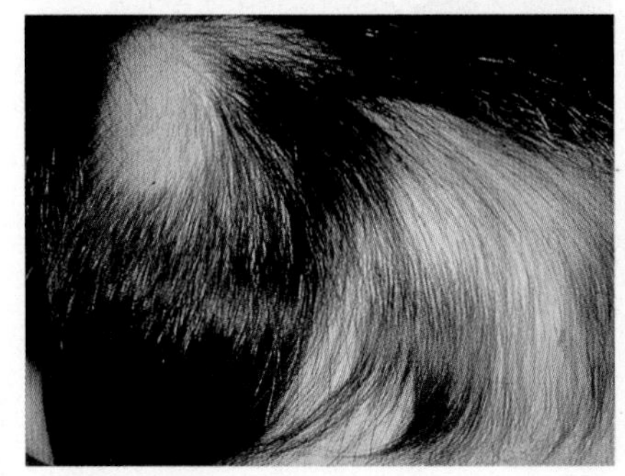

Courtesy of Robert A. Silverman, MD, Clinical Associate Professor, Department of Pediatrics, Georgetown University.

▲ Figure 11–13
Alopecia areata.

Hair Loss Treatments

Of all treatments that are said to counter hair loss, there are only two products—Minoxidil and finasteride—that have been proven to stimulate hair growth and are approved by the FDA for sale in the United States.

Minoxidil is a topical (applied to the surface of the body) medication that is put on the scalp twice a day and has been proven to stimulate hair growth. It is sold over the counter (OTC) as a nonprescription drug. Minoxidil is available for both men and women and comes in two different strengths: 2 percent regular-strength solution and 5 percent extra-strength solution. It is not known to have any serious negative side effects. The most well-known Minoxidil product on the market is Rogaine®.

Finasteride is an oral prescription medication for men only. Although finasteride is more effective and convenient than Minoxidil, possible side effects include weight gain and loss of sexual function. Women may not use this treatment, and pregnant women or those who might become pregnant are

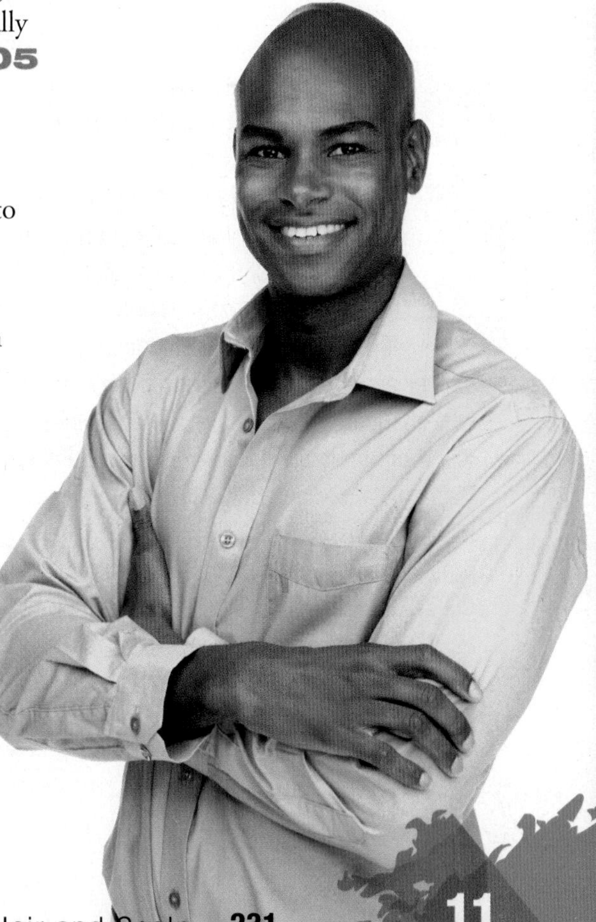

© Yuri Arcurs, 2010; used under license from Shutterstock.com.

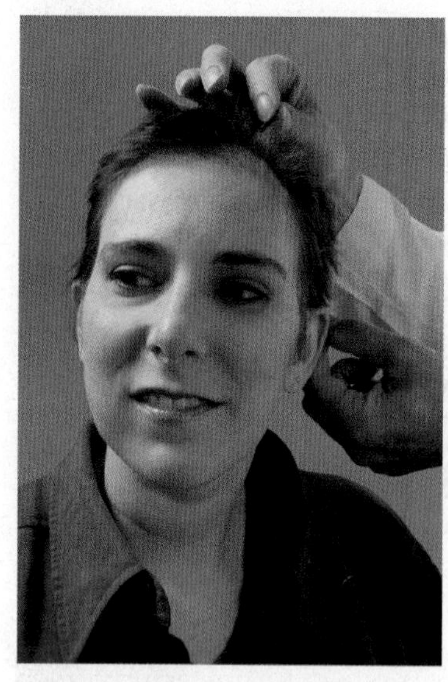

© Nancy Louie, 2010; used under license from iStockphoto.com.

cautioned not to even touch finasteride tablets because of the strong potential for birth defects.

In addition to the treatments described above, there are also several surgical options available to treat alopecia. A hair transplant is the most common permanent hair replacement technique. This process consists of removing small sections of hair, including the follicle, papilla, and hair bulb, from an area where there is a lot of hair (usually in the back) and transplanting them into the bald area. These sections grow normally in the new location. Only licensed surgeons may perform this procedure, and several surgeries are usually necessary to achieve the desired results. The cost of each surgery can range from $8,000 to over $20,000.

Hairstylists can offer a number of nonmedical options to counter hair loss. Some salons specialize in nonsurgical hair replacement systems such as wigs, toupees, hair weavings, and hair extensions. With proper training, you can learn to fit, color, cut, and style wigs and toupees. Hair weavings and hair extensions allow you to enhance a client's natural hair and create a look that boosts self-esteem. (See Chapter 19, Wigs and Hair Additions.) ☑ **LO6**

Disorders of the Hair

The following disorders of the hair range from those that are commonplace and not particularly troublesome to those that are far more unusual or distressing:

- **Canities** (kah-NIT-eez) is the technical term for gray hair. Canities results from the loss of the hair's natural melanin pigment. Other than the absence of pigment, gray hair is exactly the same as pigmented hair. The two types of canities are congenital and acquired.

  Congenital canities exists at or before birth. It occurs in albinos, who are born without pigment in the skin, hair, and eyes, and occasionally in individuals with normal hair. A patchy type of congenital canities may develop either slowly or rapidly, depending on the cause of the condition.

  Acquired canities develops with age and is the result of genetics. Although genetics is also responsible for premature canities, acquired canities may develop due to prolonged anxiety or illness.

- **Ringed hair** is a variety of canities, characterized by alternating bands of gray and pigmented hair throughout the length of the hair strand.

- **Hypertrichosis** (hi-pur-trih-KOH-sis), also known as **hirsuties** (hur-SOO-shee-eez), is a condition of abnormal growth of hair. It is characterized by the growth of terminal

FYI

An unwanted side effect of chemotherapy or radiation cancer treatments is abnormal hair loss. Look Good . . . Feel Better® (LGFB) is a free, global public service program founded in 1989 that is available in 19 countries on six continents. It teaches beauty techniques to cancer patients, helping them to boost their self-image and camouflage their hair loss. The program is open to women, men, and teenage cancer patients. More than one million women have been served by the organization since it was founded. Contact the LGFB program at 800-395-LOOK (800-395-5665), twenty-four hours a day, seven days a week, or through the Web at http://www.lookgoodfeelbetter.org.

hair in areas of the body that normally grow only vellus hair. Mustaches or light beards on women are examples of hypertrichosis.

Treatments for hypertrichosis include electrolysis, photoepilation, laser hair removal, shaving, tweezing, electronic tweezers, depilatories, epilators, threading, and sugaring (see Chapter 22, Hair Removal).

Trichoptilosis (trih-kahp-tih-LOH-sus) is the technical term for split ends (**Figure 11–14**). Hair conditioning treatments will soften and lubricate dry ends but will not repair split ends. The only way to remove split ends is by cutting them.

Trichorrhexis nodosa (trik-uh-REK-sis nuh-DOH-suh) is the technical term for knotted hair (**Figure 11–15**). It is characterized by brittleness and the formation of nodular swellings along the hair shaft. The hair breaks easily, and the broken fibers spread out like a brush along the hair shaft. Treatments include softening the hair with conditioners and moisturizers.

Monilethrix (mah-NIL-ee-thriks) is the technical term for beaded hair (**Figure 11–16**). The hair breaks easily between the beads or nodes. Treatments include hair and scalp conditioning.

Fragilitas crinium (fruh-JIL-ih-tus KRI-nee-um) is the technical term for brittle hair. The hairs may split at any part of their length. Treatments include hair and scalp conditioning and haircutting above the split to prevent further damage.

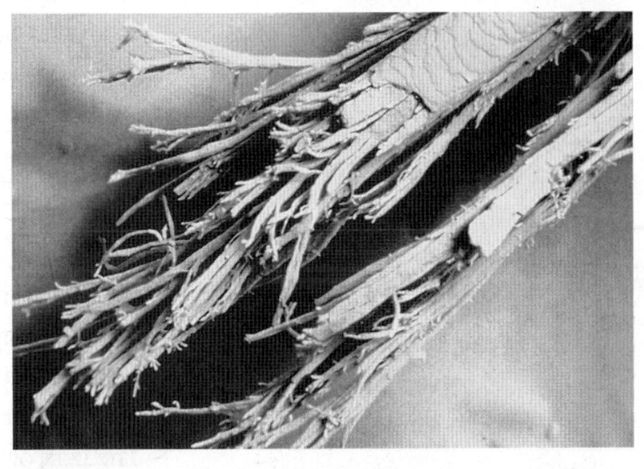

Courtesy of P&G Beauty from John Grey's, The World of Hair Care.

▲ **Figure 11–14**
Trichoptilosis.

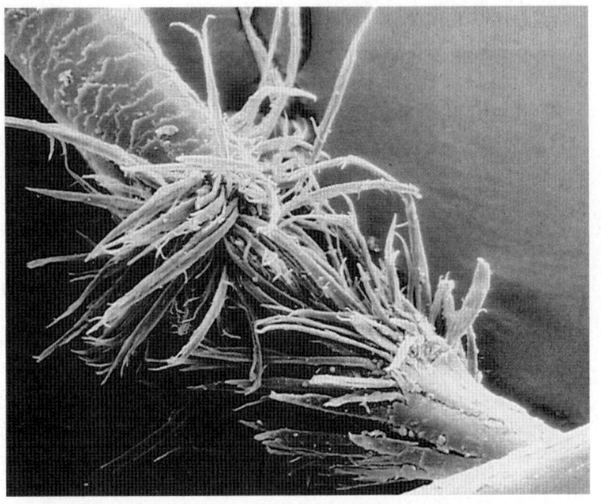

Courtesy of P&G Beauty from John Grey's, The World of Hair Care.

▲ **Figure 11–15**
Trichorrhexis nodosa.

Disorders of the Scalp

The skin is in a constant state of renewal. The outer layer of skin that covers your body is constantly being shed and replaced by new cells from below. The average person sheds about 9 pounds of dead skin each year. The skin cells of a normal, healthy scalp fall off naturally as small, dry flakes, without being noticed.

Dandruff can be easily mistaken for dry scalp because the symptoms of both conditions are a flaky, irritated scalp, but there is a difference. Dandruff commonly produces an oily scalp, but—just as the name indicates—the scalp is dry with the condition of dry scalp. The flakes from a dry scalp are much smaller and less noticeable than the larger flakes seen with dandruff. Dry scalp can result from contact dermatitis, sunburn, or extreme age, and is usually made worse by a cold, dry climate.

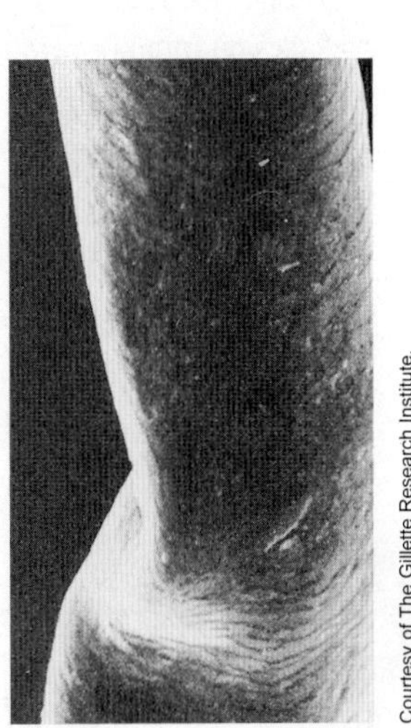

Courtesy of The Gillette Research Institute.

▲ **Figure 11–16**
Monilethrix.

CAUTION

You may find it difficult to speak with your client about a scalp disorder. After all, it is not easy to tell a client that you cannot perform a scheduled service because there may be something wrong with her scalp. If you feel that you cannot perform the service on your client and need help communicating with her about it, seek guidance from your instructor or salon manager.

If you encounter such a situation and feel you are ready to discuss the situation with your client, try this approach.

"Mrs. Smith, I noticed that your scalp looks different today. I am not licensed to diagnose any scalp disorders, but I am concerned and think you should see a physician about it as soon as possible. For your safety, I should not continue with the service you have scheduled."

Do not let your clients try to talk you into performing the service. It could put you, your other clients, and the salon at risk of spreading the scalp disorder.

Dandruff

Pityriasis (pit-ih-RY-uh-sus) is the technical term for dandruff, which is characterized by the excessive production and accumulation of skin cells. Instead of the normal, one-at-a-time shedding of tiny individual skin cells, dandruff is the shedding of an accumulation of large visible clumps of skin cells.

Although the cause of dandruff has been debated for over 150 years, current research confirms that dandruff is the result of a fungus called malassezia (mal-uh-SEEZ-ee-uh). **Malassezia** is a naturally occurring fungus that is present on all human skin but causes the symptoms of dandruff when it grows out of control. Some individuals are also more susceptible to malassezia's irritating effects. Factors such as stress, age, hormones, and poor hygiene can cause the fungus to multiply and dandruff symptoms to worsen.

Modern antidandruff shampoos contain the antifungal agents pyrithione zinc, selenium sulfide, or ketoconazole that control dandruff by suppressing the growth of malassezia. Antidandruff shampoos that contain pyrithione zinc are available in a variety of formulas for all hair types and are gentle enough to be used every day, even on color-treated hair. Frequent use of an antidandruff shampoo is essential for controlling dandruff. And although good personal hygiene and proper cleaning and disinfecting are important, dandruff is not contagious.

There are two principal types of dandruff:

- **Pityriasis capitis simplex** (pit-ih-RY-uh-sus KAP-ih-tis SIM-pleks) is the technical term for classic dandruff that is characterized by scalp irritation, large flakes, and an itchy scalp. The scales may attach to the scalp in masses, scatter loosely in the hair, or fall to the shoulders. Regular use of antidandruff shampoos, conditioners, and topical lotions are the best treatment.
- **Pityriasis steatoides** (pit-ih-RY-uh-sus stee-uh-TOY-deez) is a more severe case of dandruff characterized by an accumulation of greasy or waxy scales, mixed with sebum, that stick to the scalp in crusts. As explained in Chapter 8, Skin Disorders and Diseases, when this condition is accompanied by redness and inflammation, it is called seborrheic dermatitis. Seborrheic dermatitis also can be found in the eyebrows or beard.

You should not perform a service on anyone who has either of these conditions. A client with these conditions must be referred to a physician.

DANDRUFF Shampoo

© OlgaLIS, 2010; used under license from iStockphoto.com.

Fungal Infections (Tinea)

Tinea (TIN-ee-uh) is the technical term for ringworm. It is characterized by itching, scales, and, sometimes, painful circular lesions. Several patches may be present at one time. Tinea is caused by a fungal organism and not a parasite, as the old-fashioned term ringworm seems to suggest.

All forms of tinea are contagious and can be easily transmitted from one person to another. Infected skin scales or hairs that contain the fungi are known to spread the disease. Bathtubs, swimming pools, and uncleaned personal articles are also sources of transmission. Practicing approved cleaning and disinfection procedures will help prevent the spread of this disease in the salon.

As you read in Chapter 5, Infection Control: Principles and Practices, the most frequently encountered fungal infection resulting from hair services is tinea barbae, also known as barber's itch. It is similar to tinea capitis in appearance. You should not perform a service on anyone who has or who you suspect may have tinea barbae. A client with this condition must be referred to a physician for medical treatment.

Tinea capitis is another type of fungal infection characterized by red papules, or spots, at the opening of the hair follicles (**Figure 11–17**). The patches spread, and the hair becomes brittle. Hair often breaks off, leaving only a stump, or the hair may be shed from the enlarged open follicle.

Tinea favosa (TIN-ee-uh fah-VOH-suh), also known as **tinea favus** (TIN-ee-uh FAH-vus), is characterized by dry, sulfur-yellow, cup-like crusts on the scalp called **scutula** (SKUCH-ul-uh). Scutula has a distinctive odor. Scars from tinea favosa are bald patches that may be pink or white and shiny.

Remember: You should never perform a service on anyone who has or you suspect may have a fungal infection. If you are not certain about whether the condition is a fungal infection, be safe and refer your client to a physician.

Parasitic Infections

Scabies is a highly contagious skin disease caused by a parasite called a mite that burrows under the skin. Vesicles (blisters) and pustules (inflamed pimples with pus) usually form on the scalp from the irritation caused by this parasite. Excessive itching scratches the infected areas and makes the condition worse. Practicing approved cleaning and disinfection procedures is very important to prevent the spread of this disease.

You should not perform a service on anyone who has scabies. A client with this condition must be referred to a physician for medical treatment.

Pediculosis capitis (puh-dik-yuh-LOH-sis KAP-ih-tis) is the infestation of the hair and scalp with head lice (**Figures 11–18** and **11–19**).

did you know?

Tinea barbae (barber's itch) is the most frequently encountered infection resulting from hair services. It affects the coarse hairs in the mustache and beard area or hairs on the neck and scalp. It is usually seen on men.

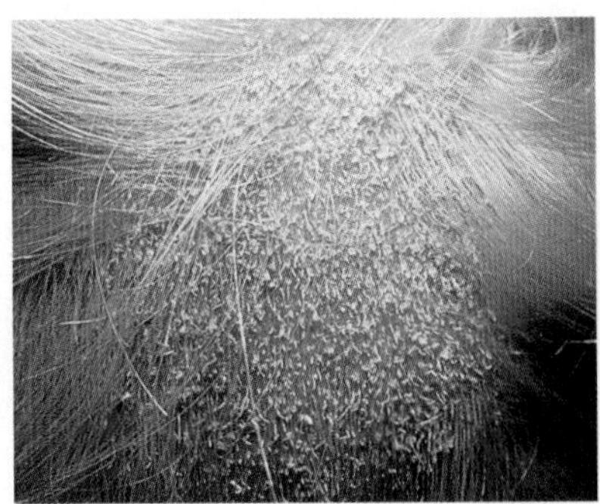

Courtesy of Robert A. Silverman, MD, Clinical Associate Professor, Department of Pediatrics, Georgetown University.

▲ Figure 11–17
Tinea capitis.

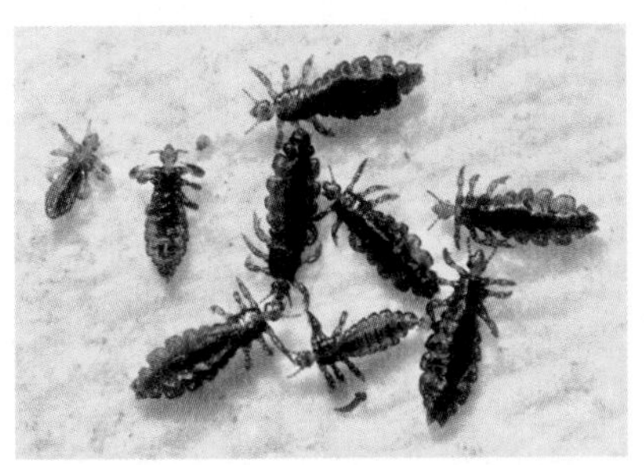

Courtesy of The National Pediculosis Association®, Inc.

▲ Figure 11–18
Head lice.

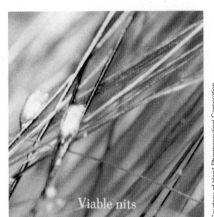

Courtesy of Hogil Pharmaceutical Corporation.

▲ Figure 11–19
Nits (lice eggs).

As these parasites feed on the scalp, it begins to itch. If the scalp is scratched, it can cause an infection. Head lice are transmitted from one person to another by contact with infested hats, combs, brushes, and other personal articles. You can distinguish head lice from dandruff flakes by looking closely at the scalp with a magnifying glass.

Properly practicing state board-approved cleaning and disinfection procedures will prevent the spread of this infestation. Several nonprescription medications are available.

You should not perform a service on anyone who has head lice. A client with this condition must be referred to a physician or a pharmacist.

Staphylococci Infections

Staphylococci are bacteria that infect the skin or scalp. The two most common types of staphylococci infections are furuncles and carbuncles.

- A **furuncle** (FYOO-rung-kul) is the technical term for a boil, an acute, localized bacterial infection of the hair follicle that produces constant pain (**Figure 11–20**). It is limited to a specific area and produces a pustule perforated by a hair.
- A **carbuncle** (KAHR-bung-kul) is an inflammation of the subcutaneous tissue caused by staphylococci. It is similar to a furuncle but is larger.

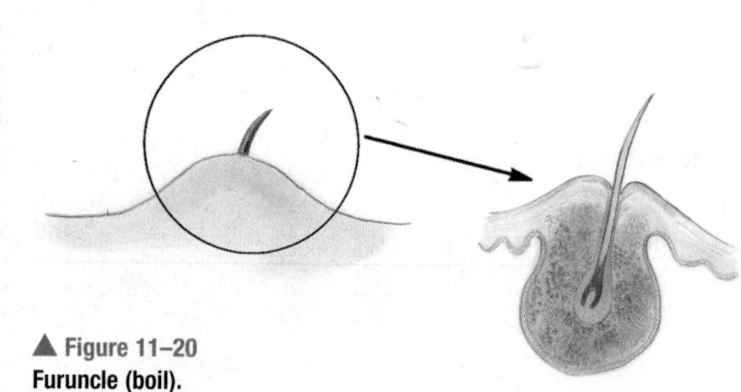

© Milady, a part of Cengage Learning.

▲ **Figure 11–20**
Furuncle (boil).

Properly practicing state board-approved cleaning and disinfection procedures will prevent the spread of these infections.

You should not perform a service on anyone who has a boil or a carbuncle. A client with either condition must be referred to a physician for medical treatment. ☑ **LO7**

Hair and Scalp Analysis

All successful salon services must begin with a thorough analysis of the condition of the client's scalp and client's hair type. Knowing the client's scalp condition and the client's hair type allows you to prepare and make decisions about the results that can be expected from the service.

Because different types of hair react differently to the same service, it is essential that a thorough analysis be performed before all salon services. Hair analysis is performed by observation using the senses of sight, touch, hearing, and smell. The four most important factors to consider in hair analysis are texture, density, porosity, and elasticity. Other factors that you should also be aware of are growth pattern and dryness versus oiliness.

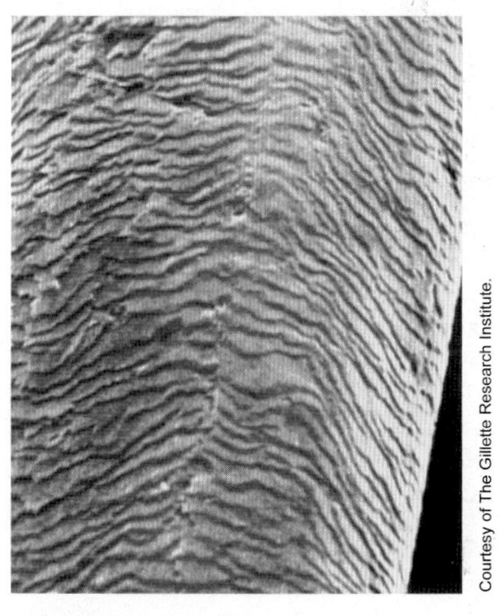
Courtesy of The Gillette Research Institute.

▲ Figure 11–21
Coarse hair.

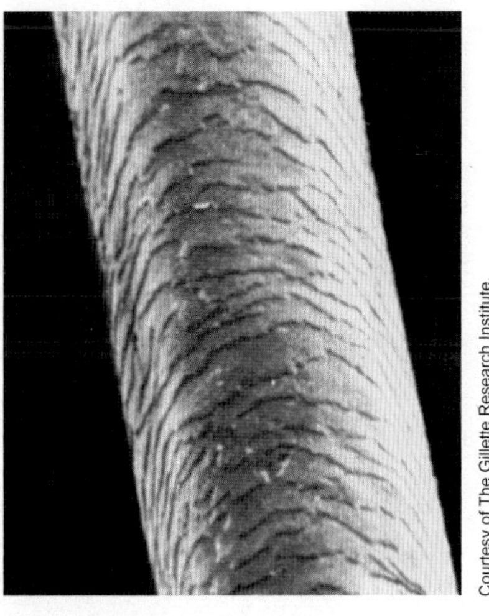
Courtesy of The Gillette Research Institute.

▲ Figure 11–22
Medium hair.

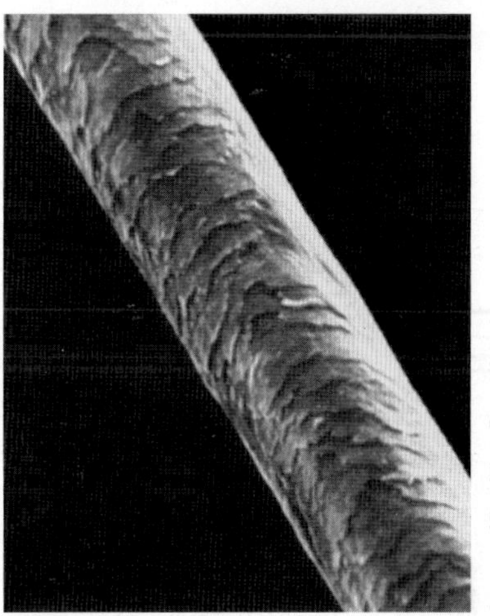
Courtesy of The Gillette Research Institute.

▲ Figure 11–23
Fine hair.

Texture

Hair texture is the thickness or diameter of the individual hair strand. Hair texture can be classified as coarse, medium, or fine (**Figures 11–21, 11–22, and 11–23**) and can vary from strand to strand on the same person's head. It is not uncommon for hair from different areas of the head to have different textures. Hair on the nape (back of the neck), crown, temples, and front hairline of the same person may have different textures.

Coarse hair texture has the largest diameter. It is stronger than fine hair, for the same reason that a thick rope is stronger than a thin rope. It is often more resistant to processing than medium or fine hair, so it usually requires more processing when you are applying products such as hair lighteners, haircolors, permanent waving solutions, and chemical hair relaxers.

Medium hair texture is the most common texture and is the standard to which other hair is compared. Medium hair does not pose any special problems or concerns.

Fine hair has the smallest diameter and is more fragile, easier to process, and more susceptible to damage from chemical services than coarse or medium hair.

As with hair cuticle analysis, hair texture can be determined by feeling a single dry strand between the fingers. Take an individual strand from four different areas of the head—front hairline, temple, crown, and nape—and hold each strand securely with one hand while feeling it with the thumb and forefinger of the other hand. With a little practice, you will be able to feel the difference between coarse, medium, and fine hair diameters (**Figure 11–24**).

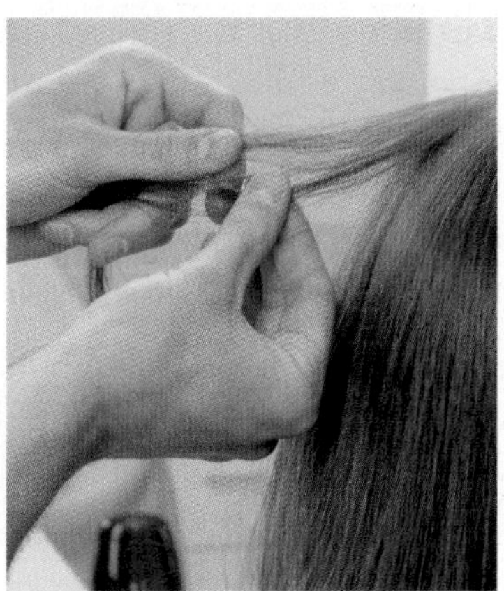
© Milady a part of Cengage Learning. Photography by Paul Castle, Castle Photography.

▲ Figure 11–24
Testing for hair texture.

FOCUS ON

RETAILING

Selling retail products increases client retention. A client who takes home a retail product is more than twice as likely to return for services. Recommending products for home use is an important part of a successful career as a hairstylist. Your client needs to know what products to use and how to use them.

A complete hair analysis will enable you to recommend the right products for your client with confidence. It is your job to know more about your client's specific needs than anyone else and to recommend the right products to satisfy those needs. Your clients consider you to be their expert in hair care, so do not be shy about analyzing their needs and making recommendations to them, since they genuinely benefit from your advice.

HAIR COLOR	AVERAGE NUMBER OF HAIRS ON HEAD
BLOND	140,000
BROWN	110,000
BLACK	108,000
RED	80,000

© Milady, a part of Cengage Learning.

Table 11–4 **Average Number of Hairs on the Head by Hair Color.**

Density

Hair density measures the number of individual hair strands on 1 square inch (2.5 square centimeters) of scalp. It indicates how many hairs there are on a person's head. Hair density can be classified as low, medium, or high (also known as thin, medium, or thick/dense). Hair density is different from hair texture—individuals with the same hair texture can have different densities.

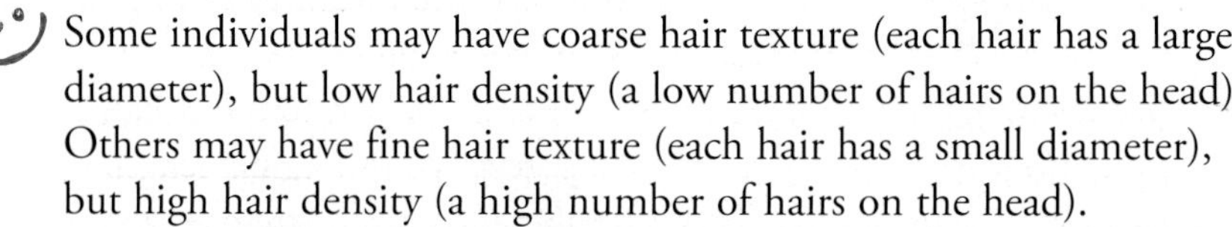

Some individuals may have coarse hair texture (each hair has a large diameter), but low hair density (a low number of hairs on the head). Others may have fine hair texture (each hair has a small diameter), but high hair density (a high number of hairs on the head).

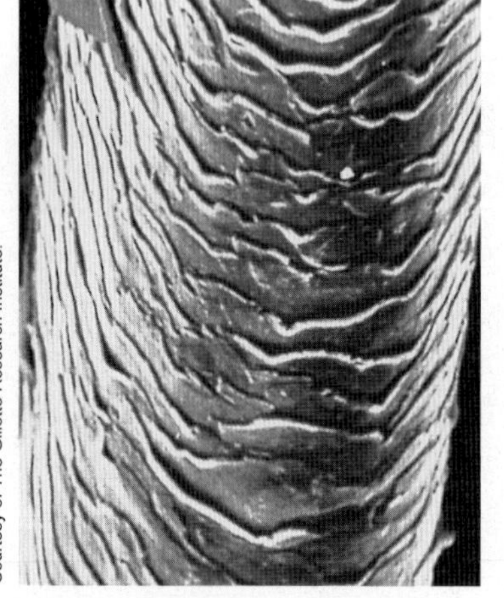

Courtesy of The Gillette Research Institute.

▲ Figure 11–25
Low porosity (resistant hair).

The average hair density is about 2,200 hairs per 1 square inch. Hair with high density (thick or dense hair) has more hairs per 1 square inch, and hair with low density (thin hair) has fewer hairs per 1 square inch. The average head of hair contains about 100,000 individual hair strands. The number of hairs on the head generally varies with the color of the hair. Blonds usually have the highest density, and people with red hair tend to have the lowest. **Table 11–4** shows hair density by hair color.

Porosity

Hair porosity is the ability of the hair to absorb moisture. The degree of porosity is directly related to the condition of the cuticle layer. Healthy hair with a compact cuticle layer is naturally resistant to being penetrated by moisture and is referred to as **hydrophobic** (hy-druh-FOHB-ik). Porous hair has a raised cuticle layer that easily absorbs moisture and is called **hydrophilic** (hy-druh-FIL-ik).

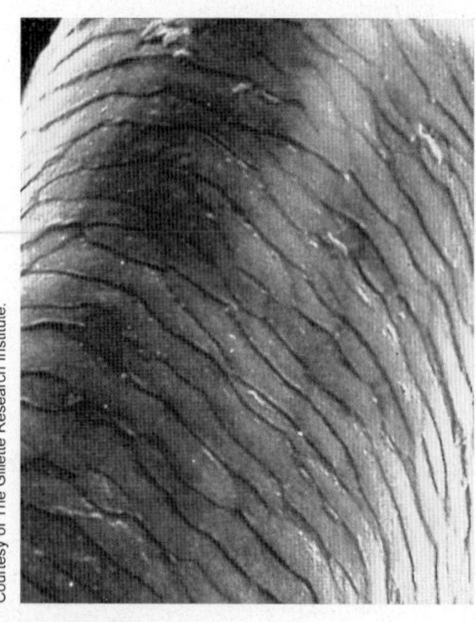

Courtesy of The Gillette Research Institute.

▲ Figure 11–26
Average porosity (normal hair).

Hair with low porosity is considered resistant (**Figure 11–25**). Chemical services performed on hair with low porosity require a more alkaline solution than those on hair with high porosity. Alkaline solutions raise the cuticle and permit uniform saturation and processing on resistant hair.

Hair with average porosity is considered to be normal hair (**Figure 11–26**). Chemical services performed on this type of hair will usually process as expected, according to the texture.

Hair with high porosity is considered overly porous hair and is often the result of previous overprocessing (**Figure 11–27**). Overly porous hair is damaged, dry, fragile, and brittle. Chemical services performed on overly porous hair require less alkaline solutions with a lower pH, which help prevent additional overprocessing and damage.

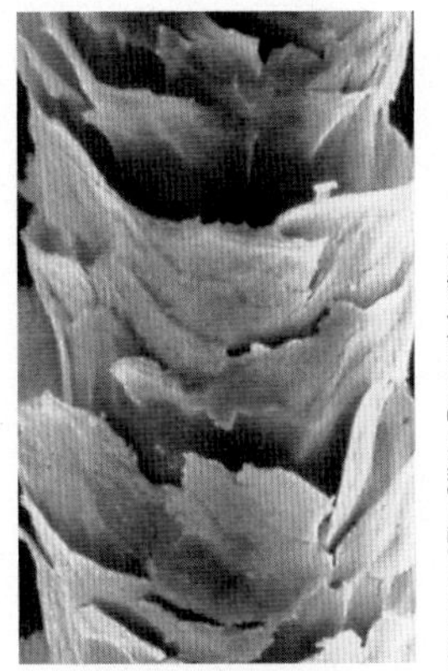
Courtesy of The Gillette Research Institute.

▲ Figure 11–27
High porosity (overly porous hair).

The texture of the hair can be an indication of its porosity, but it is only a general rule of thumb. Different degrees of porosity can be found in all hair textures. Although coarse hair normally has a low porosity and is resistant to chemical services, in some cases coarse hair will have high porosity, perhaps as the result of previous chemical services.

You can check porosity on dry hair by taking a strand of several hairs from four different areas of the head (front hairline, temple, crown, and nape). Hold the strand securely with one hand while sliding the thumb and forefinger of the other hand from the end to the scalp. If the hair feels smooth and the cuticle is compact, dense, and hard, it is considered resistant. If you can feel a slight roughness, it is considered porous. If the hair feels very rough, dry, or breaks, it is considered highly porous and may have been overprocessed (**Figure 11–28**).

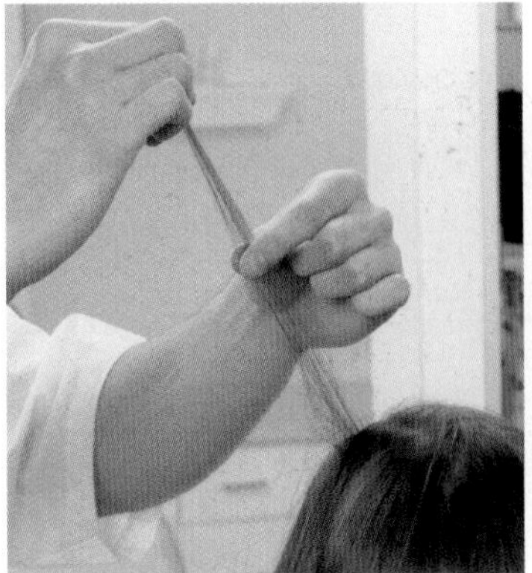
© Milady a part of Cengage Learning. Photography by Paul Castle, Castle Photography.

▲ Figure 11–28
Testing for hair porosity.

Elasticity

Hair elasticity is the ability of the hair to stretch and return to its original length without breaking. Hair elasticity is an indication of the strength of the side bonds that hold the hair's individual fibers in place. Wet hair with normal elasticity will stretch up to 50 percent of its original length and return to that same length without breaking. Dry hair stretches about 20 percent of its length.

Hair with low elasticity is brittle and breaks easily. It may not be able to hold the curl from wet setting, thermal styling, or permanent waving. Hair with low elasticity is the result of weak side bonds that usually are a result of overprocessing. Chemical services performed on hair with low elasticity require a milder solution with a lower pH to minimize further damage and prevent additional overprocessing.

Check elasticity on wet hair by taking an individual strand from four different areas of the head (front hairline, temple, crown, and nape). Hold a single strand of wet hair securely and try to pull it apart (**Figure 11–29**). If the hair stretches and returns to its original length without breaking, it has normal elasticity. If the hair breaks easily or fails to return to its original length, it has low elasticity.

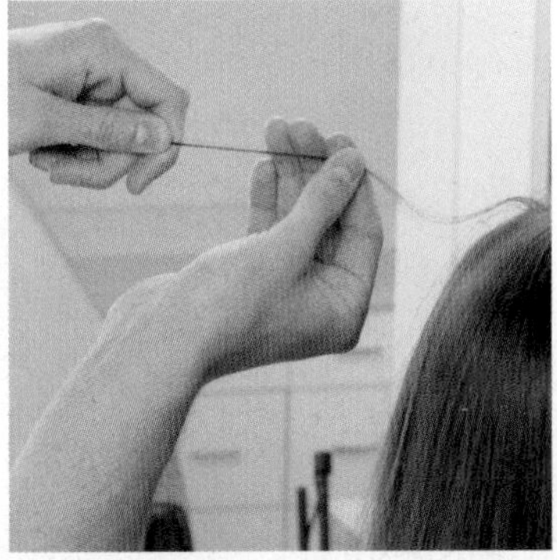
© Milady a part of Cengage Learning. Photography by Paul Castle, Castle Photography.

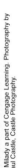

▲ Figure 11–29
Testing for hair elasticity.

ACTivity

Divide into groups of two or more in the classroom and analyze each other's hair. Hair analysis includes evaluating texture, density, porosity, and elasticity. Wave patterns, growth patterns, and the oiliness or dryness of the hair and scalp also should be noted. Follow the procedures in this textbook and use the same terminology. Write down results and present an oral report to the class. What is the most common texture among your classmates? What is the most common density?

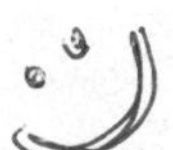

Hair Growth Patterns

As mentioned earlier in the chapter, hair growth patterns are important to identify and consider, especially when preparing to shape and style the hair. During your hair analysis, you should identify any and all hair growth patterns and take them into consideration when creating the overall look, haircut or hairstyle the client wants to achieve.

Hair follicles that grow out of the head at a perpendicular, 90-degree angle or in a straight direction from the head may cause the following growth patterns to result:

- A **hair stream** is hair flowing in the same direction, resulting from follicles sloping in the same direction. Two streams flowing in opposite directions from the head form a natural part in the hair.
- A **whorl** (WHORL) is hair that forms in a circular pattern, as on the crown of the head. A whorl normally forms in the crown with all the hair from that point growing down.
- A **cowlick** (KOW-lik) is a tuft of hair that stands straight up. Cowlicks are usually more noticeable at the front hairline but they may be located anywhere on the head.

Dry Hair and Scalp

Dry hair and scalp can be caused by inactive sebaceous glands. These conditions are aggravated by excessive shampooing or by a dry climate. The lack of natural oils (sebum) leads to hair that appears dull, dry, and lifeless. Dry hair and scalp should be treated with products that contain moisturizers and emollients.

People with dry hair and scalp should avoid frequent shampooing, along with the use of strong soaps, detergents, or products with a high alcohol content because these products could aggravate existing conditions. Dry hair should not be confused with overly porous hair that has been damaged by thermal styling, chemical services, or environmental conditions.

Oily Hair and Scalp

Oily hair and scalp, characterized by a greasy buildup on the scalp and an oily coating on the hair, are caused by improper shampooing or overactive sebaceous glands. Oily hair and scalp can be treated by properly washing with a normalizing shampoo. A well-balanced diet, exercise, regular shampooing, and good personal hygiene are essential to controlling oily hair and scalp. ☑ LO8

Healthy Hair, Happy Clients

The more you learn about the structure of hair and how to keep it healthy, the more you will understand how salon services affect different hair types. This is the key to consistent results with your services and happy clients who recommend you to their friends.

© Veronika Vasilyuk, 2010; under license fusedrom iStockphoto.com.

Review Questions

1. Name and describe the five main structures of the hair root.
2. Name and describe the three layers of the hair shaft.
3. Explain the process of keratinization.
4. What are polypeptide chains?
5. List and describe the three types of side bonds. Indicate whether they are strong or weak and why.
6. Name and describe the two types of melanin responsible for natural hair color.
7. Name and describe the two types of hair and their locations on the body.
8. What are the three phases of the hair growth cycle? What occurs during each phase?
9. What is the reason for normal daily hair loss?
10. What are the most common types of abnormal hair loss?
11. What are the only two hair loss treatments approved by the FDA?
12. Name the two main types of dandruff. Can either one be treated in the salon?
13. Which hair and scalp disorders cannot be treated in the salon?
14. What four factors about the hair should be considered in a hair analysis?

Chapter Glossary

alopecia	Abnormal hair loss.
alopecia areata	Autoimmune disorder that causes the affected hair follicles to be mistakenly attacked by a person's own immune system; usually begins with one or more small, round, smooth bald patches on the scalp.
alopecia totalis	Total loss of scalp hair.
alopecia universalis	Complete loss of body hair.
amino acids	Units that are joined together end to end like pop beads by strong, chemical peptide bonds (end bonds) to form the polypeptide chains that comprise proteins.
anagen phase	Also known as *growth phase*; phase during which new hair is produced.
androgenic alopecia	Also known as *androgenetic alopecia*; hair loss characterized by miniaturization of terminal hair that is converted to vellus hair; in men, it is known as male pattern baldness.
canities	Technical term for gray hair; results from the loss of the hair's natural melanin pigment.
carbuncle	Inflammation of the subcutaneous tissue caused by staphylococci; similar to a furuncle but larger.
catagen phase	The brief transition period between the growth and resting phases of a hair follicle. It signals the end of the growth phase.
COHNS elements	The five elements—carbon, oxygen, hydrogen, nitrogen, and sulfur—that make up human hair, skin, tissue, and nails.
cortex	Middle layer of the hair; a fibrous protein core formed by elongated cells containing melanin pigment.

Chapter Glossary

cowlick	Tuft of hair that stands straight up.
cysteine	An amino acid joined with another cysteine amino acid to create cystine amino acid.
cystine	An amino acid that joins together two peptide strands.
disulfide bond	Strong chemical side bond that joins the sulfur atoms of two neighboring cysteine amino acids to create one cystine, which joins together two polypeptide strands like rungs on a ladder.
fragilitas crinium	Technical term for brittle hair.
furuncle	Boil; acute, localized bacterial infection of the hair follicle that produces constant pain.
hair bulb	Lowest part of a hair strand; the thickened, club-shaped structure that forms the lower part of the hair root.
hair cuticle	Outermost layer of hair; consisting of a single, overlapping layer of transparent, scale-like cells that look like shingles on a roof.
hair density	The number of individual hair strands on 1 square inch (2.5 square centimeters) of scalp.
hair elasticity	Ability of the hair to stretch and return to its original length without breaking.
hair follicle	The tube-like depression or pocket in the skin or scalp that contains the hair root.
hair porosity	Ability of the hair to absorb moisture.
hair root	The part of the hair located below the surface of the epidermis.
hair shaft	The portion of hair that projects above the epidermis.
hair stream	Hair flowing in the same direction, resulting from follicles sloping in the same direction.
hair texture	Thickness or diameter of the individual hair strand.
helix	Spiral shape of a coiled protein created by polypeptide chains that intertwine with each other.
hydrogen bond	A weak, physical, cross-link side bond that is easily broken by water or heat.
hydrophilic	Easily absorbs moisture; in chemistry terms, capable of combining with or attracting water (water-loving).
hydrophobic	Naturally resistant to being penetrated by moisture.
hypertrichosis	Also known as *hirsuties*; condition of abnormal growth of hair, characterized by the growth of terminal hair in areas of the body that normally grow only vellus hair.
keratinization	Process by which newly formed cells in the hair bulb mature, fill with keratin, move upward, lose their nucleus, and die.
lanthionine bonds	The bonds created when disulfide bonds are broken by hydroxide chemical hair relaxers after the relaxer is rinsed from the hair.
malassezia	Naturally occurring fungus that is present on all human skin, but is responsible for dandruff when it grows out of control.

Chapter Glossary

medulla	Innermost layer of the hair that is composed of round cells; often absent in fine and naturally blond hair.
monilethrix	Technical term for beaded hair.
pediculosis capitis	Infestation of the hair and scalp with head lice.
peptide bond	Also known as an *end bond*; chemical bond that joins amino acids to each other, end to end, to form a polypeptide chain.
pityriasis	Technical term for dandruff; characterized by excessive production and accumulation of skin cells.
pityriasis capitis simplex	Technical term for classic dandruff; characterized by scalp irritation, large flakes, and itchy scalp.
pityriasis steatoides	Severe case of dandruff characterized by an accumulation of greasy or waxy scales mixed with sebum, that stick to the scalp in crusts.
polypeptide chain	A long chain of amino acids linked by peptide bonds.
postpartum alopecia	Temporary hair loss experienced at the conclusion of a pregnancy.
proteins	Long, coiled complex polypeptides made of amino acids.
ringed hair	Variety of canities characterized by alternating bands of gray and pigmented hair throughout the length of the hair strand.
salt bond	A weak, physical, cross-link side bond between adjacent polypeptide chains.
scutula	Dry, sulfur-yellow, cup-like crusts on the scalp in tinea favosa or tinea favus.
side bonds	Bonds that cross-link the polypeptide chains together and are responsible for the extreme strength and elasticity of human hair.
telogen phase	Also known as *resting phase*; the final phase in the hair cycle that lasts until the fully grown hair is shed.
terminal hair	Long, coarse, pigmented hair found on the scalp, legs, arms, and bodies of males and females.
tinea	Technical term for ringworm, a contagious condition caused by fungal infection and not a parasite; characterized by itching, scales, and, sometimes, painful lesions.
tinea favosa	Also known as *tinea favus*; fungal infection characterized by dry, sulfur-yellow, cup-like crusts on the scalp called scutula.
trichology	Scientific study of hair and its diseases and care.
trichoptilosis	Technical term for split ends.
trichorrhexis nodosa	Technical term for knotted hair; it is characterized by brittleness and the formation of nodular swellings along the hair shaft.
vellus hair	Also known as *lanugo hair*; short, fine, unpigmented downy hair that appears on the body, with the exception of the palms of the hands and the soles of the feet.
wave pattern	The shape of the hair strands; described as straight, wavy, curly, and extremely curly.
whorl	Hair that forms in a circular pattern on the crown of the head.

CHAPTER 12

Basics of Chemistry

Chapter Outline

Why Study Chemistry?

Chemistry

Matter

Potential Hydrogen (pH)

© Vladimir, 2010; used under license from iStockphoto.com.

Learning Objectives

After completing this chapter, you will be able to:

- ✓ **LO1** Explain the difference between organic and inorganic chemistry.
- ✓ **LO2** Describe the different states of matter: solid, liquid, and gas.
- ✓ **LO3** Describe oxidation-reduction (redox) reactions.
- ✓ **LO4** Explain the differences between pure substances and physical mixtures.
- ✓ **LO5** Explain the difference among solutions, suspensions, and emulsions.
- ✓ **LO6** Explain pH and the pH scale.

Key Terms

Page number indicates where in the chapter the term is used.

acidic solution
pg. 257

alkaline solution
pg. 257

alkalis (bases)
pg. 257

alkanolamines
pg. 255

alpha hydroxy acids (AHAs)
pg. 257

ammonia
pg. 255

anion
pg. 256

atoms
pg. 247

cation
pg. 256

chemical change
pg. 250

chemical properties
pg. 249

chemistry
pg. 246

combustion
pg. 250

compound molecules (compounds)
pg. 248

element
pg. 247

elemental molecule
pg. 248

emulsifier
pg. 253

emulsion
pg. 253

exothermic reactions
pg. 250

glycerin
pg. 255

immiscible
pg. 252

inorganic chemistry
pg. 246

ion
pg. 256

ionization
pg. 256

lipophilic
pg. 254

logarithm
pg. 257

matter
pg. 247

miscible
pg. 252

molecule
pg. 247

oil-in-water (O/W) emulsion
pg. 254

organic chemistry
pg. 246

oxidation
pg. 250

oxidation-reduction (redox)
pg. 250

oxidizing agent
pg. 250

pH
pg. 256

pH scale
pg. 257

physical change
pg. 249

physical mixture
pg. 251

physical properties
pg. 249

pure substance
pg. 251

reducing agent
pg. 250

reduction
pg. 250

reduction reaction
pg. 250

silicones
pg. 255

solute
pg. 252

solution
pg. 252

solvent
pg. 252

states of matter
pg. 248

surfactants
pg. 254

suspensions
pg. 252

thioglycolic acid
pg. 257

volatile alcohols
pg. 255

volatile organic compounds (VOCs)
pg. 256

water-in-oil (W/O) emulsion
pg. 254

What do you think about when someone mentions the word *chemistry*? Beakers of mixtures bubbling in a lab? Test tubes filled with strange-looking liquids? Petrie dishes growing fuzzy things? Most cosmetology services depend on the use of chemicals. So, studying the basics of chemistry means that you will have the knowledge you need to understand the products that you are using in the salon to give your clients the professional services they deserve.

Why Study Chemistry?

Cosmetologists should study and have a thorough understanding of chemistry because:

- Without an understanding of basic chemistry you would not be able to use professional products effectively and safely.
- Every product used in the salon and in cosmetology services contains some type of chemical.
- With an understanding of chemistry, you will be able to troubleshoot and solve common problems you may encounter with chemical services.

© Melinda Fawver, 2010; used under license from Shutterstock.com.

Chemistry

Chemistry is the science that deals with the composition, structures, and properties of matter and how matter changes under different conditions.

Organic chemistry is the study of substances that contain the element carbon. All living things or things that were once alive, whether they are plants or animals, contain carbon. Organic substances that contain both carbon and hydrogen can burn. Although the term *organic* is often used to mean safe or natural because of its association with living things, such as foods or food ingredients, not all organic substances are natural, healthy, or safe.

You may be surprised to learn that poison ivy, gasoline, motor oil, plastics, synthetic fabrics, pesticides, and fertilizers are all organic substances. All haircolor products, chemical texturizers, shampoos, conditioners, styling aids, nail enhancements, and skin care products are organic chemicals. So remember, the word *organic*, as applied to chemistry, does not mean natural or healthy; it means that the material contains both carbon and hydrogen from either natural or synthetic sources.

Inorganic chemistry is the study of substances that do not contain the element carbon, but may contain the element hydrogen. Most inorganic substances do not burn because they do not contain carbon. Inorganic substances are not, and never were, alive. Metals, minerals, glass, water, and air are inorganic substances. Pure water and oxygen are inorganic, yet they are essential to life. Hydrogen peroxide, hydroxide hair relaxers, and

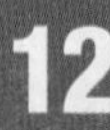

© Luchschen, 2010, used under license from Shutterstock.com.

titanium dioxide (a white pigment used to make white enhancement polymer powders and nail polish) are examples of inorganic substances. ☑ **LO1**

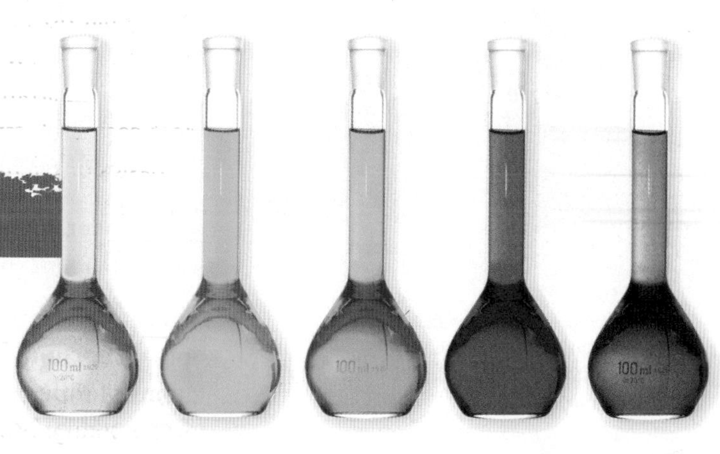

Matter

Matter is any substance that occupies space and has mass (weight). All matter has physical and chemical properties and exists in the form of a solid, liquid, or gas. Since matter is made from chemicals, everything made out of matter is a chemical.

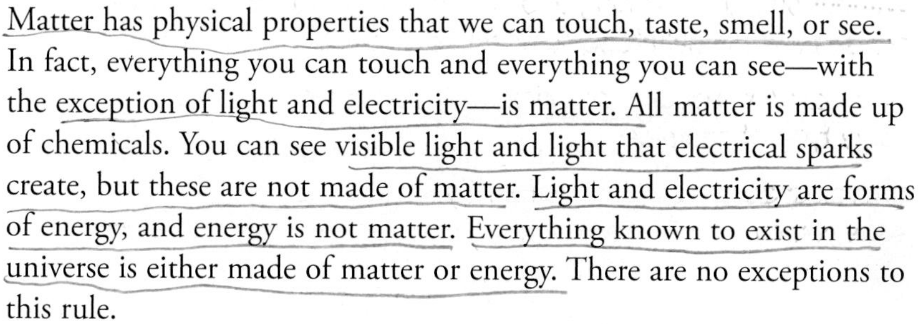

Matter has physical properties that we can touch, taste, smell, or see. In fact, everything you can touch and everything you can see—with the exception of light and electricity—is matter. All matter is made up of chemicals. You can see visible light and light that electrical sparks create, but these are not made of matter. Light and electricity are forms of energy, and energy is not matter. Everything known to exist in the universe is either made of matter or energy. There are no exceptions to this rule.

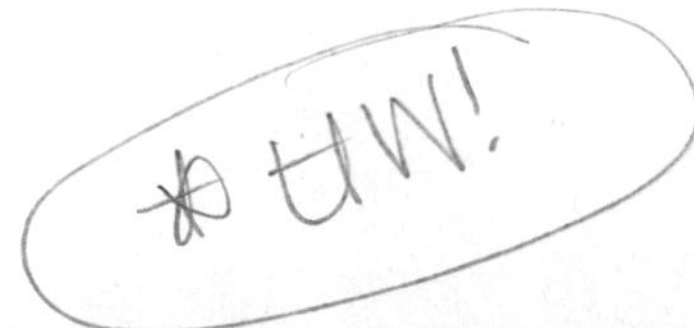

Energy does not occupy space or have mass (weight). Energy is discussed in Chapter 13, Basics of Electricity. This chapter is dedicated to matter.

Elements

An **element** is the simplest form of chemical matter. It cannot be broken down into a simpler substance without a loss of identity. There are 90 naturally occurring elements, each with its own distinct physical and chemical properties. All matter in the universe is made up of these 90 different chemical elements. Each element is identified by a letter symbol, such as *O* for oxygen, *C* for carbon, *H* for hydrogen, *N* for nitrogen, and *S* for sulfur. Symbols for all elements can be found in the Periodic Table of Elements in chemistry textbooks or by searching the Internet.

Atoms

Atoms are the smallest chemical components (often called particles) of an element. They are the structures that make up an element and have the same properties of the element. Elements are different from one another because the structure of their atoms is different. Atoms cannot be divided into simpler substances by ordinary chemical means.

Molecules

Just as words are made by combining letters, molecules are made by combining atoms. A **molecule** (MAHL-uuh-kyool) is a chemical combination of two or more atoms in definite (fixed) proportions. For example, water is made from hydrogen atoms and oxygen atoms. Carbon dioxide is made from carbon atoms and oxygen atoms.

did you know?

Using the word *chemical* to describe something does not mean it is dangerous or harmful. Water and air are 100 percent chemicals. Even your body is completely composed of chemicals.

The vast majority of chemicals you come in contact with every day are safe and harmless. When chemicals do have the potential to cause harm, manufacturers are required to describe that potential harm on the packaging or label. There is no such thing as a chemical-free product, so do not be fooled by misleading marketing claims.

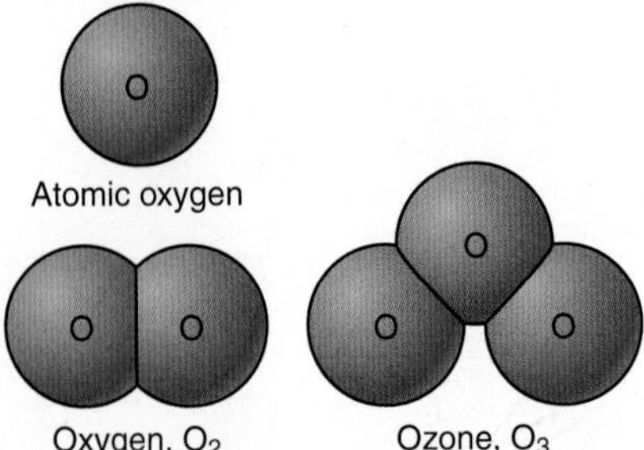

▲ **Figure 12–1**
Elemental molecules contain two or more atoms of the same element in definite (fixed) proportions.

Atmospheric oxygen and other chemical substances, such as nitrogen and water vapor, make up the air you breathe. This type of oxygen is called an **elemental molecule** (EL-uh-men-tul MAHL-uh-kyool), a molecule containing two or more atoms of the same element (in this case, oxygen) in definite (fixed) proportions. It is written as O_2. Ozone is another elemental molecule made up of oxygen. Ozone is a major component of smog and can be very dangerous. It contains three atoms of the element oxygen and is written as O_3 (**Figure 12–1**).

Compound molecules (KAHM-pownd MAHL-uh-kyools), also known as **compounds**, are a chemical combination of two or more atoms of different elements in definite (fixed) proportions (**Figure 12–2**). Sodium chloride (NaCl), common table salt, is an example of compound molecules. Each sodium chloride molecule contains one atom of the element sodium (Na) and one atom of the element chlorine (Cl).

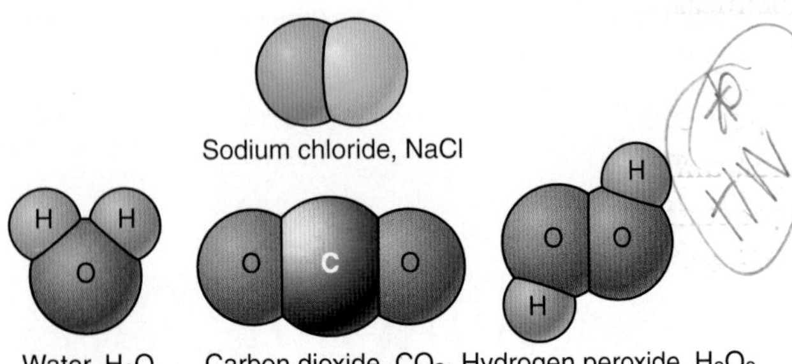

▲ **Figure 12–2**
Compound molecules contain two or more atoms of different elements in definite (fixed) proportions.

States of Matter

All matter exists in one of three different physical forms:

- Solid
- Liquid
- Gas

These three forms are called the **states of matter**. Matter (**Table 12–1**) becomes one of these states, depending on its temperature (**Figure 12–3**).

Like many other substances, water (H_2O) can exist in all three states of matter, depending on its temperature. For example, water changes according to how the temperature changes, but it is still water. When water freezes, it turns to ice. When ice melts, it turns back into water. When water boils, it turns to steam. When the steam cools, it turns back into water. The water stays the same chemical, but it becomes a different physical form. When one chemical changes its state of matter,

STATES OF MATTER

STATE	DESCRIPTION	EXAMPLES
Solid	Rigid; has a fixed shape and volume.	brush, roller, wooden nail pusher, ice
Liquid	Definite volume but takes the shape of its container.	bleach, shampoo, haircolor, water
Gas	No fixed volume or shape; takes the shape and volume of its container. Can never be liquid at normal temperatures or pressures.	propellant in hairspray, mousse, propane

Table 12–1 **States of Matter.**

© Milady, a part of Cengage Learning.

Solid

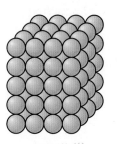

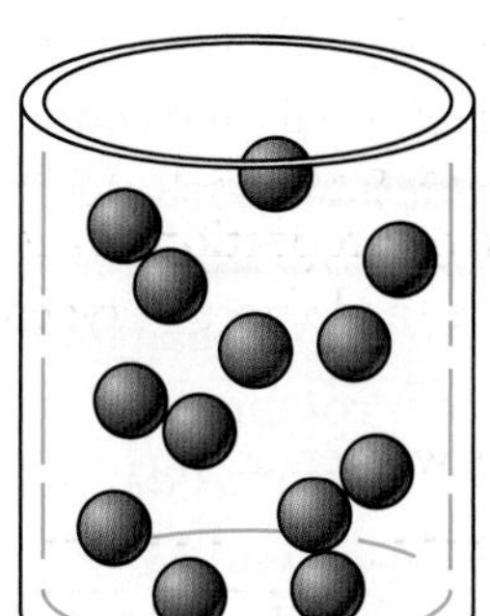

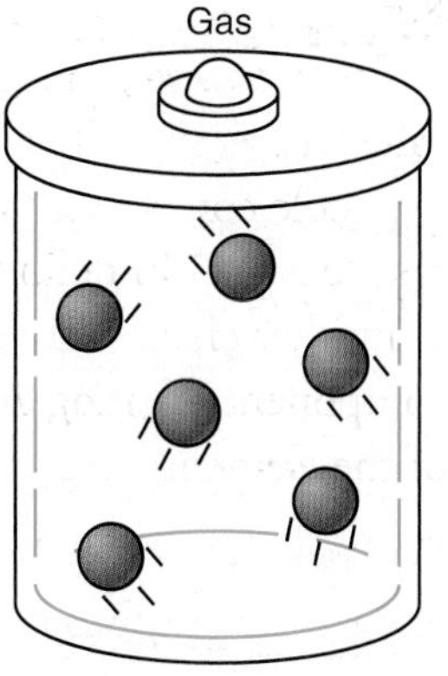

▲ **Figure 12–3**
Solid, liquid, and gas states of matter.

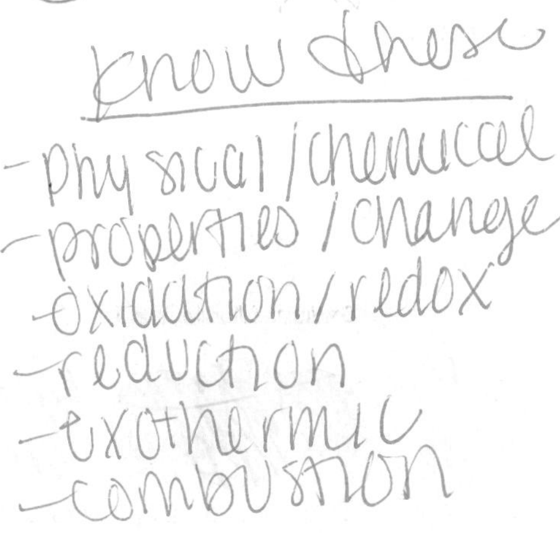

the change is called a physical change. (See Physical and Chemical Changes in this chapter.)

Vapor is a liquid that has evaporated into a gas-like state. Vapors can return to being a liquid when they cool to room temperatures, unlike a gas. Steam is an example of a vapor. Vapors are not a unique state of matter; they are liquids that have undergone a physical change. ✓ **LO2**

Physical and Chemical Properties of Matter

Every substance has unique properties that allow us to identify it. The two types of properties are physical and chemical.

Physical properties are characteristics that can be determined without a chemical reaction and that do not involve a chemical change in the substance. Physical properties include color, size, weight, hardness, and glossiness. (As described above, the state of matter that a substance becomes is an example of a physical property.)

Chemical properties are characteristics that can only be determined by a chemical reaction and a chemical change in the substance. Examples of chemical properties include the ability of iron to rust, wood to burn, or hair to change color through the use of haircolor and hydrogen peroxide.

Physical and Chemical Changes

Matter can be changed in two different ways. Physical forces cause physical changes and chemical reactions cause chemical changes.

A **physical change** is a change in the form or physical properties of a substance, without a chemical reaction or the creation of a new substance. No chemical reactions are involved in physical change and no new chemicals are formed. Solid ice undergoes a physical change when it melts into water and then converts into steam (**Figure 12–4**). A physical change occurs when a temporary haircolor is applied to the hair or nail polish is taken off the nail with a remover solvent.

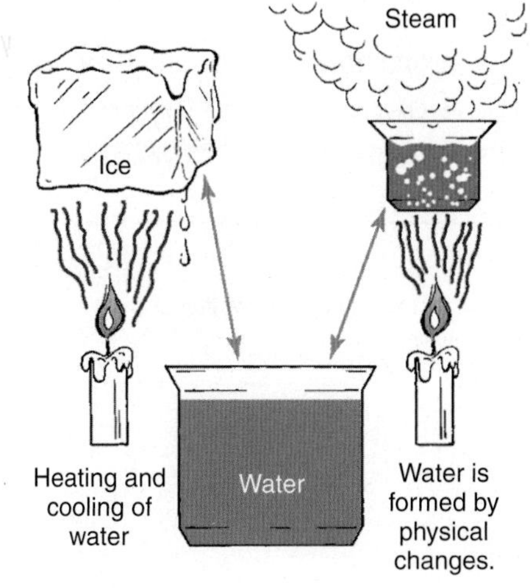

▲ **Figure 12–4**
Physical changes.

© Milady, a part of Cengage Learning.

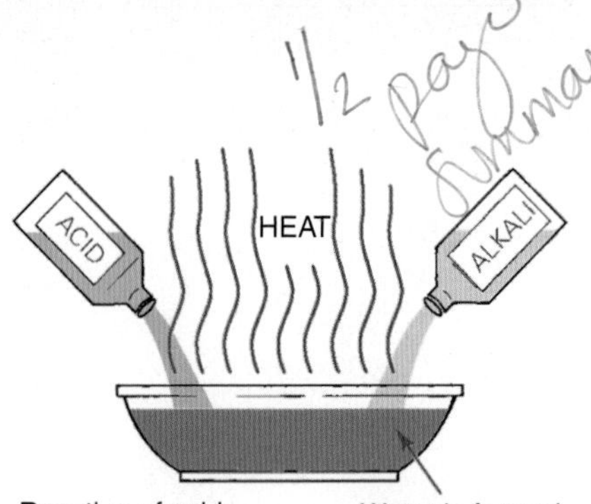

▲ **Figure 12–5**
Chemical changes.

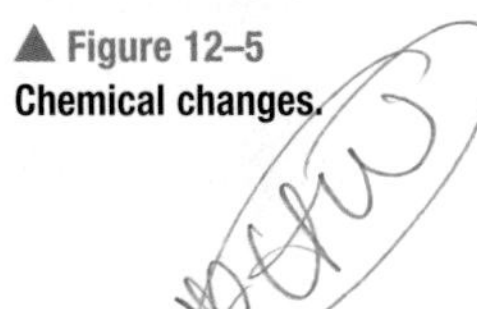

A **chemical change** is a change in the chemical composition or make-up of a substance. This change is caused by chemical reactions that create new chemical substances, usually by combining or subtracting certain elements. Those new substances have different chemical and physical properties (**Figure 12–5**). An example of a chemical change is the **oxidation** (ahk-sih-DAY-shun) of haircolor. The term *oxidation* refers to a chemical reaction that combines a substance with oxygen to produce an oxide. Another example of oxidation is wood turning into charcoal after it has burned.

Oxidation–reduction, also known as **redox** (ree-DOCS), is a chemical reaction in which the oxidizing agent is reduced (by losing oxygen) and the reducing agent is oxidized (by gaining oxygen). Even though the word order is reversed, redox is used as a contraction of the term oxidation-reduction.

An **oxidizing agent** is a substance that releases oxygen. Hydrogen peroxide (H_2O_2), which can be thought of as water with an extra atom of oxygen, is an example of an oxidizing agent. A **reducing agent** is a substance that adds hydrogen to a chemical compound or subtracts oxygen from the compound. When hydrogen peroxide is mixed with an oxidation haircolor, oxygen is subtracted from the hydrogen peroxide and the hydrogen peroxide is reduced. At the same time, oxygen is added to the haircolor and the haircolor is oxidized. In this example, haircolor is the reducing agent.

did you know?

The sugar in grapes is chemically converted into ethyl alcohol by certain types of yeast when wine is fermented in a wooden vat. Fermentation is an example of a chemical reaction.

A **reduction** is the process through which oxygen is subtracted from or hydrogen is added to a substance through a chemical reaction. This chemical reaction is called a **reduction reaction**. Oxidation and reduction (redox) reactions always occur at the same time. Redox reactions involve a transfer between the oxidizing agent and the reducing agent. The oxidizing agent is reduced, and the reducing agent is oxidized. Redox reactions can take place without oxygen because oxidation also can occur when hydrogen is subtracted from a substance (**Figure 12–6**). Redox reactions are also responsible for the chemical changes created by haircolors, hair lighteners, permanent wave solutions, and thioglycolic acid neutralizers. These chemical services would not be possible without oxidation–reduction (redox) reactions.

OXIDATION	REDUCTION
+ Oxygen	− Oxygen
− Hydrogen	+ Hydrogen

▲ **Figure 12–6**
Chart of oxidation and reduction reactions.

Under certain circumstances, chemical reactions can release a significant amount of heat. These types of chemical reactions are called **exothermic reactions** (ek-soh-THUR-mik ree-AK-shunz). In fact, all oxidation reactions are exothermic reactions. An example of an exothermic reaction is a nail product that hardens (polymerizes) to create nail enhancements. Exothermic reactions occur, but usually clients cannot feel the heat being released.

Combustion (kum-BUS-chun) is the rapid oxidation of a substance, accompanied by the production of heat and light. Lighting a match is an example of rapid oxidation. Oxidation requires the presence of oxygen; this is the reason that there cannot be a fire without air. ☑ **LO3**

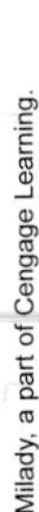
© Milady, a part of Cengage Learning.

Pure Substances and Physical Mixtures

All matter can be classified as either a pure substance or a physical mixture (blend).

A **pure substance** is a chemical combination of matter in definite (fixed) proportions. Pure substances have unique properties. All atoms, elements, elemental molecules, and compound molecules are pure substances. Distilled water is a pure substance that results from the combination of two atoms of the element hydrogen and one atom of the element oxygen in fixed proportions. Water that comes out of a faucet is not pure water.

Most substances do not exist in a pure state. Air contains many substances including nitrogen, carbon dioxide, and water vapor. This is an example of a physical mixture. A **physical mixture** is a physical combination of matter in any proportions. The properties of a physical mixture are the combined properties of the substances in the mixture. Salt water is a physical mixture of salt and water in any proportion. The properties of salt water are the properties contained in salt and in water: salt water is salty and wet. Most of the products cosmetologists and nail technicians use are physical mixtures (**Figure 12–7**).

Table 12–2 summarizes the differences between pure substances and physical mixtures. ☑ **LO4**

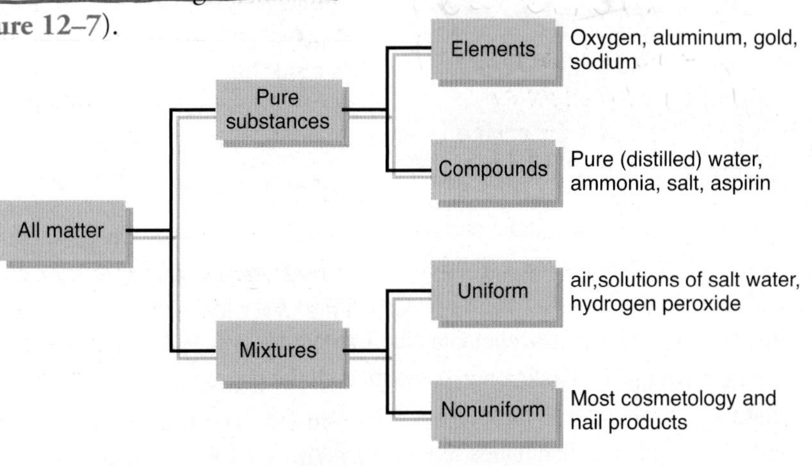

▲ **Figure 12–7**
Examples of pure substances and physical mixtures.

Solutions, Suspensions, and Emulsions

Solutions, suspensions, and emulsions are all physical mixtures. The differences among solutions, suspensions, and emulsions are

DIFFERENCES BETWEEN PURE SUBSTANCES AND PHYSICAL MIXTURES

PURE SUBSTANCES	PHYSICAL MIXTURES
United chemically	United physically
Definite (fixed) proportions	Any proportions
Unique chemical and physical properties	Combined chemical and physical properties
Salt and pure (distilled) water are examples of pure substances.	Salt water is a physical mixture.

Table 12–2 **Differences Between Pure Substances and Physical Mixtures.**

© Milady, a part of Cengage Learning.

ACTivity

Put a tablespoon of sugar in a cup of hot water. Cover it loosely with a paper towel and set it aside for a week. What happens when the water evaporates? What are the crystals that form inside the cup made from? Taste them to see whether your conclusions were right.

When sugar dissolves in water, is it a physical or chemical change?

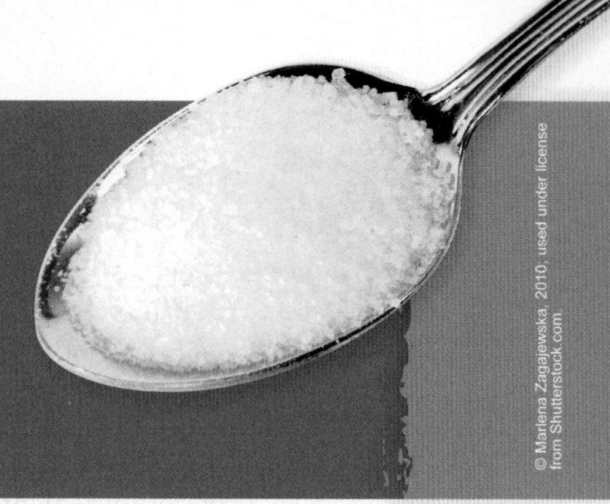

© Marlena Zagajewska, 2010, used under license from Shutterstock.com.

determined by the types of substances, the size of the particles, and the solubility of the substances.

- A **solution** is a stable physical mixture of two or more substances. The **solute** (SAHL-yoot) is the substance that is dissolved into solution. The **solvent** (SAHL-vent) is the substance that dissolves the solute and makes the solution. For example, when salt is dissolved in water, salt is the solute and water is the solvent. Water is known as a universal solvent because it has the ability to dissolve more substances than any other solvent.

did you know?

Soaps were the first synthetic surfactants. People began making soaps about 4,500 years ago by boiling oil or animal fat with wood ashes. Modern soaps are made from animal fats or vegetable oils. Traditional bar soaps are highly alkaline and combine with the minerals in hard water to form an insoluble film that coats skin and can cause hands to feel dry, itchy, and irritated. Cosmetologists who are performing nail services should be aware that soaps can leave a film on the nail plate, which could contribute to lifting of the nail enhancement. Modern synthetic surfactants have overcome these disadvantages and are superior to soaps; many are milder on the skin than soaps used in the past.

All liquids are either miscible or immiscible. **Miscible** (MIS-uh-bul) liquids are mutually soluble, meaning that they can be mixed together to form stable solutions. Water and alcohol are examples of miscible liquids, as are polish remover and water. When these substances are mixed together, they will stay mixed, forming a solution. Solutions contain small particles that are invisible to the naked eye. Solutions are usually transparent, although they may be colored. They do not separate when left still. Again, salt water is an example of a solution with a solid dissolved in a liquid. Water is the solvent that dissolves the salt (solute) and holds it in solution.

Immiscible (im-IS-uh-bul) liquids are not capable of being mixed together to form stable solutions. Water and oil are examples of immiscible liquids. These substances can be mixed together, but they will separate when left sitting still. When immiscible liquids are combined, they form suspensions.

- **Suspensions** (sus-PEN-shunz) are unstable physical mixtures of undissolved particles in a liquid. Compared with solutions, suspensions contain larger and less miscible particles. The particles are generally visible to the naked eye but are not large enough to settle quickly to the bottom. Suspensions are not usually transparent and may be colored. They are unstable and separate over time, which is why some lotions and creams can separate in the bottle and need to be shaken before they are used. Another example of a suspension is the glitter in nail polish that can separate from the polish.

Oil and vinegar salad dressing is an example of a suspension, with tiny oil droplets suspended in the vinegar. The suspension will separate when left sitting still and must be shaken before using. Calamine lotion and nail polish are other examples of suspensions.

- An **emulsion** (ee-MUL-shun) is an unstable physical mixture of two or more immiscible substances (substances that normally will not stay blended) plus a special ingredient called an emulsifier. An **emulsifier** (ee-MUL-suh-fy-ur) is an ingredient that brings two normally incompatible materials together and binds them into a uniform and fairly stable blend. Emulsions are considered to be a special type of suspension because they can separate, but the separation usually happens very slowly over a long period of time. An example of an emulsion is hand lotion. A properly formulated emulsion, stored under ideal conditions, can be stable up to three years. Since conditions are rarely ideal, all cosmetic emulsions should be used within one year of purchase. Always refer to the product's instructions and cautions for specific details.

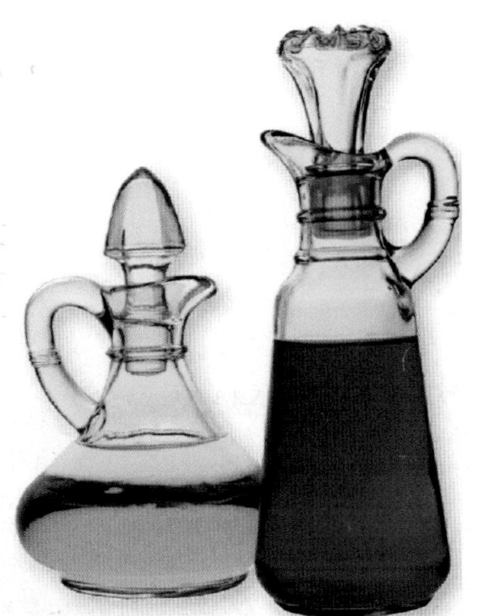

© Ed Isaacs, 2010; used under license from Shutterstock.com.

Table 12–3 offers a summary of the differences among solutions, suspensions, and emulsions.

Surfactants (sur-FAK-tants) are substances that allow oil and water to mix, or emulsify. They are one type of emulsifier. The term *surfactant* is a contraction for surface active agent. A

DIFFERENCES AMONG SOLUTIONS, SUSPENSIONS, AND EMULSIONS

SOLUTIONS	SUSPENSIONS	EMULSIONS
miscible	slightly miscible	immiscible
no surfactant	no surfactant	surfactant
small particles	larger particles	largest particles
stable mixture	unstable, temporary mixture	limited stability through an emulsifier
usually clear	usually cloudy	usually a solid color
solution of nail primer	nail polish, glitter in nail polish	shampoos, conditioners, hand lotions

© Milady, a part of Cengage Learning.

Table 12–3 Differences Among Solutions, Suspensions, and Emulsions.

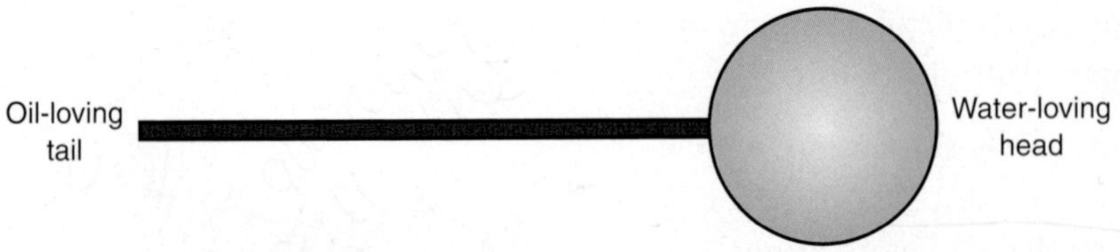

▲ Figure 12–8
A surfactant molecule.

surfactant molecule has two distinct parts (**Figure 12–8**). The head of the surfactant molecule is hydrophilic (hy-drah-FIL-ik), capable of combining with or attracting water (water-loving), and the tail is **lipophilic** (ly-puh-FIL-ik), having an affinity for or an attraction to fat and oils (oil-loving). Following the like-dissolves-like rule, the hydrophilic head dissolves in water and the lipophilic tail dissolves in oil. So a surfactant molecule mixes with and dissolves in both oil and water and temporarily joins them together to form an emulsion.

In an **oil-in-water (O/W) emulsion**, oil droplets are emulsified in water. The droplets of oil are surrounded by surfactant molecules with their lipophilic tails pointing in and their hydrophilic heads pointing out. Tiny oil droplets form the internal portion of each O/W emulsion because the oil is completely surrounded by water (**Figure 12–9**). Oil-in-water emulsions do not feel as greasy as water-in-oil emulsions because the oil is hidden and water forms the external portion of the emulsion.

In a **water-in-oil (W/O) emulsion**, water droplets are emulsified in oil. The droplets of water are surrounded by surfactants with their hydrophilic heads pointing in and their lipophilic tails pointing out (**Figure 12–10**). Tiny droplets of water form the internal portion of a W/O emulsion because the water is completely surrounded by oil. Water-in-oil emulsions feel greasier than oil-in-water emulsions because

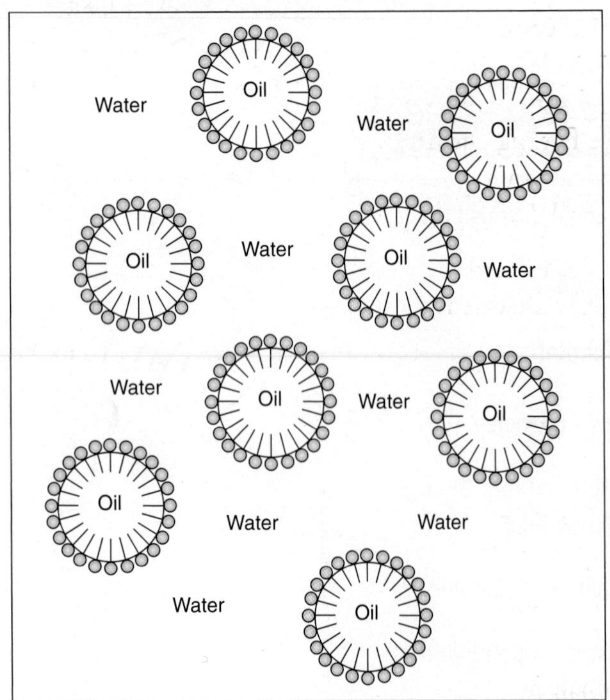

▲ Figure 12–9
Oil-in-water emulsions.

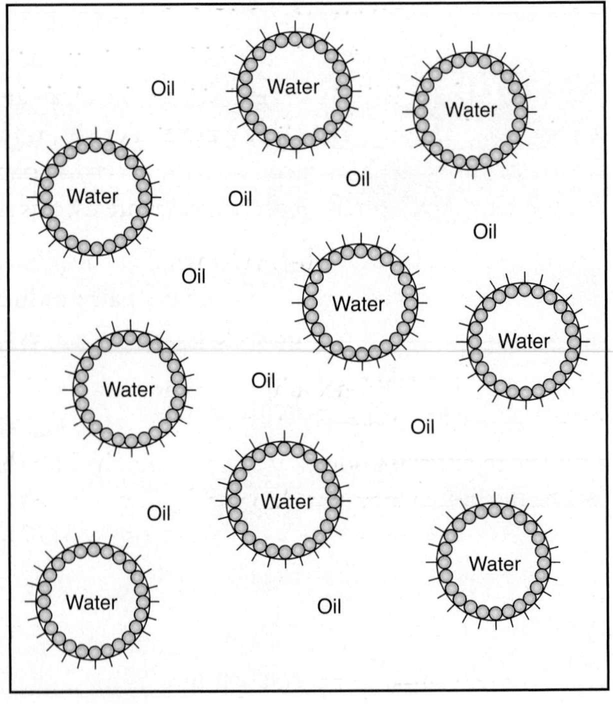

▲ Figure 12–10
Water-in-oil emulsions.

© Milady, a part of Cengage Learning.

ACTivity

Have you ever heard the saying "Oil and water don't mix"? Pour some water into a glass, then add a little cooking oil (or other oil). What happens? Stir the water briskly with a spoon and observe for a minute or two. What does the oil do?

the water is hidden and oil forms the external portion of the emulsion. Styling creams, cold creams, and foot balms are examples. ☑ **LO5**

Other Physical Mixtures

Ointments, pastes, pomades, and styling waxes are semisolid mixtures made with any combination of petrolatum (petroleum jelly), oil, and wax.

Powders are a physical mixture of one or more types of solids. Off-the-scalp powdered hair lighteners are physical mixtures. These mixtures may separate during shipping and storage and should be thoroughly mixed before each use.

Common Chemical Product Ingredients

Cosmetologists use many chemical products when performing client services. Following are some of the most common chemical ingredients used in salon products.

Volatile alcohols (VAHL-uh-tul AL-kuh-hawlz) are those that evaporate easily, such as isopropyl alcohol (rubbing alcohol) and ethyl alcohol (hairspray and alcoholic beverages). These chemicals are familiar to most people, but there are many other types of alcohols, from free-flowing liquids to hard, waxy solids. Fatty alcohols, such as cetyl alcohol and cetearyl alcohol, are nonvolatile alcohol waxes that are used as skin conditioners.

Alkanolamines (al-kan-oh-LAH-mynz) are alkaline substances used to neutralize acids or raise the pH of many hair products. They are often used in place of ammonia because they produce less odor.

Ammonia (uh-MOH-nee-uh) is a colorless gas with a pungent odor that is composed of hydrogen and nitrogen. It is used to raise the pH in hair products to allow the solution to penetrate the hair shaft. Ammonium hydroxide and ammonium thioglycolate are examples of ammonia compounds that are used to perform chemical services in a salon.

Glycerin (GLIS-ur-in) is a sweet, colorless, oily substance. It is used as a solvent and as a moisturizer in skin and body creams.

Silicones (SIL-ih-kohnz) are a special type of oil used in hair conditioners, water-resistant lubricants for the skin, and nail polish dryers. Silicones are less greasy than other oils and form a breathable

did you know?

Mayonnaise is an example of an oil-in-water emulsion of two immiscible liquids. Although oil and water are immiscible, the egg yolk in mayonnaise emulsifies the oil droplets and distributes them uniformly in the water. Without the egg yolk as an emulsifying agent, the oil and water would separate. Most of the emulsions used in a salon are oil-in-water. Haircolor, shampoos, conditioners, hand lotions, and facial creams are oil-in-water emulsions.

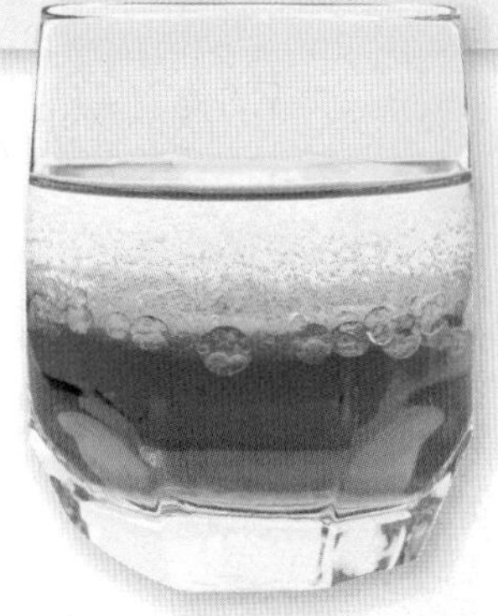

© Vasilyev A.S., 2010; used under license from Shutterstock.com.

film that does not cause comedones (blackheads). Silicones also give skin a silky, smooth feeling and great shine to hair.

Volatile organic compounds (VOCs) are compounds that contain carbon (organic) and evaporate very easily (volatile). For example, a common VOC used in hairspray is SD alcohol (ethyl alcohol). Volatile organic solvents such as ethyl acetate and isopropyl alcohol are used in nail polish, base and top coats, and polish removers.

Potential Hydrogen (pH)

Although **pH**, the abbreviation used for *potential hydrogen*, is often mentioned when talking about salon products, it is one of the least understood chemical properties. Notice that *pH* is written with a small *p* (which represents a quantity) and a capital *H* (which represents the hydrogen ion). The term *pH* represents the quantity of hydrogen ions. Understanding pH and how it affects the hair, skin, and nails is essential to understanding all salon services. For more information about the pH of products used in salon services, see Chapter 15, Scalp Care, Shampooing, and Conditioning, and Chapter 20, Chemical Texture Services.

Water and pH

Before you can understand pH, you need to learn about ions. An **ion** (EYE-on) is an atom or molecule that carries an electrical charge. **Ionization** (eye-on-ih-ZAY-shun) is the separation of an atom or molecule into positive and negative ions. An ion with a negative electrical charge is an **anion** (AN-eye-on). An ion with a positive electrical charge is a **cation** (KAT-eye-on).

© originalpunkt, 2010; used under license from Shutterstock.com.

In water, some of the water (H_20) molecules naturally ionize into hydrogen ions and hydroxide ions. The pH scale measures these ions. The hydrogen ion (H^+) is acidic. The more hydrogen ions there are in a substance, the more acidic it will be. The hydroxide ion (OH-) is alkaline. The more hydroxide ions there are in a substance, the more alkaline it will be. pH is only possible because of this ionization of water. Only products that contain water can have a pH.

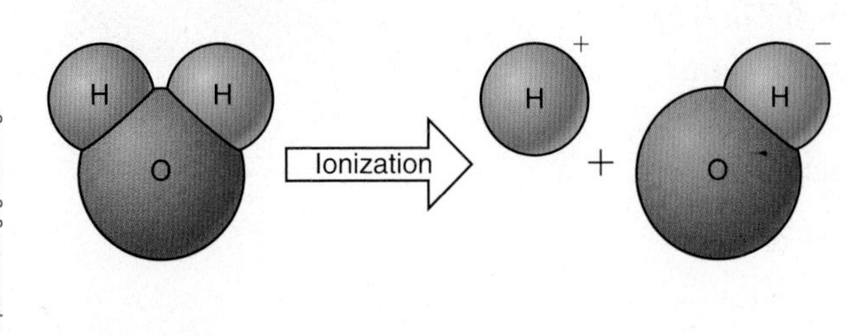

© Milady, a part of Cengage Learning.

▲ **Figure 12–11**
The ionization of water.

In pure (distilled) water, each water molecule that ionizes produces one hydrogen ion and one hydroxide ion (**Figure 12–11**). Pure water has a neutral pH because it contains the same number of hydrogen ions as hydroxide ions. It is an equal balance of 50 percent acidic and 50 percent alkaline. The pH of any substance is always a balance of both acidity and alkalinity. As acidity increases, alkalinity

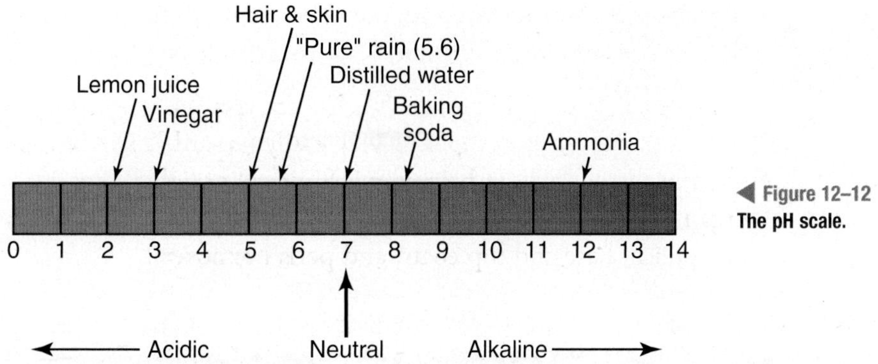

© Milady, a part of Cengage Learning.

◀ **Figure 12–12**
The pH scale.

decreases. The opposite is also true; as alkalinity increases, acidity decreases. Even the strongest acid also contains some alkalinity.

The pH Scale

A **pH scale** is a measure of the acidity and alkalinity of a substance. It has a range of 0 to 14. A pH of 7 is a neutral solution, a pH below 7 indicates an **acidic solution**, and a pH above 7 indicates an **alkaline solution** (**Figure 12–12**).

logarithm means multiples of 10

The term **logarithm** (LOG-ah-rhythm) means multiples of 10. Since the pH scale is a logarithmic scale, a change of one whole number represents a tenfold change in pH. This means, for example, that a pH of 8 is 10 times more alkaline than a pH of 7. A change of two whole numbers represents a change of 10 times 10, or a 100-fold change. So a pH of 9 is 100 times more alkaline than a pH of 7. Even a small change on the pH scale represents a large change in the pH.

pH is always a balance of both acidity and alkalinity. Pure water has a pH of 7, which is an equal balance of acid and alkaline. Although a pH of 7 is neutral on the pH scale, it is not neutral compared to the hair and skin, which have an average pH of 5. Pure (distilled) water, with a pH of 7, is 100 times more alkaline than a pH of 5, so pure water is 100 times more alkaline than your hair and skin. This difference in pH is the reason pure water can cause the hair to swell as much as 20 percent and the reason that water is drying to the skin. ☑ **LO6**

Acids and Alkalis

All acids owe their chemical reactivity to the hydrogen ion. Acids have a pH below 7.0.

Alpha hydroxy acids (AHAs) (al-FAH HY-drok-see AS-udz), derived from plants (mostly fruit), are examples of acids often used in salons to exfoliate the skin and to help adjust the pH of a lotion or cream. Acids contract and harden hair. One such acid is **thioglycolic acid** (thy-oh-GLY-kuh-lik AS-ud), a colorless liquid or white crystals with a strong unpleasant odor that is used in permanent waving solutions.

All **alkalis** (AL-kuh-lyz), also known as **bases**, owe their chemical reactivity to the hydroxide ion. Alkalis are compounds that react with

ACTivity

For a product to have a pH, it must contain water. Shampoos, conditioners, haircolor, permanent waves, relaxers, lotions, and creams have a pH. Divide into groups and research these products online to find their pH. If the information is not available online, contact the manufacturers. Make a chart and compare your findings with what your classmates found. How will the pH of these products affect the hair?

Here is a hint to save you some time: oils, waxes, nail polish, and nail monomers have no pH because they contain no water.

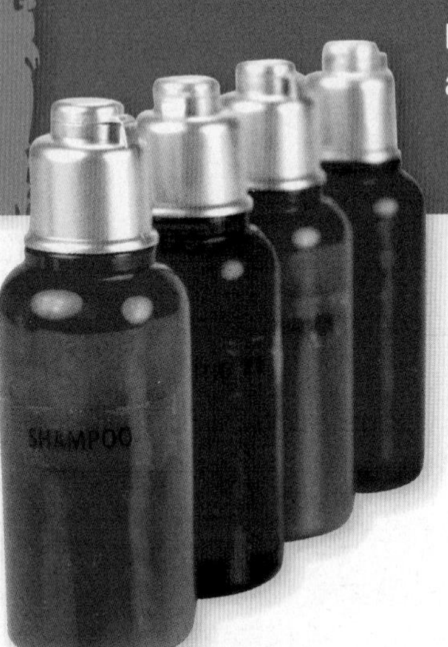

© Kitch Bain, 2010; used under license from Shutterstock.com.

acids to form salts. Alkalis have a pH above 7.0. They feel slippery and soapy on the skin. Alkalis soften and swell hair, skin, the cuticle on the nail plate, and calloused skin.

Sodium hydroxide, commonly known as lye, is a very strong alkali used in chemical hair relaxers, callous softeners, and drain cleaners. These products must be used according to manufacturer's instructions, and it is very important that you do not let the products touch or sit on the skin as they may cause injury to or a burning sensation on the skin. Sodium hydroxide products may be especially dangerous if they get into the eyes, so always wear safety glasses to avoid eye contact. Consult the product's MSDS for more specific information on safe use.

Acid-Alkali Neutralization Reactions

The same reaction that naturally ionizes water into hydrogen ions and hydroxide ions also runs in reverse. When acids and alkalis are mixed together in equal proportions, they neutralize each other to form water (**Figure 12–13**). Neutralizing shampoos and normalizing lotions used to neutralize hair relaxers work by creating an acid-alkali neutralization reaction. Liquid soaps are usually slightly acidic and can neutralize alkaline callous softener residues left on the skin after rinsing.

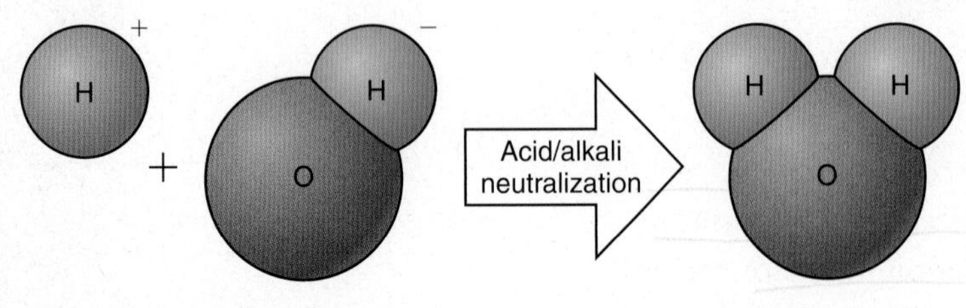

© Milady, a part of Cengage Learning.

▲ **Figure 12–13**
Acid and alkali neutralization reaction.

Chemistry Will Help You in the Salon[1]

Whether you are studying the pH of products, redox reactions, or suspensions, solutions, and emulsions, there is a lot to learn about how chemistry affects the products you use in the salon. Having a basic understanding of chemistry will help you use professional products effectively and safely in the salon.

Review Questions

1. What is chemistry?
2. What is the difference between organic and inorganic chemistry?
3. What is matter?
4. What is an element?
5. What are atoms?
6. Explain the difference between elemental molecules and compound molecules. Give examples.
7. Name and describe the three states of matter.
8. What are the physical and chemical properties of matter? Give examples.
9. What is the difference between physical and chemical change? Give examples.
10. Explain oxidation-reduction (redox).
11. Explain pure substances and physical mixtures. Give examples.
12. What are the differences among solutions, suspensions, and emulsions? Give examples.
13. Define pH and the pH scale.

Chapter Glossary

acidic solution	A solution that has a pH below 7.0 (neutral).
alkaline solution	A solution that has a pH above 7.0 (neutral).
alkalis	Also known as *bases*; compounds that react with acids to form salts.
alkanolamines	Alkaline substances used to neutralize acids or raise the pH of many hair products.
alpha hydroxy acids	Abbreviated AHAs; acids derived from plants (mostly fruit) that are often used to exfoliate the skin.
ammonia	Colorless gas with a pungent odor that is composed of hydrogen and nitrogen.
anion	An ion with a negative electrical charge.
atoms	The smallest chemical components (often called particles) of an element; structures that make up the element and have the same properties of the element.
cation	An ion with a positive electrical charge.
chemical change	A change in the chemical composition or make-up of a substance.
chemical properties	Characteristics that can only be determined by a chemical reaction and a chemical change in the substance.

Chapter Glossary

chemistry	Science that deals with the composition, structures, and properties of matter, and how matter changes under different conditions.
combustion	Rapid oxidation of a substance, accompanied by the production of heat and light.
compound molecules	Also known as *compounds;* a chemical combination of two or more atoms of different elements in definite (fixed) proportions.
element	The simplest form of chemical matter; an element cannot be broken down into a simpler substance without a loss of identity.
elemental molecule	Molecule containing two or more atoms of the same element in definite (fixed) proportions.
emulsifier	An ingredient that brings two normally incompatible materials together and binds them into a uniform and fairly stable blend.
emulsion	An unstable physical mixture of two or more immiscible substances (substances that normally will not stay blended) plus a special ingredient called an emulsifier.
exothermic reactions	Chemical reactions that release a significant amount of heat.
glycerin	Sweet, colorless, oily substance used as a solvent and as a moisturizer in skin and body creams.
immiscible	Liquids that are not capable of being mixed together to form stable solutions.
inorganic chemistry	The study of substances that do not contain the element carbon, but may contain the element hydrogen.
ion	An atom or molecule that carries an electrical charge.
ionization	The separation of an atom or molecule into positive and negative ions.
lipophilic	Having an affinity for or an attraction to fat and oils (oil-loving).
logarithm	Multiples of ten.
matter	Any substance that occupies space and has mass (weight).
miscible	Liquids that are mutually soluble, meaning that they can be mixed together to form stable solutions.
molecule	A chemical combination of two or more atoms in definite (fixed) proportions.
oil-in-water emulsion	Abbreviated O/W emulsion; oil droplets emulsified in water.
organic chemistry	The study of substances that contain the element carbon.
oxidation	A chemical reaction that combines a substance with oxygen to produce an oxide.
oxidation-reduction	Also known as *redox;* a chemical reaction in which the oxidizing agent is reduced (by losing oxygen) and the reducing agent is oxidized (by gaining oxygen).

Chapter Glossary

oxidizing agent	Substance that releases oxygen.
pH	The abbreviation used for potential hydrogen. pH represents the quantity of hydrogen ions.
pH scale	A measure of the acidity and alkalinity of a substance; the pH scale has a range of 0 to 14, with 7 being neutral. A pH below 7 is an acidic solution; a pH above 7 is an alkaline solution.
physical change	A change in the form or physical properties of a substance, without a chemical reaction or the creation of a new substance.
physical mixture	A physical combination of matter in any proportions.
physical properties	Characteristics that can be determined without a chemical reaction and that do not cause a chemical change in the substance.
pure substance	A chemical combination of matter in definite (fixed) proportions.
reducing agent	A substance that adds hydrogen to a chemical compound or subtracts oxygen from the compound.
reduction	The process through which oxygen is subtracted from or hydrogen is added to a substance through a chemical reaction.
reduction reaction	A chemical reaction in which oxygen is subtracted from or hydrogen is added to a substance.
silicones	Special type of oil used in hair conditioners, water-resistant lubricants for the skin, and nail polish dryers.
solute	The substance that is dissolved in a solution.
solution	A stable physical mixture of two or more substances.
solvent	The substance that dissolves the solute and makes a solution.
states of matter	The three different physical forms of matter—solid, liquid, and gas.
surfactants	A contraction of *surface active agents*; substances that allow oil and water to mix, or emulsify.
suspensions	Unstable physical mixtures of undissolved particles in a liquid.
thioglycolic acid	A colorless liquid or white crystals with a strong unpleasant odor that is used in permanent waving solutions.
volatile alcohols	Alcohols that evaporate easily.
volatile organic compounds	Abbreviated VOCs; compounds that contain carbon (organic) and evaporate very easily (volatile).
water-in-oil emulsion	Abbreviated W/O emulsion; water droplets are emulsified in oil.

CHAPTER 13

Basics of Electricity

Chapter Outline

Why Study Basics of Electricity?

Electricity

Electrical Equipment Safety

Electrotherapy

Other Electrical Equipment

Light Energy and Light Therapy

© William Attard McCarthy, 2010; used under license from Shutterstock.com.

Learning Objectives

After completing this chapter, you will be able to:

- ✓ **LO1** Define the nature of electricity and the two types of electric current.
- ✓ **LO2** Define electrical measurements.
- ✓ **LO3** Understand the principles of electrical equipment safety.
- ✓ **LO4** Define the main electric modalities used in cosmetology.
- ✓ **LO5** Describe other types of electrical equipment that cosmetologists use and describe how to use them.
- ✓ **LO6** Explain electromagnetic spectrum, visible spectrum of light, and invisible light.
- ✓ **LO7** Describe the types of light therapy and their benefits.

Key Terms

Page number indicates where in the chapter the term is used.

active electrode
pg. 270

alternating current (AC)
pg. 265

ampere (A, amp)
pg. 266

anaphoresis
pg. 270

anode
pg. 269

catalysts
pg. 275

cataphoresis
pg. 270

cathode
pg. 269

chromophore
pg. 276

circuit breaker
pg. 267

complete electric circuit
pg. 265

conductor
pg. 264

converter
pg. 265

desincrustation
pg. 270

direct current (DC)
pg. 265

electric current
pg. 264

electricity
pg. 264

electrode (probe)
pg. 269

electromagnetic spectrum (electromagnetic spectrum of radiation)
pg. 272

fuse
pg. 267

galvanic current
pg. 269

grounding
pg. 267

inactive electrode
pg. 270

infrared light
pg. 275

intense pulse light
pg. 277

invisible light
pg. 274

iontophoresis
pg. 270

kilowatt (K)
pg. 266

laser (light amplification stimulation emission of radiation)
pg. 276

light-emitting diode (LED)
pg. 276

light therapy (phototherapy)
pg. 275

microcurrent
pg. 270

milliampere (mA)
pg. 266

modalities
pg. 269

nonconductor (insulator)
pg. 265

ohm (O)
pg. 266

photothermolysis
pg. 276

polarity
pg. 269

rectifier
pg. 265

Tesla high-frequency current (violet ray)
pg. 271

ultraviolet light (UV light, cold light, actinic light)
pg. 275

visible spectrum of light
pg. 274

volt (V, voltage)
pg. 266

watt (W)
pg. 266

waveform
pg. 273

wavelength
pg. 273

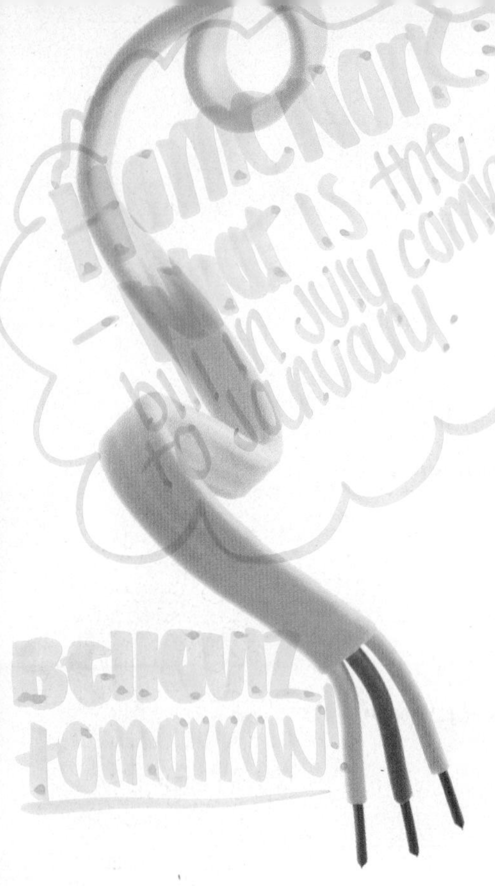

You decided to enter this field because you love cosmetology and all of the services it offers to clients: hairstyling, haircoloring, perms, facials, mani-pedis. How many of these services could you offer without using electricity? As you study this chapter, you will learn how important it is for cosmetology professionals to have a basic working knowledge of electricity.

© Titov Andriy, 2010; used under license from Shutterstock.com.

Why Study Basics of Electricity?

Cosmetologists should study and have a thorough understanding of the basics of electricity because:

- Cosmetologists use and rely upon a variety of electrical appliances. Knowing what electricity is and how it works will allow you to use it wisely and safely.
- A basic understanding of electricity will enable you to properly use and care for your equipment and tools.
- Electricity and its use impact other aspects of the salon environment, such as lighting and the temperature of styling irons. Therefore, it impacts the services you offer your clients.

Electricity

did you know?

Lightning bolts travel through the air at speeds of up to 60,000 miles per hour.

If you look at lightning on a stormy night, what you will see are the effects of electricity. If you plug a poorly wired appliance into a socket and sparks fly out of the socket, you will also see the effects of electricity. You are not really seeing electricity, however; instead, you are seeing its *visual* effects on the surrounding air. Electricity does not occupy space or have mass (weight), so it is not matter. If it is not matter, then what is it? **Electricity** (ee-lek-TRIS-ih-tee) is the movement of particles around an atom that creates pure energy. It is a form of energy that exhibits magnetic, chemical, or thermal effects when it is in motion.

An **electric current** (ee-LEK-trik KUR-unt) is the flow of electricity along a conductor. All materials can be classified as conductors or nonconductors (insulators), depending on the ease with which an electric current can be transmitted through them.

did you know?

When you touch something and get a static shock, it is a form of electricity.

A **conductor** (kahn-DUK-tur) is any material that conducts electricity. Most metals are good conductors. This means that electricity will pass through the material easily. Copper is a particularly good conductor and is used in electric wiring and electric motors. Pure (distilled) water is a poor conductor, but the ions usually found in ordinary water, such as tap water or a river or a lake, make it a good conductor. This explains why you should not swim in a lake during an electrical storm.

A **nonconductor** (nahn-kun-DUK-tur), also known as **insulator** (IN-suh-layt-ur), is a material that does not transmit electricity. Rubber, silk, wood, glass, and cement are good insulators. Electric wires are composed of twisted metal threads (the conductor) covered with a rubber or plastic coating (the nonconductor or insulator). A **complete electric circuit** (kahm-PLEET ee-LEK-trik SUR-kit) is the path of negative and positive electric currents moving from the generating source through the conductors and back to the generating source.

Types Of Electric Current

There are two types of electric current:

Direct current (dy-REKT KUR-unt), abbreviated DC, is a constant, even-flowing current that travels in one direction only and is produced by chemical means. Flashlights, mobile telephones, and cordless hairstyling tools use the direct current produced by batteries. The battery in your car stores electric energy. Without it, your car would not start in the morning. A **converter** (kun-VUR-tur) is an apparatus that changes direct current to alternating current. Converters usually have a plug and a cord. They allow you to use appliances outside of the salon or your home that normally would have to be plugged into an electric wall outlet. The mobile phone charger in a car is an example of a converter (**Figure 13–1**).

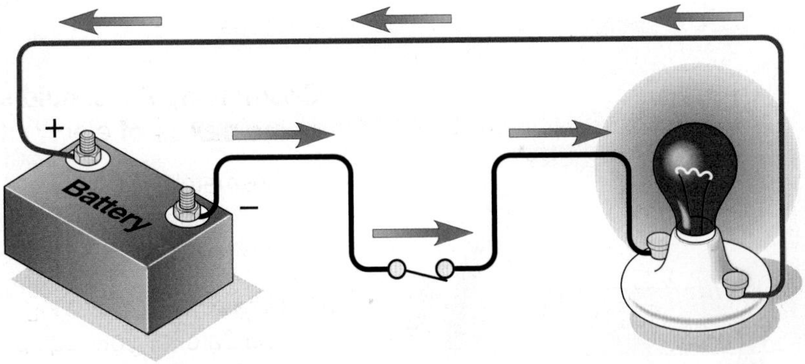

© Milady, a part of Cengage Learning.

▲ **Figure 13–1**
A complete direct current (DC) electric circuit.

Alternating current (AWL-tur-nayt-ing KUR-rent), abbreviated AC, is a rapid and interrupted current, flowing first in one direction and then in the opposite direction; it is produced by mechanical means and changes directions 60 times per second. Corded hair dryers, curling irons, electric files, and table lamps that plug into a wall outlet use alternating current. A **rectifier** (REK-ti-fy-ur) is an apparatus that changes alternating current (AC) to direct current (DC). Cordless electric clippers and mobile phone chargers use a rectifier to change the AC from an electric wall outlet to the DC needed to recharge their batteries.

did you know?

Electricity travels very fast: 186,000 miles per second. If you were to travel that fast, you could go around the world eight times in the few seconds that it takes you to turn on a light switch.

Table 13–1 outlines the differences between direct current and alternating current. ☑ **LO1**

DIRECT CURRENT (DC) AND ALTERNATING CURRENT (AC)

DIRECT CURRENT	ALTERNATING CURRENT
constant, even flow	rapid and interrupted flow
travels in one direction	travels in two directions
produced by chemical means	produced by mechanical means

© Milady, a part of Cengage Learning.

Table 13–1 **Direct Current (DC) and Alternating Current (AC).**

Electrical Measurements

The flow of an electric current can be compared to water flowing through a hose on a shampoo sink in the salon. Without pressure, neither water nor electricity would flow.

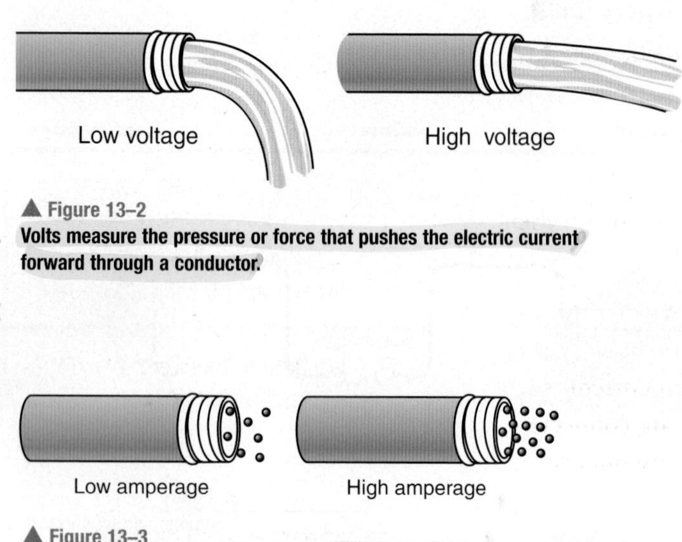

▲ **Figure 13–2**
Volts measure the pressure or force that pushes the electric current forward through a conductor.

▲ **Figure 13–3**
Amps measure the strength of the electric current.

© Milady, a part of Cengage Learning.

A **volt** (VOLT), abbreviated V and also known as **voltage** (VOL-tij), is the unit that measures the pressure or force that pushes electric current forward through a conductor (**Figure 13–2**). Car batteries are 12 volts. Normal electric wall sockets that power your hair dryer and curling iron are 120 volts. Most air conditioners and clothes dryers run on 220 volts. A higher voltage indicates more power.

An **ampere** (AM-peer), abbreviated A and also known as **amp** (AMP), is the unit that measures the strength of an electric current. Just as the sink hose must be large enough to carry the amount of water flowing through it, a wire also must be large enough to carry the amount of electricity (amps) flowing through it. A hair dryer rated at 12 amps must have a cord that is twice as thick as one rated at 6 amps; otherwise, the cord might overheat and start a fire. A higher amp rating indicates a greater number of electrons and a stronger current (**Figure 13–3**).

A **milliampere** (mil-ee-AM-peer), abbreviated mA, is $\frac{1}{1,000}$ of an ampere. The current used for facial and scalp treatments is measured in milliamperes; an ampere current would be much too strong. If used for facials and scalp treatments, ampere current would damage the skin or body.

did you know?

One kilowatt-hour will power a television for three hours, run a 100-watt bulb for twelve hours, and keep an electric clock ticking for three months.

An **ohm** (OHM), abbreviated O, is a unit that measures the resistance of an electric current. Current will not flow through a conductor unless the force (volts) is stronger than the resistance (ohms).

A **watt** (WAHT), abbreviated W, is a unit that measures how much electric energy is being used in one second. A 40-watt light bulb uses 40 watts of energy per second.

A **kilowatt** (KIL-uh-waht), abbreviated K, is 1,000 watts. The electricity in your house is measured in kilowatts per hour (kwh). A 1,000-watt (1-kilowatt) hair dryer uses 1,000 watts of energy per second. ☑ **LO2**

Electrical Equipment Safety

When working with electricity, you must always be concerned with your own safety, as well as the safety of your clients. All electrical equipment should be inspected regularly to determine whether it is in safe working order. Careless electrical connections and overloaded circuits can result in an electrical shock, a burn, or even a serious fire.

Safety Devices

A wire that is not large enough to carry the electrical current passing through it will overheat. The heating element in your hair dryer or curling iron heats up because it is not large enough to carry the electric current. Heating elements are designed to overheat and are safe when used properly, but when the electrical wires in a wall overheat, they can cause a fire. If excessive current passes through a circuit or a fuse, the circuit breaker turns off the circuit to prevent overheating.

There are two electrical safety devices that you may encounter when working in a salon:

- A **fuse** (FYOOZ) prevents excessive current from passing through a circuit. It is designed to blow out or melt when the wire becomes too hot from overloading the circuit with too much current, such as when too many appliances or faulty equipment are connected to an electricity source. To re-establish the circuit, disconnect the appliance, check all connections and insulation, insert a new fuse, then reconnect the appliance. Fuses are often found in older buildings that have not been renovated or modernized (**Figure 13–4**).
- A **circuit breaker** (SUR-kit BRAYK-ar) is a switch that automatically interrupts or shuts off an electric circuit at the first indication of an overload. Circuit breakers have replaced fuses in modern electric circuits. They have all the safety features of fuses but do not require replacement and can simply be reset by switching the circuit breaker back on. Your hair dryer has a circuit breaker located in the electric plug that is designed to protect you and your client in case of an overload or short circuit. When a circuit breaker shuts off, you should disconnect the appliance and check all connections and insulation before resetting it (**Figure 13–5**).

Grounding

Grounding (GROWND-ing) completes an electric circuit and carries the current safely away. It is another important way to promote electrical safety. All electrical appliances must have at least two rectangular electrical connections, or prongs, on the plug. This is called a two-prong plug. The two prongs supply electric current to the circuit. If you look closely at the two prongs, you will see that one is slightly larger than the other. This guarantees that the plug can be inserted only into an outlet one way and protects you and your client from an electric shock in the event of a short circuit.

For added protection, some appliances have a third circular electric connection that is a grounding pin. This is called a three-prong plug. The grounding pin is designed to guarantee a safe path of electricity

CAUTION

Underwriters Laboratories (UL) certifies the safety of electrical appliances. Curling irons, hair dryers, electric clippers, UV lamps, pedicure chairs, heating mitts, and electric files should be UL approved. This certifies that they are safe when used according to the manufacturer's directions. Always look for the UL symbol on electric appliances and take the time to read and follow the manufacturer's directions.

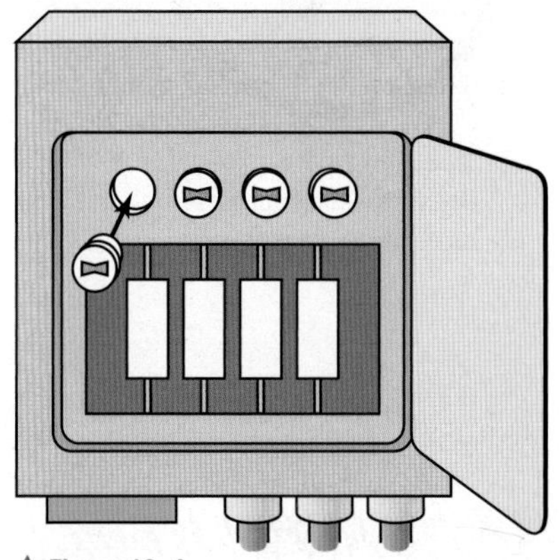

▲ Figure 13–4
Fuse box.

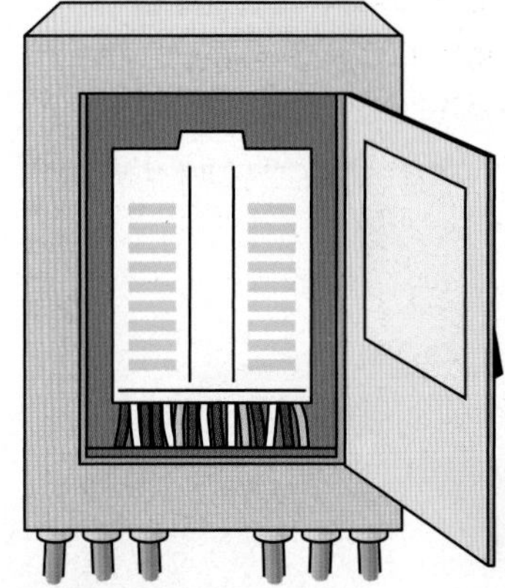

▲ Figure 13–5
Circuit breakers.

© Milady, a part of Cengage Learning.

if the plug is improperly connected. Appliances with a third circular grounding pin offer the most protection for you and your clients (**Figure 13–6**).

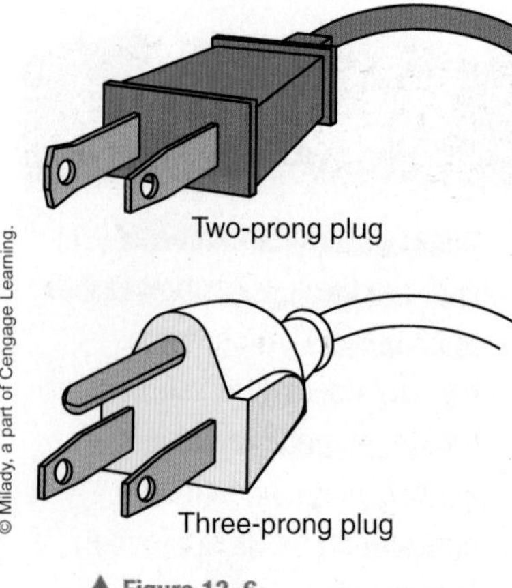

© Milady, a part of Cengage Learning.

▲ **Figure 13–6**
Two-prong and three-prong plugs.

Guidelines For Safe Use of Electrical Equipment

Salon fires are often caused by electrical problems, such as shorts in the wiring of the building or improper use of items such as appliances, extension cords, and plugs. Careful attention to electrical safety involves following recommended UL guidelines, manufacturer's directions, and the safety instructions and policies of your salon. The guidelines below will help you use electricity and electrical equipment safely.

- All the electrical appliances you use should be UL certified (**Figure 13–7**).
- Read all instructions carefully before using any piece of electrical equipment.
- Disconnect all appliances when not in use; pull on the plug, not the cord, to disconnect.
- Inspect all electrical equipment regularly.
- Keep all wires, plugs, and electrical equipment in good repair.
- Use only one plug in each outlet; overloading may cause the circuit breaker to pop. If more than one plug is needed in an area, use a power strip with a surge protector (**Figure 13–8**).

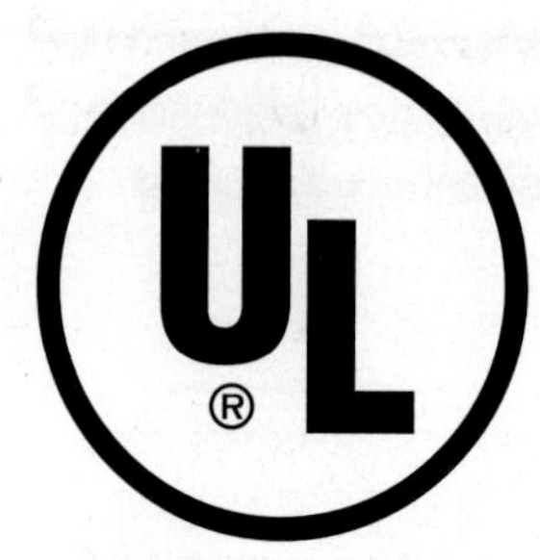

© Milady, a part of Cengage Learning.

▲ **Figure 13–7**
UL symbol, as it appears on electrical devices.

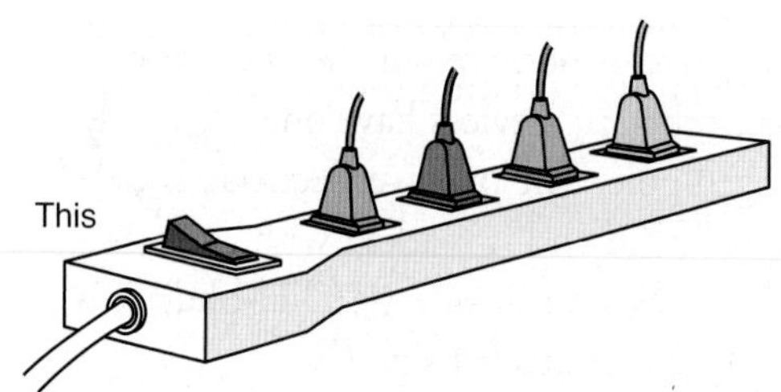

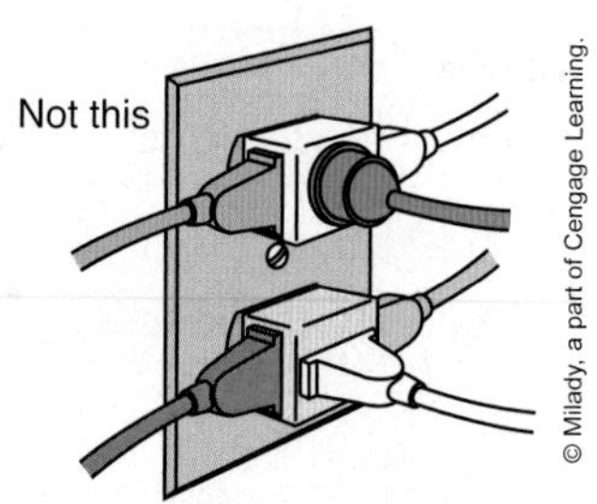

© Milady, a part of Cengage Learning.

▶ **Figure 13–8**
Use only one plug per outlet on a power strip or on the wall.

- Avoid contact, for both you and your client, with water and metal surfaces when using electricity, and do not handle electrical equipment with wet hands.
- Keep electrical cords off the floor and away from everyone's feet; getting tangled in a cord could cause you or your client to trip.
- Do not leave your client unattended while the client is connected to an electrical device.
- Do not attempt to clean around electric outlets while equipment is plugged in.
- Do not touch two metal objects at the same time if either is connected to an electric current.

© Vasilius, 2010; used under license from Shutterstock.com.

- Do not step on or place objects on electrical cords.
- Do not allow electrical cords to become twisted; this can cause a short circuit.
- Do not attempt to repair electrical appliances. If you have a problem with electric wiring or an electrical device or appliance, tell your supervisor immediately, take the device to a repair store, or call a certified electrician or repair representative to resolve the issue. ☑ LO3

CAUTION

Older buildings and homes may have two-prong wall outlets. Some equipment and tools have three-prong plugs. Never tamper with the wiring of the building or home, the wall outlets, or the plugs to make them fit your equipment and tools. Adapters are available, if it is appropriate for you to use one. Consult the manufacturer and your local hardware store about whether you can use an adapter and, if so, what type of an adapter is recommended.

Electrotherapy

The use of electrical currents to treat the skin is commonly referred to as electrotherapy (ee-lek-troh-thair-uh-pee). Currents used in electrical facial and scalp treatments are called **modalities** (MOH-dal-ih-tees). Each modality produces a different effect on the skin.

An **electrode** (ee-LEK-trohd), also known as **probe**, is an applicator for directing electric current from an electrotherapy device to the client's skin. It is usually made of carbon, glass, or metal. Each modality requires two electrodes—one negative and one positive—to conduct the flow of electricity through the body. The only exception to this rule is the Tesla high-frequency current, which is covered in more depth later in this chapter.

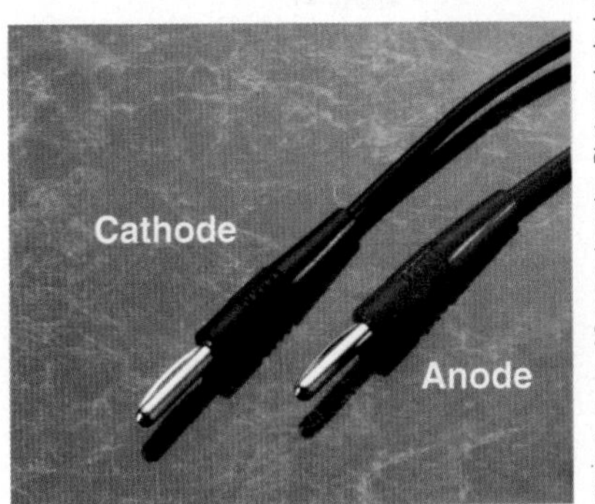

© Milady, a part of Cengage Learning. Photography by Larry Hamill.

▲ Figure 13–9
Anode and cathode.

Polarity

Polarity (poh-LAYR-ut-tee) is the negative or positive pole of an electric current. The electrodes on many electrotherapy devices have one negatively charged pole and one positively charged pole. The positive electrode is called an **anode** (AN-ohd); the anode is usually red and is marked with a *P* or a plus (+) sign. The negative electrode is called a **cathode** (KATH-ohd); it is usually black and is marked with an *N* or a minus (–) sign (**Figure 13–9**). If the electrodes are not marked, ask your instructor, salon manager, or supervisor to help you determine the positive and negative poles.

did you know?

Galvanic current is named after a doctor named Luigi Galvani who was born in Italy and lived there until his death in 1798. His studies about electric charges and how they affected the muscles of animals helped others to develop the galvanic current machines that are used in salons today.

Modalities

The main modalities used in cosmetology are galvanic current, microcurrent, and Tesla high-frequency current.

Galvanic Current

Galvanic current (gal-VAN-ik KUR-unt) is a constant and direct current, having a positive and negative pole, that produces chemical changes when it passes through the tissues and fluids of the body.

Two different chemical reactions are possible with galvanic current, depending on the polarity (positive or negative) that is used. (See

EFFECTS OF GALVANIC CURRENT	
POSITIVE POLE (ANODE) CATAPHORESIS	**NEGATIVE POLE (CATHODE) ANAPHORESIS**
produces acidic reactions	produces alkaline reactions
closes the pores	opens the pores
soothes nerves	stimulates and irritates the nerves
decreases blood supply	increases blood supply
contracts blood vessels	expands blood vessels
hardens and firms tissues	softens tissues

© Milady, a part of Cengage Learning.

Table 13–2 **Effects of Galvanic Current.**

CAUTION

Do not use negative galvanic current on skin with broken capillaries or pustular acne conditions or on clients with high blood pressure or metal implants.

Table 13–2.) The **active electrode** (AK-tiv ee-LEK-trohd) is the electrode used on the area to be treated. The **inactive electrode** (in-AK-tiv ee-LEK-trohd) is the opposite pole from the active electrode. The effects produced by the positive pole are the exact opposite of those produced by the negative pole.

Iontophoresis (eye-ahn-toh-foh-REE-sus) is the process of infusing water-soluble products into the skin with the use of electric current, such as the use of the positive and negative poles of a galvanic machine.

Cataphoresis (kat-uh-fuh-REE-sus) infuses an acidic (positive) product into deeper tissues using galvanic current from the positive pole toward the negative pole.

Anaphoresis (an-uh-for-EES-sus) infuses an alkaline (negative) product into the tissues from the negative pole toward the positive pole. **Desincrustation** (des-inkrus-TAY-shun) is a form of anaphoresis and is a process used to soften and emulsify grease deposits (oil) and blackheads in the hair follicles. Desincrustation is frequently used to treat acne, milia (small, white cyst-like pimples), and comedones (blackheads and whiteheads).

Microcurrent

Microcurrent (MY-kroh-kur-unt) is an extremely low level of electricity that mirrors the body's natural electrical impulses. Microcurrent can be used for iontophoresis, firming, toning, and soothing skin. It also can help heal inflamed tissue, such as acne.

Newer microcurrent devices have negative and positive polarity in one probe, not two probes. This allows the client to relax rather than to have to hold on to one of the probes during the service or treatment (**Figure 13–10**).

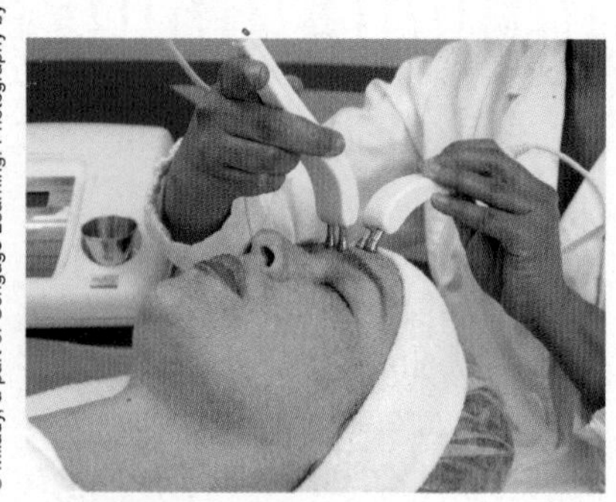

© Milady, a part of Cengage Learning. Photography by Larry Hamill.

▲ Figure 13–10
A microcurrent treatment.

Microcurrent does not travel throughout the entire body; it serves only the specific area being treated.

Microcurrent can be effective in the following ways:

- Improves blood and lymph circulation
- Produces acidic and alkaline reactions
- Opens and closes hair follicles and pores
- Increases muscle tone
- Restores elasticity
- Reduces redness and inflammation
- Minimizes healing time for acne lesions
- Improves the natural protective barrier of the skin
- Increases metabolism

When microcurrent is used during aging-skin treatments, it may give your client's skin a softer, firmer, more hydrated appearance.

CAUTION!

As with all electric current devices, microcurrent should not be used on clients with pacemakers, epilepsy, cancer, pregnancy, phlebitis, or thrombosis. It also should not be used on anyone under a physician's care for a condition that may exclude them from using certain ingredients or products or from having treatments. If you are unsure about whether it is appropriate to treat clients, ask them to obtain physician consent for the service.

Tesla High-Frequency Current

The **Tesla high-frequency current** (TES-luh HY-FREE-kwen-see KUR-ent), also known as **violet ray**, is a thermal or heat-producing current with a high rate of oscillation or vibration that is commonly used for scalp and facial treatments. Tesla current does not produce muscle contractions, and the effects can be either stimulating or soothing, depending on the method of application. The electrodes are made from either glass or metal, and only one electrode is used to perform a service (**Figure 13–11**).

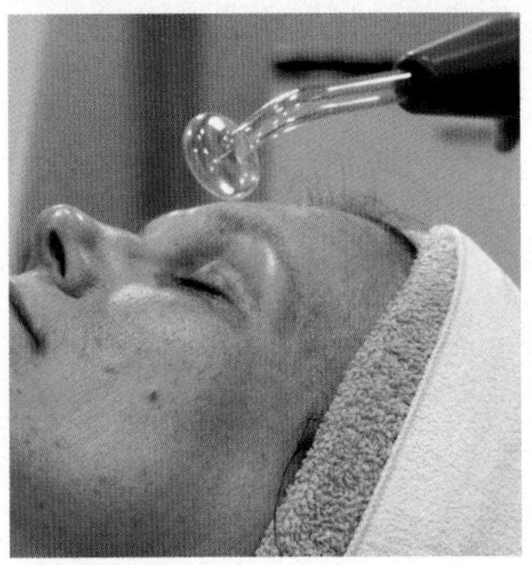

© Milady, a part of Cengage Learning.

▲ **Figure 13–11**
Applying Tesla high-frequency current with a facial electrode.

The benefits of the Tesla high-frequency current are:

- Stimulates blood circulation
- Increases elimination and absorption
- Increases skin metabolism
- Improves germicidal action
- Relieves skin congestion

As you learn more about facials and treatments, you will become familiar with the term contraindication, a condition that requires avoiding certain treatments, procedures, or products to prevent undesirable side effects. ☑ **LO4**

did you know?

The Tesla high-frequency current is named after an electrical engineer named Nikola Tesla who was born in 1856 in Croatia. He moved to the United States in 1884, where he did the majority of the work on alternating current. Tesla died in New York City in 1943.

Other Electrical Equipment

As a cosmetologist, you will be using many types of electrical equipment and tools. Here are a few of the most common electrical tools you may encounter, along with some information regarding their use:

CAUTION

Tesla high-frequency current should not be used on clients who are pregnant or who have epilepsy (seizures), asthma, high blood pressure, a sinus blockage, a pacemaker, or metal implants. The client also should avoid contact with metal, such as chair arms, jewelry, and metal bobby pins during the treatment. A burn may occur if contact is made.

- Conventional hood hair dryers or heat lamps are sources of dry heat that can be used to shorten chemical processing time. Since dry heat causes evaporation, the hair must be covered with a plastic cap to avoid drying the hair during a chemical process.
- Ionic hair dryers with the crystalline mineral tourmaline and styling irons are effective at combating static electricity and flyaway hair. When tourmaline is heated, it produces positive and negative ions that cancel the electric charges in the hair that cause static electricity. Claims that ionic dryers dry hair faster or condition hair have not been proven.
- Electric curling and flat irons are available in many types and sizes. They have built-in heating elements and plug directly into a wall outlet. Thermal styling tools now have the capacity to get extremely hot (up to 410 degrees Fahrenheit, or higher, on some styling tools). This extreme heat causes the water within the hair to boil and can severely damage hair.
- Heating caps provide a uniform source of heat and can be used with hair and scalp conditioning treatments.
- Haircolor processing machines, or accelerating machines, shorten the time it takes to process chemical hair services. These processors usually look similar to a hood dryer and dispense a hot water vapor inside the hood. A haircolor service processed with a machine at 90 degrees Fahrenheit (32 degrees Celsius) will process twice as fast as it would at a normal room temperature of 72 degrees Fahrenheit (22 degrees Celsius).
- A steamer or vaporizer produces moist, uniform heat that can be applied to the head or face. Steamers warm and cleanse the skin by increasing the flow of both oil and sweat. Some steamers also may be used for hair and scalp conditioning treatments. Estheticians often add essential oils to a facial steamer as part of a skin therapy and to enhance a client's general well-being.
- Light therapy equipment includes lasers, light-emitting diode (LED), and intense pulse light. These types of equipment are medical devices and should be used only by licensed professionals. Light therapy is described in the next section. ✓ LO5

STATE REGULATORY ALERT

Always be certain that you are in compliance with your state's regulations for licensing and use of electric current devices.

did you know?

People used to believe light traveled in straight rays, but we now know that it oscillates in wave formations, called wavelengths. The word *ray* still remains, as UV rays, UVA and UVB rays or light rays, but it represents the term *radiation*.

Light Energy and Light Therapy

The **electromagnetic spectrum** (ee-lek-troh-MAG-ne-tik SPEK-trum), also known as **electromagnetic spectrum of radiation**, is the name given to all of the forms of energy (or radiation) that exist. The forms of energy in the electromagnetic spectrum are radio waves (used by radios and televisions), microwaves (used in microwave ovens), light waves (infrared light, visible light, and ultraviolet light used for light

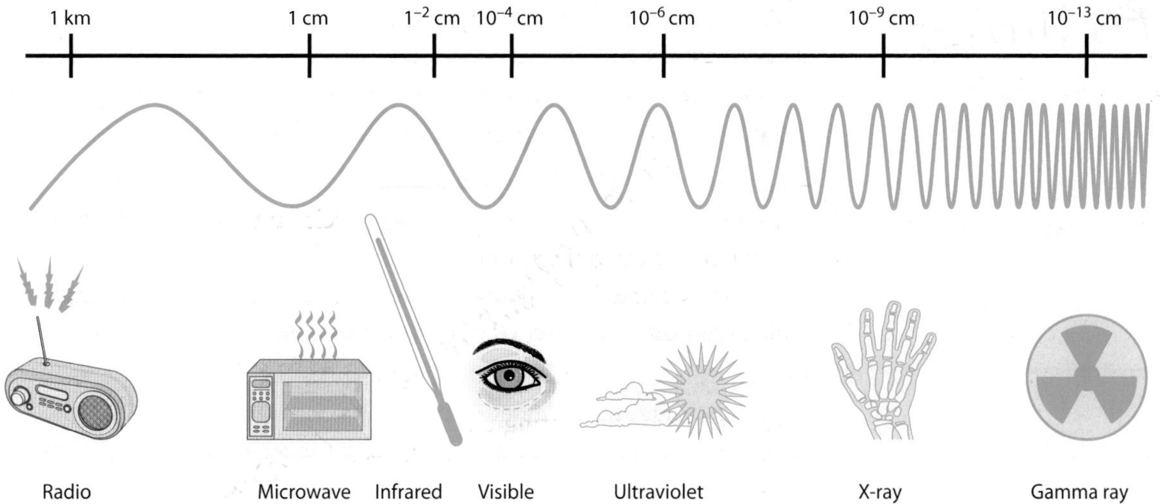

▲ **Figure 13–12**
The electromagnetic spectrum.

therapy services), X-rays (used by physicians and dentists), and gamma rays (used for nuclear power plants) (**Figure 13–12**).

Energy moves through space on waves. These waves are similar to the waves caused when a stone is dropped on the surface of water. Each type of energy has its own **wavelength**, the distance between successive peaks of electromagnetic waves. A **waveform** is the measurement of the distance between two wavelengths. Some wavelengths are long and some are short. (See **Table 13-3**, Long Wavelengths Compared With Short Wavelengths.) Long wavelengths have low frequency, meaning that the number of waves is less frequent (fewer waves) within a waveform pattern. Short wavelengths have higher frequency because the number of waves is more frequent (more waves) within a waveform pattern (**Figure 13–13**).

did you know?

Although the electric lighting in the salon is not a form of light therapy, the quality of this light can have an effect on your work and on your client's satisfaction. Fluorescent light is produced by fluorescent lamps and may be cooler (green-blue) than natural sunlight. Incandescent light is produced by standard (tungsten) light bulbs and is warmer (yellow-gold) than either natural sunlight or fluorescent light. Your client's hair and skin will appear more green-blue when viewed with fluorescent lighting and more golden when viewed with incandescent lighting.

Be careful when handling fluorescent light bulbs; they contain dangerous substances, including mercury. Avoid breaking fluorescent bulbs and dispose of used bulbs properly.

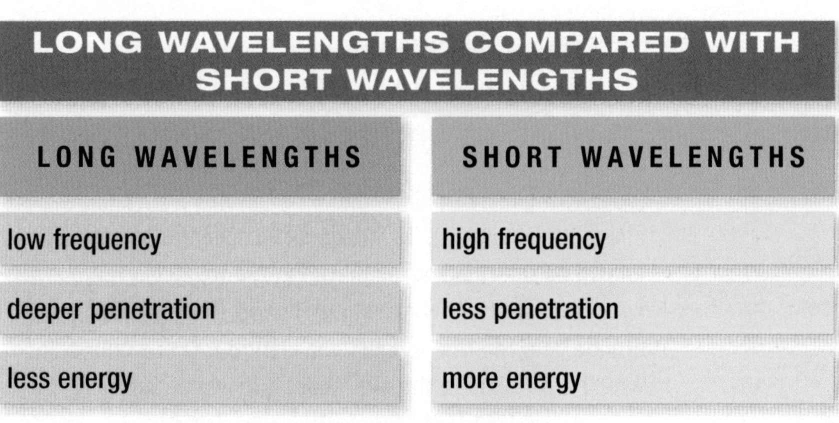

LONG WAVELENGTHS COMPARED WITH SHORT WAVELENGTHS

LONG WAVELENGTHS	SHORT WAVELENGTHS
low frequency	high frequency
deeper penetration	less penetration
less energy	more energy

Table 13–3 **Long Wavelengths Compared with Short Wavelengths.**

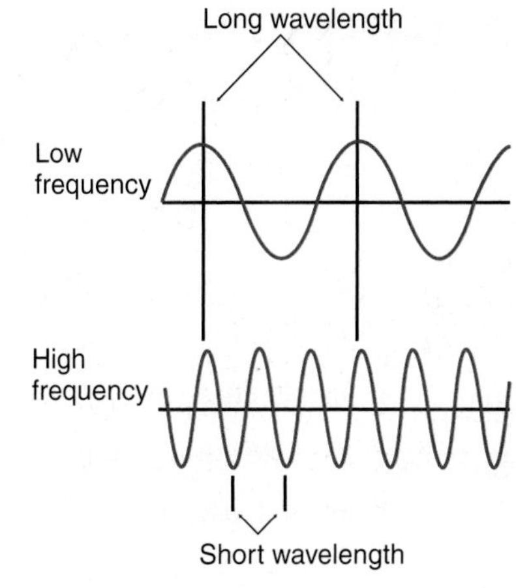

▲ **Figure 13–13**
Waveform patterns of long and short wavelengths.

© Milady, a part of Cengage Learning.

Visible Spectrum of Light

The **visible spectrum of light** is the part of the electromagnetic spectrum that can be seen. Visible light makes up only 35 percent of natural sunlight. Within the visible spectrum of light, violet has the shortest wavelength and red has the longest. The wavelength of infrared light is just below that of red light, and the wavelength of ultraviolet light is just above that of violet light.

Although they are referred to as *light*, infrared light and ultraviolet light are not really light. Ultraviolet light and infrared light, which are covered in more depth later in this chapter, are also forms of electromagnetic energy, but they are invisible because their wavelengths are beyond the visible spectrum of light. Invisible light makes up 65 percent of natural sunlight (**Figure 13–14**).

Invisible Light

Invisible light is the light at either end of the visible spectrum of light that is invisible to the naked eye. Before the visible violet light of the spectrum is ultraviolet light; it is the shortest and least penetrating light of the spectrum. Beyond the visible red light of the spectrum is infrared light, which produces heat.

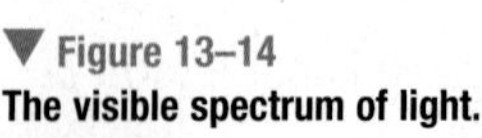

▼ **Figure 13–14**
The visible spectrum of light.

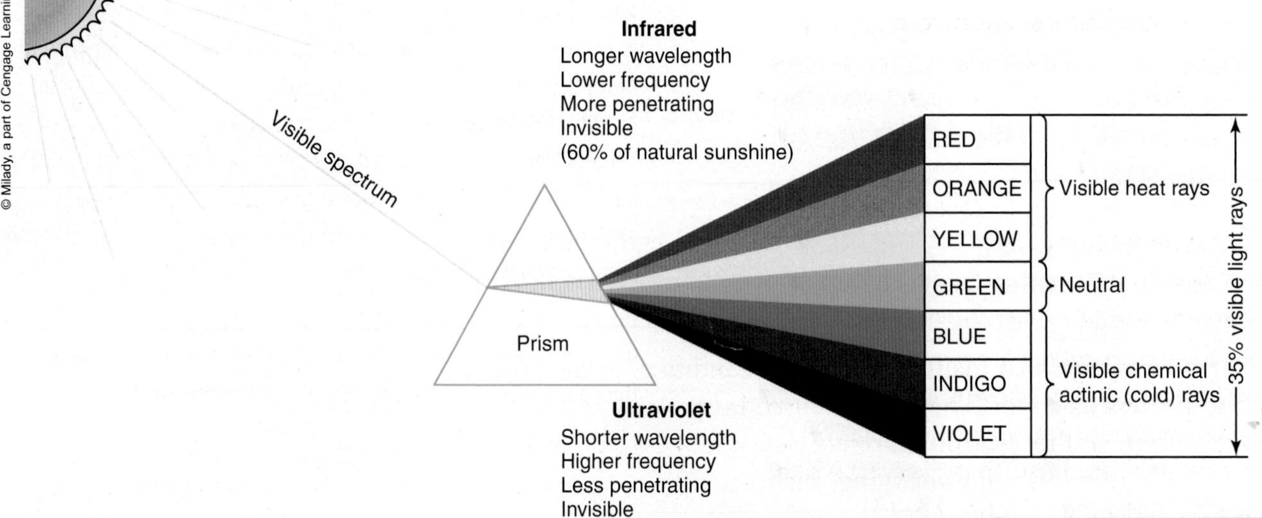

© Milady, a part of Cengage Learning.

FYI

Natural sunlight is made up of three types of light:

- Visible light = 35 percent
- Invisible infrared light = 60 percent
- Invisible ultraviolet light = 5 percent

did you know?

If light from the sun is passed through a glass prism (usually a glass or plastic prism resembles a pyramid shape after it is cut), it will appear in seven different colors, known as the rainbow, displayed in the following manner: violet (the shortest wavelength), indigo, blue, green, yellow, orange, and red (the longest wavelength). These colors, which are visible to the eye, constitute visible light.

Ultraviolet light (ul-truh-VY-uh-let LYT), abbreviated UV light and also known as **cold light** or **actinic light** (ak-TIN-ik LYT), is invisible light that has a short wavelength (giving it higher energy), is less penetrating than visible light, causes chemical reactions to happen more quickly than visible light, produces less heat than visible light, and kills some germs.

UV light prompts the skin to produce vitamin D, a fat-soluble vitamin that is good for bone growth and health. We need sunlight to survive on the planet, but overexposure to UV light can cause premature aging of the skin and skin cancer. Incidents of skin cancer have reached a near-epidemic level, with over one million new cases being diagnosed each year. It is estimated that one in five Americans will develop skin cancer and that 90 percent of those cancers will be the result of exposure to UV radiation from natural sunlight, sun lamps, and tanning beds.

There are three types of UV light:

- Ultraviolet A (UVA). Ultraviolet A light has the longest wavelength of the UV light spectrum and penetrates directly into the dermis of the skin, damaging the collagen and elastin. UVA light is the light that is often used in tanning beds.
- Ultraviolet B (UVB). Ultraviolet B light is often called the burning light because it is most associated with sunburns. Both UVA and UVB light cause skin cancers.
- Ultraviolet C (UVC). Ultraviolet C light is blocked by the ozone layer. If the Earth loses the protective layer of the ozone, life will no longer exist as we know it. We do not want to deplete the ozone layer, because it protects us from UVC radiation.

Infrared light (in-fruh-RED LYT) has longer wavelengths, penetrates more deeply, has less energy, and produces more heat than visible light. Infrared light makes up 60 percent of natural sunlight.

Infrared lamps are used mainly during hair conditioning treatments and to process haircolor. They are also used in spas and saunas for relaxation and for warming up muscles. Infrared light has been used to diminish signs of aging, such as wrinkles, to heal wounds, and to increase circulation. ☑ LO6

did you know?

Some animals can see parts of the visible spectrum that humans cannot. For example, many insects can see ultraviolet light.

CAUTION!

Although the application of UV light can be beneficial, it must be done with the utmost care in a proper manner by a qualified professional because overexposure can lead to skin damage and skin cancer. It has been used to kill bacteria on the skin and to help the body produce vitamin D. Dermatologists use UV therapy in addition to drugs for the treatment of psoriasis.

FYI

We need to strike a delicate balance with sunlight exposure. Keep in mind that tanned skin is damaged skin. Tanning will eventually cause photoaging (premature aging due to sun exposure) and irreversibly damage the skin's collagen-building properties.

Light Versus Heat and Energy

Catalysts are substances that speed up chemical reactions. Some catalysts use heat as an energy source while others use light. Whatever the energy source, catalysts absorb energy like a battery. At the appropriate time, they pass this energy to the initiator and the reaction begins.

Light Therapy

Light therapy, also known as **phototherapy**, is the application of light rays to the skin for the treatment of wrinkles, capillaries, pigmentation, or hair removal. Lasers and light therapy devices have been used for

did you know?

The wavelength of infrared light is too long to be visible to the human eye.

decades, but some of the original techniques are still valid today. Lasers are designed to focus all of the light power to a specific depth and in one direction within the skin, using the same color of light. In contrast, other light therapies have multiple depths, colors, and wavelengths and the light may be scattered. The most important point to remember about light therapy is that the equipment you use is selected based on the skin type and condition you are treating.

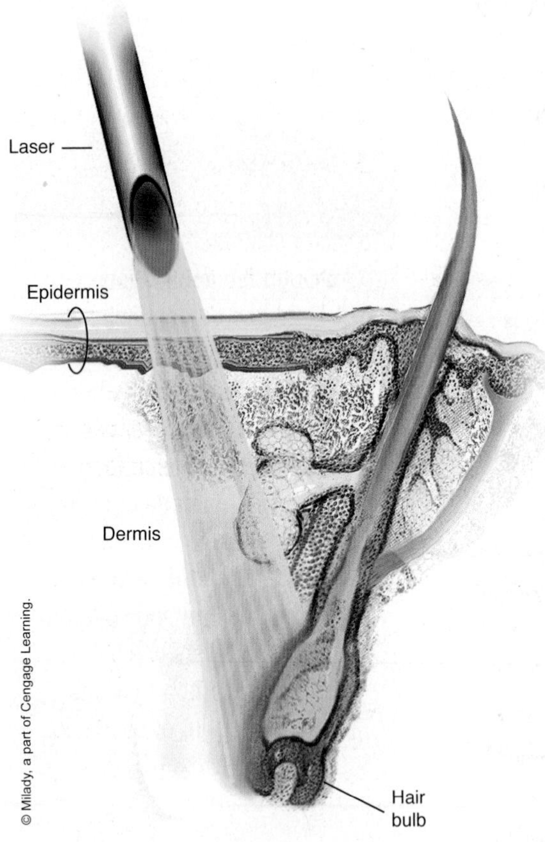

© Milady, a part of Cengage Learning.

▲ **Figure 13–15**
Some types of lasers are used for hair removal.

Lasers

Laser is an acronym for *light amplification stimulation emission of radiation*; it is a medical device that uses electromagnetic radiation for hair removal and skin treatments. There are many types of lasers used to treat a variety of skin conditions. All lasers work by selective **photothermolysis**, a process that turns the light from the laser into heat. Depending on the intended use and type, lasers can remove blood vessels, disable hair follicles, remove tattoos, or eliminate some wrinkles without destroying surrounding tissue. Lasers have been used for decades in a variety of surgical procedures (**Figure 13–15**).

Lasers work by means of a medium (solid, liquid or gas, or semiconductor) that emits light when stimulated by a power source. The medium is placed in a specifically designed chamber with mirrors located inside both ends. That chamber is stimulated by an energy source, such as electric current, which, in turn, stimulates the particles. The mirrors create light that becomes trapped and goes back and forth through the medium, gaining energy with each pass. The medium determines the wavelength of the laser and its use.

Most lasers are classified as a Level II medical device or above, which means that estheticians must be working under the supervision of a qualified physician to operate the laser.

Light-Emitting Diode (LED)

A **light-emitting diode**, abbreviated LED, is a medical device used to reduce acne, increase skin circulation, and improve the collagen content in the skin. The LED works by releasing light onto the skin to stimulate specific responses at precise depths of the skin tissue. Each color of light corresponds to a different depth—measured in one billionths of a meter, which are called nanometers—in the tissue. The LED light color seeks a color in the skin tissue known as a **chromophore**, a color component within the skin such as blood or melanin. The term chromophore is derived from the Greek term *chroma* meaning color. When the colored light reaches a specific depth in the tissue, it triggers a reaction, such as stimulating circulation or reducing bacteria.

STATE REGULATORY ALERT

Always be certain that you are in compliance with your state's regulations for the licensing and use of laser and light therapy devices.

BENEFICIAL EFFECTS OF LED THERAPY	
COLOR nm (nanometers)	**BENEFICIAL EFFECTS**
Blue light 570 nm	Reduces acne Reduces bacteria
Red light 640 nm	Increases circulation Improves collagen and elastin production Stimulates wound healing
Yellow light 590 nm	Reduces swelling and inflammation Improves lymphatic flow Detoxifies and increases circulation
Green light 525 nm	Reduces hyperpigmentation Reduces redness Calms and soothes

© Milady, a part of Cengage Learning.

Table 13–4 **Beneficial Effects of LED Therapy.**

did you know?

During space studies about 40 years ago, the National Aeronautics and Space Administration (NASA) found that LED improved the healing and growth of human tissue. These original studies have laid the foundation for light energy and LED use in skin rejuvenation.

Depending on the type of equipment used, the LED can be blue, red, yellow, or green. Blue light LED reduces acne. Red light increases circulation and improves the collagen and elastin production in the skin. Yellow light reduces swelling and inflammation and green light reduces hyperpigmentation (**Table 13-4**). Blue light LED also can be used in medical procedures performed by physicians for precancerous lesions (**Figure 13–16**).

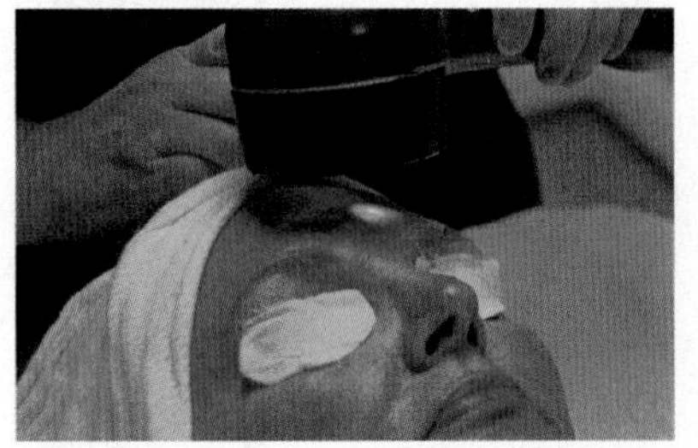

Courtesy of Revitalight.

▲ Figure 13–16
LED treatment reduces redness and improves the collagen content in skin.

As with all light therapies, it is important to be certain that you have viewed the client consultation form for any contraindications. Light therapy should not be performed on anyone who has light sensitivities (photosensitivities), phototoxic reactions, is taking antibiotics, has cancer or epilepsy, is pregnant, or is under a physician's care. If you are not sure whether you should treat certain clients, refer them to their physicians.

Intense Pulse Light

Intense pulse light is a medical device that uses multiple colors and wavelengths (broad spectrum) of focused light to treat spider veins, hyperpigmentation, rosacea and redness, wrinkles, enlarged hair follicles and pores, and excessive hair. As with most devices, multiple treatments are required. These treatments are provided only under the supervision of a qualified physician.

From dermatologists using UV therapy for treating psoriasis to estheticians using blue light therapy for acne to surgeons using lasers for advanced surgical procedures, the power of light therapy is here to stay. ☑ **LO7**

WEB RESOURCES

For more information on electricity and energy, visit the U.S. Energy Information Administration's Web site at http://www.eia.doe.gov or the Library of Congress' Web site at http://www.loc.gov and enter the search words *electricity* or *energy.*

Review Questions

1. Define electric current.
2. Explain the difference between a conductor and a nonconductor (insulator).
3. Describe the two types of electric current and give examples of each.
4. Explain the difference between a volt and an amp.
5. Define ohm.
6. Define watt and kilowatt.
7. Explain the function of a fuse.
8. What is the purpose of a circuit breaker?
9. What is the purpose of grounding?
10. List at least five steps to take for electrical safety.
11. List and describe the three main electric modalities (currents) used in cosmetology.
12. List the other types of electrical equipment that cosmetologists use and describe how to use them.
13. Define the terms electromagnetic spectrum, visible light, and invisible light.
14. Why must exposure to ultraviolet (UV) light be monitored carefully?
15. What do the acronyms laser and LED represent?
16. List and describe the three main types of light therapy.

Chapter Glossary

active electrode	Electrode of an electrotherapy device that is used on the area to be treated.
alternating current	Abbreviated AC; rapid and interrupted current, flowing first in one direction and then in the opposite direction; produced by mechanical means and changes directions 60 times per second.
ampere	Abbreviated A and also known as *amp*; unit that measures the strength of an electric current.
anaphoresis	Process of infusing an alkaline (negative) product into the tissues from the negative pole toward the positive pole.
anode	Positive electrode of an electrotherapy device; the anode is usually red and is marked with a *P* or a plus (+) sign.
catalysts	Substances that speed up chemical reactions.
cataphoresis	Process of fusing an acidic (positive) product into deeper tissues using galvanic current from the positive pole toward the negative pole.
cathode	Negative electrode of an electrotherapy device; the cathode is usually black and is marked with an *N* or a minus (–) sign.
chromophore	A color component within the skin such as blood or melanin.
circuit breaker	Switch that automatically interrupts or shuts off an electric circuit at the first indication of overload.

Chapter Glossary

complete electric circuit	The path of negative and positive electric currents moving from the generating source through the conductors and back to the generating source.
conductor	Any material that conducts electricity.
converter	Apparatus that changes direct current to alternating current.
desincrustation	A form of anaphoresis; process used to soften and emulsify grease deposits (oil) and blackheads in the hair follicles.
direct current	Abbreviated DC; constant, even-flowing current that travels in one direction only and is produced by chemical means.
electric current	Flow of electricity along a conductor.
electricity	The movement of particles around an atom that creates pure energy.
electrode	Also known as *probe*; applicator for directing electric current from an electrotherapy device to the client's skin.
electromagnetic spectrum	Also known as *electromagnetic spectrum of radiation*; name given to all of the forms of energy (or radiation) that exist.
fuse	Prevents excessive current from passing through a circuit.
galvanic current	Constant and direct current, having a positive and negative pole, that produces chemical changes when it passes through the tissues and fluids of the body.
grounding	Completes an electric circuit and carries the current safely away.
inactive electrode	Opposite pole from the active electrode.
infrared light	Infrared light has longer wavelengths, penetrates more deeply, has less energy, and produces more heat than visible light; makes up 60 percent of natural sunlight.
intense pulse light	A medical device that uses multiple colors and wavelengths (broad spectrum) of focused light to treat spider veins, hyperpigmentation, rosacea and redness, wrinkles, enlarged hair follicles and pores, and excessive hair.
invisible light	Light at either end of the visible spectrum of light that is invisible to the naked eye.
iontophoresis	Process of infusing water-soluble products into the skin with the use of electric current, such as the use of the positive and negative poles of a galvanic machine.
kilowatt	Abbreviated K; 1,000 watts.
laser	Acronym for *light amplification stimulation emission of radiation*; a medical device that uses electromagnetic radiation for hair removal and skin treatments.
light-emitting diode	Abbreviated LED; a medical device used to reduce acne, increase skin circulation, and improve the collagen content in the skin.
light therapy	Also known as *phototherapy*; the application of light rays to the skin for the treatment of wrinkles, capillaries, pigmentation, or hair removal.

Chapter Glossary

microcurrent	An extremely low level of electricity that mirrors the body's natural electrical impulses.
milliampere	Abbreviated mA; $^1/_{1,000}$ of an ampere.
modalities	Currents used in electrical facial and scalp treatments.
nonconductor	Also known as *insulator*; a material that does not transmit electricity.
ohm	Abbreviated O; unit that measures the resistance of an electric current.
photothermolysis	Process that turns the light from a medical laser device into heat.
polarity	Negative pole or positive pole of an electric current.
rectifier	Apparatus that changes alternating current (AC) to direct current (DC).
Tesla high-frequency current	Also known as *violet ray*; thermal or heat-producing current with a high rate of oscillation or vibration that is commonly used for scalp and facial treatments.
ultraviolet light	Abbreviated UV light and also known as *cold light* or *actinic light*; invisible light that has a short wavelength (giving it higher energy), is less penetrating than visible light, causes chemical reactions to happen more quickly than visible light, produces less heat than visible light, and kills germs.
visible spectrum of light	The part of the electromagnetic spectrum that can be seen. Visible light makes up only 35 percent of natural sunlight.
volt	Abbreviated V and also known as *voltage*; unit that measures the pressure or force that pushes electric current forward through a conductor.
watt	Abbreviated W; unit that measures how much electric energy is being used in one second.
waveform	Measurement of the distance between two wavelengths.
wavelength	Distance between successive peaks of electromagnetic waves.

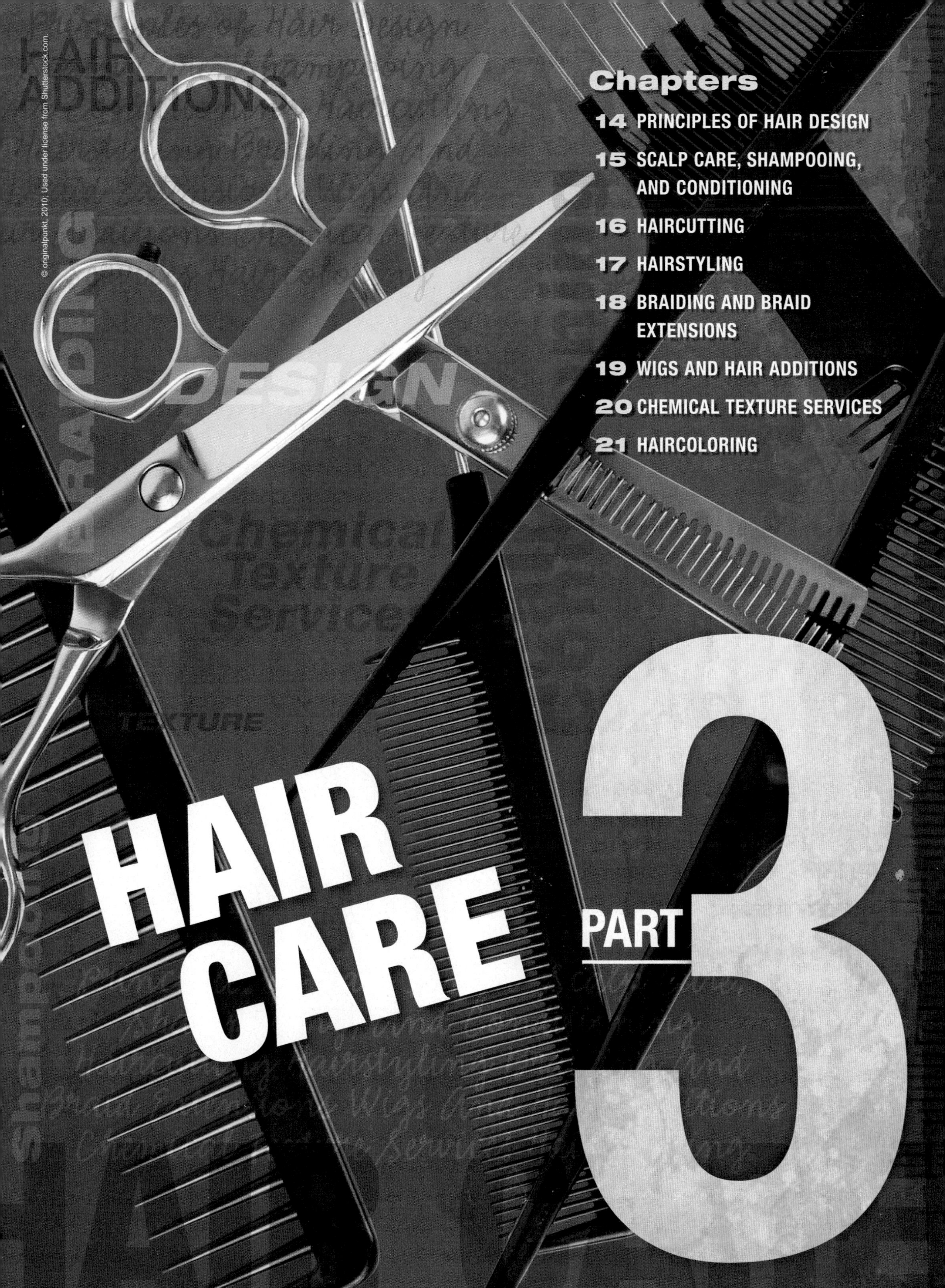

PART 3 HAIR CARE

Chapters

© originalpunkt, 2010. Used under license from Shutterstock.com.

CHAPTER 14

Principles of Hair Design

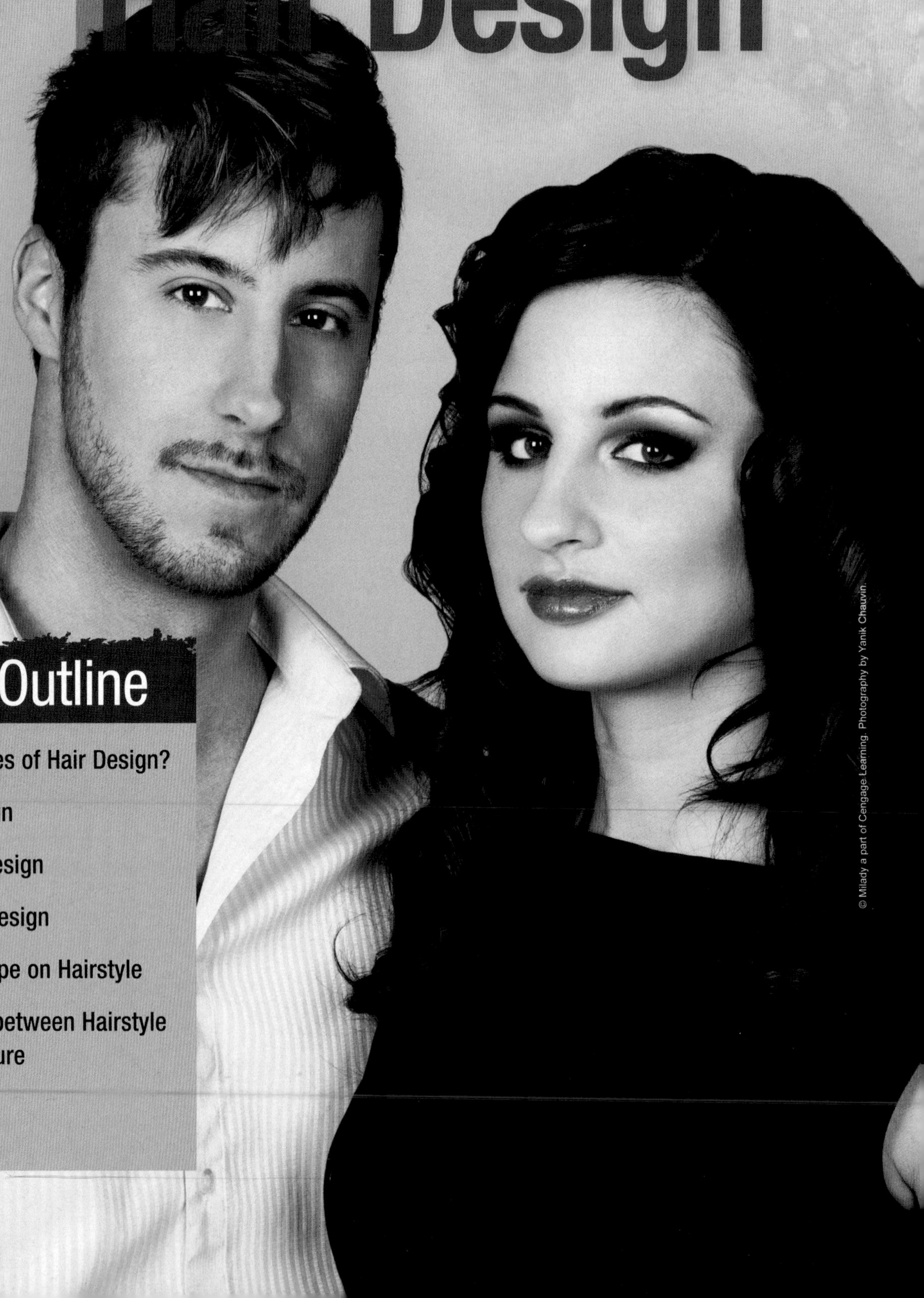

© Milady a part of Cengage Learning. Photography by Yanik Chauvin.

Chapter Outline

Learning Objectives

After completing this chapter, you will be able to:

- ✓ **LO1** Describe the possible sources of hair design inspiration.
- ✓ **LO2** List the five elements of hair design.
- ✓ **LO3** List the five principles of hair design.
- ✓ **LO4** Understand the influence of hair type on hairstyle.
- ✓ **LO5** Identify different facial shapes and demonstrate how to design hairstyles to enhance or camouflage facial features.
- ✓ **LO6** Explain design considerations for men.

Key Terms

Page number indicates where in the chapter the term is used.

asymmetrical balance
pg. 292

balance
pg. 291

bang area (fringe area)
pg. 302

concave profile
pg. 299

contrasting lines
pg. 286

convex profile
pg. 299

curved lines
pg. 286

design texture
pg. 287

diagonal lines
pg. 286

directional lines
pg. 287

emphasis (focus)
pg. 292

form
pg. 287

harmony
pg. 293

horizontal lines
pg. 285

parallel lines
pg. 286

profile
pg. 298

proportion
pg. 290

rhythm
pg. 292

single lines
pg. 286

space
pg. 287

straight profile
pg. 298

symmetrical balance
pg. 291

transitional lines
pg. 287

vertical lines
pg. 286

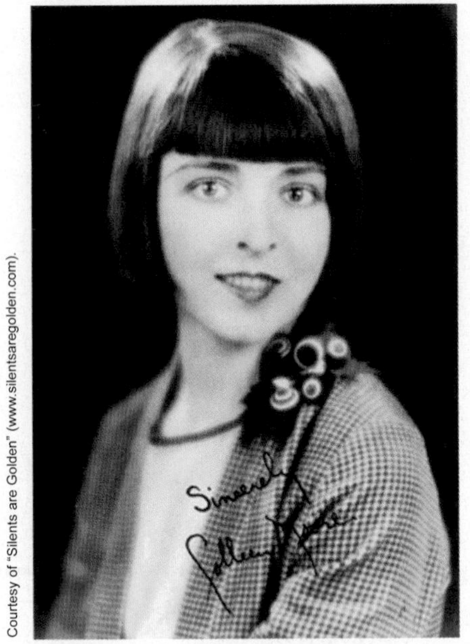

Courtesy of "Silents are Golden" (www.silentsaregolden.com).

▲ **Figure 14–1**
Colleen Moore, 1920s film star—the original flapper introduces the bob.

Design is the foundation of all artistic applications. All artists—architects, fashion designers, and interior designers, among many others—have a strong visual eye. The odds are that you do too, since you have chosen to pursue a career in the beauty industry.

Do you want to be known as a good stylist or a great one? As a stylist, your goal is to learn how to design the best hairstyle for your client. That process begins with analyzing the entire person by using the elements and principles of design to enhance positive features and minimize negative ones. An understanding of design and art principles will help you develop the artistic skill and judgment needed to create the best possible design for your client.

WHY STUDY PRINCIPLES OF HAIR DESIGN?

As a cosmetologist, you should study and have a thorough understanding of the principles of hair design because:

- You will be better able to understand why a particular hairstyle will or will not be the best choice for a client.
- The principles of design will serve as helpful guidelines to assist you in achieving your styling vision.
- You will be able to create haircuts and styles designed to help clients camouflage unattractive features while emphasizing attractive ones.

▼ **Figure14–2**
Contemporary bob.

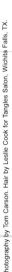

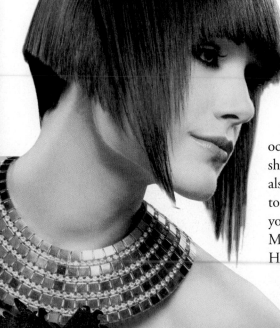

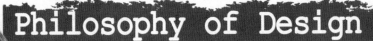

Photography by Tom Carson. Hair by Leslie Cook for Tangles Salon, Wichita Falls, TX.

Philosophy of Design

A good designer always envisions the end result before beginning. For example, when an architect designs a building, she first visualizes the final product. Then she completes drawings, and takes the necessary steps to create the design in a model.

Inspiration can come from almost anywhere, at any time. Movies, TV, magazines, videos, a person on the street—anything, anywhere—can spark the creative process. One of the best sources of inspiration can be found in nature. The rhythm and movement of ocean waves have inspired painters, poets, composers, and hairstylists. The shapes, colors, patterns, and textures of plants, animals, and minerals are also a great source of visual ideas. At times, you may find yourself looking to the past for inspiration. A hairstyle from an earlier era might inspire you to reinvent it in a way that works for today (**Figures 14–1** and **14–2**). Modern inspiration in fashion often starts on the streets and in the clubs. Hair design usually follows fashion trends to create the total look.

Once inspired, you will need to decide which tools and techniques—such as cutting shears, flat irons, permanent wave, and so forth—

are needed to achieve your design. It is always a good idea when working out a design to first practice on a mannequin head. As you develop or practice a technique, there is always the chance that your original concept will turn into something entirely different. There are no failures if the experience is a lesson learned. If you are open to change, the creative process will be exciting and satisfying.

© Milady, a part of Cengage Learning.

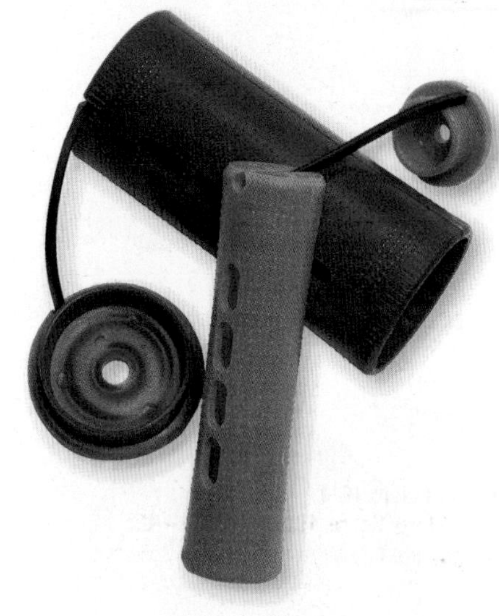

As a designer, you will need to develop a visual understanding of which hairstyles work best on different face shapes and body types. It takes time and experience to train your eye to recognize the best design decision. You cannot achieve a trained eye simply through book learning. It may help you to review these pages over and over, but do not get frustrated if it takes a while to understand this chapter. Sometimes the best teacher is time and the trial and error process that comes through experience. All good stylists have made a significant number of design mistakes in the past—great stylists learn and grow from each experience. Having a strong design foundation will help make you a great stylist. Once you have these skills, your creative juices will kick in and you can move beyond the basics.

Having a strong foundation in technique and skills will allow you to take calculated risks. It is important in this field to take those risks. Too many stylists confine themselves to the basics, where they feel safe. But "safe" can translate into "dull." If you are looking for a satisfying, long-term career, do not allow yourself to become what is known in the beauty industry as a *cookie-cutter* hair designer who learns a new haircut and then gives it to everyone who sits in his or her chair for the next month. Always explore new possibilities, and customize your design to each client's individual needs and lifestyle. Think outside of the box! Great hairstylists find inspiration everywhere by keeping an eye out for what is new in the beauty industry and by dedicating themselves to their continuing education. You can keep growing by having your eyes and mind always open to learning. ☑ **LO1**

Elements of Hair Design

To begin to understand the creative process involved in hairstyling, it is critical to learn the five basic elements of three-dimensional design. These elements are line, form, space, texture, and color.

Line

Line defines form and space. The presence of one nearly always means that the other two are involved. Lines create the shape, design, and movement of a hairstyle. The eye follows the lines in a design. They can be straight or curved. There are four basic types of lines:

Horizontal lines create width in hair design. They extend in the same direction and maintain a constant distance apart—from the floor or horizon (**Figure 14–3**).

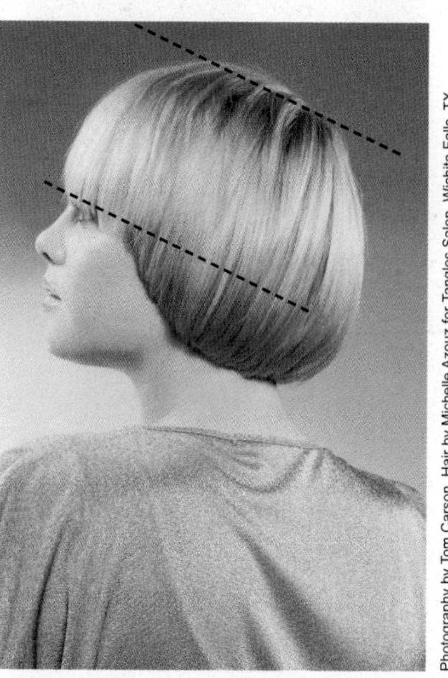

Photography by Tom Carson. Hair by Michelle Azouz for Tangles Salon, Wichita Falls, TX.

▲ **Figure 14–3**
Horizontal lines create width in a hairstyle.

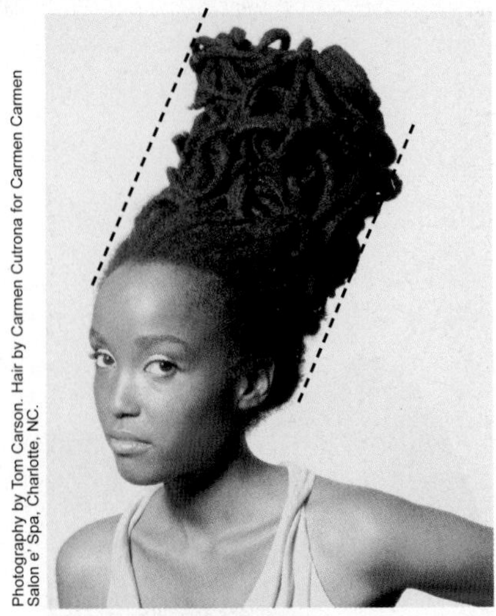

Photography by Tom Carson. Hair by Carmen Cutrona for Carmen Carmen Salon e' Spa, Charlotte, NC.

▲ **Figure 14–4**
Vertical lines in a hairstyle.

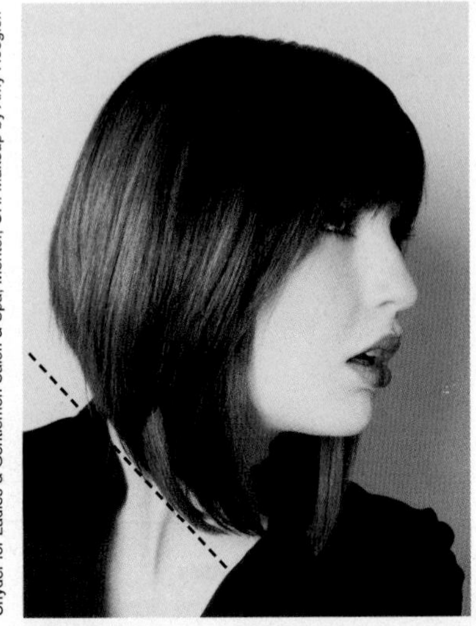

Photography by Tom Carson. Hair by Mike Pavlick, Jen Roskey, Holly Brown, & Jen Snyder for Ladies & Gentlemen Salon & Spa, Mentor, OH. Makeup by Amy Hoegler.

▲ **Figure 14–5**
Diagonal lines can create interest in a hairstyle.

Vertical lines create length and height in hair design. They make a hairstyle appear longer and narrower as the eye follows the lines up and down (**Figure 14–4**).

Diagonal lines are positioned between horizontal and vertical lines. They are often used to emphasize or minimize facial features. Diagonal lines are also used to create interest in hair design (**Figure 14–5**).

Curved lines, lines moving in a circular or semi-circular direction, soften a design. They can be large or small, a full circle, or just part of a circle (**Figure 14–6**). Curved lines may move in a clockwise or counter-clockwise direction. They can be placed horizontally, vertically, or diagonally. Curved lines repeating in opposite directions create a wave (**Figure 14–7**).

Designing with Lines

Hairstyles are created by the type of line, direction, or combination you choose:

Single lines. An example of this is the one-length hairstyle. These hairstyles are best for clients requiring the lowest maintenance when styling their hair (**Figure 14–8**).

Parallel lines are repeating lines in a hairstyle. They can be straight or curved. The repetition of lines creates more interest in the design. A finger wave is an example of a style using curved, parallel lines (**Figure 14–9**).

Contrasting lines are horizontal and vertical lines that meet at a 90-degree angle. These lines create a hard edge. Contrasting lines in a design are usually for clients able to carry off a strong look (**Figure 14–10**).

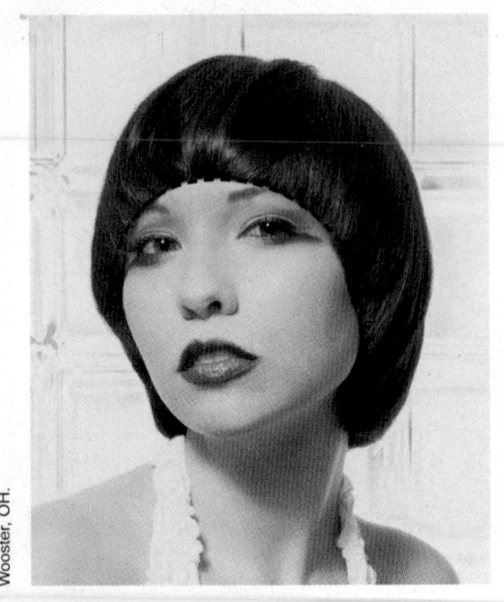

Photography by Tom Carson. Hair by Sandra Carr for Sheer Professionals, Wooster, OH.

▲ **Figure 14–6**
Curved lines can soften a hairstyle.

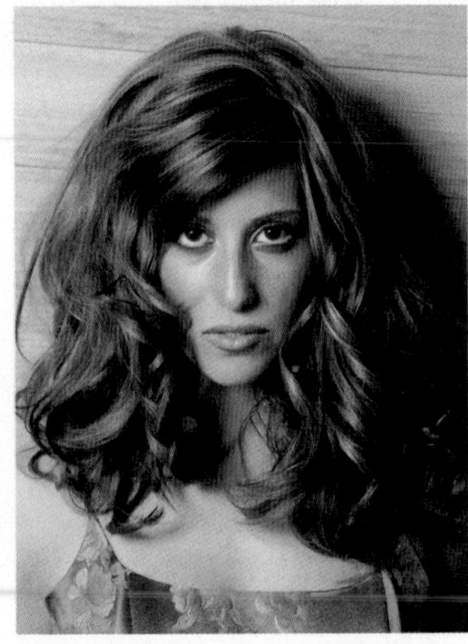

Photography by Tom Carson. Hair by Randy Currie for Currie Hair, Skin & Nails, Glen Mills, PA. Makeup by Jessica Moss.

▲ **Figure 14–7**
Wave.

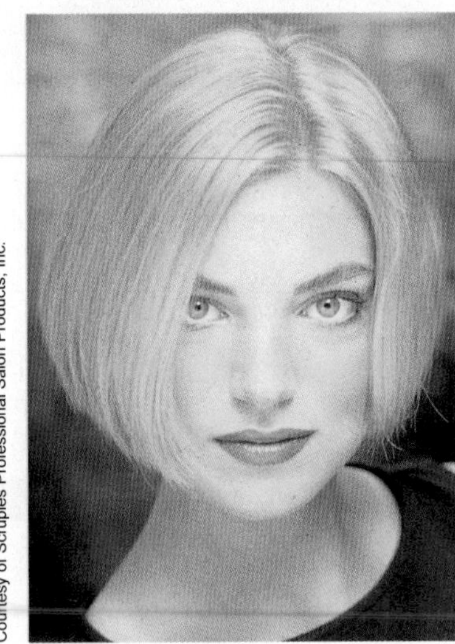

Courtesy of Scruples Professional Salon Products, Inc.

▲ **Figure 14–8**
Single-line hairstyle.

Transitional lines are usually curved lines that are used to blend and soften horizontal or vertical lines (**Figure 14–11**).

Directional lines are lines with a definite forward or backward movement.

Form

Form is the mass or general outline of a hairstyle. It is three-dimensional and has length, width, and depth. Form or mass may also be called volume. The silhouette is usually the part of the overall design that a client will respond to first. Generally, simple forms are best to use and are more pleasing to the eye. The hair form should be in proportion to the shape of the head and face, the length and width of the neck, and the shoulder line (**Figure 14–12**).

Space

Space is the area surrounding the form or the area the hairstyle occupies. We are more aware of the (positive) form than the (negative) spaces. In hair design, with every movement the relationship of the form and space change. A hairstylist must keep every angle in mind—not only of the forms being created, but of the spaces surrounding the forms as well. The space may contain curls, curves, waves, straight hair, or any combination.

Design Texture

Design texture refers to wave patterns that must be taken into consideration when designing a style for your client. All hair has a natural wave pattern—straight, wavy, curly, or extremely curly. For example, straight hair reflects light better than other wave patterns, and straight hair reflects the most light when it is cut to a single length (**Figure 14–13**). Wavy hair can be combed into waves that

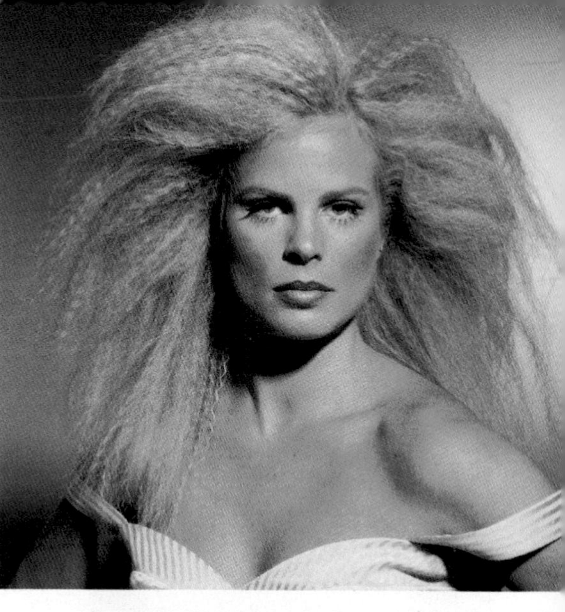

Photography by Tom Carson. Hair by Carmen Cutrona for Carmen Carmen Salon e' Spa, Charlotte, NC.

▲ **Figure 14–9**
Repeating lines in a hairstyle.

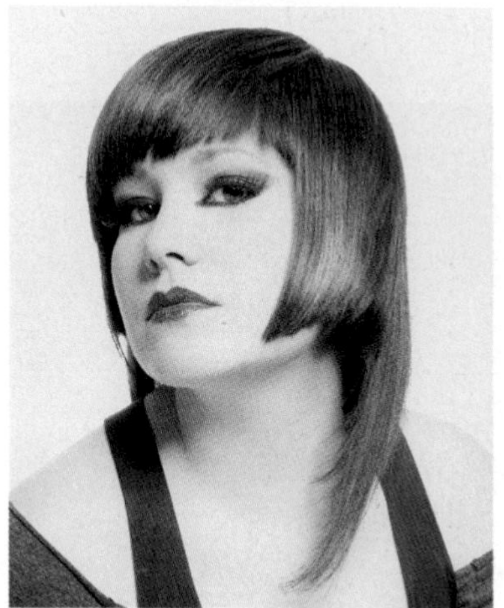

Photography by Tom Carson. Hair by Glynn Jones for Glynn Jones Salon, Alexandra, VA. Makeup by Christopher Wilson.

▲ **Figure 14–10**
Contrasting lines.

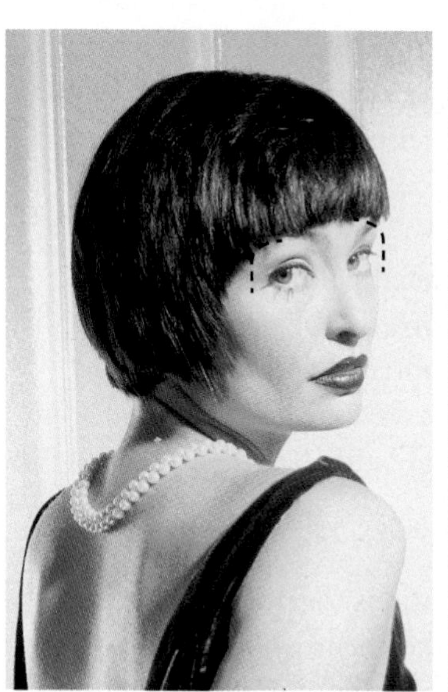

Photography by Tom Carson. Hair by Randy Currie for Currie Hair, Skin & Nails, Glen Mills, PA. Makeup by Michah Price.

▲ **Figure 14–11**
Transitional lines.

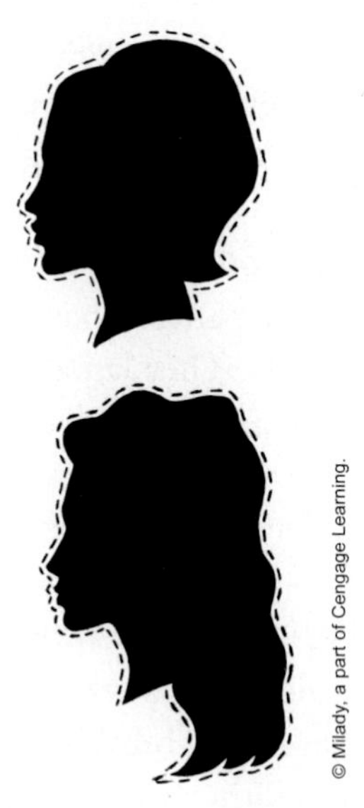

© Milady, a part of Cengage Learning.

▲ **Figure 14–12**
The outline of the hairstyle is the form.

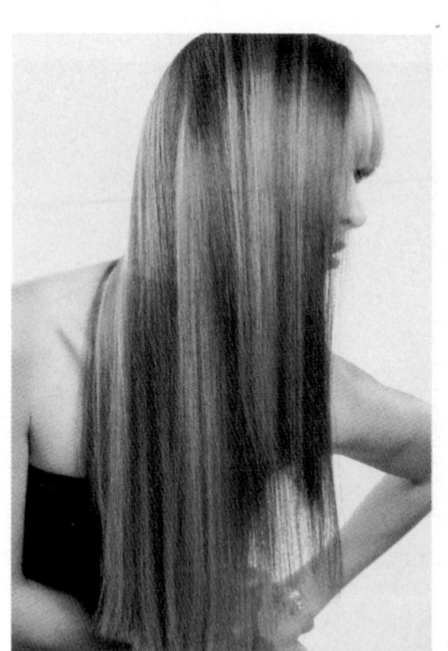

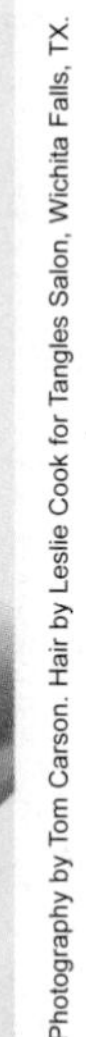

Photography by Tom Carson. Hair by Leslie Cook for Tangles Salon, Wichita Falls, TX.

▲ **Figure 14–13**
Straight hair.

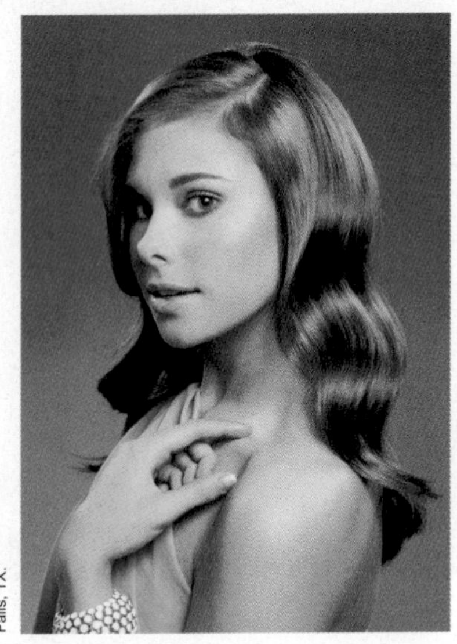

Photography by Tom Carson. Hair by Chase Williams for Tangles Salon, Wichita Falls, TX.

▲ **Figure 14–14**
Wavy hair.

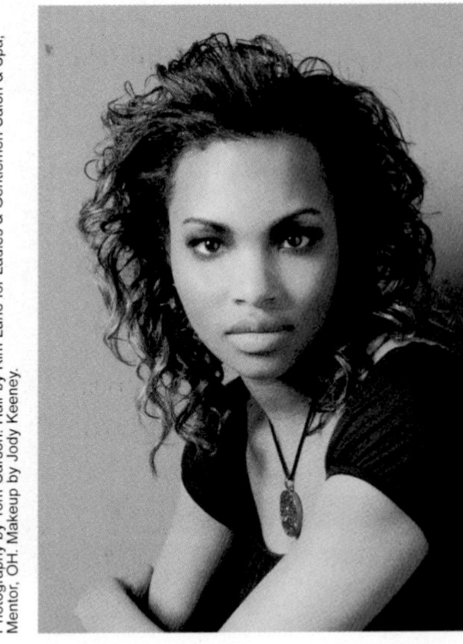

Photography by Tom Carson. Hair by Kim Lane for Ladies & Gentlemen Salon & Spa, Mentor, OH. Makeup by Jody Keeney.

▲ **Figure 14–15**
Curly hair.

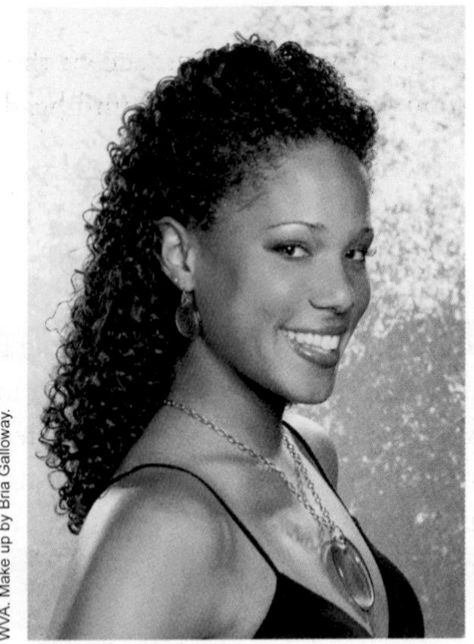

Photography by Tom Carson. Hair by Bria Galloway for Frederick's Day Spa, Wheeling, WVA. Make up by Bria Galloway.

▲ **Figure 14–16**
Very curly hair.

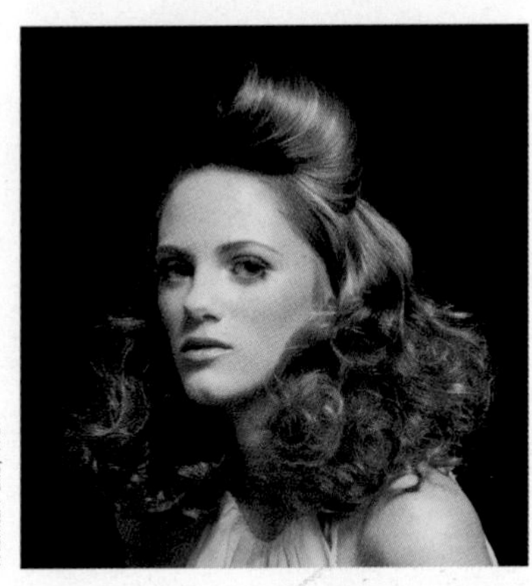

Photography by Tom Carson. Hair by Robin Cook for Tangles Salon, Wichita Falls, TX.

▲ **Figure 14–17**
Wave patterns can be altered temporarily.

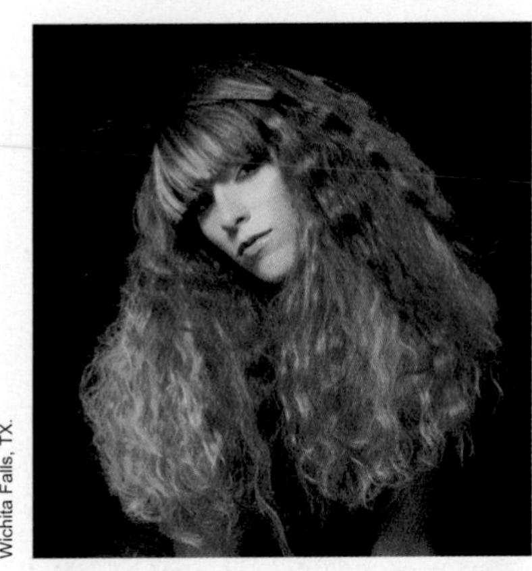

Photography by Tom Carson. Hair by Leslie Cook for Tangles Salon, Wichita Falls, TX.

▲ **Figure 14–18**
Combining wave patterns.

create horizontal lines (**Figure 14–14**). Curly hair and extremely curly hair do not reflect much light and can be coarse to the touch. Curly hair creates a larger form than straight or wavy hair does (**Figures 14–15** and **14–16**).

Creating Design Texture with Styling Tools

Texture can be created temporarily with the use of heat and/or wet styling techniques. Curling irons or hot rollers can be used to create a wave or curl.

Curly hair can be straightened with a blowdryer or flat iron (**Figure 14–17**).

Crimping irons are used to create interesting and unusual wave patterns like zigzags. Hair can also be wet-set with rollers or pincurls to create curls and waves. Finger waves, braids, and locks are another way of creating temporary textured pattern changes (**Figures 14–18** to **14–20**). You will learn more about styling techniques in subsequent chapters.

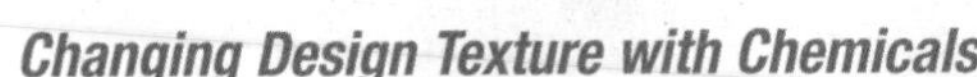

Changing Design Texture with Chemicals

Chemical wave pattern changes are considered permanent (**Figure 14–21**). They last until the new growth of hair is long enough to alter the design. Curly hair can be straightened with relaxers, and straight hair can be curled with permanent waves. These techniques are covered in detail in Chapter 20, Chemical Texture Services.

Tips for Designing with Wave Patterns

- When using many wave pattern combinations together, you create a look that is very busy. This is fine for the client who wants to achieve a multitextured look, but may be less appropriate for more conservative professionals.

- Smooth wave patterns accent the face and are particularly useful when you wish to narrow a round head shape (**Figure 14–22**).
- Curly wave patterns take attention away from the face and can be used to soften square or rectangular features (**Figure 14–23**).

Haircolor

Haircolor plays an important role in hair design, both visually and psychologically. It can be used to make all or part of the design appear larger or smaller. Haircolor can help define texture and line, and it can tie design elements together. In Chapter 21, Haircoloring, you will learn more about enhancing hair design, using haircolor as an important element.

Dimension with Color

Light colors and warm colors create the illusion of volume. Dark and cool colors recede or move in toward the head, creating the illusion of less volume. The illusion of dimension, or depth, is created when colors that are lighter and warmer alternate with those that are darker and cooler (**Figures 14–24** and **14–25**).

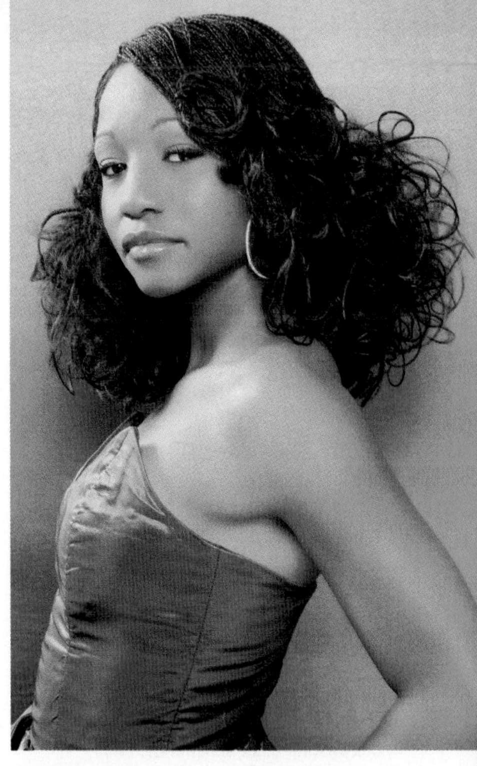

Photography by Tom Carson. Hair by Marissa Bender for The Ohio Academy Paul Mitchell Partner School, Columbus, OH.

▲ **Figure 14–19**
Fine braids create temporary waves.

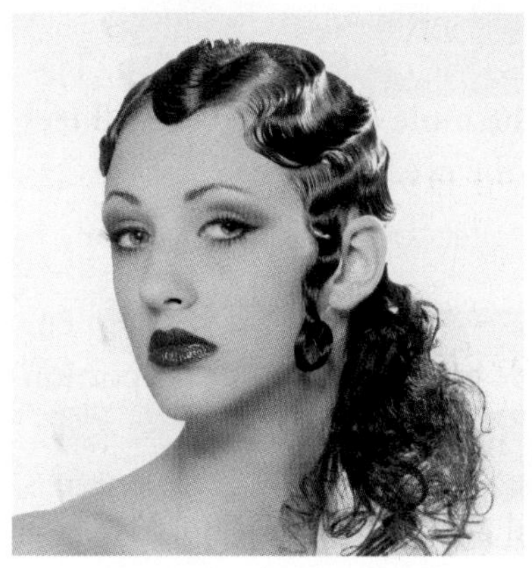

Photography by Tom Carson. Hair by Lauren Surace, Makeup by Haley Steigerwald for The Ohio Academy Paul Mitchell Partner School, Twinsburg, OH.

▲ **Figure 14–20**
Finger waves and curls.

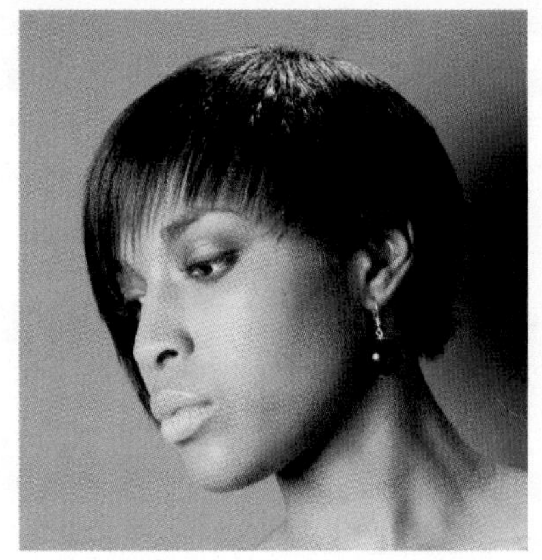

Photography by Tom Carson. Hair by Kim Lane for Ladies & Gentlemen Salon & Spa, Mentor, OH. Makeup by Jody Keeney.

▲ **Figure 14–21**
Chemically altered hairstyle.

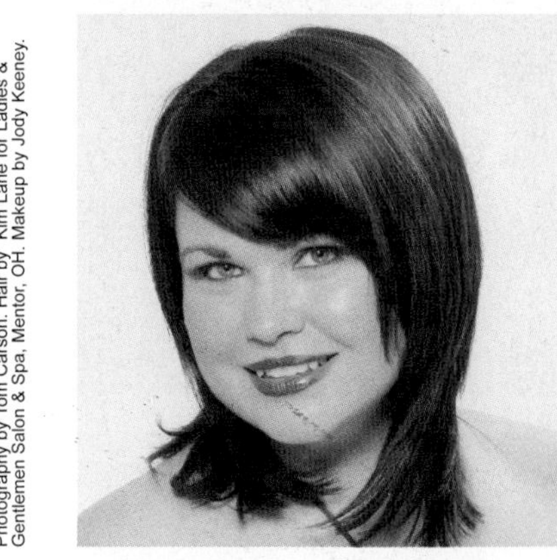

Photography by Tom Carson. Hair by Sheer Professionals, Wooster, OH.

▲ **Figure 14–22**
Straight wave patterns are flattering on the round face.

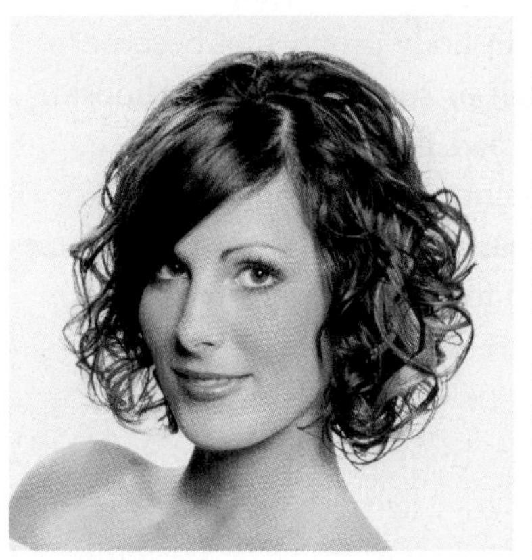

Photography by Tom Carson. Hair by Felicia Gonzales. Makeup by Cassie LaMountain for Attitudes A Salon, Toledo, OH.

▲ **Figure 14–23**
Curly wave patterns soften angular faces.

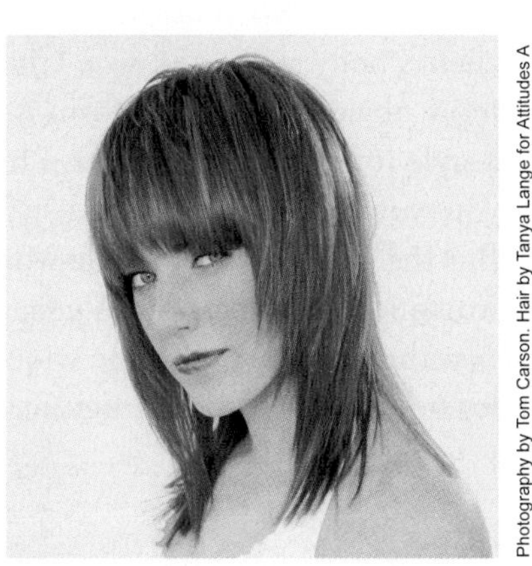

Photography by Tom Carson. Hair by Tanya Lange for Attitudes A Salon, Sylvania, OH. Makeup by Kim Bowers.

▲ **Figure 14–24**
Light colors appear closer to the surface.

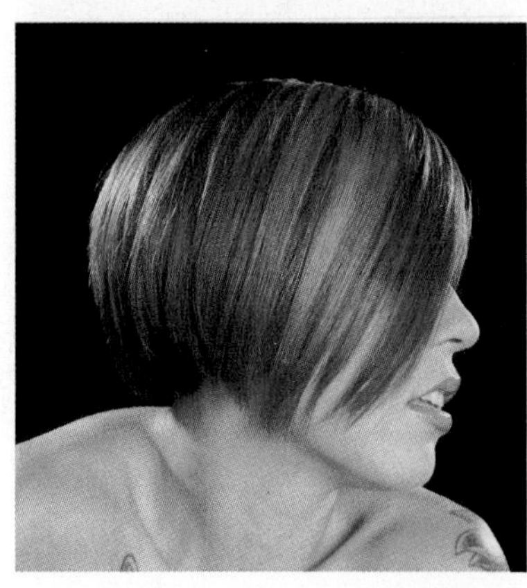

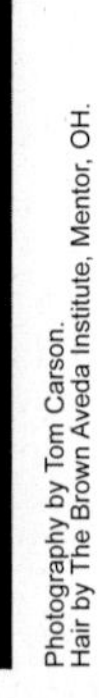

▲ **Figure 14–25**
Creating dimension with color.

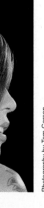

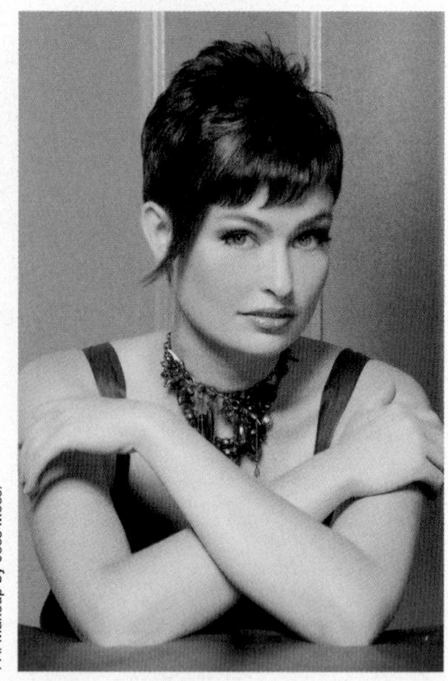

Photography by Tom Carson. Hair by Randy Currie for Currie Hair, Skin & Nail Salon, Glen Mills, PA. Makeup by Jess Moss.

▲ **Figure 14–26**
Contrasting color accents the line.

Lines wth Color

Because the eye is drawn to the lightest color, you can use a light color to draw a line in a hairstyle in the direction you want the eye to travel. A single line of color, or a series of repeated lines of color, can create a bold, dramatic accent (**Figure 14–26**).

Color Selection

When choosing a color, be sure that the tone is compatible with the skin tone of the client. If a client has a gold tone to her skin, warm haircolors are more flattering than cool haircolors. For a more conservative or natural look when using two or more colors, choose colors with similar tones within two levels of each other. When using high contrast colors in most salon situations, you should use one color sparingly. A strong contrast can create an attention-grabbing look and should only be used on clients who are trendy and can carry off a bold look (**Figure 14–27**). ☑ **LO2**

Principles of Hair Design

Five important principles in art and design—proportion, balance, rhythm, emphasis, and harmony—are also the basis of hair design. The better you understand these principles, the more confident you will feel about creating styles that are pleasing to the eye.

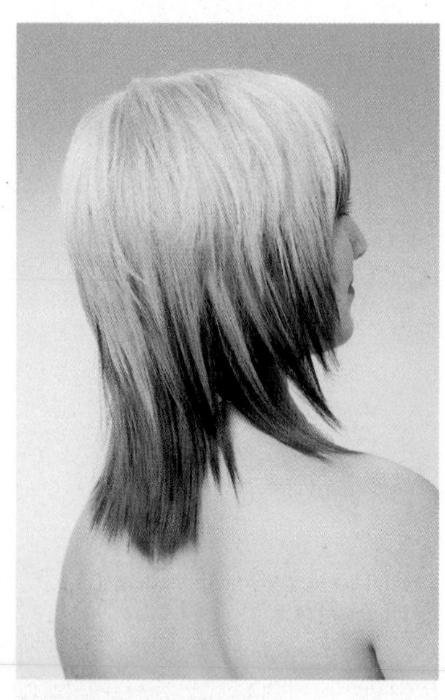

Photography by Tom Carson. Hair by Shannan DeTullio for Bella Capelli Sanctuario, Westlake, OH. Makeup by Shannan DeTullio.

▲ **Figure 14–27**
Strong color contrast.

Proportion

Proportion is the comparative relationship of one thing to another. For example, a 60-inch television set might be considered out of proportion or scale in a very small bedroom. A person with a very small chin and a very wide forehead might be said to have a head shape that is not in proportion. A well-chosen hairstyle could create the illusion of better proportion for such a client.

Body Proportion

It is essential when designing a hairstyle that you take into account the client's body shape and size. Challenges in body proportion become more obvious if the hair form is too small or too large. When choosing a style for a woman with large hips or broad shoulders, for instance, you would normally create a style with more volume (**Figure 14–28**). But the same large hair style would appear out of proportion on a petite woman (**Figure 14–29**). A general guide for classic proportion is that the hair should not be wider than the center of the shoulders, regardless of the body structure.

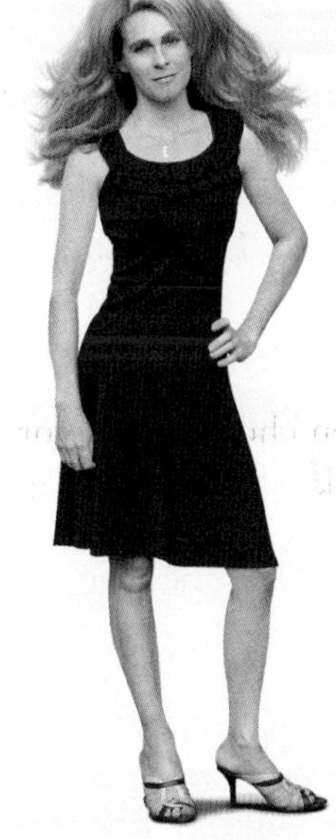

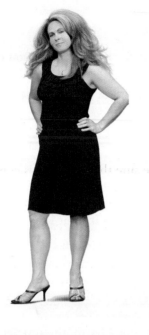

© Milady, a part of Cengage Learning.

▶ Figure 14–28
A large hairstyle balances a large body structure.

◀ Figure 14–29
A large hairstyle makes a petite woman look smaller.

Balance

Balance is establishing equal or appropriate proportions to create symmetry. In hairstyling, it can be the proportion of height to width. Balance can be symmetrical or asymmetrical. Often when you are dissatisfied with a finished hair design, it is because the style is out of balance.

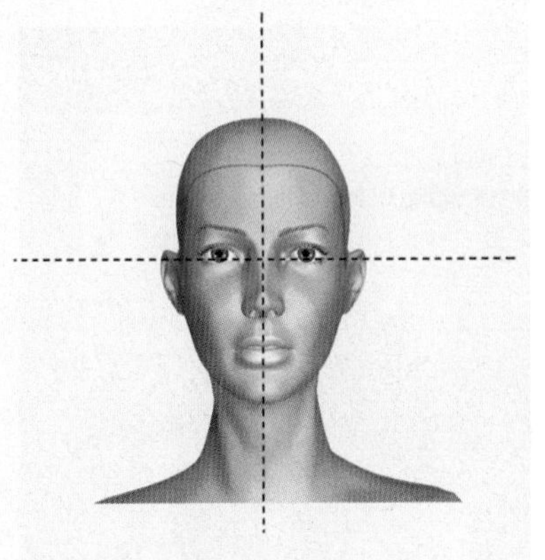

© Milady, a part of Cengage Learning.

▲ Figure 14–30
Measuring symmetry of the head.

To measure symmetry, divide the face into four equal parts. The lines cross at the central axis, the reference point for judging the balance of the hair design. You can then decide if the hairstyle looks pleasing to the eye and is in correct balance (**Figure 14–30**).

Symmetrical balance occurs when an imaginary line is drawn through the center of the face and the two resulting halves form a mirror image of one another. Both sides of the hairstyle are the same distance from the center, the same length, and have the same volume when viewed from the front (**Figures 14–31** to **14–33**).

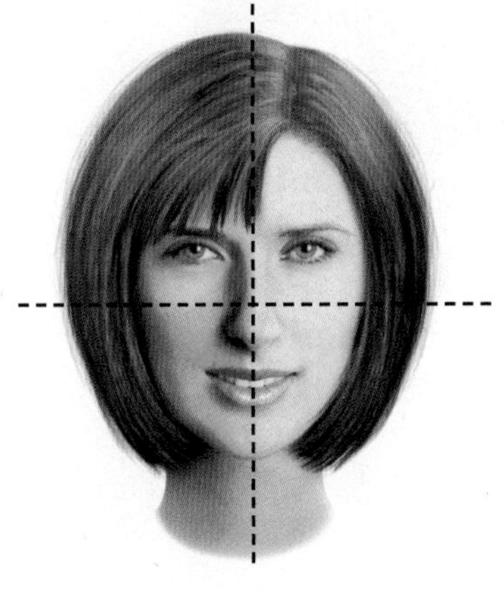

© Milady, a part of Cengage Learning.

▲ Figure 14–31
Both sides equidistant from center.

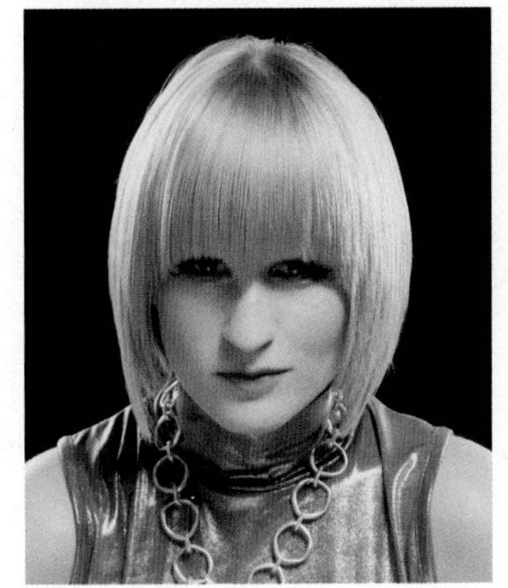

Photography by Tom Carson. Hair by Leslie Cook for Tangles Salon, Wichita Falls, TX.

▲ Figure 14–32
Perfect symmetry.

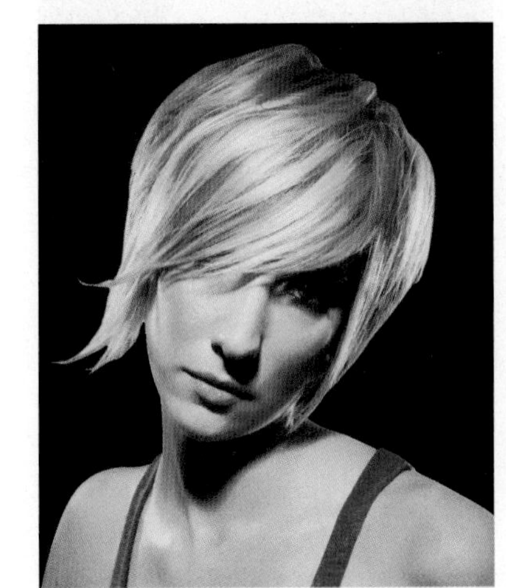

Photography by Tom Carson. Hair & makeup by Breanna Keiter for Ladies & Gentlemen Salon & Spa, Lyndhurst, OH.

▲ Figure 14–33
Symmetry with different shapes, same volume.

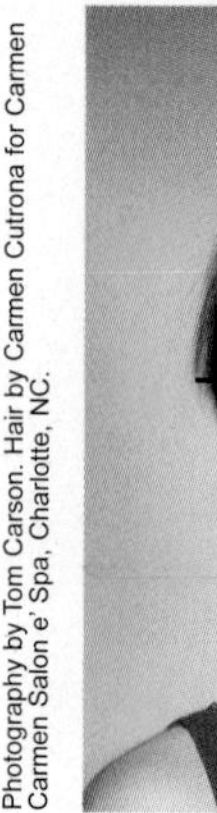
Photography by Tom Carson. Hair by Carmen Cutrona for Carmen Carmen Salon'e' Spa, Charlotte, NC.

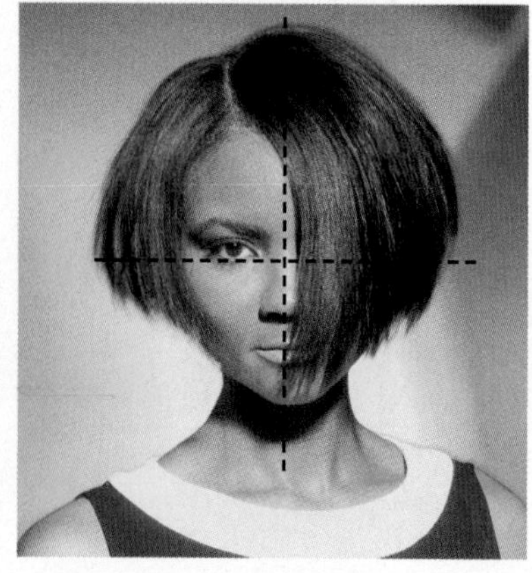

▲ **Figure 14–34**
Horizontal asymmetry.

Photography by Tom Carson. Hair by Alishia West Steigerwald for The Ohio Academy Paul Mitchell Partner School, Twinsburg, OH.

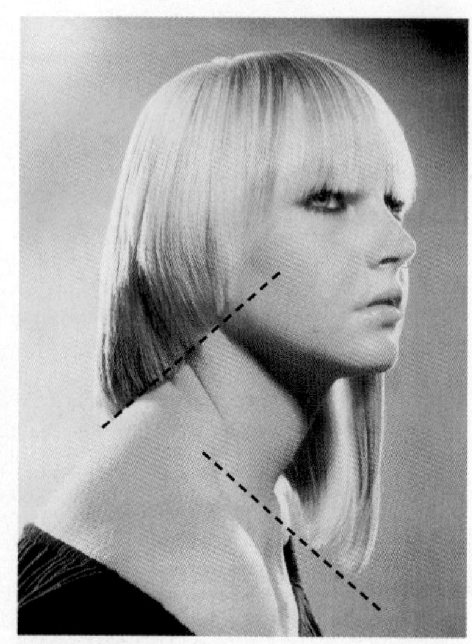

▲ **Figure 14–35**
Diagonal asymmetry.

Asymmetrical balance is established when the two imaginary halves of a hairstyle have an equal visual weight, but are positioned unevenly. Opposite sides of the hairstyle are different lengths or have a different volume. Asymmetry can be horizontal or diagonal (**Figures 14–34** and **14–35**).

Rhythm

Rhythm is a regular pulsation or recurrent pattern of movement in a design. In music or dance, rhythm can be fast or slow. In hair design, a fast rhythm moves quickly; tight curls are an example. A slow rhythm can be seen in larger shapings or long waves (**Figures 14–36** and **14–37**).

Emphasis

The **emphasis**, also known as **focus**, in a design is what draws the eye first, before it travels to the rest of the design. A hairstyle may be well balanced, with good rhythm and harmony, and yet still be boring. Create interest with an area of emphasis or focus by using the following:

- Wave patterns (**Figure 14–38**)
- Color (**Figure 14–39**)
- Change in form (**Figure 14–40**)
- Ornamentation (**Figure 14–41**)

Choose an area of the head or face that you want to emphasize. Keep the design simple so that it is easy for the eye to follow from the point of emphasis through to the rest of the style. You can have multiple points of emphasis as long as you do not use too many and as long as they are decreasing in size and importance. Remember, less is more.

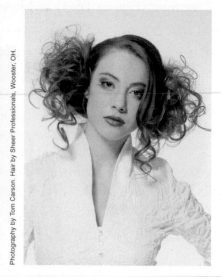

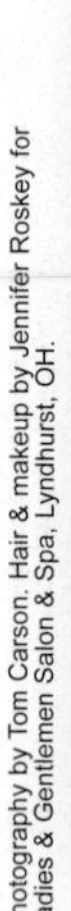
Photography by Tom Carson. Hair & makeup by Jennifer Roskey for Ladies & Gentlemen Salon & Spa, Lyndhurst, OH.

▲ **Figure 14–36**
Fast rhythm.

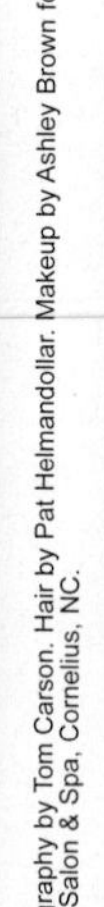
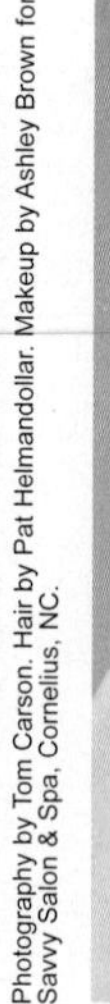
Photography by Tom Carson. Hair by Pat Helmandollar. Makeup by Ashley Brown for Savvy Salon & Spa, Cornelius, NC.

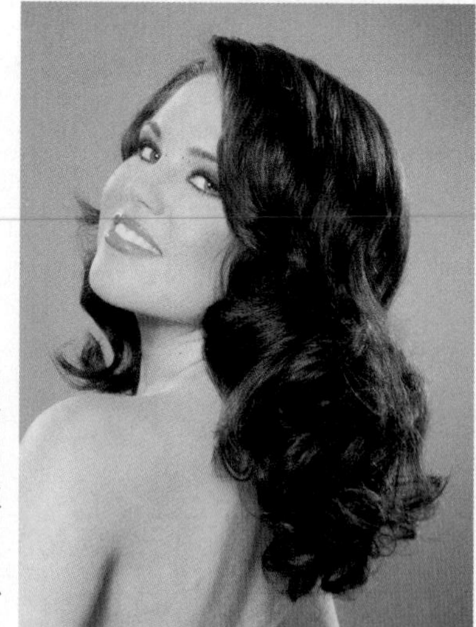
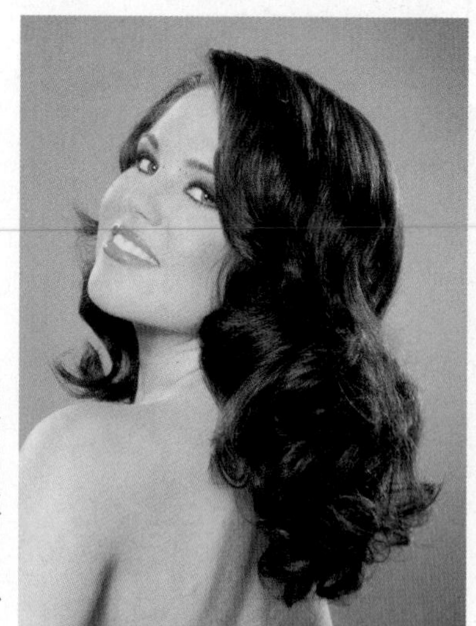

▲ **Figure 14–37**
Slow rhythm.

Photography by Tom Carson. Hair by Sheer Professionals, Wooster, OH.

▲ **Figure 14–38**
Creating emphasis with various wave patterns.

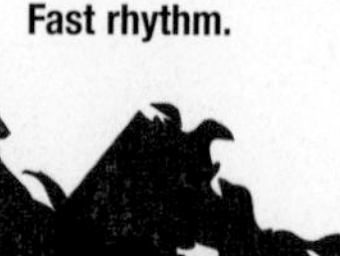

Harmony

Harmony is the creation of unity in a design and is the most important of the art principles. Harmony holds all the elements of the design together. When a hairstyle is harmonious it has the following elements:

- A form with interesting lines
- A pleasing color or combination of colors and textures
- A balance and rhythm that together strengthen the design

A harmonious design is never too busy, and it is in proportion to the client's facial and body structure. A successful harmonious design includes an area of emphasis from which the eyes move to the rest of the style.

The principles of design may be used in modern hairstyling and makeup to guide you as you decide how best to achieve a beautiful appearance for your client. The best results are obtained when each of your client's facial features is properly analyzed for its strengths and weaknesses. Your job is to accentuate a client's best features and to downplay features that do not add to the person's appearance. Every hairstyle you create for every client should be properly proportioned to body type and correctly balanced to the person's head and facial features. The hairstyle should attractively frame the client's face. An artistic and suitable hairstyle will take into account physical characteristics such as the following:

- Shape of the head, including the front view (face shape), profile, and back view
- Features (perfect as well as imperfect features)
- Body posture ☑ **LO3**

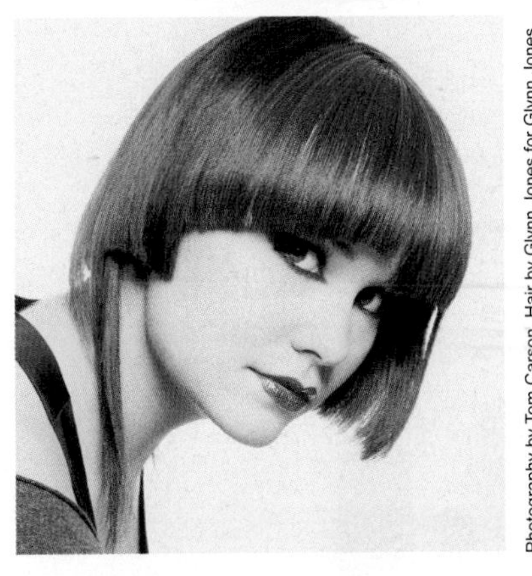

▲ **Figure 14–39**
Creating emphasis with color.

Photography by Tom Carson. Hair by Glynn Jones for Glynn Jones Salon, Alexandria, VA. Makeup by Christopher Wilson.

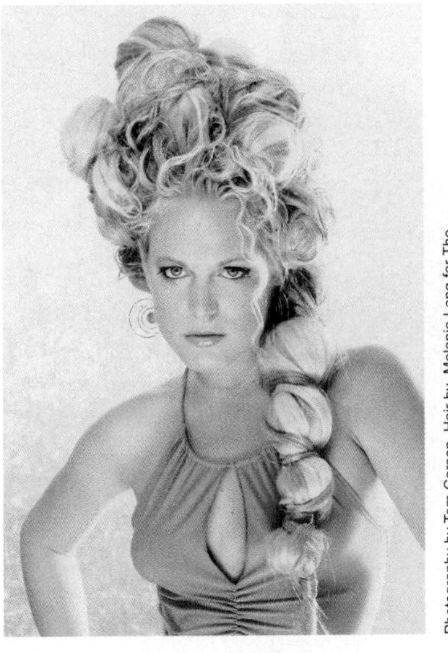

▲ **Figure 14–40**
Creating emphasis with form changes.

Photography by Tom Carson. Hair by Melanie Long for The Ohio Academy Paul Mitchell Partner School, Columbus, OH.

Influence of Hair Type on Hairstyle

Your client's hair type is a major consideration in the selection of a hairstyle. Hair type is categorized by two defining characteristics: wave patterns and hair texture.

All hair has natural wave patterns that must be taken into consideration when designing a style. These wave patterns are straight, wavy, curly, and extremely curly. Hair texture, density, and the relationship between the two are also important factors in choosing a style. The basic hair textures are: fine, medium, and coarse. Hair density, or hair per square inch, ranges from very thin to very thick.

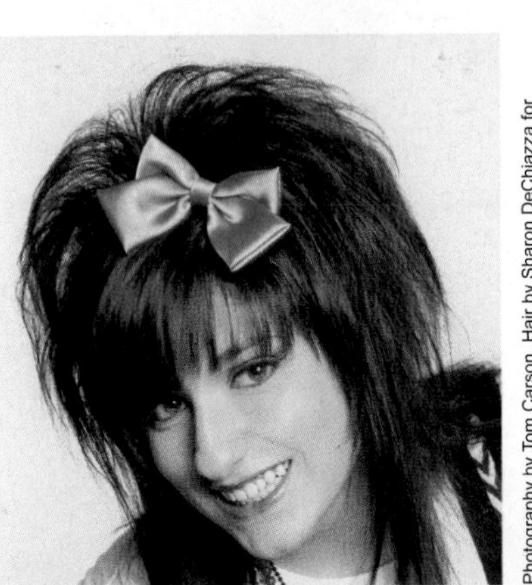

▲ **Figure 14–41**
Ornament as focal point.

Photography by Tom Carson. Hair by Sharon DeChiazza for Frederick's Day Spa, Wheeling, WVA. Makeup by Sharon DeChiazza.

Keep in mind the following guidelines for different types of hair:

- **Fine, straight hair.** This combination usually hugs the head shape due to the fact that there is no body or volume. The silhouette is small and narrow. If this is not appropriate for the client based on the facial features or body structure, think about what styling aids or chemical services can be recommended to achieve the most flattering style. Left natural, this hair type may not support many styling options.

- **Straight, medium hair.** This type of hair offers more versatility in styling. It responds well to blowdrying with various-sized brushes and has a good amount of movement. It will also respond well to rollers and thermal styling.
- **Straight, coarse hair.** This hair is hard to curl and carries more volume than the previous two types. It casts a slightly wider silhouette and responds well to thermal styling. Flat brushes are better for this hair type because of a wide diameter in the hair shaft. Blowdrying with round brushes can create too much volume for this hair type. Chemical services may also take a little longer to process.
- **Wavy, fine hair.** This type of hair can appear fuller with the appropriate haircut and style. With layering, it will look fuller, and it responds well to blowdrying and chemical services. This hair can be fragile so be careful not to overdo any of these services. If the desired result is straight hair, it will straighten easily by blowdrying, but you may sacrifice volume. If diffused, the hair will have a fuller appearance.

© Milady, a part of Cengage Learning.

- **Wavy, medium hair.** This type of hair offers the most versatility in styling. This hair can be diffused to look curly, or be easily straightened by blowdrying.
- **Wavy, coarse hair.** This hair type can produce a silhouette that is very wide, and the hair can appear unruly if it is not shaped properly. Although blowdrying can be effective with this hair type, blowdrying is often much easier for the stylist than for the client. If the client is not good at working with her own hair, try to work out a flattering shape that is easy to maintain. Clients with this hair often feel that their hair leaves them trapped between being too wavy to be left in a straight style, and not being curly enough for a curly style. A soft perm could easily bring the client to a wash-and-wear curly style. A chemical relaxer might work very well if the client prefers a straighter look.
- **Curly, fine hair.** When this hair type is worn long, it often separates, revealing the client's scalp unless the hair is thick in density. This hair type responds well to mild relaxers and to color services. Blowdrying the hair straight may be difficult unless the hair is cut into short layers. Blowdrying is not an effective solution if the client is going to be in a humid environment.
- **Curly, medium hair.** This hair type creates a wide silhouette. When left natural, this type of hair gives a soft, romantic look. The wide silhouette should be in proportion to the client's body shape and not overwhelm it. When shaping the hair, keep in mind where the

weight line of the haircut will fall. This hair responds well to relaxers and color.

- **Curly, coarse hair.** This hair needs heavy styling products to weigh it down. It is easy for this type of hair to overwhelm any client. Keep in mind while cutting this hair type that the hair will shrink considerably when dry, making it appear much shorter.
- **Very curly, fine hair.** The most flattering shape for the client must be determined before you begin styling. Keep in mind that for ease of styling, this hair type is generally best cut short. If the hair is long, the silhouette will be wide and extremely voluminous. Chemical services and hair pressing (temporary straightening) take well, but be careful because the hair may be fragile.
- **Extremely curly, medium hair.** This silhouette can get very wide, because the hair can look wider rather than longer as it grows. Chemical relaxers work very well to make the shape narrower, and hair pressing is also a good option. Thermal styling could follow the pressing. If the hair is left in its natural state, cropping it close to the head in a flattering shape is great for ease of styling and low maintenance.
- **Extremely curly, coarse hair.** This silhouette will be extremely wide. Chemical relaxing is often recommended to make it easier to style with other thermal services. This hair type is often too thick to tie back in a ponytail, so if the client does not want any chemical services and wants easy care suggest short, cropped layers to make the silhouette narrower. ☑ **LO4**

Creating Harmony between Hairstyle and Facial Structure

A client's facial shape is determined by the position and prominence of the facial bones. A good way to determine facial shape is to pull all of the client's hair completely off the face using a towel or hair band, so that you can better observe just the client's face. There are seven basic facial shapes: oval, round, square, triangle (pear-shaped), oblong, diamond, and inverted triangle (heart-shaped). To recognize each facial shape and to be able to style the hair in the most flattering

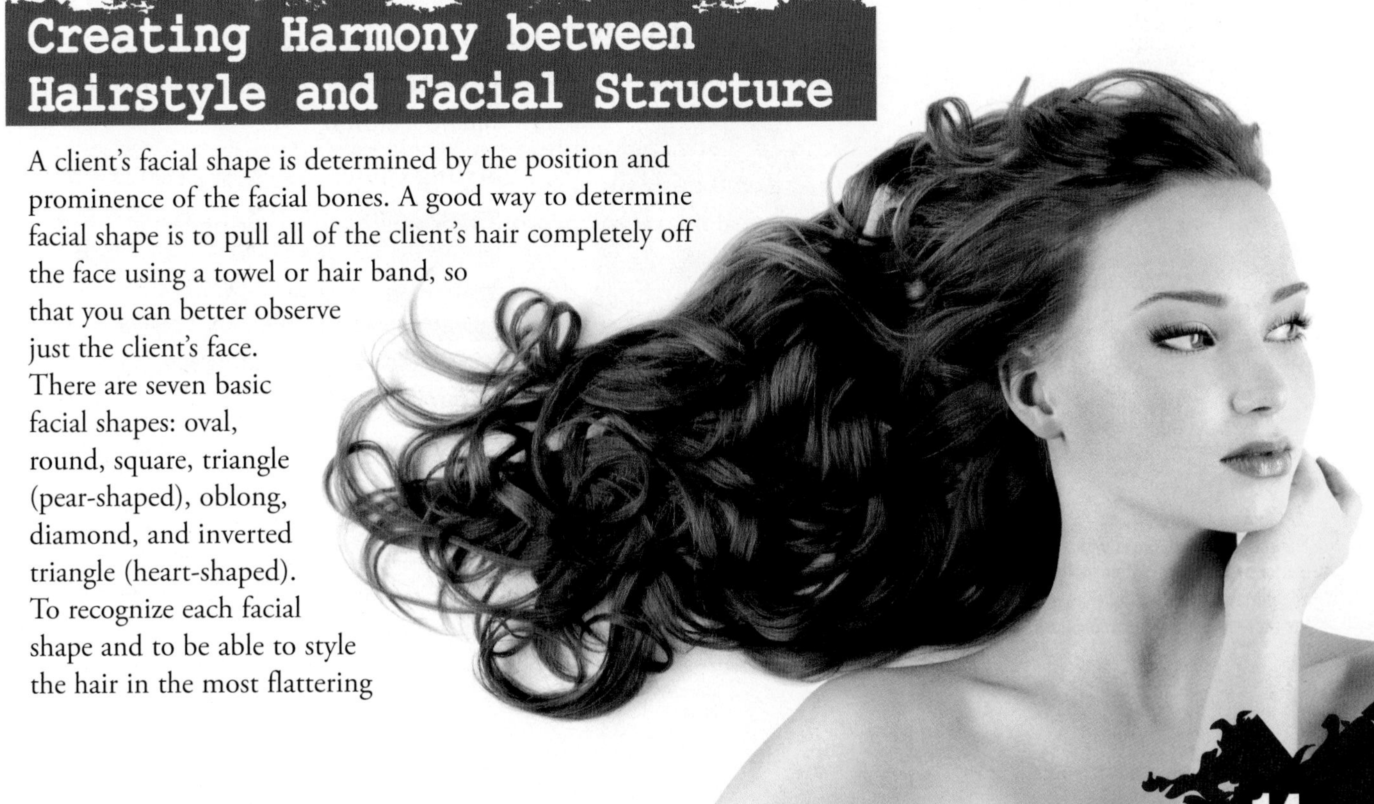

© Valua Vitaly, 2010; used under license from Shutterstock.com.

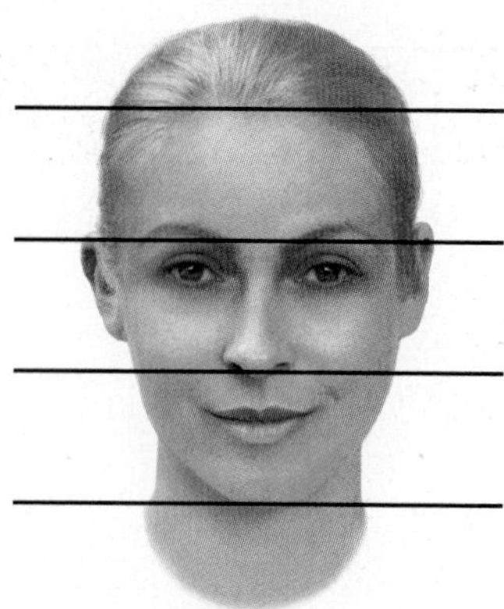

▲ Figure 14–42
Ideal facial proportions.

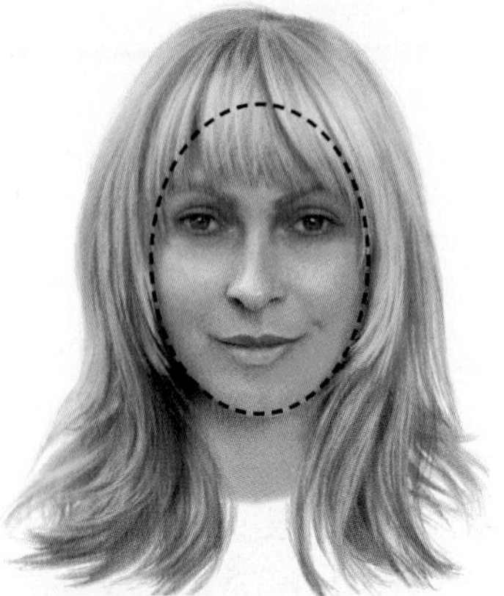

▲ Figure 14–43
The oval face shape is considered ideal and works well with any hairstyle.

design with that facial shape in mind, you should be acquainted with the characteristics of each. Remember, when designing a style for your client's facial type, you generally are trying to create the illusion of an oval shaped face.

To determine a facial shape divide the face into three zones: forehead to eyebrow, eyebrows to end of nose, and end of nose to bottom of chin.

Oval Facial Type

The contour and proportions of the oval face shape form the basis and ideals for evaluating and modifying all other facial types (**Figure 14–42**).

- **Facial contour:** The oval face is about one and a half times longer than its width across the brow. The forehead is slightly wider than the chin (**Figure 14–43**). A person with an oval face can wear any hairstyle unless there are other considerations, such as eyeglasses, length and shape of nose, or profile. (See the Special Considerations section later in this chapter.)

Round Facial Type

Facial contour: Round hairline and round chin line; wide face.

Objective: To create the illusion of length to the face, since this will make the face appear slimmer.

Styling choice: A hairstyle that has height or volume on top and closeness or no volume at the sides (**Figures 14–44a** and **b**).

Square Facial Type

Facial contour: Wide at the temples, narrow at the middle third of the face, and squared off at the jaw.

Objective: To offset or round out the square features.

Styling choice: Soften the hair around the temples and jaw by bringing the shape or silhouette close to the head form. Create volume in the area between the temples and jaw by adding width around the ear area (**Figures 14–45–a** and **b**).

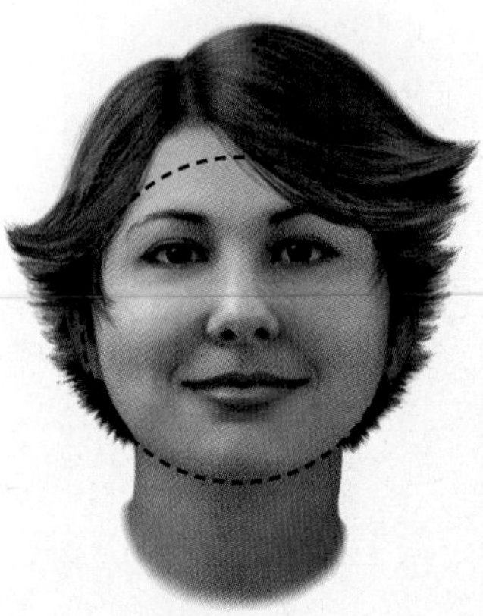

▲ Figure 14–44 a
The round face shape is widest at the center of the face. A style like this one accentuates the width at the center of the face, so is not a good choice.

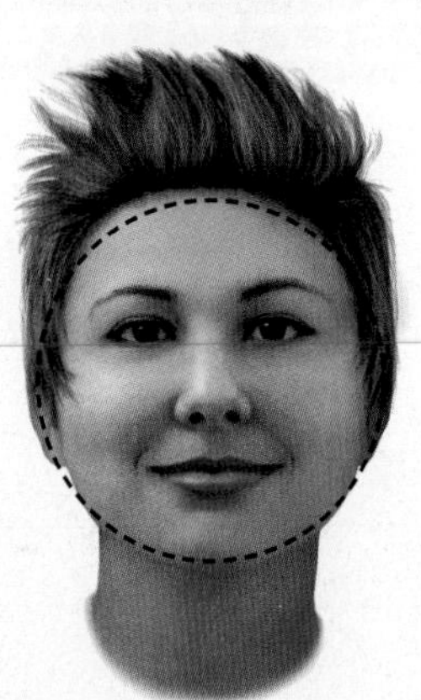

▲ Figure 14–44 b
This style helps the round face shape appear longer and more oval by using additional volume at the top of the head and decreasing volume at the temples.

© Milady, a part of Cengage Learning.

Triangular (Pear-Shaped) Facial Type

Facial contour: Narrow forehead, wide jaw and chin line.

Objective: To create the illusion of width in the forehead.

Styling choice: A hairstyle that has volume at the temples and some height at the top. You can disguise the narrowness of the forehead with a soft bang or fringe (**Figures 14–46a** and **b**).

Oblong Facial Type

Facial contour: Long, narrow face with hollow cheeks.

Objective: To make the face appear shorter and wider.

Styling choice: Keep the hair fairly close to the top of the head. Add volume on the sides to create the illusion of width. The hair should not be too long, as this will elongate the oblong shape of the face. Chin length styles are most effective for this facial type (**Figures 14–47a** and **b**).

WEB RESOURCES

Thanks to the wonders of modern computer technology we can take a facial image and try many hairstyles or haircolors with just a click of a mouse. This is a great exercise for training your eye by seeing the effect of many different styles on the same face. Have fun and be creative—it is only cyber hair! Check out http://www.dailymakeover.com for free virtual makeovers.

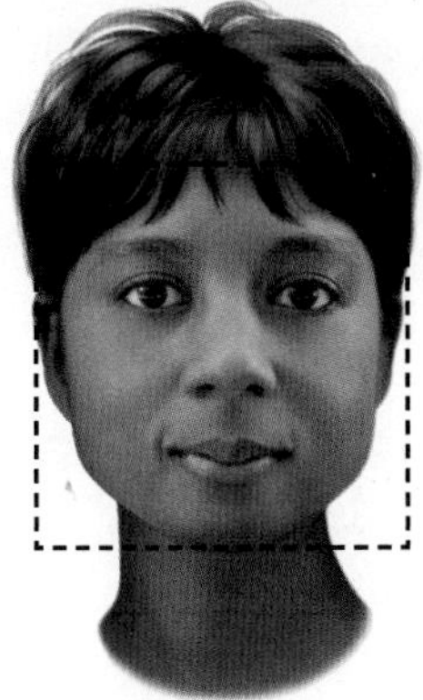

▲ **Figure 14–45 a**
The square face shape is accentuated with this hairstyle because the style has little volume and does not help to soften the squared edges of the face shape.

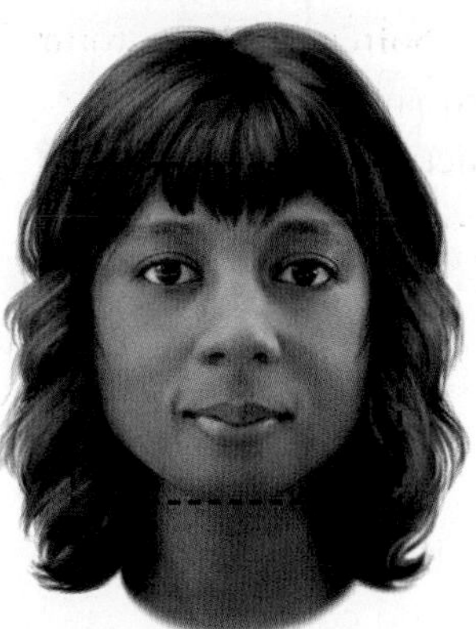

▲ **Figure 14–45 b**
With its soft waves, close-to-the-head bangs, and curls at the chin, this hairstyle has volume at the temple area. It is very flattering for the square face shape.

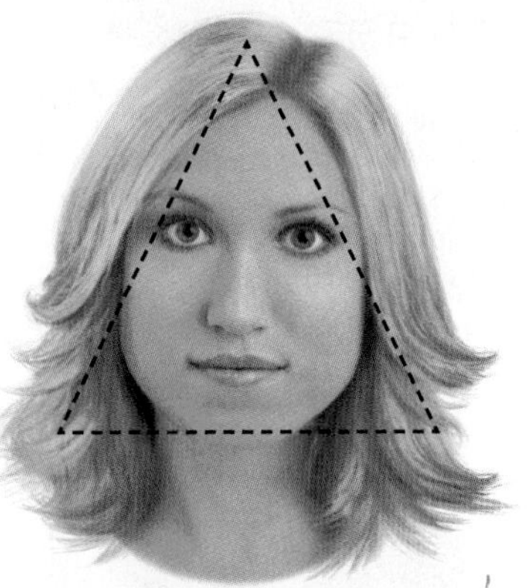

▲ **Figure 14–46 a**
This style—long, flat-on-top, and curly length—does nothing to soften the angles of a triangular face shape.

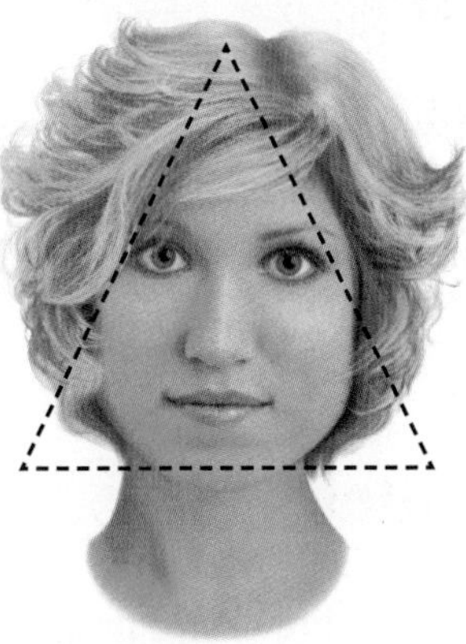

▲ **Figure 14–46 b**
A much more flattering look for the triangular face shape. This style adds fullness to the top half of the head, balancing the chin area and making the overall look more proportionate.

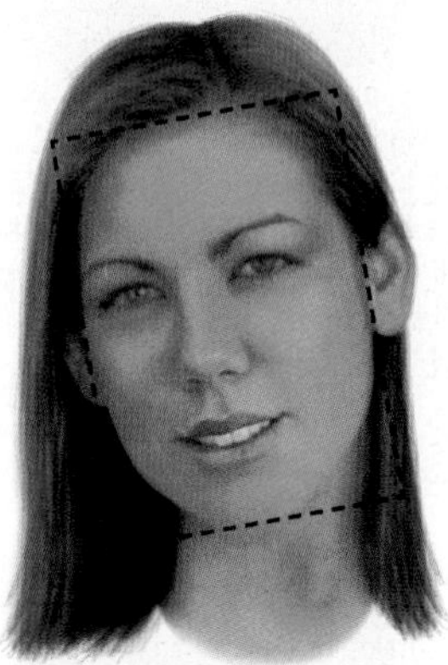

▲ **Figure 14–47 a**
With no width at the center of the hairstyle, the oblong face shape is quite obvious.

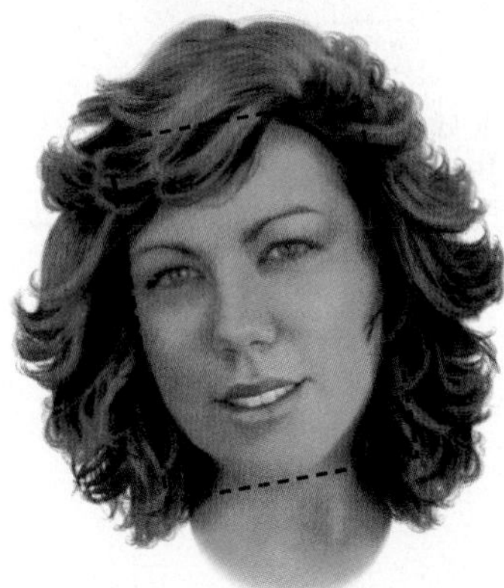

▲ **Figure 14–47 b**
Adding volume to the temple and side areas creates the appearance of width and balance for this oblong face shape.

© Milady, a part of Cengage Learning.

ACTivity

Bring to class pictures of models and celebrities from magazines and look at them with your classmates to analyze facial shapes. Which styles work or do not work? What hairstyle would you suggest if they were your clients? Why?

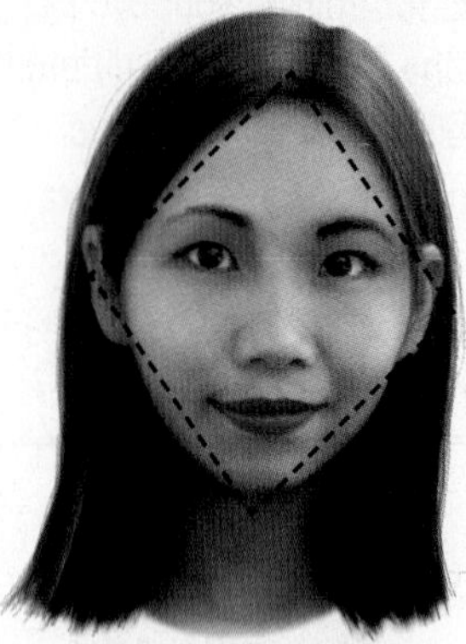

▲ Figure 14–48 a
This hairstyle accentuates the diamond face shape by being close to the head and exposing the forehead, adding to the width of the face.

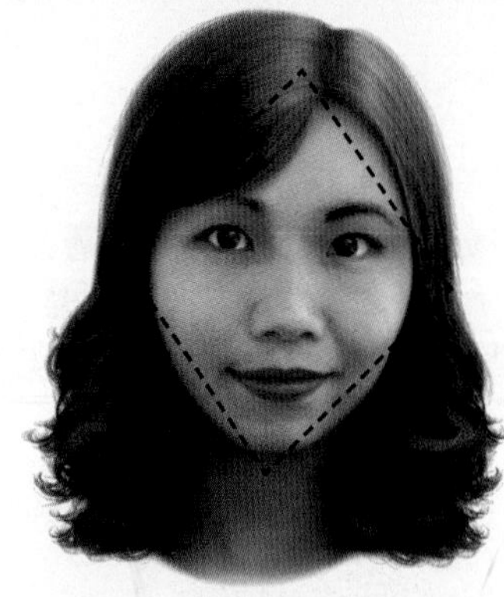

▲ Figure 14–48 b
To create the illusion of balance for a diamond face shape, keep the sides closer to the face and create volume at the top and chin area.

Diamond Facial Type

Facial contour: Narrow forehead, extreme width through the cheekbones, and narrow chin.

Objective: To reduce the width across the cheekbone line.

Styling choice: Increase the fullness across the jaw line and forehead while keeping the hair close to the head at the cheekbone line. Avoid hairstyles that lift away from the cheeks or move back from the hairline on the sides near the ear area (**Figures 14–48a** and **b**).

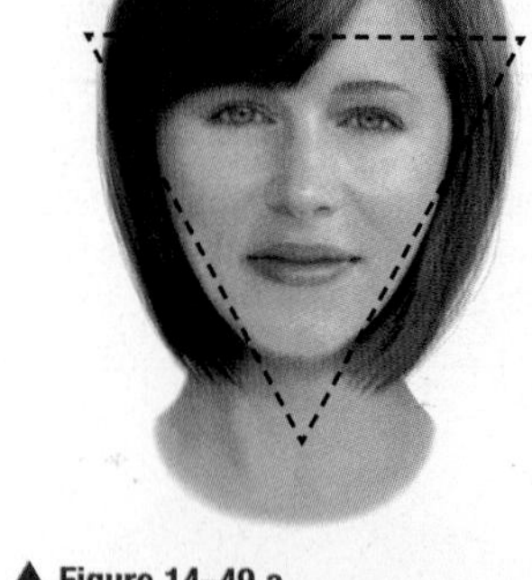

▲ Figure 14–49 a
The inverted triangle-shaped face, also called the heart-shaped face, is not flattered by a hairstyle whose lines mimic the face shape.

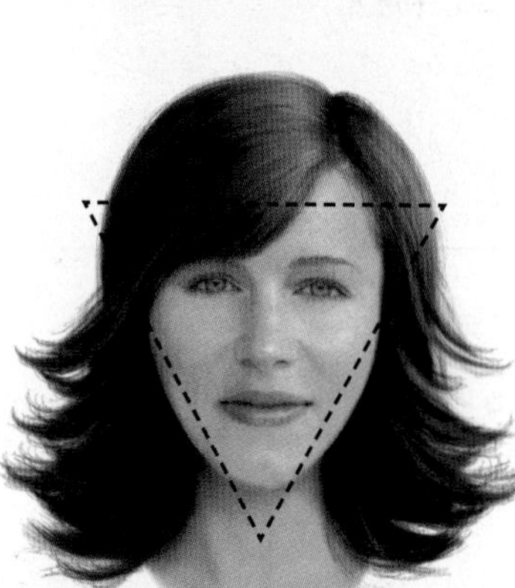

▲ Figure 14–49 b
The inverted triangle-shaped face looks best in a hairstyle that has curl and volume in the lower half of the face.

Inverted Triangle (Heart-Shaped) Facial Type

Facial contour: Wide forehead and narrow chin line.

Objective: To decrease the width of the forehead and increase the width in the lower part of the face.

Styling choice: Style the hair close to the head with no volume. A bang or fringe is recommended. Gradually increase the width of the silhouette as you style the middle third of the shape in the cheekbone area and near the ears, and keep the silhouette at its widest at the jaw and neck area (**Figures 14–49a** and **b**).

Profiles

The **profile** is the outline of the face, head, or figure seen in a side view. There are three basic profiles: straight, convex, and concave.

The **straight profile** is considered the ideal. The face when viewed in profile is neither convex (curving outward) nor concave (curving inward), although even a straight profile has a very slight curvature. Generally, all hairstyles are flattering to the straight or ideal profile (**Figure 14–50**).

© Milady, a part of Cengage Learning.

The **convex profile** has a receding forehead and chin. It calls for an arrangement of curls or bangs over the forehead. Keep the style close to the head at the nape and move hair forward in the chin area (**Figures 14–51** and **14–52**).

The **concave profile** has a prominent forehead and chin, with other features receded inward. It should be accommodated by softly styling the hair at the nape with an upward movement. Do not build hair onto the forehead (**Figures 14–53** and **14–54**).

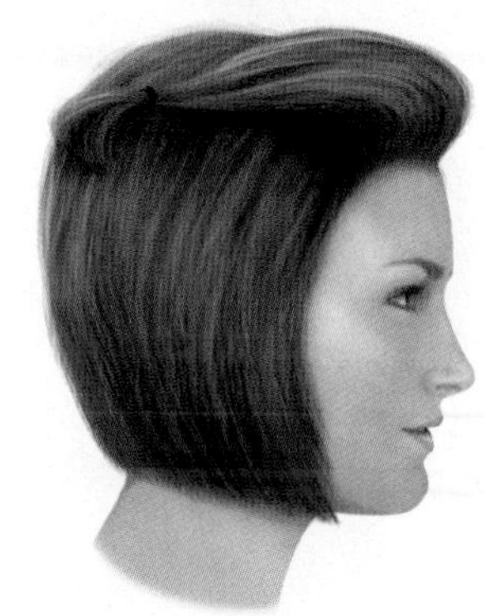

▲ Figure 14–50
Straight profile.

Special Considerations

An understanding of facial features and proportions will make it easier for you to analyze each client's face. You can then apply the design principles you have learned to help balance facial structural challenges. Dividing the face into three sections is one way to do this analysis.

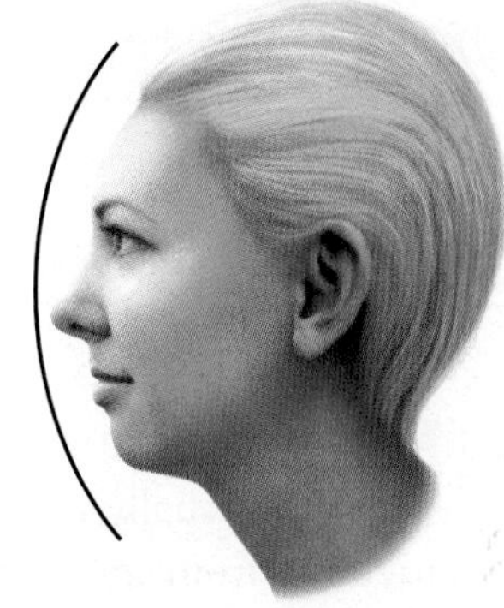

▲ Figure 14–51
Convex profile.

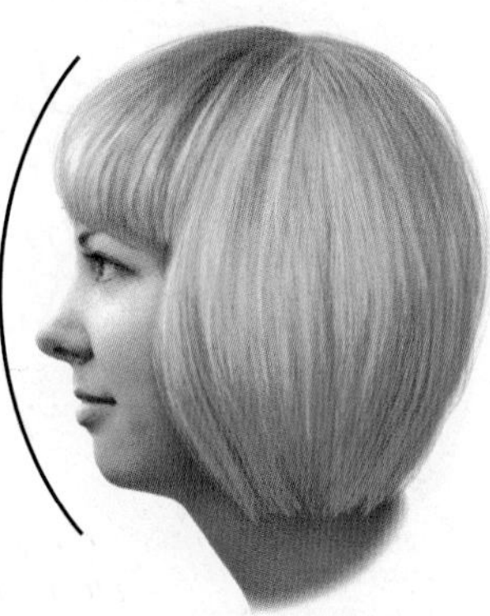

▲ Figure 14–52
Styling for a convex profile.

Top Third of the Face

- **Wide forehead:** Direct hair forward over the sides of the forehead (**Figure 14–55**).
- **Narrow forehead:** Direct hair away from the face at the forehead. Lighter highlights may be used at the temples to create the illusion of width (**Figure 14–56**).
- **Receding forehead:** Direct the bangs over the forehead with an outwardly directed volume (**Figure 14–57**).

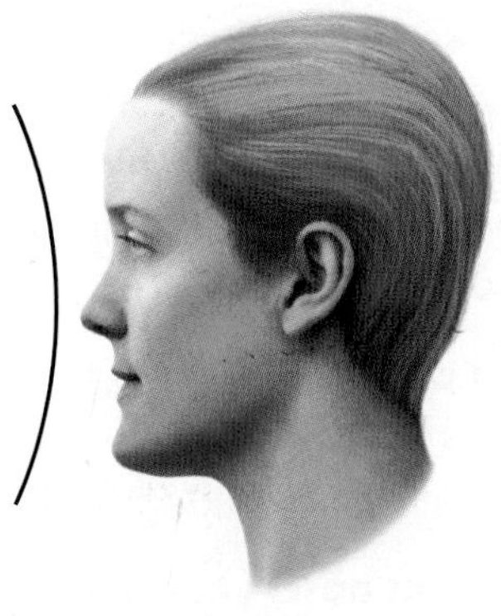

▲ Figure 14–53
Concave profile.

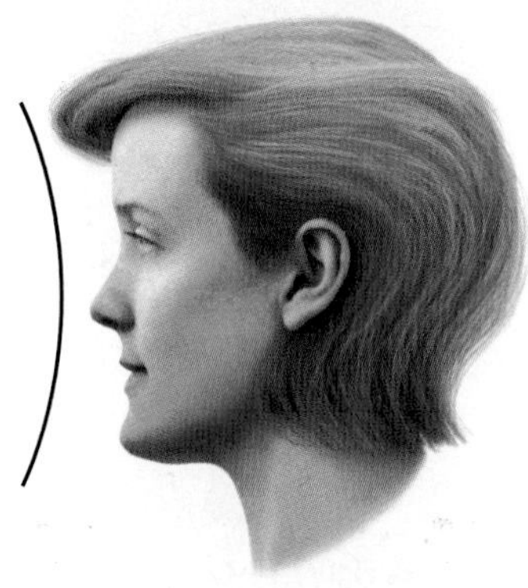

▲ Figure 14–54
Styling for a concave profile.

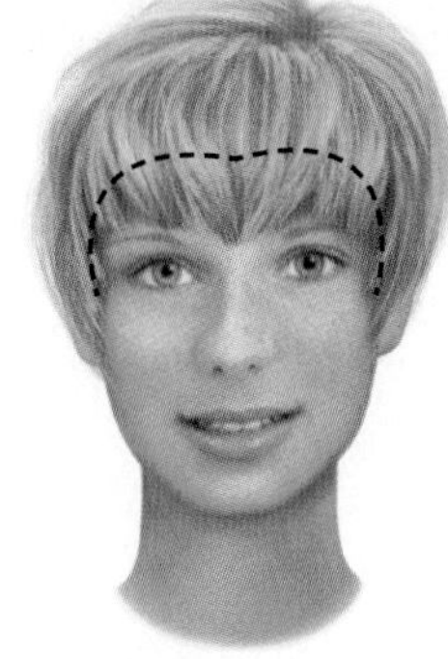

▲ Figure 14–55
Wide forehead.

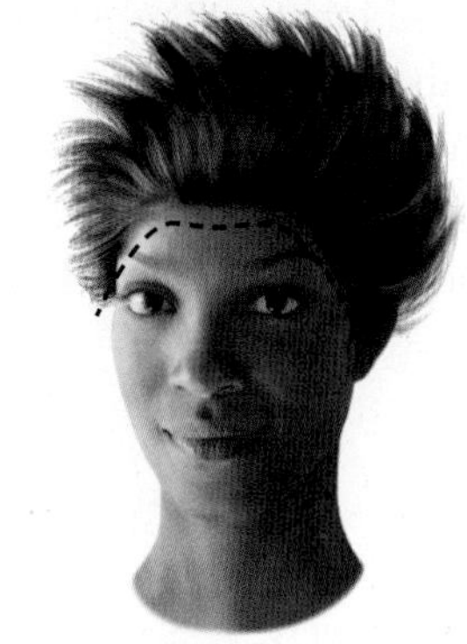

▲ Figure 14–56
Narrow forehead.

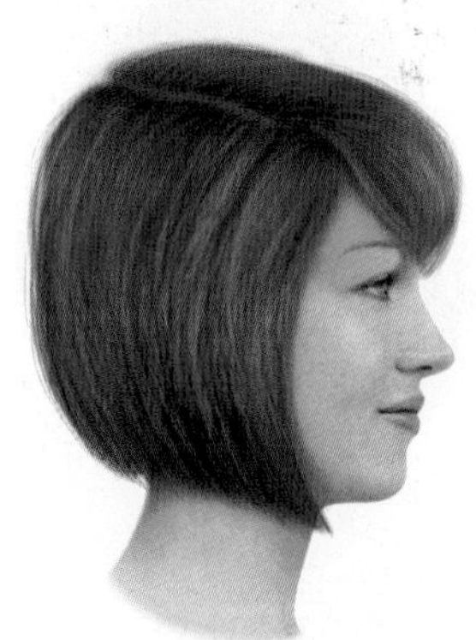

▲ Figure 14–57
Receding forehead.

© Milady, a part of Cengage Learning.

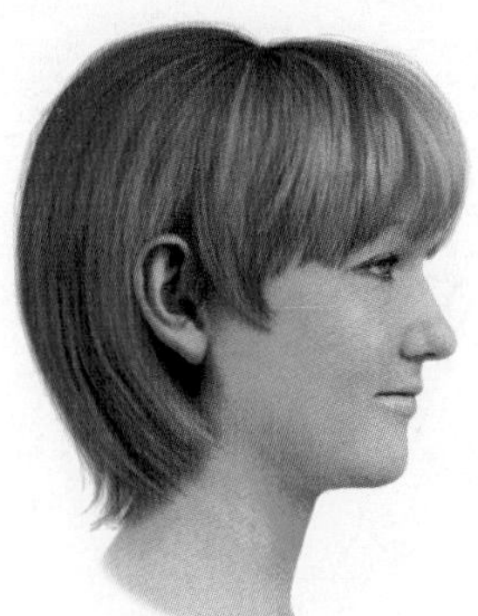

▲ Figure 14–58
Large forehead.

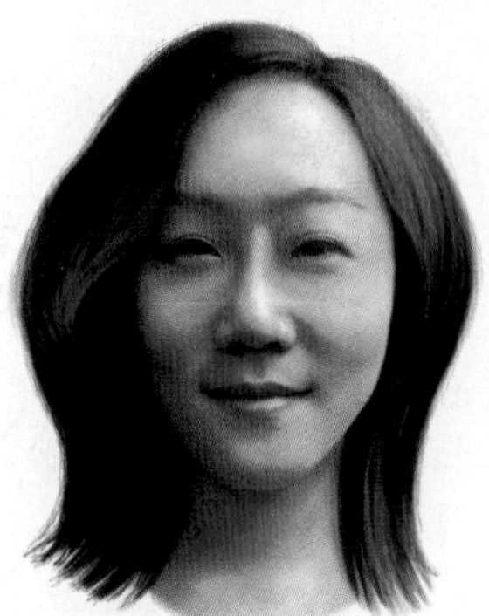

▲ Figure 14–59
Close-set eyes.

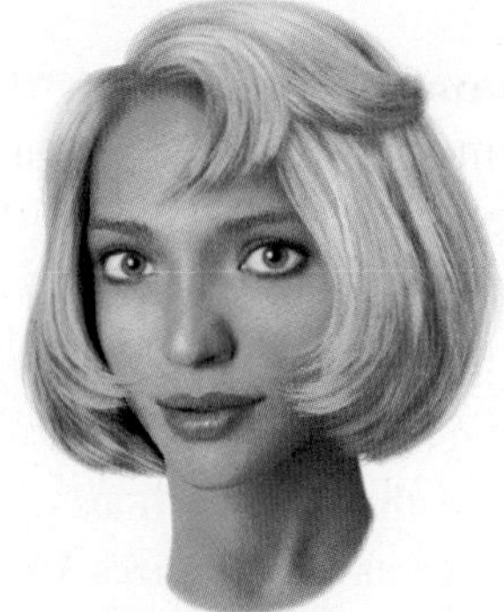

▲ Figure 14–60
Wide-set eyes.

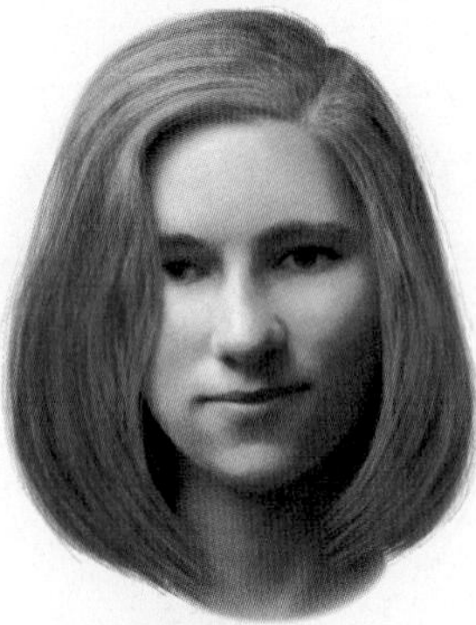

▲ Figure 14–61
Crooked nose.

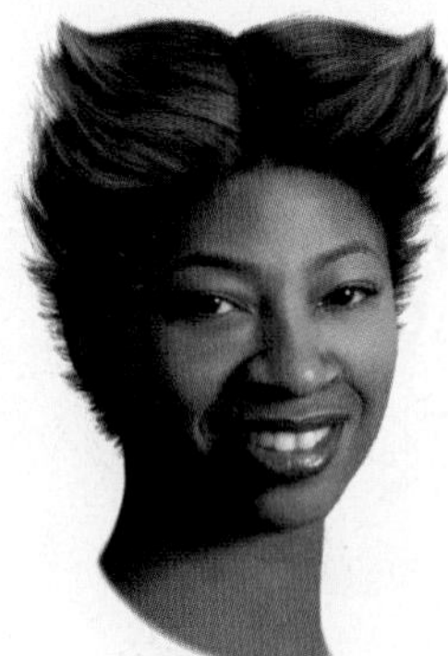

▲ Figure 14–62
Wide, flat nose.

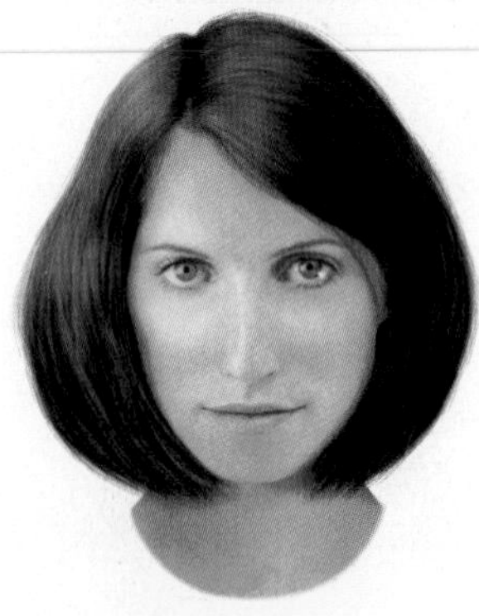

▲ Figure 14–63
Long, narrow nose.

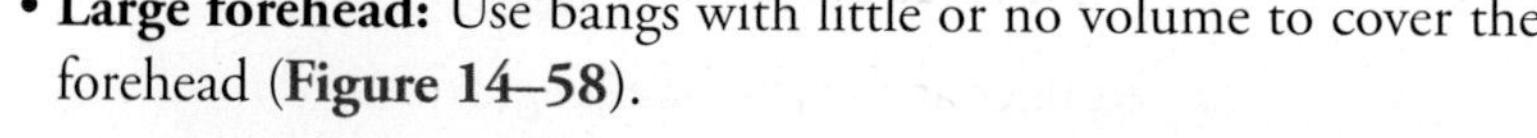

- **Large forehead:** Use bangs with little or no volume to cover the forehead (**Figure 14–58**).

Middle Third of the Face

- **Close-set eyes:** Usually found on long, narrow faces. Direct hair back and away from the face at the temples. A side movement from a diagonal back part with some height is advisable. A slight lightening of the hair at the corner of the eyes will give the illusion of width (**Figure 14–59**).
- **Wide-set eyes:** Usually found on round or square faces. Use a higher half bang to create length in the face. This will give the face the illusion of being larger and will make the eyes appear more proportional. The hair should be slightly darker at the sides than the top (**Figure 14–60**).
- **Crooked nose:** Asymmetrical, off-center styles are best, as they attract the eye away from the nose. Symmetrical styles will accentuate the fact that the face is not even (**Figure 14–61**).
- **Wide, flat nose:** Draw the hair away from the face and use a center part to help elongate and narrow the nose (**Figure 14–62**).
- **Long, narrow nose:** Stay away from styles that are tapered close to the head on the sides, with height on top. Middle parts or too much hair directed toward the face are also poor choices. These will only accentuate any long, narrow features on the face. Instead, select a style where the hair moves away from the face, creating the illusion of wider facial features (**Figure 14–63**).

© Milady, a part of Cengage Learning.

- **Small nose:** A small nose often gives a child-like look; therefore, it is best to design an age-appropriate hairstyle that would not be associated with children. Hair should be swept off the face, creating a line from nose to ear. The top hair should be moved off the forehead to give the illusion of length to the nose (**Figure 14–64**).
- **Prominent nose:** To draw attention away from the nose, bring hair forward at the forehead with softness around the face (**Figure 14–65**).

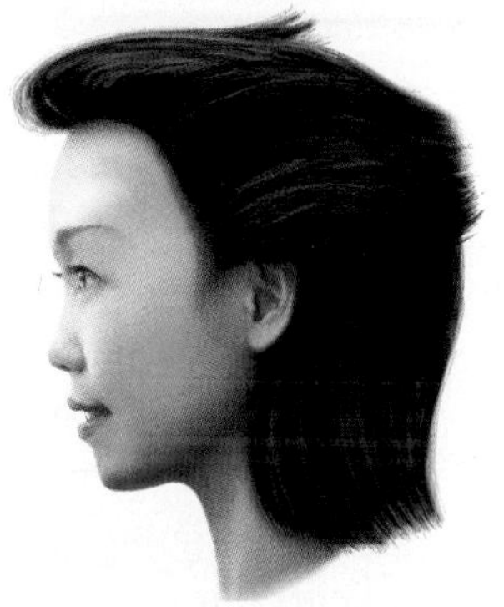

▲ Figure 14–64
Small nose.

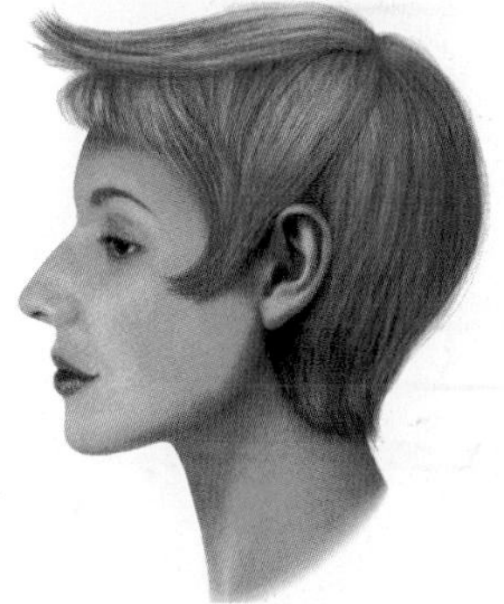

▲ Figure 14–65
Prominent nose.

Lower Third of the Face

- **Round jaw:** Use straight lines at the jaw line (**Figure 14–66**).
- **Square jaw:** Use curved lines at the jaw line (**Figure 14–67**).
- **Long jaw:** Hair should be full and fall below the jaw to direct attention away from it (**Figure 14–68**).
- **Receding chin:** Hair should be directed forward in the chin area (**Figure 14–69**).
- **Small chin:** Move the hair up and away from the face along the chin line (**Figure 14–70**).
- **Large chin:** The hair should be either longer or shorter than the chin line so as to avoid drawing attention to the chin (**Figure 14–71**).

☑ LO5

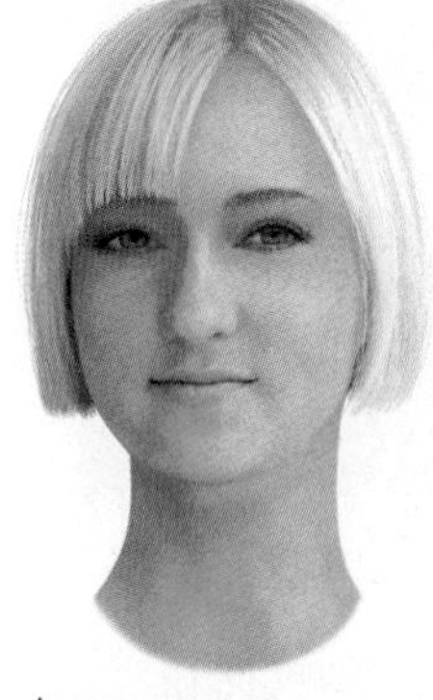

▲ Figure 14–66
Round jaw.

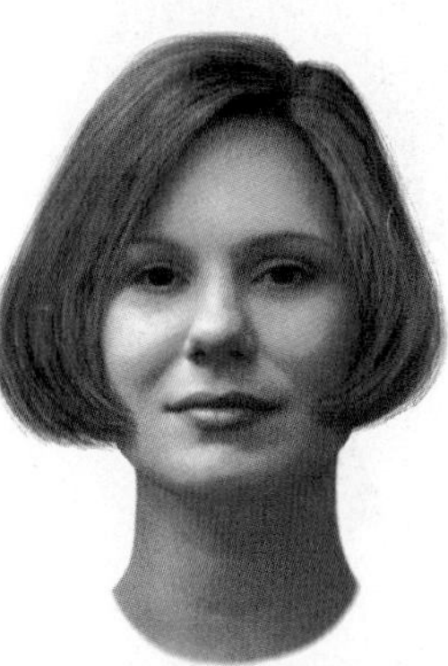

▲ Figure 14–67
Square jaw.

Head Shape

Not all head shapes are round. It is important to evaluate the head shape before deciding on a hairstyle. Design the style with volume

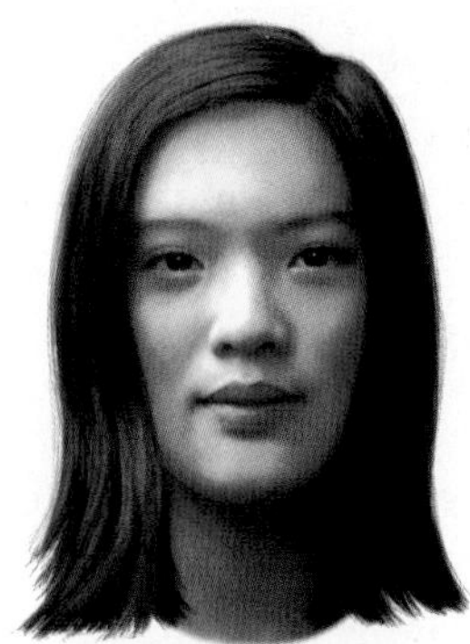

▲ Figure 14–68
Long jaw.

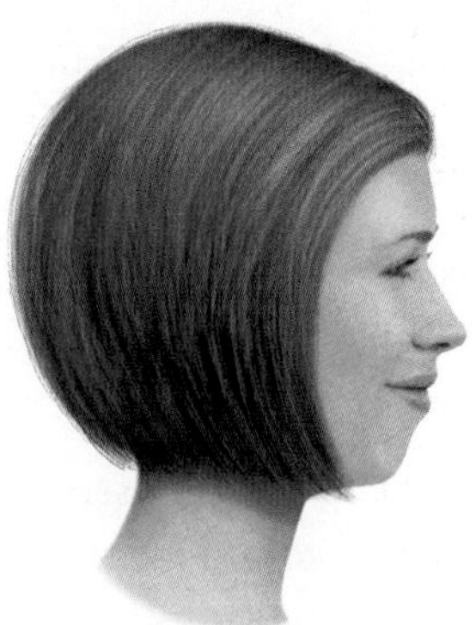

▲ Figure 14–69
Receding chin.

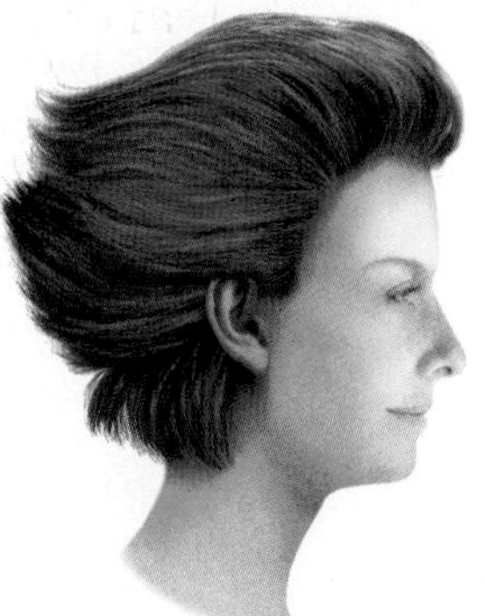

▲ Figure 14–70
Small chin.

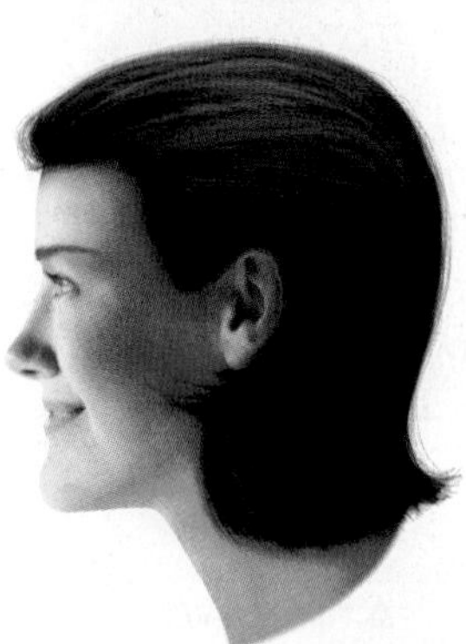

▲ Figure 14–71
Large chin.

© Milady, a part of Cengage Learning.

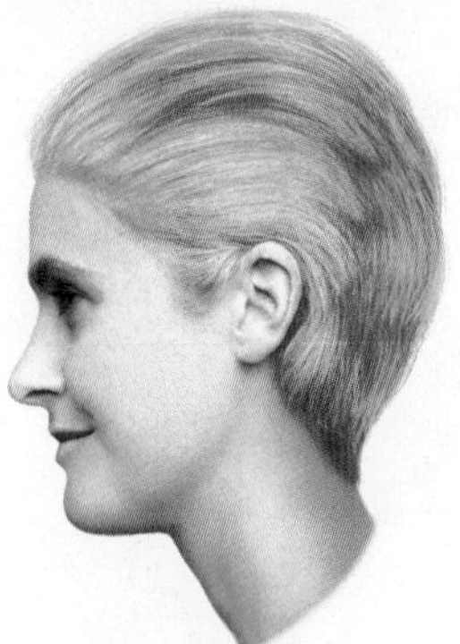

▲ Figure 14–72
Perfect oval.

in areas that are flat or small while reducing the volume of the hair in areas that are large or prominent (**Figure 14–72**).

Styling for People Who Wear Glasses

Eyeglasses have become a fashion accessory, and many people change their eyewear as often as their clothes. It is important for you to know whether your clients ever wear glasses so you can take that into account when designing the appropriate hairstyle. Keep in mind that when clients put on their glasses, the arms of the glasses (the part that rests on the ear) can push the hair at the ear and cause it to stick out.

If you are choosing a short haircut, you may want to reconsider the length of the hair around the ear, opting to either leave it a little longer or cut the hair above and around the ear. For styling purposes, choose a style in which there is enough hair covering the ear (fine hair may pop out at the ear), or direct the hair away from the face, so that the arms of the glasses are not an issue.

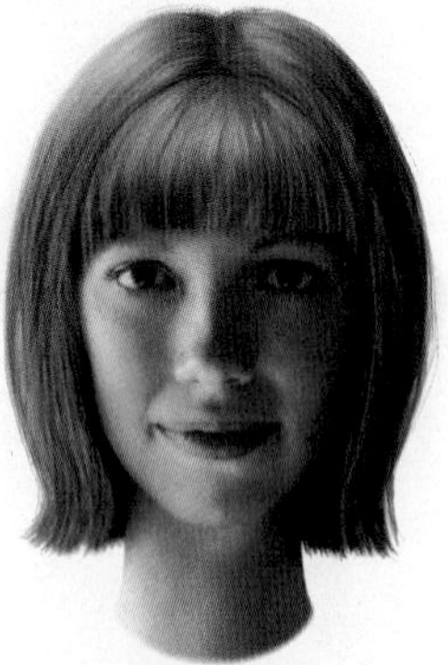

▲ Figure 14–73
Triangular part.

Hair Partings

Hair partings can be the focal point of a hairstyle. Because the eye is drawn to a part, you must be careful in the placement. When possible, it is usually best to use a natural parting. You may, however, want to create a part according to your client's head shape or facial features, or for a desired hairstyle. It is often challenging to create a hairstyle working against the natural crown parting. For best results, you might try to incorporate the natural part into the finished style. The following are suggestions for hair partings that suit the various facial types.

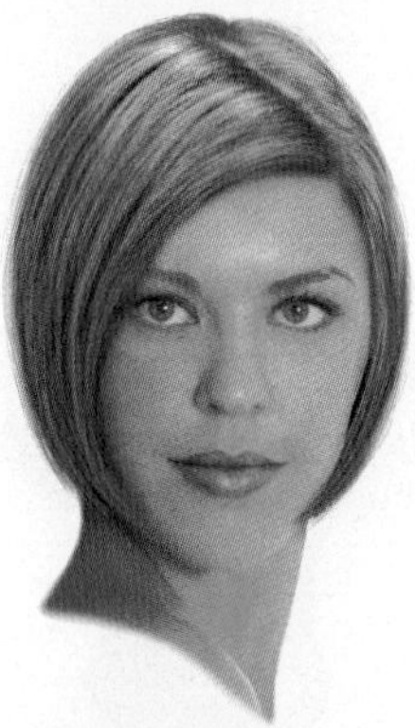

▲ Figure 14–74
Diagonal part in bangs.

Partings for the Bang (Fringe)

The **bang area**, also known as **fringe area**, is the triangular section that begins at the apex, or high point of the head, and ends at the front corners. The bang is parted in three basic ways:

- A triangular parting is the basic parting for bang sections (**Figure 14–73**).
- A diagonal parting gives height to a round or square face and width to a long, thin face (**Figure 14–74**).
- A curved part is used for a receding hairline or high forehead (**Figure 14–75**).

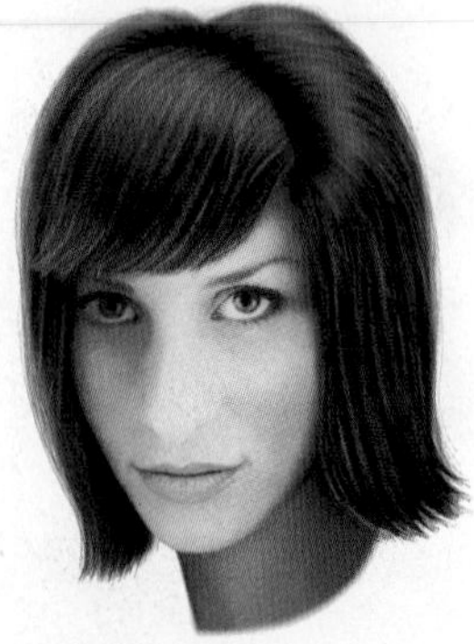

▲ Figure 14–75
Curved part.

Style Partings

There are four other partings that can be used to highlight facial features:

- Center partings are classic. They are used for an oval face, but also give an oval illusion to wide and round faces. Remember to avoid using center partings on people with prominent noses (**Figure 14–76**).

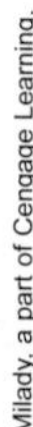

© Milady, a part of Cengage Learning.

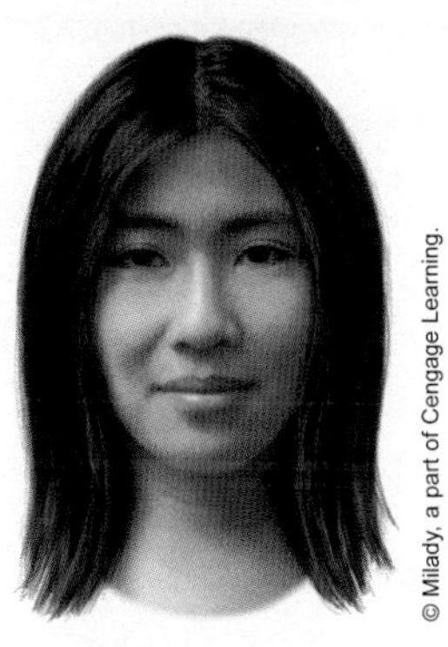
© Milady, a part of Cengage Learning.

▲ **Figure 14–76**
Center part.

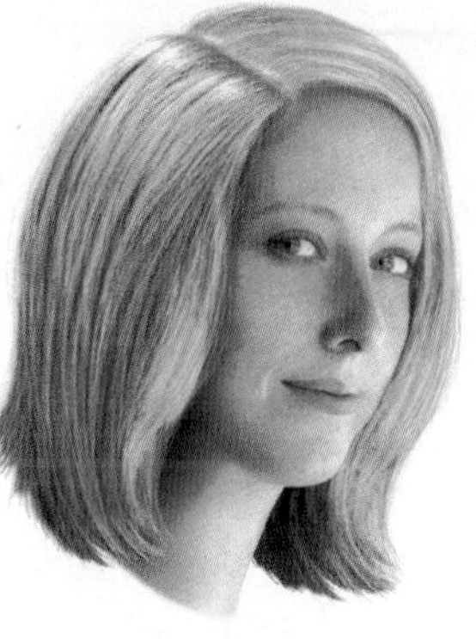
© Milady, a part of Cengage Learning.

▲ **Figure 14–77**
Side part.

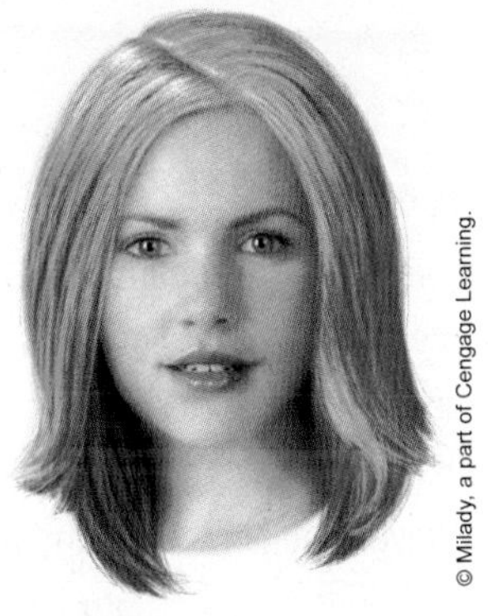
© Milady, a part of Cengage Learning.

▲ **Figure 14–78**
Diagonal part.

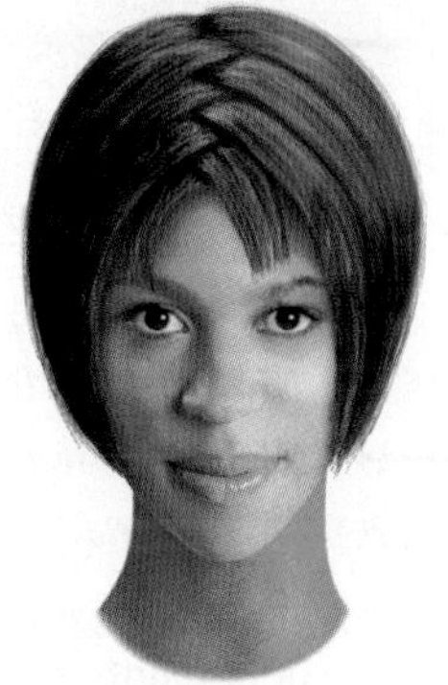
© Milady, a part of Cengage Learning.

▲ **Figure 14–79**
Zigzag part.

- Side partings are used to direct hair across the top of the head. They help develop height on top and make thin hair appear fuller (**Figure 14–77**).
- Diagonal back partings are used to create the illusion of width or height in a hairstyle (**Figure 14–78**).
- Zigzag partings create a dramatic effect (**Figure 14–79**).

Designing for Men

All the design principles and elements you have just read about work for men's hairstyles as well as for women's. Men's styles have become more individualized since the early 1960s, when the Beatles hit the music and fashion scene and greatly revolutionized men's hairstyling. Now, all hair lengths are acceptable for men, giving them more choices than ever before. As a professional, you should be able to recommend styles that are both flattering and appropriate for the client's lifestyle, career, and hair type.

Choosing Facial Hair Design

Mustaches, beards, and sideburns can be a great way for a male client to show his individual style. They can also be used to camouflage facial flaws. For example, if a man does not have a prominent chin when you look at his profile, a neatly trimmed full beard and mustache can be a good solution (**Figure 14–80**). If a man has a wide face and full cheeks, a fairly close-trimmed beard and mustache would be very thinning to the overall appearance (**Figure 14–81**).

A man who is balding with closely trimmed hair could also look very good in a closely groomed beard and mustache. Sideburns, mustaches, and beard shapes are largely dictated by current trends and fashions. No matter what the trend is, it is important that the shapes appear well groomed and are flattering to the client. ✔ **LO6**

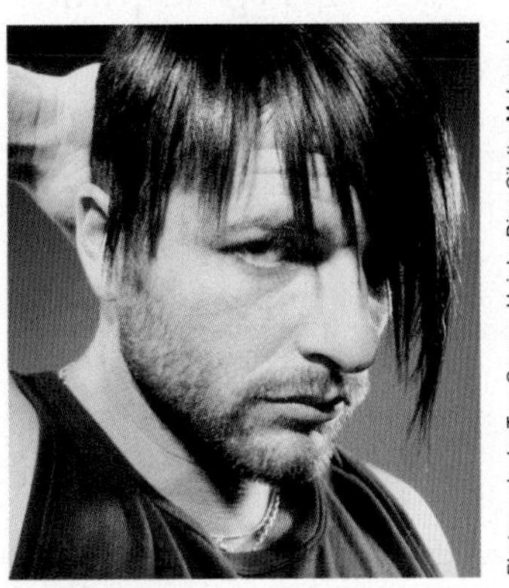
Photography by Tom Carson. Hair by Dina Cilotta. Makeup by Jodi Keeney for Ladies & Gentlemen Salon & Spa, Lyndhurst, OH.

▲ **Figure 14–80**
Full beard and mustache.

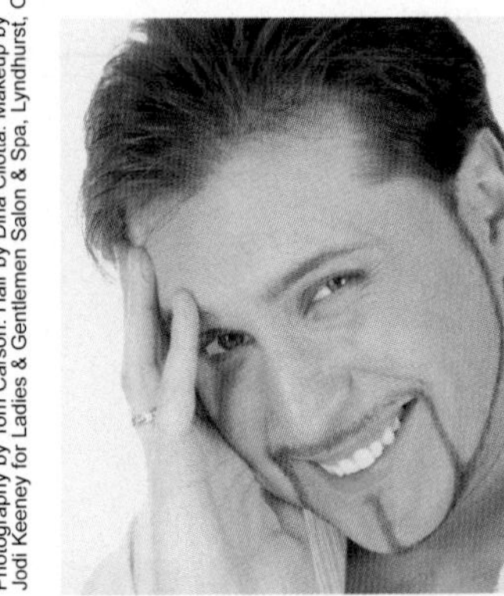
© Suravid, 2010; used under license from Shutterstock.com.

▲ **Figure 14–81**
Closely trimmed beard and mustache.

Review Questions

1. What are some of the possible sources a hair designer might use for inspiration?
2. What are the five elements of hair design?
3. What are the five principles of hair design?
4. What influence does hair type have on hairstyle?
5. List and describe the seven facial shapes and explain how hair design can be used to highlight or camouflage facial features.
6. How do the elements and principles of hair design apply to men?

Chapter Glossary

asymmetrical balance	Is established when two imaginary halves of a hairstyle have an equal visual weight, but the two halves are positioned unevenly. Opposite sides of the hairstyle are different lengths or have a different volume. Asymmetry can be horizontal or diagonal.
balance	Establishing equal or appropriate proportions to create symmetry. In hairstyling, it is the relationship of height to width.
bang area	Also known as *fringe area*; triangular section that begins at the apex, or high point of the head, and ends at the front corners.
concave profile	Curving inward; prominent forehead and chin, with other features receded inward.
contrasting lines	Horizontal and vertical lines that meet at a 90-degree angle and create a hard edge.
convex profile	Curving outward; receding forehead and chin.
curved lines	Lines moving in a circular or semi-circular direction; used to soften a design.
design texture	Wave patterns that must be taken into consideration when designing a style.
diagonal lines	Lines positioned between horizontal and vertical lines. They are often used to emphasize or minimize facial features.
directional lines	Lines with a definite forward or backward movement.
emphasis	Also known as *focus*; the place in a hairstyle where the eye is drawn first before traveling to the rest of the design.
form	The mass or general outline of a hairstyle. It is three-dimensional and has length, width, and depth.
harmony	The creation of unity in a design; the most important of the art principles. Holds all the elements of the design together.
horizontal lines	Lines parallel to the floor or horizon; create width in design.
parallel lines	Repeating lines in a hairstyle; may be straight or curved.

Chapter Glossary

profile	Outline of the face, head, or figure seen in a side view.
proportion	The comparative relation of one thing to another; the harmonious relationship among parts or things.
rhythm	A regular pulsation or recurrent pattern of movement in a design.
single lines	A hairstyle with only one line, such as the one-length hairstyle.
space	The area surrounding the form or the area the hairstyle occupies.
straight profile	Neither convex nor concave; considered the ideal.
symmetrical balance	Two halves of a style; form a mirror image of one another.
transitional lines	Usually curved lines that are used to blend and soften horizontal or vertical lines.
vertical lines	Lines that are straight up and down; create length and height in hair design.

CHAPTER 15

Scalp Care, Shampooing, and Conditioning

Chapter Outline

© Valua Vitaly, 2010; used under license from Shutterstock.com.

Learning Objectives

After completing this chapter, you will be able to:

- ✓ **LO1** Explain the two most important requirements for scalp care.
- ✓ **LO2** Describe the benefits of scalp massage.
- ✓ **LO3** Treat scalp and hair that are dry, oily, or dandruff ridden.
- ✓ **LO4** Explain the role of hair brushing to a healthy scalp.
- ✓ **LO5** Discuss the uses and benefits of the various types of shampoo.
- ✓ **LO6** Discuss the uses and benefits of the various types of conditioner.
- ✓ **LO7** Demonstrate the appropriate draping for a basic shampooing and conditioning, and draping for a chemical service.
- ✓ **LO8** Identify the Three-Part Procedure and explain why it is useful.

Key Terms

Page number indicates where in the chapter the term is used.

balancing shampoo
pg. 317

clarifying shampoo
pg. 317

color-enhancing shampoo
pg. 318

conditioner
pg. 318

conditioning shampoo (moisturizing shampoo)
pg. 317

contraindicated
pg. 309

deep-conditioning treatment (hair mask, conditioning pack)
pg. 320

deionized water
pg. 314

dry shampoo (powder shampoo)
pg. 318

hard water
pg. 314

humectants
pg. 319

medicated scalp lotion
pg. 319

medicated shampoo
pg. 317

moisturizer
pg. 315

nonstripping
pg. 317

pH-balanced shampoo
pg. 316

protein conditioner
pg. 319

scalp astringent lotion
pg. 319

scalp conditioner
pg. 319

soft water
pg. 314

spray-on thermal protector
pg. 319

When clients visit a salon for the first time, they immediately begin making judgments about the surroundings. How does the salon look? What kind of music is playing? Does the receptionist greet them with a smile and call them by name? While all of these factors are part of a good salon experience, it is what happens when the client moves into the service area that can make or break you. One of the most important experiences that a stylist provides is the shampoo, which can be heavenly, forgettable, or even a nightmare.

Often called simply "the shampoo," this first step of the service actually encompasses three different processes: scalp care and massage, shampooing, and conditioning. The shampoo can and should be a soothing, pleasurable experience that sets the mood for the entire visit.

The shampoo is an opportunity to provide the client with quality relaxation time that is free from the stresses of the day. It can be nurturing and, when done well, feel as good as a full-body massage.

Remember: If clients are happy with the shampoo experience, they are far more likely to be happy with the entire service.

WHY STUDY SCALP CARE, SHAMPOOING, AND CONDITIONING?

Cosmetologists should study and have a thorough understanding of scalp care, shampooing, and conditioning because:

- The shampoo service is the first opportunity to reinforce your position as a professional who attends to the specific, individual needs of your client.
- You will be able to examine, identify, and address hair and scalp conditions that do not require a physician's care and be able to refer clients to a physician if a more serious issue is identified.
- A thorough knowledge of hair care products will assist you in determining the best preparation for other services to be performed.
- A successful home-care regimen recommendation will keep your work looking its best for all to see.

Scalp Care and Massage

The two basic requirements for a healthy scalp are cleanliness and stimulation. Since similar manipulations are given with all scalp treatments, scalp massage is a procedure you will perform often and one that you should learn to do well. ☑ **LO1**

© Wow, 2010; used under license from Shutterstock.com.

Scalp treatments should be given with a continuous, even motion that will stimulate the scalp and help to relax the client. Do not massage or manipulate a client's scalp if abrasions are present.

Scalp treatments and massage may be performed either:

1. Before a shampoo if a scalp condition is apparent, or
2. During the shampoo (once conditioner has been applied to the hair) for relaxation.

Procedure 15-11, Scalp Massage, explains the procedure and massage manipulations that are used in all scalp massage. The difference between a *relaxation* and *treatment* massage are the products you use. Be sure to follow all of the manufacturer's directions whenever a special scalp treatment product is used. For simple relaxation, most any conditioner may be used to create a very enjoyable experience for your client.

It is this extra service that will keep your clients coming back to you. Knowing the muscles, the location of blood vessels, and the nerve points of the scalp and neck will help guide you to those areas most likely to benefit from massage movements. For details on this information, see Chapter 6, General Anatomy and Physiology. ☑ **LO2**

FYI

Before performing a service that includes a scalp massage consult the client's intake or health screening form. During the consultation acknowledge and discuss any medical condition your client listed that may be **contraindicated**, avoiding a procedure or condition that may produce undesirable side effects, for a scalp massage. Ask the client if they have discussed massage with their physician and if they have not already done so, encourage them to seek their physician's advice as to whether or not a scalp massage is advisable before performing the service.

Many clients that have high blood pressure (hypertension), diabetes, or circulatory conditions may still have massage without concern, especially if their condition is being treated and carefully looked after by a physician. Massage is, however, contraindicated for clients with severe, uncontrolled hypertension.

If your client expresses a concern about having a scalp massage and has a medical condition, have the client get a note from their physician.

If your client has any scalp sensitivity avoid using vigorous or strong massage techniques. Do not talk to your client during the scalp massage except to ask once whether your touch should be more or less firm. Talking eliminates the relaxation therapy of the scalp massage.

When making decisions about whether to perform a scalp massage on a person who has a medical condition, be conservative. When in doubt, don't include massage as part of your service.

PROCEDURE 15-11 Scalp Massage SEE PAGE 338

Normal Hair and Scalp Treatment

The purpose of a general scalp treatment is to maintain the scalp and hair in a clean and healthy condition. A hair or scalp treatment should be recommended only after a hair and scalp examination. If the client does not have the time to sit for a treatment, recommend scheduling the treatment at a later, more convenient time. If the client does request a treatment at that time, it should be given either before or after the shampoo, depending on which treatment is given.

PROCEDURE 15-3 Normal Hair and Scalp Treatment SEE PAGE 328

Dry Hair and Scalp Treatment

A dry hair and scalp treatment should be used when there is a deficiency of natural oil on the scalp and hair. Select scalp preparations containing moisturizing and emollient ingredients. Avoid the use of strong soaps, preparations containing a mineral- or sulfonated-oil base, greasy preparations, or lotions with high alcohol content. During a dry hair and scalp treatment, a scalp steamer, which resembles a hooded dryer, is used.

PROCEDURE 15-4 Dry Hair and Scalp Treatment SEE PAGE 329

Oily Hair and Scalp Treatment

Excessive oiliness is caused by overactive sebaceous glands. Manipulate the scalp and knead it to increase blood circulation to the surface. Any hardened sebum in the pores of the scalp will be removed with gentle pressing or squeezing. To normalize the function of these glands, excess sebum should be flushed out with each treatment.

PROCEDURE 15-5 Oily Hair and Scalp Treatment SEE PAGE 330

Antidandruff Treatment

Dandruff is the result of a fungus called malassezia (māl-ə-SĒ-zē-ə). Antidandruff shampoos, conditioners, and topical lotions contain antifungal agents that control dandruff by suppressing the growth of malassezia. Moisturizing salon treatments also soften and loosen scalp scales that stick to the scalp in crusts. Because of the ability of fungus to resist treatment, additional salon treatments and the frequent use of antidandruff home care should be recommended. ☑ **LO3**

PROCEDURE 15-6 Antidandruff Treatment SEE PAGE 331

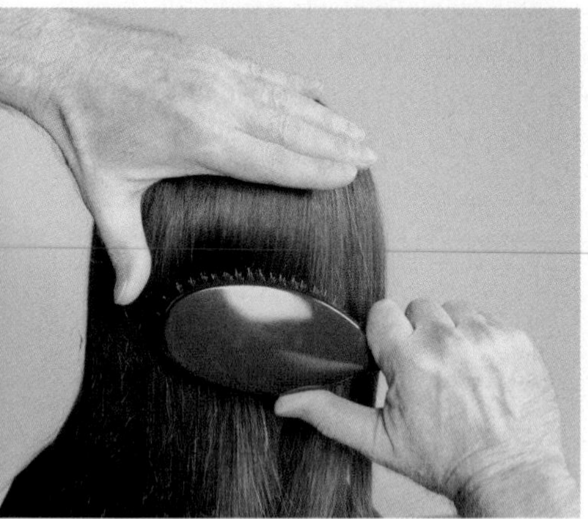

▲ **Figure 15–1**
Include a thorough hair brushing as part of every shampoo and scalp treatment.

© Milady, a part of Cengage Learning. Photography by Yanik Chauvin.

Hair Brushing

Correct hair brushing stimulates the blood circulation to the scalp; brushing helps remove dust, dirt, and hair-spray buildup from the hair and gives hair added shine. You should include a thorough hair brushing as part of every shampoo and scalp treatment, regardless of whether your client's hair and scalp are dry or oily (**Figure 15–1**). Brushing also allows the stylist to examine the scalp for abrasions and infections.

The two exceptions to hair brushing are as follows:

- Do not brush or irritate the scalp before giving a chemical service.
- Do not brush if the scalp is irritated.

© Milady, a part of Cengage Learning.

Brushing, massaging, or shampooing the scalp before a service is not recommended for:

- Single-process and double-process haircolor.
- Highlighting.
- Most chemical relaxers (follow manufacturer's directions).
- Some temporary and semipermanent haircolor (follow manufacturer's directions).

If shampooing is recommended, shampoo gently to avoid scalp irritation.

The most highly recommended hairbrushes are those made from natural bristles. Natural bristles have many tiny overlapping layers or scales, which clean and add luster to the hair. Hairbrushes with nylon bristles are shiny and smooth and are more suitable for hairstyling. ✓ **LO4**

PROCEDURE 15-7 Hair Brushing **SEE PAGE 332**

Understanding Shampoo

The shampoo provides a good opportunity to analyze the client's hair and scalp. Always check for these conditions:

- Dry, dehydrated hair
- Thinning of the hair
- Excessive hair left in the sink trap after shampooing
- Dry, tight scalp
- Oily scalp
- Abnormal flaking on the scalp
- Open wounds or scalp irritations
- Scalp disorders or diseases
- Tick or lice infestation

In salons where shampoos are performed by salon assistants, these assistants should always alert the stylist about any hair or scalp conditions, including suspected diseases or disorders. A client with

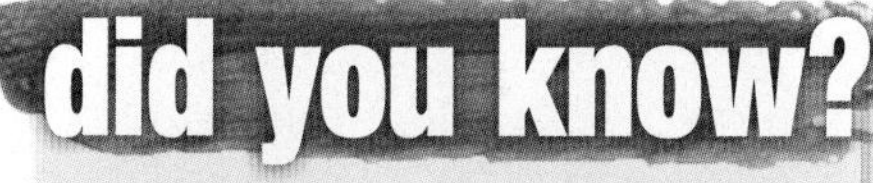

Maintaining good posture will protect you against the muscle aches, back strain, discomfort, fatigue, and other physical problems that can result from performing shampoos. The most important rule regarding posture is to always keep your shoulders back while performing the shampoo. This way, you will avoid slumping over the client. Remember, too, to hold your abdomen in, thereby lifting your upper body. Free-standing shampoo bowls allow for healthier body alignment and help reduce strain on the back and shoulders.

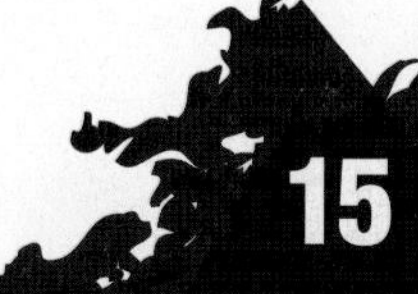

an infectious disease is never to be treated in the salon and should be referred to a physician.

Naturally, the primary purpose of a shampoo is to cleanse the hair and scalp prior to a service. This is also the time when you need to educate your client about the importance of home care and of using quality hair care products at home.

To be effective, a shampoo must remove all dirt, oils, cosmetics, and skin debris without adversely affecting either the scalp or hair. The scalp and hair need to be cleansed regularly to combat the accumulation of oils and perspiration that mix with the natural scales and dirt to create a breeding ground for disease-producing bacteria. Hair should only be shampooed as often as necessary. Excessive shampooing strips the hair of its protective oil (sebum) that, in small amounts, seals and protects the hair's cuticle. As a general rule, oily hair needs to be shampooed more often than normal or dry hair.

PROCEDURE 15-10 **Basic Shampooing and Conditioning** SEE PAGE 335

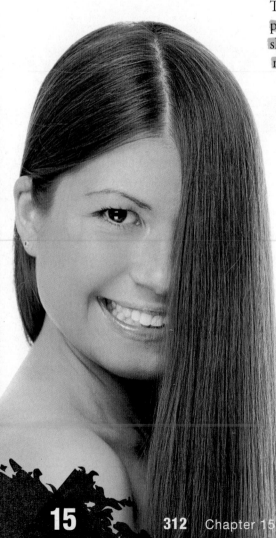

Selecting the Proper Shampoo

There are many types of shampoo available on the market. As a professional cosmetologist, you should become skilled at selecting shampoos that support the health of the hair, whether the hair is natural, color treated, fine and limp, or coarse and wiry. Always read labels and accompanying literature carefully so that you can make informed decisions about the use of various shampoos. A thorough knowledge of your products will help you recommend them as home-care items for purchase by your clients.

Select a shampoo according to the condition of the client's hair and scalp. Hair can usually be characterized as oily, dry, normal, or chemically treated. Your client might even have an oily scalp with dry hair, possibly due to overprocessing.

When selecting the shampoo product to be used, be aware of whether or not the hair has been chemically treated. Chemically treated hair (hair that has been lightened, colored, permed, chemically relaxed) and hair that has been abused by the use of harsh shampoos, or damaged by improper care and exposure to the elements such as wind, sun, cold, or heat, may require a product that is less harsh and more conditioning than virgin hair (hair that has not been chemically treated).

Using the right home-care products can make all the difference in how your clients' hair looks, feels, and behaves. It is your job to recommend and educate clients about which products they should be using, as well as how and why. Otherwise, they

© konstantynov, 2010; used under license from Shutterstock.com.

will make their own uninformed decisions, perhaps buying inferior products at the drugstore or supermarket. The wrong product choice can make a good haircut look bad, can negatively affect the client's opinion of your work, and can affect the outcome of a chemical service.

Remember: You want your clients to look their best so that they become good advertising for you.

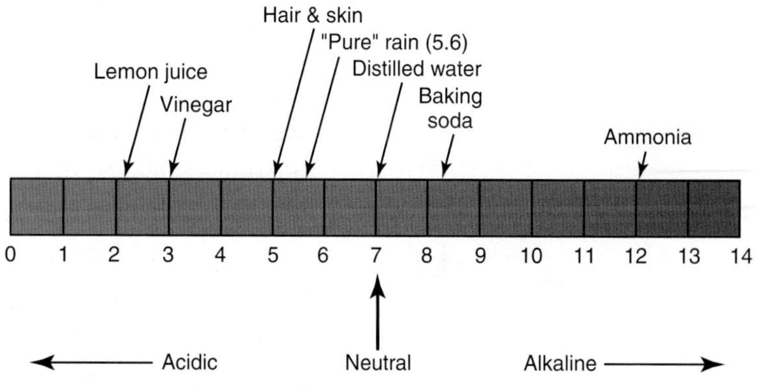

© Milady, a part of Cengage Learning.

▲ **Figure 15–2**
A review of pH as it applies to shampoo.

The pH Scale

Chapter 12, Basics of Chemistry, provides you with an overview of important chemistry basics, including pH and surfactants. Refer to that chapter as necessary. The following is a brief review of pH as it applies to shampoo (**Figure 15–2**).

Understanding pH levels will help you select the proper shampoo for your client. The amount of hydrogen in a solution, which determines whether it is alkaline or acid, is measured on a pH scale that has a range from 0 to 14. The pH of a neutral solution, one which is neither acidic nor alkaline, is 7. A shampoo that is acidic will have a pH ranging from 0 to 6.9; a shampoo that is alkaline will have a pH rating of 7.1 or higher. The more alkaline the shampoo, the stronger and harsher it is. A high-pH shampoo can leave the hair dry, brittle, and porous. A high-pH shampoo can cause fading in color treated hair. A slightly acidic shampoo more closely matches the ideal pH of hair.

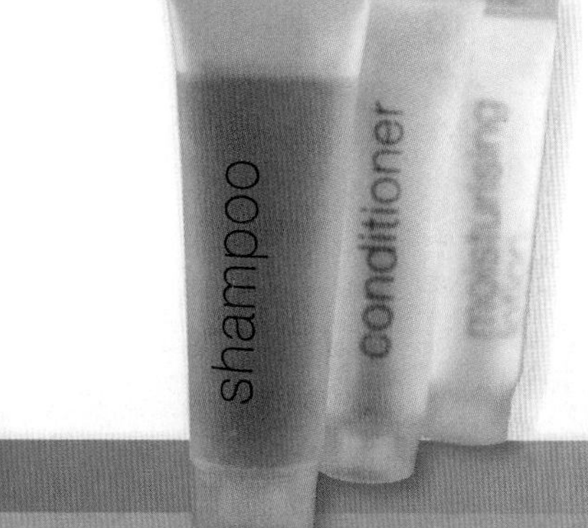

© Brett Mulcahy, 2010; used under license from Shutterstock.com.

FOCUS ON

SEVEN WAYS TO MAKE A GOOD SHAMPOO EXPERIENCE GREAT!

1. The scalp is always massaged according to the preference of the client. Some clients have a sensitive scalp and want a very light massage, while others want a firm massage. In order to service every client to the best of your ability, ask about massage preferences before beginning the procedure.
2. Always ask the client if the water feels too warm, too cool, or just right; adjust the temperature accordingly.
3. Do not allow the water or your hands to touch a woman's face during the shampoo. Allowing the client's face to get wet may remove part of her base makeup and can turn an otherwise great shampoo into an unpleasant experience.
4. It is easy to miss the nape of the neck when shampooing and rinsing, so you should always double-check this area before escorting the client to your station.
5. Throughout the shampoo, be very careful not to drench the towel that is draped around the client's neck. If the towel becomes damp, replace it with a clean, dry towel before leaving the shampoo area.
6. When blotting the hair after the shampoo, be careful once again not to touch the face. If you remove part of your client's makeup, she may feel self-conscious during her entire visit.
7. As you learn to give a great shampoo, you should also learn how to give a great relaxation massage. You may hear your clients say, "Don't stop, you can do that for hours," every time they come to you. Even though you may hear this five times a day, it is always satisfying to know that you are making your clients feel good!

The Chemistry of Water

Water is the most abundant and important element on Earth. It is classified as a universal solvent because it is capable of dissolving more substances than any other solvent known to science.

Fresh water from lakes and streams is purified by sedimentation (matter sinking to the bottom) and filtration (water passing through a porous substance, such as a filter paper or charcoal) to remove suspended clay, sand, and organic material. Before the water enters public water pipelines, small amounts of chlorine are added to kill bacteria. Boiling water at a temperature of 212 degrees Fahrenheit (100 degrees Celsius) will also destroy most microbes. Water can be further treated by distillation, a process of heating water so that it becomes a vapor, and then condensing the purified vapor so that it collects as a liquid. Distillation is often used in the manufacturing of cosmetics.

Water is of crucial importance in the cosmetology industry because it is used for shampooing, mixing solutions, and many other functions. Depending on the kinds and amounts of minerals present in water, water can be classified as either hard or soft. You will be able to make a more professional shampoo selection if you know whether the water in your salon and area is hard or soft. Most water-softener companies can supply you with a water-testing kit to determine how hard or soft your water is (soft, slightly hard, moderately hard, hard, or extremely hard).

Soft water is rainwater or chemically softened water that contains only small amounts of minerals and, therefore, allows soap and shampoo to lather freely. For this reason, it is preferred for shampooing. **Hard water** is often in well-water and contains minerals that reduce the ability of soap or shampoo to lather. Hard water may also change the results of the haircoloring service. However, a water treatment process can soften hard water.

© ifong, 2010; used under license from Shutterstock.com.

The Chemistry of Shampoo

To determine which shampoo will leave your client's hair in the best condition for the intended service, you need to understand the chemical and botanical ingredients regularly found in shampoos. Many shampoos have ingredients in common. It is often the small differences in formulation that make one shampoo better than another for a particular hair texture or condition.

Water is the main ingredient in most shampoos. Generally it is not just plain water, but purified or **deionized water**, water that has had impurities, such as calcium and magnesium and other metal ions that would make a product unstable, removed. Water is usually the first ingredient listed, which indicates that the shampoo contains more water than anything else. From there on, ingredients are listed in descending order, according to the percentage of each ingredient in the shampoo.

Surfactants

The second ingredient that most shampoos have in common is the primary surfactant (or base detergent). Surfactants are cleansing or surface active agents. A surfactant molecule has two ends: a hydrophilic or water attracting head, and a lipophilic or oil attracting tail. During the shampooing process, the hydrophilic head attracts water, and the lipophilic tail attracts oil. This creates a push/pull process that causes the oils, dirt, and deposits to roll up into little balls that can be lifted off in the water and rinsed from the hair (**Figures 15–3, 15–4, 15–5,** and **15–6**).

Other ingredients are added to the base surfactants to create a wide variety of shampoo formulas. **Moisturizer**, which is a product formulated to add moisture to dry hair or promote the retention of moisture, is a common additive along with oil, protein, preservative, foam enhancer, and perfume.

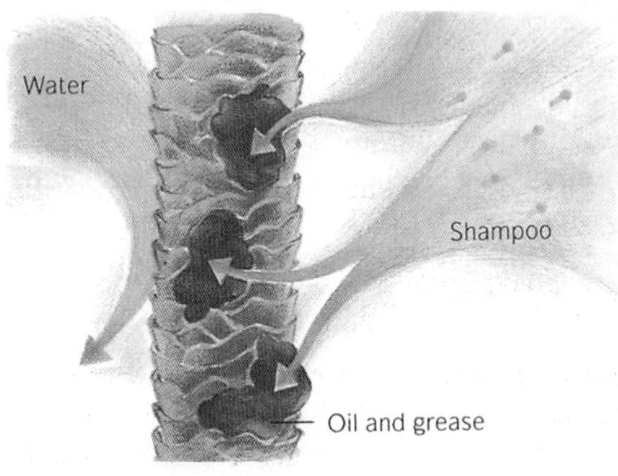

▲ Figure 15–3
The tail of the shampoo molecule is attracted to oil and dirt.

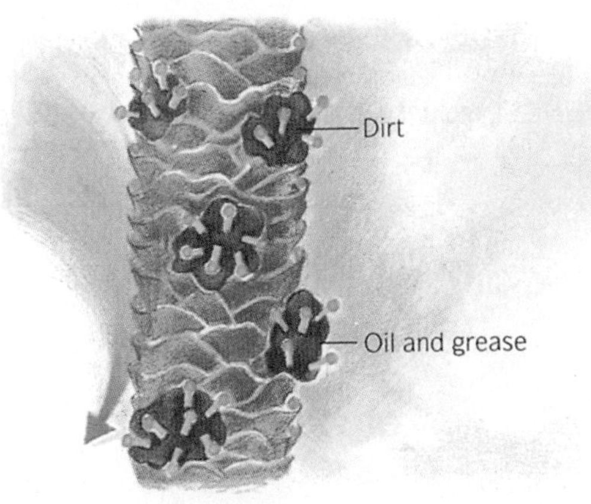

▲ Figure 15–4
Shampoo causes oils to roll up into small globules.

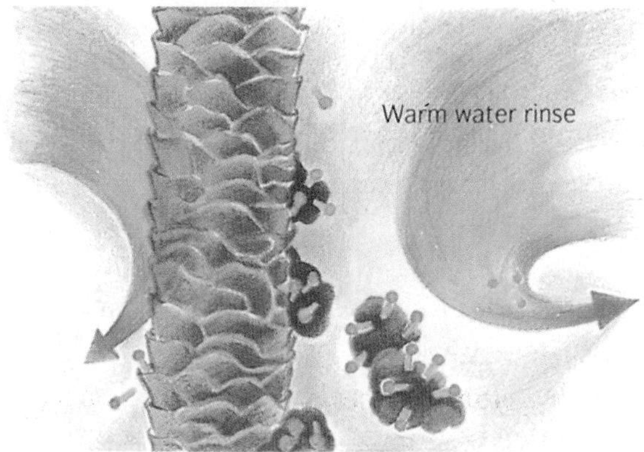

▲ Figure 15–5
The heads of the shampoo molecules attach to water molecules.

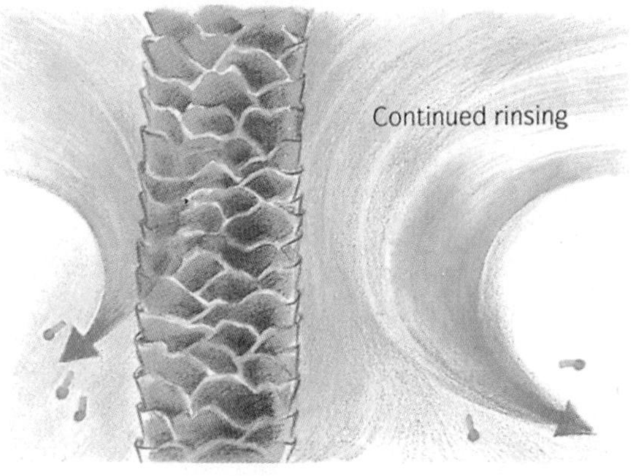

▲ Figure 15–6
Thorough rinsing washes away debris and excess shampoo.

© Milady, a part of Cengage Learning.

ACTivity

List all the hair products used in your school, along with the hair types appropriate for each. Analyze the hair of one or two classmates and recommend a particular shampoo and conditioner. List the benefits of each product for that particular "client." With your instructor's guidance, you might even try using your recommended choices on your classmates. Keep a record of what products you use, how the hair feels and behaves afterward, and your classmates' own opinions about the products.

WEB RESOURCES

To learn about the latest products and more in hair care, check out http://www.totalbeauty.com, or search the keywords *hair care products*.

Types of Shampoo

Shampoo products are the most widely purchased of all hair care products. Consumer studies show that the fastest growth items in the shampoo market are products that are retailed through professional salons. This is good news for salon professionals, but don't allow yourself to be overconfident if you want to succeed at sales. You will have to be as knowledgeable and sophisticated as possible about the products you are selling and as skilled as you can be in demonstrating their use.

Clients are increasingly well informed about beauty products from reading about them in beauty magazines and other consumer reports. Your credibility as a professional will be in question if your client is better informed than you are.

Many good shampoos exist for every type of hair and/or scalp condition. There are shampoos for dry, oily, fine, coarse, limp, lightened, permed, relaxed, or color-treated and chemically treated hair. There are shampoos that deposit a slight amount of color to color treated hair and those that cleanse hair of styling product buildup, mineral deposits, and so forth.

© block23, 2010; used under license from Shutterstock.com.

The list of ingredients is your key to determining which shampoo will leave a client's hair shiny and manageable, which will treat a scalp or hair condition, and which will prepare the hair for a chemical treatment. Now that you are familiar with pH and the chemistry of water and shampoo, here are some of the different types of shampoos.

pH-Balanced Shampoo

A **pH-balanced shampoo** is balanced to the pH of skin and hair (4.5 to 5.5). Many shampoos are pH balanced by the addition of citric, lactic, or phosphoric acid. Most experts believe that an acid pH of 4.5 to 5.5 is essential to preventing excessive dryness and hair damage during the cleansing process. Shampoos that are pH balanced help to close the hair cuticle and are recommended for hair that has been color treated or lightened.

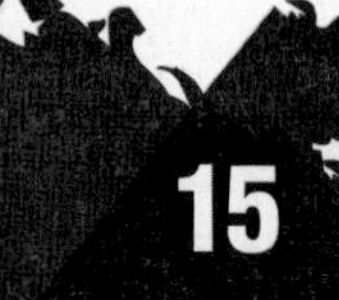

Conditioning Shampoo

Conditioning shampoo, also known as **moisturizing shampoo**, is designed to make the hair appear smooth and shiny and to improve the manageability of the hair. Protein and biotin are just two examples of conditioning agents that boost shampoos so that they can meet current grooming needs. These conditioning agents restore moisture and elasticity, strengthen the hair shaft, and add volume. They also are **nonstripping**, meaning that they do not remove artificial color from the hair.

Medicated Shampoo

Medicated shampoo contains special ingredients that are very effective in reducing dandruff or relieving other scalp conditions. Some medicated shampoos have to be prescribed by a physician. They can be quite strong and could affect the color of color-treated or lightened hair. In some cases, the shampoo must remain on the scalp for a longer period of time than other shampoos in order for the active ingredient to work. Always read and follow the manufacturer's instructions carefully.

Clarifying Shampoo

Clarifying shampoo contains an active chelating agent that binds to metals (such as iron and copper) and removes them from the hair, as well as an equalizing agent that enriches hair, helps retain moisture, and makes hair more manageable. Clarifying shampoo should be used when a buildup is evident, after swimming, and prior to all chemical services (**Figure 15–7**).

Balancing Shampoo

For oily hair and scalp, **balancing shampoo** willl wash away excess oiliness, while preventing the hair from drying out.

Dry Shampoo

Sometimes, the state of a client's health makes a wet shampoo uncomfortable or hard to manage. For instance, an elderly client may experience some discomfort at the shampoo bowl due to pressure on the

did you know?

In the 1960s, beauty pioneer Jheri Redding revolutionized the salon industry by being the first to market pH-balanced shampoos. He went around the country staging demonstrations that showed how acidic shampoos (pH below 7) outperformed alkaline shampoos. When Redding dipped a piece of litmus paper into his shampoo, it would come up a glowing orange, pink, or gold. The litmus test on his competitors' products would come up a murky purple or black. Most cosmetic chemists today agree that a low pH is good for all hair, especially chemically treated hair.

Mineral deposits
Chlorine
Styling aids and other buildup
Chelating agents
Mineral deposits attach to hair's protein while styling aids, chlorine and other oxidizers coat the cuticle.
Clarifying Treatment safely removes deposits with highly effective chelators.
Hair is left shiny, healthy-looking and ready for styling or chemical services.

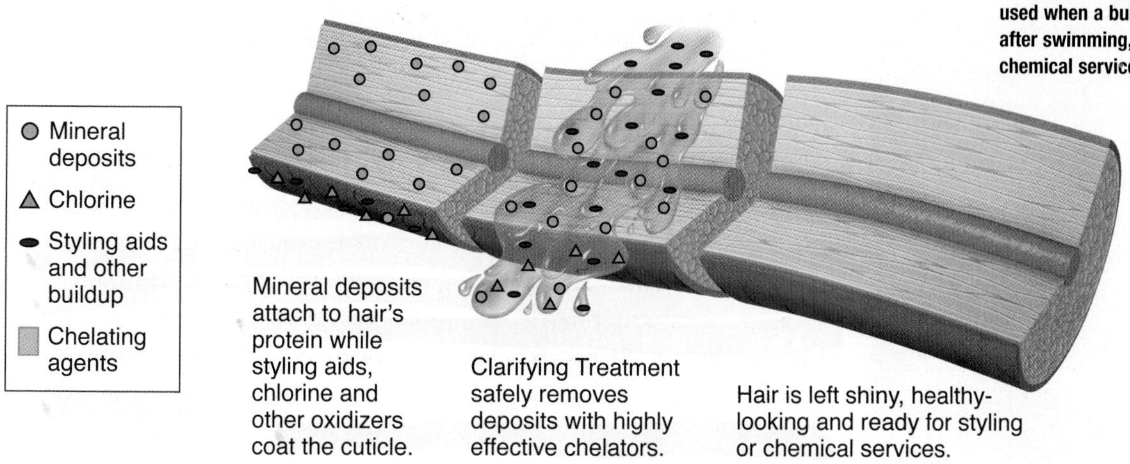

▼ **Figure 15–7**
Clarifying shampoos should be used when a buildup is evident, after swimming, and prior to all chemical services.

© Milady, a part of Cengage Learning.

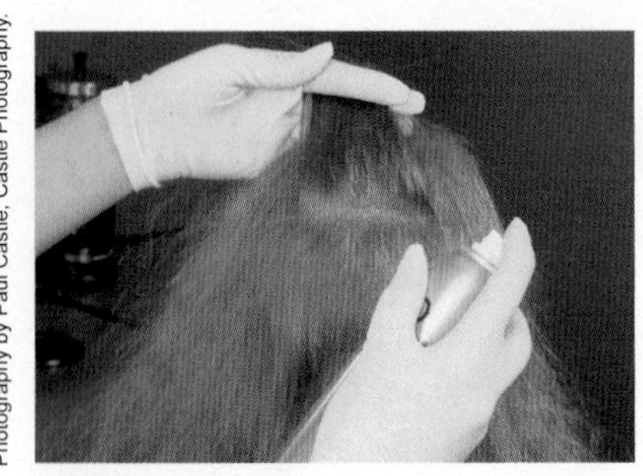

© Milady, a part of Cengage Learning. Photography by Paul Castle, Castle Photography.

▲ **Figure 15–8**
Apply the dry shampoo directly onto the scalp and out to the hair ends, then brush through with a natural-bristle brush to remove oil and dirt.

back of the neck. In such a case, it is advisable to use a **dry shampoo**, also known as **powder shampoo**, which cleanses the hair without the use of soap and water. The powder picks up dirt and oils as you brush or comb it through the hair. It also adds volume to the hair. Follow the manufacturer's instructions. Never give a dry shampoo before performing a chemical service.

A dry shampoo can be applied at the stylist's station, with the client draped as for a chemical service. Follow the manufacturer's directions, as they will vary. For the most part, you will be applying the powder directly to the hair from scalp to the ends, and then brushing through with a natural-bristle brush to remove oil and dirt (**Figure 15–8**).

FOCUS ON RETAILING

Some stylists view the shampoo as down time and use it to talk about what they did the night before. It is important to remember that your time, and your clients' time, is valuable and can be better spent. You can begin to establish your professional relationship during the shampoo by giving clients information about what you are doing and why. Let clients know what shampoo you are using and why you have selected it especially for their hair. Mention that these products are available for purchase, and emphasize their benefits. There is no need to be pushy or to worry about appearing overly assertive. Just be who you are and always be honest. When clients are concerned about the health and appearance of their hair, or when they have been unhappy with products they have been using at home, they will often make a purchase based on your advice and will thank you for your professional recommendation. You will often find that the stylist with the highest client retention also has the highest retail/home-care sales in the salon. This stylist has gained the clients' trust and professional respect.

Color-Enhancing Shampoo

Color-enhancing shampoo is created by combining the surfactant base with basic color pigment. It is similar to a temporary color rinse because it is attracted to porous hair and result in only slight color changes that are removed with plain shampooing. Color-enhancing shampoos are used to brighten, to add a slight hint of color, and to eliminate unwanted color tones, such as gold or brassiness and overly cool strands.

Shampoo for Hairpieces and Wigs

Prepared wig-cleaning solution is available for these hair enhancements (for more information on wigs and their care, see Chapter 19, Wigs and Hair Additions). ☑ **LO5**

Shampooing Clients with Special Needs

Clients with disabilities or those who are wheelchair bound will usually tell you how they prefer to be shampooed. Some clients in wheelchairs will allow you to shampoo their hair while they remain seated in their wheelchair, facing the shampoo bowl and bending forward, with a towel to protect their face. If the wheelchair is the correct height in relation to the shampoo bowl, shampoo as normal while the client remains in the wheelchair.

Sometimes a client will arrive in the salon with their hair freshly shampooed from home, and other times a dry shampoo is appropriate. The same goes for clients with other special needs. Always ask about their preferences and make their comfort and safety a priority.

Understanding Conditioner

Conditioner is a special chemical agent applied to the hair to deposit protein or moisturizer to help restore the hair's strength, to give hair body, and to protect hair against possible breakage. Conditioners are a temporary remedy or cosmetic fix for hair that feels dry or appears damaged. They can only repair hair to a certain extent; conditioners cannot improve the quality of new hair growth.

Conditioning treatments can restore luster, shine, manageability, and strength while the damaged hair grows long enough to be cut off and replaced by new, healthier hair. Because of frequent shampooing, the use of thermal styling tools and chemical services, conditioning is a must for clients who care about their hair.

Conditioners are available in the following three basic types:

- **Rinse-out conditioner.** Finishing rinses or cream rinses that are rinsed out after they are worked through the hair for detangling.
- **Treatment or repair conditioner.** Deep, penetrating conditioners that restore protein and moisture and sometimes require longer processing time or the application of heat.
- **Leave-in conditioner**. Applied to the hair and not rinsed out.

Most conditioners contain silicone along with moisture-binding **humectants** (hew-MECK-tents), substances that absorb moisture or promote the retention of moisture. Silicone reflects light and makes the hair appear shiny. Other ingredients reduce frizz or bulk up the hair. Most treatments and leave-ins contain proteins, which penetrate the cortex and reinforce the hair shaft from within.

Since the hair's cuticle is made up of overlapping scales, a healthy cuticle lies down smoothly and reflects light, giving the appearance of shiny hair. Conditioners, detangling rinses, and cream rinses, smooth the cuticle and coat the hair shaft to achieve healthier looking hair.

The cortex makes up 90 percent of the hair strand. The cortex can be penetrated with **protein conditioner**, products designed to penetrate the cortex and reinforce the hair shaft from within, to temporarily reconstruct the hair. Moisturizing conditioners also contain humectants that attract moisture from the air and are absorbed into the cortex (**Figure 15–9**).

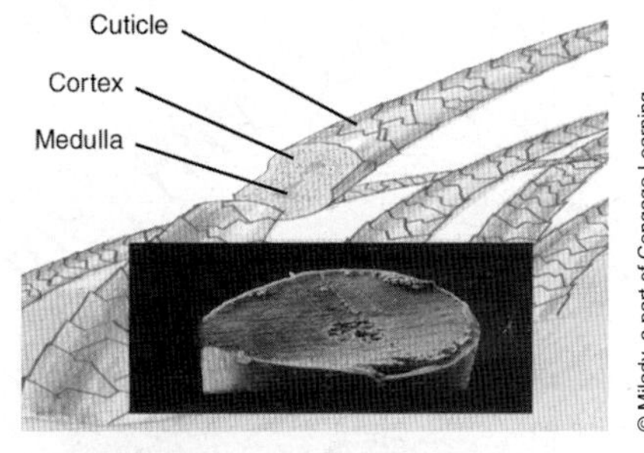

▲ **Figure 15–9**
Moisturizing conditioners contain humectants that attract moisture from the air and are absorbed into the cortex.

Other Conditioning Agents

Other conditioning agents that you need to be familiar with include the following:

- **Spray-on thermal protector** is applied to hair prior to any thermal service to protect the hair from the harmful effects of blowdrying, thermal irons, or electric rollers.
- **Scalp conditioner**, usually found in a cream base, is used to soften and improve the health of the scalp. It contains moisturizing and emollient (ee-MAHL-yunt) ingredients.
- **Medicated scalp lotion** is a conditioner that promotes healing of the scalp.
- **Scalp astringent lotion** removes oil accumulation from the scalp and are used after a scalp treatment and before styling.

Table 15–1 lists the types of products suitable for various hair types.

MATCHING PRODUCTS TO HAIR TYPES			
HAIR TYPE	**FINE**	**MEDIUM**	**COARSE**
STRAIGHT	• volumizing shampoo • detangler, if necessary • protein treatments	• ph/acid-balanced shampoo • finishing rinse • protein treatments	• moisturizing shampoo • leave-in conditioner • moisturizing treatments
WAVE, CURLY, EXTREMELY CURLY	• fine hair shampoo • light leave-in conditioner • protein • spray-on thermal protectors treatments	• ph/acid-balanced shampoo • leave-in conditioner • moisturizing treatment	• moisturizing shampoo • leave-in conditioner • protein and moisturizing treatments
DRY & DAMAGED (perms, color, relaxers, blowdrying, sun, hot irons)	• gentle cleansing shampoo • light leave-in conditioner • protein and moisturizing repair treatments • spray-on thermal protection	• shampoo for chemically treated hair • moisturizing conditioner • protein and moisturizing repair treatments	• deep-moisturizing shampoo for damaged hair • leave-in conditioner • deep-conditioning treatments and hair masks

© Milady, a part of Cengage Learning.

Table 15–1 Matching Products to Hair Types.

Deep-Conditioning Treatment

Deep-conditioning treatment, also known as **hair mask** or **conditioning pack**, is a chemical mixture of concentrated protein and intensive moisturizer. It penetrates the cuticle layer and is the chosen therapy when a moisturizing and/or protein treatment is desired.

✓ **LO6**

Draping

After the client consultation and before any professional cosmetology service can begin, the client must be appropriately draped for the service or services they are to receive. Client draping is an important aspect of every overall service because it contributes to the client's safety and comfort.

Have you ever been in a salon for a haircut and had your clothing get wet during a shampoo, because you weren't properly draped? Or worse yet, have you ever had a haircolor service and then once the service was over, realized that the haircolor was all over the collar of your shirt or somewhere else on your clothing, because the stylist didn't protect your clothing properly? Not only are these incidences annoying to the client, they are completely avoidable when the stylist takes the time to ensure a professional draping.

© digital skillet, 2010; used under license from iStockphoto.com.

There are two types of drapings that are used in the salon. They are:

1. Shampoo draping
2. Chemical service draping

A shampoo draping, sometimes called a wet draping, is a draping used when a client is in the salon for a shampoo and styling or a shampoo and haircutting service. Two terry towels are used to protect the client, one under the shampoo cape and one over the cape. Once the shampoo service is completed and before the haircutting or hairstyling service begins, the terry towels are removed and replaced with a paper neck strip, and secured with a haircutting or styling cape.

PROCEDURE 15-8 Draping for a Basic Shampoo and Conditioning SEE PAGE 333

A chemical draping is used for clients who will have a chemical service or treatment and who will not have a shampoo before the service, such as with a haircoloring, permanent wave, and chemical hair relaxing service.

In a chemical drape, the client is draped with two terry cloth towels, one under the cape and one over the cape. The towels remain as a part of the drape until the service is completed and are regularly checked for dryness and replaced by the stylist.

ACTivity

Role playing is a good way to practice recommending retail products to clients. Pair off with a classmate. One student should take the role of the stylist and the other should play a client. Your scene might go like this:

Stylist: Have you encountered any problems with your scalp or hair since your last salon visit, Mrs. Benson? Any itchiness or flaking?

Mrs. Benson: No. I don't usually have scalp problems this time of year. But in the winter I do.

Stylist: Any dryness?

Mrs. Benson: Well, ever since I started having my hair highlighted, it does feel a little drier.

Stylist: Chemical services often dry the hair. I'm going to use this shampoo for color-treated hair and finish with this moisturizing conditioner. (Show shampoo and conditioner bottles to the client and place them in her hands.)

Mrs. Benson: That sounds good. But won't the conditioner make my hair feel limp?

Stylist: I'll be using a light-weight conditioner only on your ends where you need it. It will leave your hair silky and shiny and not weigh it down. If you like it, you can purchase some before you leave. You know, using the right shampoo and conditioner will help keep your hair healthy between visits to the salon.

Mrs. Benson: Great! Let's do it!

PROCEDURE **15-9** **Draping for a Chemical Service** SEE PAGE 334

Be sure to read and follow the manufacturer's directions regarding whether or not a shampoo is required before using a particular chemical product such as haircolor. If the manufacturer requires that the client be shampooed before the color product is applied, then follow the procedure for the shampoo draping, shampoo the client gently and, before the chemical service is to begin, redrape her for a chemical service. ☑ **LO7**

Three-Part Procedure

It is easier to keep track of what you are doing, to remain organized, and to give consistent service if you break your hair care procedures into three individual parts. The Three-Part Procedure consists of: 1) pre-service, 2) actual service, and 3) post-service.

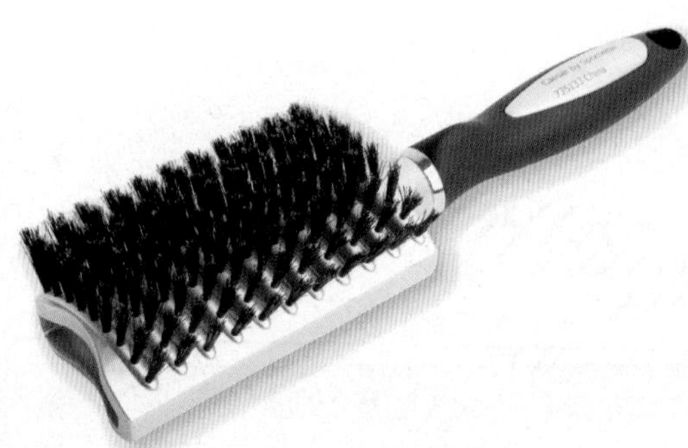

© Milady, a part of Cengage Learning.

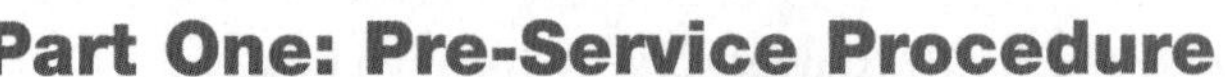

Part One: Pre-Service Procedure

The pre-service procedure is an organized step-by-step plan for the cleaning and disinfecting of your tools, implements, and materials; for setting up your station; and for meeting, greeting, and escorting your client to your service area.

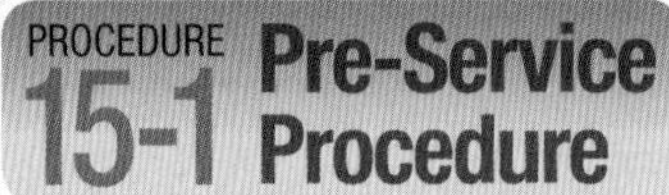

PROCEDURE **15-1** **Pre-Service Procedure** SEE PAGE 323

Part Two: Service Procedure

The service procedure is an organized, step-by-step plan for accomplishing the actual service the client has requested such as a shampoo, haircut or haircoloring.

Part Three: Post-Service Procedure

The post-service procedure is an organized step-by-step plan for caring for your client after the procedure has been completed. It details helping your client through the scheduling and payment process of the salon and provides information for you on how to prepare for the next client. ☑ **LO8**

PROCEDURE **15-2** **Post-Service Procedure** SEE PAGE 326

PROCEDURE 15-1

Pre-Service Procedure

A. Cleaning and Disinfecting

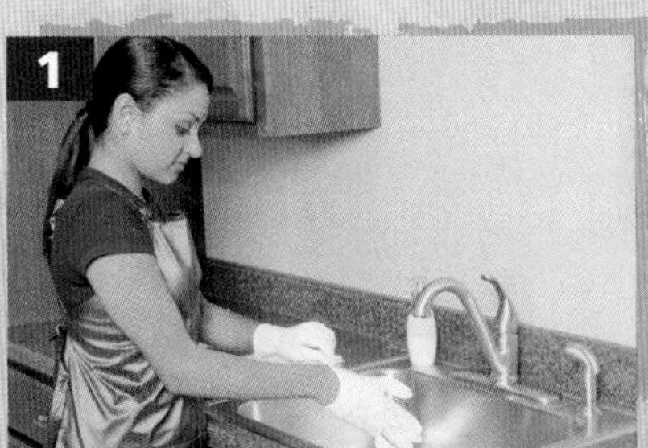

1 Put on a fresh pair of gloves while performing this pre-service to prevent possible contamination of the implements by your hands and to protect your hands from the powerful chemicals in the disinfectant solution.

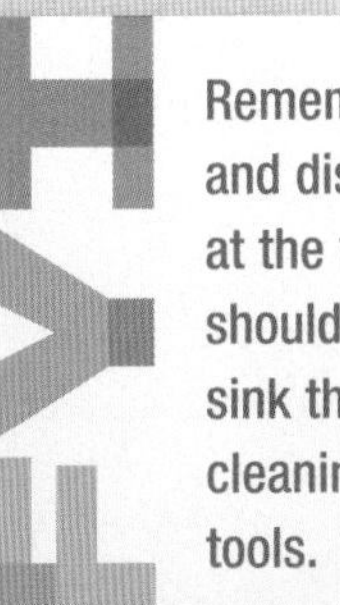

FYI Remember: Do not clean and disinfect your tools at the workstation. There should be an area near a sink that is set aside for cleaning and disinfecting tools.

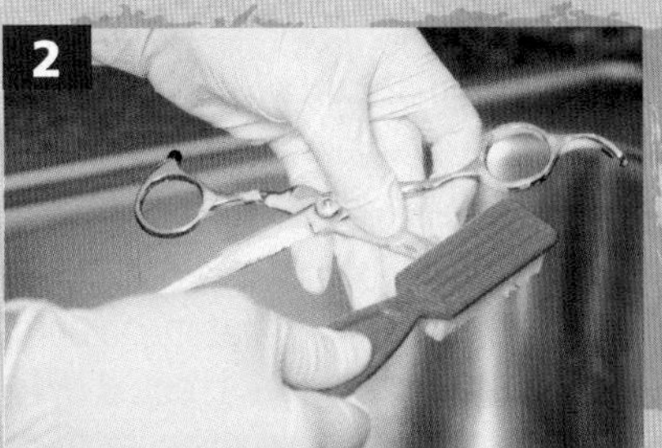

2 Clean all tools and implements such as combs, brushes, rollers, clips, scissors, and any other reusable, nonelectrical items by first rinsing them in warm running water, and then thoroughly washing them with soap, a small nylon brush, and warm water. Brush grooved items, if necessary, and open hinged tools to scrub the revealed area.

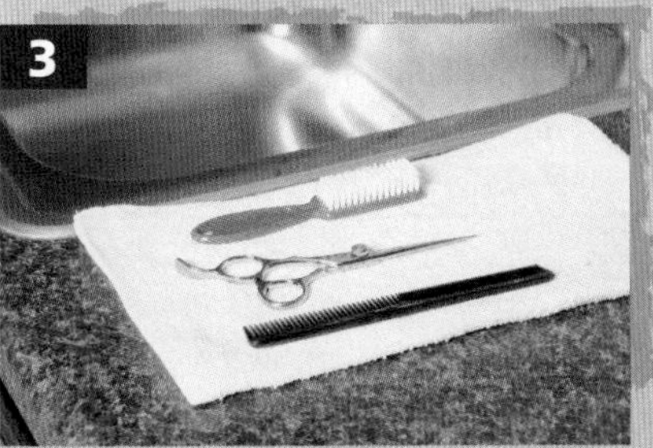

3 Rinse away all traces of soap with warm running water. The presence of soap in most disinfectants can cause them to become inactive. Dry the items thoroughly with a clean fabric or disposable towel, or allow them to air dry on a clean towel. Your implements are now properly cleaned and ready to be disinfected.

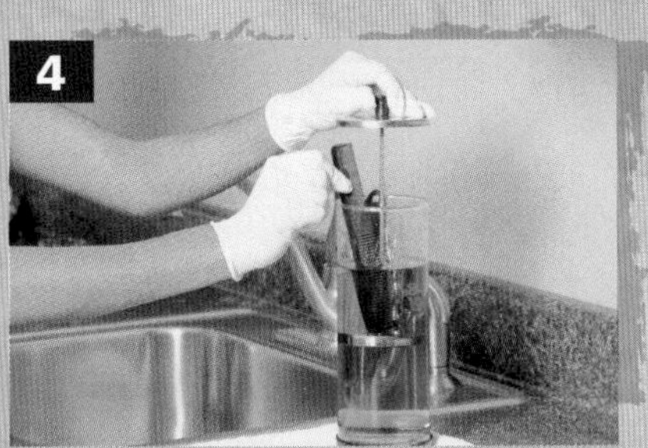

4 Immerse cleaned implements in an appropriate disinfection container holding an EPA-registered disinfectant for the required time (usually ten minutes). Remember to open hinged implements before immersing them in disinfectant solution. If the disinfectant solution is visibly dirty, the solution has been contaminated and must be replaced.

5 Remove implements, avoiding skin contact, and rinse and dry tools thoroughly.

6 Store disinfected implements in a clean, dry container until needed.

© Milady, a part of Cengage Learning. Photography by Yanik Chauvin.

Pre-Service Procedure continued

Service Tip

Take a moment and sit in your styling chair and take a good look around. Based on what you see, hear, and feel, ask yourself this question—what kind of an experience will my client have while she's here?

Asking yourself the following questions will ensure that you have done everything you can to prepare your client for a positive experience:

1. Is my station clean and organized or cluttered and messy?
2. Will the music and the temperature be comfortable for the client?
3. Am I wearing too much perfume/cologne? Am I carrying an unpleasant food or tobacco odor? Is my breath pleasant-smelling?
4. Do I see the professional I want to be when I look at myself in the mirror? Do my hair, clothing, and personal grooming look professional?
5. Do I look like I am happy and enjoying my work?
6. Is there some problem bothering me today that is affecting my ability to concentrate on the needs of my client?

Remember the old adage—*You only get one chance to make a good first impression.* Take the opportunity to stack the odds in your favor!

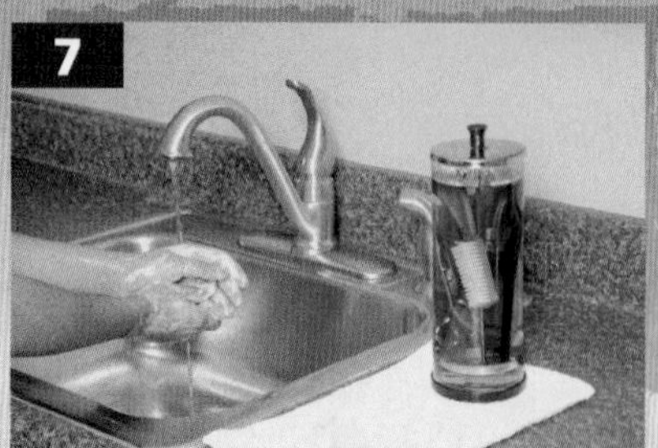

7 Remove gloves and thoroughly wash your hands with liquid soap. Then rinse and dry them with a clean fabric or disposable towel.

B. Basic Station Setup

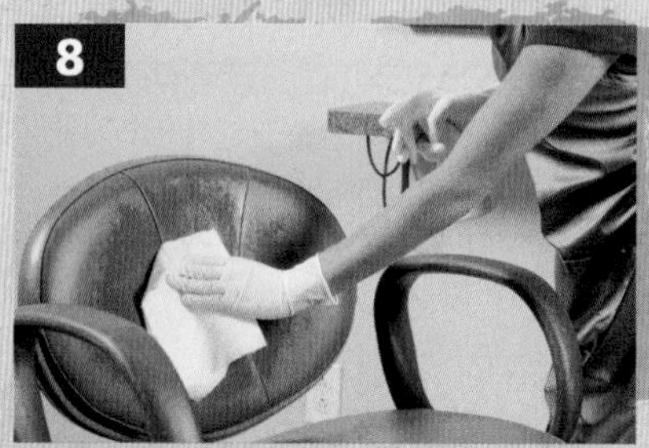

8 Put on a fresh pair of gloves and clean and disinfect your station and client chair with an approved disinfectant cleaner.

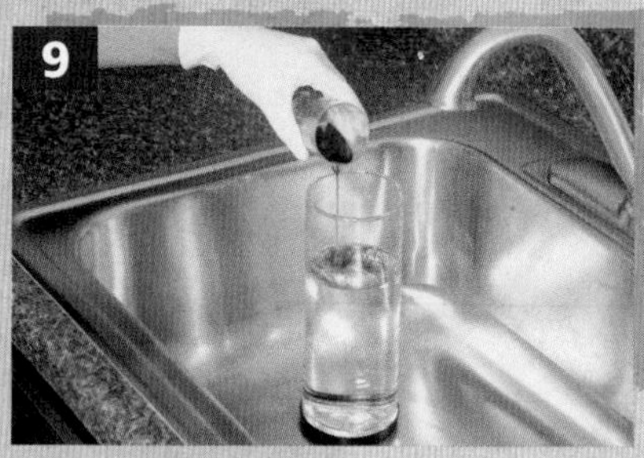

9 Ensure that your disinfection container is filled with clean disinfectant solution at least twenty minutes before your first service of the day. Use any disinfectant solution approved by your state board regulations, but make sure that you use it exactly as directed by the manufacturer. Also make sure that you change the disinfectant every day or when the solution is visibly contaminated with debris.

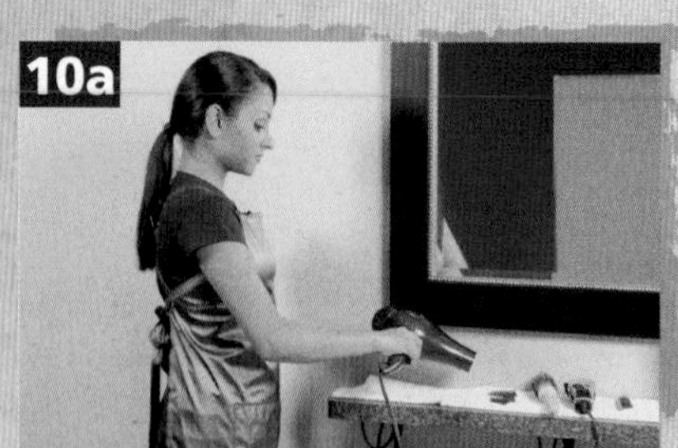

10a

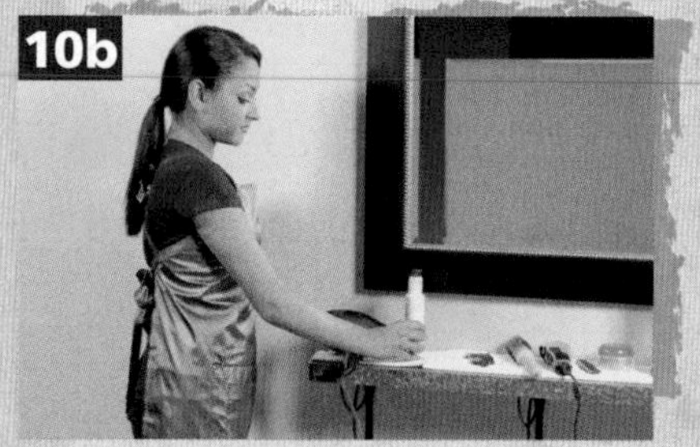

10b

10 Collect all implements and professional products that you will use during the service, along with any electrical equipment such as a blowdryer or clippers, and bring them to your station.

© Milady, a part of Cengage Learning. Photography by Yanik Chauvin.

C. Stylist Preparation

11 Review your appointment schedule for the day and resolve any potential time conflicts or challenges you perceive.

12 Retrieve the client's intake form and consultation card and review them. If the appointment is for a new client, be sure to either have a blank intake form at your station, or ensure that the receptionist will provide one to the client.

13 Organize yourself by taking care of your personal needs before the client arrives—use the restroom, get a drink of water, return a personal call—complete whatever you need to so that when your client arrives, your full attention is focused on her needs.

14 Turn off your cell phone, pager, or PDA. Be sure that you eliminate anything that can distract you from your client while she is in the salon.

15 Take a moment to clear your head of all personal concerns and issues. Take a couple of deep breaths and remind yourself that you are committed to providing your client with fantastic service and your full attention.

16 Wash your hands thoroughly before going to greet your client.

D. Greet Client

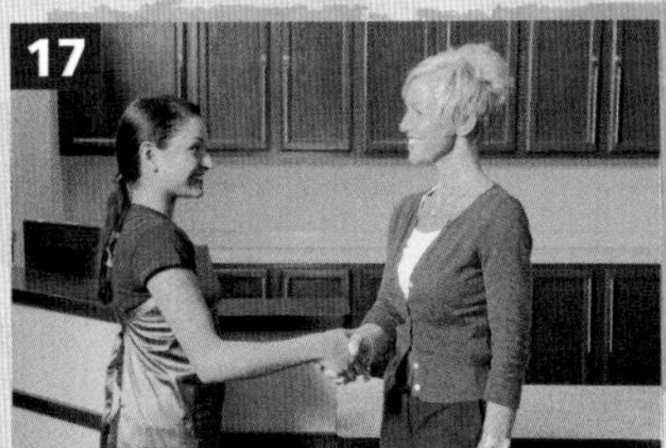

17 Greet the client in the reception area with a warm smile and in a professional manner. Introduce yourself if you have never met, and shake hands. The handshake is very important because it is your first physical contact. If the client is new, ask her for the intake form she filled out in the reception area.

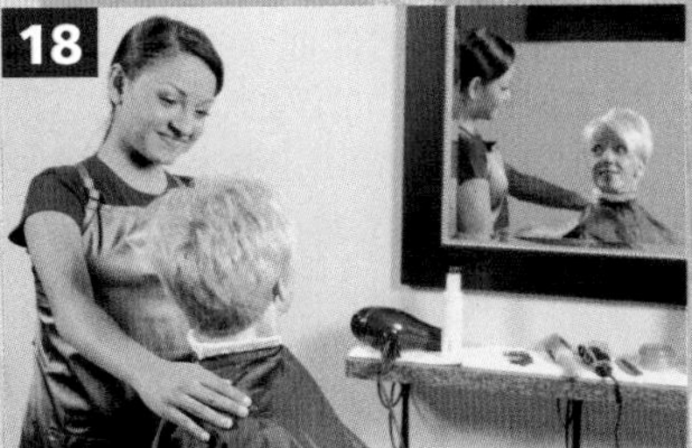

18 Escort the client to your station and invite her to take a seat. Make sure your client is comfortable before beginning the service. Remember, the client is not just a haircut, haircolor, or whatever service is scheduled, but a person with whom you want to build a relationship. By showing a client respect, you lay the foundation that establishes trust in you as a professional. An open, honest, and sincere approach is always the most effective in winning the client's trust, respect, and, ultimately, loyalty.

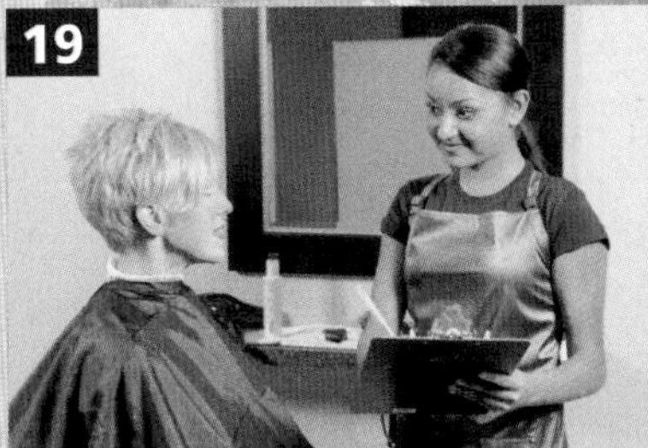

19 Perform a consultation before beginning the service. Discuss the information on the intake form and determine a course of action for the service.

© Milady, a part of Cengage Learning. Photography by Yanik Chauvin.

PROCEDURE 15-2

Post-Service Procedure

A. Advise Clients and Promote Products

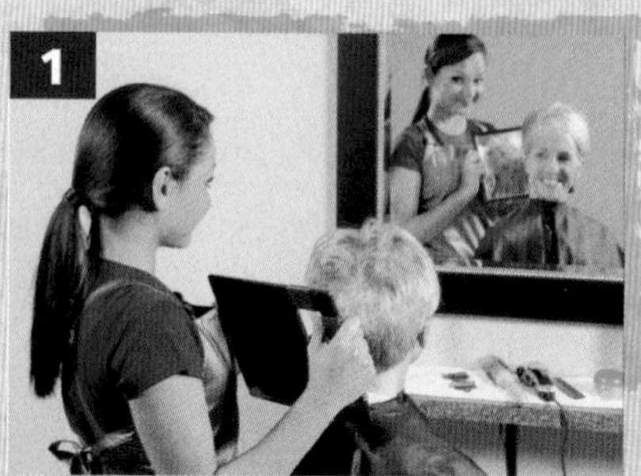

1 Before your client leaves your styling chair, show her all angles of the completed service. Determine if the client is satisfied with the outcome of your service by asking if she (or he) is pleased or has any questions or concerns to discuss. Be receptive and listen. Never be defensive. If possible, make any adjustments for total satisfaction or give an explanation as to what adjustments are achievable. Determine a plan for future visits. Give the client ideas to think over for next time.

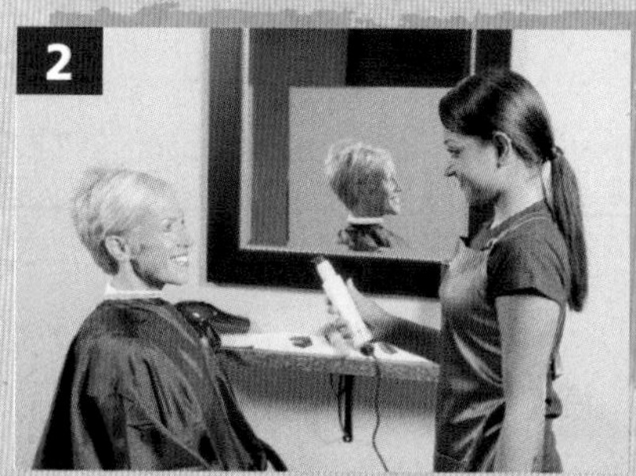

2 Advise the client about proper at-home maintenance for the service received and explain how using the recommended professional products will ensure that the hair service maintains its beauty and performance until your client returns for another visit. This is the time to discuss your retail product recommendations. Explain why the recommended products are important and how to use them.

B. Schedule Next Appointment and Thank Client

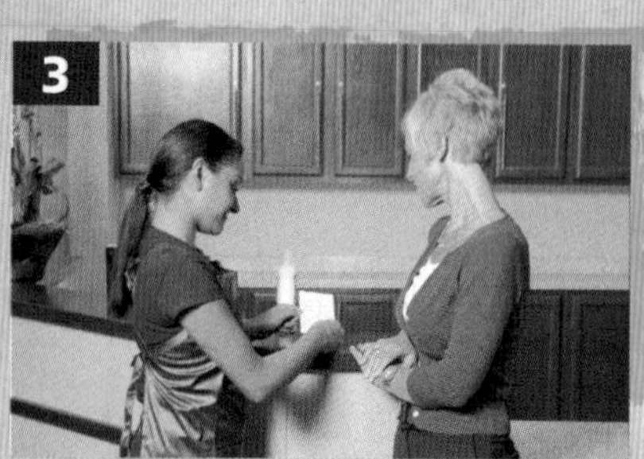

3 Escort the client to the reception desk, write up a service ticket that describes the service provided, and recommend home care and scheduling for the next visit/service. Place all the recommended professional retail home-care products on the counter for the client. Review the service ticket and the product recommendations with your client.

© Milady, a part of Cengage Learning. Photography by Yanik Chauvin.

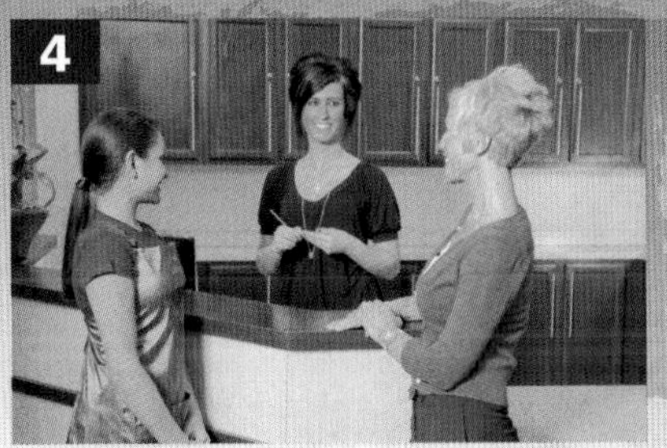

4 After the client has paid for her service and take-home products, ask her if you can schedule her next appointment for her. Set up the date, time, and services for this next appointment. Write the information on your business card and give it to the client.

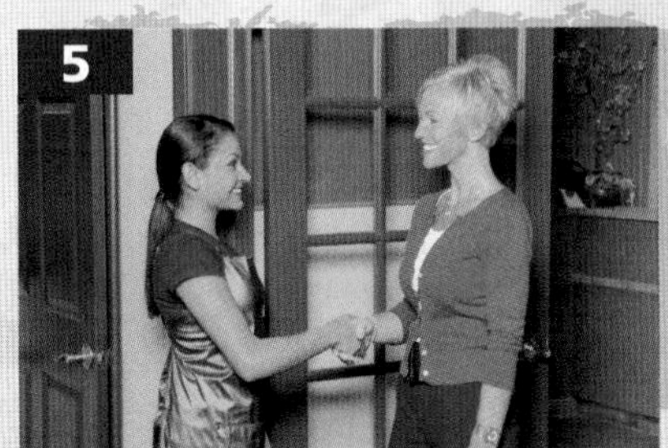

5 Thank the client for the opportunity to work with her. Express an interest in working with her again in the near future. Invite her to contact you should she have any questions or concerns about the service provided. If the client seems apprehensive, offer to call her in a day or two in order to check in with her about any issues she may encounter. Genuinely wish her well, shake her hand, and wish her a great day.

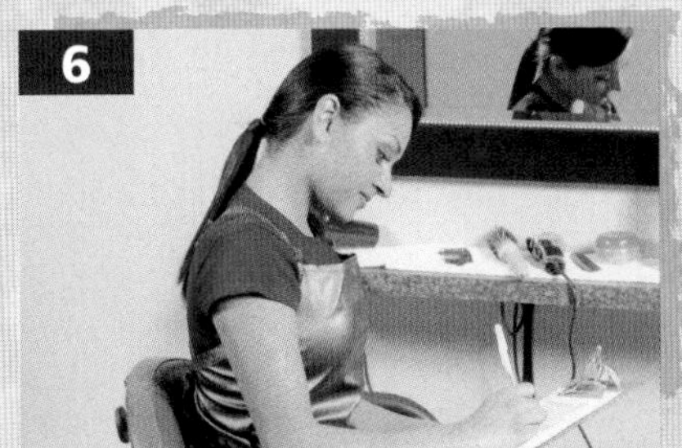

6 Once you return to your station, be sure to record service information, observations, and product recommendations on the intake form or consultation card. Be sure you return the intake form or consultation card to the proper place for filing.

C. Prepare Work Area and Implements for Next Client

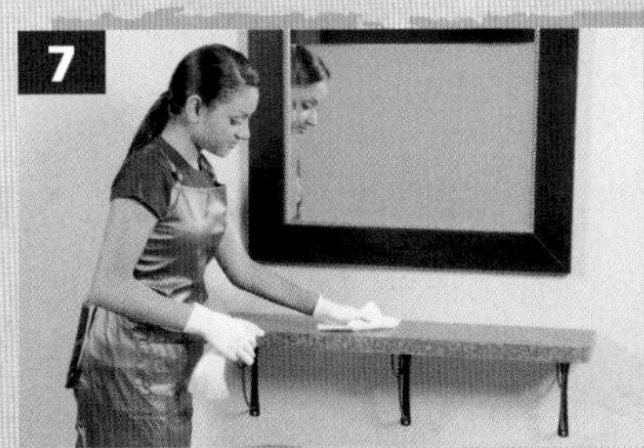

7 Put on a fresh pair of gloves and clean, then disinfect and reorganize your station, sweep and dispose of hair properly in a covered trash receptacle. Place all used towels and capes in the laundry. Close and remove any styling products or aids you used.

8 Clean and then disinfect all used tools and implements. Follow all steps for disinfecting implements described in the pre-service procedure.

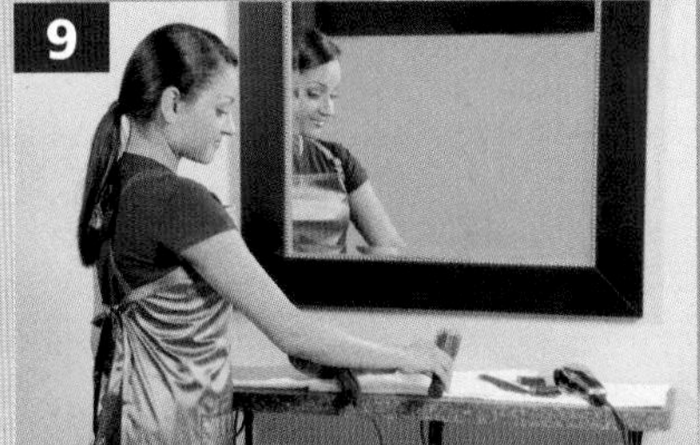

9 Reset your station with disinfected tools and the proper styling products and prepare to greet your next client.

© Milady, a part of Cengage Learning. Photography by Yanik Chauvin.

PROCEDURE 15-3

Normal Hair and Scalp Treatment

Implements and Materials

You will need all of the following implements, materials, and supplies:

- **Disposable or linen towels**
- **Hairbrush**
- **Hooded dryer**
- **Scalp lotion or conditioner**
- **Shampoo**
- **Shampoo cape**

Preparation

- Perform PROCEDURE 15-1 **Pre-Service Procedure** SEE PAGE 323

Procedure

1 Show your client to the shampoo chair and assist him or her in becoming comfortable.

2 Drape your client for a shampoo. (See Procedure 15–8, Draping for a Basic Shampooing and Conditioning.)

3 Ask the client to remove all hair ornaments, hairpins, and so on.

4 Have client remove jewelry and glasses.

5 Examine condition of scalp to be sure there are no abrasions.

6 Brush hair for five minutes. (See Procedure 15–7, Hair Brushing.)

7 Apply scalp lotion or conditioner.

8 Apply heat for about five minutes.

9 Massage scalp for ten to twenty minutes. (See Procedure 15–11, Scalp Massage.)

10 Shampoo the hair. (See Procedure 15–10, Basic Shampooing and Conditioning.)

11 Towel dry the hair.

12 Move on to the next step of the service or apply styling aids and finish the hair.

Post-Service

- Complete PROCEDURE 15-2 **Post-Service Procedure** SEE PAGE 326

PROCEDURE 15-4

Dry Hair and Scalp Treatment

Implements and Materials

You will need all of the following implements, materials, and supplies:

- **Direct high-frequency current with glass rake electrode**
- **Disposable or linen towels**
- **Hairbrush**
- **Moisturizing scalp cream**
- **Scalp preparation**
- **Shampoo**
- **Shampoo cape**
- **Scalp Steamer**

CAUTION

Do not use high-frequency current on hair treated with tonics or lotions that contain alcohol.

Preparation

- Perform PROCEDURE 15-1 **Pre-Service Procedure** **SEE PAGE 323**

Procedure

1 Show your client to the shampoo chair and assist him or her in becoming comfortable.

2 Drape your client for a shampoo. **(See Procedure 15–8, Draping for a Basic Shampooing and Conditioning.)**

3 Ask the client to remove all hair ornaments, hairpins, and so on.

4 Have client remove jewelry and glasses.

5 Examine condition of scalp to be sure there are no abrasions.

6 Brush hair for five minutes. **(See Procedure 15–7, Hair Brushing.)**

7 Apply the scalp preparation for this condition.

8 Apply the scalp steamer for seven to ten minutes, or wrap the head in warm steam towels for seven to ten minutes.

9 Shampoo with a corrective shampoo for dry hair.

10 Towel dry the hair and scalp thoroughly.

11 Apply moisturizing scalp cream sparingly with a rotary, frictional motion.

12 Stimulate the scalp with direct high-frequency current, using the glass rake electrode, for about five minutes.

13 Rinse the hair thoroughly.

14 Towel dry.

15 Move on to the next step of the service.

Post-Service

- Complete PROCEDURE 15-2 **Post-Service Procedure** **SEE PAGE 326**

PROCEDURE 15-5

Oily Hair and Scalp Treatment

Implements and Materials

You will need all of the following implements, materials, and supplies:

- **Corrective shampoo for oily hair**
- **Cotton pledget**
- **Disposable or linen towels**
- **Hairbrush**
- **Hooded dryer**
- **Infrared lamp**
- **Medicated scalp lotion**
- **Moisturizing scalp cream**
- **Scalp astringent**
- **Shampoo cape**

Preparation

- Perform PROCEDURE 15-1 **Pre-Service Procedure** **SEE PAGE 323**

Procedure

1 Show your client to the shampoo chair and assist him or her in becoming comfortable.

2 Drape your client for a shampoo. (See Procedure 15–8, Draping for a Basic Shampooing and Conditioning.)

3 Ask the client to remove all hair ornaments, hairpins, and so on.

4 Have client remove jewelry and glasses.

5 Examine condition of scalp to be sure there are no abrasions.

6 Brush hair for five minutes. (See Procedure 15–7, Hair Brushing.)

7 Apply scalp lotion. Using a cotton pledget (a tuft of cotton), apply a medicated scalp lotion to the scalp only.

8 Apply infrared lamp or heated dryer for about five minutes.

9 Massage the scalp. (See Procedure 15–11, Scalp Massage.)

10 Shampoo with a corrective shampoo for oily hair. (See Procedure 15–10, Basic Shampooing and Conditioning.)

11 Towel dry the hair.

12 Apply direct high-frequency current for three to five minutes.

13 Apply a scalp astringent and/or suitable styling aids.

Post-Service

- Complete PROCEDURE 15-2 **Post-Service Procedure** **SEE PAGE 326**

PROCEDURE 15-6

Antidandruff Treatment

Implements and Materials

You will need all of the following implements, materials, and supplies:

- **Antidandruff shampoo**
- **Disposable or linen towels**
- **Hairbrush**
- **Infrared lamp**
- **Scalp steamer**
- **Shampoo cape**

Preparation

- Perform PROCEDURE 15-1 **Pre-Service Procedure** SEE PAGE 323

Procedure

1 Show your client to the shampoo chair and assist him or her in becoming comfortable.

2 Drape your client for a shampoo. (See Procedure 15–8, Draping for a Basic Shampooing and Conditioning.)

3 Ask the client to remove all hair ornaments, hairpins, and so on.

4 Have client remove jewelry and glasses.

5 Examine condition of scalp to be sure there are no abrasions.

6 Brush hair for five minutes. (See Procedure 15–7, Hair Brushing.)

7 Apply an antidandruff conditioner or lotion.

8 Apply heat with an infrared lamp or scalp steamer for about five minutes (optional).

9 Shampoo with an antidandruff shampoo.

10 Towel dry the hair.

Service Tip

Some antidandruff treatments are alcohol-based and should not be used in conjunction with infrared lamps.

Post-Service

- Complete PROCEDURE 15-2 **Post-Service Procedure** SEE PAGE 326

PROCEDURE 15-7

Hair Brushing

Implements and Materials

You will need all of the following implements, materials, and supplies:

- **Comb**
- **Disposable or linen towels**
- **Hairbrush**
- **Shampoo cape**

Preparation

- Perform PROCEDURE 15-1 **Pre-Service Procedure** SEE PAGE 323

Procedure

1 Show your client to the shampoo chair and assist him or her in becoming comfortable.

2 Drape your client for a shampoo. (See Procedure 15–8, Draping for a Basic Shampooing and Conditioning.)

3 Ask the client to remove all hair ornaments, hairpins, and so on.

4 Have client remove jewelry and glasses.

5 Examine condition of scalp to be sure there are no abrasions.

6 Part the hair using a half-head parting.

7 Further subsection the hair 1 inch from the front hairline to crown.

8 Hold hair in nondominant hand between thumb and fingers.

9 Lay brush (held in dominant hand) with bristles down on hair close to scalp.

10 Rotate brush by turning wrist slightly and sweeping bristles full length of hair shaft.

11 Repeat brushing three times on each strand.

12 Continue brushing until entire head has been brushed.

13 Now, move on to the next portion of the service.

Post-Service

- Complete PROCEDURE 15-2 **Post-Service Procedure** SEE PAGE 326

PROCEDURE 15-8

Draping for a Basic Shampooing and Conditioning

Implements and Materials

- **Shampoo cape**
- **Two terry cloth towels**
- **Neck Strip**

Procedure

1 Once the client is comfortably seated in the shampoo chair, turn their collar to the inside of their shirt, if needed.

2 Place a terry cloth towel, folded lengthwise and diagonally, across the client's shoulders and cross the ends under the client's chin.

3 Place a shampoo cape over the towel, and fasten in the back securely, making sure it does not touch the client's skin.

4 Place another terry towel over the cape and secure it in the front.

5 Proceed with the shampoo procedure. (See Procedure 15–10, Basic Shampooing and Conditioning.)

6 Once the shampoo is completed, escort the client back to your work station.

7 Help the client to get comfortably seated and using towel two of the original draping, completely towel dry the hair. Once towel dried, pin long hair up, out of the way.

8 Remove the shampoo cape and towel one. Dispose of towels one and two properly.

9 Secure a neck strip around the client's neck. Place and fasten a cutting or styling cape over the neck strip. Fold the neck strip down over the cape so that no part of the cape touches the client's skin.

10 Proceed with the scheduled service.

PROCEDURE 15-9

Draping for a Chemical Service

Implements and Materials

- Shampoo cape
- Two terry cloth towels

Procedure

1 Once the client is comfortably seated in the shampoo or styling chair, turn their collar to the inside of their shirt, if needed.

2 Place a terry cloth towel, folded lengthwise and diagonally, across the client's shoulders and cross the ends under the client's chin.

3 Place a chemical cape over the towel, and fasten in the back securely, making sure it does not touch the client's skin.

4 Place another terry towel over the cape and secure it in the front.

5 Proceed with the chemical service. Be sure to check both towels used in the draping. If either towel becomes wet or soiled with chemicals or other product, replace it promptly.

PROCEDURE 15-10

Basic Shampooing and Conditioning

Implements and Materials

You will need all of the following implements, materials, and supplies:

- **Comb and hairbrush**
- **Conditioner**
- **Hooded dryer**
- **Plastic cap**
- **Shampoo**
- **Shampoo cape**
- **Three towels**

Preparation

- Perform PROCEDURE 15-1 **Pre-Service Procedure** **SEE PAGE 323**

Procedure

1 Show your client to the shampoo chair and assist him or her in becoming comfortable.

2 Drape your client for a shampoo. (See Procedure 15–8, Draping for a Basic Shampooing and Conditioning.)

3 Ask the client to remove all hair ornaments, hairpins, and so on.

4 Have client remove jewelry and glasses.

5 Examine condition of scalp to be sure there are no abrasions.

6 Brush hair thoroughly. (See Procedure 15–7, Hair Brushing.)

7 Assist the client in leaning back, into the shampoo bowl, making sure that her neck fits properly into the neck rest.

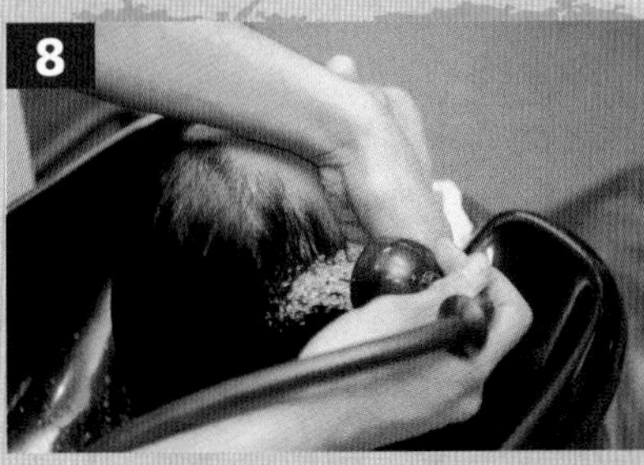

8 Turn on the water and adjust volume and temperature of water spray. Test water temperature on inner wrist; monitor by keeping fingers under spray. Saturate the hair with warm water. Lift hair and work it with free hand; protect the client's face, ears, and neck from spray.

© Milady, a part of Cengage Learning. Photography by Yanik Chauvin.

PROCEDURE 15-10

Basic Shampooing and Conditioning continued

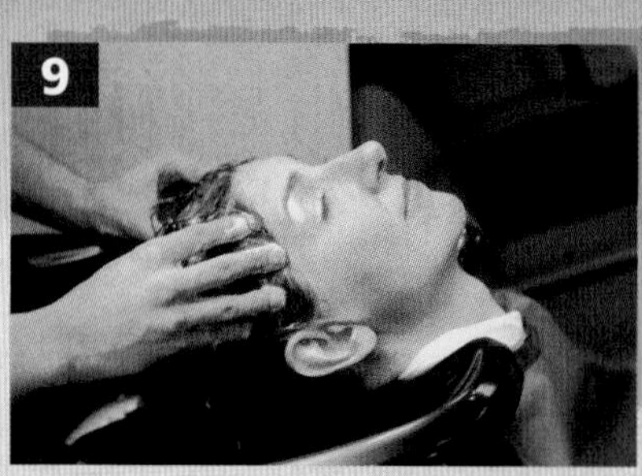

9 Apply a small amount of shampoo. Begin at the hairline, and work back and into lather using the cushions (pads) of fingertips.

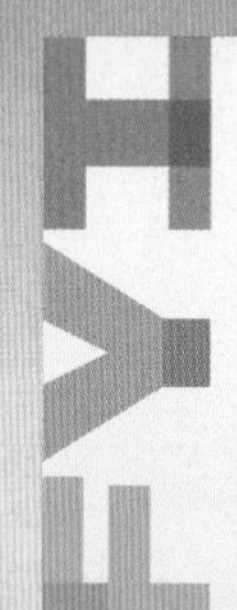

Do not use firm pressure if you will follow the shampoo with a chemical service, if the client's scalp is tender or sensitive, or if the client requests less pressure.

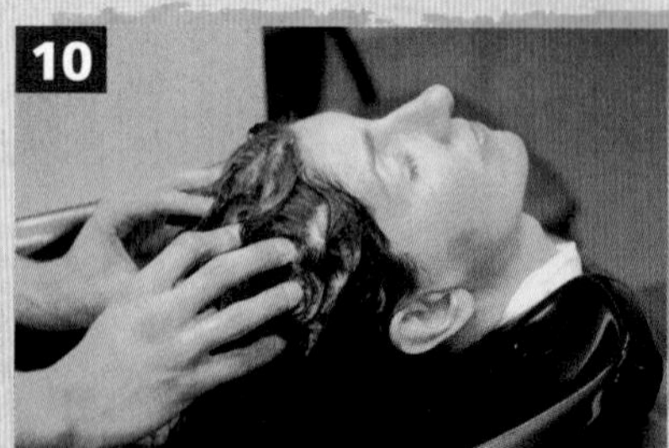

10 Begin at front hairline and work in back and forth movements until top of head is reached.

11 Continue to back of head, shifting fingers back about 1 inch at a time.

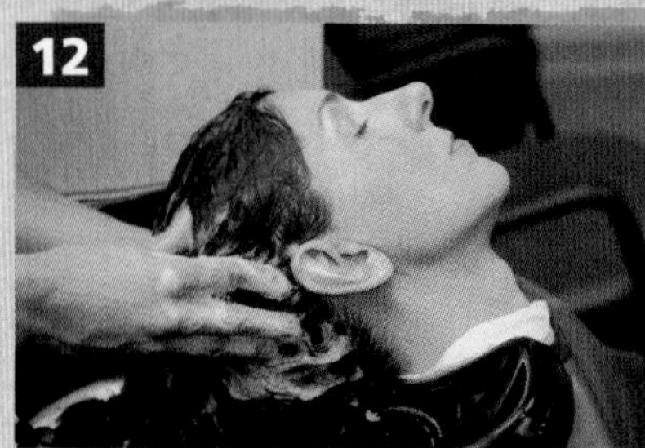

12 Lift head with either hand depending on whether you are right- or left-handed; with the nondominant hand start at top of right ear, using back and forth movement, and work to back of the head.

13 Drop fingers down about 1 inch and repeat the process until right side of head has been shampooed.

14 Beginning at the left ear, repeat the prior two steps on the left side of head.

15 Allow client's head to relax and work around hairline with thumbs in a rotary movement.

16 Repeat all steps until scalp has been thoroughly shampooed. Remove excess lather by squeezing hair gently.

17 Rinse hair thoroughly, using a strong spray of water.

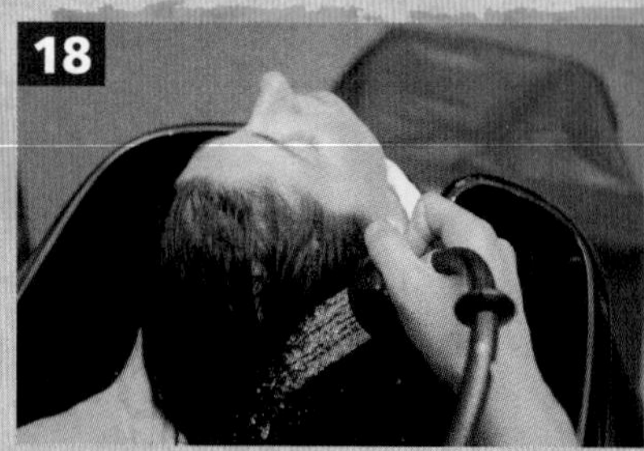

18 Lift hair at crown and back to permit spray to rinse hair until water runs clear.

19 Cup your hand along nape line and pat the hair, forcing spray against base scalp area.

20 Shampoo and rinse again if needed.

© Milady, a part of Cengage Learning. Photography by Yanik Chauvin.

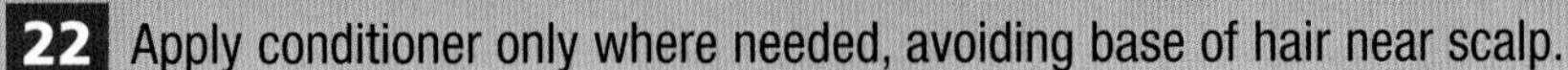

21 Gently squeeze excess water from hair.

22 Apply conditioner only where needed, avoiding base of hair near scalp.

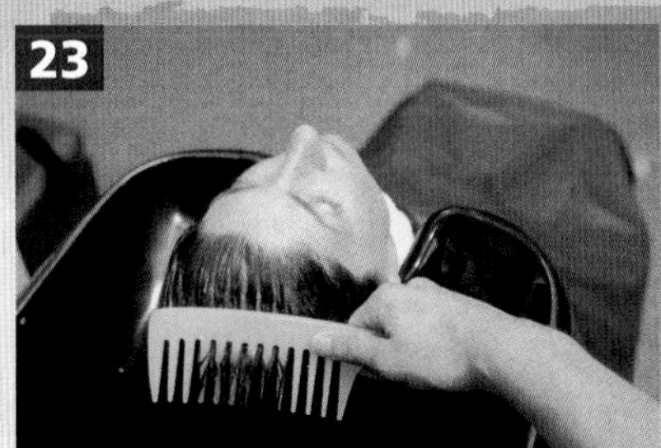

23 Gently comb conditioner through, distributing it with a wide-tooth comb.

24 Massage scalp, if applicable. (See Procedure 15–11, Scalp Massage.)

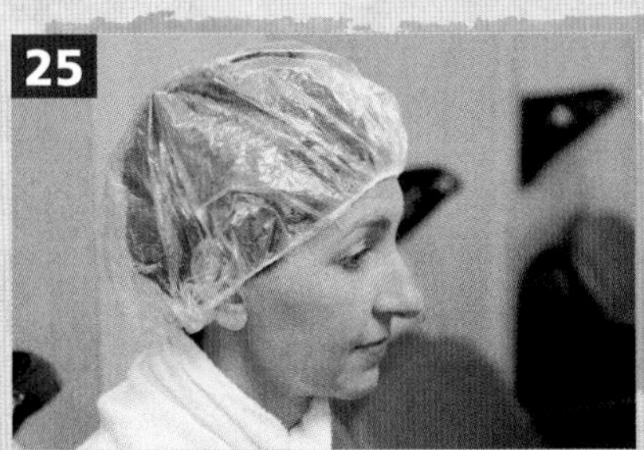

25 If conditioner is to remain on hair more than one minute, as in a deep-conditioning treatment, place a plastic cap on the client's head and sit the client upright for recommended time. If heat is required, follow manufacturer's directions.

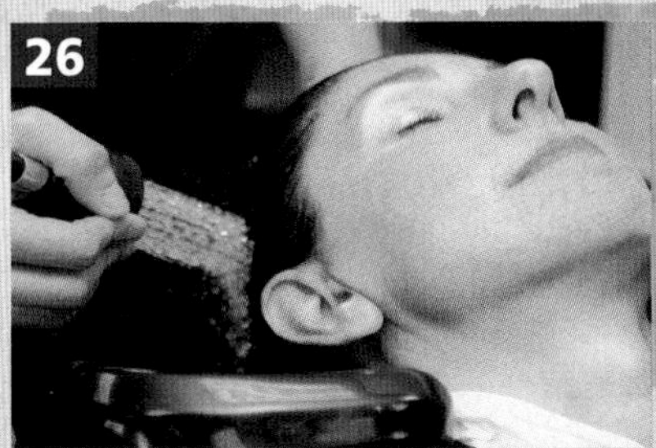

26 Rinse hair thoroughly.

27 Remove excess moisture from hair at the shampoo bowl, before the client sits up, by partially towel drying the hair and wiping excess moisture from around client's face and ears with ends of towel.

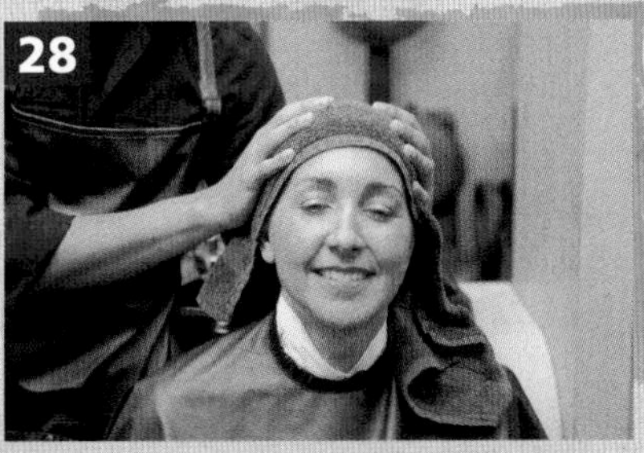

28 Lift towel and drape over client's head by placing your hands on top of towel and massaging until hair is partially dry. Ask the client to sit up.

29 Clean out shampoo bowl, removing any loose hair.

30 Escort the client back to your work station.

31 Once the client is comfortably seated, completely towel dry the hair and if needed, pin it up, out of the way. Change the drape to keep the client's clothing dry, and then comb client's hair, beginning with the ends at the nape of the neck.

32 Now you are ready to proceed with the rest of the service.

© Milady, a part of Cengage Learning. Photography by Yanik Chauvin.

Post-Service

- Complete PROCEDURE 15-2 **Post-Service Procedure** **SEE PAGE 326**

PROCEDURE 15-11

Scalp Massage

Preparation

- Perform PROCEDURE 15-1 Pre-Service Procedure SEE PAGE 323
- Perform PROCEDURE 15-10 Basic Shampooing and Conditioning SEE PAGE 335 through step 23.

Procedure

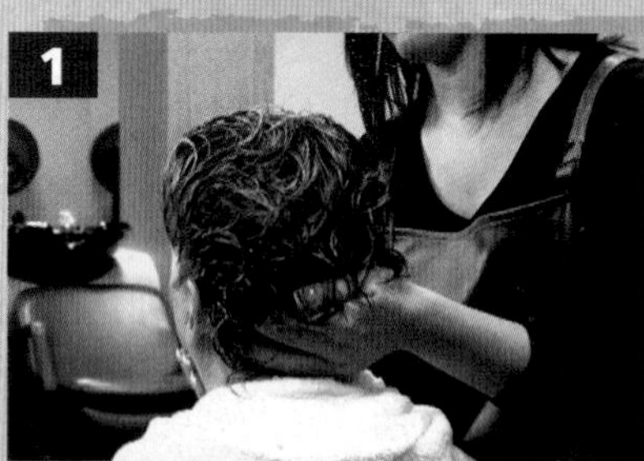

1 To begin the scalp massage cup the client's chin in your left hand. Place your right hand at the base of the skull and rotate the head gently. Reverse position of your hands and repeat.

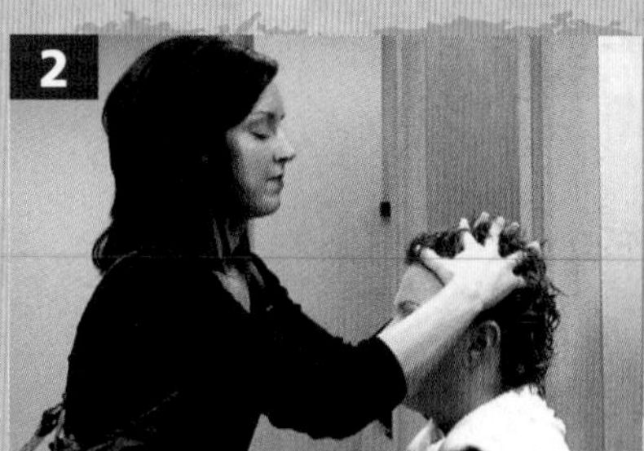

2 Place your fingertips on each side of the client's head; slide your hands firmly upward, spreading the fingertips until they meet at the top of the head. Repeat four times.

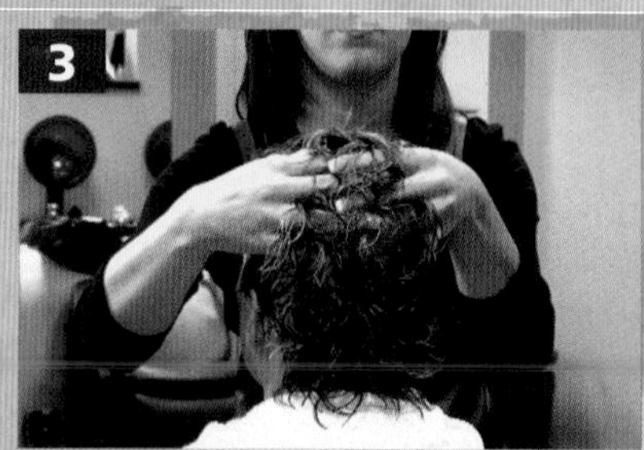

3 Place your fingertips again on each side of the client's head, this time 1 inch (2.5 cm) back from where you placed your fingertips in step 2. Slide your hands firmly upward, spreading the fingertips until they meet at the top of the head, rotate and move the client's scalp. Repeat four times.

© Milady, a part of Cengage Learning.

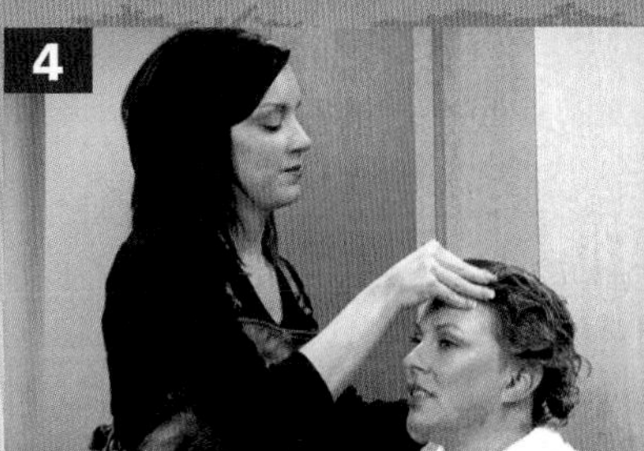

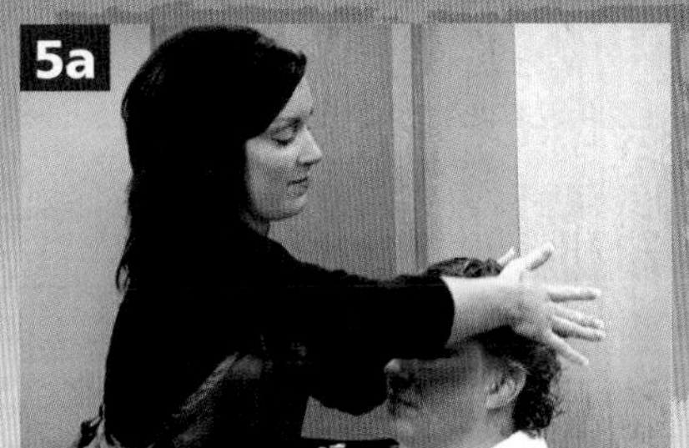

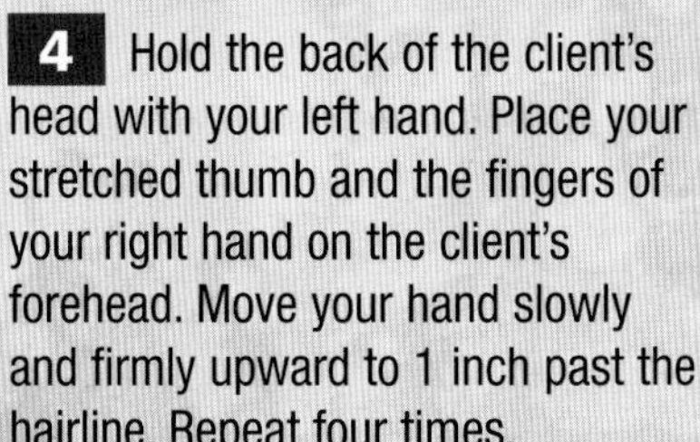

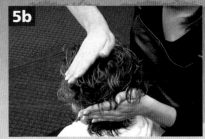

4 Hold the back of the client's head with your left hand. Place your stretched thumb and the fingers of your right hand on the client's forehead. Move your hand slowly and firmly upward to 1 inch past the hairline. Repeat four times.

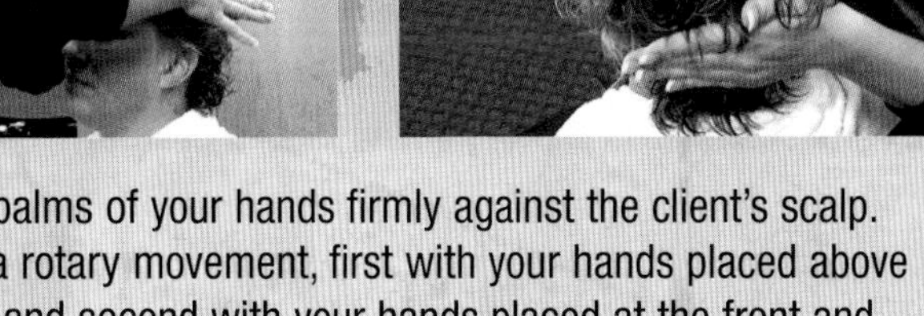

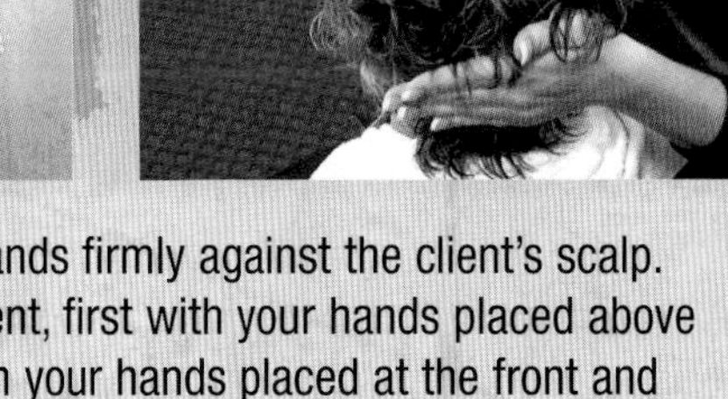

5 Place the palms of your hands firmly against the client's scalp. Lift the scalp in a rotary movement, first with your hands placed above the client's ears, and second with your hands placed at the front and back of the client's head.

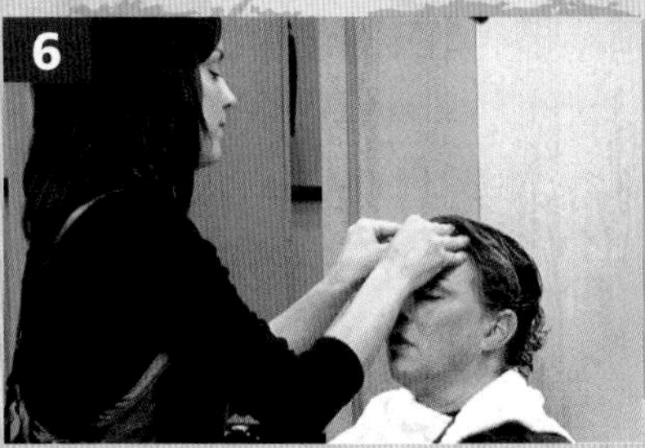

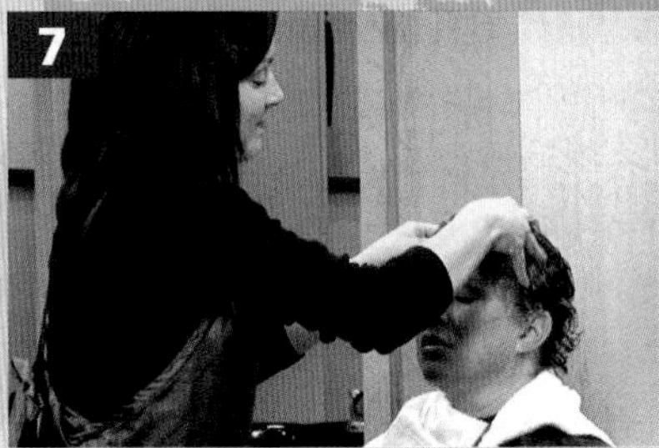

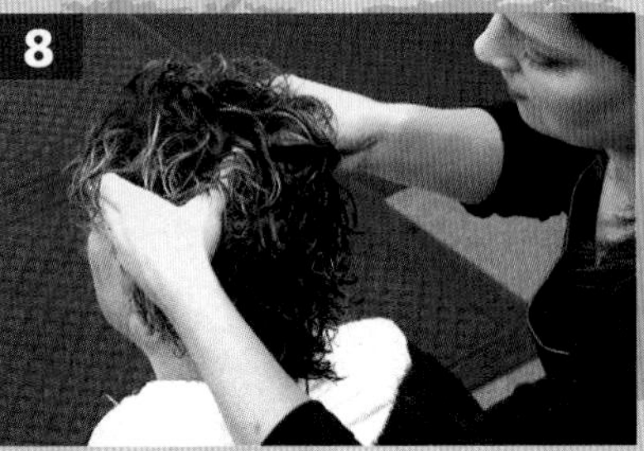

6 Place the fingers of both hands at the client's forehead. Massage around the hairline by lifting and rotating.

7 Dropping back 1 inch, repeat the preceding movement over entire front and top of the scalp.

8 Place the fingers of each hand on the sides of the client's head. Starting below the ears, manipulate the scalp with your thumbs, working upward to the crown. Repeat four times. Repeat thumb manipulations, working toward the center-back of the head.

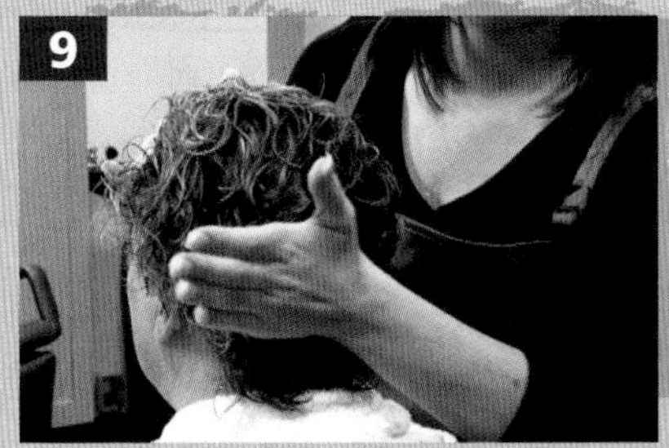

9 Place your right hand on the client's forehead. Massage from ear to ear along the base of the skull with the heel of your left hand, using a rotary movement.

10 Resume Basic Shampooing Service with step 25.

Post-Service

- Complete PROCEDURE 15-2 **Post-Service Procedure** **SEE PAGE 326**

© Milady, a part of Cengage Learning.

Review Questions

1. What are the two most important requirements for scalp care?
2. What are the benefits of scalp massage?
3. How should scalp and hair be treated if they are dry? Oily? What if dandruff is present?
4. Why is hair brushing important to maintaining a healthy scalp and hair?
5. What shampoo is appropriate for use on dandruff? On product buildup? On damaged hair?
6. What is the action of conditioner on the hair?
7. Describe the correct draping for a basic shampooing and conditioning, and for a chemical service.
8. What is the Three-Part Procedure and why is it useful?

Chapter Glossary

balancing shampoo	Shampoo that washes away excess oiliness from hair and scalp, while preventing the hair from drying out.
clarifying shampoo	Shampoo containing an active chelating agent that binds to metals (such as iron and copper) and removes them from the hair; contains an equalizing agent that enriches hair, helps retain moisture, and makes hair more manageable.
color-enhancing shampoo	Shampoo created by combining the surfactant base with basic color pigments.
conditioner	Special chemical agent applied to the hair to deposit protein or moisturizer to help restore hair strength, give hair body, or to protect hair against possible breakage.
conditioning shampoo	Also known as *moisturizing shampoo*; shampoo designed to make the hair appear smooth and shiny and to improve the manageability of the hair.
contraindicated	Avoiding a procedure or condition that may produce undesirable side effects.
deep-conditioning treatment	Also known as *hair mask* or *conditioning pack*; chemical mixture of concentrated protein and intensive moisturizer.
deionized water	Water that has had impurities, such as calcium and magnesium and other metal ions that would make a product unstable, removed.
dry shampoo	Also known as *powder shampoo*; shampoo that cleanses the hair without the use of soap and water.
hard water	Water that contains minerals that reduce the ability of soap or shampoo to lather.
humectants	Substances that absorb moisture or promote the retention of moisture.

Chapter Glossary

medicated scalp lotion	Conditioner that promotes healing of the scalp.
medicated shampoo	Shampoo containing special chemicals or drugs that are very effective in reducing dandruff or relieving other scalp conditions.
moisturizer	Product formulated to add moisture to dry hair or promote the retention of moisture.
nonstripping	Product that does not remove artificial color from the hair.
pH-balanced shampoo	Shampoo that is balanced to the pH of skin and hair (4.5 to 5.5).
protein conditioner	Product designed to penetrate the cortex and reinforce the hair shaft from within.
scalp astringent lotion	Product used to remove oil accumulation from the scalp; used after a scalp treatment and before styling.
scalp conditioner	Product, usually in a cream base, used to soften and improve the health of the scalp.
soft water	Rainwater or chemically softened water that contains only small amounts of minerals and, therefore, allows soap and shampoo to lather freely.
spray-on thermal protector	Product applied to hair prior to any thermal service to protect the hair from the harmful effects of blowdrying, thermal irons, or electric rollers.

CHAPTER 16

Haircutting

Chapter Outline

Why Study Haircutting?

Basic Principles of Haircutting

Client Consultation

Haircutting Tools

Posture and Body Position

Safety in Haircutting

Basic Haircuts

Other Cutting Techniques

Clippers and Trimmers

Procedures

© Vadym Drobot, 2010; used under license from Shutterstock.com.

Learning Objectives

After completing this chapter, you will be able to:

- ✓ **LO1** Identify reference points on the head form and understand their role in haircutting.
- ✓ **LO2** Define angles, elevations, and guidelines.
- ✓ **LO3** List the factors involved in a successful client consultation.
- ✓ **LO4** Explain the use of the various tools of haircutting.
- ✓ **LO5** Name three things you can do to ensure good posture and body position while cutting hair.
- ✓ **LO6** Perform the four basic haircuts.
- ✓ **LO7** Discuss and explain three different texturizing techniques performed with shears.
- ✓ **LO8** Explain what a clipper cut is.
- ✓ **LO9** Identify the uses of a trimmer.

Key Terms

Page number indicates where in the chapter the term is used.

angle
pg. 346

apex
pg. 345

beveling
pg. 347

blunt haircut (one-length haircut)
pg. 366

carving
pg. 377

cast
pg. 355

clipper-over-comb
pg. 381

cross-checking
pg. 367

crown
pg. 346

cutting line
pg. 347

distribution
pg. 372

elevation (projection, lifting)
pg. 347

forged
pg. 355

four corners
pg. 345

free-hand notching
pg. 377

free-hand slicing
pg. 378

graduated haircut
pg. 366

graduation
pg. 347

growth pattern
pg. 352

guideline (guide)
pg. 348

hairline
pg. 352

head form (head shape)
pg. 344

interior
pg. 348

interior guideline
pg. 370

layered haircut
pg. 366

layers
pg. 366

line
pg. 346

long-layered haircut
pg. 366

nape
pg. 346

notching
pg. 377

occipital bone
pg. 345

overdirection
pg. 349

palm-to-palm
pg. 365

parietal ridge
pg. 345

part/parting
pg. 347

perimeter
pg. 348

point cutting
pg. 376

razor-over-comb
pg. 379

razor rotation
pg. 379

reference points
pg. 344

scissor-over-comb (shear-over-comb)
pg. 375

sections
pg. 347

shrinkage
pg. 347

slicing
pg. 377

slide cutting
pg. 375

slithering (effilating)
pg. 377

stationary guideline
pg. 348

subsections
pg. 347

taper
pg. 380

tension
pg. 364

texturizing
pg. 376

traveling guideline (movable guideline)
pg. 348

uniform layers
pg. 370

weight line
pg. 366

Rapunzel, Samson, Joan of Arc, and the Beatles had just a few of the haircuts that have influenced many of us over the years. Haircuts throughout history have often reflected a change in the thinking of the time. Consider women bobbing their hair to express a newfound freedom in the 1920s or men and women whose refusal to cut their hair signaled protest during the 1960s. You will be able to give a great haircut once you have an understanding of the techniques and tools of cutting. And perhaps, one day, you will create the haircut that will rock the world.

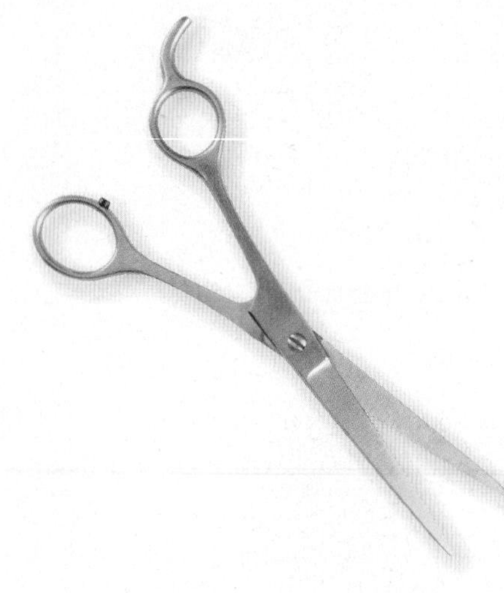

© Milady, a part of Cengage Learning. Photography by Paul Castle, Castle Photography.

WHY STUDY HAIRCUTTING?

Cosmetologists should study and have a thorough understanding of haircutting because:

- Haircutting is a basic, foundational skill upon which all other hair design is built.
- Being able to rely on your haircutting skills and techniques when creating a haircut is what will build confidence, trust, and loyalty between a cosmetologist and her clients.
- The ability to duplicate an existing haircut or create a new haircut from a photo will build a stronger professional relationship between stylist and client.
- A good haircut that is easy to style and maintain will make clients happy with their service and will build repeat services.

Basic Principles of Haircutting

Good haircuts begin with an understanding of the shape of the head, referred to as the **head form**, also known as **head shape**. Hair responds differently on various areas of the head, depending on the length and the cutting technique used. Being aware of where the head form curves, turns, and changes will help you achieve the look that you and your client are seeking.

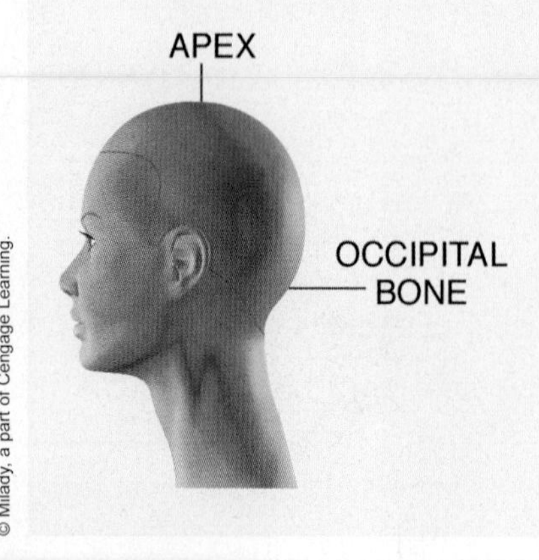

© Milady, a part of Cengage Learning.

▲ **Figure 16–1**
Reference points.

Reference Points

Reference points on the head mark where the surface of the head changes, such as the ears, jawline, occipital bone, or apex. These points are used to establish design lines (**Figure 16–1**).

An understanding of head shape and reference points will help you in the following ways:

- Finding balance within the design, so that both sides of the haircut turn out the same
- Developing the ability to create the same haircut consistently

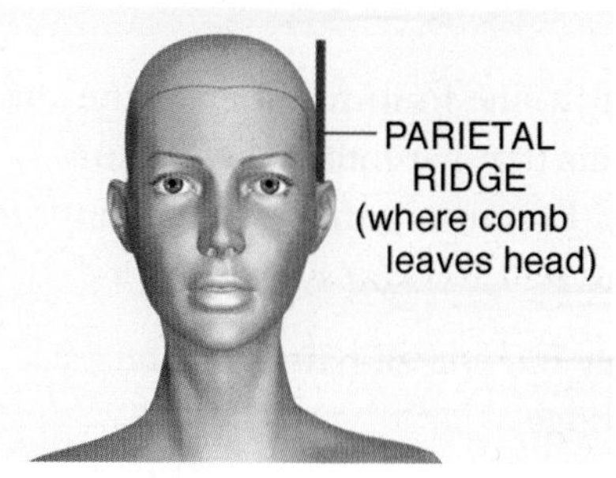

▲ **Figure 16–2**
The parietal ridge.

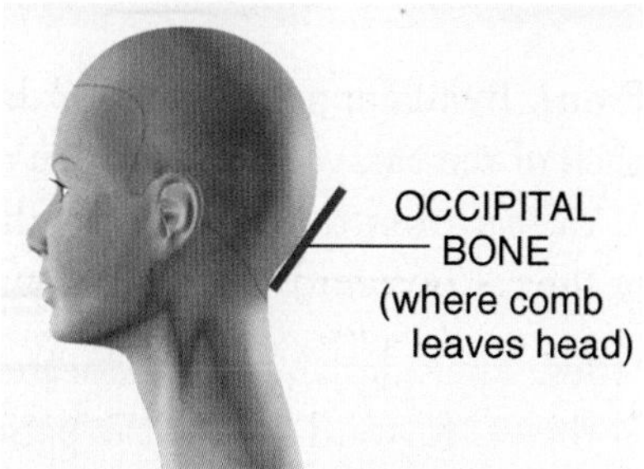

▲ **Figure 16–3**
The occipital bone.

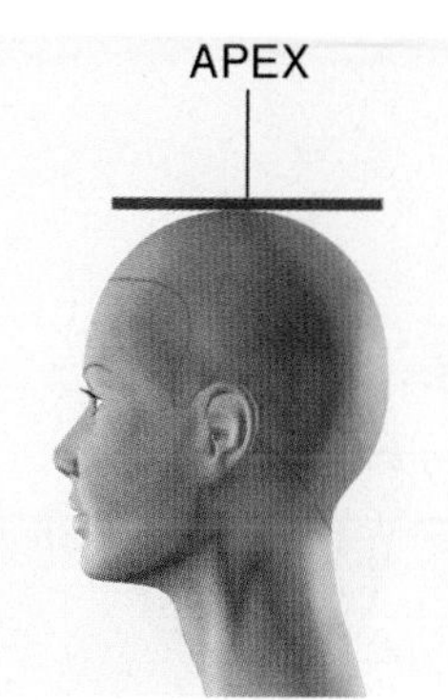

▲ **Figure 16–4**
The apex.

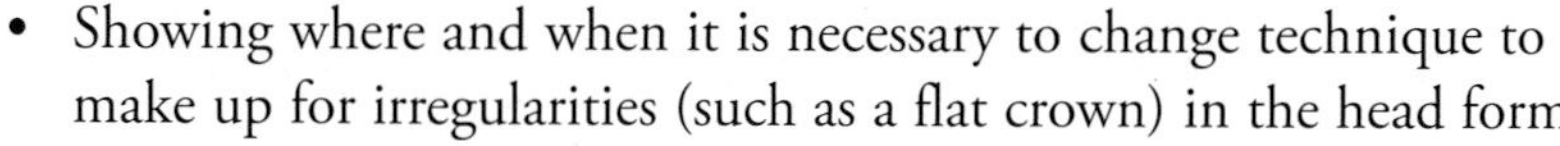

- Showing where and when it is necessary to change technique to make up for irregularities (such as a flat crown) in the head form

Standard reference points are defined below.

Parietal ridge. This is the widest area of the head, starting at the temples and ending at the bottom of the crown. This area is easily found by placing a comb flat on the side of the head: the parietal ridge is found where the head starts to curve away from the comb. The parietal ridge is also referred to as the crest area (**Figure 16–2**).

Occipital bone. The bone that protrudes at the base of the skull is the occipital bone. To find the occipital bone, simply feel the back of the skull or place a comb flat against the nape and find where the comb leaves the head (**Figure 16–3**).

Apex. This is the highest point on the top of the head. This area is easily located by placing a comb flat on the top of the head. The comb will rest on that highest point (**Figure 16–4**).

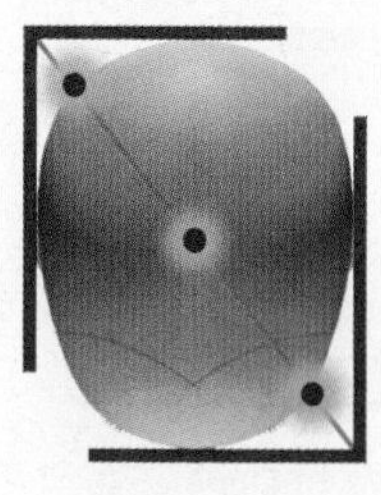

▲ **Figure 16–5**
Locating the four corners.

Four corners. These may be located in one of two ways. One is by placing two combs flat against the side and back, and then locating the back corner at the point where the two combs meet (**Figure 16–5**). The second is by making two diagonal lines crossing the apex of the head, which then point directly to the front and back corners (**Figure 16–6**).

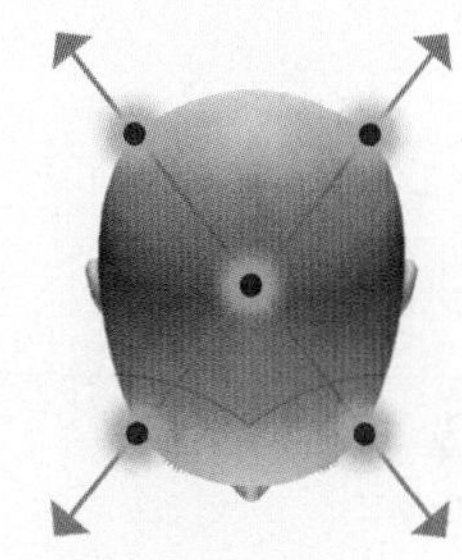

▲ **Figure 16–6**
Another way to locate the four corners.

You will not necessarily use every reference point for every haircut, but it is important to know where they are. The location of the four corners, for example, signals a change in the shape of the head from flat to round and vice versa. This change in the surface can have a significant effect on the outcome of the haircut. For example, the two front corners represent the widest points in the bang area. Cutting past these points can cause the bang to end up on the sides of the haircut once it is dry, creating an undesirable result. ☑ **LO1**

Areas of the Head

The areas of the head are described below (**Figure 16–7**).

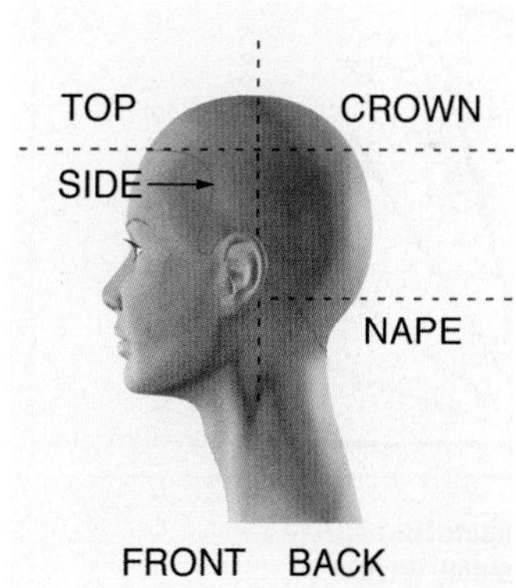

▲ **Figure 16–7**
The areas of the head.

- **Top.** By locating the parietal ridge, you can find the hair that grows on the top of the head. This hair lies on the head shape. Hair that grows below the parietal ridge, or crest, hangs because of gravity. You can locate the top by parting the hair at the parietal ridge, and continuing all the way around the head.

© Milady, a part of Cengage Learning.

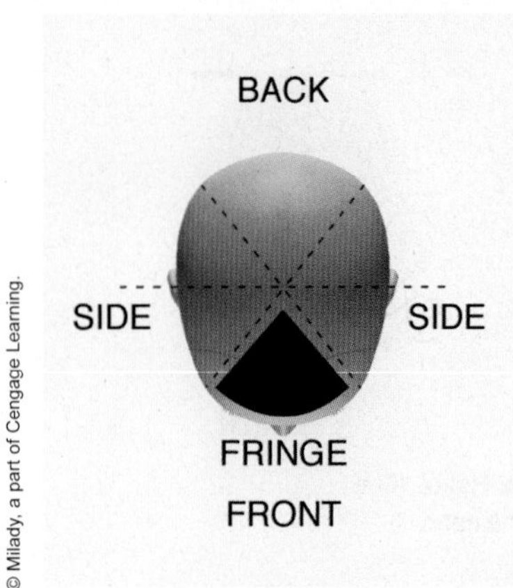

© Milady, a part of Cengage Learning.

▲ **Figure 16–8**
The bang (fringe) area.

- **Front.** By making a parting, or drawing a line from the apex to the back of the ear, you can separate the hair that naturally falls in front of the ear from the hair behind the ear. Everything that falls in front of the ear is considered the front.
- **Sides.** The sides are easy to locate. They include all hair from the back of the ear forward, below the parietal ridge.
- **Crown**. The crown is the area between the apex and the back of the parietal ridge. On many people, the crown is flat and the site of cowlicks or whorls. Because of this, it is extremely important to pay special attention to this area when haircutting.
- **Nape**. The nape is the area at the back part of the neck and consists of the hair below the occipital bone. The nape can be located by taking a horizontal parting, or by making a horizontal line across the back of the head at the occipital bone.
- **Back.** By making a parting or drawing a line from the apex to the back of the ear, you can locate the back of the head, which consists of all the hair that falls naturally behind the ear. When you have identified the front, you have also identified the back.
- **Bang area**, also known as *fringe area*. The bang area is a triangular section that begins at the apex and ends at the front corners (**Figure 16–8**). This area can be located by placing a comb on top of the head so that the middle of the comb is balanced on the apex. The spot where the comb leaves the head in front of the apex is where the bang area begins. Note that the bang area, when combed into a natural falling position, falls no farther than the outer corners of the eyes.

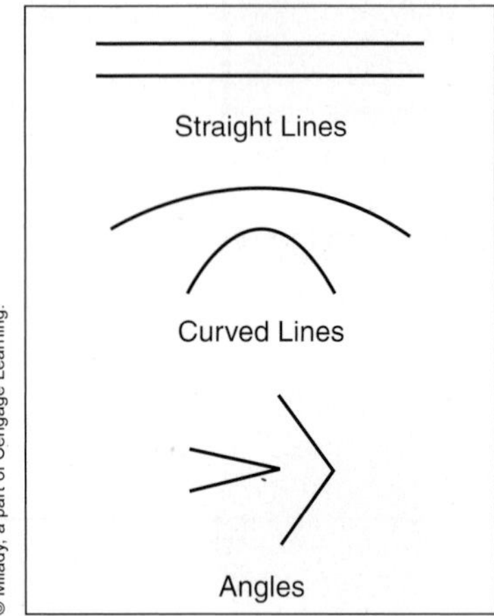

© Milady, a part of Cengage Learning.

▲ **Figure 16–9**
Lines and angles.

Lines and Angles

Every haircut is made up of lines and angles. A **line** is a thin continuous mark used as a guide. An **angle** is the space between two lines or surfaces that intersect at a given point.

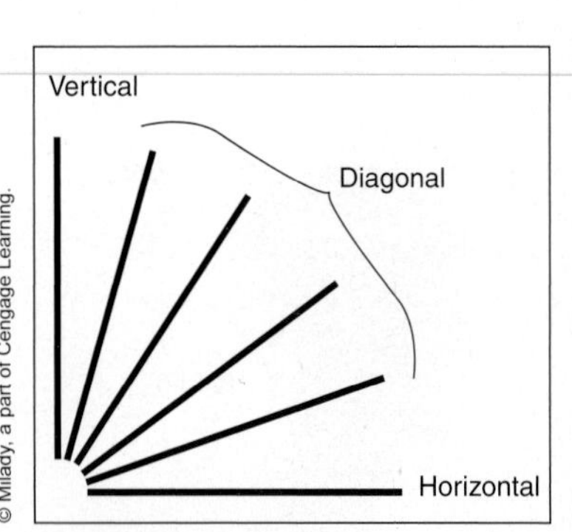

© Milady, a part of Cengage Learning.

▲ **Figure 16–10**
Horizontal, vertical, and diagonal lines.

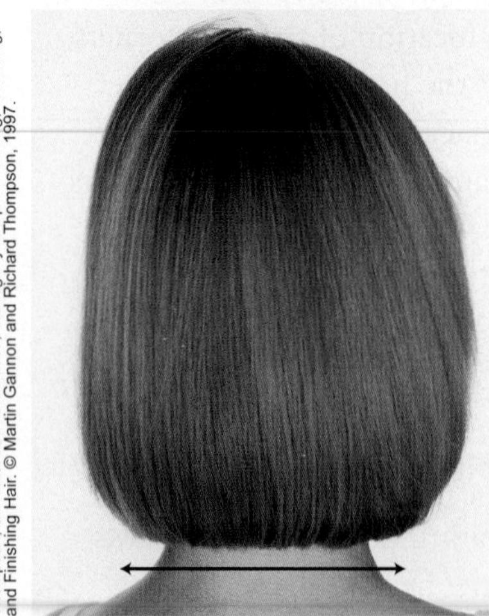

Used with the permission of the authors, Martin Gannon and Richard Thompson, as featured in their book, Mahogany: Steps to Cutting, Colouring, and Finishing Hair. © Martin Gannon and Richard Thompson, 1997.

▲ **Figure 16–11**
Horizontal line on a haircut.

The two basic lines used in haircutting are straight and curved. The head itself is made up of curved and straight lines. Cutting lines into the hair makes the hair fall into a shape (**Figure 16–9**). There are three types of straight lines in haircutting: horizontal, vertical, and diagonal (**Figure 16–10**).

- **Horizontal lines.** These are parallel to the horizon or the floor. Horizontal lines direct the eye from one side to the other. Horizontal lines build weight. They are used to create one-length and low-elevation haircuts and to add weight (**Figure 16–11**).

- **Vertical lines.** These are usually described in terms of up and down and are perpendicular to the floor; they are the opposite of horizontal. Vertical lines remove weight to create graduated or layered haircuts and are used with higher elevations (**Figure 16–12**).
- **Diagonal lines.** These are between horizontal and vertical. They have a slanting or sloping direction. Diagonal lines are used to create fullness in a haircut and to blend long layers into short layers. (See **Figure 16–13**.)
- **Beveling** and *stacking* are techniques using diagonal lines to create angles by cutting the ends of the hair with a slight increase or decrease in length. Angles are important elements in creating a strong foundation and consistency in haircutting (**Figure 16–14**) because this is how shapes are created.

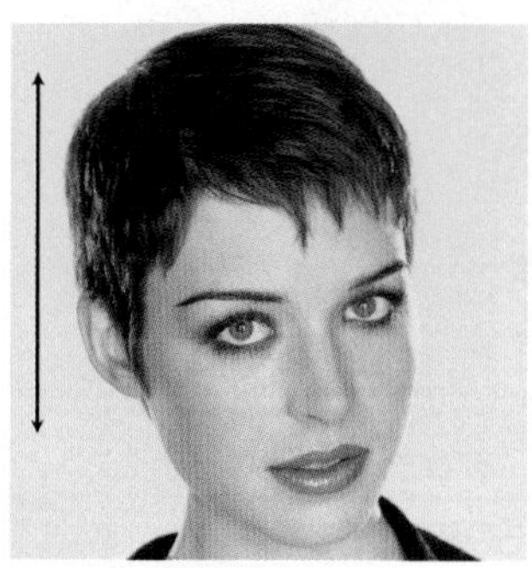

Used with the permission of the authors, Martin Gannon and Richard Thompson, as featured in their book, Mahogany: Steps to Cutting, Colouring, and Finishing Hair. © Martin Gannon and Richard Thompson, 1997.

▲ **Figure 16–12**
Vertical lines on a haircut.

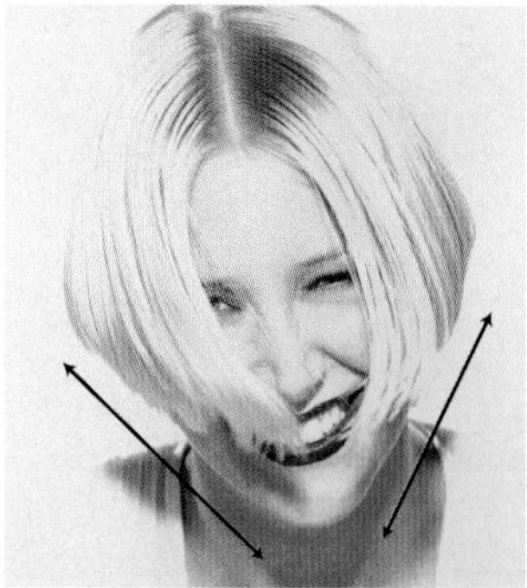

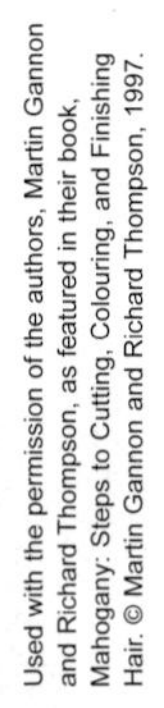

Used with the permission of the authors, Martin Gannon and Richard Thompson, as featured in their book, Mahogany: Steps to Cutting, Colouring, and Finishing Hair. © Martin Gannon and Richard Thompson, 1997.

▲ **Figure 16–13**
Diagonal lines on a haircut.

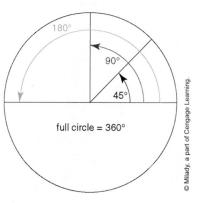

180°
90°
45°
full circle = 360°

© Milady, a part of Cengage Learning.

▲ **Figure 16–14**
Angles.

Elevation

For control during haircutting, the hair is parted into uniform working areas called **sections**. Each section may be divided into smaller partings called **subsections**. A **part** or **parting** is the line dividing the hair at the scalp, separating one section of hair from another, creating subsections. **Elevation,** also known as **projection** or **lifting**, is the angle or degree at which a subsection of hair is held, or elevated, from the head when cutting. Elevation creates **graduation** and layers, and is usually described in degrees (**Figure 16–15**). In a blunt or one-length haircut, there is no elevation (0 degrees). Elevation occurs when you lift any section of hair above 0 degrees. If a haircut is not a single length, you can be sure that elevation was used.

When a client brings in a picture of a haircut she would like, you should be able to look at the picture and determine what elevations were used. Once you understand the effects of elevation, you can create any shape you desire. The most commonly used elevations are 45 and 90 degrees. The more you elevate the hair, the more graduation you create. When the hair is elevated below 90 degrees, you are building weight. When you elevate the hair at 90 degrees or higher, you are removing weight, or layering the hair. The length of the hair also affects the end result. The weight of longer hair often makes it appear heavier or less layered. You will usually need to use less elevation on curly hair than on straighter textures, or leave the hair a bit longer because of **shrinkage**, which is when hair contracts or lifts through the action of moisture loss/drying.

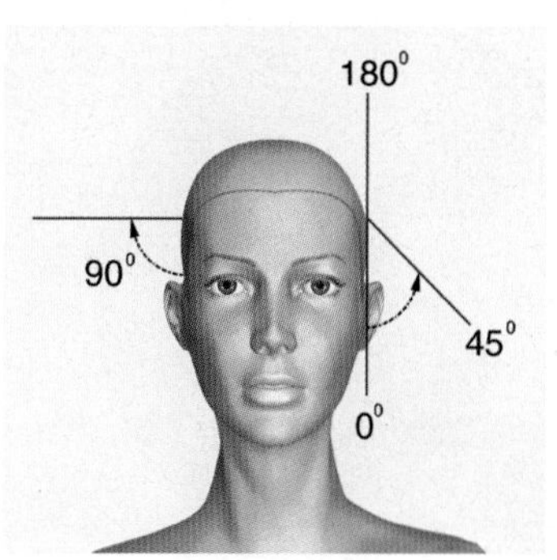

© Milady, a part of Cengage Learning.

▲ **Figure 16–15**
Angles relative to the head form.

Cutting Line

The **cutting line** is the angle at which the fingers are held when cutting the line that creates the end shape. It is also known as *cutting position*, *cutting angle*, *finger angle*, and *finger position*. The cutting line

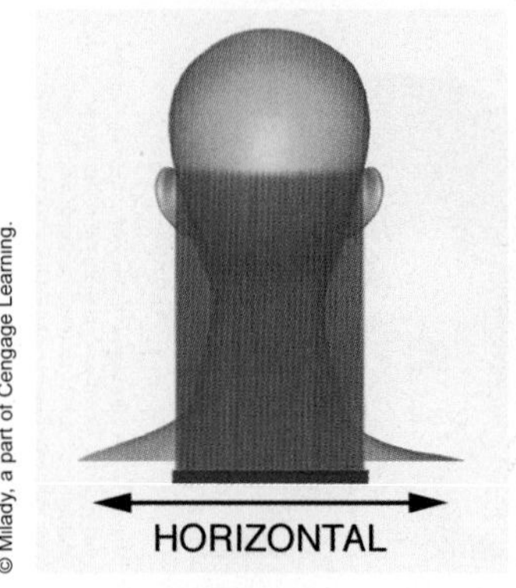

© Milady, a part of Cengage Learning.

▲ **Figure 16–16**
Horizontal cutting line.

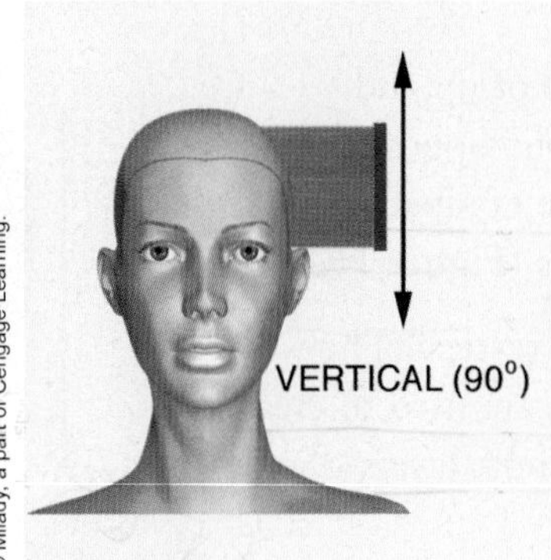

© Milady, a part of Cengage Learning.

▲ **Figure 16–17**
Vertical cutting line.

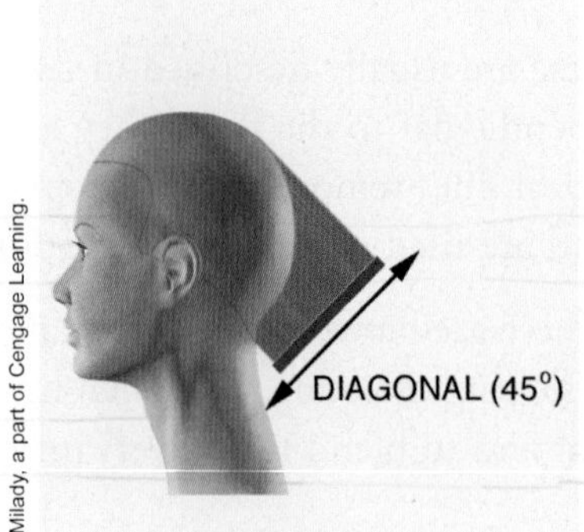

© Milady, a part of Cengage Learning.

▲ **Figure 16–18**
Diagonal cutting line.

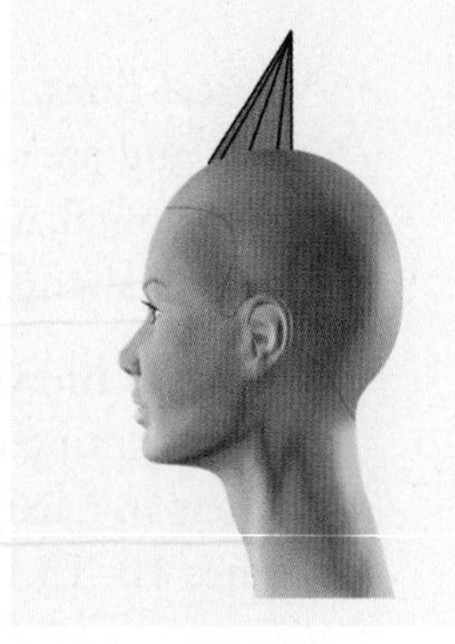
© Milady, a part of Cengage Learning.

▲ **Figure 16–19**
Stationary guideline.

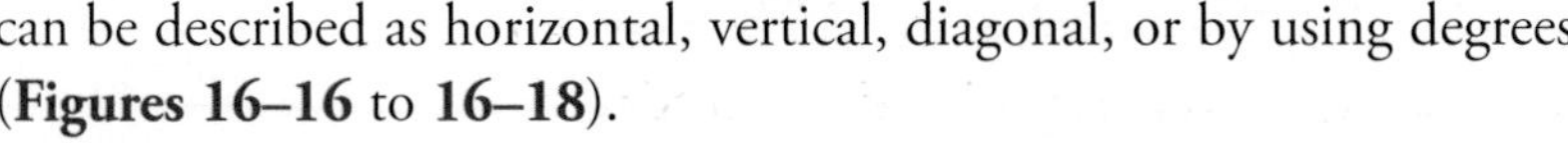
can be described as horizontal, vertical, diagonal, or by using degrees (**Figures 16–16** to **16–18**).

Guidelines

A **guideline,** also known as **guide**, is a section of hair that determines the length the hair will be cut. Guidelines are located either at the **perimeter**, the outer line, or the **interior**, inner or internal line, of the cut. The guideline is usually the first section cut when creating a shape. The two types of guidelines in haircutting are stationary and traveling.

A **stationary guideline** does not move (**Figure 16–19**). All other sections are combed to the stationary guideline and cut at the same angle and length. Stationary guidelines are used in blunt (one-length) haircuts (**Figure 16–20**), or in haircuts that use overdirection to create a length or weight increase (**Figure 16–21**).

A **traveling guideline**, also known as **movable guideline**, moves as the haircut progresses. Traveling guidelines are used when creating layered or graduated haircuts (**Figures 16–22** and **16–23**). The guideline travels with you as you work through the haircut (**Figure 16–24**). When you use a traveling guide, you take a small slice of the previous subsection and move it to the next position, or subsection, where it becomes your new guideline.

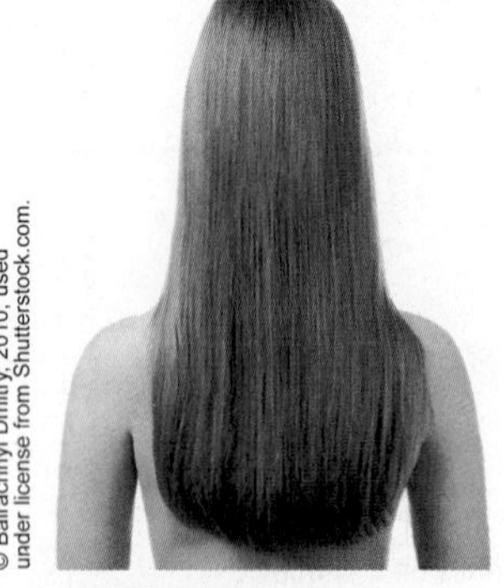
© Bairachnyi Dmitry, 2010; used under license from Shutterstock.com.

▲ **Figure 16–20**
Blunt (one-length) haircut.

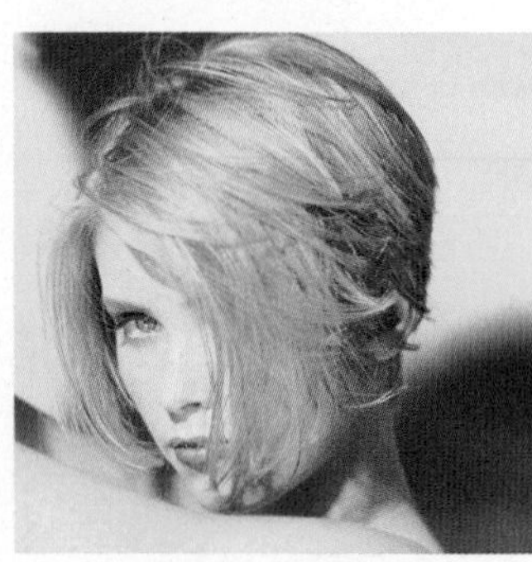
Used with the permission of the authors, Martin Gannon and Richard Thompson, as featured in their book, Mahogany: Steps to Cutting, Colouring, and Finishing Hair. © Martin Gannon and Richard Thompson, 1997.

▲ **Figure 16–21**
Graduated haircut.

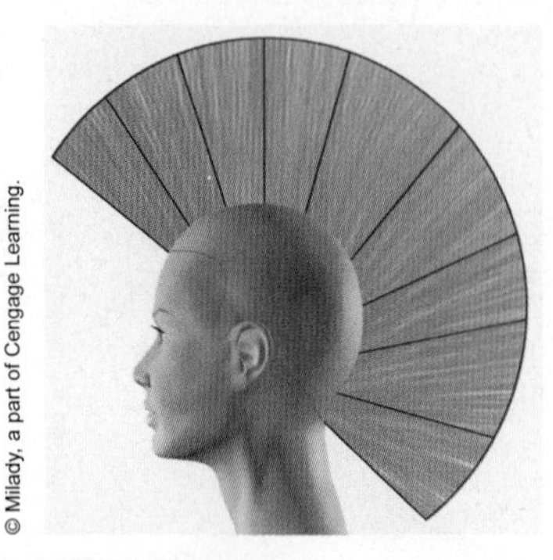
© Milady, a part of Cengage Learning.

▲ **Figure 16–22**
Traveling guideline.

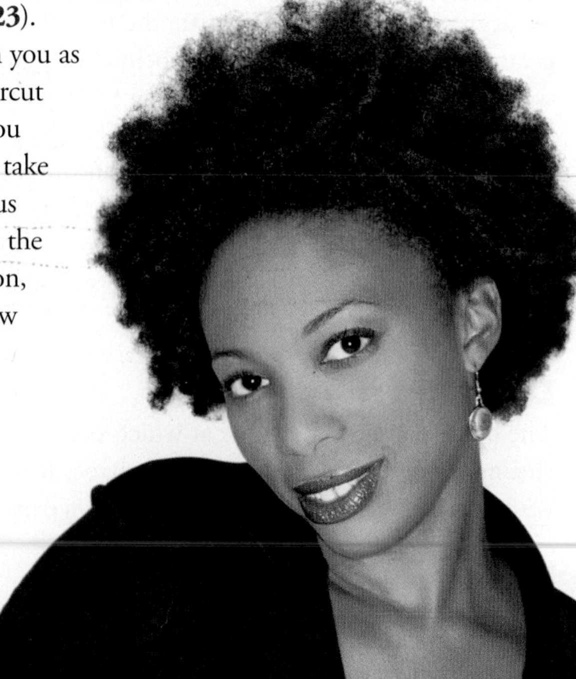
© Iofoto, 2010; used under license from Shutterstock.com.

▶ **Figure 16–23**
Uniform-layered haircut.

Used with the permission of the authors, Martin Gannon and Richard Thompson, as featured in their book, Mahogany: Steps to Cutting, Colouring, and Finishing Hair. © Martin Gannon and Richard Thompson, 1997.

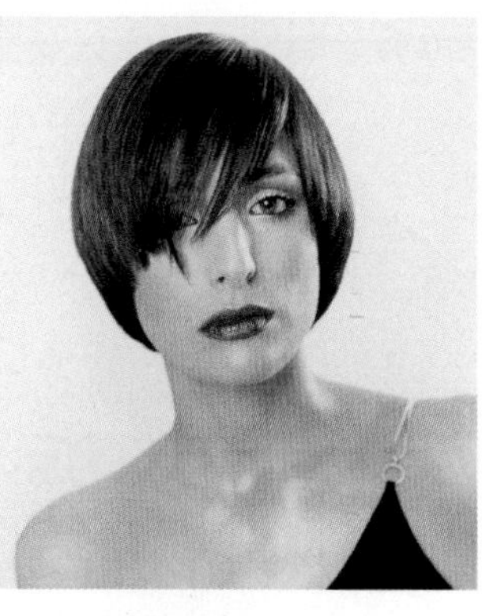

▲ **Figure 16–24**
Graduated haircut.

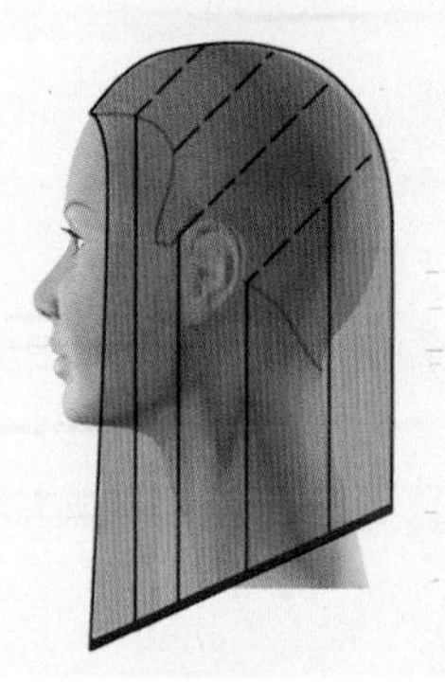

© Milady, a part of Cengage Learning.

▲ **Figure 16–25**
Blunt haircut variation: diagonal cutting line.

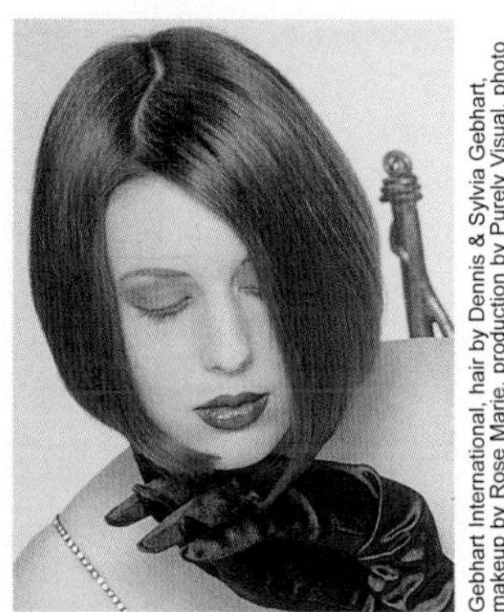

Gebhart International, hair by Dennis & Sylvia Gebhart, makeup by Rose Marie, production by Purely Visual, photo by Winterhalter.

▲ **Figure 16–26**
Finished blunt haircut variation.

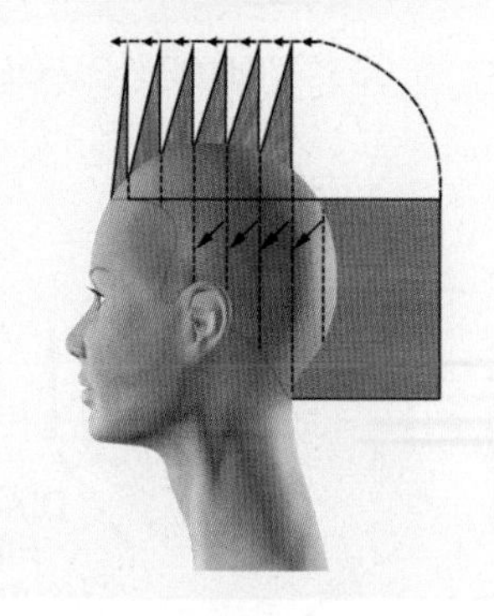

© Milady, a part of Cengage Learning.

▲ **Figure 16–27**
Layered haircut variation: vertical cutting line.

The following are just a few of the shapes that can be created by using different elevations, cutting lines, and either stationary or traveling guidelines. Keep in mind the varying amounts of weight that result from these combinations.

Figures 16–25 and **16–26** show a blunt (one-length) haircut with no elevation, a diagonal cutting line, and a stationary guideline. To achieve the layered shape in **Figures 16–27** and **16–28**, a 90-degree elevation was used, with a vertical cutting line and a traveling guideline. The shape shown in **Figures 16–29** and **16–30** was cut using a 45-degree elevation throughout the sides and back, creating a stacked effect with a diagonal (45-degree) cutting line. The top was cut using a 90-degree elevation (layered), and the entire shape was created using a traveling guideline.

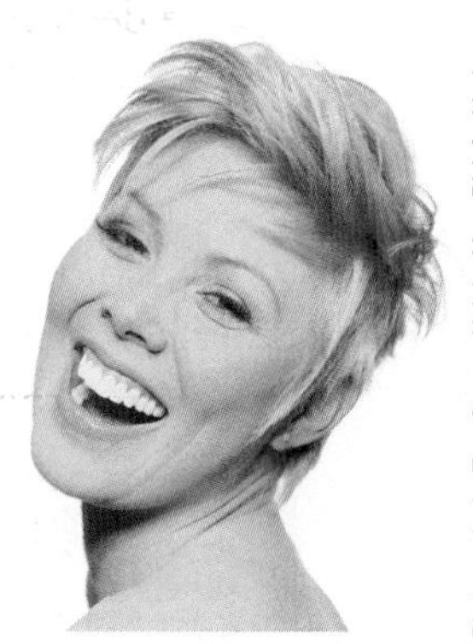

Photography by Tom Carson. Hair by Mary Rick for Vanis Salon & Day Spa, Scheveville, IN. Makeup by Amy Malone and Gretchen Wilson.

▲ **Figure 16–28**
Finished layered haircut variation.

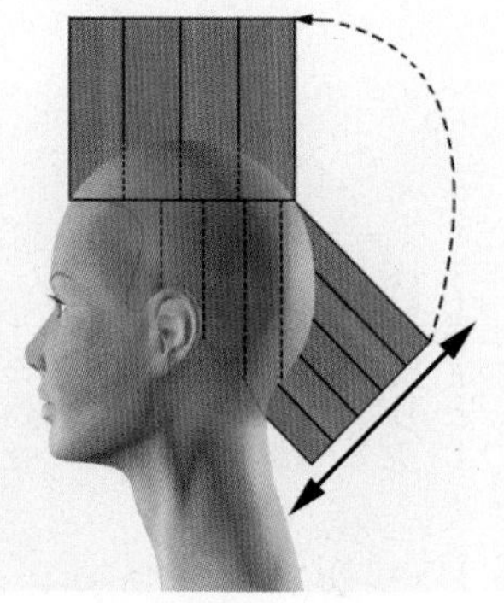

© Milady, a part of Cengage Learning.

▲ **Figure 16–29**
Graduated haircut variation: stacked effect.

Overdirection

Overdirection is best understood by comparing it to elevation. Whereas elevation is simply the degree to which you lift a section away from the head, overdirection occurs when you comb the hair away from its natural falling position, rather than straight out from the head. Overdirection is used mostly in graduated and layered haircuts, and where you want to create a length increase in the design.

For example, you are working on a layered haircut and want the hair to be longer toward the front. You can overdirect the

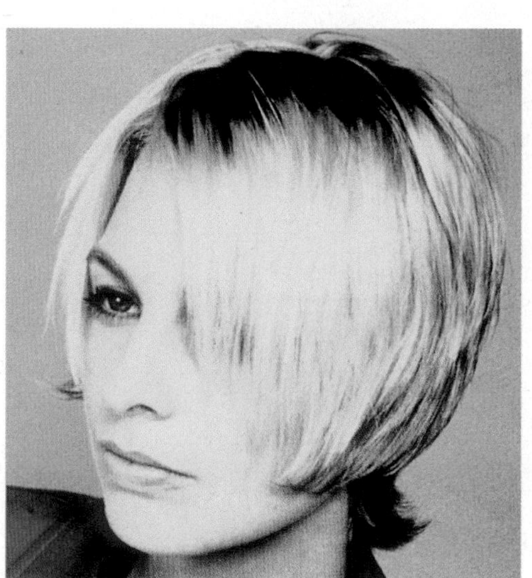

John Paul Mitchell Systems, hair by People & Schumacher, photo by Andreas Elsner.

▲ **Figure 16–30**
Finished graduated haircut variation.

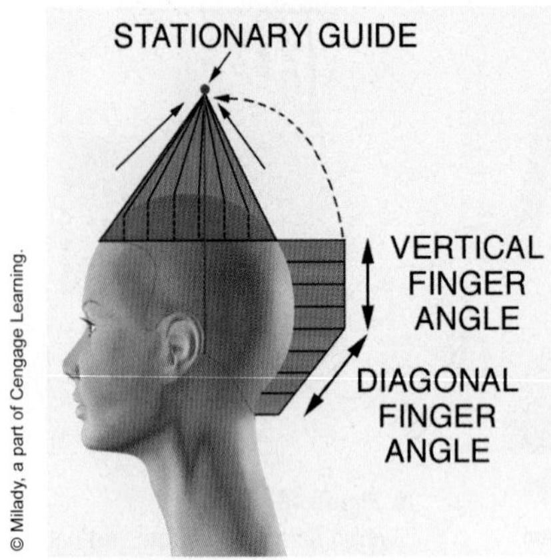

▲ Figure 16–31
Overdirection in layered haircut.

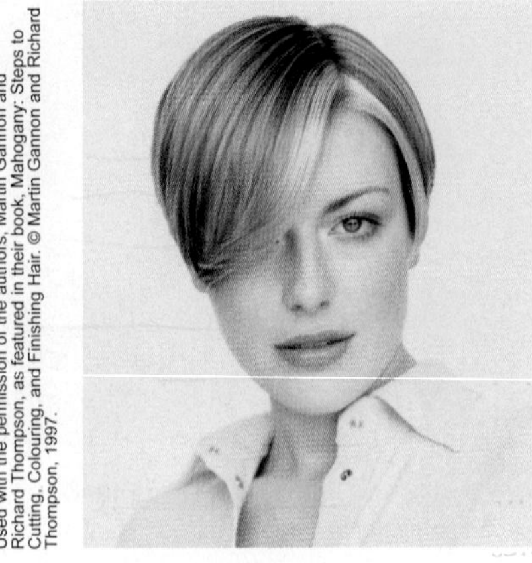

▲ Figure 16–32
Finished layered haircut.

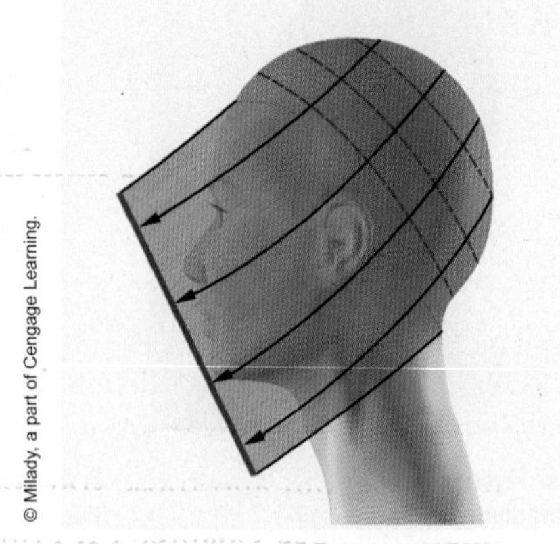

▲ Figure 16–33
Overdirection in long-layered haircut.

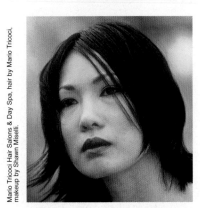

▲ Figure 16–34
Finished long-layered haircut.

sections to a stationary guideline at the back of the ear (**Figures 16–31** and **16–32**). Or, if you are creating a haircut with shorter layers around the face and longer layers in the back, you can overdirect sections to a stationary guideline at the front (**Figures 16–33** and **16–34**). ✔ **LO2**

Client Consultation

A great haircut always begins with a great consultation. A consultation is a conversation between you and your client when you find out what the client is looking for, offer suggestions and professional advice, and come to a joint decision about the most suitable haircut. If the client has a particular look in mind, you can discuss whether that look is a good choice for the client.

It can be difficult when a client asks for something that you know will not be the best look for her. This is when you will want to use gentle persuasion and positive reinforcement to offer alternative suggestions that will work with the client's hair texture, face shape, and lifestyle.

A great place to begin the consultation is to analyze the client's freshly cleansed and unstyled hair for its natural behavior. Ask the client if there is anything she would like to discuss with you about her hair. Sometimes she may ask you for your suggestions. Before recommending anything, you should consider her lifestyle and hair type. What is her lifestyle? How much time is she willing to spend on her hair every day? Does she want something that is classic or trendy? Problems may arise, for example, when a client with naturally curly hair is asking for a haircut that is really designed for straight hair. Will she be willing to take the time to blowdry it straight every day? You will need to analyze hair density and texture, growth patterns, and hairline. If the client has hair that grows straight up at the nape, and is requesting a short haircut that is soft and wispy at the nape, you should suggest other haircuts that will work with her hairline.

Face Shape

Another part of the consultation is analyzing the face shape. To analyze the shape of a client's face, pull all the hair away with a clip or wrap the hair in a towel. Look for the widest areas, the narrowest areas, and the balance of the features. A quick way to analyze a face shape is to determine if it is wide or long. Look for the features that you want to bring out and those you want to de-emphasize. See Chapter 14, Principles of Hair Design, for examples of face shapes.

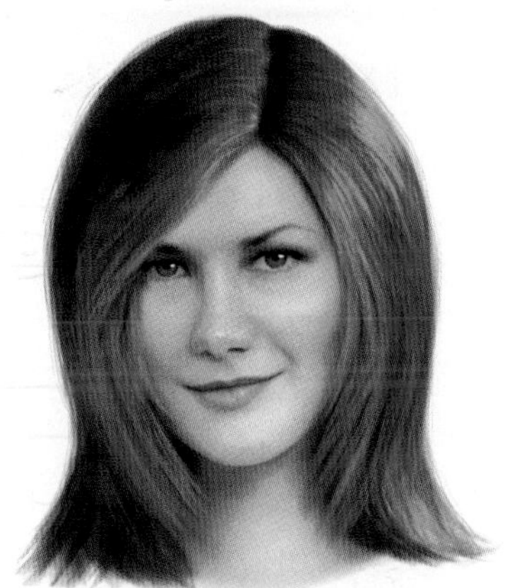

▲ **Figure 16–35**
Wide face with suitable hairstyle.

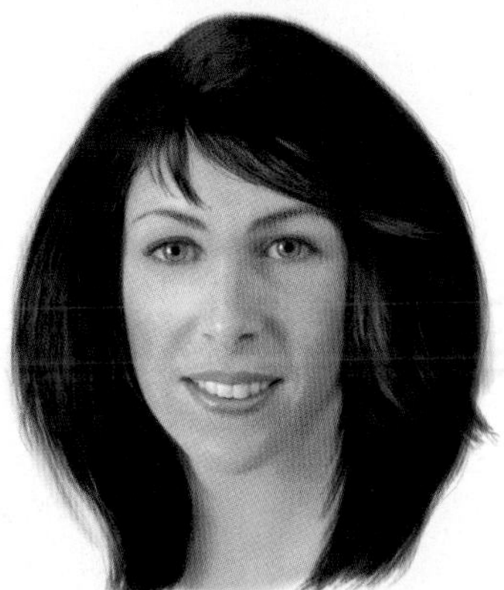

▲ **Figure 16–36**
Narrow face with suitable hairstyle.

By analyzing the face shape, you can begin to make decisions about the best haircut for the client. An important thing to remember is that weight and volume draw attention to a specific area. For example, if a client has a wide face, a hairstyle with fuller sides makes the face appear wider, whereas a narrower style will give length to the face. If the client has a long face, a hairstyle with fullness on the sides will add width. If a client has a narrow forehead, on the other hand, you can add visual width by increasing volume or weight in that area. In order to balance out face shapes or draw the eye away from certain features, you need to add or remove weight or volume in other areas. **Figures 16–35** and **16–36** illustrate two face shapes and haircuts that help create balance.

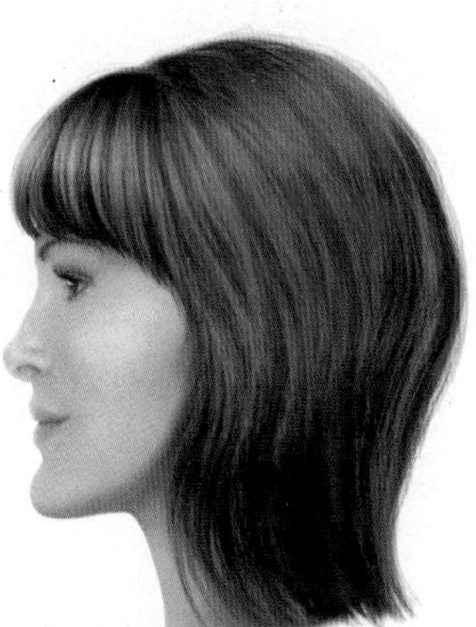

▲ **Figure 16–37**
Flattering style for client with prominent chin.

Another important point to consider is the client's profile, or how she looks from the side. Turn the chair so you can see your client's profile. Pull the hair away from the face and up and away from the neck. What do you see? Look for features to emphasize, such as a nice jawline or lovely neck. Look also for features to de-emphasize, such as a prominent or receding chin, a double chin, or an overly large nose. The haircut you choose should flatter the client by emphasizing good features and taking attention away from features that are not as flattering. For example, if a client has a prominent chin, you will want to balance the shape by adding volume or weight above or below the chin line (**Figure 16–37**). If the client has a prominent nose, you can balance the shape of the profile by adding weight and fullness to the back of the head and bang area (**Figure 16–38**).

The consultation is also the time to decide on the type of part the client will wear. Will you be working with her natural parting, a center parting, or a side parting?

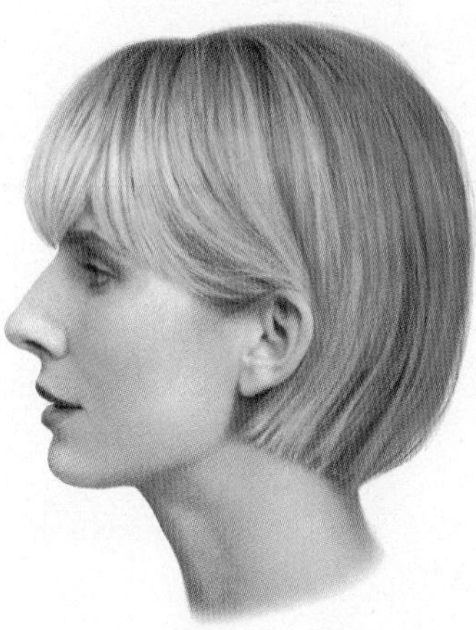

▲ **Figure 16–38**
Flattering style for client with prominent nose.

During the consultation, it is helpful to use parts of the face and body as points of reference when describing the length of the haircut. For example, you could ask, "Would you like your hair to fall chin length or shoulder length?"

Hair shrinks when it dries. Once you and the client have decided on the length, keep in mind that the hair will shrink ¼ inch (0.6 centimeters) to ½ inch (1.25 centimeters) as it dries. In other words, you need to cut wet hair ¼ to ½ inch longer than the desired length. If the hair is curly, it will shrink ½ to 2 inches (5 centimeters) or more. Be sure to check with your instructor when deciding on cutting length for curly-haired clients.

© Milady, a part of Cengage Learning.

Hair Analysis

As discussed in more detail in Chapter 11, Properties of the Hair and Scalp, there are four characteristics that determine the behavior of the hair:

- Growth patterns
- Density
- Texture
- Elasticity

Hairlines and Growth Patterns

Both the hairline and growth patterns are important to examine. The **hairline** is the hair that grows at the outermost perimeter along the face, around the ears, and on the neck. The **growth pattern** is the direction in which the hair grows from the scalp, also referred to as natural fall or natural falling position. Cowlicks, whorls, and other growth patterns affect where the hair ends up once it is dry. (See Chapter 11, Properties of the Hair and Scalp.) You may need to use less tension when cutting these areas to compensate for hair being pushed up when it dries, especially in the nape, or to avoid getting a *hole* around the ear in a one-length haircut. Another crucial area is the crown. (There may be some wild things going on up there!)

Hair Density

Hair density is the number of individual hair strands on 1 square inch of scalp. It is usually described as thin, medium, or thick.

Hair Texture

Hair texture is based on the thickness or diameter of each hair strand, usually classified as coarse, medium, and fine. A fine hair strand is much *skinnier* than a coarse hair strand. A client may, in fact, have fine-textured hair with a thick density, meaning that the individual hairs are fine, but that there are a lot of them. Or a client may have coarse texture but thin density, meaning the individual hairs are *fatter*, but they are spaced farther apart.

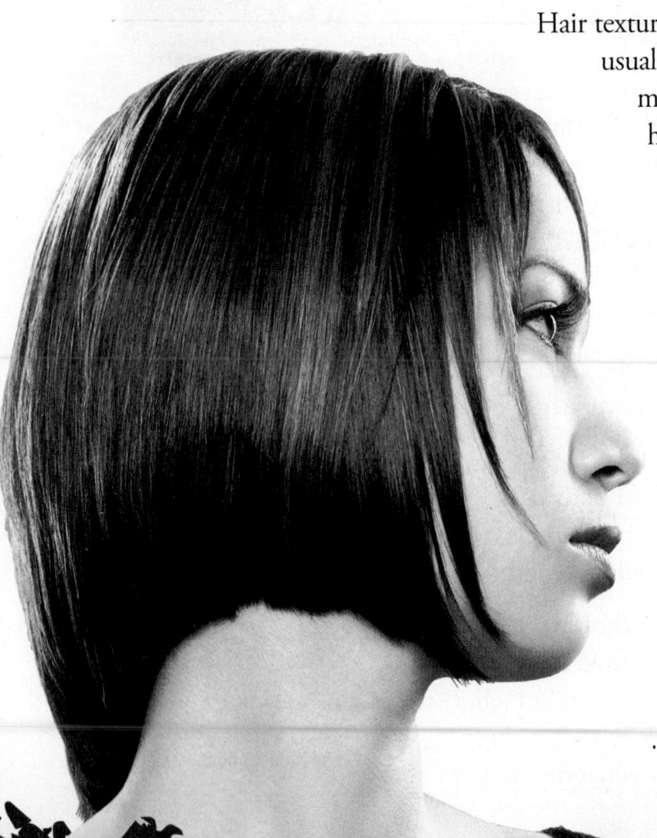

Density and texture are important because the different hair types respond differently to the same type of cutting. Some hair types need more layers, and some need more weight. For example, coarse hair tends to stick out more, especially if it is cut too short; fine hair, though, can be cut to very short lengths and still lies flat. However, if a client has fine (texture) and thin (density) hair, cutting too short can result in the scalp showing through (**Table 16–1**).

Wave Pattern

The wave pattern, or the amount of movement in the hair strand, varies from client to client, as well as within the same head of hair. A client may have

© Trinette Reed, 2010; used under license from Shutterstock.com.

DENSITY AND TEXTURE			
	DENSITY		
TEXTURE	THIN	MEDIUM	THICK
FINE	Limp, needs weight.	Great for many cuts, especially blunt and low elevation. Razor cuts are good.	Usually needs more texturizing. Suitable for many haircuts.
MEDIUM	Needs weight. Graduated shapes work well.	Great for most cuts. Hair can handle texturizing.	Many shapes are suitable. Texturizing usually necessary.
COARSE	Maintain some weight. Razor cuts not recommended.	Great for many shapes. Razor cuts appropriate if hair is in good condition.	Very short cuts do not work. Razors may frizz and *expand* hair. Maintain some length to weigh hair down.

Table 16–1 Density and Texture.

completely straight hair (no wave), wavy hair, curly hair, extremely curly hair, or anything in between.

Imagine the same haircut cut at the same length on different types of hair: fine thin hair (**Figure 16–39**), thick coarse hair (**Figure 16–40**), and medium curly hair (**Figure 16–41**). ✓ **LO3**

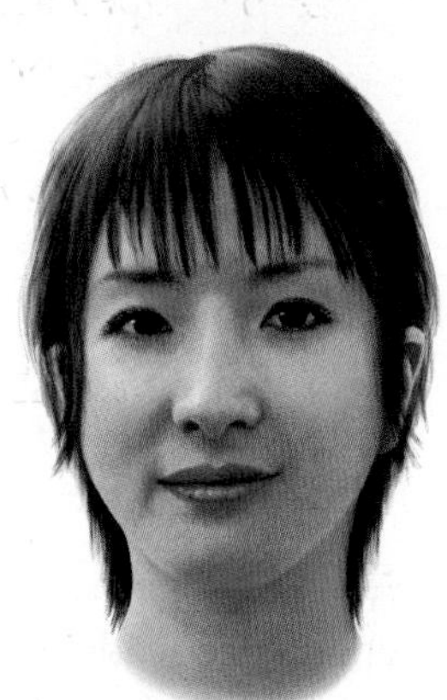

▲ Figure 16–39
Uniform-layered haircut on fine, thin hair.

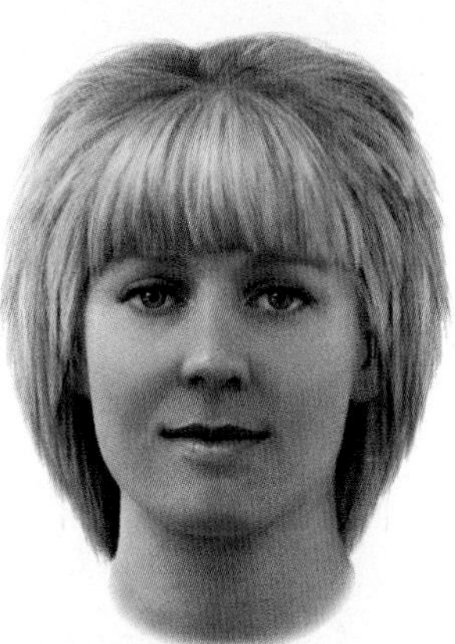

▲ Figure 16–40
Uniform-layered haircut on thick, coarse hair.

Haircutting Tools

How do you choose and use the right tools for the job? To find the answer, you will need to understand the function and characteristics of your tools, how to use them in a way that is safe for both you and your client, and how to position your body so that your energy and effectiveness are maximized and protected.

There are several tools that you will need for haircutting. Understanding these implements, and the results you can achieve with them, is necessary for creating a great haircut. To do your best work, buy and use only high-quality professional implements from a reliable manufacturer, use them properly, and take good care of them. Follow these simple suggestions, and your tools can last a lifetime.

- **Haircutting shears.** These shears, also known as *scissors,* are mainly used to cut blunt or straight lines in hair. They may also be used

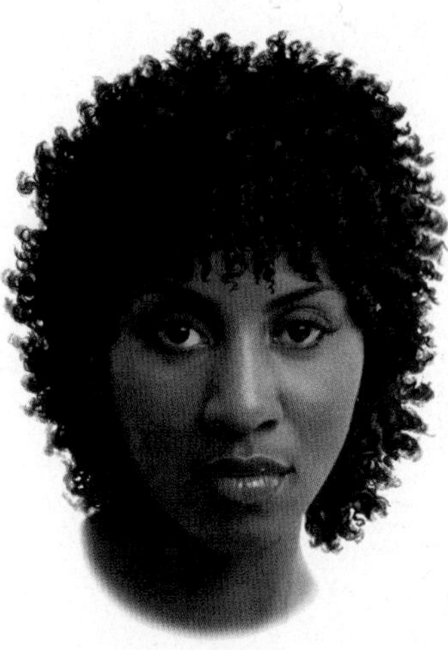

▲ Figure 16–41
Uniform-layered haircut on medium, curly hair.

© Milady, a part of Cengage Learning.

to slide cut, point cut, or to implement other texturizing techniques (discussed later in this chapter) (**Figure 16–42**).

- **Texturizing shears.** Texturizing shears are mainly used to remove bulk from the hair. They are sometimes referred to as thinning shears, tapering shears, or notching shears. Many types of thinning shears are used today, with varying amounts of teeth in the blades. A general rule of thumb is that the more teeth in the shear, the less hair is removed per cut. Notching shears are usually designed to remove more hair, with larger teeth set farther apart.
- **Razors.** Straight razors or feather blades are mainly used when a softer effect on the ends of the hair is desired. Razors can be used to create an entire haircut, to thin hair out, or to texturize in certain areas. They come in different shapes and sizes, and with or without guards (**Figures 16–43** and **16–44**).
- **Clippers.** These are mainly used when creating short haircuts, short tapers, fades, and flat tops. Clippers may be used without a guard to shave hair right to the scalp, with cutting guards of various lengths, and for the clipper-over-comb technique (**Figure 16–45**).
- **Trimmers.** These are a smaller version of clippers, and are also known as *edgers*. They are mainly used to remove excess or unwanted hair at the neckline and around the ears, and to create crisp outlines. Trimmers are generally used on men's haircuts and very short haircuts for women.
- **Sectioning clips.** These come in a variety of shapes, styles, and sizes and can be made of plastic or metal. In general, two types are used: jaw or butterfly clips and duckbill clips. Both come in large and small sizes.
- **Wide-tooth comb.** This comb is mainly used to detangle hair. The wide-tooth comb is rarely used when performing a haircut.
- **Tail comb.** This tool is mainly used to section and subsection the hair.
- **Barber comb.** This comb is mainly used for close tapers on the nape and sides when using the scissor-over-comb technique. The narrow end of the comb allows the shears to get very close to the head.
- **Styling or cutting comb.** Also referred to as an *all-purpose comb*, this tool is used for most haircutting procedures. It can be 6 to 8 inches long and has fine teeth at one end and wider teeth at the other (**Figure 16–46**). ☑ **LO4**

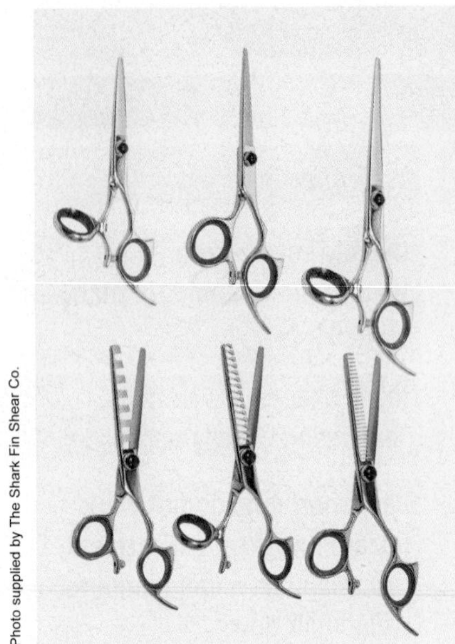

Photo supplied by The Shark Fin Shear Co.

▲ **Figure 16–42**
Haircutting and thinning shears.

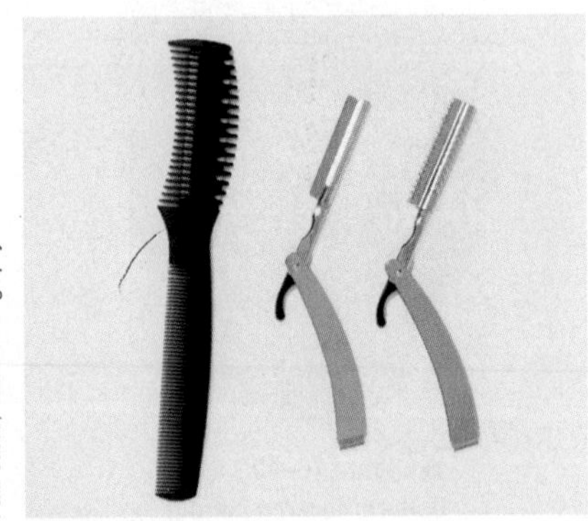

© Milady, a part of Cengage Learning. Photography by Paul Castle, Castle Photography.

▲ **Figure 16–43**
Razors.

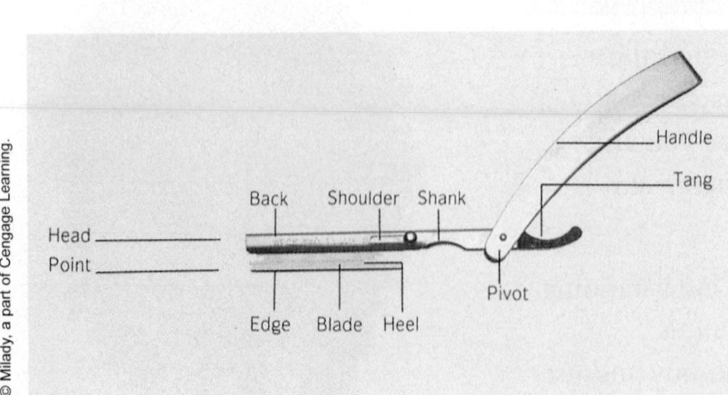

© Milady, a part of Cengage Learning.

▲ **Figure 16–44**
Parts of a razor.

All About Shears

Your haircutting shears will be one of the most important tools in your career as a professional cosmetologist. Having the right type, size, and make of shear for you—one that fits you well and is comfortable to use is vital if you are to build a career in the salon.

Steel

All professional haircutting shears are made of steel. Three countries are primarily responsible for manufacturing the steel used to make professional shears: Japan, Germany, and the United States.

It is important for a stylist to know how to gauge the hardness of the metal a shear is made from because this is how you will determine if the shear can hold a sharp edge for an extended period of time. If the metal is too soft, the shear will not hold a sharp edge and will need to be sharpened more often than a shear made with a harder metal. The gauge is called the Rockwell hardness.

Generally, a shear with a Rockwell hardness of at least 56 or 57 is ideal. A shear with a Rockwell hardness that is higher than 63 can make the shear too hard and brittle to work with; the shear could even break if dropped.

There are many different grades of steel available on the market. As the strength or hardness of the steel increases, so does the shear's ability to retain a sharp edge, which means less frequent sharpening and maintenance.

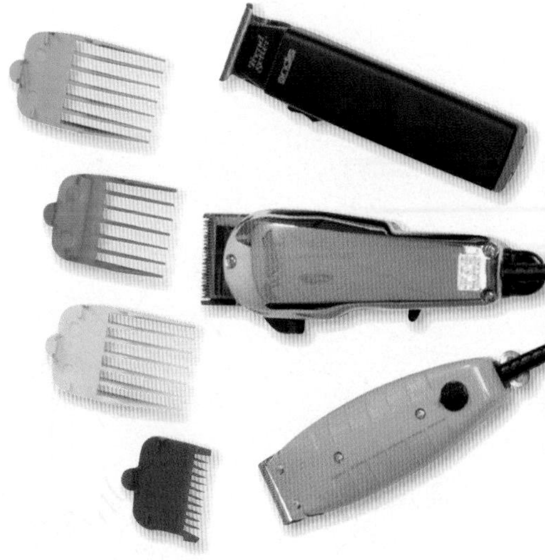

▲ **Figure 16–45**
Clippers and trimmers.

Forged versus Cast Shears

Professional shears are made in one of two ways; they are either cast or forged.

Cast shears are made by a process whereby molten steel is poured into a mold. Once the metal is cooled, it takes on the shape of the mold.

One disadvantage of a cast shear is that sometimes the casting process can create tiny pinhole bubbles that create holes or voids. If a shear with a void is dropped, it could shatter. Also, if a cast shear is bent, it cannot be bent back into shape without the risk of breaking it because cast shears are often brittle.

Cast shears are less expensive to produce than forged shears, and they are usually less expensive to purchase.

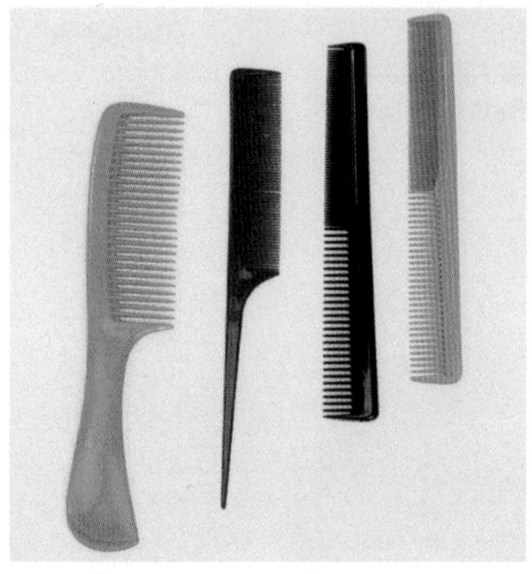

▲ **Figure 16–46**
From left to right: wide-tooth comb, tail comb, barber comb, and styling comb.

A **forged** shear is made by a process of working metal to a finished shape by hammering or pressing. The metal is heated to temperatures between 2,100 degrees Fahrenheit and 2,300 degress Fahrenheit, which expands the molecular structure of the steel so that when it is struck by a heavy object, the molecules move. After the hammering or pressing is completed, the metal is cooled in water, causing the molecules to compress. The process is repeated until the desired structure of the metal is achieved, thus making the metal much denser and harder than metal that goes through the casting process.

The forging process creates a more durable shear than the casting process. Forged shears are easier to repair if dropped or bent. With new technology in the manufacturing process, a forged shear is similar in price to a cast shear but is of much higher quality and durability. Forged shears last significantly longer than cast shears.

© Milady, a part of Cengage Learning. Photography by Paul Castle, Castle Photography.

Some forged shears have handles that are welded to the blades. These shears undergo the same forging process, but usually the blades are made with a harder metal than the handles. The benefit of this construction is that the shears can be repaired and adjusted easily by a certified technician if they are dropped or become dull.

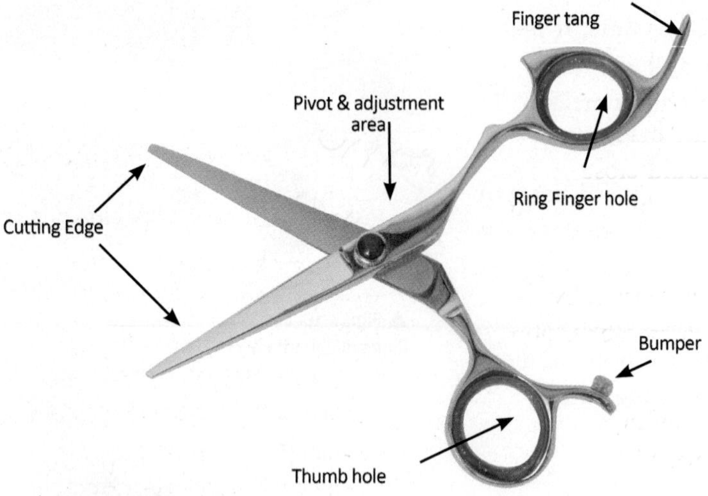

▲ **Figure 16–47**
Parts of a shear.

Photo supplied by The Shark Fin Shear Co.

Parts of a Shear

You are going to be working with a pair or pairs of haircutting shears every day and will rely on them to enable you to create great haircuts that satisfy your clients and keep them coming into the salon for your services. Therefore, you should know and understand all of the parts of a typical haircutting shear (**Figure 16–47**).

The cutting edge is the part of the blade that actually does the cutting. The pivot and the adjustment area are the parts that make your shears cut. (Your hand only directs where the shear travels.) The adjustment knob, when tightened, pulls the blades together at just the correct tension so that the hair does not fall or slide between the blades, and it also allows the hair to rest on top of the blades so that when they are closed the hair is cut on the desired line.

The finger tang gives your pinky an additional contact point so the nerves and tendons in the pinky and hand are less stressed and pressure is relieved, allowing you to relax your grip so you can hold the shear more comfortably. The finger tang also allows you to have more control over the shear.

The ring finger-hole is where you place your ring finger. Do not use your middle finger when cutting, only your ring finger should be placed in the ring finger-hole.

The thumb hole is the bottom hole and, when properly fitted, should only go to, or slightly over, the cuticle.

Shear Maintenance

To keep your shears in excellent shape and reliable, given the demanding schedule you will keep, it is important to clean and maintain your shears on a regular basis. Get into the habit of caring for your shears, and they will never let you down. You should use the following maintenance schedule, beginning now.

- **Daily cleaning and lubrication.** Use a soft cloth or towel saturated with scissor oil, and thoroughly wipe the inside of the blades of your shear after every client. This will remove your previous client's hair, reduce buildup of chemicals and debris, and keep the blades lubricated to reduce friction caused by metal-to-metal contact. Proper lubrication and blade tension will extend the life of the blades and reduce the frequency that your shear will need to be sharpened. If you own a swivel shear, lubricate the swivel joint as needed.

- **Daily tension adjustment and balancing.** Adjusting blade tension is an important task to make sure your shears are functioning correctly and to ensure that you get the best results from your shears.

If the tension is too loose, it will allow your shears to fold the hair. If it is too tight, it will cause the shears to bind and cause unnecessary wear and user fatigue. To test for tension, hold the shears with the adjustment knob facing you and the thumb handle in your left hand. With the shear perfectly straight (and the blades pointed to the left for a right-handed shear or to the right for a left-handed shear), lift up on the ring finger to open the blades halfway. Then, let the ring finger-handle go. The blades should close ⅔ of the way, or, at the end of the shear, you should have about a 1- to 2-inch gap at the tips.

If your shears need to be adjusted, you can tighten the tension by turning the adjustment knob to the right; you can loosen the tension by turning the adjustment knob to the left.

- **Weekly cleaning and lubrication.** Once a week carefully open shears to a 90-degree angle and loosen the adjustment knob enough so that the blades allow a paper towel to fit between the pivot point, then push out any hair particles or debris (be careful not to over loosen the adjustment knob or your shears could fall apart). After the area between the blades is cleaned, put one or two drops of top-quality scissor oil into the space between the blades. This removes dirt and debris from between the blades. Be careful not to put scissor oil directly under the adjustment knob, because over lubrication may cause loss of blade tension, resulting in folding and bending of the hair when cutting.

- **Disinfecting shears.** You must disinfect your shear after each client by first thoroughly cleaning the shear with soap and water and then completely immersing in an EPA-registered disinfectant spray.

Be sure to thoroughly dry the shears; however, it is not recommended that you take the shears apart by loosening the screw to dry the area. You must relubricate your blades after disinfecting them because the oil will be removed from the blades during this process.

- **Sharpening shears.** You should only sharpen your shears as needed. Do not fall into the habit of automatically having them sharpened on a three-to-six month cycle, whenever the sharpening technician comes to the salon.

Remember, the better you care for your shears, the longer the edges will last between sharpening. On average, you should be able to go one year or longer between sharpening if you follow the oiling and adjustment directions described above. When you do need to have your shears sharpened, it is best to have a factory-certified technician sharpen your shears, or to send them to the manufacturer for service.

did you know?

The only difference between a titanium shear and any other shear is its color. Titanium is simply the finish that has been applied to the surface of the steel to change the appearance of the shear. Although claims may be made that titanium makes a shear better, sharper, stronger, or harder, it actually has no bearing or benefit on the shear except to coat it in color (**Figure 16–48**).

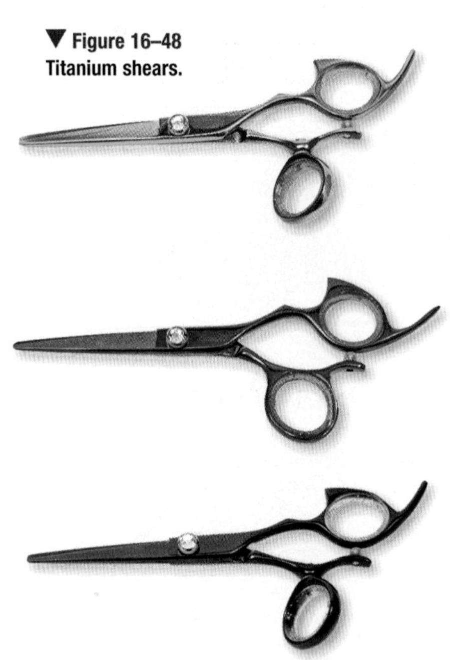

▼ **Figure 16–48** **Titanium shears.**

Photo supplied by The Shark Fin Shear Co.

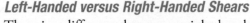

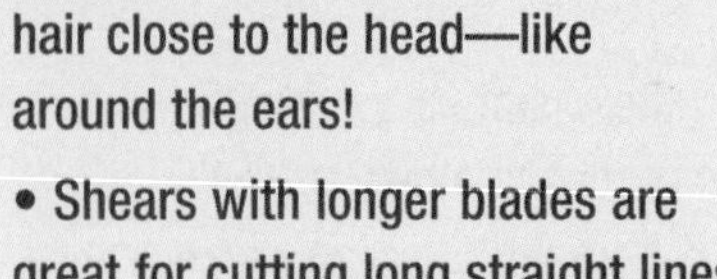

- Shears with shorter blades are great for point cutting and cutting hair close to the head—like around the ears!
- Shears with longer blades are great for cutting long straight lines into the hair—like for blunt cuts!

Left-Handed versus Right-Handed Shears

There is a difference between a right-handed and a left-handed shear. Simply taking a right-handed shear and turning it over does not make it appropriate for a left-handed cutter, because the blades of the shear need to be reversed.

It is important that you always use the correct shear for your dominant hand.

Purchasing Shears

You will purchase shears several times throughout your career, and the purchase will very likely require a substantial expenditure. Keep in mind that buying a high-quality shears is an investment in your career. Here are some things to look for in a shear you are considering for purchase:

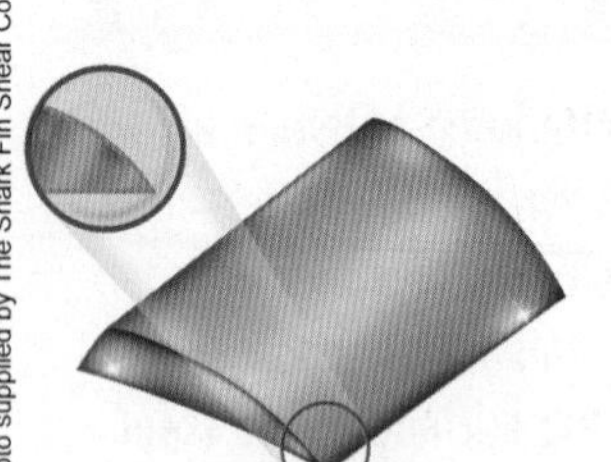
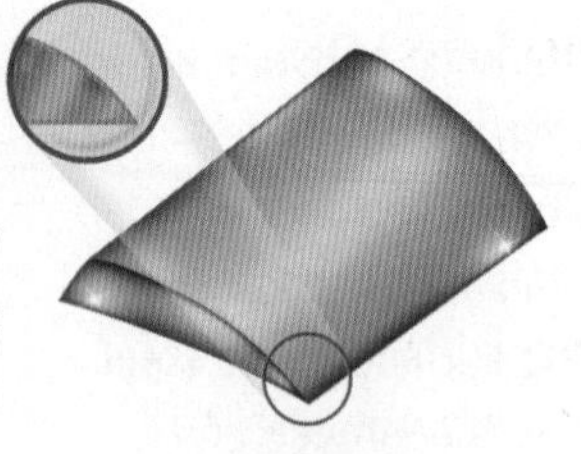

Photo supplied by The Shark Fin Shear Co.

▲ **Figure 16–49**
Convex edge; beveled edge.

- **Know how the shear was manufactured.** Remember that forged shears are of higher quality than cast shears. Even though forged shears may cost a little more, they are more structurally sound and generally last longer.
- **Ask about the steel quality.** Be sure that you know the quality of the steel that the shear is made from and the Rockwell hardness. You will want at least a *440-A* steel or higher, and as you go up the scale from *440-A* to *440-C* the steel gets harder, which means that the edges will last longer.
- **Decide on the right blade edge.** A full convex edge will give you the smoothest cut and is the sharpest edge possible (**Figure 16–49**). See **Table 16–2** for the differences in blade edges.
- **Decide on the best handle design for you.** Shears will have one of three types of handle grips, and you will need to decide which one is best for you (**Figure 16–50**). Shears with an *opposing grip* force

OPPOSING GRIP

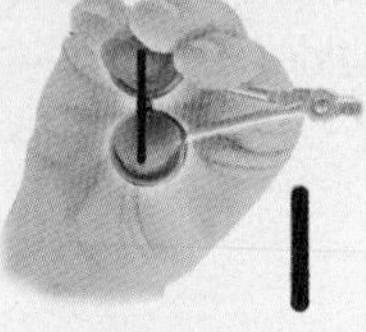

OFFSET GRIP

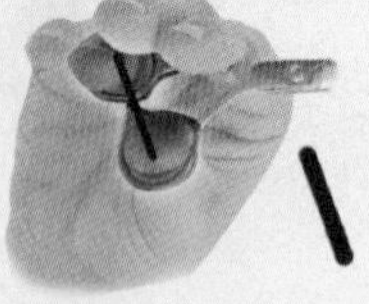

CRANE GRIP

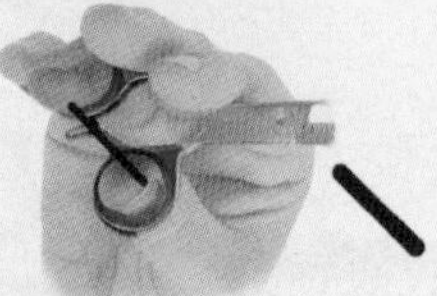

| = Line shows forward movement of thumb.

Photo supplied by The Shark Fin Shear Co.

▲ **Figure 16–50**
Opposing grip, offset grip, crane or full offset grip.

DIFFERENT BLADE EDGES	
CONVEX EDGE	**BEVELED EDGE**
Very sharp edge	Dull edge style
Smooth and quiet	Not smooth and can be noisy
Glides through the hair easily	Normally found on lower-quality shears
Best overall edge for the professional stylist	Not recommended for the professional stylist
Great for all kinds of cutting techniques, including slide cutting	Not recommended for professional salon use

© Milady, a part of Cengage Learning.

Table 16–2 Different Blade Edges.

the thumb underneath the ring finger and can create stress and pressure on the nerves and tendons of the hand. An *offset grip* moves the thumb forward, so it is resting below the ring and middle finger. A *full offset* or *crane grip* is the most anatomically correct handle design, because it positions the thumb grip under the index finger, which is how your hand is when relaxed. This position releases the pressure and stress put on the nerves and tendons of the hand and thumb.

- **Be sure the shears fit properly.** Since you will be working with your shears almost constantly, consider purchasing a shear that comes with a finger-fitting system so that the shear can be custom fitted to the exact size of your ring finger (**Figure 16–51**) and thumb diameter (**Figure 16–52**). A proper fit will ensure maximum performance, comfort, and control.
- **Hold the shears in your hands.** Since purchasing a shear is a very personal thing, you need to feel shears in your hand before you buy them. When you are ready to purchase your shears, select a vendor that has plenty of shear samples for you to try and a representative who will allow you all the time you need to make the right choice. Make sure the shear manufacturer offers a 30-day trial period, so that if you are not satisfied with the performance of the shears, you can exchange or return them for a full refund.
- **Swivel thumb shears.** The swivel shear provides great comfort and control. The swivel shear allows you to lower your

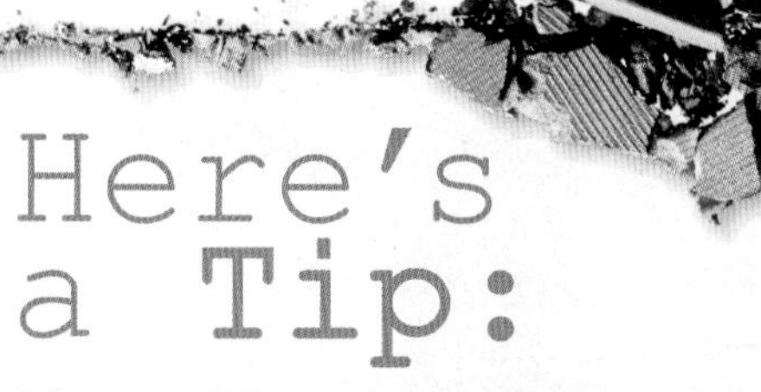

Here's a Tip:

Ask yourself these simple questions when preparing to purchase a new pair of shears:

- Do these shears fit me correctly, and do they feel comfortable?
- Do these shears feel too loose or too big? Do I feel like I have complete control of these shears?
- Do these shears come with a set of ring guards to custom fit the shear to my exact ring finger and thumb diameter (**Figure 16-51a**)?

Regardless of what anyone else says about their experience with a shear, you need to feel comfortable and satisfied with your purchase. Don't let anyone else's advice sway your choice in a shear.

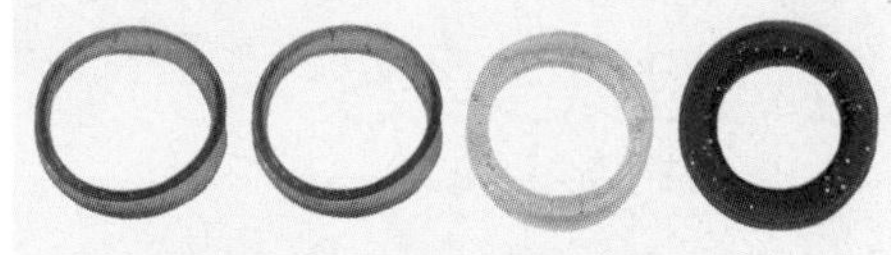

▲ **Figure 16–51a**
Custom finger-fitting system.

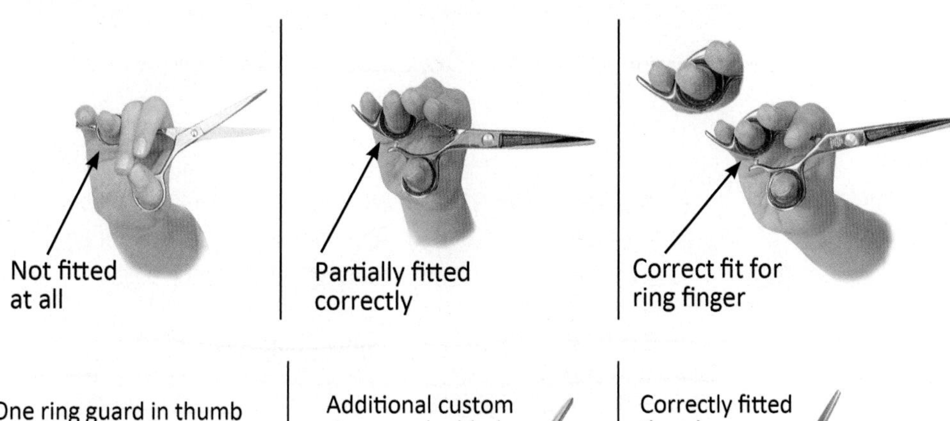

◀ **Figure 16–51**
Finger-fitting system for the ring finger.

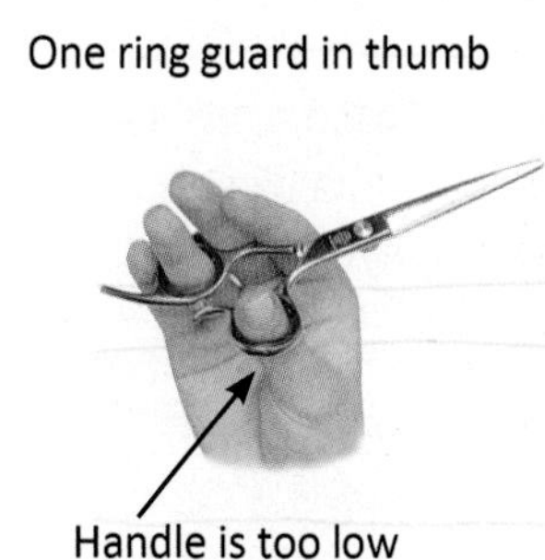

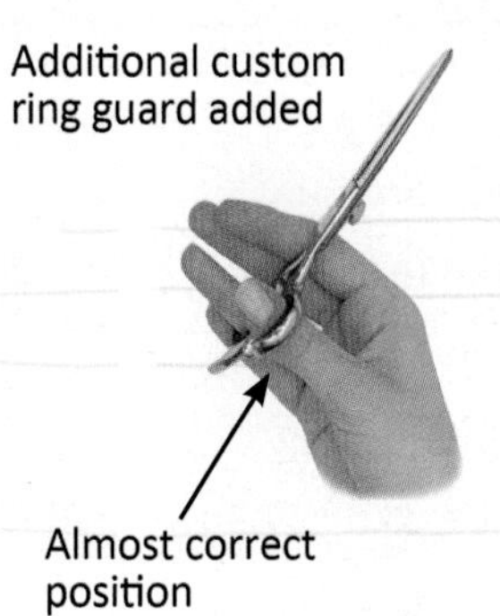

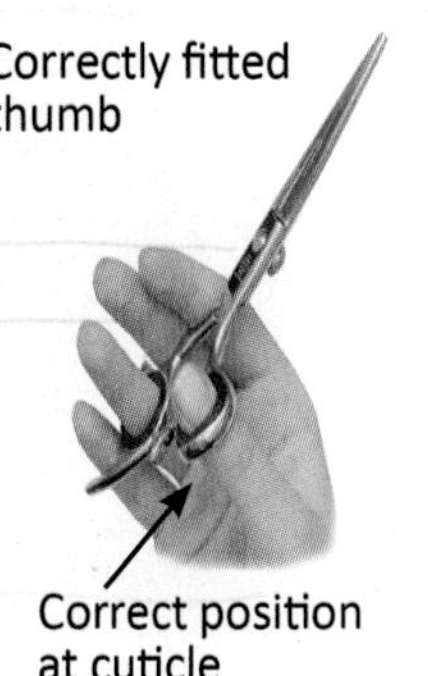

◀ **Figure 16–52**
Finger-fitting system for the thumb finger.

Photo supplied by The Shark Fin Shear Co.

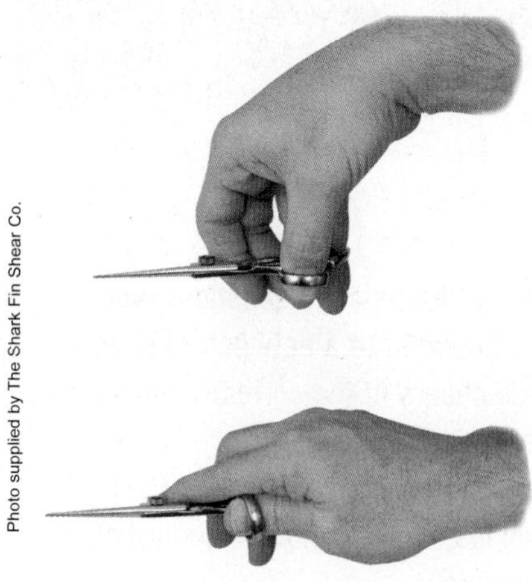

Photo supplied by The Shark Fin Shear Co.

▲ Figure 16–53
Non-swivel shear (top). Swivel shear (bottom).

shoulder and elbow and straighten the wrist while cutting, for a more relaxed working posture (**Figure 16–53**).

- **Ask about the service agreement.** Regardless of the type of shears you decide to purchase, be sure that the company you buy your shears from can service them in a timely and convenient manner. Be sure that they have a person who is certified to sharpen their shears in your area. Otherwise, you may have to send your shears away to be sharpened, ending up without them for a period of time.
- **Ask about the warranty.** Since every company offers a different warranty for their shears, make sure you know what the warranty period is and exactly what the warranty covers before you buy the shears. Make sure you are satisfied with that company's warranty policy, should you have an issue with your shears, before you decide to buy it.
- **Analyze the cost of the shears.** A pair of shears that is made from high-quality steel, is forged instead of cast, and has the kind of warranty you will need as a new cosmetologist should cost between $250 and $350. If you are buying a cast shear, you should not pay more than $200. If the price of a cast shear is higher than $200, keep looking. Better-quality forged shears are available on the market for only slightly more.
- **Determine how many pairs of shears you need.** A good rule of thumb is to have two cutting shears and one thinning or blending shear available at all times. Your second shear is

Here's a Tip:

Every type of shear has a distinct design and reason for its size, shape, and length (Table 16–3). For example, when first starting out, you might want to use a 28-tooth thinning shear or 40-tooth blending shear. These are both safe starting shears for a new cutter, because they render less dramatic cuts and are appropriate for many types of haircuts.

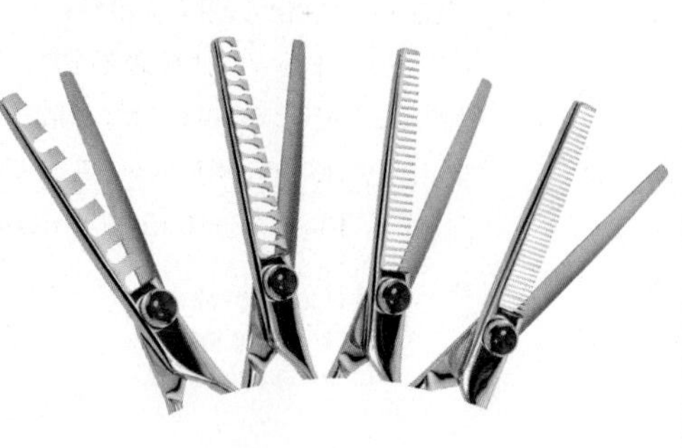

Photo supplied by The Shark Fin Shear Co.

▲ Figure 16–54
Types of texture shears.

TYPES OF TEXTURE SHEARS

TYPES OF TEXTURE SHEARS (Figure 16–54)	USES
CHUNKING SHEAR (5–9 teeth)	Great for taking out big sections (the wider the space between the blades the more pronounced the cutting will be)
TEXTURIZING SHEAR (14–19 teeth)	Adds increased blending
THINNING SHEAR (26–30 teeth)	Most universally used, consistent reduction of bulk (the closer together the teeth, the more blended the cut)
BLENDING SHEAR (38–50 teeth)	Great for scissor-over-comb cutting

© Milady, a part of Cengage Learning.

Table 16–3 Types of Texture Shears.

necessary so if anything happens to your main cutting shear, you can continue to service your clients while the damaged shear is being repaired.

Custom-Fitted Shears

Over the course of your career, you are likely to perform thousands of haircuts! Using shears that are properly fitted to your hand allows the muscles and tendons of your hand and wrist to be as relaxed as possible and will help to protect you from long-term repetitive motion injuries, such as carpal tunnel syndrome and other musculoskeletal (MUS-kyuh-lo-SKEL-uh-tul) disorders.

Prevention is the key to avoiding these problems, and a keen awareness of good work habits along with the proper tools and equipment will enhance your health and comfort. Remember, your hand's main job is to steer the shear—correct blade tension does the cutting.

Buying and using ergonomically correct and custom-fitted shears can help dramatically by:

- Allowing you to relax your grip, reducing thumb pressure while cutting, so the blades are not being forced together. This will also keep your blades sharper, longer.
- Reducing the amount of pressure on the nerves and tendons in your hand. Too much pressure of this type can result in nerve damage, carpal tunnel syndrome, or wrist, shoulder, elbow, neck, and back pain.
- Allowing the shear to do the cutting work when properly adjusted and fitted to your hand.

did you know?

The correct way to measure the length of a shear is to start at the tip of the blades and measure to where the finger rest/tang connects to the back of the ring finger-opening. Do not include the length of the tang (**Figure 16–55**).

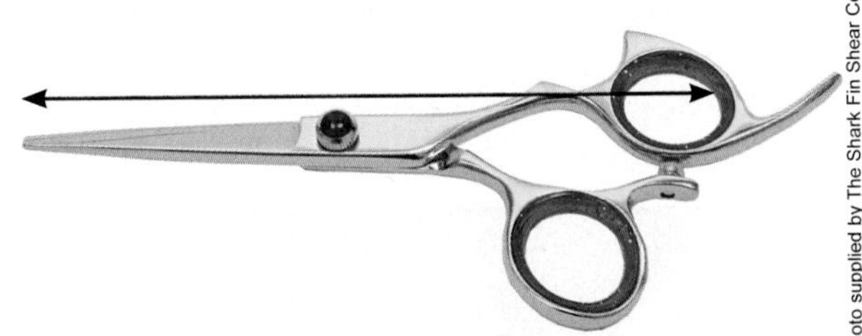

Photo supplied by The Shark Fin Shear Co.

▲ **Figure 16–55**
How to measure shears.

Fitting the Shear Correctly

Fitting the shear correctly to your hand entails four components.

1. **Fitting the ring finger.** A properly fitted shear has a ring finger-hole that rests between the first and second knuckle, far enough back on the ring finger so that your pinky is resting comfortably on the finger tang. Once you have the shear in that position, there should be only a slight bit of extra space around your finger and the finger hole. A properly fit ring finger will be centered in the middle of the finger hole.
2. **Fitting the thumb.** When your shear is properly fitted, the thumb hole will rest at or slightly over the cuticle area of your thumb, but not up to or over the knuckle. Once you have the shear at that location on your thumb, there can be a little extra space around your thumb and the thumb hole. A proper fit will have your cuticle centered underneath the center of the thumb ring guard.
3. **Relaxing your grip.** A relaxed grip allows to you to cut without any thumb pressure, so the blades are not being forced together. It reduces the amount of pressure on the nerves and tendons in your hand, which can result in damage, and it allows the shear to do the work of cutting.

did you know?

You should never lend your shears to another stylist. Everyone cuts hair using a certain amount of hand pressure. Allowing someone else—someone who uses a different level of pressure than you use—to borrow your shears can recondition the blades. The result? Your shears may not cut correctly for you.

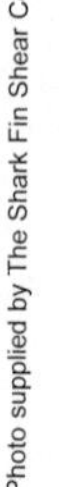

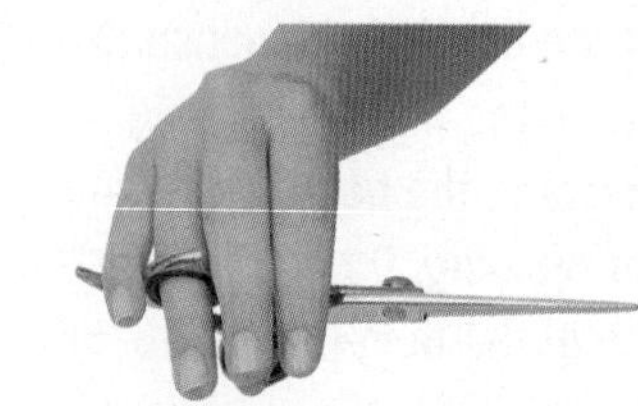

▲ **Figure 16–56**
Correct finger position and alignment.

4. Correct finger position and alignment. Correct nerve and tendon alignment while cutting hair is crucial to having a healthy career as a professional cosmetologist. Correct finger position allows your finger to stay properly aligned, which not only gives you correct nerve and tendon alignment in your hand, but also reduces the likelihood of developing hand health issues caused by improperly fitted shears. Look for a handle design that cradles your middle finger. This guarantees correct finger placement on the shear (**Figure 16–56**).

Holding Your Tools

There are two important reasons to hold your tools properly:

- A proper hold gives you the most control, and the best results when cutting hair.
- A proper hold helps you avoid muscle strain in your hands, arms, neck, and back.

© Milady, a part of Cengage Learning.

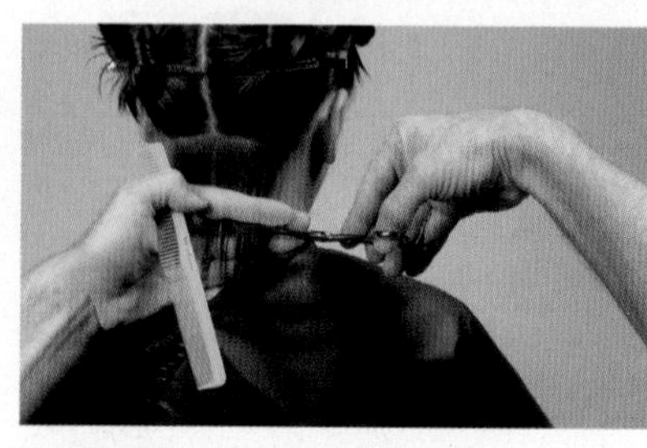

▲ **Figure 16–57**
Proper placement of ring finger and little finger.

Holding Your Shears

1. Open your right hand (left hand if you are left-handed), and place the ring finger in the finger grip of the still blade and the little finger on the finger tang (brace) (**Figure 16–57**).
2. Place the thumb in the finger grip (thumb grip) of the moving blade (**Figure 16–58**).
3. Practice opening and closing the shears. Concentrate on moving only your thumb. A great way to get the feel of this movement is to lay the still blade against the palm or forefinger of your other hand to hold it steady, while you move the other blade with your thumb (**Figure 16–59**).

Photo supplied by The Shark Fin Shear Co.

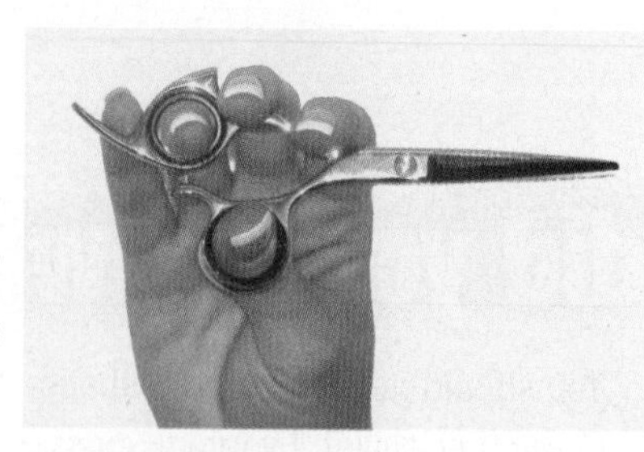

▲ **Figure 16–58**
Proper placement of thumb.

Photo supplied by The Shark Fin Shear Co.

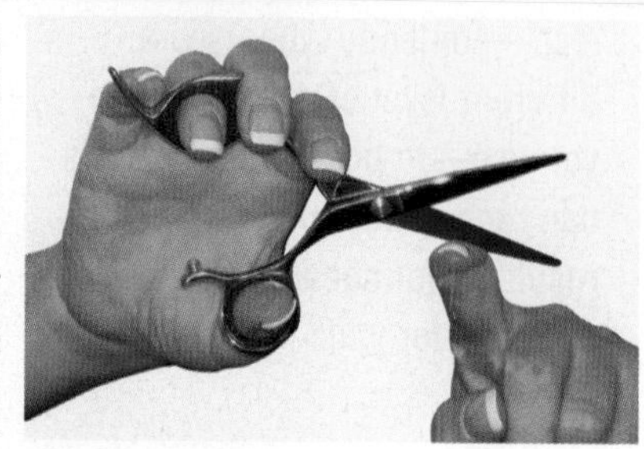

▲ **Figure 16–59**
Still and moving blades.

Holding the Shears and Comb

During the haircutting process, you will be holding the comb and shears at the same time. You may be tempted to put the comb down while cutting, but doing so will waste a lot of time. It is best to learn—from the start—to hold both tools during the entire haircut. In general, your cutting hand (dominant hand) does most of the work. It holds the shears, parts the hair, combs the hair, and cuts the hair. Your holding hand does just that: it holds the sections of hair and the comb while cutting. The holding hand helps you maintain control.

- **Palming the shears.** Remove your thumb from the thumb grip, leaving your ring and little fingers in the grip and finger rest. Curl your fingers in to palm the shears, which keeps them closed while you comb or part the hair (**Figure 16–60**). This allows you to hold the comb and the shears at the same time. While palming the shears, hold the comb between thumb, index, and middle fingers (**Figure 16–61**).
- **Transferring the comb.** After you have combed a subsection into position, you will need to free up your cutting hand. Once your fingers are in place at the correct cutting position, transfer the comb by placing it between the thumb and index finger of your holding hand (the hand

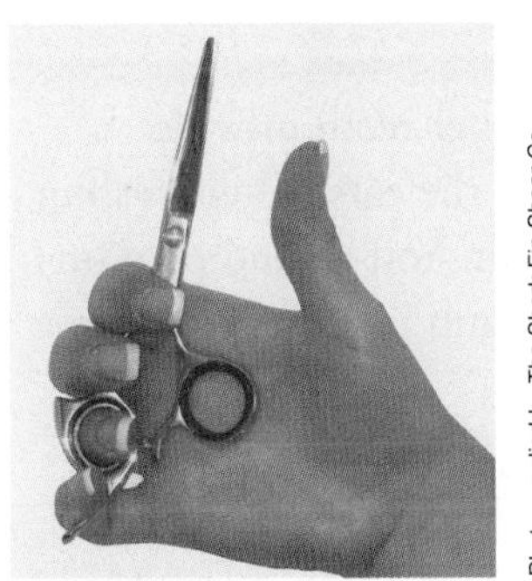
Photo supplied by The Shark Fin Shear Co.

▲ **Figure 16–60**
Palming the shears.

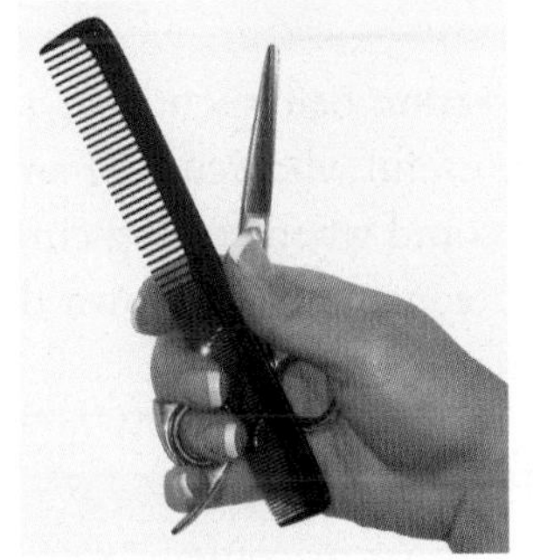
Photo supplied by The Shark Fin Shear Co.

▲ **Figure 16–61**
Holding comb and shears.

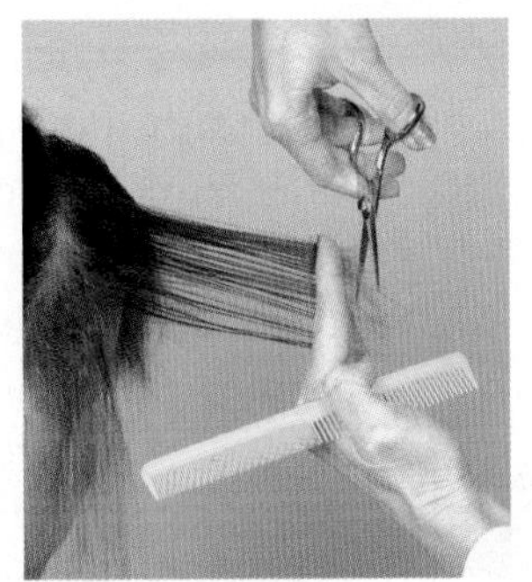
© Milady, a part of Cengage Learning.

▲ **Figure 16–62**
Transferring the comb.

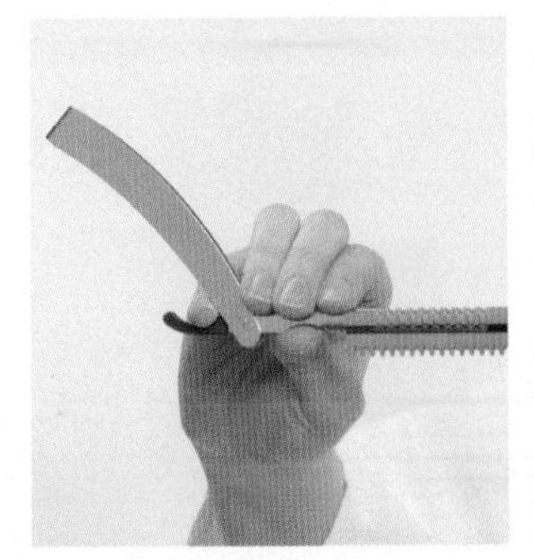
© Milady, a part of Cengage Learning. Photography by Paul Castle, Castle Photography.

▲ **Figure 16–63**
Holding razor properly.

holding the subsection) (**Figure 16–62**). You are now ready to cut the subsection.

Holding the Razor

The straight razor, or feather blade, is a versatile tool that can be used for an entire haircut, or just for detailing and texturizing. Holding and working with a razor feels very different from holding and working with shears. The more you practice holding and palming the razor, the more comfortable you will become with this tool. There are two methods for holding the razor for cutting.

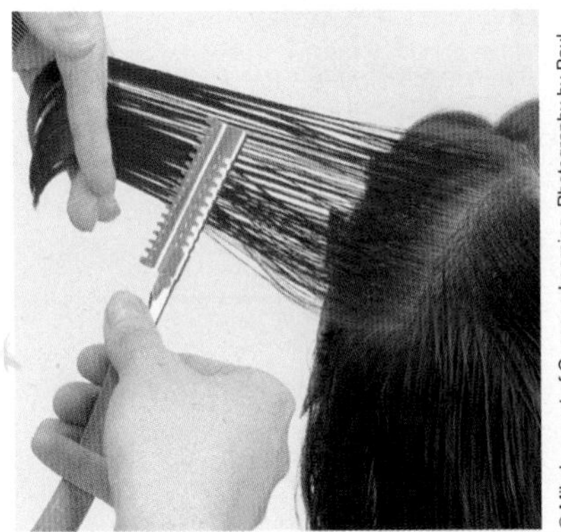
© Milady, a part of Cengage Learning. Photography by Paul Castle, Castle Photography.

▲ **Figure 16–64**
Holding razor for cutting.

Method A

1. Open the razor so that the handle is higher than the shank. Place the thumb on the thumb grip, and the index, middle, and ring fingers on the shank.
2. Place the little finger in the tang, underneath the handle (**Figure 16–63**).
3. When cutting a subsection, position the razor on top of the subsection, the part facing you, for maximum control (**Figure 16–64**).

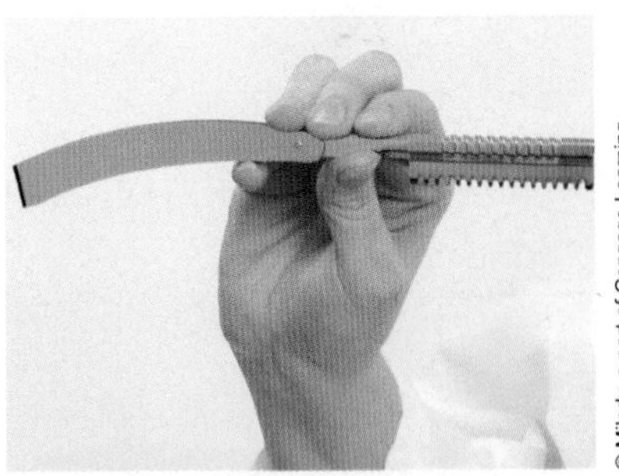
© Milady, a part of Cengage Learning. Photography by Paul Castle, Castle Photography.

▲ **Figure 16–65**
Alternate method of holding razor.

Method B

1. Open the razor until the handle and shank form a straight line.
2. Place the thumb on the grip and wrap the fingers around the handle (**Figure 16–65**).

Just as you need to be able to hold the comb and the shears in your cutting hand while working, you also need to palm the razor so that you can comb and section hair during a haircut. Curl your ring finger and little finger to palm the razor. Hold the comb between your thumb and the index and middle fingers (**Figure 16–66**). Most accidents with razors happen when combing the hair, not when cutting the hair, because of a loose grip when palming. Be sure to practice keeping a firm grip on the razor with the ring and little fingers, which keeps the open blade from sliding and cutting your hand while you comb the hair.

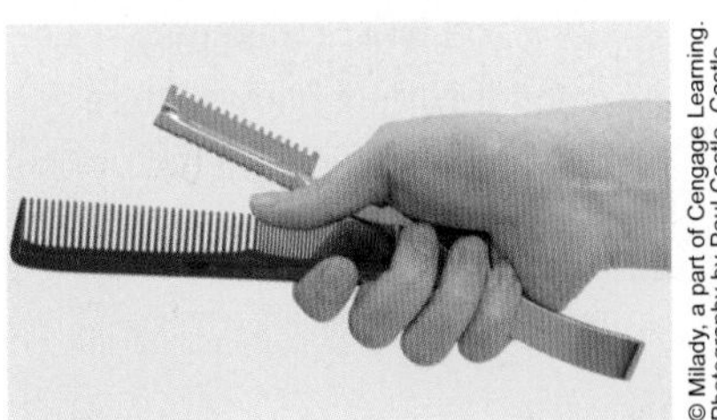
© Milady, a part of Cengage Learning. Photography by Paul Castle, Castle Photography.

▲ **Figure 16–66**
Palming the razor.

Handling the Comb

Both the wide and fine teeth of the comb are regularly used when cutting hair. The wide teeth are used for combing and parting hair, while the

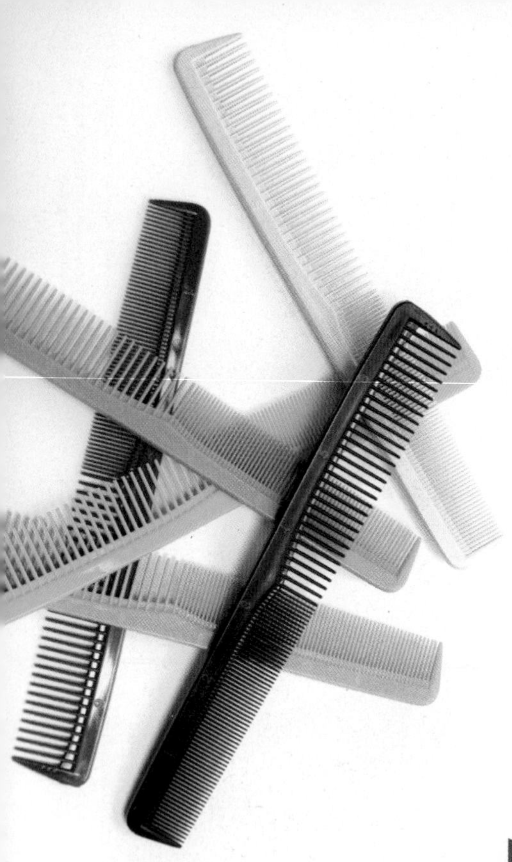

finer teeth comb the section before cutting. The finer teeth provide more tension, and are useful when cutting around the ears, when dealing with difficult hairlines, and when cutting curly hair. You should plan on spending some time practicing how to turn the comb in your hand while palming the shears.

© Milady, a part of Cengage Learning. Photography by Paul Castle, Castle Photography.

Tension

Tension in haircutting is the amount of pressure applied when combing and holding a subsection. Tension is created by stretching or pulling the subsection.

Tension ranges from minimum to maximum. You control tension with your fingers when you hold the subsection of hair between them. Consistent tension is important for constant, even results in a haircut. Use maximum tension on straight hair when you want precise lines. With curly or wavy hair, less tension is better, because a lot of tension will result in the hair shrinking even more than usual as it dries. Minimum tension should be used around the ears and on hairlines with strong growth patterns.

Posture and Body Position

It is important to be aware of your habits of posture (how you stand and sit) and body position (how you hold your body when cutting hair). As a working cosmetologist, you will be spending many hours on your feet, and you may want to consider using a cutting stool and wearing proper footwear as preventive measures. Good posture and body position will help you avoid future back problems and ensure better haircutting results. The correct body position will help you move more efficiently during the haircut, and help you maintain more control over the process.

- **Position the client.** Not only is your body position important, but so is your client's. Make sure that your client is sitting up straight and that her legs are not crossed. Gentle reminders as the haircut progresses may be necessary. Remember, you can move the client by turning the chair or raising/lowering of the chair, whichever gives you the option of keeping your body in the same place, or by angling the client's chair so you can see what you are doing in the mirror.
- **Center your weight.** When working, keep your body weight centered and firm. When standing, keep your knees slightly bent rather than locked. Instead of bending at the waist, try bending one knee if you need to lean slightly one way or the other. When sitting, keep both feet on the floor.
- **Work in front of your section.** When cutting hair, a general rule of thumb is to stand or sit directly in front of the area you are cutting. By doing this, you keep your body weight centered, and you will automatically find yourself moving around the head during a haircut. If you want to sit or stand in the same place, or be able to view what you are doing in the mirror, you need to move the client's chair. As

CAUTION

Back and wrist strain may result if correct body posture and hand position are not maintained while cutting.

much as possible, keep to the general rule of always standing in front of the area you are working on, and positioning your hands according to the cutting line. ☑ **LO5**

Hand Positions for Different Cutting Angles

- **Cutting over your fingers.** There are some situations in which you will be cutting over your fingers or on top of your knuckles. This hand position is used most often when cutting uniform or increasing layers (**Figure 16–67**).
- **Cutting below the fingers.** When cutting a blunt haircut or a heavier graduated haircut, it is customary to use a horizontal cutting line. In this case, you will be cutting below your fingers, or on the inside of your knuckles (**Figure 16–68**).
- **Cutting palm-to-palm.** When cutting with a vertical or diagonal cutting line, cutting palm-to-palm is the best way to maintain control of the subsection, especially with regard to elevation and overdirection. Cutting palm-to-palm means that the palms of both hands are facing each other while cutting. This is different from cutting on the top of your fingers or knuckles. Cutting palm-to-palm also helps to prevent strain on your back as you work (**Figures 16–69** and **16–70**).

Learning how to control your shears is important because many techniques, such as scissor-over-comb and point cutting, are difficult to learn and perform if you hold the shears improperly.

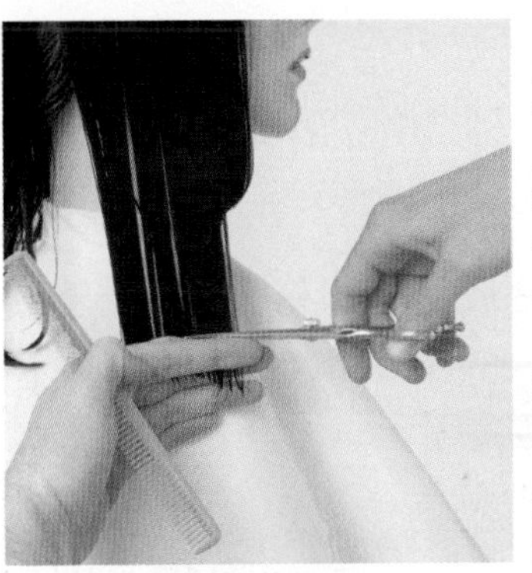
© Milady, a part of Cengage Learning. Photography by Paul Castle, Castle Photography.

▲ **Figure 16–67**
Cutting over the fingers.

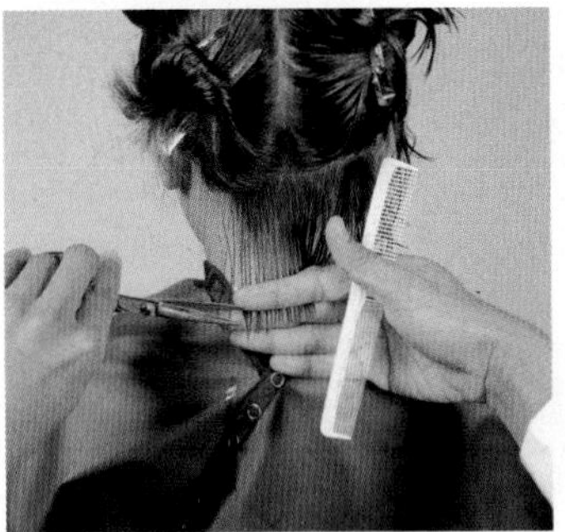
© Milady, a part of Cengage Learning. Photography by Yanik Chauvin.

▲ **Figure 16–68**
Cutting below the fingers.

Safety in Haircutting

It is absolutely essential for you to keep in mind that when you are cutting hair, accidents can happen. You will be handling sharp tools and instruments, and you must always protect yourself and your client by following the proper precautions.

Always palm the shears and the razor when combing or parting the hair. This keeps the points of the shears closed and pointed away from the client while combing and prevents you from cutting yourself or the client. Palming the shears also reduces strain on the index finger and thumb while combing the hair.

Do not cut past the second knuckle when cutting below your fingers, or when cutting palm-to-palm. The skin is soft and fleshy past the second knuckle and is easy to cut.

When cutting around the ears, take extra care not to accidentally cut the ear. Cuts on the ears can produce large amounts of blood!

When cutting the bangs (fringe), or any area close to the skin, balance the shears by placing the tip of the index finger of your left hand (your right hand if you cut left-handed) on the pivot screw and the knuckles

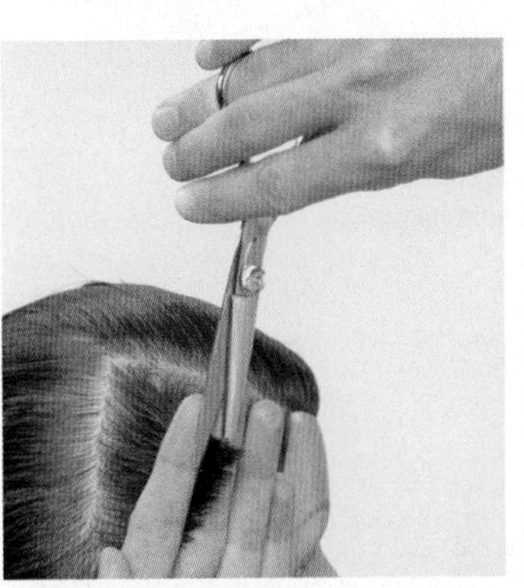
© Milady, a part of Cengage Learning. Photography by Paul Castle, Castle Photography.

▲ **Figure 16–69**
Cutting palm-to-palm, vertical cutting line.

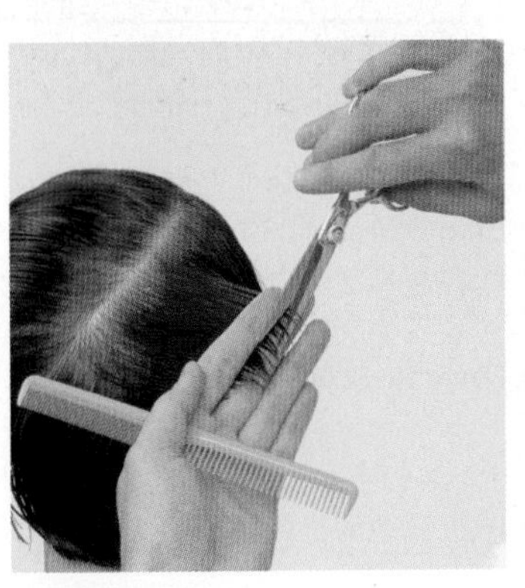
© Milady, a part of Cengage Learning. Photography by Paul Castle, Castle Photography.

▲ **Figure 16–70**
Cutting palm-to-palm, diagonal cutting line.

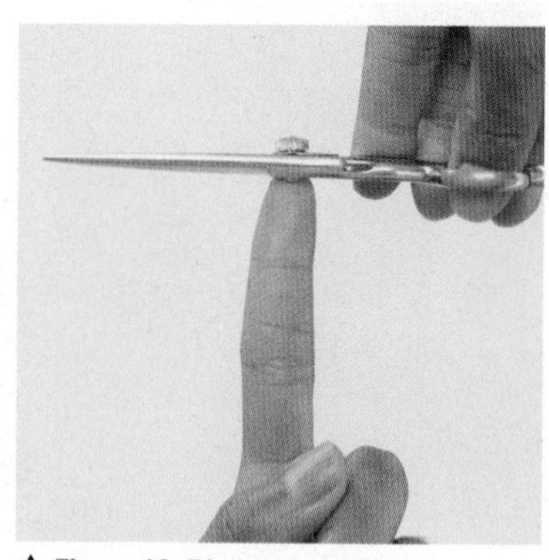

© Milady, a part of Cengage Learning. Photography by Paul Castle, Castle Photography.

▲ **Figure 16–71**
Balancing scissors.

of your left hand against the skin (**Figure 16–71**). This helps prevent clients from being accidentally poked with the shears if they move suddenly. This also helps to balance your shears and cut a cleaner line.

When working with a razor, learn with a guard. You should never practice holding, palming, or cutting with the razor without a guard unless directed and supervised by your instructor. Take extra care when removing and disposing of the razor blade. Discard used blades in a puncture-proof container.

Basic Haircuts

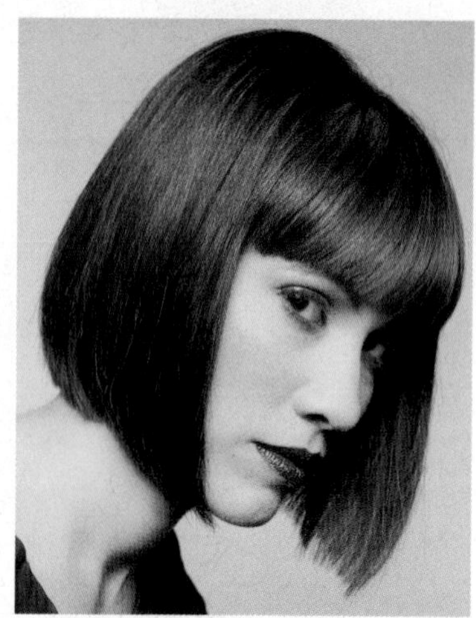

Photograph by Tom Carson. Hair by Laura Dorelli for Vanis Salon & Day Spa, Scheveville, IN. Makeup by Amy Malone and Gretchen Wilson.

▲ **Figure 16–72**
Blunt haircut.

The art of haircutting is made up of variations on four basic haircuts: blunt, graduated, layered, and long layered. An understanding of these basic haircuts is essential before you can begin experimenting with other cuts and effects.

In a **blunt haircut**, also known as a **one-length haircut**, all the hair comes to a single hanging level, forming a weight line. The **weight line** is a visual line in the haircut, where the ends of the hair hang together. The blunt cut is also referred to as a zero-elevation cut or no-elevation cut, because it has no elevation or overdirection. It is cut with a stationary guide. The cutting line can be horizontal, diagonal, or rounded. Blunt haircuts are excellent for finer and thinner hair types, because all the hair is cut to one length, therefore making it appear thicker (**Figure 16–72**).

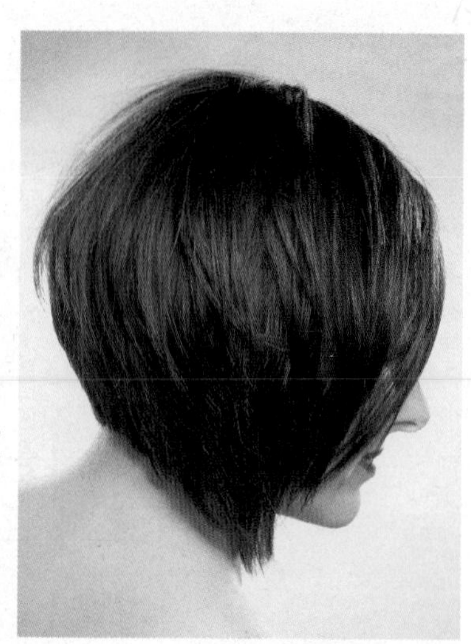

Photography by Tom Carson. Hair by Antonio Morosi, hair stylist for Above and Beyond Salon, Vermillion, Ohio. Laura Hall, Color for Above and Beyond Salon, Vermillion, Ohio. Makeup by Laura Hall.

▲ **Figure 16–73 Graduated haircut.**

A **graduated haircut** is a graduated shape or wedge. This is caused by cutting the hair with tension, low to medium elevation, or overdirection. The most common elevation is 45 degrees. In a graduated haircut, there is a visual buildup of weight in a given area. The ends of the hair appear to be stacked. There are many variations and effects you can create with graduation simply by adjusting the degree of elevation, the amount of overdirection, or your cutting line (**Figure 16–73**).

A **layered haircut** is a graduated effect achieved by cutting the hair with elevation or overdirection. The hair is cut at higher elevations, usually 90 degrees and above. Layered haircuts generally have less weight than graduated haircuts. In a graduated haircut, the ends of the hair appear closer together. In a layered haircut, the ends appear farther apart. **Layers** create movement and volume in the hair by releasing weight. A layered haircut can be created with a traveling guide, a stationary guide, or both (**Figure 16–74**).

Another basic haircut is the **long-layered haircut**. The hair is cut at a 180-degree angle. This technique gives more volume to hairstyles and can be combined with other basic haircuts. The resulting shape will have shorter layers at the top and increasingly longer layers toward the perimeter (**Figure 16–75**).

By using these four basic concepts, you can create any haircut you want. Every haircut is made up of one, two, or three of these basic techniques. Add a little texturizing, slide cutting, or scissor-over-comb, and you have advanced haircutting. Advanced haircutting is simply learning the basics and then applying them in any combination to create unlimited shapes and effects.

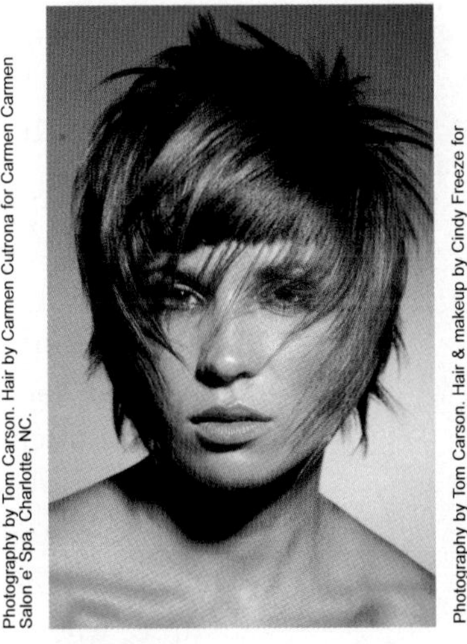
Photography by Tom Carson. Hair by Carmen Cutrona for Carmen Carmen Salon e' Spa, Charlotte, NC.

▲ Figure 16–74
Layered haircut.

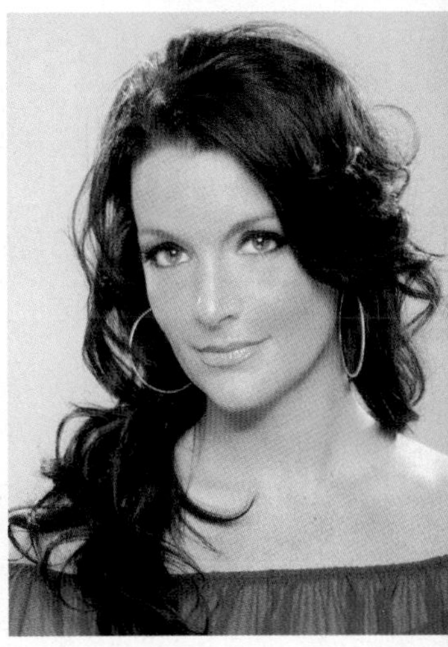
Photography by Tom Carson. Hair & makeup by Cindy Freeze for Kathy Adams Salon, Buford, GA.

▲ Figure 16–75
Long-layered haircut.

The Blunt Haircut

The blunt haircut—also known as a *bob*, *one-length*, *one-level*, *pageboy*, or *bowl haircut*, is an all-time classic. Although the line of the cut appears to be simple, the success of the cut relies on precision, which can be anything but simple when working with a variety of hair types, growth patterns, and animated clients.

The client's head should be upright and straight for this cut. If you tilt the head forward, the hair will not fall into its natural position. If you cut a blunt haircut with the head forward, you will make two discoveries: (1) the line will not fall as you cut it, and (2) you will have created some graduation where you did not intend to.

FOCUS ON

GENERAL HAIRCUTTING TIPS

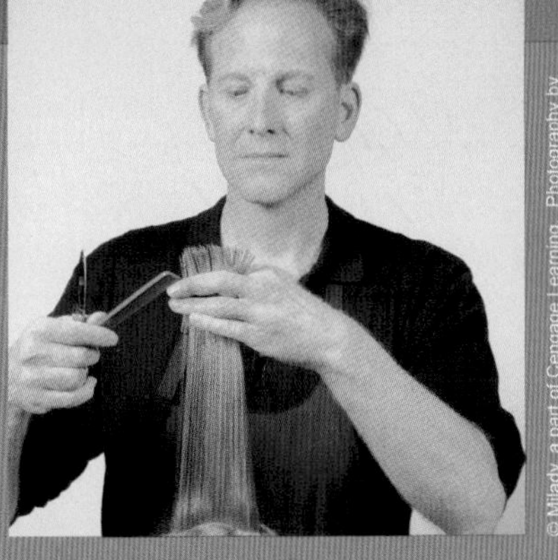
© Milady, a part of Cengage Learning. Photography by Yanik Chauvin.

▲ Figure16–76
Cross-checking.

- Always make consistent and clean partings, which will give an even amount of hair to each subsection and produce more precise results.
- Take extra care when working in the crown and neckline, which sometimes have very strong growth patterns. These areas are potential danger zones.
- Another danger zone is the hair that grows around the ear or hangs over the ear in a finished haircut. Allow for the ear sticking out by either keeping more weight in this area, or cutting with minimal tension.
- Always use consistent tension. Tension may range from maximum to minimum. You can maintain light tension by using the wide teeth of the comb, and by not pulling the subsection too tightly. Use consistent tension for the entire section of hair.
- Pay attention to head position. If the head is not upright, it may alter the amount of elevation and overdirection.
- Maintain an even amount of moisture in the hair. Dry hair responds to cutting differently than wet hair and may give you uneven results in the finished haircut.
- Always work with your guideline. If you cannot see the guide, your subsection is too thick. Go back and take a smaller subsection before cutting. Using a subsection that is too big can result in a mistake that may be too big to fix. If a mistake is made while using a smaller subsection, the mistake is also smaller and therefore easier to correct.
- Always cross-check the haircut. Cross-checking is parting the haircut in the opposite way that you cut it to check for precision of line and shape. For example, if you use vertical partings in a haircut, cross-check the lengths with horizontal partings (Figure 16–76).
- Use the mirror to see your elevation. You can also turn the client sideways so that you can see one side in the mirror while working on the opposite side. This helps create even lines and maintains visual balance while working.
- Check both sides. Always check that both sides are even by standing in front of your client.
- Cutting curly hair. Remember that curly hair shrinks more than straight hair, anywhere from ½ to 2 inches or more (1.25 to 5 centimeters). Always leave the length longer than the desired end result.

FOCUS ON

TIPS FOR BLUNT HAIRCUTS

- Always cut with minimal or no tension.
- Work with the natural growth patterns of the hair, keeping the client's head upright.
- Always comb the section twice before cutting to ensure that you have combed the hair clean from the parting to the ends. If using the wide teeth of the comb while cutting, always comb the section first with the fine teeth, then turn the comb around, and re-comb with the wide teeth.
- Always maintain an even amount of moisture in the hair.
- Pay close attention to growth patterns in the crown and hairline.
- Take precautions to allow for the ears sticking out to avoid creating a hole.

Blunt haircuts may be performed by either holding the sections between the fingers or using the comb to hold the hair with little or no tension. If the hair length is past the shoulders, sections need to be held between the fingers with minimal tension. For very long hair, it is often useful to have the client stand while you sit on a cutting stool as you work.

When cutting a blunt cut, be aware of the crown area, sometimes called the danger zone, because this is where irregular growth patterns are most often found. The crown can be challenging when you are doing blunt haircuts. Look at the scalp to see the natural growth pattern. You may want to cut this area at the very end of the haircut, or cut it slightly longer than the guideline. Once the hair is dry, you can see where it falls, and then match the length to the guideline.

Another danger zone is around the ears. Because ears do not lie flat against the head, you need to take special steps to keep an even cutting line. Always work with very little tension or no tension around the ears, unless you are working with shorter layers.

Blunt cuts can be designed with or without bangs (fringe), on straight or curly hair, and with a short, medium, or long length.

PROCEDURE 16-1 **Blunt Haircut with Fringe** SEE PAGE 384

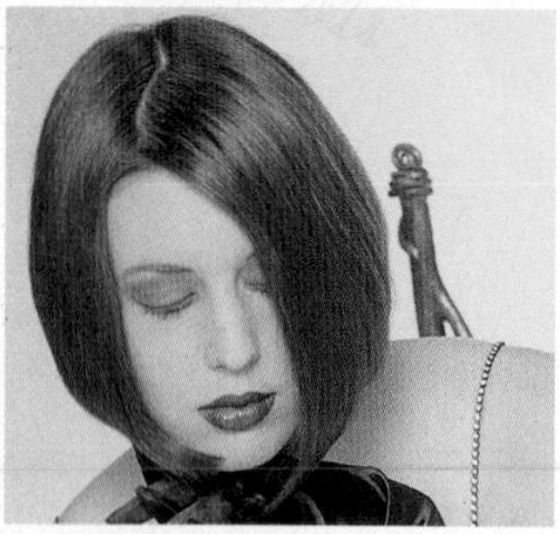

Other Blunt Haircuts

The blunt haircut is the basis for many other classic cuts.

In a classic A-line bob, a diagonal cutting line (finger angle) is used (**Figure 16–77**).

Photography by Tom Carson. Hair by Yellow Strawberry Global Salon, Sarasota, FL.

▲ **Figure 16–77**
A-line haircut.

In this longer blunt haircut (**Figure 16–78**), the bang has been left long and was cut with a horizontal finger angle. When blunt cutting longer hair, hold the hair between the fingers with very little tension.

Figure 16–79 illustrates a blunt haircut on curly hair. Note how the hair naturally graduates itself when it dries.

In a classic pageboy, the perimeter is curved, using a combination of horizontal and curved lines (**Figure 16–80**).

Graduated (45-Degree) Haircut

In this basic haircut, you will be working with a vertical cutting line and a 45-degree elevation, as well as a 90-degree elevation. Although you will use a center part, keep in mind that this haircut can also work with a side part or a bang. You will be using a stationary guideline and a traveling guideline.

Remember, a stationary guideline is a guideline that does not move. All other sections are combed toward the guideline and are cut to match it. A traveling guideline moves with you as you work through the haircut.

Photography by Tom Carson. Hair by Leslie Cook for Tangles Salon, Wichita Falls, TX.

▲ **Figure 16–78**
Longer blunt haircut with one-length fringe.

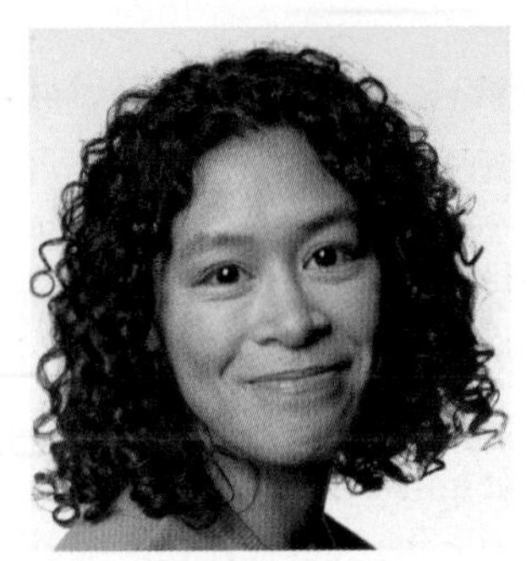
Getty Images.

▲ **Figure 16–79**
Blunt haircut on curly hair.

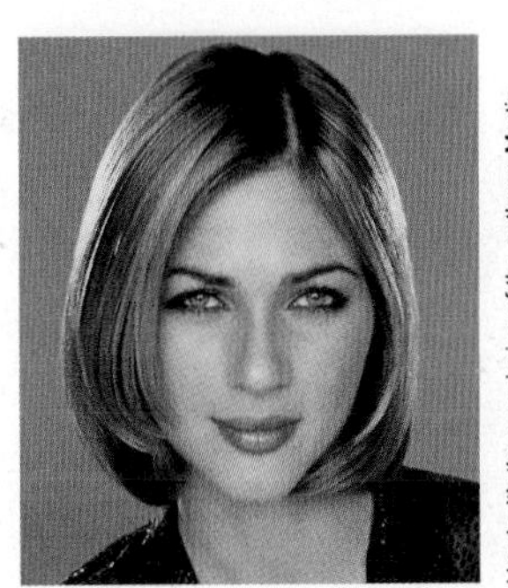
Used with the permission of the authors, Martin Gannon and Richard Thompson, as featured in their book, Mahogany: Steps to Cutting, Colouring, and Finishing Hair. © Martin Gannon and Richard Thompson, 1997.

▲ **Figure 16–80**
Classic blunt haircut.

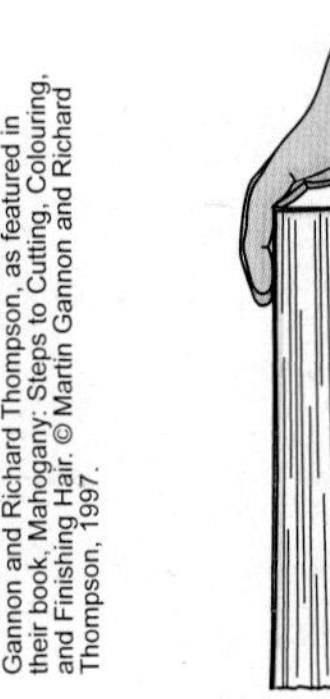
© Milady, a part of Cengage Learning.

▲ **Figure 16–81**
Straight or blunt hanging line.

Here's a great way to understand what a graduated haircut looks like. Hold a telephone book by the spine with the pages hanging down. The edges of the pages make a straight line, just like a blunt haircut (**Figure 16–81**). Now turn the book the other way, open it in the middle, and let the pages flop down on either side. The edges of the pages make a beveled line, just like a graduated haircut (**Figure 16–82**).

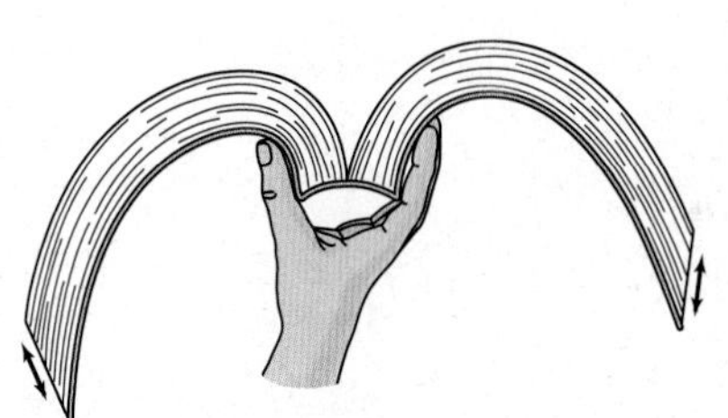
© Milady, a part of Cengage Learning.

▲ **Figure 16–82**
Beveled or graduated hanging line.

Here is another type of graduated haircut, created with different cutting angles. In the classic graduated bob made popular by Vidal Sassoon, diagonal sections and finger angles are used to create a rounded or beveled effect. This haircut begins in the back, using a 45-degree elevation throughout, and gradually incorporates the sides and top. If you find that the hairline grows up or toward the center, you can use the scissor-over-comb technique to blend it (**Figures 16–83** and **16–84**).

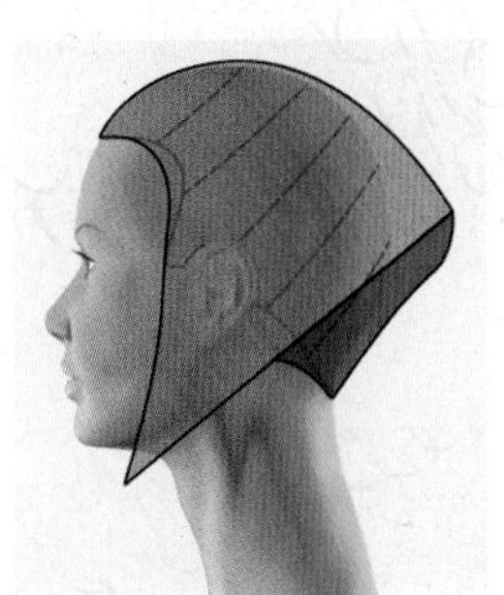
© Milady, a part of Cengage Learning.

▲ **Figure 16–83**
Graduated design.

In the example in **Figures 16–85**, **16–86**, and **16–87**, you can see a shorter shape that has rounded weight. This haircut is created using diagonal partings that connect at the back of the ear. In front of the ear, the diagonal partings point down toward the face. Behind the ear, the diagonal partings point down toward the back. The sides are elevated and overdirected to the back of the ear, producing more length toward the face. The back is cut using a traveling guideline, with each section overdirected to the previous section.

PROCEDURE 16-2 Graduated Haircut SEE PAGE 392

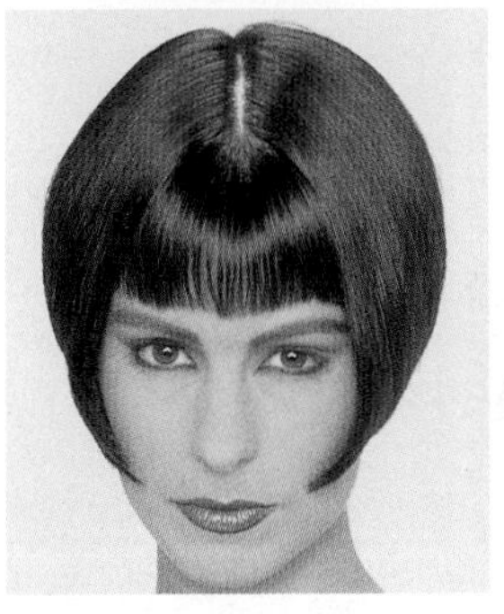
Hair by Brian & Sandra Smith, makeup by Rose Marie, wardrobe by Victor Paul, photo by Taggart/Winterhalter, production by Purely Visual.

▲ **Figure 16–84**
Finished graduated design.

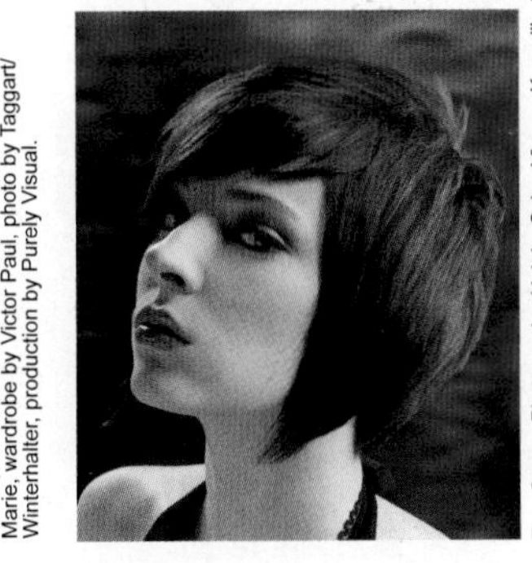
Tom Carson Photography. Hair by Salon Visage, Knoxville, TN.

▲ **Figure 16–85**
Finished graduated haircut: side view.

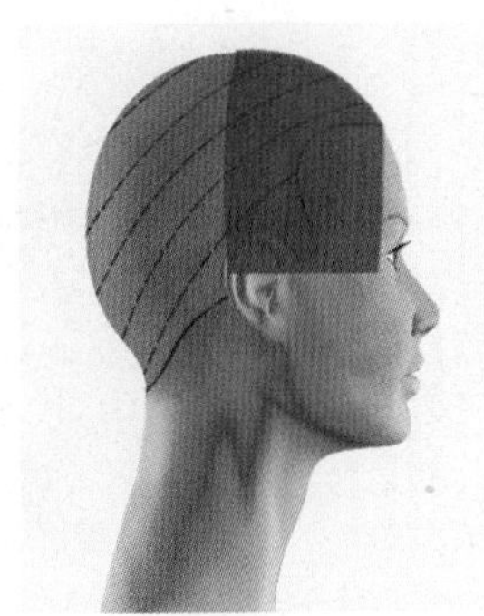
© Milady, a part of Cengage Learning.

▲ **Figure 16–86**
Classic (round) graduated haircut: design.

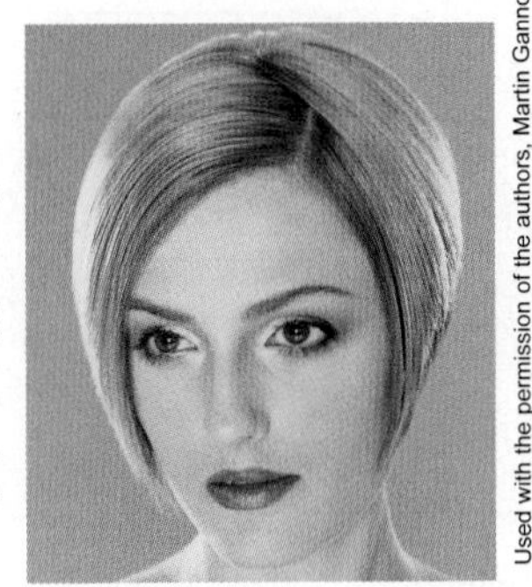
Used with the permission of the authors, Martin Gannon and Richard Thompson, as featured in their book, Mahogany: Steps to Cutting, Colouring, and Finishing Hair. © Martin Gannon and Richard Thompson, 1997.

▲ **Figure 16–87**
Finished classic (round) graduated haircut.

FOCUS ON

TIPS FOR GRADUATED HAIRCUTS

- Heavier graduated haircuts (those cut with lower elevations) work well on hair that tends to expand when dry. Coarse textures and curly hair will appear to graduate more than straight hair. Keep your elevation below 45 degrees when working on these hair types.
- Fine hair is great for graduation. Because graduation builds weight, you can make thin or fine hair appear thicker and fuller. However, if hair is both fine and thin, avoid creating heavy weight lines. Softer graduation, using diagonal partings, will create a softer weight line. If hair has medium density but is fine in texture, it is safe to elevate more because there is enough density to support it.
- Check the neckline carefully before cutting the nape short. If the hairline grows straight up, you may want to leave the length longer and the graduation lower, so that it falls below the hairline. You can also blend in a tricky hairline by using the scissor-over-comb technique, which is explained later in this chapter.
- Always use the fine teeth of the comb and maintain even tension to ensure a precise line.

The Uniform-Layered (90-Degree) Haircut

The third basic haircut is the layered haircut created with **uniform layers**, all the hair is elevated to 90 degrees from the scalp and cut at the same length. Your guide for this haircut is an interior traveling guideline. An **interior guideline** is inside the haircut rather than on the perimeter. The resulting shape will appear soft and rounded, with no built-up weight or corners. The perimeter of the hair will fall softly, because the vertical sections in the interior reduce weight (**Figure 16–88**).

PROCEDURE 16-3 Uniform-Layered Haircut SEE PAGE 401

Other Examples of Layered Haircuts

There are many variations on the basic layered haircut.

If you follow the uniform-layering technique but cut the hair much shorter, to 1 inch (2.5 centimeters) or so, you will create a *pixie*, *cro*, or *Caesar* haircut. This hairstyle is flattering on both men and women (**Figure 16–89**).

If you follow the same method but keep the corners by holding your fingers vertically and not following the head form, you can create a square shape, which is common in a man's basic haircut (**Figures 16–90** and **16–91**).

You can create a layered haircut with longer perimeter lengths, otherwise known as a *shag*, by cutting the top area the same as you do for uniform layers and then elevating the side and back sections straight up (180 degrees), blending them into the top lengths (**Figures 16–92** and **16–93**).

In the long-layered haircut, you will use increased layering, which features progressively longer layers. Your guide is an interior guide, beginning at the top of the head. All remaining hair will be elevated up (180 degrees) to match the guide. ☑ **LO6**

© Tyler Olson, 2010; used under license from Shutterstock.com.

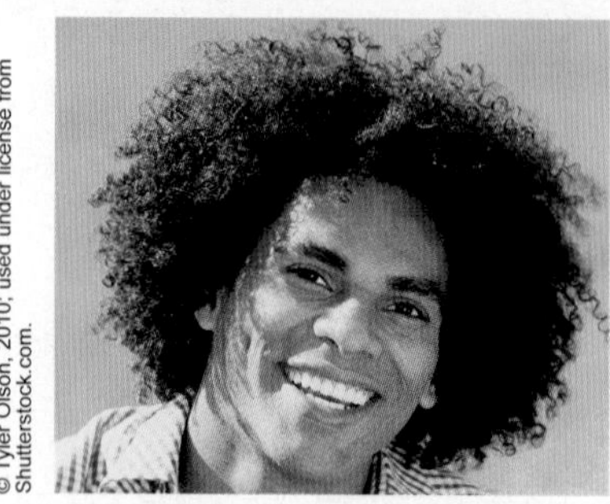

▲ **Figure 16–88**
A uniform-layered haircut.

Used with the permission of the authors, Martin Gannon and Richard Thompson, as featured in their book, Mahogany: Steps to Cutting, Colouring, and Finishing Hair. © Martin Gannon and Richard Thompson, 1997.

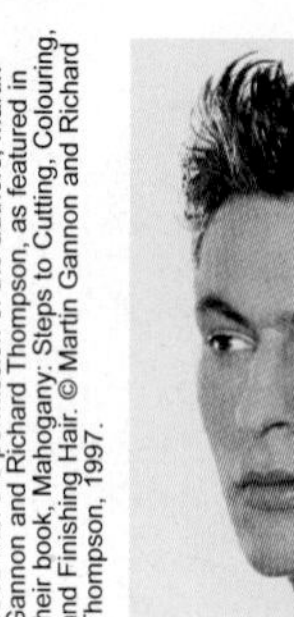

▲ **Figure 16–89**
Short crop, men's haircut.

© Milady, a part of Cengage Learning.

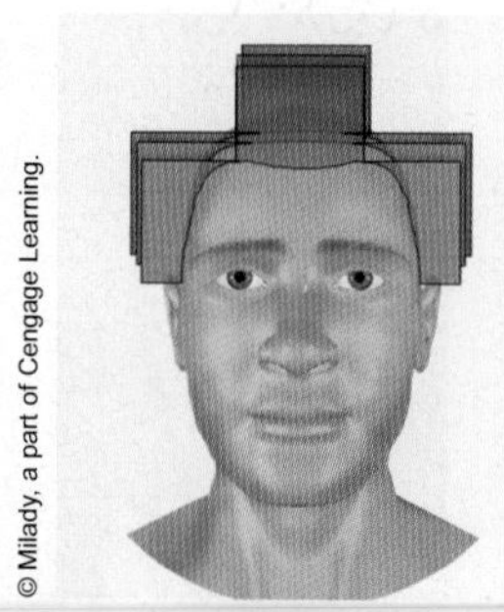

▲ **Figure 16–90**
Basic men's haircut design.

© Milady, a part of Cengage Learning. Photography by Paul Castle, Castle Photography.

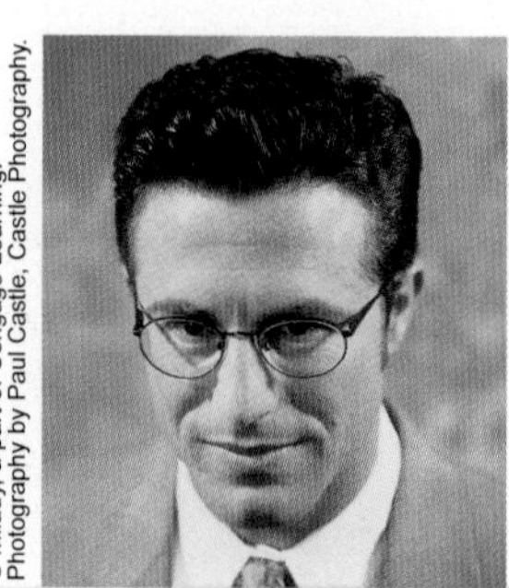

▲ **Figure 16–91**
Basic men's haircut.

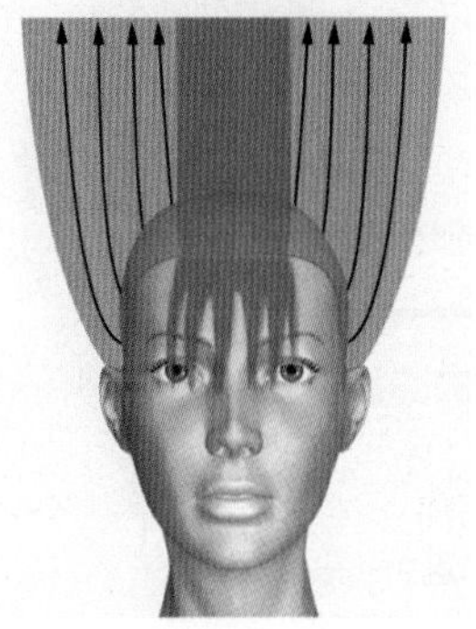

© Milady, a part of Cengage Learning.

▲ **Figure 16–92**
Long-layered design.

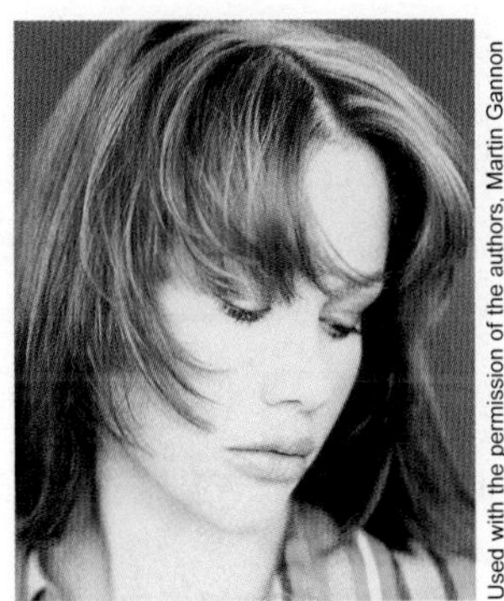

Used with the permission of the authors, Martin Gannon and Richard Thompson, as featured in their book, Mahogany: Steps to Cutting, Colouring, and Finishing Hair. © Martin Gannon and Richard Thompson, 1997.

▲ **Figure 16–93**
Long-layered haircut.

PROCEDURE 16-4 Long-Layered (180-Degree) Haircut SEE PAGE 408

Other Cutting Techniques

To go beyond the basic haircut, there are many techniques you can use to create different effects in hair. You can make wild hairlines calm down. You can make thick hair behave like thinner hair or fine hair appear to be fuller. You can create more movement, and add or reduce volume. You can also compensate for various growth patterns that exist on the same head of hair.

Cutting Curly Hair

Curly hair can be a challenge to cut. Once you gain confidence, curly hair can be a lot of fun to style. However, it is important to understand how curly hair behaves after it has been cut and dried. Although you can apply any cutting technique to curly hair, you will get very different results than you get when cutting straight hair. Curl patterns can range from slightly wavy to extremely curly, and curly-haired clients may have fine, medium, or coarse textures with a density ranging from thin to thick.

Examples of Basic Haircuts on Curly Hair

Let us take a look at some basic haircuts and how they work on curly hair. In **Figure 16–94**, note how the hair appears stacked, even though it was cut with a blunt technique. Although the hair was not elevated, it appears graduated. Note how the volume in the graduated haircut (**Figure 16–95**) is above the ears. The hair shrinks as it dries, resulting in a weight line that has graduated itself

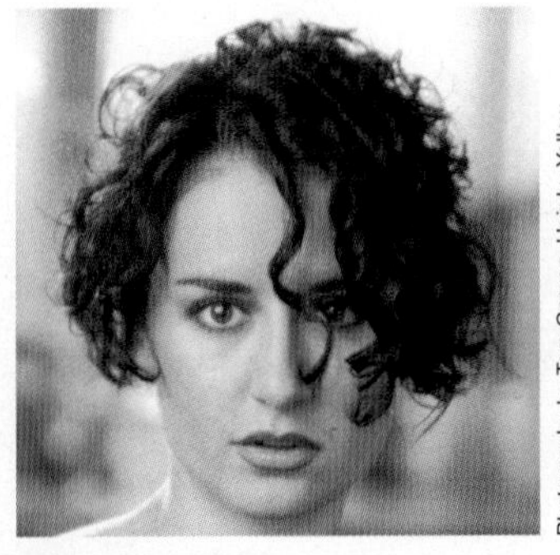

Photography by Tom Carson. Hair by Yellow Strawberry Global Salon, Sarasota, FL.

▲ **Figure 16–94**
Blunt haircut on curly hair.

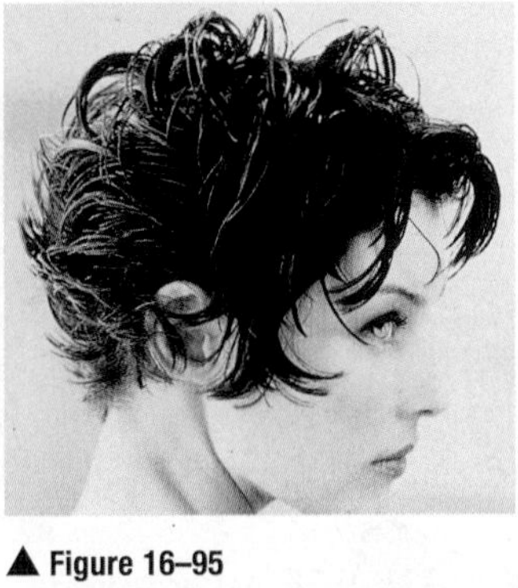

John Paul Mitchell Systems, hair by Jeanne Braa, photo by Alberto Tolot.

▲ **Figure 16–95**
Graduated haircut on curly hair.

FOCUS ON

TIPS FOR LAYERED HAIRCUTS

- Cut the interior first. Then go back to the perimeter edges and cut stronger lines, cut out around the ears, and texturize where needed.
- When layering short hair, you will achieve the best results on medium to thicker densities. Cutting thin hair too short can expose the scalp.
- Coarse hair tends to stick out if cut shorter than 3 inches. This hair texture needs the extra length to hold it down.
- When working on longer layered shapes in which you want to maintain thickness at the bottom, remember to keep the top sections longer. Cutting the top layers too short will take too much hair away from the rest of the haircut, and may leave you with a collapsed shape that is stringy at the bottom.
- If the client has hair past the shoulder blades, use slide cutting (explained later in this chapter) to connect the top sections to the lengths. This will maintain maximum length and weight at the perimeter of the haircut.

FOCUS ON

TIPS FOR CUTTING CURLY HAIR

- Curly hair can appear shorter after it dries because of a shrinking effect. The curlier the hair, the more it will shrink. For every ¼ inch (0.6 centimeters) you cut when the hair is wet, it will shrink up to 1 inch (2.5 centimeters) when dry. Always keep this in mind when consulting with your client.
- So as not to cut curly hair shorter than desired, use minimal tension and/or the wide teeth of your comb when cutting and be sure not to stretch the hair as you cut it.
- Maintain a consistent dampness of the hair while cutting.
- Curly hair naturally graduates itself. If the shape you want to create has strong angles, you need to elevate less than when working with straight hair.
- Curly hair when dry has more volume than straight hair. This means that you will generally need to leave lengths longer, which ultimately helps weigh the hair down and keeps the shape from ending up too short.
- In general, a razor should not be used on curly hair. Doing so weakens the cuticle and causes the hair to frizz.
- Choose your texturizing techniques carefully. Avoid using the razor, and work mostly with point cutting and free-hand notching to remove bulk and weight (these techniques are discussed later in this chapter).

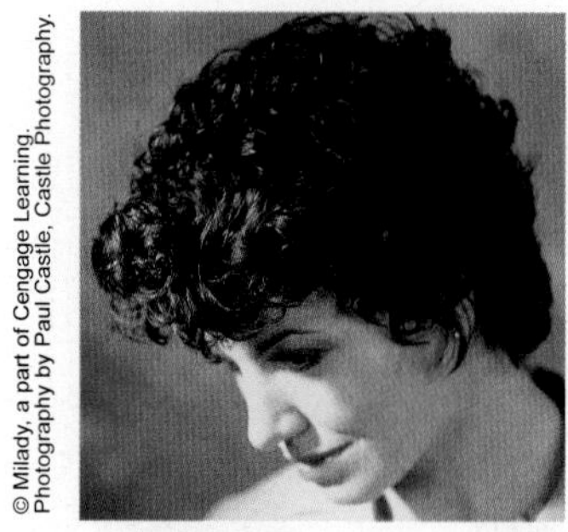
© Milady, a part of Cengage Learning. Photography by Paul Castle, Castle Photography.

▲ **Figure 16–96**
Uniform-layered haircut on curly hair.

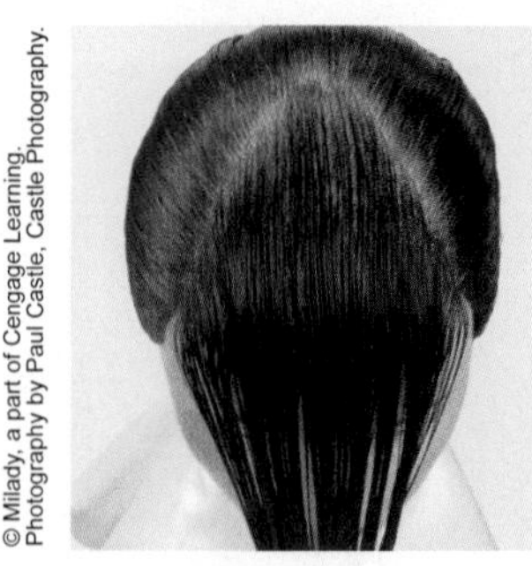
© Milady, a part of Cengage Learning. Photography by Paul Castle, Castle Photography.

▲ **Figure 16–97**
Bang area.

even higher. In the next example (**Figure 16–96**), note the round shape. This is a uniform-layered cut on curly hair.

Cutting the Bangs (Fringe)

Because much of our haircutting history comes from England, you will sometimes hear the word *fringe* used instead of *bangs*. The two words mean the same thing. The bang or fringe area includes the hair that lies between the two front corners, or approximately between the outer corners of the eyes (**Figure 16–97**).

It is important to work with the natural **distribution**, where and how hair is moved over the head, when locating the bang area. Every head is different, and you need to make sure that you cut only the hair that falls in that area. Otherwise, you can end up with short pieces falling where they don't belong, ruining the lines of the haircut. When creating bangs (fringe), you do not always cut all of the hair in this area, but you only cut more if you are blending into the sides or the top.

Let us have a look at a few types of bangs.

In **Figures 16–98** and **16–99**, the bang is cut using a stationary guide, elevating at 90-degrees straight up from the head form.

A short bang makes a strong statement. In **Figures 16–100** and **16–101**, short bangs are combined with a shorter layered

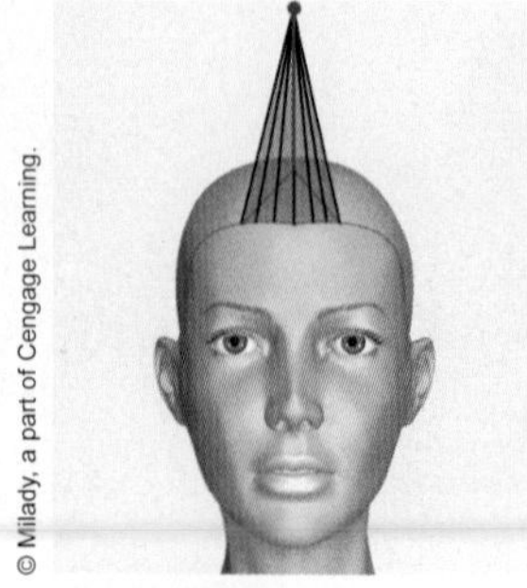
© Milady, a part of Cengage Learning.

▲ **Figure 16–98**
Layered bang design.

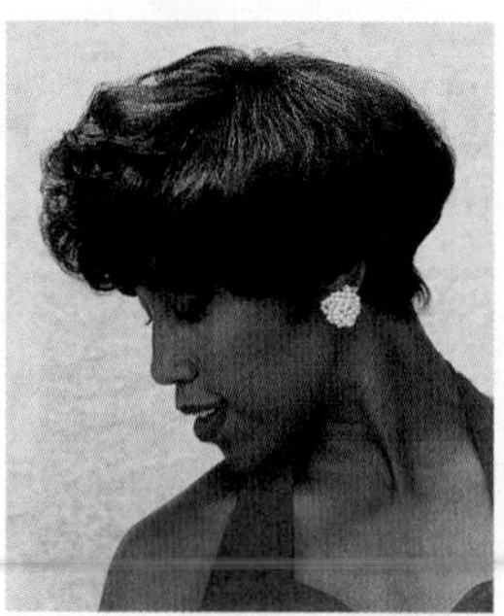
© Milady, a part of Cengage Learning. Photography by Paul Castle, Castle Photography.

▲ **Figure 16–99**
Layered bang cut.

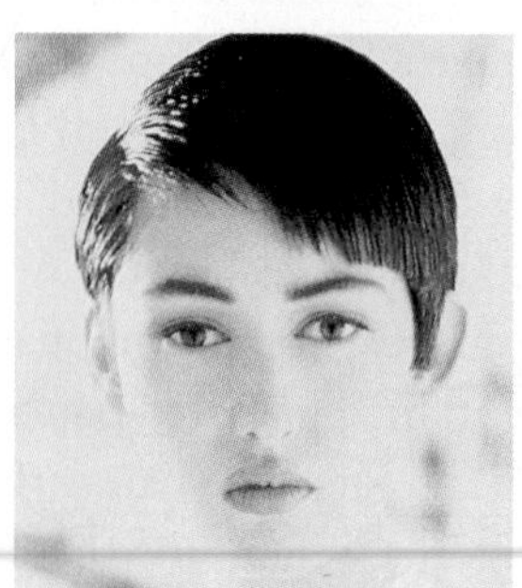
Used with the permission of the authors, Martin Gannon and Richard Thompson, as featured in their book, Mahogany: Steps to Cutting, Colouring, and Finishing Hair. © Martin Gannon and Richard Thompson, 1997.

▲ **Figure 16–100**
Short, curved bang design.

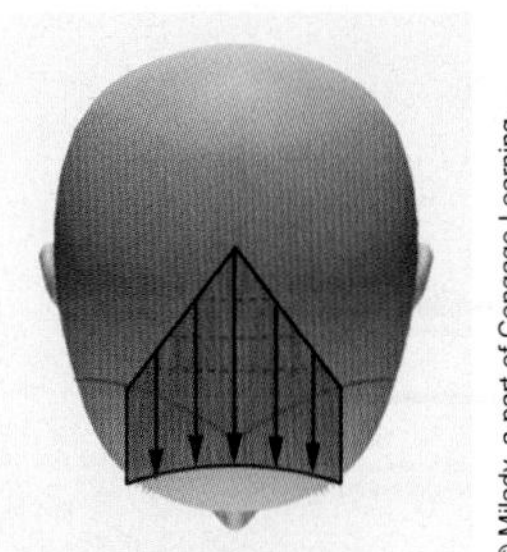
© Milady, a part of Cengage Learning.

▲ **Figure 16–101**
Short, curved bang cut.

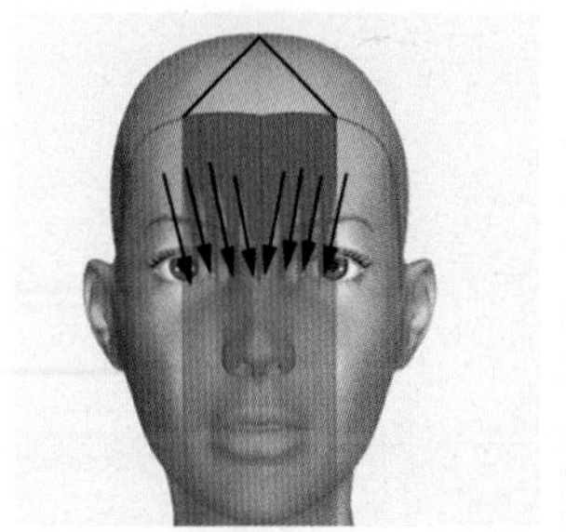
© Milady, a part of Cengage Learning.

▲ **Figure 16–102**
Long bang design.

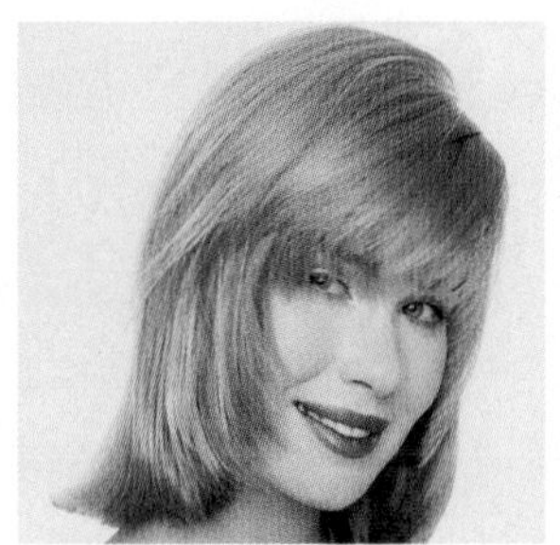
Used with the permission of the authors, Martin Gannon and Richard Thompson, as featured in their book, Mahogany: Steps to Cutting, Colouring, and Finishing Hair. © Martin Gannon and Richard Thompson, 1997.

▲ **Figure 16–103**
Long bang cut.

haircut. Note that the line is curved. It has been cut with low elevation, so that it remains more solid and not too heavy.

In **Figures 16–102** and **16–103**, the bang is very long and was cut with the slide cutting technique to create a wispy effect.

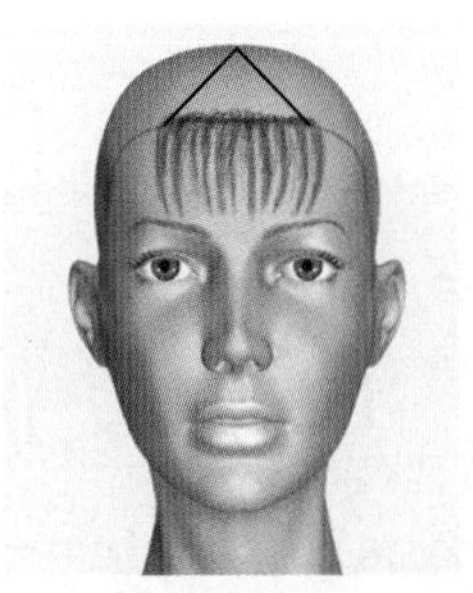
© Milady, a part of Cengage Learning.

▲ **Figure 16–104**
Wispy bang design.

Sometimes only a few pieces are cut in the bang area, which keeps the hair out of the face. In this case, you will not be cutting all the hair in the bang area. You will cut only a small portion of this area and might even use a razor for that purpose (**Figures 16–104** and **16–105**).

Depending on the haircut, a bang can be blended or not. If you are working with a blunt haircut and the bang is one length, you usually will not need to blend it in. If you are working with layered or graduated shapes, you may want to blend the length of the bang into the sides and/or the top (**Figures 16–106** and **16–107**).

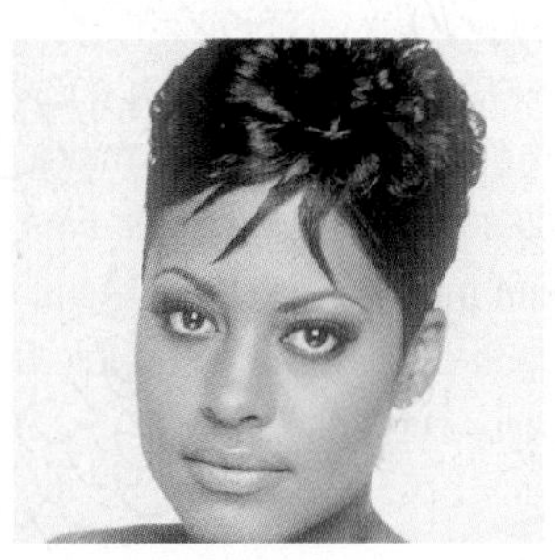
John Paul Mitchell Systems, The Relaxer Workshop, photo by Sean Cokes.

▲ **Figure 16–105**
Wispy bang cut.

Razor Cutting

A razor cut gives a totally different result than other haircutting techniques. For instance, a razor cut gives a softer appearance than a shear cut. The razor is a great option when working with medium to fine hair textures. When you work with shears, the ends of the hair are cut blunt. When working with a razor, the ends are cut at an angle, and the line is not blunt. This produces softer shapes with more visible separation, or a feathered effect, on the ends. With the razor, there is only one blade cutting the hair, and it is a much finer blade than the shears. With shears, there are two blades that close on the hair, creating blunt ends (**Figure 16–108**).

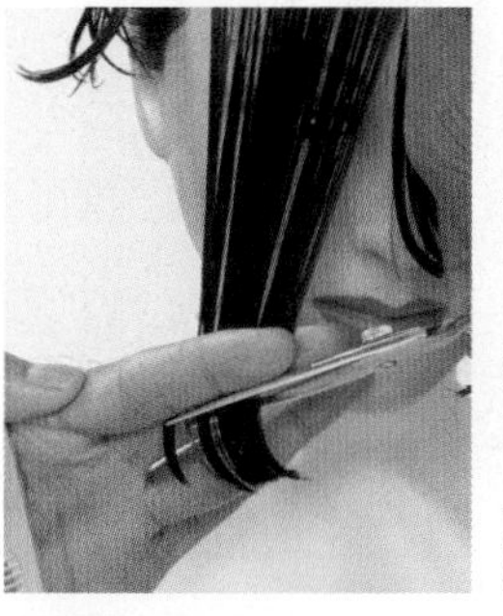
© Milady, a part of Cengage Learning, Photography by Paul Castle, Castle Photography.

▲ **Figure 16–106**
Blend bang to sides.

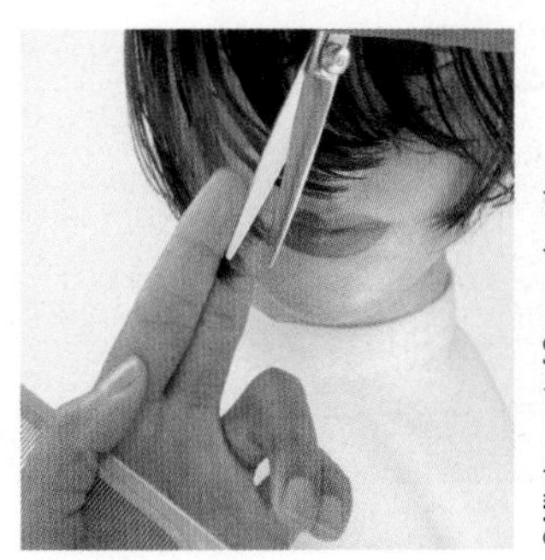
© Milady, a part of Cengage Learning, Photography by Paul Castle, Castle Photography.

▲ **Figure 16–107**
Blend bang to layered top.

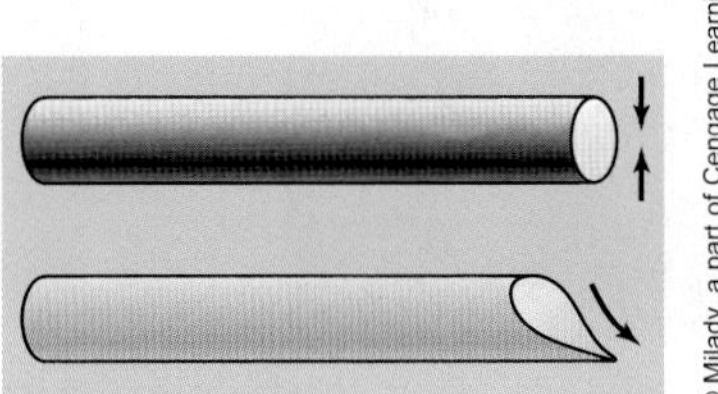
© Milady, a part of Cengage Learning.

▲ **Figure 16–108**
Shear-cut and razor-cut strands.

FOCUS ON

RAZOR CUTTING TIPS

- Always check with your instructor before performing a razor cut. Make sure that the hair is in good condition. For best results do not use a razor on curly hair, coarse wiry hair, or overprocessed, damaged hair.
- Always use a guard.
- Always use a new blade. Working with a dull blade pulls the client's hair and puts added stress on the hair. Discard used blades in a puncture-proof container.
- Keep the hair wet. Cutting dry hair with a razor can make the hair frizz and pull the client's hair.
- Always work with the razor at an angle. Never force the razor through the hair.

CAUTION

Always check with your instructor to see if the hair type you are working on is suitable for the razor. Coarse, wiry, curly, or damaged hair is not suitable for razor cuts. The razor may tend to make these hair types frizzier. Fine and medium hair textures in good condition are suitable for razor cuts.

Any haircut you can create with shears can also be done with the razor. You can cut horizontal, vertical, and diagonal lines. The main difference is that the guide is above your fingers, whereas with shears the guide is usually below your fingers. Razor cutting is an entirely different technique from cutting with shears. The best way to become comfortable with the razor is to practice. Before cutting with a razor, review how to properly hold the razor in the "Haircutting Tools" section of this chapter.

There are two commonly used methods for cutting with a razor. In the first method, the razor is kept parallel to the subsection (**Figure 16–109**). This technique is used to thin the ends of the hair, and the entire length of the blade is used. The other approach is to come into the subsection with the blade at an angle (about 45 degrees). Here you are using about one-third of the blade to make small strokes as you work through the subsection (**Figure 16–110**). If the blade is not entering the hair at an angle and you attempt to push the razor through the hair, you place added stress on the hair and risk losing control of the hair (**Figure 16–111**). Always remember that the blade needs to be at an angle when entering the hair.

When cutting a section, you move from top to bottom or side to side, depending on the section and finger angle. Examples of razor techniques

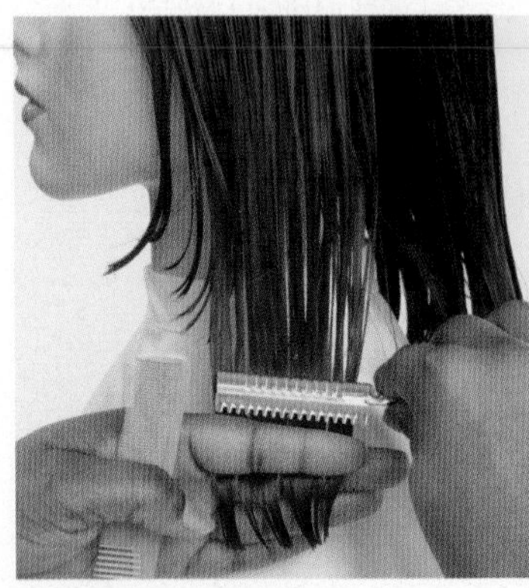

▲ **Figure 16–109**
Razor cutting parallel to subsection.

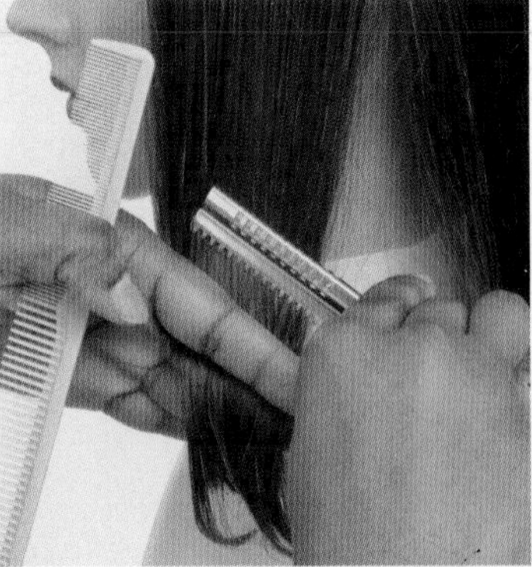

▲ **Figure 16–110**
Razor cutting at a 45-degree angle.

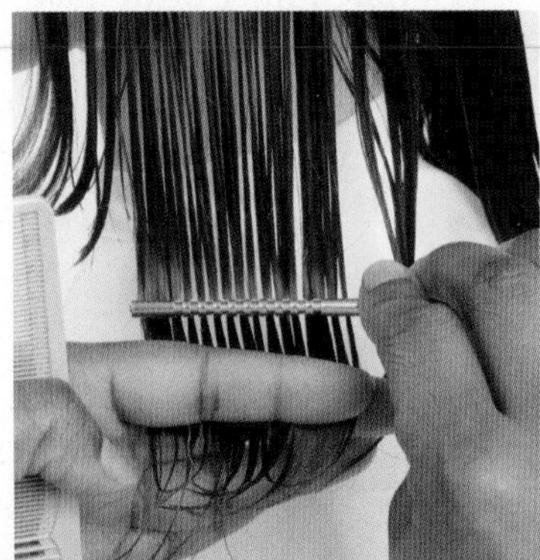

▲ **Figure 16–111**
Incorrect razor angle.

© Milady, a part of Cengage Learning. Photography by Paul Castle, Castle Photography.

and hand positions on a vertical and horizontal subsection, respectively, are found in **Figures 16–112** and **16–113**.

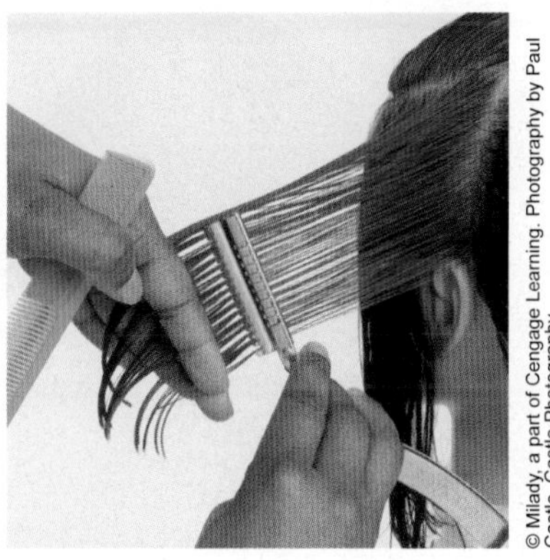
© Milady, a part of Cengage Learning. Photography by Paul Castle, Castle Photography.

▲ Figure 16–112
Hand position on vertical section.

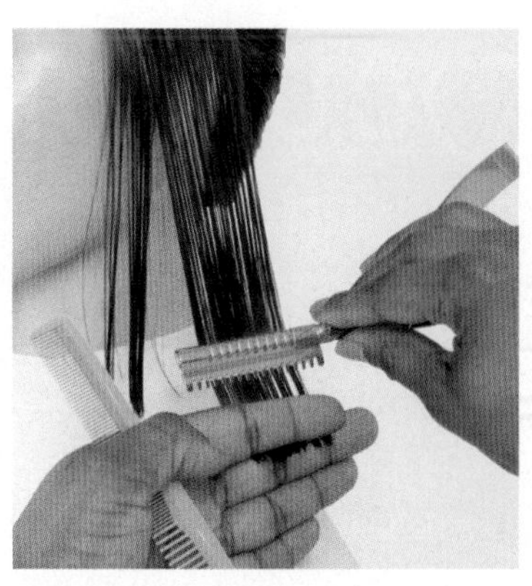
© Milady, a part of Cengage Learning. Photography by Paul Castle, Castle Photography.

▲ Figure 16–113
Hand position on horizontal section.

Slide Cutting

Slide cutting is a method of cutting or thinning the hair in which the fingers and shears glide along the edge of the hair to remove length. It is useful for removing length, blending shorter lengths to longer lengths, and texturizing. Slide cutting is a perfect way to layer very long hair and keep weight at the perimeter. Rather than opening and closing the shears, you keep them partially open as you slide along the edge of the section. This technique should only be performed on wet hair with very sharp shears.

There are two methods of holding the subsection when slide cutting. It is important to visualize the line you wish to cut before you begin (**Figure 16–114**). In one method, you hold the subsection with tension beyond the cutting line (**Figure 16–115**). In the other method, you place your shears on top of your knuckles, and then use both hands to move simultaneously out the length to the ends.

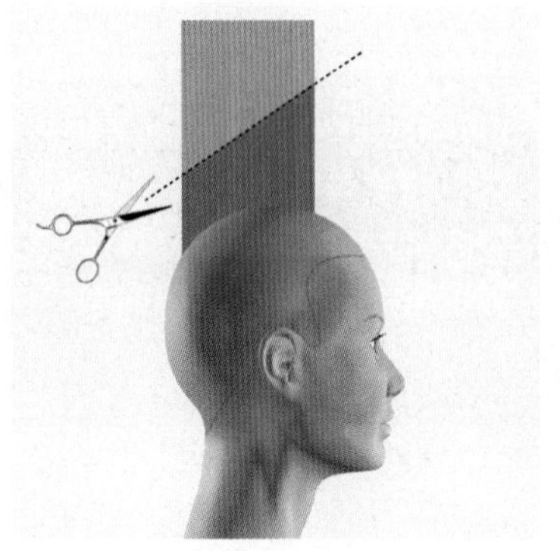
© Milady, a part of Cengage Learning.

▲ Figure 16–114
Visualize your cutting line first.

Scissor-Over-Comb

Scissor-over-comb, also known as **shear-over-comb**, is a barbering technique that has crossed over into cosmetology. In this technique, you hold the hair in place with the comb while using the tips of the shears to remove length. Scissor-over-comb is used to create very short tapers and allows you to cut from an extremely short length to longer lengths. In most cases, you start at the hairline and work your way up to the longer lengths.

It is best to use this technique on dry hair, because then you can see exactly how much hair you are cutting—and that helps you maintain control.

Lift (elevate) the hair away from the head using the comb, and allow the comb to act as your guide. Do not hold the hair between your fingers. Let the shear and comb move simultaneously up the head. It is important that one blade stays still and remains parallel to the spine of the comb as you move the thumb blade to close the shears. Try to cut with an even rhythm. Stopping the motion may cause steps or visible weight lines in the hair. Practice moving the comb and scissors simultaneously, keeping the bottom blade still and opening and closing the shears with your thumb (**Figure 16–116**).

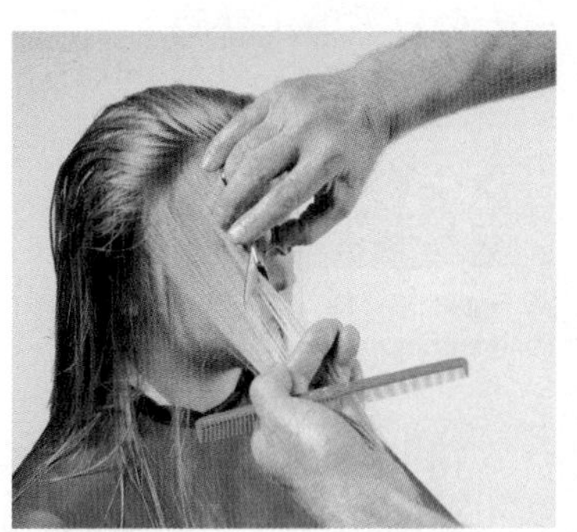
© Milady, a part of Cengage Learning. Photography by Paul Castle, Castle Photography.

▲ Figure 16–115
Slide cutting.

The basic steps when working with the scissor-over-comb technique are summarized below.

1. Stand or sit directly in front of the section you are working on. The area that you are cutting should be at eye level.

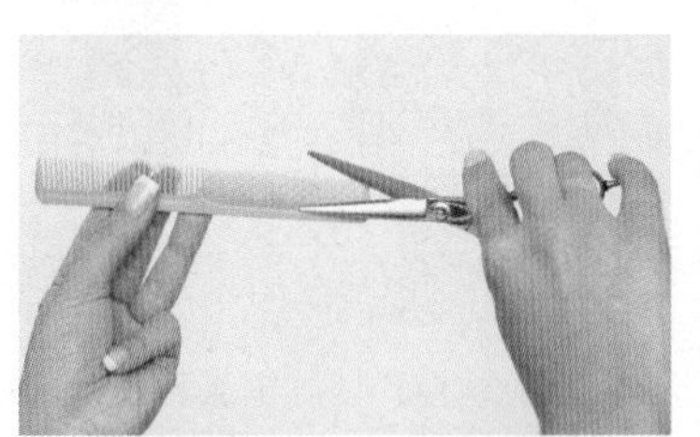
© Milady, a part of Cengage Learning. Photography by Paul Castle, Castle Photography.

▲ Figure 16–116
Scissor-over-comb technique.

FOCUS ON

SCISSOR-OVER-COMB TIPS

- Work with small areas at a time (no wider than the blade).
- Always start at the hairline and work up toward the length. You can run the comb through a previously cut section on your way up to a new area.
- Cross-check by working across the area diagonally.
- Use a barber comb to cut areas very close (usually on sideburns and hairlines where the hair is cut close to the scalp). Switch to a regular cutting comb as you work up into the longer lengths.

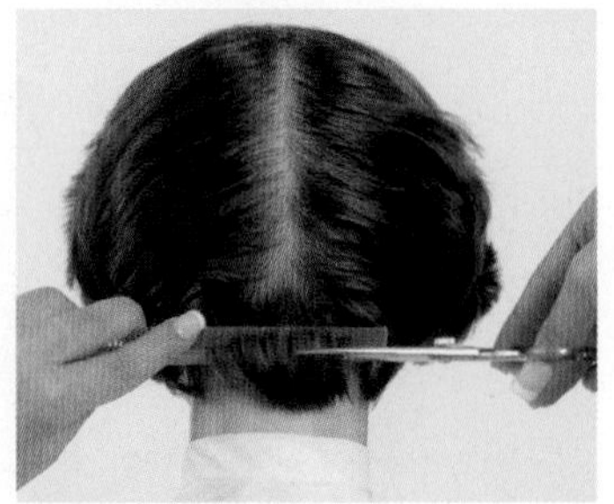
© Milady, a part of Cengage Learning. Photography by Paul Castle, Castle Photography.

▲ **Figure 16–117**
Comb position.

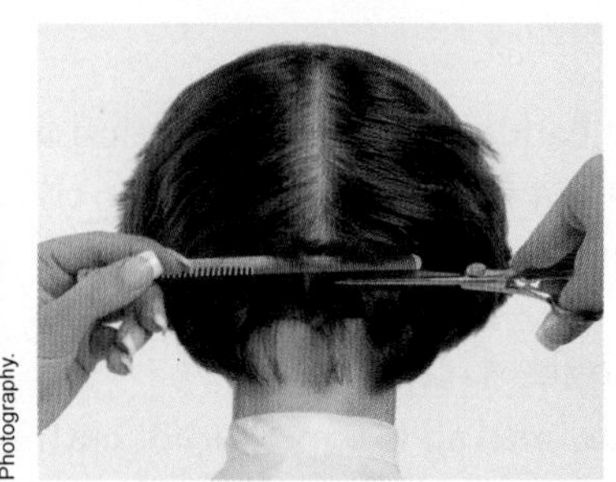
© Milady, a part of Cengage Learning. Photography by Paul Castle, Castle Photography.

▲ **Figure 16–118**
Reaching the weight line.

2. Place the comb, teeth first, into the hairline and turn the comb so that the teeth are angled away from the head (**Figure 16–117**).
3. With the still blade of the scissor parallel to the spine of the comb, begin moving the comb up the head, continually opening and closing the thumb blade smoothly and quickly.
4. Angle the comb farther away from the head as you reach the area you are blending to avoid cutting into the length (weight) (**Figure 16–118**).

Texturizing

Texturizing is a technique often used in today's haircuts. **Texturizing** is the process of removing excess bulk without shortening the length. It can also be used to cut for effect within the hair length, causing wispy or spiky results. The term *texturize* should not be confused with hair texture, which is the diameter of the hair strand itself.

Texturizing techniques can be used to add or remove volume, to make hair move, and to blend one area into another. It can also be used to compensate for different densities that exist on the same head of hair.

Texturizing can be done with cutting shears, thinning shears, or a razor.

There are many texturizing techniques, and a number of them will be explained in this section. You will need to practice all the techniques so that you can use them to create specific effects as needed.

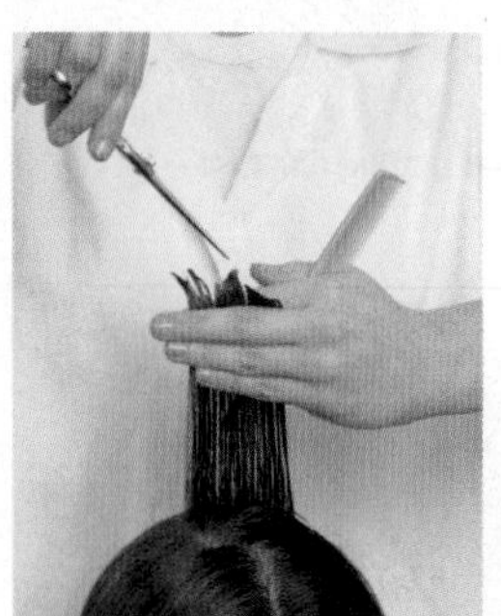
© Milady, a part of Cengage Learning. Photography by Paul Castle, Castle Photography.

▲ **Figure 16–119**
Point cutting.

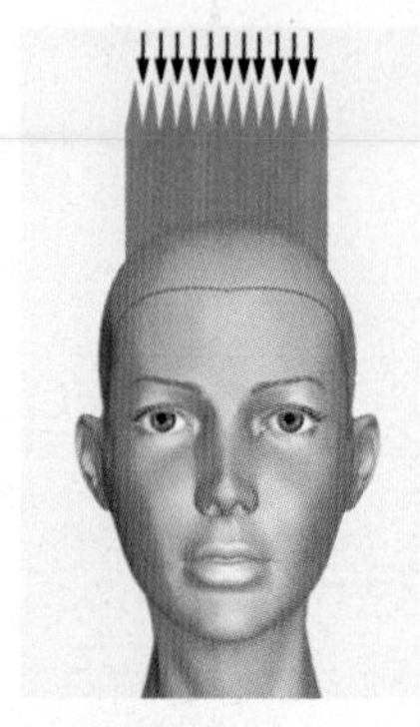
© Milady, a part of Cengage Learning.

▲ **Figure 16–120**
Point cutting with vertical angle of shears.

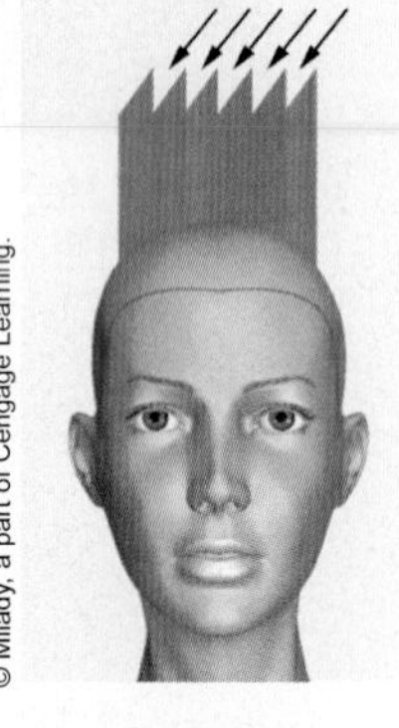
© Milady, a part of Cengage Learning.

▲ **Figure 16–121**
Point cutting with diagonal angle of shears.

Texturizing with Shears

Point cutting is a technique performed on the ends of the hair using the tips, or points, of the shears. This can be done on wet or dry hair. It is very easy to do on dry hair because the hair stands up and away from your fingers. Hold the hair 1 to 2 inches (2.5 to 5 centimeters) from the ends. Turn your wrist so that the tips of the scissors are pointing into the ends. Open and close the scissors by moving your thumb as you work across the section. As you close the scissors, move them away from your fingers to avoid cutting yourself. Move them back in toward your fingers as you open them (**Figure 16–119**). Basically, you are cutting points in the hair. A more vertical angle of the shears removes less hair (**Figure 16–120**). The more diagonal the angle of the shears, the more hair is taken away and the chunkier the effect (**Figure 16–121**).

Notching is another version of point cutting. Notching is more aggressive and creates a chunkier effect. Notching is done toward the ends. Hold the section about 3 inches (7.5 centimeters) from the ends. Place the tips of your shears about 2 inches (5 centimeters) from the ends. Close your shears as you quickly move them out toward the ends. If you are working on very thick hair, you can repeat the motion every ⅛ inch (0.3 centimeters). On medium to fine hair, place your notches farther apart. This technique can be done on wet or dry hair (**Figure 16–122**).

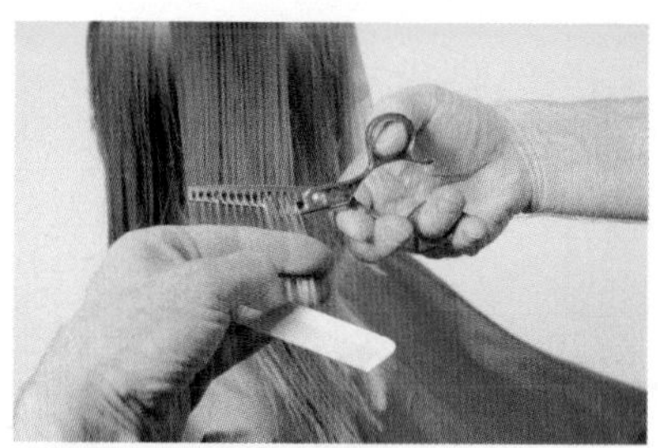

▲ Figure 16–122
Notching with notching shears.

Free-hand notching also uses the tips of the shears. Do not slide the shears, but simply snip out pieces of hair at random intervals. This technique is generally used on the interior of the section, rather than at the ends. It works well on curly hair, where you do not want to add too many layers, but instead want to release the curl and remove some density (**Figure 16–123**).

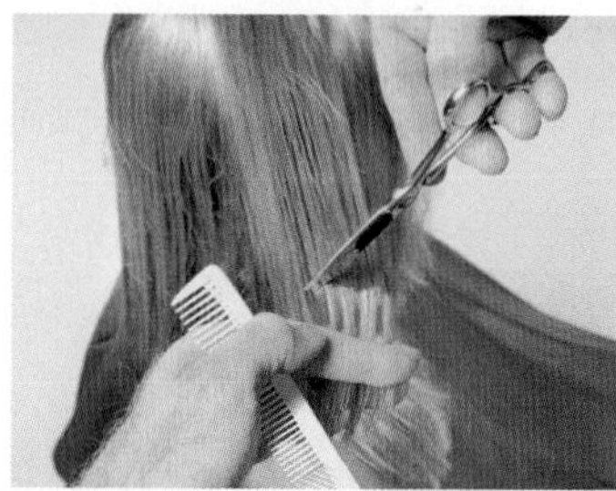

▲ Figure 16–123
Free-hand notching with cutting shears.

Slithering, also known as **effilating**, is the process of thinning the hair to graduated lengths with shears. In this technique, the hair strand is cut by a sliding movement of the shears, with the blades kept partially opened (**Figure 16–124**). Slithering reduces volume and creates movement.

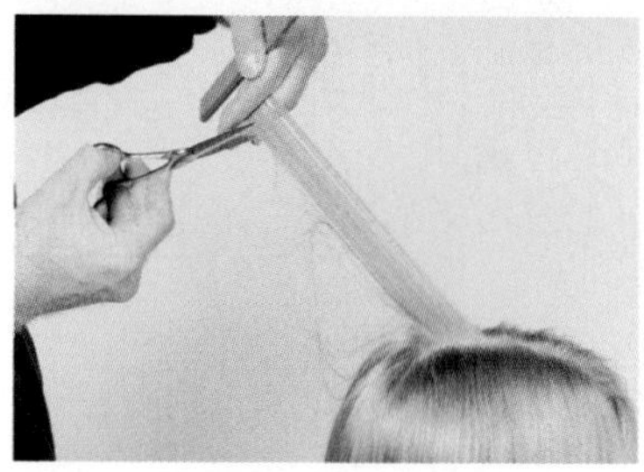

▲ Figure 16–124
Slithering.

Slicing is a technique that removes bulk and adds movement through the lengths of the hair. When slicing, twist the section of hair to be cut and never completely close the scissors. Use only the portion of the blades near the pivot. This prevents removing large pieces of hair (**Figures 16–125** and **16–126**). This technique can be performed within a subsection or on the surface of the hair with haircutting or texturizing shears (**Figures 16–127** and **16–128**). To slice an elevated subsection, work with either wet or dry hair. When slicing on the surface of the haircut, it is best to work on dry hair, because you can see exactly how much hair you are taking away.

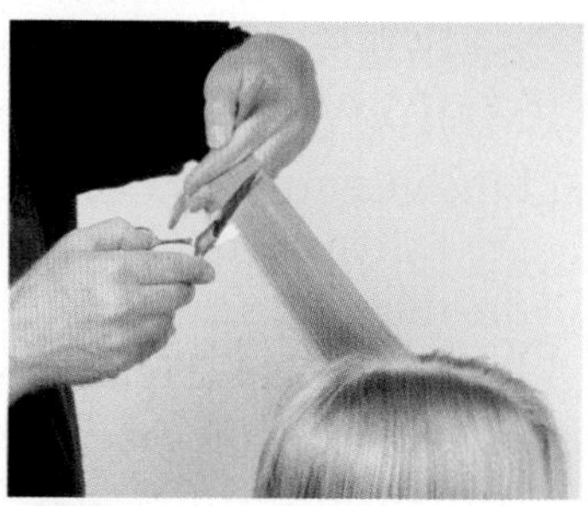

▲ Figure 16–125
Ideal open position.

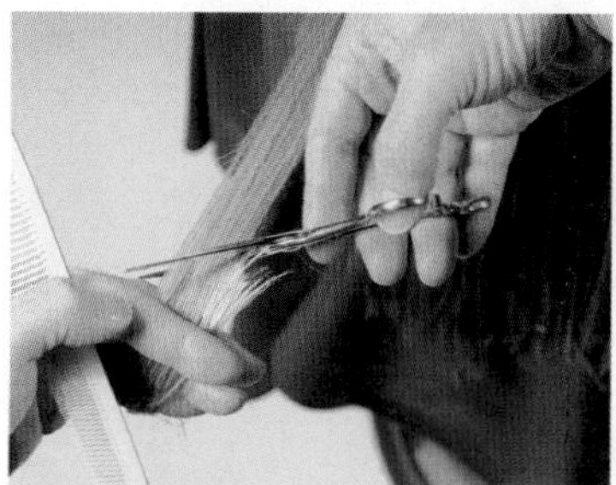

▲ Figure 16–126
Slicing with shears.

Carving is a version of slicing that creates a visual separation in the hair. It works best on short hair (1½ to 3 inches or 3.75 to 7.5 centimeters in length). This technique is done by placing the still blade into the hair and resting it on the scalp. Move the shears through the hair, gently opening and partially closing the scissors as you move, thus carving

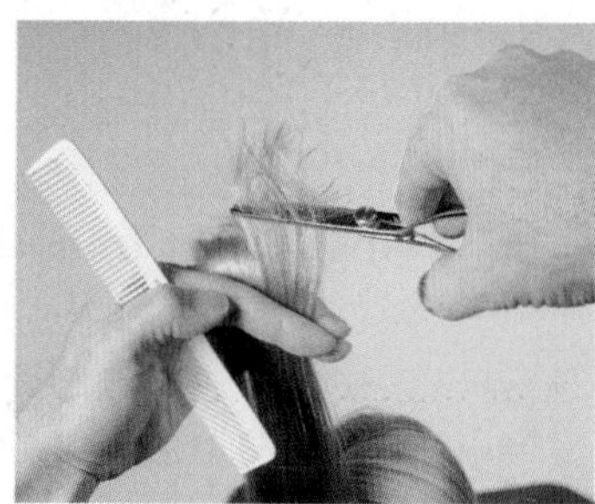

▲ Figure 16–127
Slicing through a subsection with texturizing shears.

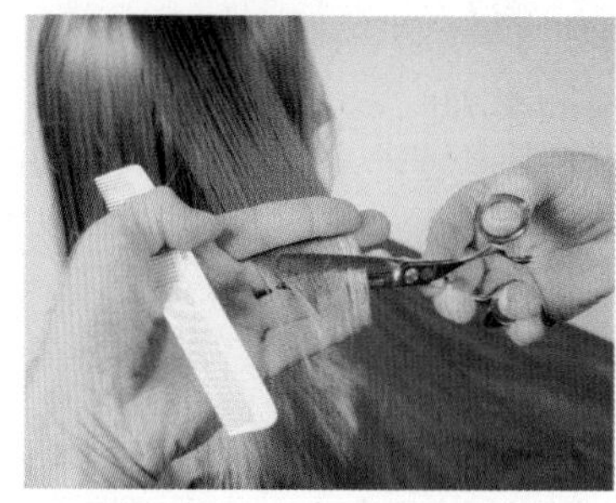

▲ Figure 16–128
Slicing through the surface with texturizing shears.

© Milady, a part of Cengage Learning. Photography by Yanik Chauvin.

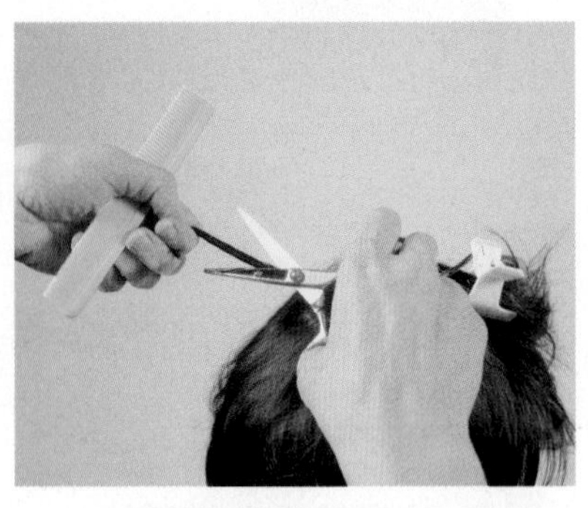

© Milady, a part of Cengage Learning. Photography by Yanik Chauvin.

▲ **Figure 16–129**
Slicing a twisted section of hair to remove bulk.

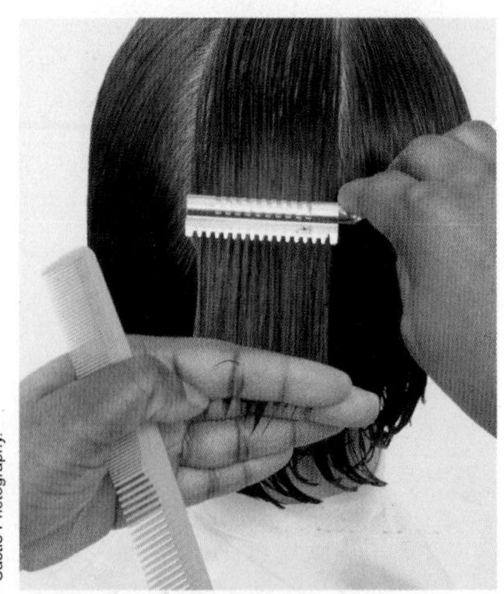

© Milady, a part of Cengage Learning. Photography by Paul Castle, Castle Photography.

▲ **Figure 16–130**
Thinning out a midsection.

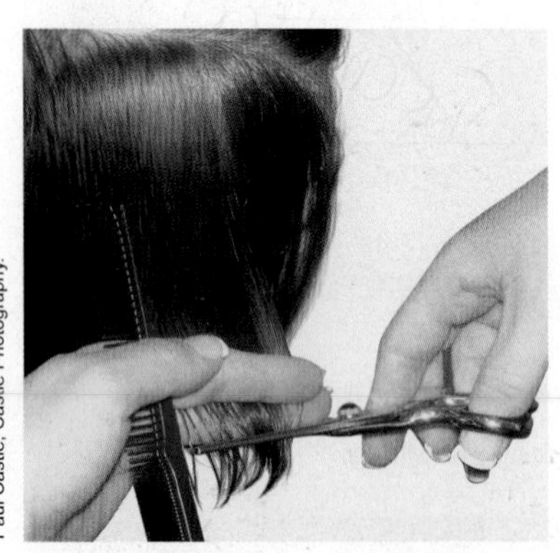

© Milady, a part of Cengage Learning. Photography by Paul Castle, Castle Photography.

▲ **Figure 16–131**
Thinning out the ends.

out areas (**Figure 16–129**). The more horizontal your scissors, the more hair you remove; the more vertical, the less hair you remove.

When carving the ends, you can add texture and separation to the perimeter of a haircut by holding the ends of a small strand of hair between your thumb and index fingers, and carving on the surface of that strand. Begin carving about 3 inches from the ends toward your fingers.

Texturizing with the Razor

- **Removing weight.** You can use the razor to thin out the ends of the hair. On damp hair, hold the section out from the head with your fingers at the ends. Place the razor flat to the hair, 2 to 3 inches (5 to 7.5 centimeters) away from your fingers. Gently stroke the razor, removing a thin sheet of hair from the area (**Figure 16–130**). This tapers the ends of the section. This technique can be used on any area of the haircut where this effect is desired.
- **Free-hand slicing**. This technique can be used throughout the section or at the ends, and should be done on wet hair. When working on the midshaft of the subsection, comb the hair out from the head, and hold it with your fingers close to the ends. With the tip of the razor, slice out pieces of hair. The more vertical the movement, the less hair you remove; the more horizontal the movement, the more hair you remove. This technique releases weight from the subsection, allowing it to move more freely.

Texturizing with Thinning Shears and Razor

- **Removing bulk (thinning).** Thinning shears were originally created for the purpose of thinning hair and blending. Many clients are afraid of the word *thinning*. A better choice of words would be *removing bulk* or *removing weight*. When using the thinning shears for this purpose, it is best to follow the same sectioning as used in the haircut. Comb the subsection out from the head and cut it with the thinning scissors, at least 4 to 5 inches (10 to 12.5 centimeters) from the scalp (**Figure 16–131**). On longer lengths, you may need to repeat the process again as you move out toward the ends. On coarse hair textures, stay farther away from the scalp, as sometimes the shorter hairs will poke through the haircut. On blunt haircuts, avoid thinning the top surfaces, because you may see lines where the hair is cut with the thinning shears. When working on curly hair, it is best to use the free-hand notching technique rather than thinning shears.
- **Removing weight from the ends.** You can also use thinning shears to remove bulk from the ends. This process works well on many hair textures. It can be used on both thin and thick hair, and it helps taper the perimeter of both graduated and blunt haircuts. Elevating each subsection out from the head, place the thinning shears into the hair at an angle and close the shears a few times as you work out toward the ends (**Figure 16–132**).

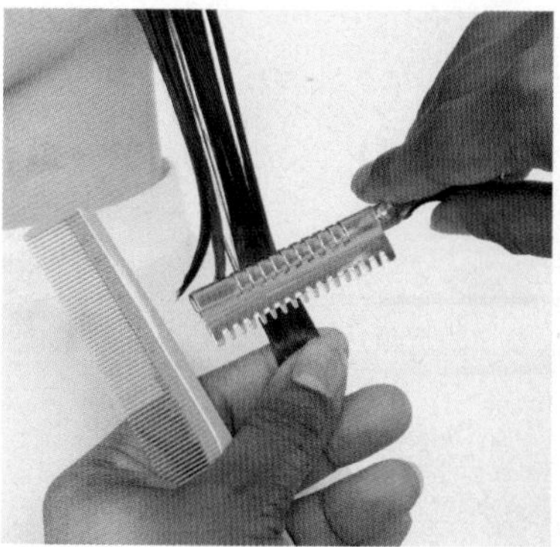

▲ Figure 16–132
Tapering the ends with the razor.

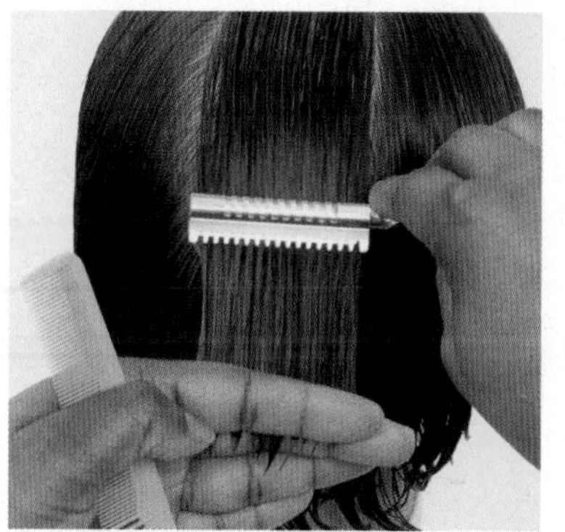

▲ Figure 16–133
Slicing the midshaft.

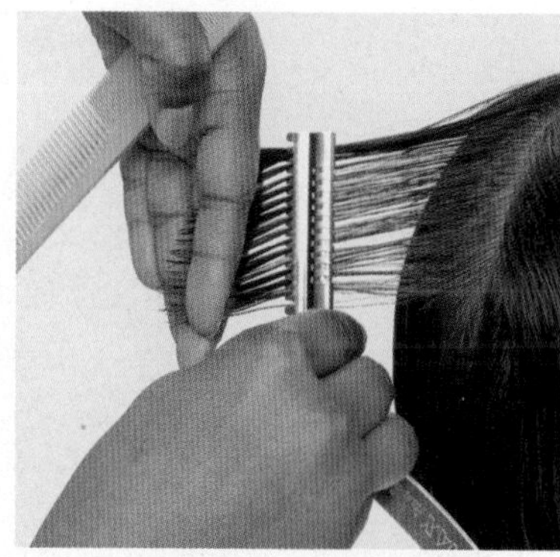

▲ Figure 16–134
Slicing the perimeter.

- **Scissor-over-comb with thinning shears.** Practicing the scissor-over-comb technique with the thinning shears is a good way to master this technique. This technique is useful for blending weight lines on fine textured hair, and can also be used on thick and coarse textured hair that is cut very short, especially at the sides and the nape. This technique will help the hair lie closer to the head.
- **Other thinning shear techniques.** Any texturizing technique that can be performed with regular haircutting shears may also be performed with the thinning shears. When working on very fine or thin hair, try using the thinning shears for carving, point cutting, and slicing. This will help avoid over texturizing and removing too much weight.
- **Free-hand slicing with razor.** You can also use free-hand slicing on the ends of the hair to produce a softer perimeter or to create separation throughout the shape (**Figure 16–133**). In this case, hold the ends of a small piece of hair in your fingertips. Beginning about 3 inches from your fingers, slice down one side of the piece toward your fingers (**Figure 16–134**).
- **Razor-over-comb**. In this technique, the comb and the razor are used on the surface of the hair. Using the razor on the surface softens weight lines and causes the area to lie closer to the head. This technique is used mainly on shorter haircuts. To perform this technique, place the comb into the hair, with the teeth pointing down, a few inches above the area on which you will be working. Make small, gentle strokes on the surface of the hair with the razor. Move the comb down as you move the razor down (**Figure 16–135**). This is a great technique for tapering in the nape area or softening weight lines.
- **Razor rotation** is very similar to razor-over-comb. The difference is that with razor rotation you make small circular motions. Begin by combing the hair in the direction you will be moving in. Place the razor on the surface of the hair. Then allow the comb to follow the razor through the area just cut. Then comb back into the section or

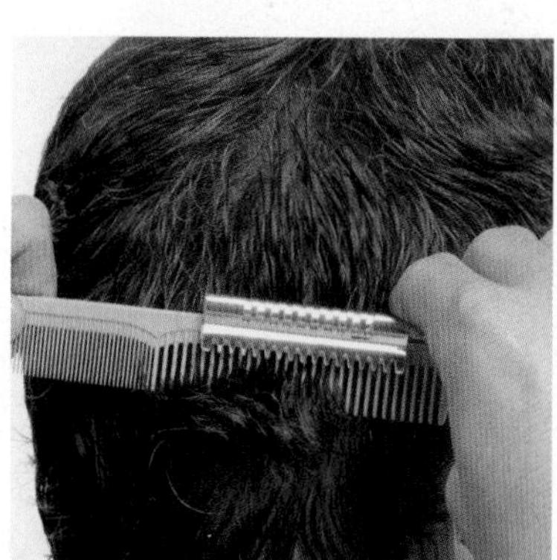

▲ Figure 16–135
Razor-over-comb technique.

© Milady, a part of Cengage Learning. Photography by Paul Castle, Castle Photography.

CAUTION

When thinning or texturizing hair, remember that you can always go back and remove more hair if necessary. Once the hair has been cut, it is impossible to replace, and you may have difficulty achieving the desired hairstyle.

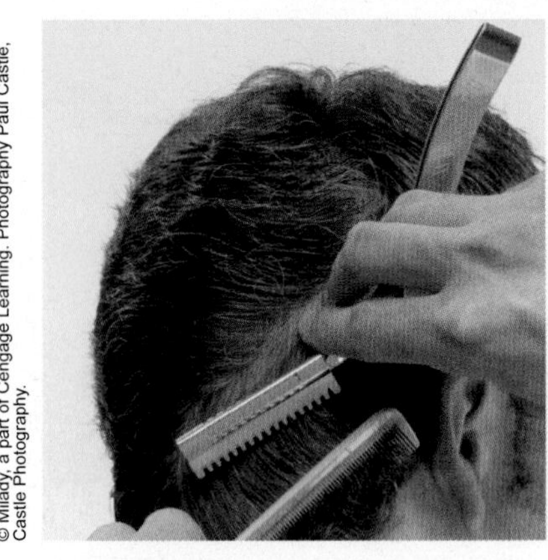

© Milady, a part of Cengage Learning. Photography Paul Castle, Castle Photography.

▲ **Figure 16–136**
Razor rotation.

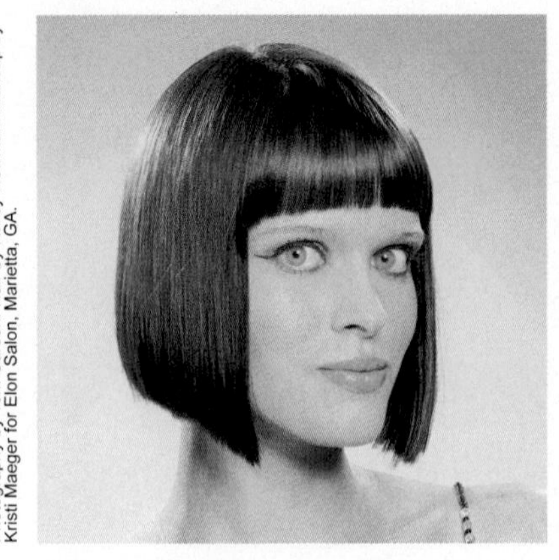

Photography by Tom Carson. Hair by Kelley Newman. Makeup by Kristi Maeger for Elon Salon, Marietta, GA.

▲ **Figure 16–137**
Blunt haircut before texturizing.

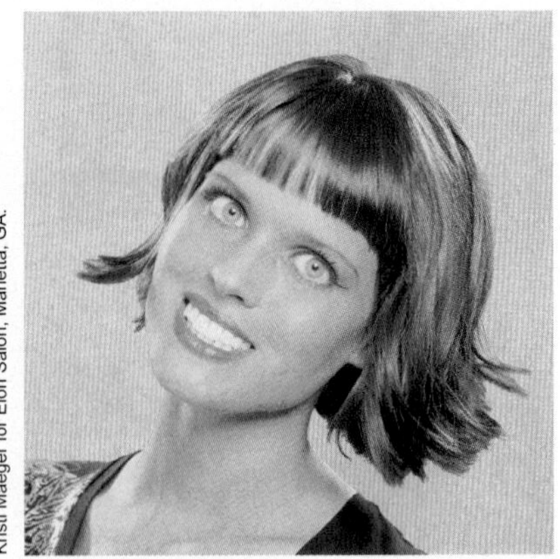

Photography by Tom Carson. Hair by Kelley Newman. Makeup by Kristi Maeger for Elon Salon, Marietta, GA.

▲ **Figure 16–138**
Texturized blunt haircut.

onto a new section. This helps soften the texture of the area and gives direction to the haircut (**Figure 16–136**).

Basic Haircuts Enhanced with Texturizing Techniques

Examine these three basic haircuts and see how texturizing techniques have changed the appearance of each haircut.

- **Figure 16–137** shows a blunt haircut before free-hand razor slicing, and **Figure 16–138** shows the same haircut after free-hand razor slicing has been used.
- **Figure 16–139** shows a graduated haircut before free-hand scissors slicing, and **Figure 16–140** shows the same haircut after free-hand scissors slicing.
- **Figure 16–141** shows a uniform-layered haircut before texturizing, and **Figure 16–142** shows the same haircut after notching on the ends and free-hand notching on the interior. ☑ **LO7**

Clippers and Trimmers

Other types of tools that all stylists should be familiar with are clippers and trimmers, which offer solutions for many haircutting challenges.

Clippers are electric or battery-operated tools that cut the hair by using two moving blades held in place by a metal plate with teeth. The blade action is faster than the eye can see. Clippers are mainly used for cutting shorter haircuts, and can be used to create a **taper**, hair that is cut very short and close to the hairline and that gradually gets longer as you move up the head. While men have been getting clipper cuts for many years, today clippers are being used more and more in women's haircutting. Clippers can be used as follows:

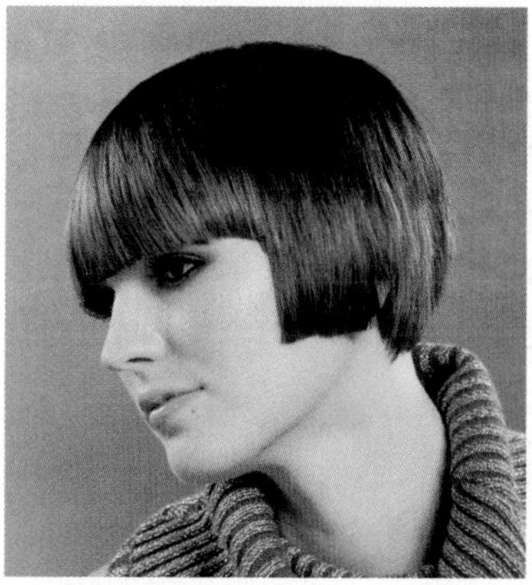

Photography by Tom Carson. Hair by Michelle Azouz for Tangles Salon, Wichita Falls, TX.

▲ **Figure 16–139**
Graduated haircut before texturizing.

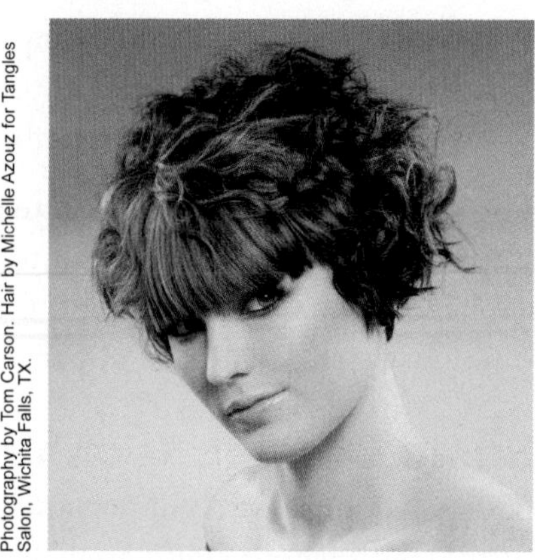

Photography by Tom Carson. Hair by Michelle Azouz for Tangles Salon, Wichita Falls, TX.

▲ **Figure 16–140**
Texturized graduated haircut.

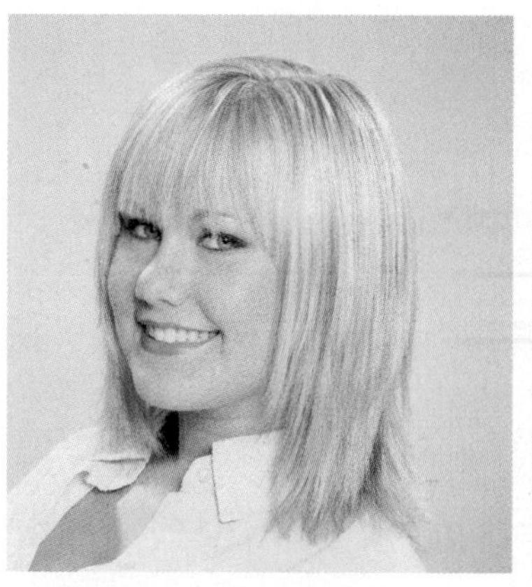

Photography by Tom Carson. Hair by Vickie Poole. Makeup by Nico for Elon Salon, Marietta, GA.

▲ **Figure 16–141**
Uniform-layered haircut before texturizing.

- Without length guards, to remove hair completely (great for cleaning up necklines and around the ears).
- Without length guards, to taper hairlines from extremely short lengths into longer lengths, using the **clipper-over-comb** technique (this technique is very similar to scissor-over-comb, except that the clippers move side to side across the comb rather than bottom to top).
- With length guards, attachments that fit over the blade plate and vary in size from 1/8 inch to 1 inch for short, layered cuts.

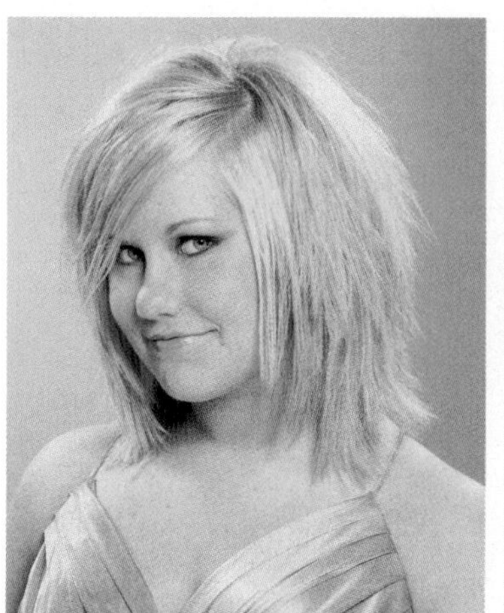

Photography by Tom Carson. Hair by Vickie Poole. Makeup by Nico for Elon Salon, Marietta, GA.

▲ **Figure 16–142**
Texturized uniform-layered haircut.

Tools for Clipper Cutting

There are several tools to have on hand. When clipper cutting, you will not need to use each tool for every haircut, but it is still important to understand when these tools are needed.

- **Clippers.** Clippers come in different shapes and sizes. They can be used with or without attachments. Trimmers, also called *edgers*, are usually cordless, smaller-sized clippers. They are mainly used to clean the necklines and around the ears (**Figure 16–143**). Clean your clippers and trimmers with a clipper brush after each use. Apply one drop of clipper oil to the top of the blades while the clipper is running. Disinfect the detachable blade and heel after each use as well. Always follow the manufacturer's instructions for care and cleaning.
- **Length guard attachments.** When attached to the clippers, length guards allow you to cut all the hair evenly to that exact length. They range from 1/8- to 1-inch (.3 to 2.5 centimeters) wide, and can be used in different combinations to create different lengths.
- **Haircutting shears.** Used mainly for removing length and detailing the haircut.
- **Thinning shears.** Also called *blending* or *tapering scissors*, these are great for removing excess bulk and for blending one area with another.

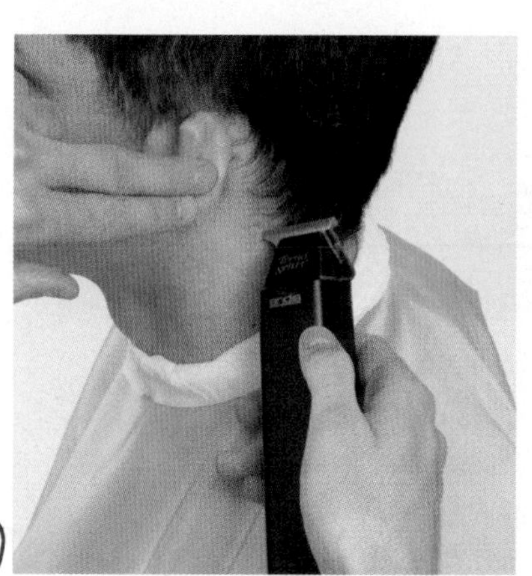

© Milady, a part of Cengage Learning. Photography by Paul Castle, Castle Photography.

▲ **Figure 16–143**
Trimmer cutting around the ear.

FOCUS ON

TIPS FOR CLIPPER CUTTING

- Always work against the natural growth patterns, especially in the nape. This ensures that you are lifting the hair away from the head and cutting the hair evenly.
- Always work with small sections. When using the clipper-over-comb technique, do not try to cut all the way across the entire length of the comb. The area you are cutting should be no wider than 3 inches.
- When using the clipper-over-comb technique, the angle of the comb determines the length. If the comb is consistently held parallel to the head, you will cut the hair the same length as you move up the head. If the comb is angled away from the head as you move, you begin to increase length. ✓ LO8

CAUTION

When trimming facial hair, have clients keep their eyes closed and remain still and silent until you are finished.

- **Combs.** With a regular cutting comb, the wider-spaced teeth are intended for combing and cutting. The finer-spaced teeth are used for detailing, scissor-over-comb, and clipper-over-comb techniques.

The classic barbering comb is often used in the nape, at the sides, and around the ears, and allows you to cut the hair very short and close to the head. The wide-tooth comb is used when cutting thicker and longer lengths, where detailing is not required.

Basic Clipper Techniques

Basic techniques with clippers include clipper-over-comb and clipper cutting with length guard attachments.

Clipper-Over-Comb

The clipper-over-comb technique allows you to cut the hair very close to the scalp and create a flat top or square shape. The way you use the comb is the same as when you are working with scissor-over-comb. The main difference is that the clippers move across the comb, which requires that you keep the comb in position as you cut. The angle at which you hold the comb determines the amount of hair that is removed.

Clippers are more accurate when used on dry to slightly damp hair. Use the lever switch on the clipper or a numbered attachment to vary the distance that the clipper is held from the head.

Tips for working with the clipper-over-comb technique follow. This technique will be illustrated in the procedure for the men's basic clipper cut later in this chapter.

1. Stand directly in front of the section on which you are working. The area you are cutting should be at eye level.
2. Place the comb, teeth first, into the hairline, and turn the comb so that the teeth are angled slightly away from the head. Always work against the growth patterns of the hair to ensure that you are lifting the hair away from the head and cutting evenly.
3. Hold the comb stationary and cut the length against the comb, moving the clippers from right to left. (If you are left-handed, you will move the clippers left to right.)
4. Although your movements should be fluid, remember to stop momentarily to cut the section. Remove the comb from the hair and begin the motion again, using the previously cut section underneath as your guideline. Continue working up the head toward the weight or length.

Clipper Cutting with Attachments

Using the length guard attachments is a quick and easy way to create short haircuts. With practice, clipper cutting with attachments allows you to create many different shapes. For example, you can use the ¼-inch guard on the nape and sides. Then you can switch to the

½-inch guard as you reach the parietal area, which will maintain more length at the parietal area. This technique produces a square shape.

Men's Basic Clipper Cut

In this cut, the hair is cropped close along the bottom and sides and becomes longer as you travel up the head. The distance between the comb and the scalp determines the amount of hair to be cut. The clipper can be positioned horizontally, vertically, or diagonally.

PROCEDURE 16-5 Men's Basic Clipper Cut SEE PAGE 413

Using Trimmers

- **Using trimmers around the ears.** When cutting a clean line around the ears, use both hands to hold the edger sideways. Using just the outer edge on the skin, arc the edger up and around the ear (**Figure 16–144**). As you reach the area behind the ear, use the comb to hold the hair in place, and continue with the arcing motion (**Figure 16–145**).
- **Using trimmers at the neckline.** Clean up the hair on the neck that grows below the design line (**Figure 16–146**). Trimmers also help create more defined lines at the perimeter (**Figure 16–147**).

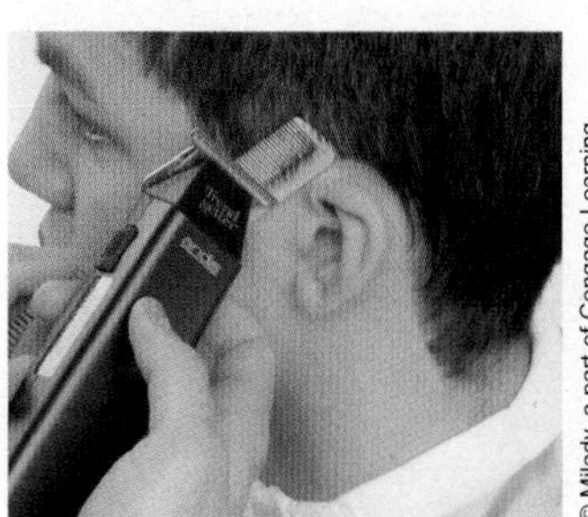
© Milady, a part of Cengage Learning. Photography by Paul Castle, Castle Photography.

▲ **Figure 16–144**
Arcing trimmer at front of the ear.

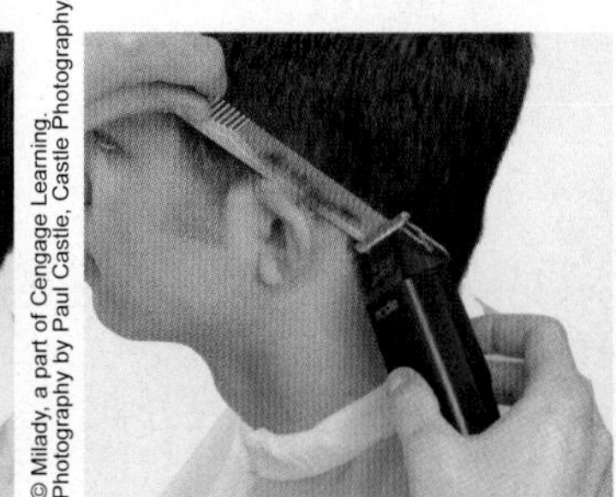
© Milady, a part of Cengage Learning. Photography by Paul Castle, Castle Photography.

▲ **Figure 16–145**
Arcing trimmer at back of the ear with comb.

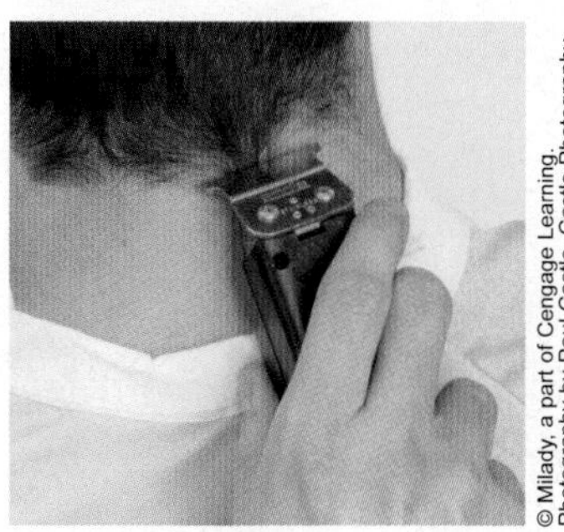
© Milady, a part of Cengage Learning. Photography by Paul Castle, Castle Photography.

▲ **Figure 16–146**
Cleaning up neck hair.

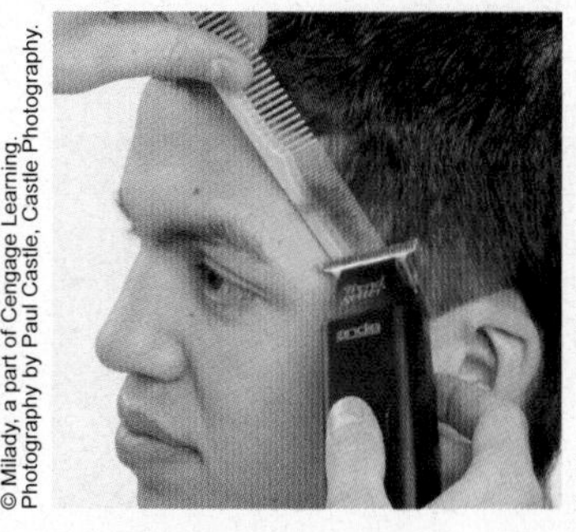
© Milady, a part of Cengage Learning. Photography by Paul Castle, Castle Photography.

▲ **Figure 16–147**
Edging line at side perimeter.

Trimming Facial Hair

Clippers and trimmers can be used to trim beards and mustaches as well. The technique is very similar to scissor-over-comb and clipper-over-comb. When removing length, use the comb to control the hair, and always cut against the comb (**Figure 16–148**). You can also use the length guard attachments to trim a beard to the desired length (**Figure 16–149**). If you choose to use haircutting shears to trim facial hair, you may want to keep a less expensive pair for this purpose, because facial hair is very coarse and may dull your haircutting shears.

Some male clients have long eyebrows or excess hair in or on their ears. When performing a haircut or trimming facial hair, always check the ears and eyebrows, then ask the client if he would like you to remove any excess hair you may find. Carefully snip away the hair with your shears or trimmers, using complete focus. ☑ **LO9**

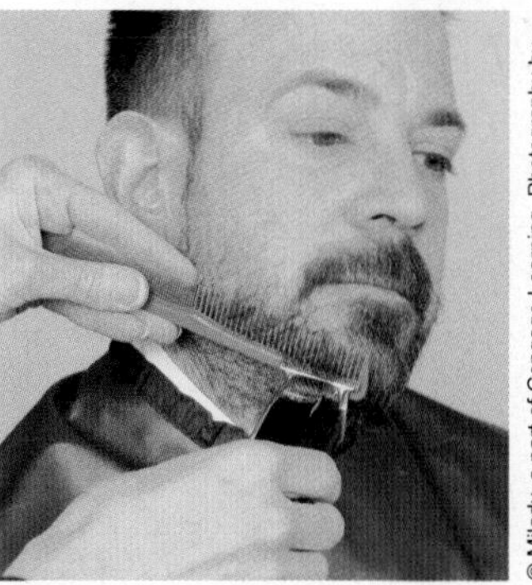
© Milady, a part of Cengage Learning. Photography by Yanik Chauvin.

▲ **Figure 16–148**
Trimming beard with clipper-over-comb.

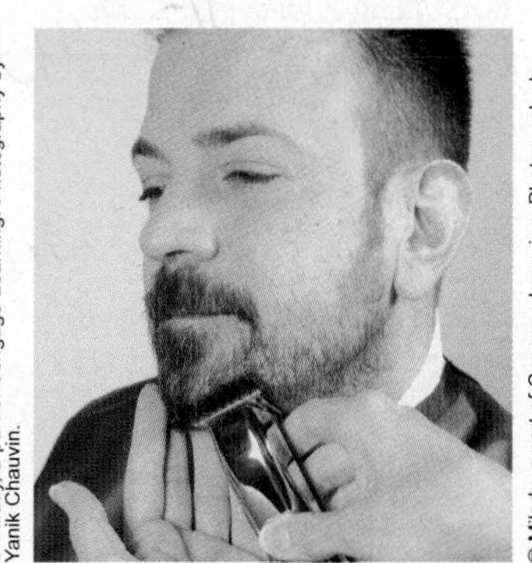
© Milady, a part of Cengage Learning. Photography by Yanik Chauvin.

▲ **Figure 16–149**
Trimming beard with clipper and guard.

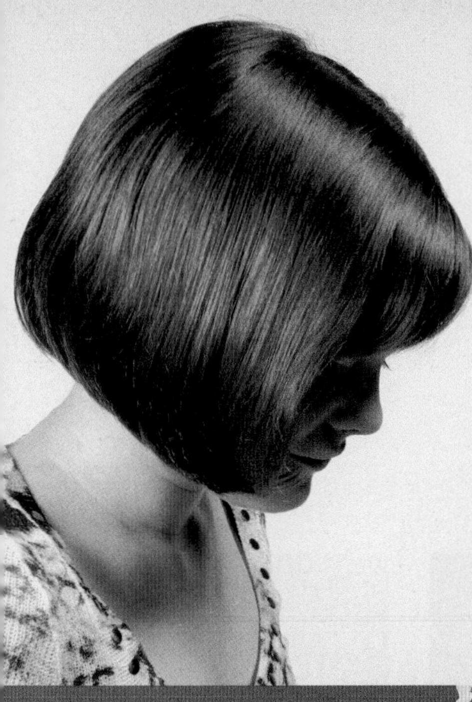

PROCEDURE 16-1 Right Handed

Blunt Haircut with Fringe

Implements and Materials

You will need all of the following implements, materials, and supplies:

- **Cutting cape**
- **Cutting or styling comb**
- **Haircutting shears**
- **Neck strip**
- **Sectioning clips**
- **Shampoo and conditioner**
- **Shampoo cape**
- **Spray bottle with water**
- **Towels**
- **Wide-tooth comb**

Preparation

- Perform PROCEDURE 15-1 **Pre-Service Procedure** **SEE PAGE 323**

Procedure

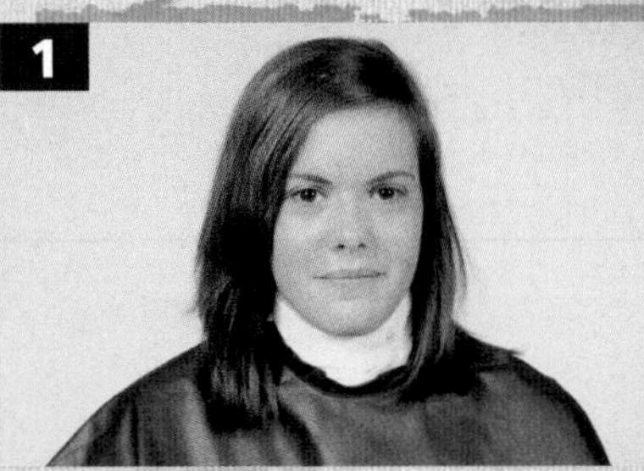

1 Drape your client for a shampoo.

2 Shampoo and condition the hair as necessary.

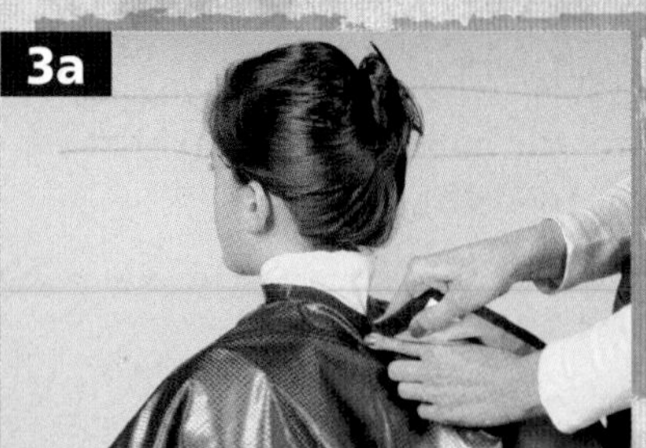

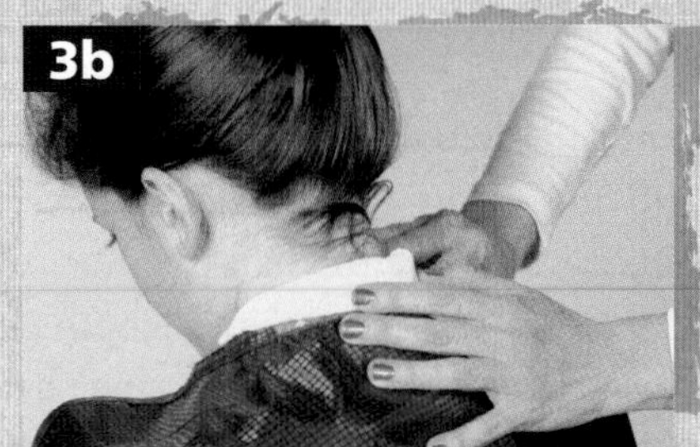

3 Escort the client back to the styling chair. Secure a neck strip around the client's neck. Place a cape over the neck strip and fasten in the back. Fold the neck strip down over the cape so that no part of the cape touches the client's skin.

4 Detangle the hair with the wide-tooth comb.

5 To find the natural part, comb the hair back from the hairline and push the hair gently forward with the palm of the hand. Use the comb and other hand to separate the hair where it parts, or, if the natural part doesn't work for your finished style, part it the way the client will be wearing it.

© Milady, a part of Cengage Learning. Photography by Yanik Chauvin.

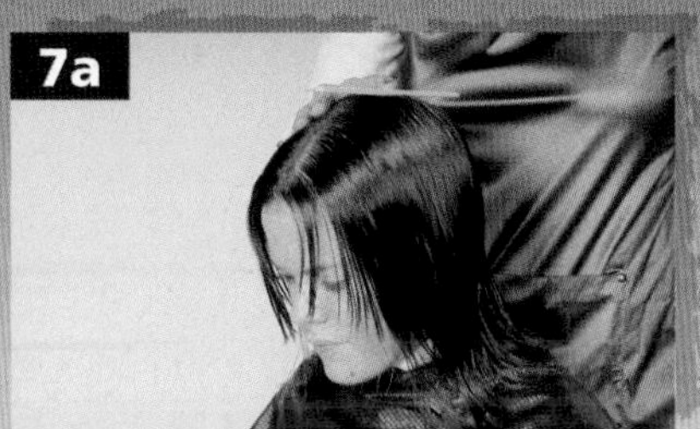

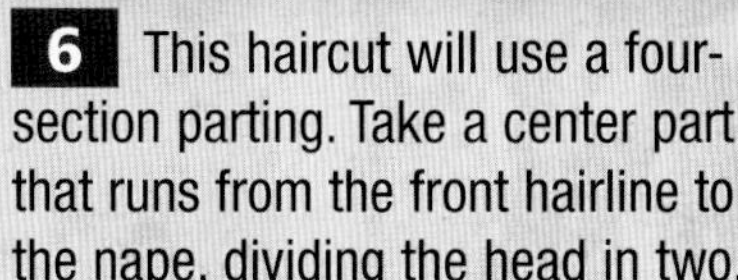

6 This haircut will use a four-section parting. Take a center part that runs from the front hairline to the nape, dividing the head in two.

7 Find the apex of the head. Take a parting that runs from the apex to the back of the ear on both sides and clip. You have now divided the head into four sections.

---

8 Beginning at the nape, on the right side, take a horizontal parting ¼ to ½ inch (0.6 to 1.25 centimeters) from the hairline, depending on the density of the hair. This creates the first subsection.

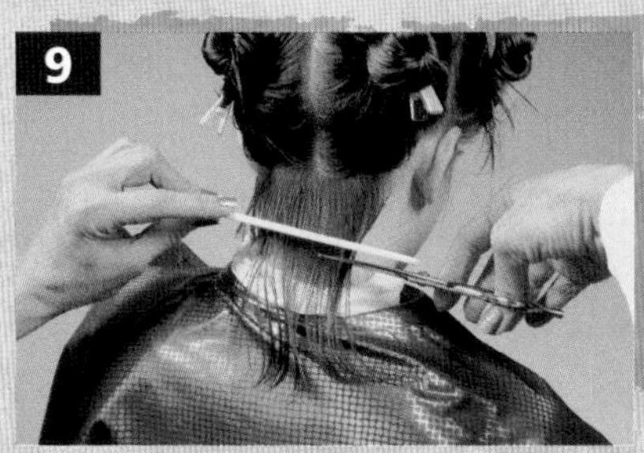

9 With the client's head upright, comb the subsection in a natural fall from scalp to ends. With your dominant hand, comb the subsection again, stopping just above the cutting line. Make sure the comb is horizontal and just above the cutting line (desired length). Cut the subsection straight across against the comb, remembering to keep your shears horizontal and parallel to the floor. Repeat on the left side, using the length of your first subsection as a guide. Check to make sure your cutting line is straight before moving on. You have now created your guideline for the entire haircut.

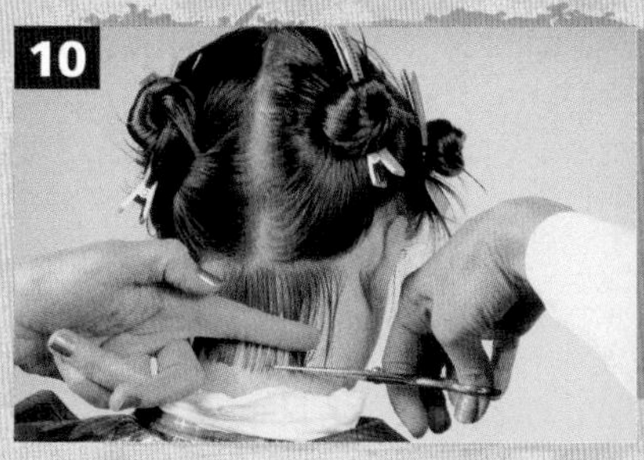

10 If the hairline lies down nicely, an alternate way of cutting a blunt line in the nape is to comb down the subsection and hold the hair against the skin with the edge of your nondominant hand. Cut the guideline below your hand, making sure that your shears are horizontal and parallel to the floor.

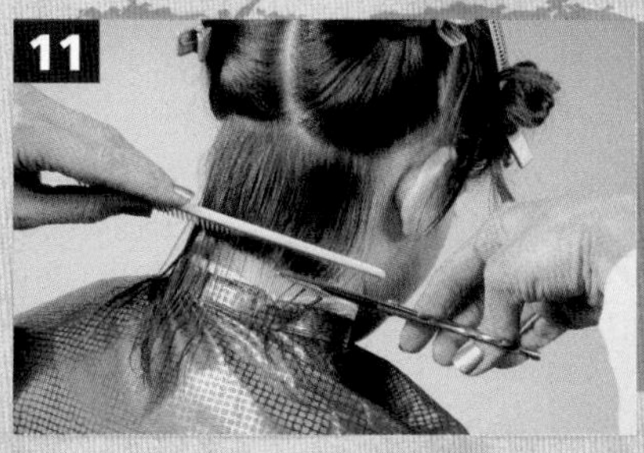

11 Returning to the right side, take another horizontal parting, creating a subsection the same size as your previous subsection. As a rule, you should be able to see the guideline through the new subsection. If you cannot see the guide, take a smaller subsection. Comb the hair down in a natural fall, and cut the length to match the guide. Repeat on the left side.

Service Tip

The density (thickness) of the hair will determine the size of the subsection. The thicker the hair, the narrower the subsection; the thinner the hair, the wider the subsection. In other words, to create narrower subsections, your partings need to be closer together. To create wider subsections, your partings should be farther apart. If there is too much hair in one subsection, it becomes difficult to see your guideline and to control the hair, because the hair is pushed away as you close the shears, producing an uneven line.

© Milady, a part of Cengage Learning. Photography by Yanik Chauvin.

PROCEDURE 16-1

Blunt Haircut with Fringe: Right-Handed continued

Service Tip

Using the comb to control the hair allows you to cut with very little tension. This allows the hair to do what it naturally wants to do, and still maintain a clean line.

12 Continue working up the back of the head, alternating from the right section to the left section, using ½-inch subsections.

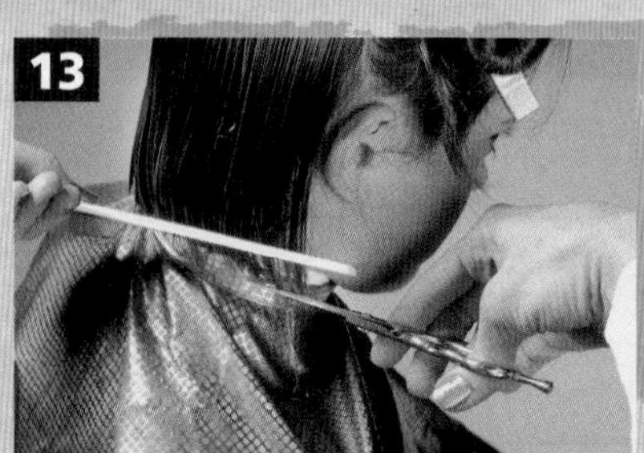

13 When you reach the crown area (danger zone), pay close attention to the natural fall of the hair. Comb the hair into its natural falling position, and cut with little or no tension to match the guide. You have now completed the back of the haircut.

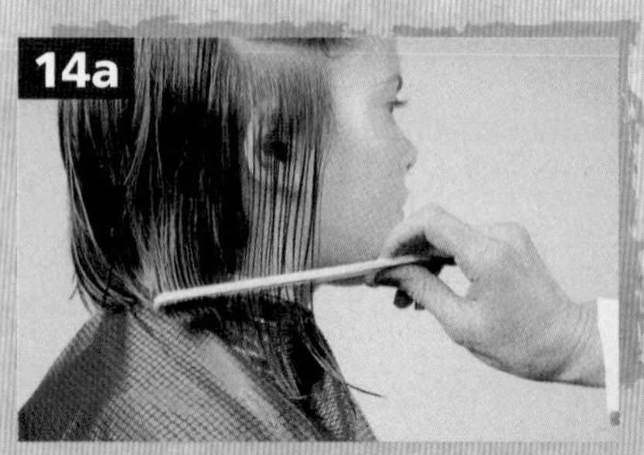

14 Now move to the sides of the haircut. Beginning on the right side, take a horizontal parting and part off a portion from the back area, and use it to cut the side guideline to match in length. This will help you maintain consistency with the blunt line when connecting the back to the sides. Be sure to take a subsection that is large enough to give you an even amount of hair at the cutting line, allowing for the ears sticking out. Comb the hair from scalp to ends, release the subsection, and allow the hair to hang in a natural fall. Using the wide teeth, place the comb back into the subsection just below the ear. Slide the comb down to just above the cutting line. Holding the comb parallel to the floor, cut the hair straight across just below the comb, connecting the line to the back. Repeat on the left side.

15 When working on the right side, your shears will be pointing toward the back. To maintain consistency in your line, take smaller subsections, connecting at the ear first, and gradually moving forward with the line until you reach the face.

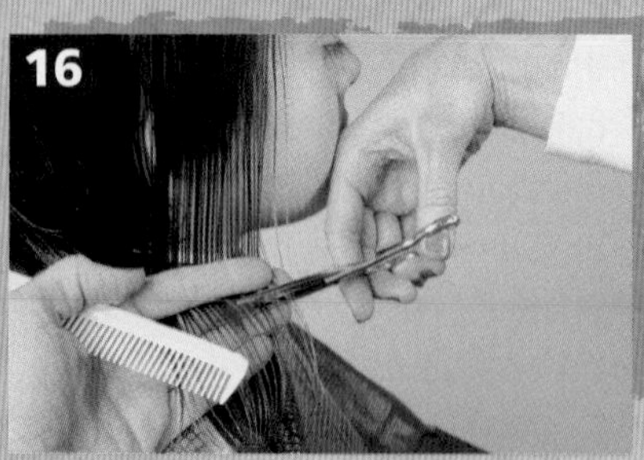

16 An alternative approach for cutting the right side is to turn your wrist so that your palm is facing upward and your shears are pointed toward the back of the head. This requires that you position your body slightly behind the section you are working on, with your elbow straight down. Either method gives a consistent result in your line.

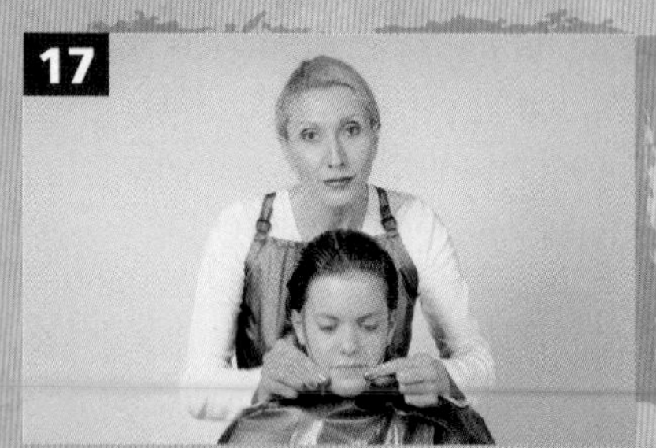

17 Before moving on, check that both sides of the haircut are even. Stand behind the client and check the lengths on both sides while looking in the mirror. Make any needed adjustments.

© Milady, a part of Cengage Learning. Photography by Yanik Chauvin.

18 Continue working up the right side with horizontal partings, until all the hair has been cut to match the guide. When cutting the hair that falls along the face, make sure to comb the hair so it lies on the side, not the front, of the face. Repeat on the left side.

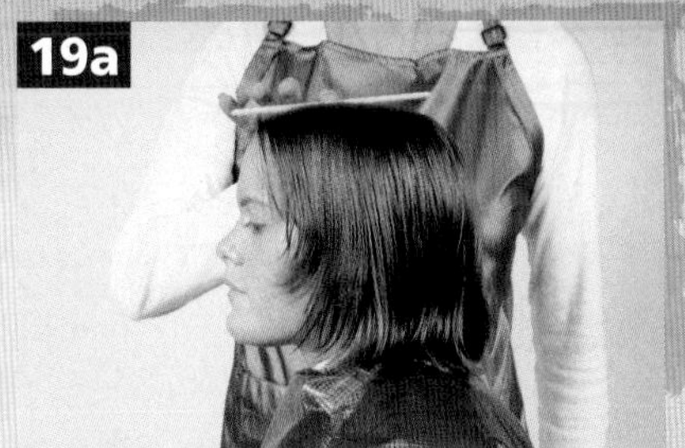
19a

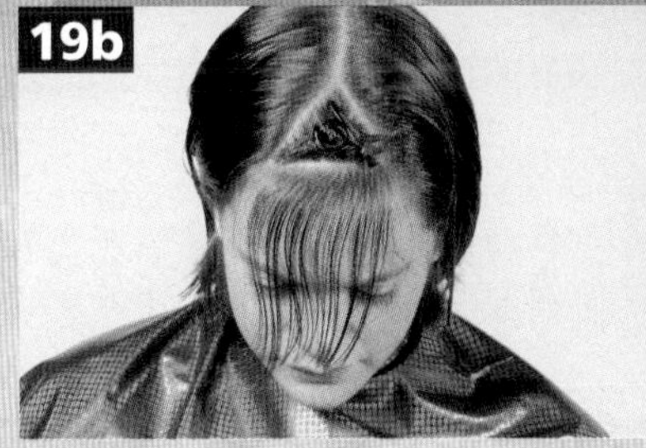
19b

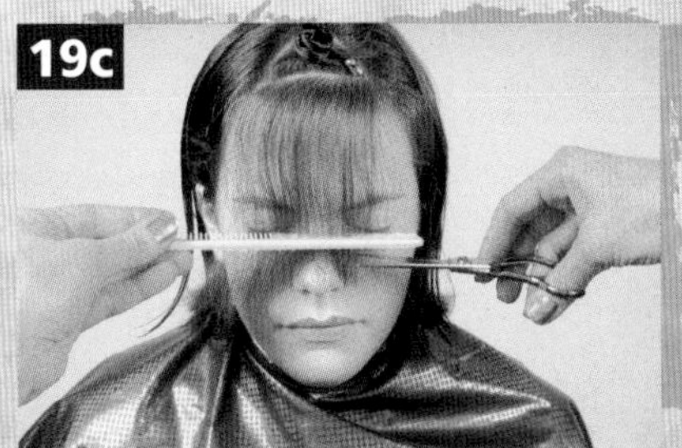
19c

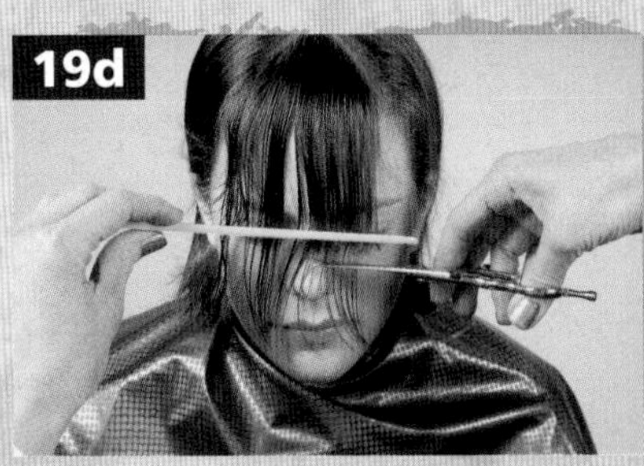
19d

19 Now, move directly in front of your client to cut the bangs (fringe) area. Begin by parting the hair down the middle and, using your cutting comb, find the apex of the front of the head. Make a triangular parting from the apex to the center of each eye. Leave a ½-inch subsection at the forehead and clip the rest of the hair back. Now, ask your client to close her eyes and, using your cutting comb, comb the section to the bridge of the nose and cut the bang (fringe) guideline. Next, part off ½-inch subsections and, without tension, cut to match the guideline length. Continue in this manner until the bangs are completely cut.

20 Sweep up cut hair from the floor and dispose of properly.

21 In order to get a true reading of the haircut, it is best to perform a smooth blowdry, with very little lift at the scalp.

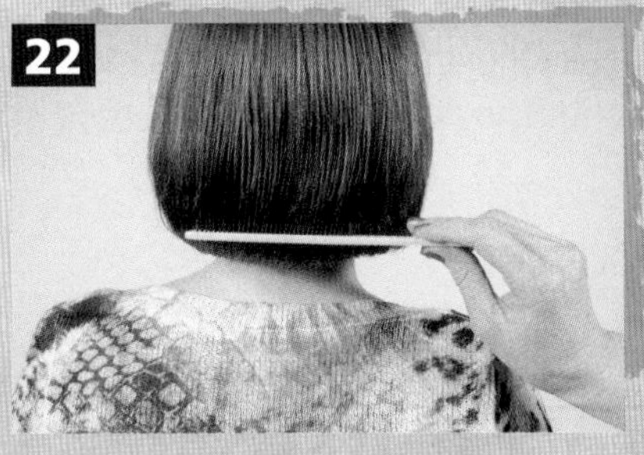
22

22 Once the haircut is dry, have the client stand. Check the line in the mirror. You should see an even, horizontal line all the way around the head. This is the time to clean up any hair at the neckline and check where the hair falls when dry. Use the wide teeth of the comb to connect the crown area. If this section was left longer during the haircut, now is the time to connect it into the line.

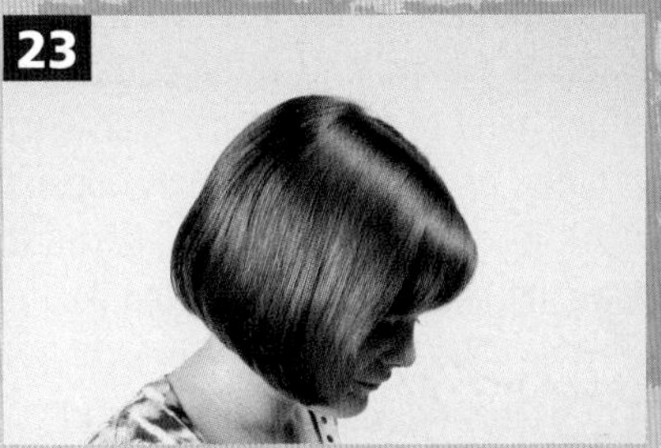
23

23 Finished look.

Service Tip

When cutting the bangs or fringe, be sure the hair is either slightly damp or completely dry. Also, when combing and preparing to cut the hair at the fringe, do not use tension, allow for the natural lift of the hair.

Post-Service

- Complete PROCEDURE 15-2 **Post-Service Procedure** SEE PAGE 326

© Milady, a part of Cengage Learning. Photography by Yanik Chauvin.

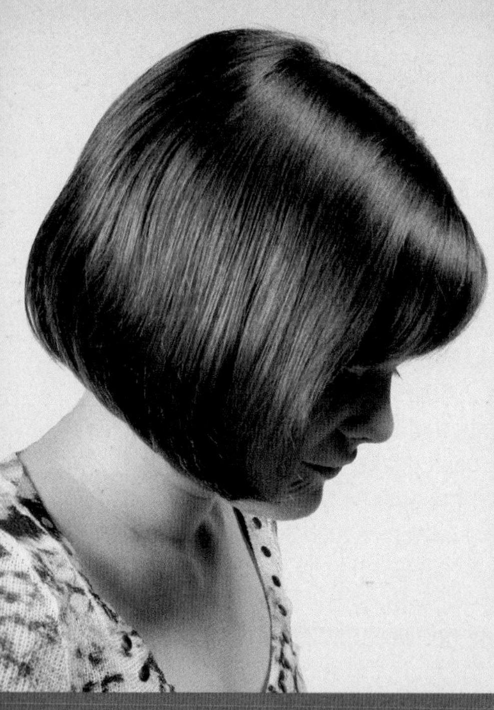

PROCEDURE 16-1 Left Handed

Blunt Haircut with Fringe

Implements and Materials

You will need all of the following implements, materials, and supplies:

- **Cutting cape**
- **Cutting or styling comb**
- **Haircutting shears**
- **Neck strip**
- **Sectioning clips**
- **Shampoo and conditioner**
- **Shampoo cape**
- **Spray bottle with water**
- **Towels**
- **Wide-tooth comb**

Preparation

- Perform PROCEDURE 15-1 **Pre-Service Procedure** **SEE PAGE 323**

Procedure

1 Drape your client for a shampoo.

2 Shampoo and condition the hair as necessary.

3 Escort the client back to the styling chair. Secure a neck strip around the client's neck. Place a cape over the neck strip and fasten in the back. Fold the neck strip down over the cape so that no part of the cape touches the client's skin.

4 Detangle the hair with the wide-tooth comb.

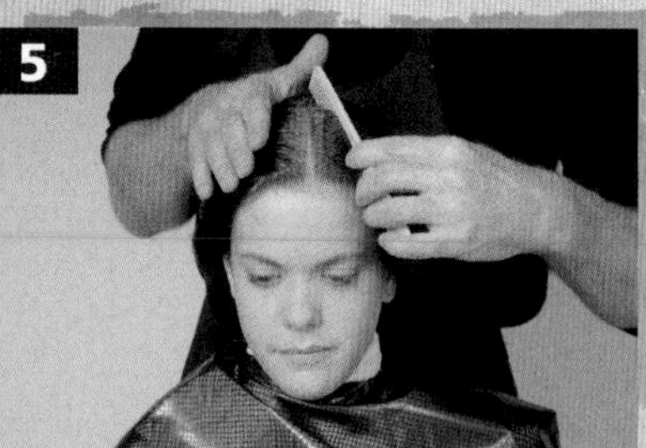

5 To find the natural part, comb the hair back from the hairline and push the hair gently forward with the palm of the hand. Use the comb and other hand to separate the hair where it parts, or, if the natural part doesn't work for your finished style, part it the way the client will be wearing it.

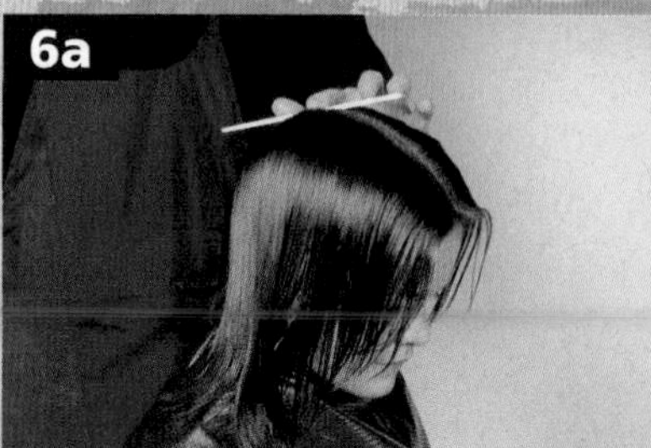

6a This haircut will use a four-section parting. Take a center part that runs from the front hairline to the nape, dividing the head in two.

© Milady, a part of Cengage Learning. Photography by Yanik Chauvin.

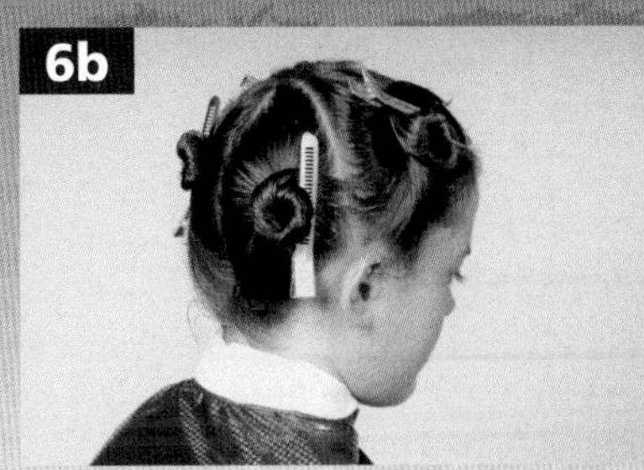

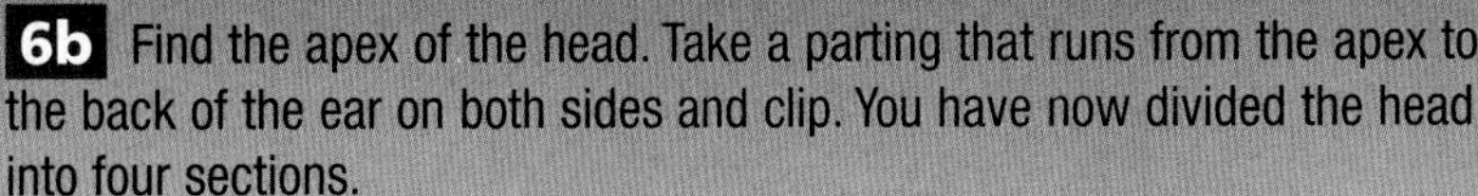

6b Find the apex of the head. Take a parting that runs from the apex to the back of the ear on both sides and clip. You have now divided the head into four sections.

7 Beginning at the nape, on the left side, take a horizontal parting ¼ to ½ inch (0.6 to 1.25 centimeters) from the hairline, depending on the density of the hair. This creates the first subsection.

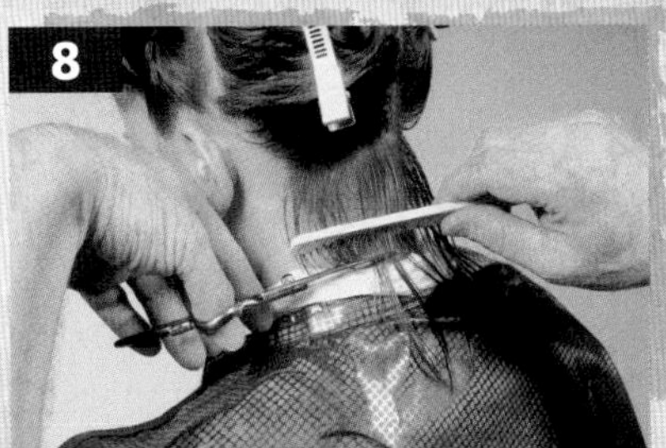

8 With the client's head upright, comb the subsection in a natural fall from scalp to ends. With your dominant hand, comb the subsection again, stopping just above the cutting line. Make sure the comb is horizontal and just above the cutting line (desired length). Cut the subsection straight across against the comb, remembering to keep your shears horizontal and parallel to the floor. Repeat on the right side, using the length of your first subsection as a guide. Check to make sure your cutting line is straight before moving on. You have now created your guideline for the entire haircut.

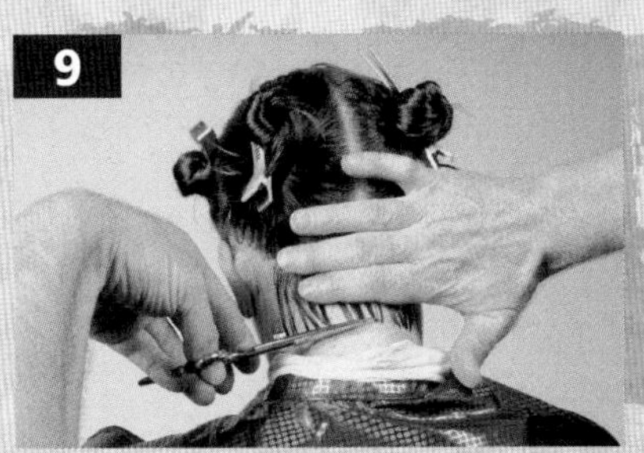

9 If the hairline lies down nicely, an alternate way of cutting a blunt line in the nape is to comb down the subsection and hold the hair against the skin with the edge of your nondominant hand. Cut the guideline below your hand, making sure that your shears are horizontal and parallel to the floor.

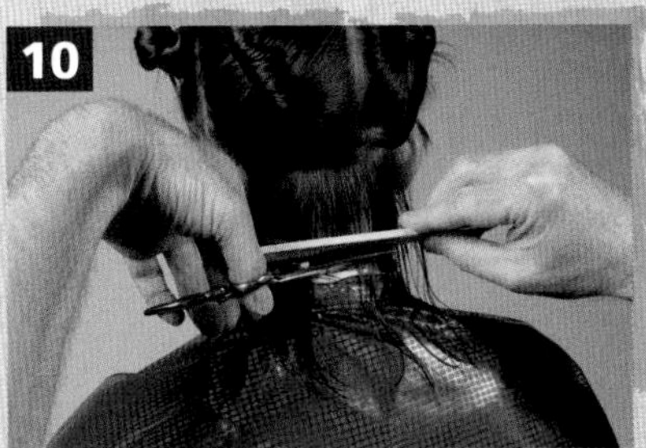

10 Take another horizontal parting, creating a subsection the same size as your previous subsection. As a rule, you should be able to see the guideline through the new subsection. If you cannot see the guide, take a smaller subsection. Comb the hair down in a natural fall, and cut the length to match the guide. Repeat on the right side.

11 Continue working up the back of the head, alternating from the left section to the right section, using ½-inch subsections.

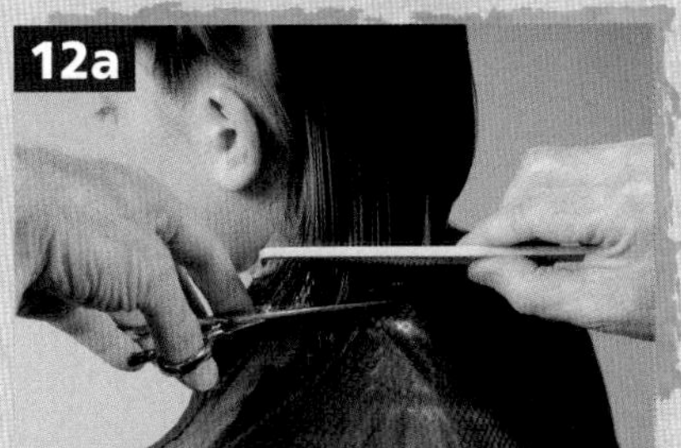

12a When you reach the crown area (danger zone), pay close attention to the natural fall of the hair. Comb the hair into its natural falling position, and cut with little or no tension to match the guide.

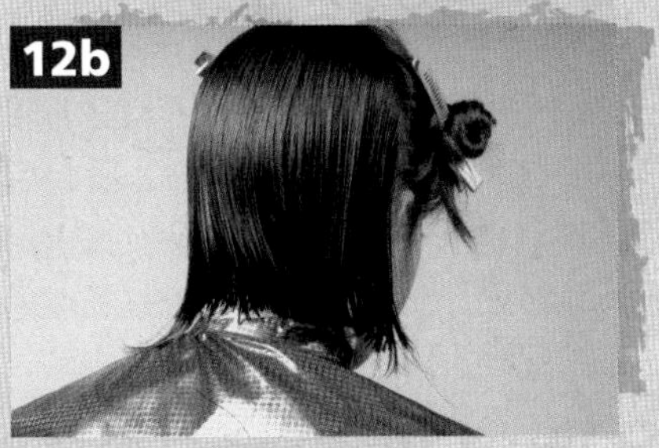

12b You have now completed the back of the haircut.

© Milady, a part of Cengage Learning. Photography by Yanik Chauvin.

Blunt Haircut with Fringe: Left-Handed continued

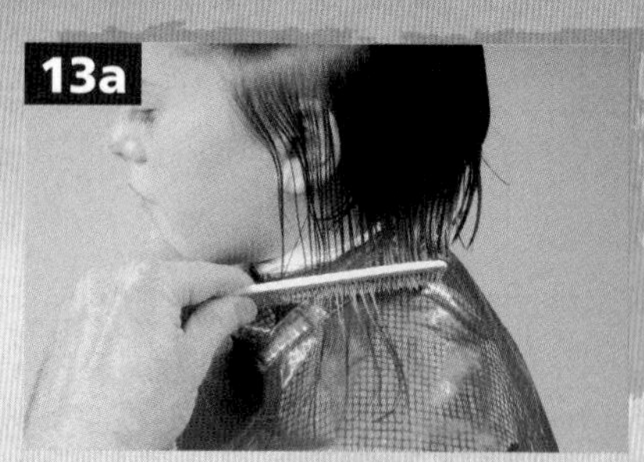

13a Now move to the sides of the haircut. Beginning on the left side, take a horizontal parting and part off a portion from the back area, and use it to cut the side guideline to match in length. This will help you maintain consistency with the blunt line when connecting the back to the sides. Be sure to take a subsection that is large enough to give you an even amount of hair at the cutting line, allowing for the ears sticking out. Comb the hair from scalp to ends, release the subsection, and allow the hair to hang in a natural fall. Using the wide teeth, place the comb back into the subsection just below the ear. Slide the comb down to just above the cutting line.

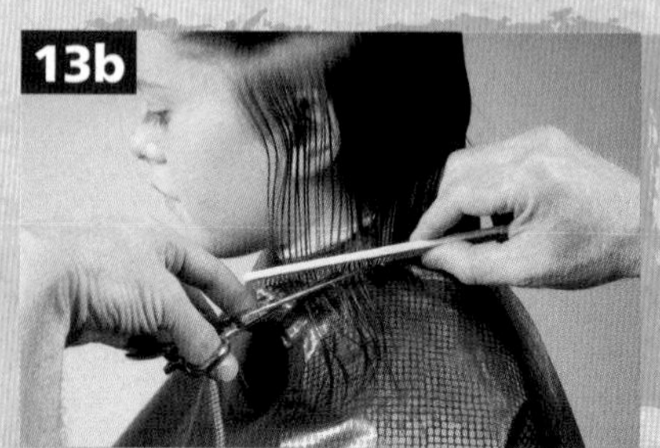

13b Holding the comb parallel to the floor, cut the hair straight across just below the comb, connecting the line to the back. Repeat on the right side.

14 When working on the left side, your shears will be pointing toward the back. To maintain consistency in your line, take smaller subsections, connecting at the ear first, and gradually moving forward with the line until you reach the face.

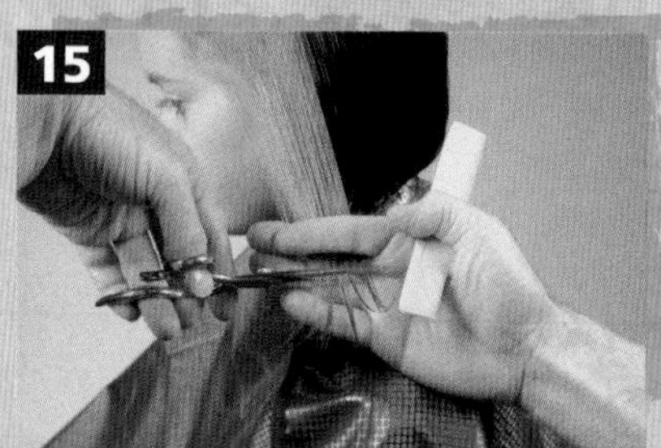

15 An alternative approach for cutting the left side is to turn your wrist so that your palm is facing upward and your shears are pointed toward the back of the head. This requires that you position your body slightly behind the section you are working on, with your elbow straight down. Either method gives a consistent result in your line.

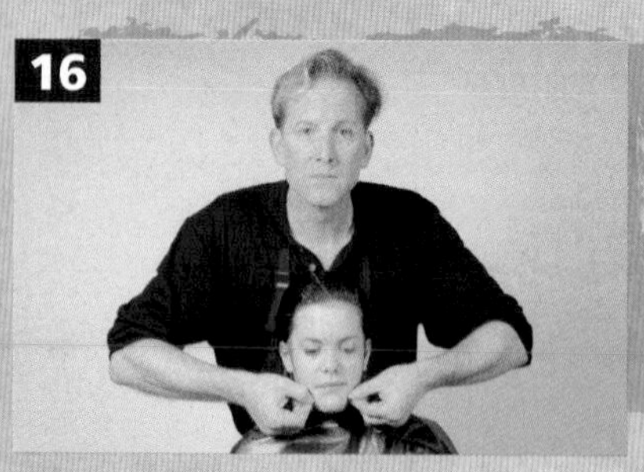

16 Before moving on, check that both sides of the haircut are even. Stand behind the client and check the lengths on both sides while looking in the mirror. Make any needed adjustments.

17 Continue working up the left side with horizontal partings, until all the hair has been cut to match the guide. When cutting the hair that falls along the face, make sure to comb the hair so it lies on the side, not the front, of the face. Repeat on the right side.

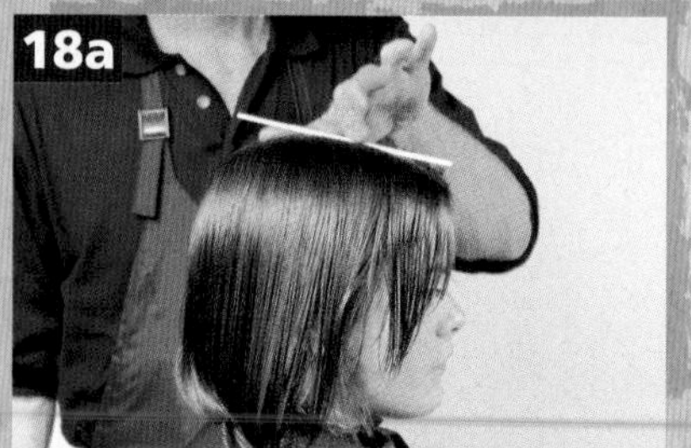

18a Now, move directly in front of your client to cut the bangs (fringe) area. Begin by parting the hair down the middle and, using your cutting comb, find the apex of the front of the head.

© Milady, a part of Cengage Learning. Photography by Yanik Chauvin.

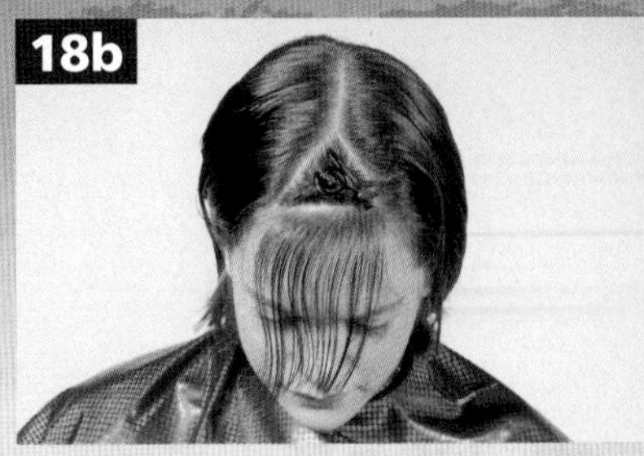

18b Make a triangular parting from the apex to the center of each eye. Leave a ½-inch subsection at the forehead and clip the rest of the hair back.

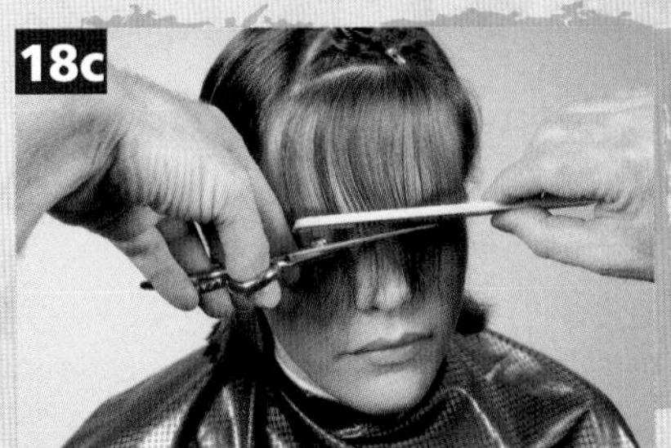

18c Now, ask your client to close her eyes and using your cutting comb, comb the section to the bridge of the nose and cut the bang (fringe) guideline.

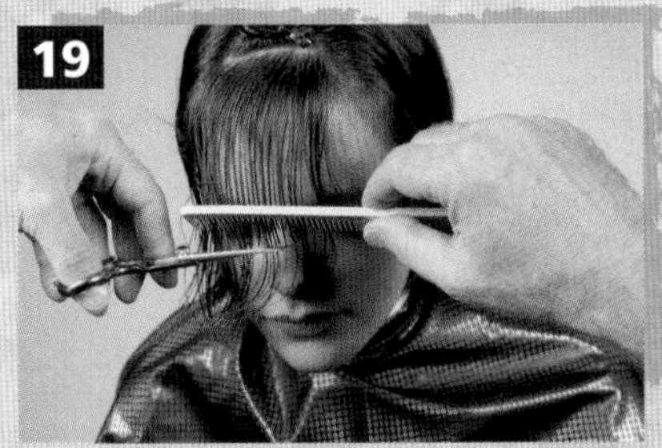

19 Next, part off ½-inch subsections and, without tension, cut to match the guideline length. Continue in this manner until the bangs are completely cut.

20 Sweep up cut hair from the floor and dispose of properly.

21 In order to get a true reading of the haircut, it is best to perform a smooth blowdry, with very little lift at the scalp.

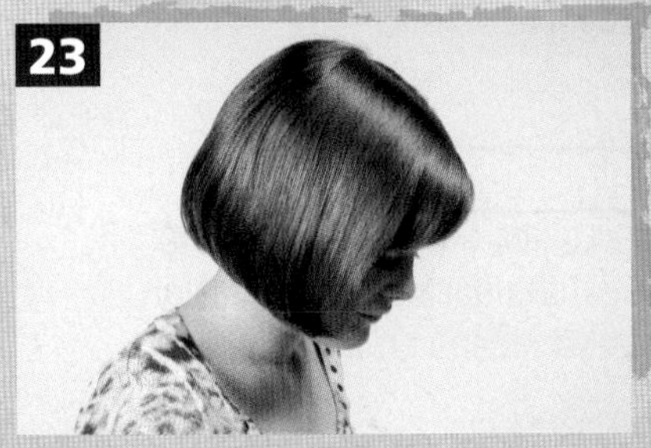

22 Once the haircut is dry, have the client stand. Check the line in the mirror. You should see an even, horizontal line all the way around the head. This is the time to clean up any hair at the neckline and check where the hair falls when dry. Use the wide teeth of the comb to connect the crown area. If this section was left longer during the haircut, now is the time to connect it into the line.

23 Finished look.

© Milady, a part of Cengage Learning. Photography by Yanik Chauvin.

Post-Service

- Complete PROCEDURE 15-2 **Post-Service Procedure** **SEE PAGE 326**

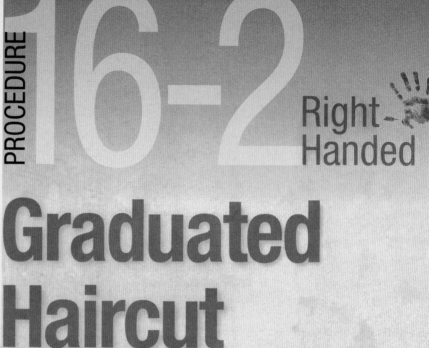

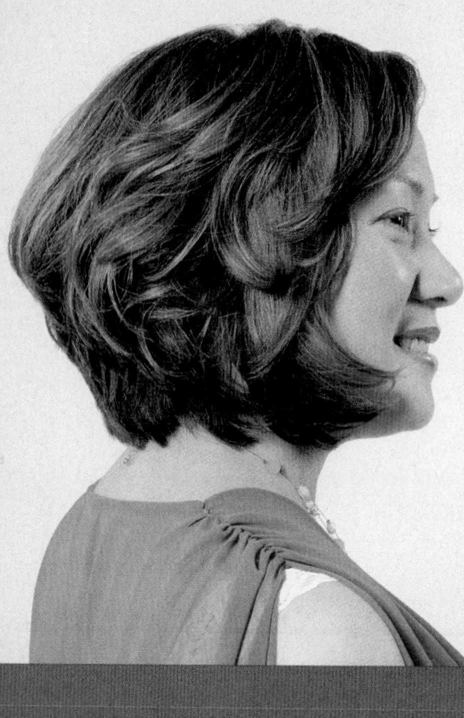

PROCEDURE 16-2 Right-Handed

Graduated Haircut

Implements and Materials

You will need all of the following implements, materials, and supplies:

- **Cutting cape**
- **Cutting or styling comb**
- **Haircutting shears**
- **Neck strip**
- **Sectioning clips**
- **Shampoo and conditioner**
- **Shampoo cape**
- **Spray bottle with water**
- **Towels**
- **Wide-tooth comb**

Preparation

- Perform PROCEDURE 15-1 **Pre-Service Procedure** **SEE PAGE 323**

Procedure

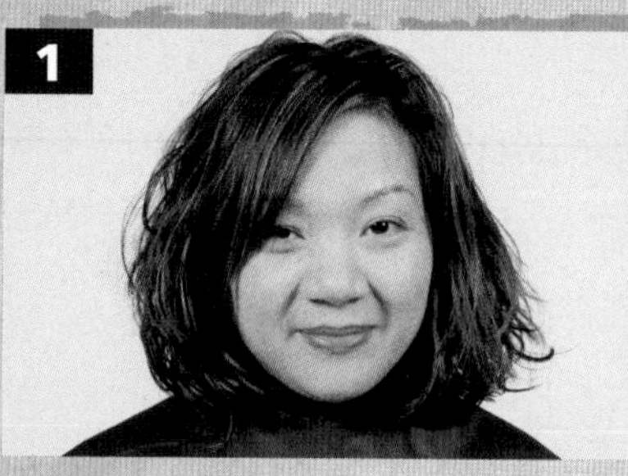

1 Drape your client for a shampoo.

2 Shampoo and condition the hair as necessary.

3 Escort the client back to the styling chair. Secure a neck strip around the client's neck. Place a cape over the neck strip and fasten in the back. Fold the neck strip down over the cape so that no part of the cape touches the client's skin.

4 Detangle the hair with the wide-tooth comb.

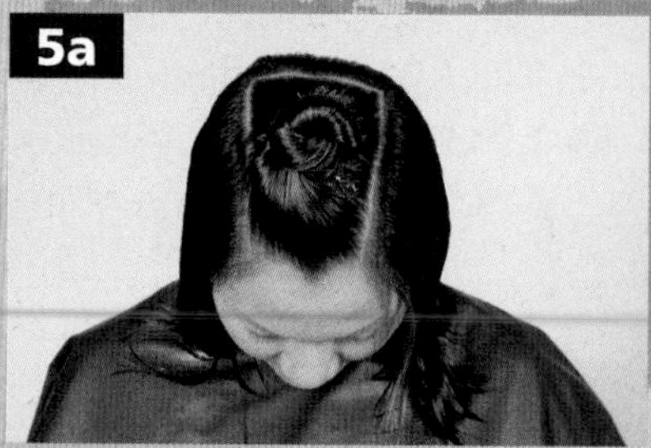

5a This haircut will use a six-section parting. Begin with a part from the front hairline just above the middle of each eyebrow back to the crown area, and clip the hair in place.

© Milady, a part of Cengage Learning. Photography by Yanik Chauvin.

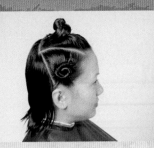

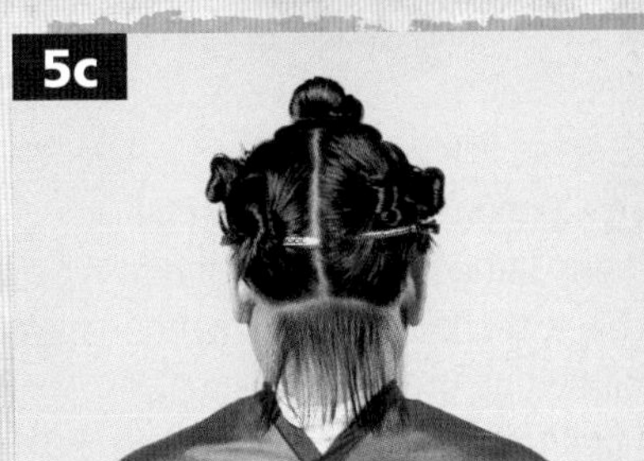

5b Establish another part from the crown area where section one ends to the back of each ear, forming side-sections two and three. Clip these sections in place.

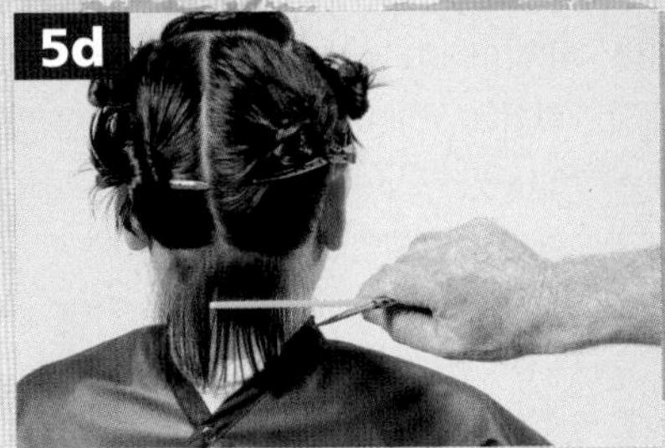

5c Part the hair down the center of the back to form sections four and five.

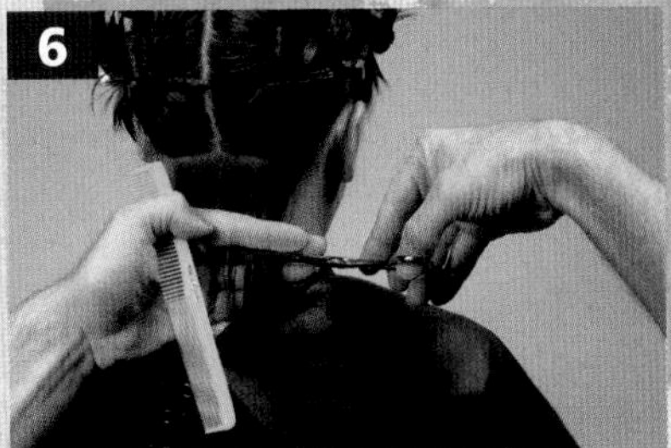

5d Take a horizontal part from one ear to the other across the nape area about 1 inch (2.5 centimeters) above the hairline. This section (six) is your horizontal guide section.

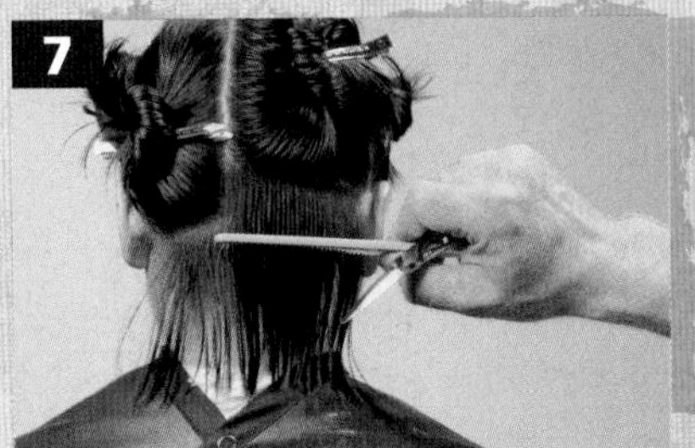

6 Establish your guideline by the right side of the guide to the desired length. Use a horizontal cutting line parallel to the fingers. Cut the left side of the nape section the same length as the right guideline.

7 Working upward in the left back section, measure and part off the first horizontal section approximately 1-inch wide.

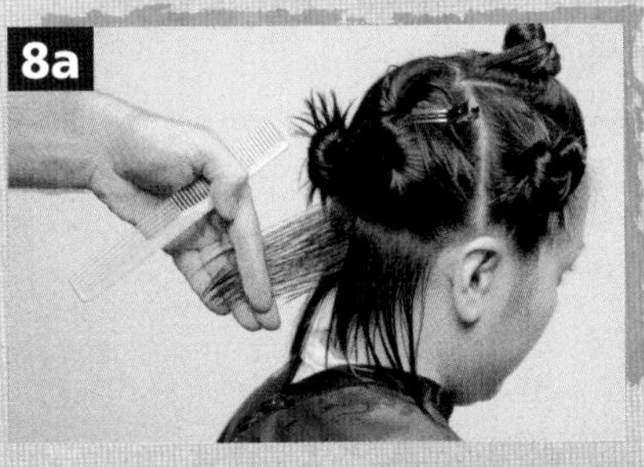

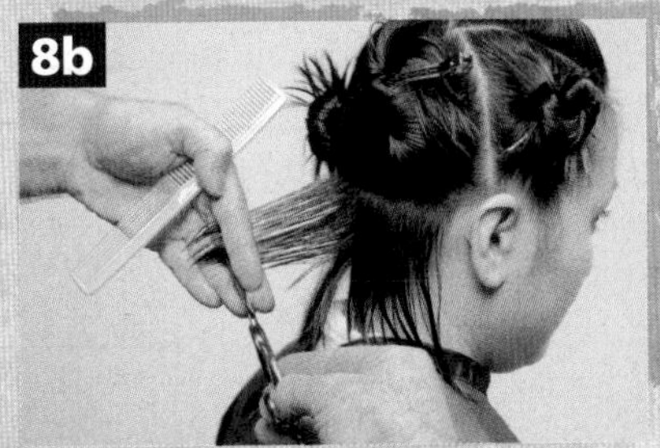

8 Beginning at the center part, establish a vertical subsection approximately ½-inch (1.25 centimeters) wide. Extend the subsection down to include the nape guideline. Comb the subsection smooth at a 45-degree angle to the scalp. Hold your fingers at a 90-degree angle to the strand and cut.

9 Proceed to cut the entire horizontal section by parting off vertical subsections and cutting in the same manner. Check each section vertically and horizontally throughout the haircut. Each completed section will serve as a guideline for the next section.

© Milady, a part of Cengage Learning. Photography by Yanik Chauvin.

PROCEDURE 16-2 Graduated Haircut: Right-Handed continued

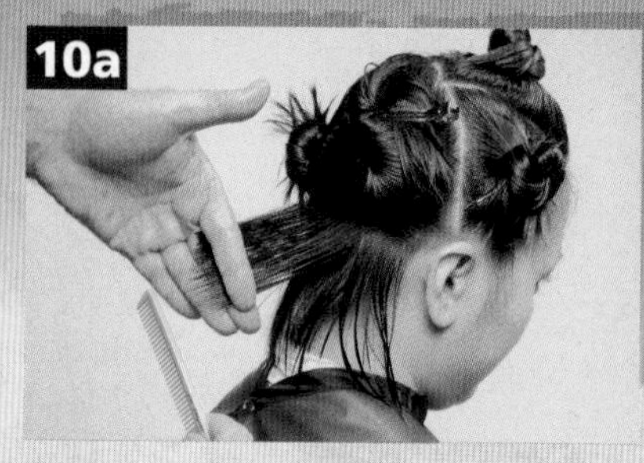

10a Beginning at the center, create another vertical subsection that extends down and includes the previously cut strands. Comb the hair smoothly at a 45-degree elevation to the head.

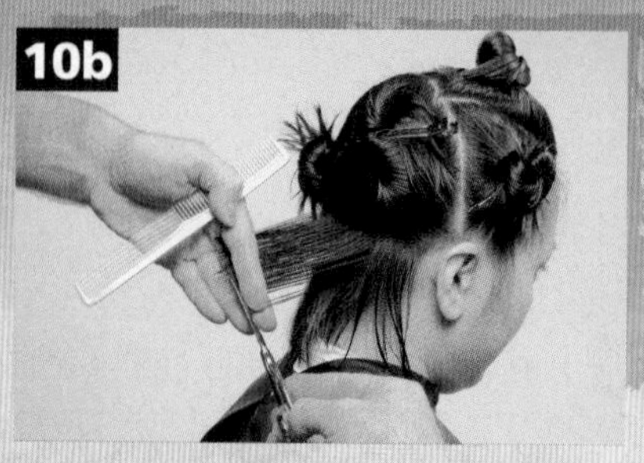

10b Hold the fingers and shears at a 90-degree angle to the subsection and cut. Cut the entire horizontal section this way. Make sure the second section blends evenly with the previously cut section.

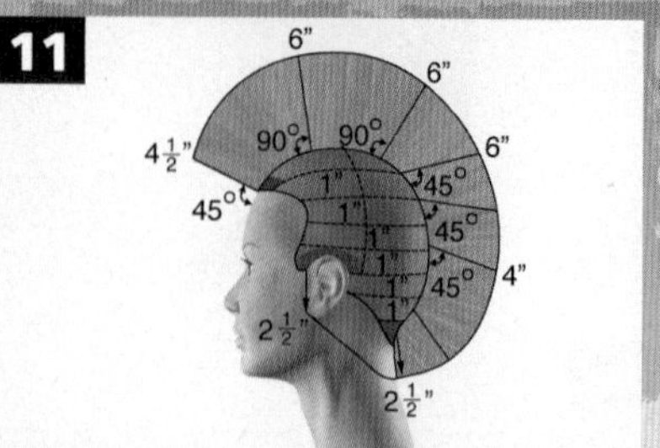

11 Continue taking horizontal sections throughout the right and left back sections, and follow the same cutting procedure. The hair will gradually become longer as it reaches the apex. For example, if your nape guide was 2½-inches (6.25 centimeters) long, your upper crown section will be approximately 6-inches (15 centimeters) long.

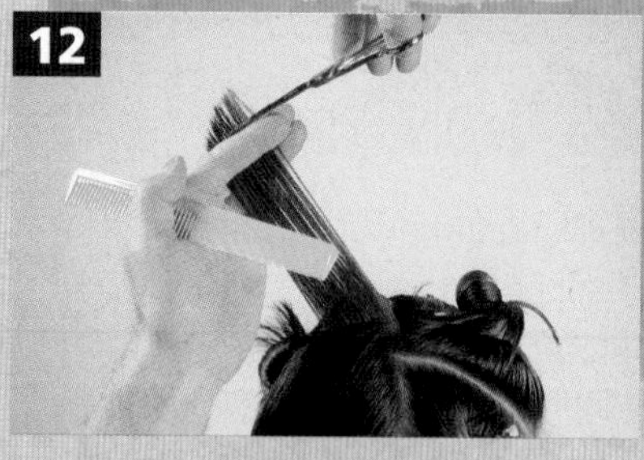

12 Cut the crown. Maintain the length in the upper crown by holding each vertical subsection throughout the crown area at a 90-degree angle while cutting. After checking the back and crown for even blending, proceed to the left side section.

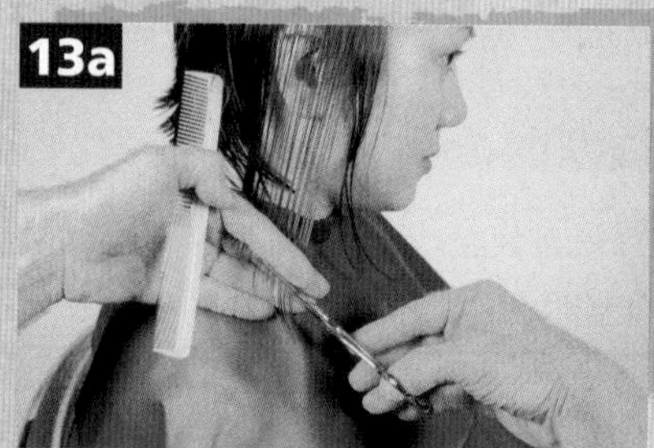

13a Establish a narrow guide section on the right side at the hairline approximately ½-inch wide. Cut side guideline to match the length in the nape. Move to the left side of the head and establish a matching guideline there.

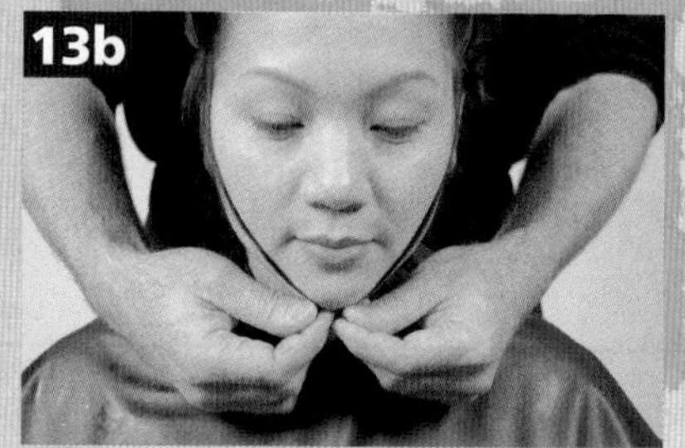

13b This will help you to be sure that both side sections will be the same length when the right side section is cut later.

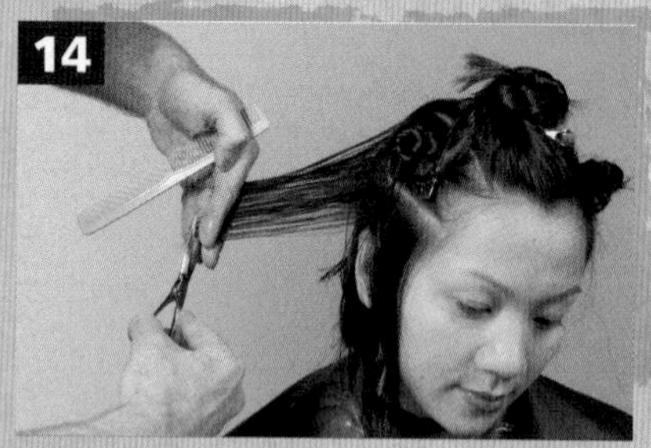

14 To cut the next section, establish a ½-inch parting that curves and follows the hairline above the ear back to the nape section. Smoothly comb the section, including the side guideline and part of the nape section.

15 Holding the hair with little or no tension, cut the hair from the nape guide to the side guide. Note that the fingers are held at a slight angle to connect the two guides.

© Milady, a part of Cengage Learning. Photography by Yanik Chauvin.

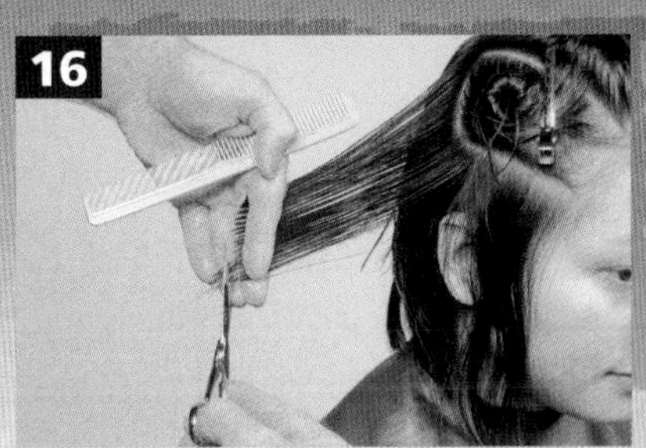

16 Establish a horizontal section on the side, taking hair from the side and the crown area. The width of this section will vary because of the irregular hairline around the ear. This is how you will blend the side and back sections of the cut.

17 To begin cutting the side section, start at the ear, part a ½-inch vertical subsection (include the underlying guideline and a small portion of the nape section), and cut section.

18 Continue following the same cutting procedure. Take vertical subsections, comb smooth, elevate at a 45-degree angle from the head, holding the fingers at a 90-degree angle to the hair. Cut the section even with the side guideline and nape section. Be sure to hold the vertical subsections straight out from the head at 45 degrees, not pulled to the right or left.

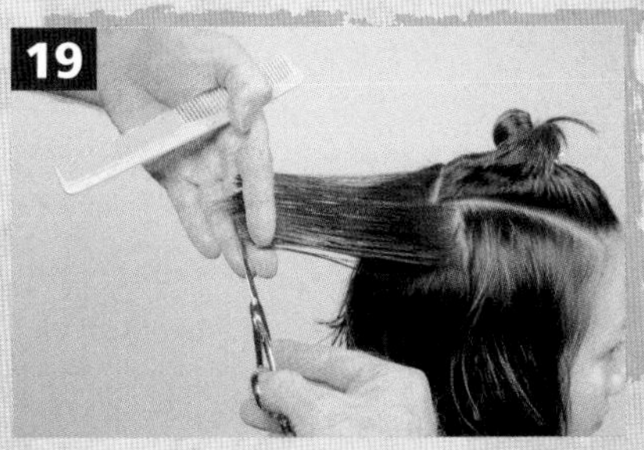

19 When the left side section is complete, the hair in the uppermost part of the section should be the same length as that in the upper crown area. In the final 1-inch section, comb the vertical subsections and hold them at a 90-degree angle to the head. Position your fingers at 90 degrees to the head and cut parallel to your fingers. Check the completed section horizontally to make sure the ends are even.

20 Move to the right side of the head and cut the hair in the same manner as you did on the left side, using the previously established guide. Once the back and both sides are complete, move to the bang and top areas.

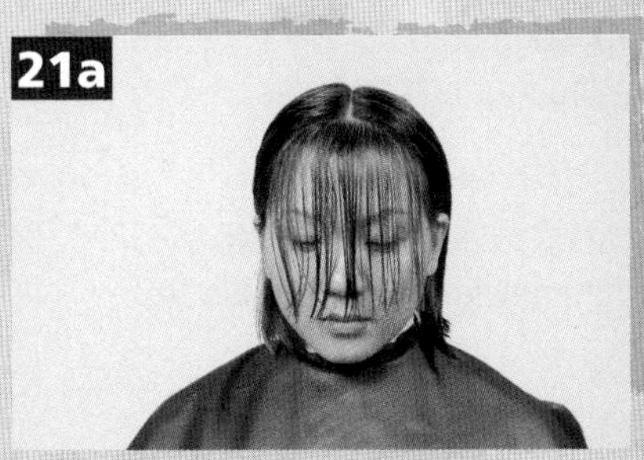

21a You can create a variety of bang (fringe) designs by cutting the bang length close to that of the side guideline. Create a bang guide section along the hairline about ½-inch wide.

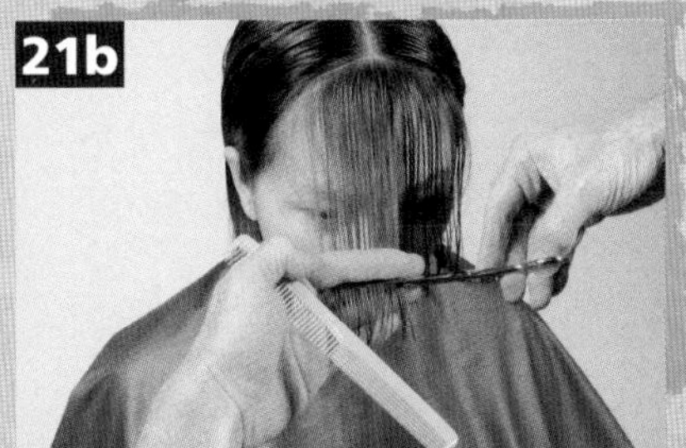

21b Starting at the center part and working on the left side of the forehead, cut to the desired length.

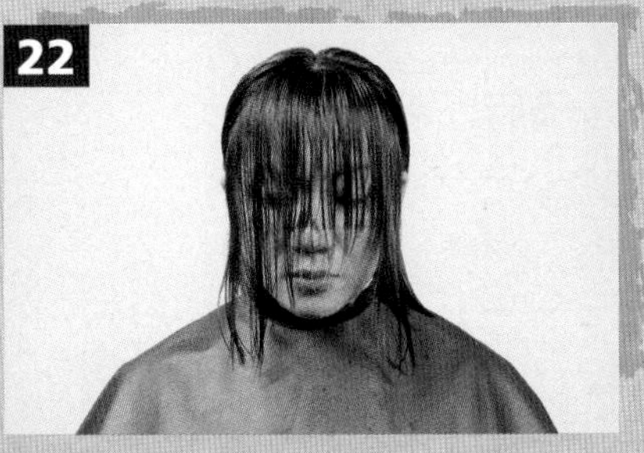

22 Bring down another ½-inch section and cut this subsection of the bang section at a low elevation, to the guideline.

© Milady, a part of Cengage Learning. Photography by Yanik Chauvin.

Graduated Haircut: Right-Handed continued

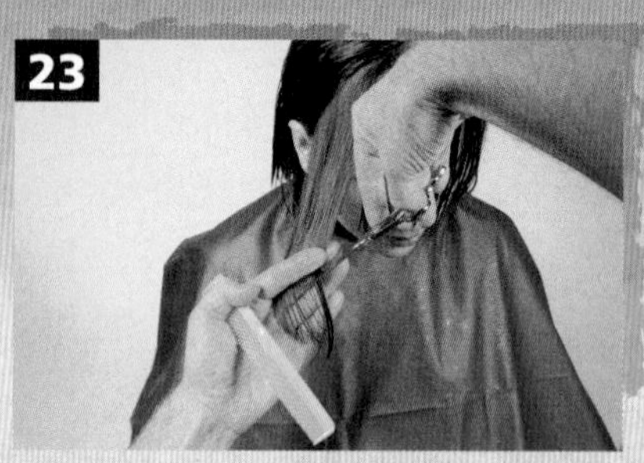

23 Now take a vertical parting along the hairline that connects the guideline from the bang and the guideline from in front of the ear. Slide your hand slowly, keeping both guidelines in your grasp, and stop when you have only about a ¼ inch of both guidelines in your hand. Connecting the two guidelines will determine the angle of the cut. Complete the guideline on both sides of the head.

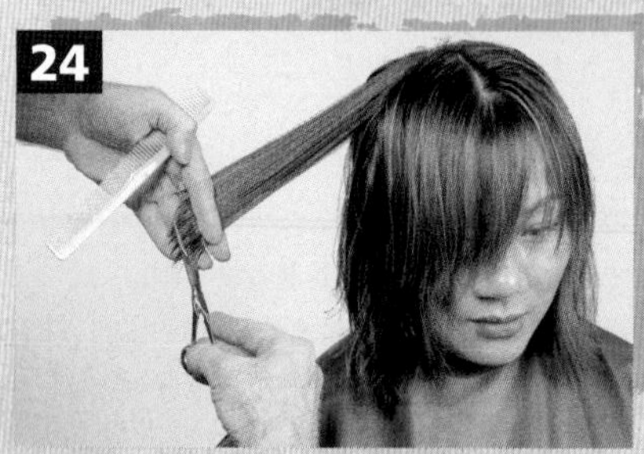

24 Using the guideline you established in step 23, take ½-inch subsections and cut the top section at a 45-degree angle, blending with the sides.

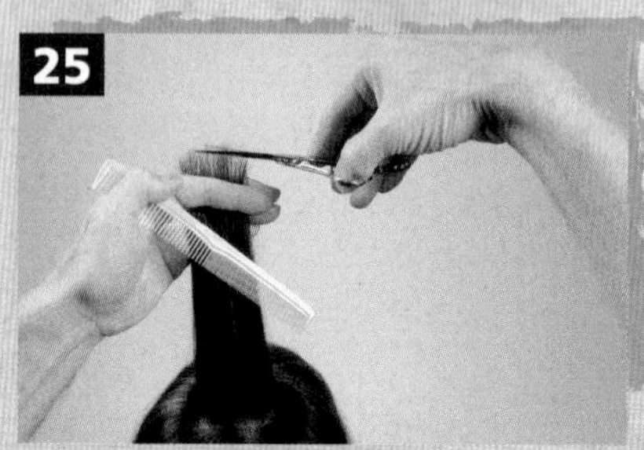

25 Finish the top section by taking ½-inch vertical subsections parallel to the center part. Hold the hair up from the head at a 90-degree angle. Include hair from the crown and bang area, and cut to blend the section with the two pre-cut sections. Continue cutting in this manner until the remainder of the top section is cut. Hold the hair up from the head at a 90-degree angle and check the completed cut. Trim any uneven ends. The bang guide gradually increases in length to the pre-established length in the top and crown areas.

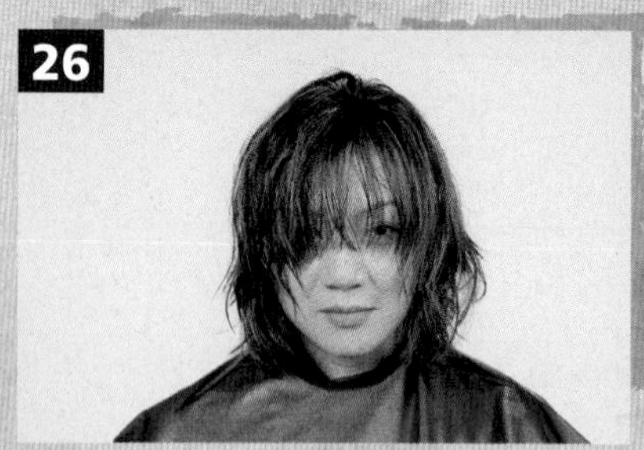

26 Once the cut is completed, use your hands to put the hair into place. Blowdry the haircut and view the design, movement, and ends to be sure they are evenly blended.

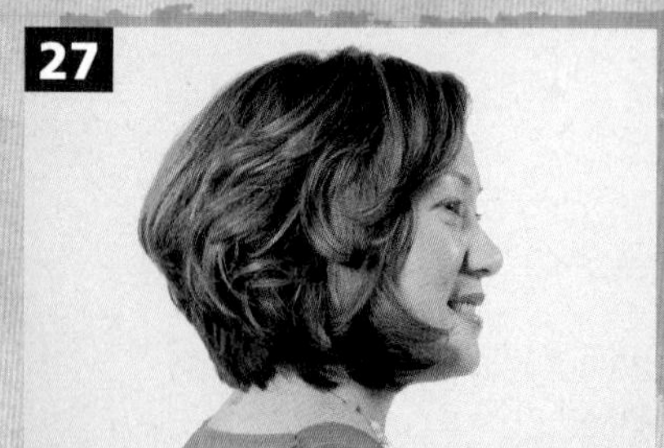

27 Finished look.

Post-Service

- Complete PROCEDURE 15-2 **Post-Service Procedure** SEE PAGE 326

© Milady, a part of Cengage Learning. Photography by Yanik Chauvin.

PROCEDURE 16-2 Left Handed

Graduated Haircut

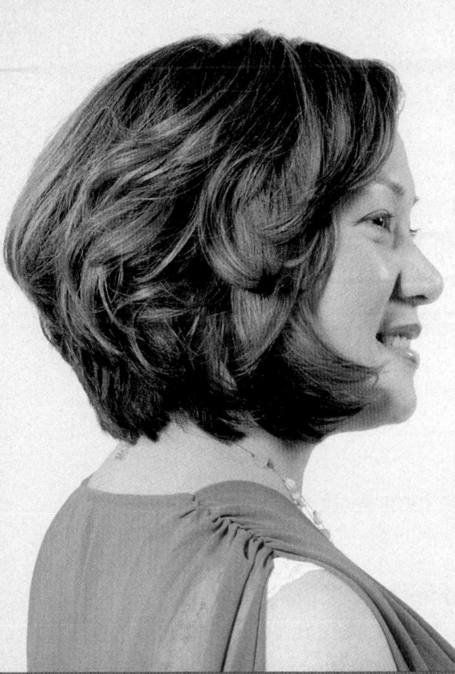

Implements and Materials

You will need all of the following implements, materials, and supplies:

- **Cutting cape**
- **Cutting or styling comb**
- **Haircutting shears**
- **Neck strip**
- **Sectioning clips**
- **Shampoo and conditioner**
- **Shampoo cape**
- **Spray bottle with water**
- **Towels**
- **Wide-tooth comb**

© Milady, a part of Cengage Learning. Photography by Yanik Chauvin.

Preparation

- Perform PROCEDURE 15-1 **Pre-Service Procedure** **SEE PAGE 323**

Procedure

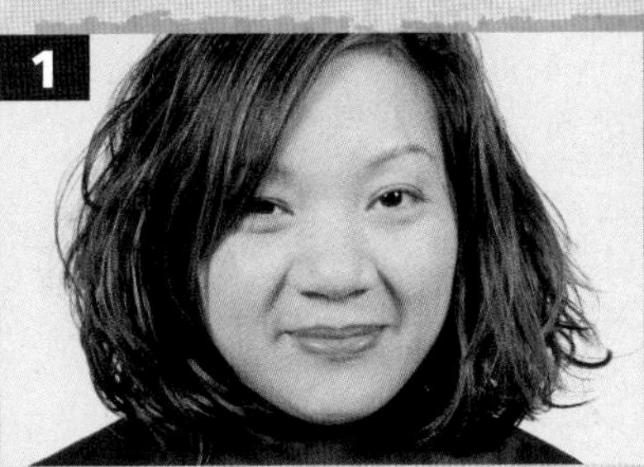

1 Drape your client for a shampoo.

2 Shampoo and condition the hair as necessary.

3 Escort the client back to the styling chair. Secure a neck strip around the client's neck. Place a cape over the neck strip and fasten in the back. Fold the neck strip down over the cape so that no part of the cape touches the client's skin.

4 Detangle the hair with the wide-tooth comb.

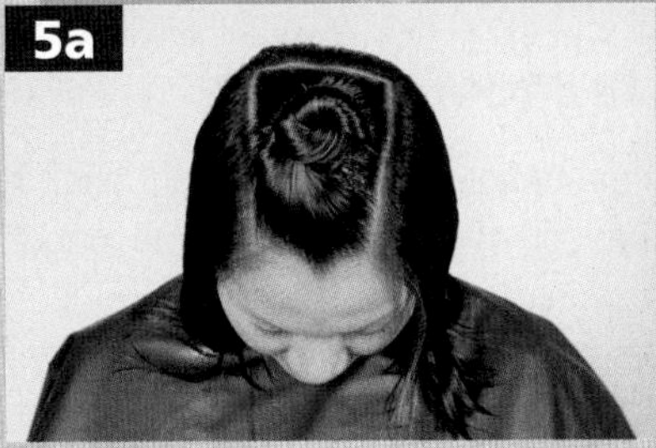

5a This haircut will use a six-section parting. Begin with a part from the front hairline just above the middle of each eyebrow back to the crown area, and clip the hair in place.

Graduated Haircut: Left-Handed continued

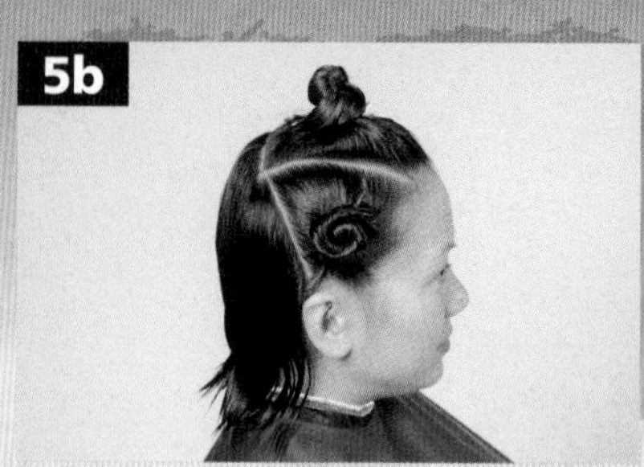
5b

5b Establish another part from the crown area where section one ends to the back of each ear, forming side-sections two and three. Clip these sections in place.

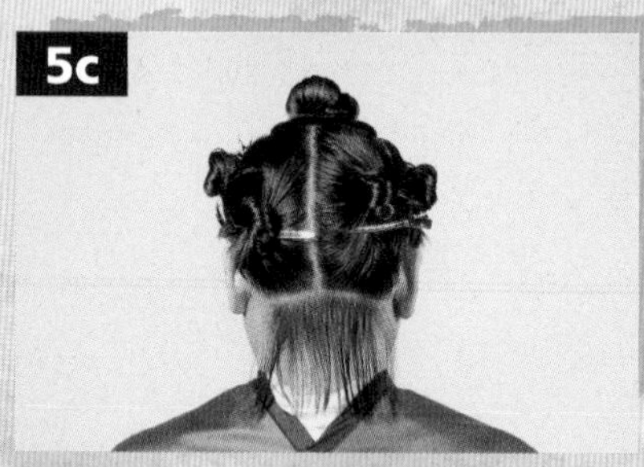
5c

5c Part the hair down the center of the back to form sections four and five.

5d Take a horizontal part from one ear to the other across the nape area about 1 inch (2.5 centimeters) above the hairline. This section (six) is your horizontal guide section.

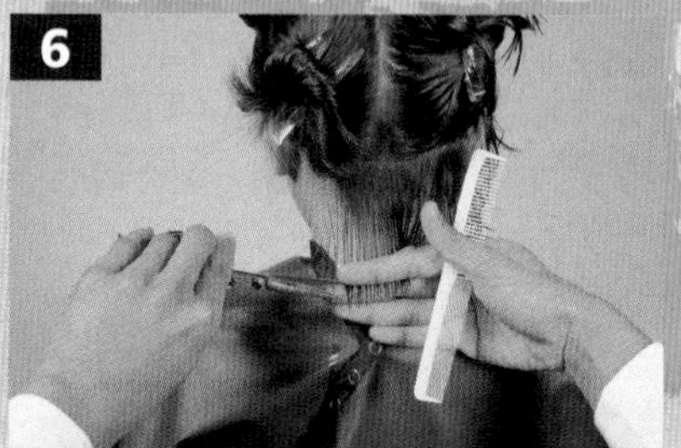
6

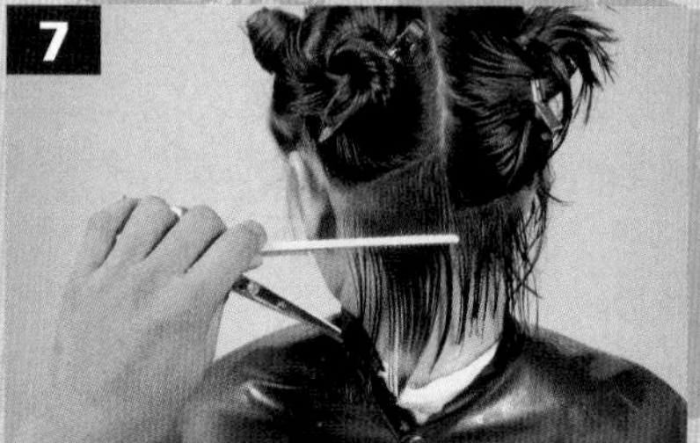
7

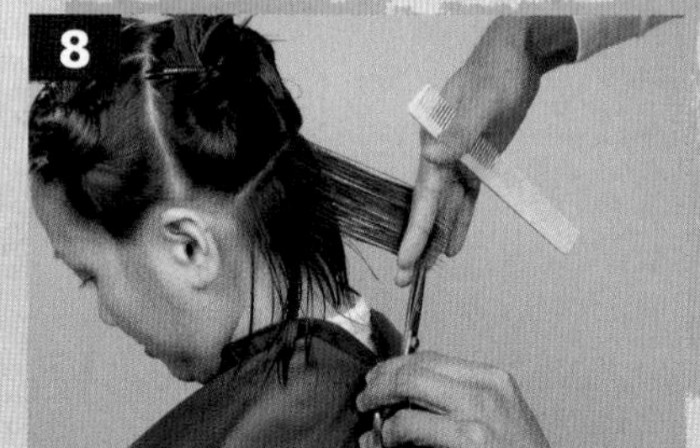
8

6 Establish your guideline by cutting the left side of the nape to the desired length. Use a horizontal cutting line parallel to the fingers. Cut the right side of the nape section the same length as the guideline.

7 Working upward in the left back section, measure and part off the first horizontal section approximately 1-inch wide.

8 Beginning at the center part, establish a vertical subsection approximately ½-inch (1.25 centimeters) wide. Extend the subsection down to include the nape guideline. Comb the subsection smooth at a 45-degree angle to the scalp. Hold your fingers at a 90-degree angle to the strand and cut.

9 Proceed to cut the entire horizontal section by parting off vertical subsections and cutting in the same manner. Check each section vertically and horizontally throughout the haircut. Each completed section will serve as a guideline for the next section.

10 Part off another horizontal section approximately 1-inch wide. Beginning at the center, create another vertical subsection that extends down and includes the previously cut strands. Comb the hair smoothly at a 45-degree elevation to the head. Hold the fingers and shears at a 90-degree angle to the subsection and cut. Cut the entire horizontal section this way. Make sure the second section blends evenly with the previously cut section.

11 Continue taking horizontal sections throughout the left and right back sections, and follow the same cutting procedure. The hair will gradually become longer as it reaches the apex. For example, if your nape guide was 2½-inches (6.25 centimeters) long, your upper crown section will be approximately 6-inches (15 centimeters) long.

© Milady, a part of Cengage Learning. Photography by Yanik Chauvin.

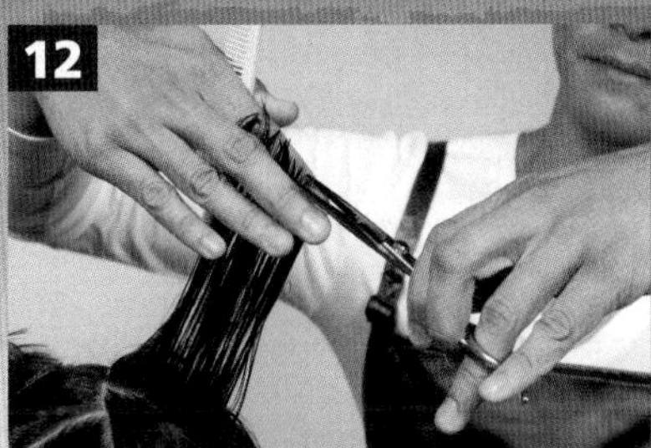

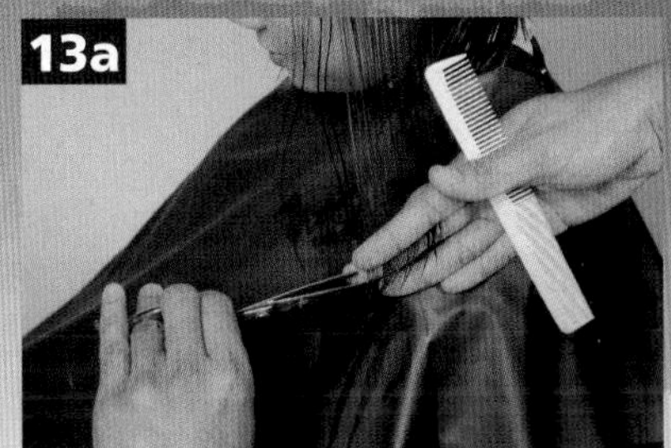

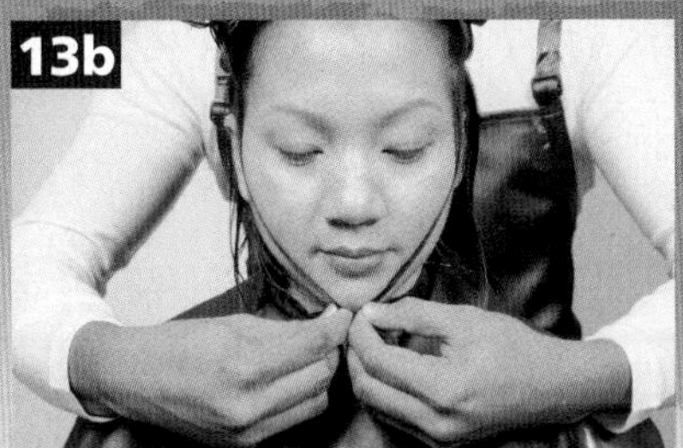

12 Maintain the length in the upper crown by holding each vertical subsection throughout the crown area at a 90-degree angle while cutting. After checking the back and crown for even blending, proceed to the right side section.

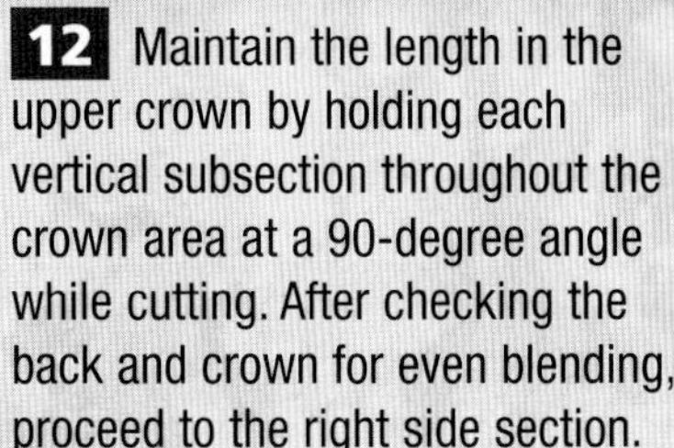

13a Establish a narrow guide section on the left side at the hairline approximately ½-inch wide. Cut side guideline to match the length in the nape.

13b Move to the right side of the head and establish a matching guideline there. This will help you to be sure that both side sections will be the same length when the right side section is cut later.

---

14 To cut the next section, establish a ½-inch parting that curves and follows the hairline above the ear back to the nape section. Smoothly comb the section, including the side guideline and part of the nape section.

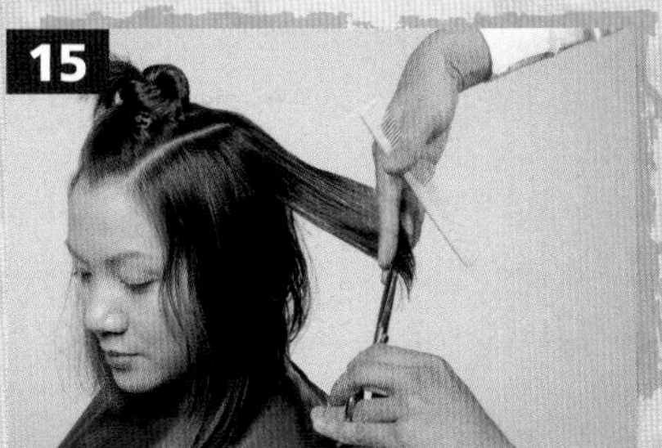

15 Holding the hair with little or no tension, cut the hair from the nape guide to the side guide. Note that the fingers are held at a slight angle to connect the two guides.

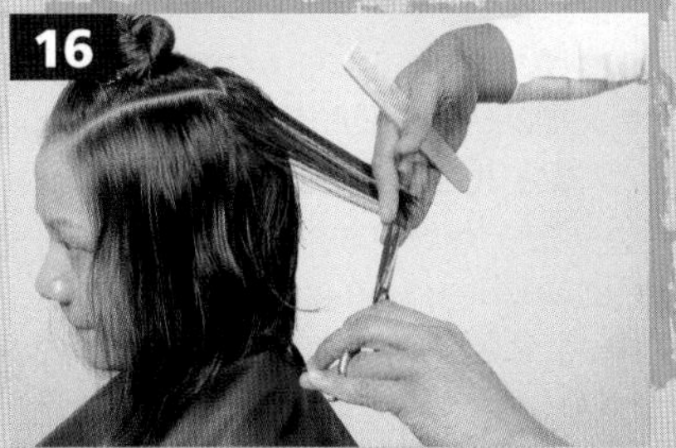

16 Establish a horizontal section on the left side, taking hair from the side and the crown area. The width of this section will vary because of the irregular hairline around the ear. This is how you will blend the side and back sections of the cut.

17 To begin cutting the side section, start at the ear, part a ½-inch vertical subsection (include the underlying guideline and a small portion of the nape section), and cut section.

18 Continue following the same cutting procedure. Take vertical subsections, comb smooth, elevate at a 45-degree angle from the head, holding the fingers at a 90-degree angle to the hair. Cut the section even with the side guideline and nape section. Be sure to hold the vertical subsections straight out from the head at 45 degrees, not pulled to the right or left.

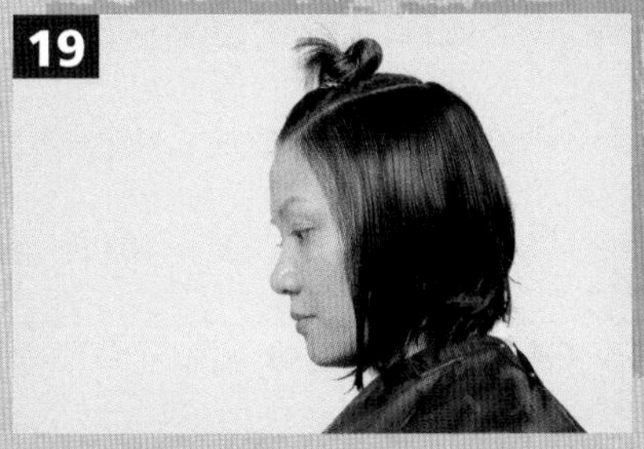

19 When the left side section is complete, the hair in the uppermost part of the section should be the same length as that in the upper crown area. In the final 1-inch section, comb the vertical subsections and hold them at a 90-degree angle to the head. Position your fingers at 90 degrees to the head and cut parallel to your fingers. Check the completed section horizontally to make sure the ends are even.

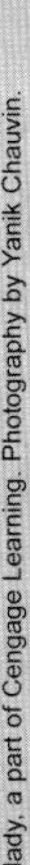
© Milady, a part of Cengage Learning. Photography by Yanik Chauvin.

Graduated Haircut: Left-Handed continued

20 Move to the right side of the head and cut the hair in the same manner as you did on the left side, using the previously established guide. Once the back and both sides are complete, move to the bang and top areas.

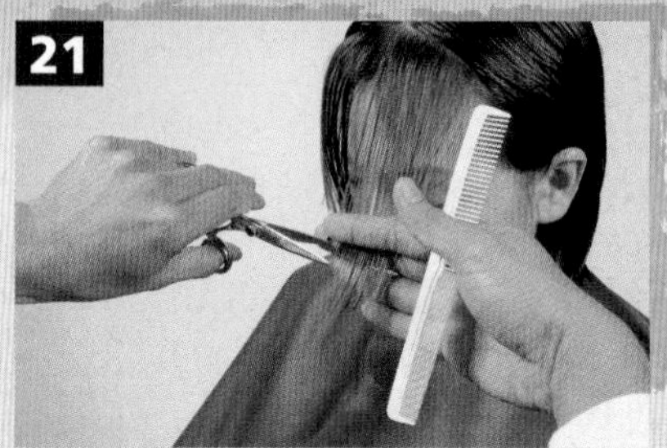
21

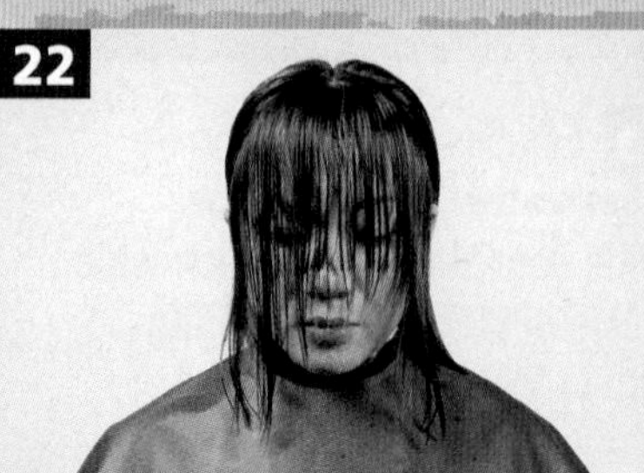
22

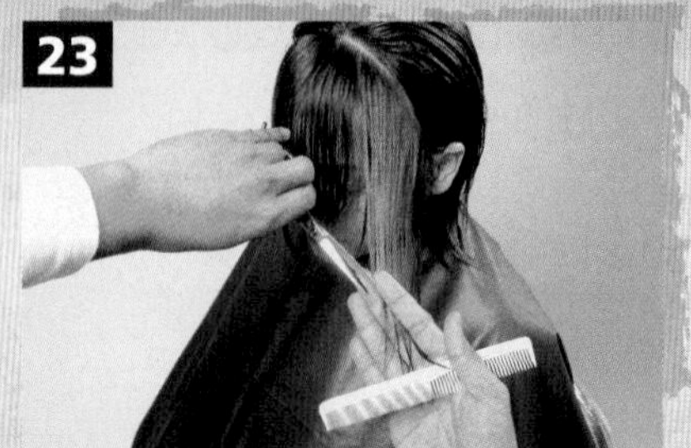
23

21 You can create a variety of bang (fringe) designs by cutting the bang length close to that of the side guideline. Create a bang guide section along the hairline about ½-inch wide. Starting on the right side of the forehead, cut to the desired length. Finish cutting the bang guide on the left side.

22 Bring down another ½-inch section and cut this subsection of the bang section at a low elevation, to the guideline.

23 Now take a vertical parting along the hairline that connects the guideline from the bang and the guideline from in front of the ear. Slide your hand slowly, keeping both guidelines in your grasp, and stop when you have only about a ¼ inch of both guidelines in your hand. Connecting the two guidelines will determine the angle of the cut. Complete the guideline on both sides of the head.

---

24 Using the guideline you established in the previous step, take ½-inch subsections and cut the top section at a 45-degree angle, blending with the sides.

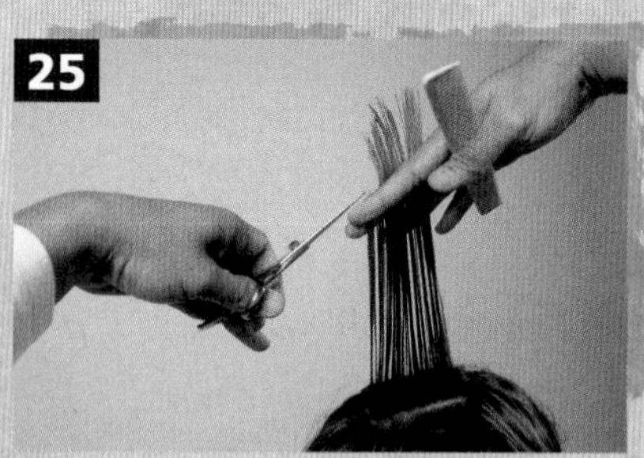
25

25 Finish the top section by taking ½-inch vertical subsections parallel to the center part. Hold the hair up from the head at a 90-degree angle. Include hair from the crown and bang area, and cut to blend the section with the two precut sections. Continue cutting in this manner until the remainder of the top section is cut. Hold the hair up from the head at a 90-degree angle and check the completed cut. Trim any uneven ends. The bang guide gradually increases in length to the pre-established length in the top and crown areas.

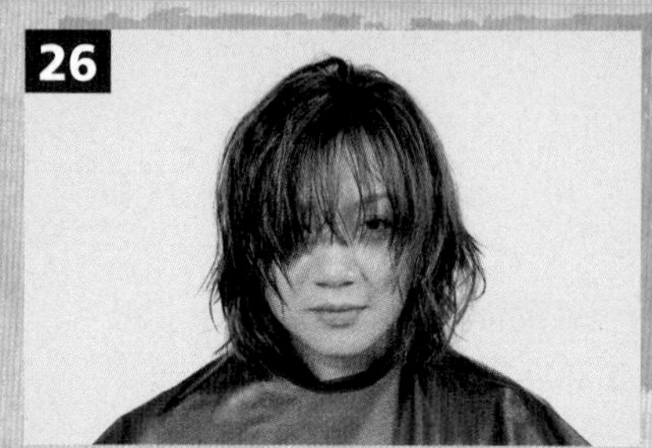
26

26 Once the cut is completed, use your hands to put the hair into place. Blowdry the haircut and view the design, movement, and ends to be sure they are evenly blended.

27 Finished look.

Post-Service

- Complete PROCEDURE 15-2 **Post-Service Procedure** SEE PAGE 326

© Milady, a part of Cengage Learning. Photography by Yanik Chauvin.

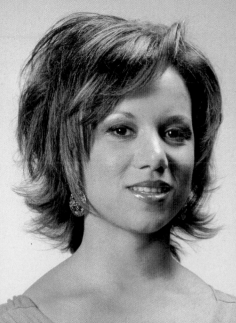

PROCEDURE 16-3 Right-Handed

Uniform-Layered Haircut

Implements and Materials

You will need all of the following implements, materials, and supplies:

- **Cutting cape**
- **Cutting or styling comb**
- **Haircutting shears**
- **Neck strip**
- **Sectioning clips**
- **Shampoo and conditioner**
- **Shampoo cape**
- **Spray bottle with water**
- **Towels**
- **Wide-tooth comb**

© Milady, a part of Cengage Learning. Photography by Yanik Chauvin.

Preparation

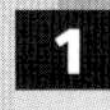

- Perform PROCEDURE 15-1 **Pre-Service Procedure** **SEE PAGE 323**

Procedure

1

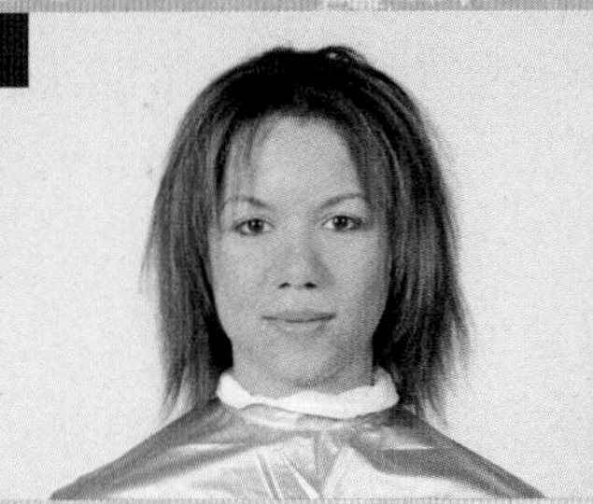

1 Drape your client for a shampoo.

2 Shampoo and condition the hair as necessary.

3 Escort the client back to the styling chair. Secure a neck strip around the client's neck. Place a cape over the neck strip and fasten in the back. Fold the neck strip down over the cape so that no part of the cape touches the client's skin.

4 Detangle the hair with the wide-tooth comb.

PROCEDURE 16-3

Uniform-Layered Haircut: Right-Handed

continued

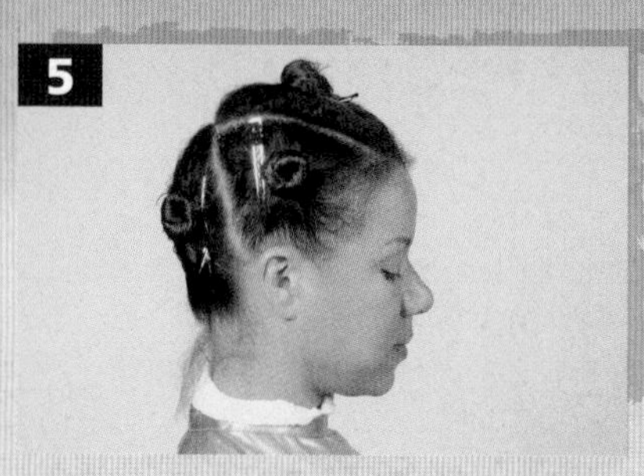

5

5 This haircut will use a five-section parting. Begin with a part from the front hairline just above the middle of each eyebrow back to the crown area, and clip the hair in place. Establish another part from the crown area where section one ends to the back of each ear, forming side sections two and three. Clip these sections in place. Part the hair down the center of the back to form sections four and five.

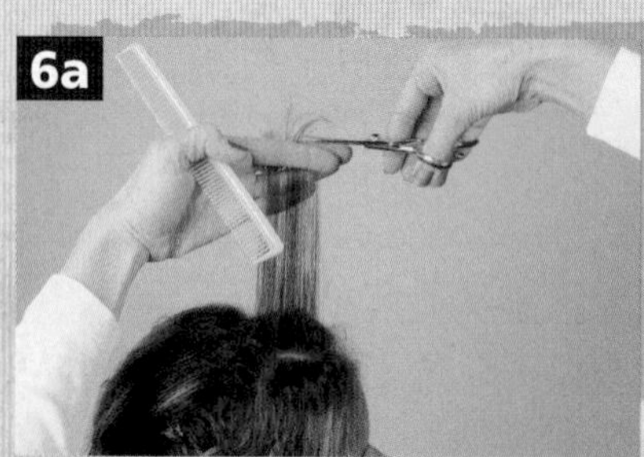

6a

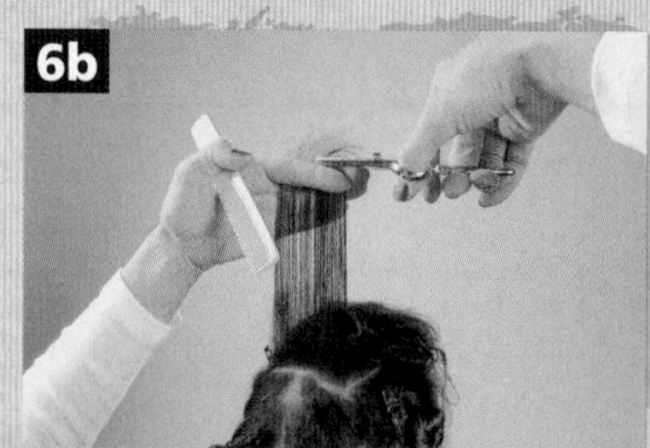

6b

6 To create the guideline, take two partings ½ inch (1.25 centimeters) apart, creating a section that runs from the front hairline to the bottom of the nape. Comb all other hair out of the way.

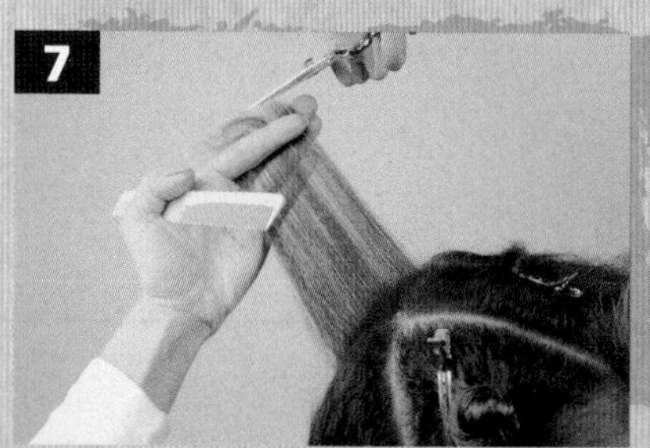

7

7 Beginning at the crown, comb the section straight out from the head, keeping your fingers parallel to the head form, and cut to the desired length. Continue working forward to the front hairline, making sure to stand to the side of the client.

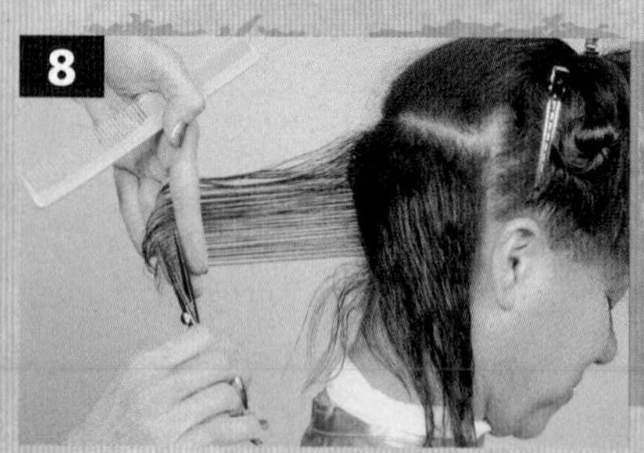

8

8 Continue cutting the guideline from the crown to the nape, rounding off any corners as you go along and making sure that your fingers are parallel to the head form.

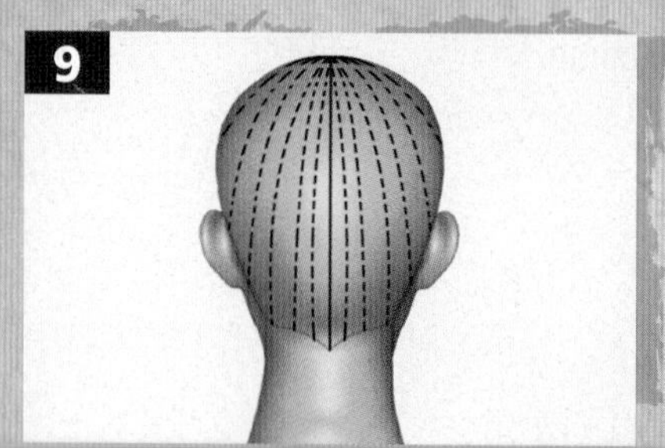

9

9 To maintain control and consistency while working through the haircut, separate the sides from the back by parting the hair from the apex to the back of the ear. Work through the back areas first. The parting pattern will be wedge shaped, where each section begins at the same point in the crown and is slightly wider at the bottom of the nape.

© Milady, a part of Cengage Learning. Photography by Yanik Chauvin.

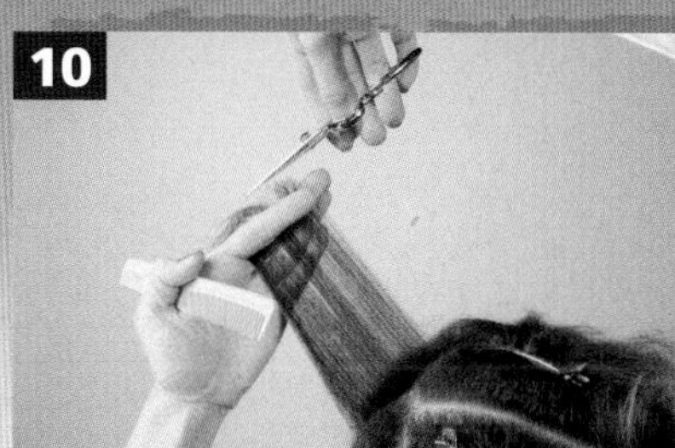

10 Work through the client's right side first. Take a vertical parting that begins at the crown and connects with the guideline, creating a vertical section that ends at the hairline. Keep the sections small to maintain control. Beginning at the crown and using the previously cut guideline, comb the new section to the guide, and elevate the hair straight out from the head, with no overdirection. Cut the line by keeping your fingers parallel to the head and matching the guideline.

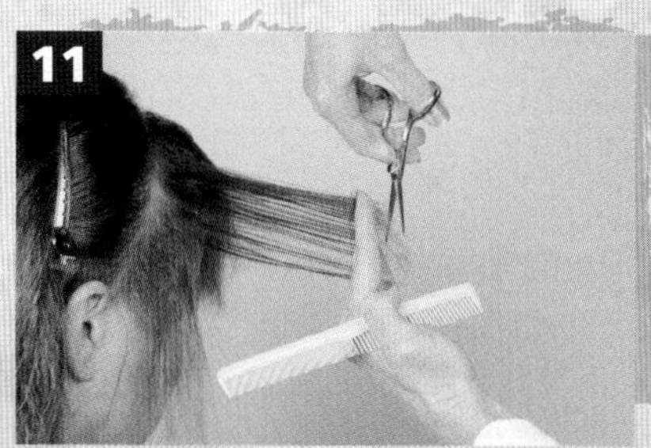

11 Continue working with a traveling guideline to the back of the ear. Repeat on the left side. When working on the left side of the back, shift your hand position so that you are now holding the section with the tips of your fingers pointing upwards and the tips of your shears pointing downwards. Part from the front of the ear to the front of the other ear, including the top and side areas.

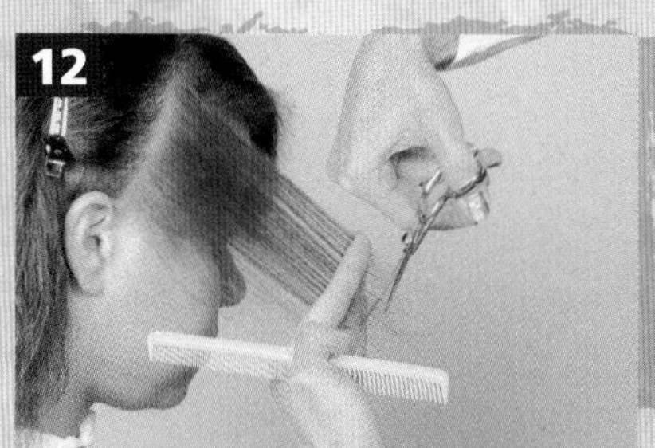

12 Now move to the side and top section. Take a section at the front hairline above the ear and begin to blend the top with the side section.

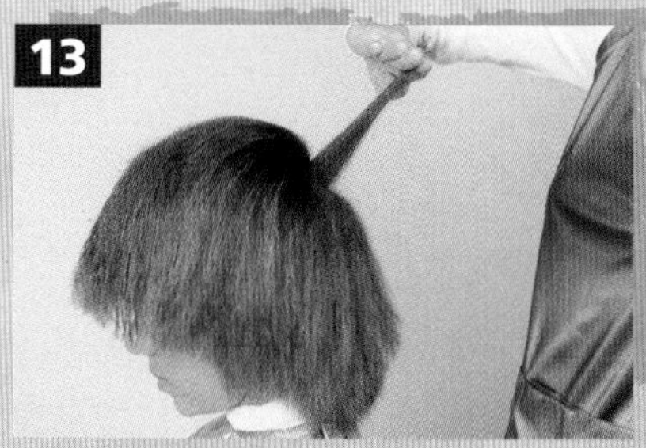

13 Continue cutting until the top and side sections are blended.

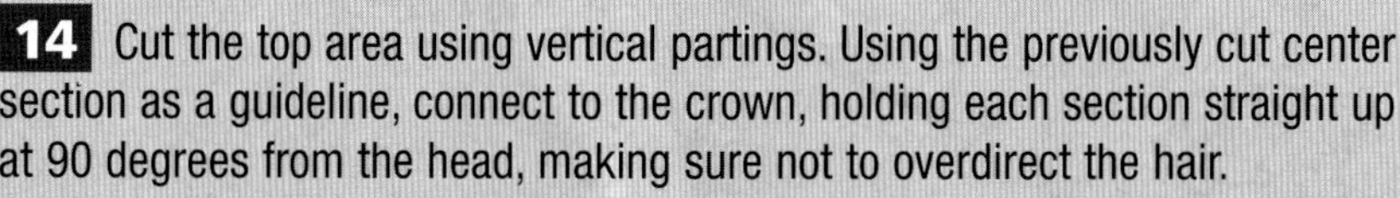

14 Cut the top area using vertical partings. Using the previously cut center section as a guideline, connect to the crown, holding each section straight up at 90 degrees from the head, making sure not to overdirect the hair.

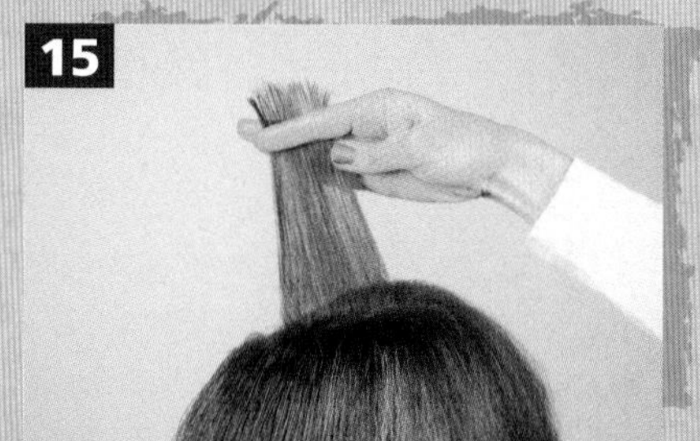

15 Cross-check the top, using horizontal partings and elevating the hair 90 degrees from the head.

© Milady, a part of Cengage Learning. Photography by Yanik Chauvin.

PROCEDURE 16-3

Uniform-Layered Haircut: Right-Handed continued

16 Now move to the right side. Work from the back of the ear toward the face, using vertical sections, and connect to the previous section at the back of the ear and the top. Comb the hair straight out from the head at 90 degrees, removing any corners as you go. Repeat on the left side. Cross-check the side sections.

17 Cross-check the side sections, using horizontal partings and combing the hair straight out at 90 degrees.

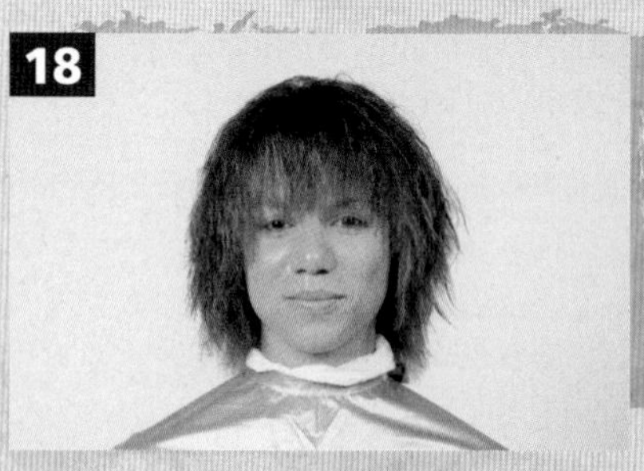

18 Comb the hair down. Note the soft perimeter and rounded head shape.

19 Blowdry and style the haircut using a vent brush to encourage movement.

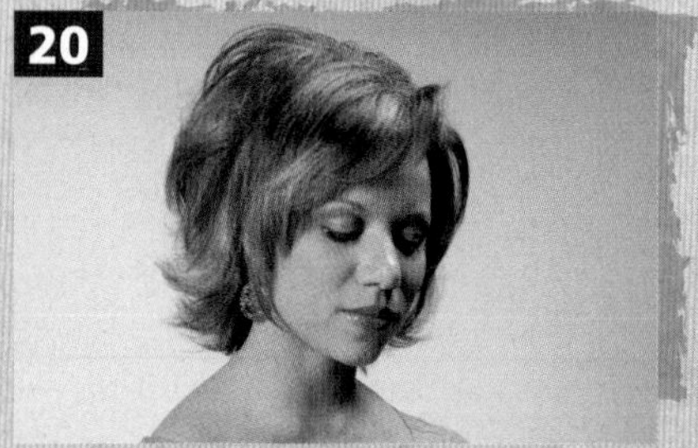

20 Finished look.

Post-Service

- Complete PROCEDURE 15-2 **Post-Service Procedure** SEE PAGE 326

© Milady, a part of Cengage Learning. Photography by Yanik Chauvin.

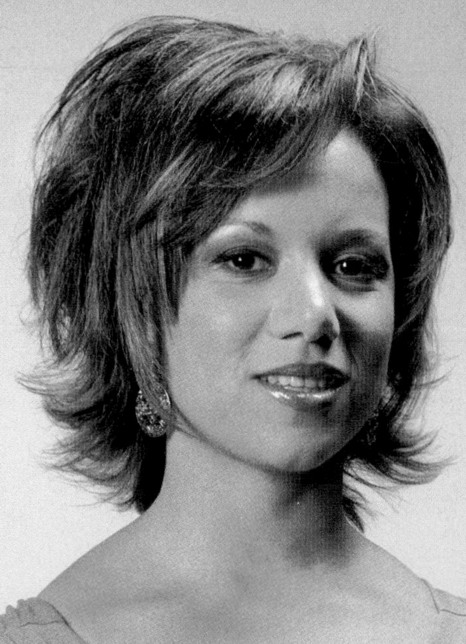

PROCEDURE 16-3 Left Handed

Uniform-Layered Haircut

Implements and Materials

You will need all of the following implements, materials, and supplies:

- **Cutting cape**
- **Cutting or styling comb**
- **Haircutting shears**
- **Neck strip**
- **Sectioning clips**
- **Shampoo and conditioner**
- **Shampoo cape**
- **Spray bottle with water**
- **Towels**
- **Wide-tooth comb**

© Milady, a part of Cengage Learning. Photography by Yanik Chauvin.

Preparation

- Perform PROCEDURE 15-1 **Pre-Service Procedure** **SEE PAGE 323**

Procedure

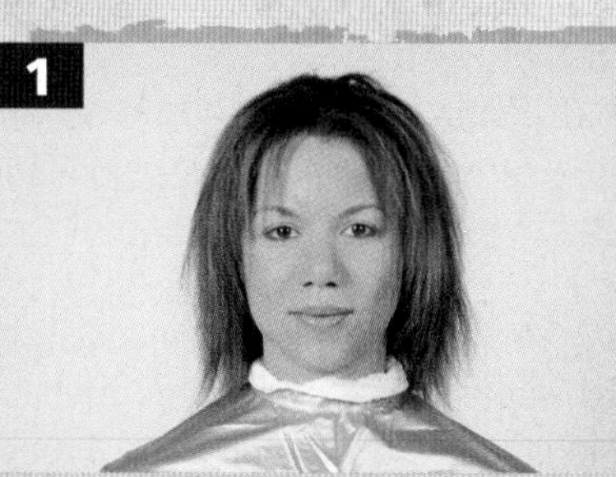

1 Drape your client for a shampoo.

2 Shampoo and condition the hair as necessary.

3 Escort the client back to the styling chair. Secure a neck strip around the client's neck. Place a cape over the neck strip and fasten in the back. Fold the neck strip down over the cape so that no part of the cape touches the client's skin.

4 Detangle the hair with the wide-tooth comb.

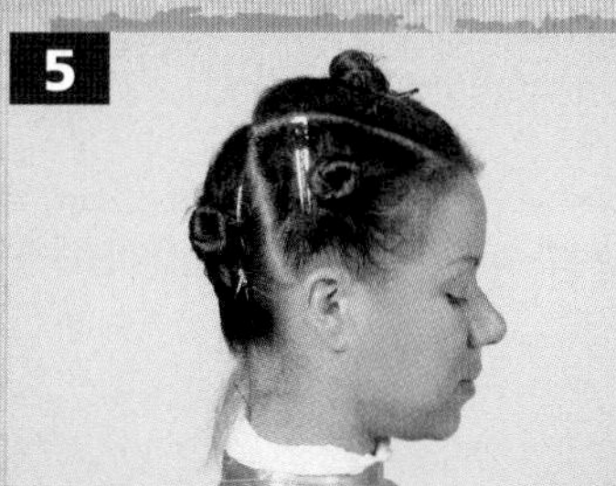

5 This haircut will use a five-section parting. Begin with a part from the front hairline just above the middle of each eyebrow back to the crown area, and clip the hair in place. Establish another part from the crown area where section one ends to the back of each ear, forming side sections two and three. Clip these sections in place. Part the hair down the center of the back to form sections four and five.

Uniform-Layered Haircut: Left-Handed continued

6 To create the guideline, take two partings ½ inch (1.25 centimeters) apart, creating a section that runs from the front hairline to the bottom of the nape. Comb all other hair out of the way.

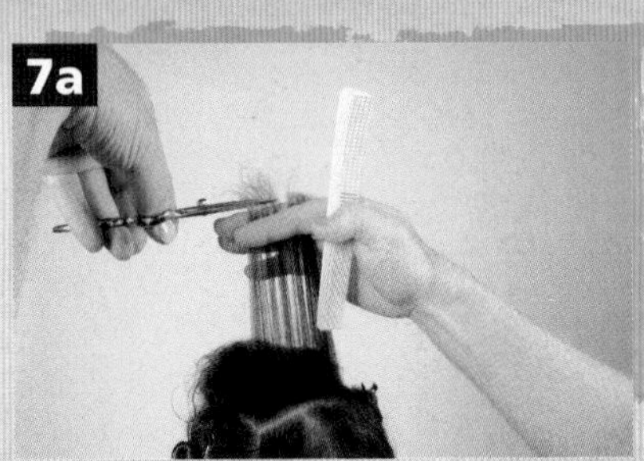

7a Beginning at the crown, comb the section straight out from the head, keeping your fingers parallel to the head form, and cut to the desired length.

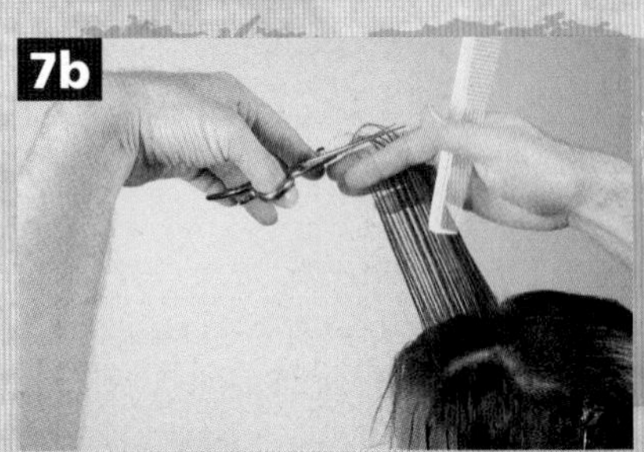

7b Continue working forward to the front hairline, making sure to stand to the side of the client.

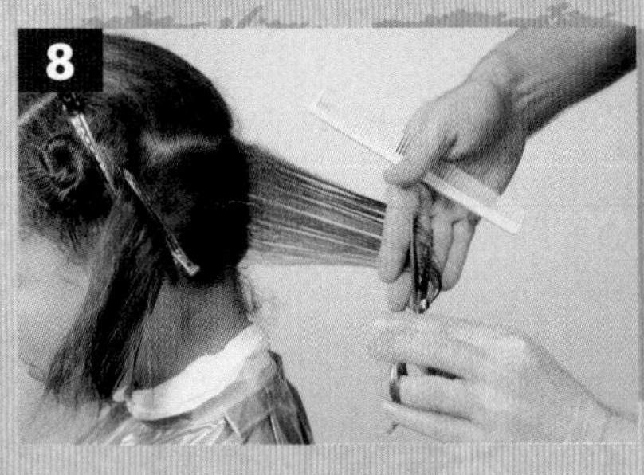

8 Continue cutting the guideline from the crown to the nape, rounding off any corners as you go along and making sure that your fingers are parallel to the head form.

9 To maintain control and consistency while working through the haircut, separate the sides from the back by parting the hair from the apex to the back of the ear. Work through the back areas first. The parting pattern will be wedge shaped, where each section begins at the same point in the crown and is slightly wider at the bottom of the nape.

10 Work through the client's left side first. Take a vertical parting that begins at the crown and connects with the guideline, creating a vertical section that ends at the hairline. Keep the sections small to maintain control. Beginning at the crown and using the previously cut guideline, comb the new section to the guide, and elevate the hair straight out from the head, with no overdirection. Cut the line by keeping your fingers parallel to the head and matching the guideline.

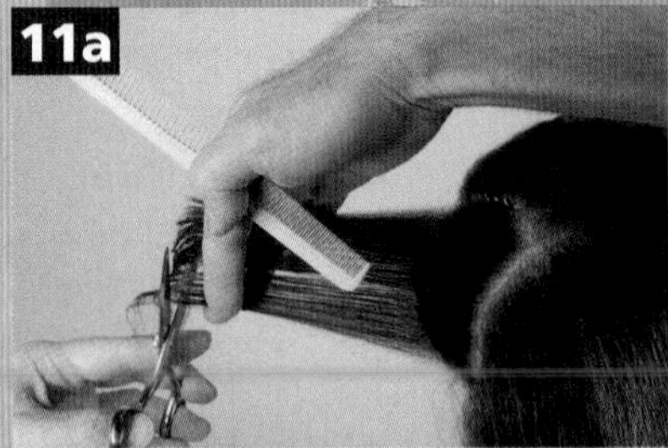

11a Continue working with a traveling guideline to the back of the ear.

© Milady, a part of Cengage Learning. Photography by Yanik Chauvin.

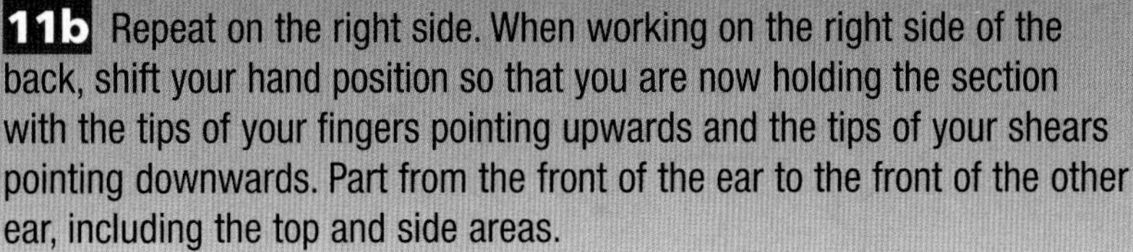

11b Repeat on the right side. When working on the right side of the back, shift your hand position so that you are now holding the section with the tips of your fingers pointing upwards and the tips of your shears pointing downwards. Part from the front of the ear to the front of the other ear, including the top and side areas.

12 Now move to the side and top section. Take a section at the front hairline above the ear and begin to blend the top with the side section.

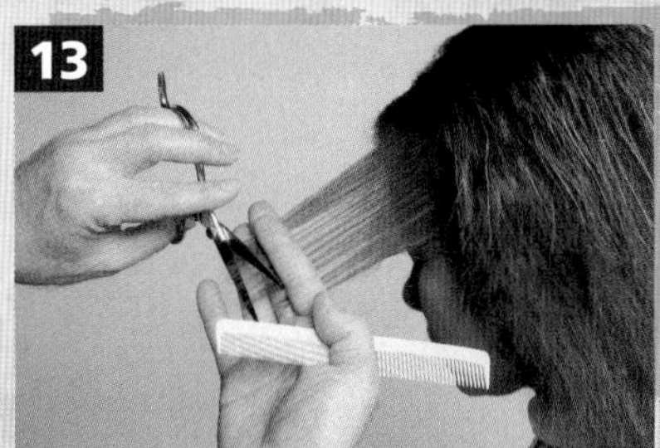

13 Continue cutting until the top and side sections are blended.

14 Using the previously cut center section as a guideline, connect to the crown, holding each section straight up at 90 degrees from the head, making sure not to overdirect the hair. Cross-check the cut hair in the crown area.

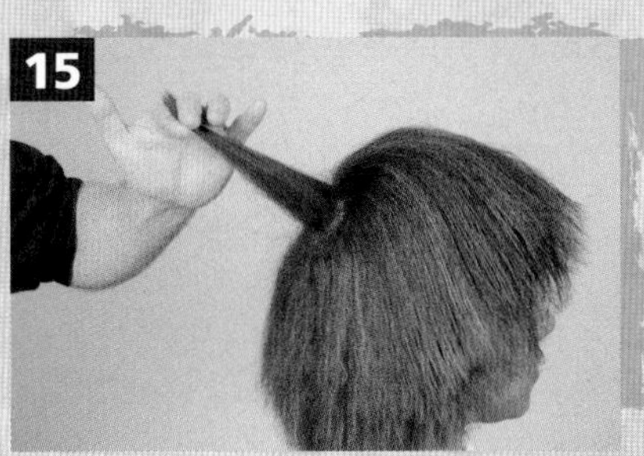

15 Cross-check the top, using horizontal partings and elevating the hair 90 degrees from the head.

16 Now move to the right side. Work from the back of the ear toward the face, using vertical sections, and connect to the previous section at the back of the ear and the top. Comb the hair straight out from the head at 90 degrees, removing any corners as you go. Repeat on the left side. Cross-check the side sections.

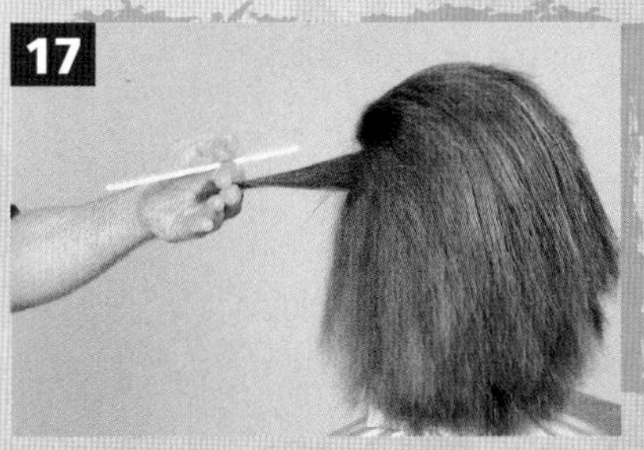

17 Cross-check the side sections, using horizontal partings and combing the hair straight out at 90 degrees.

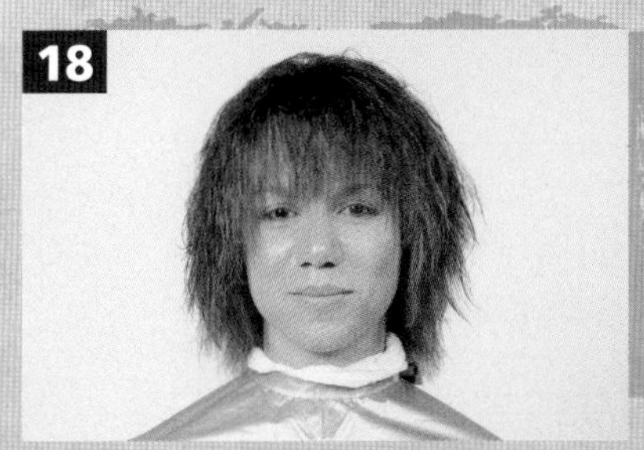

18 Comb the hair down. Note the soft perimeter and rounded head shape.

19 Blowdry and style the haircut using a vent brush to encourage movement.

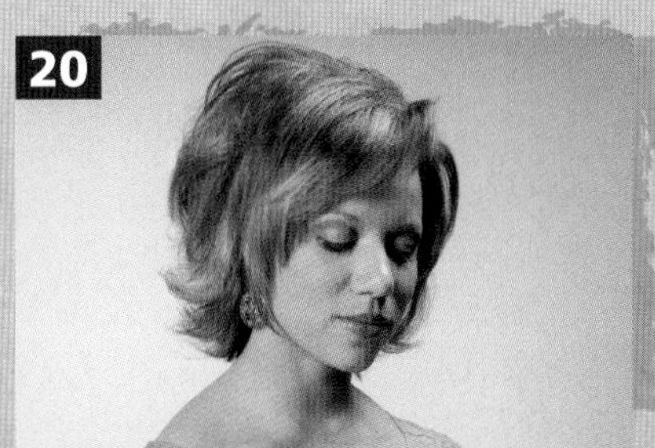

20 Finished look.

Post-Service

- Complete PROCEDURE 15-2 **Post-Service Procedure** **SEE PAGE 326**

© Milady, a part of Cengage Learning. Photography by Yanik Chauvin.

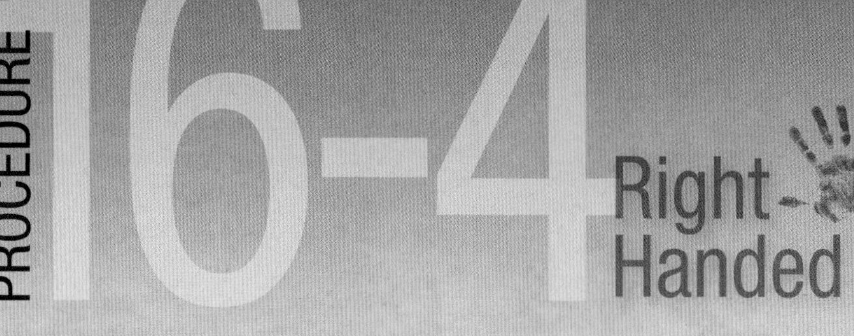

Long-Layered (180-Degree) Haircut

Implements and Materials

You will need all of the following implements, materials, and supplies:

- **Cutting cape**
- **Cutting or styling comb**
- **Haircutting shears**
- **Neck strip**
- **Sectioning clips**
- **Shampoo and conditioner**
- **Shampoo cape**
- **Spray bottle with water**
- **Towels**
- **Wide-tooth comb**

Preparation

- Perform PROCEDURE 15-1 **Pre-Service Procedure** **SEE PAGE 323**

Procedure

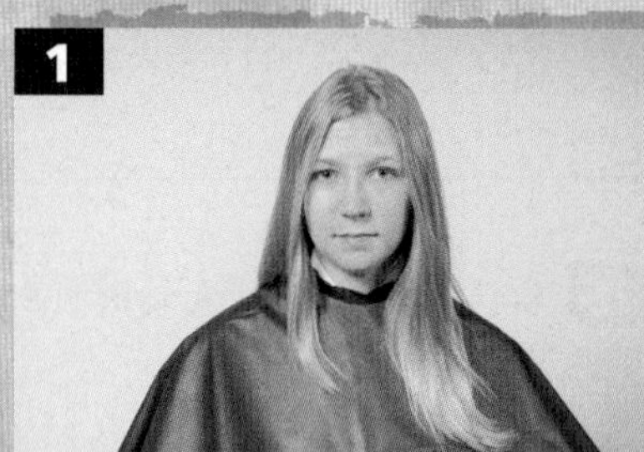

1 Drape your client for a shampoo.

2 Shampoo and condition the hair as necessary.

3 Escort the client back to the styling chair. Secure a neck strip around the client's neck. Place a cape over the neck strip and fasten in the back. Fold the neck strip down over the cape so that no part of the cape touches the client's skin.

4 Detangle the hair with the wide-tooth comb.

© Milady, a part of Cengage Learning. Photography by Yanik Chauvin.

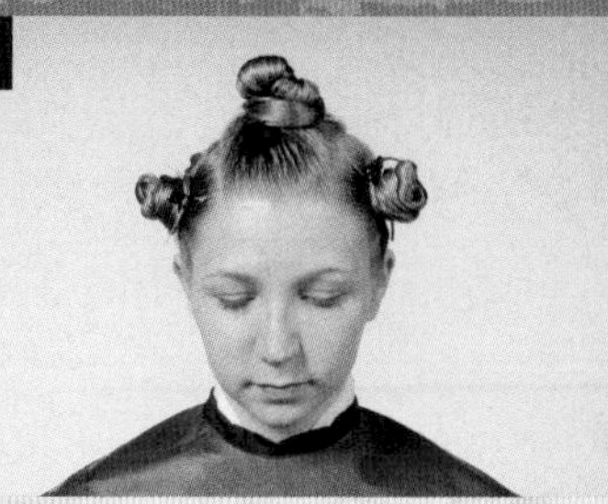

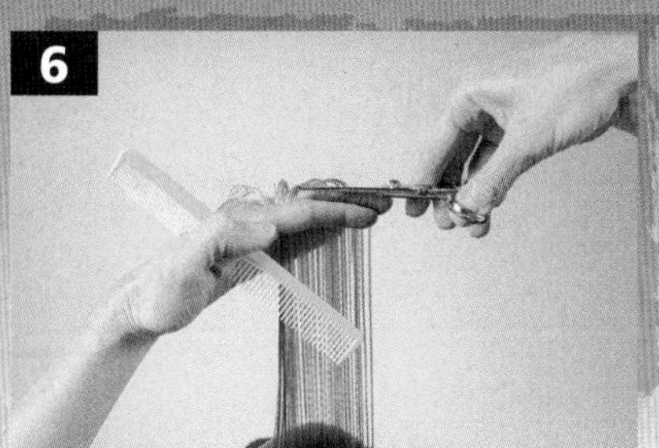

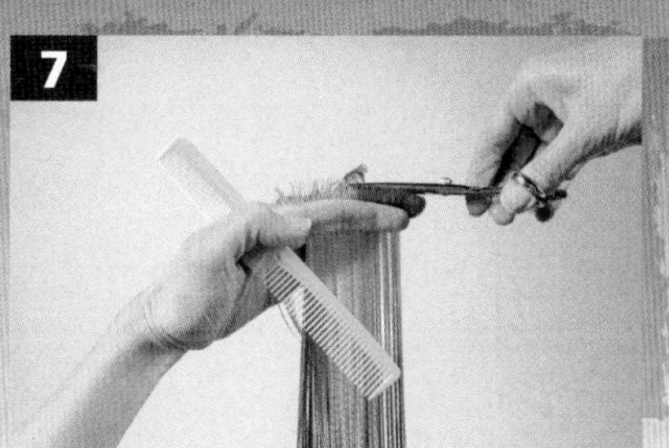

5 Part the hair into five sections, as in step 5 of Procedure 16-3.

6 Begin at the top of the crown by taking a ½-inch (1.25 centimeters) subsection across the head. Comb straight up from the head form and cut straight across.

7 Work to the front of the top section by taking a second ½-inch subsection. Direct the first subsection (guideline) to the second one and cut to the same length.

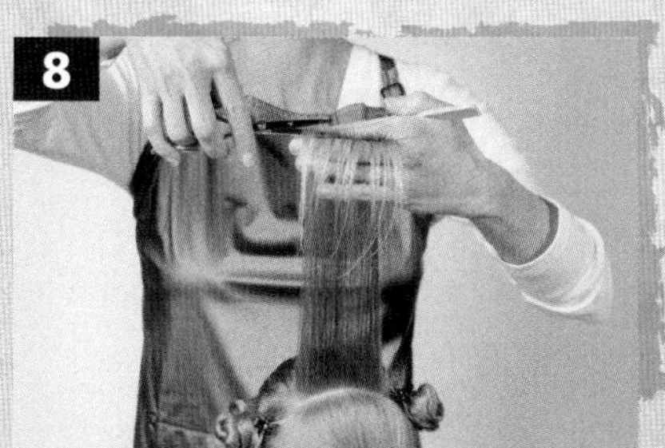

8 Continue, using the previously cut subsection as your guideline to cut a new ½-inch subsection throughout the top section.

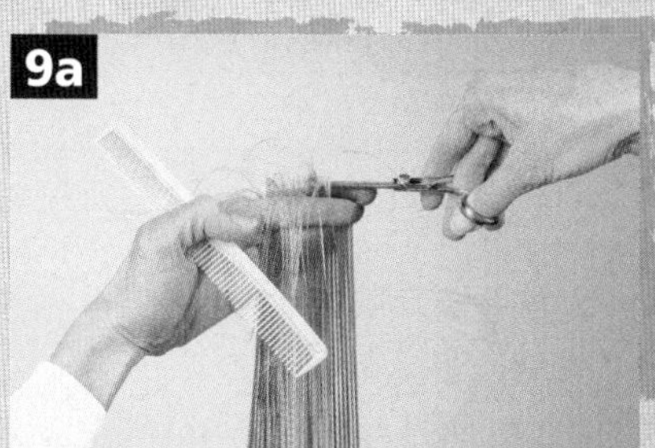

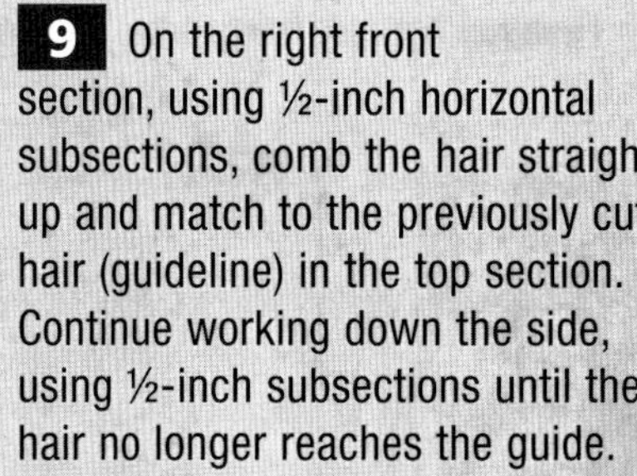

9 On the right front section, using ½-inch horizontal subsections, comb the hair straight up and match to the previously cut hair (guideline) in the top section. Continue working down the side, using ½-inch subsections until the hair no longer reaches the guide.

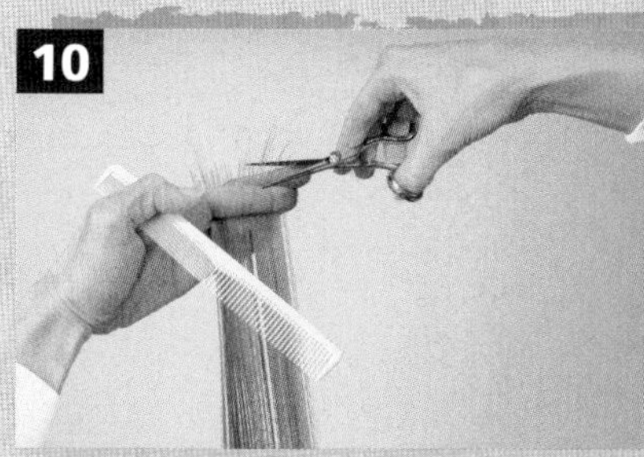

10 Repeat on the left side.

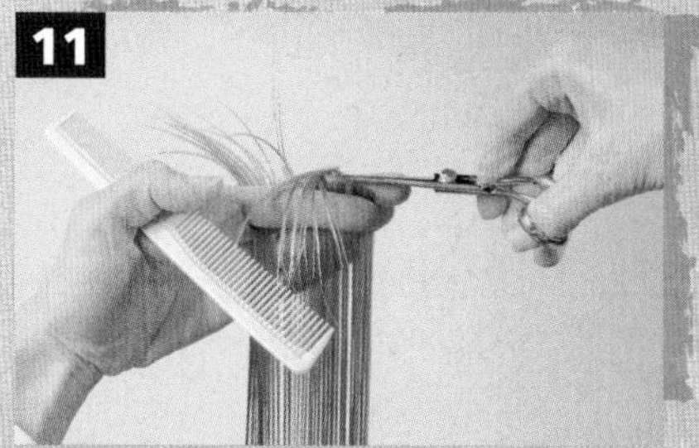

11 Complete the back sections.

12 Continue cutting using ½-inch horizontal subsections and working from top to bottom until the hair no longer reaches the guideline.

© Milady, a part of Cengage Learning. Photography by Yanik Chauvin.

PROCEDURE 16-4

Long-Layered (180-Degree) Haircut: Right-Handed continued

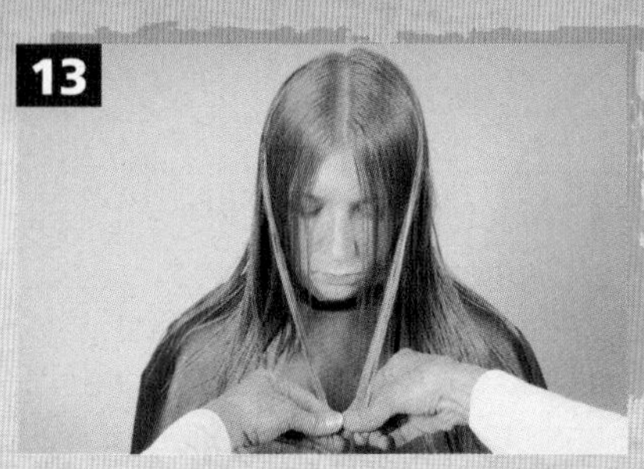

13 Check to be sure both sides are the same length.

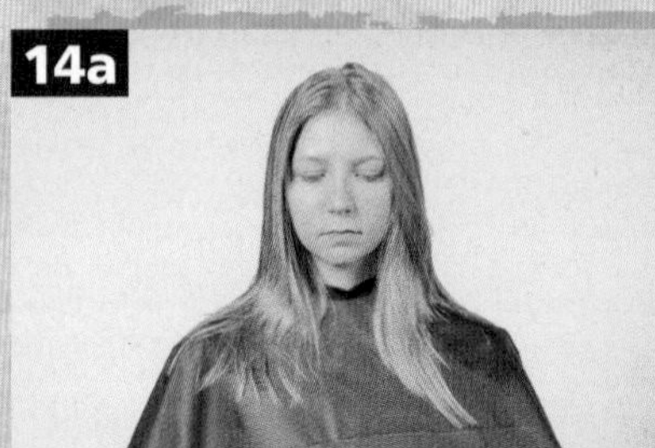

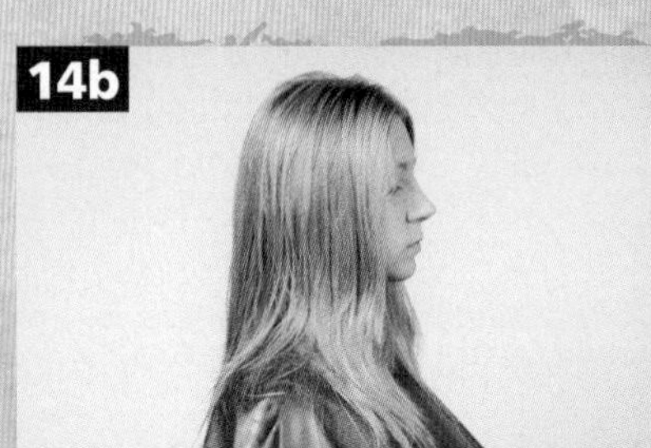

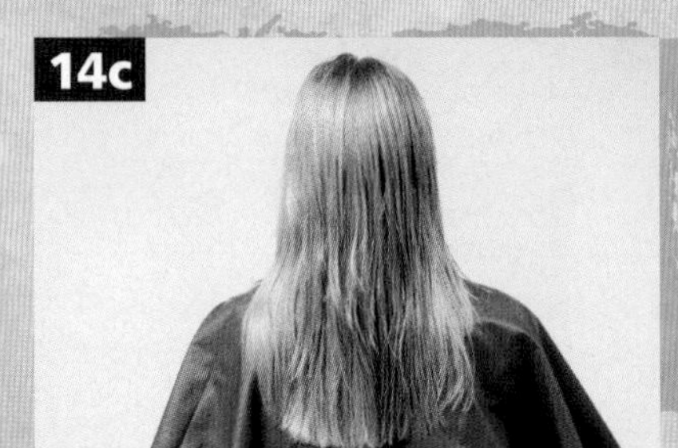

14 Finished haircut: front, side, and back.

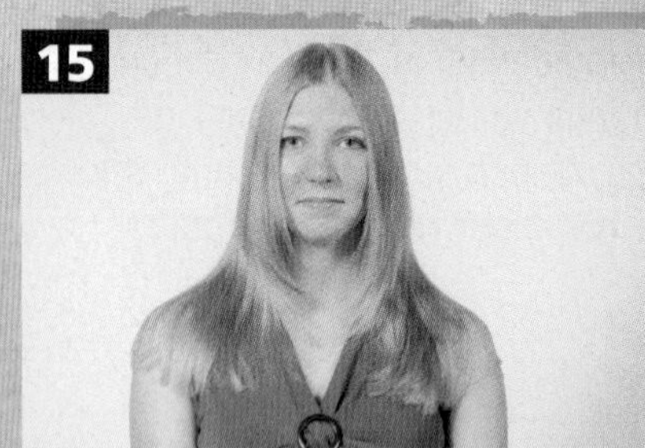

15 Finished look.

Post-Service

- Complete PROCEDURE 15-2 Post-Service Procedure SEE PAGE 326

© Milady, a part of Cengage Learning. Photography by Yanik Chauvin.

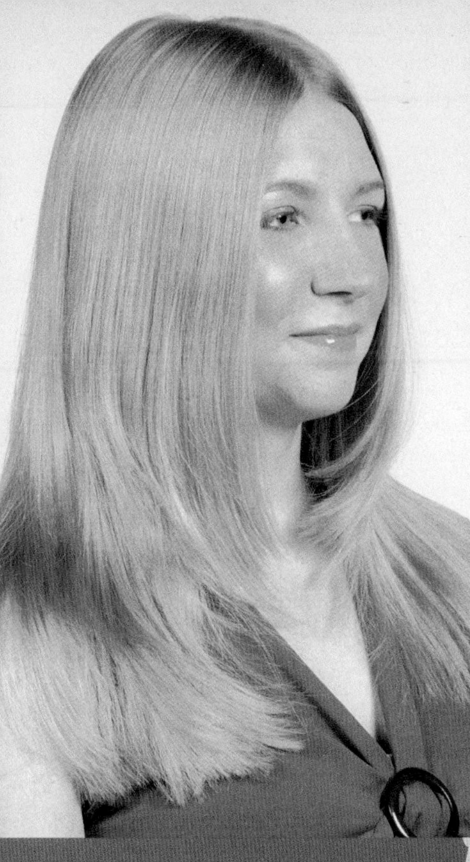

PROCEDURE 16-4 Left Handed

Long-Layered (180-Degree) Haircut

Preparation

- Perform PROCEDURE 15-1 Pre-Service Procedure SEE PAGE 323

Procedure

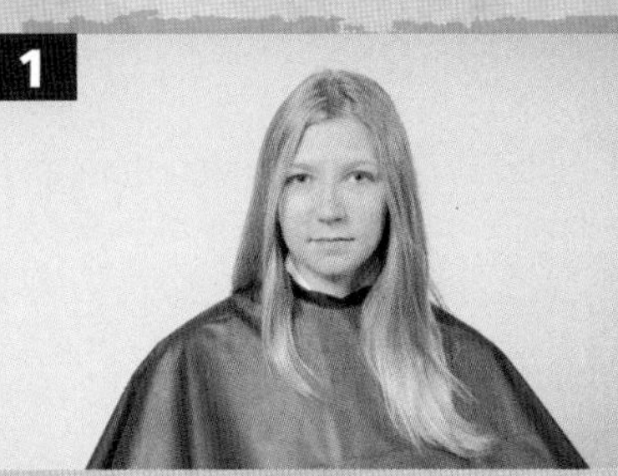

1 Drape your client for a shampoo.

2 Shampoo and condition the hair as necessary.

3 Escort the client back to the styling chair. Secure a neck strip around the client's neck. Place a cape over the neck strip and fasten in the back. Fold the neck strip down over the cape so that no part of the cape touches the client's skin.

4 Detangle the hair with the wide-tooth comb.

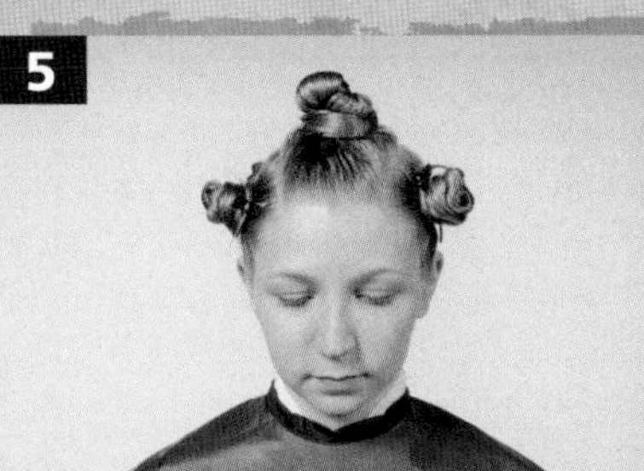

5 Part the hair into five sections, as in step 5 of Procedure 16-3.

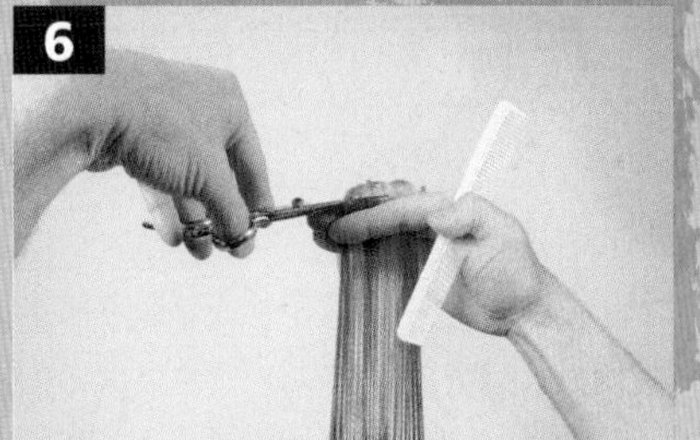

6 Begin at the top of the crown by taking a ½-inch (1.25 centimeters) subsection across the head. Comb straight from the head form and cut straight across.

Implements and Materials

You will need all of the following implements, materials, and supplies:

- **Cutting cape**
- **Cutting or styling comb**
- **Haircutting shears**
- **Neck strip**
- **Sectioning clips**
- **Shampoo and conditioner**
- **Shampoo cape**
- **Spray bottle with water**
- **Towels**
- **Wide-tooth comb**

© Milady, a part of Cengage Learning. Photography by Yanik Chauvin.

Long-Layered (180-Degree) Haircut: Left-Handed continued

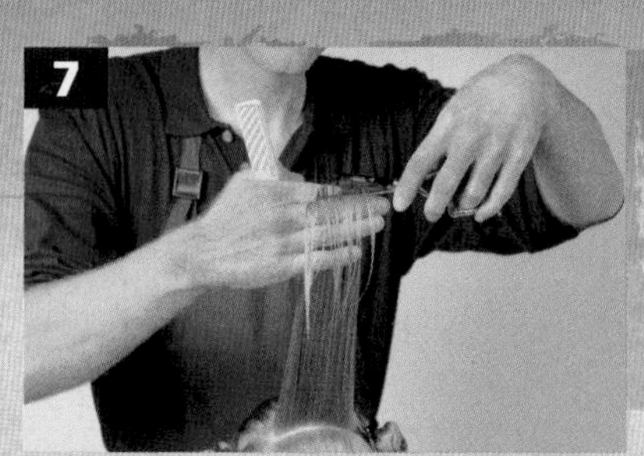

7 Work to the front of the top section by taking a second ½-inch subsection. Direct the first subsection (guideline) to the second one and cut to the same length.

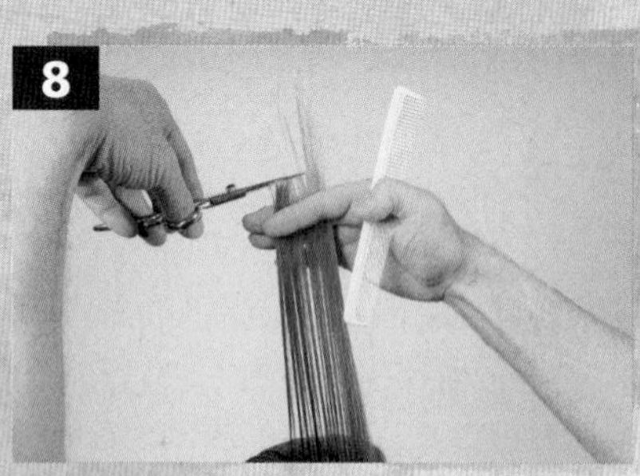

8 Continue, using the previously cut subsection as your guideline to cut a new ½-inch subsection throughout the top section.

9 On the left front section, using ½-inch horizontal subsections, comb the hair straight up and match to the previously cut hair (guideline) in the top section. Continue working down the side, using ½-inch subsections until the hair no longer reaches the guide.

10 Repeat on the right side.

11 Complete the back sections.

12 Continue cutting, using ½-inch horizontal subsections and working from top to bottom until the hair no longer reaches the guideline.

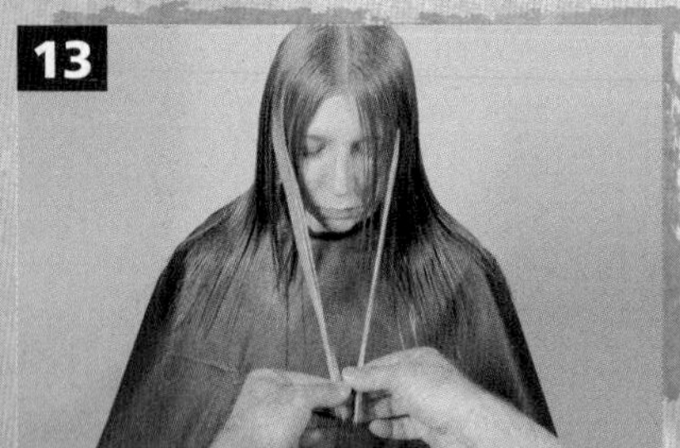

13 Check to be sure both sides are the same length.

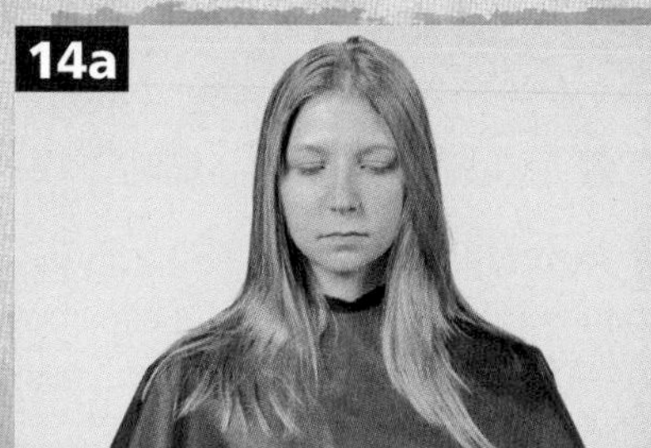

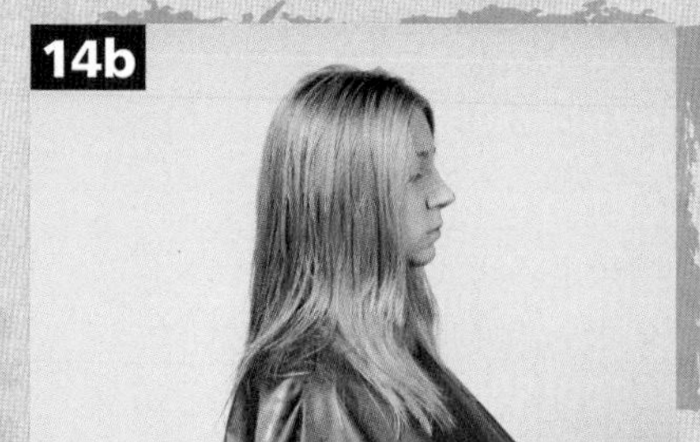

14 Finished haircut: front, side, and back.

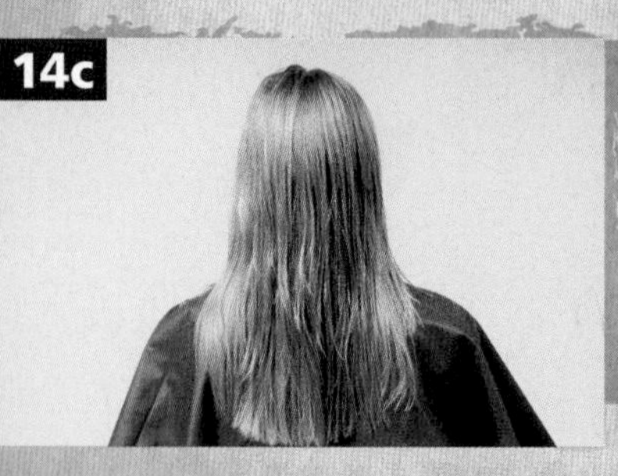

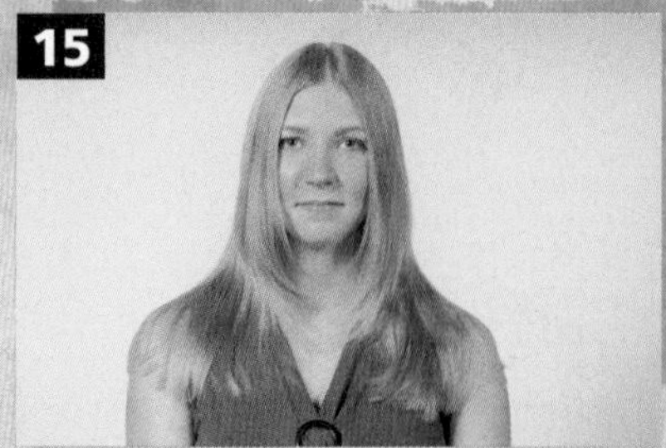

15 Finished look.

Post-Service

- Complete

PROCEDURE 15-2 **Post-Service Procedure**

SEE PAGE 326

© Milady, a part of Cengage Learning. Photography by Yanik Chauvin.

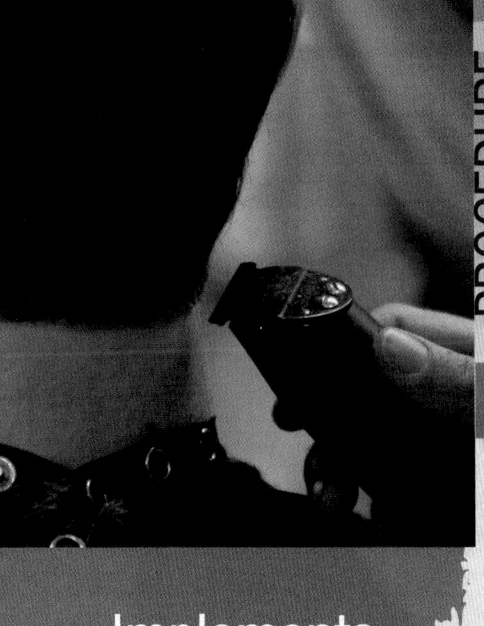

PROCEDURE 16-5

Men's Basic Clipper Cut

Implements and Materials

You will need all of the following implements, materials, and supplies:

- **Barber comb**
- **Clipper**
- **Cutting cape**
- **Haircutting comb**
- **Haircutting shears**
- **Low-number guard attachment (optional)**
- **Neck strip**
- **Shampoo and conditioner**
- **Spray bottle with water**
- **Towels**
- **Trimmer**
- **Wide-tooth comb**

© Milady, a part of Cengage Learning. Photography by Paul Castle. Castle Photography.

Preparation

- Perform PROCEDURE 15-1 Pre-Service Procedure SEE PAGE 323

Procedure

1 Drape your client for a shampoo.

2 Shampoo and condition the hair as necessary.

3 Escort the client back to the styling chair. Secure a neck strip around the client's neck. Place a cape over the neck strip and fasten in the back. Fold the neck strip down over the cape so that no part of the cape touches the client's skin.

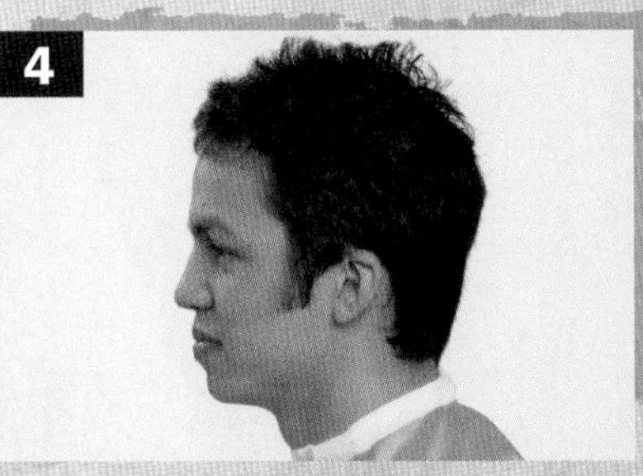

4 Towel dry and detangle the hair with the wide-tooth comb.

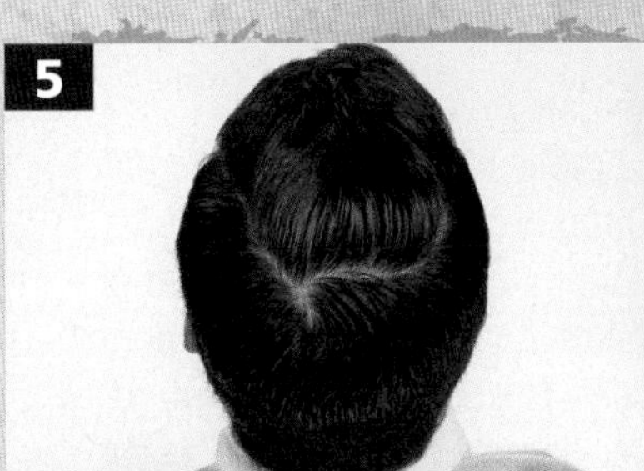

5 Make a horseshoe parting about 2 inches (5 centimeters) below the apex of the head, beginning and ending at the front hairline. Comb the hair above the part forward.

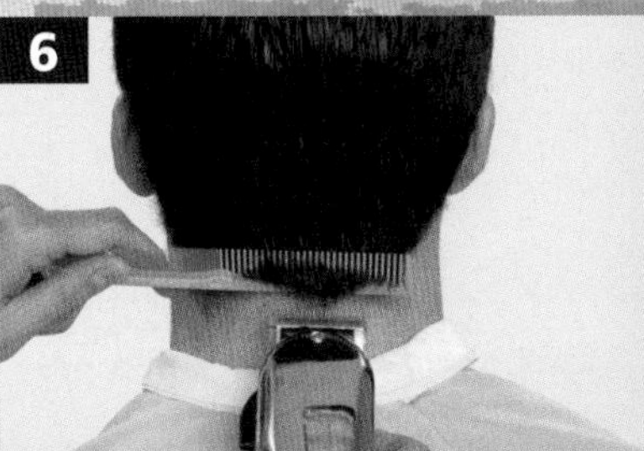

6 Starting in the nape area, place the haircutting comb against the scalp, teeth up. Angle the comb against the scalp from 0 to 45 degrees, allowing for the natural contour of the head. Cut the hair that extends through the teeth of the comb.

Men's Basic Clipper Cut continued

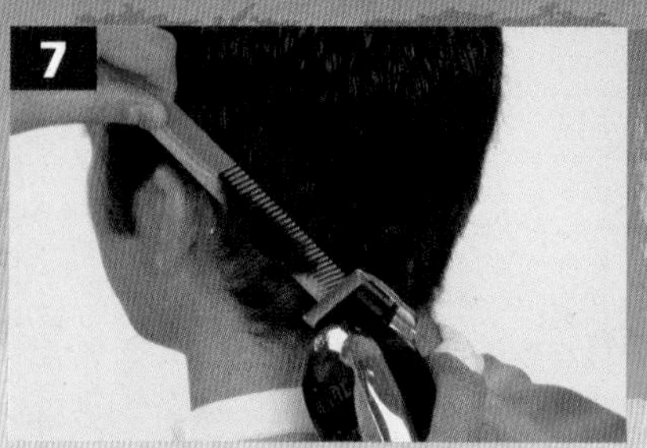

7 Repeat step 6 as you move up the back of the head. Blend the lengths over the curve of the head by cross-cutting horizontally, from side to side. Shape the back center area first, from the nape to the parietal ridge. Then, still using the clipper-over-comb technique, cut both sides of the back from ear to ear.

8 Carefully blend the lengths over the curve of the head by cross-cutting.

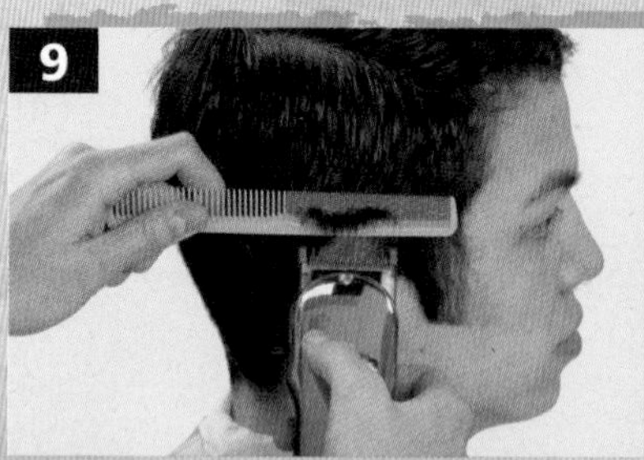

9 Using a low-number length attachment on the clipper, cut up each side from the sideburn to the parietal ridge. The hair length will be very close to the scalp. If the client wants longer sides, the weight on the top will need to be blended.

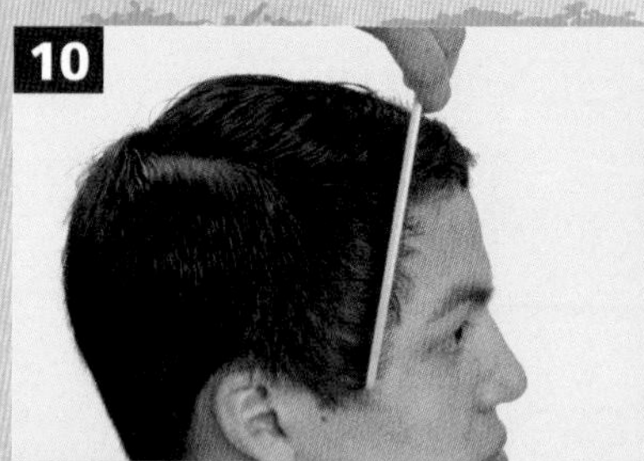

10 Measure the distance between the eyebrows and the natural hairline to establish a guideline for the length in the crown area if the client wishes to keep hair out of the eyes.

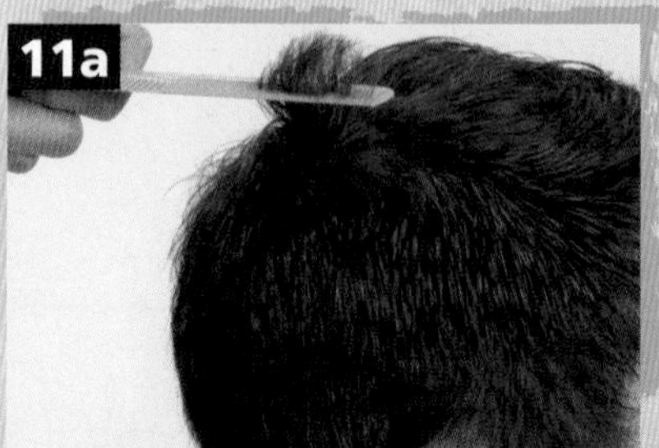

11a Cut a narrow guideline at the crown end of the horseshoe parting. Determine the length by the forehead measurement. Beginning at the crown end, cut the top area with the clipper to the exact length of the initial crown guideline.

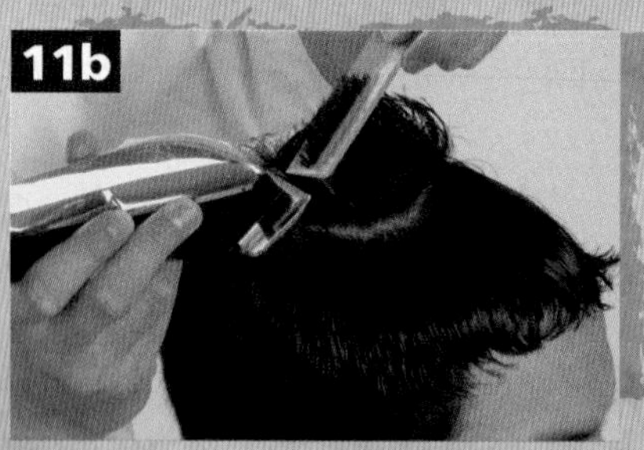

11b As you move toward the forehead, overdirect the hair back toward the guideline in order to increase the length at the forehead.

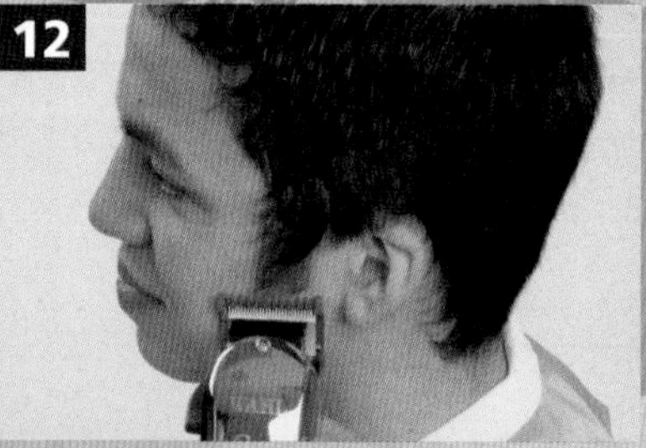

12 Using the clipper and attachment, shorten and shape the hair around the ears and sideburns. To blend or outline the perimeter of the haircut, you may use a clipper or trimmer. The scissor-over-comb or clipper-over-comb technique, using the front teeth of a barber comb, may also be used here.

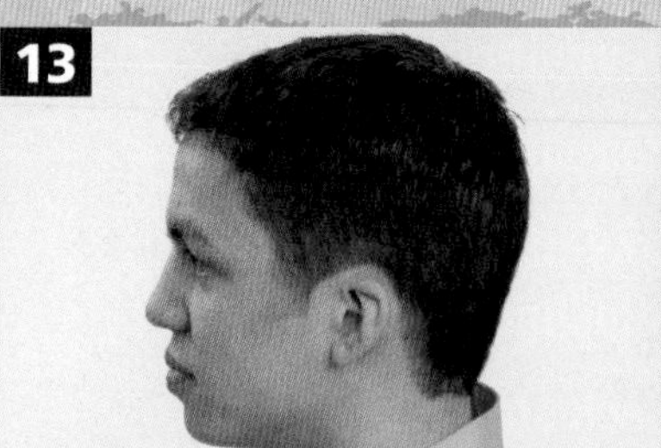

13 Finished look.

© Milady, a part of Cengage Learning. Photography by Paul Castle, Castle Photography.

Post-Service

- Complete PROCEDURE 15-2 Post-Service Procedure SEE PAGE 326

Review Questions

1. What are reference points and what is their function?
2. What are angles, elevations, and guidelines?
3. What are important considerations to discuss with a client during a haircutting consultation?
4. What is a razor, haircutting shear, styling or cutting comb, and texturizing shear used for?
5. What are three things you can do to ensure good posture and body position while cutting hair?
6. Name and describe the four basic types of haircuts.
7. Name and describe three different texturizing techniques performed with shears.
8. What is a clipper cut?
9. How is a trimmer used?

Chapter Glossary

angle	Space between two lines or surfaces that intersect at a given point.
apex	Highest point on the top of the head.
beveling	Haircutting technique using diagonal lines by cutting hair ends with a slight increase or decrease in length.
blunt haircut	Also known as a *one-length haircut*; haircut in which all the hair comes to one hanging level, forming a weight line or area; hair is cut with no elevation or overdirection.
carving	Haircutting technique done by placing the still blade into the hair and resting it on the scalp, and then moving the shears through the hair while opening and partially closing the shears.
cast	Method of manufacturing shears; a metal-forming process whereby molten steel is poured into a mold and, once the metal is cooled, takes on the shape of the mold.
clipper-over-comb	Haircutting technique similar to scissor-over-comb, except that the clippers move side to side across the comb rather than bottom to top.
cross-checking	Parting the haircut in the opposite way from which you cut it in order to check for precision of line and shape.
crown	Area of the head between the apex and back of the parietal ridge.
cutting line	Angle at which the fingers are held when cutting, and, ultimately, the line that is cut; also known as *finger angle*, *finger position*, *cutting position*, or *cutting angle*.
distribution	Where and how hair is moved over the head.
elevation	Also known as *projection* or *lifting*; angle or degree at which a subsection of hair is held, or lifted, from the head when cutting.
forged	Process of working metal to a finished shape by hammering or pressing.

Chapter Glossary

four corners	Points on the head that signal a change in the shape of the head, from flat to round or vice versa.
free-hand notching	Haircutting technique in which pieces of hair are snipped out at random intervals.
free-hand slicing	Haircutting technique used to release weight from the subsection, allowing the hair to move more freely.
graduated haircut	Graduated shape or wedge; an effect or haircut that results from cutting the hair with tension, low to medium elevation, or overdirection.
graduation	Elevation occurs when a section is lifted above 0 degrees.
growth pattern	Direction in which the hair grows from the scalp; also referred to as natural fall or natural falling position.
guideline	Also known as *guide*; section of hair, located either at the perimeter or the interior of the cut, that determines the length the hair will be cut. Usually the first section that is cut to create a shape.
hairline	Hair that grows at the outermost perimeter along the face, around the ears, and on the neck.
head form	Also known as *head shape*; shape of the head, which greatly affects the way the hair falls and behaves.
interior	Inner or internal part.
interior guideline	Guideline that is inside the haircut rather than on the perimeter.
layered haircut	Graduated effect achieved by cutting the hair with elevation or overdirection; the hair is cut at higher elevations, usually 90 degrees or above, which removes weight.
layers	Create movement and volume in the hair by releasing weight.
line	Thin continuous mark used as a guide; can be straight or curved, horizontal, vertical, or diagonal.
long-layered haircut	Haircut in which the hair is cut at a 180-degree angle; the resulting shape has shorter layers at the top and increasingly longer layers toward the perimeter.
nape	Back part of the neck; the hair below the occipital bone.
notching	Haircutting technique, a version of point cutting, in which the tips of the scissors are moved toward the hair ends rather than into them; creates a chunkier effect.
occipital bone	Bone that protrudes at the base of the skull.
overdirection	Combing a section away from its natural falling position, rather than straight out from the head, toward a guideline; used to create increasing lengths in the interior or perimeter.
palm-to-palm	Cutting position in which the palms of both hands are facing each other.
parietal ridge	Widest area of the head, usually starting at the temples and ending at the bottom of the crown.

Chapter Glossary

part/parting	Line dividing the hair at the scalp, separating one section of hair from another, creating subsections.
perimeter	Outer line of a hairstyle.
point cutting	Haircutting technique in which the tips of the shears are used to cut *points* into the ends of the hair.
razor-over-comb	Texturizing technique in which the comb and the razor are used on the surface of the hair.
razor rotation	Texturizing technique similar to razor-over-comb, done with small circular motions.
reference points	Points on the head that mark where the surface of the head changes or the behavior of the hair changes, such as ears, jawline, occipital bone, apex, and so on; used to establish design lines that are proportionate.
scissor-over-comb	Also known as *shear-over-comb*; haircutting technique in which the hair is held in place with the comb while the tips of the scissors are used to remove the lengths.
sections	To divide the hair by parting into uniform working areas for control.
shrinkage	When hair contracts or lifts through the action of moisture loss or drying.
slicing	Haircutting technique that removes bulk and adds movement through the lengths of the hair; the shears are not completely closed, and only the portion of the blades near the pivot is used.
slide cutting	Method of cutting or thinning the hair in which the fingers and shears glide along the edge of the hair to remove length.
slithering	Also known as *effilating*; process of thinning the hair to graduated lengths with shears; cutting the hair with a sliding movement of the shears while keeping the blades partially opened.
stationary guideline	Guideline that does not move.
subsections	Smaller sections within a larger section of hair, used to maintain control of the hair while cutting.
taper	Haircutting effect in which there is an even blend from very short at the hairline to longer lengths as you move up the head; *to taper* is to narrow progressively at one end.
tension	Amount of pressure applied when combing and holding a section, created by stretching or pulling the section.
texturizing	Haircutting technique designed to remove excess bulk without shortening the length; changing the appearance or behavior of the hair through specific haircutting techniques using shears, thinning shears, or a razor.
traveling guideline	Also known as *movable guideline*; guideline that moves as the haircutting progresses, used often when creating layers or graduation.
uniform layers	Hair is elevated to 90 degrees from the scalp and cut at the same length.
weight line	Visual line in the haircut where the ends of the hair hang together.

CHAPTER 17

Hairstyling

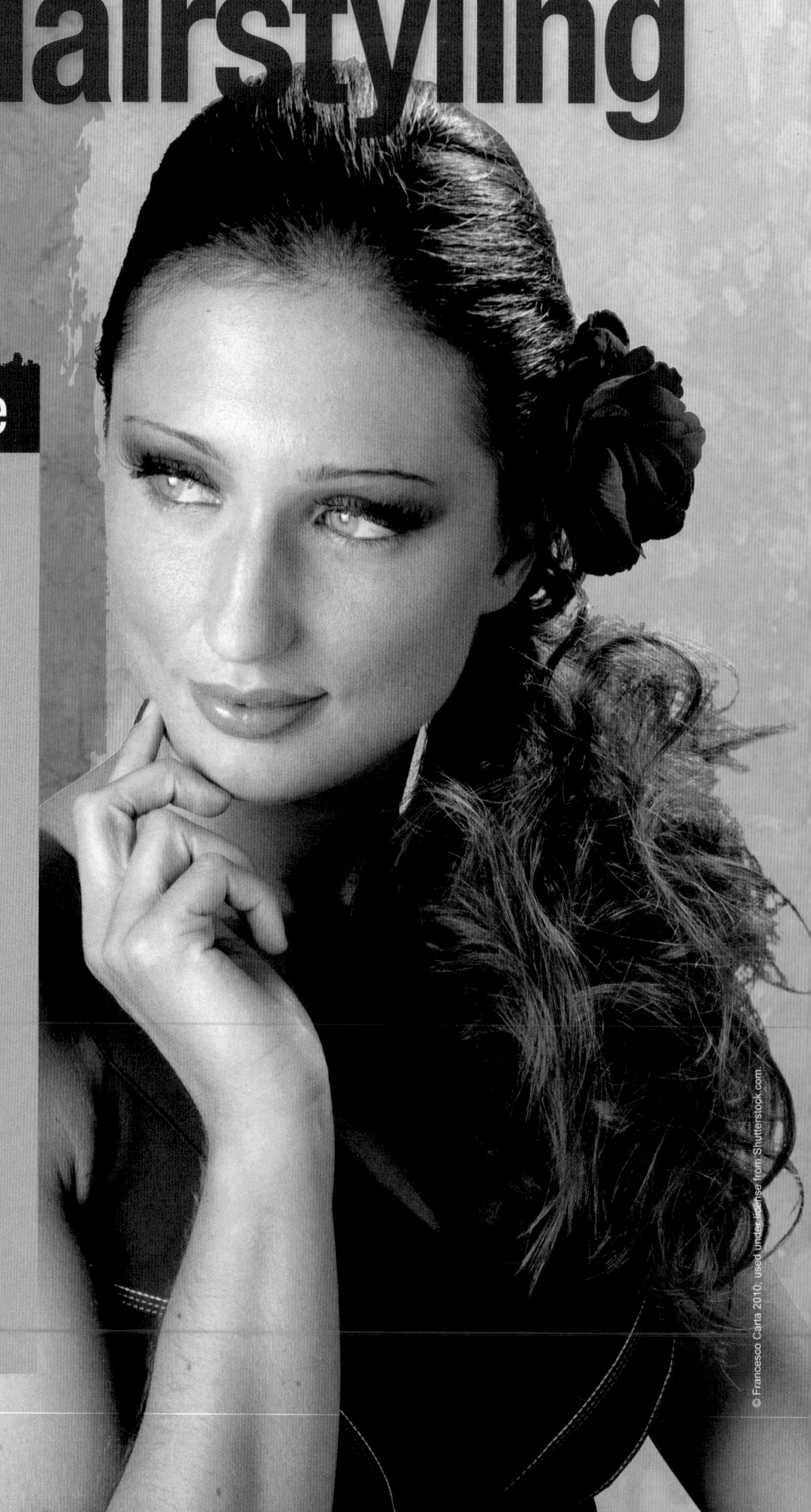
© Francesco Carta 2010; used under license from Shutterstock.com.

Chapter Outline

Why Study Hairstyling?

Client Consultation

Wet Hairstyling Basics

Finger Waving

Pin Curls

Roller Curls

Comb-Out Techniques

Hair Wrapping

Blowdry Styling

Thermal Hairstyling

Thermal Hair Straightening (Hair Pressing)

Styling Long Hair

Formal Styling

The Artistry of Hairstyling

Procedures

After completing this chapter, you will be able to:

- ✓ **LO1** Demonstrate finger waving, pin curling, roller setting, and hair wrapping.
- ✓ **LO2** Demonstrate various blowdry styling techniques.
- ✓ **LO3** Demonstrate the proper use of thermal irons.
- ✓ **LO4** Demonstrate various thermal iron manipulations and explain how they are used.
- ✓ **LO5** Describe the three types of hair pressing.
- ✓ **LO6** Demonstrate the procedures for soft pressing and hard pressing.
- ✓ **LO7** Demonstrate three basic techniques of styling long hair.

Key Terms

Page number indicates where in the chapter the term is used.

backbrushing (ruffing)
pg. 429

backcombing (teasing, ratting, matting, French lacing)
pg. 429

barrel curls
pg. 425

base
pg. 422

blowdry styling
pg. 431

carved curls (sculptured curls)
pg. 425

cascade curls (stand-up curls)
pg. 425

circle
pg. 423

closed-center curls
pg. 423

concentrator
pg. 431

curl (circle)
pg. 427

diffuser
pg. 431

double press
pg. 442

end curls
pg. 439

finger waving
pg. 421

foam (mousse)
pg. 433

full-base curls
pg. 440

full-stem curl
pg. 423

gel
pg. 433

hair pressing
pg. 441

hair spray (finishing spray)
pg. 434

hair wrapping
pg. 431

half base
pg. 427

half-base curls
pg. 440

half-stem curl
pg. 423

hard press
pg. 442

indentation
pg. 428

knot (chignon)
pg. 446

liquid gels (texturizers)
pg. 434

medium press
pg. 441

no-stem curl
pg. 423

off base
pg. 427

off-base curls
pg. 440

on base (full base)
pg. 427

open-center curls
pg. 423

pleat (classic French twist)
pg. 446

pomade (wax)
pg. 434

ribboning
pg. 424

ridge curls
pg. 425

rod
pg. 436

shaping
pg. 423

shell
pg. 436

skip waves
pg. 425

soft press
pg. 441

spiral curl
pg. 439

stem
pg. 422

straightening gel
pg. 434

temper
pg. 444

thermal irons
pg. 435

thermal waving and curling (Marcel waving)
pg. 435

twist
pg. 446

updo
pg. 446

volume-base curls
pg. 439

volumizers
pg. 434

waving lotion
pg. 421

The art of hairstyling or dressing the hair has always changed in direct relation to the fashion, art, and life of the times. When you compare the ornate hair fantasies of Marie Antoinette and her court prior to the French Revolution to the sleek bobs with finger waves and pin curls of flappers during the 1920s and 1930s, when streamline modern or art deco was the rage, you can see how a person's hairstyle reflects the period in which they live (**Figure 17–1**).

With ready-to-wear clothing came wash-and-wear hair, misleading many hairstylists to believe that finishing a style was no longer necessary. With the exception of styling for formal occasions, many stylists have passed this important part of the hair experience into the hands of the client. It is our professional responsibility to educate clients about at-home maintenance and styling options for their hair. No matter how great the haircut or haircolor, a client will often judge your work by the finished style.

Historical and technical knowledge of hairstyling will prepare you for the constant cyclical changes of fashion. Inspiration is often found in the past. Think retro—because what is out of style today may be back in style tomorrow. By learning the basic styling techniques, you will be ready and able to create what dreams are made of and to hear a satisfied client happily say, "This is what I always wanted."

Why Study Hairstyling?

Cosmetologists should study and have a thorough understanding of hairstyling because:

- Hairstyling is an important, foundational skill that allows the professional to articulate creativity and deliver a specific outcome desired by the client.
- Clients rely on you to teach them about their hair and how to style it so they can have a variety of options based on their lifestyle and fashion needs. You are the expert!
- The client looks to you for that special style desired for that special day.
- Hairstyling skills will enable you to help clients to be as contemporary as they would like to be, allowing them to keep up with the trends.

▼ Figure 17–1
Today, many women wear beautiful and dramatic finger-wave styles for special occasions.

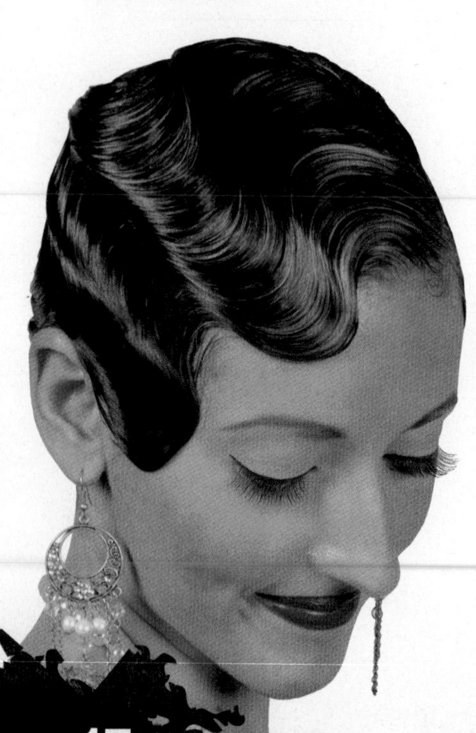

© Milady, a part of Cengage Learning. Photography by Yanik Chauvin.

Client Consultation

The client consultation is always the first step in the hairstyling process. Have your client look through magazines to find styles that she likes, or better yet, show her your portfolio of hairstyles. A picture is worth a thousand words. When deciding the best hairstyle, take into consideration all that you have learned in Chapter 14, Principles of Hair Design, regarding face shape, hair type, and lifestyle.

Often, you will be called upon as a creative problem solver. What if, on the client's last visit to another salon, she asked for a hairstyle that was not right for her hair? Because the stylist did not suggest something more appropriate, the outcome was disastrous. Now you are being asked to fix the problem. If you can come up with an alternative style, one that is both flattering and easy to manage, she may become one of your most loyal clients.

Wet Hairstyling Basics

Wet hairstyling tools include the following items:

- Combs
- Brushes
- Rollers (plastic)
- Clips (duckbill, sectioning, finger waving, double prong, and single prong)
- Pins (bobby pins and hairpins)
- Clamps (sectioning clamps) (**Figure 17–2**)

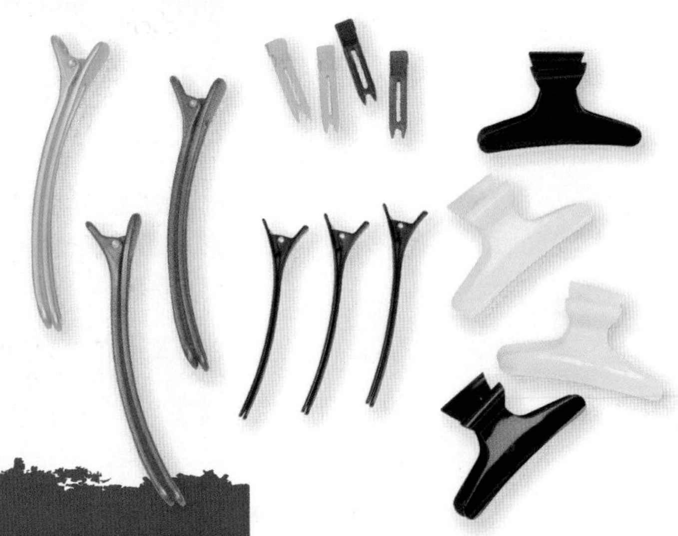

© Milady, a part of Cengage Learning.

▲ Figure 17–2
Clips (duckbill, sectioning, double prong) and sectioning clamps.

Finger Waving

Finger waving is the process of shaping and directing the hair into an S pattern through the use of the fingers, combs, and waving lotion. Finger waving was all the rage in the 1920s and 1930s, which may have you wondering why you are being asked to learn this technique today. The answer is that many women today are influenced by the movie stars and celebrities they see wearing gorgeous, dramatic finger waves!

From Madonna to Tyra Banks, well-known celebrities have embraced the elegance of the finger-wave style for the red carpet and other special, highly televised and photographed events. Clients will ask you for the very same look for their own special occasions, and you need to be prepared! In addition to its use in today's fashions, finger waving teaches you the technique of moving and directing hair. It also provides valuable training in molding hair to the curved surface of the head and is an excellent introduction to hairstyling.

Finger-Waving Lotion

Waving lotion is a type of hair gel that makes the hair pliable enough to keep it in place during the finger-waving procedure. It is traditionally made from karaya (kuh-Ry-uh) gum, taken from trees found in Africa and India. Karaya gum is diluted for use on fine hair, or it can be used in a more concentrated consistency on medium or coarse hair. A good waving lotion is harmless to the hair and does not flake when it dries. Be sure not to use too much of it at any one time. You will know if you have used too much, because the hair will be too wet and the waving lotion will drip. Liquid styling gels are also commonly used in conjunction with finger waving, and in many cases they have replaced traditional karaya gum products.

Other Methods of Finger Waving

Instead of completing one side before beginning the other, you may want to complete the first ridge on one side of the head, and then move to the other side to form the first ridge on that side. After joining the two, you can repeat the process in this manner until you are finished with the entire head.

In vertical finger waving, the ridges and waves run up and down the head. Horizontal finger waves are sideways and parallel around the head. The procedure is the same for both.

PROCEDURE 17-1 **Preparing Hair for Wet Styling** SEE PAGE 448

PROCEDURE 17-2 **Horizontal Finger Waving** SEE PAGE 450

Pin Curls

Pin curls serve as the basis for patterns, lines, waves, curls, and rolls that are used in a wide range of hairstyles. You can use them on all types of hair, including straight, permanent waved, or naturally curly hair. Pin curls work best when the hair is layered and smoothly wound. This makes springy and long-lasting curls with good direction and definition.

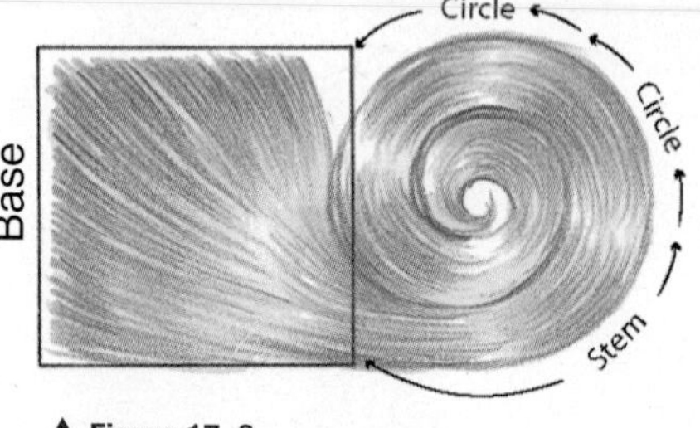

▲ **Figure 17–3**
Parts of a curl.

© Milady, a part of Cengage Learning.

Parts of a Curl

Pin curls are made up of three principal parts: base, stem, and circle (**Figure 17–3**).

The **base** is the stationary (non-moving) foundation of the curl, which is the area closest to the scalp, the panel of hair on which the roller is placed.

The **stem** is the section of the pin curl between the base and first arc (turn) of the circle that gives the curl its direction and movement, the hair between the scalp and the first turn of the roller.

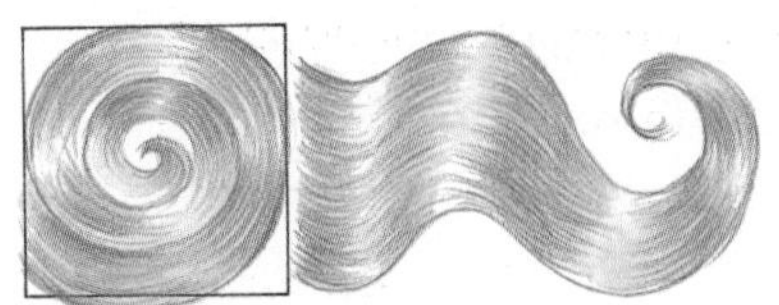

▲ **Figure 17–4**
No-stem curl unwound.

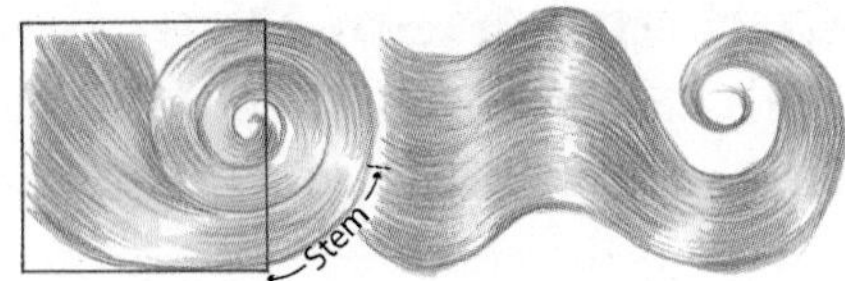

▲ **Figure 17–5**
Half-stem curl opened out.

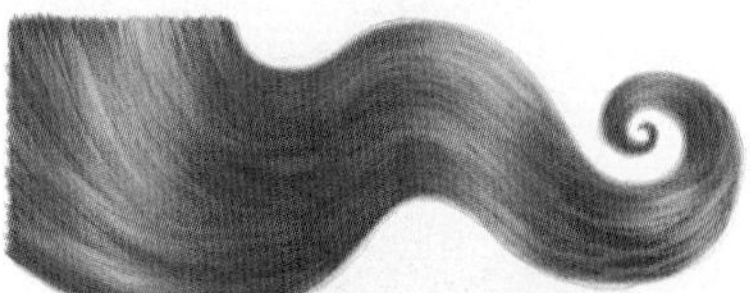

▲ **Figure 17–6**
Full-stem curl opened out.

The **circle** is the part of the curl that forms a complete circle and ultimately the wave. The size of the circle determines the width of the wave and its strength.

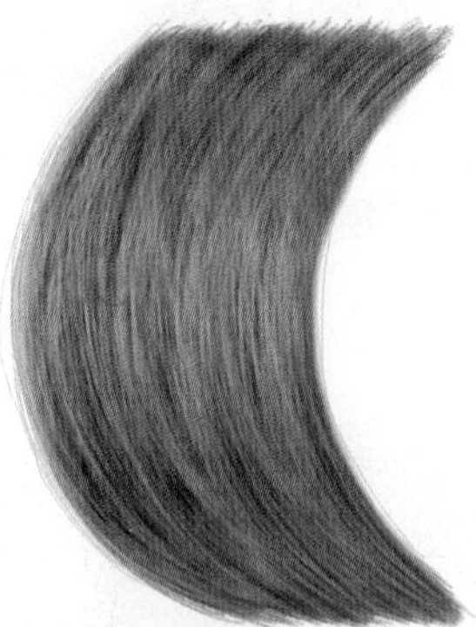

▲ **Figure 17–7**
Closed and open ends of a curl.

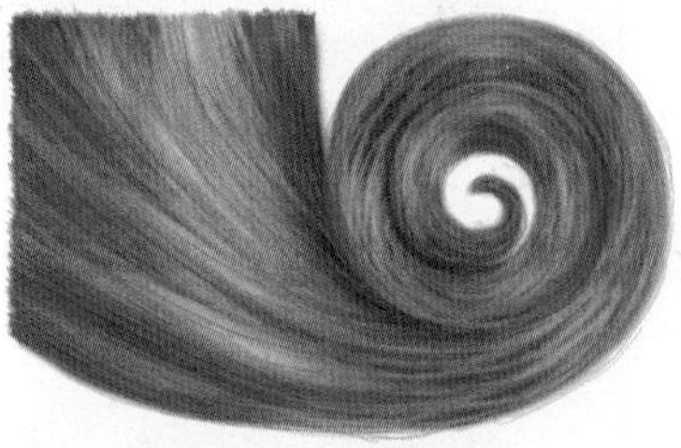

Mobility of a Curl

The stem determines the amount of mobility, or movement, in a section of hair. Curl mobility is classified as: no stem, half stem, and full stem.

- The **no-stem curl** is placed directly on the base of the curl. It produces a tight, firm, long-lasting curl and allows minimum mobility (**Figure 17–4**).
- The **half-stem curl** permits medium movement; the curl (circle) is placed half off the base. It gives good control to the hair (**Figure 17–5**).
- The **full-stem curl** allows for the greatest mobility. The curl is placed completely off the base. The base may be a square, triangular, half-moon, or rectangular section, depending on the area of the head in which the full-stem curls are used. It gives as much freedom as the length of the stem will permit. If it is exaggerated, the hair near the scalp will be flat and almost straight. It is used to give the hair a strong, definite direction (**Figure 17–6**).

▲ **Figure 17–8**
Curl in the shaping.

Shaping for Pin Curl Placements

A **shaping** is a section of hair that is molded in a circular movement in preparation for the formation of curls. Shapings are either open- or closed-end. Always begin a pin curl at the open end, or convex side, of a shaping (**Figures** 17–7 and **17–8**).

Open- and Closed-Center Curls

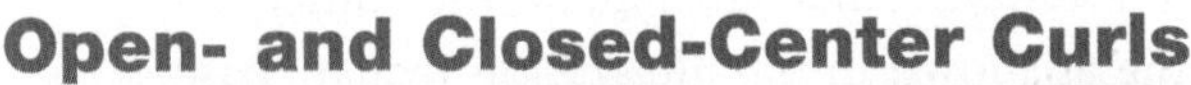

Open-center curls produce even, smooth waves and uniform curls. **Closed-center curls** produce waves that get smaller toward the end. They are good for fine hair, or if a fluffy curl is desired. Note the difference in the waves produced by pin curls with open centers and those with closed centers. The width of the curl determines the size of the wave. If you make pin curls with the ends outside the curl, the resulting wave will be narrower near the scalp and wider toward the ends (**Figures 17–9** and **17–10**).

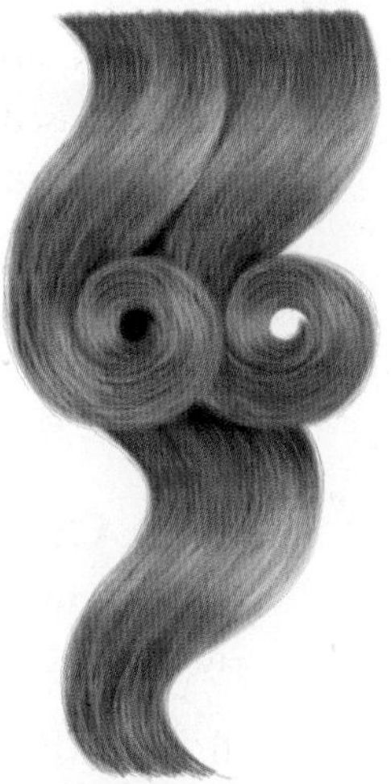

▲ **Figure 17–9**
Curl with open center.

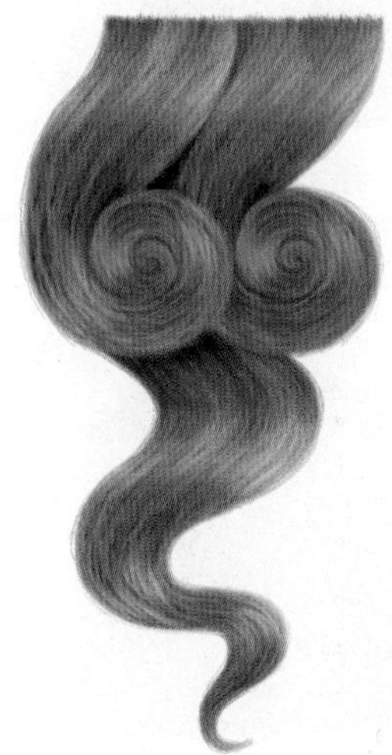

▲ **Figure 17–10**
Curl with closed center.

© Milady, a part of Cengage Learning.

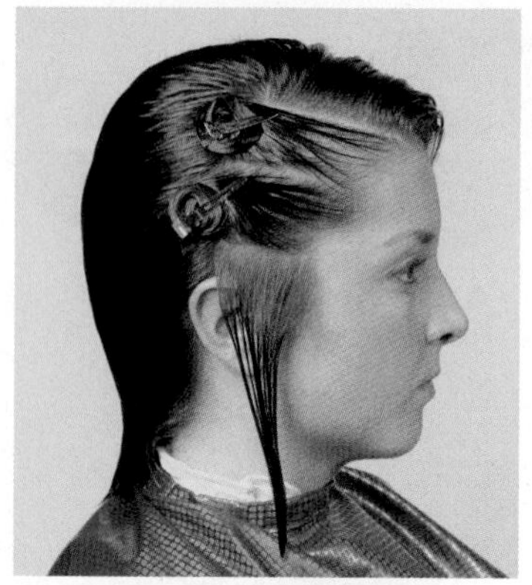
▲ Figure 17–11
Rectangular base pin curls.

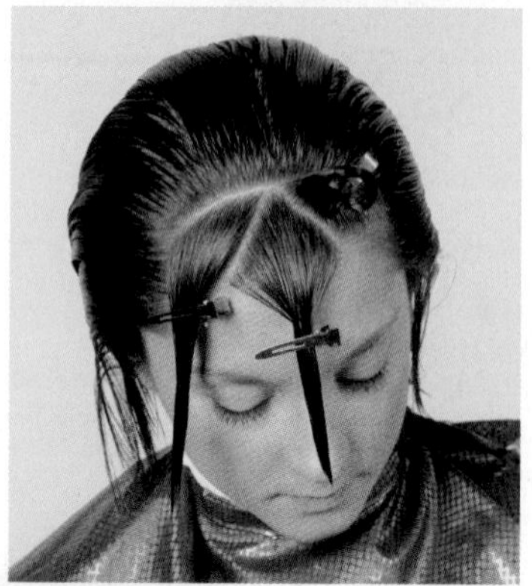
▲ Figure 17–12
Triangular base pin curls.

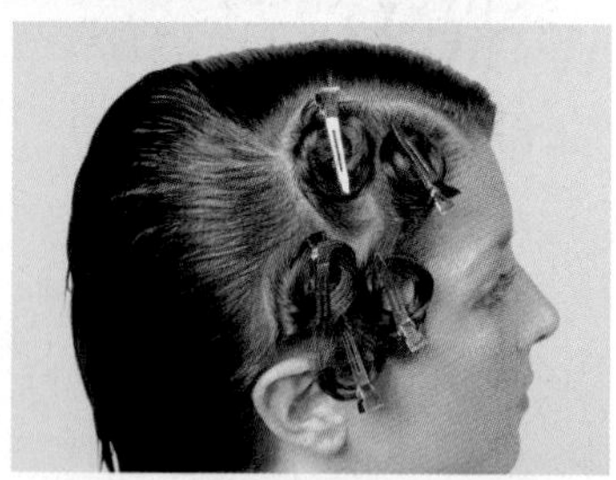
▲ Figure 17–13
Arc base pin curls.

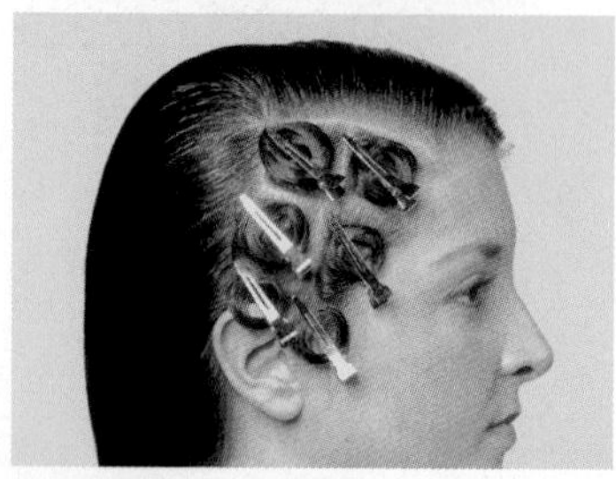
▲ Figure 17–14
Square base pin curls.

Curl and Stem Direction

Curls may be turned toward the face, away from the face, upward, downward, or diagonally. The finished result will be determined by the stem's direction.

The terms clockwise curls and counterclockwise curls are used to describe the direction of pin curls. Curls formed in the same direction as the movement of the hands of a clock are known as clockwise curls. Curls formed in the opposite direction are known as counterclockwise curls.

Pin Curl Bases or Foundations

Before you begin to make pin curls, divide the wet hair into sections or panels. Then subdivide each section into the type of base required for the various curls. The most commonly shaped base is the arc base (half-moon or C shaped). Others are rectangular, triangular, or square.

To avoid splits in the finished hairstyle, you must use care when selecting and forming the curl base. When the sections of hair are as close to equal as possible, you will get curls that are similar to one another. Each curl must lie flat and smooth on its base. If it is too far off the base, the curl will lie loose away from the scalp. The shape of the base, however, does not affect the finished curl.

- Rectangular base pin curls are usually recommended at the side front hairline for a smooth, upswept effect (**Figure 17–11**). To avoid splits in the comb out, the pin curls must overlap.
- Triangular base pin curls are recommended along the front or facial hairline to prevent breaks or splits in the finished hairstyle. The triangular base allows a portion of the hair from each curl to overlap the next, and this style can be combed into a wave without splits (**Figure 17–12**).
- Arc base pin curls, also known as half-moon or C shaped base curls, are carved out of a shaping. Arc base pin curls give good direction and may be used at the hairline or in the nape (**Figure 17–13**).
- Square base pin curls are suitable for curly hairstyles without much volume or lift. They can be used on any part of the head and will comb out with lasting results. To avoid splits in the comb out, stagger the sectioning as shown in the illustration (square base, brick-lay fashion) (**Figure 17–14**).

Pin Curl Techniques

Various methods are used to make pin curls. We will illustrate several methods below, but your instructor might demonstrate other methods that are equally effective.

One important technique to learn is called **ribboning** (RIB-un-ing), which involves forcing the hair between the thumb and the back of

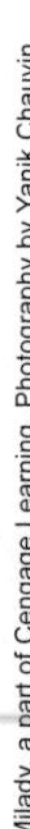
© Milady, a part of Cengage Learning. Photography by Yanik Chauvin.

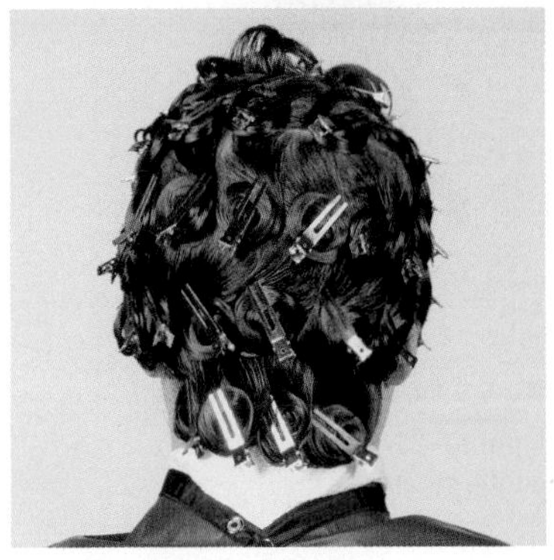

▲ Figure 17–15
Setting pattern for wave.

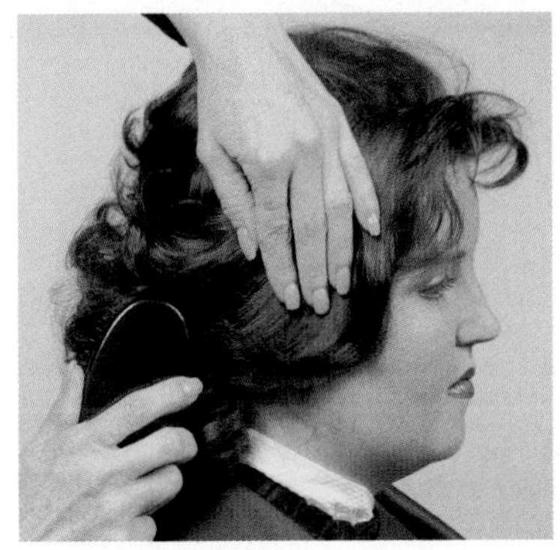

▲ Figure 17–16
Comb out of wave setting.

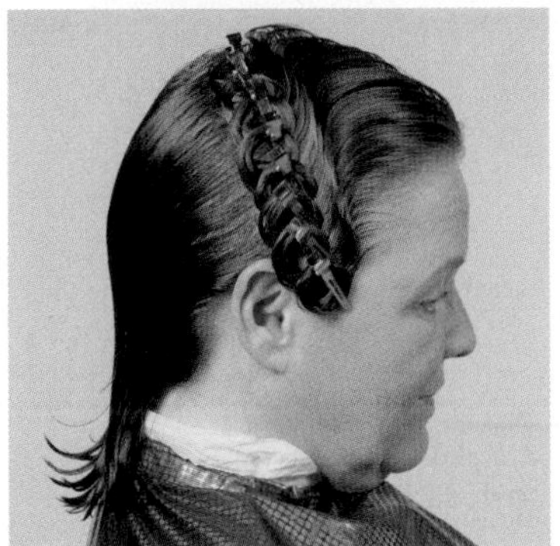

▲ Figure 17–17
Setting pattern for ridge curl.

the comb to create tension. You can also ribbon hair by pulling the strands while applying pressure between your thumb and index finger out toward the ends of the strands.

Carved or Sculptured Curls

Pin curls sliced from a shaping and formed without lifting the hair from the head are referred to as **carved curls**, also known as **sculptured curls**.

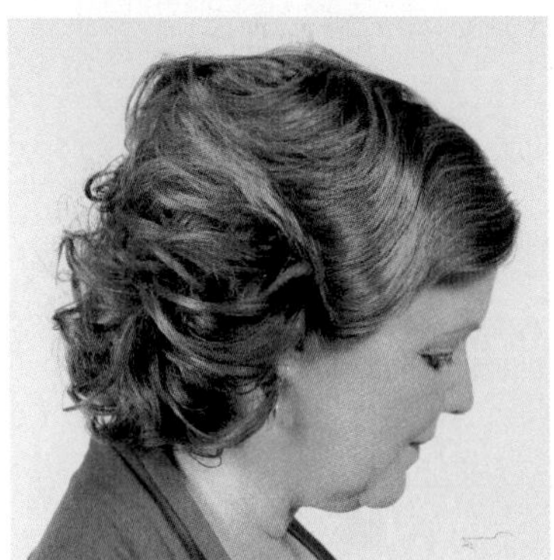

▲ Figure 17–18
Comb out for ridge curl.

Designing with Pin Curls

- To create a wave, use two rows of pin curls. Set one row clockwise and the second row counterclockwise (**Figures 17–15** and **17–16**).
- **Ridge curls** are pin curls placed immediately behind or below a ridge to form a wave (**Figures 17–17** and **17–18**).
- **Skip waves** are two rows of ridge curls, usually on the side of the head. Skip waves create a strong wave pattern with well-defined lines between the waves. This technique represents a combination of finger waving and pin curls (**Figures 17–19** and **17–20**).
- **Barrel curls** have large center openings and are fastened to the head in a standing position on a rectangular base. They have the same effect as stand-up pin curls. A barrel curl's effect is similar to that of a roller, but does not have the same tension as a roller when it is set.

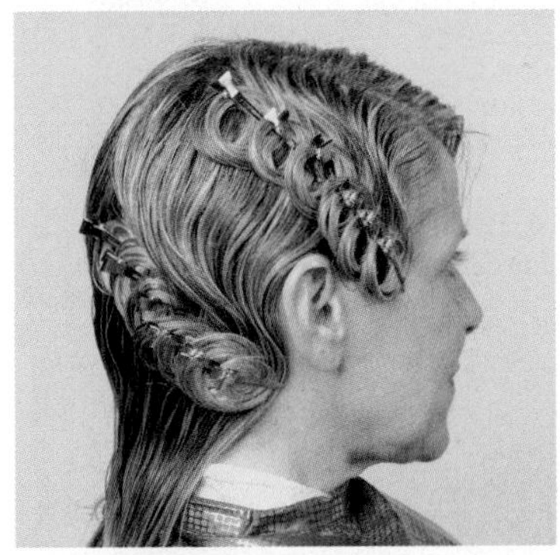

▲ Figure 17–19
Setting pattern for skip wave.

Creating Volume with Pin Curls

One of the best things about pin curls is they can add volume to the hair. Two types of pin curls that are particularly effective for adding volume are the following:

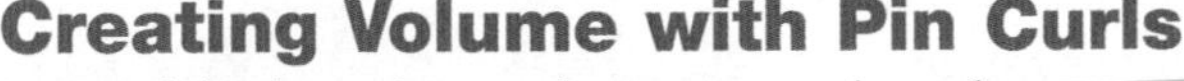

- **Cascade curls**, also known as **stand-up curls**, are used to create height in the hair design. They are fastened to the head in a standing position to allow the hair to flow upward and then downward. The size of the

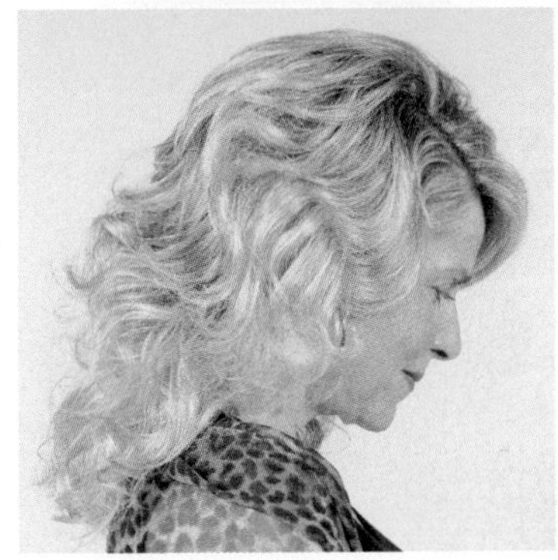

▲ Figure 17–20
Comb out of skip wave setting.

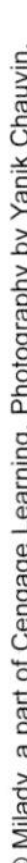

© Milady, a part of Cengage Learning. Photography by Yanik Chauvin.

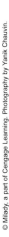

© Milady, a part of Cengage Learning. Photography by Yanik Chauvin.

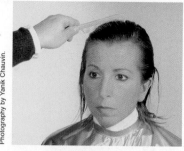

▲ **Figure 17–21**
Comb, divide, and smooth section.

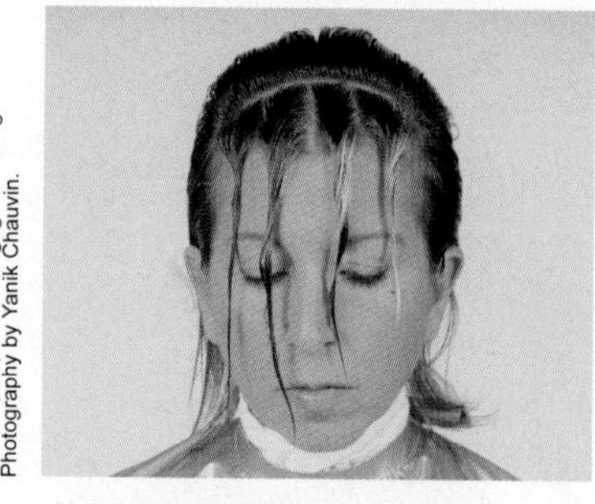
© Milady, a part of Cengage Learning. Photography by Yanik Chauvin.

▲ **Figure 17–22**
Divide section into strands.

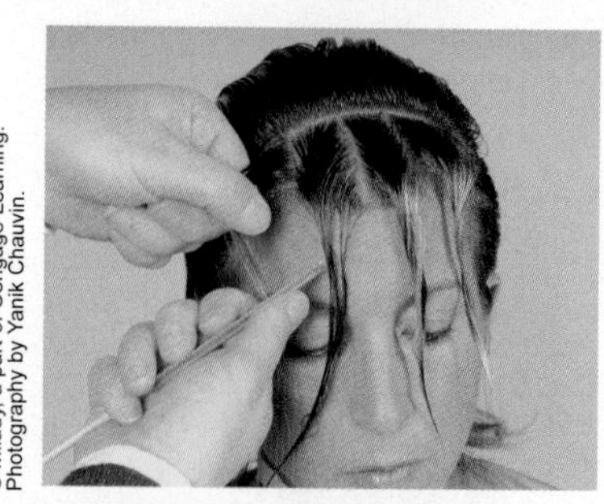
© Milady, a part of Cengage Learning. Photography by Yanik Chauvin.

▲ **Figure 17–23**
Ribbon the strand.

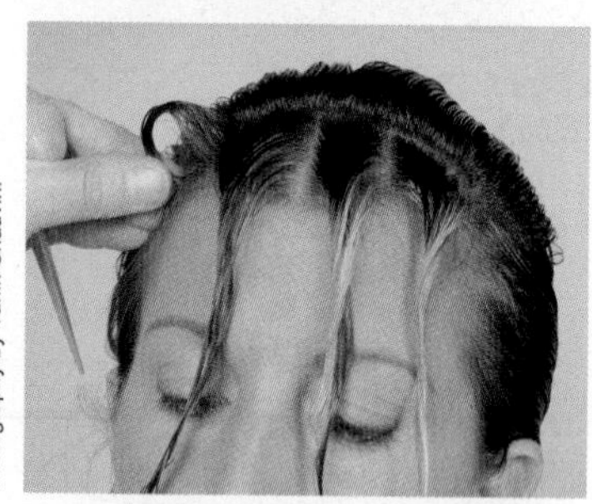
© Milady, a part of Cengage Learning. Photography by Yanik Chauvin.

▲ **Figure 17–24**
Direct the strand.

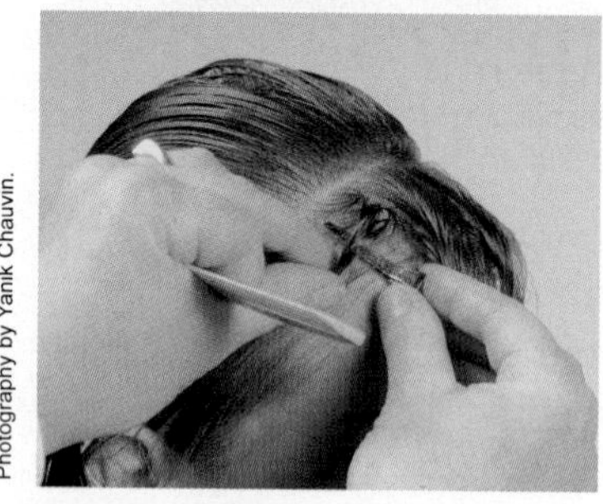
© Milady, a part of Cengage Learning. Photography by Yanik Chauvin.

▲ **Figure 17–25**
Anchor curl at base.

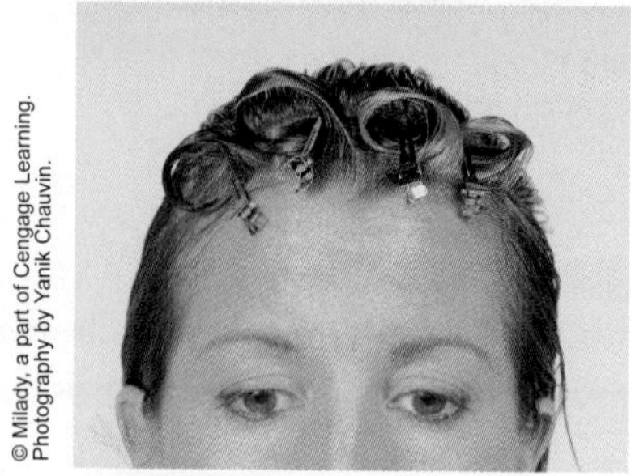
© Milady, a part of Cengage Learning. Photography by Yanik Chauvin.

▲ **Figure 17–26a**
Top setting.

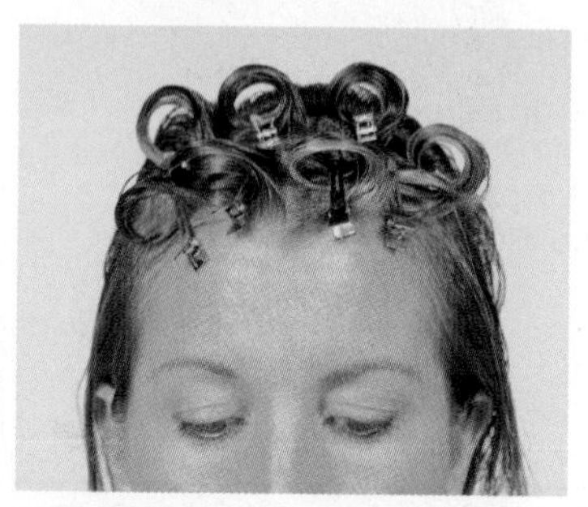
© Milady, a part of Cengage Learning. Photography by Yanik Chauvin.

▲ **Figure 17–26b**
Top setting.

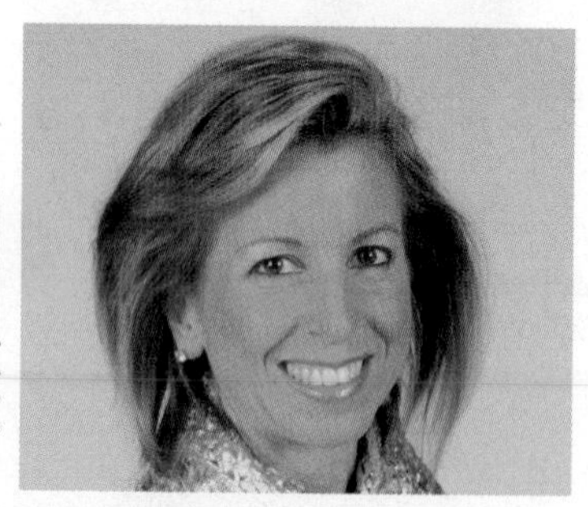
© Milady, a part of Cengage Learning. Photography by Yanik Chauvin.

▲ **Figure 17–27**
Comb out as you would a roller set.

curl determines the amount of height in the comb out (**Figures 17–21** through **17–27**).

PROCEDURE 17-3 Carved or Sculpted Curls **SEE PAGE 457**

Roller Curls

Rollers are used to create many of the same effects as stand-up pin curls.

Rollers have the following advantages over pin curls:

- Because a roller holds the equivalent of two to four stand-up curls, the roller is a much faster way to set the hair.
- The hair is wrapped around the roller with tension, which gives a stronger and longer-lasting set.
- Rollers come in a variety of shapes, widths, and sizes, which broadens the creative possibilities for any style (**Figure 17–28**).

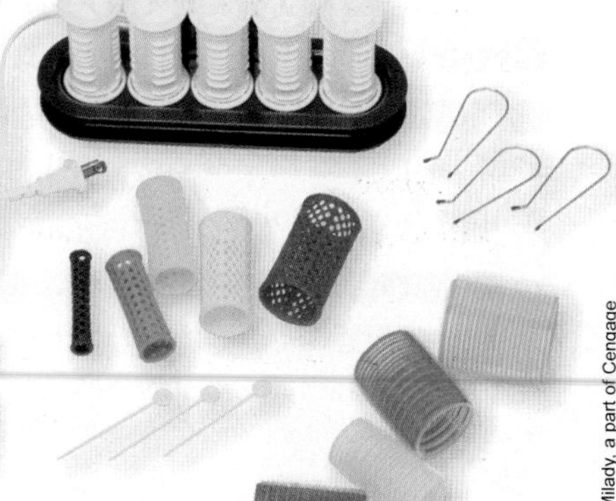
© Milady, a part of Cengage Learning. Photography by Paul Castle, Castle Photography.

▶ **Figure 17–28**
Rollers: plastic, mesh, hot, and Velcro.

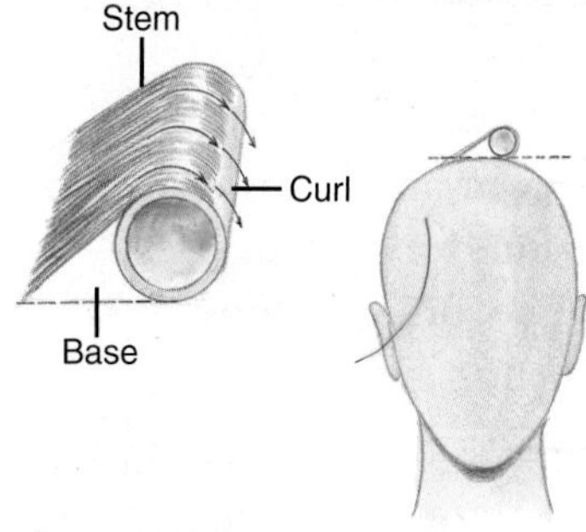

▲ **Figure 17–29**
Parts of a roller curl.

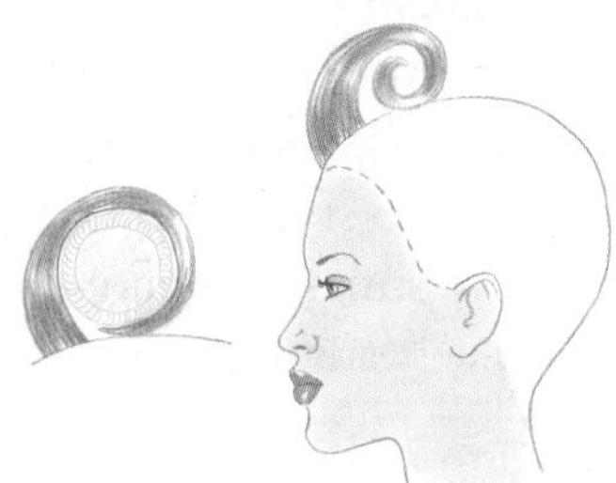

▲ **Figure 17–30**
C-shaped curl.

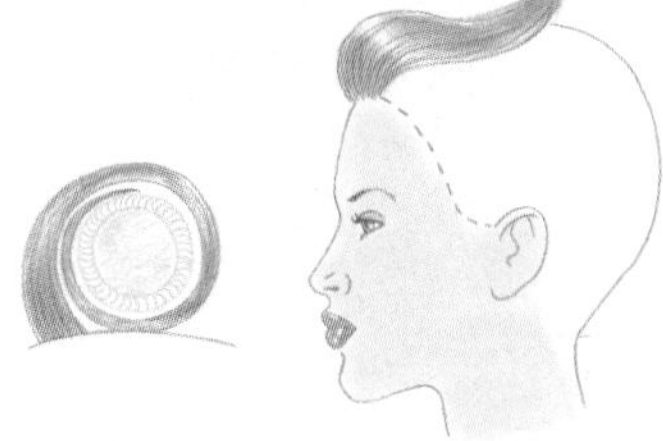

▲ **Figure 17–31**
Wave.

Parts of a Roller Curl

It is important for you to be able to identify the three parts of a roller curl (**Figure 17–29**).

- The **base** is the panel of hair on which the roller is placed. The base should be the same length and width as the roller. The type of base affects the volume.
- The **stem** is the hair between the scalp and the first turn of the roller. The stem gives the hair direction and mobility.
- The **curl,** also known as **circle**, is the hair that is wrapped around the roller. It determines the size of the wave or curl.

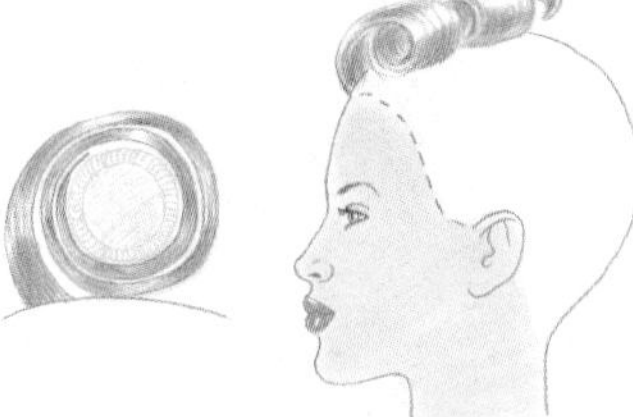
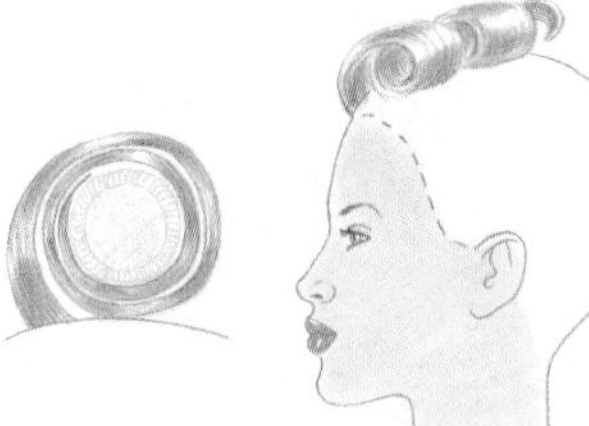

▲ **Figure 17–32**
Curl.

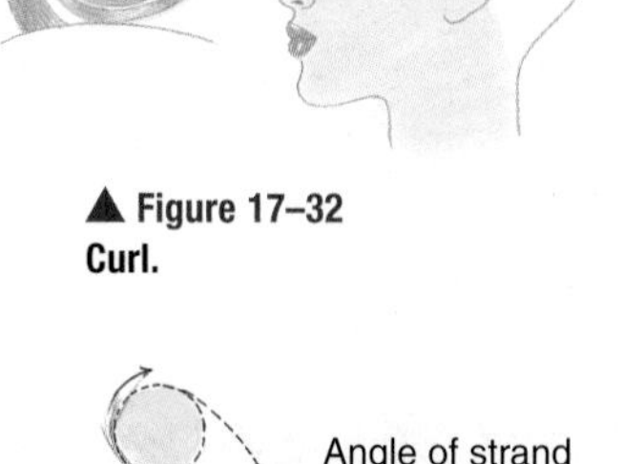
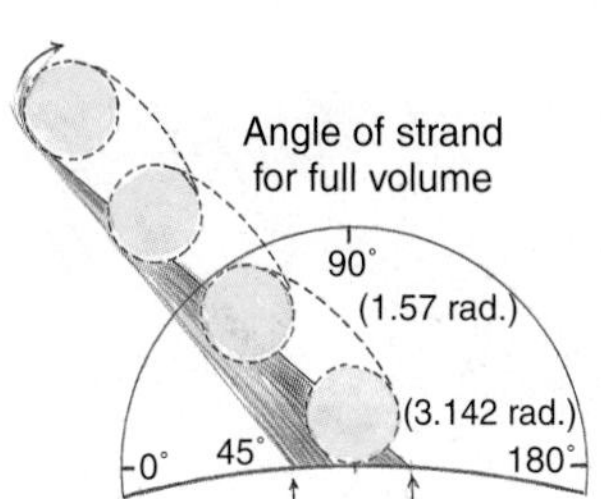
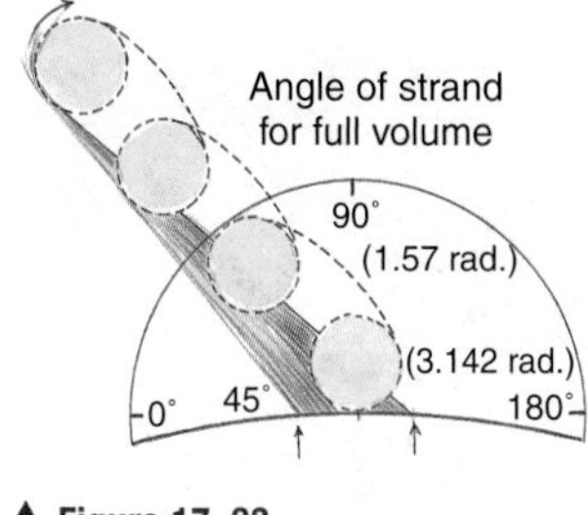

▲ **Figure 17–33**
On-base roller: full volume.

Choosing Your Roller Size

The relationship between the length of the hair and the size of the roller will determine whether the result will be a C shape, wave, or curl. These three shapes are created as follows:

- One complete turn around the roller will create a C-shape curl (**Figure 17–30**).
- One and a half turns will create a wave (**Figure 17–31**).
- Two and a half turns will create curls (**Figure 17–32**).

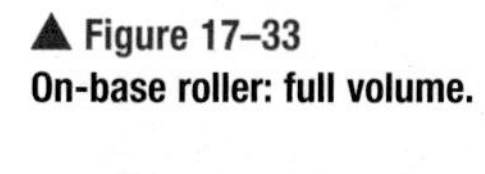
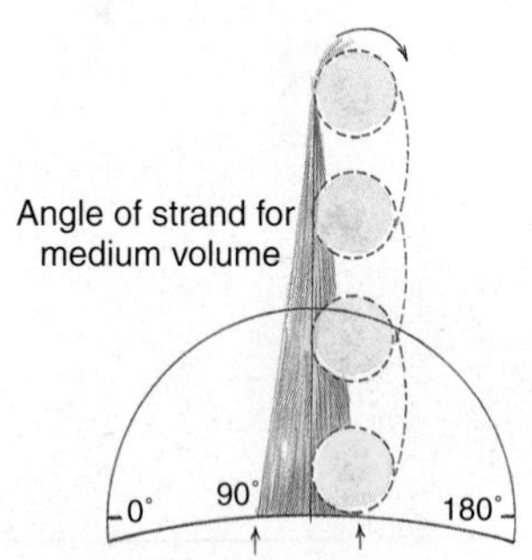

▲ **Figure 17–34**
Half-base roller: medium volume.

Roller Placement

The amount of volume that is achieved depends on the size of the roller and how it sits on its base. The general rule of thumb is that the larger the roller, the greater the volume. There are three kinds of bases.

- **On base**, also known as **full base.** For full volume, the roller sits directly on its base. Overdirect (higher than 90 degrees) the strand slightly in front of the base, and roll the hair down to the base. The roller should fit on the base (**Figure 17–33**).
- **Half base.** For medium volume, the roller sits halfway on its base and halfway behind the base. Hold the strand straight up (90 degrees) from the head and roll the hair down (**Figure 17–34**).
- **Off base.** For the least volume, the roller sits completely off the base. Hold the strand 45 degrees down from the base and roll the hair down (**Figure 17–35**).

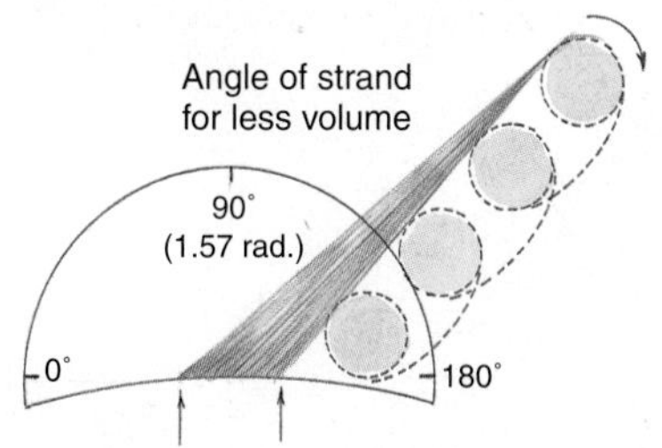

▲ **Figure 17–35**
Off-base roller: less volume.

© Milady, a part of Cengage Learning.

Roller Direction

The placement of rollers on the head usually follows the movement of the finished style. For versatility in styling, a downward directional wrap gives options to style in all directions—under, out, forward, or back—while still maintaining volume. To reduce volume, bringing movement closer to the head, use indentation curl placement.

Indentation is the point where curls of opposite directions meet, forming a recessed area. This is often found in flip styles or in bangs (fringes) with a dip or wave movement. Indentation can be achieved using rollers, curling irons, or a round brush.

PROCEDURE 17-4 **Wet Set with Rollers** SEE PAGE 461

Hot Rollers

Hot rollers are to be used only on dry hair. They are heated either electrically or by steam, and they are a great time saver in the salon. Follow the same setting patterns as with wet setting, but allow the hot roller to stay on the hair for about ten minutes. A thermal protector can be sprayed on the hair before setting. The result is a curl that is weaker than a wet-set curl, but stronger and longer lasting than can be achieved using a curling iron. Spray-on products are available for application to each section of hair to create a stronger set.

Velcro Rollers

Velcro rollers are not allowed by the state board of some states and provinces because they are difficult to clean and disinfect properly. Check with your regulatory agency to determine if you can use them in your state.

Like hot rollers, Velcro rollers are used only on dry hair. Using them on wet hair will snag and pull the hair. If you have a client who needs more body than can be achieved with a round brush, but less volume than a hot roller or wet set will produce, try Velcro rollers. When they are used after blowdrying, Velcro rollers may provide just the amount of volume you need.

Velcro rollers need to stay in the hair for only five to ten minutes, depending on how much set you want in the hair. Follow the same setting patterns as with wet setting, but keep in mind that no clipping is necessary to secure the roller. The Velcro fabric grips the hair well and stays in place on its own.

Mist the entire head with hair spray, and then either place the client under a hooded dryer for five to ten minutes, or use the diffuser attachment on your blowdryer for the recommended time to give a soft set to the hair. For an even softer look, do not apply heat after the rollers are put in, simply have your client sit for a few minutes. This would be a good time to instruct the client on how she can repeat the process at home in order to maintain the style.

© Junial Enterprises, 2010; used under license from Shutterstock.com.

Always remove any hair from Velcro and electric rollers after use. See Chapter 5, Infection Control: Principles and Practices, for instructions on disinfecting rollers.

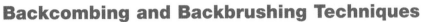

Comb-Out Techniques

A good set leads to a good comb out (**Figure 17–36**). For successful finishes, learn how to shape and mold the hair, and then practice fast, simple, and effective methods for comb outs (**Figure 17–37**). If you follow a well-structured system of combing out hairstyles, you will save time and get more consistent results.

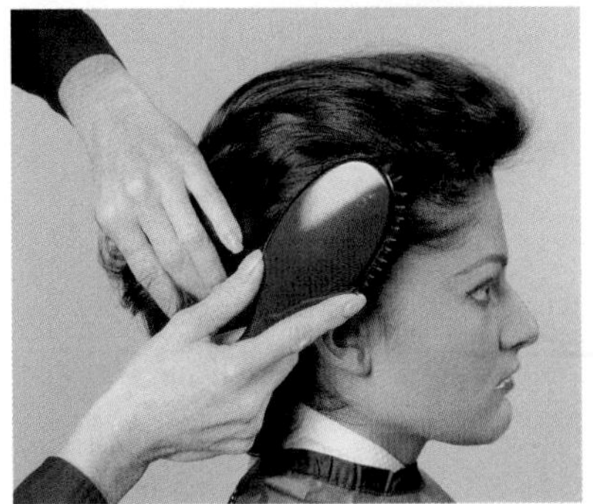

▲ **Figure 17–36**
Brush out the hair.

Backcombing and Backbrushing Techniques

Backcombing and backbrushing are the best ways to lift and increase volume, as well as to remove indentations caused by roller setting. **Backcombing** also known as **teasing**, **ratting**, **matting**, or **French lacing**, involves combing small sections of hair from the ends toward the scalp, causing shorter hair to mat at the scalp and form a cushion or base. **Backbrushing**, also known as **ruffing** (RUF-ing), is used to build a soft cushion or to mesh two or more curl patterns together for a uniform and smooth comb out.

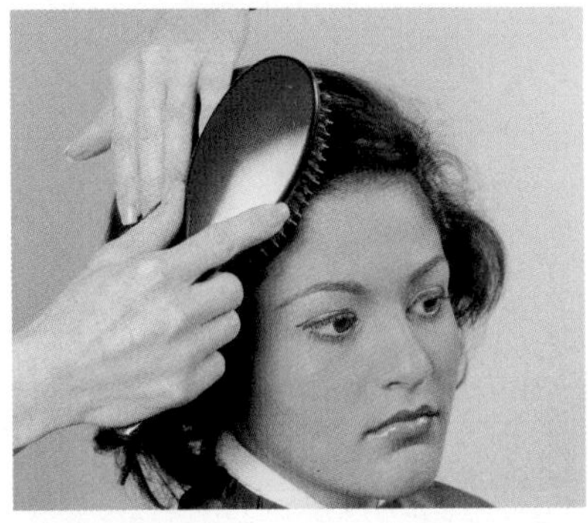

▲ **Figure 17–37**
Direct hair into desired pattern.

During the 1950s and 1960s, women typically had their hair wet set and combed out, and the set would last an entire week with backcombing and backbrushing. Now these techniques are used for styling updos or for adding a little height to a hairstyle after hot-roller setting or blowdrying.

Backcombing Technique

1. **Section hair.** Starting in the front, pick up a section of hair no more than 1 inch thick and no more than 2- to 3-inches (5 to 7.5 centimeters) wide.
2. **Insert comb.** Insert the fine teeth of your comb into the hair at a depth of about 1½ inches (3.75 centimeters) from the scalp (**Figure 17–38**).
3. **Press comb down.** Press the comb gently down toward the scalp, sliding it down and out of the hair. Repeat this process, working up the section until the desired volume is achieved (**Figure 17–39**).
4. **Create a cushion.** If you wish to create a cushion (base), the third time you insert the comb, use the same sliding motion but firmly push the hair down to the scalp. Slide the comb out of the hair(**Figure 17–40**).

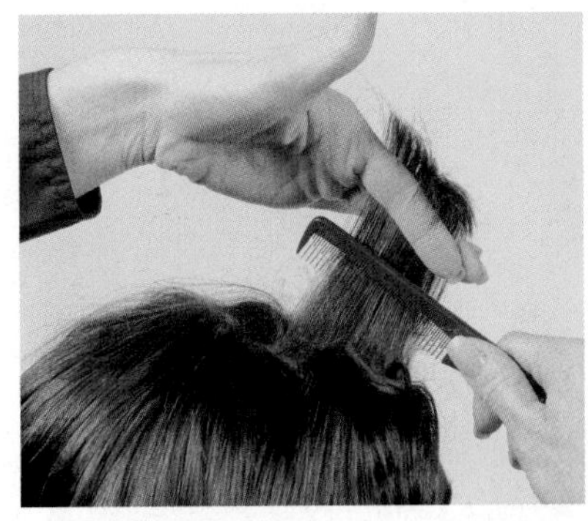

▲ **Figure 17–38**
Insert comb.

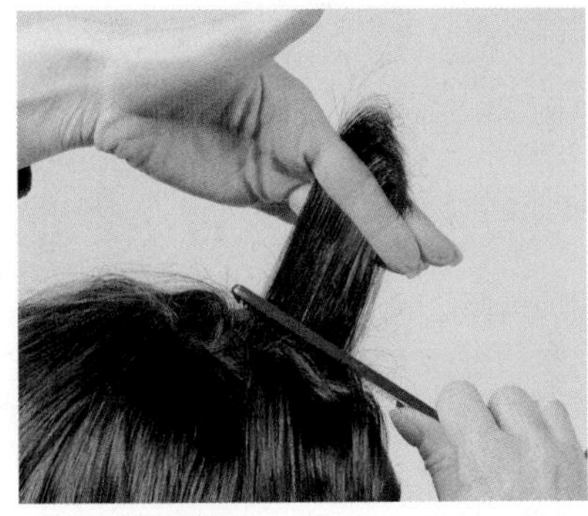

▲ **Figure 17–39**
Press comb down.

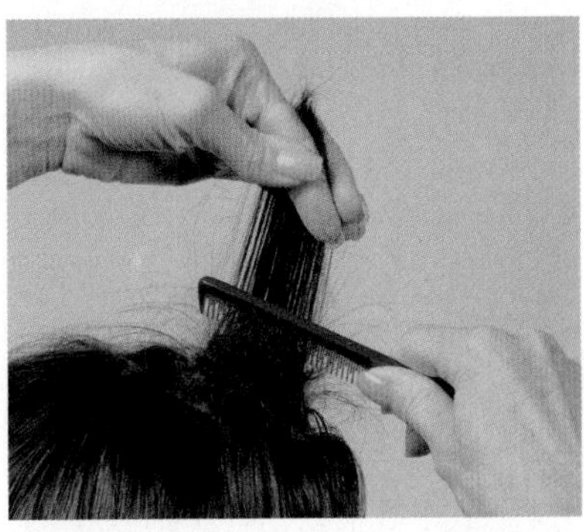

▲ **Figure 17–40**
Create base of backcombed hair.

© Milady, a part of Cengage Learning. Photography by Yanik Chauvin.

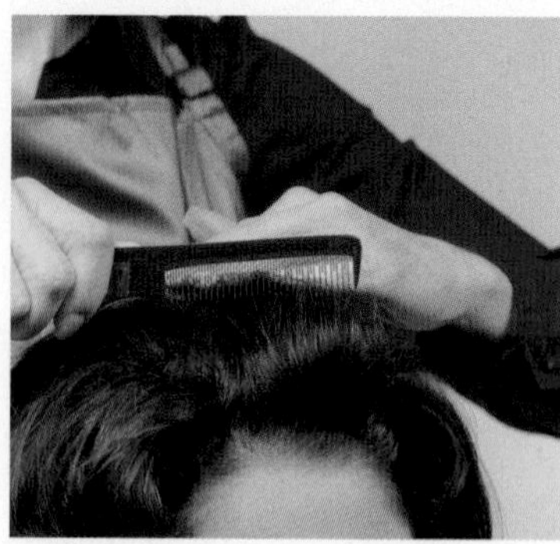

▲ Figure 17–41
Smoothing hair with comb.

5. **Repeat for volume.** Repeat this process, working up the strand until the desired volume is achieved.
6. **Smooth hair.** To smooth hair that is backcombed, hold the teeth of a comb (or the bristles of a brush) at a 45-degree angle pointing away from you, and lightly move the comb over the surface of the hair (**Figure 17–41**).

Backbrushing Technique

1. **Hold strand.** Pick up and hold a strand straight out from the scalp.
2. **Place brush.** Maintaining a slight amount of slack in the strand, place a teasing brush or a grooming brush near the base of the strand. Push and roll the inner edge of the brush with the wrist until it touches the scalp.
3. **Roll brush.** For interlocking to occur, the brush must be rolled (**Figure 17–42**).
4. **Turn brush.** Remove the brush from the hair with a turn of the wrist, peeling back a layer of hair (**Figure 17–43**). The hair will be interlocked to form a soft cushion at the scalp.
5. **Blend hair.** You can create softness and evenness of flow by blending, smoothing, and combing (**Figure 17–44**). Avoid exaggerations and overemphasis. Finished patterns should reflect rhythm, balance, and smoothness of line.
6. **Complete styling.** Final touches make hairstyles look professional, so take your time. After completing the comb out, you can use the tail of a comb to lift areas where the shape and form are not as full as you want them to be (**Figure 17–45**). Every touch during the final stage must be very lightly done. When you have completed your finishing touches, check the entire set for structural balance and then lightly spray the hair with a finishing spray (**Figure 17–46**).

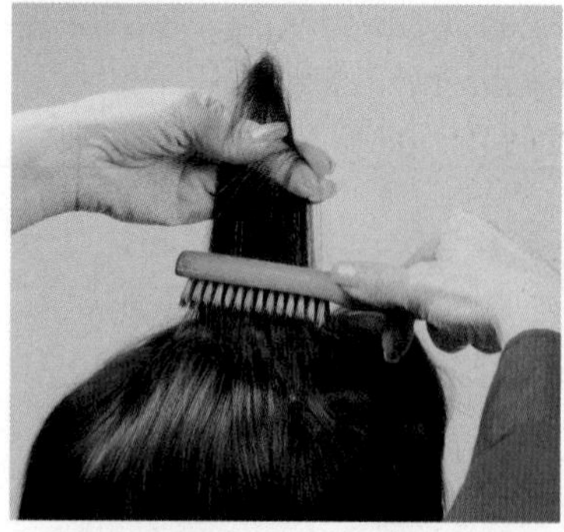

▲ Figure 17–42
Roll brush.

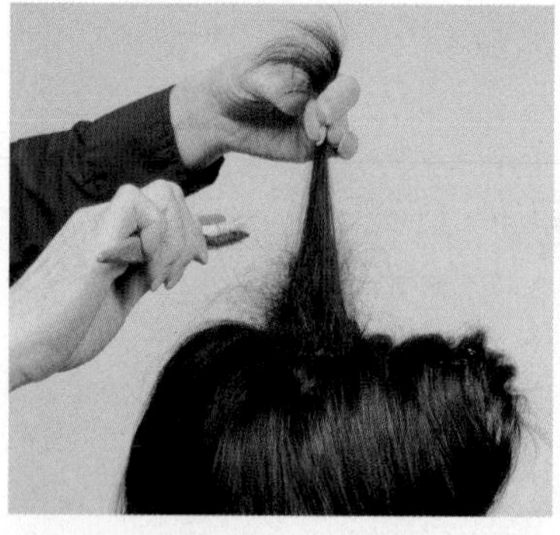

▲ Figure 17–43
Remove brush.

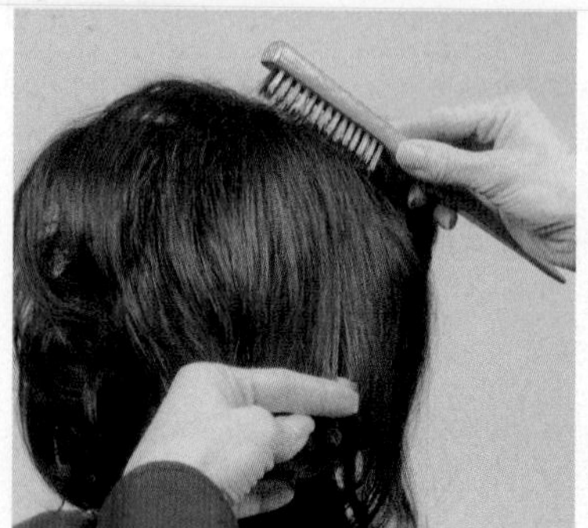

▲ Figure 17–44
Blend sections with backcombing.

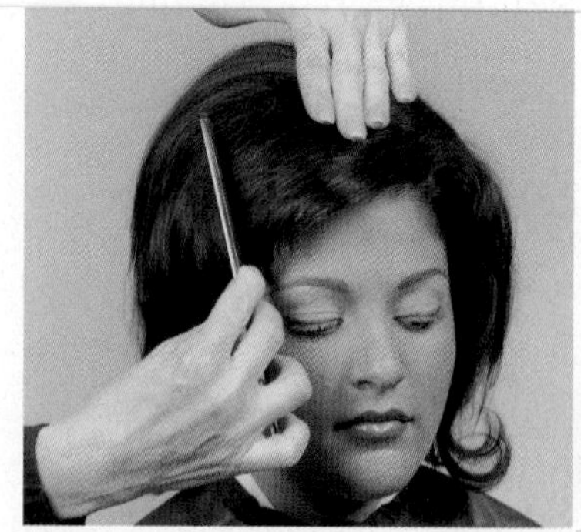

▲ Figure 17–45
Finished style.

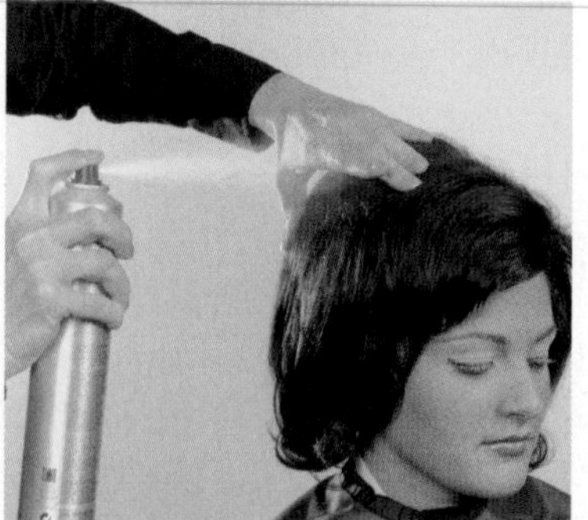

▲ Figure 17–46
Apply finishing spray to complete style.

© Milady, a part of Cengage Learning. Photography by Yanik Chauvin.

Hair Wrapping

Hair wrapping is a technique used to keep curly hair smooth and straight while retaining a beautiful shape. Curly hair can be wrapped around the head to give it a smooth, rounded contour, resulting in an effect that is similar to that attained with rollers. When wrapping hair, very little volume is attained because the hair at the scalp is not lifted. If height is desired, you can place large rollers directly at the crown, with the remainder of the hair wrapped around the head.

Wrapping can be done on wet or dry hair. On curly hair, wet wrapping creates a smooth, sleek look. When working with very curly hair, press it first, then do a dry hair wrapping.

PROCEDURE 17-5 Hair Wrapping SEE PAGE 463 ✓ LO1

Here's a Tip

Wondering when to use a hood dryer versus a blowdryer to complete your styling? A hood dryer is best used for any kind of wet set—finger waves, pin curls, or rollers. A wet set will last longer than a blown dry style for many people. A blowdry will give a softer result and often takes less time. Choose the best technique in order to achieve the look you want, given the styling techniques you have used.

Blowdry Styling

Blowdry styling is the technique of drying and styling damp hair in one operation, and it has revolutionized the hairstyling world. Today, women desire hairstyles that require the least possible time and effort to maintain. The selection of styling tools, techniques, and products must relate to the client's lifestyle. Is the client capable of styling her own hair, and how much time will she have to do it? As the stylist, you are responsible for guiding and educating the client through this process. To do so, you must first learn all about the tools and products available to you. Remember, the client's first impression of the haircut you have provided will be determined by the quality of the blowdry.

CAUTION

Blowdryers can get very hot! Do not hold the blowdryer too close to the hair or scalp, or you may burn your client.

Tools for Blowdry Styling

The following are the basic tools used for blowdrying techniques.

The Blowdryer

A blowdryer is an electrical appliance designed for drying and styling hair. Its main parts are a handle, slotted nozzle, small fan, heating element, and speed/heat controls. Some blowdryers also come with cooling buttons which are used to help set the hair. The temperature control switch helps to produce a steady stream of air at the desired temperature. The blowdryer's nozzle attachment, or **concentrator**, is a directional feature that creates a concentrated stream of air.

The **diffuser** is an attachment that causes the air to flow more softly, and helps to accentuate or keep textural definition (**Figure 17–47**).

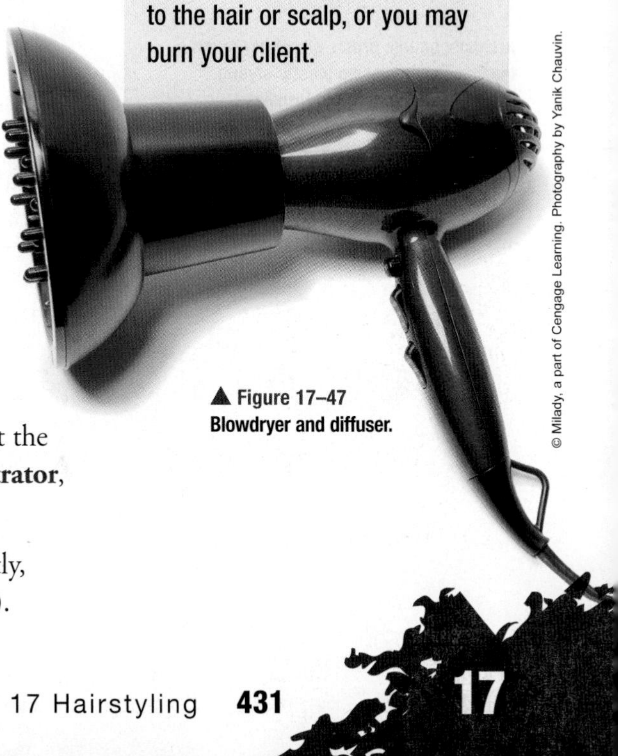

▲ **Figure 17–47** Blowdryer and diffuser.

© Milady, a part of Cengage Learning. Photography by Yanik Chauvin.

To keep your blowdryer as safe and effective as possible, always make sure that it is perfectly clean and free of dirt, oil, and hair before use. Dirt or hair in the blowdryer can cause extreme heat and thus burn the hair. The air intake at the back of the dryer must also be kept clear at all times. If the intake is covered and air cannot pass through freely, the dryer element will burn out prematurely.

© Milady, a part of Cengage Learning. Photography by Paul Castle, Castle Photography.

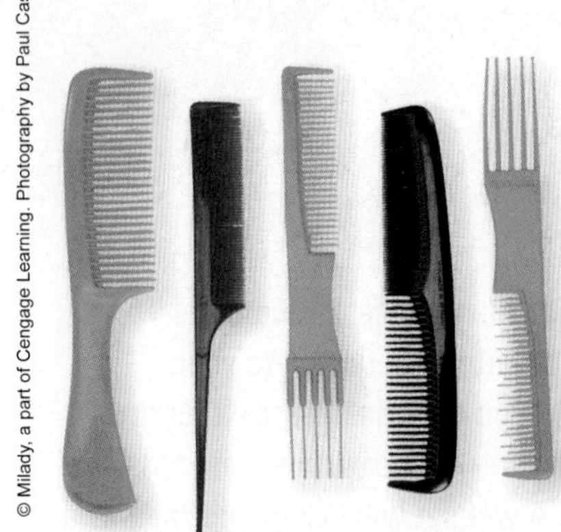

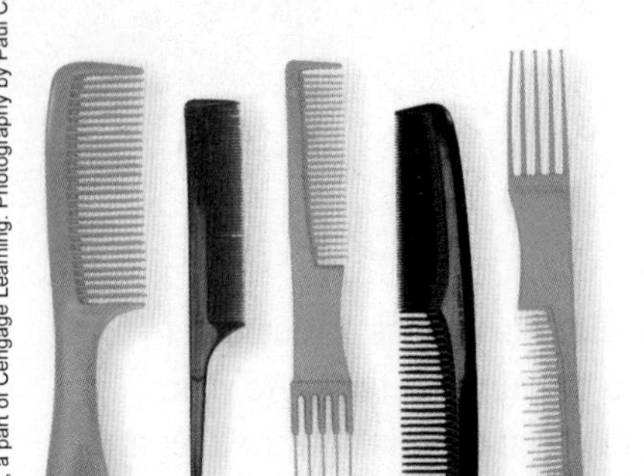

▲ **Figure 17–48**
From left to right: wide-tooth comb, fine-tooth tail comb, styling comb with metal pins, finger-wave comb, teasing comb.

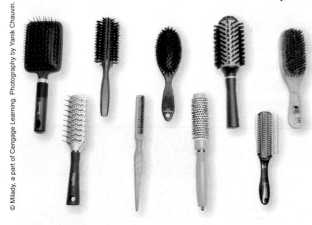

Combs and Picks

Combs and picks are designed to distribute and part the hair. They come in a wide variety of sizes and shapes to adapt to many styling options (**Figure 17–48**). The length and spacing of the teeth vary from one comb to another. Teeth that are closely spaced remove definition from the curl and create a smooth surface; widely spaced teeth shape larger sections of hair for a more textured surface. Combs with a pick at one end lift the hair away from the head.

Brushes

When choosing a styling brush, take into account the texture, length, and styling needs of the hair that you are working with. Brushes come in many sizes, shapes, and materials (**Figure 17–49**).

© Milady, a part of Cengage Learning. Photography by Yanik Chauvin.

▲ **Figure 17–49**
Brushes: paddle brush, grooming brush, teasing brush, classic plastic styling brush, vent brush, round brushes.

- A classic styling brush is a half-round, rubber-based brush. These brushes typically have either seven or nine rows of round-tipped nylon bristles. They are heat resistant, antistatic, and ideal for smoothing and untangling all types of hair. While they are perfect for blowdrying precision haircuts, where little volume is desired, they are less suitable for smooth, classic looks.
- Paddle brushes, with their large, flat bases, are well suited for mid-length to longer-length hair. Some have ball-tipped nylon pins and staggered pin patterns that help keep the hair from snagging.
- Grooming brushes are generally oval, with a mixture of boar and nylon bristles. The boar bristles help distribute the scalp oils over the hair shaft, giving it shine. The nylon bristles stimulate the circulation of blood to the scalp. Grooming brushes are particularly useful for adding polish and shine to fine to medium hair, and they are great for combing out updos.
- Vent brushes, with their ventilated design, are used to speed up the blowdrying process, and they are ideal for blowdrying fine hair and adding lift at the scalp.
- Round brushes come in various diameters. The client's hair should be long enough to wrap twice around the brush. Round brushes often have natural bristles, sometimes with nylon mixed in for better grip. Smaller brushes add more curl; larger brushes straighten the hair and bevel the ends of the hair. Medium round brushes can be used to lift the hair at the scalp. Some round brushes have metal cylinder bases so that the heat

from the blowdryer is transferred to the metal base, creating a stronger curl that is similar to those produced with an electric roller. Always use the cooling button on the blowdryer before releasing the section to set the hair into the new shape.

- A teasing brush is a thin, nylon styling brush that has a tail for sectioning, along with a narrow row of bristles. Teasing brushes are perfect for backcombing hair, and the sides of the bristles are ideal for smoothing it into the desired style.

© M. Antonis, 2010; used under license from Shutterstock.com.

Sectioning Clips

Sectioning clips are usually metal or plastic and have long prongs to hold wet or dry sections of hair in place. It is important to keep the wet hair you are not working on sectioned off in clips so that it does not sit over the dry hair. This is particularly important when drying long hair.

Styling Products

Styling products can be thought of as liquid tools. They give a style more hold, and they can be used to either increase or decrease the amount of curl. They can also be used to add shine. When used correctly, styling products greatly enhance a style.

With so many styling products on the market, stylists need to carefully consider their options before applying one of these products to a client's hair. First, how long does the style need to hold? Under what environmental conditions—dryness, humidity, wind, sun—will the client be wearing the style? You also must consider the type of hair—fine, coarse, straight, curly—when deciding on a product. Heavier products work by causing strands of hair to cling together, adding more pronounced definition, but they can also weigh the hair down, especially fine hair. Styling products range from a light hold to a very firm hold. Determine the amount of support desired and choose accordingly.

Types of Styling Products

Foam, also known as **mousse**, is a light, airy, whipped styling product that resembles shaving foam. It builds moderate body and volume into the hair. Massage it into damp hair to highlight textural movement, or blowdry it straight for styles when body without texture is desired. Foam is good for fine hair because it does not weigh the hair down. It will hold for six to eight hours in dry conditions. Conditioning foams are excellent for drier, more porous hair.

Gel is a thickened styling preparation that comes in a tube or bottle. Gels create the strongest control for slicked or molded styles, and they add distinct texture definition when spread with the fingers. When hair is brushed out, gel creates long-lasting body. Firm hold gel formulations may overwhelm fine hair because of the high resin content. This is not a concern if fine hair is molded into the lines of the style and is not brushed through when dry.

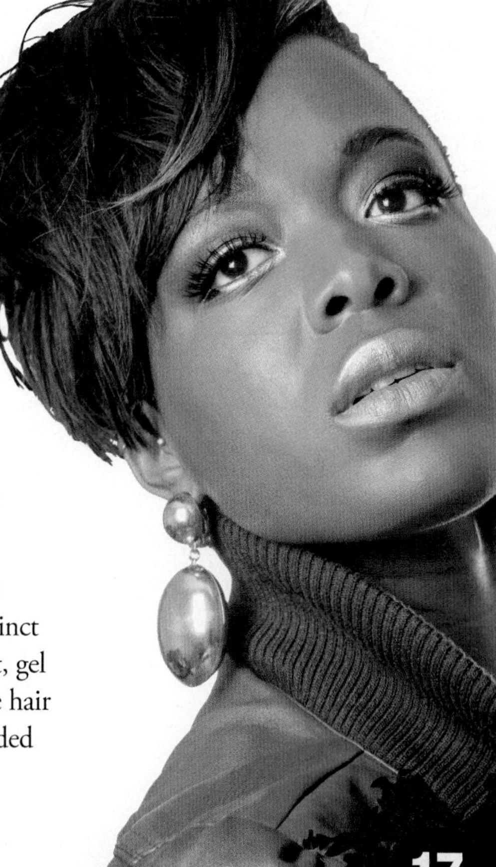

© Martin Dry, 2010; used under license from Shutterstock.com.

Liquid gels, also known as **texturizers**, are similar to firm hold gels except that they are lighter and less viscous (more liquid) in form. They allow for easy styling, defining, and molding. With brushing, they add volume and body to the style. Good for all hair types, they offer firmer, longer hold for fine hair with the least amount of heaviness, and they give a lighter, more moderate hold for normal or coarse hair types. Home-care recommendations regarding styling products represent a natural retailing opportunity in the salon. As you style the client's hair, talk about the products you are using to achieve the desired look and why you have chosen them. Have the client hold the product while you demonstrate its uses and benefits. Most clients are eager to learn any and all styling secrets. By discussing and recommending professional products as you use them, you not only enlighten your client, you also enhance the salon's reputation and help sell its products.

When **straightening gel** is applied to damp hair (ranging from wavy to extremely curly) and blown dry, it creates a smooth, straight look that provides the most hold in dry outdoor conditions. Straightening gel counters frizz by coating the hair shaft and weighing it down. This is a temporary solution that will last only from shampoo to shampoo. Also, styles that use straightening gel may come undone in extremely humid conditions.

When sprayed into the base of fine, wet hair that is then blown dry, **volumizers** add volume, especially at the base. When a vent brush or round brush is used and the hair is not stretched too tightly around the brush, even more volume can be achieved. You may want to add a light gel or mousse to the rest of the hair for more hold, but be careful to avoid the base of hair that has already been treated with volumizer.

Pomade, also known as **wax**, adds considerable weight to the hair by causing strands to join together, showing separation in the hair. Used on dry hair, pomade makes the hair very easy to mold, allowing greater manageability. It should be used sparingly on fine hair because of the weight. As a man's grooming product, pomade is excellent on short hair.

Silicone adds gloss and sheen to the hair while creating textural definition. Nonoily silicone products are excellent for all hair types, either to provide lubrication and protection to the hair during blowdrying, or to finish a style by adding extra shine. When applied like hair spray, silicone spray–shines add gloss without weight, so they are useful for all hair types.

Hair spray, also known as **finishing spray**, is applied in the form of a mist to hold a style in position. It is the most widely used hairstyling product. Available in both aerosol and pump containers, and in a variety of holding strengths, it is useful for all hair types. Finishing spray is used when the style is complete and will not be disturbed.

PROCEDURE 17-6 Blowdrying Short, Layered, Curly Hair to Produce Smooth and Full Finish SEE PAGE 465

© Factoria Singular, 2010; used under license from iStockphoto.com.

PROCEDURE 17-7 Blowdrying Short, Curly Hair in Its Natural Wave Pattern SEE PAGE 469

PROCEDURE 17-8 Diffusing Long, Curly or Extremely Curly Hair in Its Natural Wave Pattern SEE PAGE 471

PROCEDURE 17-9 Blowdrying Straight or Wavy Hair for Maximum Volume SEE PAGE 472

PROCEDURE 17-10 Blowdrying Blunt or Long-Layered, Straight to Wavy Hair into a Straight Style SEE PAGE 476

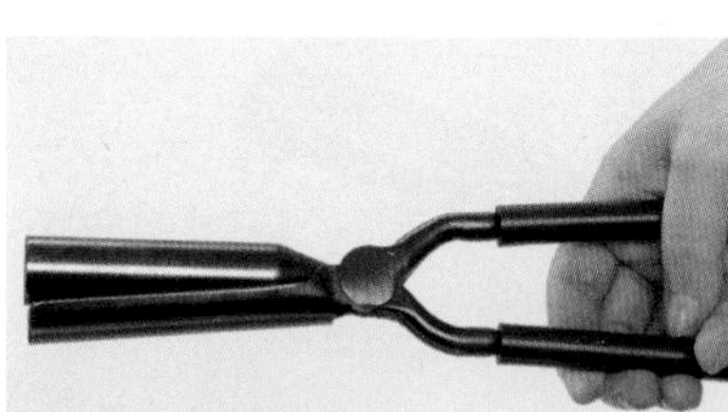

© Milady, a part of Cengage Learning. Photography by Paul Castle, Castle Photography.

▲ **Figure 17–50**
Conventional thermal (Marcel) iron.

Graduated Haircuts

Graduated haircuts have either long-layered or short-layered interiors. To blowdry graduated haircuts, use the same basic blowdrying techniques presented in the previous sections, choosing the technique that best suits the length of the hair you are working on. ☑ **LO2**

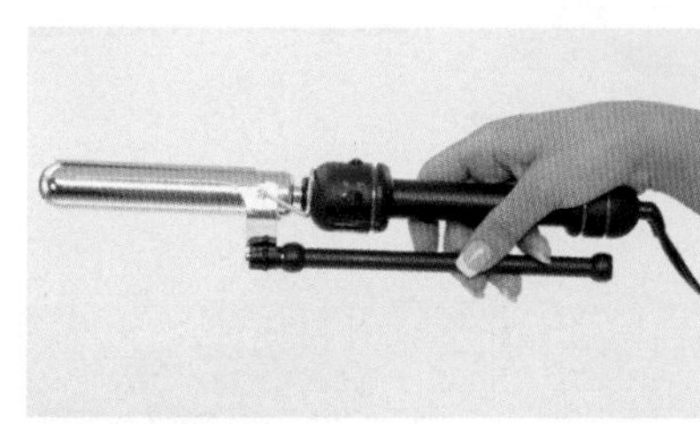

© Milady, a part of Cengage Learning. Photography by Paul Castle, Castle Photography.

▲ **Figure 17–51**
Electric thermal iron.

Thermal Hairstyling

Thermal waving and curling, also known as **Marcel waving**, are methods of waving and curling straight or pressed dry hair using thermal irons and special manipulative techniques (**Figure 17–50**). Thermal irons, which can be either electrical or stove heated, have been modernized so successfully that they are more popular today than ever before. Manipulative techniques are basically the same for electric irons or stove-heated irons.

Thermal Irons

Thermal irons are implements made of quality steel that are used to curl dry hair. They provide an even heat that is completely controlled by the stylist. Electric curling irons have cylindrical barrels ranging from ½ inch to 3 inches in diameter (**Figure 17–51**). Nonelectrical thermal irons are favored by many stylists who cater to clients with excessively curly hair because of the larger range of barrel or rod sizes and higher heat capabilities. Nonelectric thermal irons are heated in a specially designed electric or gas stove (**Figure 17–52**).

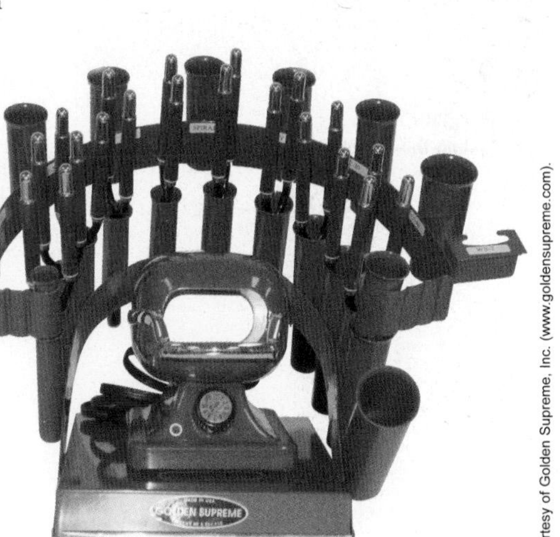

Courtesy of Golden Supreme, Inc. (www.goldensupreme.com).

▲ **Figure 17–52**
A modern stove-heated thermal iron and stove.

▶ Figure 17–53
The parts of a thermal iron.

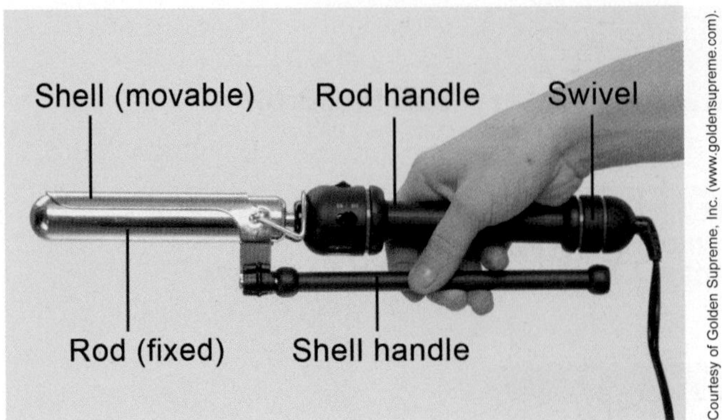

Courtesy of Golden Supreme, Inc. (www.goldensupreme.com).

All thermal irons have four basic parts: (1) rod handle, (2) shell handle, (3) barrel or **rod** (round, solid prong), and (4) **shell** (the clamp that presses the hair against the barrel or rod) (**Figure 17–53**).

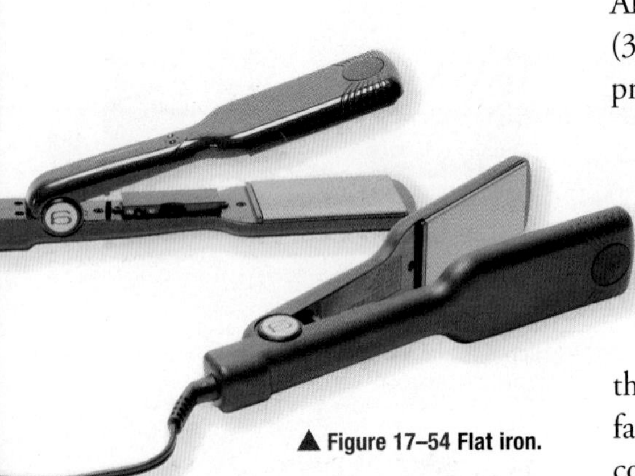

▲ Figure 17–54 Flat iron.

© Milady, a part of Cengage Learning. Photography by Yanik Chauvin.

Flat Irons

Flat irons have two hot plates ranging in size from ½ inch to 3 inches across (**Figure 17–54**). Flat irons with straight edges are used to create smooth, straight styles, even on very curly hair.

Flat irons with beveled edges can be manipulated to bend or cup the ends. The edge nearest the stylist is called the inner edge; the one farthest from the stylist is called the outer edge. Modern technology is constantly improving electric curling and flat irons by adding infinite heat settings for better control, constant heat even on high settings, ergonomic grips, and lightweight designs for ease of handling.

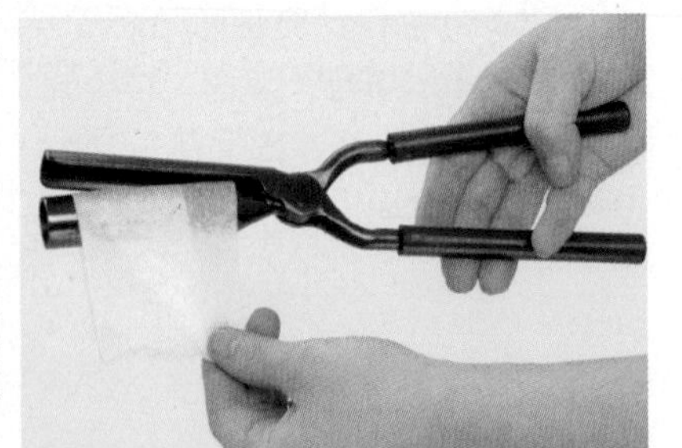

© Milady, a part of Cengage Learning. Photography by Paul Castle, Castle Photography.

▲ Figure 17–55
Testing the heat of a thermal iron.

Testing Thermal Irons

After heating the iron to the desired temperature, test it on a piece of tissue paper or a white cloth. Clamp the heated iron over this material and hold for five seconds. If it scorches or turns brown, the iron is too hot (**Figure 17–55**). Let it cool a bit before using. An overly hot iron can scorch the hair and might even discolor white hair. Remember that fine, lightened, or badly damaged hair withstands less heat than normal hair.

Care of Thermal Irons

Before cleaning a thermal iron, be sure to check the manufacturer's directions for care and cleaning. One way to remove dirt, oils, and product residue is to dampen a towel or rag and wipe down the barrel of the iron with a soapy solution containing a few drops of ammonia. If you are using a nonelectrical thermal iron, immerse the barrel in this solution. Do not clean your iron when it is turned on or when it is still cooling from a previous styling service.

Comb Used with Thermal Irons

The comb should be about 7-inches (17.5 centimeters) long, should be made of hard rubber or another nonflammable substance, and should have fine teeth to firmly hold the hair.

Hold the comb between the thumb and all four fingers of the non-dominant hand, with the index finger resting on the backbone of the comb for better control and one end of the comb resting against the outer edge of the palm. This position ensures a strong hold and a firm movement (**Figure 17–56**).

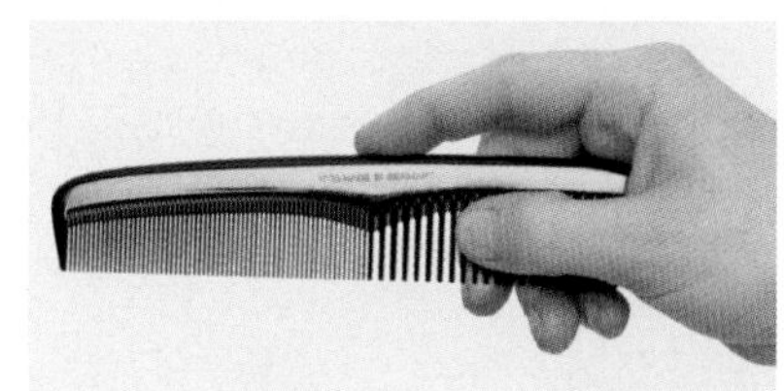

▲ **Figure 17–56**
Holding the comb.

Manipulating Thermal Irons

Hold the iron in a comfortable position that gives you complete control. Grasp the handles of the iron in your dominant hand, far enough away from the joint to avoid the heat. Place your three middle fingers on the back of the lower handle, your little finger in front of the lower handle, and your thumb in front of the upper handle.

The best way to practice manipulative techniques with thermal irons is by rolling the cold iron in your hand, first forward and then backward. This rolling movement should be done without any sway or motion in the arm; only the fingers are used as you roll the handles in each direction (**Figure 17–57**).

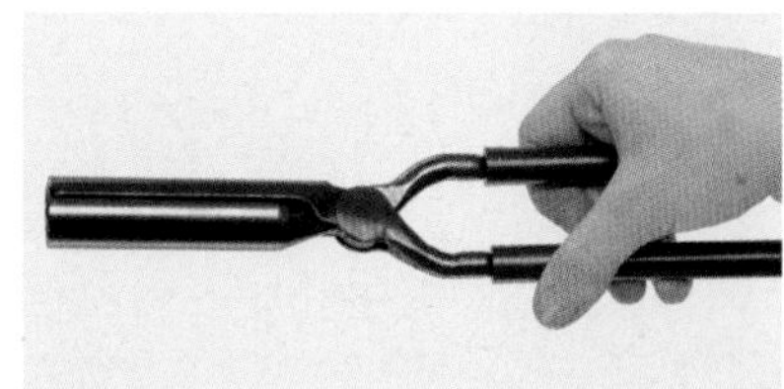

▲ **Figure 17–57**
Rolling the iron.

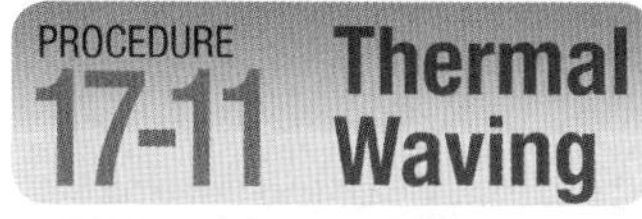

SEE PAGE 481 ☑ LO3

Temperature

There is no single correct temperature used for the iron when thermal curling or thermal waving the hair. The temperature setting for an iron depends on the texture of the hair, whether it is fine or coarse, and whether it has been lightened or tinted. Hair that has been lightened or tinted, as well as white hair, should be curled and waved with a gentle heat. As a rule, coarse and gray hair can withstand more heat than fine hair.

CAUTION

When using thermal irons on chemically straightened hair, be cautious and test the heat of the iron to avoid causing breakage.

Thermal Curling with Electric Thermal Irons

A modern thermal iron and a hard rubber comb are all you need to give your client curls. Thermal curling, which requires no setting gels or lotions, may be used to great advantage on the following hair types:

- **Straight hair.** Thermal curling permits quick styling because it eliminates the need for rollers (which are placed in wet hair) and a long hair drying process.
- **Pressed hair.** Thermal curling permits styling the hair without the danger of its returning to its former extremely curly condition, and it prepares the hair for any desired style.
- **Wigs and hairpieces (human hair).** Thermal curling presents a quick and effective method for styling.

Curling Iron Manipulations

The following is a series of basic manipulative movements for using curling irons. Most other curling iron movements are variations of these

© Milady, a part of Cengage Learning. Photography by Paul Castle, Castle Photography.

basic movements (**Figures 17–58** through **17–64**). Some stylists prefer to use just the little finger, or the little finger plus the ring finger, for this purpose. Either method is correct. The method of holding the iron is a matter of personal preference. Choose the one that gives you the most ease, comfort, and control.

If you want to get really good at using curling irons, the key is to practice manipulating them. Always practice with cold irons. The following four exercises are designed to help you learn the most effective ways to use an iron.

- Because it is important to develop a smooth rotating movement, practice turning the iron while opening and closing it at regular intervals. Practice rotating the iron in both directions—downward (toward you) and upward (away from you) (**Figure 17–65**).
- Practice releasing the hair by opening and closing the iron in a quick, clicking movement.
- Practice guiding the hair strand into the center of the curl as you rotate the iron. This movement ensures that the end of the strand is firmly in the center of the curl (**Figure 17–66**).
- Practice removing the curl from the iron by drawing the comb to the left and the rod to the right (**Figure 17–67**). Use the comb to protect the client's scalp from burns.

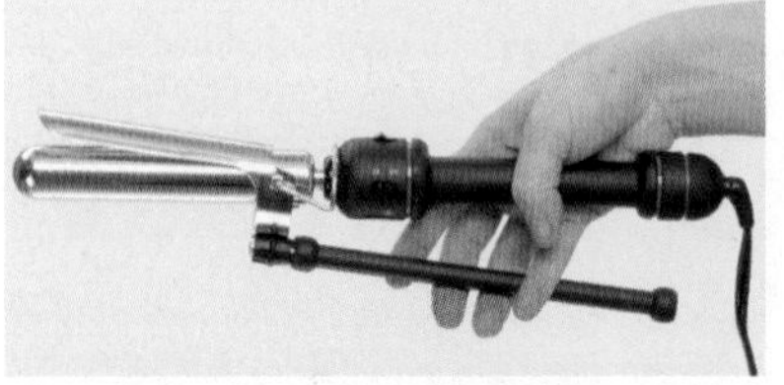

▲ **Figure 17–58**
Use the little finger to open the clamp.

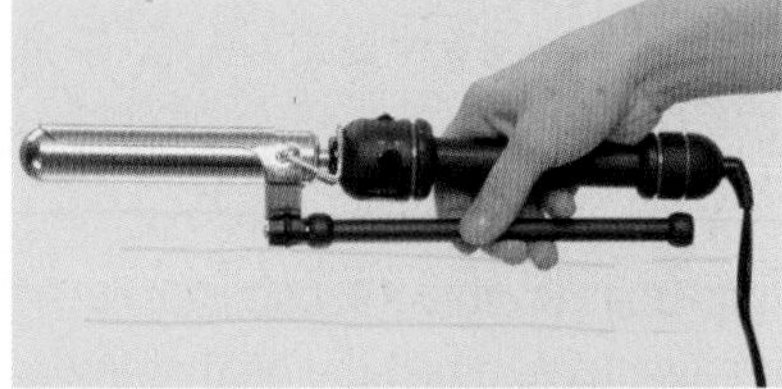

▲ **Figure 17–59**
Use your three middle fingers to close and manipulate the iron.

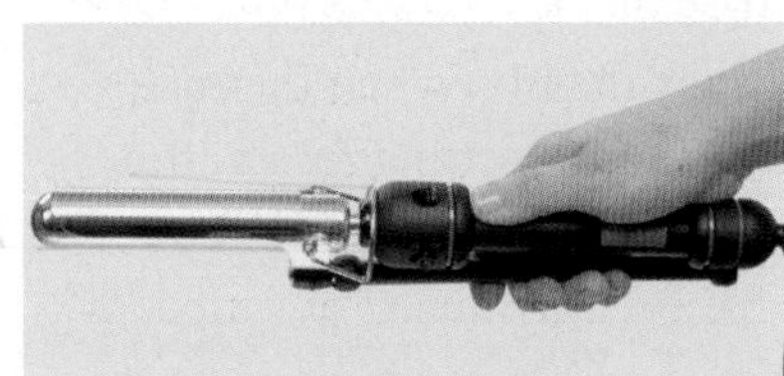

▲ **Figure 17–60**
Shift thumb when manipulating the iron.

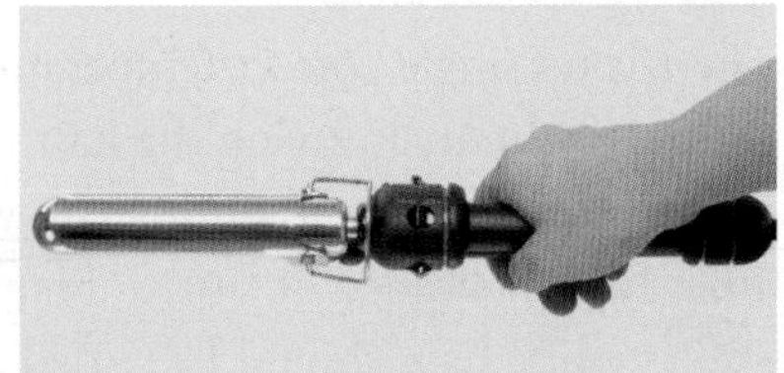

▲ **Figure 17–61**
Close shell and make a one-quarter turn downward.

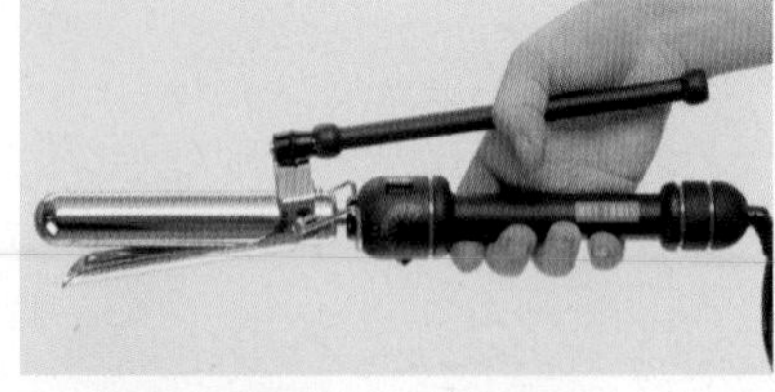

▲ **Figure 17–62**
Iron has made a half turn. Use thumb to open clamp and relax hair tension.

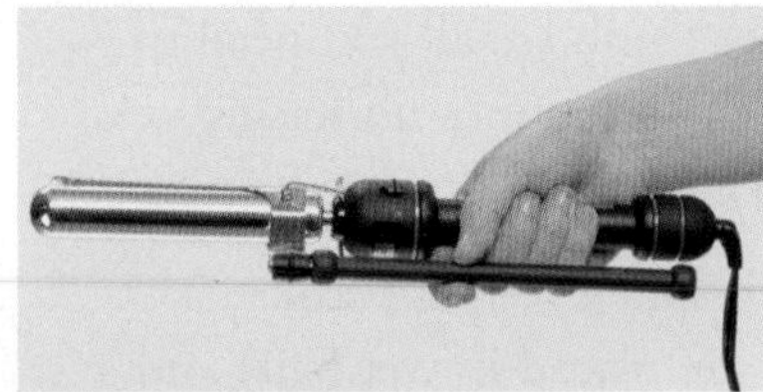

▲ **Figure 17–63**
Rotate iron to three quarters of a complete turn.

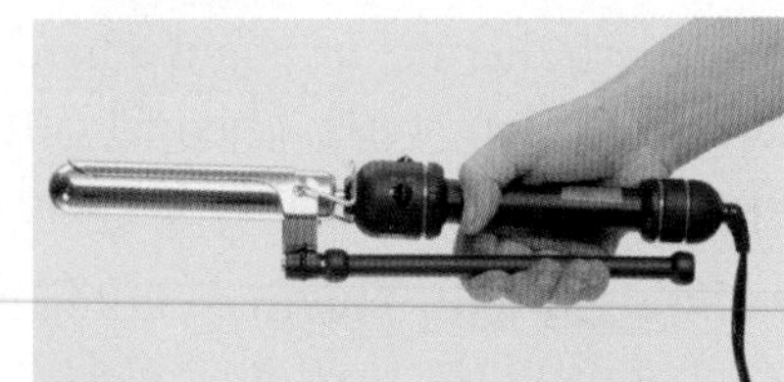

▲ **Figure 17–64**
Full turn.

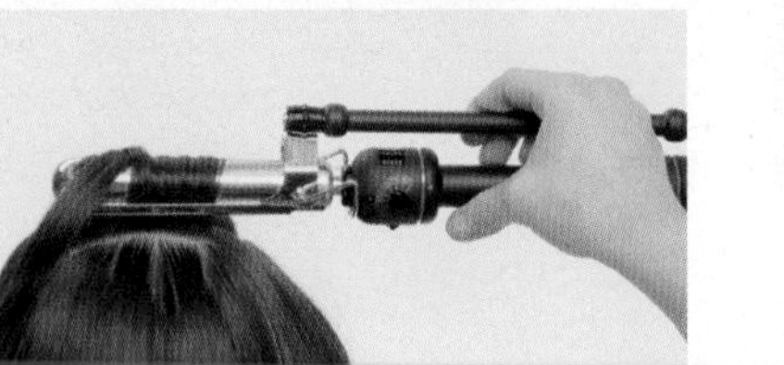

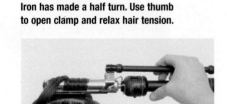

▲ **Figure 17–65**
Rotate while opening and closing the iron.

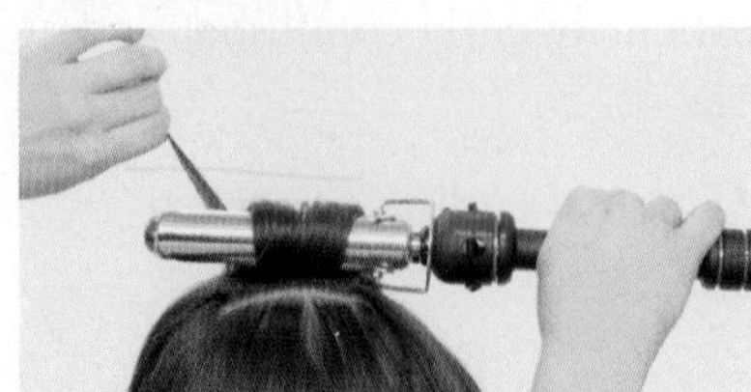

▲ **Figure 17–66**
Guide the hair strand into the center of curl while rotating the iron.

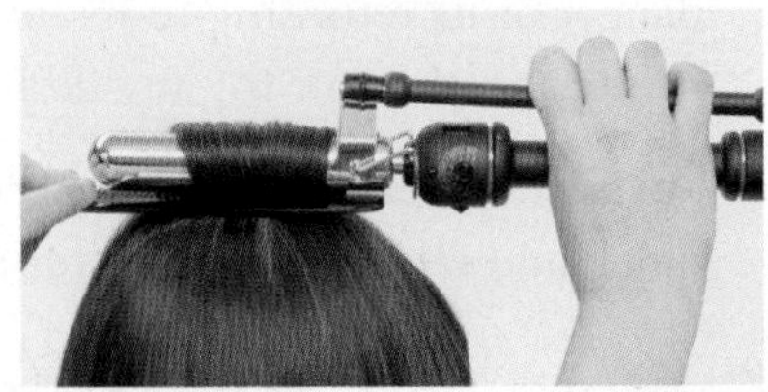

▲ **Figure 17–67**
Remove curl using the comb as you guide.

© Milady, a part of Cengage Learning. Photography by Paul Castle, Castle Photography.

PROCEDURE **17-12 Curling Short Hair**

SEE PAGE 487

PROCEDURE **17-13 Curling Medium-Length Hair**

SEE PAGE 489

PROCEDURE **17-14 Curling Hair Using Two Loops or Figure 8**

SEE PAGE 491

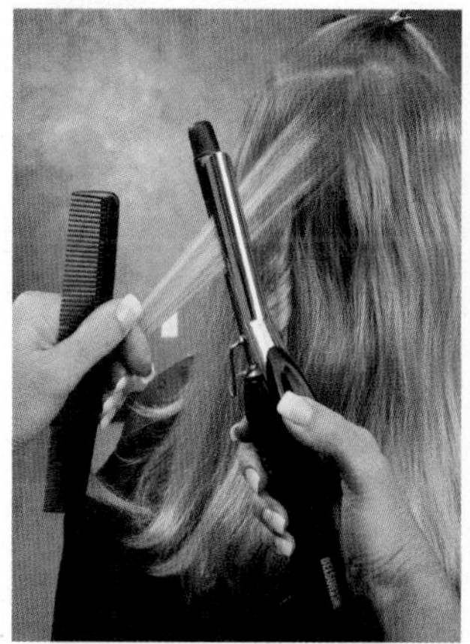

▲ Figure 17–68
Insert iron at an angle.

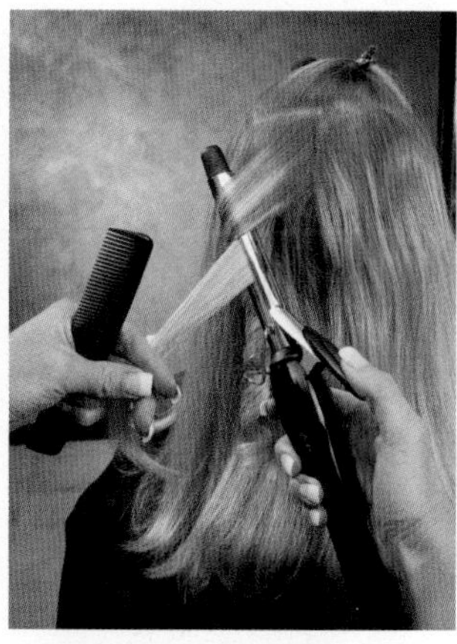

▲ Figure 17–69
Rotate iron until hair is wound.

Other Types of Curls

There are a number of other curls used for styling purposes. The **spiral curl** is a method of curling the hair by winding a strand around the rod. It creates hanging curls suitable for medium to long hairstyles. To create a spiral curl, part the hair into as many sections as there will be curls and comb smooth. Holding one section, insert the iron at an angle, with the bowl (groove) on top near the base of the strand, and rotate the iron until all the hair is wound (**Figures 17–68** and **17–69**). Hold the curl in this position for four to five seconds, and remove the iron in the usual manner (**Figures 17–70** and **17–71**).

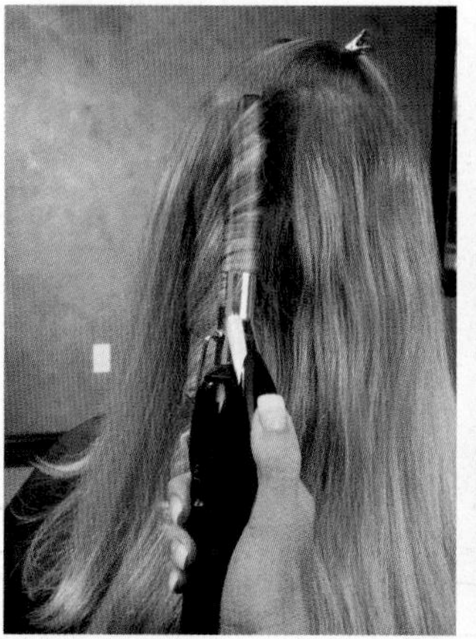

▲ Figure 17–70
Hold curl in position.

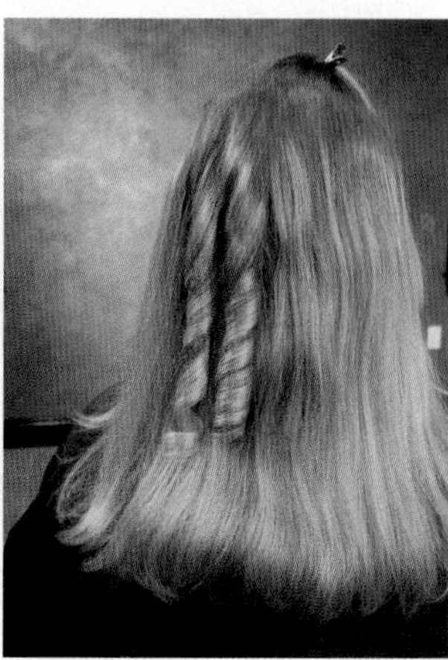

▲ Figure 17–71
Finished spiral curl.

End curls can be used to give a finished appearance to hair ends. Long, medium-length, or short hair may be styled with end curls. The hair ends can be turned under or over, as desired. The position and direction of the curling iron determine whether the end curls will turn under or over (**Figures 17–72** and **17–73**).

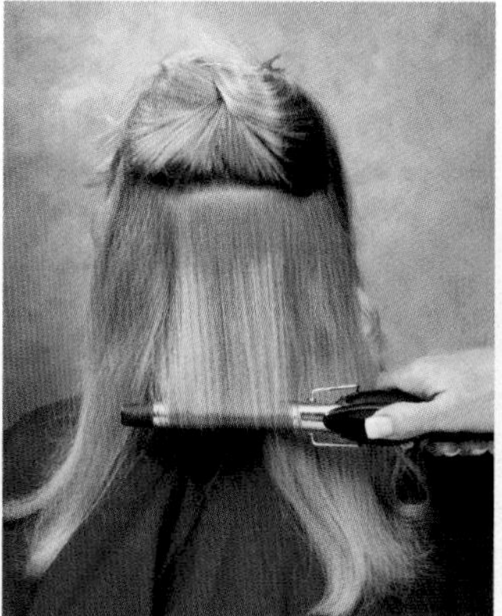

▲ Figure 17–72
Turn iron under.

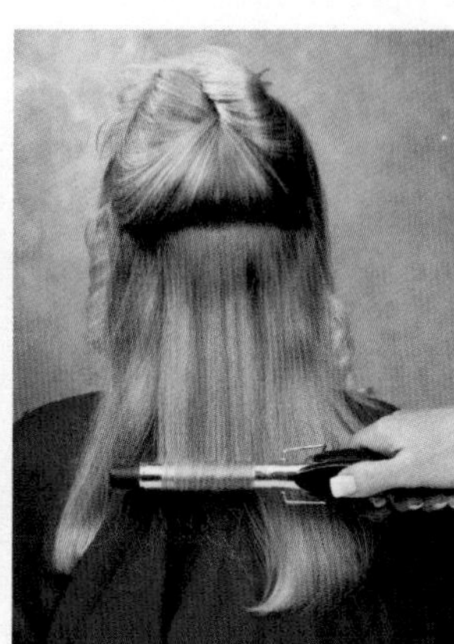

▲ Figure 17–73
Turn iron over.

Volume Thermal Iron Curls

Volume thermal iron curls are used to create volume or lift in a finished hairstyle. The degree of lift desired determines the type of volume curls to be used.

Volume-Base Thermal Curls

Volume-base curls provide maximum lift or volume, since the curl is placed very high on its base. Section off the base as described. Hold the curl strand at a 135-degree angle. Slide the iron over the strand about ½ inch (1.25 centimeters) from the scalp. Wrap the strand over the rod with medium tension.

© Milady, a part of Cengage Learning. Photography by Paul Castle, Castle Photography.

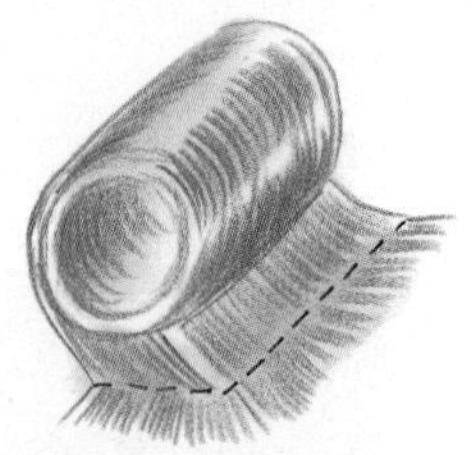
© Milady, a part of Cengage Learning.

▲ **Figure 17–74**
Volume-base curl.

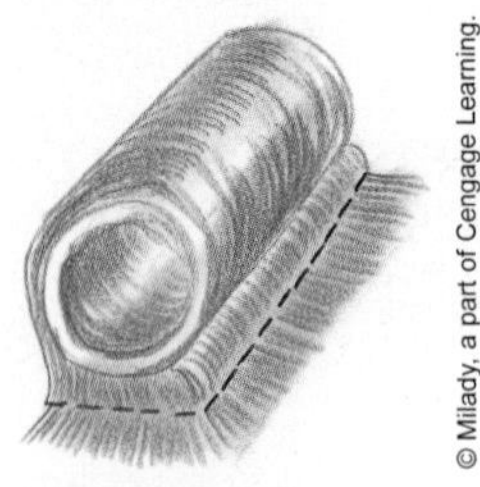
© Milady, a part of Cengage Learning.

▲ **Figure 17–75**
Full-base curl.

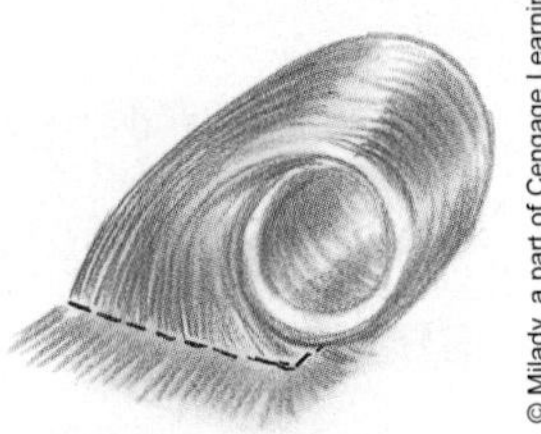
© Milady, a part of Cengage Learning.

▲ **Figure 17–76**
Half-base curl.

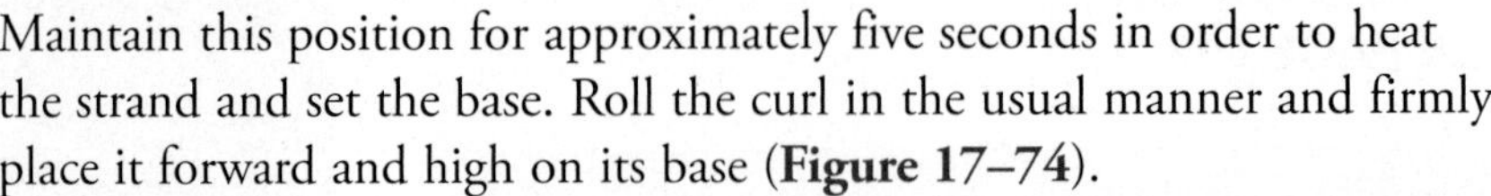

Maintain this position for approximately five seconds in order to heat the strand and set the base. Roll the curl in the usual manner and firmly place it forward and high on its base (**Figure 17–74**).

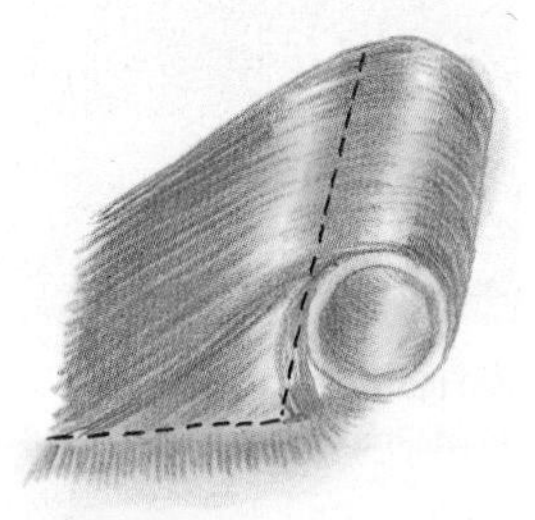
© Milady, a part of Cengage Learning.

▲ **Figure 17–77**
Off-base curl.

Full-Base Thermal Curls

Full-base curls sit in the center of their base and provide a strong curl with full volume. Section off the base as described. Hold the hair strand at a 125-degree angle. Slide the iron over the hair strand about ½ inch (1.25 centimeters) from the scalp. Wrap the strand over the rod with medium tension. Maintain this position for about five seconds to heat the strand and set the base. Roll the curl in the usual manner, and place it firmly in the center of its base (**Figure 17–75**).

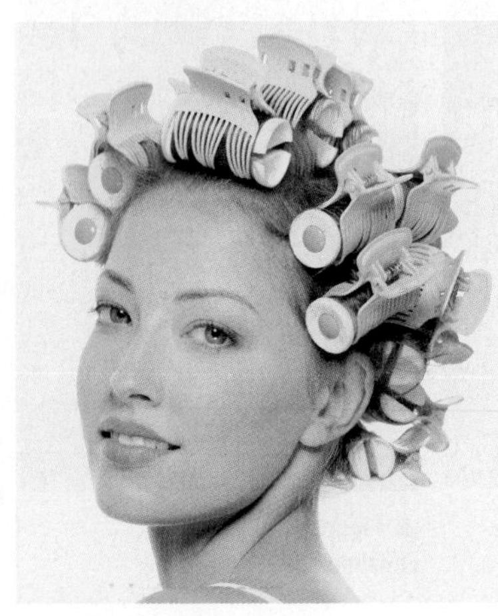
© Valua Vitaly, 2010; used under license from Shutterstock.com.

▲ **Figure 17–78**
Model in thermal rollers.

Half-Base Thermal Curls

Half-base curls sit half off their base and provide a strong curl with moderate lift or volume. Section off the base as described. Hold the hair at a 90-degree angle. Slide the iron over the hair strand about ½ inch (1.25 centimeters) from the scalp. Wrap the strand over the rod with medium tension. Maintain this position for about five seconds to heat the strand and set the base. Roll the curl in the usual manner, and place it half off its base (**Figure 17–76**).

Off-Base Thermal Curls

Off-base curls are placed completely off their base and offer a curl option with only slight lift or volume. Section off the base as described previously, holding the hair at a 70-degree angle. Slide the iron over the hair strand about ½ inch (1.25 centimeters) from the scalp. Wrap the strand over the rod with medium tension. Maintain this position for about five seconds to heat the strand and set the base. Roll the curl in the usual manner, and place it completely off its base (**Figure 17–77**).

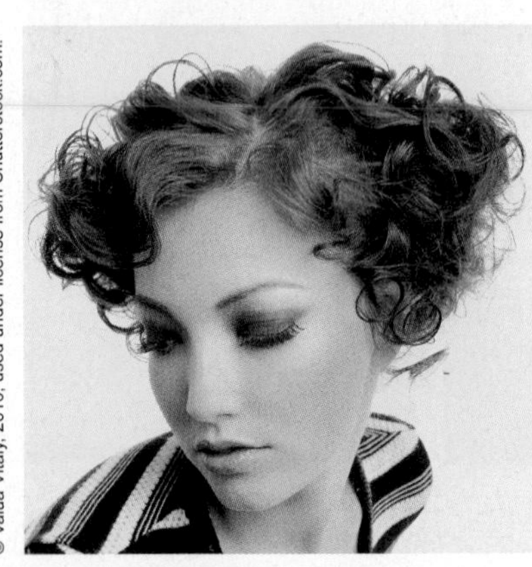
© Valua Vitaly, 2010; used under license from Shutterstock.com.

▲ **Figure 17–79**
Finished thermal-curled short hairstyle.

Finished Thermal Curl Settings

For best results when giving a thermal setting, clip each curl in place until the whole head has been curled and is ready for styling (**Figure 17–78**). Brush the hair, working up from the neckline and pushing the waves into place as you progress over the entire head. If the hairstyle is to be finished with curls, do the bottom curls last (**Figures 17–79** through **17–81**). ☑ **LO4**

Using Thermal Irons Safely

Here are some guidelines for the safe use of thermal irons:

- Use thermal irons only after receiving instruction in their use.
- Keep thermal irons clean.
- Do not overheat thermal irons, because this can damage their ability to hold heat uniformly.
- Test the temperature of the iron on tissue paper or a white cloth before placing it on the hair in order to prevent burning the hair.
- Handle thermal irons carefully to avoid burning yourself or the client.
- Place hot irons in a safe place to cool. Do not leave them where someone might accidentally come into contact with them and be burned.
- When heating a conventional iron, do not place the handles too close to the heater. Your hand might be burned when removing the iron.
- Make sure the iron is properly balanced in the heater, or it might fall and be damaged or injure someone.
- Use only hard rubber or nonflammable combs. Celluloid combs must not be used in thermal curling, as they are flammable.
- Do not use metal combs; they can become hot and burn the scalp.
- Place a comb between the scalp and the thermal iron when curling or waving hair to prevent burning the scalp.
- The client's hair must be clean and completely dry to ensure a good thermal curl or wave.
- Do not allow the hair ends to protrude over the iron; this causes fishhooks (hair that is bent or folded).
- When ironing lightened, tinted, or relaxed hair, always use a gentle heat setting.

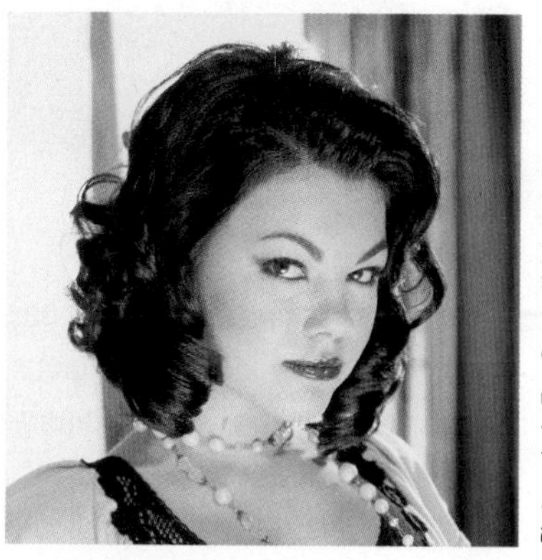

Photography by Tom Carson. Hair by Julie Beauchesne for Je Beau International, Manchester, NH.

▲ **Figure 17–80**
Finished thermal-curled medium-length hairstyle.

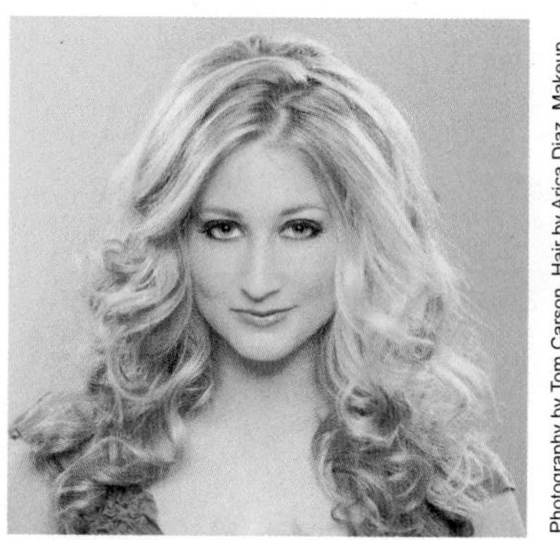

Photography by Tom Carson. Hair by Arica Diaz. Makeup by Melisa McDonald for Kathy Adams Salon, Buford, GA.

▲ **Figure 17–81**
Finished thermal-curled long hairstyle.

Thermal Hair Straightening (Hair Pressing)

Thermal hair straightening, or pressing, is a popular service that is very profitable in the salon. When properly done, **hair pressing** temporarily straightens extremely curly or unruly hair by means of a heated iron or comb. A pressing generally lasts until the hair is shampooed. (Permanent or chemical hair straightening is covered in Chapter 20, Chemical Texture Services.) Hair pressing also prepares the hair for additional services, such as thermal curling and croquignole (KROH-ken-yohl) thermal curling (the two-loop or Figure 8 technique). A good hair pressing leaves the hair in a natural and lustrous condition, and it is not harmful to the hair (**Figure 17–82**).

▼ **Figure 17–82**
Pressed hairstyle.

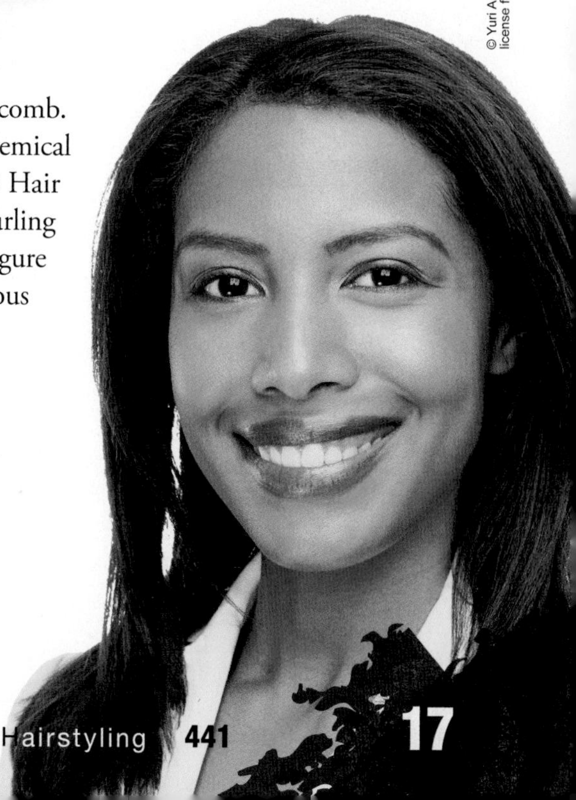

© Yuri Arcurs, 2010; used under license from Shutterstock.com.

There are three types of hair pressing:

- **Soft press,** which removes about 50 to 60 percent of the curl, is accomplished by applying the thermal pressing comb once on each side of the hair.
- **Medium press,** which removes about 60 to 75 percent of the curl, is accomplished by applying the thermal pressing comb once on each side of the hair, using slightly more pressure.

CAUTION

Under no circumstances should hair pressing be performed on a client who has a scalp abrasion, a contagious scalp condition, a scalp injury, or chemically damaged hair. Chemically relaxed hair should not be pressed.

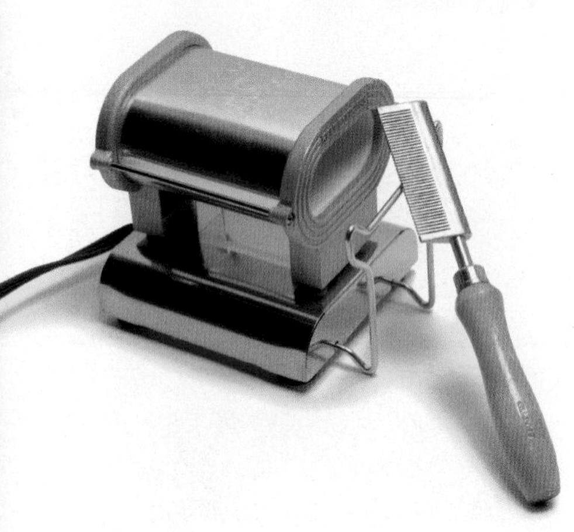

© Milady, a part of Cengage Learning. Photography by Yanik Chauvin.

- **Hard press,** which removes 100 percent of the curl, is accomplished by applying the thermal pressing comb twice on each side of the hair. A hard press can also be done by first passing a hot thermal iron through the hair. This is called a **double press.** ☑ **LO5**

Analysis of Hair and Scalp

Before you press a client's hair, you will need to analyze the condition of the hair and scalp. (You may wish to review the steps of "Hair and Scalp Analysis" in Chapter 11, Properties of the Hair and Scalp.) If the client's hair and scalp are not healthy, you should give appropriate advice concerning corrective treatments.

In the case of scalp skin disease, it is not the cosmetologist's job to diagnose the condition, but rather to advise the client to see a dermatologist.

If the hair shows signs of neglect or abuse caused by faulty pressing, lightening, or tinting, recommend a series of conditioning treatments. Failure to correct dry and brittle hair can result in hair breakage during hair pressing. Burned hair strands cannot be conditioned.

Remember to check your client's hair for elasticity and porosity. Under normal conditions, if a client's hair has good elasticity, it can be stretched to about 50 percent of its original length before breaking. If the porosity is normal, the hair will return to its natural wave pattern when it is wet or moistened.

A careful analysis of the client's hair and scalp should cover the following points:

- Wave pattern
- Length
- Texture (coarse, medium, or fine)
- Feel (wiry, soft, or silky)
- Elasticity
- Color (natural, faded, streaked, gray, tinted, or lightened)
- Condition of hair (normal, brittle, dry, oily, damaged, or chemically treated)
- Condition of scalp (normal, flexible, or tight)

It is important that the cosmetologist be able to recognize individual differences in hair texture, porosity, elasticity, and scalp flexibility. Guided by this information, the cosmetologist can determine how much pressure the hair and scalp can handle without hair breakage, hair loss, or burning from a pressing comb that is too hot.

Hair Texture

Variations in hair texture have to do with the diameter of the hair (coarse, medium, or fine) and the feel of the hair (wiry, soft, or silky). Touching the client's hair and asking about specific hair characteristics will help you determine the best way to treat the hair.

Coarse, extremely curly hair has qualities that make it difficult to press. Coarse hair has the greatest diameter, and during the pressing process it requires more heat and pressure than medium or fine hair.

Medium curly hair is the type of hair that cosmetologists deal with most often in the beauty salon. No special problem is presented by this type of hair, and this hair type is the least resistant to pressing.

Fine hair requires special care. To avoid hair breakage, use less heat and pressure than you would use on other hair textures.

Wiry, curly hair may be coarse, medium, or fine, and it feels stiff, hard, and glassy. Because of the compact construction of its cuticle cells, hair of this type is very resistant to hair pressing and requires more heat and pressure than other types of hair.

Scalp Condition

The condition of the client's scalp can be classified as normal, tight, or flexible. If the scalp is normal, proceed with an analysis of hair texture and elasticity. If the scalp is tight and the hair coarse, press the hair in the direction in which it grows to avoid injury to the scalp. If the scalp is flexible, remember to use enough tension to press the hair satisfactorily.

Service Notes

Be sure to record the results of your hair and scalp analysis, as well as all pressing treatments, on the client's intake form or service record card.

During your client consultation, question the client about any lightener, tint, gradual colors (metallic), or other chemical treatment that have been used on her hair. As with all services, a release statement should be signed by the client prior to hair pressing in order to protect the school, the salon, and the stylist from liability due to accidents or damage.

Conditioning Treatments

Effective conditioning treatments involve special cosmetic preparations for the hair and scalp, thorough brushing, and scalp massage. The application of a conditioning treatment usually results in better hair pressing.

A tight scalp can be made more flexible by the systematic use of scalp massage and hair brushing. The client benefits because there is better circulation of blood to the scalp.

© Milady, a part of Cengage Learning.

Pressing Combs

There are two types of pressing combs: regular and electric. Both should be constructed of good quality stainless steel or brass. The handle is usually made of wood, because wood does not readily absorb heat.

The space between the teeth of the comb varies with the size and style of the comb. Closely spaced teeth provide a smooth press. As spacing gets wider, the press gets less smooth.

Pressing combs also vary in size. Shorter combs are used to press short hair; longer combs are used to press long hair.

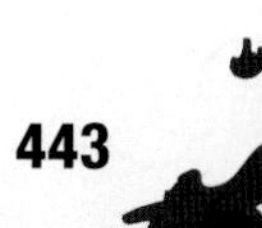

Tempering The Comb

It may be a good idea to **temper** a new brass pressing comb so that it will hold heat evenly along its entire length and provide consistent results. To temper a new pressing comb, heat the comb until it is extremely hot. Coat the comb in petroleum or pressing oil. Let it cool down naturally, and then rinse under hot running water to remove the oil.

Tempering the pressing comb also allows you to burn off any polish the manufacturer may have used to coat the comb. If the polish is not burned off, the comb may stick to the hair, causing scorching and breakage.

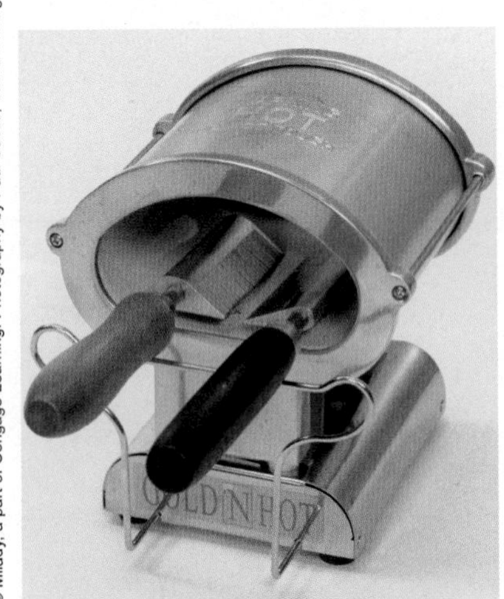

© Milady, a part of Cengage Learning. Photography by Paul Castle, Castle Photography.

▲ Figure 17–83
Electric heater for pressing combs.

Heating the Comb

Depending on what they are made of, pressing combs vary in their ability to accept and retain heat. Regular pressing combs may be designed as electrical appliances or to be heated in electric or gas stoves (**Figure 17–83**). When heating a pressing comb in a gas stove, point the teeth faceup and keep the handle away from the fire.

After heating the comb to the proper temperature, test it on a piece of light paper. If the paper becomes scorched, allow the comb to cool slightly before applying it to the hair.

Electric pressing combs are available in two forms. One comes with an on/off switch; the other is equipped with a thermostat that indicates high or low degrees of heat.

Straightening comb attachments are available for purchase to fit the nozzle of a standard hand-held blowdryer. While these attachments are less damaging than either an electric comb or an oven-heated comb, they may also be less effective at pressing the hair.

Cleaning the Comb

The pressing comb will perform more efficiently if it is kept clean. Wipe the comb clean of loose hair, grease, and dust before and after every use. Once all loose hair and clinging dirt are removed, the comb's intense heat keeps it sterile.

With a stove-heated pressing comb (nonelectrical), remove the carbon by rubbing the outside surface and between the teeth with a fine steel-wool pad or fine sandpaper. Then place the metal portion of the comb in a hot baking soda solution for about one hour. Rinse and dry the comb thoroughly. The metal will acquire a smooth and shiny appearance.

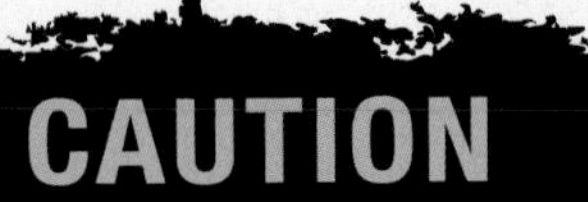

In case of a scalp burn, immediately apply 1 percent gentian (JEN-chun) violet jelly.

Pressing Oil or Cream

Prepare the hair for a pressing treatment by first applying pressing oil or cream. Both of these products offer the following benefits:

- Make hair softer
- Prepare and condition the hair for pressing
- Help protect the hair from burning or scorching
- Help prevent hair breakage

- Condition the hair after pressing
- Add sheen to pressed hair
- Help hair stay pressed longer

PROCEDURE 17-15 Soft Pressing for Normal Curly Hair SEE PAGE 493

Hard Press

A hard press is only recommended when the results of a soft or medium press are not satisfactory. The entire comb press procedure is repeated. Pressing oil should be added to hair strands only if necessary. A hard press is also known as a double comb press. ☑ **LO6**

Touch-Ups

Touch-ups are sometimes necessary when the hair becomes curly again due to perspiration, dampness, or other conditions. The process is the same as for the original pressing treatment, with the shampoo omitted.

Reminders and Hints for All Pressing Procedures

Good judgment should be used to avoid damage, with consideration always given to the texture of the hair and the condition of the scalp. The client's safety is ensured only when the stylist observes every precaution and takes special care during the actual hair pressing. Listed below are rules of thumb for hair pressing:

- Avoid excessive heat or pressure on the hair and scalp.
- Avoid too much pressing oil on the hair (it attracts dirt and makes the hair look greasy and artificial).
- Avoid perfumed pressing oil near the scalp if the client has allergies.
- Avoid overly frequent hair pressing.
- Keep the comb clean at all times.
- Avoid overheating the pressing comb if using a stove.
- Test the temperature of the heated comb on a white cloth or paper before applying it to the hair.
- Adjust the temperature of the pressing comb to the texture and condition of the client's hair.
- Use the heated comb carefully to avoid burning the skin, scalp, or hair.
- Prevent the smoking or burning of hair during the pressing treatment by drying the hair completely after it is shampooed and by avoiding excessive application of pressing oil.
- Use a moderately warm comb to press short hair on the temples andback of the neck. You may also use a temple comb, which is about half the size of a regular pressing comb.

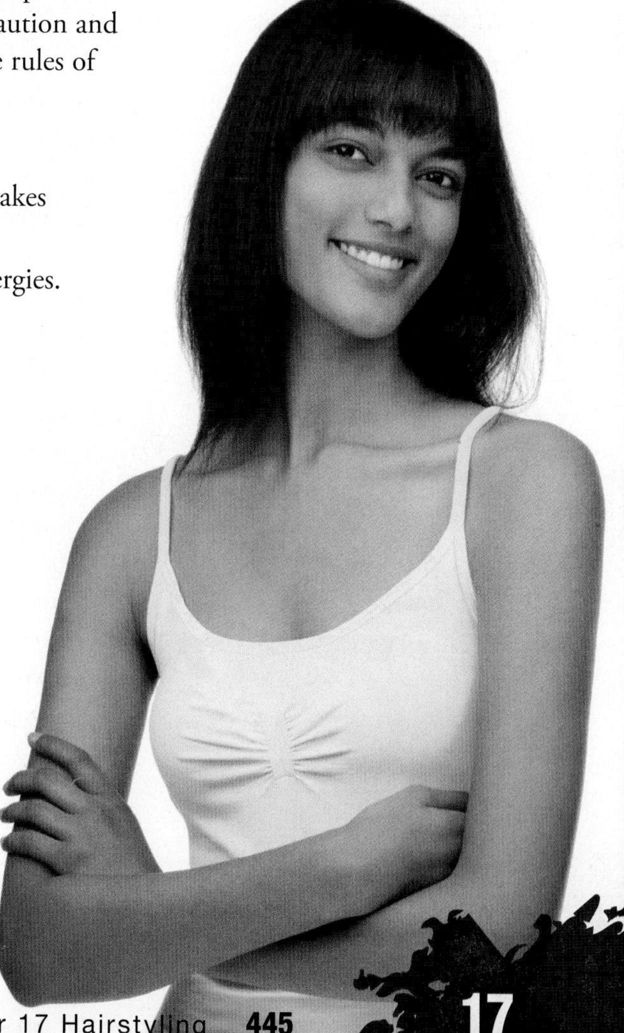

© Yuri Arcurs 2010; used under license from Shutterstock.com.

CAUTION

Two general types of injuries can occur in hair pressing:

- Injuries that are the immediate result of hair pressing and that cause physical damage include burned hair that breaks off, burned scalp that causes either temporary or permanent hair loss, and burns on the ears and neck that form scars.
- Injuries that are not immediately evident but can cause physical damage later include a skin rash if the client is allergic to pressing oil and the breaking and shortening of the hair due to frequent hair pressings.

Special Considerations

You should take certain precautions and safeguards when dealing with the following special situations:

- **Pressing fine hair.** Follow the same procedure as for normal hair, while avoiding the use of a hot pressing comb or too much pressure. To avoid hair breakage, apply less pressure to the hair near the ends. After completely pressing the hair, style it.
- **Pressing short, fine hair.** Extra care must be taken at the hairline. When the hair is extra short, the pressing comb should not be too hot because the hair is fine and will burn easily. A hot comb can also cause painful burns and may result in scars. In the event of an accidental burn, immediately apply 1 percent gentian violet jelly to the burn.
- **Pressing coarse hair.** Apply enough pressure so that the hair remains straightened.
- **Pressing tinted, lightened, or gray (unpigmented) hair.** This hair requires special care. Lightened or tinted hair might require conditioning treatments, depending on the extent to which it has been damaged. Gray hair may be particularly resistant. To obtain good results on gray hair, use a moderately heated pressing comb applied with light pressure. Avoid excessive heat as discoloration or breakage can occur.

Styling Long Hair

An **updo** is a hairstyle with the hair arranged up and off the shoulders and secured with implements such as hairpins, bobby pins, and elastics. Clients usually request updos for special occasions such as weddings, proms, and evening events. A few classic updo techniques—knot, twist, and pleat—are described below. Once these techniques are mastered, any placement or combination of them can give a unique update to a classic look. When executing an updo, always inspect the shape you are building from every angle to make sure that it is well balanced and well proportioned.

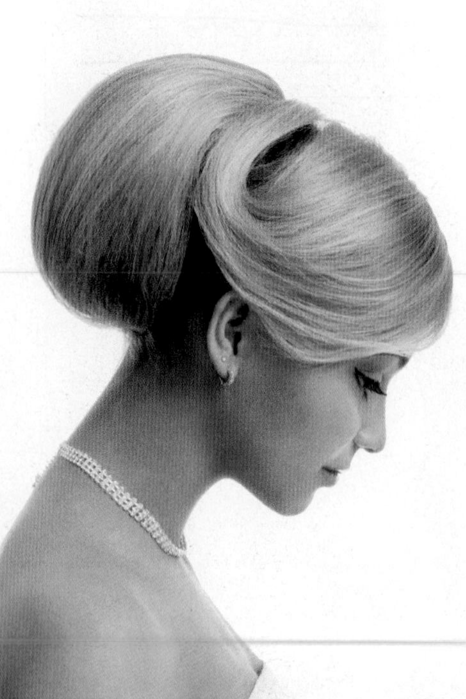

- **Knot.** A truly classic style, the knot, also known as **chignon** (SHEEN-yahn), has been popular for centuries. It is created out of a simple ponytail and can be dressed up with flowers or ornaments, or kept simple. If the client's hair is very straight and silky, you may want to first set the hair for ten minutes in electric rollers, or the style will not last. If the hair is wavy or curly, blowdry the hair straight. If it is extremely curly, you could press the hair first or leave it natural for a textured-looking chignon.
- **Twist.** This elegant, sleek look can go anywhere. If you are working on straight, fine hair, you may want to first set the hair in electric or Velcro rollers to give it more body.
- **Pleat.** This traditional updo is usually used for weddings and black-tie events and is also known as **classic French twist**. The pleat (which

© Valua Vitaly, 2010; used under license from iStockphoto.com.

means "folded" in French) is much more severe and controlled than the basic twist, and you can be more creative with the directional placement. ☑ **LO7**

Formal Styling

Client Consultation

As always, consult with the client first to make sure you understand what she has in mind. Have magazines available that show a lot of updos, such as bridal magazines, or keep a folder of pictures clipped from magazines at your station that show current styles. If you are doing a pre-wedding consultation with a bride, ask the bride to bring her headpiece so that she can try several styles and see how they look. Take photographs to help her decide which style she likes best. Always suggest classic, timeless styles for brides and leave the latest trend for the bridesmaids. This suggestion will be appreciated years later. Keep a photo of the chosen style so that you can duplicate it for the bride's big day.

PROCEDURE **17-16 Knot or Chignon** SEE PAGE 496

PROCEDURE **17-17 Twist** SEE PAGE 498

PROCEDURE **17-18 Pleat** SEE PAGE 500

The Artistry of Hairstyling

Hairstyling offers a cosmetologist a wonderful artistic outlet. Once you master the basic styles presented in this chapter and the foundational techniques these styles require, you will have the technical abilities to experiment and create your own unique and attractive looks.

Styling trends change quickly. In order to offer your clients the latest looks, you may want to consider having a mannequin at home. This will enable you to practice creating the looks you see in magazines and to try out new styling ideas and techniques. Remember, every client's hair presents creative possibilities!

© Zoom Team, 2010; used under license from iStockphoto.com.

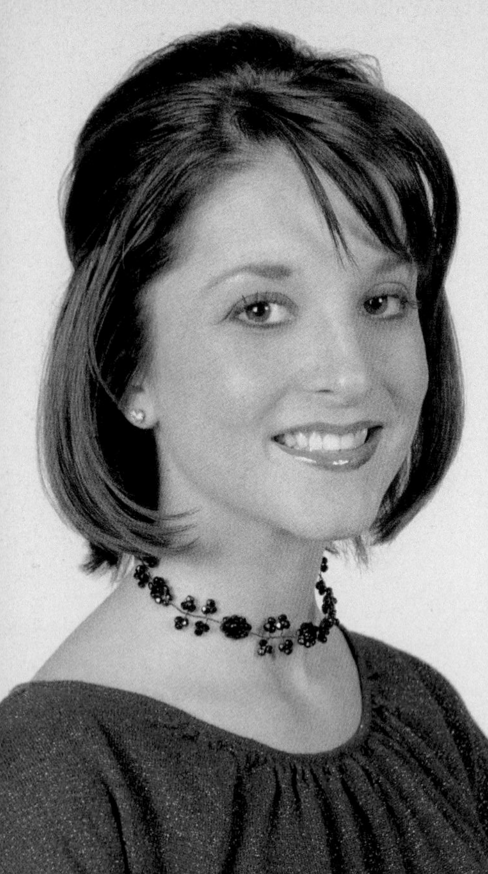

PROCEDURE 17-1

Preparing Hair for Wet Styling

Implements and Materials

You will need all of the following implements, materials, and supplies:

- **Conditioner**
- **Neck strip**
- **Plastic cape**
- **Shampoo**
- **Towels**

Preparation

- Perform PROCEDURE 15-1 **Pre-Service Procedure** **SEE PAGE 323**

Procedure

1 Drape the client for a shampoo service.

2 Shampoo the client's hair, and condition if necessary.

3 Towel dry the hair.

4 Remove any tangles with a wide-tooth comb, starting at the ends and working up to the scalp.

5 Part the hair, using the client's natural part if that works with your hair design, or create a part anywhere on the head if that better suits the final design.

© Milady, a part of Cengage Learning. Photography by Yanik Chauvin.

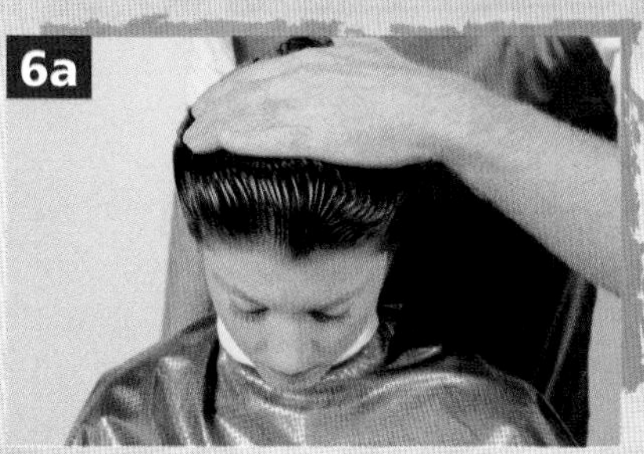

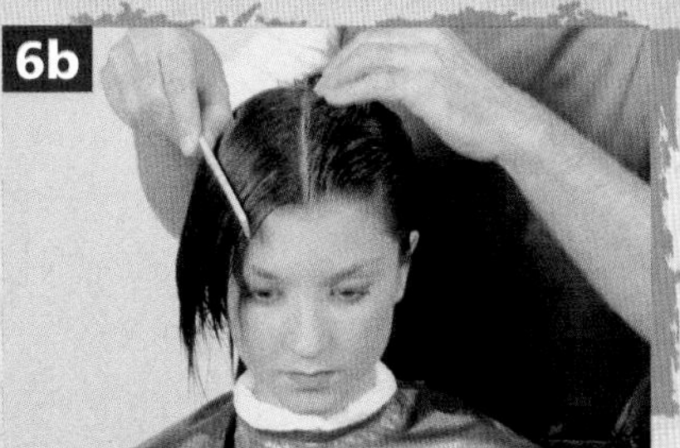

6 To find the client's natural part, comb wet hair straight back from the hairline, and push the hair gently forward with the palm of the hand. Use your comb and other hand to separate the hair where it parts.

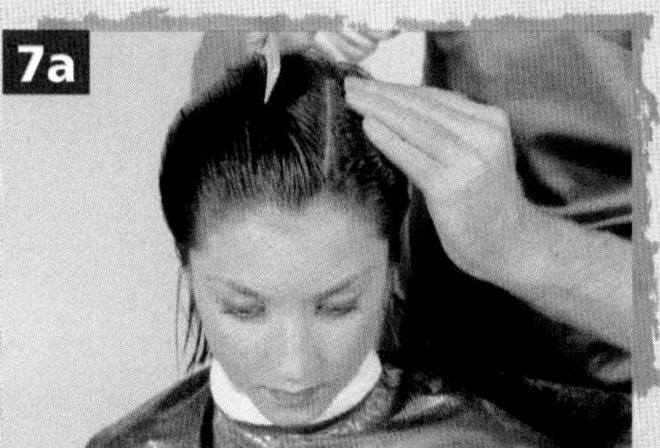

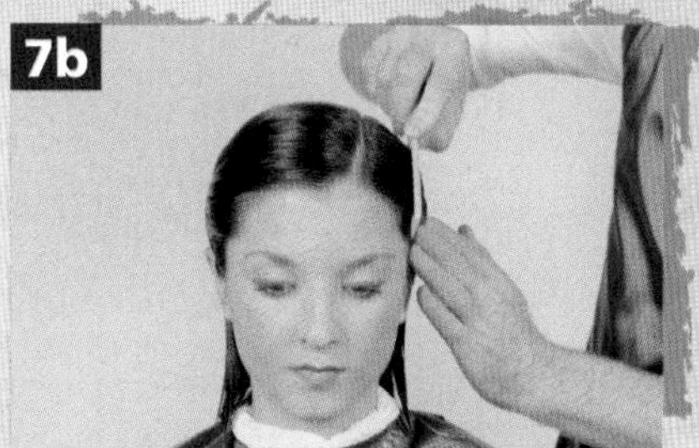

7 To create a part, lay the wide-tooth end of a styling comb flat at the hairline, and draw the comb back to the end of the desired part. Hold the hair with the index finger on one side of the part. Pull the rest of the hair down with the comb.

8 You are now ready to move on to the next aspect of the service.

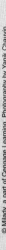

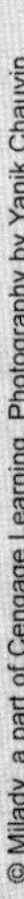
© Milady, a part of Cengage Learning. Photography by Yanik Chauvin.

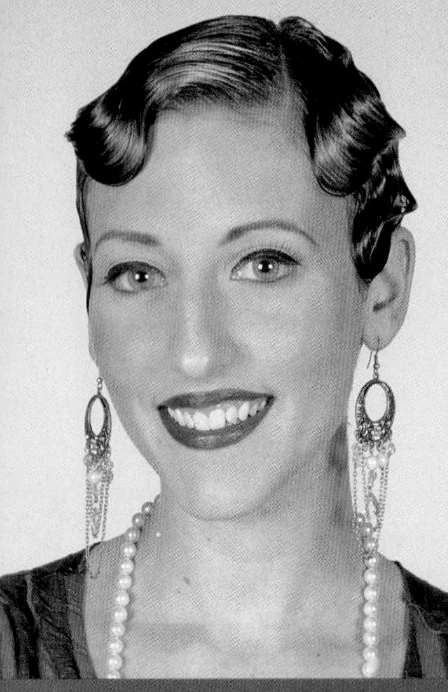

PROCEDURE 17-2 Right-Handed

Horizontal Finger Waving

Implements and Materials

You will need all of the following implements, materials, and supplies:

- **Conditioner**
- **Finishing products such as shine or hair spray**
- **Hairnet**
- **Hairpins**
- **Neck strip**
- **Plastic cape**
- **Shampoo**
- **Styling comb**
- **Towels**
- **Waving lotion or styling gel**

Preparation

- Perform PROCEDURE 15-1 **Pre-Service Procedure** **SEE PAGE 323**

Procedure

1 Drape the client for a shampoo service.

2 Shampoo the client's hair, and condition if necessary.

3 Towel dry the hair.

4

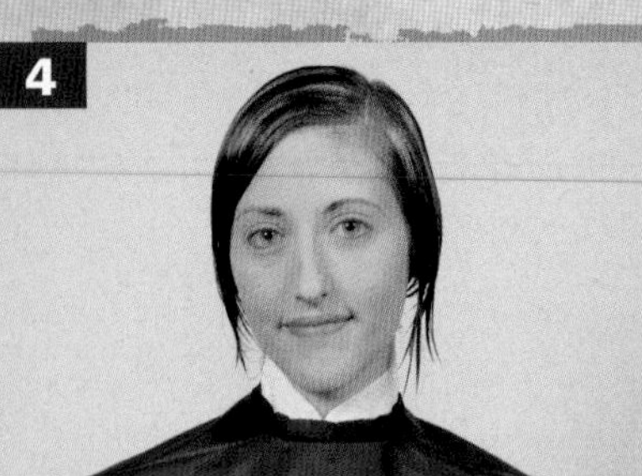

4 Remove any tangles with a wide-tooth comb, starting at the ends and working up to the scalp.

5 Part the hair, comb it smooth, and arrange it according to the planned style. Using the wide teeth of the comb will allow the hair to move more easily. Always follow the natural growth pattern when combing and parting the hair.

© Milady, a part of Cengage Learning. Photography by Yanik Chauvin.

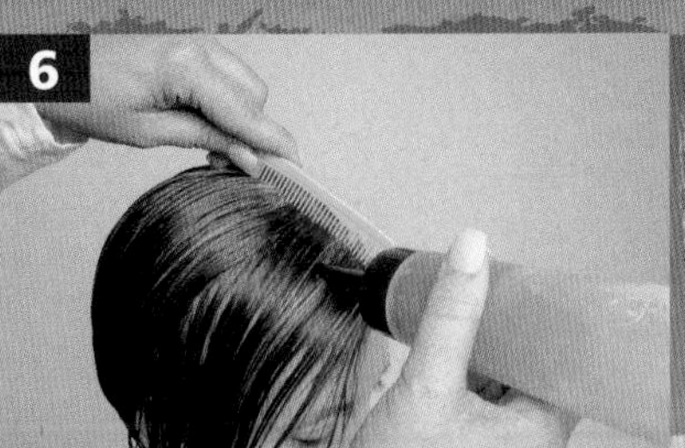

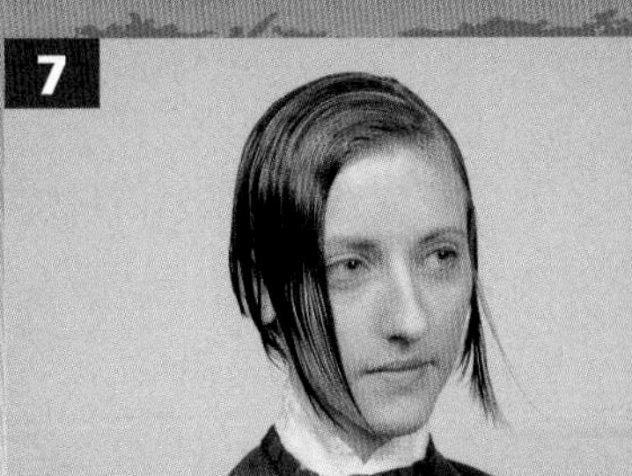

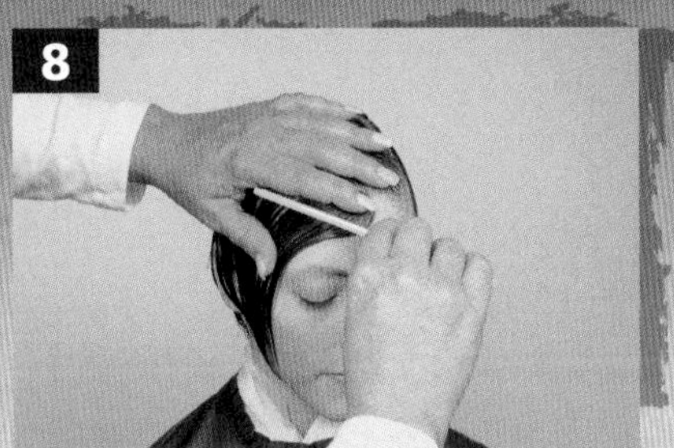

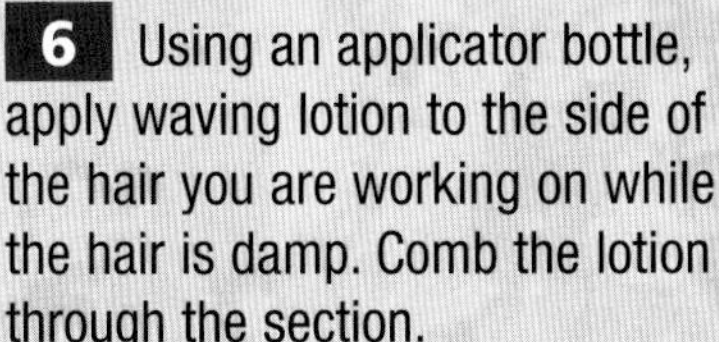

6 Using an applicator bottle, apply waving lotion to the side of the hair you are working on while the hair is damp. Comb the lotion through the section.

7 Begin the first wave on the right side of the head. Using the index finger of your left hand as a guide, shape the top hair with a comb into the beginning of the S-shaping, using a circular movement. Starting at the hairline, work toward the crown in 1½- to 2-inch (3.7 to 5 centimeters) sections at a time.

8 To form the first ridge, place the index finger of your left hand directly above the position for the first ridge. With the teeth of the comb pointing slightly upward, insert the comb directly under the index finger. Draw the comb forward about 1 inch (2.5 centimeters) along the fingertip.

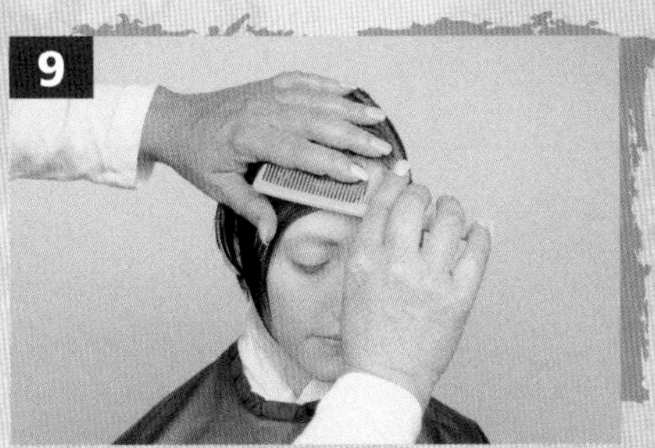

9 With the teeth still inserted in the ridge, flatten the comb against the head in order to hold the ridge in place.

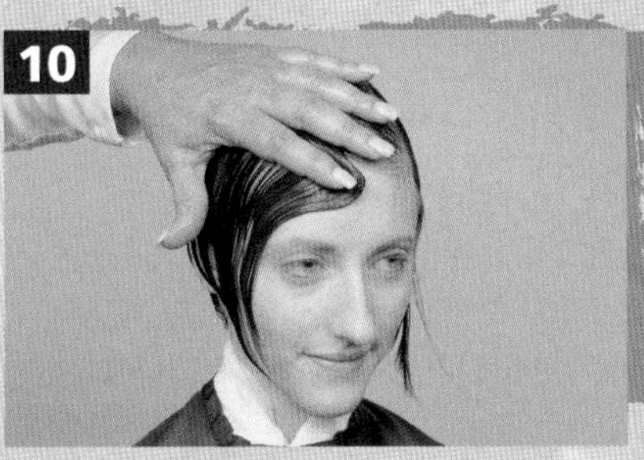

10 Remove your left hand from the client's head and place your middle finger above the ridge with your index finger on the teeth of the comb. Draw out the ridge by closing the two fingers and applying pressure to the head. Do not try to increase the height or depth of a ridge by pinching or pushing with your fingers; such movements will create overdirection of the ridge and uneven hair placement.

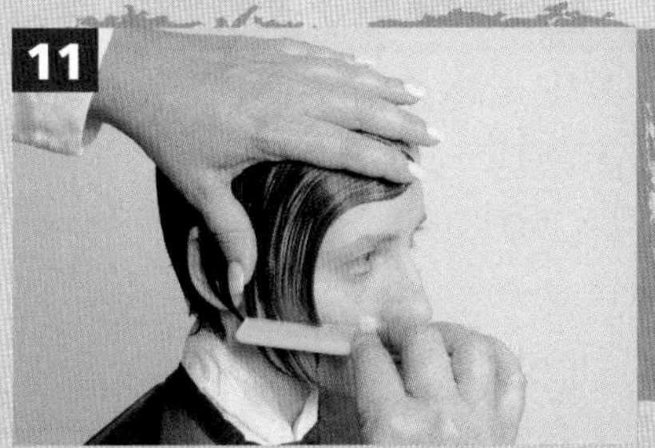

11 Without removing the comb, turn the teeth downward, and comb the hair in a semicircular direction to form a dip in the hollow part of the wave.

© Milady, a part of Cengage Learning. Photography by Yanik Chauvin.

PROCEDURE 17-2 Horizontal Finger Waving: Right-Handed continued

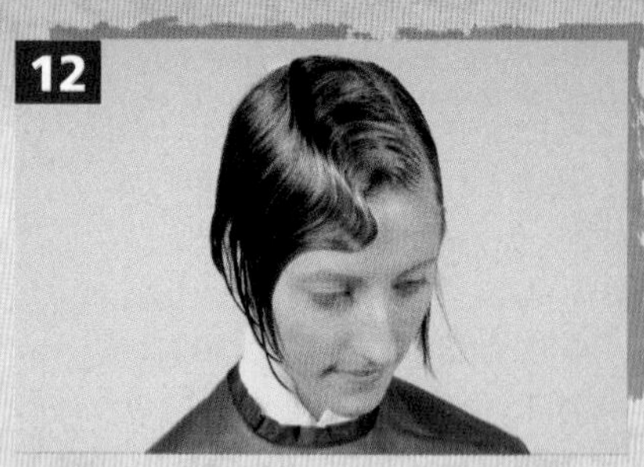

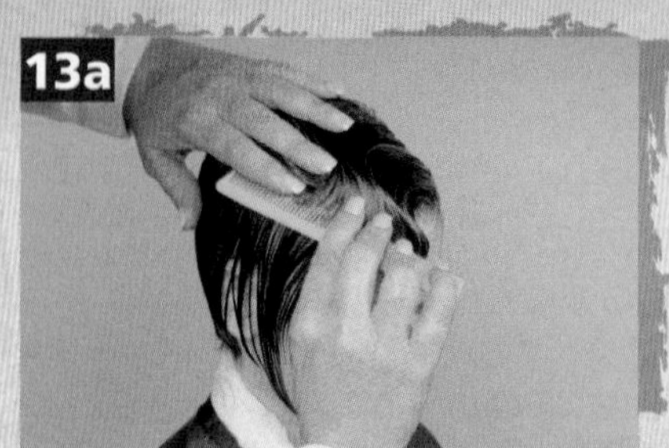

12 Follow this procedure, section by section, until the crown has been reached, where the ridge phases out. The ridge and wave of each section should match evenly, without showing separations in the ridge or in the hollow part of the wave.

13 To form the second ridge, begin at the crown area. The movements are the reverse of those followed in forming the first ridge. Draw the comb from the tip of the index finger toward the base. All movements are followed in a reverse pattern until the hairline is reached, completing the second ridge.

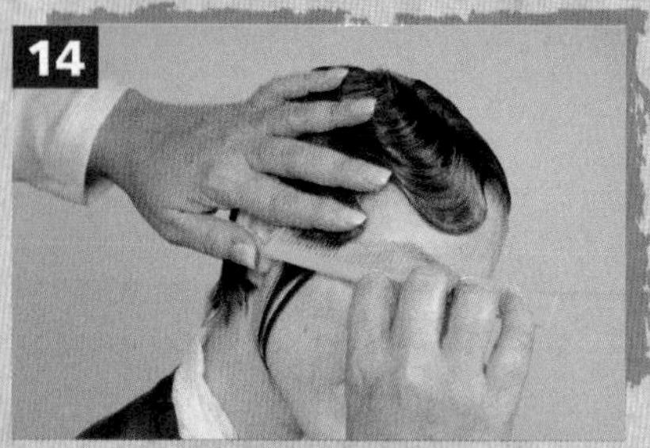

14 Movements for the third ridge closely follow those used to create the first ridge. However, the third ridge is started at the hairline and is extended back toward the back of the head.

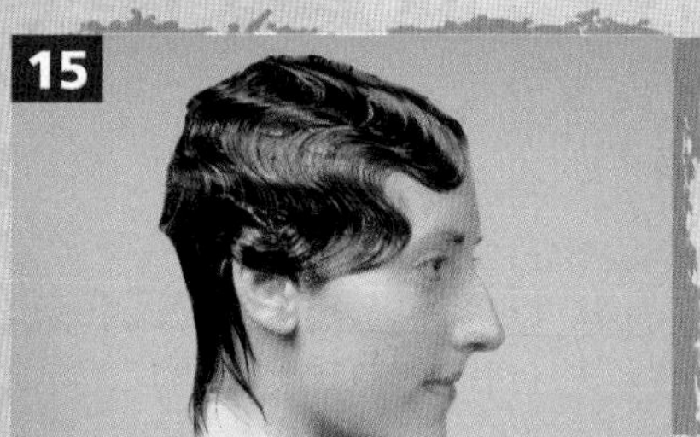

15 Continue alternating directions until the side of the head has been completed.

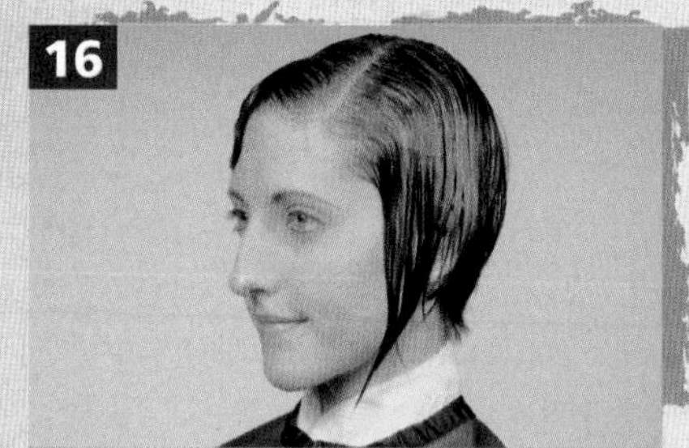

16 Use the same procedure for the left (light) side of the head as you used for finger waving the right (heavy) side of the head. First, shape the hair by combing it in the direction of the first wave.

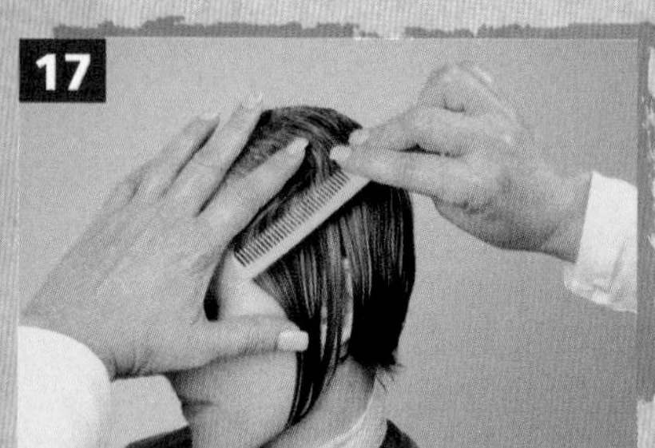

17 Starting at the hairline, form the first ridge, and work section by section, until the second ridge of the opposite side is reached.

© Milady, a part of Cengage Learning. Photography by Yanik Chauvin.

18 Both the ridge and the wave must blend, without splits or breaks, with the ridge and wave on the right side of the head.

19 Move to the left side and start with the ridge and wave in the back of the head and proceed, section by section, toward the left side of the face.

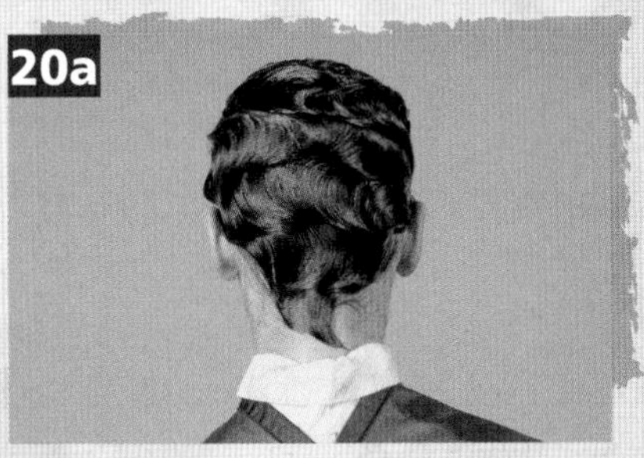
20a

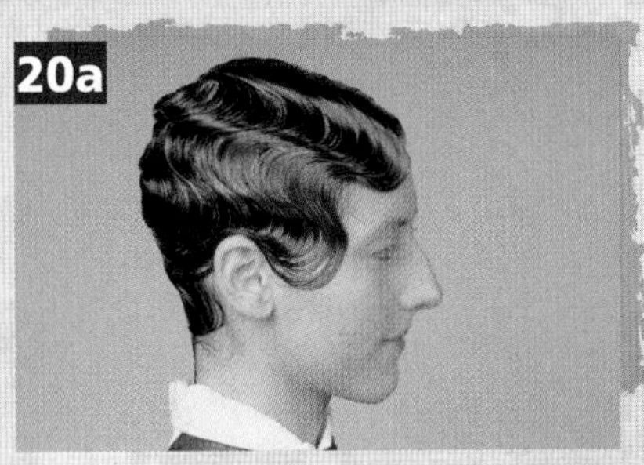
20a

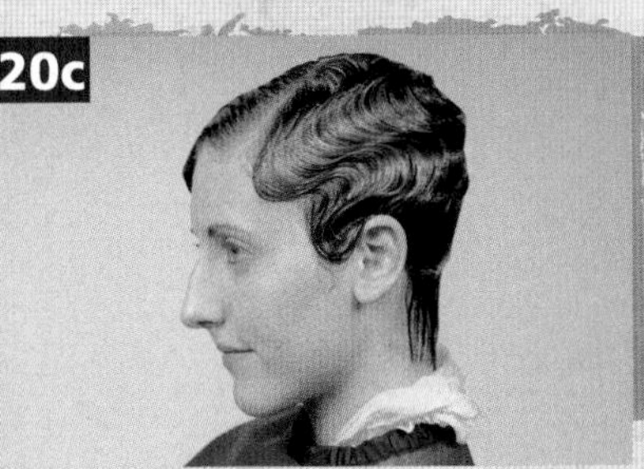
20c

20 Continue working back and forth until the entire head is completed.

21 Place a net over the hair, secure it with hairpins or clips if necessary, and protect the client's forehead and ears with cotton, gauze, or paper protectors while under the hood dryer. Adjust the dryer to medium heat and allow the hair to dry thoroughly.

22 Remove the client from under the dryer and let the hair cool down. Remove all clips or pins and the hairnet from the hair.

23 Comb out or brush the hair into a soft, waved hairstyle. Add a finishing spray for hold and shine. For a retro look, do not comb or brush the hair, but do consider adding a hair ornament such as a rhinestone clip in the hollow portion of a wave.

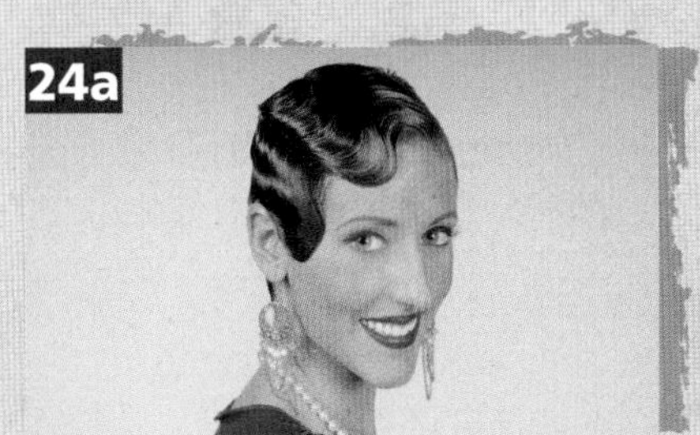
24a

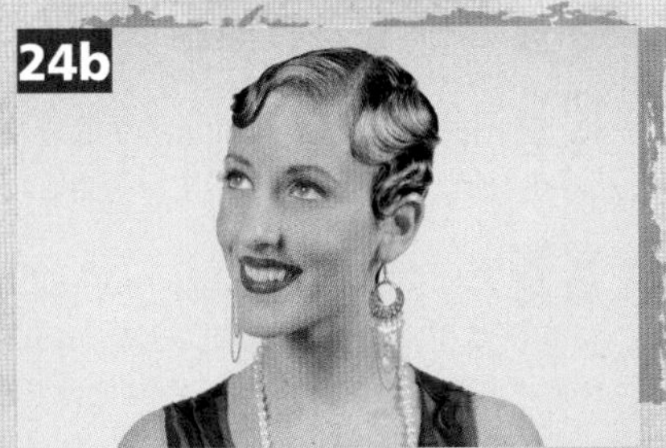
24b

24 Finished look.

© Milady, a part of Cengage Learning. Photography by Yanik Chauvin.

Post-Service

- Complete PROCEDURE 15-2 **Post-Service Procedure** **SEE PAGE 326**

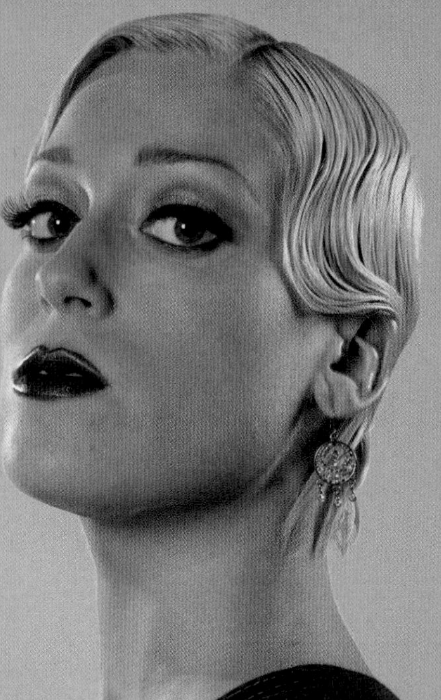

PROCEDURE 17-2 Left Handed

Horizontal Finger Waving

Implements and Materials

You will need all of the following implements, materials, and supplies:

- **Conditioner**
- **Finishing products such as shine or hair spray**
- **Hairnet**
- **Hairpins**
- **Neck strip**
- **Plastic cape**
- **Shampoo**
- **Styling comb**
- **Towels**
- **Waving lotion or styling gel**

Preparation

- Perform PROCEDURE 15-1 **Pre-Service Procedure** **SEE PAGE 323**

Procedure

1 Drape the client for a shampoo service.

2 Shampoo the client's hair, and condition if necessary.

3 Towel dry the hair.

4 Remove any tangles with a wide-tooth comb, starting at the ends and working up to the scalp.

5 Part the hair, comb it smooth, and arrange it according to the planned style. Using the wide teeth of the comb will allow the hair to move more easily. Always follow the natural growth pattern when combing and parting the hair.

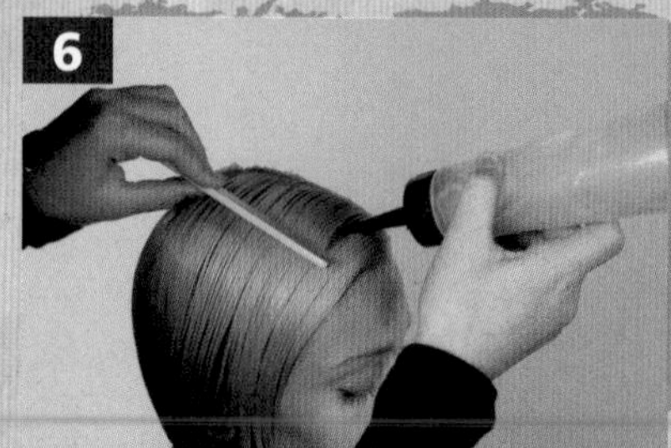

6 Using an applicator bottle, apply waving lotion to the side of the hair you are working on while the hair is damp. Comb the lotion through the section.

© Milady, a part of Cengage Learning. Photography by Yanik Chauvin.

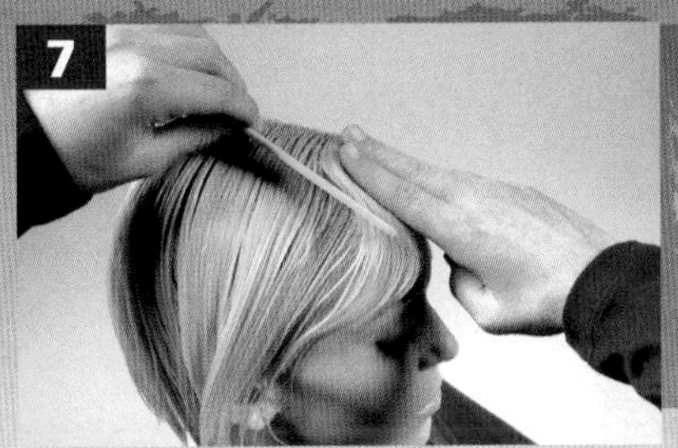

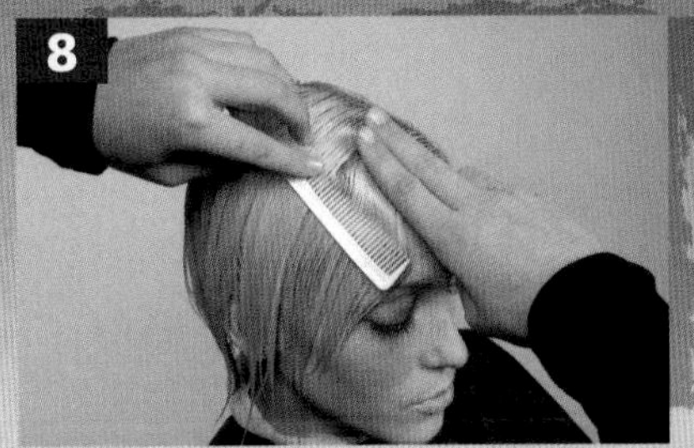

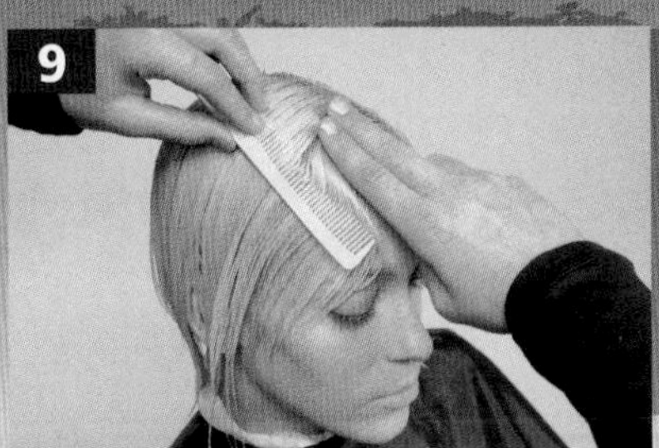

7 Begin the first wave on the right side of the head. Using the index finger of your right hand as a guide, shape the top hair with a comb into the beginning of the S-shaping, using a circular movement. Starting at the hairline, work toward the crown in 1½- to 2-inch (3.7 to 5 centimeters) sections at a time.

8 To form the first ridge, place the index finger of your right hand directly above the position for the first ridge. With the teeth of the comb pointing slightly upward, insert the comb directly under the index finger. Draw the comb forward about 1 inch (2.5 centimeters) along the fingertip.

9 With the teeth still inserted in the ridge, flatten the comb against the head in order to hold the ridge in place.

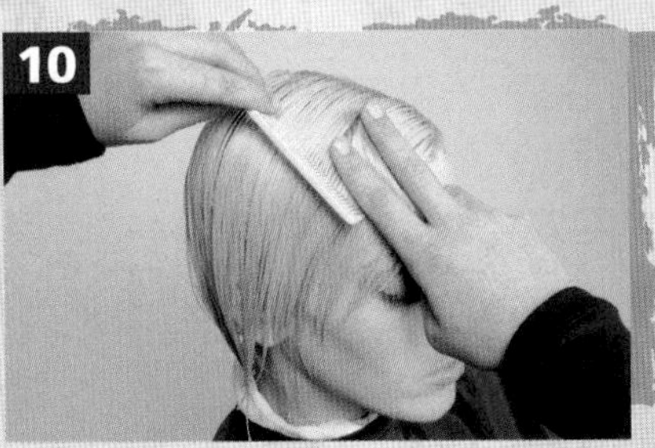

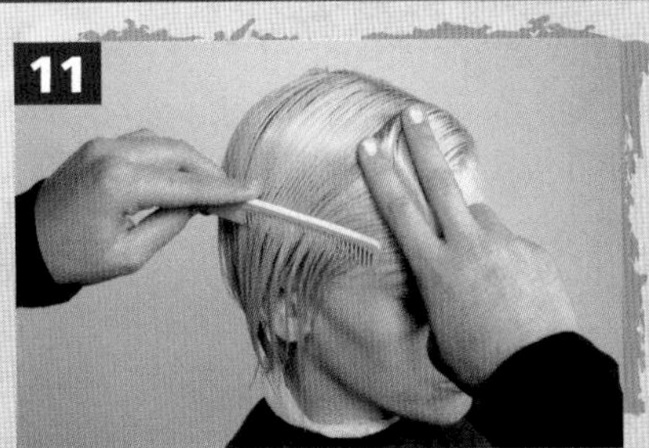

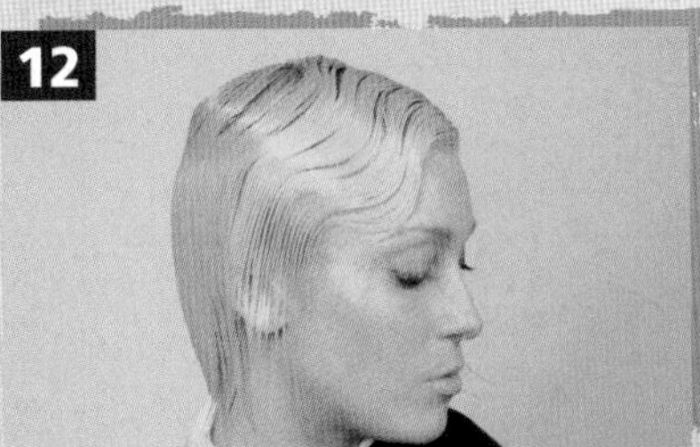

10 Remove your right hand from the client's head and place your middle finger above the ridge with your index finger on the teeth of the comb. Draw out the ridge by closing the two fingers and applying pressure to the head. Do not try to increase the height or depth of a ridge by pinching or pushing with your fingers; such movements will create overdirection of the ridge and uneven hair placement.

11 Without removing the comb, turn the teeth downward, and comb the hair in a semicircular direction to form a dip in the hollow part of the wave.

12 Follow this procedure, section by section, until the crown has been reached, where the ridge phases out. The ridge and wave of each section should match evenly, without showing separations in the ridge or in the hollow part of the wave.

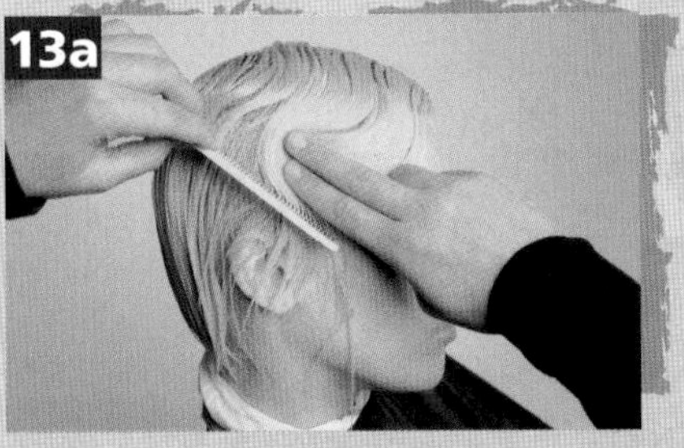

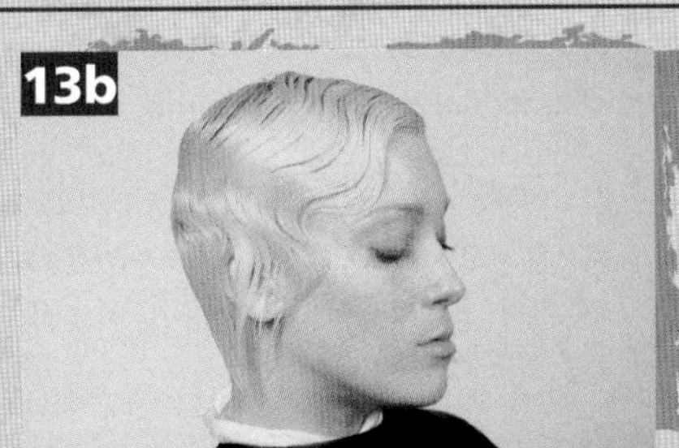

13 To form the second ridge, begin at the crown area. The movements are the reverse of those followed in forming the first ridge. Draw the comb from the tip of the index finger toward the base. B. All movements are followed in a reverse pattern until the hairline is reached, completing the second ridge.

14 Movements for the third ridge closely follow those used to create the first ridge. However, the third ridge is started at the hairline and is extended back toward the back of the head.

© Milady, a part of Cengage Learning. Photography by Yanik Chauvin.

PROCEDURE 17-2

Horizontal Finger Waving: Left-Handed continued

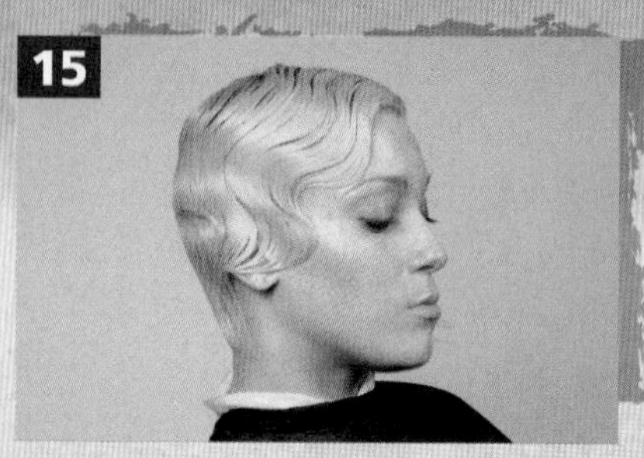

15 Continue alternating directions until the right side of the head has been completed.

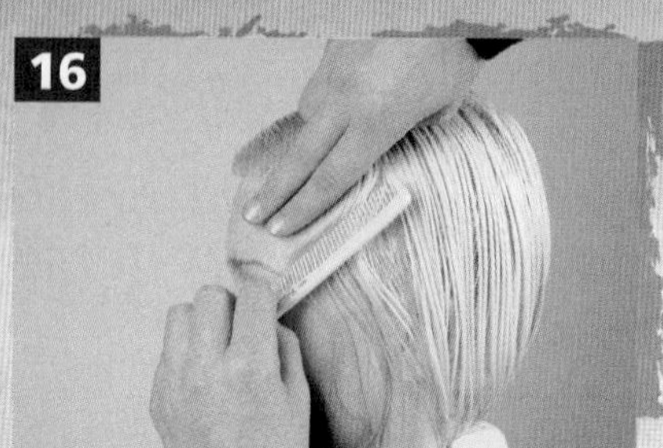

16 Use the same procedure for the left (light) side of the head as you used for finger waving the right (heavy) side of the head. First, shape the hair by combing it in the direction of the first wave.

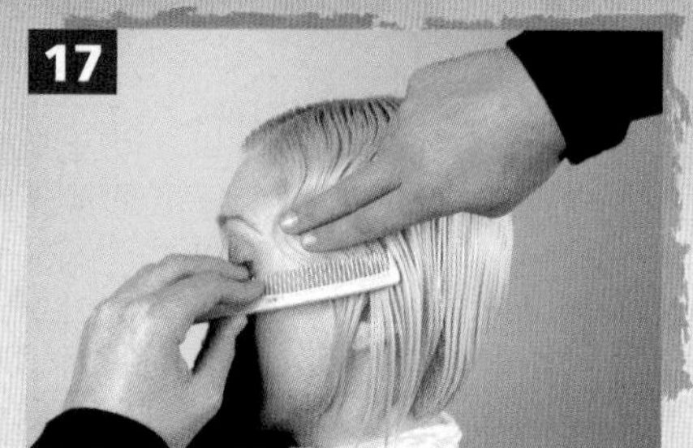

17 Starting at the hairline, form the first ridge, and work section by section, until the second ridge of the opposite side is reached.

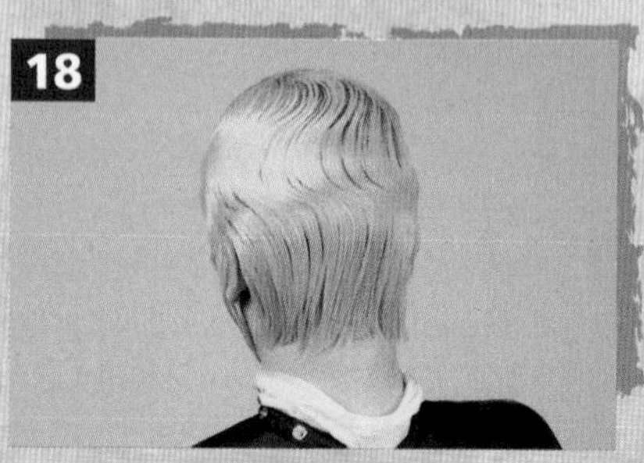

18 Both the ridge and the wave must blend, without splits or breaks, with the ridge and wave on the right side of the head.

19 Move to the left side and start with the ridge and wave in the back of the head and proceed, section by section, toward the left side of the face.

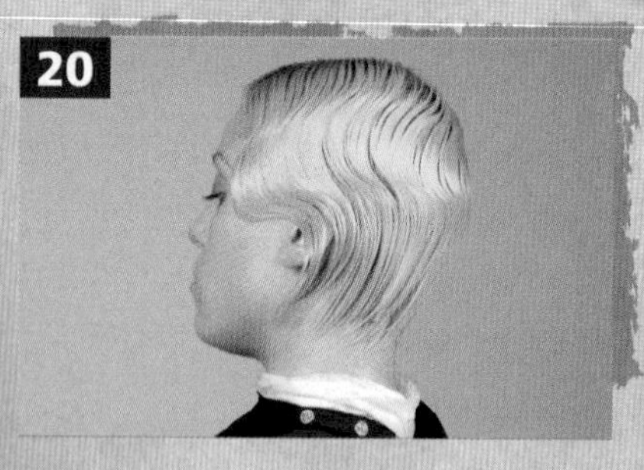

20 Continue working back and forth until the entire head is completed.

21 Place a net over the hair, secure it with hairpins or clips if necessary, and protect the client's forehead and ears with cotton, gauze, or paper protectors while under the hood dryer. Adjust the dryer to medium heat and allow the hair to dry thoroughly.

22 Remove the client from under the dryer and let the hair cool down. Remove all clips or pins and the hairnet from the hair.

23 Comb out or brush the hair into a soft, waved hairstyle. Add a finishing spray for hold and shine. For a retro look, do not comb or brush the hair, but do consider adding a hair ornament such as a rhinestone clip in the hollow portion of a wave.

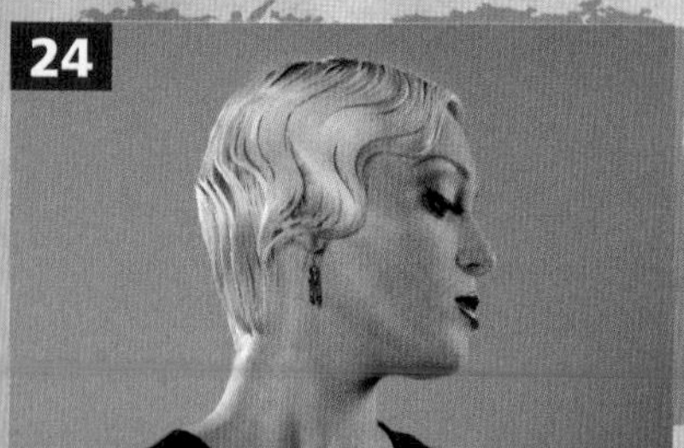

24 Finished look.

Post-Service

- Complete PROCEDURE 15-2 **Post-Service Procedure** SEE PAGE 326

© Milady, a part of Cengage Learning. Photography by Yanik Chauvin.

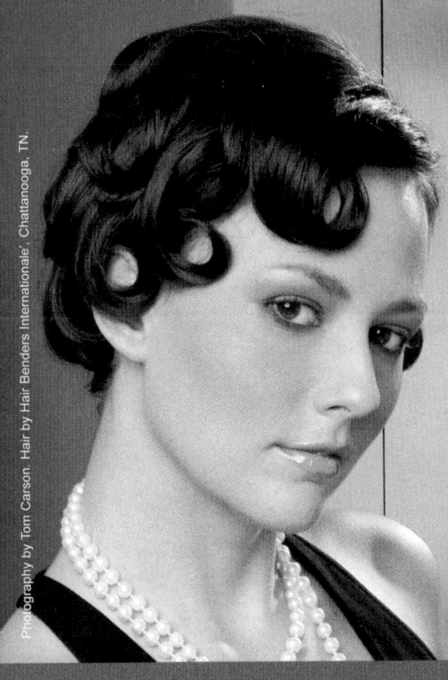

Photography by Tom Carson. Hair by Hair Benders Internationale', Chattanooga, TN.

PROCEDURE 17-3 Right-Handed

Carved or Sculpted Curls

Implements and Materials

You will need all of the following implements, materials, and supplies:

- **Conditioner**
- **Double- or single-prong clips**
- **Finishing products such as shine or hair spray**
- **Neck strip**
- **Plastic cape**
- **Setting lotion**
- **Shampoo**
- **Styling comb**
- **Towels**

Preparation

- Perform PROCEDURE 15-1 **Pre-Service Procedure** **SEE PAGE 323**

Procedure

1 Drape the client for a shampoo service.

2 Shampoo the client's hair, and condition if necessary.

3 Towel dry the hair.

4 Remove any tangles with a wide-tooth comb, starting at the ends and working up to the scalp.

5 Apply a gel or setting lotion and comb the hair smooth.

6 Part the hair either using the client's natural part, if that works with your hair design, or create a part anywhere on the head if that better suits the final design.

7

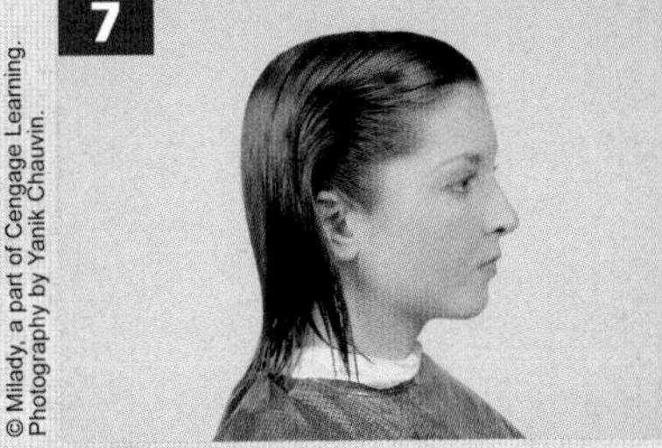

© Milady, a part of Cengage Learning. Photography by Yanik Chauvin.

7 Form the first shaping.

PROCEDURE 17-3

Carved or Sculpted Curls: Right-Handed continued

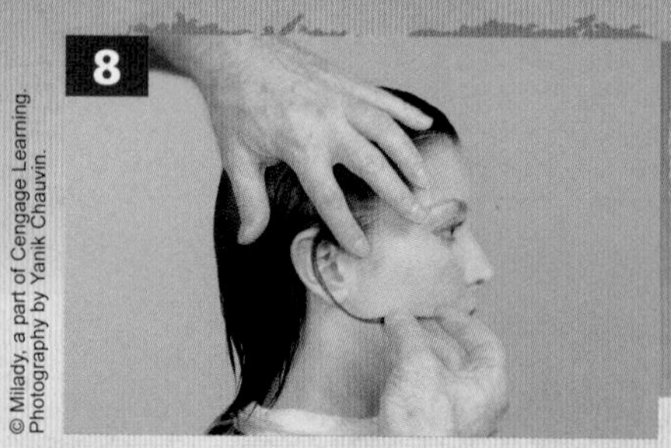

© Milady, a part of Cengage Learning. Photography by Yanik Chauvin.

8 Start making curls at the open end of the shaping. Slice a strand to create the first curl. Point your left index finger down and hold the strand in place.

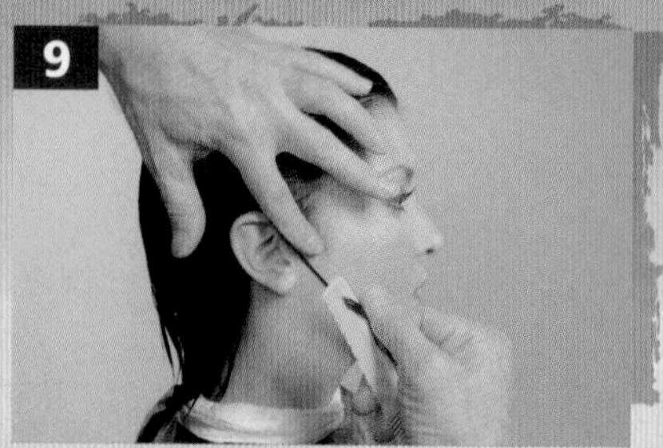

© Milady, a part of Cengage Learning. Photography by Yanik Chauvin.

9 Ribbon the strand.

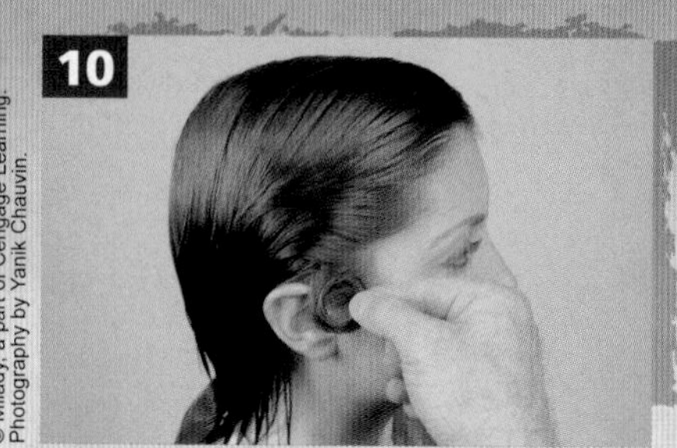

© Milady, a part of Cengage Learning. Photography by Yanik Chauvin.

10 Wind the curl forward, keeping the hair ends inside the center of the curl.

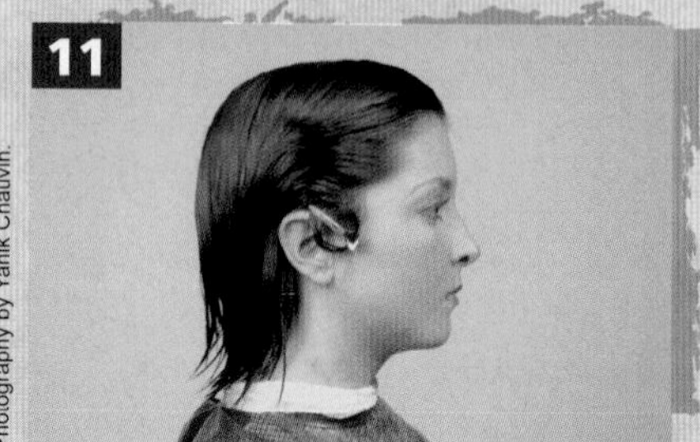

© Milady, a part of Cengage Learning. Photography by Yanik Chauvin.

11 Hold the curl in the shaping and anchor it with a clip.

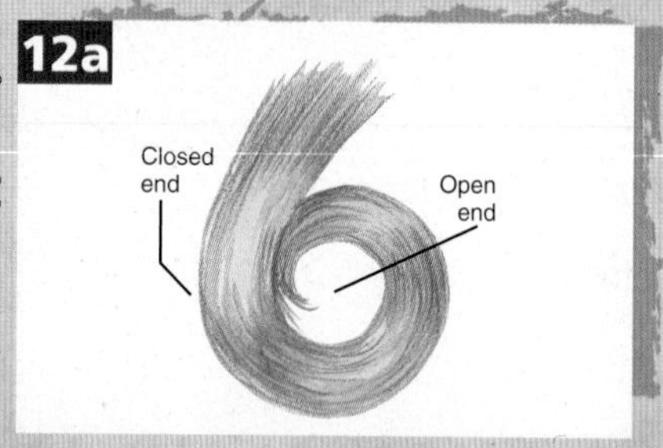

© Milady, a part of Cengage Learning.

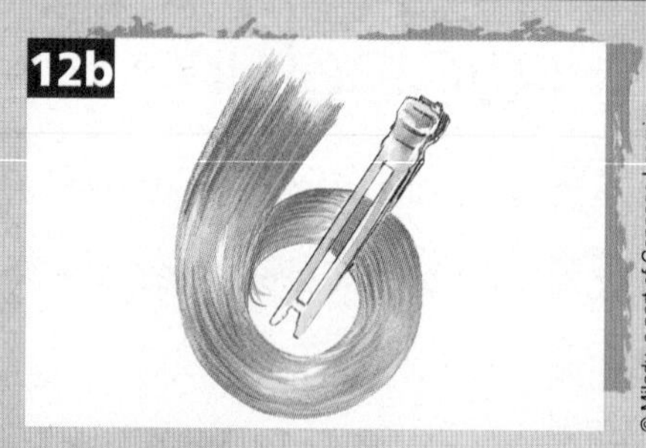

© Milady, a part of Cengage Learning.

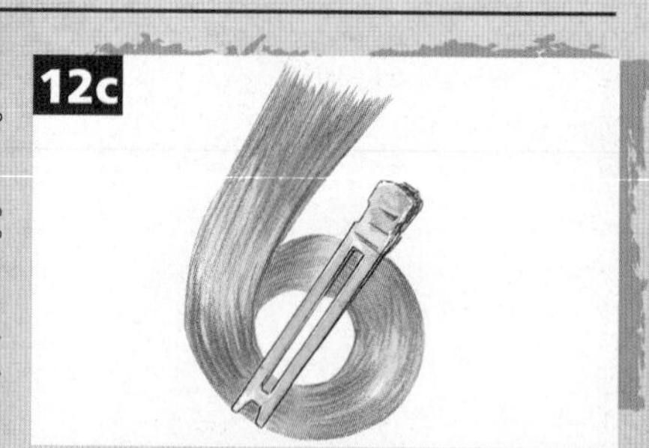

© Milady, a part of Cengage Learning.

12 To anchor pin curls, start at the open end of the curl. This is the side opposite the stem. The clip should enter the circle parallel to the stem. Open the clip, and place one prong above and one prong below one side of the circle. The upper prong should enter the hair in the center of the circle. The curl should be in the gap between the prongs. To avoid an indentation (dent) in the curl, do not pin across the circle.

13 If any clips touch the skin, place cotton between the skin and the clip to keep the skin from burning when the client is placed under the hood dryer.

14 Once the hair is dry, complete the style.

Post-Service

- Complete PROCEDURE 15-2 **Post-Service Procedure** **SEE PAGE 326**

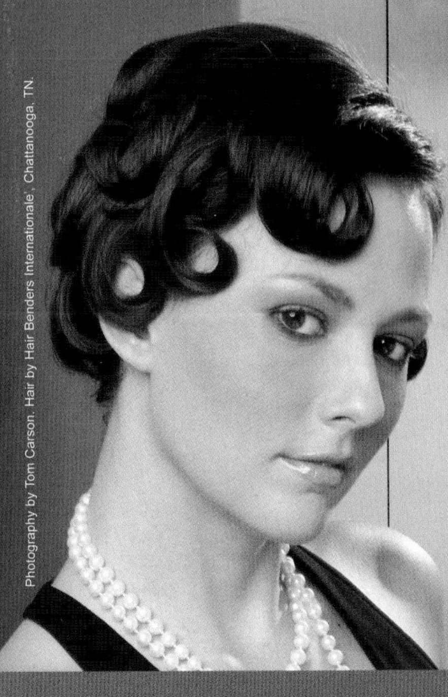
Photography by Tom Carson. Hair by Hair Benders International, Chattanooga, TN.

PROCEDURE 17-3 Left Handed

Carved or Sculpted Curls

Implements and Materials

You will need all of the following implements, materials, and supplies:

- **Conditioner**
- **Double- or single-prong clips**
- **Finishing products such as shine or hair spray**
- **Neck strip**
- **Plastic cape**
- **Setting lotion**
- **Shampoo**
- **Styling comb**
- **Towels**

Preparation

- Perform PROCEDURE 15-1 **Pre-Service Procedure** **SEE PAGE 323**

Procedure

1 Drape the client for a shampoo service.

2 Shampoo the client's hair, and condition if necessary.

3 Towel dry the hair.

4 Remove any tangles with a wide-tooth comb, starting at the ends and working up to the scalp.

5 Apply a gel or setting lotion and comb the hair smooth.

6 Part the hair either using the client's natural part, if that works with your hair design, or create a part anywhere on the head if that better suits the final design.

7

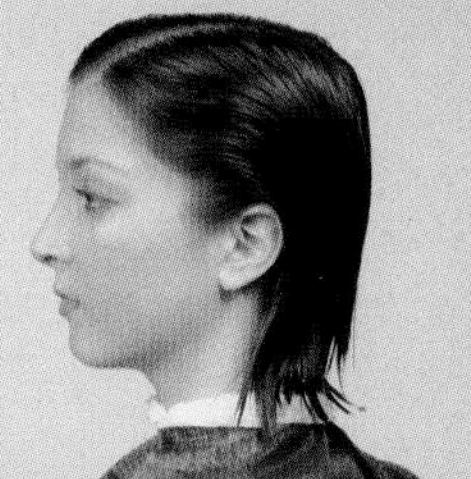
© Milady, a part of Cengage Learning. Photography by Yanik Chauvin.

7 Form the first shaping.

Carved or Sculpted Curls: Left-Handed continued

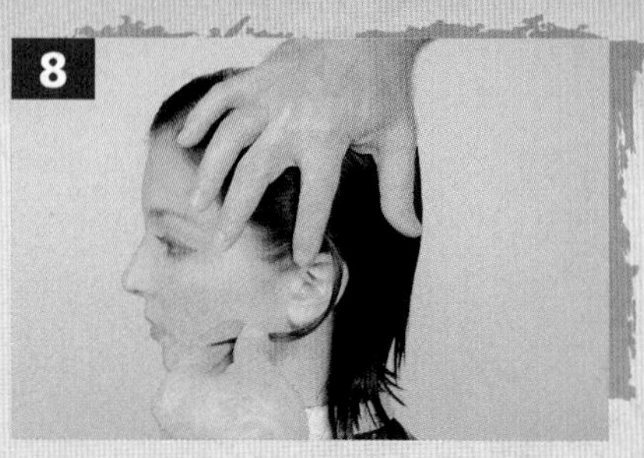

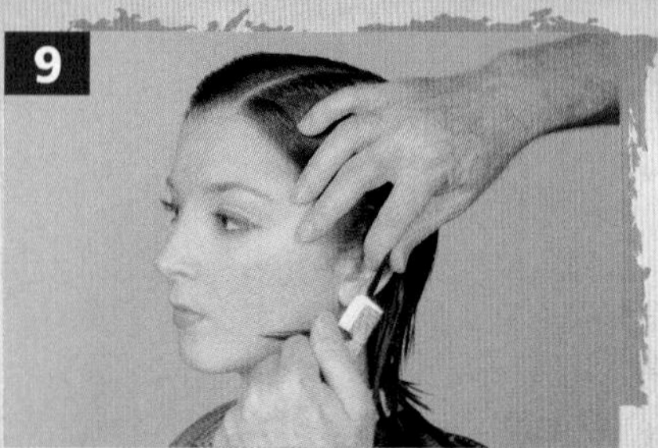

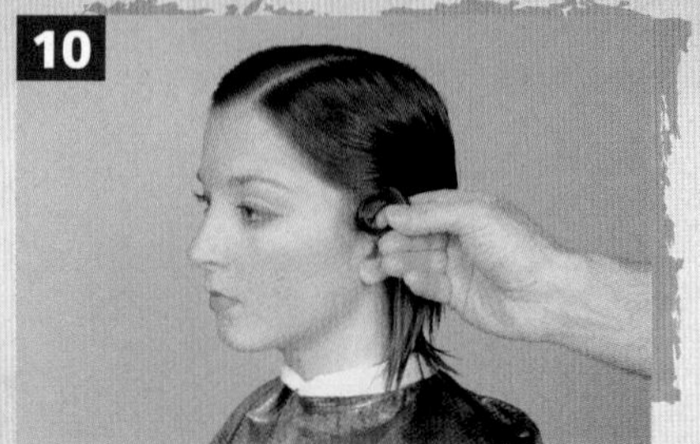

8 Start making curls at the open end of the shaping. Slice a strand to create the first curl. Point your left index finger down and hold the strand in place.

9 Ribbon the strand.

10 Wind the curl forward, keeping the hair ends inside the center of the curl.

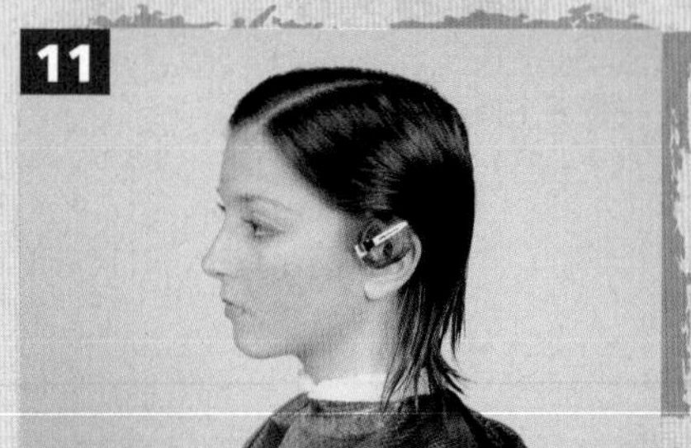

11 Hold the curl in the shaping and anchor it with a clip.

12 To anchor pin curls, start at the open end of the curl. This is the side opposite the stem. The clip should enter the circle parallel to the stem. Open the clip, and place one prong above and one prong below one side of the circle. The upper prong should enter the hair in the center of the circle. The curl should be in the gap between the prongs. To avoid an indentation (dent) in the curl, do not pin across the circle.

13 If any clips touch the skin, place cotton between the skin and the clip to keep the skin from burning when the client is placed under the hood dryer.

14 Once the hair is dry, complete the style.

Post-Service

- Complete PROCEDURE 15-2 **Post-Service Procedure** SEE PAGE 326

© Milady, a part of Cengage Learning. Photography by Yanik Chauvin.

PROCEDURE 17-4

Wet Set with Rollers

Implements and Materials

You will need all of the following implements, materials, and supplies:

- **Clips (double or single prong)**
- **Conditioner**
- **Finishing products such as shine or hair spray**
- **Neck strip**
- **Plastic cape**
- **Plastic rollers of various sizes**
- **Setting or styling lotion**
- **Shampoo**
- **Tail comb**
- **Towels**

© Milady, a part of Cengage Learning. Photography by Paul Castle, Castle Photography.

Preparation

- Perform PROCEDURE 15-1 **Pre-Service Procedure** SEE PAGE 323

Procedure

1 Drape the client for a shampoo service.

2 Shampoo the client's hair, and condition if necessary.

3 Towel dry the hair.

4 Remove any tangles with a wide-tooth comb, starting at the ends and working up to the scalp.

5 Comb the hair in the direction of the setting pattern. Shapings may be used to accent the design.

6 Starting at the front hairline, part off a section the same length and width as the roller.

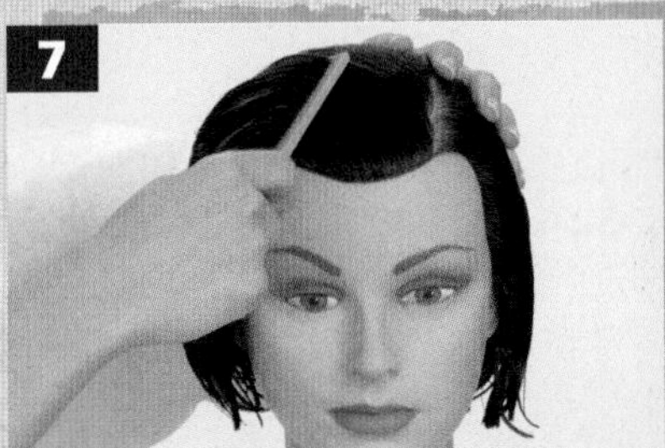

7 Choose the type of base according to the desired volume. Comb the hair out from the scalp to the ends, using the fine teeth of the comb. Repeat several times to make sure that the hair is smooth.

Wet Set with Rollers continued

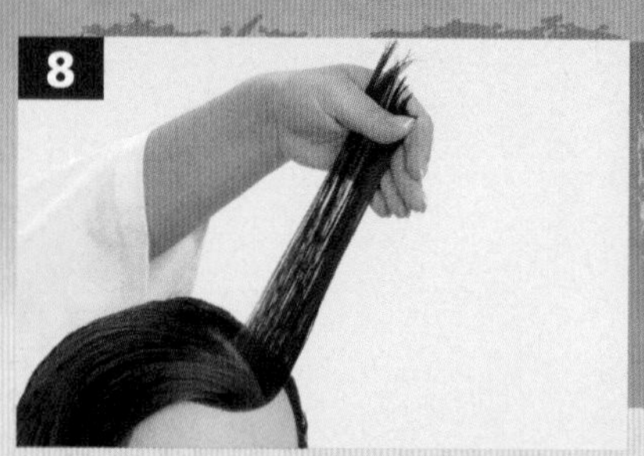

8 Hold the hair with tension between the thumb and middle finger of the left hand. Place the roller below the thumb of the left hand. Do not bring the ends of the hair together. Wrap the ends of the hair smoothly around the roller until the hair catches and does not release.

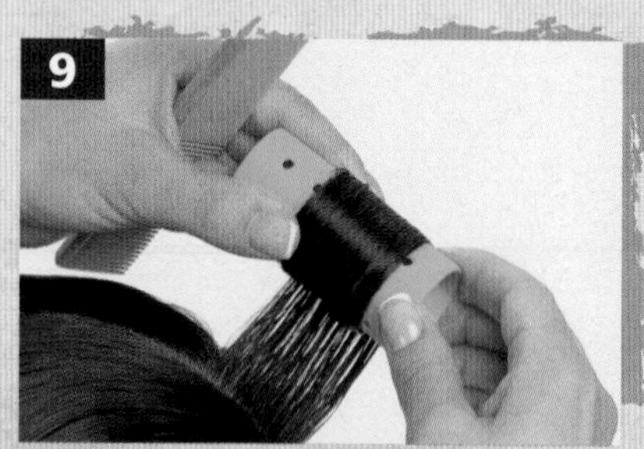

9 Place the thumbs over the ends of the roller and roll the hair firmly to the scalp.

Service Tip

Some stylists find using a tail comb is easier for creating sections and subsections.

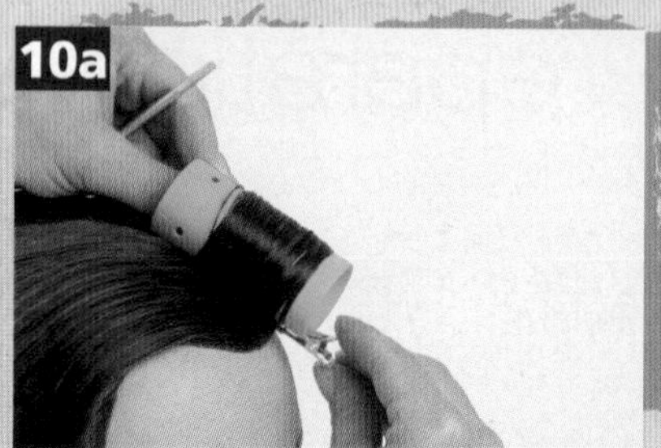

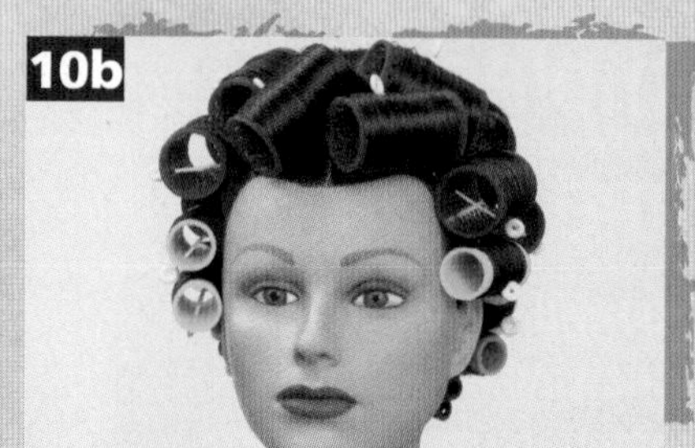

10 Clip the roller securely to the scalp hair. Roll the remainder of the hair according to the desired style.

11 Place the client under a hood dryer. Set the dryer at a temperature that is comfortable for the client.

Service Tip

When clipping the roller, make sure you secure the roller properly to the head. A loose roller will lose its tension, resulting in a weak set. If the clip is placed at an angle against the hair, the sharp metal edge can cause the hair to break. Hold the roller against the scalp, maintaining the tension. Open the clip and slide it into the center of the roller. Place one end under the roller and one end inside the roller.

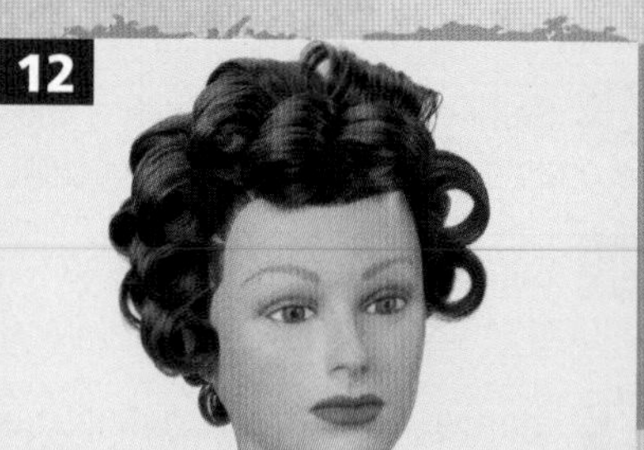

12 When the hair is dry, allow it to cool, then remove the rollers.

13 Comb out and style the hair as desired.

Post-Service

- Complete PROCEDURE 15-2 Post-Service Procedure SEE PAGE 326

© Milady, a part of Cengage Learning. Photography by Paul Castle, Castle Photography.

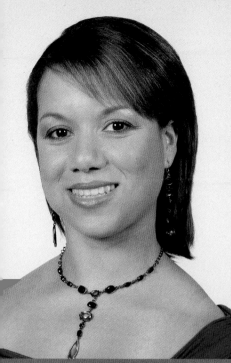

PROCEDURE 17-5

Hair Wrapping

Implements and Materials

You will need all of the following implements, materials, and supplies:

- **Boar-bristle brush**
- **Bobby pins**
- **Comb**
- **Duckbill clips**
- **Gel or silicone shine product**
- **Neck strip**

© Milady, a part of Cengage Learning. Photography by Yanik Chauvin.

Preparation

- Perform PROCEDURE 15-1 Pre-Service Procedure SEE PAGE 323

Procedure

1 Drape the client for a shampoo service.

2 Shampoo the client's hair, and condition if necessary.

3 Towel dry the hair.

4 Remove any tangles with a wide-tooth comb, starting at the ends and working up to the scalp.

5 Apply a light gel before wrapping wet hair.

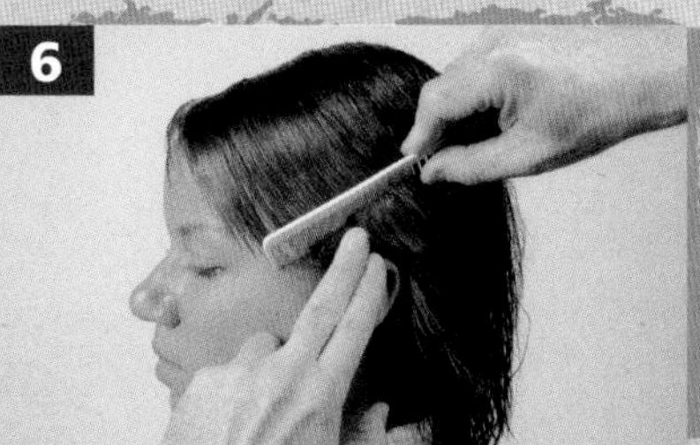

6

6 If necessary, place one hand on the top of the head to hold it still. Use a comb or brush in a circular motion to wrap the hair on the outer perimeter of the head. Do not brush or push the hair to the back; instead, brush the hair clockwise around the head. Think of the head as a roller. Your job is to smooth the hair in a circular motion around it.

PROCEDURE 17-5 Hair Wrapping continued

Service Tip

When wrapping dry hair, use a silicone shine product instead of using a gel. This will provide a glossy comb out.

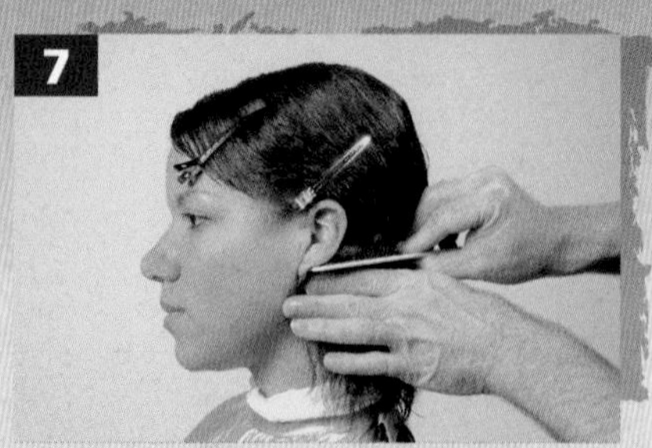

7 Use duckbill clips to keep the hair in place while wrapping.

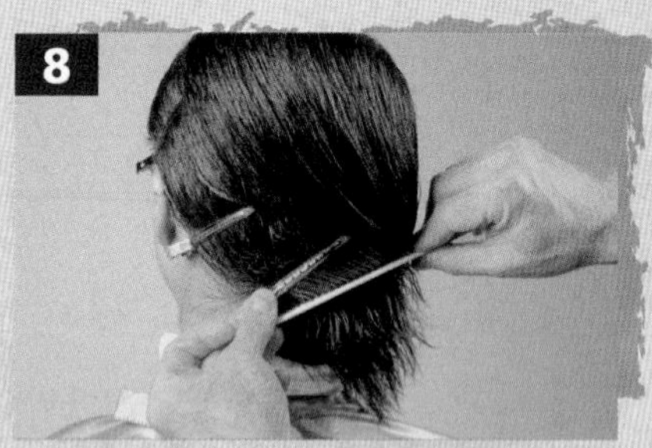

8 Continue wrapping the hair in a clockwise direction around the head. Follow the comb or brush with your hand, smoothing down the hair and keeping it tight to the head as you proceed.

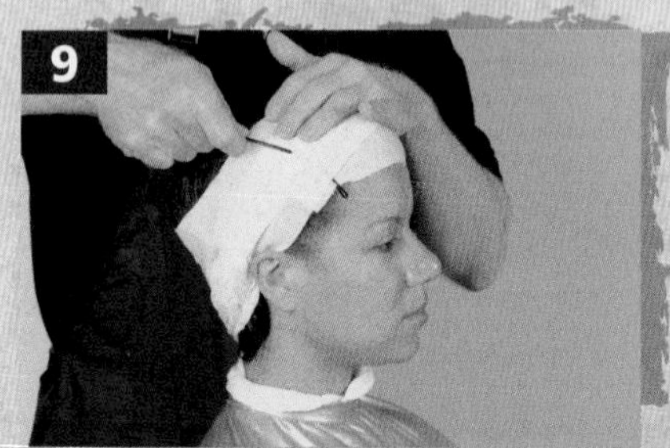

9 When all the hair is wrapped, stretch a neck strip around the head so that it overlaps at the ends. Secure the wrapped strip with a bobby pin and remove the clips.

10 Place the client under a hooded dryer until the hair is completely dry, usually forty-five minutes to one hour, depending on the hair length. If you have been working on dry hair, leave the hair wrapped for about seventeen minutes. The longer the hair is wrapped, the smoother it will be.

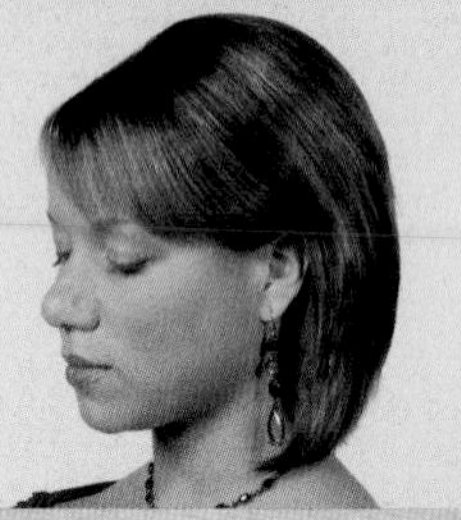

11 Finished look.

Post-Service

- Complete PROCEDURE 15-2 Post-Service Procedure SEE PAGE 326

© Milady, a part of Cengage Learning. Photography by Yanik Chauvin.

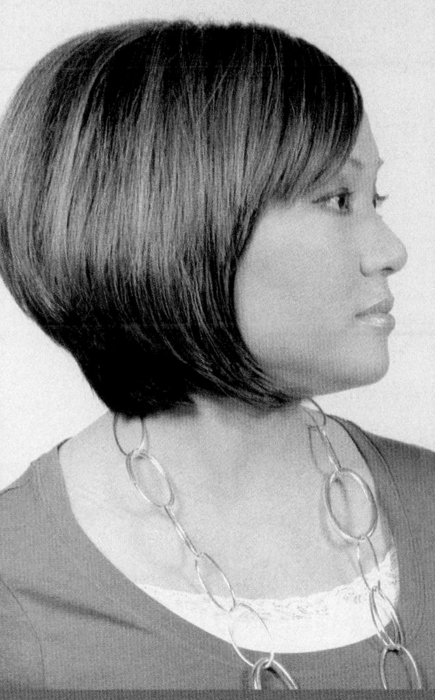

PROCEDURE 17-6 Right-Handed

Blowdrying Short, Layered, Curly Hair to Produce Smooth and Full Finish

Implements and Materials

You will need all of the following implements, materials, and supplies:

- **Blowdryer with attachments**
- **Finishing products such as shine or hair spray**
- **Neck strip**
- **Round brush**
- **Sectioning clips**
- **Styling cape**
- **Styling product**
- **Wide-tooth comb**

Preparation

- Perform PROCEDURE 15-1 **Pre-Service Procedure** SEE PAGE 323

Procedure

1 Drape the client for a shampoo service.

2 Shampoo the client's hair, and condition if necessary.

3 Towel dry the hair.

4 Remove any tangles with a wide-tooth comb, starting at the ends and working up to the scalp.

5 Place a clean neck strip on the client, and drape with a cutting or styling cape.

6 Distribute styling product through the hair with your fingers, and comb through with a wide-tooth comb.

7

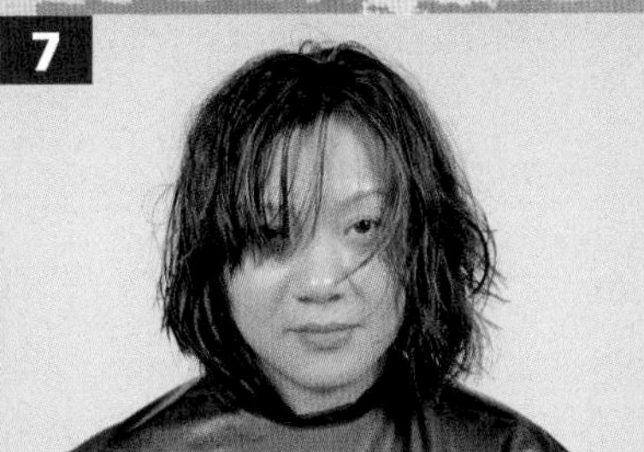

7 Using the comb, mold the hair into the desired shape while still wet.

8 For volume and lift similar to that provided by a roller set, use a small round brush. Apply a mousse or spray volumizer at the base. Section and part the hair according to the amount of volume desired.

© Milady, a part of Cengage Learning. Photography by Yanik Chauvin.

PROCEDURE 17-6 Blowdrying Short, Layered, Curly Hair to Produce Smooth and Full Finish: Right Handed continued

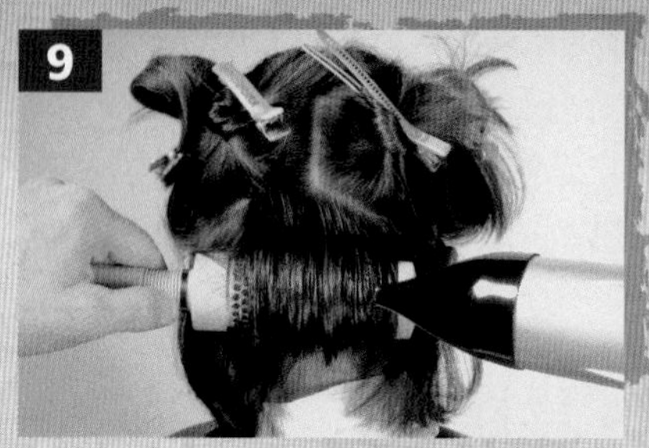

9 The degree of lift determines the type of volume you will achieve. Using the techniques that you have learned in roller setting, dry each section either full base or half base. For maximum lift, insert the brush on base and direct the hair section up at a 125-degree angle. Roll the hair down to the base with medium tension. Direct the stream of air from the blowdryer over the curl and away from the scalp in a back and forth motion.

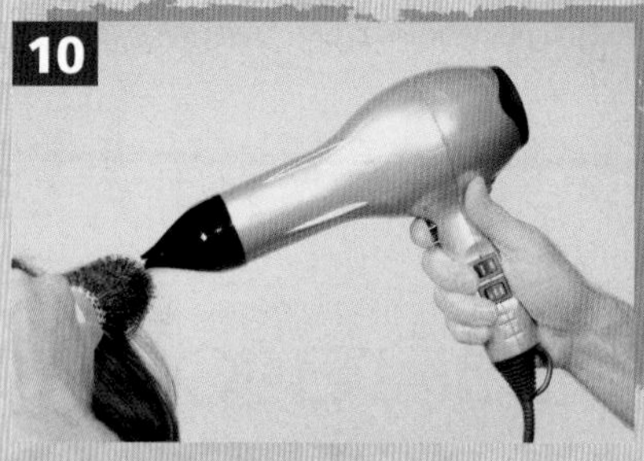

10 When the section is completely dry, press the cooling button and cool the section to strengthen the curl formation.

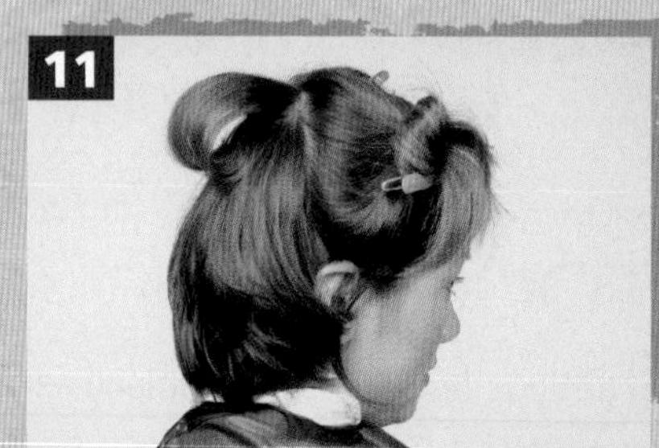

11 Release the curl by unwinding the section from the brush. (Pulling it out could cause the hair to get tangled in the brush.)

12 For less lift at the scalp, begin by holding the section at a 70- to 90-degree angle, following the same procedure.

13 Make sure that the scalp and hair are completely dry before combing out the style, or the shape will not last. Finish with hair spray.

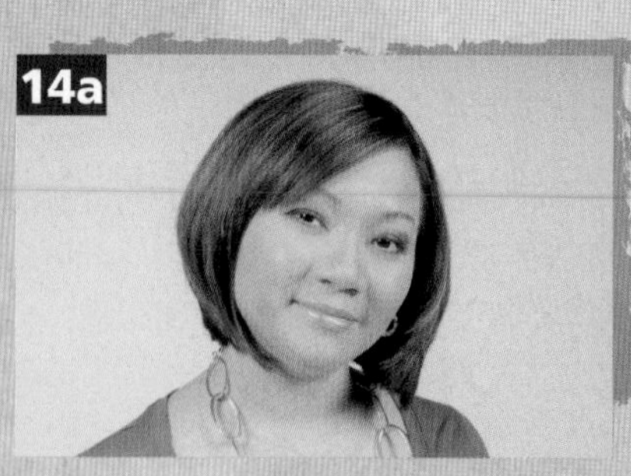

14a

14b

14 Finished look.

Service Tip

Never hold the blowdryer too long in one place. Always direct the hot air away from the client's scalp to avoid scalp burns. Direct it from the scalp toward the ends of the hair. The hot air should flow in the direction in which the hair is wound; improper technique will rough up the hair cuticle and give the hair a frizzy appearance.

Move the blowdryer in a constant back and forth motion unless you are using the cooling button to cool a section.

Because hair stretches easily when it is wet, partially towel dry the hair before blowdrying. This is especially important when you are working with damaged or chemically treated hair. This is not necessary if you are cutting the hair before you blowdry it, as the hair will already be partially dry due to the amount of time it takes to cut it.

Post-Service

- Complete PROCEDURE 15-2 Post-Service Procedure SEE PAGE 326

© Milady, a part of Cengage Learning. Photography by Yanik Chauvin.

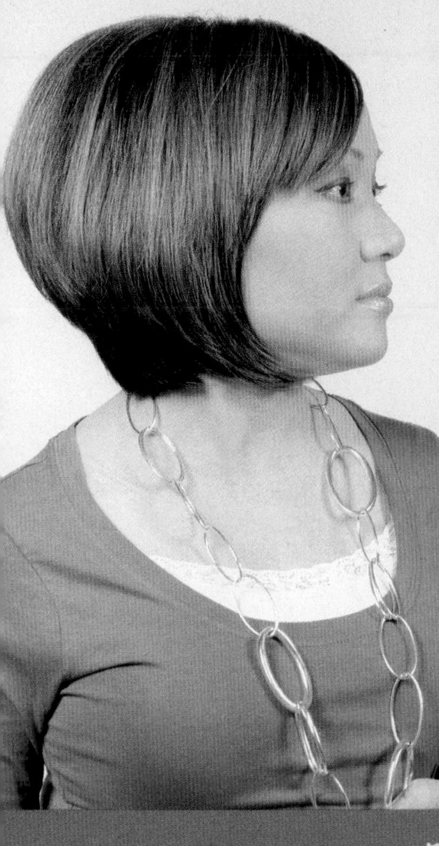

PROCEDURE 17-6 Left Handed

Blowdrying Short, Layered, Curly Hair to Produce Smooth and Full Finish

Implements and Materials

You will need all of the following implements, materials, and supplies:

- **Blowdryer with attachments**
- **Finishing products such as shine or hair spray**
- **Neck strip**
- **Round brush**
- **Sectioning clips**
- **Styling cape**
- **Styling product**
- **Wide-tooth comb**

© Milady, a part of Cengage Learning. Photography by Yanik Chauvin.

Preparation

- Perform PROCEDURE 15-1 Pre-Service Procedure SEE PAGE 323

Procedure

1 Drape the client for a shampoo service.

2 Shampoo the client's hair, and condition if necessary.

3 Towel dry the hair.

4 Remove any tangles with a wide-tooth comb, starting at the ends and working up to the scalp.

5 Place a clean neck strip on the client, and drape with a cutting or styling cape.

6 Distribute styling product through the hair with your fingers, and comb through with a wide-tooth comb.

7 Using the comb, mold the hair into the desired shape while still wet.

8 For volume and lift similar to that provided by a roller set, use a small round brush. Apply a mousse or spray volumizer at the base. Section and part the hair according to the amount of volume desired.

PROCEDURE 17-6

Blowdrying Short, Layered, Curly Hair to Produce Smooth and Full Finish: Left-Handed continued

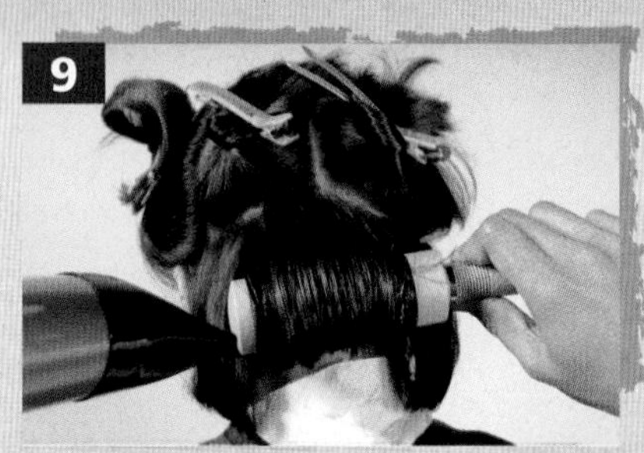

9 The degree of lift determines the type of volume you will achieve. Using the techniques that you have learned in roller setting, dry each section either full base or half base. For maximum lift, insert the brush on base and direct the hair section up at a 125-degree angle. Roll the hair down to the base with medium tension. Direct the stream of air from the blowdryer over the curl and away from the scalp in a back and forth motion.

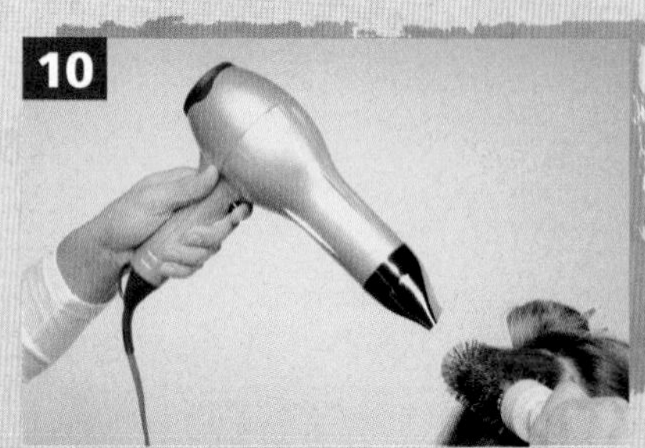

10 When the section is completely dry, press the cooling button and cool the section to strengthen the curl formation.

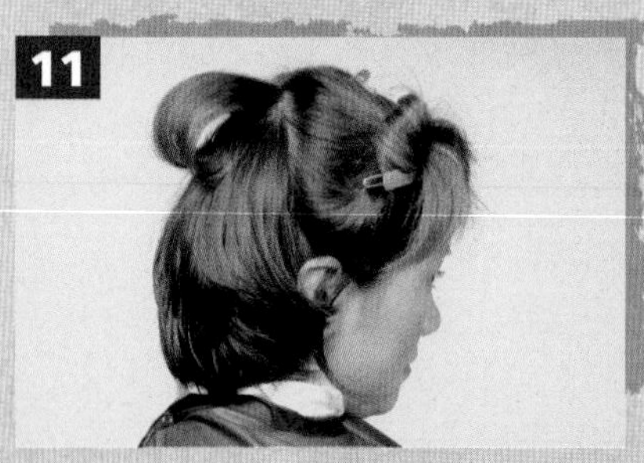

11 Release the curl by unwinding the section from the brush. (Pulling it out could cause the hair to get tangled in the brush.)

12 For less lift at the scalp, begin by holding the section at a 70- to 90-degree angle, following the same procedure.

13 Make sure that the scalp and hair are completely dry before combing out the style, or the shape will not last. Finish with hair spray.

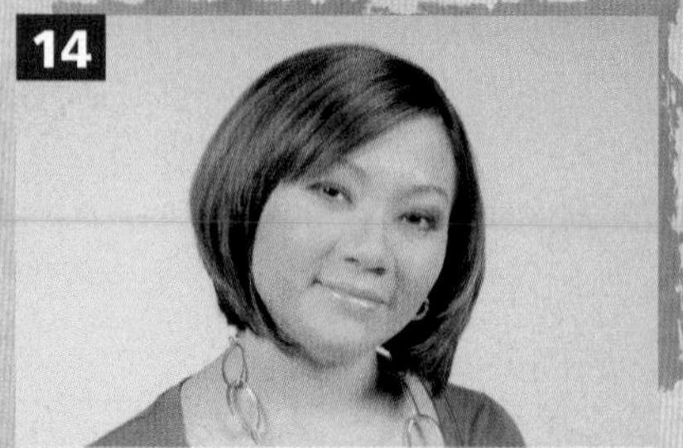

14 Finished look.

Post-Service

- Complete PROCEDURE 15-2 Post-Service Procedure SEE PAGE 326

© Milady, a part of Cengage Learning. Photography by Yanik Chauvin.

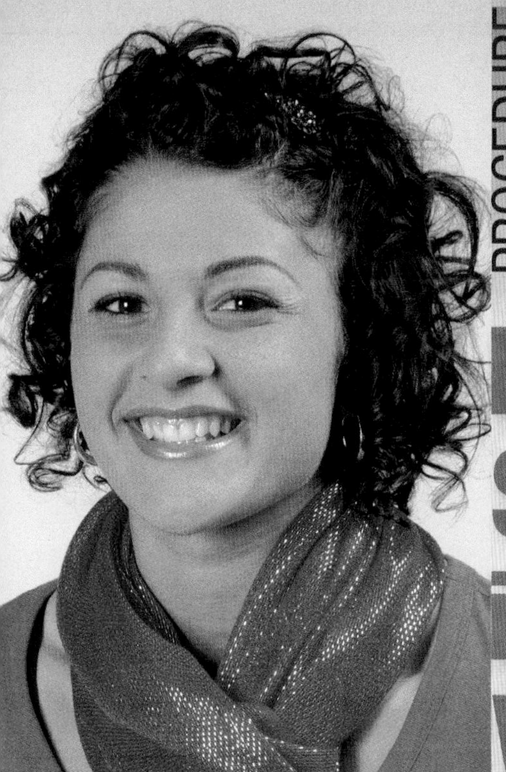

PROCEDURE 17-7

Blowdrying Short, Curly Hair in Its Natural Wave Pattern

Implements and Materials

You will need all of the following implements, materials, and supplies:

- **Blowdryer with attachments**
- **Finishing products such as shine or hair spray**
- **Neck strip**
- **Round brush**
- **Sectioning clips**
- **Styling cape**
- **Styling product**
- **Wide-tooth comb**

© Milady, a part of Cengage Learning. Photography by Yanik Chauvin.

Preparation

- Perform PROCEDURE 15-1 **Pre-Service Procedure** **SEE PAGE 323**

Procedure

1 Drape the client for a shampoo service.

2 Shampoo the client's hair, and condition if necessary.

3 Towel dry the hair.

4 Remove any tangles with a wide-tooth comb, starting at the ends and working up to the scalp.

5 Place a clean neck strip on the client, and drape with a cutting or styling cape.

6 Apply a liquid gel on the client's hair.

7 Attach the diffuser to the blowdryer.

PROCEDURE 17-7

Blowdrying Short, Curly Hair in Its Natural Wave Pattern continued

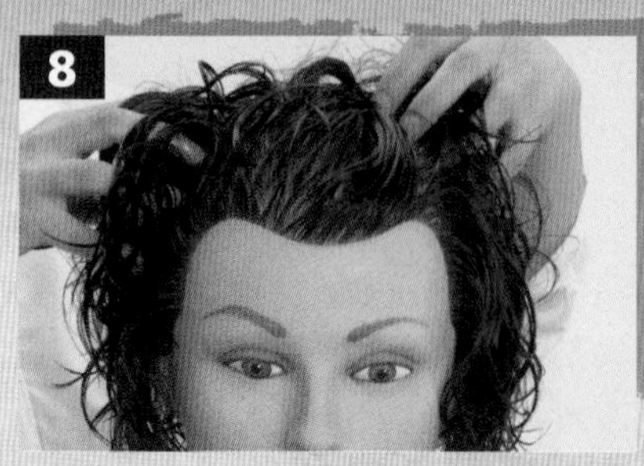

8 With a wide-tooth comb or your fingers, encourage the hair into the desired shape.

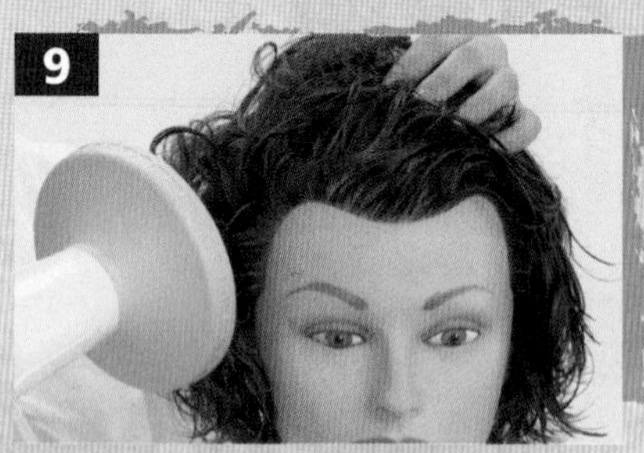

9 Diffuse the hair gently, pressing the diffuser on and off the hair without over-manipulating the hair, until each area of the head is dry.

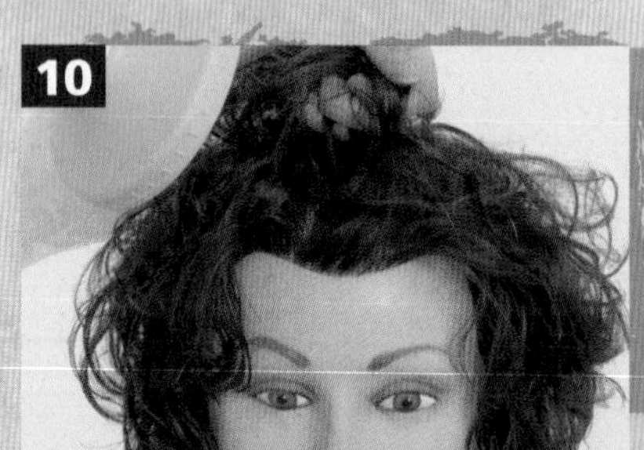

10 To relax or soften the curl, slowly and gently run your fingers through the curl when the hair is almost dry.

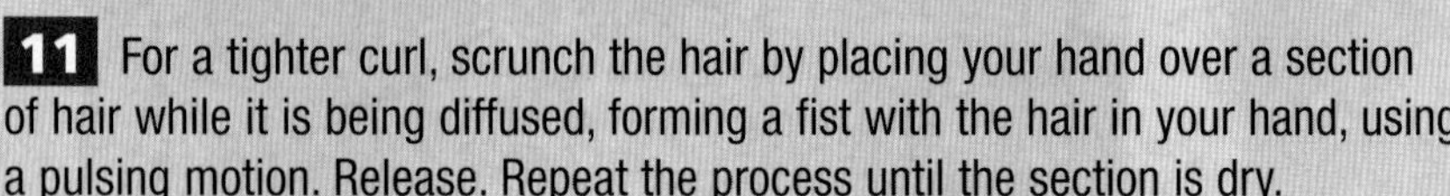

11 For a tighter curl, scrunch the hair by placing your hand over a section of hair while it is being diffused, forming a fist with the hair in your hand, using a pulsing motion. Release. Repeat the process until the section is dry.

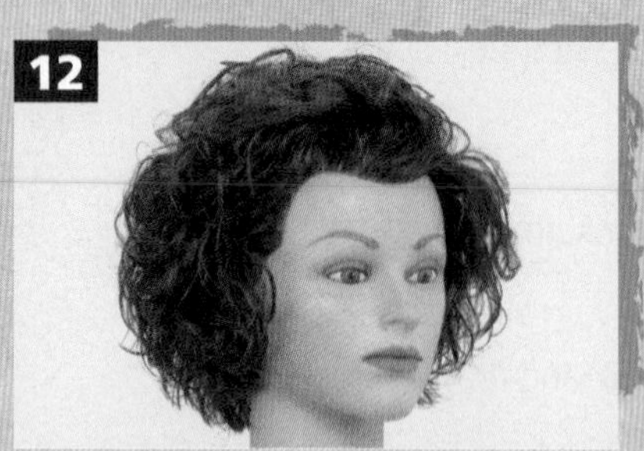

12 For more shine, finish the look with a silicone spray product.

© Milady, a part of Cengage Learning. Photography by Paul Castle, Castle Photography.

Post-Service

- Complete PROCEDURE 15-2 **Post-Service Procedure** SEE PAGE 326

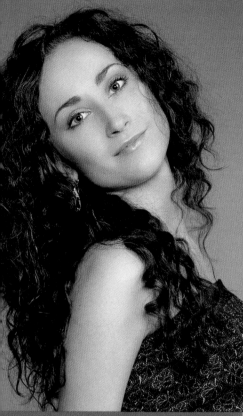

PROCEDURE 17-8

Diffusing Long, Curly, or Extremely Curly Hair in Its Natural Wave Pattern

© Konstantynov, 2010; used under license from Shutterstock.com.

Implements and Materials

You will need all of the following implements, materials, and supplies:

- **Blowdryer with attachments**
- **Neck strip**
- **Round brush**
- **Sectioning clips**
- **Styling and finishing products**
- **Styling cape**
- **Wide-tooth comb**

Preparation

- Perform PROCEDURE 15-1 Pre-Service Procedure SEE PAGE 323

Procedure

1 Drape the client for a shampoo service.

2 Shampoo the client's hair, and condition if necessary.

3 Towel dry the hair.

4 Remove any tangles with a wide-tooth comb, starting at the ends and working up to the scalp.

5 Place a clean neck strip on the client, and drape with a cutting or styling cape.

6 Distribute styling product through the hair with your fingers, and comb through with a wide-tooth comb.

7 For easier control, section the hair and work on one section at a time.

© Milady, a part of Cengage Learning. Photography by Paul Castle, Castle Photography.

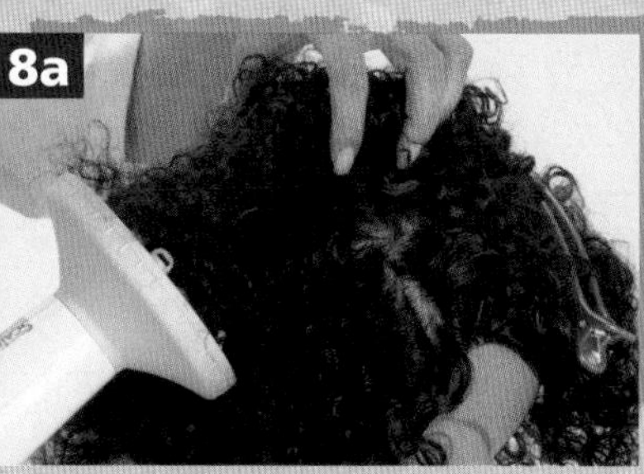

8a

8b

© Milady, a part of Cengage Learning. Photography by Paul Castle, Castle Photography.

8 Attach the diffuser to the blowdryer and diffuse the hair by letting the hair sit on top of the diffuser and pulsing the dryer toward the scalp and then away, repeating until the section is dry. Alternatively, gently run the section being dried through your fingers and bring the diffuser toward your hand.

Post-Service

- Complete PROCEDURE 15-2 Post-Service Procedure SEE PAGE 326

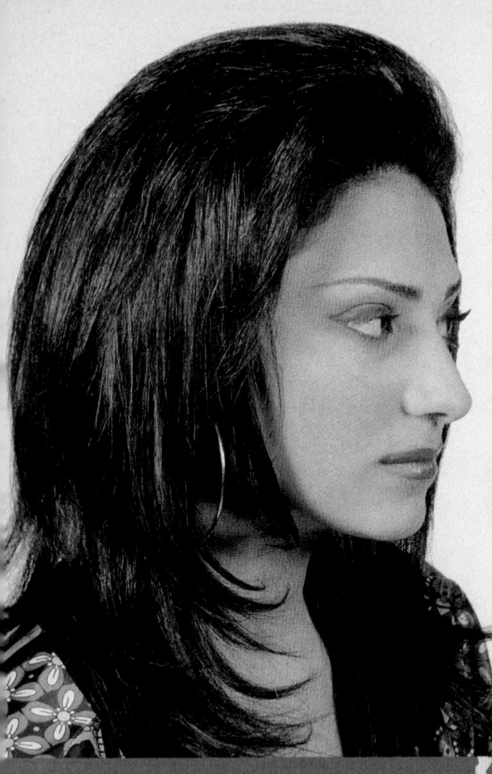

PROCEDURE 17-9 Right-Handed

Blowdrying Straight or Wavy Hair for Maximum Volume

Implements and Materials

You will need all of the following implements, materials, and supplies:

- **Blowdryer with attachments**
- **Neck strip**
- **Sectioning clips**
- **Styling and finishing product**
- **Styling cape**
- **Vent or classic styling brush**
- **Wide-tooth comb**

Preparation

- Perform PROCEDURE 15-1 **Pre-Service Procedure** **SEE PAGE 323**

Procedure

1 Drape the client for a shampoo service.

2 Shampoo the client's hair, and condition if necessary.

3 Towel dry the hair.

4 Remove any tangles with a wide-tooth comb, starting at the ends and working up to the scalp.

5 Place a clean neck strip on the client, and drape with a cutting or styling cape.

6 Apply a mousse, volumizing spray, or lightweight gel.

7 Using a vent brush or classic styling brush, distribute the hair into the desired shape.

© Milady, a part of Cengage Learning. Photography by Yanik Chauvin.

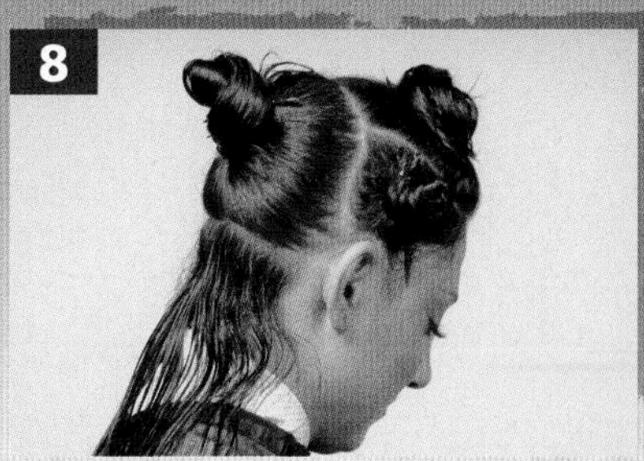

8 Build your shape from the bottom up, working from the nape up toward the crown. When you begin at the nape, hold the wet hair above the nape in a sectioning clip.

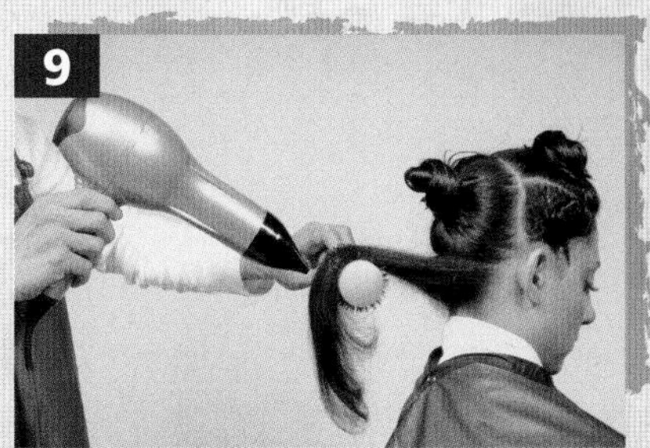

9 While turning the brush downward and away from the scalp, allow the brush to pick up a section of hair and begin drying. Direct the airflow toward the top of the brush, moving in the desired direction.

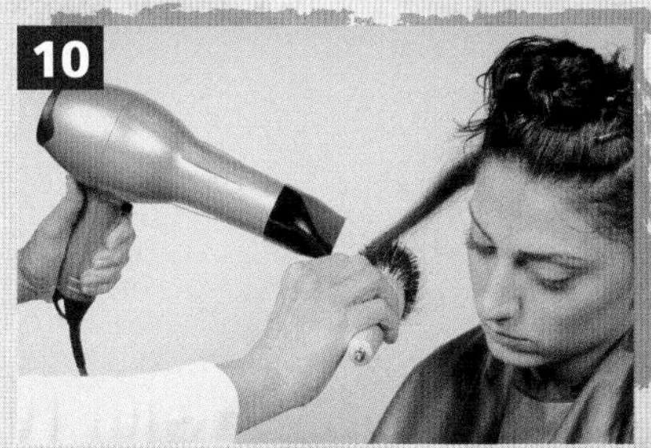

10 Work in sections, lifting and drying the sections and then brushing them in the desired direction when they are completely dry. Repeat over the entire head, directing the hair at the sides either away or forward. The bang area can be dried either onto the forehead or away from the face.

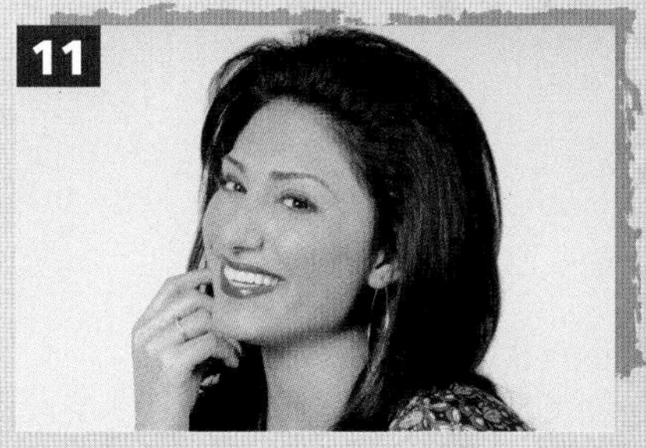

11 Finished look.

Post-Service

- Complete PROCEDURE 15-2 **Post-Service Procedure** **SEE PAGE 326**

© Milady, a part of Cengage Learning. Photography by Yanik Chauvin.

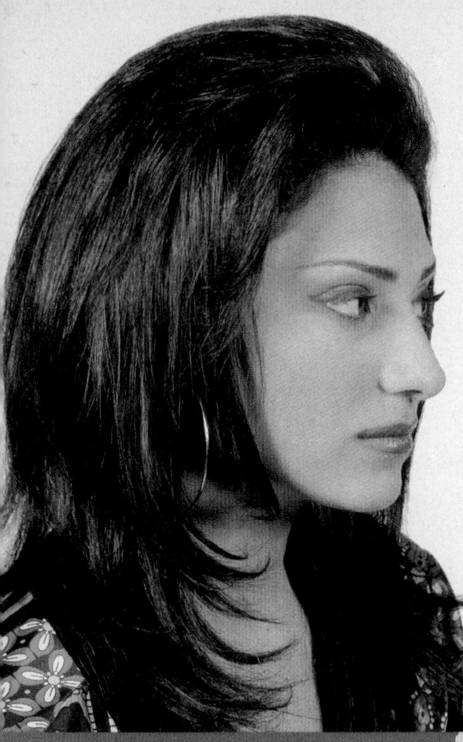

PROCEDURE 17-9 Left Handed

Blowdrying Straight or Wavy Hair for Maximum Volume

Implements and Materials

You will need all of the following implements, materials, and supplies:

- **Blowdryer with attachments**
- **Neck strip**
- **Sectioning clips**
- **Styling and finishing product**
- **Styling cape**
- **Vent or classic styling brush**
- **Wide-tooth comb**

Preparation

- Perform PROCEDURE 15-1 **Pre-Service Procedure** **SEE PAGE 323**

Procedure

1 Drape the client for a shampoo service.

2 Shampoo the client's hair, and condition if necessary.

3 Towel dry the hair.

4 Remove any tangles with a wide-tooth comb, starting at the ends and working up to the scalp.

5 Place a clean neck strip on the client, and drape with a cutting or styling cape.

6 Apply a mousse, volumizing spray, or lightweight gel.

7 Using a vent brush or classic styling brush, distribute the hair into the desired shape.

© Milady, a part of Cengage Learning. Photography by Yanik Chauvin.

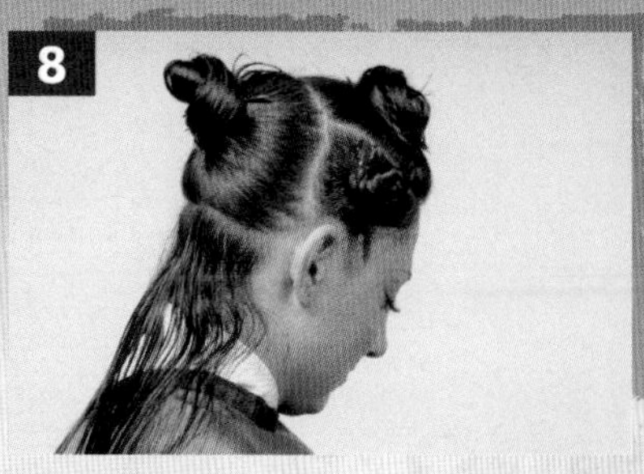

8 Build your shape from the bottom up, working from the nape up toward the crown. When you begin at the nape, hold the wet hair above the nape in a sectioning clip.

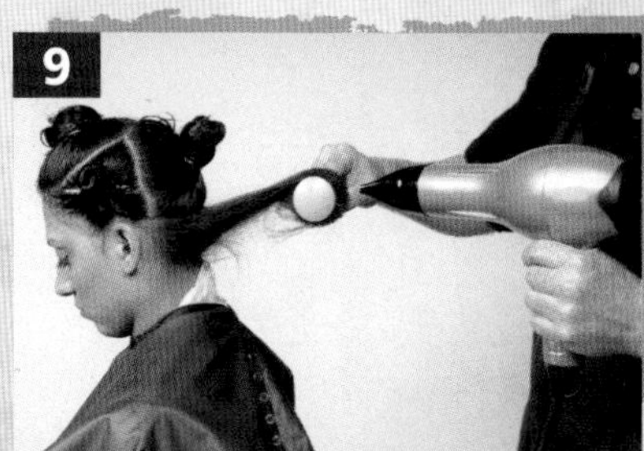

9 While turning the brush downward and away from the scalp, allow the brush to pick up a section of hair and begin drying. Direct the airflow toward the top of the brush, moving in the desired direction.

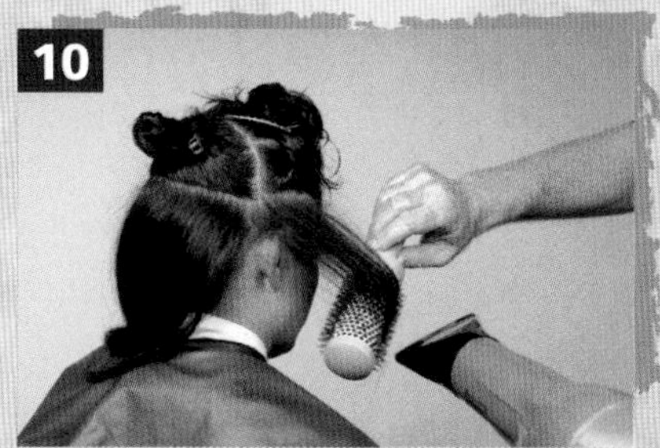

10 Work in sections, lifting and drying the sections and then brushing them in the desired direction when they are completely dry. Repeat over the entire head, directing the hair at the sides either away or forward. The bang area can be dried either onto the forehead or away from the face.

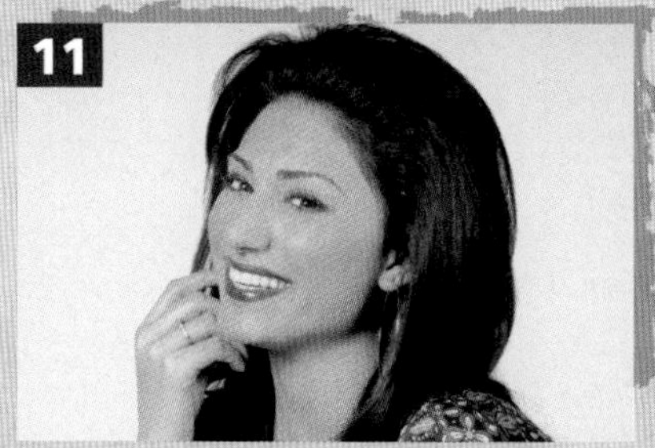

11 Finished look.

Post-Service

- Complete PROCEDURE 15-2 **Post-Service Procedure** **SEE PAGE 326**

© Milady, a part of Cengage Learning. Photography by Yanik Chauvin.

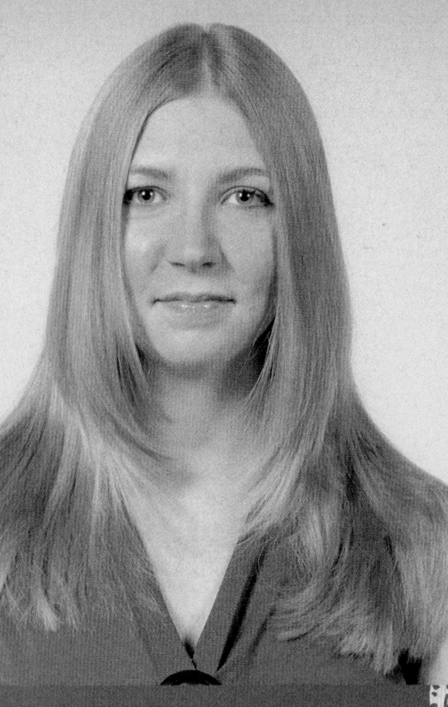

PROCEDURE 17-10 Right-Handed

Blowdrying Blunt or Long-Layered, Straight to Wavy Hair into a Straight Style

Implements and Materials

You will need all of the following implements, materials, and supplies:

- **Blowdryer with attachments**
- **Neck strip**
- **Round brush**
- **Sectioning clips**
- **Styling and finishing products**
- **Styling cape**
- **Wide-tooth comb**

Preparation

- Perform PROCEDURE 15-1 **Pre-Service Procedure** **SEE PAGE 323**

Procedure

1 Drape the client for a shampoo service.

2 Shampoo the client's hair, and condition if necessary.

3 Towel dry the hair.

4 Remove any tangles with a wide-tooth comb, starting at the ends and working up to the scalp.

5 Place a clean neck strip on the client, and drape with a cutting or styling cape.

6 Apply a light gel or a straightening gel.

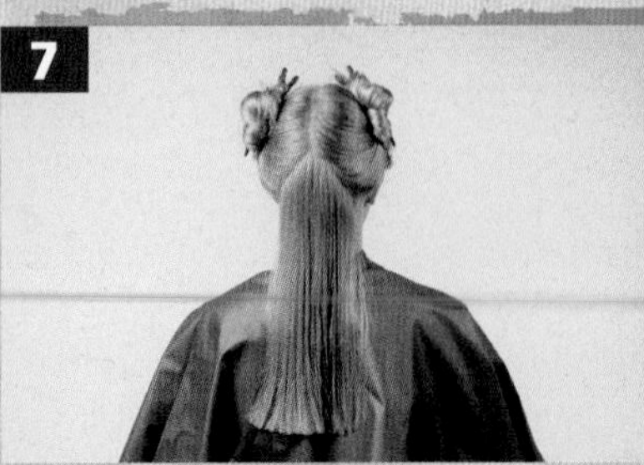

7 Attach the nozzle or concentrator attachment to the blowdryer for more controlled styling. Part and section the hair so that only the section you are drying is not in clips.

© Milady, a part of Cengage Learning. Photography by Yanik Chauvin.

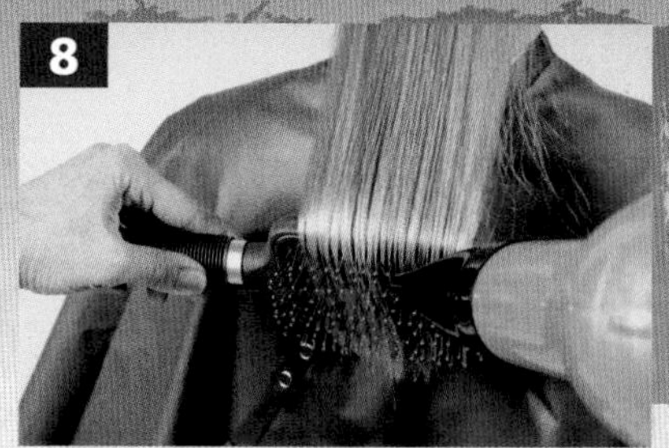

8 Using 1-inch subsections, start your first section at the nape of the neck and use a classic styling brush to dry the hair straight and smooth. Place the brush under the first section and hold the hair low.

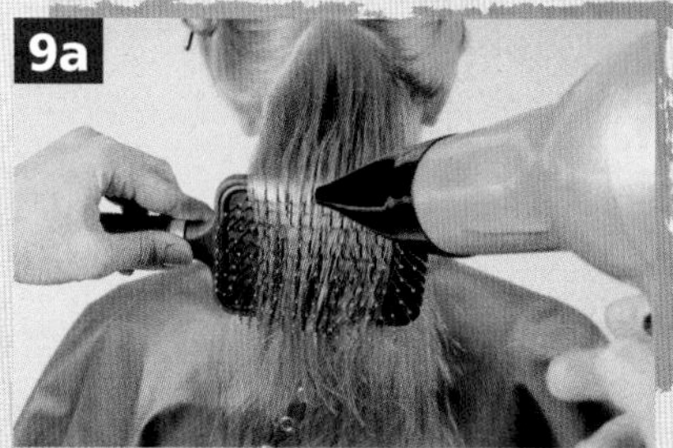

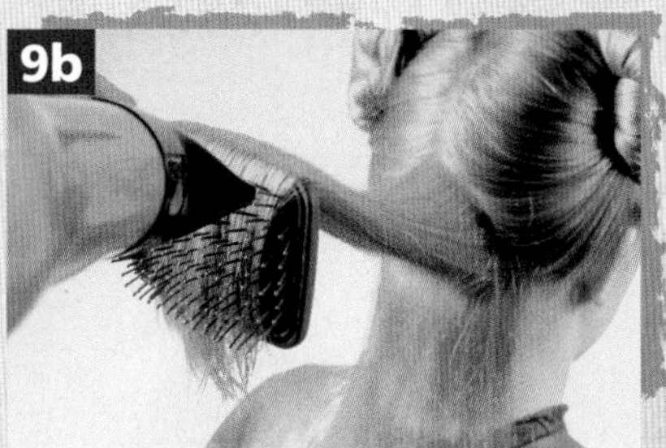

9 Follow the brush with the nozzle of the dryer, while bending the ends of the hair in the desired direction, either under or flipped outward. Continue using the same technique, working up to the occipital area in 1-inch sections. To keep the shape flat and straight, use low elevation. For more lift and volume, hold the section straight out from the head or overdirect upward.

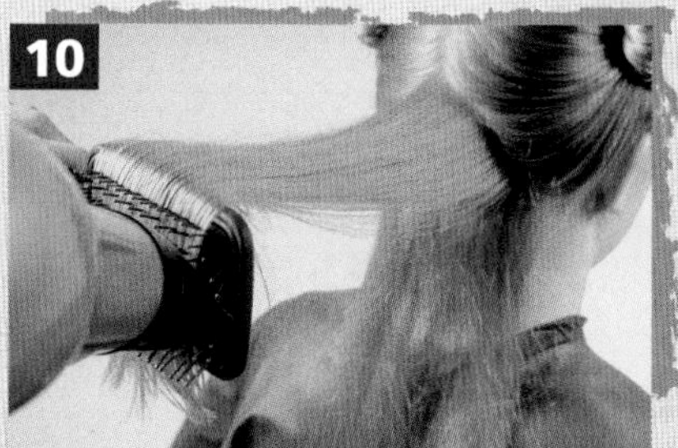

10 Work up to the crown, continuing to take 1-inch sections. On the longer sections toward the top of the crown, you can switch to a paddle brush, using the curve of the brush to add bend to the ends of the hair.

11 After each section is blown dry, follow by using the cooling button on the blowdryer to help set each section and to keep it smooth. For a fuller look, switch to a round brush.

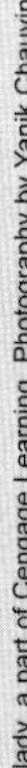
© Milady, a part of Cengage Learning. Photography by Yanik Chauvin.

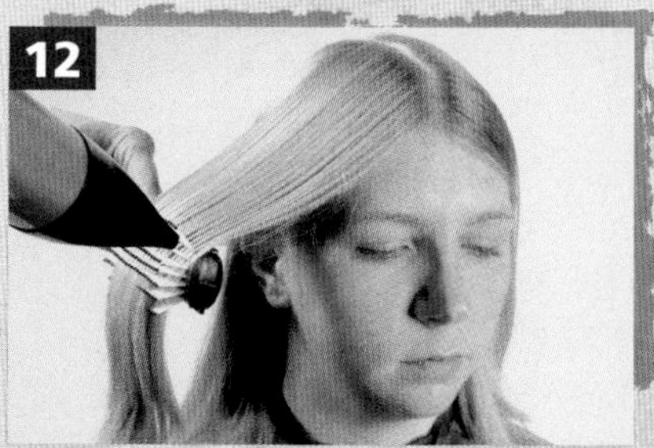

12 Continue by subdividing the hair on the side, and start with the section above the ear. Continue working in 1-inch sections. Hold at a low elevation and follow with the nozzle of the dryer facing toward the ends. Bend the ends under by turning the brush under for a rounded edge, or outward for a flipped edge.

Blowdrying Blunt or Long-Layered, Straight to Wavy Hair into a Straight Style: Right-Handed continued

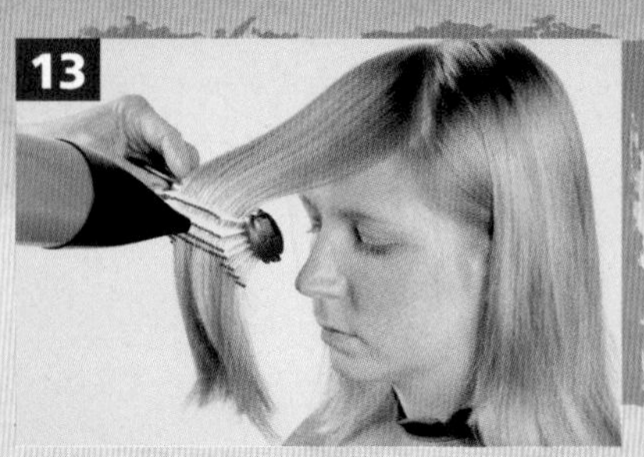

13 Work in the same manner across the top of the head. If there is a bang, dry it in the desired direction. To dry the bang straight and onto the forehead, point the nozzle of the dryer down over the bang and dry it straight, using your fingers or a classic styling brush to direct the hair.

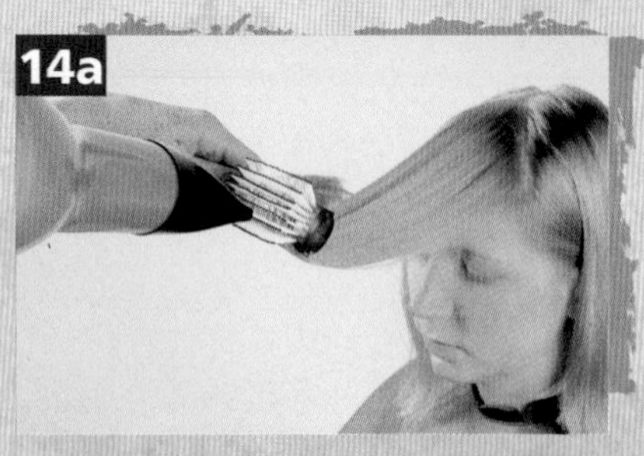

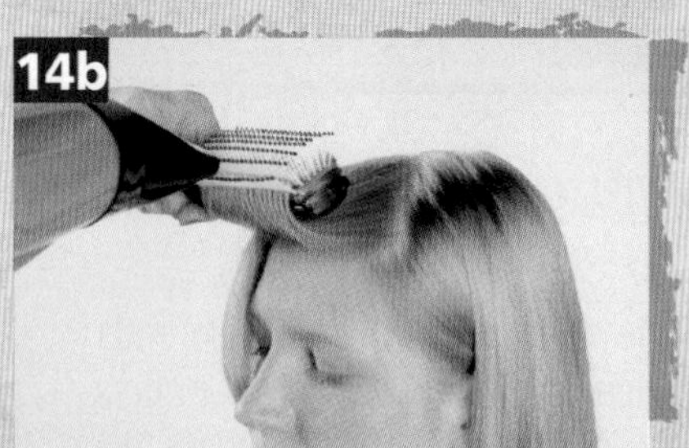

14 To direct the bang away from the face, brush the bang back and push the hair slightly forward with the brush, creating a curved shaping. Place the dryer on a slow setting and point the nozzle toward the brush. When dry, the bang will fall away from the face and slightly to the side, for a soft look.

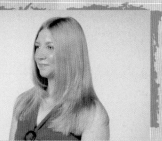

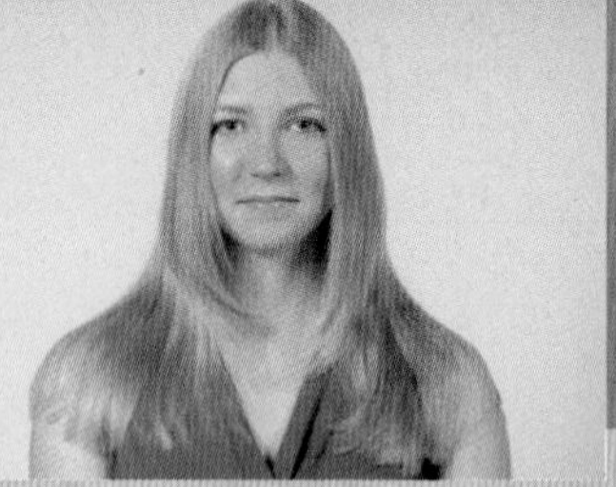

15 Finished look.

Post-Service

- Complete PROCEDURE 15-2 **Post-Service Procedure** SEE PAGE 326

© Milady, a part of Cengage Learning. Photography by Yanik Chauvin.

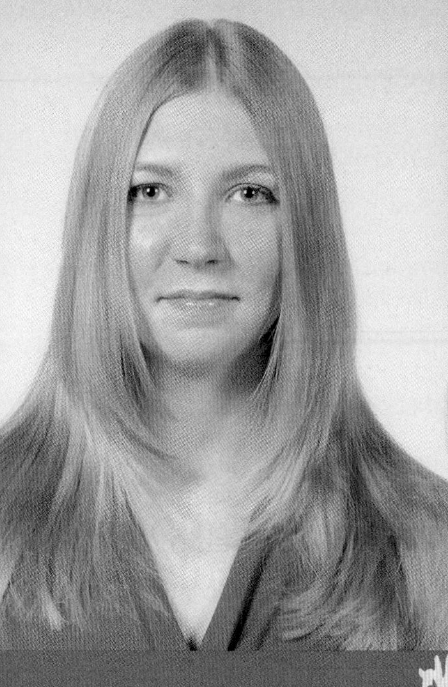

PROCEDURE 17-10 Left Handed

Blowdrying Blunt or Long-Layered, Straight to Wavy Hair into a Straight Style

Implements and Materials

You will need all of the following implements, materials, and supplies:

- **Blowdryer with attachments**
- **Neck strip**
- **Round brush**
- **Sectioning clips**
- **Styling and finishing products**
- **Styling cape**
- **Wide-tooth comb**

© Milady, a part of Cengage Learning. Photography by Yanik Chauvin.

Preparation

- Perform PROCEDURE 15-1 **Pre-Service Procedure** **SEE PAGE 323**

Procedure

1 Drape the client for a shampoo service.

2 Shampoo the client's hair, and condition if necessary.

3 Towel dry the hair.

4 Remove any tangles with a wide-tooth comb, starting at the ends and working up to the scalp.

5 Place a clean neck strip on the client, and drape with a cutting or styling cape.

6 Apply a light gel or a straightening gel.

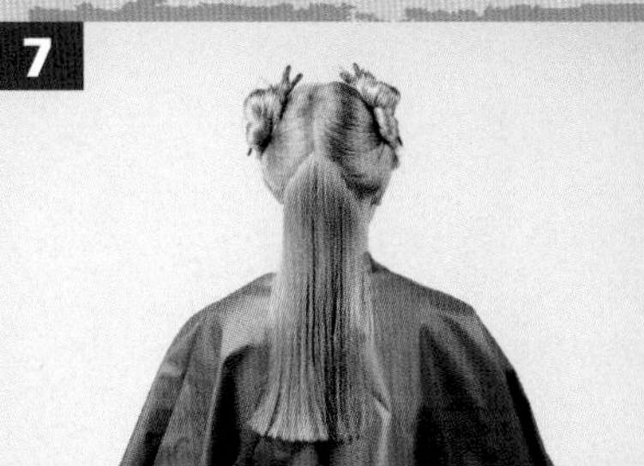

7 Attach the nozzle or concentrator attachment to the blowdryer for more controlled styling. Part and section the hair so that only the section you are drying is not in clips.

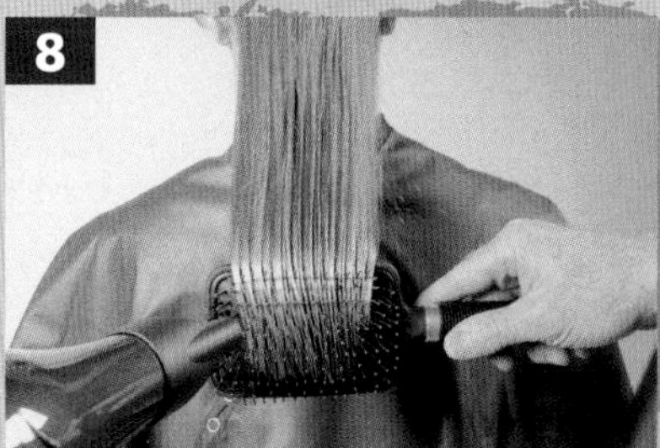

8 Using 1-inch subsections, start your first section at the nape of the neck and use a classic styling brush to dry the hair straight and smooth. Place the brush under the first section and hold the hair low.

Blowdrying Blunt or Long-Layered, Straight to Wavy Hair into a Straight Style: Left-Handed continued

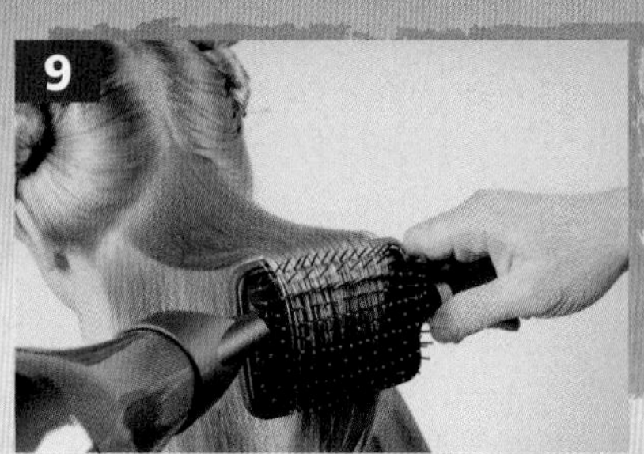

9 Follow the brush with the nozzle of the dryer, while bending the ends of the hair in the desired direction, either under or flipped outward. Continue using the same technique, working up to the occipital area in 1-inch sections. To keep the shape flat and straight, use low elevation. For more lift and volume, hold the section straight out from the head or overdirect upward.

10 Work up to the crown, continuing to take 1-inch sections. On the longer sections toward the top of the crown, you can switch to a paddle brush, using the curve of the brush to add bend to the ends of the hair.

11 After each section is blown dry, follow by using the cooling button on the blowdryer to help set each section and to keep it smooth. For a fuller look, switch to a round brush.

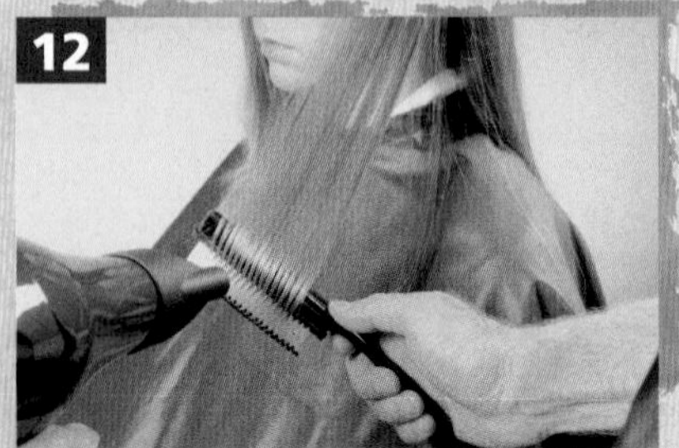

12 Continue by subdividing the hair on the side, and start with the section above the ear. Continue working in 1-inch sections. Hold at a low elevation and follow with the nozzle of the dryer facing toward the ends. Bend the ends under by turning the brush under for a rounded edge, or outward for a flipped edge.

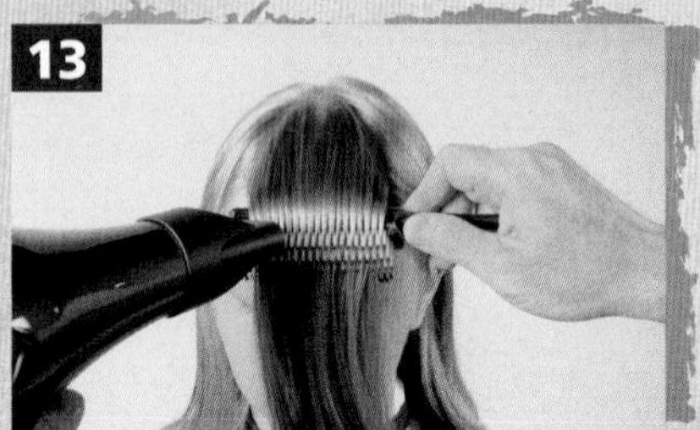

13 Work in the same manner across the top of the head. If there is a bang, dry it in the desired direction. To dry the bang straight and onto the forehead, point the nozzle of the dryer down over the bang and dry it straight, using your fingers or a classic styling brush to direct the hair.

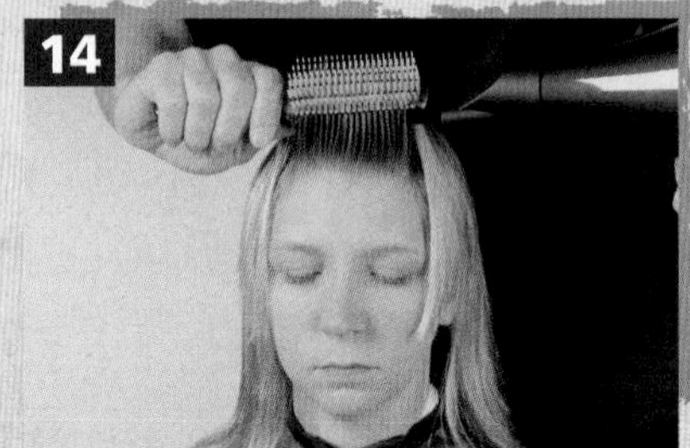

14 To direct the bang away from the face, brush the bang back and push the hair slightly forward with the brush, creating a curved shaping. Place the dryer on a slow setting and point the nozzle toward the brush. When dry, the bang will fall away from the face and slightly to the side, for a soft look.

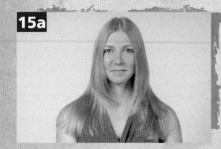

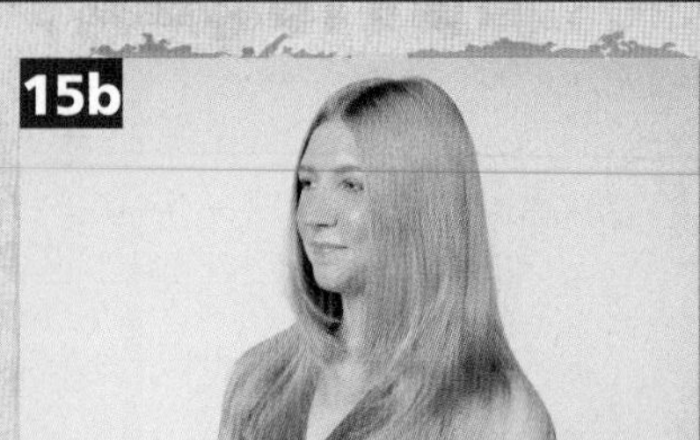

15 Finished look.

© Milady, a part of Cengage Learning. Photography by Yanik Chauvin.

Post-Service

- Complete PROCEDURE 15-2 **Post-Service Procedure** SEE PAGE 326

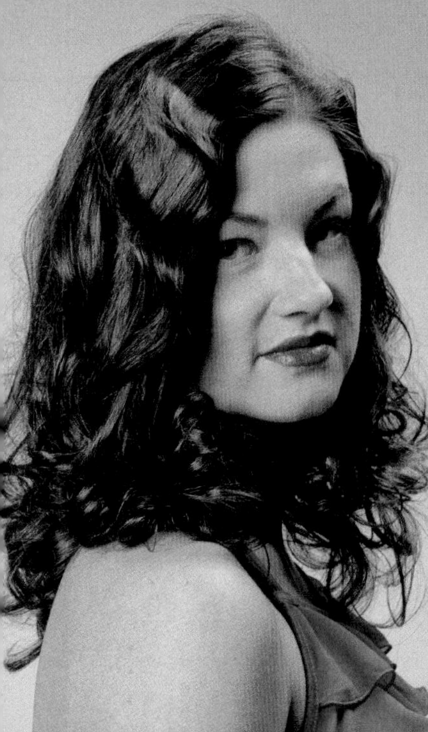

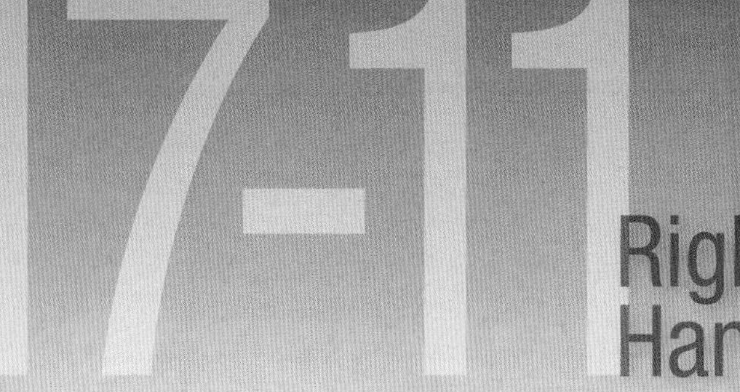

PROCEDURE 17-11

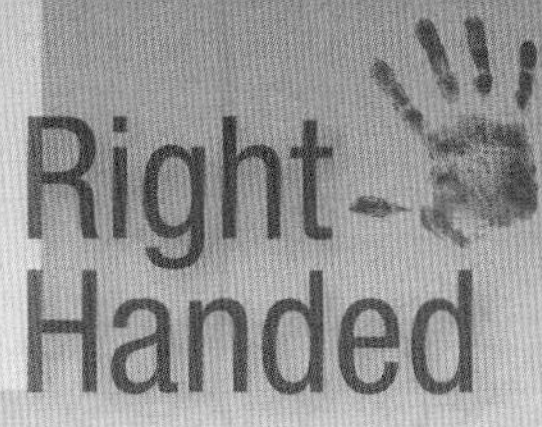

Right-Handed

Thermal Waving

Implements and Materials

You will need all of the following implements, materials, and supplies:

- **Conventional (Marcel) or electric irons**
- **Hard rubber comb (fine toothed)**
- **Shampoo**
- **Styling cape and neck strip**

© Milady, a part of Cengage Learning. Photography by Yanik Chauvin.

Preparation

- Perform PROCEDURE 15-1 Pre-Service Procedure SEE PAGE 323

Procedure

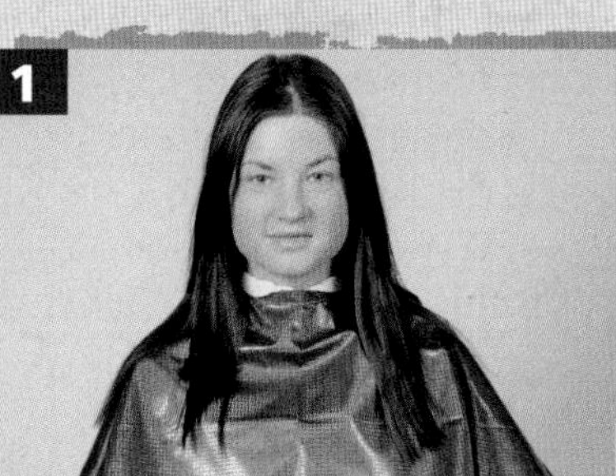

1 Drape the client for a shampoo service.

2 Shampoo the client's hair, and condition if necessary.

3 Towel dry the hair.

4 Remove any tangles with a wide-tooth comb, starting at the ends and working up to the scalp.

5 Dry the client's hair completely.

6 Drape the client for a dry hair service.

7 Heat the iron.

Thermal Waving: Right-Handed continued

8 Before beginning the waves, comb the hair in the general shape desired by the client. The natural growth will determine whether or not the first wave will be a left-moving wave or a right-moving wave. The procedure described here is for a left-moving wave.

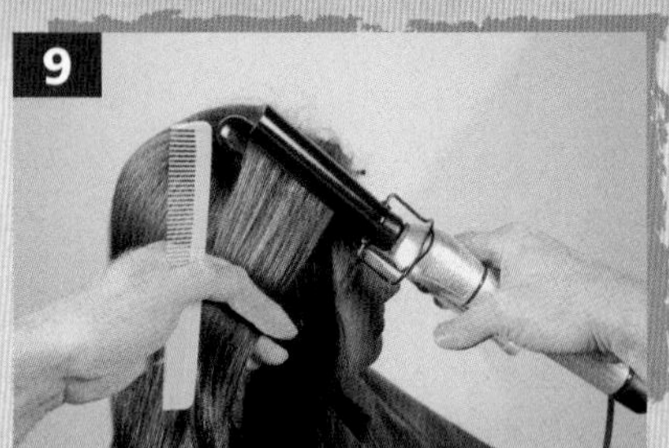

9 With the comb, pick up a strand of hair about 2 inches (5 centimeters) in width. Insert the iron in the hair with the groove facing upward.

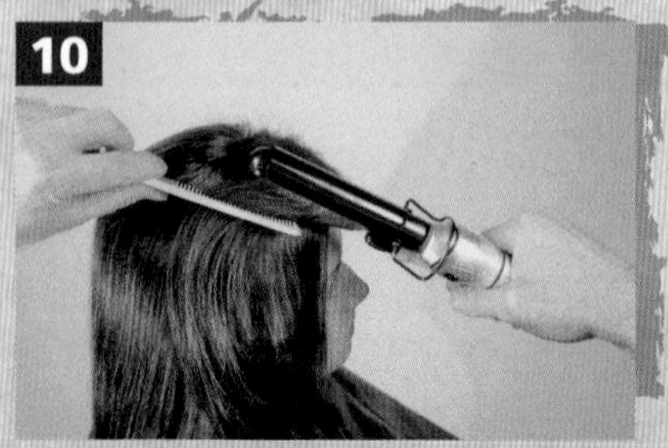

10 Close the iron and give it a ¼-inch turn forward (away from you). At the same time, draw the hair with the iron about ¼ inch (.625 centimeters) to the left, and direct the hair ¼ inch (.625 centimeters) to the right with the comb.

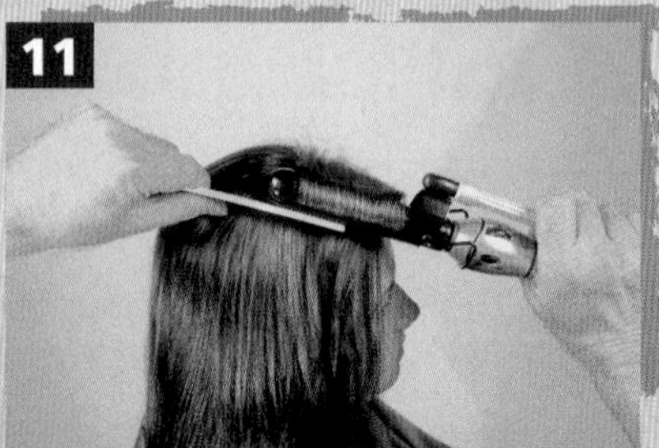

11 Roll the iron one full turn forward and away from you. When doing this, keep the hair uniform with the comb. You will find that the hair has rolled on a slight slant on the prong of the iron. Keep this position for a few seconds in order to allow the hair to become sufficiently heated throughout.

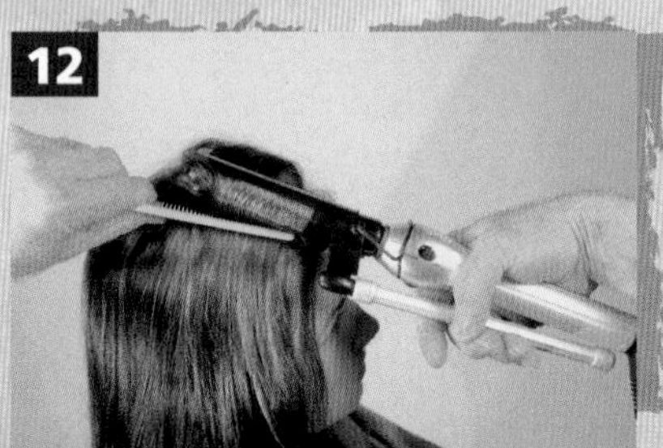

12 Reverse the movement by simply unrolling the hair from the iron and bringing it back into its first resting position. When this movement is completed, you will find the comb resting somewhat away from the iron.

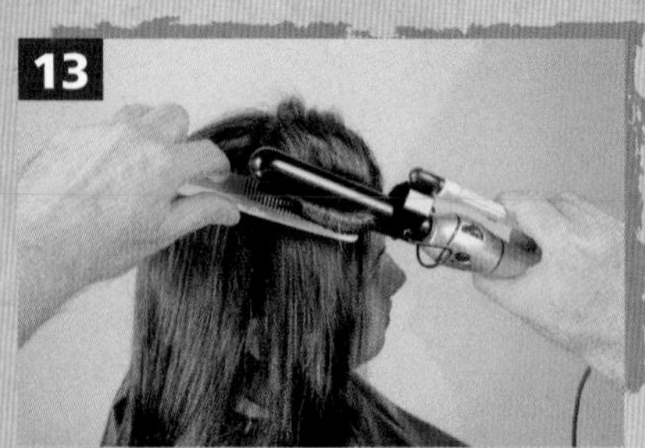

13 Open the iron with your little finger and place it just below the ridge or crest by swinging the rod of the iron toward you, and then closing it. The outer edge of the groove should be directly underneath the ridge just produced by the inner ridge.

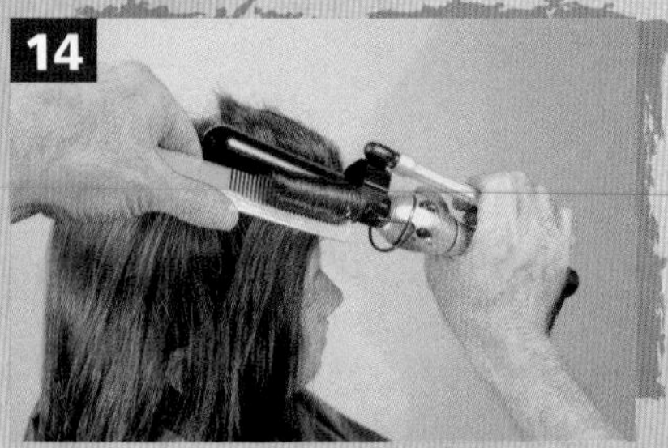

14 Keeping the iron perfectly still, direct the hair with the comb upward about 1 inch (2.5 centimeters), thus forming the hair into a half circle. Remember that you should not move the comb from the position explained in step 12.

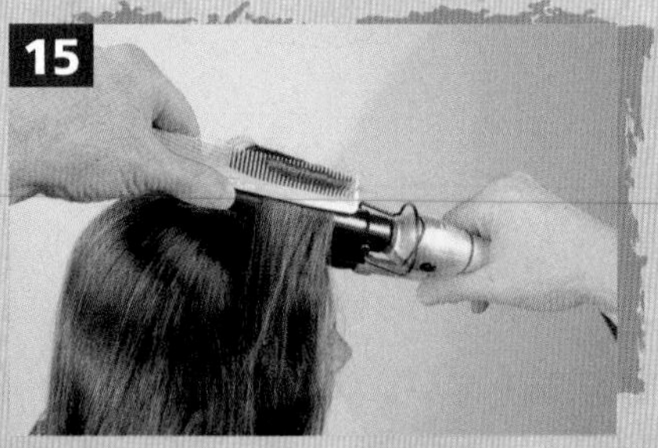

15 Without opening the iron, roll it a half-turn forward and away from you. In this movement, keep the comb perfectly still and unchanged.

© Milady, a part of Cengage Learning. Photography by Yanik Chauvin.

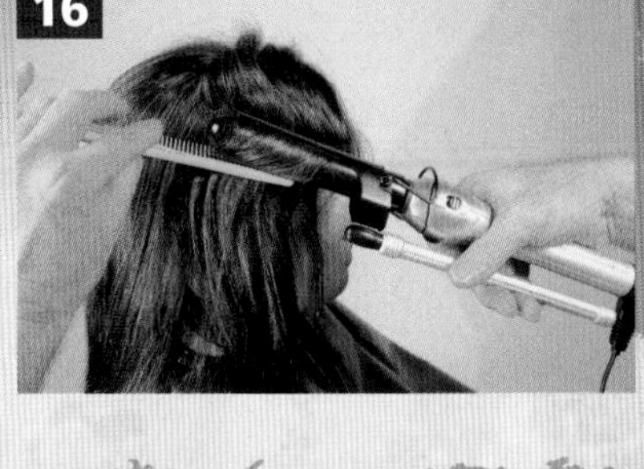

16 Slide the iron down about 1 inch (2.5 centimeters). This movement is accomplished by opening the iron slightly, gripping it loosely, and then sliding it down the strand.

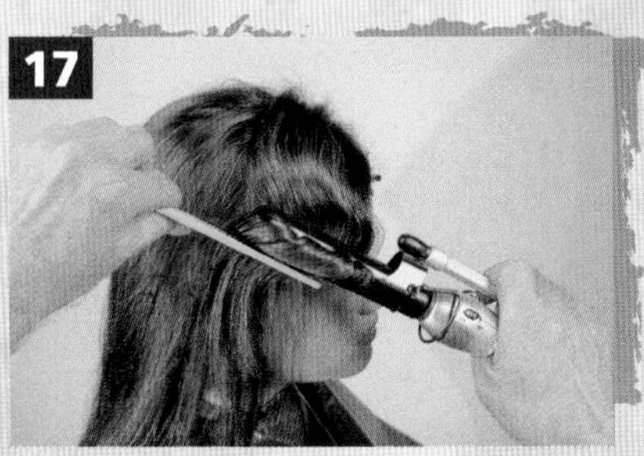

17 After completing step 16, you will find the iron and comb in the correct position to make the second ridge. This is the beginning of a right-moving wave, in which the hair is directed opposite to that of a left-moving wave.

18 After completely waving one strand of hair, wave the next strand to match. Pick up the strand in the comb and include a small section of the waved strand to guide you as you form a new wave. When waving the second strand of hair, be sure to use the same comb and iron movements you used when waving the first strand of hair. This will make the waves match.

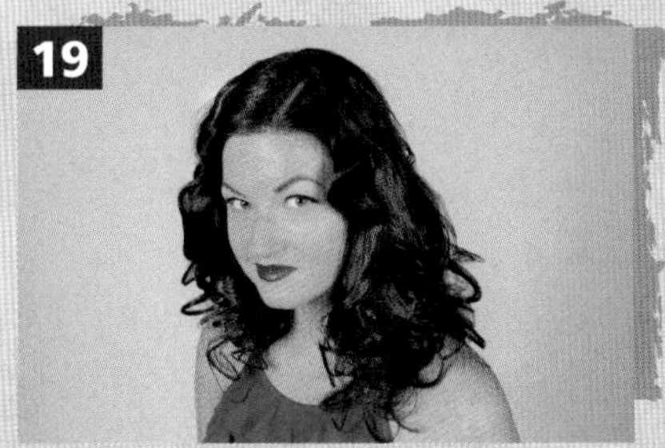

19 Finished look.

Post-Service

- Complete PROCEDURE **15-2 Post-Service Procedure** **SEE PAGE 326**

© Milady, a part of Cengage Learning. Photography by Yanik Chauvin.

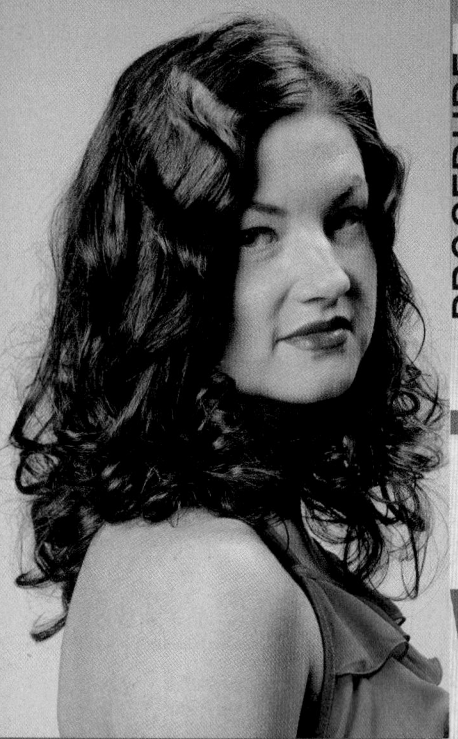

PROCEDURE 17-11

Left Handed

Thermal Waving

Implements and Materials

You will need all of the following implements, materials, and supplies:

- **Conventional (Marcel) or electric irons**
- **Hard rubber comb (fine toothed)**
- **Shampoo**
- **Styling cape and neck strip**

Preparation

- Perform PROCEDURE 15-1 Pre-Service Procedure SEE PAGE 323

Procedure

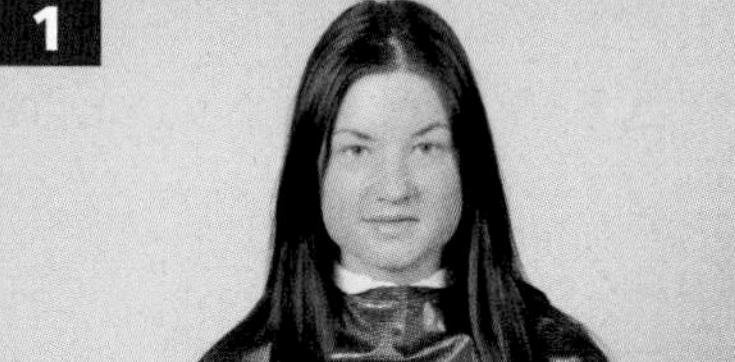

1 Drape the client for a shampoo service.

2 Shampoo the client's hair, and condition if necessary.

3 Towel dry the hair.

4 Remove any tangles with a wide-tooth comb, starting at the ends and working up to the scalp.

5 Dry the client's hair completely.

6 Drape the client for a dry hair service.

7 Heat the iron.

© Milady, a part of Cengage Learning. Photography by Yanik Chauvin.

8 Before beginning the waves, comb the hair in the general shape desired by the client. The natural growth will determine whether or not the first wave will be a left-moving wave or a right-moving wave. The procedure described here is for a left-moving wave.

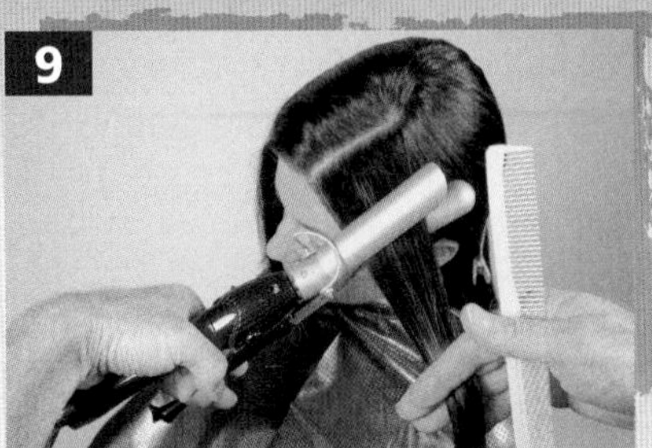

9 With the comb, pick up a strand of hair about 2 inches (5 centimeters) in width. Insert the iron in the hair with the groove facing upward.

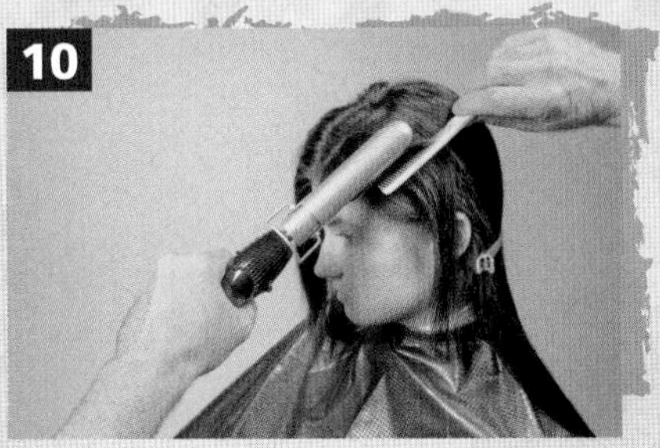

10 Close the iron and give it a ¼-inch turn forward (away from you). At the same time, draw the hair with the iron about ¼ inch (.625 centimeters) to the left, and direct the hair ¼ inch (.625 centimeters) to the right with the comb.

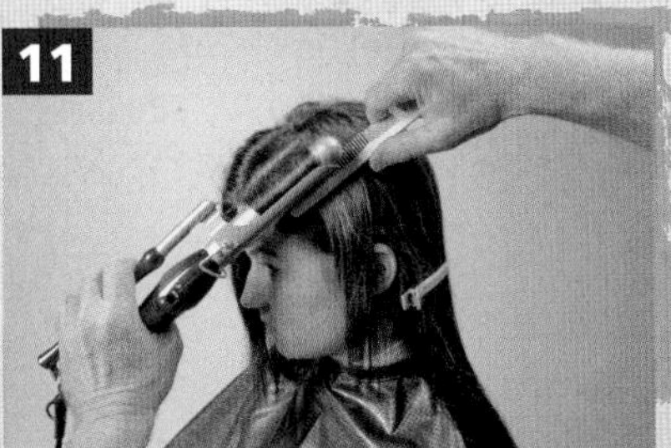

11 Roll the iron one full turn forward and away from you. When doing this, keep the hair uniform with the comb. You will find that the hair has rolled on a slight slant on the prong of the iron. Keep this position for a few seconds in order to allow the hair to become sufficiently heated throughout.

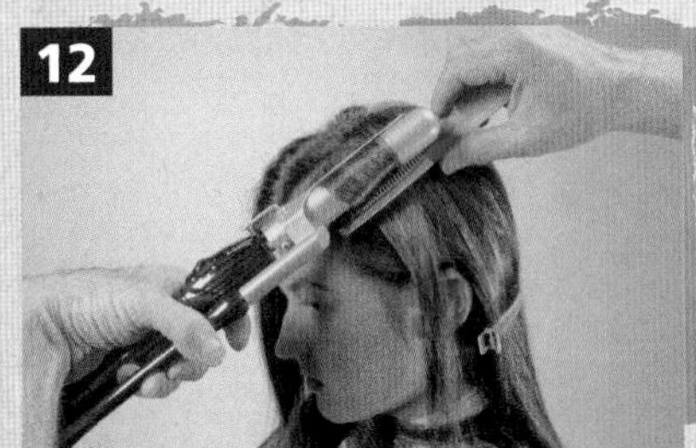

12 Reverse the movement by simply unrolling the hair from the iron and bringing it back into its first resting position. When this movement is completed, you will find the comb resting somewhat away from the iron.

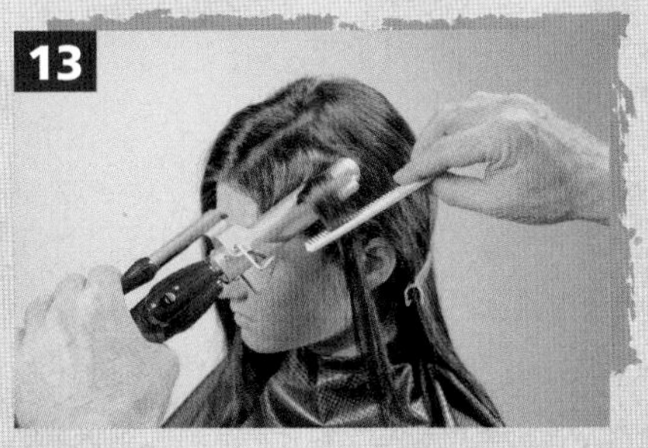

13 Open the iron with your little finger and place it just below the ridge or crest by swinging the rod of the iron toward you, and then closing it. The outer edge of the groove should be directly underneath the ridge just produced by the inner ridge.

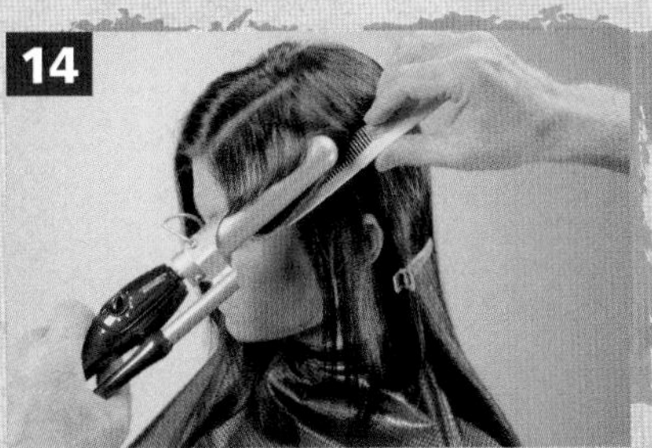

14 Keeping the iron perfectly still, direct the hair with the comb upward about 1 inch (2.5 centimeters), thus forming the hair into a half circle. Remember that you should not move the comb from the position explained in step 12.

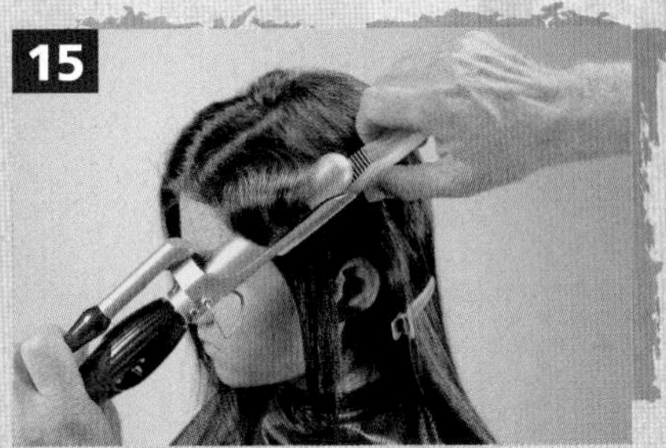

15 Without opening the iron, roll it a half-turn forward and away from you. In this movement, keep the comb perfectly still and unchanged.

© Milady, a part of Cengage Learning. Photography by Yanik Chauvin.

PROCEDURE 17-11

Thermal Waving: Left-Handed continued

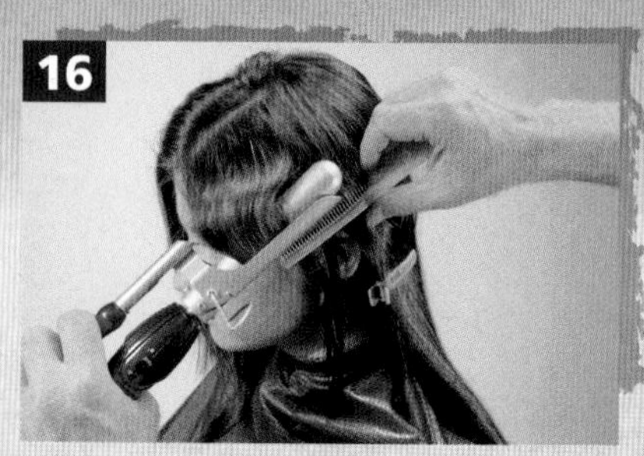

16 Slide the iron down about 1 inch (2.5 centimeters). This movement is accomplished by opening the iron slightly, gripping it loosely, and then sliding it down the strand.

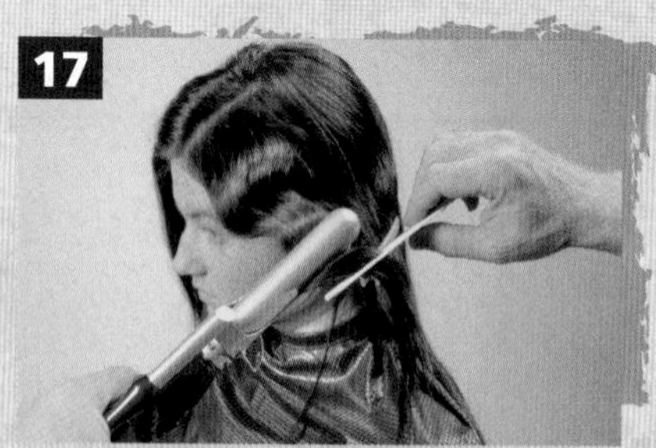

17 After completing step 16, you will find the iron and comb in the correct position to make the second ridge. This is the beginning of a right-moving wave, in which the hair is directed opposite to that of a left-moving wave.

18 After completely waving one strand of hair, wave the next strand to match. Pick up the strand in the comb and include a small section of the waved strand to guide you as you form a new wave. When waving the second strand of hair, be sure to use the same comb and iron movements you used when waving the first strand of hair. This will make the waves match.

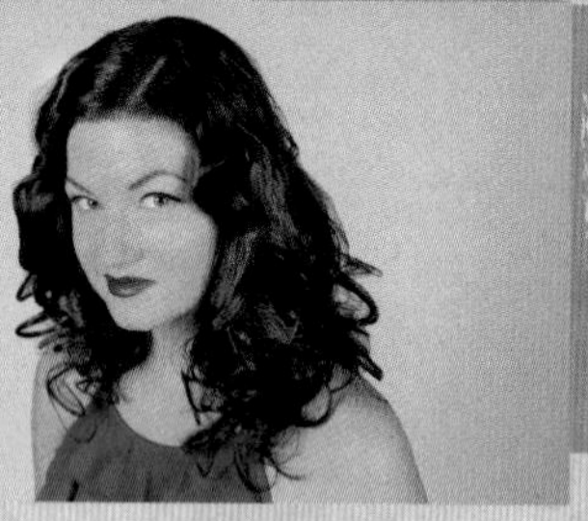

19 Finished look.

Post-Service

- Complete PROCEDURE 15-2 **Post-Service Procedure** SEE PAGE 326

© Milady, a part of Cengage Learning. Photography by Yanik Chauvin.

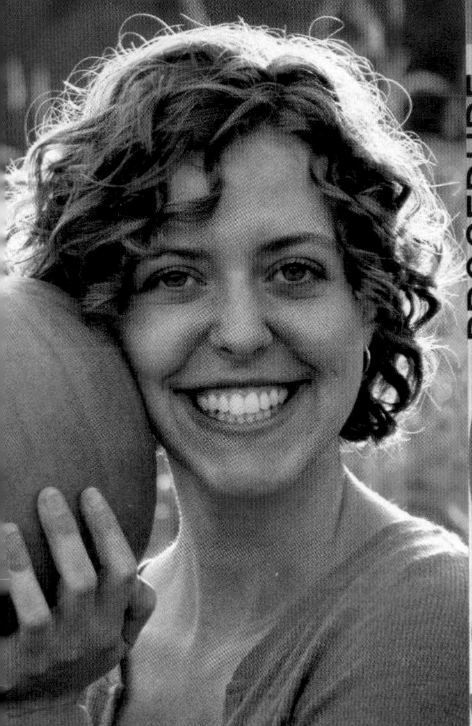

PROCEDURE 17-12

Curling Short Hair

Implements and Materials

You will need all of the following implements, materials, and supplies:

- **Conventional (Marcel) or electric irons**
- **Hard rubber comb (fine toothed)**
- **Shampoo**
- **Styling cape and neck strip**

© Carly Rose Hennigan, 2010; used under license from Shutterstock.com.

Preparation

- Perform PROCEDURE 15-1 **Pre-Service Procedure** **SEE PAGE 323**

Procedure

1 Drape the client for a shampoo service.

2 Shampoo the client's hair, and condition if necessary.

3 Towel dry the hair.

4 Remove any tangles with a wide-tooth comb, starting at the ends and working up to the scalp.

5 Dry the client's hair completely and divide the head into five sections. The first section should be about 2½-inches (6.25 centimeters) wide and extend from the center of the forehead to the nape of the neck. Divide the two side panels in half, from the top parting to the neck, to create four additional sections.

6 Heat thermal iron (large or jumbo size).

7 Begin by sectioning and parting the base of each curl to match the size of the curl desired. It is important to consider hair length, density, and texture. The base is usually about 1½ inches to 2 inches (3.75 centimeters to 5 centimeters) in width and ½ inch (1.25 centimeters) in depth.

8 After sectioning off the base, comb the hair smooth and straight out from the scalp. Loose hairs may result in an uneven and ragged curl.

Curling Short Hair continued

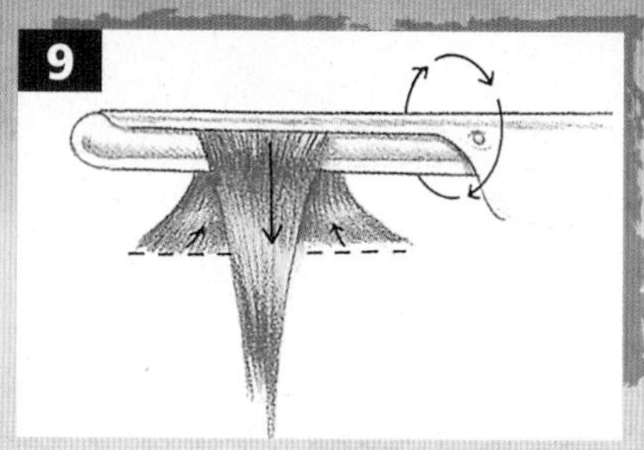

9 After the iron has been heated to the desired temperature, pick up a strand of hair and comb it smooth. With the groove on top, insert the iron about 1 inch (2.5 centimeters) from the scalp, and pull the hair over the rod in the direction of the curl. Hold for a few seconds to form a base.

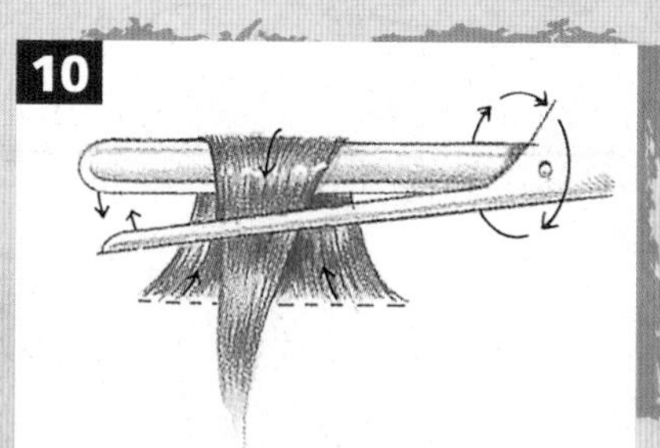

10 Hold the ends of the hair strand with your thumb and two fingers of your left hand (right hand if you are left-handed), using a medium degree of tension. Turn the iron downward (toward you) with your right hand.

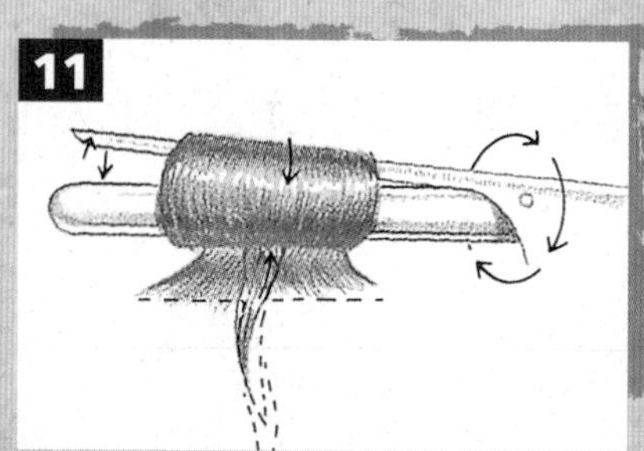

11 Open and close the iron rapidly as you turn in order to prevent binding. Guide the ends of the strand into the center of the curl as you rotate the iron.

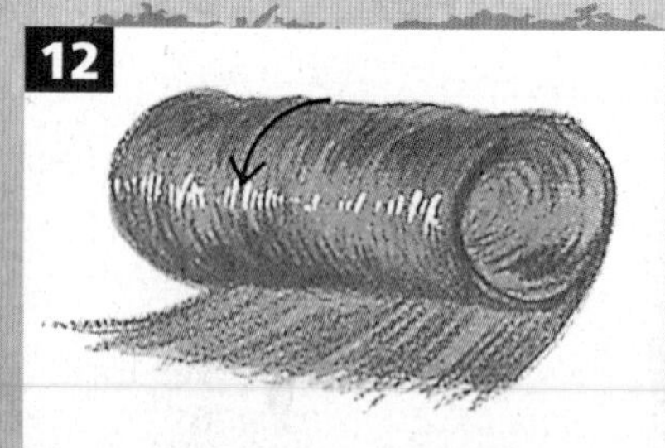

12 The result of this procedure will be a smooth, finished curl, with the ends firmly fixed in the center. Remove the iron from the curl.

Post-Service

- Complete PROCEDURE 15-2 **Post-Service Procedure** SEE PAGE 326

© Milady, a part of Cengage Learning.

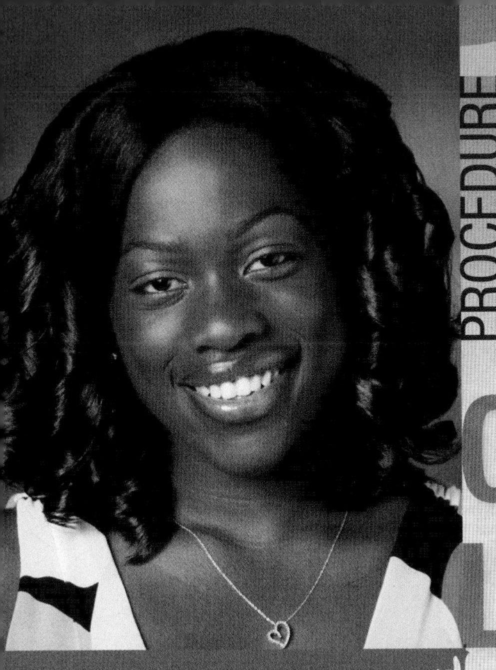

PROCEDURE 17-13

Curling Medium-Length Hair

© Cris Calhoun, 2010; used under license from Shutterstock.com.

Implements and Materials

You will need all of the following implements, materials, and supplies:

- **Conventional (Marcel) or electric irons**
- **Hard rubber comb (fine toothed)**
- **Shampoo**
- **Styling cape and neck strip**

Preparation

- Perform PROCEDURE 15-1 **Pre-Service Procedure** **SEE PAGE 323**

Procedure

1 Drape the client for a shampoo service.

2 Shampoo the client's hair, and condition if necessary.

3 Towel dry the hair.

4 Remove any tangles with a wide-tooth comb, starting at the ends and working up to the scalp.

5 Dry the client's hair completely.

6 Heat thermal iron (large or jumbo size).

7 Section and form the base of the curl as described for short hair.

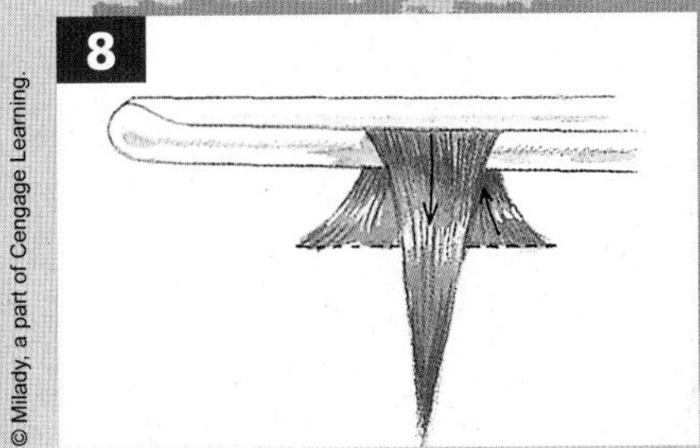

© Milady, a part of Cengage Learning.

8 Insert the hair into the open iron at the scalp. Pull the hair over the rod in the direction of the curl and close the shell. Hold the iron in this position for about five seconds to heat the hair, and then slide it upward to 1 inch (2.5 centimeters) from the scalp. The shell must be on top.

Curling Medium-Length Hair continued

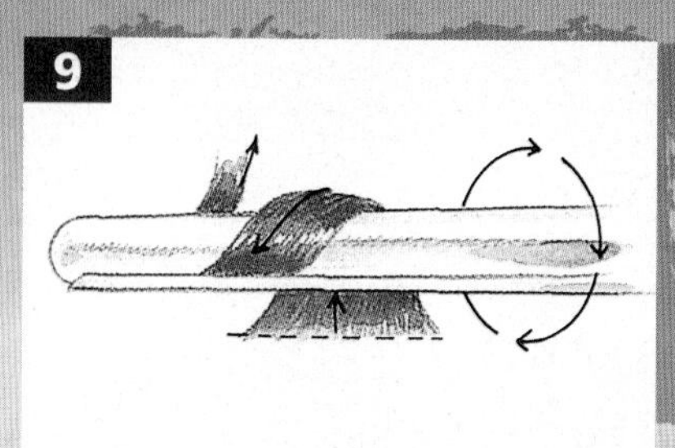

9 Turn the iron downward a half revolution. Then, pull the end of the strand over the rod to the left, directing the strand toward the center of the curl.

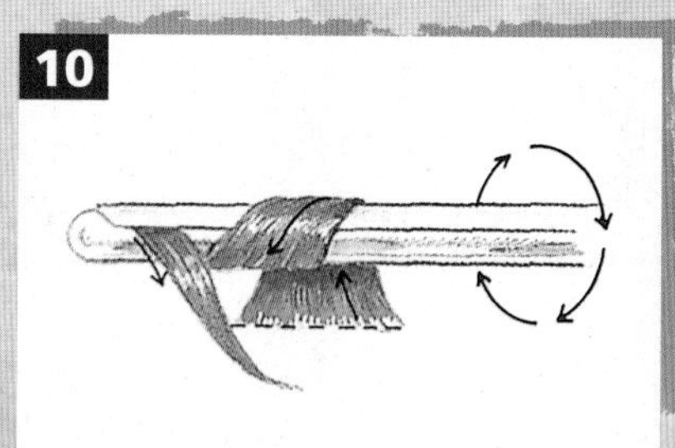

10 Complete the revolution of the iron, and continue directing the ends toward the center.

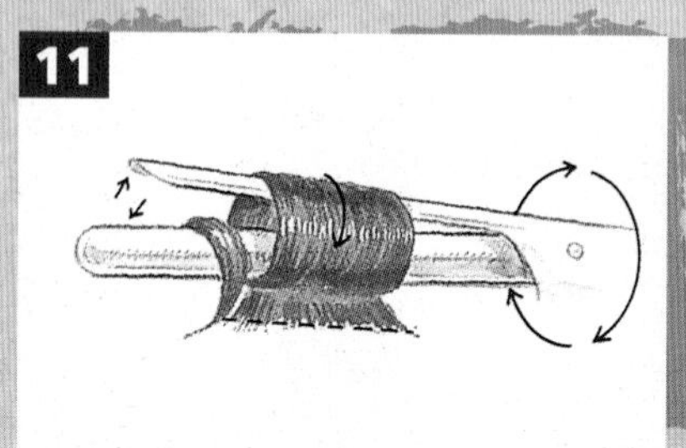

11 Make another complete revolution of the iron. The entire strand has now been curled with the exception of the ends. Enlarge the curl by opening the shell. Insert the ends of the curl into the opening created between the shell and the rod.

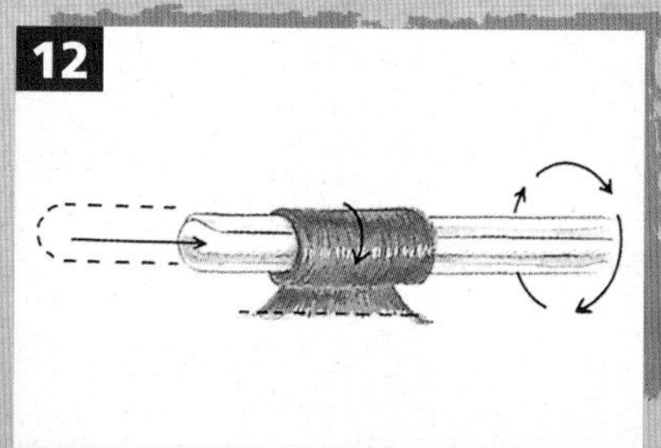

12 Close the shell and slide the iron toward the handles. This technique will move the ends of the strand into the center of the curl. Rotate the iron several times to even out the distribution of the hair in the curl.

13 When the curl is formed and the ends are freed from between the rod and the shell, make one complete revolution of the iron inside the curl. This smoothes the ends and loosens the hair away from the iron. Use the comb to help remove the curl from the iron. Slowly draw the iron in one direction while drawing the hair in the opposite direction with the comb. To protect the client during the curling process, keep the comb between the scalp and the iron.

Post-Service

- Complete PROCEDURE 15-2 **Post-Service Procedure** SEE PAGE 326

© Milady, a part of Cengage Learning.

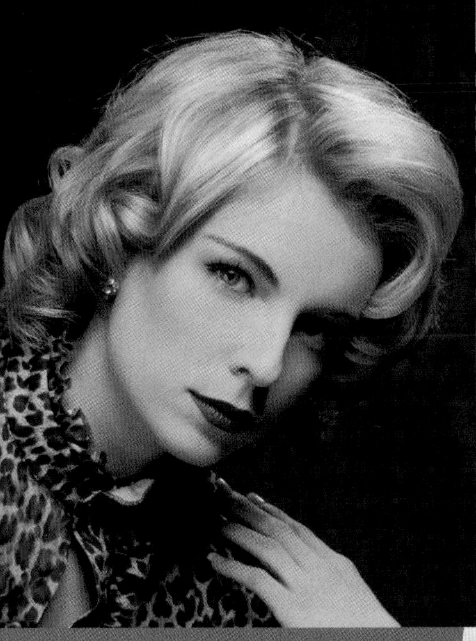

PROCEDURE 17-14

Curling Hair Using Two Loops or Figure 8

© Photography by Tom Carson. Hair by Bob Steele Salon, Atlanta, GA.

Implements and Materials

You will need all of the following implements, materials, and supplies:

- **Conventional (Marcel) or electric irons**
- **Hard rubber comb (fine toothed)**
- **Shampoo**
- **Styling cape and neck strip**

Preparation

- Perform PROCEDURE 15-1 **Pre-Service Procedure** **SEE PAGE 323**

Procedure

1 Drape the client for a shampoo service.

2 Shampoo the client's hair, and condition if necessary.

3 Towel dry the hair.

4 Remove any tangles with a wide-tooth comb, starting at the ends and working up to the scalp.

5 Dry the client's hair completely.

6 Heat thermal iron (large or jumbo size).

7 Section and form the base of the curl as described for short hair.

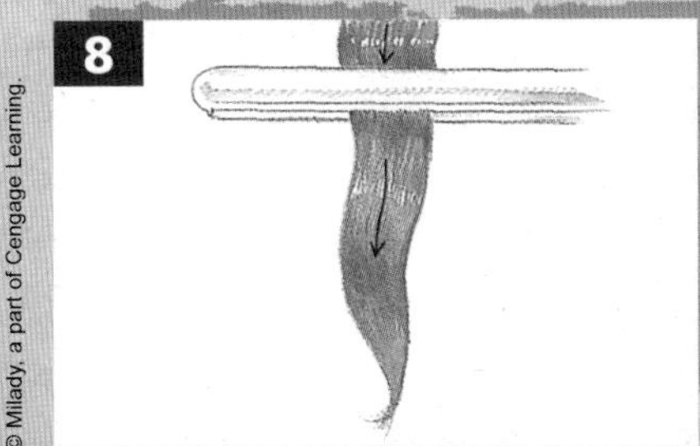

© Milady, a part of Cengage Learning.

8 Insert the hair into the open iron about 1 inch (2.5 centimeters) from the scalp. Pull the hair over the rod in the direction in which the curl is to move and close the shell. Hold the iron in this position for about five seconds, in order to heat the hair. Hold the strand of hair with a medium degree of tension.

Curling Hair Using Two Loops or Figure 8 continued

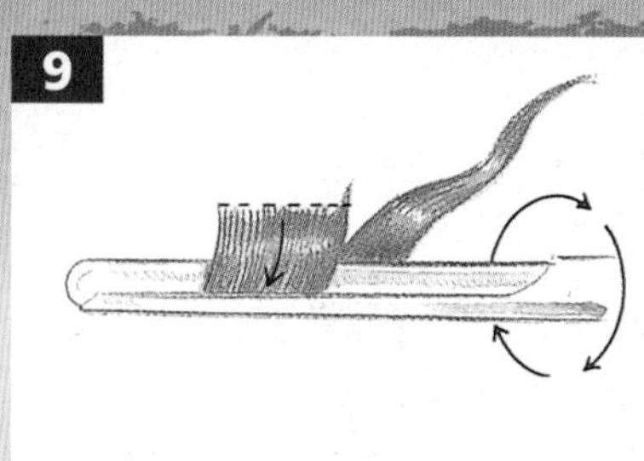
© Milady, a part of Cengage Learning.

9 Roll the iron under; click and roll it until the groove is facing you.

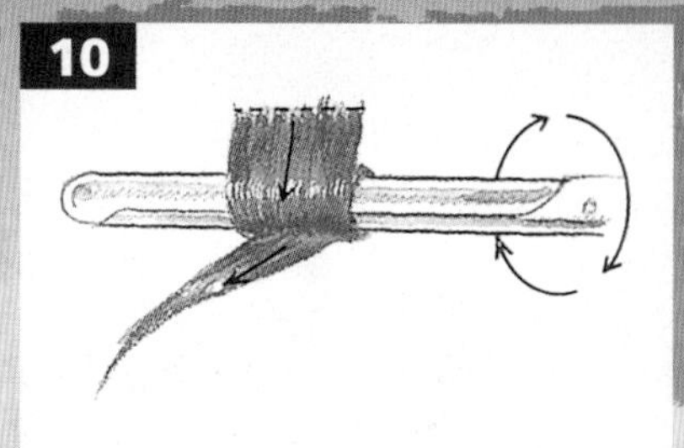
© Milady, a part of Cengage Learning.

10 With the left hand, pick up the ends of the hair.

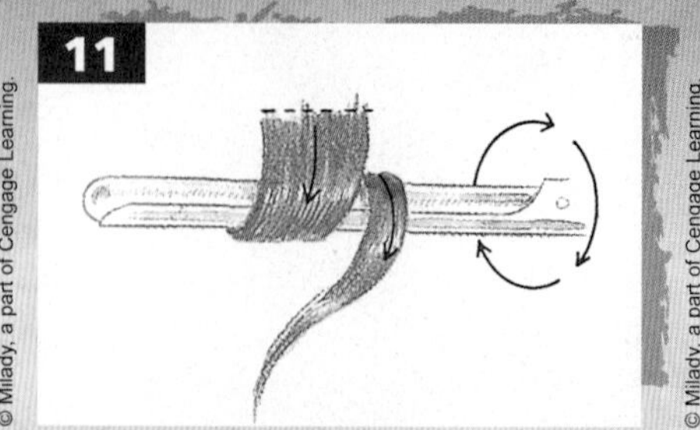
© Milady, a part of Cengage Learning.

11 Continue to roll and click the iron, keeping it the same distance from the scalp.

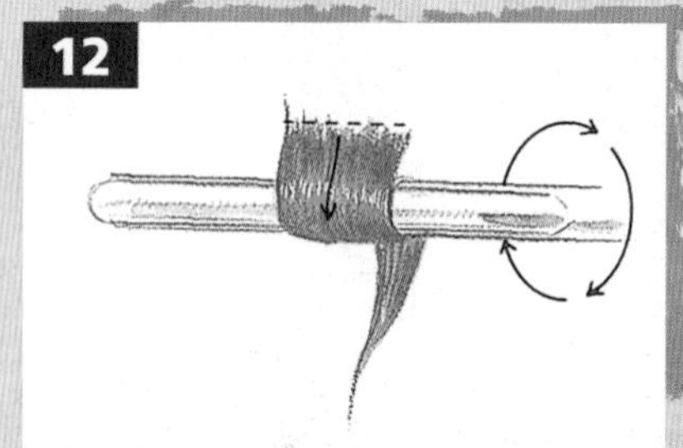
© Milady, a part of Cengage Learning.

12 Draw the hair strand toward the tip of the iron.

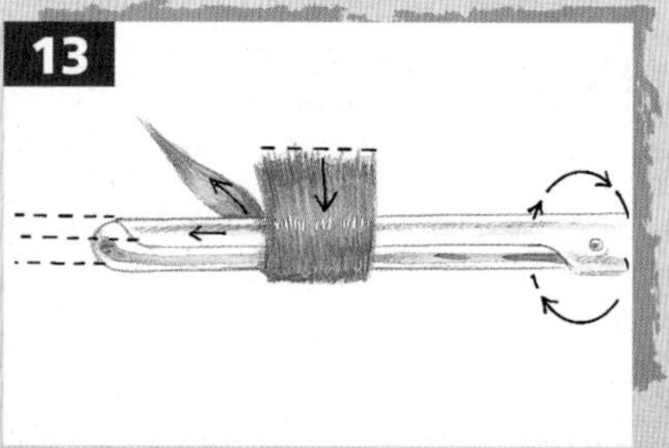
© Milady, a part of Cengage Learning.

13 Draw the strand a little to the right and, at the same time, push the iron slightly to the left.

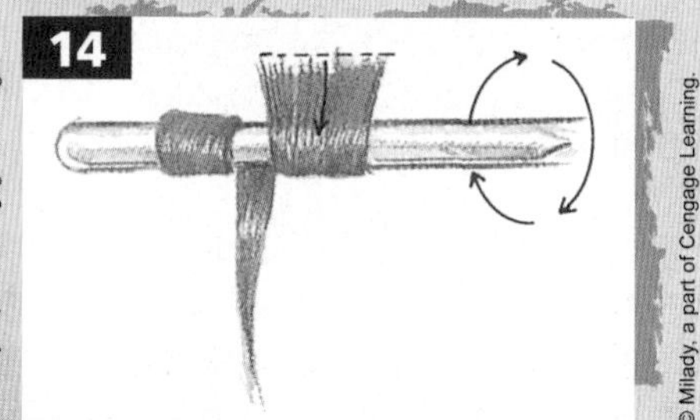
© Milady, a part of Cengage Learning.

14 By pushing the iron forward and pushing the hair with the left hand, you will form two loops around the closed iron, with the ends of the strand extending out between the loops.

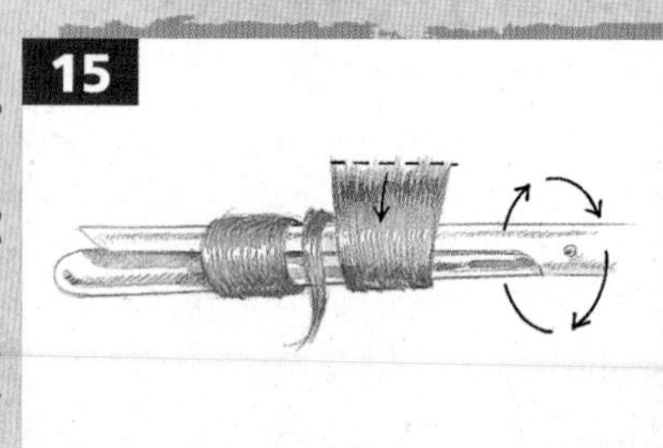
© Milady, a part of Cengage Learning.

15 Roll under and click the iron until the ends of the hair disappear.

16 Rotate the iron several times to even out the distribution of the hair in the curl and to facilitate the movement of the curl off the iron.

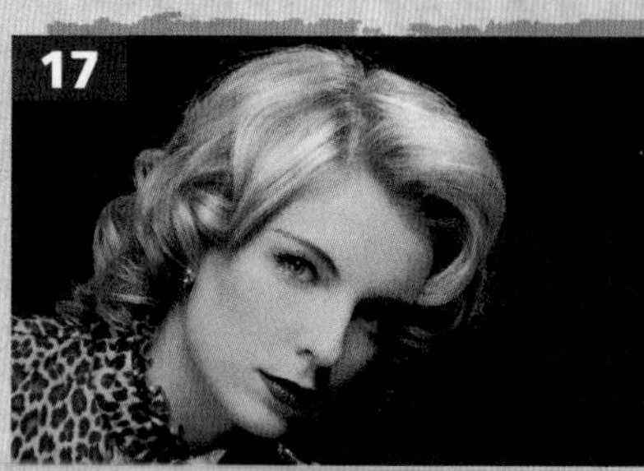
© Photography by Tom Carson. Hair by Bob Steele Salon, Atlanta, GA.

17 Finished look.

Post-Service

- Complete PROCEDURE 15-2 Post-Service Procedure SEE PAGE 326

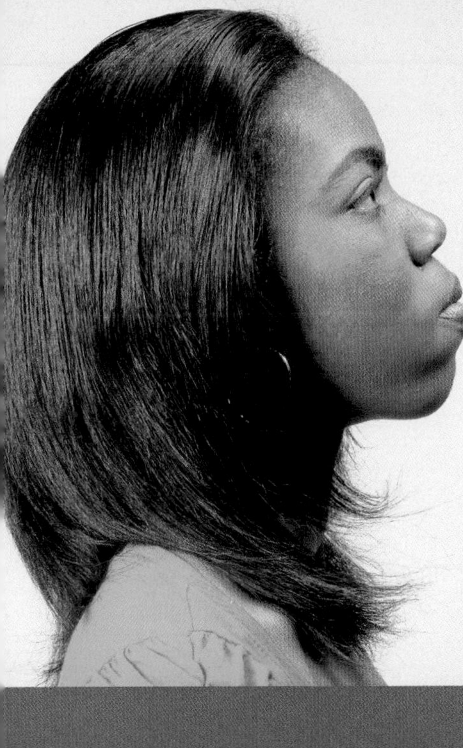

PROCEDURE 17-15

Soft Pressing for Normal Curly Hair

Implements and Materials

You will need all of the following implements, materials, and supplies:

- **Clips**
- **Hairbrush and comb**
- **Neck strip**
- **Pomade**
- **Pressing comb**
- **Pressing oil or cream**
- **Shampoo**
- **Shampoo and styling capes**
- **Spatula**
- **Thermal iron**
- **Towels**

© Milady, a part of Cengage Learning. Photography by Yanik Chauvin.

Preparation

- Perform PROCEDURE 15-1 Pre-Service Procedure SEE PAGE 323

Procedure

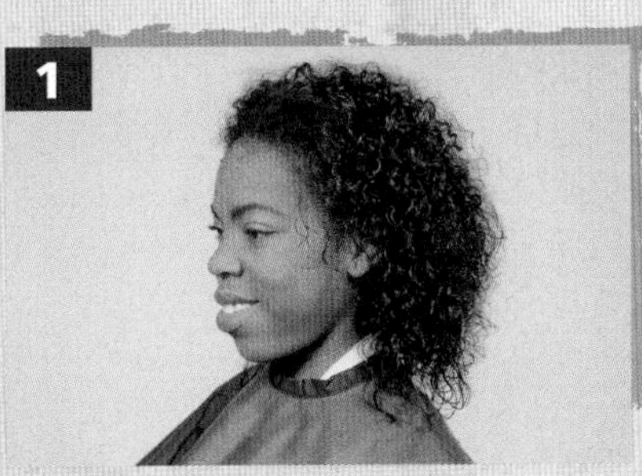

1 Shampoo, rinse, and towel dry the client's hair.

2 Drape the client for thermal styling, using a neck strip and styling cape.

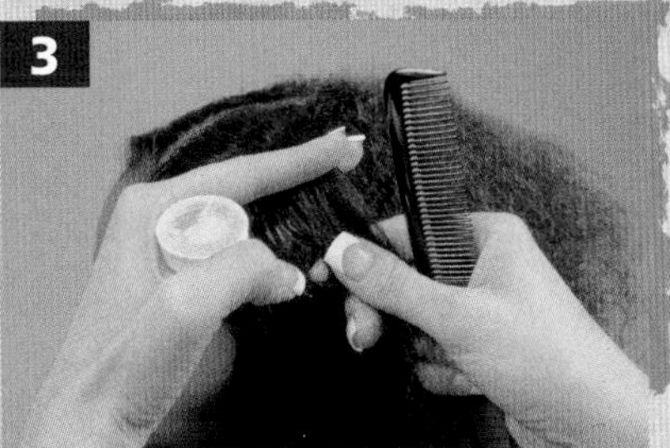

3 Apply pressing oil or cream. (Some stylists prefer to apply pressing oil or cream to the hair after it has been completely dried.)

4 Dry hair thoroughly. (Blowdrying will leave the hair more manageable than hood drying.)

Soft Pressing for Normal Curly Hair continued

Service Tip

Subdivide the sections into 1-inch to 1½-inch (2.5 to 3.75 centimeters) partings, depending on the texture and density of the hair. For medium textured hair of average density, use subsections of average size. For coarse hair with greater density, use smaller sections to ensure complete heat penetration and effectiveness. For thin or fine hair with sparse density, use larger sections.

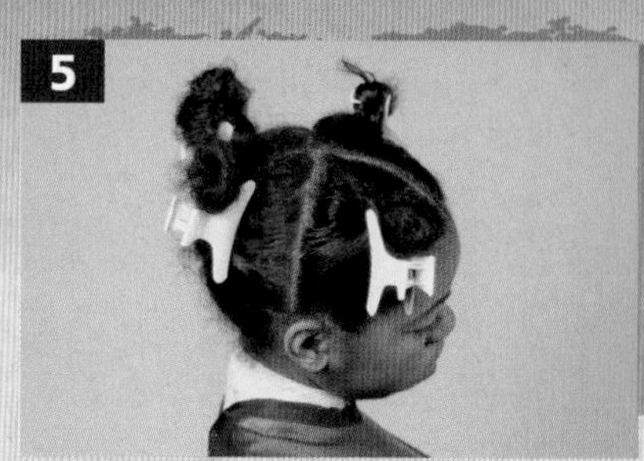

5 Comb and divide the hair into four main sections and pin them up.

6 Heat the pressing comb.

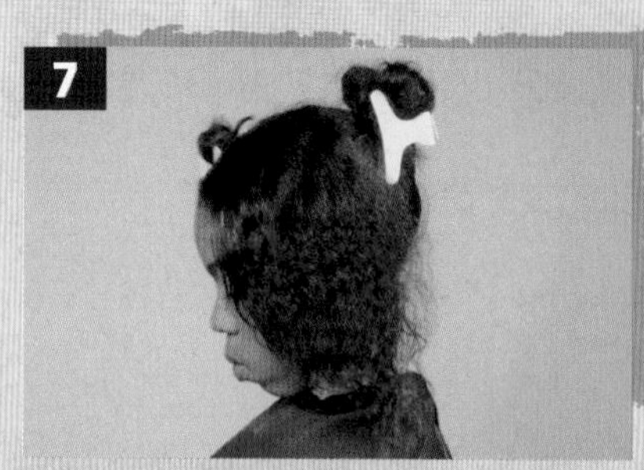

7 Unpin one section of the hair at a time and subdivide into smaller partings. Beginning at the right side of the head, work from front to back (some stylists prefer to start at the back of the head and work forward).

8 If necessary, apply pressing oil evenly and sparingly over the small hair sections.

Service Tip

The steps in this procedure show one way of many possible ways to give a hair-pressing treatment. Keep in mind that you can adjust the procedure according to the methods your instructor demonstrates.

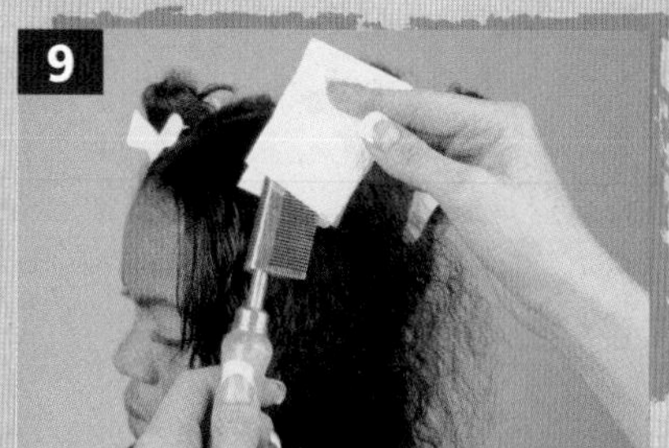

9 Test the temperature of the heated pressing comb on a white cloth or white paper to determine heat intensity before you place it on the hair.

10 Lift the end of a small hair section with the index finger and thumb of the left hand and hold it upward, away from the scalp.

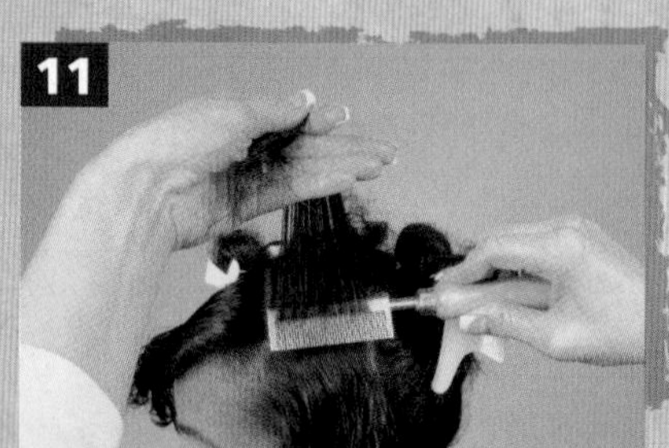

11 Holding the pressing comb in the right hand, insert the teeth of the comb into the top side of the hair section.

© Milady, a part of Cengage Learning. Photography by Yanik Chauvin.

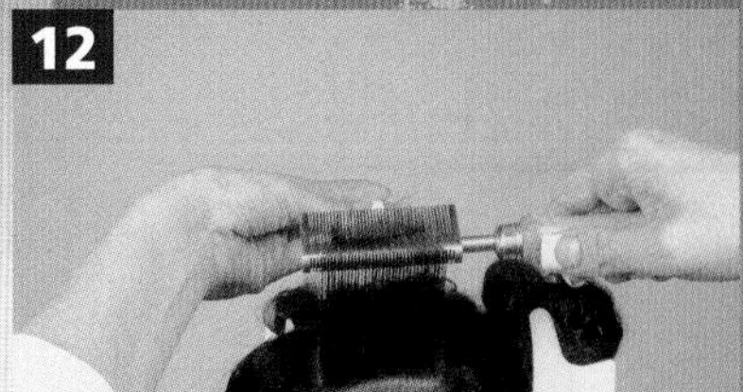

12 Draw out the pressing comb slightly, and make a quick turn so that the hair strand wraps itself partly around the comb. The back rod of the comb actually does the pressing.

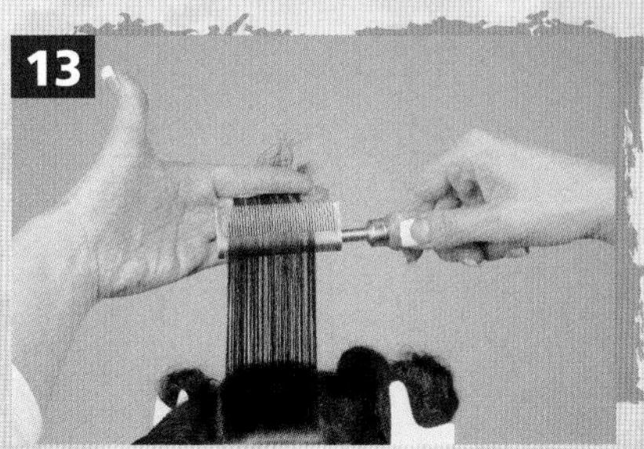

13 Press the comb slowly through the hair strand until the ends of the hair pass through the teeth of the comb.

14 Bring each completed hair section over to the opposite side of the head.

15 Continue on both sections on the right side of the head, and then do the same on both sections on the left side of the head.

16 Apply a little pomade to the hair near the scalp and brush it through the hair. The hair can be curled with a curling iron at this time.

17 Style and comb the hair according to the client's wishes.

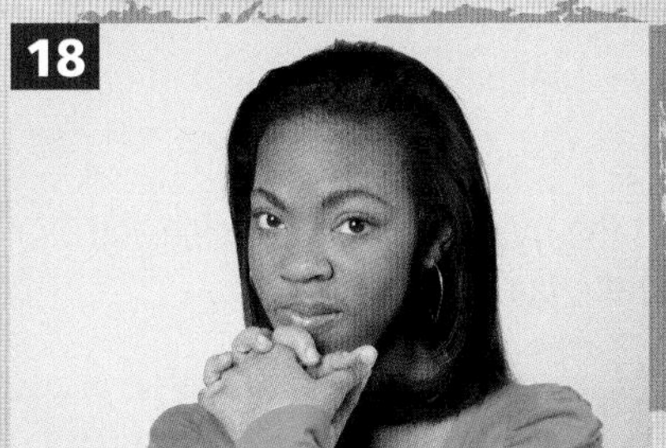

18 Finished look.

© Milady, a part of Cengage Learning. Photography by Yanik Chauvin.

Post-Service

- Complete PROCEDURE 15-2 **Post-Service Procedure** **SEE PAGE 326**

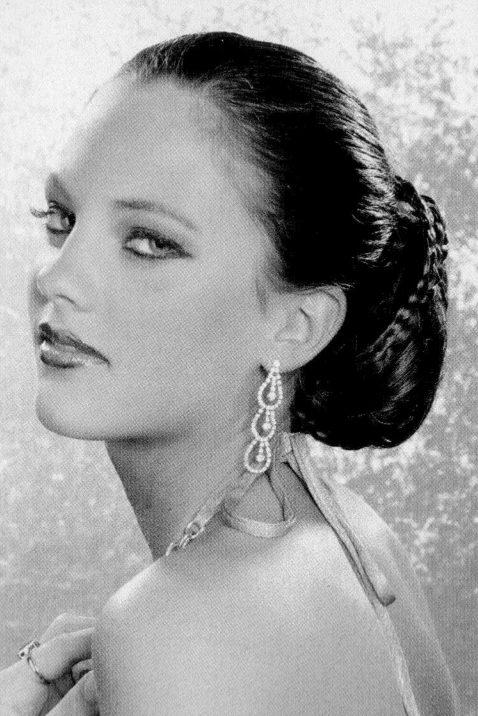

PROCEDURE 17-16

Knot or Chignon

Photography by Tom Carson. Hair by Tina Fall for Frederick's Day Spa, Wheeling, WVA. Makeup by Tina Fall.

Implements and Materials

You will need all of the following implements, materials, and supplies:

- **Bobby pins, hairpins**
- **Bristle brush**
- **Curling iron**
- **Elastics**
- **Electric or Velcro rollers**
- **Finishing spray**
- **Grooming or teasing brush**
- **Hair spray**
- **Neck strip**
- **Styling cape**
- **Tail comb**

Preparation

- Perform PROCEDURE 15-1 **Pre-Service Procedure** **SEE PAGE 323**

Procedure

1 Drape the client; shampoo and towel dry the hair.

2 Redrape the client with a neck strip and styling cape.

3 Apply the appropriate styling product that will give the hair a lot of hold. Blowdry the hair, smoothing it with a brush for a sleek finish.

4 Set hair in electric or Velcro rollers, depending on the amount of curl or volume you may need.

5 Using a grooming bristle brush, part the hair on whichever side you choose, and brush it into a low ponytail at the nape.

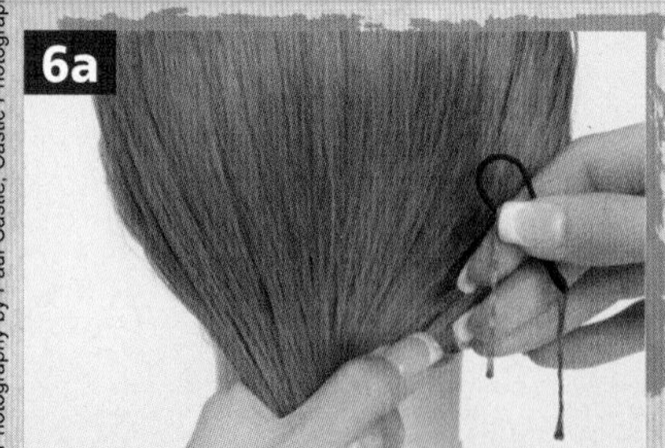

© Milady, a part of Cengage Learning. Photography by Paul Castle, Castle Photography.

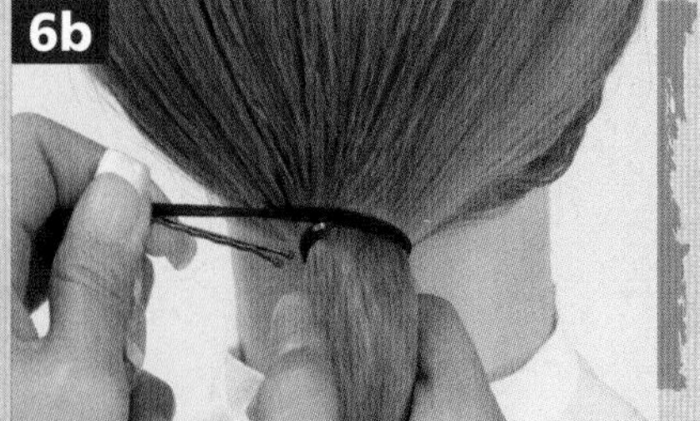

© Milady, a part of Cengage Learning. Photography by Paul Castle, Castle Photography.

6 Secure the ponytail with an elastic band, keeping the hair as smooth as possible. Use the side of the bristles to smooth the hair. Place two bobby pins onto the band and spread them apart, one on each side. Place one bobby pin in the base of the ponytail. Stretch the band around the ponytail base. Place the second bobby pin in the base. Lock the two pins together.

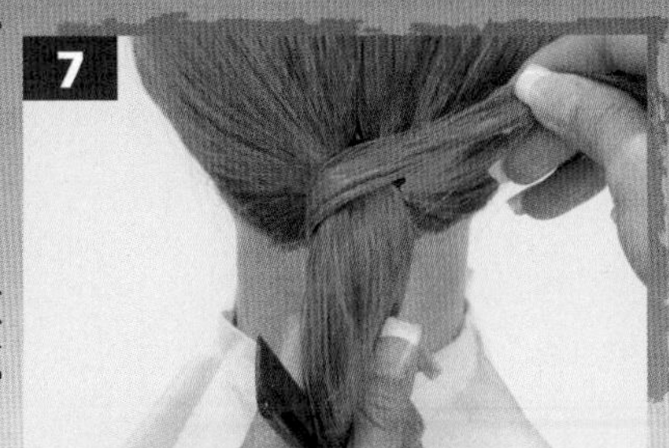

© Milady, a part of Cengage Learning. Photography by Paul Castle. Castle Photography.

7 Part a small section of hair from the underside of the ponytail, wrap it around the ponytail to cover the elastic, and secure with a bobby pin underneath.

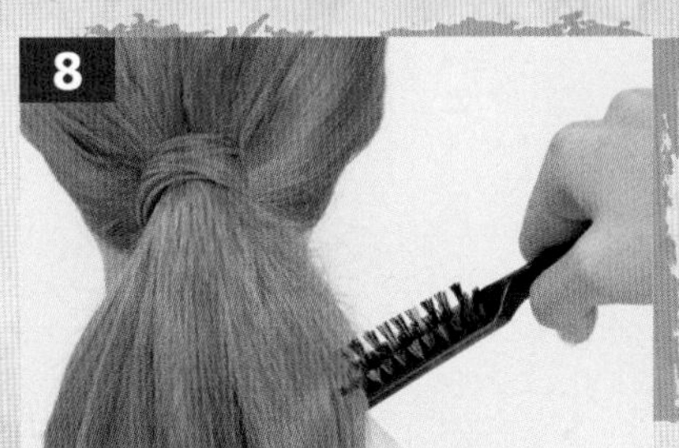

© Milady, a part of Cengage Learning. Photography by Paul Castle. Castle Photography.

8 Smooth out the ponytail and hold it with one hand, and then begin backbrushing from underneath the ponytail with your other hand. Gently smooth out the ponytail after backbrushing, using the sides of the bristles.

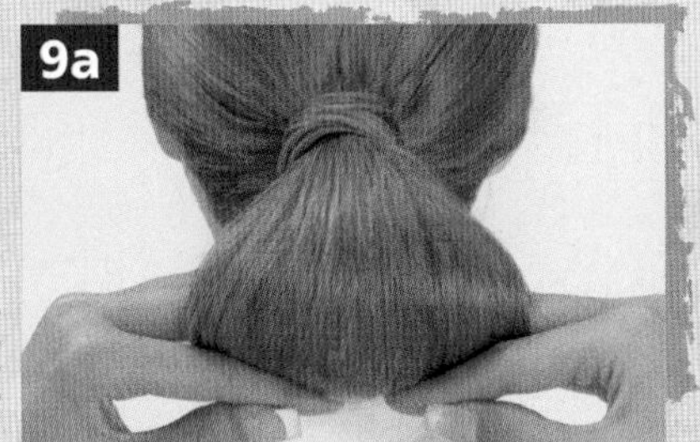

© Milady, a part of Cengage Learning. Photography by Paul Castle. Castle Photography.

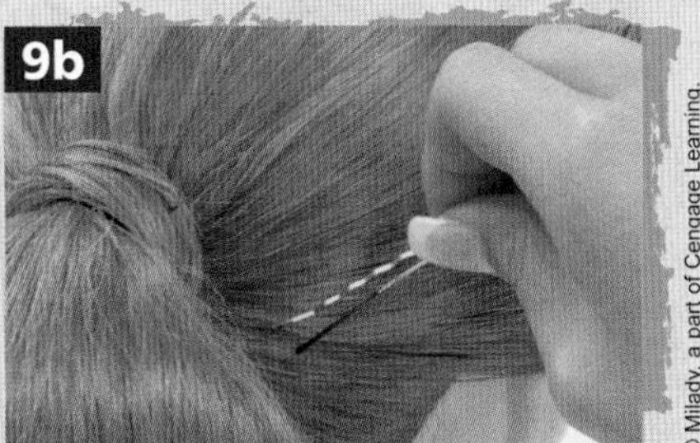

© Milady, a part of Cengage Learning. Photography by Paul Castle. Castle Photography.

9 Roll the hair under and toward the head to form the chignon. Secure on the left and right undersides of the roll with bobby pins.

Service Tip

Performing an updo on hair that has been washed the previous day is often recommended. Freshly washed hair can be very slippery and difficult to work with. Many stylists also choose to set the hair in hot rollers prior to doing an updo. The curl allows the hair to be more easily manipulated into rolls or loops and creates a fuller shape.

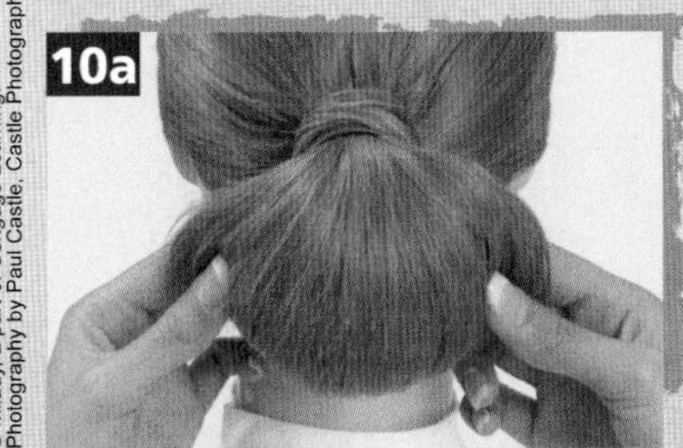

© Milady, a part of Cengage Learning. Photography by Paul Castle. Castle Photography.

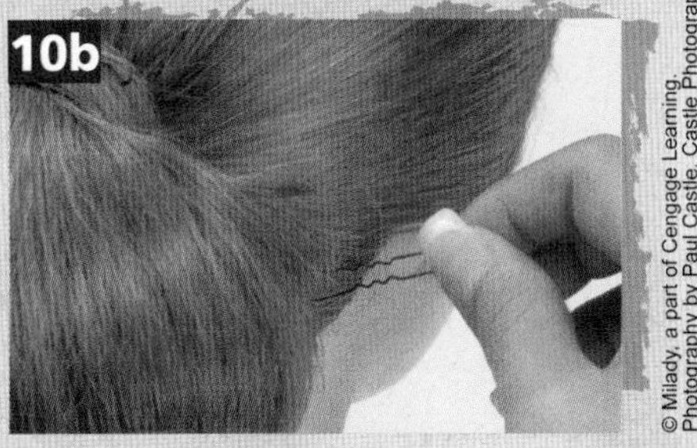

© Milady, a part of Cengage Learning. Photography by Paul Castle. Castle Photography.

10 Fan out both sides by spreading the chignon with your fingers. Secure with hairpins, pinning close to the head. Use bobby pins if more hold is needed.

11 Finish with a strong hair spray, and add flowers or ornaments if desired.

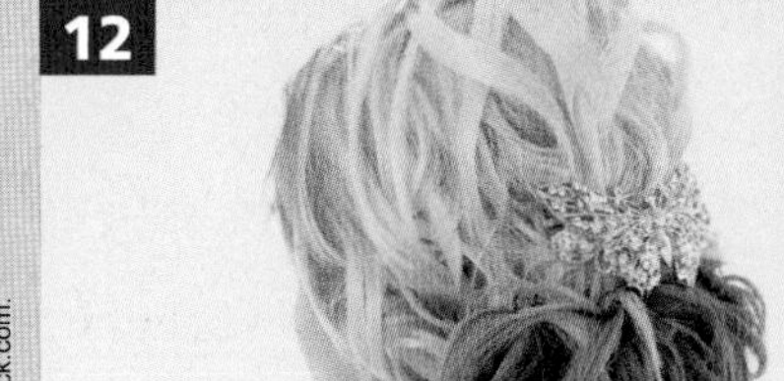

© gbphoto, 2010; used under license from Shutterstock.com.

12 Finished look.

Post-Service

- Complete PROCEDURE 15-2 **Post-Service Procedure** **SEE PAGE 326**

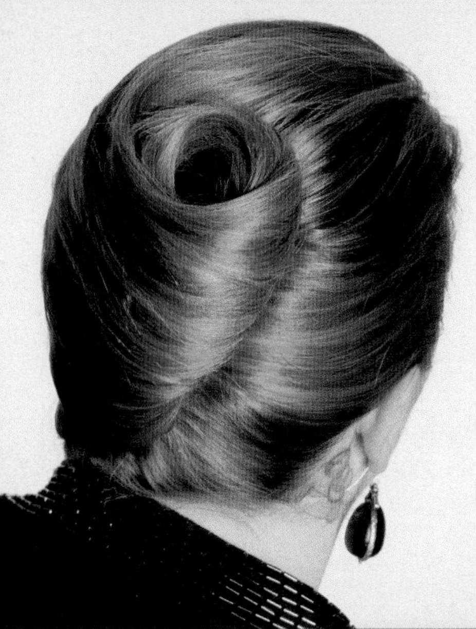

PROCEDURE 17-17

Twist

Photography by Wilson Black. Salon,TC Salon Spa; Hair, Frank Shipman; Makeup, Jennifer Bashour; Model, Jill Benway.

Implements and Materials

You will need all of the following implements, materials, and supplies:

- **Bobby pins, hairpins**
- **Bristle brush**
- **Curling iron**
- **Elastics**
- **Electric or Velcro rollers**
- **Finishing spray**
- **Grooming or teasing brush**
- **Neck strip**
- **Styling cape**
- **Tail comb**
- **Working hair spray**

Preparation

- Perform PROCEDURE 15-1 Pre-Service Procedure SEE PAGE 323

Procedure

1 Drape the client; shampoo and towel dry the hair.

2 Redrape the client with a neck strip and styling cape.

3 Apply the appropriate styling product that will give the hair a lot of hold. Blowdry the hair, smoothing it with a brush for a sleek finish.

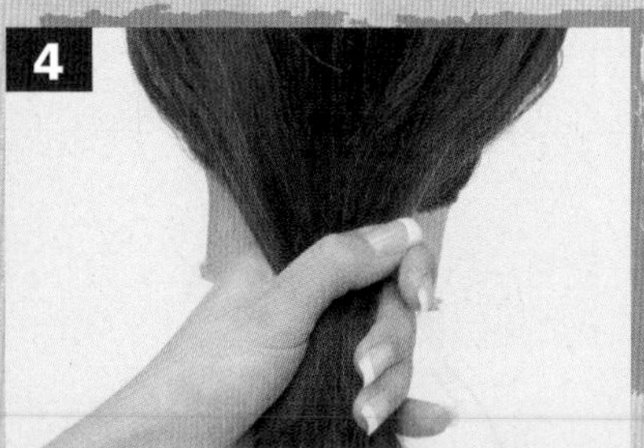

4

© Milady, a part of Cengage Learning. Photography by Paul Castle, Castle Photography.

4 Brush all the hair smoothly into a ponytail at the occipital bone.

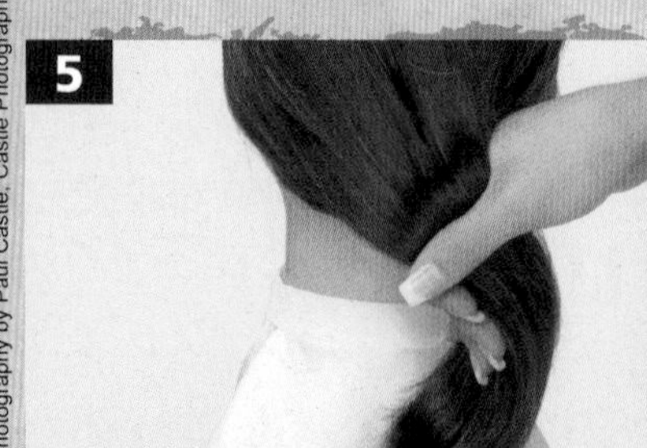

5

© Milady, a part of Cengage Learning. Photography by Paul Castle, Castle Photography.

5 With your free hand, reach in front of the hand that is holding the ponytail, with the thumb pointing down toward the client's nape.

© Milady, a part of Cengage Learning. Photography by Paul Castle, Castle Photography.

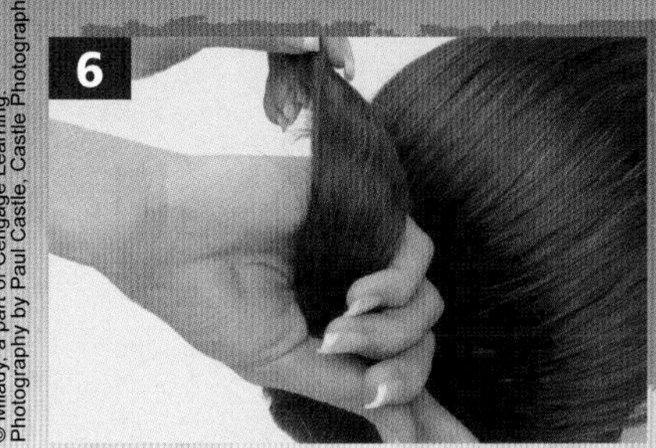

6 Grab the ponytail with your thumb still pointing down and twist the hair in the direction in which your palm is facing, moving the hair inward and upward.

© Milady, a part of Cengage Learning. Photography by Paul Castle, Castle Photography.

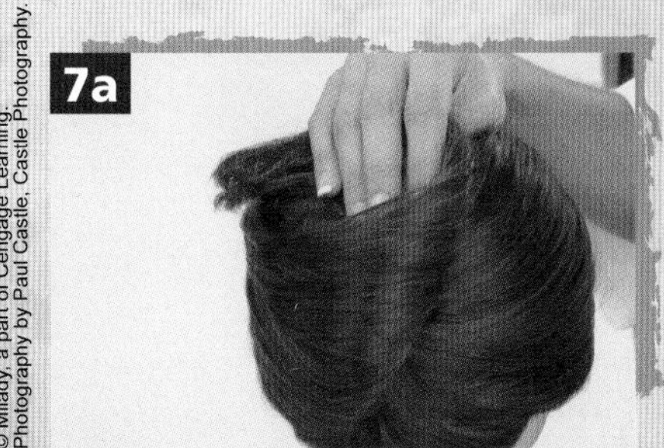

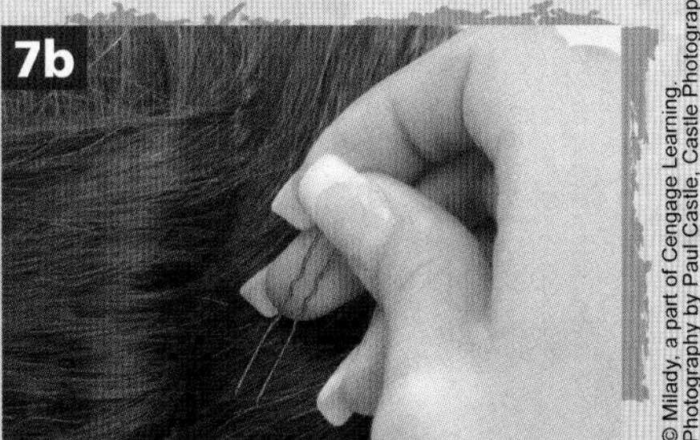

© Milady, a part of Cengage Learning. Photography by Paul Castle, Castle Photography.

7 As you move toward the crown, twist the hair into a funnel shape and secure the twist with hairpins by pinning into the seam, making sure not to expose the pins.

© Milady, a part of Cengage Learning. Photography by Paul Castle, Castle Photography.

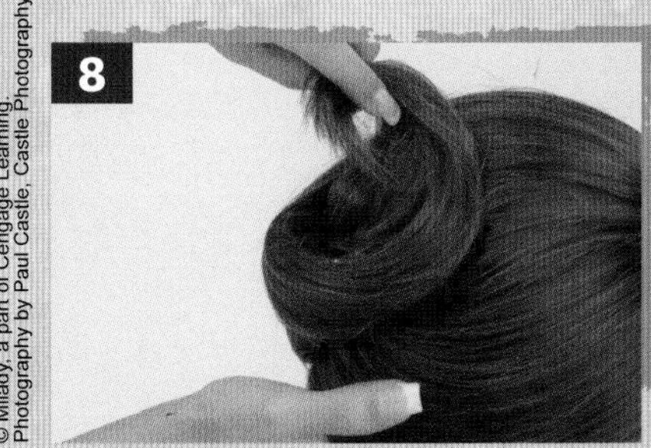

8 Tuck the ends into the top of the funnel of the twist near the crown.

9 For a less formal or younger look, let the hair ends fan out and fall loosely over the sides of the twist, instead of tucking them into the top of the twist. Another option is to form curls, loops, or knots with the hair at the top of the twist.

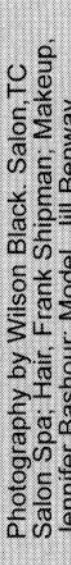

Photography by Wilson Black. Salon,TC Salon Spa; Hair, Frank Shipman; Makeup, Jennifer Bashour; Model, Jill Benway.

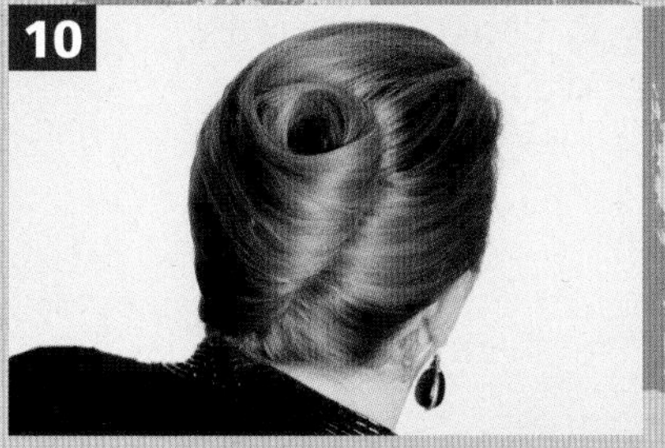

10 Finished look.

Post-Service

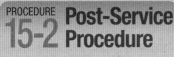

- Complete PROCEDURE **15-2 Post-Service Procedure** **SEE PAGE 326**

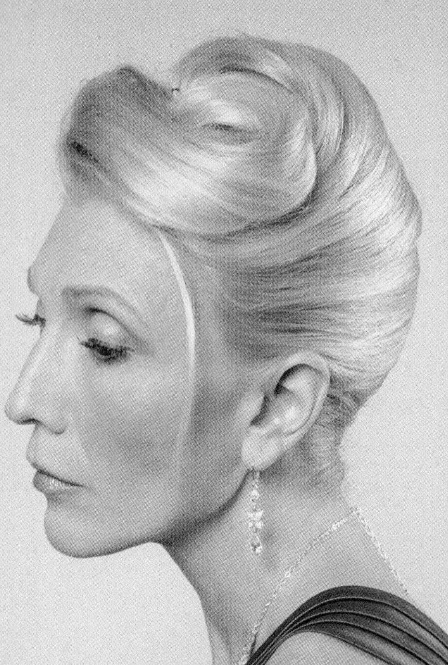

PROCEDURE 17-18

Pleat

Implements and Materials

You will need all of the following implements, materials, and supplies:

- **Bobby pins, hairpins**
- **Bristle brush**
- **Curling iron**
- **Elastics**
- **Electric or Velcro rollers**
- **Finishing spray**
- **Grooming or teasing brush**
- **Hair spray**
- **Neck strip**
- **Styling cape**
- **Tail comb**

Preparation

- Perform PROCEDURE 15-1 **Pre-Service Procedure** **SEE PAGE 323**

Procedure

1

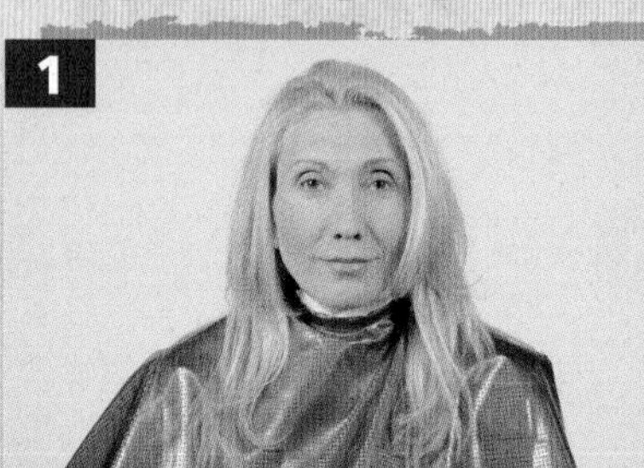

1 Drape the client; shampoo and towel dry the hair.

2 Redrape the client with a neck strip and styling cape.

3 Apply the appropriate styling product that will give the hair a lot of hold. Blowdry the hair, smoothing it with a brush for a sleek finish.

4 Set the hair with a wet set or, if you wish to save time, electric rollers or thermal irons.

5

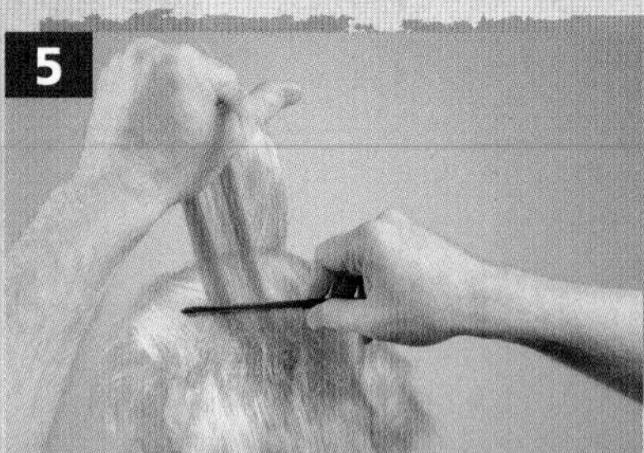

5 Once completely dry, backcomb hair.

6

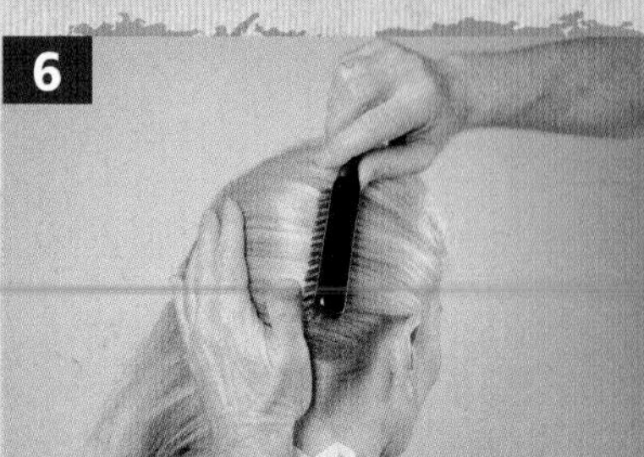

6 Using a grooming brush or a teasing brush, gently smooth all the hair of the back section to one side of the head. (In this example all the hair will move to the left.) Hold the hair to that side by reaching over the client's head with your free hand.

© Milady, a part of Cengage Learning. Photography by Yanik Chauvin.

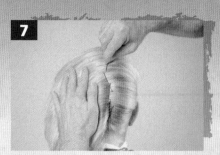

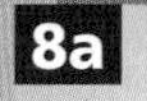

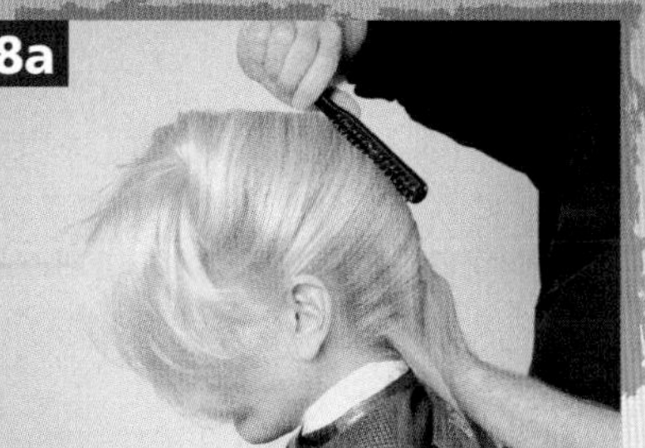

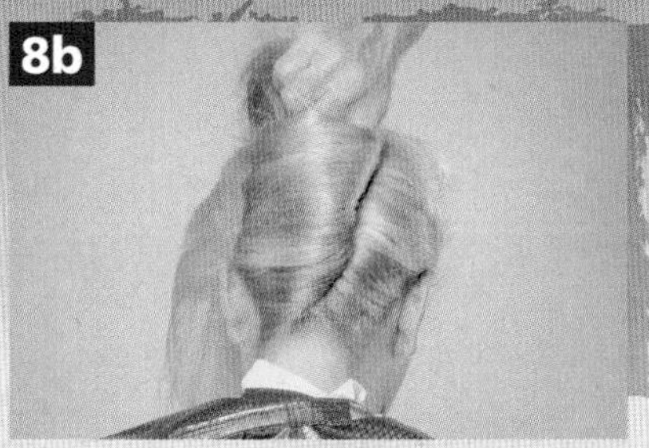

7 Begin pinning the hair at the center of the nape. Move upward with the bobby pins while having the client hold her head completely upright, overlapping the pins by crisscrossing them to lock into place. Repeat until you reach the back of the crown.

8 With the brush, bring the hair from the left side over the center line (where the bobby pins were placed) and smooth; twist from the center of the nape. Move upward and inward, tucking the ends into the fold as you move up, to create a funnel shape. Secure with hairpins vertically down into the seam as you work up, hiding the pins in the seam.

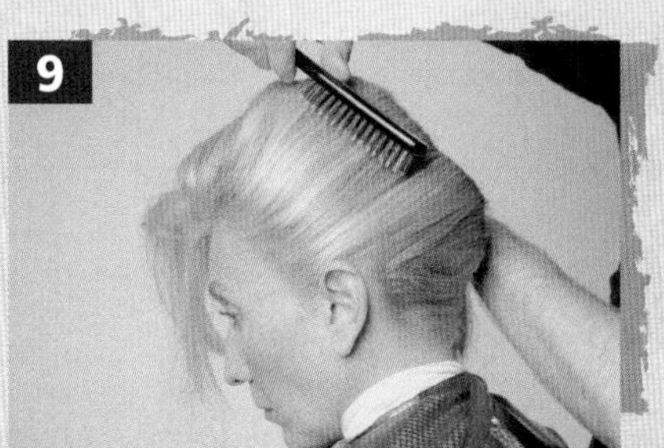

9 Move to a side section and lightly backbrush the section. Bring the side section up to last completed section and blend into the fold. Secure with a bobby pin at the top of the side section, leaving the ends out.

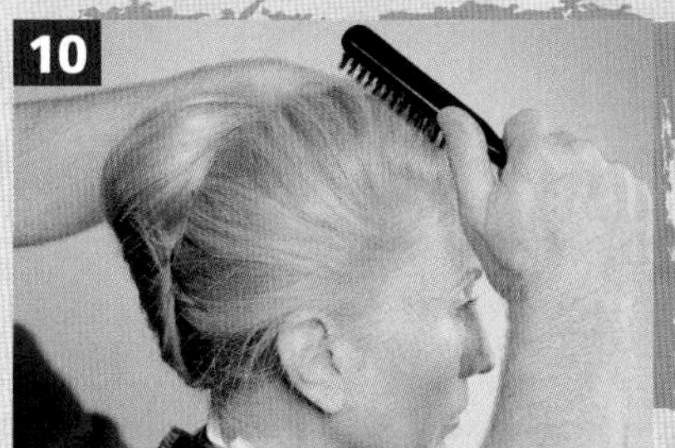

10 Repeat on the other side. Fold over while smoothing and pin downward.

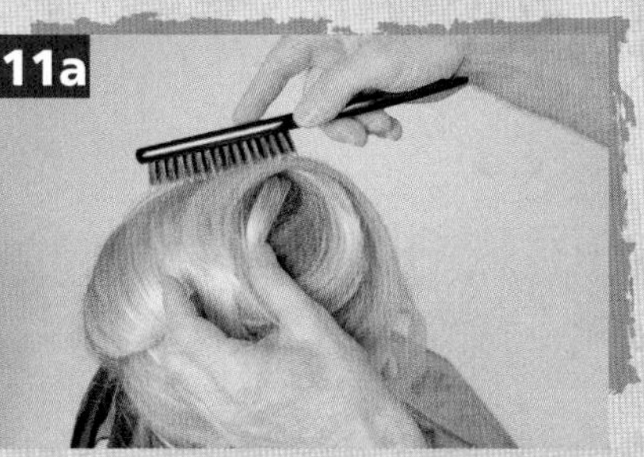

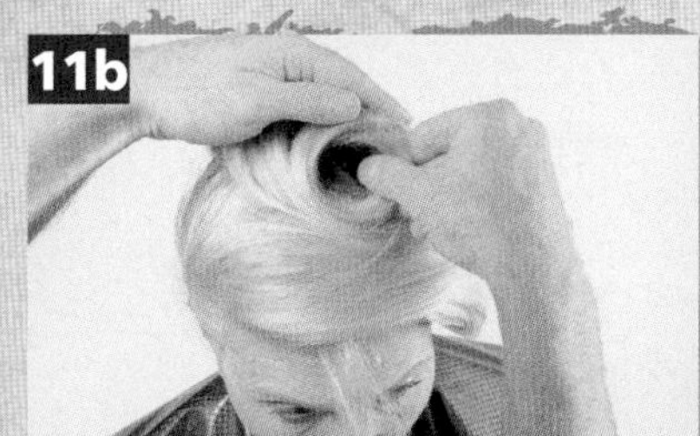

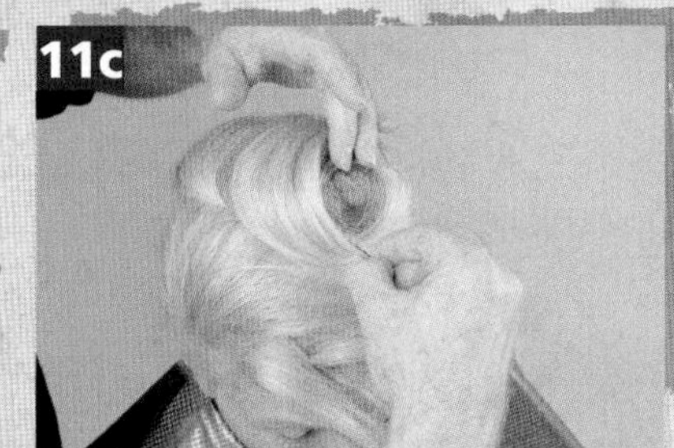

11 Backbrush and smooth the remaining side section on the right into the remaining section on the left, just above the top of the twist. Swirl and join this new joined section of hair into the open end of the twist. Use a tail comb or the tail of the backcombing brush to smooth and curl ends into the twist and pin. Take care not to expose the pin.

© Milady, a part of Cengage Learning. Photography by Yanik Chauvin.

PROCEDURE 17-18 Pleat continued

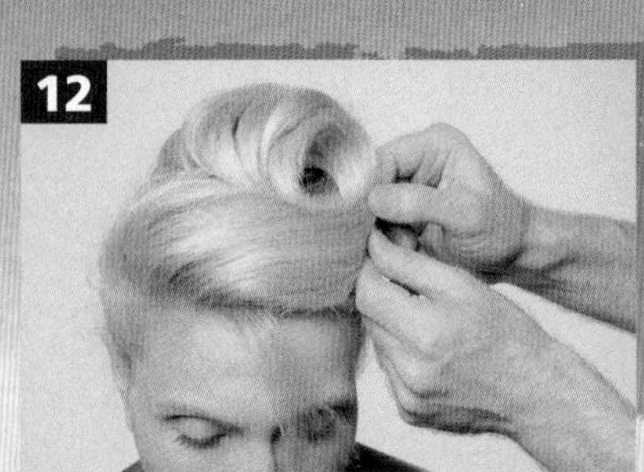

12 Style the section in the bangs as you wish. This section could also be brought back and added to the crown if your client is more comfortable with all her hair off her face. Or you can sweep the hair loosely to the side and leave the ends hanging softly down. Here is where your creativity comes into play as you make the best design decision for your client.

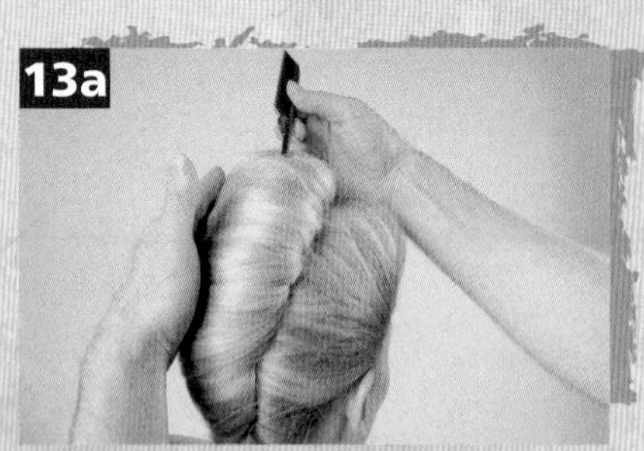

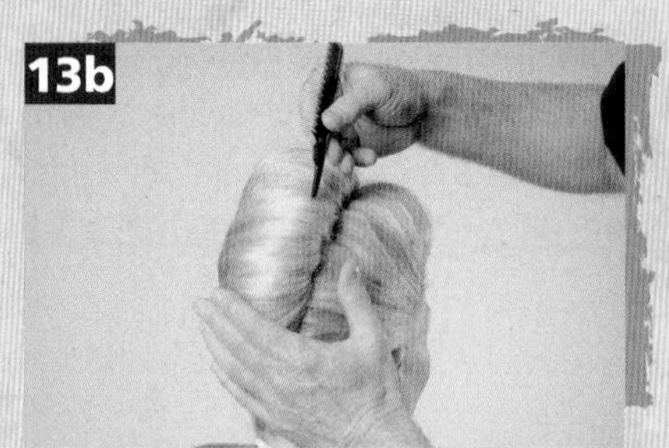

13 Spray finished style with a firm hold hair spray, and check to make sure there are no exposed pins. Use a tail comb to balance the shape of the pleat.

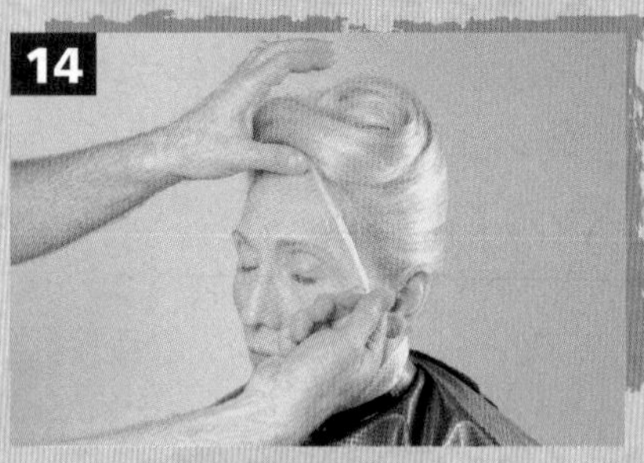

14 Finish the bangs.

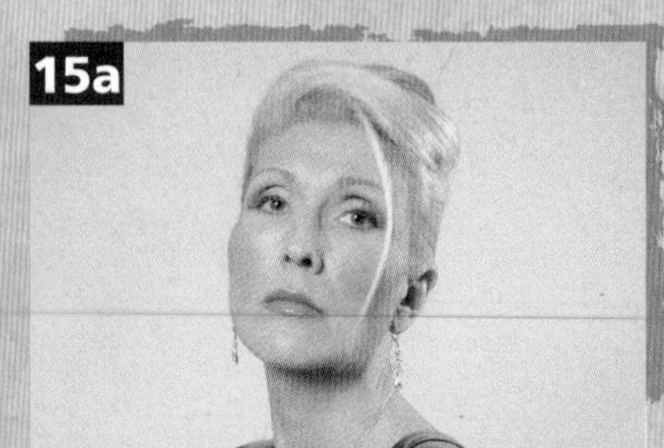

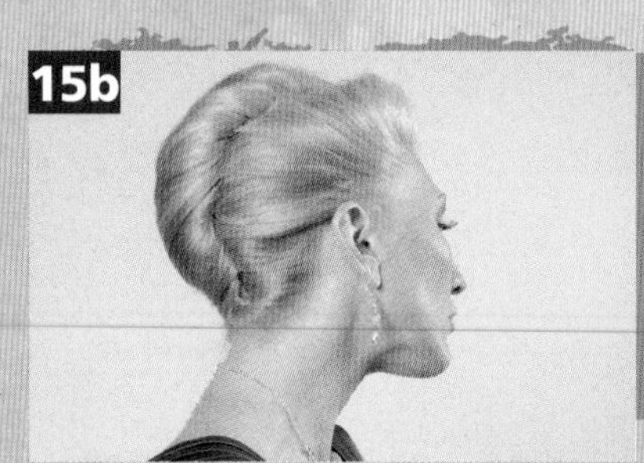

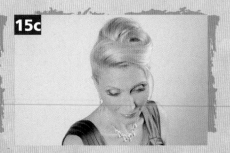

15 Finished look.

Post-Service

- Complete PROCEDURE 15-2 Post-Service Procedure SEE PAGE 326

© Milady, a part of Cengage Learning. Photography by Yanik Chauvin.

Review Questions

1. What is the purpose of finger waving?
2. What are the three parts of a pin curl?
3. Name the four pin curl bases and their uses.
4. Describe the three kinds of roller curl bases and the uses of each.
5. What is the purpose of backcombing and backbrushing?
6. How can you avoid burning the client's scalp during blowdrying?
7. List and describe the various styling products used in blowdry styling.
8. How is volume achieved with thermal curls?
9. List at least 10 safety measures that must be followed when using thermal irons.
10. Name and describe the three types of hair presses.
11. How do you test the pressing comb before beginning a service?
12. What are the considerations in a hair and scalp analysis prior to hair pressing?
13. Under what circumstances should hair not be pressed?
14. List at least four safety measures that must be followed when pressing the hair.

Chapter Glossary

backbrushing	Also known as *ruffing*; technique used to build a soft cushion or to mesh two or more curl patterns together for a uniform and smooth comb out.
backcombing	Also known as *teasing, ratting, matting,* or *French lacing*; combing small sections of hair from the ends toward the scalp, causing shorter hair to mat at the scalp and form a cushion or base.
barrel curls	Pin curls with large center openings, fastened to the head in a standing position on a rectangular base.
base	Stationary, or nonmoving, foundation of a pin curl (the area closest to the scalp); the panel of hair on which a roller is placed.
blowdry styling	Technique of drying and styling damp hair in a single operation.
carved curls	Also known as *sculptured curls*; pin curls sliced from a shaping and formed without lifting the hair from the head.
cascade curls	Also known as *stand-up curls*; pin curls fastened to the head in a standing position to allow the hair to flow upward and then downward.
circle	The part of the pin curl that forms a complete circle; also, the hair that is wrapped around the roller.
closed-center curls	Pin curls that produce waves that get smaller toward the end.
concentrator	Nozzle attachment of a blowdryer; directs the air stream to any section of the hair more intensely.
curl	Also known as *circle*; the hair that is wrapped around the roller.

Chapter Glossary

diffuser	Blowdryer attachment that causes the air to flow more softly and helps to accentuate or keep textural definition.
double press	Technique of passing a hot curling iron through the hair before performing a hard press.
end curls	Used to give a finished appearance to hair ends either turned under or over.
finger waving	Process of shaping and directing the hair into an S pattern through the use of the fingers, combs, and waving lotion.
foam	Also known as *mousse*; a light, airy, whipped styling product that resembles shaving foam and builds moderate body and volume into the hair.
full-base curls	Thermal curls that sit in the center of their base; strong curls with full volume.
full-stem curl	Curl placed completely off the base; allows for the greatest mobility.
gel	Thickened styling preparation that comes in a tube or bottle and creates a strong hold.
hair pressing	Method of temporarily straightening extremely curly or unruly hair by means of a heated iron or comb.
hair spray	Also known as *finishing spray*; a styling product applied in the form of a mist to hold a style in position; available in a variety of holding strengths.
hair wrapping	A technique used to keep curly hair smooth and straight.
half base	Position of a curl or a roller that sits halfway on its base and halfway behind the base, giving medium volume and movement.
half-base curls	Thermal curls placed half off their base; strong curls with moderate lift or volume.
half-stem curl	Curl placed half off the base; permits medium movement and gives good control to the hair.
hard press	Technique that removes 100 percent of the curl by applying the pressing comb twice on each side of the hair.
indentation	The point where curls of opposite directions meet, forming a recessed area.
knot	Also known as *chignon*; a technique used for formal hairstyling that creates the look of a knot or bun.
liquid gels	Also known as *texturizers*; styling products that are lighter and less viscous than firm hold gels, used for easy styling, defining, and molding.
medium press	Technique that removes 60 to 75 percent of the curl by applying a thermal pressing comb once on each side of the hair, using slightly more pressure than in the soft press.
no-stem curl	Curl placed directly on its base; produces a tight, firm, long-lasting curl and allows minimum mobility.
off base	The position of a curl or a roller completely off its base for maximum mobility and minimum volume.
off-base curls	Thermal curls placed completely off their base, offering only slight lift or volume.
on base	Also known as *full base*; position of a curl or roller directly on its base for maximum volume.

Chapter Glossary

open-center curls	Pin curls that produce even, smooth waves and uniform curls.
pleat	Also known as *classic French twist*; a technique used for formal hairstyling that creates a look of folded hair.
pomade	Also known as *wax*; styling products that add considerable weight to the hair by causing strands to join together, showing separation in the hair.
ribboning	Technique of forcing the hair between the thumb and the back of the comb to create tension.
ridge curls	Pin curls placed immediately behind or below a ridge to form a wave.
rod	Round, solid prong of a thermal iron.
shaping	Section of hair that is molded in a circular movement in preparation for the formation of curls.
shell	The clamp that presses the hair against the barrel or rod of a thermal iron.
skip waves	Two rows of ridge curls, usually on the side of the head.
soft press	Technique of pressing the hair to remove 50 to 60 percent of the curl by applying the thermal pressing comb once on each side of the hair.
spiral curl	Method of curling the hair by winding a strand around the rod.
stem	Section of the pin curl between the base and first arc (turn) of the circle that gives the curl its direction and movement; the hair between the scalp and the first turn of the roller.
straightening gel	Styling product applied to damp hair that is wavy, curly, or extremely curly and then blown dry; relaxes the hair for a smooth, straight look.
temper	A process used to condition a new brass pressing comb so that it heats evenly.
thermal irons	Implements made of quality steel that are used to curl dry hair.
thermal waving and curling	Also known as *Marcel waving*; methods of waving and curling straight or pressed dry hair using thermal irons and special manipulative curling techniques.
twist	A technique used for formal hairstyling that creates a look of conical shape.
updo	Hairstyle in which the hair is arranged up and off the shoulders.
volume-base curls	Thermal curls placed very high on their base; provide maximum lift or volume.
volumizers	Styling products that add volume, especially at the base, when wet hair is blown dry.
waving lotion	Type of hair gel that makes the hair pliable enough to keep it in place during the finger-waving procedure.

CHAPTER 18

Braiding and Braid Extensions

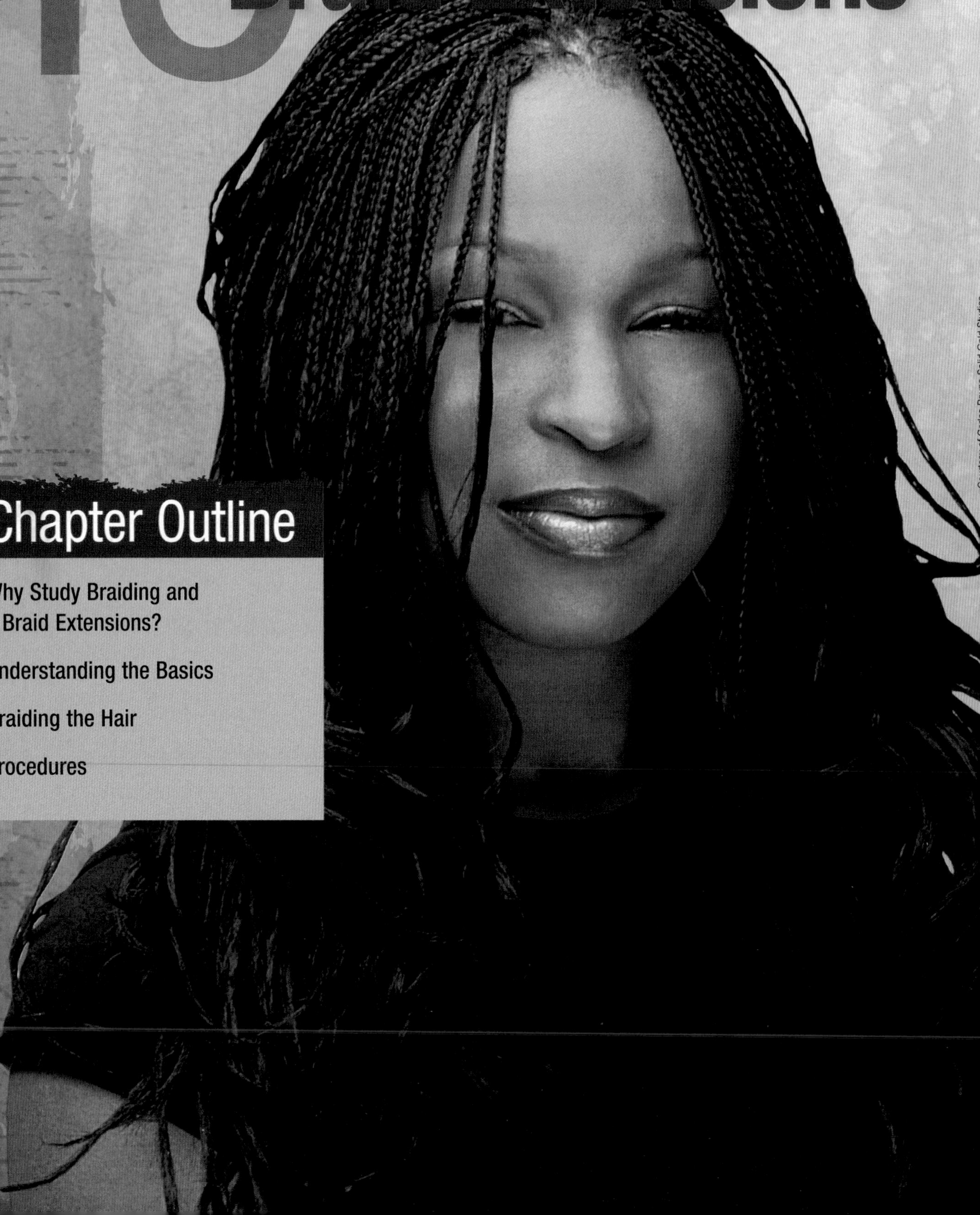

Courtesy of Carlos Payne-Solid Gold Studios.

Chapter Outline

Learning Objectives

After completing this chapter, you will be able to:

✓ **LO1** Explain how to prepare the hair for braiding.

✓ **LO2** Demonstrate the procedure for cornrowing.

Key Terms

Page number indicates where in the chapter the term is used.

cornrows (canerows)
pg. 516

fishtail braid
pg. 515

invisible braid (inverted braid, French braid)
pg. 514

locks (dreadlocks)
pg. 518

natural hairstyling
pg. 509

overhand technique
pg. 514

rope braid
pg. 514

single braids (box braids, individual braids)
pg. 515

twisting
pg. 510

underhand technique (plaiting)
pg. 514

visible braid
pg. 514

weaving
pg. 510

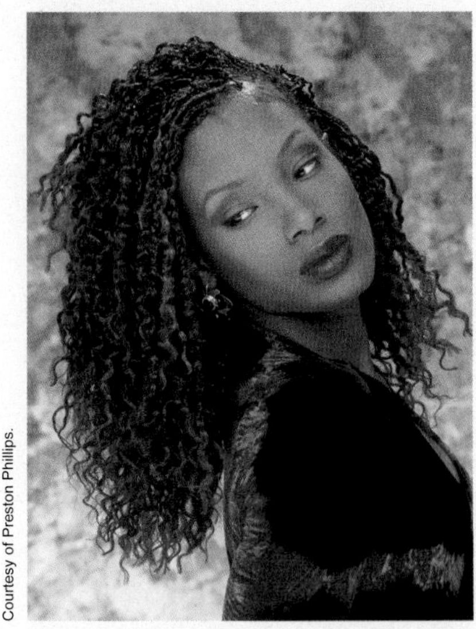

Courtesy of Preston Phillips.

▲ **Figure 18–1**
A contemporary braiding style.

From its origins in Africa to its widespread use today, hair braiding has always played a significant role in grooming and beauty practices. In some African tribes, the statement made by a person's braiding went beyond mere appearance or fashion. Different styles of braiding signified a person's social status within the community. The more important a person was, the more elaborate his or her braiding would be. Today, braiding styles continue to communicate important signals about a person's self-esteem and self-image (**Figure 18–1**).

Hair braiding reached its peak of social and esthetic significance in Africa, where it has always been regarded as an art form to be handed down from generation to generation. This art form can require an enormous investment of time, with some elaborate styles taking up to an entire day to complete. Because braiding is so time consuming, it is regarded in many African cultures as an opportunity for women to socialize and form relationships.

WHY STUDY BRAIDING AND BRAID EXTENSIONS?

Cosmetologists should study and have a thorough understanding of the importance of braiding and braid extensions because:

- These services are very popular and consumers are interested in wearing styles specific to their hair texture.
- These techniques provide an opportunity for stylists to express their artistic abilities and to add another high-ticket service to their current service menu!
- All professional cosmetologists should be prepared to work with every type of hair and hairstyle trends within every culture.
- Working with braid extensions exposes cosmetologists to the fundamental techniques of adding hair extensions, which is another lucrative service for the stylist and the salon.

Historically, the first highly decorative braids were seen among African tribes. Many of these tribes, such as the Zulu, were and still are identified by their distinctive hairstyles. As early as 3000 BC, Egyptian women wore braids or plaits decorated with shells, sequins, and glass or gold beads. Ancient paintings from India show women with long, heavy braids. Additional evidence shows that the Anasazi, who (circa AD 100) populated what is now the American Southwest, also favored braids, as did later Native Americans.

The revival of cultural hairstyles in the 1960s and 1970s resulted in the banning of wearing braids in many professions and even high schools, which in turn lead to lawsuits. Suppression was followed by acceptance and mainstream adaptation, and today, braids are as acceptable as any other hairstyle in most modern workplaces.

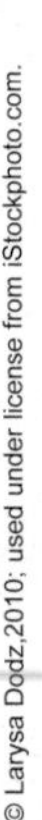

© Larysa Dodz,2010; used under license from iStockphoto.com.

Braiding salons have sprung up in many areas in the United States. These salons practice what is commonly known as **natural hairstyling**, which uses no chemicals or dyes, and does not alter the natural curl or coil pattern of the hair. While the origins of natural hairstyling are rooted in African-American heritage, people of all ethnicities appreciate its beauty and versatility. In the twenty-first century, natural hairstyling has brought a diverse approach to hair care. Natural hairstyling can be elaborate, simple, traditional or trendy. In all cases, offering your clients many different styles of braiding can inspire your creativity as a hair artist, and create a greater sense of client loyalty.

Some braided styles take many hours to complete. These more complex styles are not disposable hairdos to be casually brushed out. In fact, with proper care, a braided hair design can last up to three months, with six to eight weeks being preferable. The investment in time and money is high for both the client and stylist. After you spend hours braiding a client's hair, the last thing you want is to have the client reject it and demand that all the braids be removed. Giving your clients a thorough and detailed consultation is the best way to avoid misunderstandings and ensure a happy ending to every natural-styling service. Always fill out a client card during the initial consultation, and update it every time the client returns.

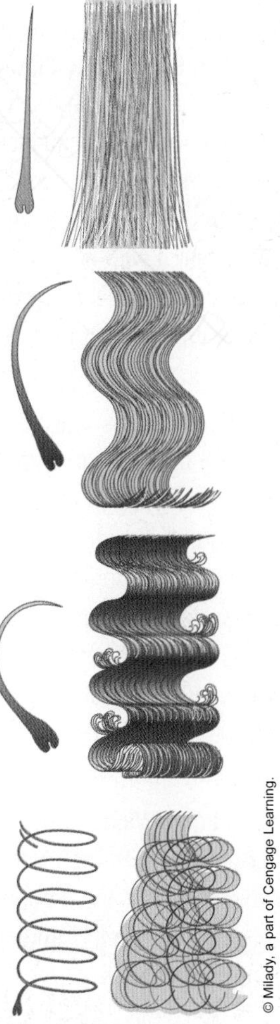
© Milady, a part of Cengage Learning.

▲ **Figure 18–2**
Wave pattern or coil configuration.

Understanding the Basics

Before exploring the various braiding techniques, it is important to have a good grasp of braiding basics. During the consultation, you will be analyzing the condition of your client's hair and scalp, paying particular attention to the hair's texture (**Figure 18–2**).

Hair Analysis: What Is Different

In braiding and other natural hairstyling, texture refers to the following three qualities.

- **Diameter of the hair.** Is the hair coarse, medium, or fine?
- **Feel.** Does the hair feel oily, dry, hard, soft, smooth, coarse, or wiry?
- **Wave pattern or coil configuration.** Is the hair straight, wavy, curly, or coiled? A coil is a very tight curl. It is spiral in formation and, when lengthened or stretched, resembles a series of loops. For the purposes of this chapter, the term *textured hair* refers to hair with a tight coil pattern.

In addition to texture, consider the following:

- **Density.** Look for areas where the hair is thin.
- **Condition.** Check for damage and breakage from previous braids or chemical services.

FYI

Within the natural hairstyling/braiding world, hair is referred to as *natural* or *virgin* if it has never had any chemical treatments. Some people use these terms even more narrowly, adding "no exposure to thermal styling tools" to the definition. Techniques used in natural hairstyling include braiding of extensions; ***twisting***, overlapping two strands to form a candy cane effect; ***weaving***, interweaving a weft or faux hair with natural hair; wrapping; and locking to create what are called African locks or dreadlocks.

Some states have separate natural hairstyling licenses. Furthermore, state regulatory agencies may define the term *natural hairstyling* in different ways. Stylists who hold only braiding, natural hairstyling, or locktician (sometimes spelled loctician) licenses—as opposed to full cosmetology licenses—cannot perform chemical services, such as coloring, perming, or straightening the hair.

For African-Americans, braided styles are a proud acknowledgment of their cultural heritage. However, their use is not limited to African-Americans. People today borrow and enjoy styles and traditions from many different cultures.

- **Length.** Make sure that the hair is physically long enough to execute the braiding style.
- **Scalp health.** Check the condition of the scalp to ensure that it is healthy and properly cared for.

Carefully checking the hair and scalp is essential for a good outcome. If the hair has extremely thin areas, for instance, the braid thickness will be noticeably different in these areas. In addition, damaged hair should not be braided since it will further stress the hair. Because everyone has thinner, finer hair around the hairline, you should never choose styles that place excessive tension in this area.

Tools for Braiding

Artists are only as good as their tools, and this adage applies equally to cutting, coloring, and creating natural hairstyles. No matter what length and texture the hair might be, certain tools are essential in order to master various braiding techniques (**Figures 18–3** and **18–4**).

- **Boar-bristle brush (natural hairbrush).** Best for stimulating the scalp as well as removing dirt and lint from locks. Nylon-bristle brushes are not as durable, and many snag the hair. However, soft nylon brushes may be an option for fine, soft hair around the hairline.
- **Square paddle brush.** This brush is good for releasing tangles, knots, and snarls in short, textured hair and long, straight hair. Square paddle brushes are pneumatic because they have a cushion of air in the head that makes the bristles collapse when they encounter too much resistance. This is key to preventing breakage in fragile African-American hair.
- **Vent brush.** This brush has a single or double row of widely spaced pins with protective tips to prevent tearing and breaking the hair. Vent brushes are used to gently remove tangles on wet wavy or dry curly hair, as well as on human hair extensions. Always check the protective tips before using a vent brush on the hair. If even one is missing, discard the brush.
- **Wide-toothed comb.** These are available in a variety of shapes and designs, and they glide through hair with little snarling. The teeth, which range in width from medium to large, have long rounded tips to avoid scratching the scalp. The distance between the teeth is the most important feature of this comb; larger spacing allows textured hair to move between the rows of teeth with ease.
- **Double-toothed comb (detangling comb).** This tool separates the hair as it combs, making it an excellent detangling comb for wet curly hair.

© Valua Vitaly 2010; used under license from Shutterstock.com.

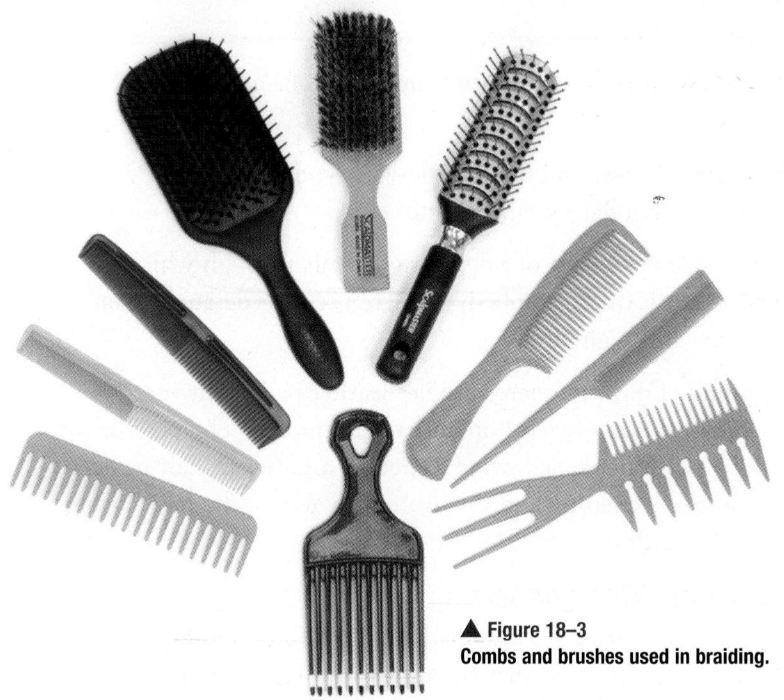

▲ **Figure 18–3**
Combs and brushes used in braiding.

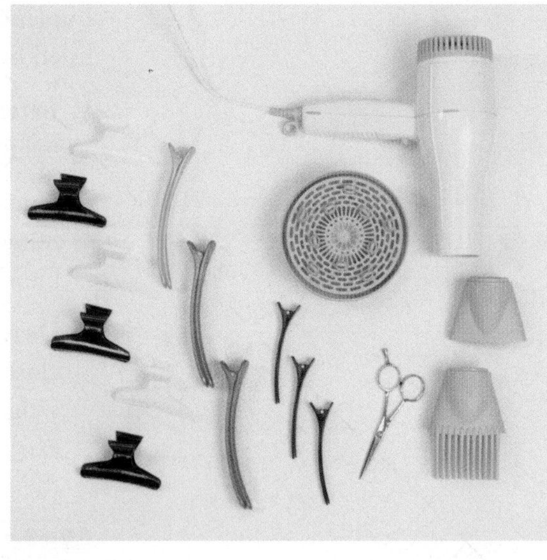

▲ **Figure 18–4**
Clips, blowdryer, diffuser concentrator, nozzle, and scissors.

- **Tail comb.** A tail comb is excellent for design parting, sectioning large segments of hair, and opening and removing braids.
- **Finishing comb.** Usually 8 to 10 inches in length, finishing combs are used while cutting. They work well on fine or straight hair.
- **Cutting comb.** This tool is used for cutting small sections. It should be used only after the hair is softened and elongated with a blowdryer.
- **Pick with rounded teeth.** This tool is useful for lifting and separating textured hair. It has long, widely spaced teeth and is commonly made of metal, plastic, or wood.
- **Blowdryer with pick nozzle.** A pick nozzle loosens the curl pattern in textured hair for braiding styles, and it dries, stretches, and softens textured hair. Use a hard-plastic pick nozzle because metal attachments become too hot.
- **Diffuser.** Dries hair without disturbing the finished look and without dehydrating the hair.
- **Five-inch scissors.** This tool is used for creating shapes and finished looks, and for trimming bangs (fringes) and excess extension material.
- **Long clips.** These are used for separating hair into large sections.
- **Butterfly and small clips.** These clips can be used to separate hair into large or small sections.
- **Hood dryer.** Use a hood dryer to remove excess moisture before blowdrying hair.
- **Small rubber bands or string.** Use these to secure the ends.

STATE REGULATORY ALERT

Lockticians specialize in creating and grooming locks. Although some states may require them to hold a braider's license, they are not braiders. Even if a locktician's license is the only license you hold, state and federal regulations require you take specific preventive measures against the spread of germs and infectious disease.

All surfaces and tools in the salon must be cleaned and disinfected after every client. You should always check with your state's regulatory agency regarding specific requirements in your state.

© Milady, a part of Cengage Learning. Photography by Paul Castle, Castle Photography.

Implements and materials you will need for extensions are listed below.

- **Extension fibers.** These come in a variety of types: Kanekalon®, nylon, rayon, human hair, yarn, lin, and yak.
- **Hackle.** A hackle is a board of fine, upright nails through which human hair extensions are combed; they are used for detangling or blending colors and highlights.
- **Drawing board.** Drawing boards are flat leather pads with very close, fine teeth that sandwich human hair extensions. The pads are weighed down with books, allowing a specific amount of hair to be extracted without loosening and disturbing the rest of the hair during the process of braiding.

Materials for Extensions

A wide variety of fibers are available for the purpose of extending hair. It is important to keep in mind that the fibers you use will largely determine how successful and durable the extension will be. Although it may seem like a good idea to buy the least expensive product, in the long run this may not prove to be the most economical solution, especially if you are buying hair fabric in large quantities. You may get stuck with a lot of material, for instance, that does not give you the results you desire. When buying a new product, buy in small quantities and test the fiber on a mannequin before using it on a client.

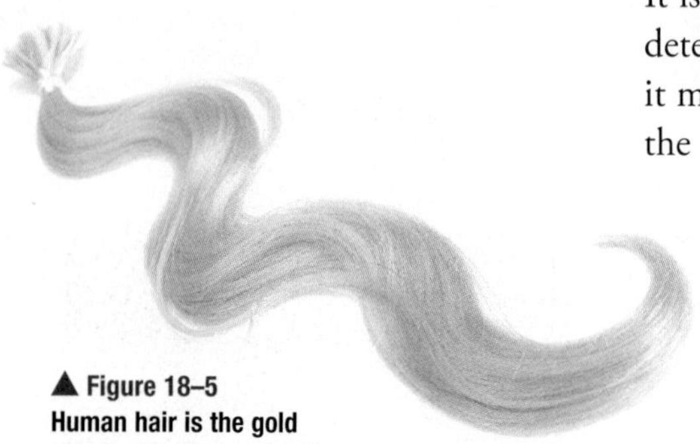

▲ Figure 18–5
Human hair is the gold standard for hair extensions.

The following materials are most commonly used for hair extensions:

- **Human hair.** Human hair is the gold standard for hair extensions. Unfortunately, the human hair market can be a confusing and sometimes deceptive business. Most human hair is imported from Asia, with little information about how it was processed, or even if it is 100 percent human hair. This makes it very important to deal only with suppliers you know and trust (**Figure 18–5**).
- **Kanekalon.** A manufactured, synthetic fiber of excellent quality, Kanekalon is made in a wide variety of types, with different names, colors and textures. Many companies that offer synthetic hair goods use a line or brand made of Kanekalon. Some Kanekalon fibers are high-heat resistant, some are especially made for braided styles, and others mimic human hair as closely as possible. Durable, soft, and less inclined to tangle than many other synthetics, Kanekalon holds up to shampooing and styling. This durability is one of the reasons it is an extremely popular fiber for use in hair additions and extensions (**Figure 18–6**).
- **Nylon or rayon synthetic.** This product is less expensive than many other synthetics and is available in varying qualities. It reflects light and leaves the hair very shiny. A drawback of nylon and rayon is that

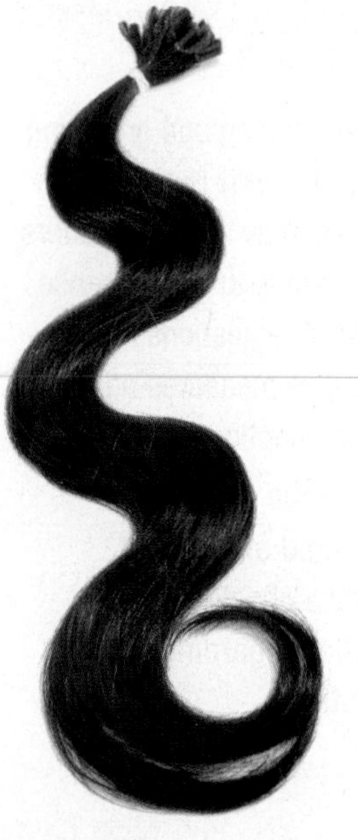

▲ Figure 18–6
Kanekalon is a top-of-the-line synthetic fiber used for hair extensions.

© Milady, a part of Cengage Learning. Photography by Paul Castle, Castle Photography. Products from Cinderella Hair.

both of these fibers have been known to cut or break the surrounding natural hair. In addition, repeated shampooing will make these extensions less durable, and they may melt if high heat, such as that from a hot blowdryer, is applied.

- **Yarn.** Traditional yarn used to make sweaters and hats is now being used to adorn hair. It can be made of cotton or a nylon blend, and is very inexpensive and easy to find. Yarn is light, soft, and detangles easily. It is available in many colors, does not reflect light, and gives the braid a matte finish. While yarn may expand when shampooing, it will not slip from the base, making it durable for braids. Be careful when you purchase yarn because some products may appear jet black in the store but actually show a blue or green tint in natural light.
- **Lin.** This beautiful wool fiber imported from Africa has a matte finish and comes only in black and brown. Lin comes on a roll and can be used in any length and size. Keep in mind that this cotton-like fabric is very flammable.
- **Yak.** This strong fiber comes from the domestic ox found in the mountains of Tibet and Central Asia. Yak hair is shaved and processed to be used alone or blended with human hair. Mixing human hair with yak hair helps to remove the manufactured shine (**Figure 18–7**).

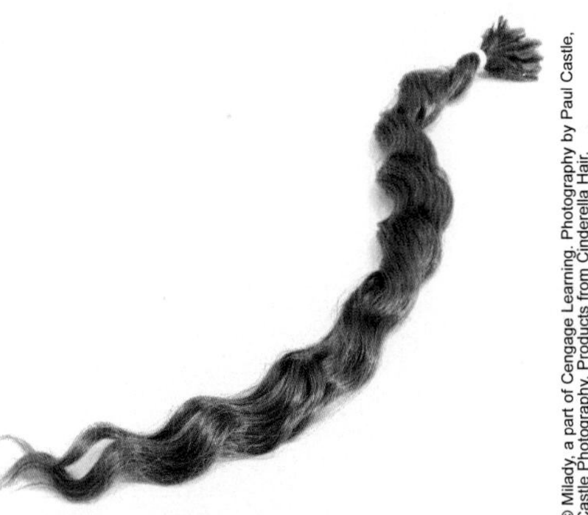

© Milady, a part of Cengage Learning. Photography by Paul Castle, Castle Photography. Products from Cinderella Hair.

▲ Figure 18–7
Yak blends beautifully with human hair.

Working with Wet or Dry Hair

In general, it is best to braid curly hair when it is dry. If curly hair is braided wet, it shrinks and recoils as it dries, which may create excess pulling and scalp tension. In turn, the tension can lead to breakage or hair loss from pulling or twisting. If you are using a style that requires your client's hair to be wet while you manipulate it, you must allow for shrinkage in order to avoid damage to the hair and scalp.

Straight, resistant hair is best braided slightly damp or very lightly coated with a wax or pomade to make it more pliable. After you shampoo the client's hair, towel blot the hair without rubbing or tension, using several towels if necessary. Apply a leave-in conditioner to make combing the hair easier. Begin combing at the ends of the hair strand and gently work out the tangles while moving upward toward the scalp. Use a wide-toothed or detangling comb for this purpose, and then blowdry the hair. Wax, pomades, pastes, or lotions can be used to hold the hair in place for a finished look. Brush the hair with a large paddle brush, beginning at the ends, just as you did with the comb.

Textured hair presents certain challenges when styling. It is very fragile both wet and dry. Because most braiding styles require the hair to be dry, blowdrying is the most effective way to prepare the hair for the braiding service. Not only does blowdrying quickly dry the hair, it softens it in the process, making it more manageable for combing and

CAUTION

While braiding is one of the most beautiful expressions in professional hairstyling, placing excessive tension on the hair can lead to a condition called *traction alopecia*. This condition is particularly prevalent among African-American women and children. It begins with scalp irritation and excessive flakiness, and eventually leads to hair loss, particularly around the hairline. Wearing excessively tight braids (tight enough to pull the hair or impede circulation to the scalp) over a prolonged period of time can lead to permanent hair loss. Keep in mind that while braids are beautiful, they must be without excessive tension to avoid long-term follicle damage.

sectioning. Blowdrying also loosens and elongates the wave pattern, while stretching the hair-shaft length. This is great for short hair, allowing for easier pick up and manipulation of the hair. Make sure to control the hair while blowdrying to prevent frizzing! ☑ **LO1**

PROCEDURE **18-1 Preparing Textured Hair for Braiding** **SEE PAGE 520**

Braiding the Hair

Braiding styles can be broadly classified as visible and invisible. A **visible braid** is a three-strand braid that is created with an underhand technique. An **underhand technique**, also known as **plaiting**, is one in which the left section goes under the middle strand, then the right section goes under the middle strand. This technique is often used for cornrowing because many braiders believe it creates less tangling.

Interestingly, the underhand technique has nothing to do with holding the palms up or down.

An **invisible braid**, also known as an **inverted braid** or **French braid**, is a three-strand braid that is produced with an **overhand technique.** In an overhand technique, the first side section goes over the middle one, then the other side section goes over the middle strand. You can start with either the right or left section; what is key is that the side sections go *over* the middle section (**Figure 18–8**).

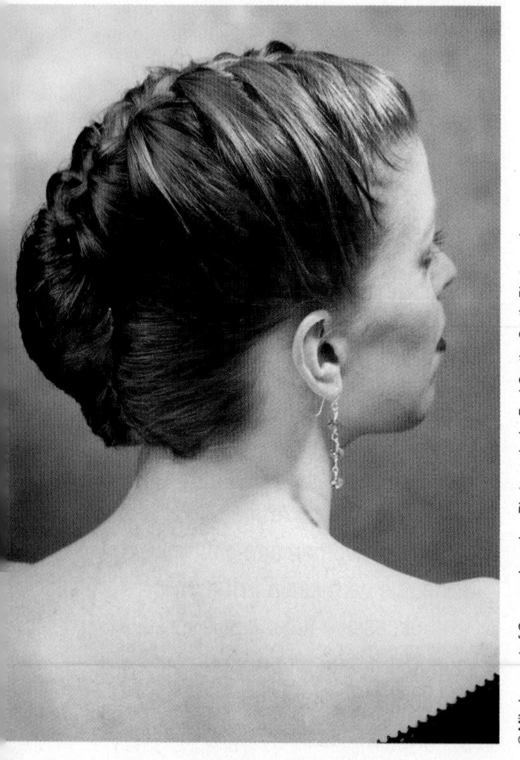
© Milady, a part of Cengage Learning. Photography by Paul Castle, Castle Photography.

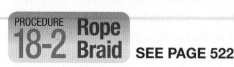

▲ **Figure 18–8**
Braided French twist.

The following discussion and procedures will provide you with a basic overview of foundational braiding styles. These techniques are important to master because all of the more advanced and trendy braiding techniques build upon these. Once you have become proficient with these techniques, your creativity—along with additional training and practice—will allow you to create some of the most complex and beautiful styles you and your clients can imagine.

The procedures begin with the most basic and move on to more complex techniques, including braided extensions.

Rope Braid

The **rope braid** is created with two strands that are twisted around each other. This braid can be done on hair that is all one length or on long, layered hair. Remember to pick up and add hair to both sides before you twist the right side over the left.

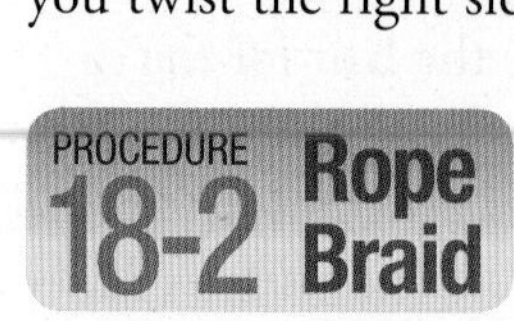

SEE PAGE 522

Fishtail Braid

The **fishtail braid** is a simple, two-strand braid in which hair is picked up from the sides and added to the strands as they are crossed over each other. It is best done on non-layered hair that is at least shoulder length.

PROCEDURE **18-3 Fishtail Braid** SEE PAGE 524

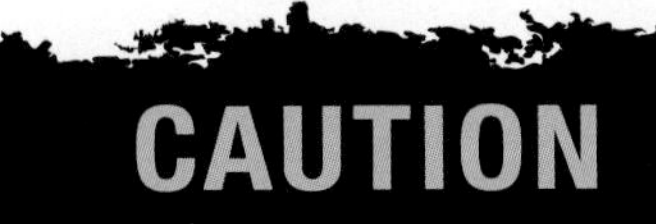

CAUTION

If you notice a scalp disorder during the hair and scalp analysis you perform prior to braiding, be sure to advise your client to seek medical attention.

Invisible Braid

The invisible braid uses an overhand pick-up technique. It can be done on or off the scalp and with or without extensions. This style is ideal for long hair, but it can also be executed successfully on shorter hair with long layers. If you are dealing with straight, layered hair, apply a light coating of wax or pomade to the hair to help hold shorter strands in place. Procedure 18–4 demonstrates one braid down the back of the head.

PROCEDURE **18-4 Invisible Braid** SEE PAGE 526

Single Braids

Single braids, also known as **box braids** and **individual braids**, are free-hanging braids, with or without extensions, that can be executed using either an underhand or overhand technique. Single braids can be used with all hair textures and in a variety of ways. For instance, two or three single braids added to a ponytail or chignon can be a lovely evening look.

The partings or subsections for single braids can be square, triangular, or rectangular. The parting determines where the braid is placed, and how it moves. Single braids can move in any direction, so make sure to braid in the direction you want them to go. As you are braiding, you are styling and shaping the finished look. The procedure for medium-to-large single braids uses the underhand technique.

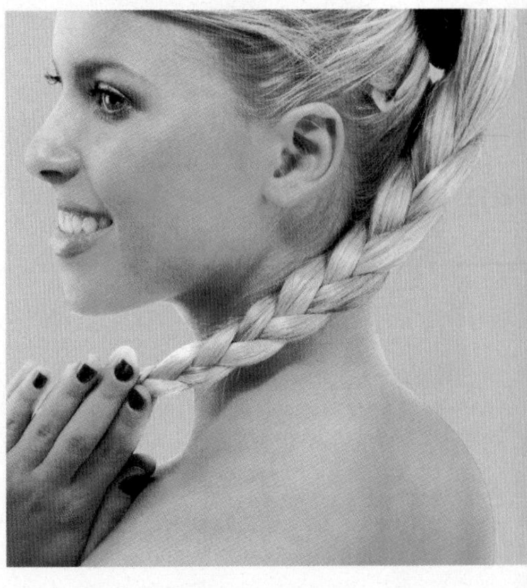

© Eduard Titov 2010; used under license from Shutterstock.com.

Extensions for single braids come in a wide range of sizes and lengths, and are integrated into the natural hair using the three-strand underhand technique. Fiber for extensions can be selected from synthetic hair, yarn, or human hair; the selection is vital in determining the finished style. Braiding must be consistent and close together.

As part of the consultation step, open the package of extension fibers and show them to the client to verify that the color is correct. Remove the fibers from the package and, if necessary, cut them to the desired length. Place half the extension fibers in the bottom portion of the drawing board and sandwich them with the upper portion of board. To secure the hair extensions, place a heavy object on top of the board, such as a large book. This allows you to easily extract the appropriate amount of fibers for the braids. Hair extensions can also be separated and dispensed by a free-hand method.

PROCEDURE **18-5** **Single Braids without Extensions** SEE PAGE 528

PROCEDURE **18-6** **Single Braids with Extensions** SEE PAGE 530

Cornrows

Cornrows, also known as **canerows**, are narrow rows of visible braids that lie close to the scalp and are created with a three-strand, on-the-scalp braiding technique. Consistent and even partings are the foundation of beautiful cornrows. Learning to create these partings requires patience and practice. Using a mannequin to practice will help develop your speed, accuracy, and finger and wrist dexterity.

Cornrows are worn by men, women, and children, and can be braided on hair of various lengths and textures. For long, straight hair, large cornrows are a fashionable and elegant hairstyle. Designer cornrows have become increasingly popular, with elaborate designs that demonstrate the stylist's skill and creative expression. The flat, contoured styles can last several weeks when applied without extensions, and up to two months when applied with extensions.

Cornrows with Extensions (Feed-in Method)

Extensions can be applied to cornrows or individual braids with the feed-in method. In this method, the braid is built up strand by strand. Excess amounts of extension material can place too much weight on the fragile areas of the hairline and will tighten and pull the hair to leave an unrealistic finished look. By properly applying the correct tension when using the feed-in method, the braid stylist can avoid an artificial look and prevent breakage.

The traditional cornrow is flat, natural, and contoured to the scalp. The parting is important because it defines the finished style. The feed-in method creates a tapered or narrow base at the hairline. Small pieces or strips of extension hair are added to fill in the base, bringing the adjoining braids closer together. This technique takes longer to perform than traditional cornrowing. However, a cornrow achieved by the feed-in method will last longer and look more natural, without placing excessive tension on the hairline. There are several different ways to start a cornrow and feed in extension pieces.

During the cornrow process, when picking up hair at the base, the hair directly underneath the previous revolution must be incorporated

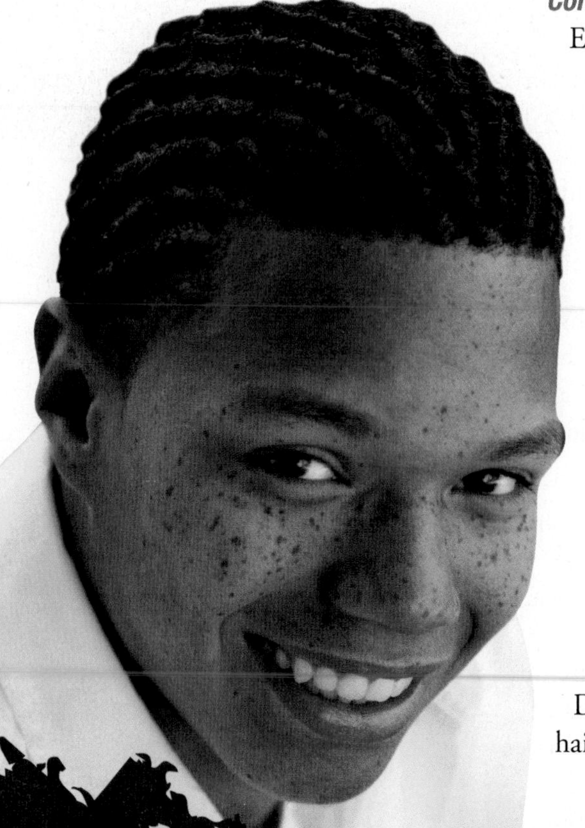

© Tracy Whiteside, 2010; used under license from Shutterstock.com.

ACTivity

Braids can be created in different lengths and styled into a variety of updos that suit your client's facial shape. Working with classmates, determine one another's facial shape, based on the following major types. Then, experiment with artistic ways to create updos and interwoven braided styles that work with the different types of facial shapes.

- An oval face is egg-shaped, and most any braided style suits this facial shape.
- The elongated face is a too-long oval and requires a style with more width at the sides.
- A round face is wide at the cheeks and will benefit from a style with height, such as one in which braids are gathered high on top and secured below the crown in back.
- A square face has a strong, square jaw line, which is minimized by allowing longer braids to frame the face.
- Heart-shaped faces are wide at the forehead and narrow at the chin and jaw.
- Pear-shaped faces are the opposite: narrow at the forehead and wide at the chin and jaw. For heart-shaped faces, use bangs or sweep braids across the forehead; for the pear shape, do the opposite by bringing at least some braids forward to create the illusion of a narrower chin line.

When styling braids for updos, you can coil them around the head, sweep up and intertwine some sections and then secure them with a braid or band, and even create a side chignon to draw attention away from an elongated face. Use the head shape to guide your style choices, and secure groups of braids by wrapping two or three other braids around them. With some styles, your biggest challenge will be discovering ways to hold up heavy braids (**Figure 18–9**).

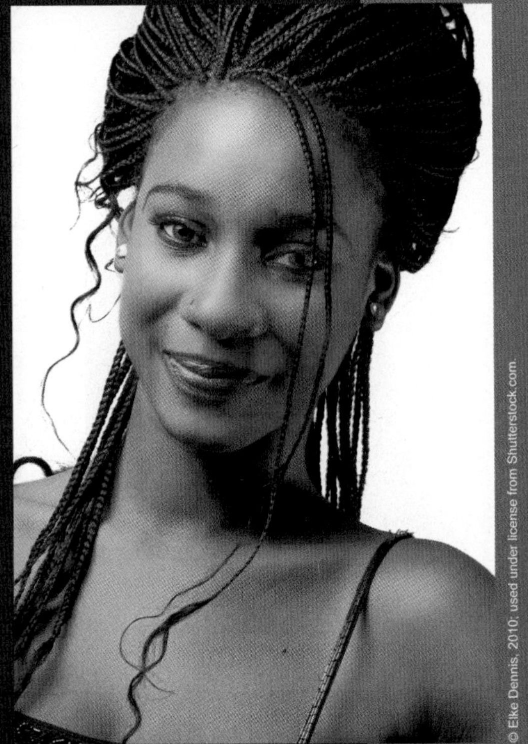

© Elke Dennis, 2010; used under license from Shutterstock.com.

▲ Figure 18–9
Upswept braids elongate a slightly wide face shape.

into the braid. The hair that you pick up must never come from another panel or from a lower part of the braid. The same is true when executing any braid technique. Overextending or misplacing the beginning of the extension leaves the hair exposed and unsupported, which can lead to breakage and hair loss in that area. This is particularly true when adding extensions at the hairline. If the extension is not made secure by two or three revolutions before picking up, it may shift away from the point of entry. ☑ **LO2**

PROCEDURE 18-7 **Basic Cornrows** SEE PAGE 533

PROCEDURE 18-8 **Cornrows with Extensions** SEE PAGE 535

© Milady, a part of Cengage Learning.

Tree Braids

Tree braiding is a newer way to add hair for a longer look. The client's hair is braided along with an extension, but the finished look shows mostly faux hair. Braiders report that tree braids take about four hours, making them faster than some other techniques. Tree braiding techniques are still evolving, and there are many ways to do them.

Some braiders add individual strands of hair, which are braided along with the natural hair and tied in place about half an inch from the root area. In this technique, a few very short braids can be seen standing up along the front hairline, then the hair extension (long and unbraided) flows freely to create the look of naturally long, straight hair.

Tree braids can also be created by adding long, loose pieces of hair to cornrows. After a few sections are braided together, a small section of the extension is pulled out and left to hang free. This technique continues all along the cornrow. When the look is completed, the free-hanging sections of the extensions completely conceal the cornrows, creating the look of naturally long, straight or wavy hair, depending on the texture of the extensions.

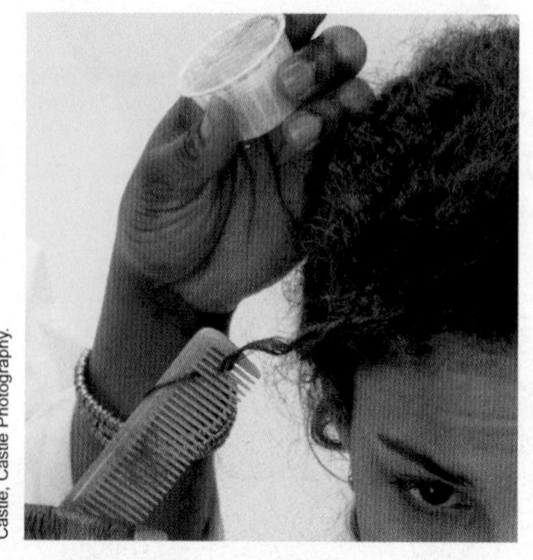

© Milady, a part of Cengage Learning. Photography by Paul Castle, Castle Photography.

▲ **Figure 18–10**
Spiral the hair with the comb.

Locks

Locks, also known as **dreadlocks**, are separate networks of curly, textured hair that have been intertwined and meshed together. Hair locking is done without the use of chemicals. The hair locks in several slow phases, which can take from six months to a year depending on the length, density, and coil pattern of the hair (**Figure 18–10** and **Table 18–1**).

DEVELOPMENTAL PHASES OF LOCKS

PHASE	CHARACTERISTICS
PHASE 1	Hair is soft and is coiled into spiral configurations. The coil is smooth and the end is open. The coil has a shiny or a glossy texture.
PRELOCK STAGE, PHASE 2	Hair begins to interlace and mesh. The separate units begin to puff up and expand in size. The units are no longer glossy or smooth.
SPROUTING STAGE, PHASE 3	A bulb can be felt at the end of each lock. Interlacing continues.
GROWING STAGE, PHASE 4	Hair begins to regain length. Lock may still be frizzy, but also solid in some areas.
MATURATION STAGE, PHASE 5	Locks are closed at the ends, dense and dull, and do not reflect light.

© Milady, a part of Cengage Learning.

Table 18–1 Developmental Phases of Locks.

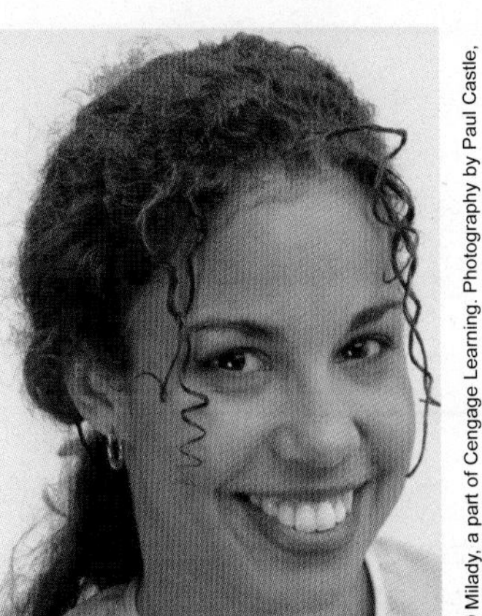

© Milady, a part of Cengage Learning. Photography by Paul Castle, Castle Photography.

▲ **Figure 18–11**
Finished coils.

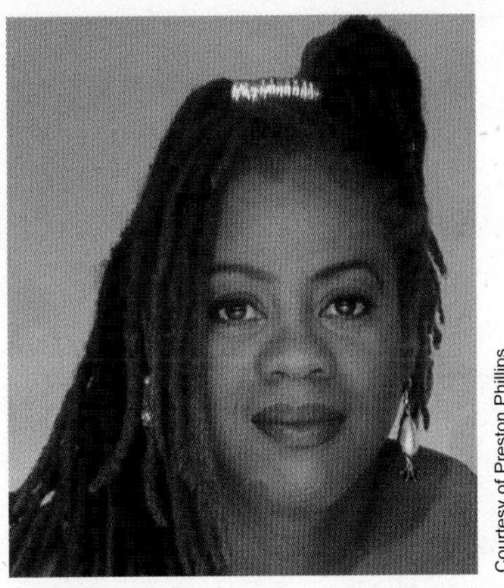

Courtesy of Preston Phillips.

▲ **Figure 18–12**
Locks.

Locks are more than just a hairstyle; they are a cultural expression. There are several ways to cultivate locks, such as double twisting, wrapping with cord, coiling, palm rolling, and braiding. Locks will also form themselves in textured hair that is not combed or brushed out. As demonstrated by the Rastafarians of Jamaica, leaving coily hair to take its own natural course will cause it to intertwine and lock. Cultivated African locks have symmetry and balance.

The three basic methods of locking are:

- **The comb technique.** Particularly effective during the early stages of locking while the coil is still open, this method involves placing the comb at the base of the scalp and, with a rotating motion, spiraling the hair into a curl. With each revolution, the comb moves down until it reaches the end of the hair shaft. It offers a tight coil and is excellent on short (1-inch to 3-inch) hair (**Figures 18–11** and **18–12**).
- **The palm roll.** This method is the gentlest on the hair, and it works through all the natural stages of locking. Palm rolling takes advantage of the hair's natural ability to coil. This method involves applying gel to dampened subsections, placing the portion of hair between the palms of both hands, and rolling in a clockwise or counterclockwise direction (**Figure 18–13**). With each revolution, as you move down the coil shaft, the entire coil is formed (**Figure 18–14**). Partings can be directional, horizontal, vertical, or brick-layered. Decorative designs and sculpting patterns are some of the creative options you can choose.
- **Braids or extensions.** Another effective way to start locks involves sectioning the hair for the desired size of lock and single braiding the hair to the end. Synthetic hair fiber, human hair fiber, or yarn can be added to a single braid to form a lock. After several weeks, the braid will grow away from the scalp, at which time the palm roll method can be used to cultivate the new growth to form a lock.

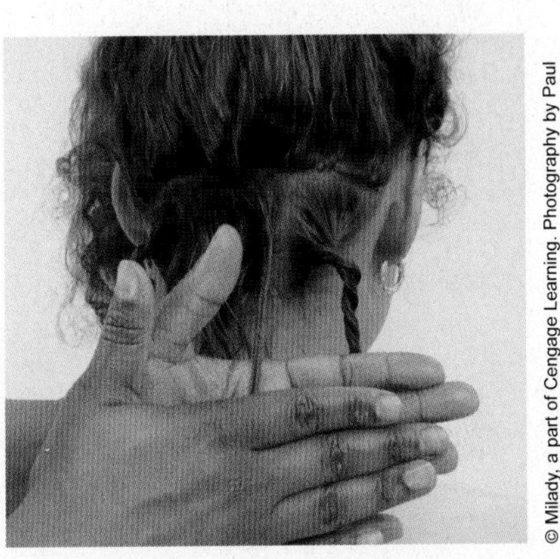

© Milady, a part of Cengage Learning. Photography by Paul Castle, Castle Photography.

▲ **Figure 18–13**
Roll the hair between the palms.

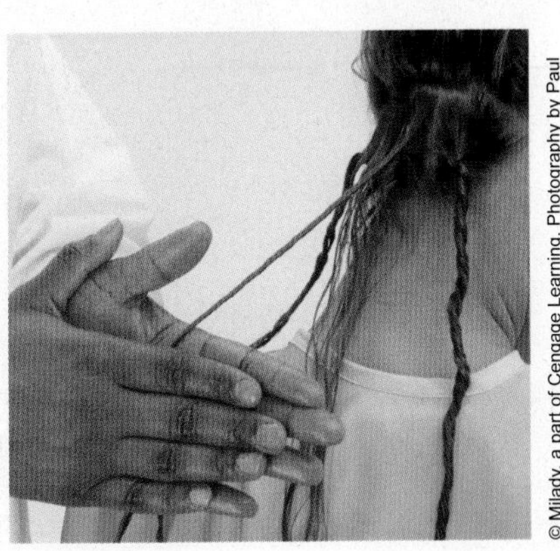

© Milady, a part of Cengage Learning. Photography by Paul Castle, Castle Photography.

▲ **Figure 18–14**
Roll down the coil shaft.

Shaping dreadlocks takes patience and commitment on the part of clients. In the beginning, clients must have frequent professional hair shapings to ensure a good outcome.

PROCEDURE 18-1

Preparing Textured Hair for Braiding

Implements and Materials

You will need all of the following implements, materials, and supplies:

- **Blowdrying cream or lotion with oil or glycerin base**
- **Butterfly clips**
- **Conditioner (protein or moisturizing)**
- **Detangling solution (four parts water to one part cream rinse or oil) in spray bottle**
- **Neck strip**
- **Shampoo**
- **Shampoo cape**
- **Tail comb with large rounded teeth**
- **Towels**

Preparation

- Perform PROCEDURE 15-1 Pre-Service Procedure SEE PAGE 323

Procedure

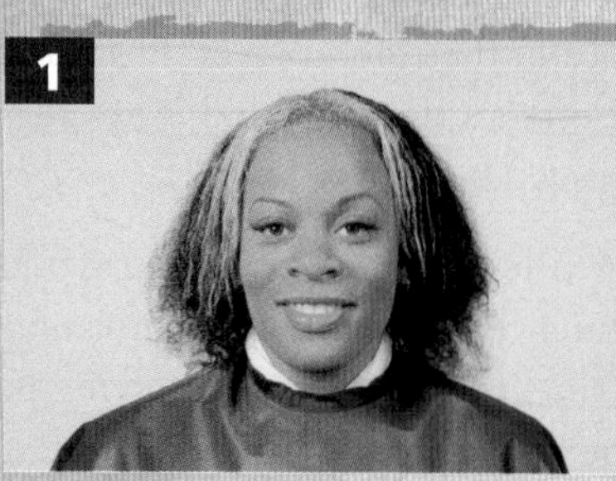

1 Drape the client for a shampoo. If necessary, comb and detangle the hair.

2 Shampoo, rinse, apply conditioner, and rinse thoroughly.

3 Gently towel dry the hair.

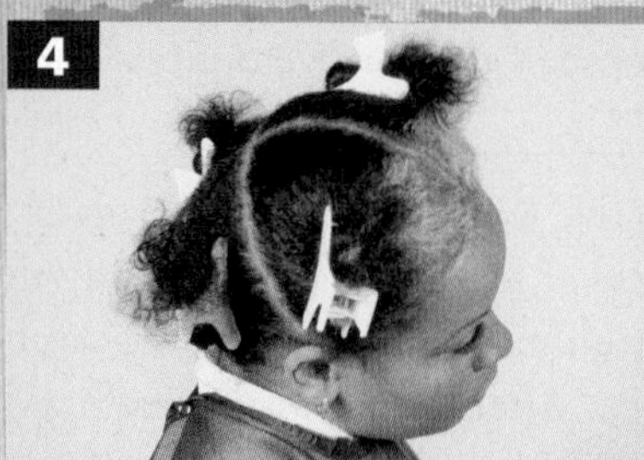

4 Part damp hair from ear to ear across crown. Use butterfly clips to separate front section from back section.

5 Part the back of head into four to six sections. For thick textured hair, make more sections to allow for increased ease and control. For thinner hair, use fewer sections. The front half of the head, where hair is less dense, can be sectioned in three or more sections. Separate the sections with clips.

© Milady, a part of Cengage Learning. Photography by Yanik Chauvin.

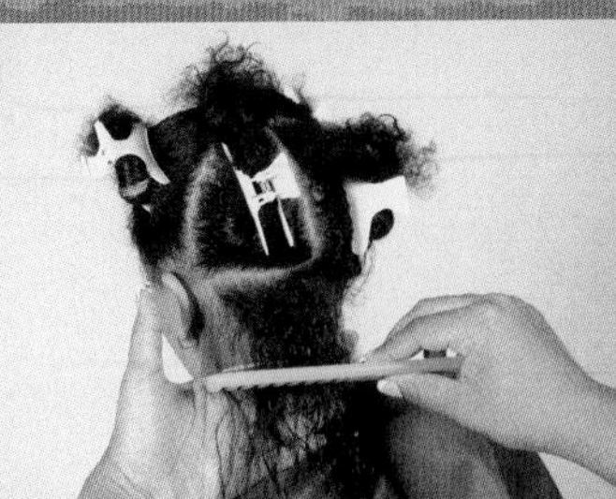

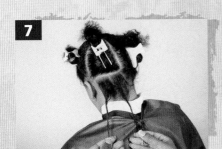

6 Beginning on left section in the back, start combing the ends of the hair first, working your way up to the base of the scalp. As you go along, lightly spray each section with detangling solution if needed. The combing movement should be fast and rhythmic, without creating tension on the scalp. Use a picking motion to comb through the hair.

7 After combing thoroughly, divide the section into two equal parts and twist them together to the end to hold the section in place.

8 Continue with the other sections of the hair until the entire head is sectioned.

9 Place client under a medium-heat hood dryer for five to ten minutes to remove excess moisture.

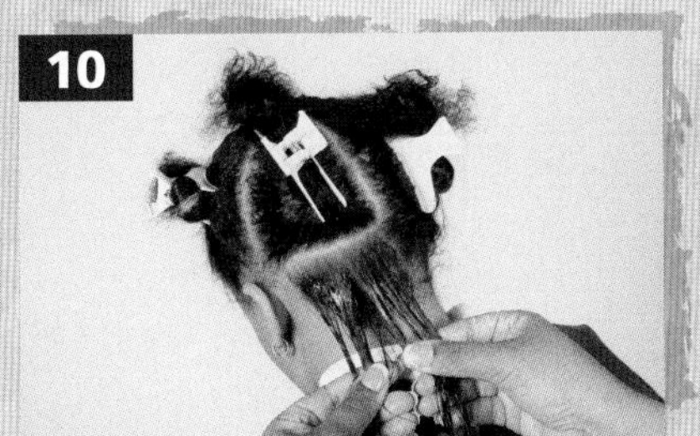

10 Open one of the combed sections. Using fingers, apply blowdrying cream to hair from scalp to ends.

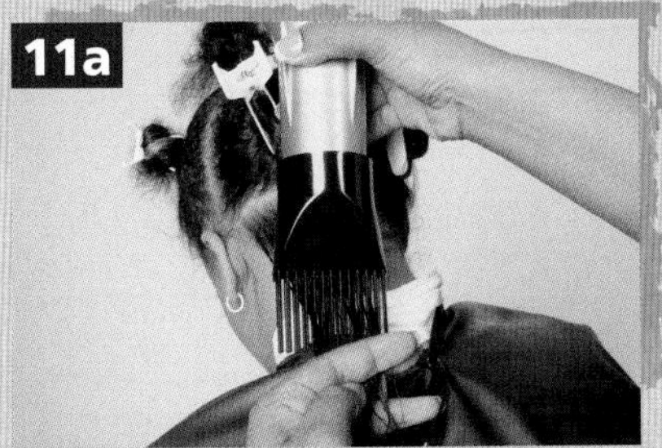

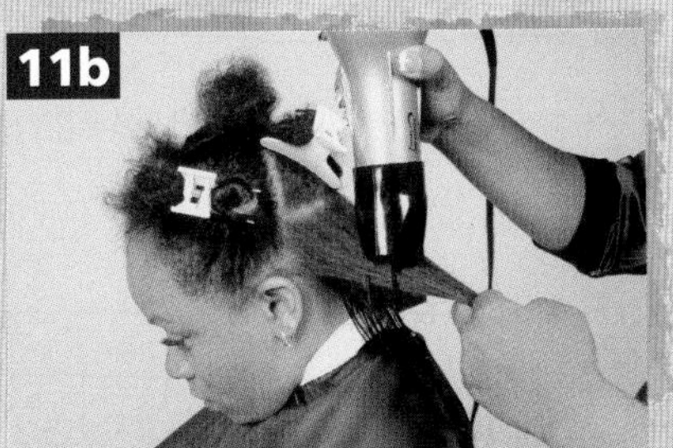

11 Using a pick nozzle attachment on a blowdryer, hold hair down and away from client's head as you begin drying. Use comb-out motion with the pick, always pointing the nozzle away from client. As ends relax and stretch, continue to use the pick nozzle to comb through and smooth sections. Use moderate tension, and direct air flow down the hair shaft to smooth and seal the cuticle. Blowing directly on scalp can cause a burn or discomfort. When the blow-out is completed, the hair is ready to braid.

Post-Service

- Complete PROCEDURE **15-2 Post-Service Procedure** SEE PAGE 326

© Milady, a part of Cengage Learning. Photography by Yanik Chauvin.

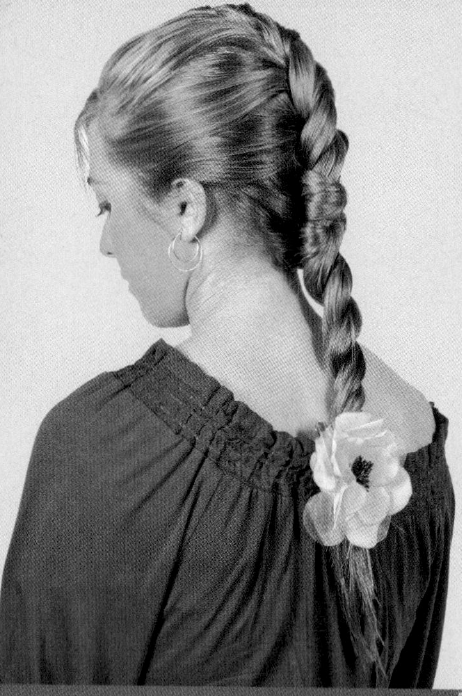

PROCEDURE 18-2

Rope Braid

Implements and Materials

You will need all of the following implements, materials, and supplies:

- **Blowdrying cream or lotion with oil or glycerin base**
- **Butterfly clips**
- **Conditioner (protein or moisturizing)**
- **Detangling solution in spray bottle**
- **Hair accessories or ornamentation (if desired)**
- **Neck strip**
- **Rubber bands, fabric-covered elastics, or other implements for securing the ends**
- **Shampoo**
- **Shampoo cape**
- **Styling and finishing products**
- **Tail comb with large rounded teeth**
- **Towels**

Preparation

- Perform PROCEDURE 15-1 **Pre-Service Procedure** **SEE PAGE 323**

Procedure

1 Drape the client for a shampoo. If necessary, comb and detangle the hair.

2 Shampoo, rinse, apply conditioner, and rinse thoroughly.

3 Gently towel dry the hair, then blowdry it completely.

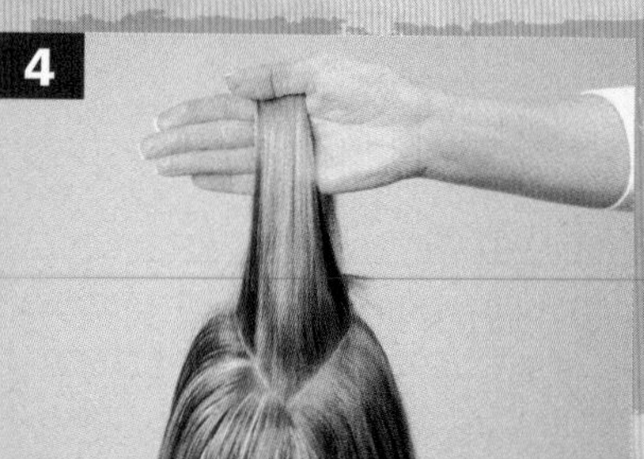

4

4 Take a triangular section of hair from the front. If client has bangs (fringe), begin behind the bangs.

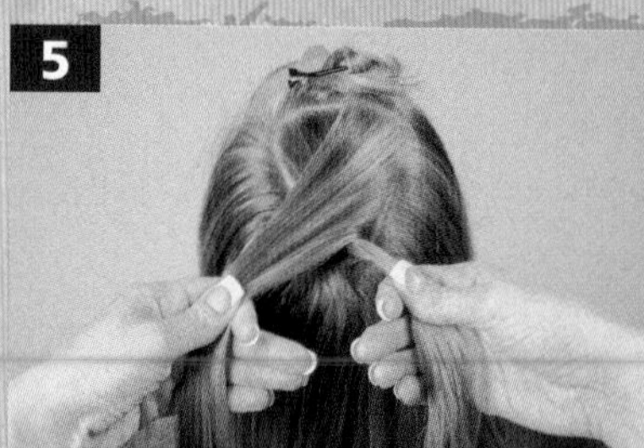

5

5 Divide the section into two equal strands. Cross the right strand over the left strand.

© Milady, a part of Cengage Learning. Photography by Yanik Chauvin.

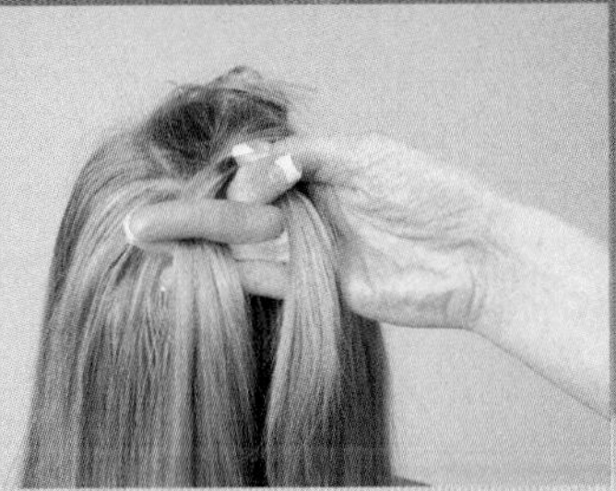

6 Put both strands in right hand with index finger in between and palm facing upward.

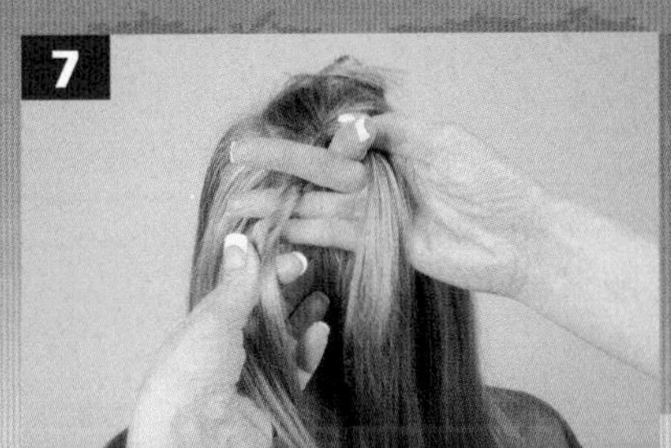

7 Twist the left strand two times clockwise (toward the center).

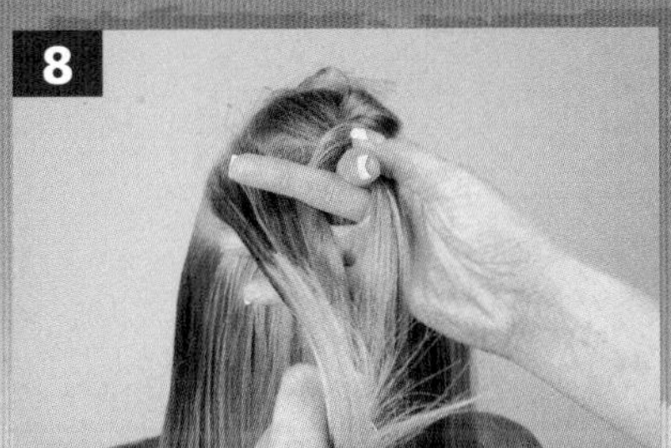

8 Pick up a 1-inch section from the left side. Add this section to the left strand.

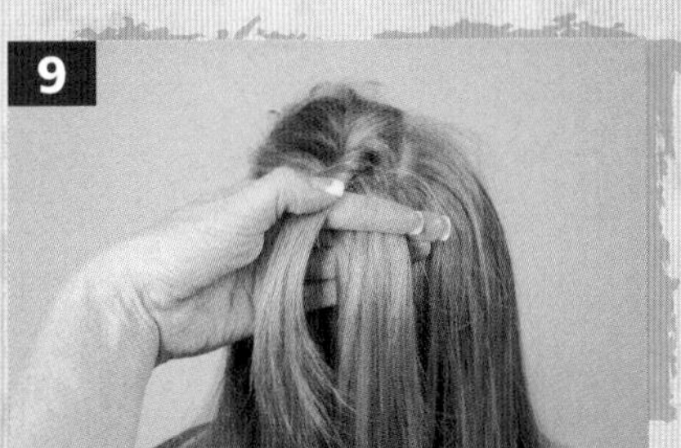

9 Put both strands in your left hand with the index finger in between and your palm up.

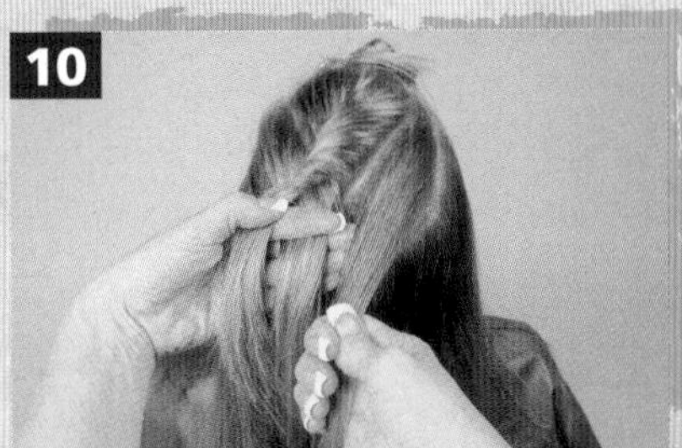

10 Pick up a 1-inch section from the right side and add it to the right strand.

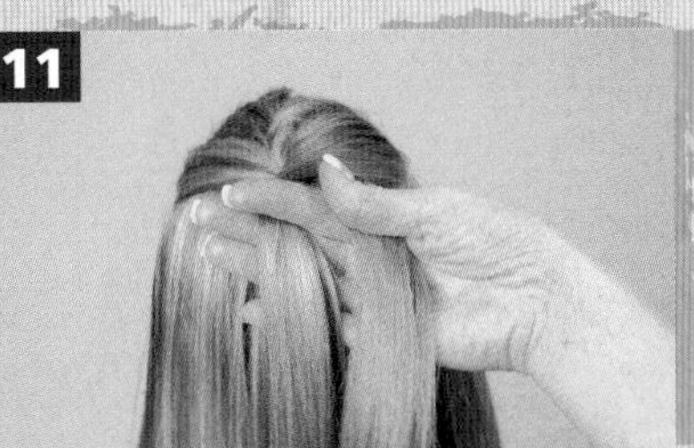

11 Put both strands in your right hand with your index finger in between and your palm up.

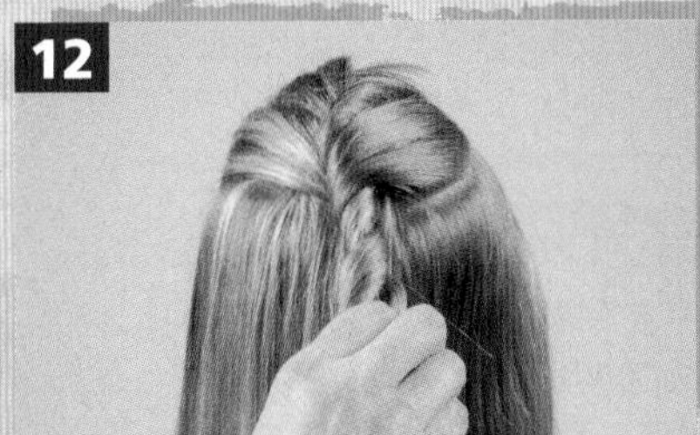

12 With your hand in this position, twist toward the left (toward the center) until your palm is facing down.

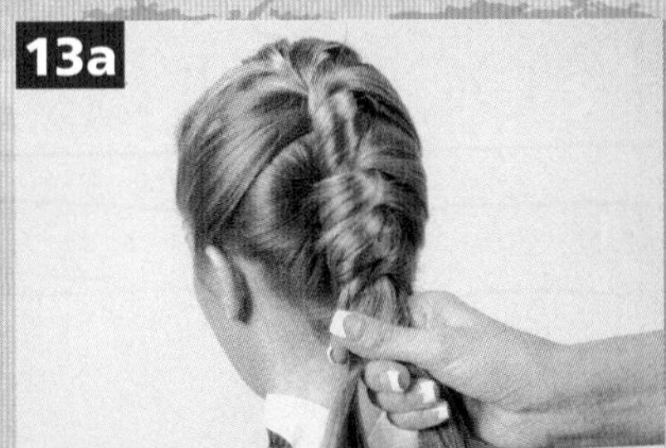

13a Work toward the nape until the style is complete.

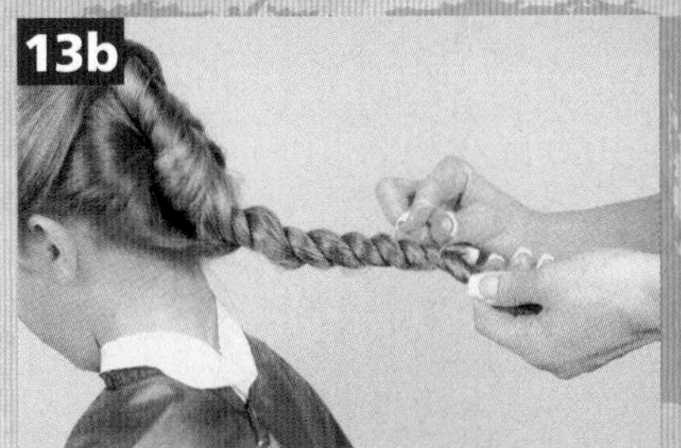

13b Secure with a rubber band.

14 When you run out of sections to pick up, another option is to create a rope ponytail with the remaining hair. Twist the left strand clockwise (away from the center) two or three times. Place the strands in your right hand, index finger in between and palm up. Twist the palm down (toward the center), right hand over left.

15 Repeat these steps until you reach the end of the hair. Secure ends with a rubber band.

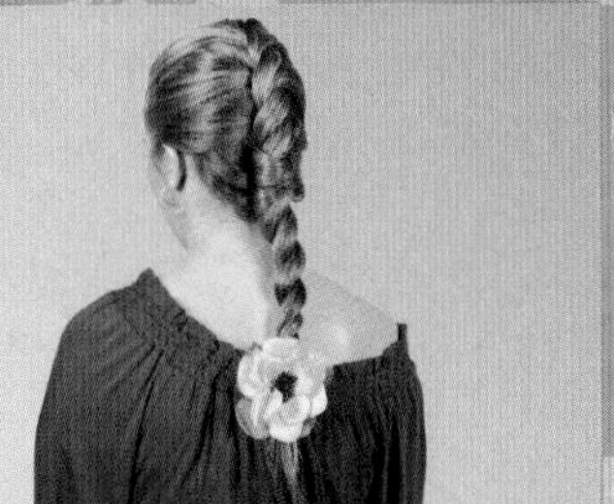

16 Finished look.

© Milady, a part of Cengage Learning. Photography by Yanik Chauvin.

Post-Service

- Complete PROCEDURE 15-2 **Post-Service Procedure** SEE PAGE 326

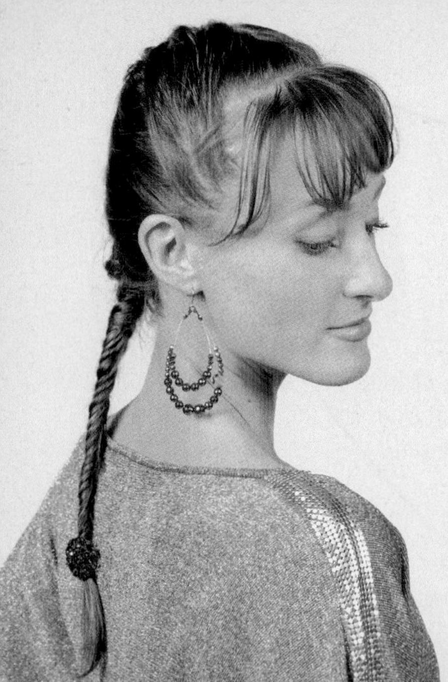

PROCEDURE 18-3

Fishtail Braid

Implements and Materials

You will need all of the following implements, materials, and supplies:

- **Blowdrying cream or lotion with oil or glycerin base**
- **Butterfly clips**
- **Conditioner (protein or moisturizing)**
- **Detangling solution in spray bottle**
- **Hair accessories or ornamentation (if desired)**
- **Neck strip**
- **Rubber bands, fabric-covered elastics, or other implements for securing the ends**
- **Shampoo**
- **Shampoo cape**
- **Styling and finishing products**
- **Tail comb with large rounded teeth**
- **Towels**

Preparation

- Perform PROCEDURE 15-1 **Pre-Service Procedure** **SEE PAGE 323**

Procedure

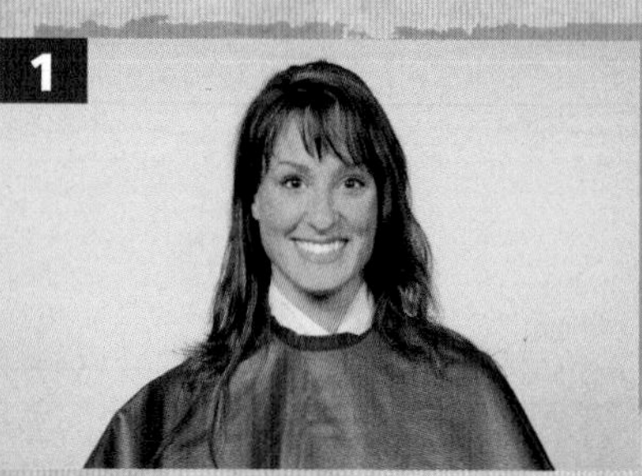

1 Drape the client for a shampoo. If necessary, comb and detangle the hair.

2 Shampoo, rinse, apply conditioner, and rinse thoroughly.

3 Gently towel dry the hair, then blowdry it completely.

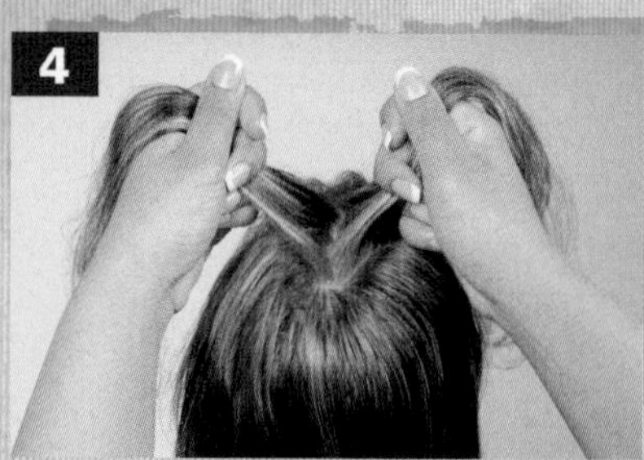

4 Take a triangular section from the front. If the client has bangs (fringe), begin behind the bangs. Divide this section into two equal strands.

© Milady, a part of Cengage Learning. Photography by Yanik Chauvin.

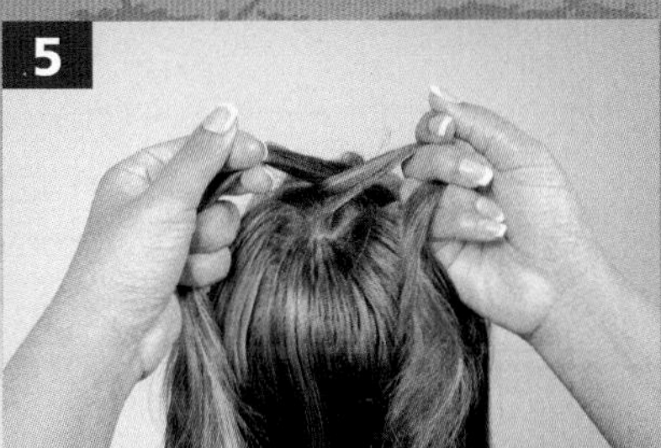

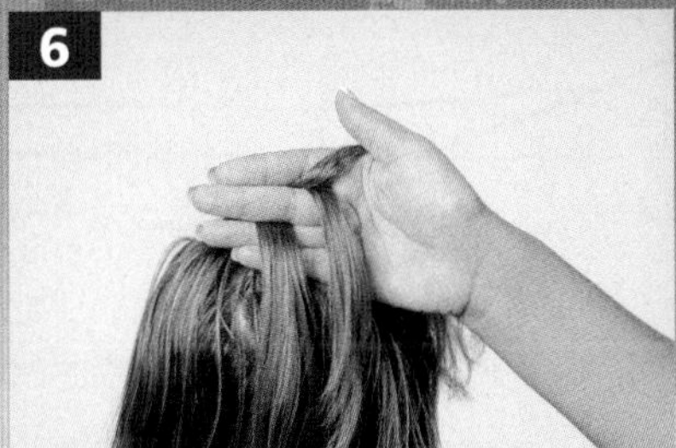

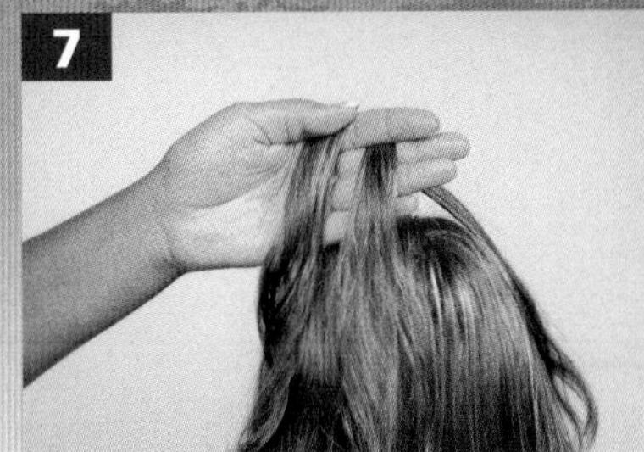

5 Cross the right strand over the left strand. Place both strands in the right hand, index finger in between and palm up.

6 Cross this section over the left strand and add it to the right strand.

7 Place two outer strands in the left hand, index finger in between and palm up.

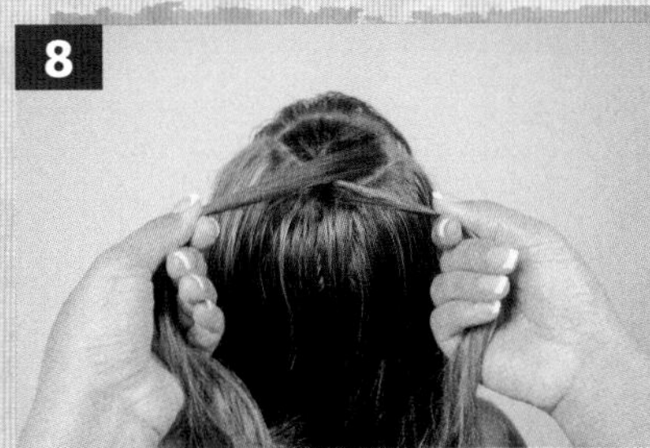

8 Cross this section over the right strand and add it to the left strand. You have now completed an X shape.

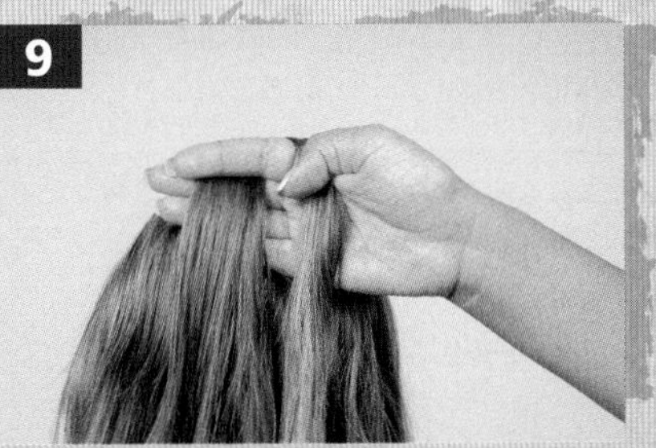

9 Put both strands in the right hand, as in step 5.

10 Move your hand down toward the nape with each new section picked up.

11 When you run out of sections, secure the hair with an elastic band to hold.

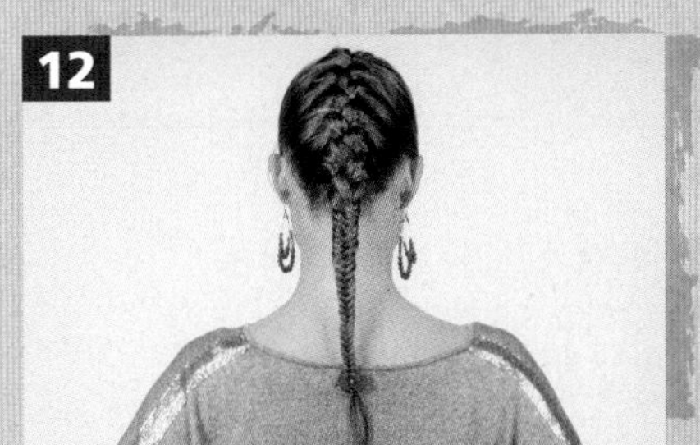

12 Finished look.

© Milady, a part of Cengage Learning. Photography by Yanik Chauvin.

Post-Service

- Complete PROCEDURE 15-2 **Post-Service Procedure** SEE PAGE 326

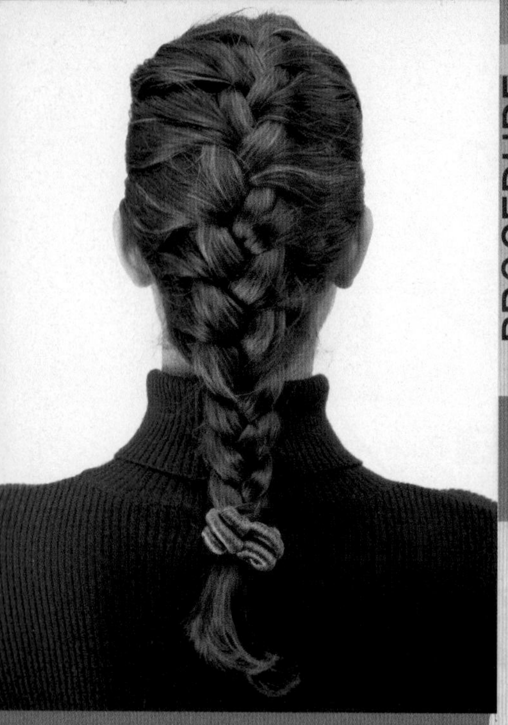

PROCEDURE 18-4

Invisible Braid

Implements and Materials

You will need all of the following implements, materials, and supplies:

- **Blowdrying cream or lotion with oil or glycerin base**
- **Butterfly clips**
- **Conditioner (protein or moisturizing)**
- **Detangling solution in spray bottle**
- **Hair accessories or ornamentation (if desired)**
- **Neck strip**
- **Rubber bands, fabric-covered elastics, or other implements for securing the ends**
- **Shampoo**
- **Shampoo cape**
- **Styling and finishing products**
- **Tail comb with large rounded teeth**
- **Towels**

Preparation

- Perform PROCEDURE 15-1 **Pre-Service Procedure** **SEE PAGE 323**

Procedure

1 Drape the client for a shampoo. If necessary, comb and detangle the hair.

2 Shampoo, rinse, apply conditioner, and rinse thoroughly.

3 Gently towel dry the hair, then blowdry it completely.

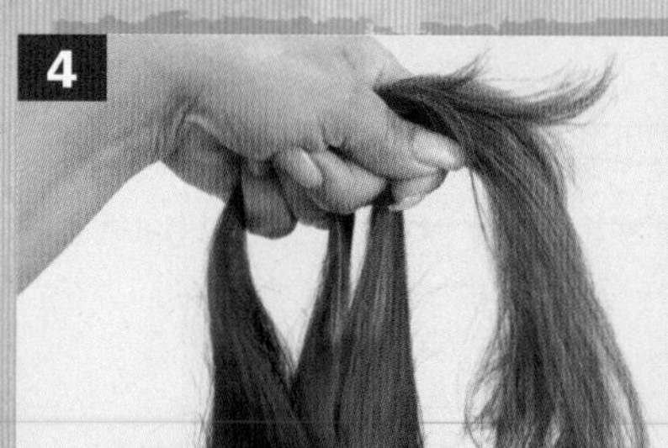
4

4 At crown of head, take a triangular section of hair and place it in your left hand. Divide the section into three equal strands, two in your left hand, and one in your right hand.

5 Place your fingers close to the scalp for a tight stitch. For a looser stitch, move away from the scalp. Cross the right strand (1) over the center strand (2). Strand 1 is now in the new center, and strand 2 is now on the right.

6 Cross the left strand (3) over the center section and place it in your right hand.

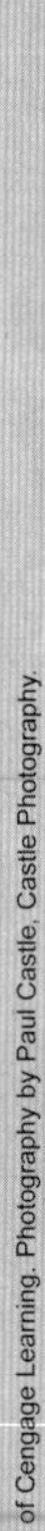
© Milady, a part of Cengage Learning. Photography by Paul Castle, Castle Photography.

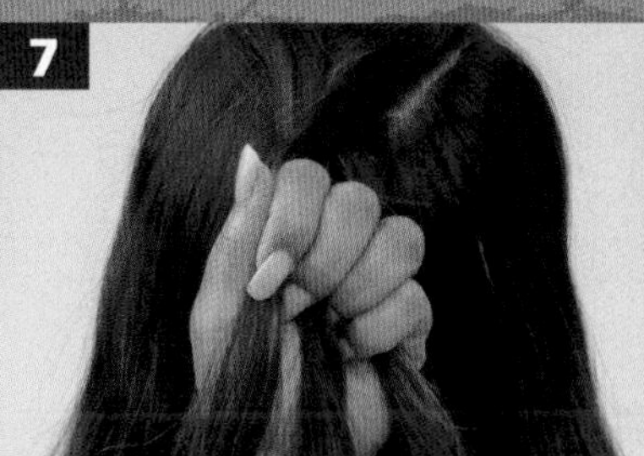

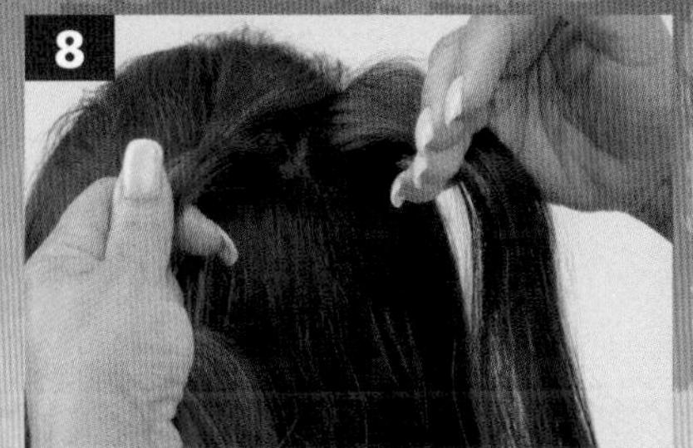

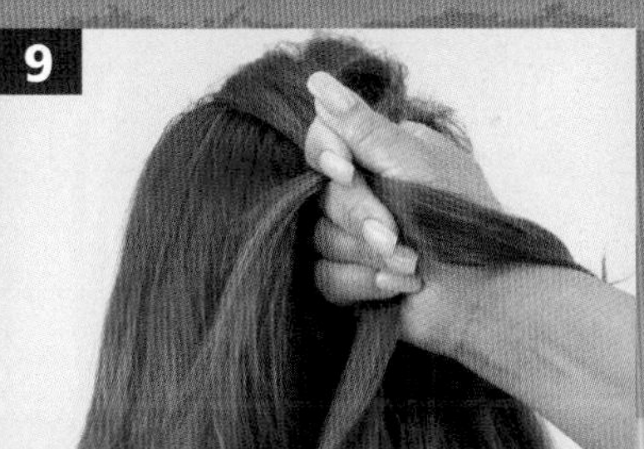

7 Place all three strands in your left hand with your fingers separating the strands.

8 With your right hand, pick up a 1-inch x 1-inch section of hair on the right side. Add to strand 2 in your left hand.

9 Take the combined strands in your right hand and cross them over the center strand. Place all the strands in your right hand.

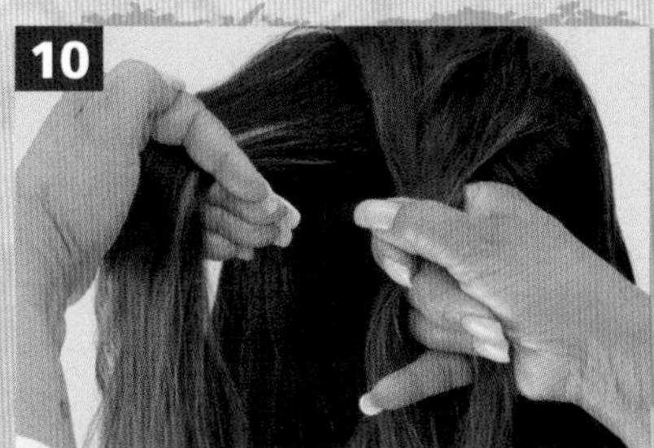

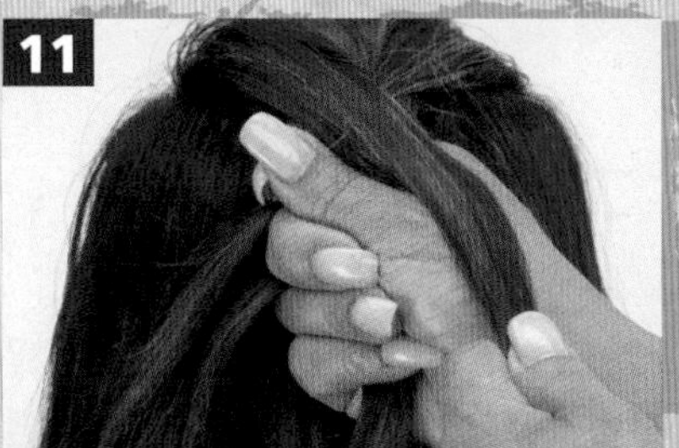

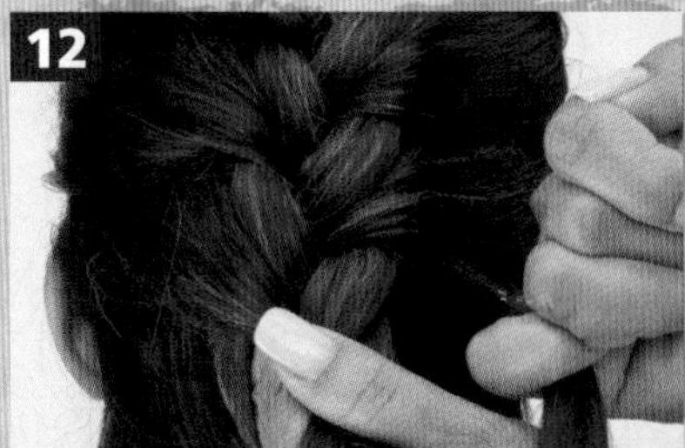

10 With your left hand, pick up a 1-inch section on the left side. Add this section to the left outer strand (1) in your right hand.

11 Take the combined strands and cross them over the center strand.

12 Place all three sections in your left hand, pick up the right side, and add to the outer strand (3).

---

13 Remember that the outer strands are added to and then crossed over the center. Continue these movements until the braid is complete. Secure the braid with a rubber band, then with

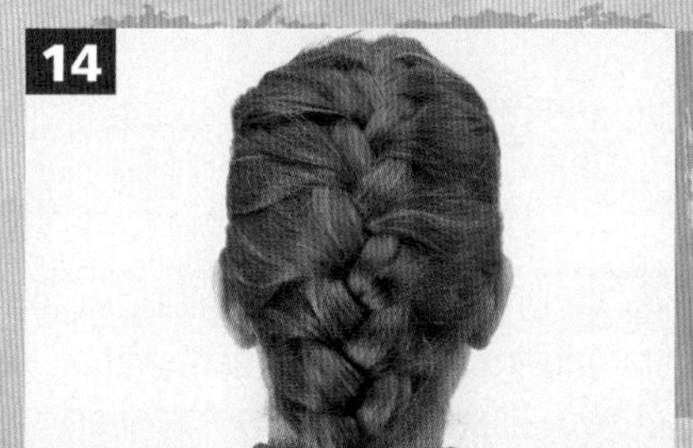

14 Finished look.

© Milady, a part of Cengage Learning. Photography by Paul Castle, Castle Photography.

Post-Service

- Complete PROCEDURE 15-2 **Post-Service Procedure** **SEE PAGE 326**

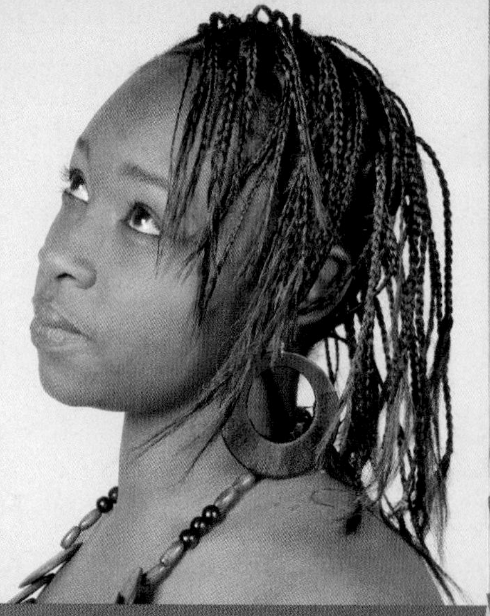

PROCEDURE 18-5

Single Braids without Extensions

Implements and Materials

You will need all of the following implements, materials, and supplies:

- **Blowdrying cream or lotion with oil or glycerin base**
- **Bobby pins**
- **Butterfly clips**
- **Conditioner (protein or moisturizing)**
- **Detangling solution in spray bottle**
- **Hair accessories or ornamentation (if desired)**
- **Light essential oil**
- **Neck strip**
- **Oil sheen**
- **Rubber bands, fabric-covered elastics, or other implements for securing the ends**
- **Shampoo**
- **Shampoo cape**
- **Styling and finishing products**
- **Tail comb with large rounded teeth**
- **Towels**

Preparation

- Perform PROCEDURE 15-1 **Pre-Service Procedure** **SEE PAGE 323**

Procedure

1 Drape the client for a shampoo. If necessary, comb and detangle the hair.

2 Shampoo, rinse, apply conditioner, and rinse thoroughly.

3 Gently towel dry the hair, then blowdry it completely.

4 Apply a light essential oil to the scalp and massage the oil into the scalp and throughout the hair.

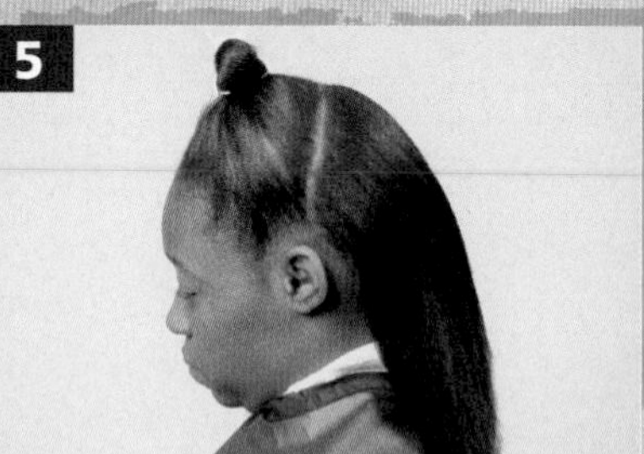

5 Divide the hair in half by parting from ear to ear across the crown. Clip away the front section.

6 Based on the style that you and the client have selected, determine the size and direction of the base of the braid.

© Milady, a part of Cengage Learning. Photography by Yanik Chauvin.

7 Part a diagonal section in the back of the head about 1-inch wide, taking into account the texture and length of the client's hair.

8 Divide the section into three even strands. Place your fingers close to the base. Cross the left strand under the center strand and then cross the right strand under.

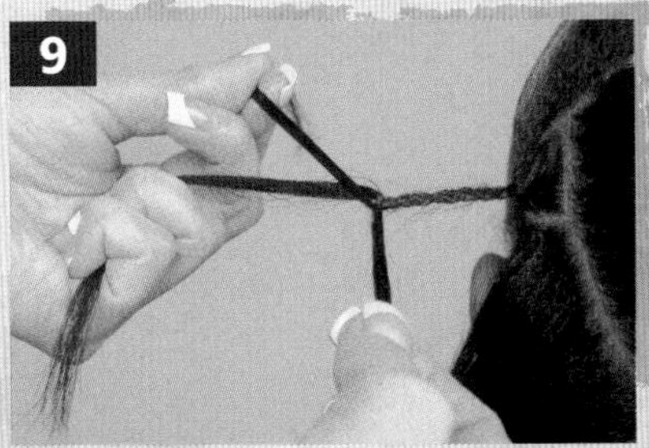

9 Pass the outer strands under the center strands, moving down the braid to the end. Secure the end as desired.

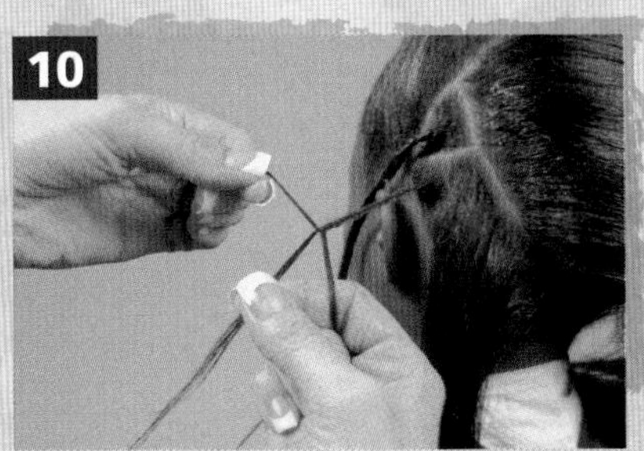

10 Move to the next subsection. Working systematically, repeat the braiding movement by passing the alternating outside strands under the center strand. Maintain an even tension on all strands.

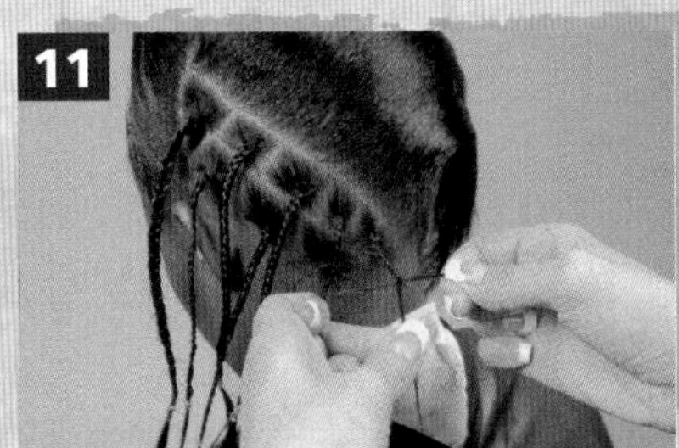

11 Move across the back, and take the next diagonal parting. Continue procedure until the entire back is completed.

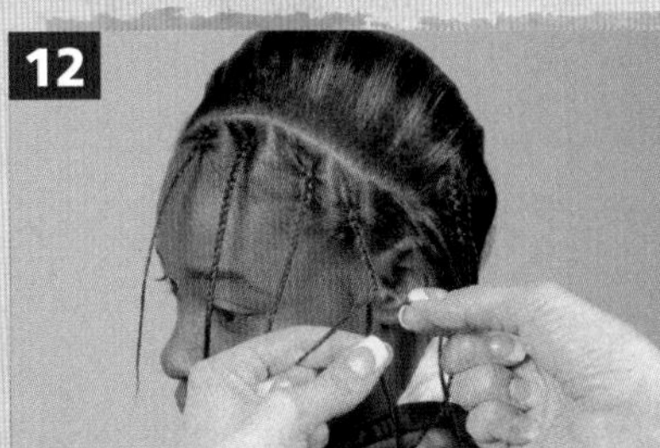

12 Then, move to the front and repeat the procedure in the front section.

13 Try to build up speed and accuracy to create straight and even braids. Rubber bands are optional to finish each braid.

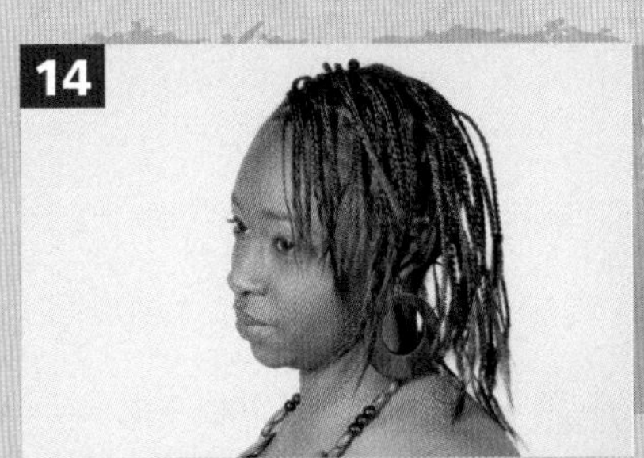

14 Apply an oil sheen product as desired by your client for a shiny finished look.

© Milady, a part of Cengage Learning. Photography by Yanik Chauvin.

Post-Service

- Complete PROCEDURE 15-2 **Post-Service Procedure** SEE PAGE 326

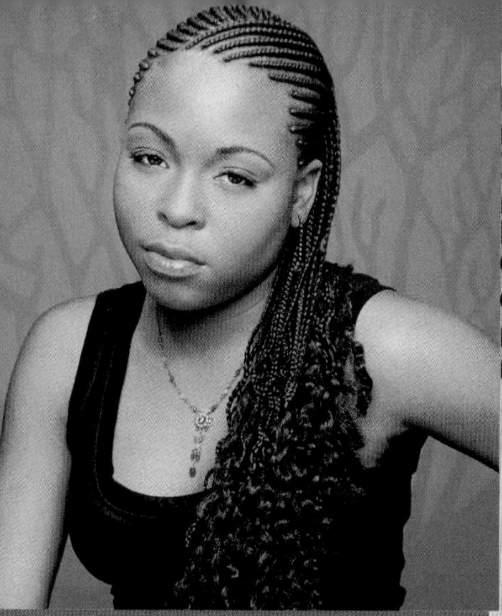

Courtesy of Carlos Payne-Solid Gold Studios.

PROCEDURE 18-6 Single Braids with Extensions

Implements and Materials

You will need all of the following implements, materials, and supplies:

- **Blowdrying cream or lotion with oil or glycerin base**
- **Bobby pins**
- **Butterfly clips**
- **Conditioner (protein or moisturizing)**
- **Detangling solution in spray bottle**
- **Drawing board**
- **Extension fibers**
- **Hair accessories or ornamentation (if desired)**
- **Neck strip**
- **Oil sheen**
- **Rubber bands, fabric-covered elastics, or other implements for securing the ends**
- **Shampoo**
- **Shampoo cape**
- **Styling and finishing products**
- **Tail comb with large rounded teeth**
- **Towels**

Preparation

- Perform PROCEDURE 15-1 **Pre-Service Procedure** **SEE PAGE 323**

Procedure

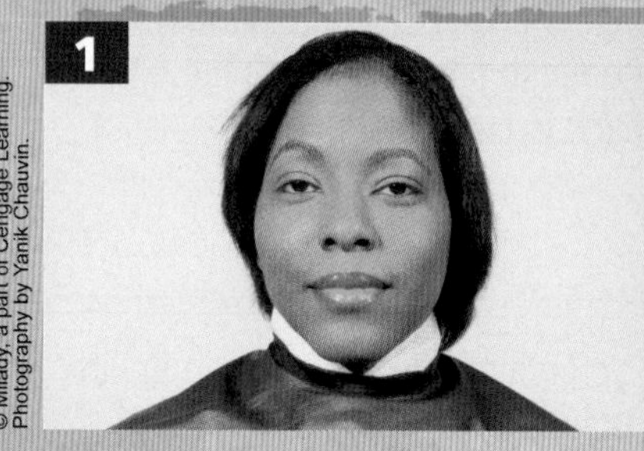

© Milady, a part of Cengage Learning. Photography by Yanik Chauvin.

1 Drape the client for a shampoo. If necessary, comb and detangle the hair before shampooing.

2 Shampoo and comb, then blowdry the hair completely

3 Prepare the extension fibers.

4 Apply a light essential oil to the scalp and massage the oil into the scalp and throughout the hair.

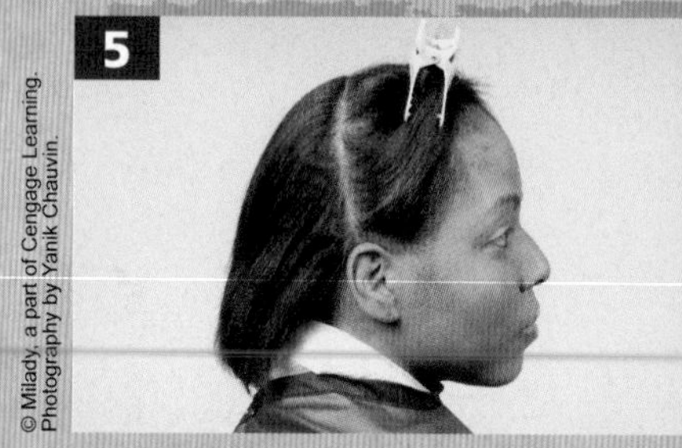

© Milady, a part of Cengage Learning. Photography by Yanik Chauvin.

5 Part the hair across the crown from ear to ear. Clip away the front section.

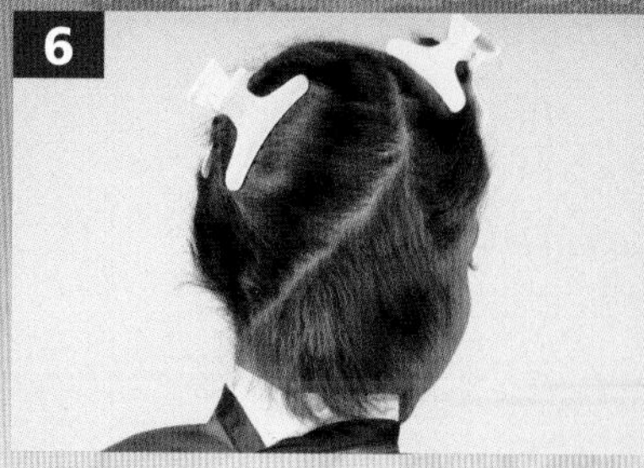

6 Part a diagonal section in the back of the head, at about a 45-degree angle, from the ear to the nape of the neck. For a medium-size braid, this section can be from ¼-inch (0.6 centimeters) to 1-inch (2.5 centimeters) wide, depending on the texture and length of the client's hair.

7 Using vertical parts to separate the base into subsections, create a diamond-shaped base.

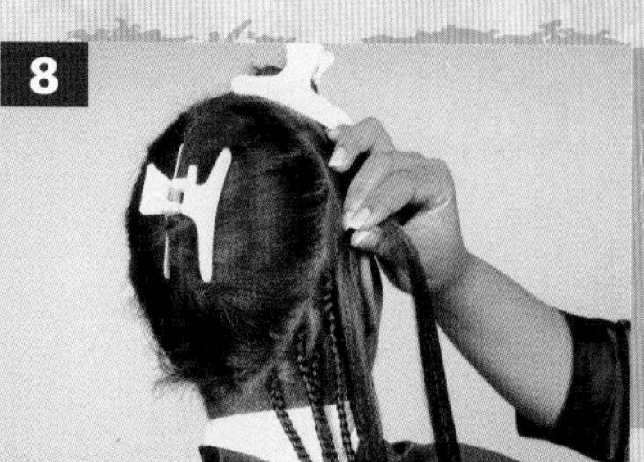

8 Select the appropriate amount of extension fibers from the drawing board. The extension should always be proportional to the section that it is being applied to. For tapered ends, gently pull extension fibers at both sides so that the ends are uneven. Then fold the fibers in half.

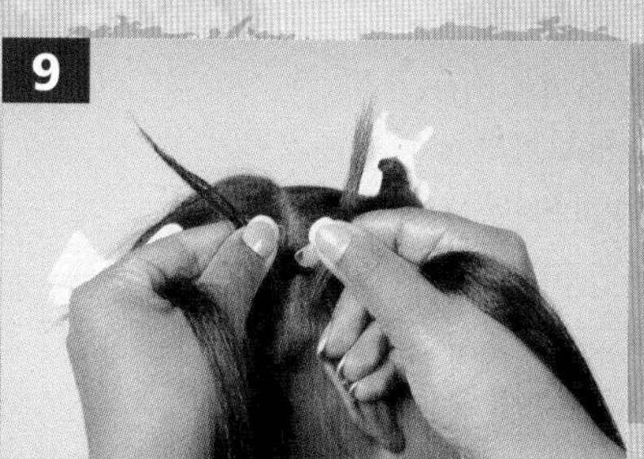

9 Divide the natural hair into three equal sections. Place the folded extension on top of the natural hair, on the outside and center portions of the braid. If desired, wrap one side of the extension two or three revolutions around the base of the natural hair and re-divide into three equal sections.

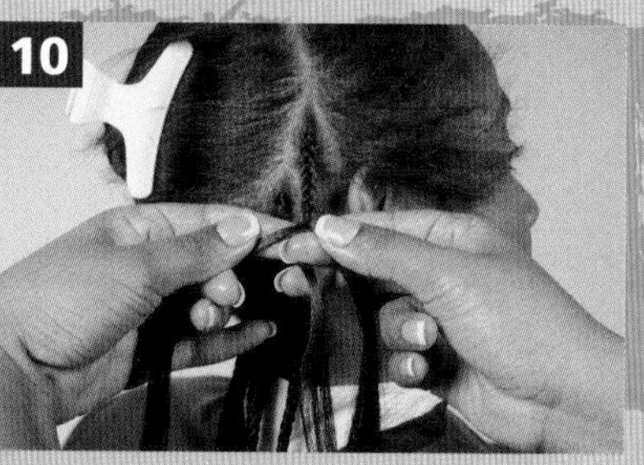

10 Once the extension is in place, begin the underhand braiding technique. Remember that the outer strands should cross under the center strand. Each time you pass an outer strand under the center strand, bring the center strand over tightly so that the outside strand stays securely in the center. As you move down the braid, keep your fingers close to the stitch, so that the braid remains tight and straight.

11 Continue braid to the desired length. Small rubber bands can be used to hold the ends in place, or you can tie them off with string and cut off the ends of the string. Other optional finishes, such as singeing (heat sealing), are considered advanced methods and require special training.

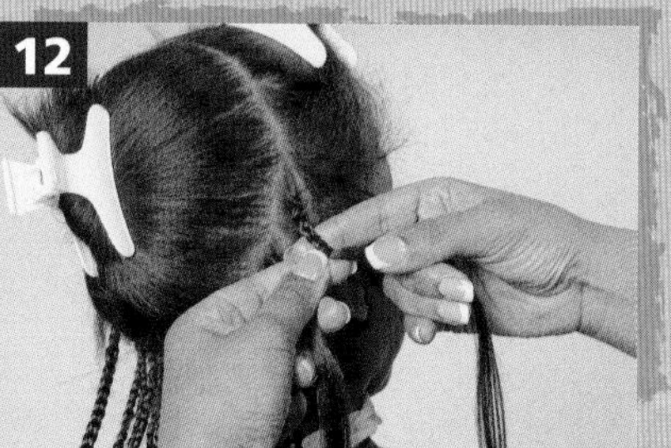

12 The next section should be above the previous section on a diagonal part, moving toward the ear.

© Milady, a part of Cengage Learning. Photography by Yanik Chauvin.

Single Braids with Extensions continued

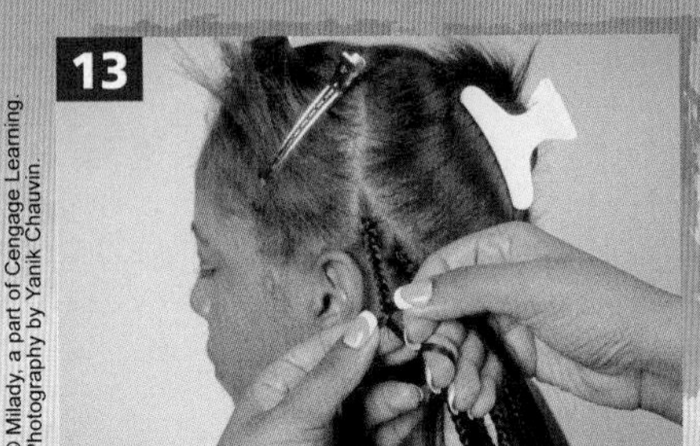

© Milady, a part of Cengage Learning. Photography by Yanik Chauvin.

13 After several sections have been completed, alternate the direction of the diagonal partings so that a V-shaped pattern forms in the back of the head.

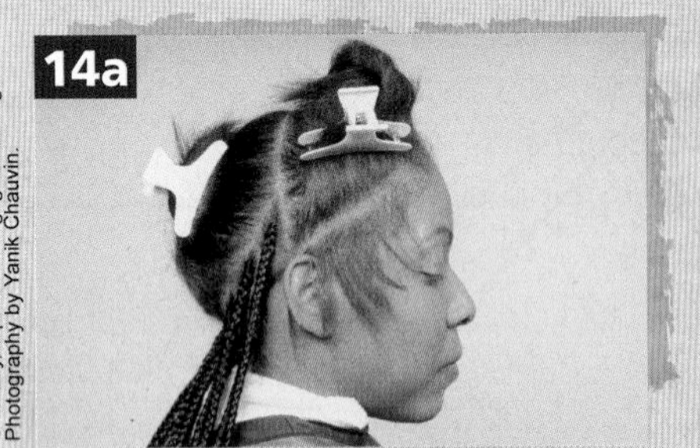

© Milady, a part of Cengage Learning. Photography by Yanik Chauvin.

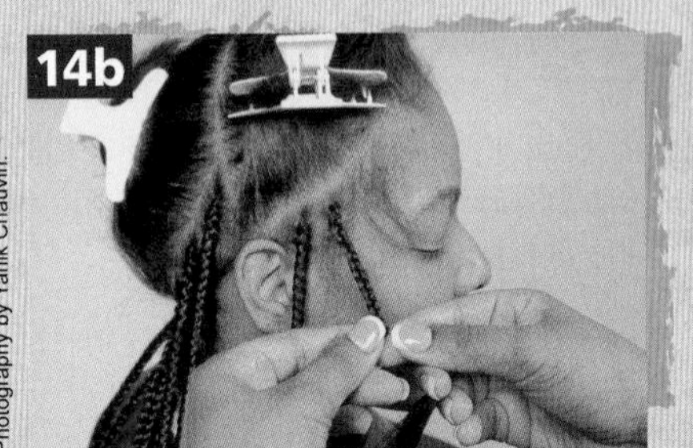

© Milady, a part of Cengage Learning. Photography by Yanik Chauvin.

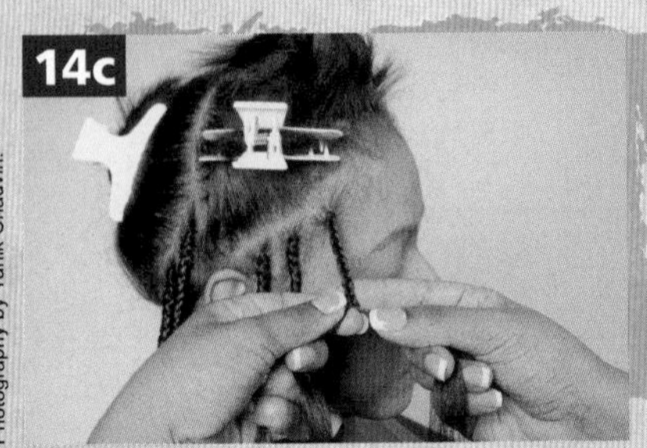

© Milady, a part of Cengage Learning. Photography by Yanik Chauvin.

14 Once the back is finished, create a diagonal or horizontal parting above the ear in the front. As you get closer to the hairline, be aware of the amount of extension hair that is applied to the hairline. Do not add excessive amounts of fiber into a fragile hairline. The fiber should always be proportionate to the hair to which it is being applied.

15 After the entire head has been braided, remove all loose hair ends from the braid shaft with scissors.

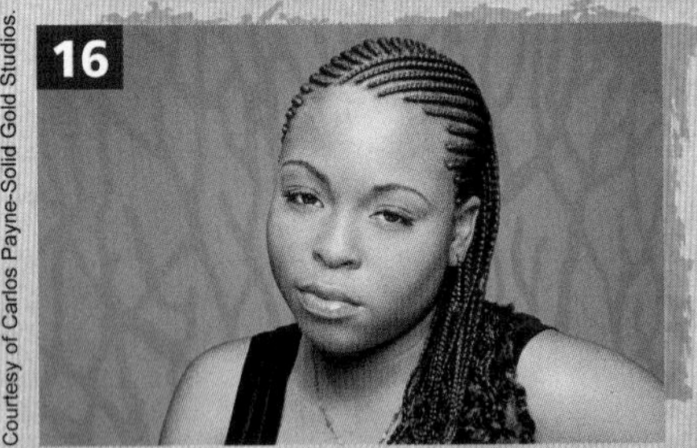

Courtesy of Carlos Payne-Solid Gold Studios.

16 If using human hair, spray hair ends with water to activate the wave in the extensions. The finished braids will look quite natural.

Post-Service

- Complete PROCEDURE 15-2 **Post-Service Procedure** SEE PAGE 326

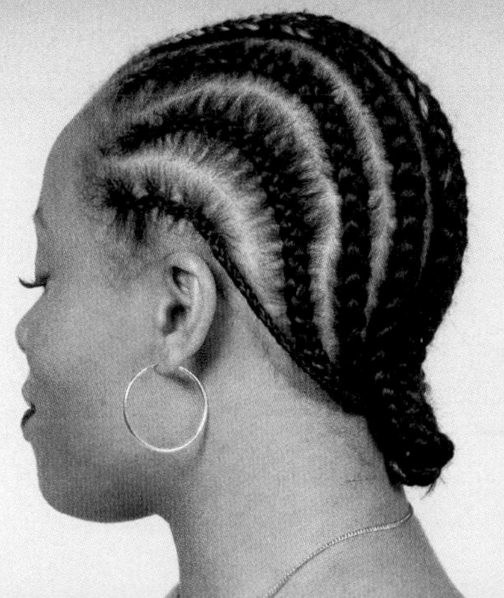

PROCEDURE 18-7

Basic Cornrows

Implements and Materials

You will need all of the following implements, materials, and supplies:

- **Blowdrying cream or lotion with oil or glycerin base**
- **Bobby pins**
- **Butterfly clips**
- **Conditioner (protein or moisturizing)**
- **Detangling solution in spray bottle**
- **Drawing board**
- **Extension fibers**
- **Hair accessories or ornamentation (if desired)**
- **Neck strip**
- **Oil sheen**
- **Rubber bands, fabric-covered elastics, or other implements for securing the ends**
- **Shampoo**
- **Shampoo cape**
- **Styling and finishing products**
- **Tail comb with large rounded teeth**
- **Towels**

© Milady, a part of Cengage Learning. Photography by Yanik Chauvin.

Preparation

- Perform PROCEDURE 15-1 **Pre-Service Procedure** **SEE PAGE 323**

Procedure

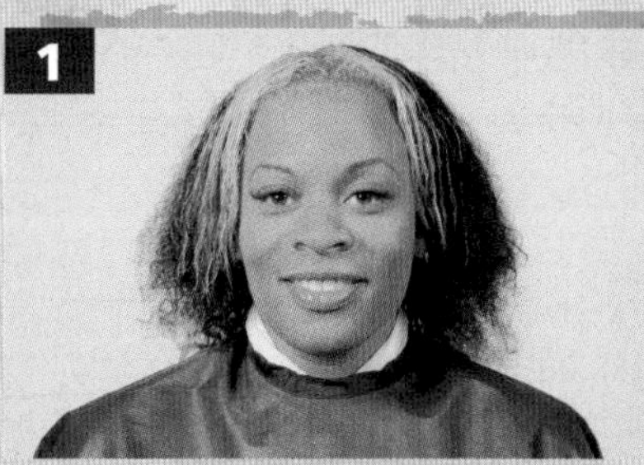

1 Drape the client for a shampoo. If necessary, comb and detangle the hair before shampooing.

2 Shampoo and comb, then blowdry the hair completely.

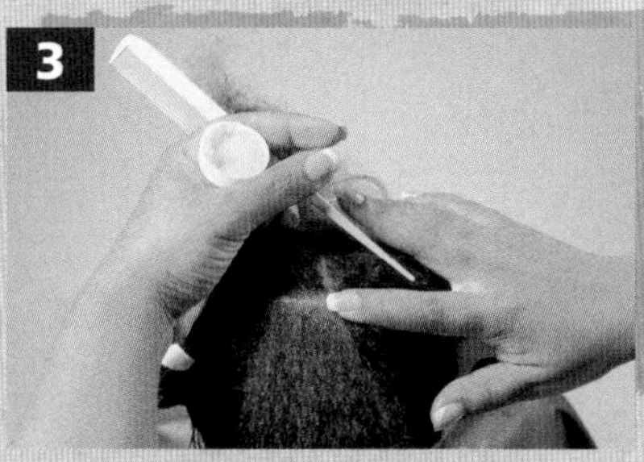

3 Depending on desired style, determine the correct size and direction of the cornrow base. With tail comb, part hair into 2-inch sections (or smaller, depending on the desired style) and apply a light essential oil to the scalp. Massage oil throughout scalp and hair.

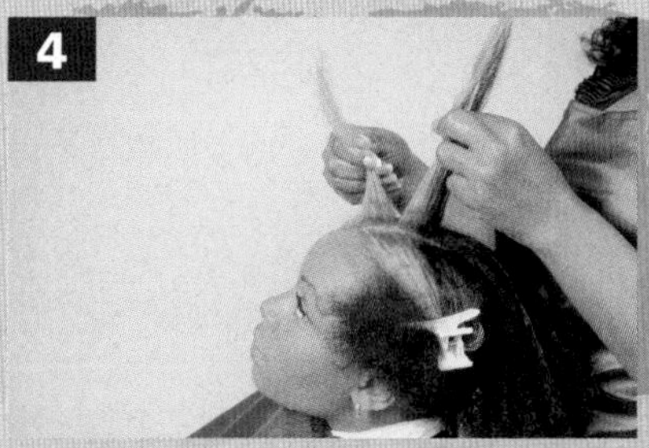

4 Start by taking two even partings to form a neat row for the cornrow base. With a tail comb, part the hair into a panel, using butterfly clips to keep the other hair pinned to either side.

PROCEDURE 18-7

Basic Cornrows continued

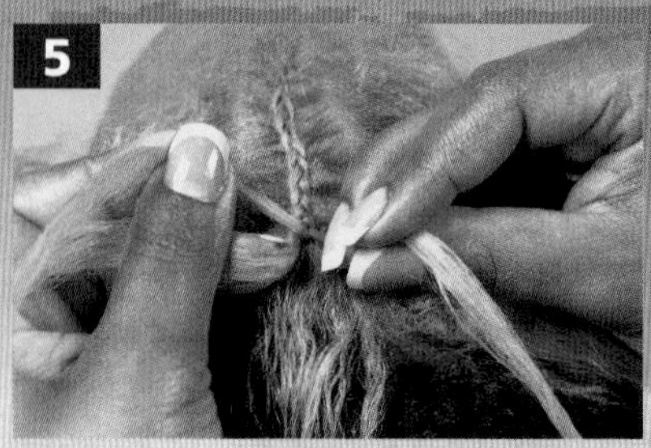

5 Divide the panel into three even strands. To ensure consistency, make sure that strands are the same size. Place fingers close to the base. Cross the left strand (1) under the center strand (2). The center strand is now on the left and the former left strand (1) is the new center.

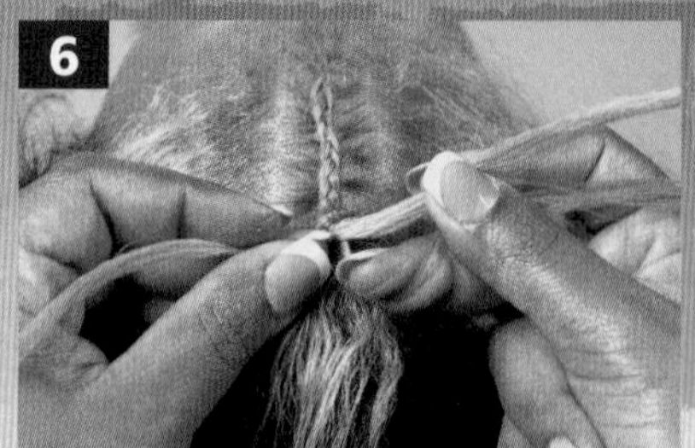

6 Cross the right strand (3) under the center strand (1). Passing the outer strands under the center strand this way creates the underhand cornrow braid.

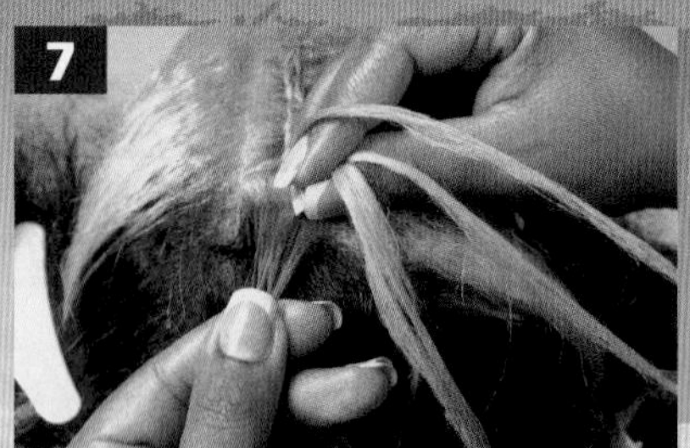

7 With each crossing under or revolution, pick up from the base of the panel a new strand of equal size and add it to the outer strand before crossing it under the center strand.

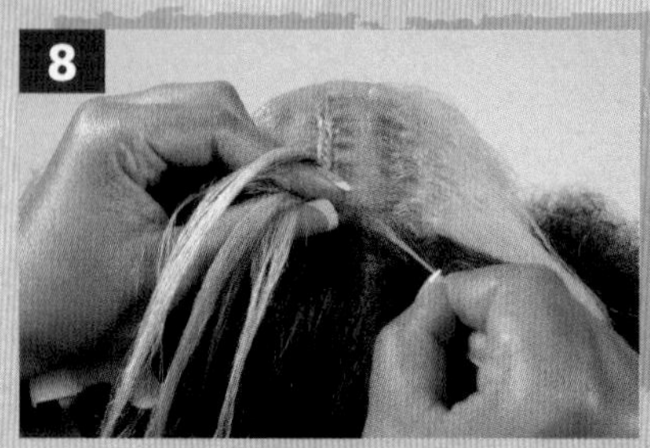

8 As you move along the braid panel, pick up a strand from the scalp with each revolution, and add it to the outer strand before crossing it under, alternating the side of the braid on which you pick up the hair.

9 As new strands are added, the braid will become fuller. Braid to the end.

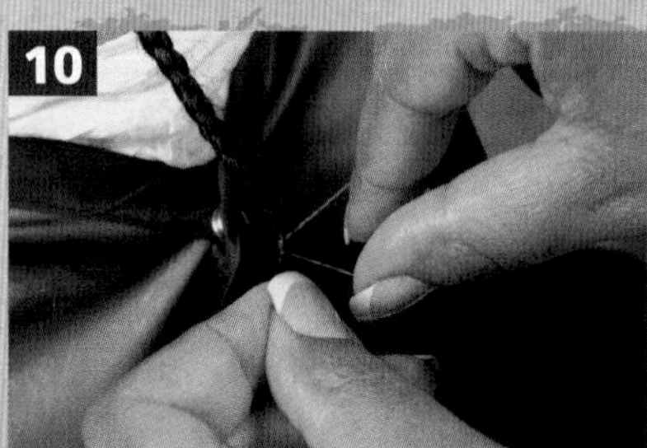

10 Simply braiding to the ends can finish the cornrow; small rubber bands can be used to hold the ends in place. Other optional finishes, such as singeing (heat sealing), are considered advanced methods and require special training.

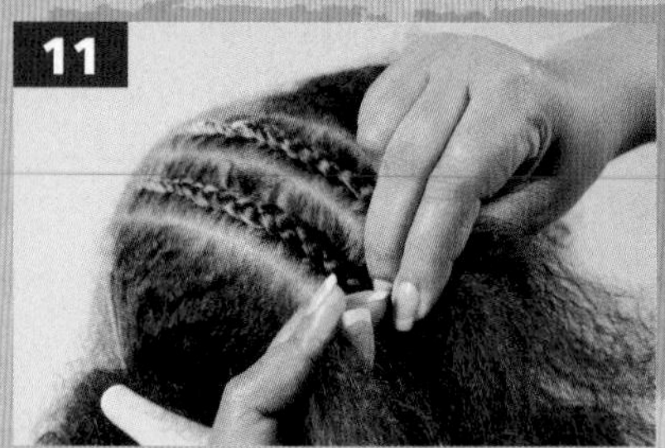

11 Braid the next panel in the same direction and in the same manner. Keep the partings clean and even.

12 Repeat until all the hair is braided, and apply oil sheen for shine.

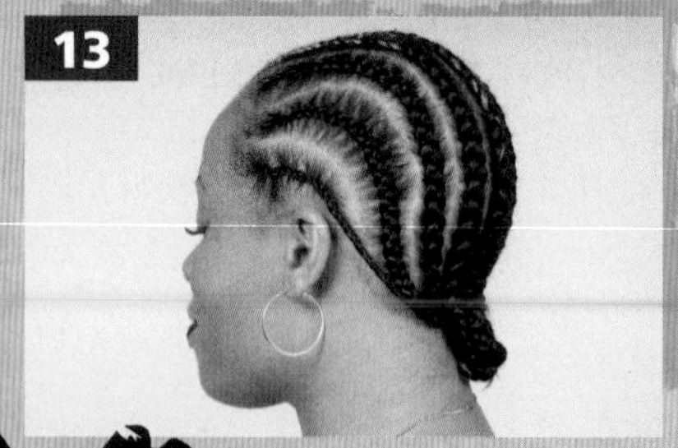

13 Finished look.

Post-Service

- Complete PROCEDURE 15-2 **Post-Service Procedure** SEE PAGE 326

© Milady, a part of Cengage Learning. Photography by Yanik Chauvin.

PROCEDURE 18-8

Cornrows with Extensions

Implements and Materials

You will need all of the following implements, materials, and supplies:

- **Blowdrying cream or lotion with oil or glycerin base**
- **Bobby pins**
- **Butterfly clips**
- **Conditioner (protein or moisturizing)**
- **Detangling solution in spray bottle**
- **Drawing board**
- **Extension fibers**
- **Hair accessories or ornamentation (if desired)**
- **Neck strip**
- **Oil sheen**
- **Rubber bands, fabric-covered elastics, or other implements for securing the ends**
- **Shampoo**
- **Shampoo cape**
- **Styling and finishing products**
- **Tail comb with large rounded teeth**
- **Towels**

Preparation

- Perform PROCEDURE 15-1 Pre-Service Procedure SEE PAGE 323

Procedure

1 Drape the client for a shampoo. If necessary, comb and detangle the hair.

2 Shampoo and comb, then blowdry it completely.

3 Prepare the extension fibers.

4 Apply a light essential oil to the scalp and massage the oil into the scalp and throughout the hair.

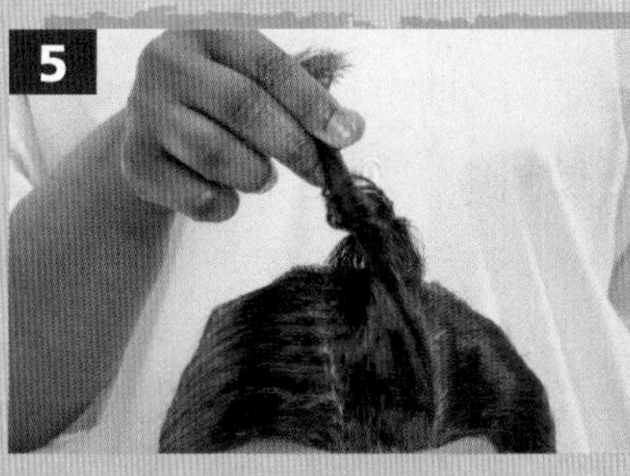

5 Starting at the hairline, part off a cornrow base in the desired direction. No extension is added at the starting point. If the hair extension is required because of a thinning hairline, apply minute amounts, as small as 5 to 10 strands. Divide the natural hair into three equal strands.

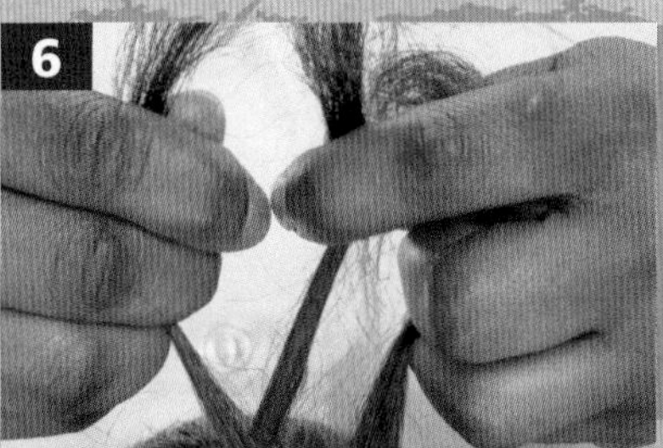

6 With the first revolution, cross left strand 1 under center strand 2.

© Milady, a part of Cengage Learning. Photography by Paul Castle, Castle Photography.

Cornrows with Extensions continued

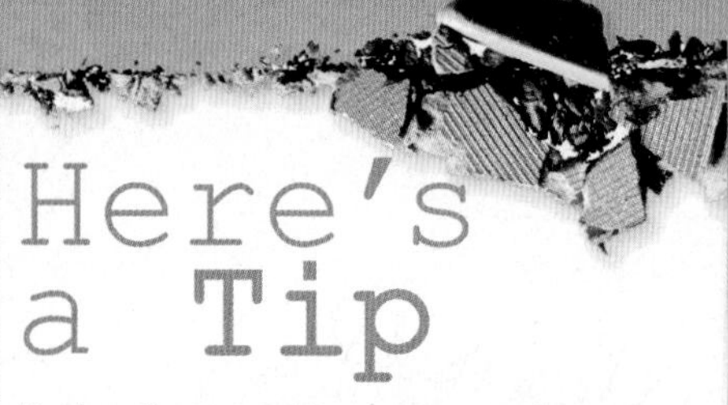

Here's a Tip

During the cornrow process, when picking up hair at the base, the hair directly underneath the previous revolution must be incorporated into the braid. The hair that you pick up must never come from another panel or from a lower part of the braid. The same is true when executing any braid technique. Overextending or misplacing the beginning of the extension leaves the hair exposed and unsupported, which can lead to breakage and hair loss in that area. This is particularly true when adding extensions at the hairline. If the extension is not made secure by two or three revolutions before picking up, it may shift away from the point of entry.

For a professional finish, always trim any ends that may stick up through the braid. Holding your scissors flat, move up the shaft as you trim, making sure that you avoid cutting into the braid.

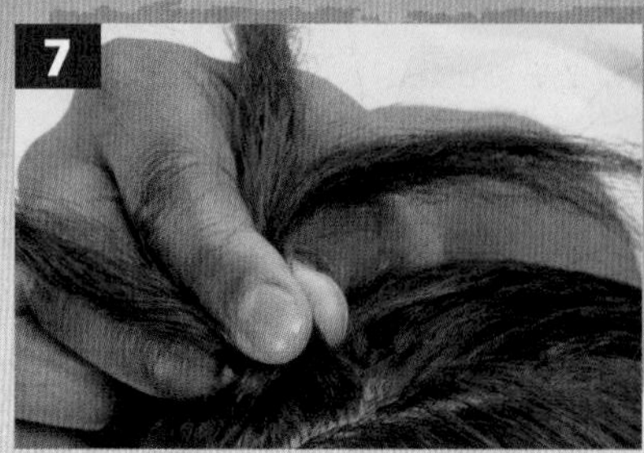

7 On the second revolution, the right strand 3 crosses under strand 1, which is now in the center. Pick up a small portion of natural hair and add it to the outer strand during the revolution.

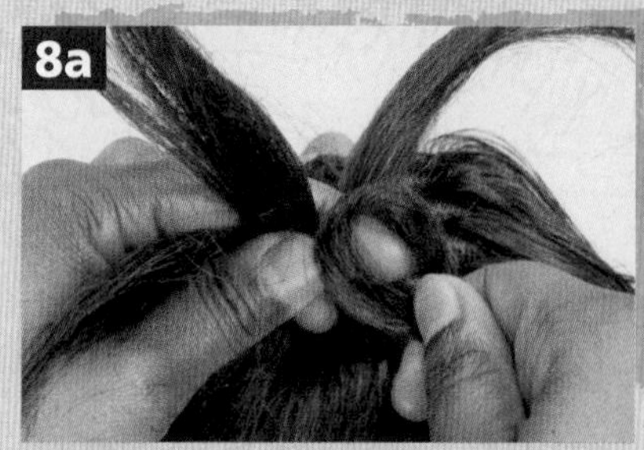

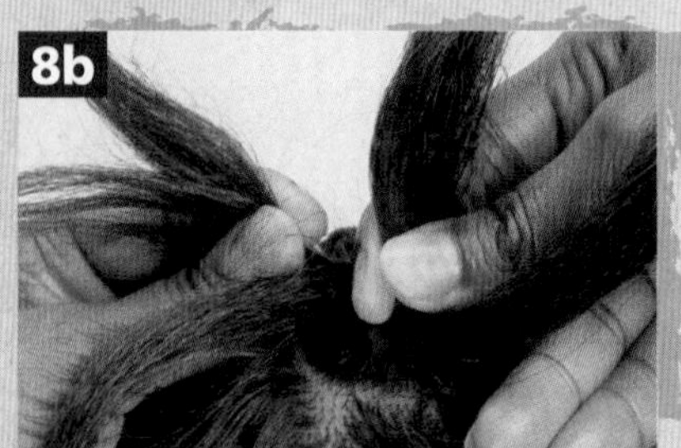

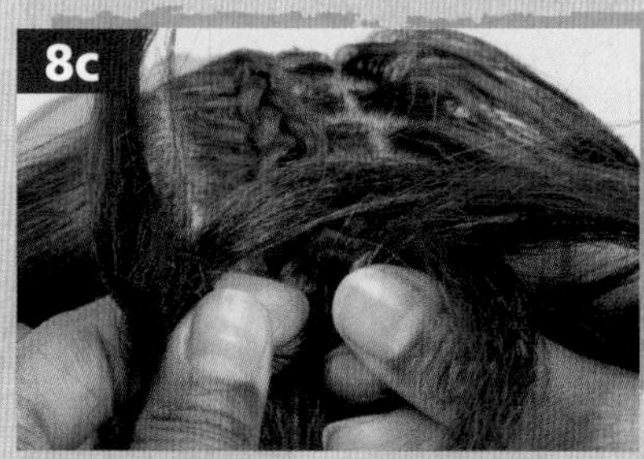

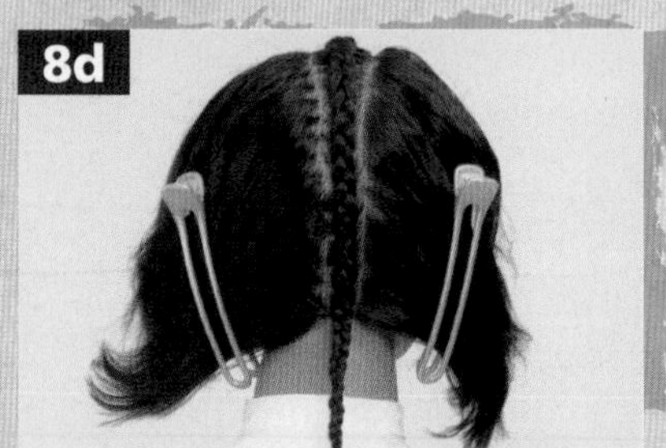

8 After several revolutions and pick-ups of the natural hair, you can introduce small amounts of extension fiber, perhaps 10 to 20 fibers. To avoid bulk or knots, the amount of extension should be proportionately less than the size of the base. Fold the fibers in the middle and tuck the point in between two adjoining strands of natural hair. The folded fibers will form two portions, which are added to the center and outer strands before the next pick-up and revolution. Do not forget to continue picking up natural hair with each revolution in order to execute the cornrow. Work to the end.

9 Repeat the procedure in the same manner until all the hair is braided.

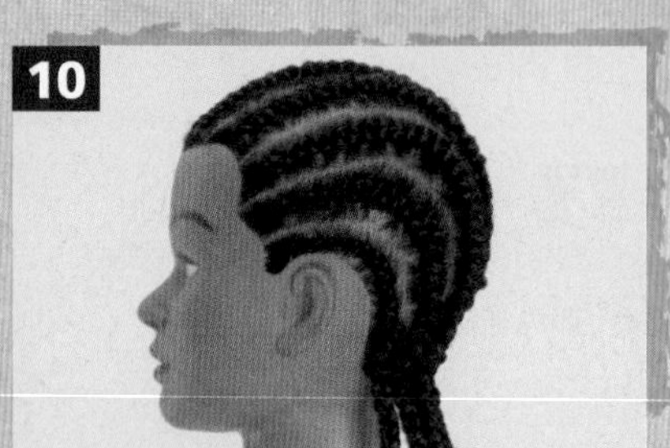

10 Finished look.

Post-Service

- Complete PROCEDURE 15-2 **Post-Service Procedure** SEE PAGE 326

© Milady, a part of Cengage Learning. Photography by Paul Castle, Castle Photography.

Review Questions

1. What is the most effective way to prepare hair for braiding?
2. What are the steps in creating basic cornrows?

Chapter Glossary

cornrows	Also known as *canerows*; narrow rows of visible braids that lie close to the scalp and are created with a three-strand, on-the-scalp braiding technique.
fishtail braid	Simple two-strand braid in which hair is picked up from the sides and added to the strands as they are crossed over each other.
invisible braid	Also known as *inverted braid* or *French braid*; a three-strand braid that is produced with an overhand technique.
locks	Also known as *dreadlocks*; separate networks of curly, textured hair that have been intertwined and meshed together.
natural hairstyling	Hairstyling that uses no chemicals or dyes and does not alter the natural curl or coil pattern of the hair.
overhand technique	A technique in which the first side section goes over the middle one, then the other side section goes over the middle strand.
rope braid	Braid created with two strands that are twisted around each other.
single braids	Also known as *box braids* or *individual braids*; free-hanging braids, with or without extensions, that can be executed using either an underhand or an overhand technique.
twisting	Overlapping two strands to form a candy cane effect.
underhand technique	Also known as *plaiting*; a technique in which the left section goes under the middle strand, then the right section goes under the middle strand.
visible braid	Three-strand braid that is created using an underhand technique.
weaving	Interweaving a weft or faux hair with natural hair.

CHAPTER 19

Wigs and Hair Additions

Chapter Outline

Why Study Wigs and Hair Additions?

Human versus Synthetic Hair

Wigs

Hairpieces

Hair Extensions

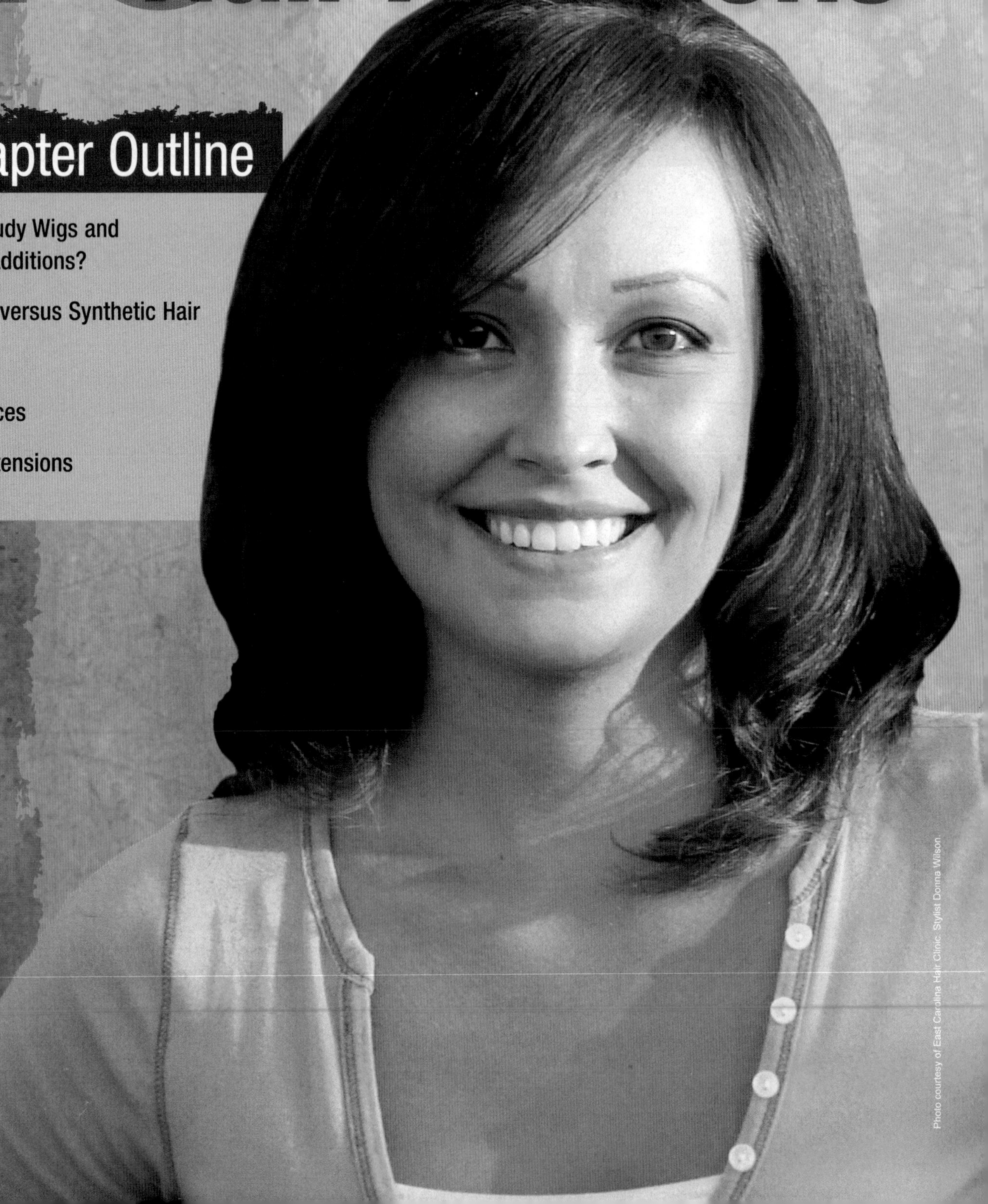

Photo courtesy of East Carolina Hair Clinic. Stylist Donna Wilson

Learning Objectives

After completing this chapter, you will be able to:

- ✓ **LO1** Explain the differences between human hair and synthetic hair.
- ✓ **LO2** Describe the two basic categories of wigs.
- ✓ **LO3** Describe several types of hairpieces and their uses.
- ✓ **LO4** Explain several different methods of attaching hair extensions.

Key Terms

Page number indicates where in the chapter the term is used.

block
pg. 546

bonding
pg. 556

braid-and-sew method
pg. 554

cap wigs
pg. 544

capless wigs (caps)
pg. 544

fallen hair
pg. 544

fusion bonding
pg. 557

hair extensions
pg. 553

hairpiece
pg. 544

hand-tied wigs (hand-knotted wigs)
pg. 545

integration hairpiece
pg. 551

machine-made wigs
pg. 545

semi-hand-tied wigs
pg. 545

toupee
pg. 551

turned hair (Remi hair)
pg. 543

wefts
pg. 544

wig
pg. 544

From the beginning of recorded history, wigs have played an important role in the world of fashion. The ancient Egyptians shaved their heads with bronze razors and wore heavy black wigs to protect themselves from the sun. In ancient Rome, women wore wigs made from the prized blond hair of barbarians captured from the north. In eighteenth-century England, men wore wigs, called *perukes,* to indicate that they were in the army or navy, or engaged in the practice of law.

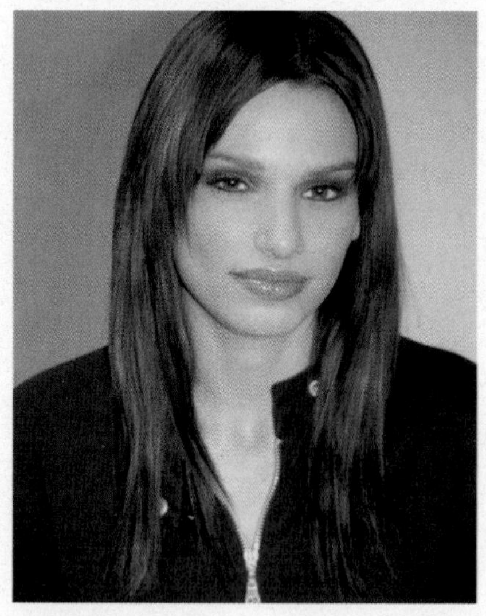

▲ **Figure 19–1**
Client before getting hair extensions.

In today's fashion-conscious world, wigs and hair additions (a category that includes hairpieces and hair extensions) play an incredibly important role. Working with hair additions can be either a simple retail effort or a highly specialized field. Most clients buy wigs off-the-shelf or on the Internet, and rarely have them custom fitted anymore, although there are some opportunities for stylists to cut, color, and care for wigs. Toupees are often custom-made and fitted, using hair-type matches and a perfect mold or exact measurements of the head. Working with toupees takes years of specialized training, which is why much of the toupee business is found in hair replacement centers.

Hair additions range from clip-on hairpieces that salons retail, such as ponytails, chignons, bangs, and even extensions, to elaborately applied extensions in which addition strands are attached individually. In the newest technique, single strands of hair are meticulously hand-tied onto individual strands of the client's hair. In any case, moving beyond clip-in hair additions requires specialized training (**Figures 19–1** and **19–2**).

Each hair extension manufacturer has its own attachment method, and normally you must take the manufacturer's class to be allowed to purchase that manufacturer's extensions. Inventory can be a hefty investment. Even carrying clip-on extensions requires stocking a range of styles and colors, but with every woman in Hollywood wearing them, the demand is high.

The income that hair addition services represent ranges from a small amount for a clip-on ponytail or bang to thousands of dollars for human-hair extensions that are fusion bonded strand-by-strand to the client's hair. Additionally, hair-loss clients and medical clients, such as cancer patients, have very particular needs for hair additions, which you can learn if you choose to specialize.

Because there are many options that require additional training, this chapter gives you a simple, basic overview of the many alternatives available in the world of hair additions. It is a gratifying and lucrative specialty open to any cosmetologist who furthers his or her education.

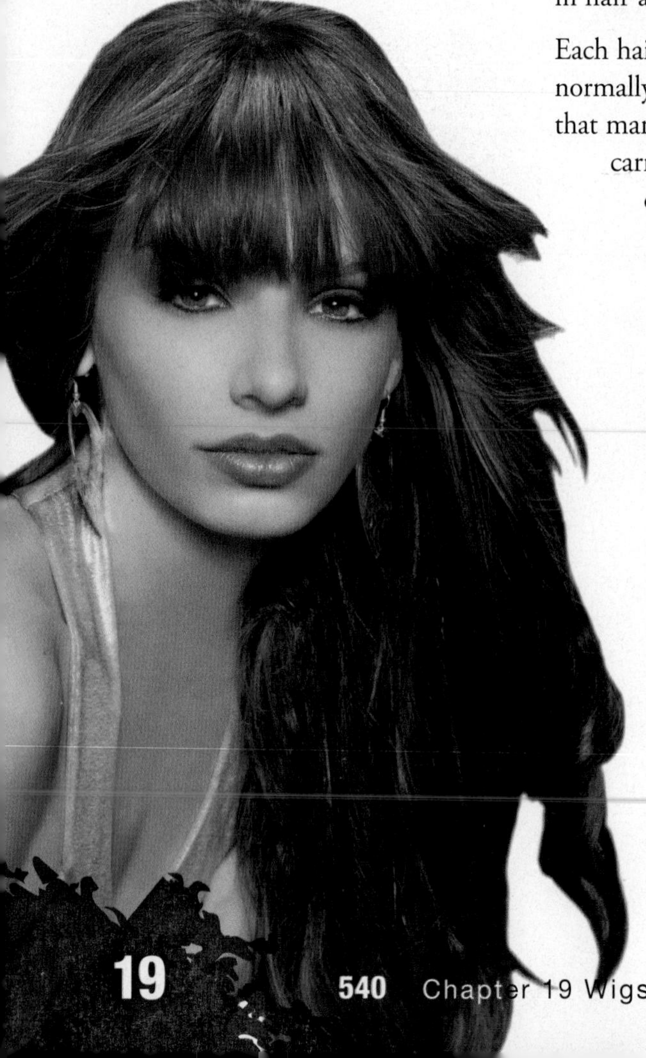

◀ **Figure 19–2**
The same client, transformed with clip-in extensions.

Courtesy of www.GarlandDrake.com. Photography by Dixie Dixon, Makeup by Kay Castro, Hairstyling by Tony Greenleaf, all for Garland Drake.

WHY STUDY WIGS AND HAIR ADDITIONS?

Cosmetologists should study and have a thorough understanding of wigs and hair additions because:

- The market for products and services related to faux hair has expanded to every consumer group, from baby boomers with fine and thinning hair to young trendsetters.
- Hair extensions, additions, and customized wigs can be some of the most lucrative services in the salon.
- Each manufacturer has its own systems, but if you understand the fundamentals, you can easily work with any company on the market.
- The skills you develop will open many doors, from working behind the scenes on Broadway shows to working with celebrities, who today invariably wear faux hair.

did you know?

In 1989 the Cosmetic, Toiletry, and Fragrance Association (CTFA) founded the CTFA Foundation, a charitable organization, and established the Look Good . . . Feel Better program to help cancer patients deal with hair loss. For more information about working with or helping clients with hair loss due to illness, visit the Look Good . . . Feel Better Web site at http://www.lookgoodfeelbetter.org or call 1-800-395-LOOK.

Human versus Synthetic Hair

What is the fastest way to tell if a strand of hair is a synthetic product or real human hair? Pull the strand out of the wig or hairpiece and burn it with a match. Human hair will burn slowly, giving off a distinctive odor. A strand of synthetic fiber, on the other hand, will either ball up and melt, extinguishing itself (a characteristic of a synthetic like Kanekalon®), or it will continue to flame and burn out very quickly (typical of polyester). In either case, it will not give off an odor.

How can you determine whether real hair or synthetic hair is best for your client? Both have advantages and disadvantages.

Advantages of Human Hair

- More realistic appearance.
- Greater durability.
- Same styling and maintenance requirements as natural hair. Human hair can be custom colored and permed to suit the client, and it tolerates heat from a blowdryer, curling iron, or hot rollers (**Figure 19–3**).

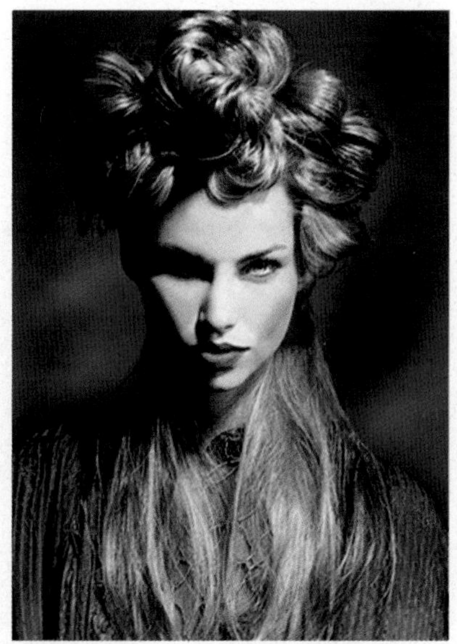

Hair by Vivienne Mackinder, Photograph by Jill Wachter.

▲ **Figure 19–3 Human hair additions can add a dramatic touch.**

Disadvantages of Human Hair

- Human hair reacts to the climate the way that natural hair does. Depending on what type of hair it is, it may frizz or lose its curl in humid weather.
- After shampooing, the hair needs to be reset. This can be a challenge for the client who intends to maintain the hair at home.
- The color will oxidize, meaning that it will fade with exposure to light.

- The hair will break and split if mistreated by harsh brushing, backcombing, or excessive use of heat.

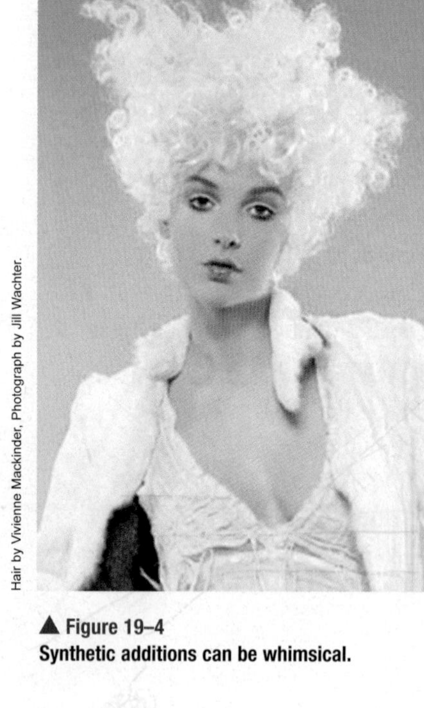

Hair by Vivienne Mackinder, Photograph by Jill Wachter.

▲ **Figure 19–4**
Synthetic additions can be whimsical.

Advantages of Synthetic Hair

- Over the years, the technology used to produce synthetic fibers has greatly improved. Wigs, hairpieces, and extensions made of modacrylic are particularly strong and durable. Top-of-the-line synthetics like Kanekalon®, a modacrylic fiber, simulate protein-rich hair, with a natural, lustrous look and feel. These synthetics are so realistic they can even fool stylists (**Figure 19–4**).
- Synthetic hair is a great value. Not only is it very realistic, but it is less expensive than human hair. Both style and texture are set into the hair. Ready-to-wear synthetic hair is very easy for the client to maintain at home. Shampooing in cold water will not change the style, nor will exposure to extreme humidity.
- Most synthetic wigs, hairpieces, and extensions are cut according to the latest styles with the cut, color, and texture already set, so all that is required is some detailing, custom trimming, or attachment of the extensions.
- The colors are limitless, ranging from natural to wild fantasy shades. Price is a factor when it comes to color and texture. The cheaper synthetic wigs and hair additions tend to be more solid in color (less tone-on-tone) and the fiber is coarser (polyester based). The higher-end products are a mix of many shades, containing highlights and lowlights for a natural effect.
- Synthetic colors will not fade or oxidize, even when exposed to long periods in the sun.

Disadvantages of Synthetic Hair

- Synthetic hair cannot be exposed to extreme heat (curling irons, hot rollers, or the high heat of blowdryers). However, some synthetic hair is coated with a protein base and can tolerate low heat (lower than 390 degrees Fahrenheit or 200 degrees Celsius). Always check with the manufacturer and perform a test strand on a small section of the actual synthetic piece.
- Coloring synthetic fibers is not recommended because traditional haircolor will not work on them.
- Sometimes synthetic hair is so shiny that it may not look natural. Also, if the hair is thick, it will look unnatural on a fine-haired client.
- Price often has a lot to do with how natural synthetic hair looks. In other words, the most natural-looking synthetic pieces can be expensive. ☑ **LO1**

© Mayer George Vladimirovich, 2010; used under license from Shutterstock.com.

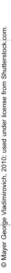

Quality and Cost

There are pros and cons for both human hair and synthetic hair. The bottom line in both cases is that you get what you pay for.

Ultimately, your success in working with any hair addition will be determined by the quality of the product itself. Do not be fooled by imitations. Inexpensive wigs, hairpieces, and extensions may be great for fun moments or to practice cutting on, but in other situations they can look tacky and unattractive.

The more expensive wigs, hairpieces, and extensions are those made of human hair. Pricing varies as follows:

- European hair is at the top of the line. Virgin hair is the most costly; color-treated hair is second in cost.
- Hair from India and Asia, the two regions that provide most of the human hair commercially available, are next in cost. Indian hair is usually available in lengths from 12 inches to 16 inches. Asian hair is available in lengths of 12 inches to 28 inches. Indian hair is usually wavy; Asian hair is usually straight.
- Human hair mixed with animal hair is next in expense. The animal hair may be angora, horse, yak, or sheep. Yak hair is taken from the animal's belly and is the purest of whites. Its natural color lends itself to adding fantasy colors, which attract teenagers. Mixed-hair products are often used in theatrical or fashion settings.
- Human hair mixed with synthetic hair finishes the list. The mix is often half human hair and half synthetic hair. These wigs and hairpieces blend the advantages and disadvantages of both, and can be a good option if chosen in the best color and texture for the client.

There are several important questions to ask when selecting a hair addition for the client:

- Is the addition made of human hair, animal hair, a mix of both, or is it synthetic or a synthetic blend?
- Is the hair colored, or in its natural state (virgin hair)?
- If the hair is human hair, is it graded in terms of strength, elasticity, and porosity?
- Is the cuticle intact? Cuticle-intact hair is more expensive, because the hair has been turned. **Turned hair,** also known as **Remi hair,** is hair in which the root end of every single strand is sewn into the base, so that the cuticles of all hair strands move in the same direction: down. The hair is in better condition, and it is much easier to work with because it doesn't tangle easily. Turning is a tedious, time-consuming process that increases the cost of the hair addition.

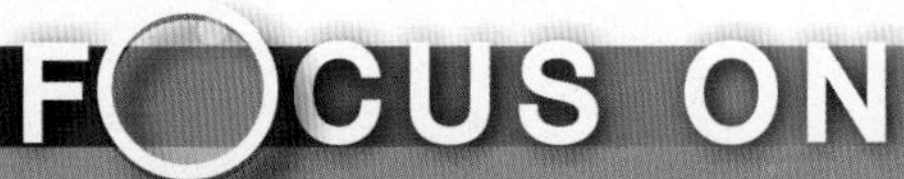

COST

To the average consumer, the deals at the local beauty supply store may look good. But that apparent deal could be a mix of animal hair and human hair, and one washing could mat the wig into a big ball. The most realistic hair additions, such as those used in film work, cost thousands of dollars. Your client will not necessarily need something of this grade, but you must still pay attention to quality. As a professional, you must educate your client and recommend only well-made products. Remember, when you recommend a product, you put your reputation on the line.

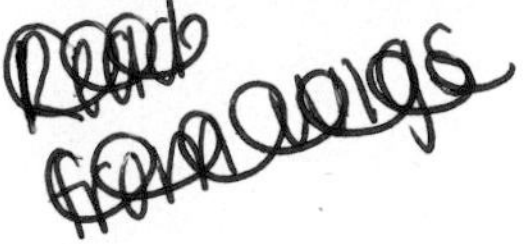

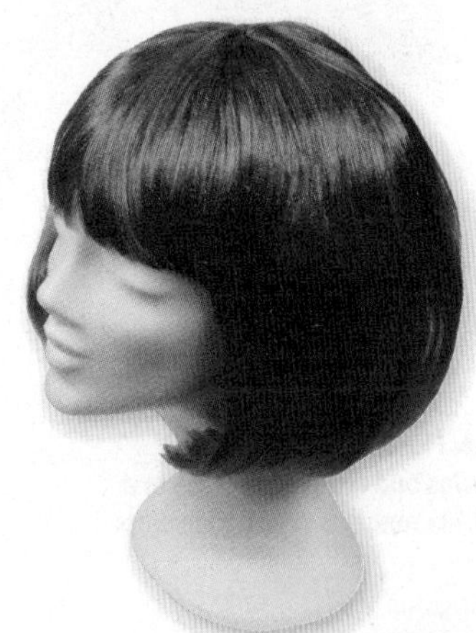

© Alena Dvorakova, 2010; used under license from iStockphoto.com.

- Is it **fallen hair** (the opposite of Remi hair), hair that has been shed from the head and gathered from a hairbrush, as opposed to hair that has been cut? Fallen hair is not turned, so the cuticles of the strands will move in different directions. This makes it tangle. In what is called Remi refined hair, the cuticle is partially removed, so that it will not lock and mat. This hair tends to be less expensive than Remi hair.
- Is the hair tangle-free? If the cuticle has been removed, this often means you cannot condition the hair, because it will tend to mat.
- What is the condition of the hair? Has it been bleached? Can it be colored? Has it been colored with metallic dye?
- Will the hair match the client's hair? Is it similar in type and texture? Is the color-match close enough?
- Can the hair be permed?
- If the client is going to maintain her hair at home, will the hair addition last a reasonable amount of time? (Additions should last four to six months in continual use.)

Wigs

A **wig** can be defined as an artificial covering for the head consisting of a network of interwoven hair. When a client wears a wig, the client's hair is completely concealed (100 percent coverage). If a hair addition does not fully cover the head, it is either a **hairpiece,** which is a small wig used to cover the top or crown of the head, or a hair attachment of some sort (**Figure 19–5**).

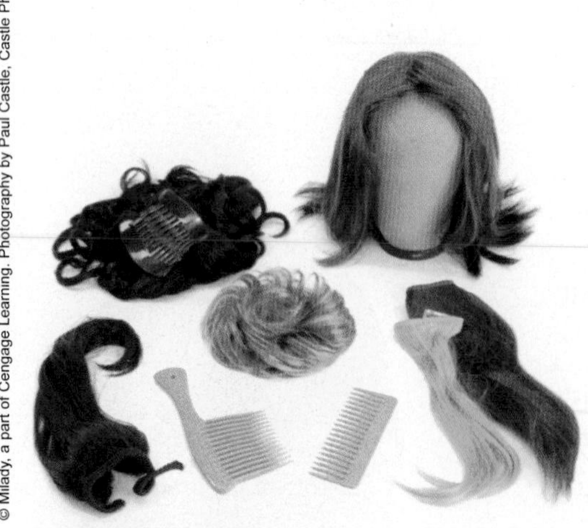

© Milady, a part of Cengage Learning. Photography by Paul Castle, Castle Photography.

▲ **Figure 19–5**
Wigs and hairpieces come in a wide range of styles and colors.

Types of Wigs

There are two basic categories of wigs: cap and capless.

Cap wigs are constructed with an elasticized, mesh-fiber base to which the hair is attached. They are made in several sizes and require special fittings. More often than not, cap wigs are hand-knotted. The front edge of a cap wig is made of a material that resembles the client's scalp, along with a lace extension and a wire support that is used at the temples for a snug, secure fit. Hair is hand-tied under the net (under-knotted) to conceal the cap edge. The side and back edges contain wire supports, elastic, and hooks for a secure fit. Latex molded cap wigs are also available; these are prostheses for clients with special needs.

Capless wigs, also known as **caps**, are machine-made from human or artificial hair. The hair is woven into **wefts,** which are long strips of hair with a threaded edge. Rows of wefts are sewn to elastic strips in a circular pattern to fit the head shape. Capless wigs are more popular than cap wigs as they are ready-to-wear and less expensive.

The capless wig is a frame of connected wefts with open areas. To understand the construction of a capless wig, compare a nylon stocking to a fishnet stocking: one has a closed framework (the cap wig), and the other is open (capless). Due to their construction and airiness, capless wigs are extremely light and comfortable to wear (**Figure 19–6**).

In general, capless wigs are healthier, because they allow the scalp to breathe and because they prevent excess perspiration. A cap wig is best for clients with extremely thin hair and for clients with no hair because capless wigs will allow a bald scalp to show through. There are many new innovations that make wigs more comfortable and practical than ever, like lace front wigs, which have an incredibly natural-looking hairline. Today's wigs are so well designed and fashionable that many are bought off-the-shelf for immediate wear. ☑ **LO2**

FOCUS ON

CLIENT CARE

Although many clients wear wigs for fun and versatility, others have experienced hair loss due to a serious illness or treatments such as chemotherapy. Be attuned to your client's emotional state about his or her well-being, and be sensitive to the possibility that some clients will need a private consultation.

Methods of Construction

- **Hand-tied wigs,** also known as **hand-knotted wigs**, are made by inserting individual strands of hair into mesh foundations and knotting them with a needle. Hand-tying is done particularly around the front hairline and at the top of the head. These wigs have a natural, realistic look and are wonderful for styling. The hand-tied method most closely resembles actual human hair growth, with flexibility at the roots. There is no definite direction to the hair, and it can be combed in almost any direction.
- **Semi-hand-tied wigs** are constructed with a combination of synthetic hair and hand-tied human hair. Reasonably priced, they offer a natural appearance and good durability.
- **Machine-made wigs,** the least expensive option, are made by feeding wefts through a sewing machine, then stitching them together to form the base and shape of the wig. They have the disadvantage of the wefting direction, which restricts styling options. Another favorable characteristic of these wigs is their bounce-back quality; even after shampooing, the style returns.

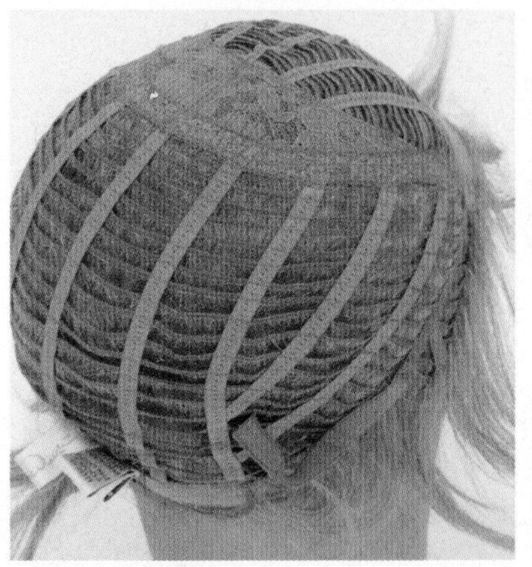

© Milady, a part of Cengage Learning. Photography by Paul Castle, Castle Photography.

▲ **Figure 19–6**
A capless wig.

It is important to be aware of the artificial growth patterns of a wig. Wig construction will determine the direction in which you style the hair. The most flexible and versatile of all patterns is the hand-tied wig. Machine-made wigs are sewn in a specific direction, offering no versatility. If the client likes the style, this is a good thing; if not, the wig is not right for the client.

Taking Wig Measurements

In recent years, working with wigs has become a specialty among salon professionals. As a result, salons have become less and less likely to carry an inventory of wigs, or even to carry a wig catalogue. However, it is advantageous to have a basic understanding of wigs. Here is an overview: The creation of a custom-made wig begins with taking the client's measurements. Use a soft tape measure, keeping it close to the head without pressure. Always keep a written record of the client's head measurements, and forward a copy to the wig dealer or manufacturer. Each manufacturer has its own form to fill out, which notes the measurements required. Most manufacturers ask for precise specifications of hair shade, quality of hair, length of hair, and type of hair part and pattern. Higher-end companies ask you to include a sample of the client's hair with the order.

If the wig is ready-to-wear, no measuring will be needed because it can be adjusted by tightening or loosening the straps or the elastic in the nape. Ready-to-wear wigs are more common today. But still, many wigs need to be adjusted to the head and custom styled or trimmed to suit the client.

Blocking the Wig

A **block** is a head-shaped form, usually made of canvas-covered cork or Styrofoam, on which the wig is secured for fitting, coloring, and sometimes styling. Canvas blocks are available in six sizes, from 20 inches (50 centimeters) to 22 inches (56.25 centimeters). The block is best attached to your work area with a swivel clamp, which allows for greater control. However, today most wigs are cut and finished while on the client, and then cleaned and stored on a drying rack. A block is best used for practicing on a wig.

Putting on the Wig

One of the most important steps in the wig service is instructing the client on how to put on the wig. Start by educating the client on the correct method for preparing her hair. The client's skill at securing her hair under the wig cap and making it flat and even will determine how well the wig sits on her head. If the wig does not fit properly—for instance if it is too large and does not have tightening straps or elastic—you can create a small fold or tuck and sew the wig along the inside to create a seam. To shorten the wig from front to nape and remove bulk, create a horizontal tuck or fold across the back. To remove width at the back, create a vertical tuck and sew it in place. Keep in mind that sewing the wig to create a customized fit is a highly specialized art.

Cutting Wigs

When cutting a wig, generally your goal is to make the hair look more realistic. As you know, natural hair has many lengths. Even when hair is cut to one length, internally there are various stages of hair growth. Hair that is one-month old and hair that is years-old exist on the same head. The stylist should try to achieve this natural look in the wig. The most effective way to do this is to taper the ends when cutting the wig. The more solid the shape, the more unnatural the hair will look.

© Vika Valter, 2010; used under license from iStockphoto.com.

When cutting and trimming wigs, you can follow the basic methods of haircutting—blunt, layered, and graduated—using the same sectioning and elevations as on a real head of hair. Or you may do what many top stylists prefer to do, which is to cut free-form on dry hair. The wig should be placed on the block for cutting, but the comb out and finishing should be done on the client's head.

If you use free-form cutting, always work toward the weight. Vertical sections create lightness. Diagonal sections create a rounder beveled edge. Horizontal sections build heavier weight (**Figures 19–7** to **19–9**).

To use this visual approach, begin by cutting a small section and observe how the hair falls. Your next step will be based on how the hair responds.

Draw a diagram of the silhouette or have handy a photo image for reference. These will work as a kind of blueprint for you to follow.

Free-form cutting is usually done on dry hair, which allows you to see more easily how the hair will fall. When the hair is wet, it can be hard to judge how the hair will fall.

To practice wig cutting, buy two inexpensive ready-to-wear wigs in the same style. Take a photo for reference purposes. Draw a diagram of the sections, indicating how you are going to cut the wigs. This way, you can rehearse your plan before even picking up the shears.

Begin your practice with the shadow cut. Trim the wigs following the original design that has been precut into the wig, but cut the first wig wet. Then air-dry it and evaluate the style. Trim the second wig, following the same style, but this time cut it dry. Take photos of both results, and evaluate the looks you have achieved with both dry and wet cutting.

You will discover that the wet cutting method was more controlled and technical, while the dry cutting method was freer and more abstract. Often, the more abstract method results in a cut that looks more realistic.

Repeat the above exercise with a razor, thinning shears, and standard haircutting shears using the tapering method only. Compare the results.

Styling the Wig

The important thing to remember when you are styling a wig is that you must never lose sight of the big picture. Some stylists get overly involved in the wig, as if it is a creation that exists apart from the client. This is the wrong approach. A great stylist works with the total person, not just the head. When you have finished styling the wig, step back and ask the client to stand up and walk around so that you can check for balance and proportion and make corrections accordingly.

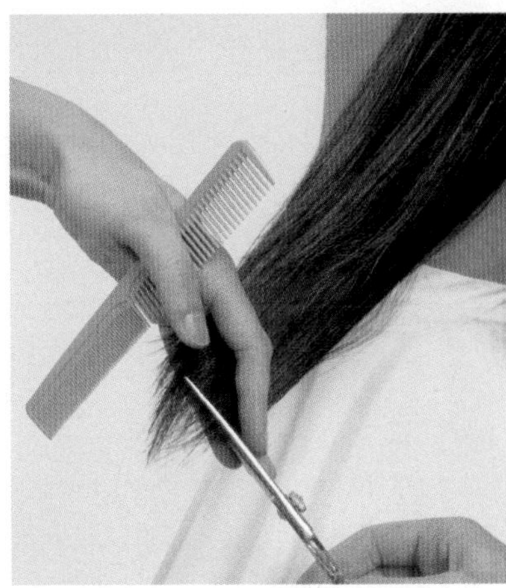

▲ **Figure 19–7**
Free-form cutting with vertical sections.

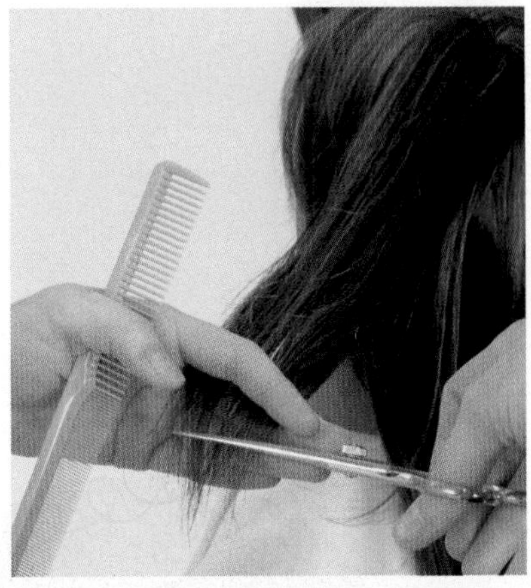

▲ **Figure 19–8**
Free-form cutting with diagonal sections.

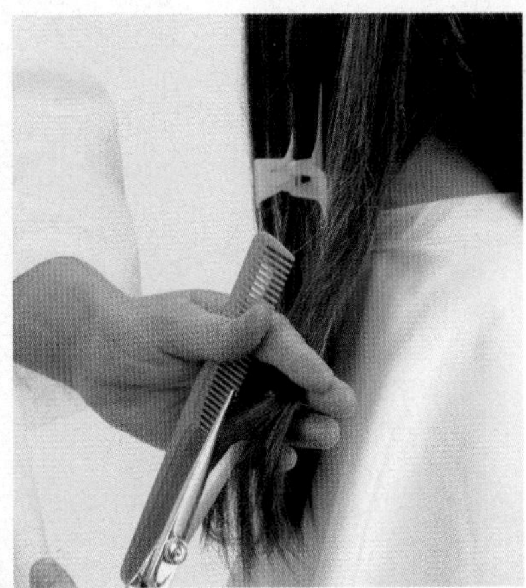

▲ **Figure 19–9**
Free-form cutting with horizontal sections.

© Milady, a part of Cengage Learning. Photography by Paul Castle, Castle Photography.

Most of the hair you will be working with is chemically treated, so it needs to be handled gently. You will achieve the best styling results by following these guidelines:

- When using heat on human hair, always set the styling tool on low.
- Treat the hair gently; do not pull it or otherwise treat it carelessly.
- Traditionally, brushes made with natural boar bristles have been regarded as best for use on human hair. The brush's soft bristles are preferable to sharp-edged synthetic bristles, which can damage hair. Today, however, you will find many synthetic brushes that have smooth, rounded plastic teeth, more like combs, and they are excellent and economical choices. Keep in mind that the key with any brush or comb is to be gentle because hair can be easily damaged.

Use a block when necessary for coloring, perming, setting, and basic cut outlining. The comb-out and finishing touches for most modern cuts should be completed on the client's head in order to achieve proper balance and personalization (**Figure 19–10**).

Remember that most clients come into the salon looking for a natural look. Making a wig look believable is very challenging, and to do it well is truly an art form. The areas that must appear the most convincing are the crown, the part, and the hairline. Sometimes, crowns and parts look more natural when they are flat to the head; other times a more natural look is attained by adding volume to these areas. This will be determined by the style. A general rule is to follow the direction of the knotting and weave, as preset by the wig maker. If you fight the direction, the results may look odd.

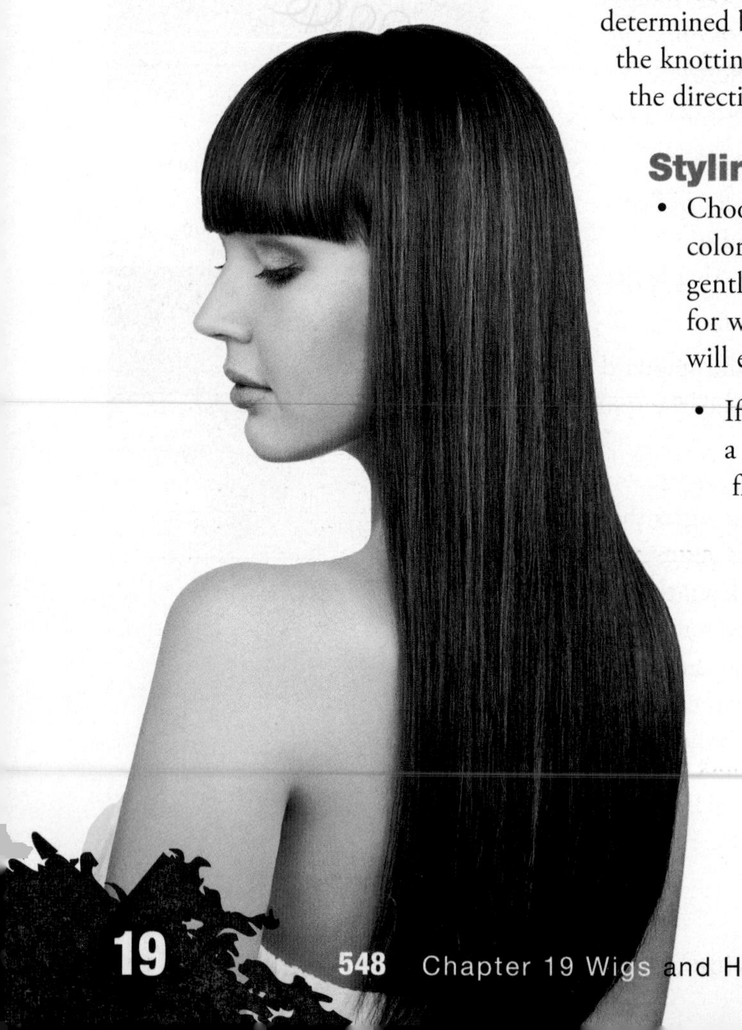

▼ Figure 19–10
A natural-looking style.

© Ipatov, 2010; used under license from Shutterstock.com.

Styling Tips for the Hairline

- Choose styling products that have been formulated for color-treated hair. These will work the best, and they are gentlest to human hair. There are also specialized products for wigs. Just remember that whatever you put into the hair will eventually have to be shampooed out.
- If the wig does not have a natural-looking hairline or a lace front, backcomb gently around the hairline. The fluffy effect softens the hairline.
- Release the client's hair around the hairline, and cut and blend it into the wig hair.
- The best test to gauge how realistic the wig looks is to use the wind test. This test simulates the wind blowing the client's hair away from her face. Gently blow around the client's face with a blowdryer set at cool and low. Observe how the hairline looks. Does it seem realistic? If so, point out the results to the

client, who may be feeling insecure about whether the wig looks natural enough (**Figure 19–11**).

When styling a wig, do not try to make it look perfect. Little imperfections help achieve a realistic look. Use your hands rather than a brush for a more natural look (**Figure 19–12**). Do not plaster the hair down, because it will look artificial.

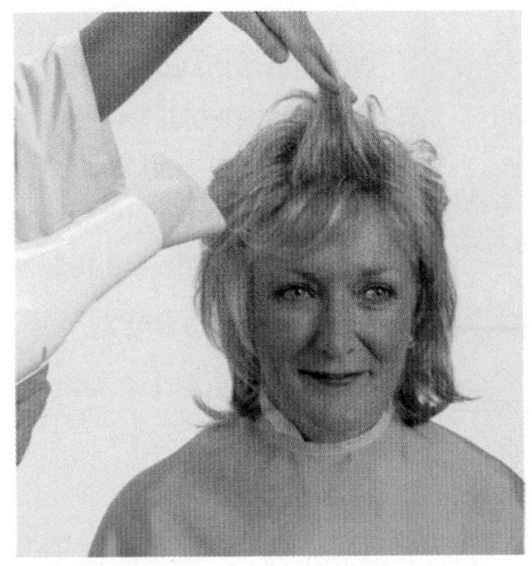

▲ Figure 19–11
The wind test.

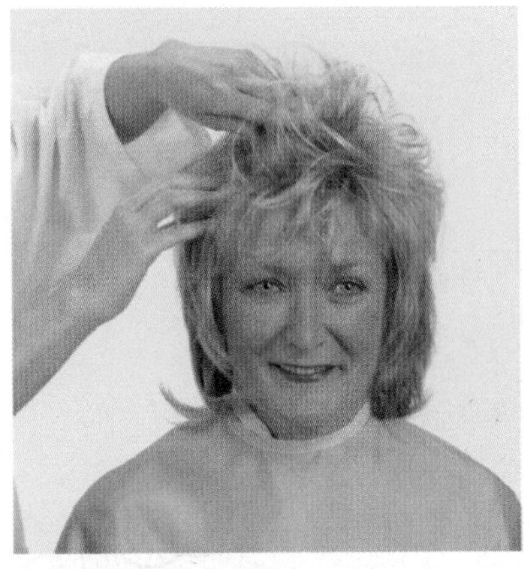

▲ Figure 19–12
Style with the fingers for a natural look.

Cleaning the Wig

Clients who bought off-the-shelf wigs may bring them to a salon for cleaning, reshaping, and styling. To clean any wig, always follow the manufacturer's instructions. If shampooing is recommended, use a gentle shampoo, such as one you would use for color-treated hair, or use shampoo specially developed for wigs. Avoid any harsh shampoos with a sulfur base, such as dandruff shampoos. Soak, then gently squeeze the wig and use a drying rack for drying. If you are cleaning a wig made of human hair, you should also condition it.

Coloring Wigs and Hair Additions

All synthetic haircolors used for wigs and hairpieces are standardized according to the 70 colors on the haircolor ring used by wig and hairpiece manufacturers. The colors range from black to pale blond. Because most commercially available hair originates in either India or China, the most common natural color level is 1, or black. It is very difficult to lift level 1 to level 10. (See Chapter 21, Haircoloring, for a discussion of hair color levels.) At the other end of the spectrum is white yak hair, which is an excellent base for adding color. Yak hair is especially good to use with fantasy colors that appeal to some younger clients.

If you are going to custom color the hair, use hair that has been decolorized (bleached) through the lifting process, not with metallic dyes. Be sure to check with the manufacturer.

The principles that guide the coloring of natural hair also apply to the art of coloring wigs and hair extensions. As in all disciplines, you must first learn the rules before you break them. Good colorists are not afraid to make mistakes, because they have worked hard to learn the basics and know how to correct mistakes.

When coloring a wig, first check to see if the cuticle is intact. Hair in which the cuticle is absent is very porous and will react to color in an extreme manner. Always strand-test the hair prior to a full-color application. Use semipermanent, demipermanent, glaze, rinse, or color mousse products. Use permanent haircolor on human hair wigs unless the hair is porous, in which case semipermanent color is the better choice. (See Chapter 21, Haircoloring, for more detail.)

When coloring a human-hair wig or hair addition, conduct regular color checks every five to ten minutes. Remember that the hair you are working on did not come from one head, but from many different

CAUTION

Harsh handling will damage wig hair, and—unlike hair on the human head—wig hair will not grow back. If you treat a wig carelessly, it will have a short life, so remember to be gentle.

© Milady, a part of Cengage Learning. Photography by Paul Castle, Castle Photography.

FYI

Working with wigs and toupees requires special tools, many of which are sold by the wig manufacturers. Special tools needed for wigs include the following:

- Boar-Bristle Brush
- Cloth Measuring Tape
- Duckbill Clips
- Hair and Bobby Pins
- Neck Strip
- Specialized Needle and Thread
- Specialized Shampoos and Conditioners for Wigs
- T-shaped Pins
- Wig Block
- Wig Caps

Special tools needed for toupees include the following:

- Block
- Clips
- Specialized Adhesive
- Specialized Needle and Thread
- Specialized Shampoos and Conditioners
- Specialized Tape
- T-shaped Pins

heads, so it may be unpredictable. Often, it is easier to color the client's hair to match a hair addition than to color the addition itself.

Perming Wigs and Hair Additions

If you want to perm human hair to match the client's natural wave pattern, you need to know how the hair was colored. Was it decolorized (bleached) or dyed with metallic dye? Do not perm hair that has been colored with a metallic dye.

The permanent wave must be performed with the hair additions off the client's head. For wigs and hairpieces, cover the head form with plastic to protect it from the chemical solutions, pin the wig securely to the head form, and perm as you would a natural head of hair. Perm extensions as they lie flat. (See Chapter 20, Chemical Texture Services, for perming procedures.)

Hairpieces

In eighteenth-century France, women wore towering hairdos complete with extensions and various apparatuses such as springs to adjust the height. Some of these coiffures were 3-feet high and had elaborate visual elements worked into them such as model ships or gardens. These styles were often untouched for weeks at a time. The bad news is that they sometimes attracted vermin. The moral of this story is that sometimes it is best not to get swept up in current trends or passing fashions. Always be aware of the strength of classic design. Keep it simple, remembering that less is more, and try not to let yourself get carried away.

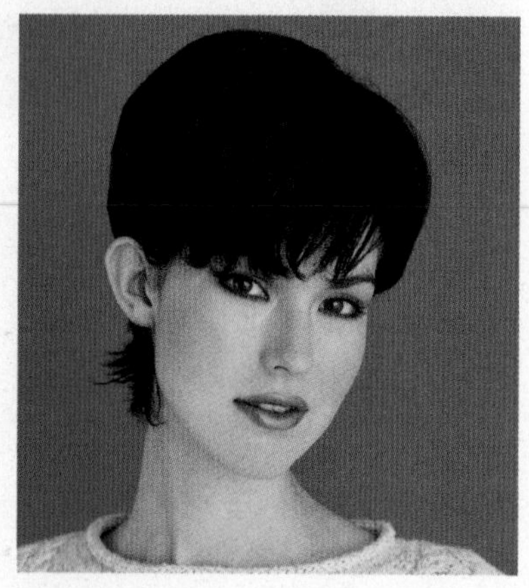

Photography from the Gabor Collection, supplied by Eva Gabor International.

▲ **Figure 19–13**
Hairpieces can look very natural.

Hairpieces are an important area of hair additions (**Figure 19–13**). They sit on top of the client's head, covering a portion of it, or clip onto another area, such as the nape. They are usually attached by temporary methods. (They are not worn during sleep.) Some, like wiglets that conceal a thinning top, can also be attached with a braid-and-sew technique.

There are many different types of hairpieces, including integration pieces (which are attached with a semipermanent method), toupees (which can be complex and challenging to work with), and fashion hairpieces. Fashion hairpieces include falls, half wigs (falls on a cap that attaches with combs an inch or so behind the hairline and can be used with a headband or with the natural hair combed straight back to conceal the attachment site), wiglets, chignons, bandeaus (falls with a headband attached), cascades (clip-on top curls), ponytails, bangs, and fillers (which add volume to fine hair). Many of the newest fashion hairpieces simply clip on with pressure-sensitive clips, claw clips, or combs. Here, only the major types are covered, to give you a general overview. Working with hair additions and hair replacement systems is a specialized art, and many manufacturers have their own attachment systems and training.

The client's hair can be prepared in a number of ways before the hairpiece is attached. It can be tied into a ponytail or bun or twisted into a French twist. It can be blended with the hairpiece or serve as a base for it.

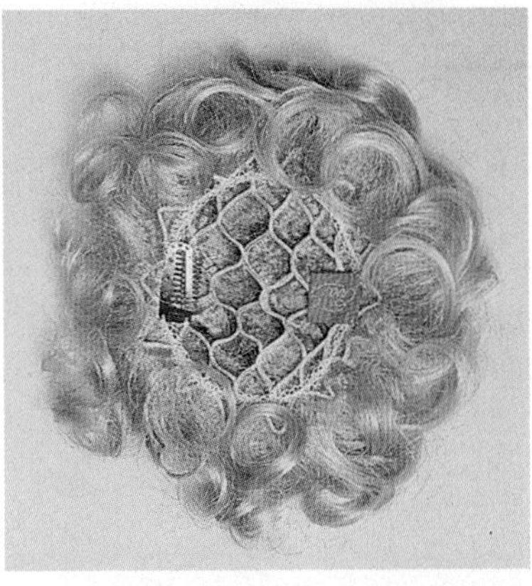

▲ Figure 19–14
Integration hairpiece.

Integration Hairpieces

An **integration hairpiece** is a hairpiece that has openings in the base, through which the client's own hair is pulled to blend with the (natural or synthetic) hair of the hairpiece. These hairpieces are very lightweight, natural-looking products that add length and volume to the client's hair. If your client is wearing hair extensions and would like a change, the integration hairpiece can be a good alternative. It is also recommended for clients with thinning hair, but not for those with total hair loss, as the scalp is likely to show through (**Figures 19–14** and **19–15**).

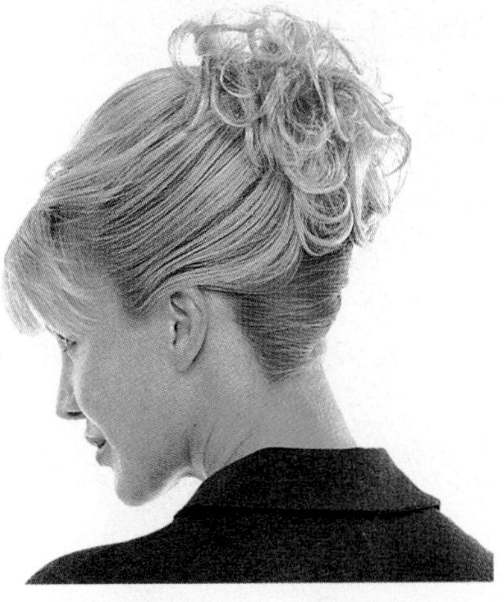

▲ Figure 19–15
An integration hairpiece is easy to wear.

Toupees

While men usually are the clients for toupees, women can also wear these hairpieces. A **toupee** is a small wig used to cover the top and crown of the head. The fine-net base is usually the most appropriate material for the client with severe hair loss. There are two ways to attach toupees: temporary (tape or clips) or semipermanent (tracks, adhesive, or sewing).

Most wearers of toupees prize the confidence gained from wearing an authentic-looking hairpiece and are prepared to pay a high price for it. The best toupees are custom designed. The top manufacturers offer in-depth instruction for those interested in learning this specialty service (**Figures 19–16** and **19–17**).

Fashion Hairpieces

Fashion hairpieces are a great salon product for special occasions or for use as fashion accessories. They include ponytails, chignons, cascades, streaks, bangs, falls/half wigs, and clip-in hair extensions.

These hairpieces vary in size and usually are constructed on a stiff net base. They are attached, temporarily, with hairpins, clips, combs, bobby pins, or elastic. Three of these attachment methods are illustrated here.

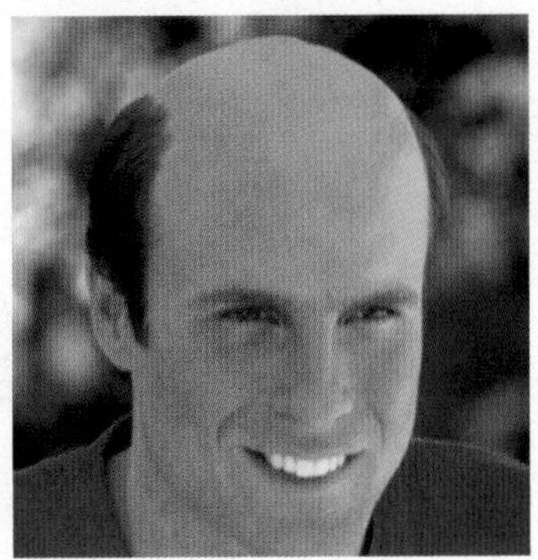

▲ Figure 19–16
Male hair-enhancement client.

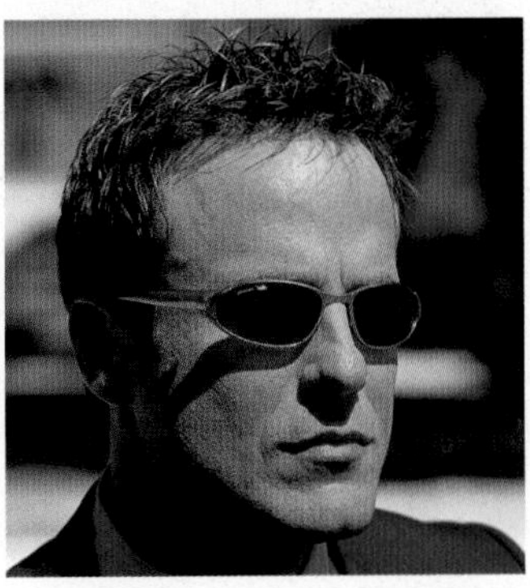

▲ Figure 19–17
The same client fitted with a toupee.

Photography from the Gabor Collection, supplied by Eva Gabor International.

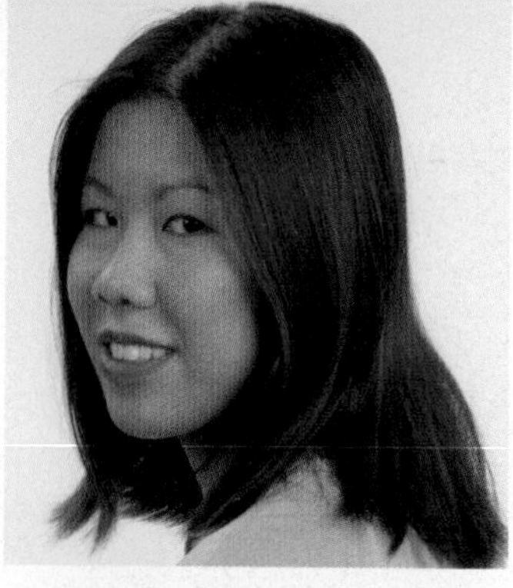

▲ **Figure 19–18**
Client before fitting with a wraparound ponytail.

- The wraparound ponytail is a long length of wefted hair that covers 10 to 20 percent of the head. It is used as a simple ponytail or in chignons. It is particularly useful for the client who can just get her own hair into a ponytail (**Figures 19–18** to **19–22**).
- A cascade of curls is attached with combs (**Figures 19–23** to **19–27**).
- A hair wrap is mounted on an elastic loop. It is further secured to the client's own hair with hairpins (**Figures 19–28** to **Figure 19–31**). ☑ **LO3**

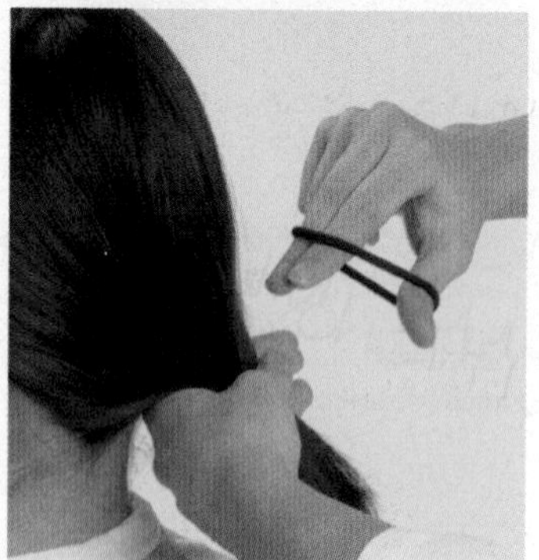

▲ **Figure 19–19**
Client's own ponytail.

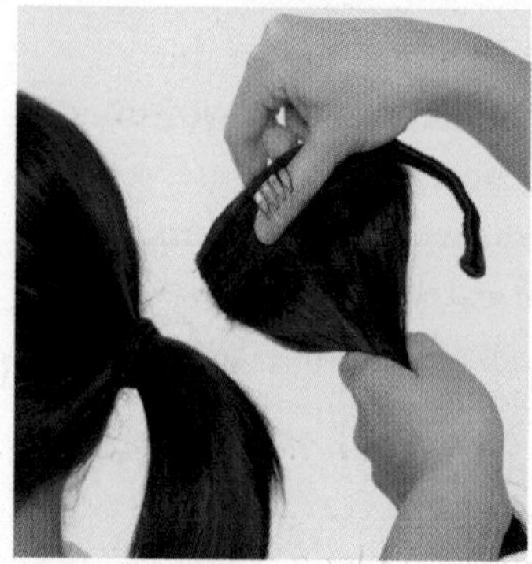

▲ **Figure 19–20**
Attaching the hairpiece.

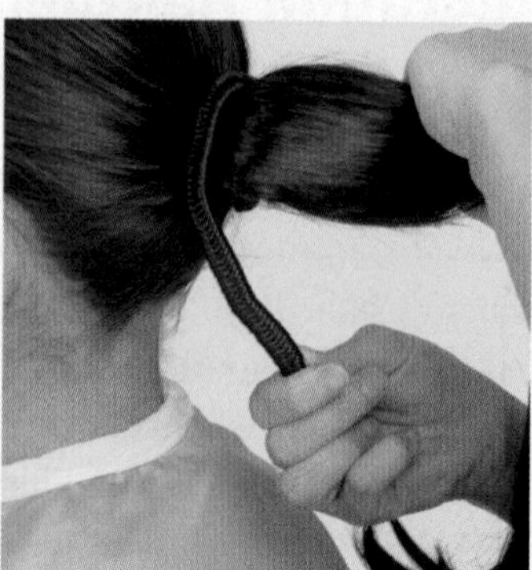

▲ **Figure 19–21**
Wrapping the band around the ponytail base.

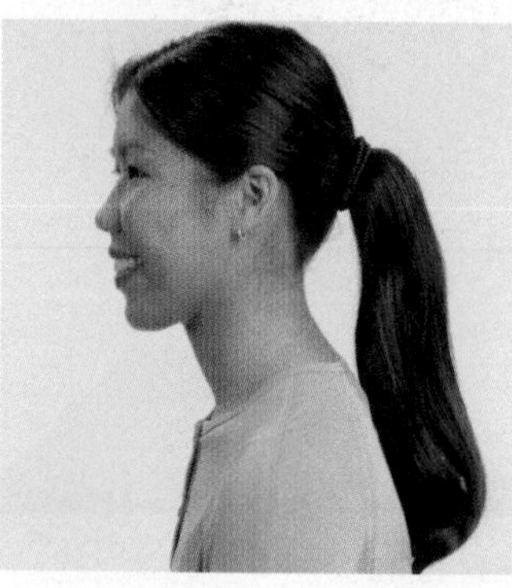

▲ **Figure 19–22**
Same client with a new, much longer ponytail.

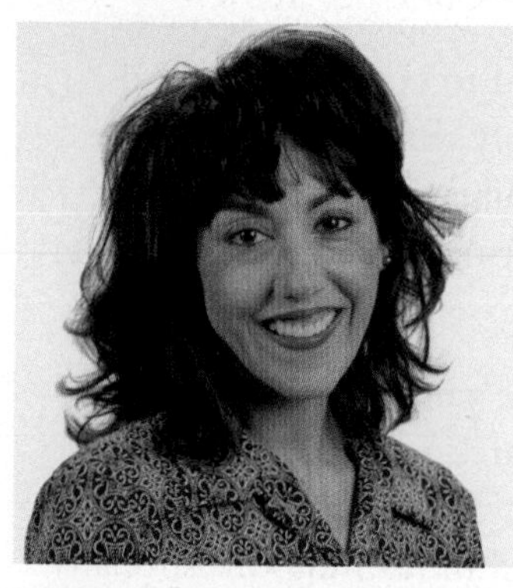

▲ **Figure 19–23**
Client before fitting with comb-attached curls.

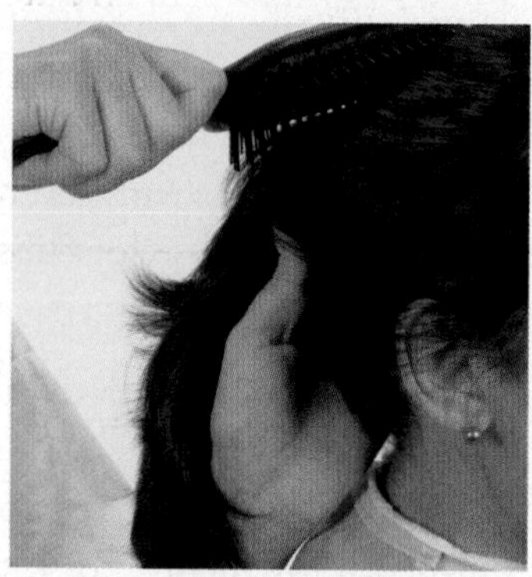

▲ **Figure 19–24**
Brushing the client's hair into a ponytail.

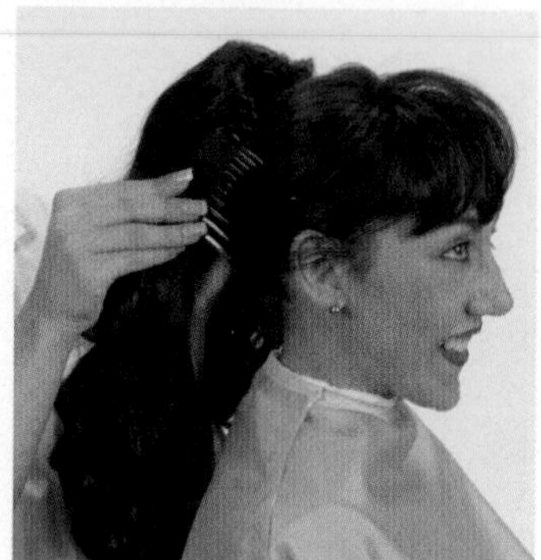

▲ **Figure 19–25**
Attaching the combs.

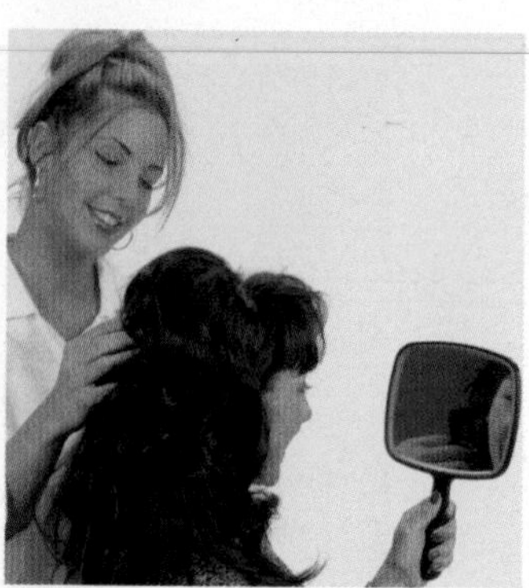

▲ **Figure 19–26**
Adjusting the hairpiece.

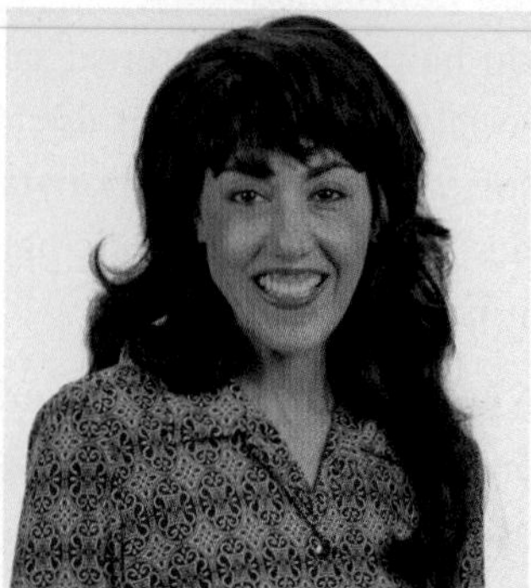

▲ **Figure 19–27**
Cascade of curls.

© Milady, a part of Cengage Learning. Photography by Paul Castle, Castle Photography.

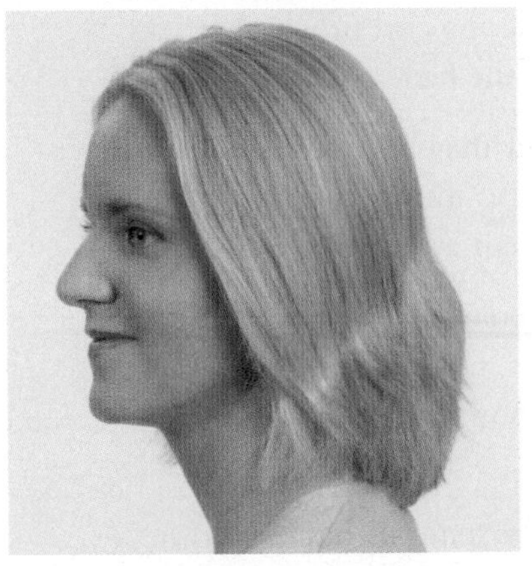

▲ Figure 19–28
Client before fitting with a hair wrap.

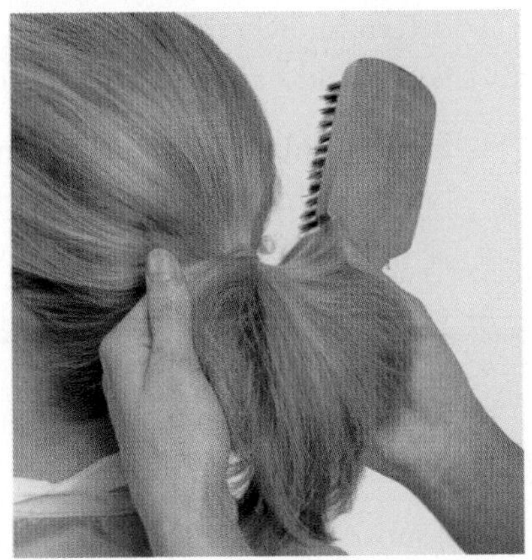

▲ Figure 19–29
Brushing client's hair into a ponytail.

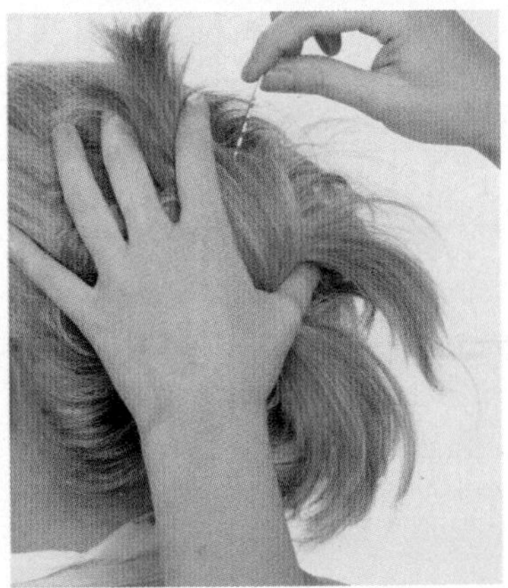

▲ Figure 19–30
Securing the hairpiece with hairpins.

Hair Extensions

Hair extensions are hair additions that are secured to the base of the client's natural hair in order to add length, volume, texture, or color. Extensions can be human hair, synthetic hair, or a blend of the two. They are either wefts of hair or strands (small bundles of hair); the latter are attached one-by-one and are usually pre-bonded or keratin-tipped. Unless they are clip-in extensions, they are applied with semipermanent attachment methods.

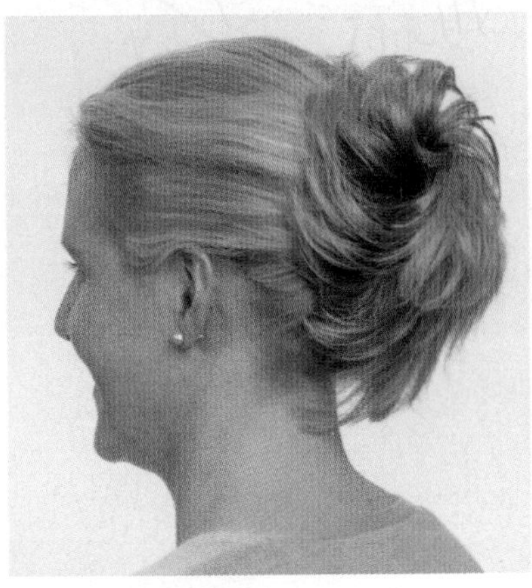

▲ Figure 19–31
An easy, dressed-up look.

Hair extensions represent an increasingly popular salon service, not only for clients who are looking for something different but also for those who have naturally fine hair or who suffer from hair loss. Hair extensions are extremely popular among celebrities, who never seem to have thin hair and who seem to magically grow their hair long overnight.

Manufacturers generally offer their own method of training in the attachment of hair extensions, but there are certain general guidelines to keep in mind:

- Start by deciding whether you are adding length, thickness, or both.
- Know which final style you are striving to achieve, and map it out. Sketch or visualize a placement pattern.
- As a general rule of thumb, stay 1 inch (2.5 centimeters) away from the hairline at the front, sides, and nape, and 1 inch away from the part.
- With very thin hair, you must be careful that the base does not show through.
- Curly hair tends to expand and can give the illusion of being thicker than it really is. When working with curly hair, you will need to

© Milady, a part of Cengage Learning. Photography by Paul Castle, Castle Photography.

FOCUS ON

SHARPENING YOUR SKILLS

In order to achieve a natural look, it is crucial that you blend the client's hair with the hairpiece. You must match both the color and the wave pattern. If the client has naturally wavy hair, it is wise to find a hairpiece with a wave pattern that matches the client's. To match the color, use the color ring. Most hairpieces come in many colors, so it is relatively easy to match to the client's hair. You cannot color a synthetic hairpiece, so any custom coloring to achieve a match must be performed on the client's hair.

determine whether you are matching the curl or whether you wish to add another curl pattern to the hair.

- Straight thin hair and curly thin hair may have similar density, but curly hair will appear thicker. This means you may not need to put as many extensions in curly hair as in straight hair.

As you now know, there are many different ways to attach hair additions. When it comes to extensions, methods include braid-and-sew, simple bonding (also known as *fusion bonding*), linking, and tube shrinking.

The most important professional approaches to hair addition and extension services should be practiced—always in the following order:

1. Safety for the client's own hair.
2. Comfort—there should be no pulling or pinching; avoid excess tension on the natural hair.
3. Security—make certain the additions will not fall off. If they are attached with a semipermanent method such as braid-and-sew, bonding, or fusion bonding be certain that they will last several weeks before they are removed or require readjustment to accommodate the natural hair's growth.
4. Style and fashion.

Braid-and-Sew Attachment Method

In the **braid-and-sew method,** hair extensions are secured to client's own hair by sewing braids or a weft onto an on-the-scalp braid or cornrow, which is sometimes called the track (**Figure 19–32**). The wefts can also be attached by creating a track, using fiber filler. The filler and hair from the scalp are braided together, using an underhand braiding technique. The filler helps grip the client's own hair and creates a longer-lasting braid, to which you attach the weft. The angle of the track determines how the hair will fall. You may position braids or tracks horizontally, vertically, diagonally, or along curved lines that follow the contours of the head. The braid-and-sew method can also be used to attach hairpieces.

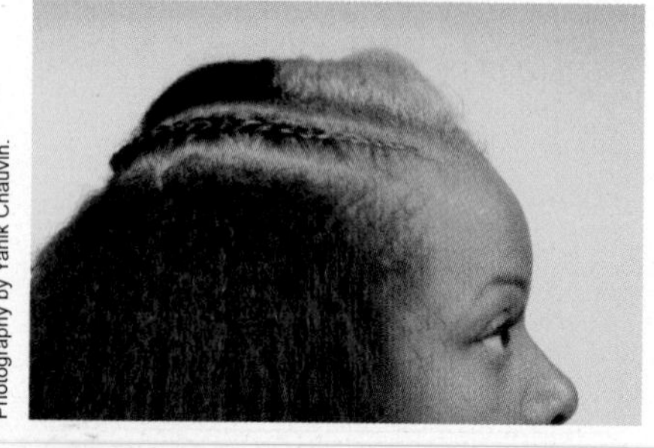

© Milady, a part of Cengage Learning. Photography by Yanik Chauvin.

▲ **Figure 19–32**
Cornrow braid.

Partings are determined according to the style you have chosen. The size of the sections is determined by the amount of hair that will be added to the head. Plan the tracks or braids so that the ends will be hidden. It is best to position them 1 inch (2.5 centimeters) behind the hairline to ensure proper coverage.

When sewing on the extension, use only a blunt, custom-designed needle, either straight or curved. These blunt ends will help avoid damage to the hair and will protect you and the client as well. Extensions can be sewn to the track using a variety of stitches.

- **Lock stitch.** Cut a length of thread that is double the length of the weft being sewn. Pass the needle through the weft to connect

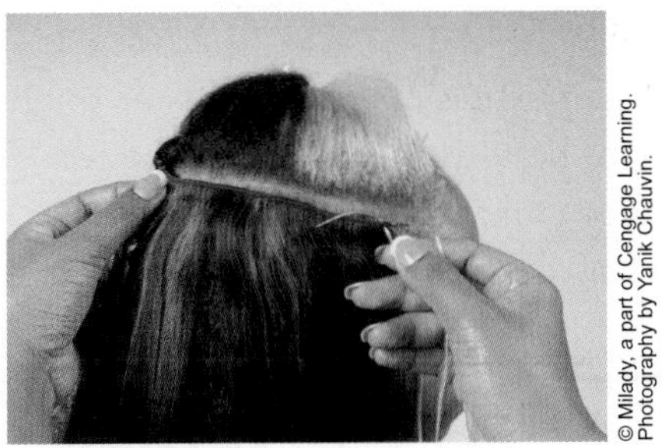
© Milady, a part of Cengage Learning. Photography by Yanik Chauvin.

▲ **Figure 19–33**
Sew weft to braid.

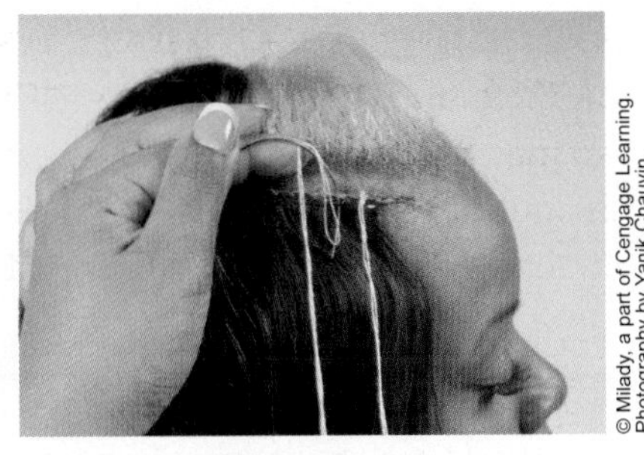
© Milady, a part of Cengage Learning. Photography by Yanik Chauvin.

▲ **Figure 19–34**
Wrap thread around needle.

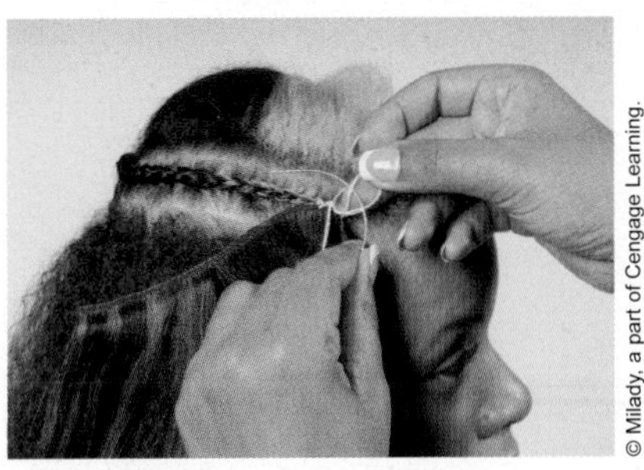
© Milady, a part of Cengage Learning. Photography by Yanik Chauvin.

▲ **Figure 19–35**
Form lock stitch.

it to the track (**Figure 19–33**). Pull the thread through to create a loop. Pass the needle though the loop and wrap the thread around the needle (**Figure 19–34**). Pull the loop tight to form a lock stitch to secure the ends of the weft to the track (**Figure 19–35**). This stitch can also be used over the entire length of the track in evenly spaced stitches.

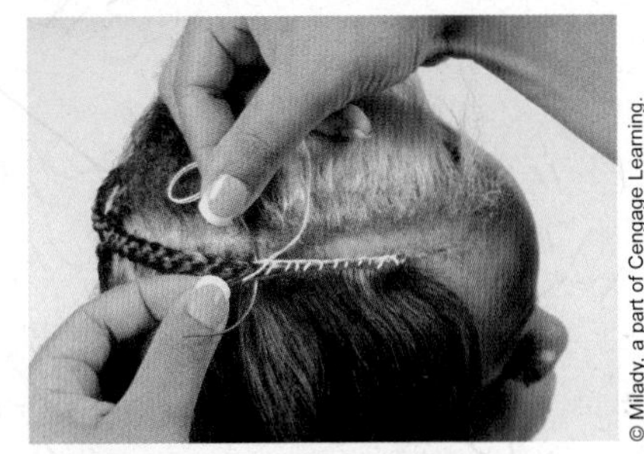
© Milady, a part of Cengage Learning. Photography by Yanik Chauvin.

▲ **Figure 19–36**
Finished overcast stitches.

- **Double-lock stitch.** This stitch is much like the lock stitch, but the thread is wound around the needle twice to create the double lock. It is used in the same ways as the lock stitch.
- **Overcast stitch.** This simple, quick stitch can be used to secure the entire length of the weft to the track. Pass the needle under both the track and the weft, and then bring it back over to make a new stitch (**Figure 19–36**). Moving along the track, repeat the stitch until you reach the end of the track. Complete with a lock stitch for security (**Figure 19–37**).

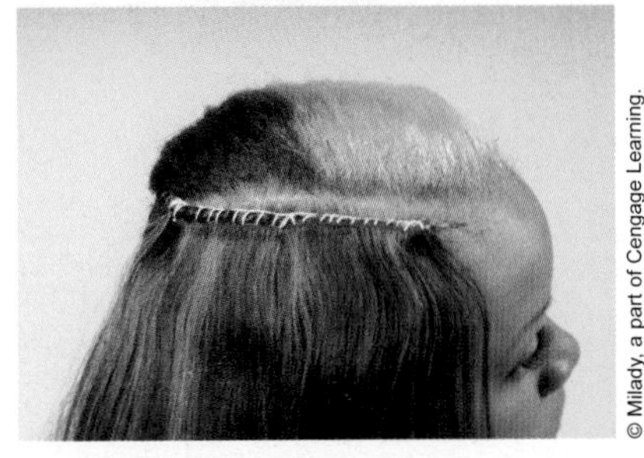
© Milady, a part of Cengage Learning. Photography by Yanik Chauvin.

▲ **Figure 19–37**
Completed line of overcast stitching.

Advantages of the braid-and-sew method include the fact that, if done correctly, it is a very safe technique (**Figures 19–38** and **19–39**).

It requires no special equipment, and with practice, you can do it fairly quickly. Drawbacks include the fact that if there is too much tension on the braid, the client's real hair can be damaged. Also, this technique is not appropriate for clients who have extremely damaged hair, clients who have baby-fine hair (because breakage can occur), or clients who don't keep their scalps clean.

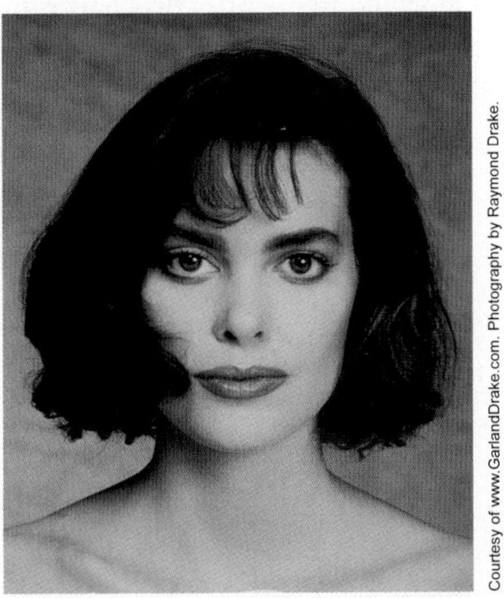
Courtesy of www.GarlandDrake.com. Photography by Raymond Drake.

▶ **Figure 19–38**
Before braid-and-sew extensions.

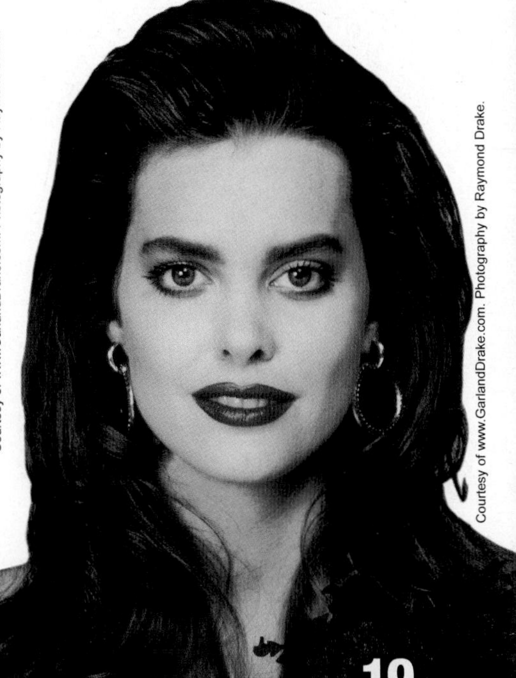
Courtesy of www.GarlandDrake.com. Photography by Raymond Drake.

▶ **Figure 19–39**
After braid-and-sew extensions.

Bonding Method

In the **bonding** method of attaching hair extensions, hair wefts or single strands are attached with an adhesive or bonding agent. The adhesive is applied to the weft with an applicator gun. This gun is not like those available in crafts stores; it is a tool created specifically for bonding.

For bonding, the natural hair should be at least 4-inches long. Bonded hair sits snugly on the head, and is fast to apply. There is, however, a certain degree of slippage. Generally, the bonding product lasts from two to four weeks, depending on factors such as the frequency of shampooing, the oiliness or dryness of the scalp, and the quality of the products used. This means that the client will need to be on a maintenance program that requires salon visits as often as every two weeks.

The bonding procedure generally begins by sectioning off the hair at the nape. Measure the first weft against the parting, ¼ inch to ½ inch (0.6 to 1.25 centimeters) from the hairline (**Figure 19–40**). Lay the weft on a flat surface and carefully apply adhesive along the base (**Figure 19–41**). Use a consistent amount of adhesive—too much will ooze on the head, and too little will fail to adhere. Lightly press the weft against the clean parting (**Figure 19–42**). Hold for approximately twenty seconds, gently tugging to make sure that the weft has adhered. (You may use a blowdryer, set on low to medium heat, to help seal the bond.) Proceed to the next section, working upward on the head, until the desired length and volume are achieved.

© Camilla Wisbauer, 2010; used under license from iStockphoto.com.

Care must be taken when bonding to avoid working too close to the crown and the parting, or the weft will show through. Working 1 inch (2.5 centimeters) away from the hairline will also keep the wefts from showing. Remember that hair is not a static material; it has a natural swing, and it moves. When the wind blows, it should be the hairline that shows, not the wefts.

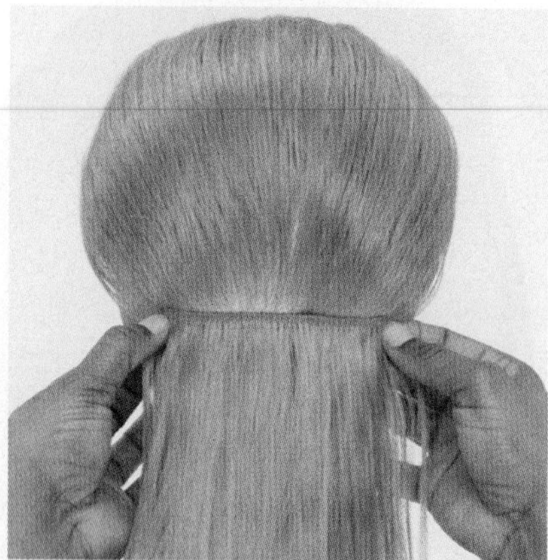

▲ **Figure 19–40**
Measure weft against parting.

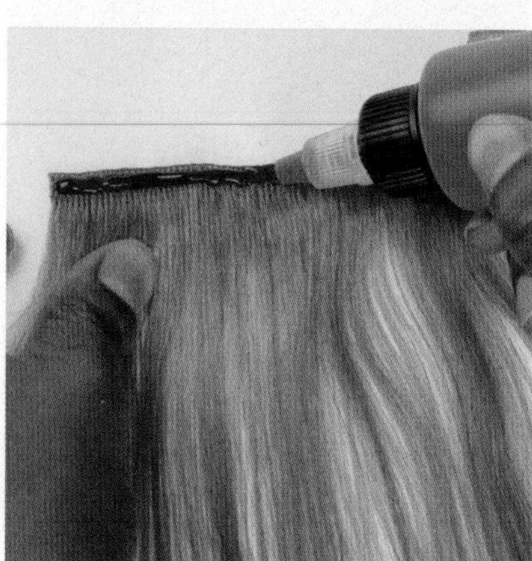

▲ **Figure 19–41**
Apply adhesive to base of weft.

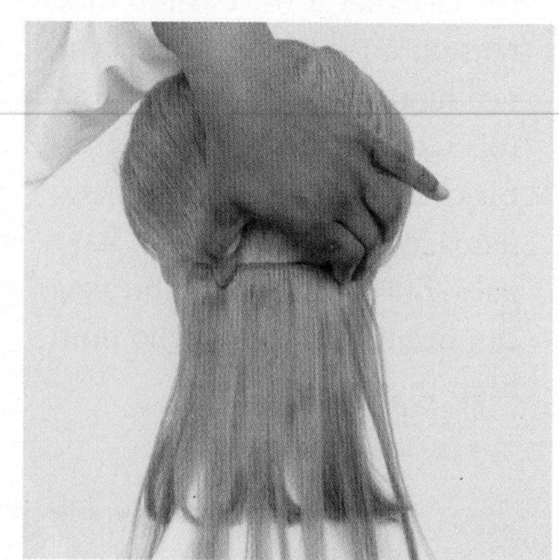

▲ **Figure 19–42**
Press weft to parting.

© Milady, a part of Cengage Learning. Photography by Paul Castle, Castle Photography.

Bonded wefts are removed by dissolving the adhesive bond with oil or bond remover. The same technique can be used with loose hair or wefts that are cut into very small sections. This is called strand bonding.

Two advantages of bonding are that it can be offered at a very affordable price and the service does not take much longer than the average haircut appointment. Also, the client can shampoo with the wefts in, as long as it is done gently. One drawback of bonding is that some clients may have an allergic reaction to the ingredients in the bonding adhesive. Always perform a patch test prior to the application of bonded extensions, especially when using a latex-based adhesive. Also, bonding is not appropriate for clients who have severely damaged hair, or those who do not have enough natural hair to hide the wefts. The wefts cannot be exposed to oils or they will slide off. In general, bonding should *not* be used to attach wefts that are longer than 12 inches to avoid excessive heaviness and the possibility of pulling on the client's natural hair and scalp.

Fusion Bonding Method

In the **fusion bonding** method of attaching extensions, extension hair is bonded to the client's own hair with a bonding material that is activated by the heat from a special tool. This method, while expensive and extremely time-consuming, harmonizes with the client's natural hair with no uncomfortable or unattractive attachment sites. The bonds are light and comfortable to wear, the hair moves like real hair, and the hair is easy to maintain (**Figures 19–43** and **19–44**). The attachment lasts up to four months, almost twice as long as other methods. Removal is quick and painless. The fusion method requires certification training, because it is manufacturer specific.

Some fusion-bonding procedures involve wrapping a keratin-based strip around both the client's hair and the extension or applying the bond to the extension first with a special gun-applicator. Today, many of the extensions or addition strands are pre-tipped or keratin-tipped. In fusion bonding, natural strands along a parting are selected and then isolated with a hair shield (**Figure 19–45**).

Courtesy of www.GarlandDrake.com. Photography by Raymond Drake.

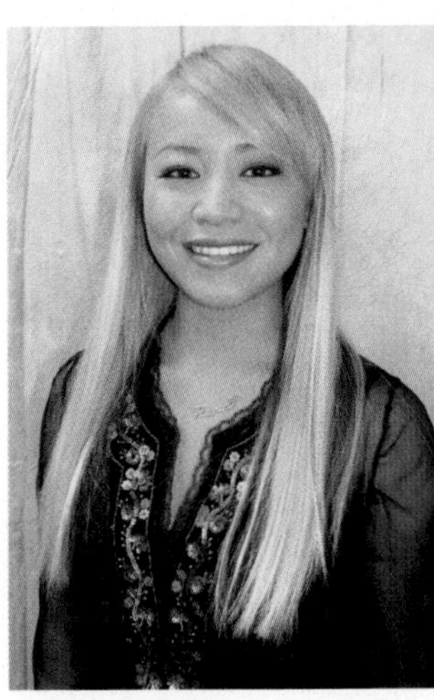

▲ **Figure 19–43**
Before fusion bonding.

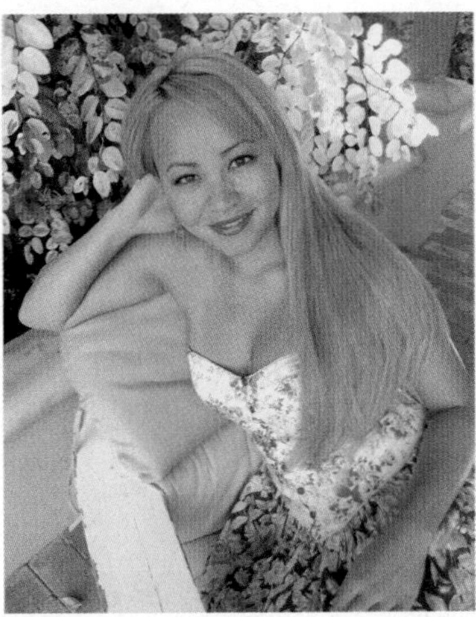

▲ **Figure 19–44**
Fusion-bonded extensions.

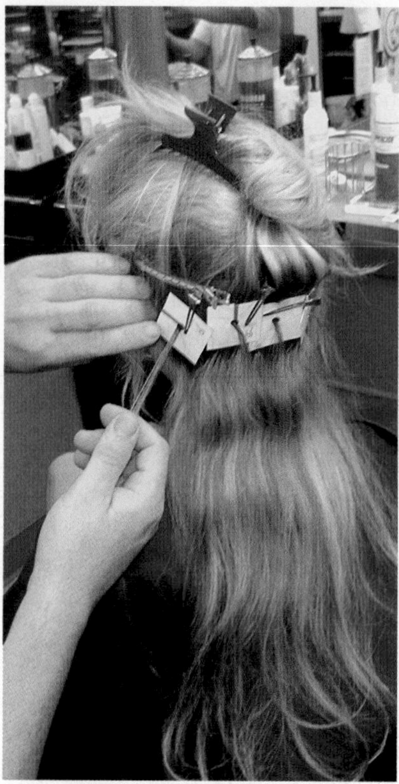

▲ Figure 19–45
Select strands.

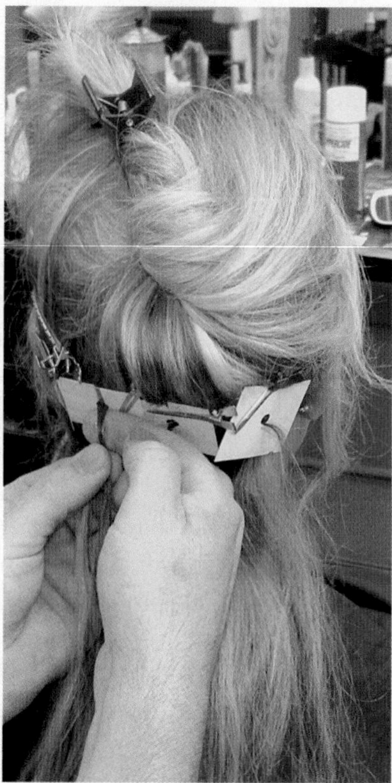

▲ Figure 19–46
Position pre-tipped strand with natural hair.

The extension strand is positioned under the natural hair and near the base (**Figure 19–46**).

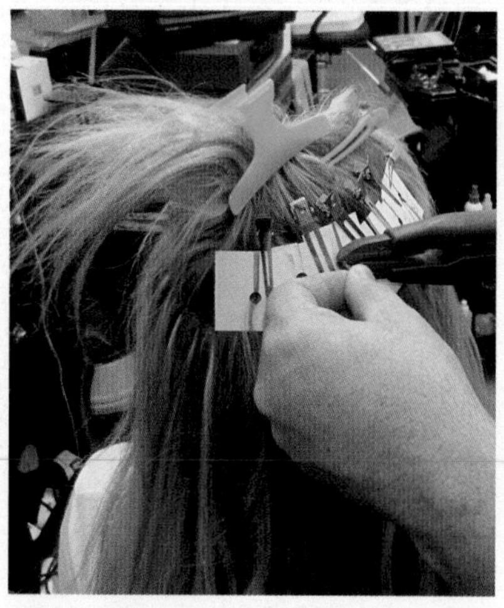

▲ Figure 19–47
Apply heating tool to bond.

The heating element is applied until the bonding agent on the pre-tipped strand has softened (**Figure 19–47**).

Then bond is rolled between the fingers, creating a bead that captures and holds both the natural hair and the extension strand (**Figure 19–48**).

One advantage of fusion bonding is that the client's hair will dry more quickly than when bonding full wefts because there is less bulk. By using extensions in slightly different colors, you can create the illusion of depth and dimension or a highlighted effect. This method also allows for styling versatility. Drawbacks include the fact that the technique is time consuming and the fact that the pre-tipped extensions are expensive. Some suppliers will take back the extension hair and re-tip it, which saves costs and reduces waste; others will not. Applying the adhesive or bonding material yourself avoids this issue, but can be messier and even more time consuming.

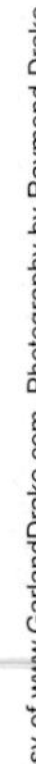

Linking

In linking, a hook is used to pick up a small amount of hair off a parting. A link is slid on close to the scalp with a special tool. Then, an extension or special addition strand is inserted into the link (**Figure 19–49**). Once the extension and the natural hair are captured in the link, the link is pinched flat with pliers. Removed properly with a removal tool (pliers), the extensions can be reused.

To use a linking method of attachment, the natural hair should be at least five-inches long. Advantages are styling versatility and the fact that the integrity of the natural hair can be maintained, if the procedure is done properly. Drawbacks are that this method is expensive and time consuming. Also, the metal links can oxidize (rust).

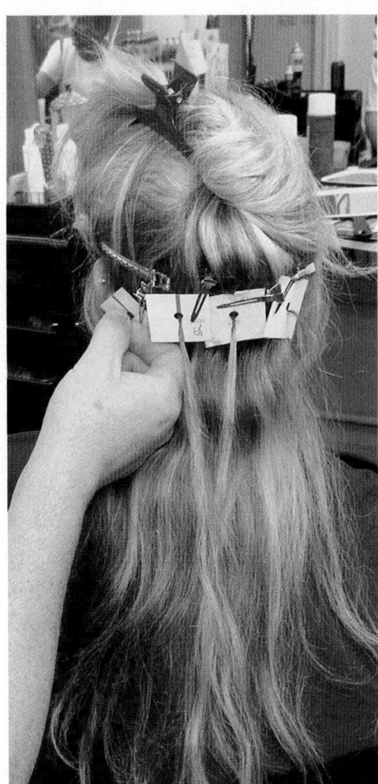

▲ **Figure 19–48**
Roll the bond between your fingers.

Tube Shrinking

In tube shrinking, the client's hair and the addition strand are inserted into a tube, which is then heated to shrink it. This method requires special tools and training.

As with all semipermanent attachment methods for hair extensions, various problems can arise. Usually, these problems are caused by the stylist or the client and not the material. Stylists must follow a logical placement pattern carefully, pay attention to natural growth patterns, and provide complete home-care instructions. Clients must follow home-care instructions carefully to keep the hair neat and clean. They must also return to the salon regularly for maintenance. ☑ **LO4**

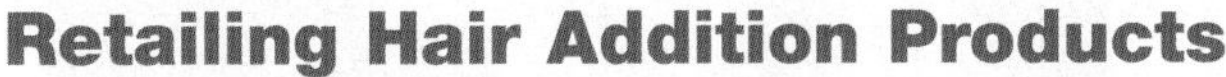

Retailing Hair Addition Products

Simple hairpieces are a great retail product for the salon. They can be displayed in fun, creative ways. Because they are fairly easy to attach and remove, they almost sell themselves, particularly to younger, more adventurous clients. Retailing hair additions and related home-care products can mean substantial additional income for you. Offering hair-addition services can be lucrative for the highly trained stylist.

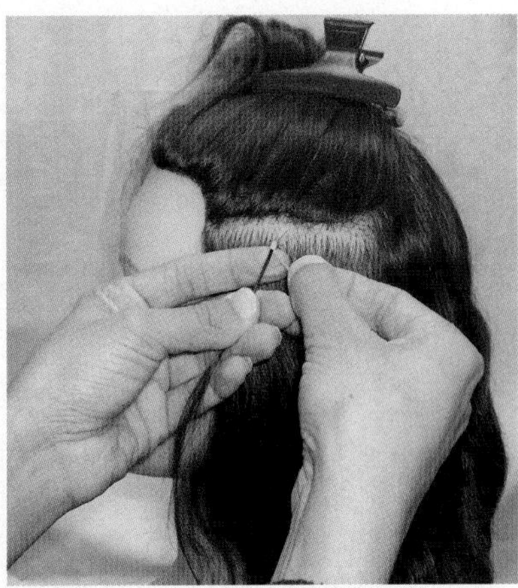

▲ **Figure 19–49**
Linking.

Courtesy of www.GarlandDrake.com. Photography by Raymond Drake.

Whether retailing hair goods or offering hair-addition services, keep the following guidelines in mind:

- Identify the client's needs.
- Explain why it would be worthwhile for the client to make the investment.
- Describe the features and benefits of the products you recommend.
- Discuss product performance and cost.
- Choose high-quality hairpieces and extensions.
- Always believe in your recommendations and stand by your products.
- Price services according to time spent on the service, materials, your expertise, and what the local market will bear.

To be the best, work only with the best. Work with one or two companies that offer a good range of human and synthetic hair, high-quality products, good customer service, and first-rate support, as well as product education through training, seminars, and videos. Always stick with companies that stand by their products.

A Final Thought: Practice, Practice, Practice

Working with hair additions can be one of the most exciting, challenging, and lucrative areas of cosmetology. But to become skilled at this work, you need to take specialized, formal training and practice continually. The more you do, the better you will become. The better you become, the more you will be able to help people look good and feel good about themselves. There is a great satisfaction in being able to do this, particularly when working with people who have suffered the trauma of hair loss and may have given up hope that they could look good again (**Figures 19–50** and **19–51**).

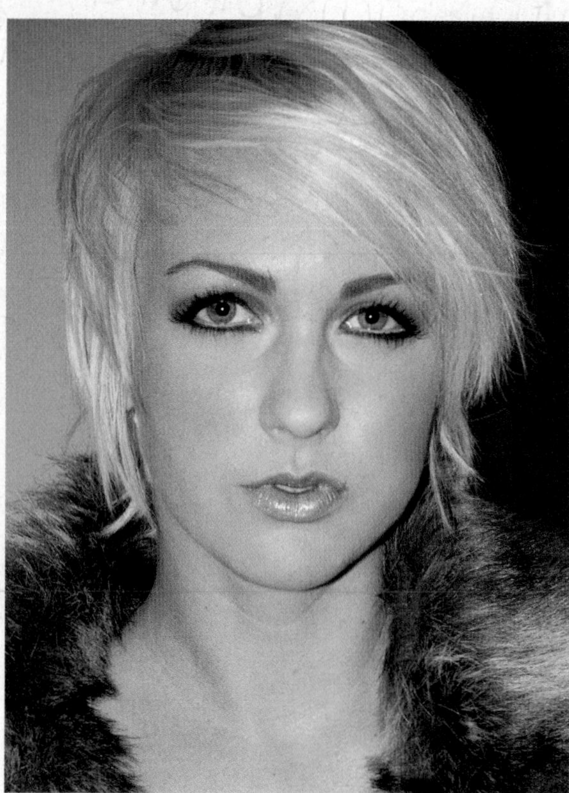

▲ **Figure 19–50**
Before hair extensions.

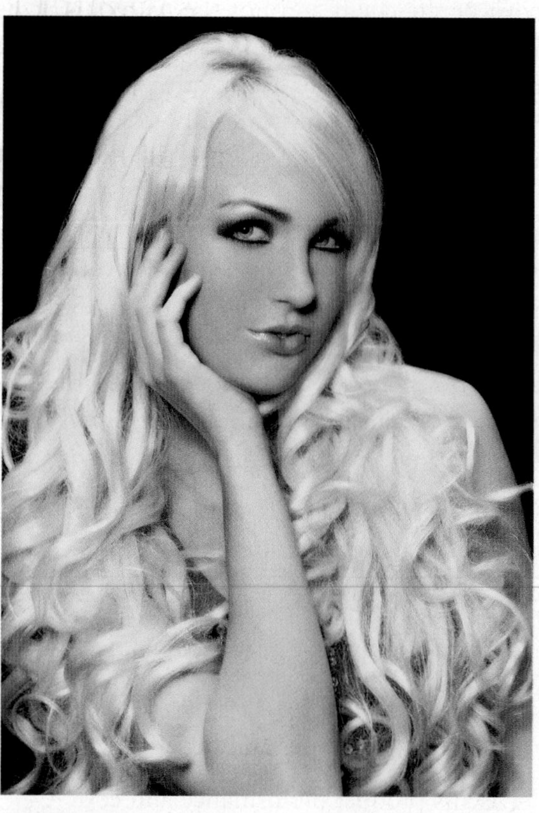

▲ **Figure 19–51**
Post-extension transformation.

Courtesy of www.GarlandDrake.com. Photography by Dixie Dixon, Makeup by Kay Castro, Hairstyling by Tony Greenleaf, all for Garland Drake.

Review Questions

1. What are the main advantages and disadvantages of human hair and synthetic hair?
2. What are the two basic categories of wigs?
3. What are three types of hairpieces and how are they used?
4. What are five methods for attaching hair extensions? Describe each one.

Chapter Glossary

block	Head-shaped form, usually made of canvas-covered cork or Styrofoam, on which the wig is secured for fitting, cleaning, coloring, and styling.
bonding	Method of attaching hair extensions in which hair wefts or single strands are attached with an adhesive or bonding agent.
braid-and-sew method	Attachment method in which hair extensions are secured to client's own hair by sewing braids or a weft onto an on-the-scalp braid or cornrow, which is sometimes called the track.
cap wigs	Wigs constructed of elasticized, mesh-fiber bases to which the hair is attached.
capless wigs	Also known as *caps*; machine-made from human or artificial hair which is woven into rows of wefts. Wefts are sewn to elastic strips in a circular pattern to fit the head shape.
fallen hair	Hair that has been shed from the head or gathered from a hairbrush, as opposed to hair that has been cut; the cuticles of the strands will move in different directions (opposite of turned or Remi hair).
fusion bonding	Method of attaching extensions in which extension hair is bonded to the client's own hair with a bonding material that is activated by heat from a special tool.
hair extensions	Hair additions that are secured to the base of the client's natural hair in order to add length, volume, texture, or color.
hairpiece	Small wig used to cover the top or crown of the head, or a hair attachment of some sort.
hand-tied wigs	Also known as *hand-knotted wigs*; wigs made by inserting individual strands of hair into mesh foundations and knotting them with a needle.
integration hairpiece	Hairpiece that has openings in the base through which the client's own hair is pulled to blend with the hair (natural or synthetic) of the hairpiece.
machine-made wigs	Wigs made by machine by feeding wefts through a sewing machine, and then sewing them together to form the base and shape of the wig.
semi-hand-tied wigs	Wigs constructed with a combination of synthetic hair and hand-tied human hair.
toupee	Small wig used to cover the top or crown of the head.
turned hair	Also called *Remi hair*; the root end of every single strand is sewn into the base, so that the cuticles of all hair strands move in the same direction: down.
wefts	Long strips of human or artificial hair with a threaded edge.
wig	Artificial covering for the head consisting of a network of interwoven hair.

CHAPTER 20

Chemical Texture Services

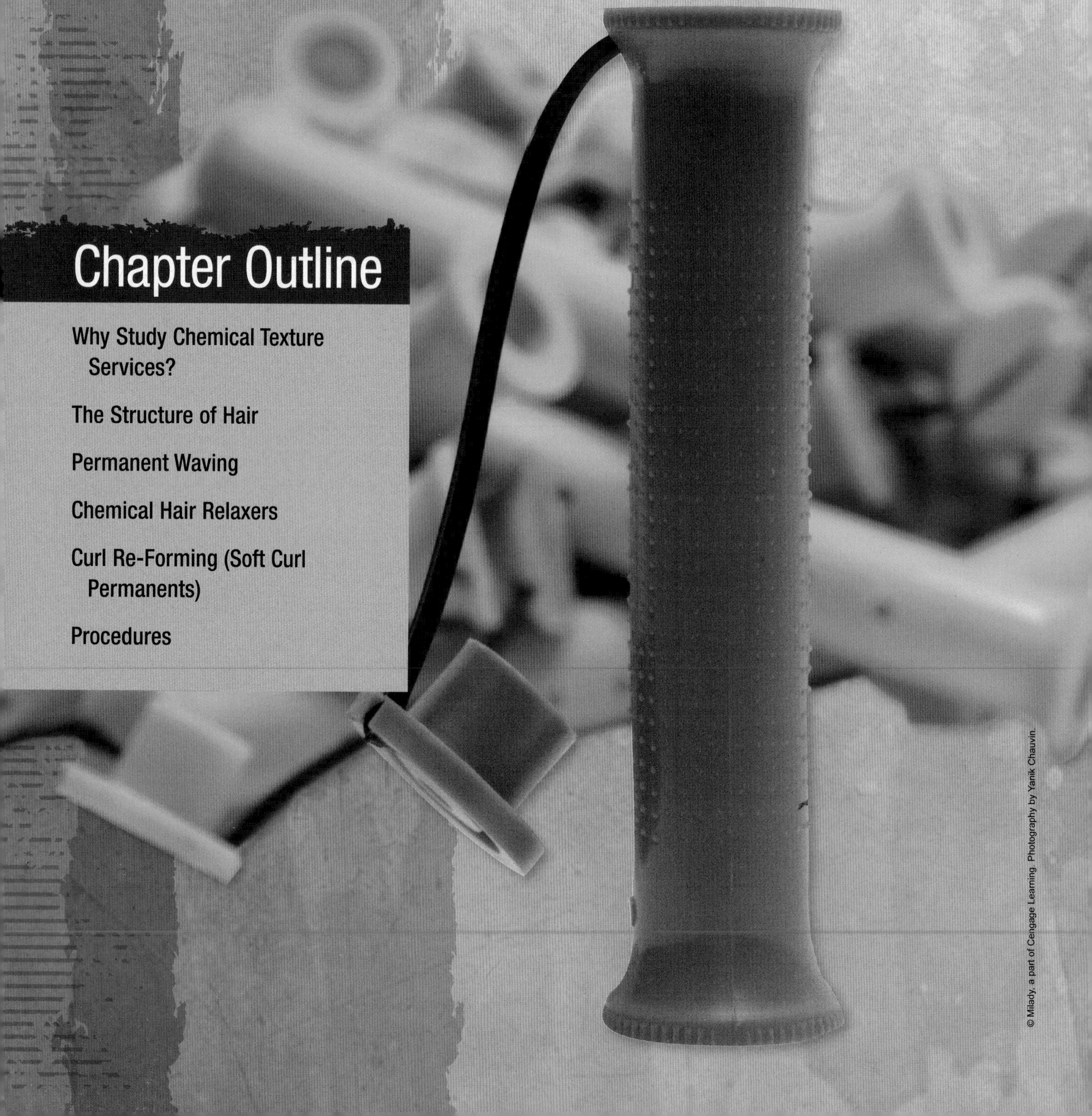

Chapter Outline

© Milady, a part of Cengage Learning. Photography by Yanik Chauvin.

Learning Objectives

After completing this chapter, you will be able to:

- ✓ **LO1** Explain the structure and purpose of each of the hair's layers.
- ✓ **LO2** Explain chemical actions that take place during permanent waving.
- ✓ **LO3** Explain the difference between an alkaline wave and a true acid wave.
- ✓ **LO4** Explain the purpose of neutralization in permanent waving.
- ✓ **LO5** Describe how thio relaxers straighten the hair.
- ✓ **LO6** Describe how hydroxide relaxers straighten the hair.
- ✓ **LO7** Describe curl re-forming and what it is best used for.

Key Terms

Page number indicates where in the chapter the term is used.

acid-balanced waves
pg. 574

alkaline waves (cold waves)
pg. 573

amino acids
pg. 566

ammonia-free waves
pg. 575

ammonium thioglycolate (ATG)
pg. 572

base control
pg. 579

base cream (protective base cream)
pg. 587

base direction
pg. 570

base placement
pg. 569

base relaxers
pg. 587

base sections
pg. 569

basic permanent wrap (straight set wrap)
pg. 579

bookend wrap
pg. 568

bricklay permanent wrap
pg. 580

chemical hair relaxing
pg. 583

chemical texture services
pg. 564

concave rods
pg. 568

croquignole perm wrap
pg. 570

curvature permanent wrap
pg. 580

double flat wrap
pg. 568

double-rod wrap (piggyback wrap)
pg. 571

end papers (end wraps)
pg. 568

endothermic waves
pg. 575

exothermic waves
pg. 574

glyceryl monothioglycolate (GMTG)
pg. 573

half off-base placement
pg. 570

hydroxide neutralization
pg. 587

hydroxide relaxers
pg. 585

keratin proteins
pg. 566

lanthionization
pg. 585

loop rod (circle rod)
pg. 568

low-pH waves
pg. 575

metal hydroxide relaxers
pg. 585

no-base relaxers
pg. 587

normalizing lotions
pg. 589

off-base placement
pg. 570

on-base placement
pg. 569

peptide bonds (end bonds)
pg. 566

permanent waving
pg. 567

polypeptide chains
pg. 566

single flat wrap
pg. 568

soft bender rods
pg. 568

soft curl permanent
pg. 591

spiral perm wrap
pg. 570

straight rods
pg. 568

thio neutralization
pg. 578

thio relaxers
pg. 583

thio-free waves
pg. 575

true acid waves
pg. 573

viscosity
pg. 583

weave technique
pg. 580

Chemical hair texture services give you the ability to permanently change the hair's natural wave pattern and offer your client a variety of styling options that would not be possible otherwise. Texture services can be used to curl straight hair, straighten overly curly hair, or to soften coarse, straight hair and make it more manageable (**Figure 20–1**).

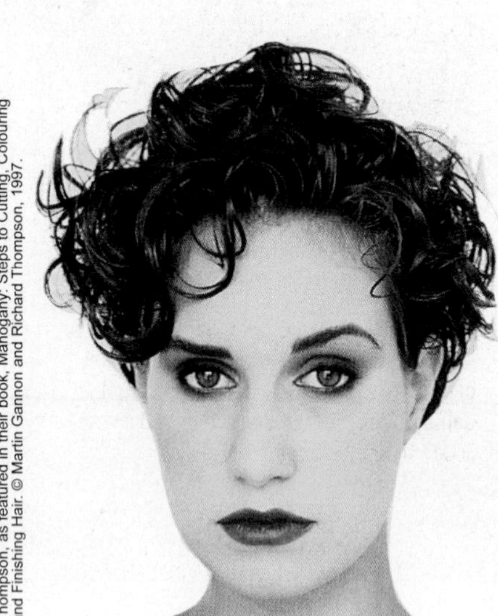

Photo used with the permission of the authors, Martin Gannon and Richard Thompson, as featured in their book, Mahogany: Steps to Cutting, Colouring and Finishing Hair. © Martin Gannon and Richard Thompson, 1997.

▲ **Figure 20–1**
Permanent waving is one kind of chemical texture service.

WHY STUDY CHEMICAL TEXTURE SERVICES?

Cosmetologists should study and have a thorough understanding of chemical texture services because:

- Chemical texture services are problem solvers for stylists and clients in that they change the texture of the hair and can allow a person to wear just about any conceivable hair texture.
- Knowing how to perform these services accurately and professionally will help build a trusting and loyal clientele.
- They are among the most lucrative services in the salon, and many retail products are specific to the hair's condition and the chemical service to which it has been exposed.
- Without a thorough understanding of chemistry, cosmetologists could damage the hair.

Chemical texture services are hair services that cause a chemical change that alters the natural wave pattern of the hair. They include the following:

- Permanent waving: adding wave or curl to the hair
- Relaxing: removing curl, leaving the hair smooth and wave-free
- Curl re-forming (soft curl permanents): loosening overly curly hair, such as when tight curls are turned into loose curls or waves

Because of the large number of people who wish to smooth their curls or give their straight hair more body, mastering the techniques in this chapter will allow you to greatly expand your potential as a stylist.

The Structure of Hair

Because all chemical texture procedures involve chemically and physically changing the structure of the hair, this chapter begins by reviewing the structure and purpose of each layer of the hair, characteristics of hair that were first discussed in Chapter 11, Properties of the Hair and Scalp.

- **Cuticle.** Tough exterior layer of the hair. It surrounds the inner layers and protects the hair from damage. Although the cuticle is not directly involved in the texture or movement of the hair, texture chemicals must penetrate through the cuticle to their target in the cortex in order to be effective (**Figures 20–2** and **20–3**).

- **Cortex**. Middle layer of the hair, located directly beneath the cuticle layer. The cortex is responsible for the incredible strength and elasticity of human hair. Breaking the side bonds of the cortex makes it possible to change the natural wave pattern of the hair.
- **Medulla**. Innermost layer of the hair, often called the *pith* or *core* of the hair. The medulla does not play a role in chemical texture services and may be missing in fine hair.

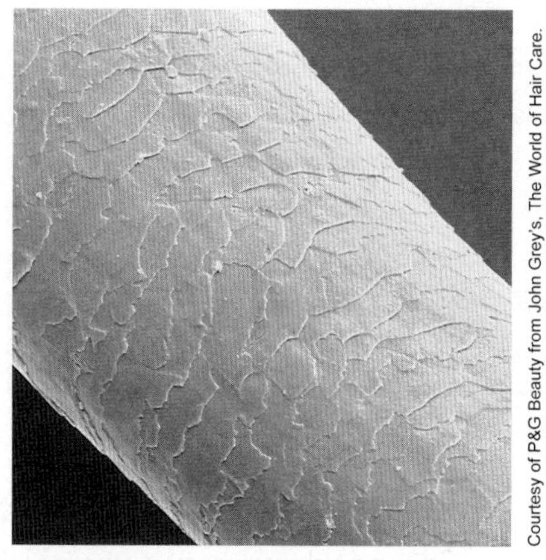

Courtesy of P&G Beauty from John Grey's, The World of Hair Care.

▲ **Figure 20–2**
A healthy cuticle is compact and lies tight against the hair strand. It protects the hair from damage and makes it appear smooth and shiny.

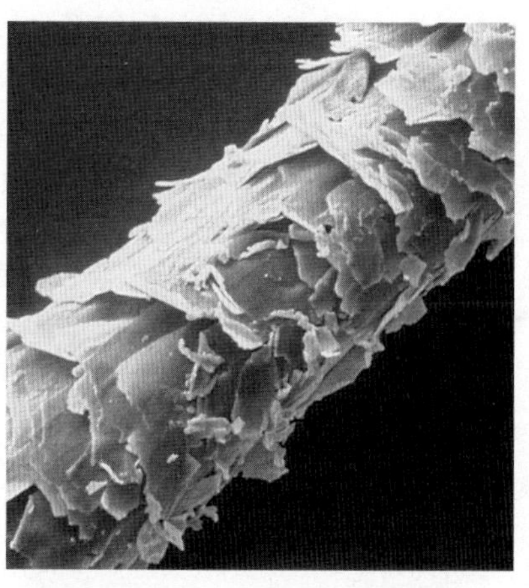

Courtesy of P&G Beauty from John Grey's, The World of Hair Care.

▲ **Figure 20–3**
A damaged cuticle is chipped and does not lie tight against the hair shaft. Because it cannot adequately protect the hair against damage, the hair becomes rough, dull, and prone to split ends and breakage.

For more detailed information on the hair's structure, see Chapter 11, Properties of the Hair and Scalp. ☑ **LO1**

Importance of pH in Texture Services

In Chapter 12, Basics of Chemistry, you learned that pH is an abbreviation used for potential hydrogen. The symbol pH represents the quantity of hydrogen ions. The pH scale measures the acidity and alkalinity of a substance by measuring the quantity of hydrogen ions it contains. The pH scale has a range from 0 to 14. A pH of 7 is neutral, a pH below 7 is acidic, and a pH above 7 is alkaline. The natural pH of hair is between 4.5 and 5.5. Chemical texturizers raise the pH of the hair to an alkaline state in order to soften and swell the hair shaft. This action opens the cuticle layer and allows the solution to reach the cortex layer, where restructuring takes place. Coarse, resistant hair with a strong, compact cuticle layer requires a highly alkaline chemical solution. Porous, damaged, or chemically treated hair requires a less alkaline solution.

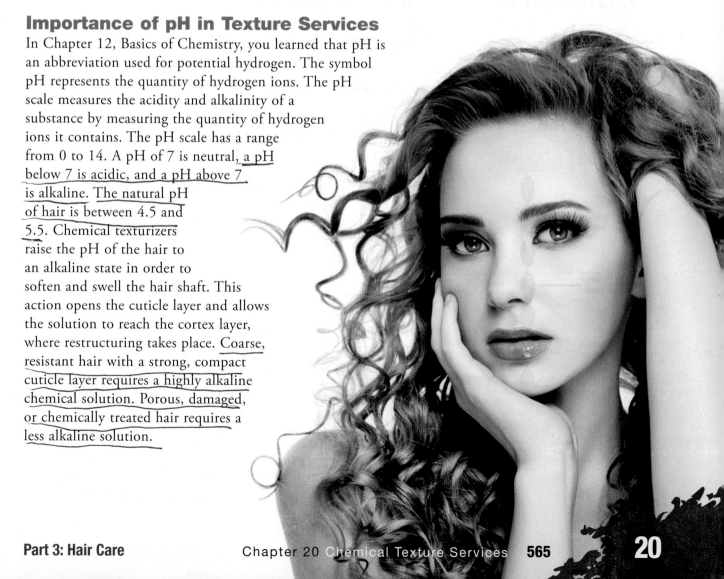

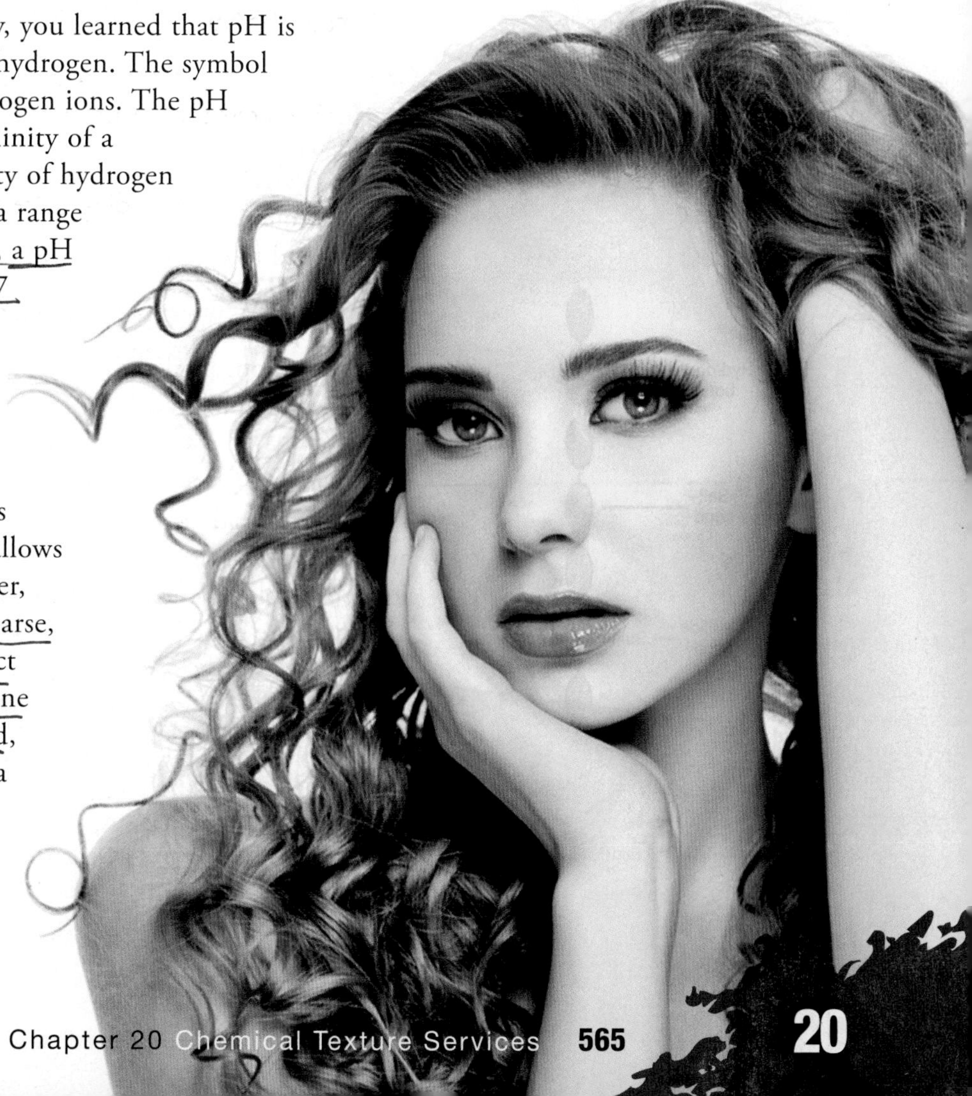

© Valua Vitaly, 2010; used under license from Shutterstock.com.

The Amino Acid Content of Hair

All the protein structures of hair are made from these eighteen amino acids:

Cysteic acid	Aspartic acid	Threonine
Arginine	Serine	Glutamic acid
Proline	Glycine	Alanine
Valine	Cystine	Methionine
Isoleucine	Leucine	Tyrosine
Phenylalanine	Lysine	Histidine

▲ **Figure 20–4**
Amino acids are the building blocks of proteins.

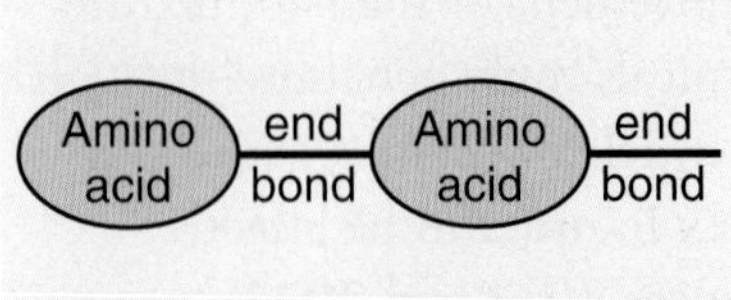

▲ **Figure 20–5**
Peptide bonds (end bonds) link amino acids together in long chains.

Basic Building Blocks of Hair

To understand how a chemical texturizer changes the structure of hair, it is important to understand the basic building blocks of hair (**Figures 20–4** through **20–8**).

- **Amino acids** are compounds made up of carbon, oxygen, hydrogen, nitrogen, and sulfur.
- **Peptide bonds**, also known as **end bonds**, are chemical bonds that join amino acids together, end to end in long chains, to form a polypeptide chain.
- **Polypeptide chains** are long chains of amino acids joined together by peptide bonds.
- **Keratin proteins** are long, coiled polypeptide chains.
- **Side bonds** are disulfide, salt, and hydrogen bonds that cross-link polypeptide chains together.

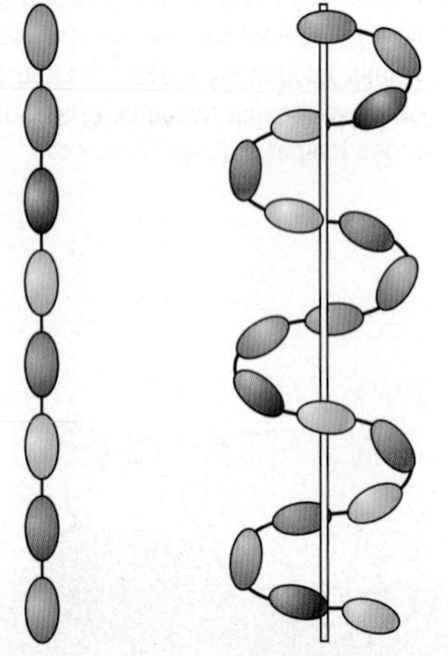

▲ **Figure 20–6**
Polypeptide chains are formed when amino acids link together.

▲ **Figure 20–7**
Keratin proteins are long, coiled peptide chains.

Keratin Proteins

Keratin p[illegible]s are made of long chains of amino acids linked [illegible] end like beads. The amino acid chains are linked [illegible]ide bonds (end bonds). These chains of amino acids [illegible] bonds are called polypeptides. Keratin proteins [illegible] coiled, polypeptide chains, which in turn are [illegible]no acids.

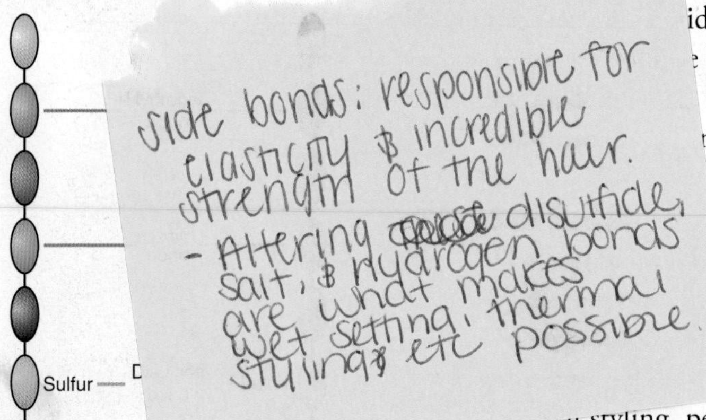

[illegible] up of millions of polypeptide chains cross-linked [illegible]de bonds: disulfide, salt, and hydrogen. Side bonds [illegible]he elasticity and incredible strength of the hair. [illegible] types of side bonds is what makes wet setting, [illegible] styling, permanent waving, curl re-forming, and chemical hair relaxing possible (**Figure 20–9**).

Sulfur
side bonds: responsible for elasticity & incredible strength of the hair.
- Altering disulfide, salt, & hydrogen bonds are what makes wet setting, thermal styling & etc possible.

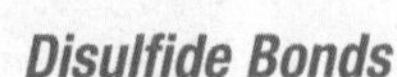

▲ **Figure 20–8**
Side bonds cross-link polypeptide chains together.

Disulfide Bonds

Disulfide bonds are strong chemical side bonds formed when the sulfur atoms in two adjacent protein chains are joined together. Disulfide bonds are not broken by water, and although the amount of heat used in conventional thermal styling does not break disulfide

© Milady, a part of Cengage Learning.

bonds, they can be broken by the extreme heat produced by some thermal styling tools or boiling water. The chemical and physical changes in disulfide bonds make permanent waving, curl re-formin and chemical hair relaxing possible. Although there are far fewer disulfide bonds than hydrogen or salt bonds, they are the stronge of the three side bonds, accounting for about one-third of the h overall strength.

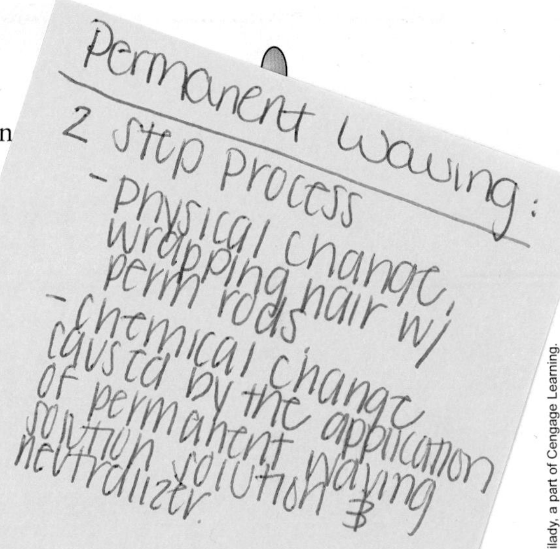

Permanent Waving:
2 step process
- physical change, wrapping hair w/ perm rods
- chemical change caused by the application of permanent waving solution & neutralizer.

© Milady, a part of Cengage Learning.

only

Salt Bonds

Salt bonds are relatively weak physical side bonds that are th of an attraction between negative and positive electrical cha bonds); they are easily broken by changes in pH, and they when the pH returns to normal. Hydrogen bonds can be water, whereas salt bonds are broken by changes in pH. L salt bonds are far weaker than disulfide bonds, the hair has so ma bonds that they account for about one-third of the hair's total strength.

Hydrogen Bonds

Hydrogen bonds are weak physical side bonds that are also the result of an attraction between opposite electrical charges; they are easily broken by water (wet setting) or heat (thermal styling), and they re-form as the hair dries or cools. Although individual hydrogen bonds are very weak, there are so many of them that they, too, account for about one-third of the hair's total strength.

Permanent Waving

Permanent waving is a two-step process whereby the hair undergoes a physical change caused by wrapping the hair on perm rods, and then the hair undergoes a chemical change caused by the application of permanent waving solution and neutralizer. Because chemical changes are involved, you should always perform an elasticity test before perming the hair (**Figure 20–10**).

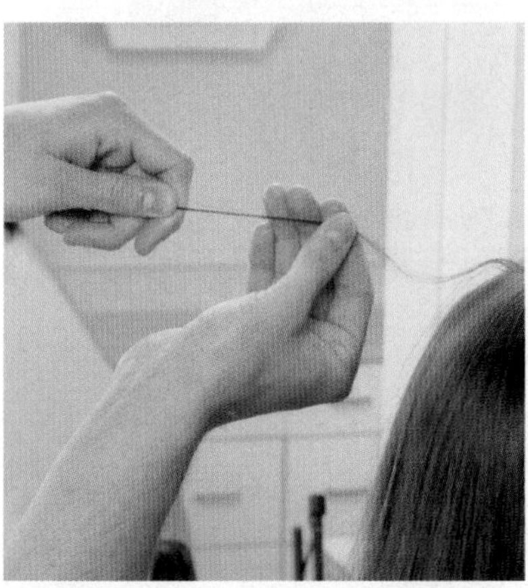

© Milady, a part of Cengage Learning. Photography by Paul Castle, Castle Photography.

▲ Figure 20–10

Perm. wave
wet set: breaks hydrogen bonds
perm wave: breaks disulfide bonds.

Perm Wrap

A perm wrap is essentially a wet set on perm rods instead of rolle The major difference between a wet set and a permanent wave is type of side bonds that are broken. A wet set breaks hydrogen bo whereas a permanent wave breaks disulfide bonds, which are much stronger and more resistant.

In permanent waving, the size of the rod determines the size of the curl. The shape and type of curl are determined by the shape and type of rod and by the wrapping method used (**Figure 20–11**). Selecting the correct perm rod and wrapping method is key to creating a successful permanent. Perm rods come in a wide variety of sizes and shapes that can be combined with different wrapping methods to provide an exciting range of styling options.

© Milady, a part of Cengage Learning.

▲ **Figure 20–11**
The diameter of the rod determines the size of the curl.

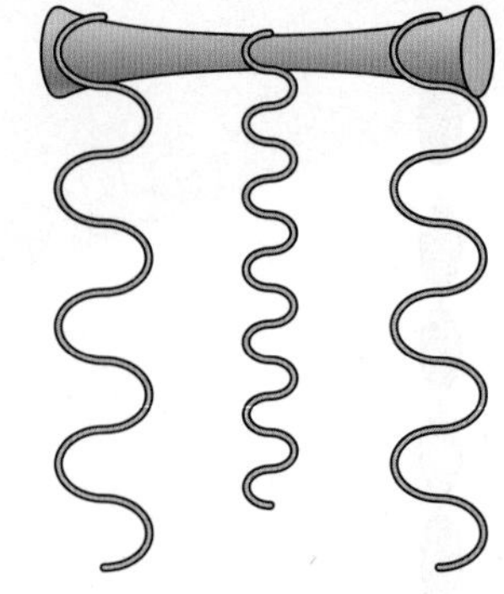

© Milady, a part of Cengage Learning.

▲ Figure 20–12
Concave rods create curl that it tightest in the center.

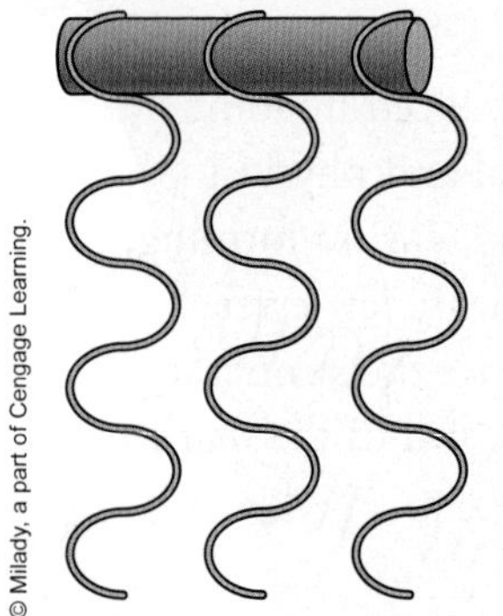

© Milady, a part of Cengage Learning.

▲ Figure 20–13
Straight rods create curl that is tightest on the ends and looser towards the scalp.

Types of Rods

Concave rods are the most common type of perm rod; they have a smaller diameter in the center that increases to a larger diameter on the ends. Concave rods produce a tighter curl in the center, and a looser curl on either side of the strand (**Figure 20–12**).

Straight rods are equal in diameter along their entire length or curling area. This produces a uniform curl along the entire width of the strand (**Figure 20–13**).

Both concave and straight rods come in different lengths to accommodate different sections on the head. Short rods, for instance, can be used for wrapping small and awkward sections where long rods would not fit.

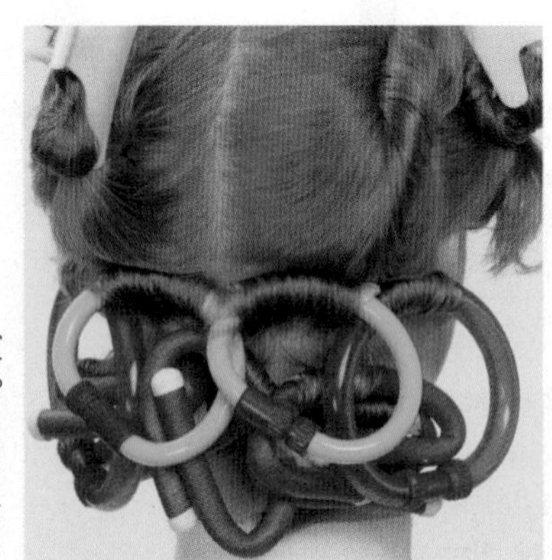

© Milady, a part of Cengage Learning. Photography by Paul Castle, Castle Photography.

▲ Figure 20–14
Loop rods atop soft bender rods.

Soft bender rods are usually about 12-inches (30.5 centimeters) long with a uniform diameter along the entire length of the rod. These soft foam rods have a flexible wire inside that permits them to be bent into almost any shape (**Figure 20–14**).

The **loop rod**, also known as **circle rod**, is usually about 12-inches (30.5 centimeters) long with a uniform diameter along the entire length of the rod. After the hair is wrapped, the rod is secured by fastening the ends together to form a loop (**Figure 20–15**).

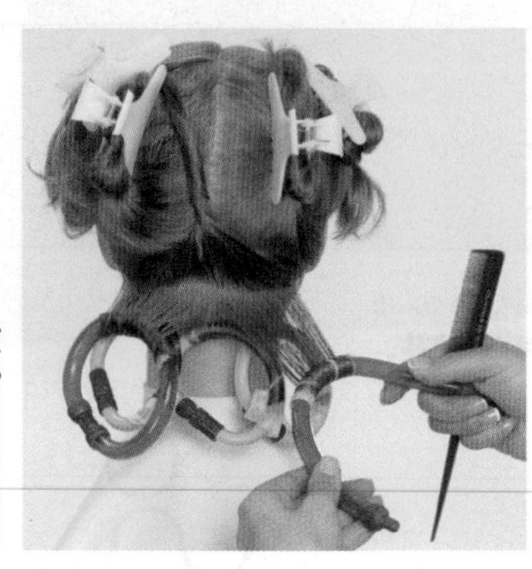

© Milady, a part of Cengage Learning. Photography by Paul Castle, Castle Photography.

▲ Figure 20–15
Loop rods.

Today, many perms are performed with large rollers, rag rollers or other tools, in order to achieve large, loose curls and waves. Larger tools are also used for root perms, in which only the base of the hair is permed in order to create volume and lift without curl.

End Papers

End papers, also known as **end wraps**, are absorbent papers used to control the ends of the hair when wrapping and winding hair on the perm rods. End papers should extend beyond the ends of the hair to keep them smooth and straight and prevent fishhooks, or hair that is bent up at the ends. The most common end paper techniques are the double flat wrap, single flat wrap, and bookend single paper wrap.

- The **double flat wrap** is a perm wrap in which one end paper is placed under and another is placed over the strand of hair being wrapped. Both papers extend past the hair ends. This wrap provides the most control over the hair ends and also helps keep them evenly distributed over the entire length of the rod (**Figure 20–16**).

- The **single flat wrap** is similar to the double flat wrap but uses only one end paper, placed over the top of the strand of hair (**Figure 20–17**).

- The **bookend wrap** uses one end paper folded in half over the hair ends like an envelope. The bookend wrap eliminates excess paper and

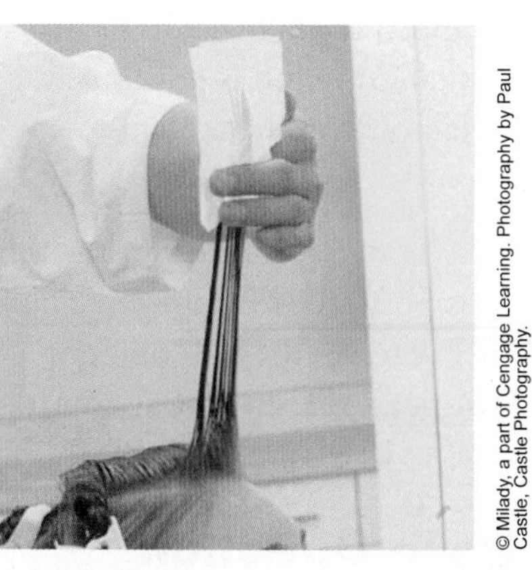
© Milady, a part of Cengage Learning. Photography by Paul Castle, Castle Photography.

▲ Figure 20–16
Double flat wrap.

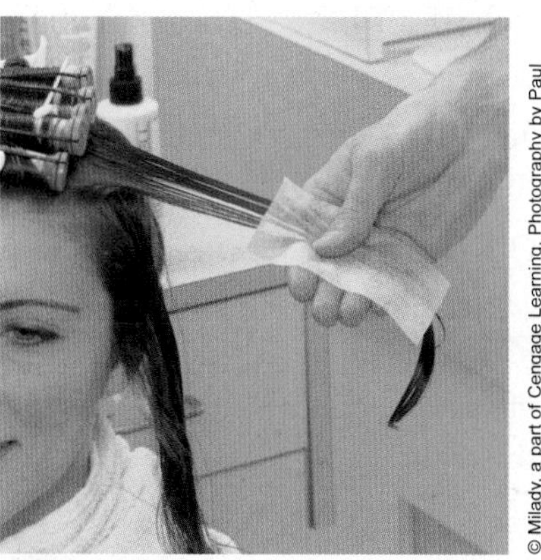
© Milady, a part of Cengage Learning. Photography by Paul Castle, Castle Photography.

▲ Figure 20–17
Single flat wrap.

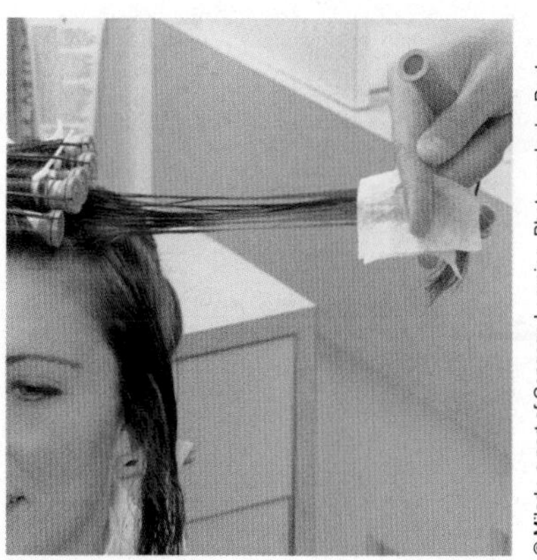
© Milady, a part of Cengage Learning. Photography by Paul Castle, Castle Photography.

▲ Figure 20–18
Bookend wrap.

can be used with short rods or with very short lengths of hair. When using this wrap method, be careful to distribute the hair evenly over the entire length of the rod. Avoid bunching the hair in the fold of the paper—hair should be in the center—to produce an even curl (**Figure 20–18**).

Here's a Tip

Keeping the hair evenly damp throughout wrapping helps the end papers cling to the hair and helps with the distribution of solutions, including water.

Sectioning for a Perm

All perm wraps begin by sectioning the hair into panels. The size, shape, and direction of these panels vary, based on the wrapping pattern and the type and size of the rod being used. **Base sections** are subsections of panels into which the hair is divided for perm wrapping; one rod is normally placed on each base section (**Figure 20–19**). The size of each base section is usually the length and width of the rod being used.

Base Placement

Base placement refers to the position of the rod in relation to its base section; base placement is determined by the angle at which the hair is wrapped. Rods can be wrapped on base, half off base, or off base.

For **on-base placement**, the hair is wrapped at a 45-degree angle beyond perpendicular to its base section, and the rod is positioned on its base (**Figure 20–20**). Although on-base placement may result in greater volume at the scalp area, any increase in volume will be lost as soon as the hair begins to grow out. Caution should be used with on-base placement, because the additional stress and tension can mark or break the hair.

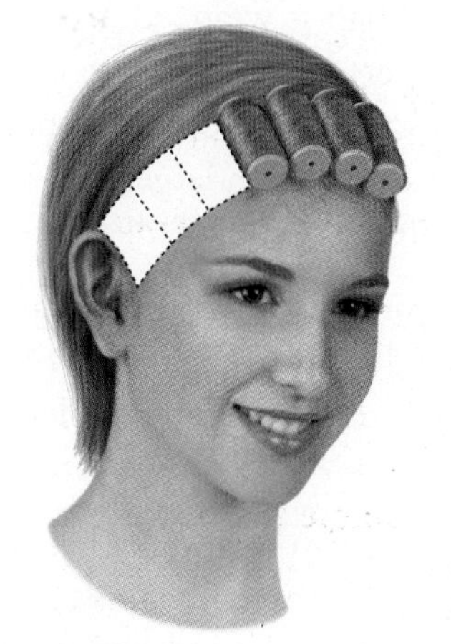
© Milady, a part of Cengage Learning.

▲ Figure 20–19
All perm wraps section the hair into panels. These panels are then divided into base sections.

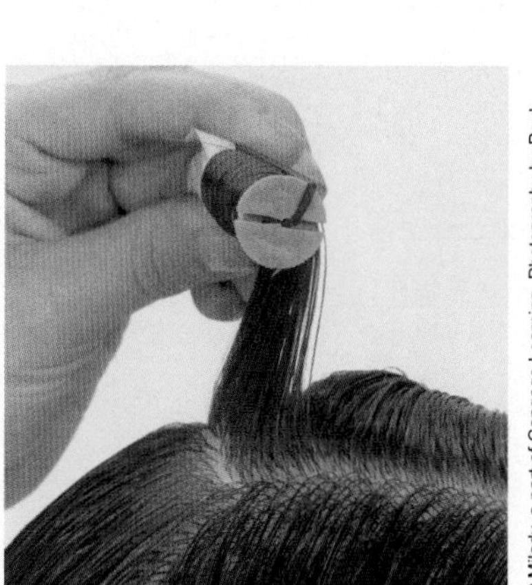
© Milady, a part of Cengage Learning. Photography by Paul Castle, Castle Photography.

▲ Figure 20–20
On-base placement.

CAUTION

Using a base section that is wider than the perm rod can create an uneven curl pattern and undue tension on the hair.

In **half off-base placement**, the hair is wrapped at an angle of 90 degrees or perpendicular to its base section, and the rod is positioned half off its base section (**Figure 20–21**). Half off-base placement minimizes stress and tension on the hair.

Off-base placement refers to wrapping the hair at 45 degrees below the center of the base section, so that the rod is positioned completely off its base (**Figure 20–22**). Off-base placement creates the least amount of volume and results in a curl pattern that begins farthest away from the scalp.

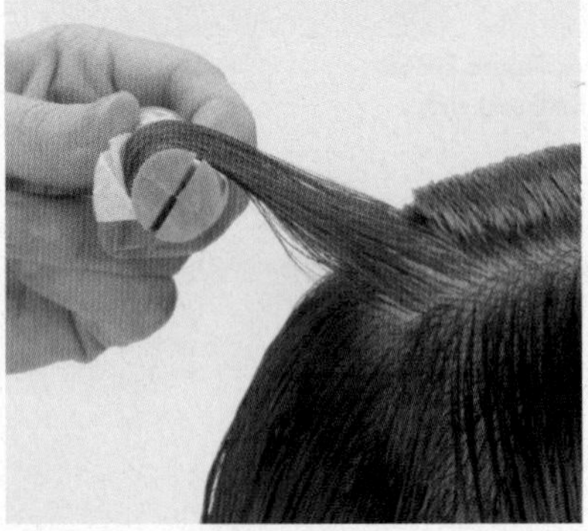

© Milady, a part of Cengage Learning. Photography by Paul Castle, Castle Photography.

▲ **Figure 20–21**
Half off-base placement.

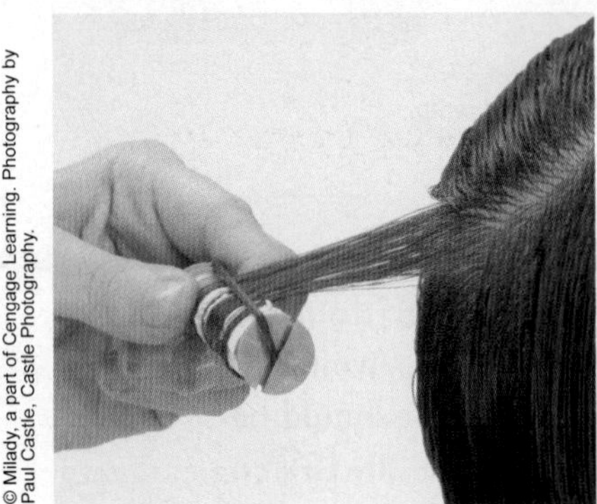

© Milady, a part of Cengage Learning. Photography by Paul Castle, Castle Photography.

▲ **Figure 20–22**
Off-base placement.

Base Direction

Base direction refers to the angle at which the rod is positioned on the head: horizontally, vertically, or diagonally (**Figure 20–23a** and **b**); *base direction* also refers to the directional pattern in which the hair is wrapped. Although directional wraps can be wrapped backward, forward, or to one side, it is important to remember that wrapping with the natural direction of hair growth causes the least amount of stress to the hair. Wrapping against the natural growth pattern can produce a band mark or breakage at the base of the curl.

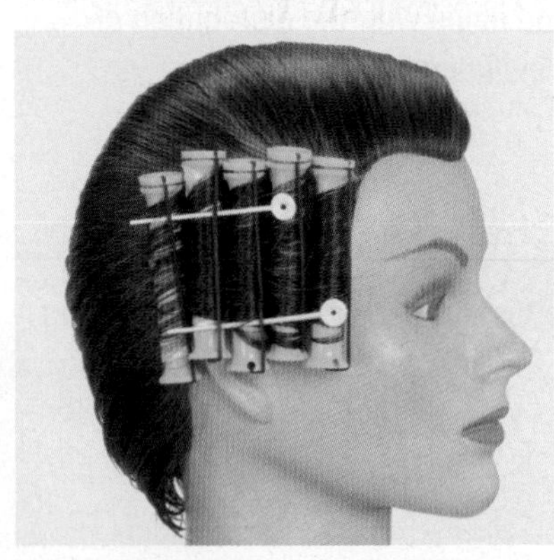

© Milady, a part of Cengage Learning. Photography by Paul Castle, Castle Photography.

▲ **Figure 20–23a**
Vertical base direction.

Wrapping Techniques

There are two basic methods of wrapping the hair around the perm rod: croquignole perm wrap and spiral perm wrap.

A **croquignole perm wrap** (KROH-ken-ohl) is wrapped from the ends to the scalp in overlapping concentric layers (**Figure 20–24**). Because the hair is wrapped perpendicular to the length of the rod, each new layer of hair is wrapped on top of the previous layer, increasing the size (diameter) of the curl with each new overlapping layer, because each layer is rolled on top of the previous ones. This produces a tighter curl at the ends, and a larger curl at the scalp. Longer, thicker hair increases this effect.

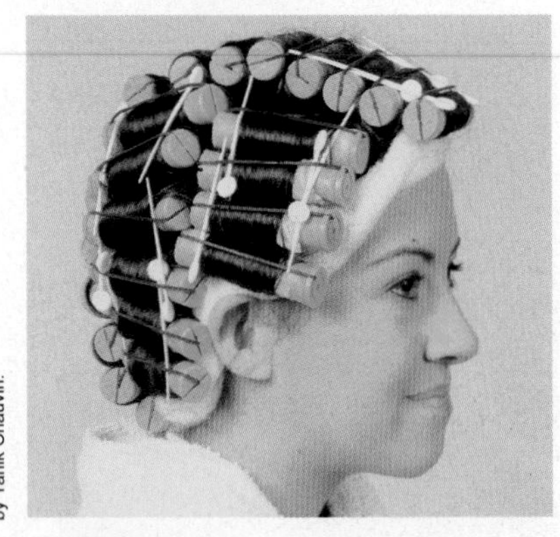

© Milady, a part of Cengage Learning. Photography by Yanik Chauvin.

▲ **Figure 20–23b**
Horizontal base direction.

In a **spiral perm wrap** the hair is wrapped at an angle other than perpendicular to the length of the rod (**Figure 20–25**), which causes the hair to spiral along the length of the rod, like the stripes on a candy cane.

A spiral perm wrap may partially overlap the preceding layers. As long as the angle remains constant, any overlap will be uniform along the length of the rod and the strand of hair (**Figure 20–26**). This wrapping technique causes the size (diameter) of the curl to remain

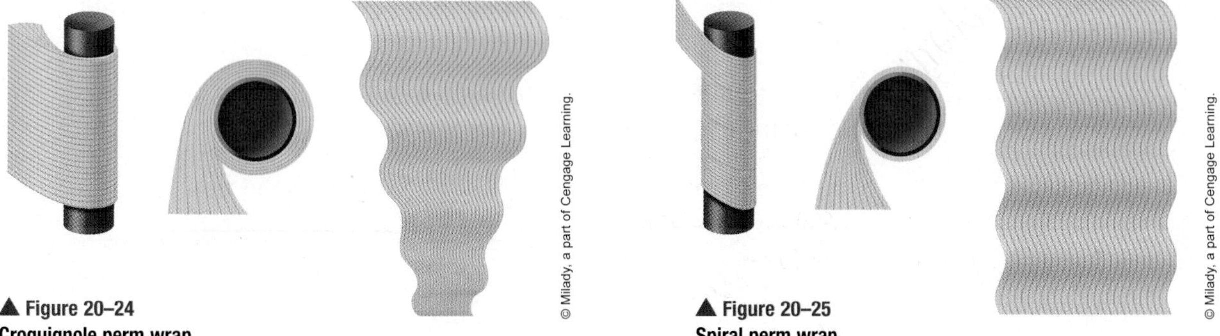
▲ Figure 20–24
Croquignole perm wrap.

© Milady, a part of Cengage Learning.

▲ Figure 20–25
Spiral perm wrap.

© Milady, a part of Cengage Learning.

constant along the entire length of the strand and produces a uniform curl from the scalp to the ends.

For extra-long hair, you may need to use a **double-rod wrap**, also known as **piggyback wrap**, in which the hair is wrapped on one rod from the scalp to midway down the hair shaft (**Figure 20–27**), and another rod is used to wrap the remaining hair strand in the same direction. This allows for better penetration of the processing solution and for a tighter curl near the scalp than that provided by a conventional croquignole wrap.

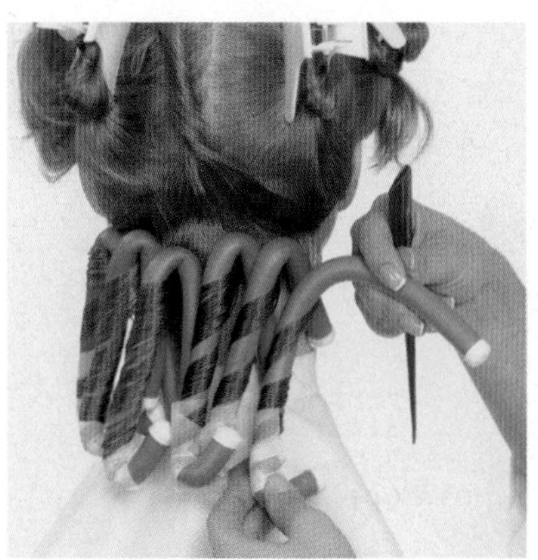
▲ Figure 20–26
Spiral wrap on bender rods.

© Milady, a part of Cengage Learning. Photography by Paul Castle, Castle Photography.

The Chemistry Of Permanent Waving

Alkaline permanent waving solutions soften and swell the hair, and they open the cuticle, permitting the solution to penetrate into the cortex. **Figure 20–28** illustrates hair saturated with alkaline permanent waving solution (pH 9.4) for five minutes. Note the swelling of the cuticle layer. In **Figure 20–29**, hair from the same sample has been saturated with acid-balanced permanent waving solution (pH 7.5) for five minutes. Note that there is far less swelling of the cuticle layer.

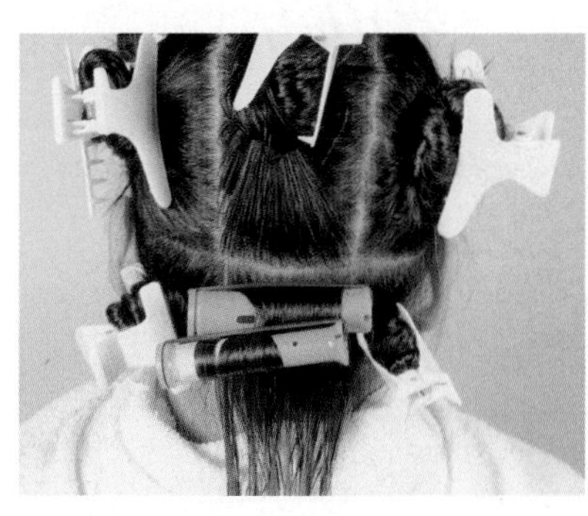
▲ Figure 20–27
Piggyback wrap.

© Milady, a part of Cengage Learning. Photography by Yanik Chauvin.

Reduction Reaction

Once in the cortex, the waving solution breaks the disulfide bonds through a chemical reaction called reduction. A reduction reaction involves either the addition of hydrogen or the removal of oxygen. The reduction reaction in permanent waving is due to the addition of hydrogen.

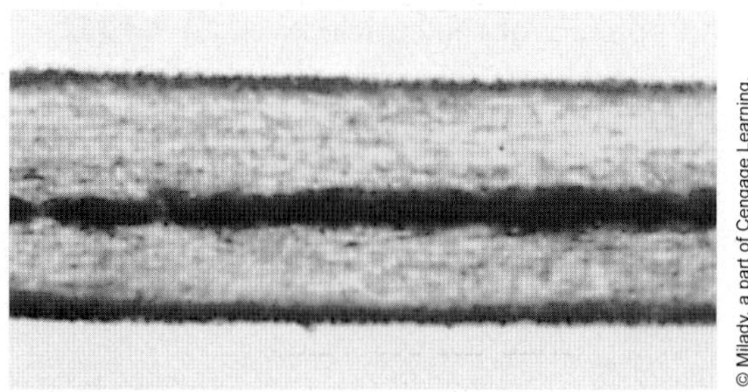
▲ Figure 20–28
Hair that has been saturated with alkaline waving solution (9.4 pH) for five minutes.

© Milady, a part of Cengage Learning.

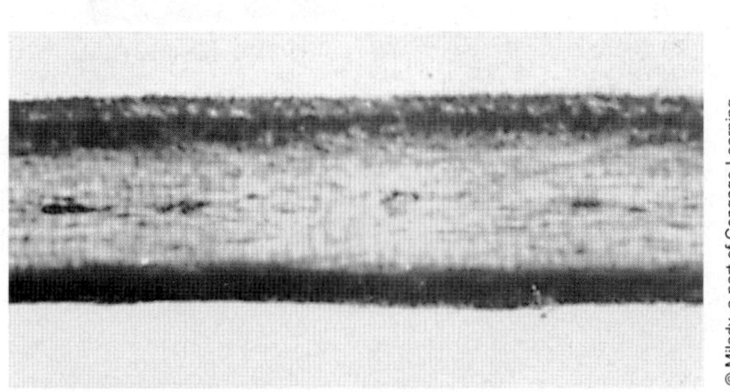
▲ Figure 20–29
Hair that has been saturated with acid-balanced waving solution (7.5 pH) for five minutes.

© Milady, a part of Cengage Learning.

The chemical process of permanent waving involves the following reactions:

- A disulfide bond joins the sulfur atoms in two adjacent polypeptide chains.
- Permanent wave solution breaks a disulfide bond by adding a hydrogen atom to each of its sulfur atoms.
- The sulfur atoms attach to the hydrogen from the permanent waving solution, breaking their attachment to each other.
- Once the disulfide bond is broken, the polypeptide chains can form into their new curled shape. Reduction breaks disulfide bonds (**Figure 20–30**) and oxidation reforms them.

All permanent wave solutions contain a reducing agent. The reducing agent commonly referred to as *thio* is used in permanent waving solutions. It contains a *thiol* (THY-ohl), which is a particular group of compounds, along with carboxylic acid.

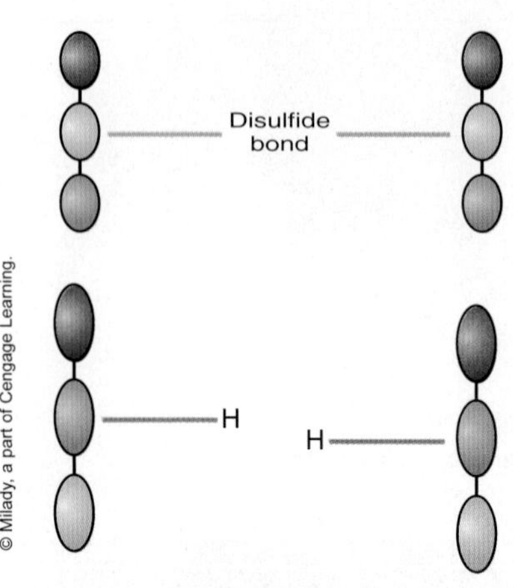

© Milady, a part of Cengage Learning.

▲ **Figure 20–30**
A reduction reaction breaks disulfide bonds during the permanent waving process.

Thioglycolic acid (thy-oh-GLY-kuh-lik), a colorless liquid with a strong, unpleasant odor, is the most common reducing agent in permanent wave solutions. The strength of the permanent waving solution is determined primarily by the concentration of thio. Stronger perms have a higher concentration of thio, which means that more disulfide bonds are broken compared to weaker perms.

Because acids do not swell the hair nor penetrate into the cortex, it is necessary for manufacturers to add an alkalizing agent. The addition of ammonia to thioglycolic acid produces a new chemical called **ammonium thioglycolate (ATG)** (uh-MOH-nee-um thy-oh-GLY-kuh-layt), which is alkaline and is the active ingredient or reducing agent in alkaline permanents.

The degree of alkalinity (pH) is a second factor in the overall strength of the waving solution. Coarse hair with a strong, resistant cuticle layer needs the additional swelling and penetration that is provided by a more alkaline waving solution.

By contrast, porous hair, or hair with a damaged cuticle layer, is easily penetrated and could be damaged by a highly alkaline permanent waving solution. The alkalinity of the perm solution should correspond to the resistance, strength, and porosity of the cuticle layer. ☑ **LO2**

Types of Permanent Waves

A variety of permanent waves are available in salons today (**Figure 20–31**). Brief descriptions of the most commonly used perms follow.

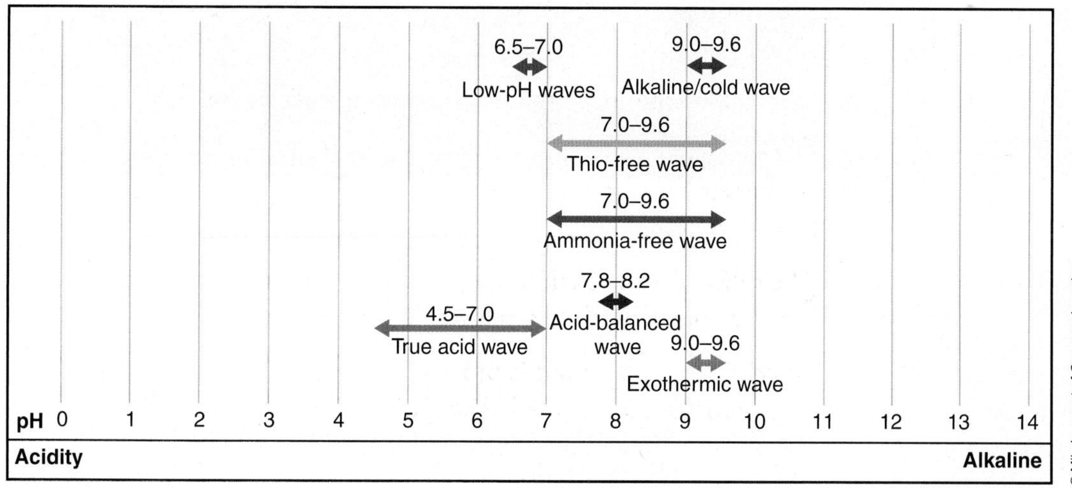

▲ **Figure 20–31**
Depending on the type and formulation, perm solutions can vary from being slightly acidic to highly alkaline.

Alkaline Waves or Cold Waves

Alkaline waves, also known as **cold waves**, were developed in 1941, have a pH between 9.0 and 9.6, use ammonium thioglycolate (ATG) as the reducing agent, and process at room temperature without the addition of heat.

Acid Waves

Glyceryl monothioglycolate (**GMTG**) (GLIS-ur-il mon-oh-thy-oh-GLY-koh-layt) is the main active ingredient in true acid and acid-balanced waving lotions. It has a low pH. Although it is the primary reducing agent in all acid waves, it may not be the only one. Most acid waves also contain ATG, just like a cold wave. Although the low pH of acid waves may seem ideal, repeated exposure to GMTG is known to cause allergic sensitivity in both hairstylists and clients.

True Acid Waves

All acid waves have three separate components: permanent waving solution, activator, and neutralizer. The activator tube contains GMTG, which must be added to the permanent waving solution immediately before using. The first true acid waves were introduced in the early 1970s. **True acid waves** have a pH between 4.5 and 7.0 and require heat to process; they process more slowly than alkaline waves and do not usually produce as firm a curl as alkaline waves. GMTG, which has a low pH, is the active ingredient.

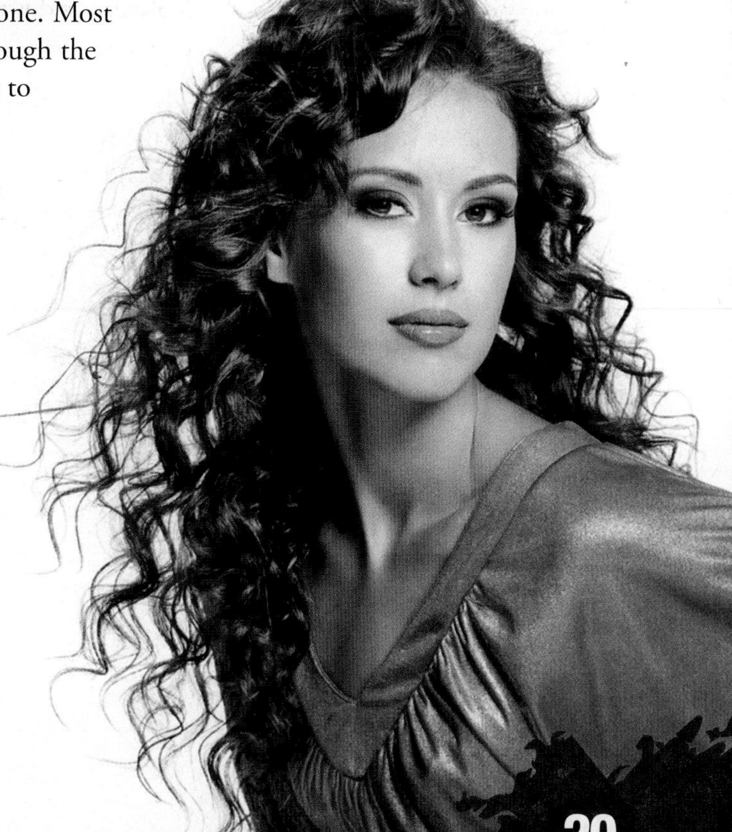

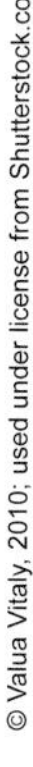
© Valua Vitaly, 2010; used under license from Shutterstock.com.

ACTivity

Get some pH test strips and test various liquids, including acid waves, acid-balanced waves, lemon juice, and more. Track your results.

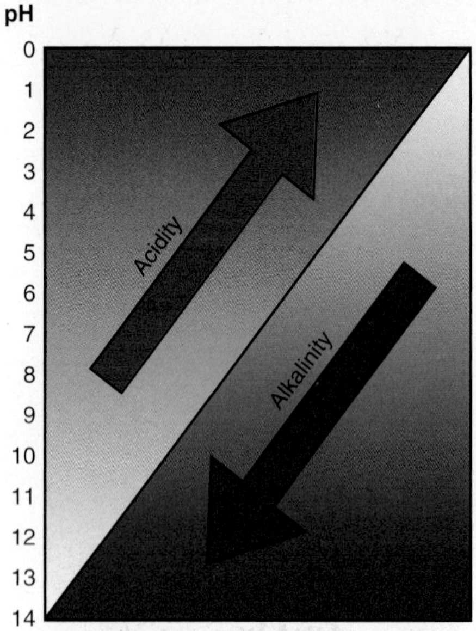

© Milady, a part of Cengage Learning.

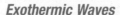

▲ **Figure 20–32**
Acidity increases as alkalinity decreases and alkalinity increases as acidity decreases.

Since acidic solutions contract the hair, you may be wondering how a true acid wave, with a pH below 7.0, can cause the hair to swell. Although a pH of 7.0 is neutral on the pH scale, a pH of 5.0 is neutral for hair. The pH of any substance is always a balance of both acidity and alkalinity. Even the strongest acid also contains some alkalinity. (To review the pH scale, see Chapter 12, Basics of Chemistry.) Acidity increases when alkalinity decreases, and alkalinity increases when acidity decreases (**Figure 20–32**).

Because every step in the pH scale represents a tenfold change in pH, a pH of 7.0 is 100 times more alkaline than the pH of hair (5.0). Even pure water with a pH of 7.0 can damage the hair and cause it to swell. ☑ **LO3**

Acid-Balanced Waves

In order to permit processing at room temperature and produce a firmer curl, the strength and pH of acid waves have increased steadily over the years. Most of the acid waves found in today's salons have a pH between 7.8 and 8.2. Modern acid waves are actually **acid-balanced waves**, which are permanent waves that have a 7.0 or neutral pH; because of their higher pH, they process at room temperature, do not require the added heat of a hair dryer, process more quickly, and produce firmer curls than true acid waves.

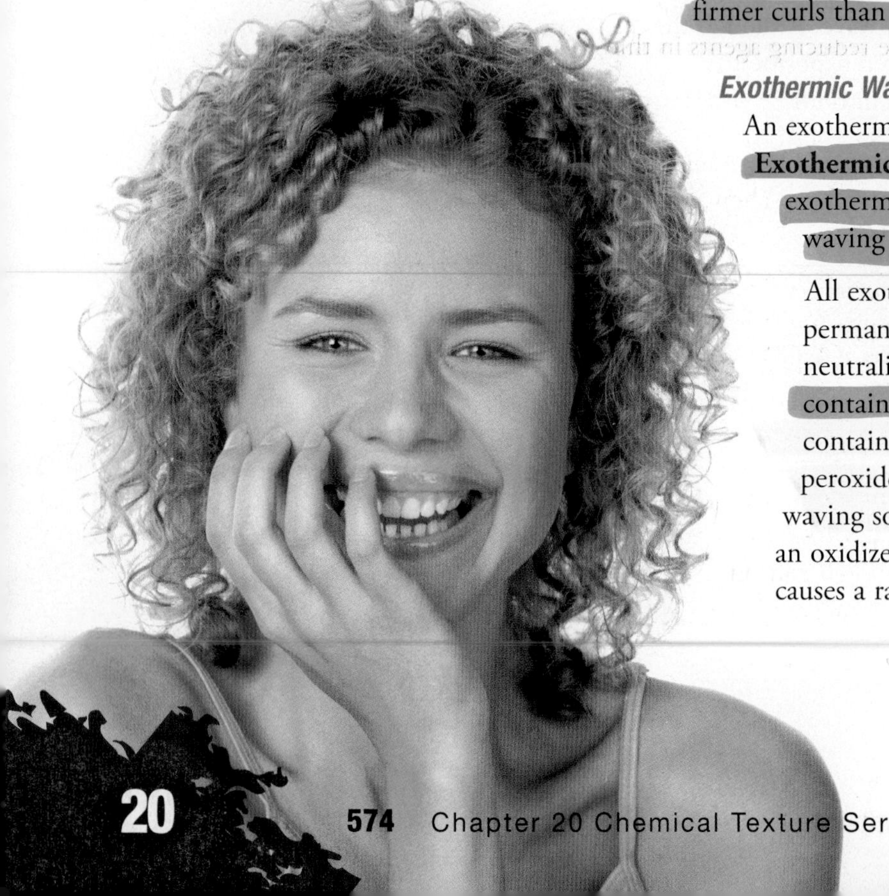

Exothermic Waves

An exothermic chemical reaction produces heat. **Exothermic waves** (Eks-oh-THUR-mik) create an exothermic chemical reaction that heats up the waving solution and speeds up the processing.

All exothermic waves have three components: permanent waving solution, activator, and neutralizer. The permanent waving solution contains thio, just as in a cold wave. The activator contains an oxidizing agent (usually hydrogen peroxide) that must be added to the permanent waving solution immediately before use. Mixing an oxidizer with the permanent waving solution causes a rapid release of heat and an increase in the

© Christo, 2010; used under license from Shutterstock.com.

temperature of the solution. The increased temperature increases the rate of the chemical reaction, which shortens the processing time.

Endothermic Waves

An endothermic chemical reaction is one that absorbs heat from its surroundings. **Endothermic waves** (en-duh-THUR-mik) are activated by an outside heat source, usually a conventional hood-type hair dryer.

Endothermic waves will not process properly at room temperature. Most true acid waves are endothermic and require the added heat of a hair dryer.

Ammonia-Free Waves

Ammonia-free waves are perms that use an ingredient that does not evaporate as readily as ammonia, so there is very little odor associated with their use.

Aminomethylpropanol (uh-MEE-noh-meth-yl-pro-pan-all), or AMP, and monoethanolamine (mahn-oh-ETH-an-all-am-een), or MEA, are examples of alkanolamines that are used in permanent waving solutions as a substitute for ammonia. Even though these solutions may not smell as strong as ammonia, they can still be every bit as alkaline and just as damaging. Remember: Ammonia free does not necessarily mean damage free.

Thio-Free Waves

Thio-free waves use an ingredient other than ATG, such as cysteamine (SIS-tee-uhmeen) or mercaptamine (mer-KAPT-uh-meen), as the primary reducing agent. Even though these thio substitutes are not technically ATG, they are still thio compounds.

Although thio free is often marketed as damage free, that is not necessarily true. At a high concentration, the reducing agents in thio-free waves can be just as damaging as thio.

Low-pH Waves

The use of sulfates, sulfites, and bisulfites presents an alternative to ATG known as **low-pH waves**. Sulfites work at a low pH. They have been used in perms for years, but they have never been very popular. Permanents based on sulfites are very weak and do not provide a firm curl, especially on strong or resistant hair. Sulfite permanents are usually marketed as body waves or alternative waves.

Selecting the Right Type of Perm

It is extremely important to select the right type of perm for each client. Each client's hair has a distinct texture and condition, so individual needs must always be addressed. After a thorough consultation, you should be able to determine which type of permanent is best suited to

CAUTION

Accidentally mixing the contents of the activator tube with the neutralizer instead of the permanent waving solution will cause a violent chemical reaction that can cause injury, especially to the eyes.

CAUTION

The ingredients, strength, and pH of permanent wave solutions from different manufacturers may vary considerably, even within the same category. Always check the manufacturer's instructions and the products Material Safety Data Sheet (MSDS) for accurate, detailed information.

PERMANENT WAVE CATEGORIES			
PERM TYPE	**ACTIVE INGREDIENT**	**PROCESS**	**RECOMMENDED HAIR TYPE**
alkaline/cold wave pH: 9.0 to 9.6	ammonium thioglycolate (ATG)	room temperature	coarse, thick, or resistant
exothermic wave pH: 9.0 to 9.6	ammonium thioglycolate (ATG)	exothermic	coarse, thick, or resistant
true acid wave pH: 4.5 to 7.0	glyceryl monothioglycolate (GMTG)	endothermic	extremely porous or very damaged hair
acid-balanced wave pH: 7.8 to 8.2	glyceryl monothioglycolate (GMTG)	room temperature	porous or damaged hair
ammonia-free wave pH: 7.0 to 9.6	monoethanolamine (MEA)/ aminomethylpropanol (AMP)	room temperature	porous to normal
thio-free wave pH: 7.0 to 9.6	mercaptamine/ cysteamine	room temperature	porous to normal
low-pH waves pH: 6.5 to 7.0	ammonium sulfite/ ammonium bisulfite	endothermic	normal, fine, or damaged

© Milady, a part of Cengage Learning.

Table 20–1 Permanent Wave Categories.

your client's hair type, condition, and desired results. **Table 20–1** lists the most common types of permanent waves along with recommended hair type for each. These are only general guidelines. Just because a perm is indicated for use on color-treated hair does not mean it is safe for damaged or bleached hair. Also, hair that has been treated with a semipermanent color, which coats the hair, is not as porous as hair treated with permanent color; it is actually more resistant.

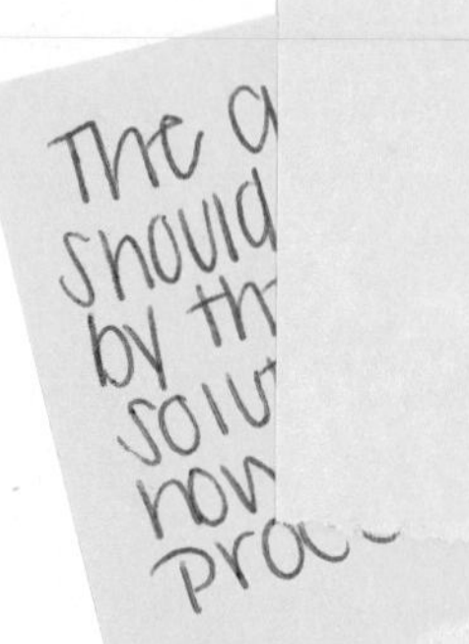

Permanent Wave Processing

The strength of any permanent wave is based on the concentration of its reducing agent. In turn, the amount of processing is determined by the strength of the permanent wave solution. If a weak permanent wave solution s used on coarse hair, there may not be enough hydrogen ions to break the ecessary number of disulfide bonds, no matter how long the permanent rocesses. But the same weak solution may be exactly right for fine hair with wer disulfide bonds. On the other hand, a strong solution, which releases any hydrogen atoms, may be perfect for coarse hair, but too damaging for fine hair. The amount of processing should be determined by the strength of the solution, not necessarily how long the perm processes.

In permanent waving, most of the processing takes place as soon as the solution penetrates the hair, within the first five to ten minutes. The additional processing time allows the polypeptide chains to shift into their new configuration.

If you find that your client's hair has been overprocessed, it probably happened within the first five to ten minutes of the service, and a weaker permanent waving solution should have been used. If the hair is not sufficiently processed after ten minutes, it may require a reapplication of waving solution. Resistant hair requires a stronger solution, a higher pH, and a more thorough saturation.

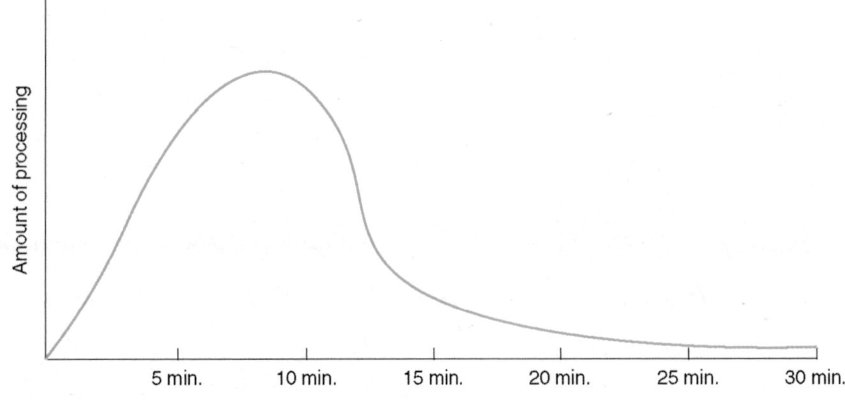

▲ **Figure 20–33**
Average processing times.

Thorough saturation of the hair is essential to proper processing in all permanent waves—especially those applied on resistant hair. Regardless of the strength or pH of the solution, resistant hair may not become completely saturated with just one application of waving solution. You may need to apply the solution slowly and repeatedly until the hair looks wet and stays wet!

Overprocessed Hair

A thorough saturation with a stronger (more alkaline) solution will break more disulfide bonds and process the hair more, but processing the hair more does not necessarily translate into more curl. A properly processed permanent wave should break and rebuild approximately 50 percent of the hair's disulfide bonds (**Figure 20–33**).

If too many disulfide bonds are broken, the hair may not have enough strength left to hold the desired curl. Weak hair equals a weak curl.

Contrary to what many people believe, overprocessed hair does not necessarily mean hair that is overly curly. If too many disulfide bonds are broken, the hair will be too weak to hold a firm curl. Overprocessed hair usually has a weak curl or may even be completely straight. Since the hair at the scalp is usually stronger than the hair at the ends, overprocessed hair is usually curlier at the scalp and straighter at the ends (**Figure 20–34**). If the hair is overprocessed, further processing will make it straighter.

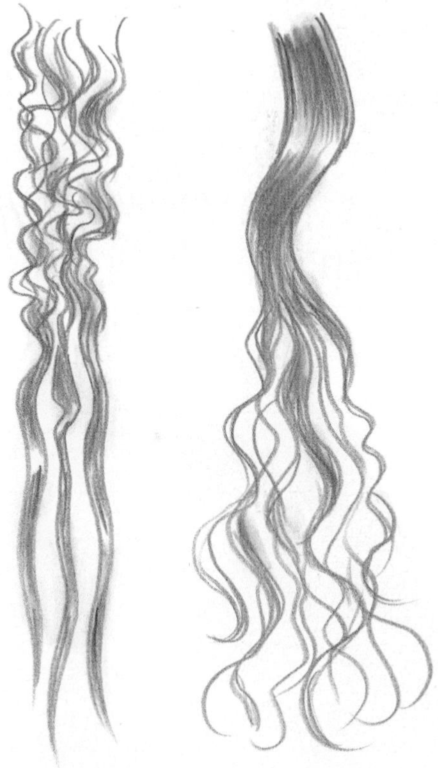

▲ **Figure 20–34**
Overprocessed hair.

▲ **Figure 20–35**
Underprocessed hair.

Underprocessed Hair

As the title suggests, underprocessed hair is the exact opposite of overprocessed hair. If too few disulfide bonds are broken, the hair will not be sufficiently softened and will not be able to hold the desired curl.

Underprocessed hair usually has a very weak curl, but it may also be straight. Since the hair at the scalp is usually stronger than the ends, underprocessed hair is usually straighter at the scalp and curlier at the ends (**Figure 20–35**). If the hair is underprocessed, processing it more will make it curlier.

© Milady, a part of Cengage Learning.

Permanent Waving (Thio) Neutralization

In permanent waving, **thio neutralization** stops the action of the waving solution and rebuilds the hair into its new curly form. Neutralization performs two important functions:

- Any waving solution that remains in the hair is deactivated (neutralized).
- Disulfide bonds that were broken by the waving solution are rebuilt.

The neutralizers used in permanent waving are oxidizers. In fact, the term neutralizer is not accurate because the chemical reaction involved is actually oxidation. The most common neutralizer is hydrogen peroxide. Concentrations vary between 5 volume (1.5 percent) and 10 volume (3 percent).

Thio Neutralization: Stage One

The first function of permanent waving (thio) neutralization is the deactivation, or neutralization, of any waving lotion that remains in the hair after processing and rinsing. The chemical reaction involved is called oxidation.

Properly rinsing the hair after the permanent has processed removes any remaining perm solution, prior to applying the neutralizer. Oxidative reactions can also lighten hair color, especially at an alkaline pH. To avoid scalp irritation and unwanted lightening of hair color, always rinse perm solution from the hair for at least five minutes, and then blot the hair with towels to remove as much moisture as possible. Excess water left in the hair reduces the effectiveness of the neutralizer.

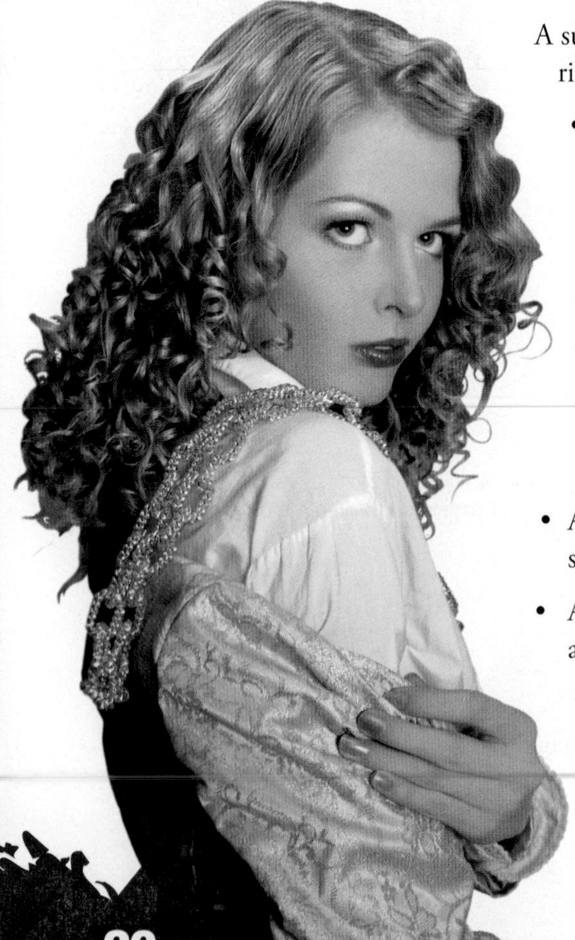

A successful perm takes time, patience, and expertise. Proper rinsing and blotting are important!

- Always rinse the hair with warm water, never hot water.
- Always use a gentle stream of water, never a strong blast of water.
- Never apply pressure to the rods while rinsing out the solution.
- Always rinse the most fragile areas first (typically the temple area).
- Always check the nape area to ensure that you are thoroughly rinsing the bottom rods.
- Always rinse for at least the time recommended by the manufacturer.
- Always smell the hair after the recommended time has elapsed; if it still smells like perm solution, continue rinsing until the odor is gone.
- Always gently blot the hair with a dry towel; never firmly or aggressively blot the hair.
- Always check for excess moisture, especially at the nape of the neck where water tends to accumulate (pull of gravity), prior to neutralizing the hair.
- Always adjust any rods that have become loose or have drifted out of alignment prior to applying the neutralizer.

© Tassh, 2010; used under license from Shutterstock.com.

Some manufacturers recommend the application of a pre-neutralizing conditioner after rinsing and blotting, just before application of the neutralizer. An acidic liquid protein conditioner can be applied to the hair and dried under a warm hair dryer (hair is uncovered) for five minutes or more prior to neutralization. This added step is especially beneficial for very damaged hair, because it strengthens the hair prior to neutralization. Always follow the manufacturer's directions and the procedures approved by your instructor.

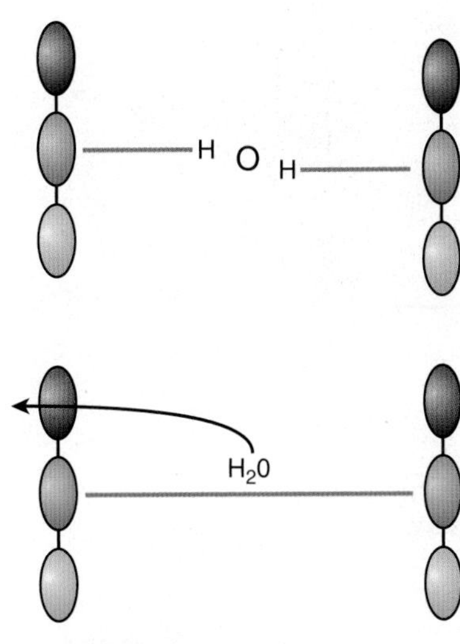

▲ **Figure 20–36**
Oxidation reaction of thio neutralizers.

Thio Neutralization: Stage Two

As discussed previously, permanent waving solution breaks disulfide bonds by adding hydrogen. Thio neutralization rebuilds the disulfide bonds by removing the hydrogen that was added by the permanent waving solution. The hydrogen atoms are strongly attracted to the oxygen in the neutralizer and release their bond with the sulfur atoms and join with the oxygen (**Figure 20–36**). Each oxygen atom joins with two hydrogen atoms to rebuild one disulfide bond, forming a water molecule. The water is removed in the final rinse. Side bonds are then re-formed into their new shape as different pairs (**Figure 20–37**). ☑ **LO4**

Permanent Waving Procedures

The information presented earlier in the chapter on sectioning, base control, base direction, perm rods, wrapping techniques, and wrapping patterns should be used with permanent waving procedures.

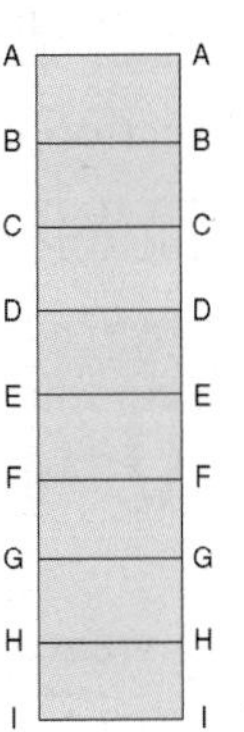

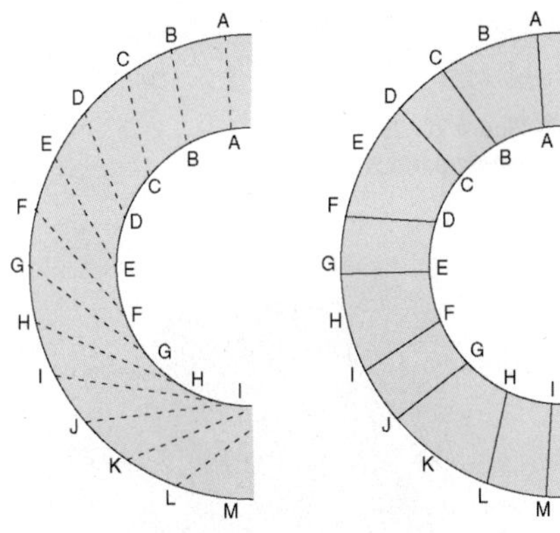

▲ **Figure 20–37**
New disulfide pairs.

Preliminary Test Curls

Preliminary test curls help you determine how your client's hair will react to a perm. It is advisable to take preliminary test curls if the hair is damaged or if there is any uncertainty about the results. Preliminary test curls provide the following information:

- Correct processing time for the best curl development
- Results you can expect from the type of perm solution you have selected
- Curl results for the rod size and wrapping technique you are planning to use

PROCEDURE 20-1 Preliminary Test Curl for a Permanent Wave SEE PAGE 593

Wrapping Patterns

These basic wrapping patterns may be combined in different ways to create a wide variety of specialized perm wraps that provide an unlimited number of styling options.

The **basic permanent wrap**, also known as **straight set wrap**, is a wrapping pattern in which all the rods within a panel move in the same direction and are positioned on equal-sized bases; all the base sections are horizontal and are the same length and width as the perm rod. The **base control** is the position of the

© Milady, a part of Cengage Learning.

tool in relation to its base section, determined by the angle at which the hair is wrapped (**Figure 20–38**).

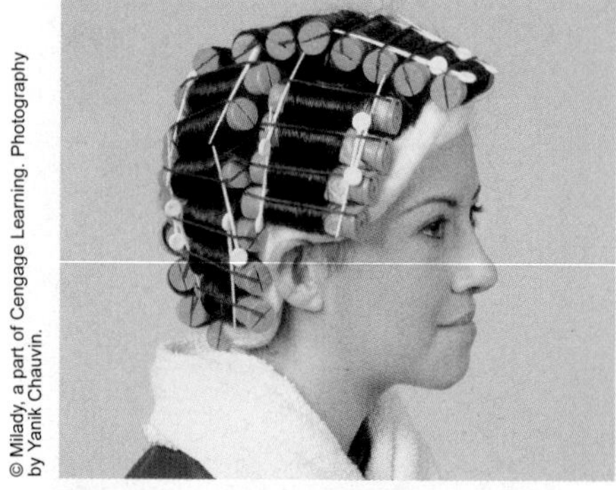
© Milady, a part of Cengage Learning. Photography by Yanik Chauvin.

▲ **Figure 20–38**
Basic perm wrapping pattern.

PROCEDURE 20-2 Permanent Wave and Processing Using a Basic Permanent Wrap SEE PAGE 595

In the **curvature permanent wrap**, partings and bases radiate throughout the panels to follow the curvature of the head. This wrapping pattern uses pie-shaped base sections in the curvature areas (**Figure 20–39**).

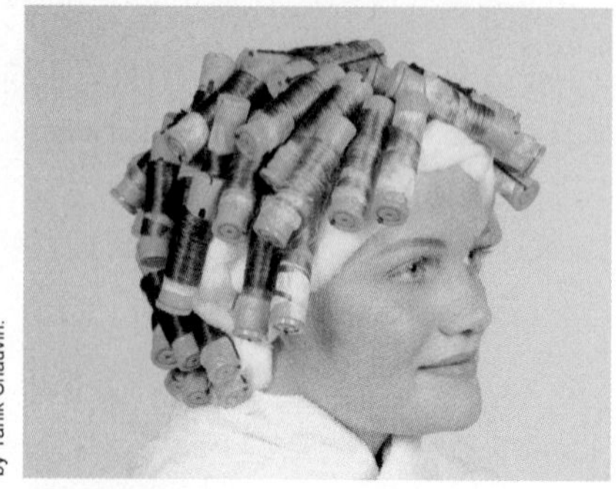
© Milady, a part of Cengage Learning. Photography by Yanik Chauvin.

▲ **Figure 20–39**
Curvature perm wrapping pattern.

PROCEDURE 20-3 Permanent Wave and Processing Using a Curvature Permanent Wrap SEE PAGE 598

The **bricklay permanent wrap** is similar to the actual technique of bricklaying; base sections are offset from each other row by row, to prevent noticeable splits, and to blend the flow of the hair. Different bricklay patterns use different starting points (front hairline, occipital area, and crown), and these starting points affect the directional flow of the hair. The bricklay perm wrap can be used with various combinations of sectioning, base control, base direction, wrapping techniques, and perm rods (**Figure 20–40**).

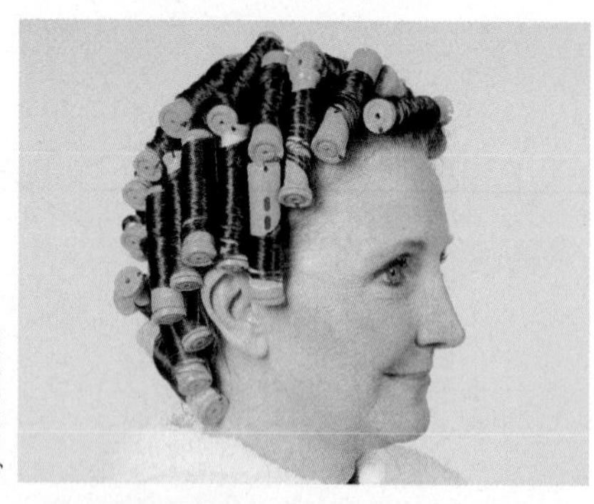
© Milady, a part of Cengage Learning. Photography by Yanik Chauvin.

▲ **Figure 20–40**
Bricklay perm wrapping pattern.

PROCEDURE 20-4 Permanent Wave and Processing Using a Bricklay Permanent Wrap SEE PAGE 601

The **weave technique** uses zigzag partings to divide base areas. It can be used throughout the entire perm wrap or only in selected areas. This technique is very effective for blending between perm rods with opposite base directions. It can also be used to create a smooth transition from the rolled areas into the unrolled areas of a partial perm. The weave technique can be used with a variety of base directions, wrapping patterns, and perm rods (**Figure 20–41**).

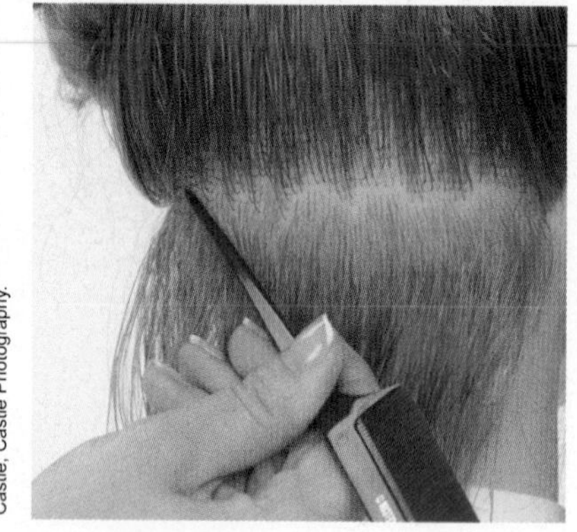
© Milady, a part of Cengage Learning. Photography by Paul Castle, Castle Photography.

▲ **Figure 20–41**
Weave technique.

PROCEDURE 20-5 Permanent Wave And Processing Using a Weave Technique SEE PAGE 603

The double-rod wrap technique (piggyback wrap), discussed earlier, is a wrap technique whereby extra-long hair is wrapped on one rod from the scalp to midway down the hair shaft. Another rod is then used to wrap the remaining hair strand in the same direction. The upper half of the strand is wrapped around one rod, and then the lower half of the same strand is wrapped around a second rod in an alternate direction and stacked (piggybacked) on top of the first.

PROCEDURE 20-6 Permanent Wave and Processing Using a Double-Rod or Piggyback Technique SEE PAGE 605

The double-rod wrap technique doubles the number of rods used. Using more rods increases the amount of curl in the finished perm, making this technique especially effective on long hair. Rods of various diameters may be used to create different effects. The double-rod wrap technique can also be used with a variety of base directions, wrapping patterns, and perm rods.

In a spiral perm wrap, the hair is wrapped at an angle other than perpendicular to the length of the rod. This wrapping technique produces a uniform curl from the scalp to the ends. Longer, thicker hair will benefit most from this effect (**Figure 20–42**).

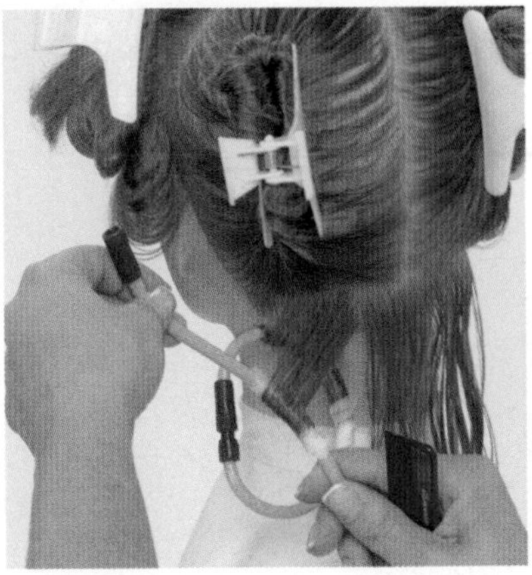

© Milady, a part of Cengage Learning. Photography by Paul Castle, Castle Photography.

▲ **Figure 20–42**
Spiral perm wrap.

PROCEDURE 20-7 Permanent Wave and Processing Using a Spiral Wrap Technique SEE PAGE 607

The spiral wrapping technique can be used with a variety of base sections, base directions, and wrapping patterns. Base sections may be either horizontal or vertical and do not affect the finished curl. Conventional rods, bendable soft foam rods, and loop rods can all be used for this technique, depending on the length of the rod and the length of the hair.

Partial Perms

If your client wants a perm but does not wish the entire head of hair to be curled, a partial perm may be the answer. Partial perms also allow you to give a perm when some of the hair is too short to roll on rods (**Figure 20–43**).

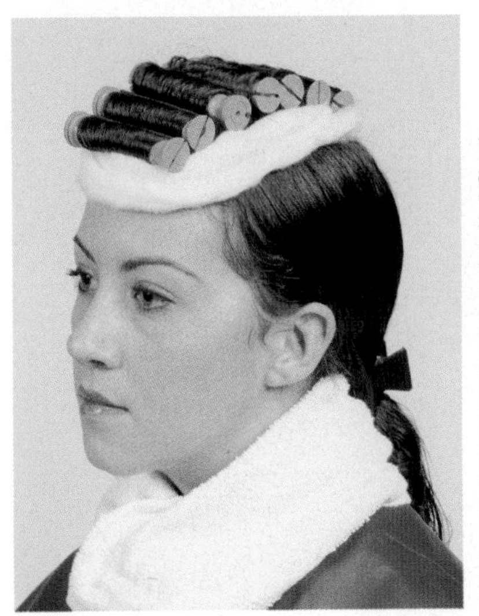

© Milady, a part of Cengage Learning. Photography by Yanik Chauvin.

▲ **Figure 20–43**
Partial perm wrap.

Partial perms can be used for:

- Male and female clients who have long hair on the top and crown but very short hair with tapered sides and nape.
- Clients who only need volume and lift in certain areas.
- Clients who desire a hairstyle with curls along the perimeter but a smooth, sleek crown.

Partial perms rely on the same techniques and wrapping patterns as those used with other perms, but there are additional considerations:

- In order to make a smooth transition from the rolled section to the unrolled section, use a larger rod for the last rod next to an unrolled section.
- Applying waving solution to unrolled hair may straighten it or make it difficult to style. To protect the unrolled hair, apply a protective barrier cream to the unrolled section before applying the waving lotion.

Perms for Men

Do not assume that perms are only for women. Many male clients are looking for the added texture, fullness, style, and low maintenance that only a perm can provide. Perms help thin hair look fuller, make straight or coarse hair more manageable, and help control stubborn cowlicks. Although men's and women's hairstyles may be different, the techniques for permanent waving are essentially the same.

Safety Precautions for Permanent Waving

- Always protect your client's clothing. Have the client change into a gown, use a waterproof shampoo cape, and double drape with towels to absorb accidental spills.
- Do not give a permanent to any client who has experienced an allergic reaction to a previous permanent.
- Always examine the scalp before the perm service. Do not proceed if there are any skin abrasions or signs of scalp disease.
- Do not perm hair that is excessively damaged or shows signs of breakage.
- Do not attempt to perm hair that has been previously treated with hydroxide relaxers.
- If there is a possibility that metallic haircolor has been previously used on the hair, perform a test for metallic salts.
- Always apply protective barrier cream around the client's hairline and ears prior to applying permanent waving solution.
- Do not dilute or add anything to the waving lotion or neutralizer unless specified in the manufacturer's directions.
- Keep waving lotion out of the client's eyes. In case of accidental exposure, rinse thoroughly with cool water.
- Always follow the manufacturer's directions.
- Wear gloves when applying solutions.
- Immediately replace cotton or towels that have become wet with solution.
- Do not save any opened, unused waving solution or neutralizer. When not used promptly, these chemicals may change in strength and effectiveness.

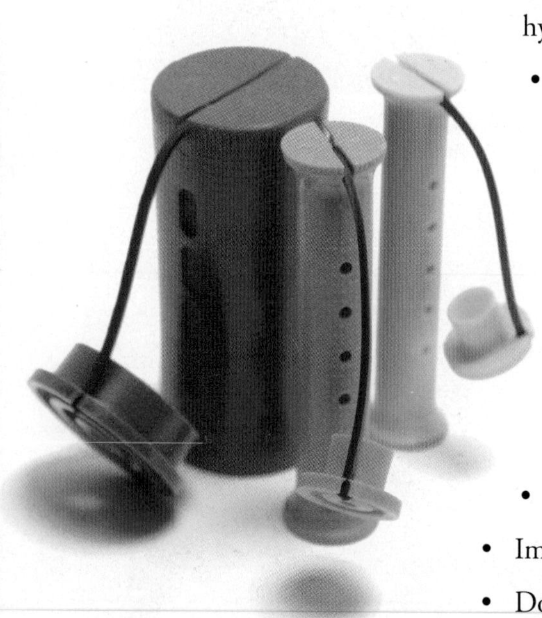

© Milady, a part of Cengage Learning.

Hair that has been permanently waved should be shampooed and conditioned with products formulated for chemically treated hair.

Metallic Salts

Some home haircoloring products contain metallic salts that are not compatible with permanent waving. Metallic salts leave a coating on the hair that may cause uneven curls, severe discoloration, or hair breakage.

Metallic salts are more commonly found in men's haircolors that are sold for home use. Haircolor restorers and progressive haircolors that darken the hair gradually with repeated applications are the most likely to contain metallic salts. If you suspect that metallic salts may be present on the hair, perform the following test.

In a glass or plastic bowl, mix 1 ounce of 20-volume peroxide with 20 drops of 28-percent ammonia. Immerse at least 20 strands of hair in the solution for thirty minutes. If metallic salts are not present, the hair will lighten slightly and you may proceed with the service. If metallic salts are present, the hair will lighten rapidly. The solution may get hot and give off an unpleasant odor, indicating that you should not proceed with the service.

Chemical Hair Relaxers

Chemical hair relaxing is a process or service that rearranges the structure of curly hair into a straighter or smoother form. Whereas permanent waving curls straight hair, chemical hair relaxing straightens curly hair (**Figure 20–44**).

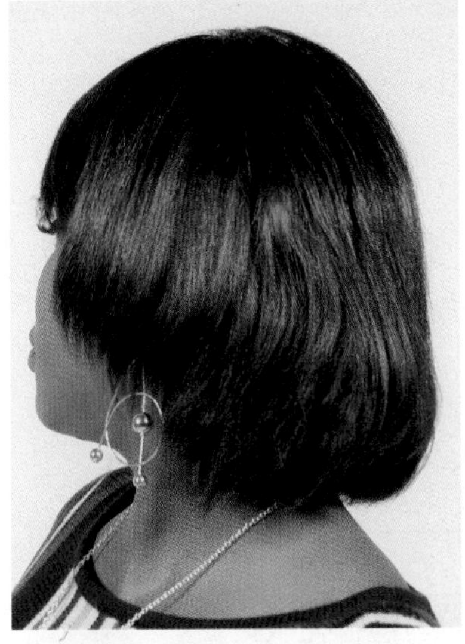

© Milady, a part of Cengage Learning. Photography by Yanik Chauvin.

▲ **Figure 20–44**
Relaxed hair.

Other than their objectives being quite different, the permanent wave and relaxer services are very similar. In fact, the chemistry of thio relaxers and permanent waving is exactly the same. And even though the chemistry of hydroxide relaxers and permanent waving may be different, all relaxers and all permanents change the shape of the hair by breaking disulfide bonds.

The two most common types of chemical hair relaxers are thio (ammonium thioglycolate) and sodium hydroxide.

Extremely Curly Hair

Extremely curly hair grows in long twisted spirals, or coils. Cross-sections are highly elliptical and vary in shape and thickness along their lengths. Compared to straight or wavy hair, which tends to possess a fairly regular and uniform diameter along a single strand, extremely curly hair is irregular, exhibiting varying diameters along a single strand.

The thinnest and weakest sections of the hair strands are located at the twists. These sections are also bent at an extremely sharp angle and will be stretched the most during relaxing. A chain is only as strong as its weakest link, and hair is only as strong as its weakest section. Hair breaks at its weakest point. Extremely curly hair usually breaks at the twists because of the inherent weakness in that section and because of the extra physical force that is required to straighten it.

CAUTION

Relaxers are extremely alkaline and can literally melt or dissolve hair if used incorrectly. Most relaxers contain the same ingredients used in depilatories (products used for temporary hair removal).

Thio Relaxers

Thio relaxers use the same ATG that is used in permanent waving, but at a higher concentration and a higher pH (above 10). Thio relaxers are also thicker, with a higher **viscosity**, the measurement of the thickness or thinness of a liquid that affects how the fluid flows, making them more suitable for application as a relaxer.

Thio relaxers break disulfide bonds and soften hair, just as in permanents. After enough bonds are broken, the hair is straightened into its new shape, and the relaxer is rinsed from the hair. Blotting comes next, followed by a neutralizer. The chemical reactions of thio relaxers are identical to those in permanent waving. ☑ **LO5**

Thio Neutralization

The neutralizer used with thio relaxers is an oxidizing agent, usually hydrogen peroxide, just as in permanents. The oxidation reaction caused by the neutralizer rebuilds the disulfide bonds that were broken by the thio relaxer.

Thio Relaxer Application

The application steps for thio relaxers are the same as those for hydroxide relaxers, although the neutralization procedure is different. Relaxer may be applied with bowl and brush, applicator bottle, or the back of a hard rubber comb. Although all thio relaxers follow the same procedures, different application methods are used for virgin relaxers and retouch relaxers.

The same implements and materials as for virgin hydroxide relaxers are used, but thio relaxer, pre-neutralizing conditioner, and thio neutralizer are substituted for hydroxide products.

You will follow the same preparation steps as for virgin hydroxide relaxers. A light shampoo before a thio relaxer is optional. Do not forget to perform an analysis of the client's hair and scalp. Test the hair for elasticity and porosity on several areas of the head. If the hair has poor elasticity, do not perform a relaxer service.

PROCEDURE 20-8 Applying Thio Relaxer to Virgin Hair **SEE PAGE 610**

PROCEDURE 20-9 Thio Relaxer Retouch **SEE PAGE 612**

Japanese Thermal Straighteners

Japanese thermal straightening, sometimes called thermal reconditioning or TR, combines use of a thio relaxer with flat ironing. When first introduced, they were called thermal ionic reconstructors. Each manufacturer has slightly different procedures. Generally, after the hair is shampooed and conditioned, the straightener is applied to sections, distributed evenly, and processed until the desired degree of curl or frizz reduction is reached. Then the hair is rinsed thoroughly for about ten minutes, conditioned and blown dry until it is completely dry. Next, each section is flat ironed; several passes of the flat

© R McKown, 2010; used under license from Shutterstock.com.

iron are required for each section. (The added heat and mechanical pressing helps to make these formulas more effective than standard thio relaxers.) The hair is then neutralized and blown dry.

The service can take several hours and is not always appropriate for extremely curly hair or some color-treated hair. Thermal reconditioning is considered a specialty, and many manufacturers require certification in their particular procedure.

CAUTION

Hair that has been treated with a hydroxide relaxer is unfit for permanent waving and will not hold a curl. The disulfide bonds have been permanently broken and can never be re-formed.

Hydroxide Relaxers

The hydroxide ion is the active ingredient in all **hydroxide relaxers**, which are very strong alkalis with a pH over 13. Sodium hydroxide, potassium hydroxide, lithium hydroxide, and guanidine hydroxide are all types of hydroxide relaxers, which can swell the hair up to twice its normal diameter.

Hydroxide relaxers are not compatible with thio relaxers, permanent waving, or soft curl perms because they use a different chemistry. Thio relaxers use thio to break the disulfide bonds. The high pH of a thio relaxer is needed to swell the hair, but it is the thio that breaks the disulfide bonds.

Hydroxide relaxers have a pH that is so high that the alkalinity alone breaks the disulfide bonds. The average pH of the hair is 5.0, and many hydroxide relaxers have a pH over 13.0. Since each step in the pH scale represents a tenfold change in concentration, a pH of 13.0 is 100 million (100,000,000) times more alkaline than a pH of 5.0 (**Figure 20–45**).

CAUTION

Application of a thio relaxer or thio permanent on hair that has been treated with a hydroxide relaxer will not properly relax or curl the hair, and it may cause extreme damage. Hair that has been treated with hydroxide relaxers is unfit for thio relaxers and for soft curl permanents.

Hydroxide relaxers break disulfide bonds differently than in the reduction reaction of thio relaxers. In **lanthionization** (lan-thee-oh-ny-ZAY-shun), the process by which hydroxide relaxers permanently straighten hair, the relaxers remove a sulfur atom from a disulfide bond and convert it into a lanthionine bond. A disulfide bond consists of two bonded sulfur atoms. Lanthionine bonds contain only one sulfur atom. The disulfide bonds that are broken by hydroxide relaxers are broken permanently and can never be re-formed. That is why hair that has been treated with a hydroxide relaxer is unfit for permanent waving and will not hold a curl.

Types of Hydroxide Relaxers

Metal hydroxide relaxers are ionic compounds formed by a metal—sodium (Na), potassium (K), or lithium (Li)—which is combined with oxygen (O) and hydrogen (H). Metal hydroxide relaxers include sodium

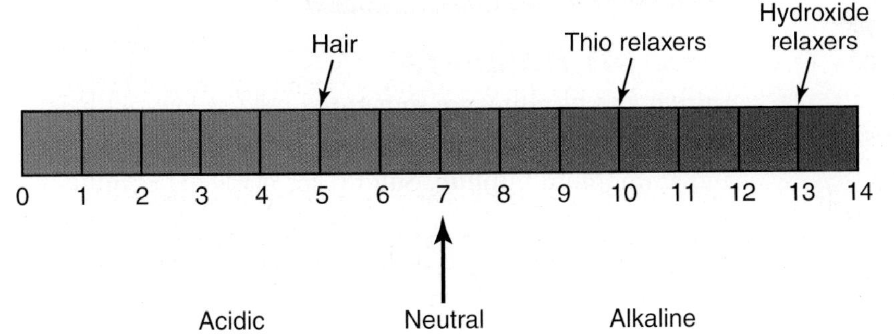

◀ **Figure 20–45**
pH of thio and hydroxide relaxers.

© Milady, a part of Cengage Learning.

CAUTION

Make sure that the client has not had haircoloring containing metallic salts, such as gradual or progressive haircolors, before applying either thio or hydroxide relaxers to the hair. Extreme damage or breakage can occur.

When combining a relaxing service with a permanent or demipermanent haircoloring service, it is always preferable to relax the hair first and color it two weeks later. This is the best way to protect the integrity of the hair and to prevent the relaxing product from lightening the haircolor. Also keep in mind that—although many manufacturers call their demipermanent products *no lift*—all demipermanent haircoloring uses low volumes of peroxide or other alkalizing agents, such as MEA, as well as oxidizing agents other than hydrogen peroxide. In other words (like the term *no lye*), the term *no ammonia* does not mean that no chemicals are used.

Never use bleaches or high-lift color products on relaxed hair. This combination has resulted in many lawsuits.

You can use a semipermanent product on the same day as relaxing because these colors contain no ammonia or peroxide. Relax the hair first, check the hair's condition, and then apply the semipermanent color, following the manufacturer's guidelines.

When in doubt, test the hair's strength, and then do a strand test for the color. Accomplished colorists say they use demipermanent and even permanent color products on the same day as relaxing the hair, and some manufacturers claim their coloring products allow this; however, same-day chemical services are advanced techniques that depend on the hair's condition, the experience of the stylist, and the specific products used.

Same-day chemical services always compromise the hair's integrity to some degree, whether you are combining hydroxide-based chemicals and haircolor or thio-based chemicals and color. For instance, same-day coloring and Japanese Thermal Straightening, done incorrectly, can result in extreme hair breakage, as many Internet postings attest.

hydroxide (NaOH), potassium hydroxide (KOH), and lithium hydroxide (LiOH).

Although calcium hydroxide (CaOH) is sometimes added to hydroxide relaxers, it is not used by itself to relax hair.

All metal hydroxide relaxers contain only one component and are used exactly as they are packaged in the container; no mixing is used. The hydroxide ion is the active ingredient in all hydroxide relaxers. There is no significant difference in the performance of these metal hydroxide relaxers.

Lye-Based Relaxers

Sodium hydroxide (NaOH) relaxers are commonly called lye relaxers. Sodium hydroxide is the oldest, and still the most common, type of chemical hair relaxer. Sodium hydroxide is also known as lye or caustic soda. Sodium hydroxide is the same chemical that is used in drain cleaners and chemical hair depilatories.

No-Lye Relaxers

Lithium hydroxide (LiOH) and potassium hydroxide (KOH) relaxers are often advertised and sold as *no mix–no lye* relaxers. Although technically they are not lye, their chemistry is identical, and there is very little difference in their performance.

Guanidine (GWAN-ih-deen) hydroxide relaxers are also advertised and sold as no-lye relaxers. Although technically they are not lye, the hydroxide ion is still the active ingredient. Guanidine hydroxide relaxers contain two components that must be mixed immediately prior to use. These relaxers straighten hair completely, with less scalp irritation than other hydroxide relaxers. Most guanidine hydroxide relaxers are recommended for sensitive scalps, and they are sold over the counter for home use. Although they reduce scalp irritation, they do not reduce hair damage. They swell the hair slightly more than other hydroxide relaxers, and they are also more drying, especially after repeated applications. ☑ **LO6**

Low-pH Relaxers

Sulfites and bisulfites are sometimes used as low-pH hair relaxers. The most commonly used are ammonium sulfite and ammonium bisulfite. Sulfites are marketed as mild alternative relaxers, and are compatible with thio relaxers but not compatible with hydroxide relaxers. They do not completely straighten extremely curly hair. Low-pH relaxers are intended for use on color-treated, damaged, or fine hair. See Table 20–2 on page 589 for a summary of the types and uses of relaxers.

Base and No-Base Relaxers

Hydroxide relaxers are usually sold in base and no-base formulas. **Base cream**, also known as **protective base cream**, is an oily cream used to protect the skin and scalp during hair relaxing. **Base relaxers** require the application of a protective base cream to the entire scalp prior to the application of the relaxer.

No-base relaxers do not require the application of a protective base cream. They contain a protective base cream that is designed to melt at body temperature. As the relaxer is applied, body heat causes the protective base cream to melt and settle out onto the scalp in a thin, oily, protective coating. No-base relaxers are an improvement only on the protection that is provided to the skin by the oils in all hydroxide relaxers. For added protection, protective base cream may be applied to the entire hairline and around the ears, even with no-base relaxers.

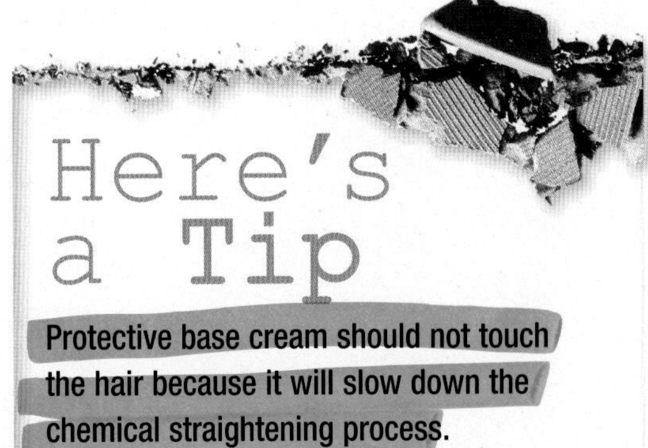

Protective base cream should not touch the hair because it will slow down the chemical straightening process.

Relaxer Strengths

Most chemical hair relaxers are available in three strengths: mild, regular, and super. The difference in strength of hydroxide relaxers parallels the concentration of hydroxide.

- Mild-strength relaxers are formulated for fine, color-treated, or damaged hair.
- Regular-strength relaxers are intended for normal hair texture with a medium natural curl.
- Super-strength relaxers should be used for maximum straightening on very coarse, extremely curly, and resistant hair.

When in doubt, always choose the gentler alternative: mild instead of regular or regular instead of super.

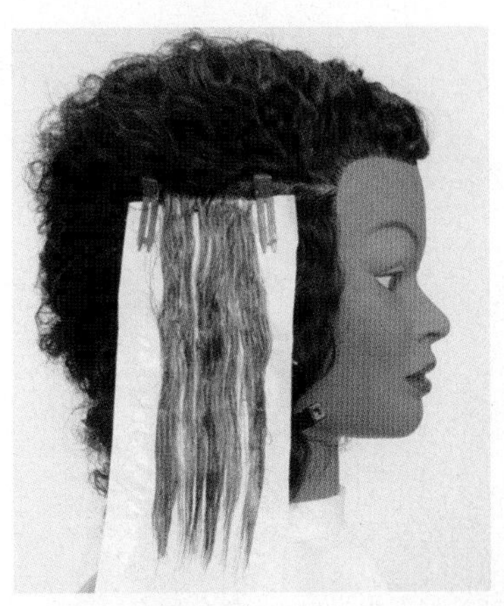

▲ Figure 20–46
Sufficiently relaxed strand.

Periodic Strand Testing

Periodic strand testing during processing will help to tell you when the hair is sufficiently relaxed. After the relaxer is applied, stretch the strands to see how fast the natural curls are being removed. You may also smooth and press the strand to the scalp using the back of the comb, the applicator brush, or your finger. Be gentle! If the strand remains smooth, it is sufficiently relaxed. If the curl returns, continue processing. Processing time will vary according to the strength of the relaxer, hair type and condition, and the desired results (**Figures 20–46** and **20–47**).

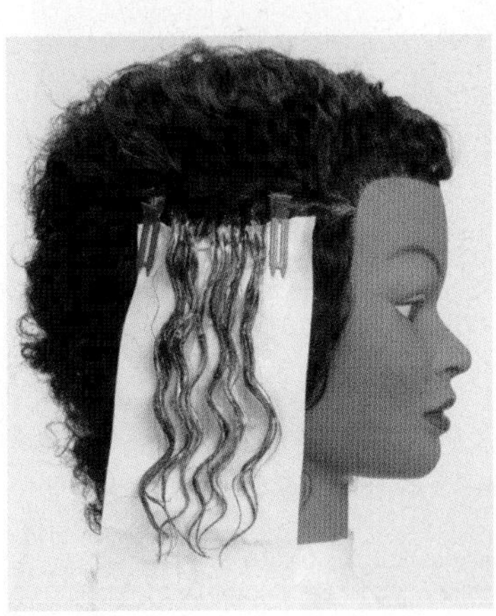

▲ Figure 20–47
Insufficiently relaxed strand.

Hydroxide Neutralization

Unlike thio neutralization, **hydroxide neutralization** is an acid–alkali neutralization that neutralizes (deactivates) the alkaline residues left in the hair by a hydroxide relaxer and lowers the pH of the hair and scalp;

© Milady, a part of Cengage Learning. Photography by Paul Castle, Castle Photography.

hydroxide relaxer neutralization does not involve oxidation or rebuilding disulfide bonds. The pH of hydroxide relaxers is so high that the hair remains at an extremely high pH, even after thorough rinsing. Although rinsing is important, rinsing alone does not neutralize (deactivate) the relaxer, nor does it restore the normal acidic pH of the hair and scalp.

As described in Chapter 12, Basics of Chemistry, acids neutralize alkalis. Therefore, the application of an acid-balanced shampoo or a normalizing lotion neutralizes any remaining hydroxide ions to lower the pH of the hair and scalp. Some neutralizing shampoos intended for use after hydroxide relaxers have a built-in pH indicator that changes color to show when the pH of the hair has returned to normal.

The neutralization of a hydroxide relaxer does not rebuild the disulfide bonds. Since the disulfide bonds that have been broken by hydroxide relaxers cannot be re-formed by oxidation, application of a neutralizer that contains an oxidizing agent will not be of any benefit and will only damage the hair.

Hydroxide Relaxer Procedures

Although the same procedure is used for all hydroxide relaxers, application methods vary according to previous use of texture services.

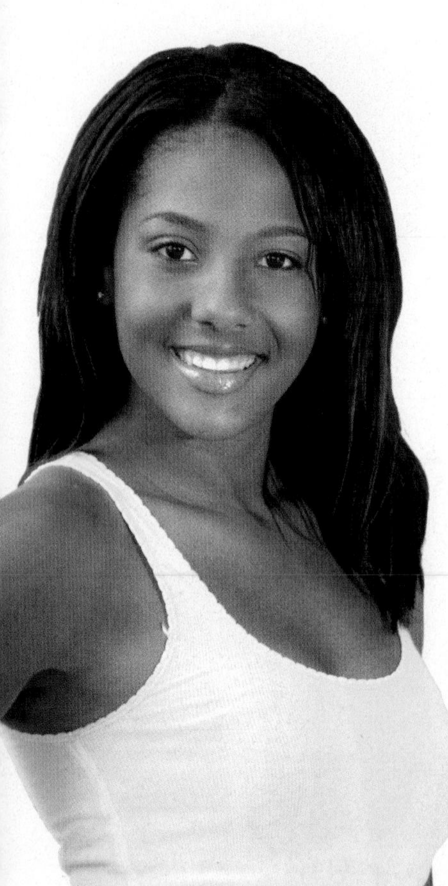

- A virgin relaxer application should be used for hair that has not had previous chemical texture services. Since the scalp area and the porous ends will usually process more quickly than the middle of the strand, the application for a virgin relaxer starts ¼-inch (0.6 centimeters) to ½-inch (1.25 centimeters) away from the scalp and includes the entire strand up to the porous ends. To avoid overprocessing and scalp irritation, do not apply relaxer to the hair closest to the scalp or to the ends until the last few minutes of processing.

PROCEDURE 20-10 Applying Hydroxide Relaxer to Virgin Hair SEE PAGE 614

- A retouch relaxer application should be used for hair that has had previous chemical texture services. The application for a retouch relaxer starts ¼-inch to ½-inch away from the scalp and includes only the new growth. To avoid overprocessing and scalp irritation, do not apply relaxer to the hair closest to the scalp until the last few minutes of processing. If the previously relaxed hair requires additional straightening, relaxer may be applied during the last few minutes of processing.

PROCEDURE 20-11 Hydroxide Relaxer Retouch SEE PAGE 617

- A texturizing or retexturizing service uses a hydroxide relaxer to reduce the curl pattern by degrees. The procedure for texturizing is similar to that for relaxing, only the product is gently combed through, using a

© Flashon Studio, 2010; used under license from Shutterstock.com.

large-toothed comb. This allows you to observe the curl pattern as it releases and halt processing when the desired degree of curl reduction is achieved.

- Option A: Some manufacturers recommend the use of a normalizing lotion after rinsing out the relaxer and prior to shampooing. **Normalizing lotions** are conditioners with an acidic pH that restore the hair's natural pH after a hydroxide relaxer and prior to shampooing. Option B: Many manufacturers include a normalizing or neutralizing shampoo that must be used after rinsing out the relaxer. It is an acidic shampoo designed to restore the natural pH of hair and scalp. Often, it includes a color signal that turns pink if any relaxer residue remains in the hair.

After a thorough consultation, you should be able to determine which type of relaxer is best suited to your client's hair type, condition, and desired results. **Table 20–2** lists the most common types of relaxers along with selected advantages and disadvantages for each.

Keratin Straightening Treatments

Keratin straightening treatments (also called smoothing treatments or Brazilian keratin treatments) are available to salon professionals and are widely used. Keratin straightening treatments contain silicone polymers and formalin or similar ingredients, which release formaldehyde gas when heated to high temperatures. Some keratin straightening treatments marketed as *formaldehyde free* have been found to contain formalin; some other formulas simply use different aldehydes. Do not confuse these treatments with simple *keratin conditioning treatments*. Keratin alone will not straighten hair.

Keratin straightening treatments work by fixing the keratin in place in a semipermanent manner; they do not break bonds. Once the treatment

ACTIVE INGREDIENT	SELECTING THE CORRECT RELAXER			
	pH	MARKETED AS	ADVANTAGES	DISADVANTAGES
sodium hydroxide	12.5–13.5	lye relaxer	very effective for extremely curly hair	may cause scalp irritation and damage the hair
lithium hydroxide and potassium hydroxide	12.5–13.5	no-mix, no-lye relaxer	very effective for extremely curly hair	may cause scalp irritation and damage the hair
guanidine hydroxide	13–13.5	no-lye relaxer	causes less skin irritation than other hydroxide relaxers	more drying to hair with repeated use
ammonium thioglycolate	9.6–10.0	thio relaxer, no-lye relaxer	compatible with soft curl permanents	strong, unpleasant ammonia smell
ammonium sulfite/ ammonium bisulfite	6.5–8.5	low-pH relaxer, no-lye relaxer	less damaging to hair	does not sufficiently relax extremely curly hair

© Milady, a part of Cengage Learning.

Table 20–2 Selecting the Correct Relaxer.

is applied, the hair is blown dry, and a flat iron set at 450 degrees Fahrenheit is used on narrow sections, one by one, to polymerize a coating on the hair. Each section is flat ironed several times, and the procedure takes about two hours or more for longer or very dense hair. Formalin is reactive to proteins and creates a chemical link or bridge with them when heated, so as to release formaldehyde.

Depending on the size of the salon, the type of ventilation system in place, and the number of technicians simultaneously performing the service, the formaldehyde released during the process has the potential to exceed the maximum concentration allowed by OSHA (Occupational Safety and Health Administration) of 0.75 parts per million (ppm) over an eight-hour period. Local source capture ventilation is recommended, particularly because the flat ironing takes place so close to the client's and stylist's face and because the stylist may be exposed for long periods of time. Because the coating breaks down over time, the client can be exposed to released vapors even when the treatment itself is complete. This is why it is usually recommended that the client wait at least seventy-two hours after the treatment before taking a shower. Within this time period, the steam and heat from the shower can accelerate release of the vapors.

Generally, keratin straightening treatments eliminate up to 95 percent of frizz and curl and last three to five months. They are not usually appropriate for extremely curly, tightly coiled hair. Although this is an advanced treatment, no certification is actually required; nevertheless, most manufacturers do offer specialized training in both the service and the all-important after care.

It is essential to conduct a detailed consultation before performing a keratin straightening service, so the client will understand what to expect from the service, based upon condition of hair, chemical history, and degree of curl.

You will need to discuss the following:

- The client's recent hair history, including all chemical treatments that may still be on the hair and the products used.
- Home-care maintenance during the three-day (seventy-two hour) period after the service is performed, as described below:
  - Usually the hair may not be shampooed for three days (seventy-two hours) after the service.
  - With most systems, the client should avoid getting any moisture into hair for seventy-two hours. If the hair gets damp, blowdry immediately and go over lightly with a flat iron on low heat setting.
  - The client should wear her hair down, and she should not use pins, clips, ponytail holders, or sunglasses to hold the hair back.
- Determine the length and density of the client's hair before quoting a price.

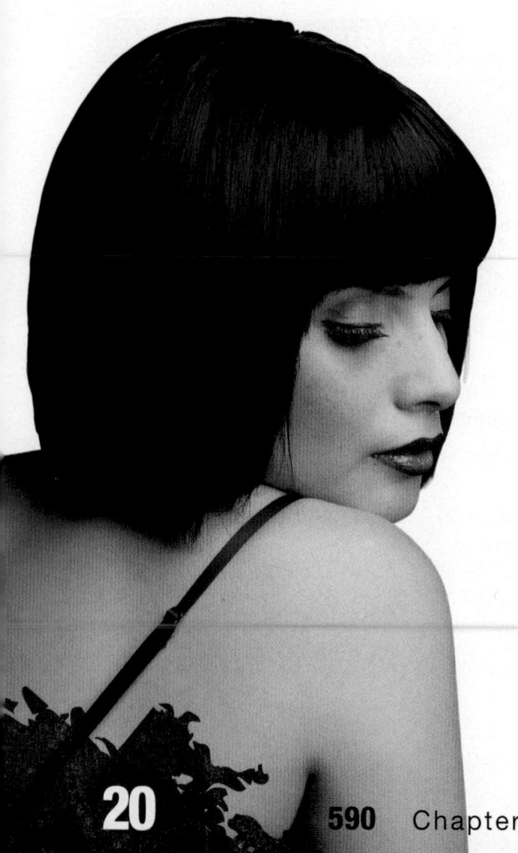

© Nutech21, 2010; used under license from Shutterstock.com.

PreConditioning before a Keratin Straightening Treatments

Preconditioning is meant to equalize the porosity of the hair, taking it to a healthier level. For hair that is extremely overprocessed, damaged, or very curly, shampoo and deep condition prior to beginning the service.

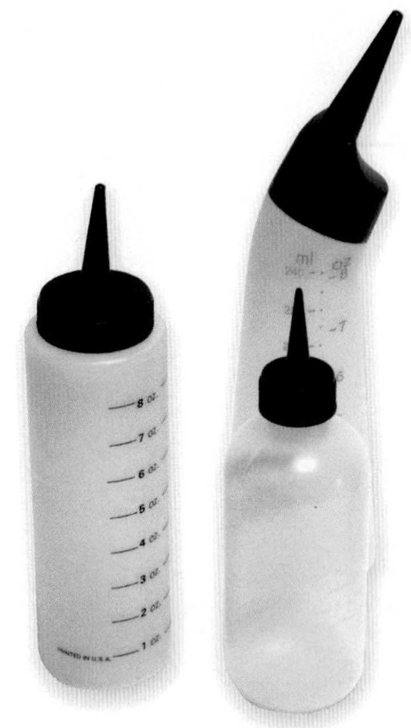

© Milady, a part of Cengage Learning.

Permanent Color/Highlights and Keratin Straightening Treatments

Clients may have a permanent haircolor or highlighting service before the keratin straightening treatments is applied. For those clients, be sure to use a regular/mild shampoo during the haircolor service. Follow the manufacturer's directions regarding the use of a clarifying shampoo before the treatment product is applied.

Do not use a clarifying product on a client that has 70 percent or more highlights.

Toners or Demi-Gloss and Keratin Straightening Treatments

If the client wishes to have a demi-gloss treatment, it should be done at least three to five days after the keratin treatment to prevent color loss and to avoid wetting the newly straightened hair. However, since keratin straightening treatments do coat the hair, a strand test may show that the product you've chosen will not cover the existing cuticle coating to the desired degree.

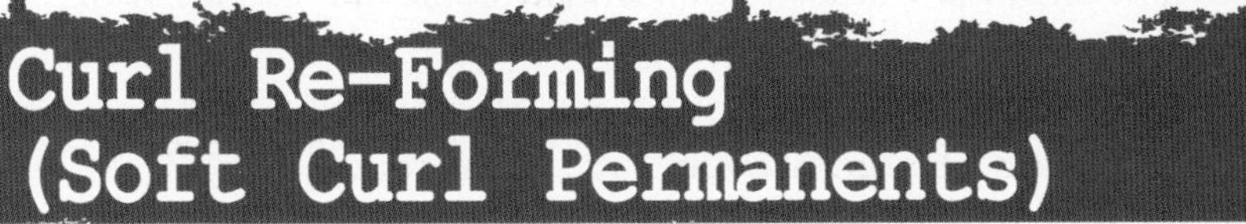

Curl Re-Forming (Soft Curl Permanents)

Curl re-forming does not straighten the hair; it simply makes the existing curl larger and looser. A **soft curl permanent** is a combination of a thio relaxer and a thio permanent that is wrapped on large rods to make existing curl larger and looser. Often, it is simply called a curl. In some markets, it is called a perm, but in others, the word *perm* is used for a permanent relaxing service. Always make sure you clarify what is meant by this term. Soft curl permanents use ATG and oxidation neutralizers, just as thio permanent waves do.

PROCEDURE 20-12 **Curl Re-Forming (Soft Curl Perm)** SEE PAGE 620 ☑ LO7

Safety Precautions for Hair Relaxing and Curl Re-Forming

- Perform a thorough hair analysis and client consultation prior to the service.
- Examine the scalp for abrasions. Do not proceed with the service if redness, swelling, or skin lesions are present.
- Keep accurate and detailed client records of the services performed and the results achieved.

- Have the client sign a release statement indicating that he or she understands the possible risks related to the service.
- Do not apply a hydroxide relaxer on hair that has been previously treated with a thio relaxer.
- Do not apply a thio relaxer or soft curl perm on hair that has been previously treated with a hydroxide relaxer.
- Do not chemically relax hair that has been treated with a metallic dye.
- Do not relax overly damaged hair. Suggest instead a series of reconstruction treatments.
- Do not shampoo the client prior to the application of a hydroxide relaxer.
- The client's hair and scalp must be completely dry and free from perspiration prior to the application of a hydroxide relaxer.
- Apply a protective base cream to avoid scalp irritation.
- Wear gloves during the relaxer application.
- Protect the client's eyes.
- If any solution accidentally gets into the client's eye, flush the eye immediately with cool water and refer the client to a doctor.
- Do not allow chemical relaxers to accidentally come into contact with the client's ears, scalp, or skin.
- Perform periodic strand tests to see how fast the natural curls are being removed.
- Avoid scratching the scalp with your comb or fingernails.
- Do not allow the application of a relaxer retouch to overlap onto previously relaxed hair.
- Never use a strong relaxer on fine or damaged hair. It may cause breakage.
- Do not attempt to remove more than 80 percent of the natural curl.
- Thoroughly rinse the chemical relaxer from the hair. Failure to rinse properly can cause excessive skin irritation and hair breakage.
- Use a normalizing lotion to restore the hair and scalp to their normal acidic pH.
- Use a neutralizing shampoo with a color indicator to guarantee that the hair and scalp have been restored to their normal pH.
- Use a conditioner and wide-tooth comb to eliminate excessive stretching when combing out tangles.
- Do not use hot irons or excessive heat on chemically relaxed hair.

Performing texture services involves using powerful chemicals, which must be handled with the utmost caution. If you act responsibly and perfect your techniques, your services will be in great demand.

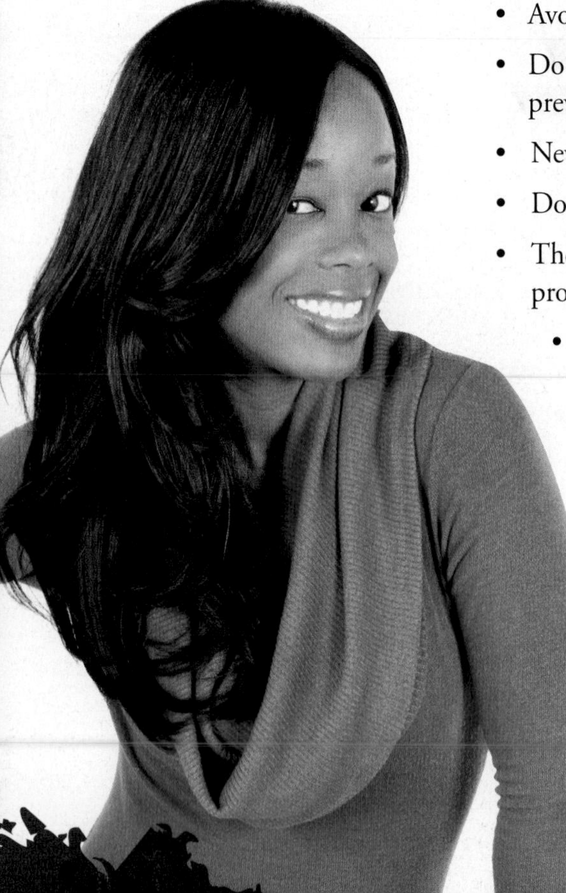

© Julia Lutgendorf, 2010; used under license from Shutterstock.com.

PROCEDURE 20-1

Preliminary Test Curl for a Permanent Wave

Implements and Materials

You will need all of the following implements, materials, and supplies:

- **Acid-balanced shampoo (optional)**
- **Applicator bottles**
- **Conditioner (optional)**
- **Cotton coil or rope**
- **Disposable gloves**
- **End papers**
- **Neutralizer**
- **Neutralizing bib**
- **Perm rods**
- **Perm solution**
- **Plastic clips for sectioning**
- **Plastic tail comb**
- **Pre-neutralizing conditioner (optional)**
- **Protective barrier cream**
- **Roller picks**
- **Shampoo cape**
- **Spray bottle**
- **Styling comb**
- **Timer**
- **Towels**

Preparation

- Perform PROCEDURE 15-1 **Pre-Service Procedure** SEE PAGE 323

Procedure

1 Drape the client for shampoo.

2 Gently shampoo and towel-dry hair. Avoid irritating the client's scalp. Re-drape the client for a chemical service.

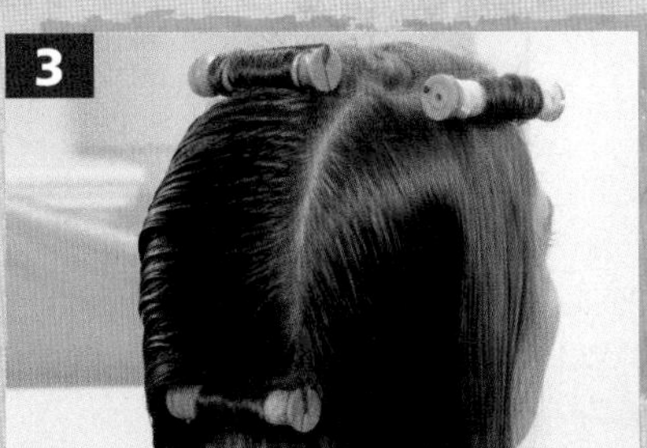

3 Wrap one rod in each different area of the head (top, side, and nape).

4 Wrap a coil of cotton around each rod.

© Milady, a part of Cengage Learning. Photography by Paul Castle, Castle Photography.

Preliminary Test Curl for a Permanent Wave continued

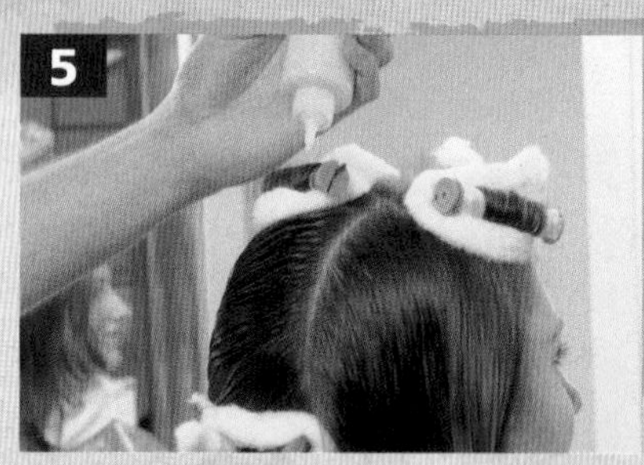

5 Apply waving lotion to the wrapped curls. Do not allow waving lotion to come into contact with unwrapped hair.

6 Set a timer, and process according to the manufacturer's directions.

7 Check each test curl frequently for proper curl development. Unfasten the rod and unwind the curl about one to two turns of the rod. Do not allow the hair to become loose or completely unwound. Gently move the rod toward the scalp to encourage the hair to fall loosely into the wave pattern.

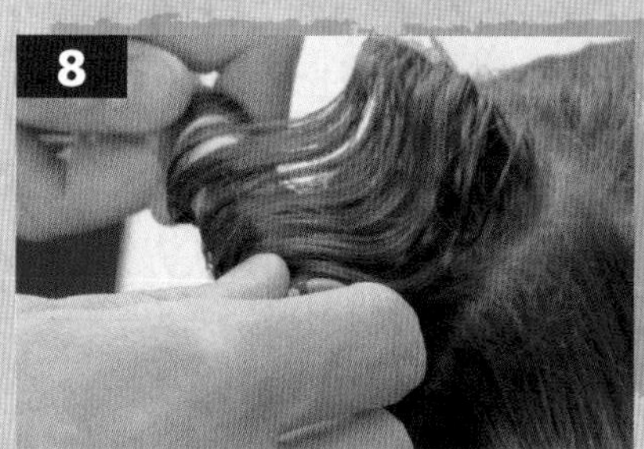

8 Curl development is complete when a firm S is formed that reflects the size of the rod used. Different hair textures will have slightly different S formations. The wave pattern for fine, thin hair may be weak, with little definition. The wave pattern for coarse, thick hair is usually stronger and better defined.

9 When the curl has been formed, rinse thoroughly with warm water for at least five minutes, blot thoroughly, apply neutralizer, and process according to the manufacturer's directions. Gently dry the hair and evaluate the results. Do not proceed with the permanent if the test curls are extremely damaged or overprocessed. If the test curl results are satisfactory, proceed with the perm, but do not re-perm these preliminary test curls. Rinse and process the test rods, but wait to remove them with the rest of the rods after the perm is completed.

Post-Service

- Complete PROCEDURE 15-2 **Post-Service Procedure** SEE PAGE 326

© Milady, a part of Cengage Learning. Photography by Paul Castle, Castle Photography.

PROCEDURE 20-2

Permanent Wave and Processing Using a Basic Permanent Wrap

Implements and Materials

You will need all of the following implements, materials, and supplies:

- **Acid-balanced shampoo (optional)**
- **Applicator bottles**
- **Conditioner (optional)**
- **Cotton coil or rope**
- **Disposable gloves**
- **End papers**
- **Neutralizer**
- **Neutralizing bib**
- **Perm rods**
- **Perm solution**
- **Plastic clips for sectioning**
- **Plastic tail comb**
- **Pre-neutralizing conditioner (optional)**
- **Protective barrier cream**
- **Roller picks**
- **Shampoo cape**
- **Spray bottle**
- **Styling comb**
- **Timer**
- **Towels**

© Milady, a part of Cengage Learning. Photography by Paul Castle, Castle Photography.

Preparation

- Perform PROCEDURE 15-1 Pre-Service Procedure SEE PAGE 323

Procedure

1 After completing the pre-service procedure, seat the client. If the manufacturer's directions indicate a shampoo is necessary before the service, then drape the client for a shampoo and gently shampoo and towel-dry hair. Avoid irritating the client's scalp.

2 Re-drape the client for a chemical service.

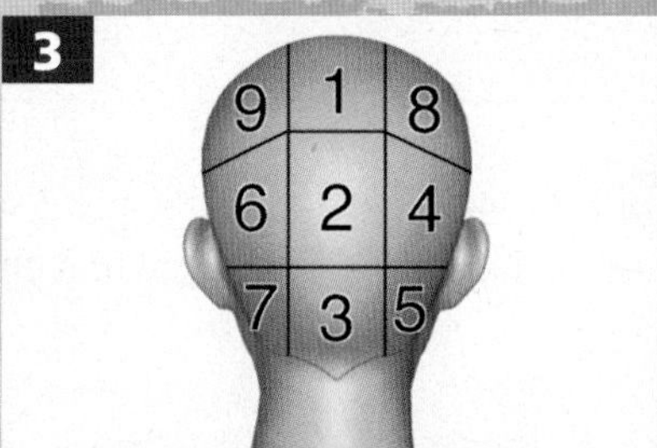

3 Divide the hair into nine panels. Use the length of the rod to measure the width of the panels. Remember to keep the hair evenly damp as you wrap.

PROCEDURE 20-2

Permanent Wave and Processing Using a Basic Permanent Wrap continued

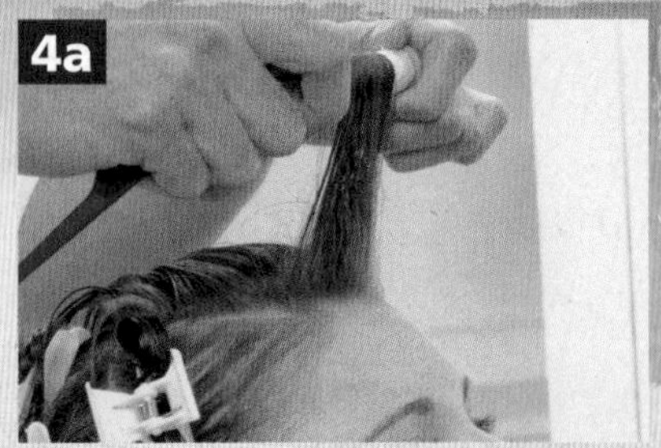

4a Begin wrapping at the front hairline or crown. Make a horizontal parting the same size as the rod. Using two end papers, roll the hair down to the scalp in the direction of hair growth, and position the rod half off base.

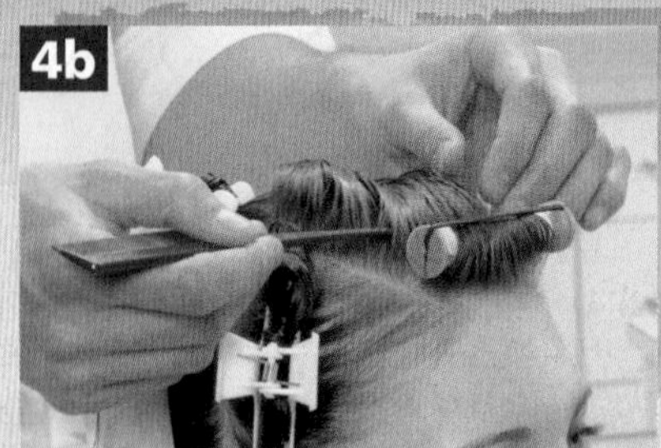

4b The band should be smooth, not twisted, and should be fastened straight across the top of the rod. Excessive tension may cause band marks or hair breakage.

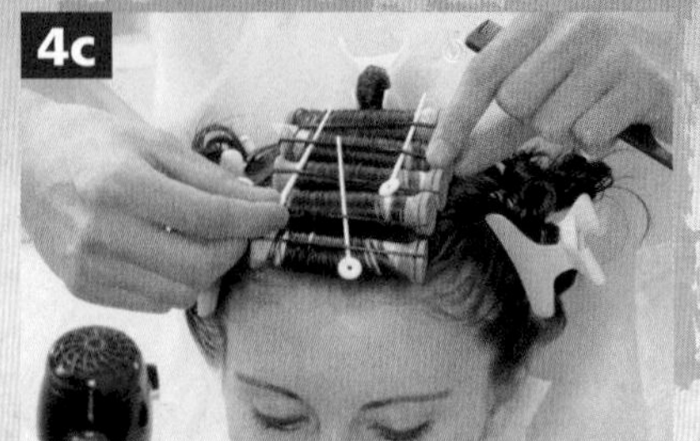

4c Continue wrapping the remainder of the first panel using the same technique. Option: Insert roller picks to stabilize the rods and eliminate any tension caused by the band.

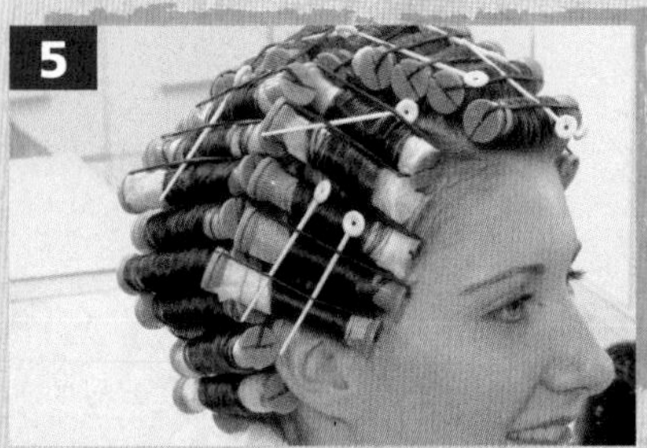

5 Continue wrapping the remaining eight panels in numerical order, holding the hair at a 90-degree angle.

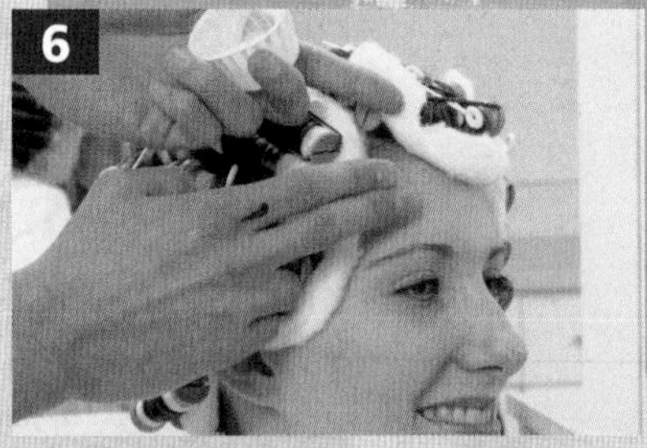

6 Apply protective barrier cream to the hairline and the ears. Apply a coil of cotton around the entire hairline and offer the client a towel to blot any drips. Put on gloves.

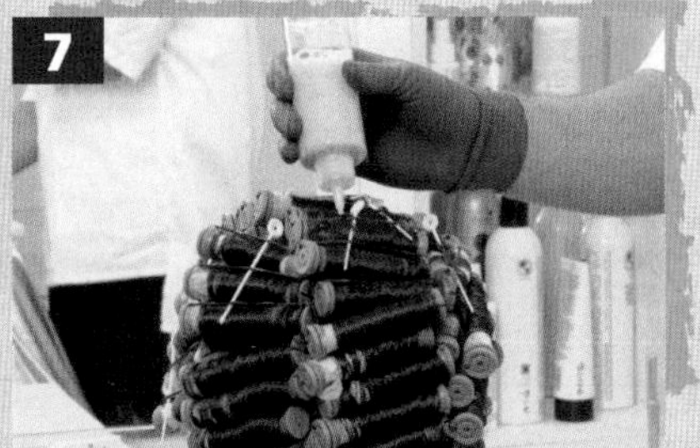

7 Slowly and carefully apply the perm solution to each rod. Ask the client to lean forward while you apply solution to the back area; ask the client to lean back as you apply solution to the front and sides. Avoid splashing and dripping. Continue to apply the solution slowly until each rod is completely saturated. Apply solution to the most resistant area first.

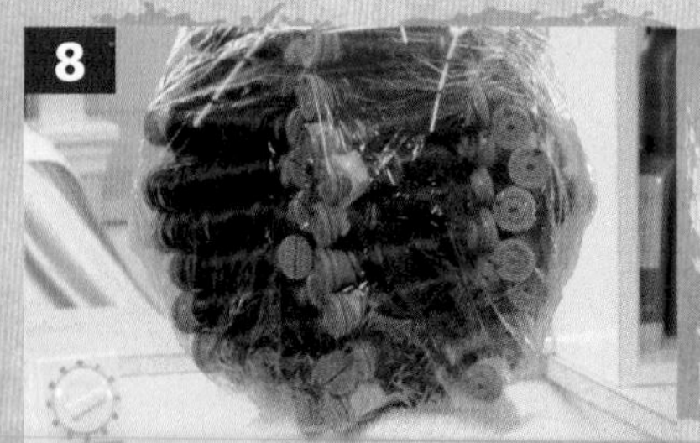

8 If a plastic cap is used, punch a few holes in the cap and cover all the hair completely. Do not allow the plastic cap to touch the client's skin.

© Milady, a part of Cengage Learning.

9 Check cotton and towels. If they are saturated with solution, replace them.

10 Process according to the manufacturer's directions. Processing time varies according to the strength of the solution, hair type and condition, and desired results. As a general rule, processing usually takes less than twenty minutes at room temperature.

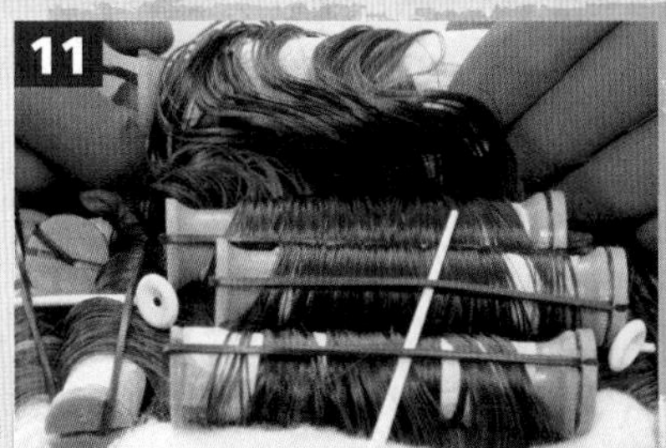

11 Check frequently for curl development. Unwind the rod and check the S pattern formation described in the preliminary test curl procedure. Check a different rod each time!

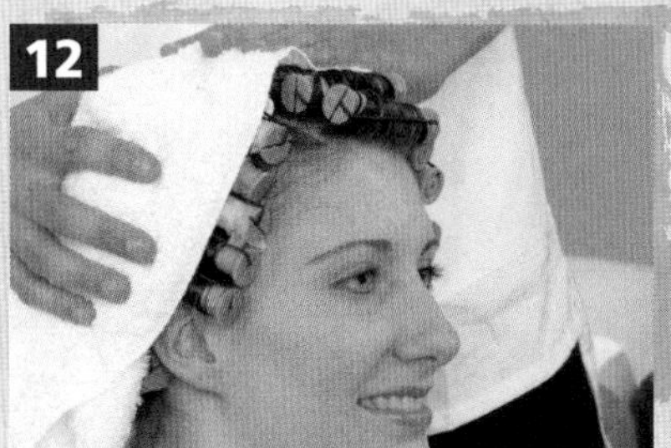

12 When processing is completed, rinse the hair thoroughly for at least five minutes. Then, towel-blot each rod to remove excess moisture. Option: Some manufacturers recommend the application of a pre-neutralizing conditioner after rinsing and blotting and before applying the neutralizer. Always follow the manufacturer's directions and the procedures approved by your instructor.

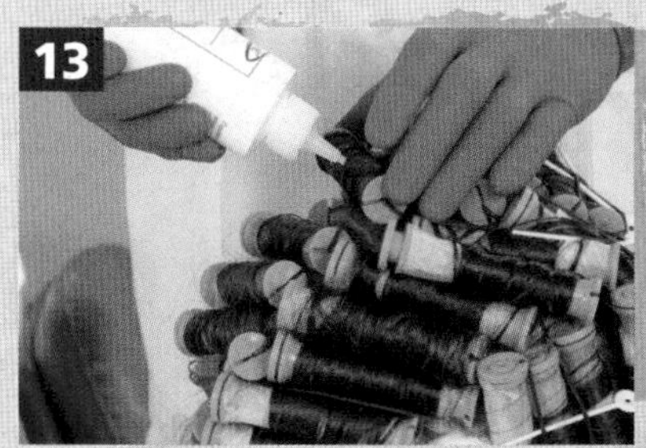

13 Apply the neutralizer slowly and carefully to the hair on each rod. Ask the client to lean forward while you apply solution to the back area, and then to lean back as you apply solution to the front and sides. Avoid splashing and dripping. Continue to apply the neutralizer until each rod is completely saturated.

14 Set a timer for the amount of time specified by the manufacturer.

15 Rinse thoroughly. Option: Shampoo and condition. Always follow the manufacturer's directions and the procedures approved by your instructor.

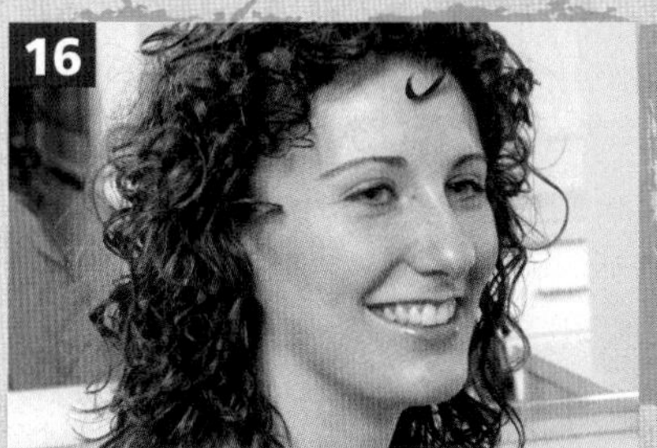

16 Style the hair as desired.

© Milady, a part of Cengage Learning. Photography by Paul Castle, Castle Photography.

Post-Service

- Complete PROCEDURE 15-2 **Post-Service Procedure** SEE PAGE 326

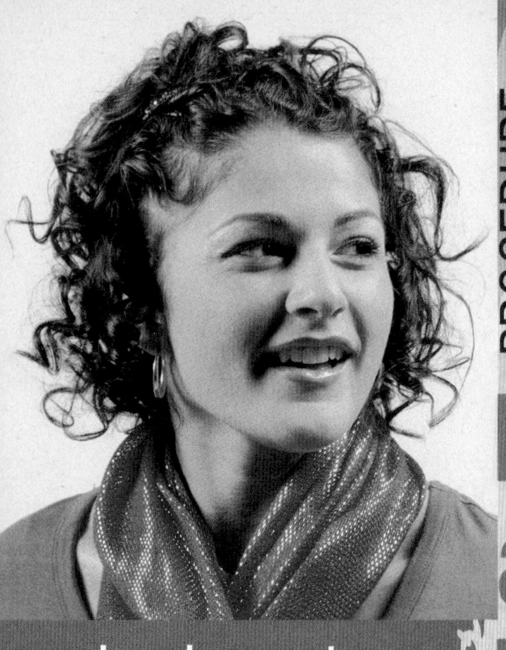

PROCEDURE 20-3

Permanent Wave and Processing Using a Curvature Permanent Wrap

Implements and Materials

You will need all of the following implements, materials, and supplies:

- Acid-balanced shampoo (optional)
- Applicator bottles
- Conditioner (optional)
- Cotton coil or rope
- Disposable gloves
- End papers
- Neutralizer
- Neutralizing bib
- Perm rods
- Perm solution
- Plastic clips for sectioning
- Plastic tail comb
- Pre-neutralizing conditioner (optional)
- Protective barrier cream
- Roller picks
- Shampoo cape
- Spray bottle
- Styling comb
- Timer
- Towels

Preparation

- Perform PROCEDURE 15-1 Pre-Service Procedure SEE PAGE 323

Procedure

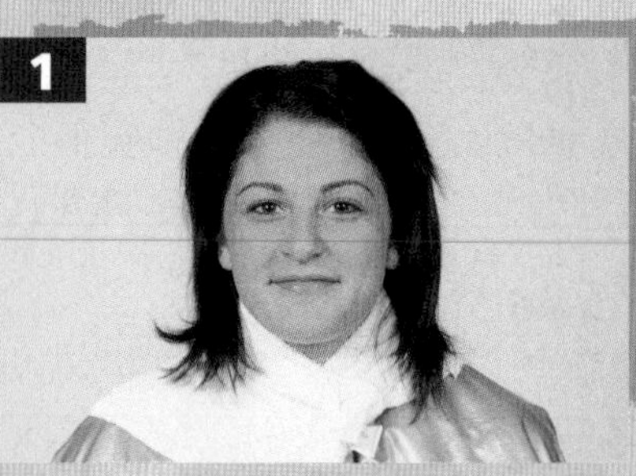

1 After completing the pre-service procedure, seat the client. If the manufacturer's directions indicate a shampoo is necessary before the service, then drape the client for a shampoo and gently shampoo and towel-dry hair. Avoid irritating the client's scalp.

2 Re-drape the client for a chemical service.

© Milady, a part of Cengage Learning. Photography by Yanik Chauvin.

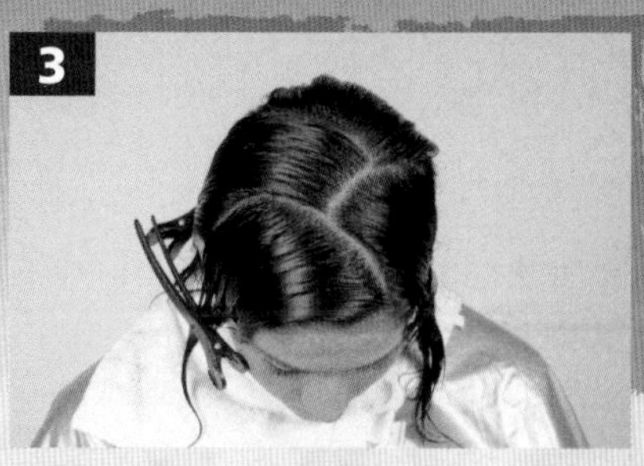

3 Begin sectioning at the front hairline on one side of the part. Comb the hair in the direction of growth. Alternate from side to side as you section out all the curvature panels over the entire head. Sectioning the panels in advance creates a road map that provides direction and gives continuity to the wrapping pattern.

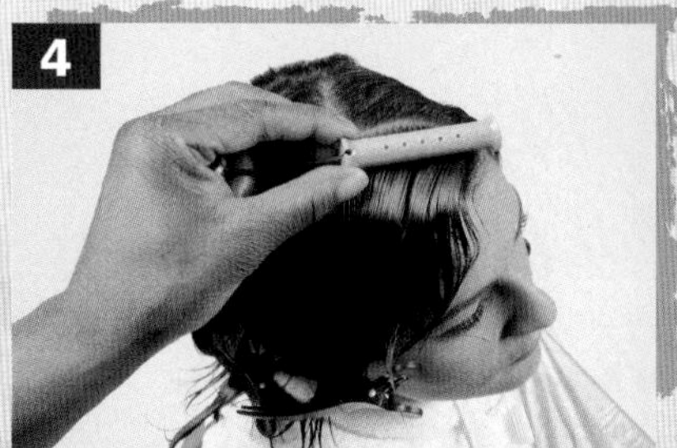

4 Section out individual panels to match the length of the rod.

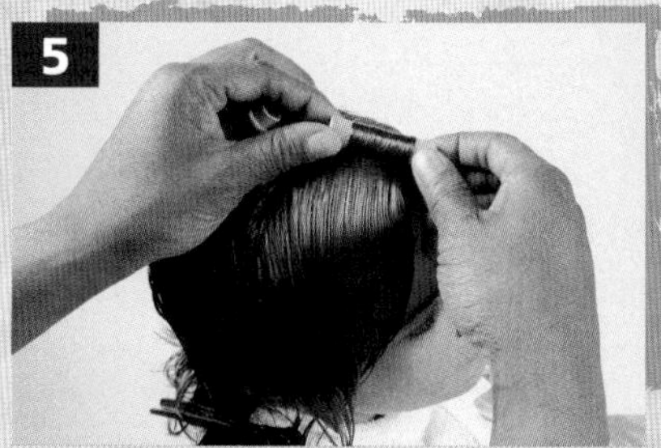

5 Begin wrapping the first panel at the front hairline on one side of the part. Comb out a base section the same width as the diameter of the rod. The base direction should point away from the face. Hold the hair at a 90-degree angle to the head. Using two end papers, roll the hair down to the scalp and position the rod half off base.

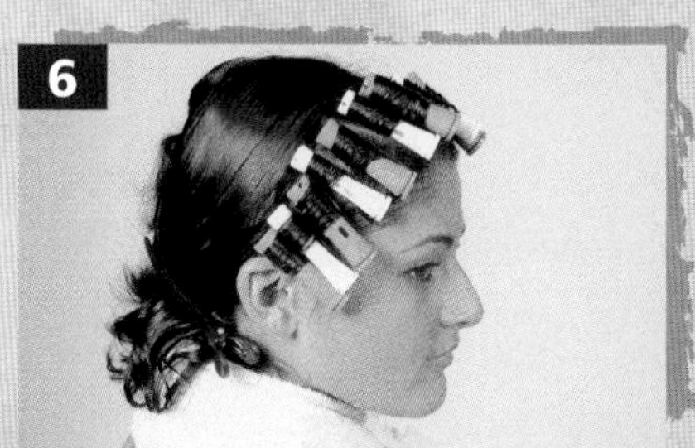

6 The remaining base sections in the panel should be wider on the outside of the panel (the side farthest away from the face). Continue wrapping the rest of the rods in the panel, alternating rod diameters.

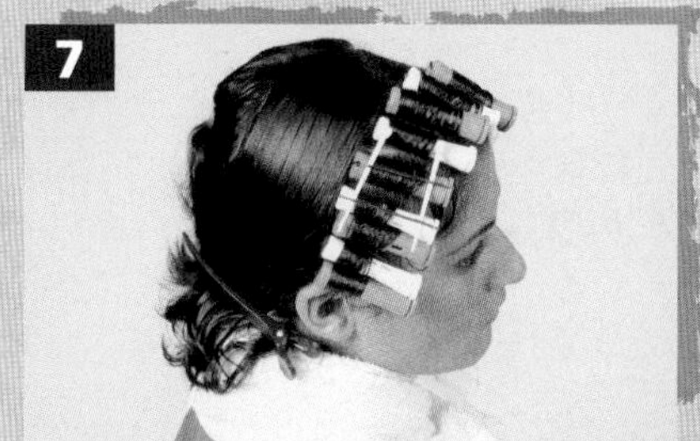

7 Insert picks to stabilize the rods and eliminate any tension caused by the band.

8 When you reach the last rod at the hairline, comb the hair flat at the base and change the base direction. Direct the rod up and toward the base, keeping the base area flat.

© Milady, a part of Cengage Learning. Photography by Yanik Chauvin.

Permanent Wave and Processing Using a Curvature Permanent Wrap continued

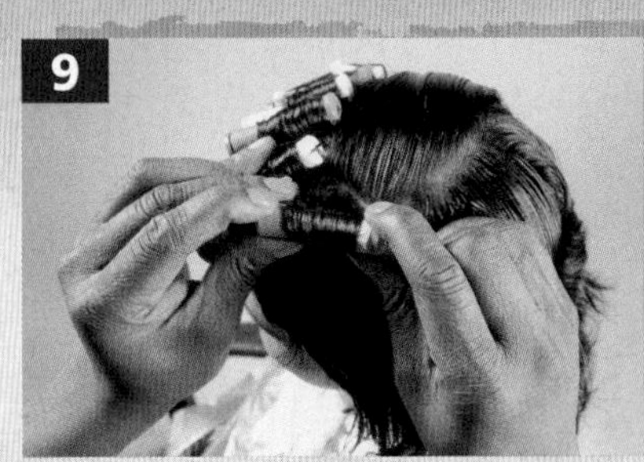

9 Continue by wrapping panel two, which is the front panel on the other side of the part. Repeat the same procedure as on the first panel.

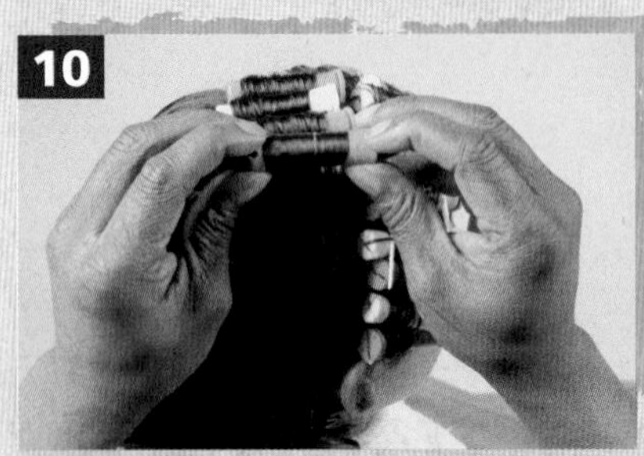

10 Continue with the third panel, which is the panel behind and next to the first panel. Repeat the same procedure until you reach the last two rods at the hairline. Comb the hair flat at the base and change the base direction. Direct the last two rods up and toward the base, keeping the base area flat.

11 Continue with the fourth panel, on the opposite side of the head, behind and next to the second panel. Repeat the same procedure you used with the third panel. Maintain consistent dampness as you work by remisting the hair with water if necessary.

12 Follow the same procedure with the fifth panel. The base direction should remain consistent with the pattern already established. The base direction in the back flows around and contours to the perimeter hairline area.

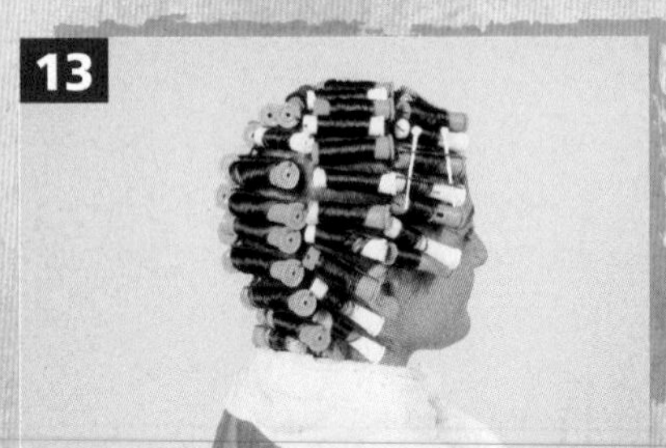

13 All panels should fit the curvature of the head and should blend into the surrounding panels.

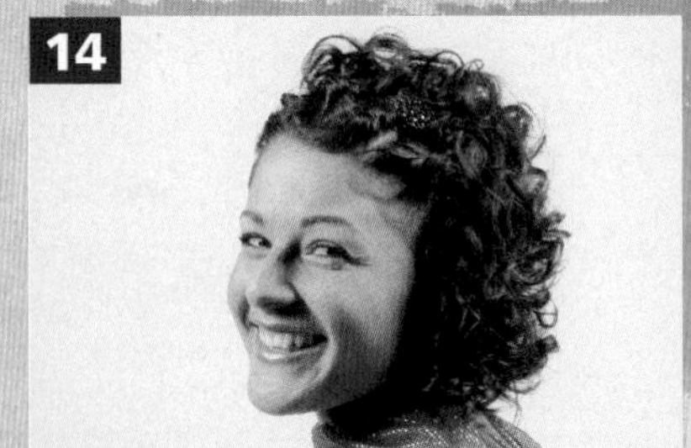

14 Process and style the hair.

Post-Service

- Complete PROCEDURE 15-2 **Post-Service Procedure** SEE PAGE 326

© Milady, a part of Cengage Learning. Photography by Yanik Chauvin.

PROCEDURE 20-4

Permanent Wave and Processing Using a Bricklay Permanent Wrap

Implements and Materials

You will need all of the following implements, materials, and supplies:

- Acid-balanced shampoo (optional)
- Applicator bottles
- Conditioner (optional)
- Cotton coil or rope
- Disposable gloves
- End papers
- Neutralizer
- Neutralizing bib
- Perm rods
- Perm solution
- Plastic clips for sectioning
- Plastic tail comb
- Pre-neutralizing conditioner (optional)
- Protective barrier cream
- Roller picks
- Shampoo cape
- Spray bottle
- Styling comb
- Timer
- Towels

© Milady, a part of Cengage Learning. Photography by Yanik Chauvin.

Preparation

- Perform PROCEDURE 15-1 Pre-Service Procedure SEE PAGE 323

Procedure

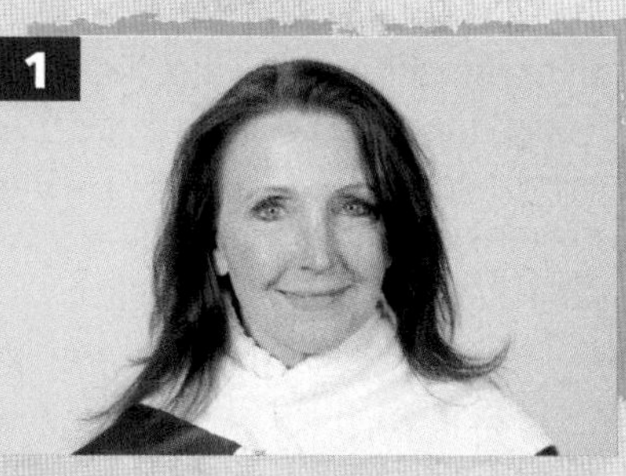

1 After completing the pre-service procedure, seat the client. If the manufacturer's directions indicate a shampoo is necessary before the service, then drape the client for a shampoo and gently shampoo and towel-dry hair. Avoid irritating the client's scalp.

2 Re-drape the client for a chemical service.

3 Begin sectioning at the front hairline on one side of the part. Comb the hair in the direction of growth, and then section out individual panels to match the length of the rod.

PROCEDURE 20-4

Permanent Wave and Processing Using a Bricklay Permanent Wrap continued

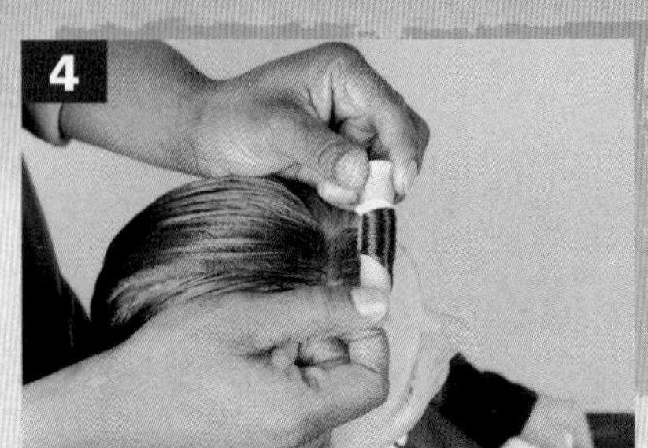

4 Begin by parting out a base section parallel to the front hairline that is the length and width of the rod being used. The base direction is back, away from the face. Hold the hair at a 90-degree angle to the head. Using two end papers, roll the hair down to the scalp and position the rod half off base.

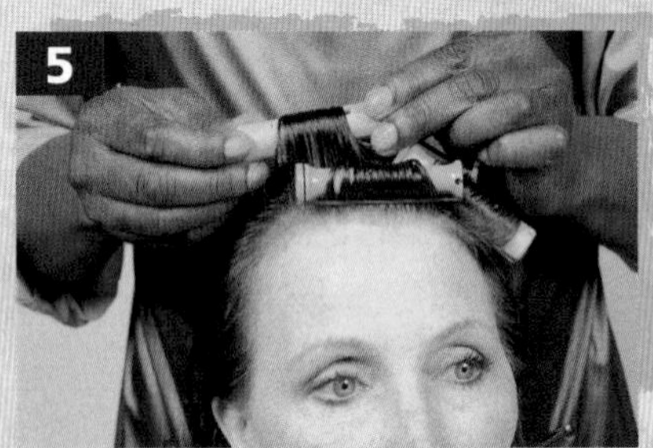

5 In the second row directly behind the first rod, part out two base sections for two rods offset from the center of the first rod. Hold the hair at a 90-degree angle to the head. Using two end papers, roll the hair down to the scalp and position the rods half off base.

6 Insert picks to stabilize rods and eliminate any tension caused by the band.

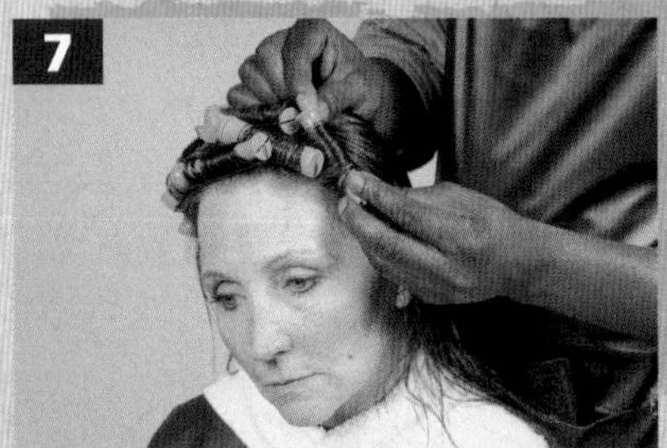

7 On the third row, part out a base section at the point where the two rods meet in the previous row. Complete the third row in this manner. This same pattern is used throughout the entire wrap.

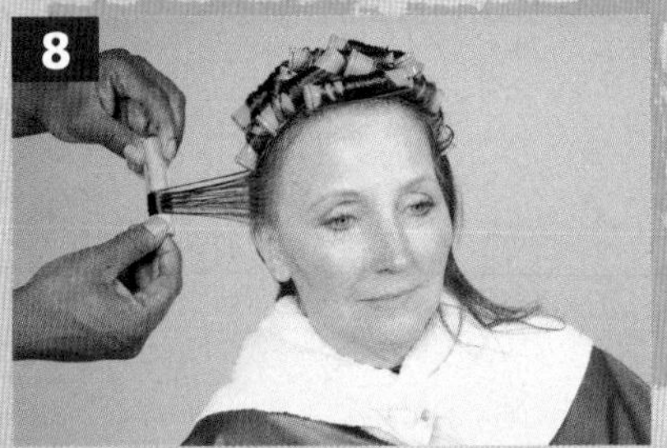

8 Continue to part out rows that radiate around the curve of the head through the crown area. Maintain even dampness as you work. Extend rows around and down to the side hairline, parting out base sections at the center of the point where the two rods meet in the previous row.

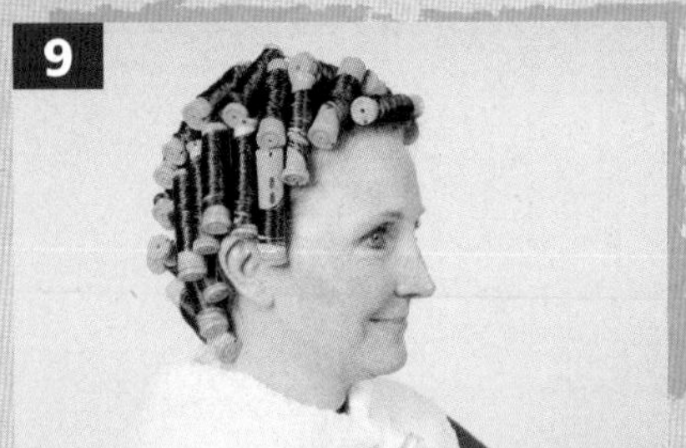

9 Stop the curving rows after you have finished wrapping the crown area. Part out horizontal sections throughout the back of the head, and continue with the bricklay pattern. You may need to change the length of the rods from row to row to maintain the pattern.

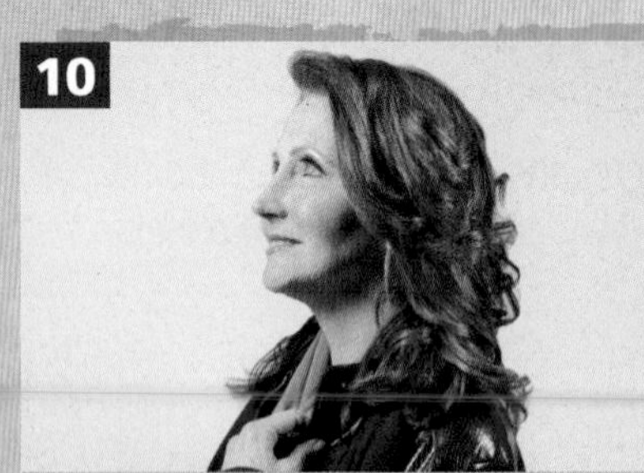

10 Process and style the hair.

Post-Service

- Complete PROCEDURE 15-2 **Post-Service Procedure** SEE PAGE 326

© Milady, a part of Cengage Learning. Photography by Yanik Chauvin.

PROCEDURE 20-5

Permanent Wave and Processing Using a Weave Technique

Implements and Materials

You will need all of the following implements, materials, and supplies:

- Acid-balanced shampoo (optional)
- Applicator bottles
- Conditioner (optional)
- Cotton coil or rope
- Disposable gloves
- End papers
- Neutralizer
- Neutralizing bib
- Perm rods
- Perm solution
- Plastic clips for sectioning
- Plastic tail comb
- Pre-neutralizing conditioner (optional)
- Protective barrier cream
- Roller picks
- Shampoo cape
- Spray bottle
- Styling comb
- Timer
- Towels

Preparation

- Perform PROCEDURE 15-1 Pre-Service Procedure SEE PAGE 323

Procedure

1 After completing the pre-service procedure, seat the client. If the manufacturer's directions indicate a shampoo is necessary before the service, then drape the client for a shampoo and gently shampoo and towel-dry hair. Avoid irritating the client's scalp.

2 Re-drape the client for a chemical service.

3 Begin sectioning at the front hairline on one side of the part. Comb the hair in the direction of growth, and then section out individual panels to match the length of the rod.

PROCEDURE 20-5

Permanent Wave and Processing Using a Weave Technique continued

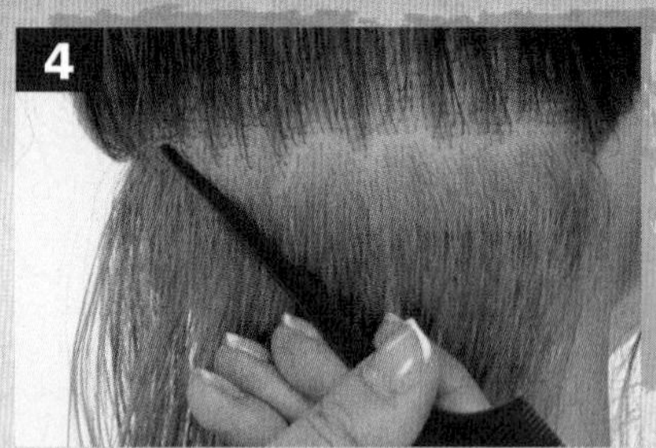

4 Part out one base section the same size as two rods. Comb the entire base section at a 90-degree angle to the head, and use a tail comb to make a zigzag parting along the length of the base section.

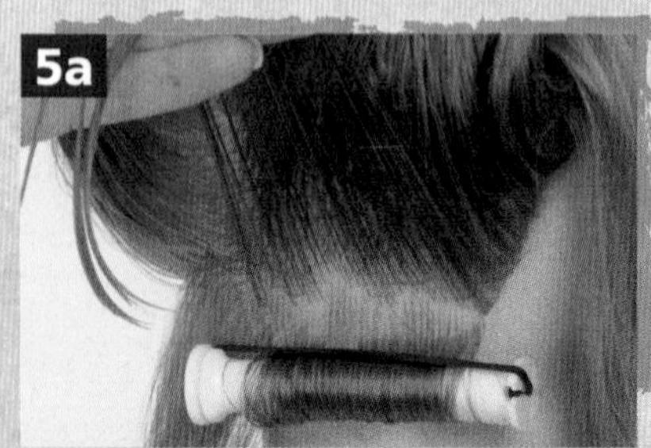

5a Using two end papers, roll half of the strand down to the scalp. Maintain even dampness as you work, remisting the hair with water if necessary.

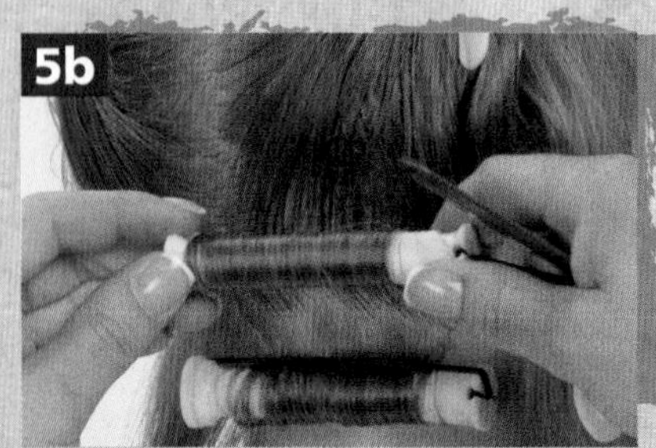

5b Comb the remaining half of the base section at a 90-degree angle, use two end papers, and roll the strand down to the scalp.

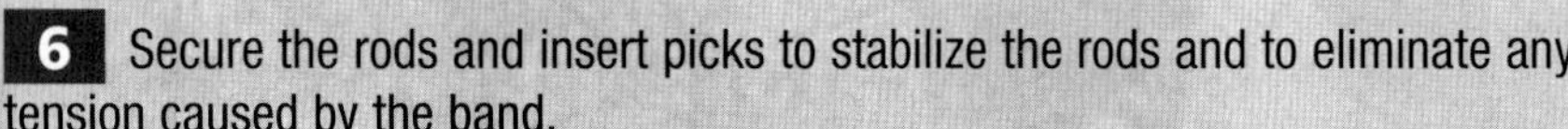

6 Secure the rods and insert picks to stabilize the rods and to eliminate any tension caused by the band.

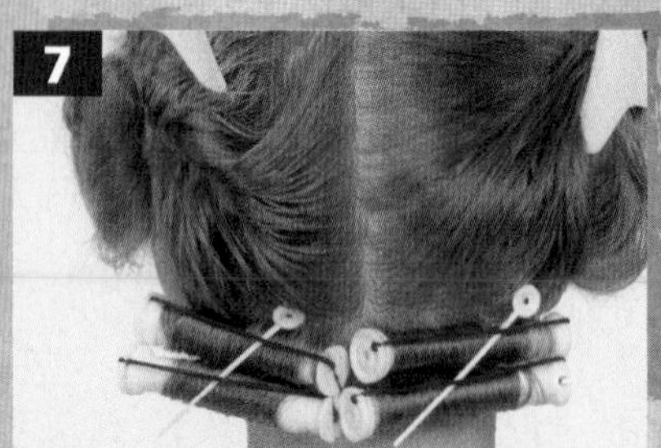

7 Continue with the same procedure in any sections where the effect is desired.

8 Process and style the hair.

Post-Service

- Complete PROCEDURE 15-2 Post-Service Procedure SEE PAGE 326

© Milady, a part of Cengage Learning. Photography by Paul Castle, Castle Photography.

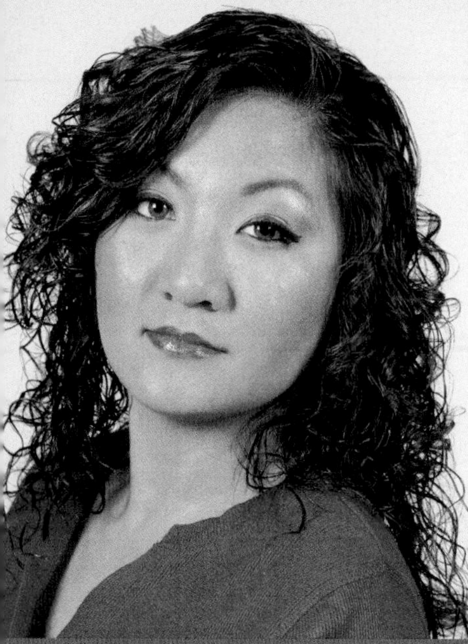

PROCEDURE 20-6

Permanent Wave and Processing Using a Double-Rod or Piggyback Technique

Implements and Materials

You will need all of the following implements, materials, and supplies:

- **Acid-balanced shampoo (optional)**
- **Applicator bottles**
- **Conditioner (optional)**
- **Cotton coil or rope**
- **Disposable gloves**
- **End papers**
- **Neutralizer**
- **Neutralizing bib**
- **Perm rods**
- **Perm solution**
- **Plastic clips for sectioning**
- **Plastic tail comb**
- **Pre-neutralizing conditioner (optional)**
- **Protective barrier cream**
- **Roller picks**
- **Shampoo cape**
- **Spray bottle**
- **Styling comb**
- **Timer**
- **Towels**

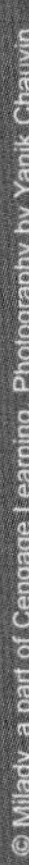
© Milady, a part of Cengage Learning. Photography by Yanik Chauvin.

Preparation

- Perform PROCEDURE 15-1 Pre-Service Procedure SEE PAGE 323

Procedure

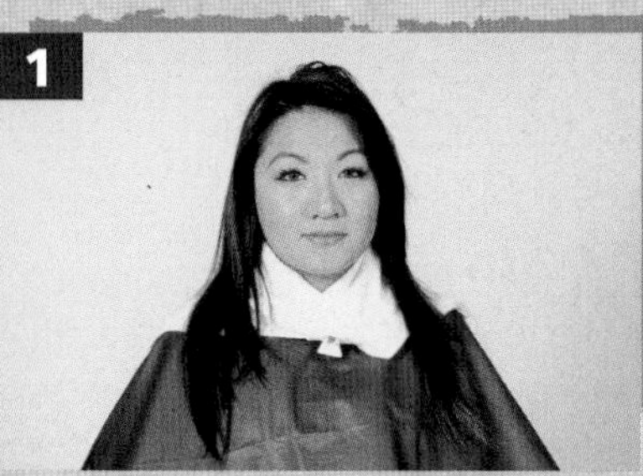

1 After completing the pre-service procedure, seat the client. If the manufacturer's directions indicate a shampoo is necessary before the service, then drape the client for a shampoo and gently shampoo and towel-dry hair. Avoid irritating the client's scalp.

2 Re-drape the client for a chemical service.

3 Begin sectioning at the front hairline on one side of the part. Comb the hair in the direction of growth, and then section out individual panels to match the length of the rod.

Permanent Wave and Processing Using a Double-Rod or Piggyback Technique continued

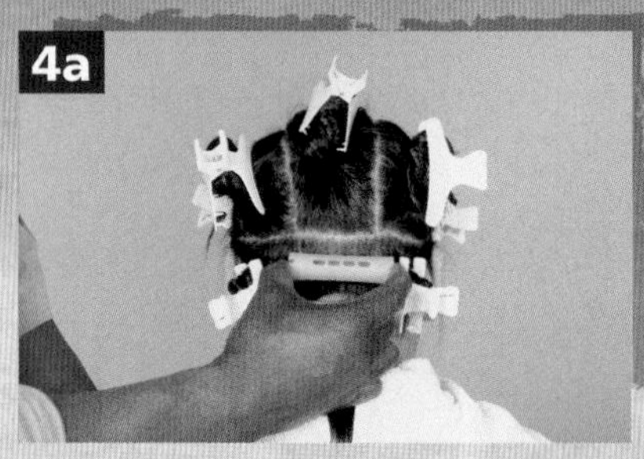

4a Begin by placing the base rod in the middle of the strand.

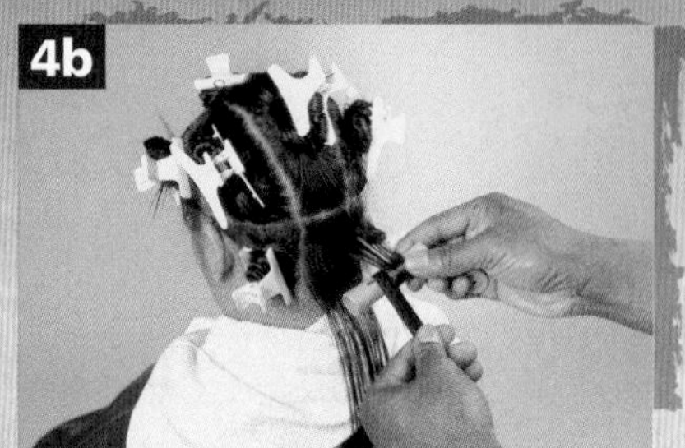

4b Wrap the end of the strand one revolution around the rod while holding it to one side.

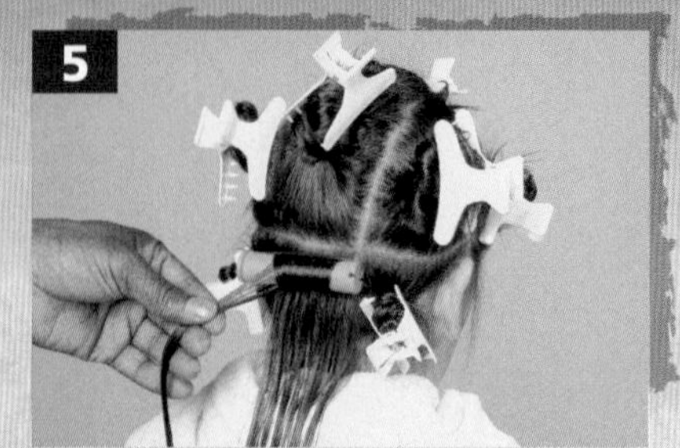

5 Roll the rod up to the base area, letting the loose ends follow as you roll.

6 Insert picks to stabilize the rods and to eliminate any tension caused by the band.

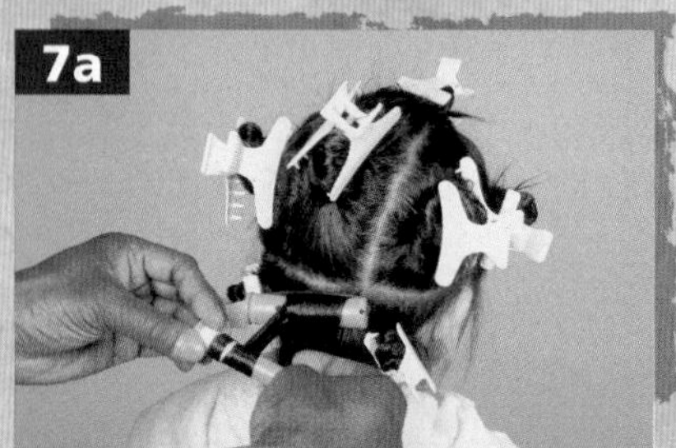

7a Place two end papers on the ends of the strand, position the rod, and roll from the ends toward the base.

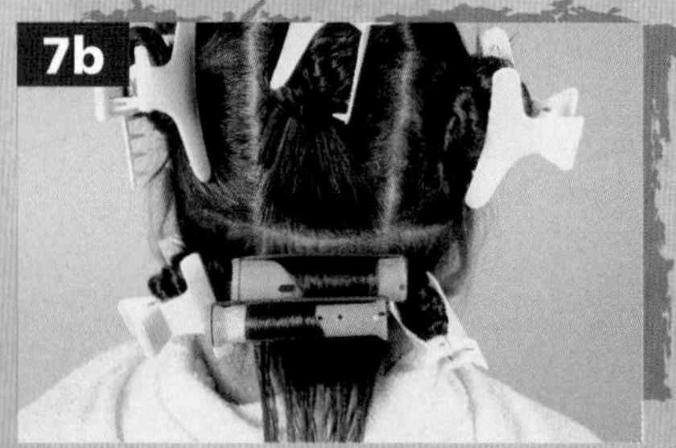

7b Secure the end rod on top of the base rod.

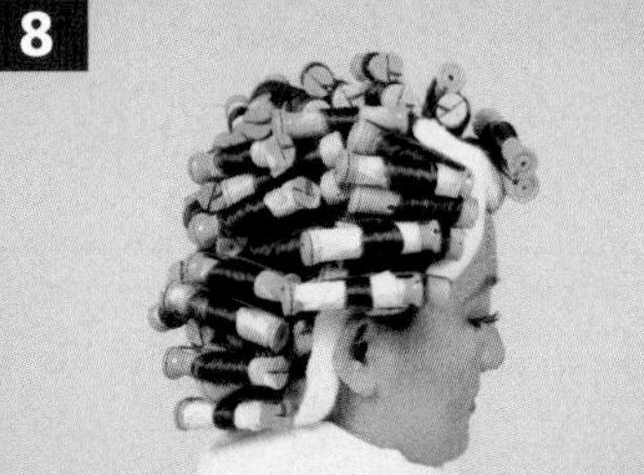

8 Maintain consistent dampness as you work, remisting the hair with water if necessary. Continue with the same procedure in any sections where the effect is desired.

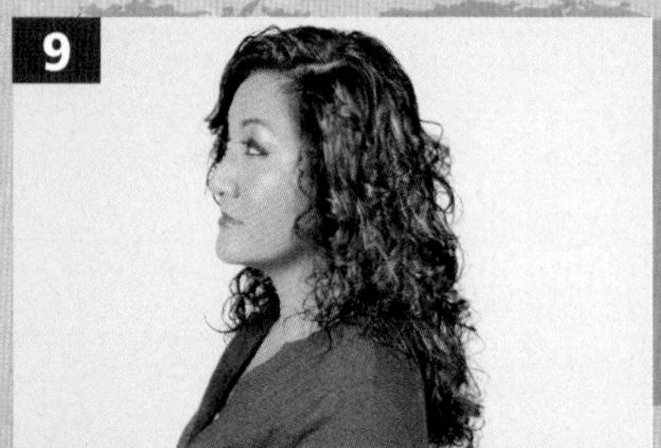

9 Process and style the hair.

Post-Service

- Complete PROCEDURE 15-2 **Post-Service Procedure** SEE PAGE 326

© Milady, a part of Cengage Learning. Photography by Yanik Chauvin.

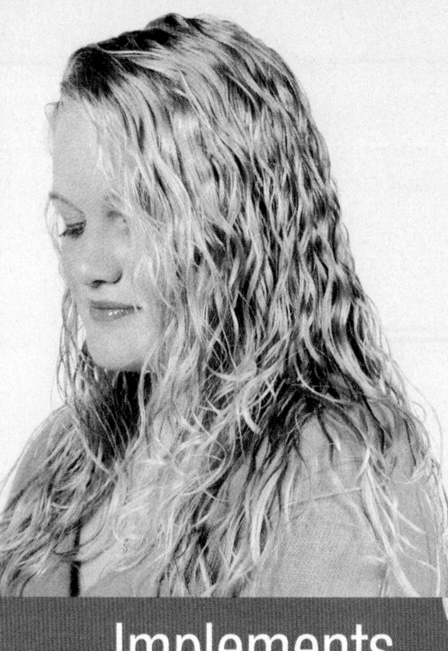

PROCEDURE 20-7

Permanent Wave and Processing Using a Spiral Wrap Technique

Implements and Materials

You will need all of the following implements, materials, and supplies:

- **Acid-balanced shampoo (optional)**
- **Applicator bottles**
- **Conditioner (optional)**
- **Cotton coil or rope**
- **Disposable gloves**
- **End papers**
- **Neutralizer**
- **Neutralizing bib**
- **Perm rods**
- **Perm solution**
- **Plastic clips for sectioning**
- **Plastic tail comb**
- **Pre-neutralizing conditioner (optional)**
- **Protective barrier cream**
- **Roller picks**
- **Shampoo cape**
- **Spray bottle**
- **Styling comb**
- **Timer**
- **Towels**

© Milady, a part of Cengage Learning. Photography by Yanik Chauvin.

Preparation

- Perform PROCEDURE 15-1 **Pre-Service Procedure** **SEE PAGE 323**

Procedure

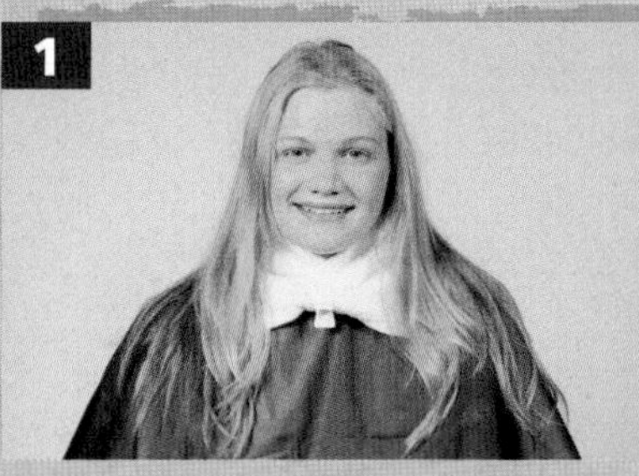

1 After completing the pre-service procedure, seat the client. If the manufacturer's directions indicate a shampoo is necessary before the service, then drape the client for a shampoo and gently shampoo and towel-dry hair. Avoid irritating the client's scalp.

2 Re-drape the client for a chemical service.

3 Begin sectioning at the front hairline on one side of the part. Comb the hair in the direction of growth, and then section out individual panels to match the length of the rod.

PROCEDURE 20-7

Permanent Wave and Processing Using a Spiral Wrap Technique continued

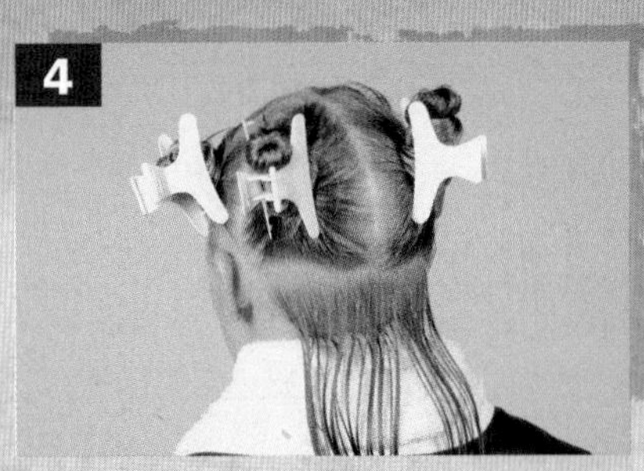

4 Part the hair into four panels, from the center of the front hairline to the center of the nape, and from ear to ear. Section out a fifth panel from ear to ear in the nape area.

5 Section out the first row along the hairline in the nape area. Comb the remainder of the hair up, and secure it out of the way.

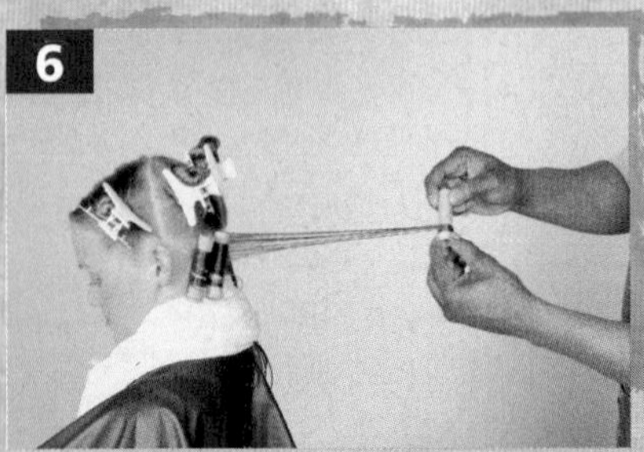

6 Part out the first base section on one side of the first row. Hold the hair at a 90-degree angle to the head. Using one or two end papers, begin wrapping at one end of the rod. Starting the wrap from the right or left side of the rod will orient the curl in that direction.

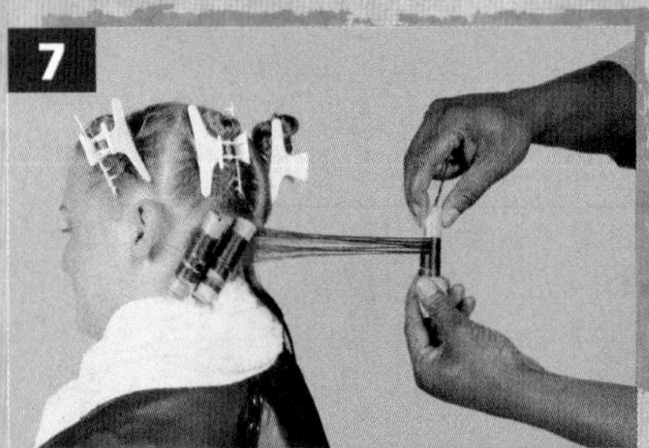

7 Roll the first two full turns at a 90-degree angle to the rod to secure the ends of the hair, and then start spiraling the hair on the rod by changing the angle to an angle other than 90 degrees.

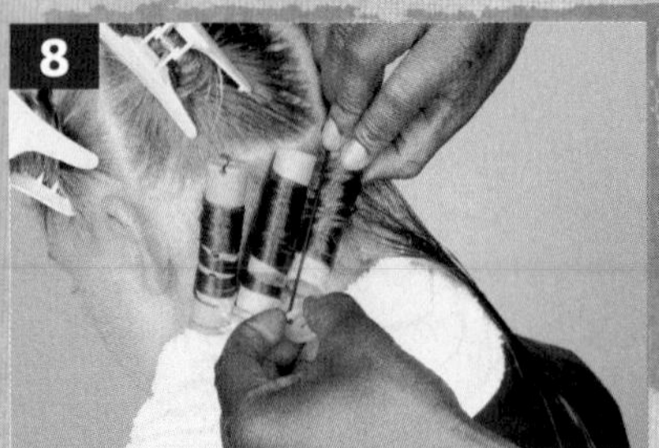

8 Continue to spiral the hair toward the other end of the rod. Roll the hair down to the scalp, position the rod half off base, and secure it by fastening the ends of the rod together.

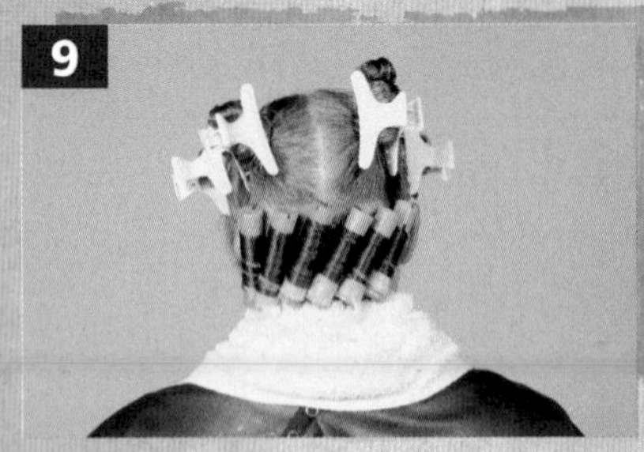

9 Continue wrapping with the same technique, in the same direction, until the first row is completed.

© Milady, a part of Cengage Learning. Photography by Yanik Chauvin.

10 Section out the second row above and parallel to the first row. Comb the remainder of the hair up, and secure it to keep it out of the way.

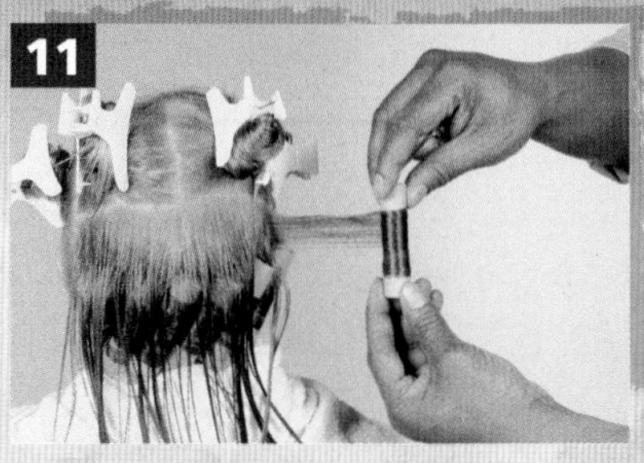

11 Begin wrapping at the opposite side from the side where the first row began, and move in the direction opposite the direction established in the first row.

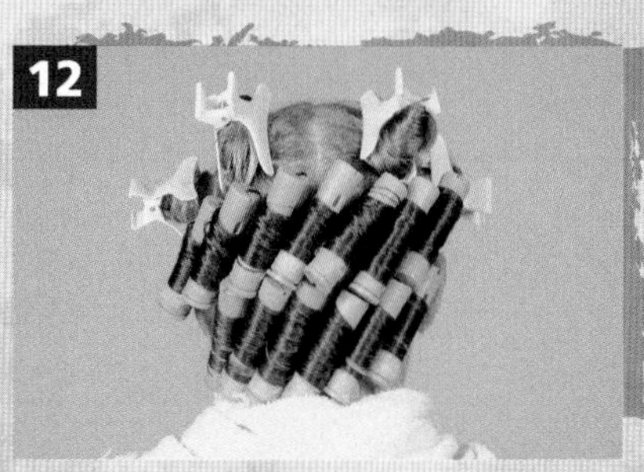

12 Follow the same procedure to wrap the second row, but begin wrapping each rod at the opposite end established in the first row. Maintain consistent dampness as you work, misting the hair with water if necessary. Continue wrapping with the same technique, in the same direction, until the second row is completed.

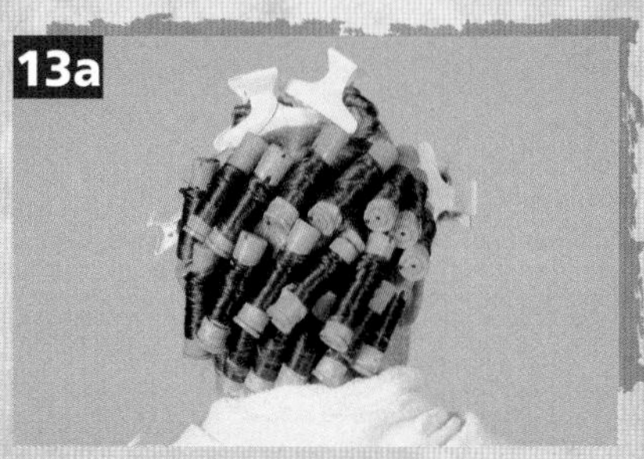

13a Section out the third row above and parallel to the second row. Follow the same wrapping procedure, alternating the rows from left to right as you move up the head. This will alternate the orientation of the curl throughout the head.

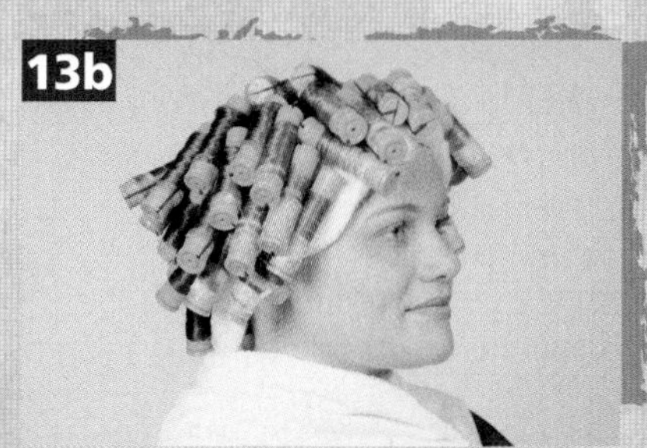

13b Complete wrapping.

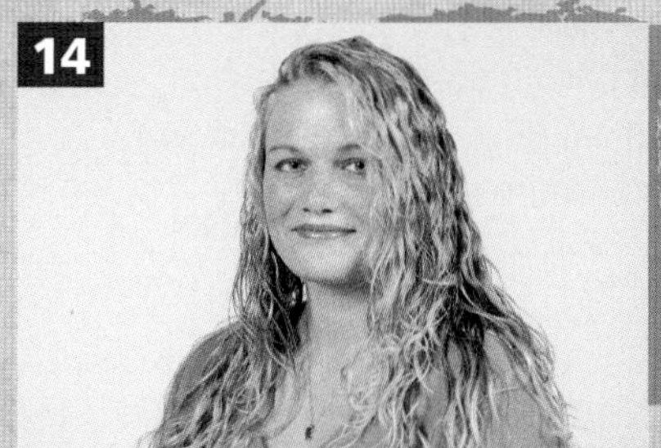

14 Process and style the hair.

© Milady, a part of Cengage Learning. Photography by Yanik Chauvin.

Post-Service

- Complete **PROCEDURE 15-2 Post-Service Procedure** SEE PAGE 326

PROCEDURE 20-8

Applying Thio Relaxer to Virgin Hair

Implements and Materials

You will need all of the following implements, materials, and supplies:

- **Acid-balanced shampoo**
- **Bowl and applicator brush**
- **Conditioner**
- **Disposable gloves**
- **Hard rubber comb**
- **Plastic clips**
- **Pre-neutralizing conditioner**
- **Protective base cream**
- **Shampoo cape**
- **Spray bottle**
- **Styling comb**
- **Thio neutralizer**
- **Thio relaxer**
- **Timer**
- **Towels**

Preparation

- Perform PROCEDURE 15-1 **Pre-Service Procedure** **SEE PAGE 323**

Procedure

1 Perform an analysis of the hair and scalp. Perform tests for porosity and elasticity.

2 Drape the client for a chemical service. To avoid scalp irritation, do not shampoo the hair prior to a thio relaxer. *The hair and scalp must be completely dry prior to the application of a thio relaxer.*

3 Part the hair into four sections, from the center of the front hairline to the center of the nape, and from ear to ear. Clip the sections up to keep them out of the way.

4 Apply protective base cream to the hairline and ears. Option: Take ¼-inch to ½-inch (0.6 to 1.25 centimeters) horizontal partings, and apply a protective base cream to the entire scalp. Always follow the manufacturer's directions, and the procedures approved by your instructor.

5 Wear gloves on both hands. Begin application in the most resistant area, usually at the back of the head. Make ¼-inch to ½-inch (0.6 to 1.25 centimeters) horizontal partings, and apply the relaxer to the top of the strand first, and then to the underside. Apply the relaxer with an applicator brush, or with the back of the comb, or with your fingers. Apply relaxer ¼-inch to ½-inch (0.6 to 1.25 centimeters) away from the scalp, and up to the porous ends. To avoid scalp irritation, do not allow the relaxer to touch the scalp until the last few minutes of processing.

6 Continue applying the relaxer, working your way down the section toward the hairline.

7 Continue the same application procedure with the remaining sections. Finish the most resistant sections first.

8 After the relaxer has been applied to all sections, use the back of the comb or your hands to smooth each section. Never comb the relaxer through the hair.

9 Process according to the manufacturer's directions. Perform periodic strand tests. Processing usually takes less than twenty minutes at room temperature. Always follow manufacturer's processing directions.

10 During the last few minutes of processing, work the relaxer down to the scalp and through the ends of the hair, using additional relaxer as needed. Carefully smooth all sections using an applicator brush, your fingers, or the back of the comb.

11 Rinse thoroughly with warm water to remove all traces of the relaxer.

12 Shampoo at least three times with an acid-balanced shampoo. It is essential that all traces of the relaxer be removed from the hair. Optional: Apply the pre-neutralizing conditioner, and comb it through to the ends of the hair. Leave it on for approximately five minutes and then rinse. Always follow the manufacturer's directions and the procedures approved by your instructor.

13 Blot excess water from the hair.

14 Apply thio neutralizer in ¼- to ½-inch (0.6 to 1.25 centimeters) sections throughout the hair and smooth with your hands or the back of the comb.

15 Process the neutralizer according to the manufacturer's directions.

16 Rinse thoroughly, shampoo, condition, and style.

Post-Service

- Complete PROCEDURE 15-2 **Post-Service Procedure** SEE PAGE 326

PROCEDURE 20-9

Thio Relaxer Retouch

Implements and Materials

You will need all of the following implements, materials, and supplies:

- **Acid-balanced shampoo**
- **Bowl and applicator brush**
- **Conditioner**
- **Disposable gloves**
- **Hard rubber comb**
- **Plastic clips**
- **Pre-neutralizing conditioner**
- **Protective base cream**
- **Shampoo cape**
- **Spray bottle**
- **Styling comb**
- **Thio neutralizer**
- **Thio relaxer**
- **Timer**
- **Towels**

Preparation

- Perform PROCEDURE 15-1 **Pre-Service Procedure** **SEE PAGE 323**

Procedure

1 Perform an analysis of the hair and scalp. Perform tests for porosity and elasticity.

2 Drape the client for a chemical service. To avoid scalp irritation, do not shampoo the hair prior to a thio relaxer. *The hair and scalp must be completely dry prior to the application of a thio relaxer retouch.*

3 Divide the hair into four sections, from the center of the front hairline to the center of the nape, and from ear to ear. Clip sections up to keep them out of the way.

4 Wear gloves on both hands. Apply a protective base cream to the hairline and ears, unless you are using a no-base relaxing product. Option: Take ¼-inch to ½-inch horizontal (0.6 to 1.25 centimeters) partings and apply protective base cream to the entire scalp.

5 Begin application of the relaxer in the most resistant area, usually at the back of the head. Make ¼-inch to ½-inch (0.6 to 1.25 centimeters) horizontal partings, and apply the relaxer to the top of the strand. Apply the relaxer as close to the scalp as possible, but do not touch the scalp with the product. Only allow the relaxer to touch the scalp itself during the last few minutes of processing. To avoid overprocessing or breakage, do not overlap the relaxer onto the previously relaxed hair.

6 Continue applying the relaxer, using the same procedure and working your way down the section toward the hairline.

7 Continue the same application procedure with the remaining sections, finishing the most resistant sections first.

8 After the relaxer has been applied to all sections, use the back of the comb, the applicator brush, or your hands to smooth each section.

9 Process according to the manufacturer's directions. Perform periodic strand tests. Processing usually takes less than twenty minutes at room temperature. Always follow the manufacturer's processing directions.

10 During the last few minutes of processing, gently work the relaxer down to the scalp.

11 If the ends of the hair need additional relaxing, work the relaxer through to the ends for the last few minutes of processing. Do not relax ends during each retouch; doing this will cause overprocessing. Option: A cream conditioner may be applied to relaxed ends to protect from overprocessing caused by overlapping.

12 Rinse thoroughly with warm water to remove all traces of the relaxer.

13 Shampoo at least three times with an acid-balanced shampoo. It is essential that all traces of the relaxer be removed from the hair. Optional: Apply the pre-neutralizing conditioner, and comb it through to the ends of the hair. Leave it on for approximately five minutes and then rinse. Always follow the manufacturer's directions and the procedures approved by your instructor.

14 Blot excess water from hair.

15 Apply thio neutralizer in ¼- to ½-inch (0.6 to 1.25 centimeters) sections throughout the hair and smooth with your hands or the back of the comb.

16 Process the neutralizer according to the manufacturer's directions.

17 Rinse thoroughly, shampoo, condition, and style.

Post-Service

- Complete PROCEDURE 15-2 **Post-Service Procedure** SEE PAGE 326

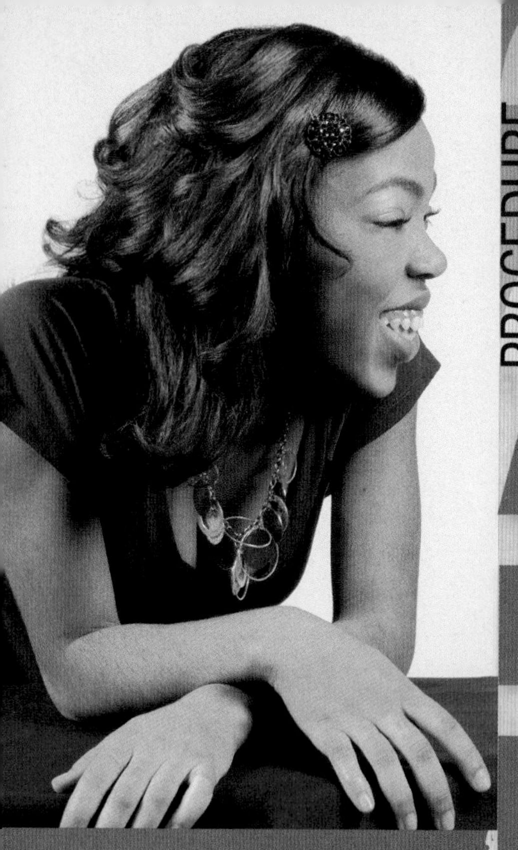

PROCEDURE 20-10

Applying Hydroxide Relaxer to Virgin Hair

Implements and Materials

You will need all of the following implements, materials, and supplies:

- **Acid-balanced shampoo**
- **Bowl and applicator brush**
- **Conditioner**
- **Disposable gloves**
- **Hard rubber comb**
- **Hydroxide neutralizer**
- **Hydroxide relaxer**
- **Plastic clips**
- **Protective base cream**
- **Shampoo cape**
- **Spray bottle**
- **Styling comb**
- **Timer**
- **Towels**

Preparation

- Perform PROCEDURE 15-1 **Pre-Service Procedure** **SEE PAGE 323**

Procedure

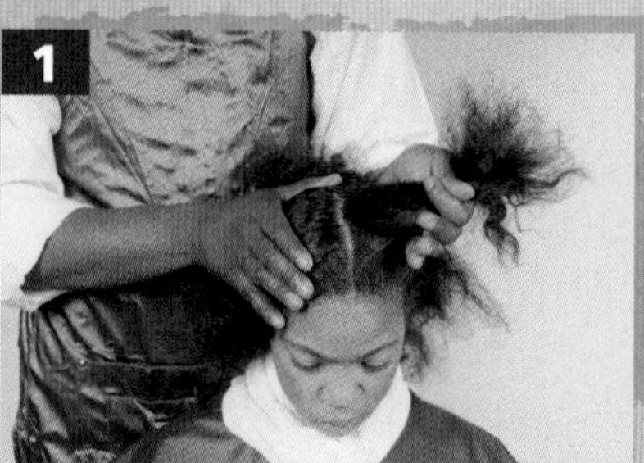

1 Perform an analysis of the hair and scalp. Perform tests for porosity and elasticity.

2 Drape the client for a chemical service. To avoid scalp irritation, do not shampoo the hair. *The hair and scalp must be completely dry prior to the application of a hydroxide relaxer.*

© Milady, a part of Cengage Learning. Photography by Yanik Chauvin.

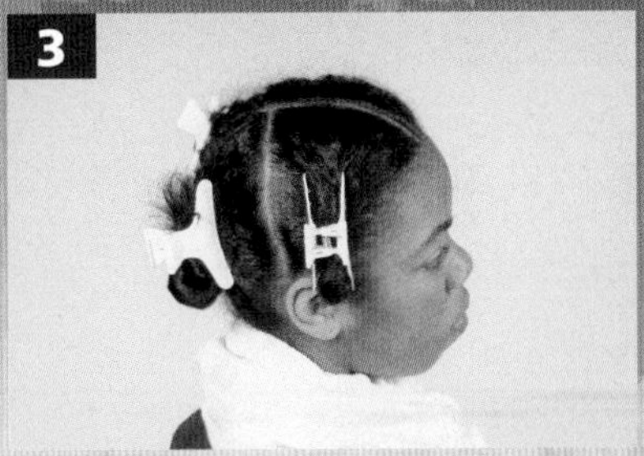

3 Part the hair into four sections, from the center of the front hairline to the center of the nape, and from ear to ear. Clip the sections up to keep them out of the way.

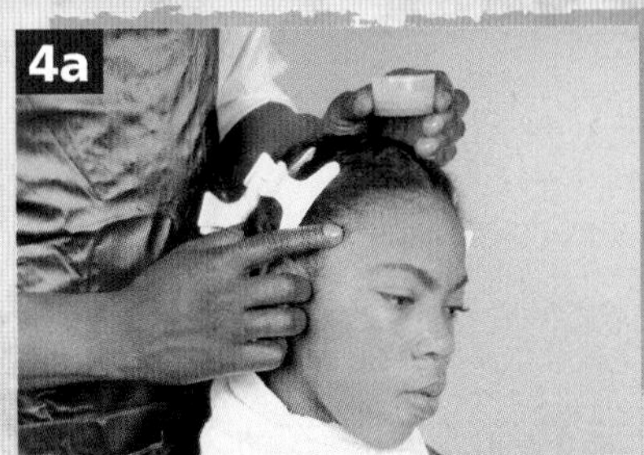

4a Apply protective base cream to the hairline and ears.

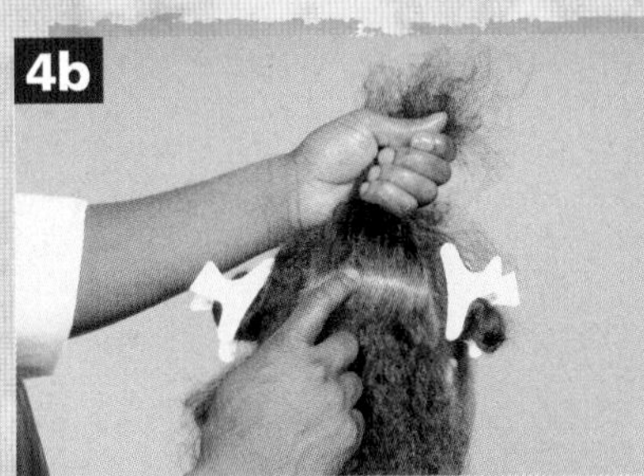

4b Option: Take ¼-inch to ½-inch (0.6 to 1.25 centimeters) horizontal partings, and apply a protective base cream to the entire scalp. Always follow the manufacturer's directions and the procedures approved by your instructor.

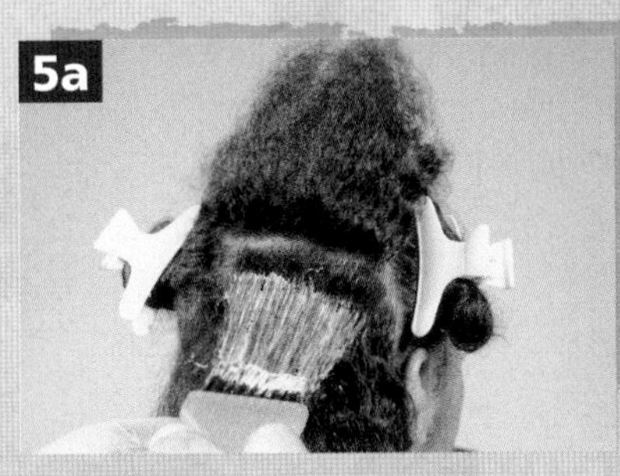

5a Wear gloves on both hands. Begin application in the most resistant area, usually at the back of the head. Make ¼-inch to ½-inch horizontal partings, and apply the relaxer to the top of the strand first.

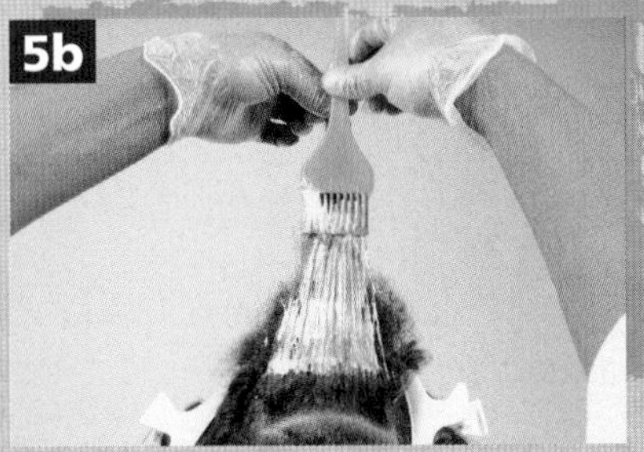

5b And then apply relaxer to the underside. Apply the relaxer with an applicator brush, or the back of the comb, or your fingers. Apply relaxer ¼-inch to ½-inch away from the scalp, and up to the porous ends. To avoid scalp irritation, do not allow the relaxer to touch the scalp until the last few minutes of processing.

6 Continue applying the relaxer, working your way down the section toward the hairline. Continue the same application procedure with the remaining sections. Finish the most resistant sections first.

© Milady, a part of Cengage Learning. Photography by Yanik Chauvin.

Applying Hydroxide Relaxer to Virgin Hair continued

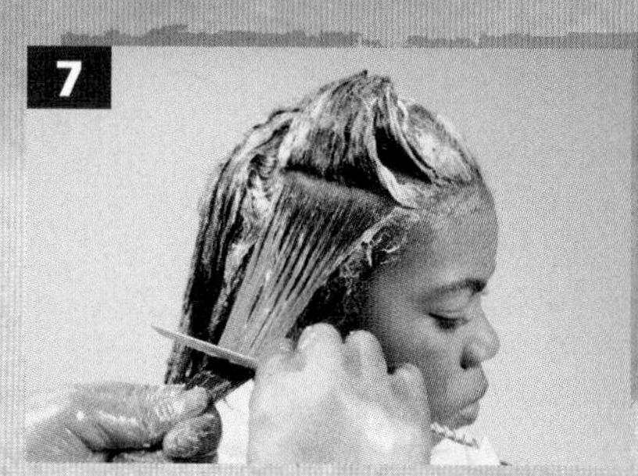

7 After the relaxer has been applied to all sections, use the back of the comb or your hands to smooth each section. Never comb the relaxer through the hair.

8 Process according to the manufacturer's directions. Perform periodic strand tests. Processing usually takes less than twenty minutes at room temperature. Always follow manufacturer's processing directions.

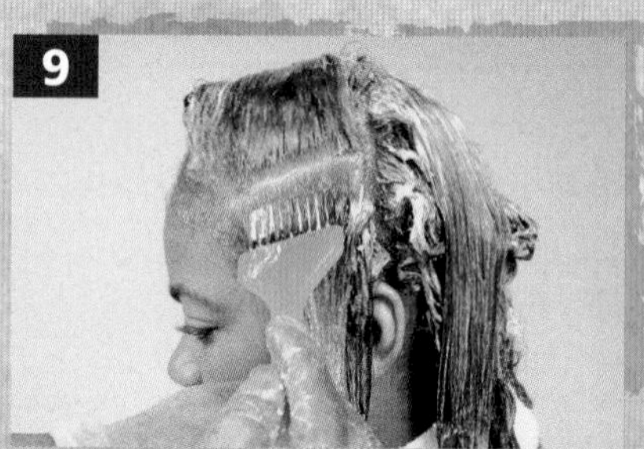

9 During the last few minutes of processing, work the relaxer down to the scalp and through the ends of the hair, using additional relaxer as needed. Carefully smooth all sections, using an applicator brush, fingers, or back of the comb.

10 Rinse thoroughly with warm water to remove all traces of the relaxer.

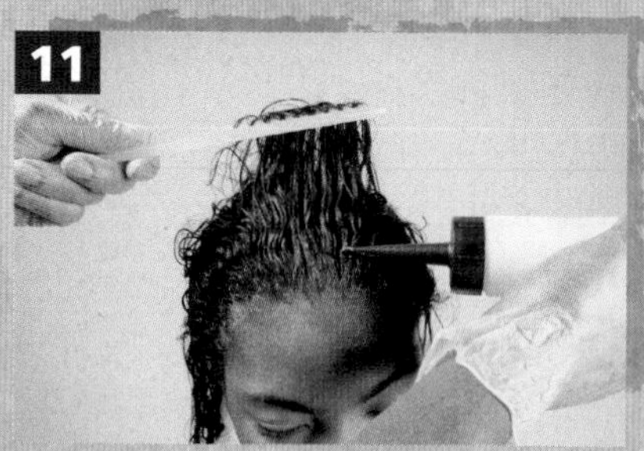

11 Optional: Apply the normalizing lotion and comb it through to the ends of the hair. Leave it on for approximately five minutes and then rinse thoroughly. (Always follow the manufacturer's directions and the procedures approved by your instructor.)

12 Shampoo at least three times with an acid-balanced neutralizing shampoo. It is essential that all traces of the relaxer be removed from the hair. Option: If you are using a neutralizing shampoo with a color indicator, a change in color will indicate when all traces of the relaxer are removed and the natural pH of the hair and scalp has been restored.

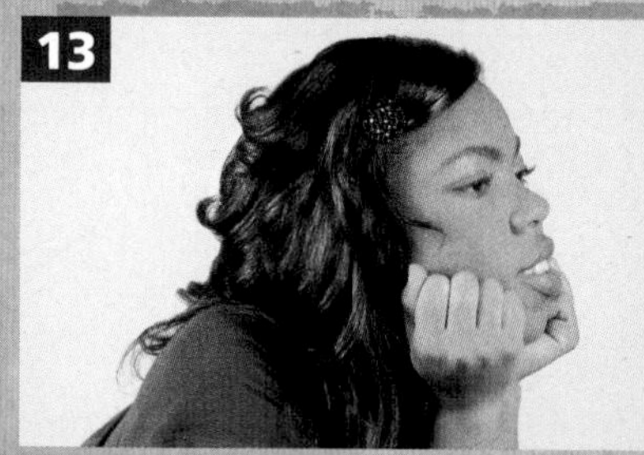

13 Rinse thoroughly, condition, and style as desired.

Post-Service

- Complete PROCEDURE 15-2 **Post-Service Procedure** SEE PAGE 326

© Milady, a part of Cengage Learning. Photography by Yanik Chauvin.

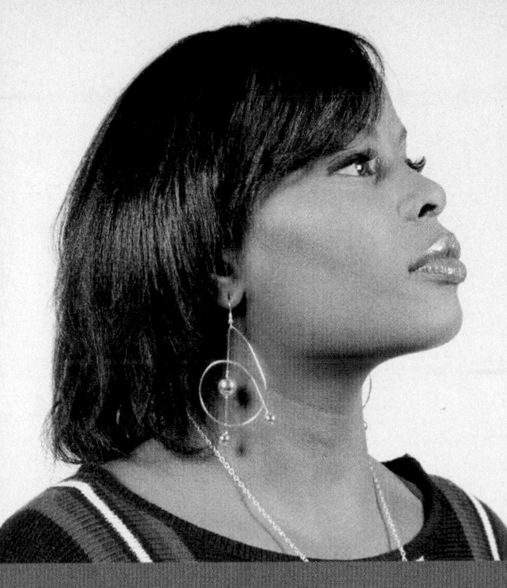

PROCEDURE 20-11

Hydroxide Relaxer Retouch

Implements and Materials

You will need all of the following implements, materials, and supplies:

- Acid-balanced shampoo
- Bowl and applicator brush
- Conditioner
- Disposable gloves
- Hard rubber comb
- Hydroxide neutralizer
- Hydroxide relaxer
- Plastic clips
- Protective base cream
- Shampoo cape
- Spray bottle
- Styling comb
- Timer
- Towels

© Milady, a part of Cengage Learning. Photography by Yanik Chauvin.

Preparation

- Perform PROCEDURE 15-1 Pre-Service Procedure SEE PAGE 323

Procedure

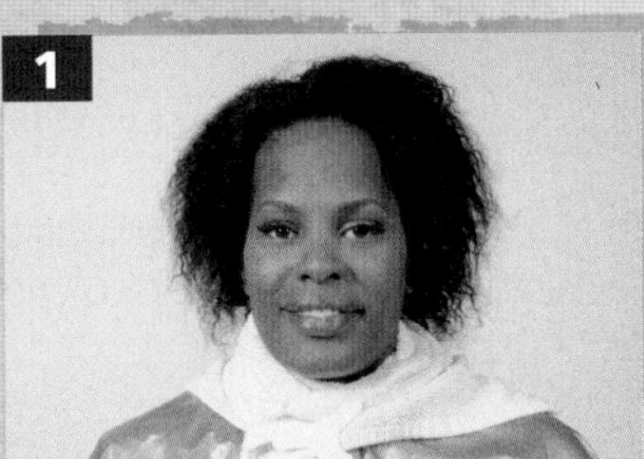

1 Perform an analysis of the hair and scalp. Perform tests for porosity and elasticity.

2 Drape the client for a chemical service. To avoid scalp irritation, do not shampoo the hair. *The hair and scalp must be completely dry prior to the application of a hydroxide relaxer retouch.*

3 Divide the hair into four sections, from the center of the front hairline to the center of the nape, and from ear to ear. Clip sections up to keep them out of the way.

Hydroxide Relaxer Retouch continued

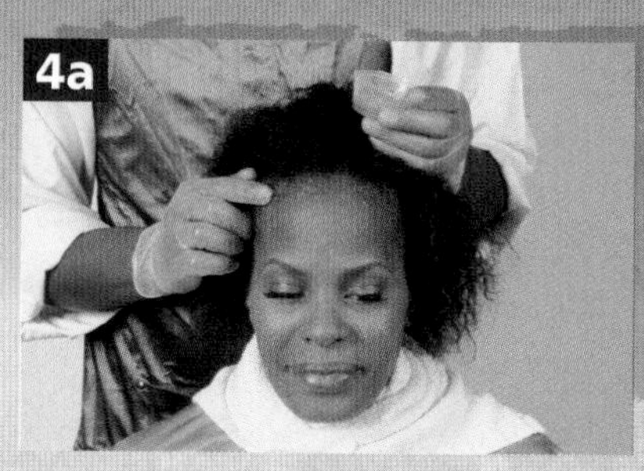

4a Wear gloves on both hands. Apply a protective base cream to the hairline and ears, unless you are using a no-base relaxing product.

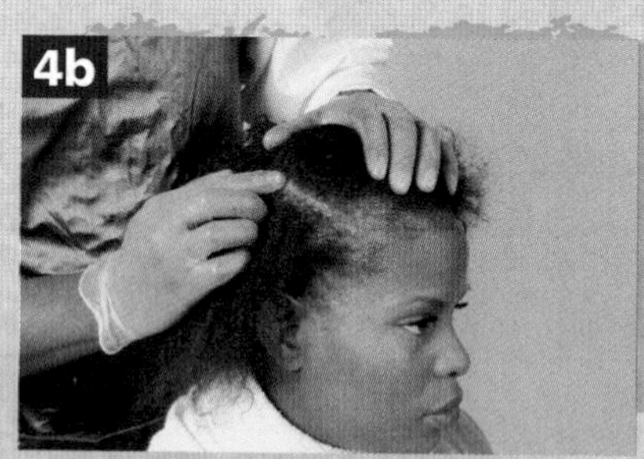

4b Option: Take ¼-inch to ½-inch horizontal (0.6 to 1.25 centimeters) partings and apply protective base cream to the entire scalp.

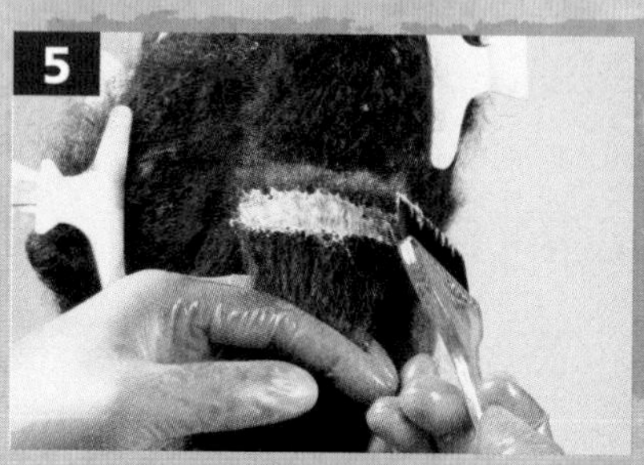

5 Begin application of the relaxer in the most resistant area, usually at the back of the head. Make ¼-inch to ½-inch (0.6 to 1.25 centimeters) horizontal partings, and apply the relaxer to the top of the strand. Apply the relaxer as close to the scalp as possible, but do not touch the scalp with the product. Only allow the relaxer to touch the scalp itself during the last few minutes of processing. To avoid overprocessing or breakage, do not overlap the relaxer onto the previously relaxed hair.

6 Continue applying the relaxer, using the same procedure and working your way down the section toward the hairline.

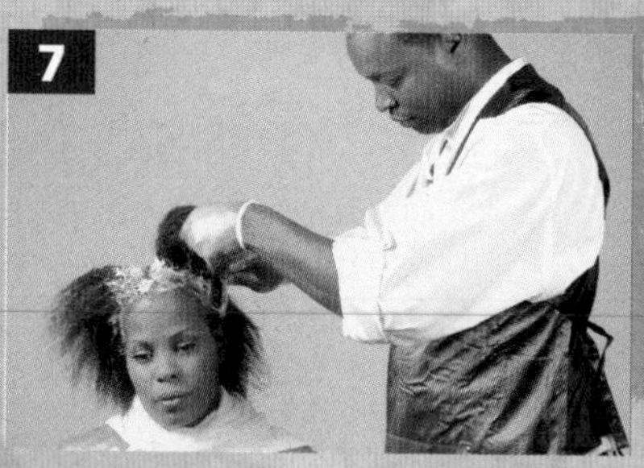

7 Continue the same application procedure with the remaining sections, finishing the most resistant sections first.

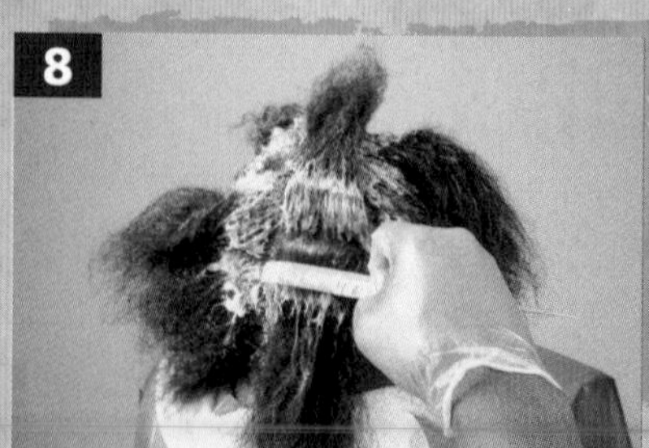

8 After the relaxer has been applied to all sections, use the back of the comb, the applicator brush, or your hands to smooth each section.

© Milady, a part of Cengage Learning. Photography by Yanik Chauvin.

9 Process according to the manufacturer's directions. Perform periodic strand tests. Processing usually takes less than twenty minutes at room temperature. Always follow the manufacturer's processing directions.

10 During the last few minutes of processing, gently work the relaxer down to the scalp.

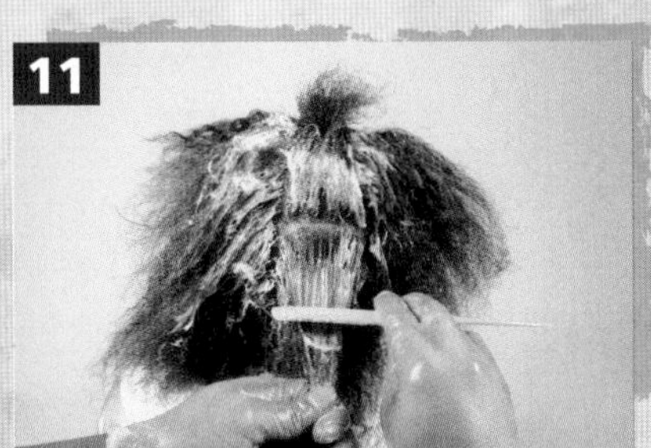
11

11 If the ends of the hair need additional relaxing, work the relaxer through to the ends for the last few minutes of processing. Do not relax ends during each retouch; doing this will cause overprocessing. Option: A cream conditioner may be applied to relaxed ends to protect from overprocessing caused by overlapping.

12 Rinse thoroughly with warm water to remove all traces of the relaxer.

13 Shampoo at least three times with an acid-balanced neutralizing shampoo. It is essential that all traces of the relaxer be removed from the hair.

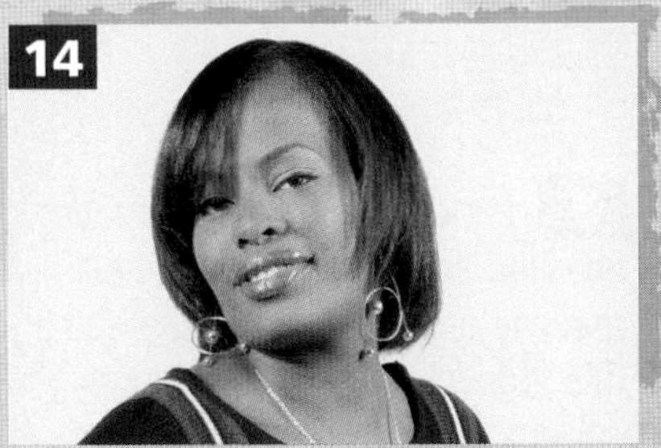
14

14 Style the hair as desired.

Post-Service

• Complete 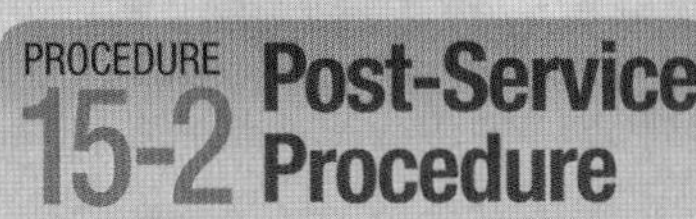

SEE PAGE 326

© Milady, a part of Cengage Learning. Photography by Yanik Chauvin.

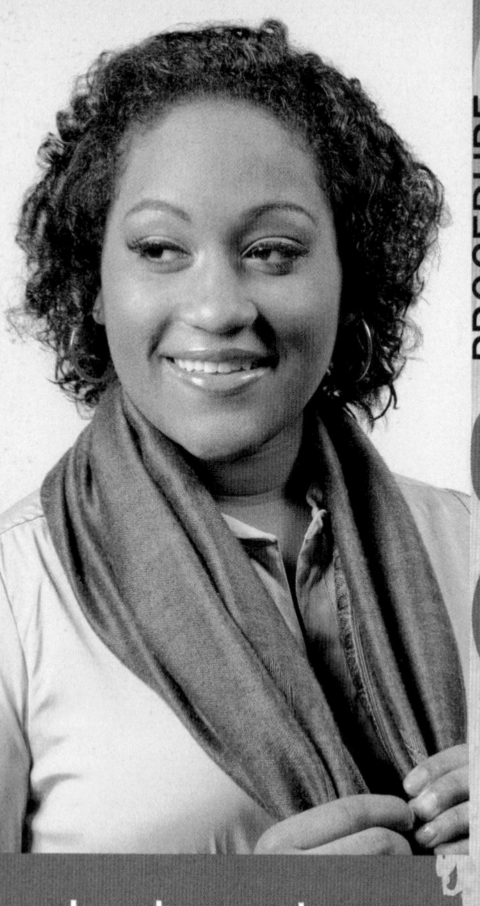

PROCEDURE 20-12 Curl Re-Forming (Soft Curl Perm)

Implements and Materials

You will need all of the following implements, materials, and supplies:

- **Acid-balanced shampoo**
- **Applicator bottles**
- **Applicator brush**
- **Conditioner**
- **Disposable gloves**
- **Plastic or glass bowl**
- **Pre-neutralizing conditioner (optional)**
- **Protective base cream**
- **Thio cream relaxer (curl rearranger)**
- **Thio curl booster**
- **Thio neutralizer**

Preparation

- Perform PROCEDURE 15-1 Pre-Service Procedure SEE PAGE 323

Procedure

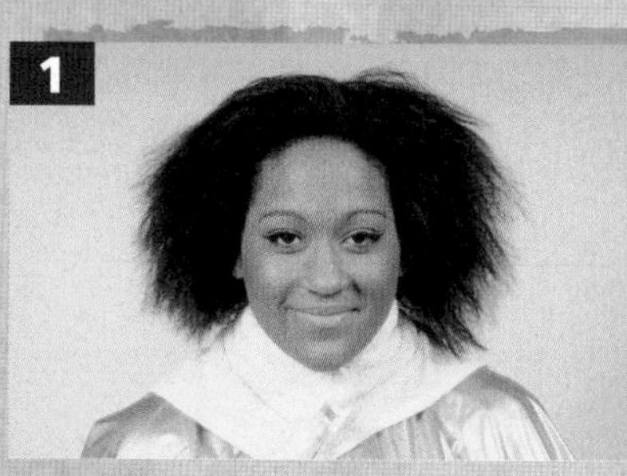

1 Perform an analysis of the hair and scalp. Perform tests for porosity and elasticity. Remember, this procedure requires that the hair and scalp be completely dry.

2 Drape the client for a chemical service. Follow steps 1–12 of Procedure 20–10, Applying Hydroxide Relaxer to Virgin Hair.

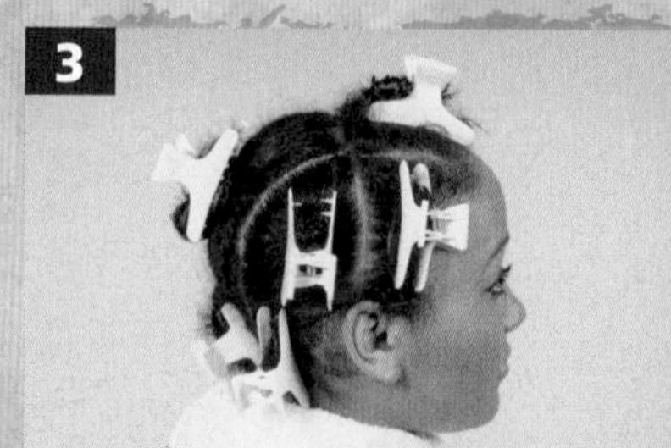

3 After rinsing the hair, towel blot and part it into nine panels. Use the length of the rod to measure the width of the panels. Roll hair on the appropriate-sized perm rods.

© Milady, a part of Cengage Learning. Photography by Yanik Chauvin.

CAUTION

Hair that has been treated with hydroxide relaxers must not be treated with thio relaxers or soft curl permanents.

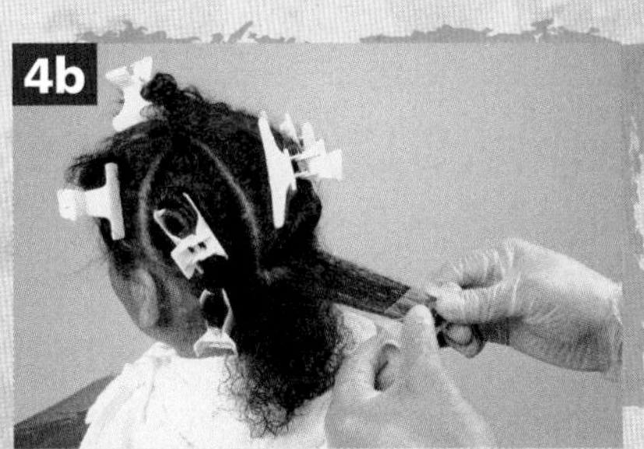

4a Wear gloves on both hands and begin wrapping at the most resistant area. Apply and distribute the thio curl booster to each panel as you wrap the hair.

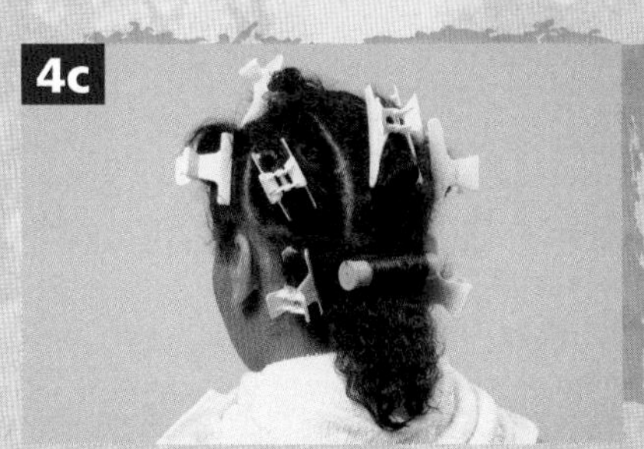

4b Make a horizontal parting the same size as the rod. Hold the hair at a 90-degree angle to the head. Using two end papers, roll the hair down to the scalp.

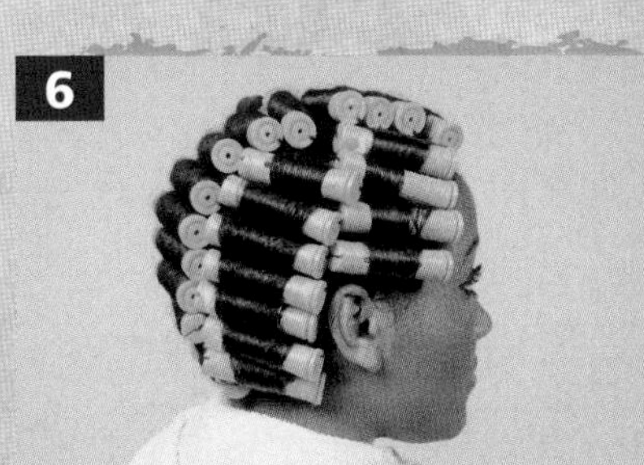

4c Position the rod half off base. Option: Insert roller picks to stabilize the rods and eliminate any tension caused by the band.

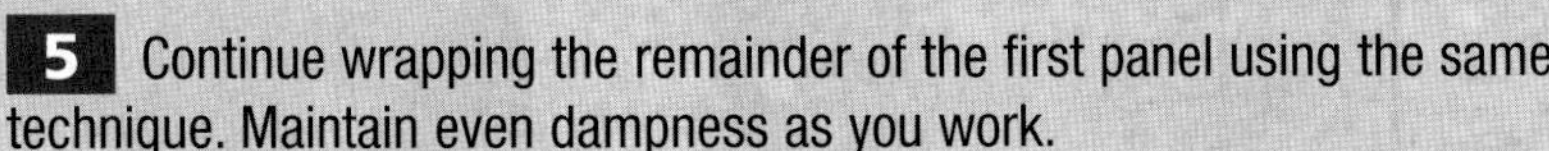

5 Continue wrapping the remainder of the first panel using the same technique. Maintain even dampness as you work.

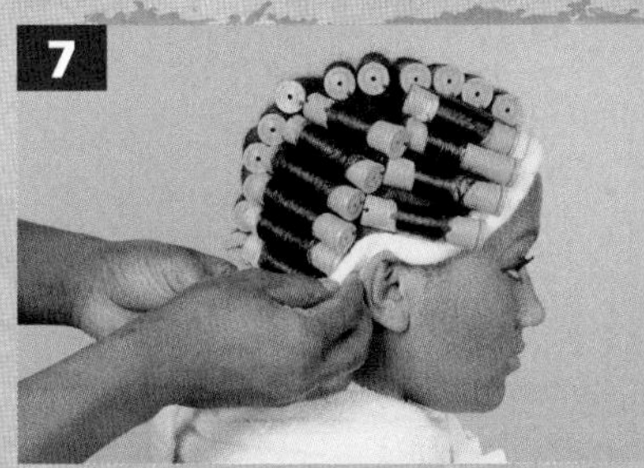

6 Continue wrapping the remaining eight panels in numerical order using the same technique.

7 Place cotton around the hairline and neck and apply thio curl booster to all the curls until they are completely saturated.

© Milady, a part of Cengage Learning. Photography by Yanik Chauvin.

Curl Re-Forming (Soft Curl Perm) continued

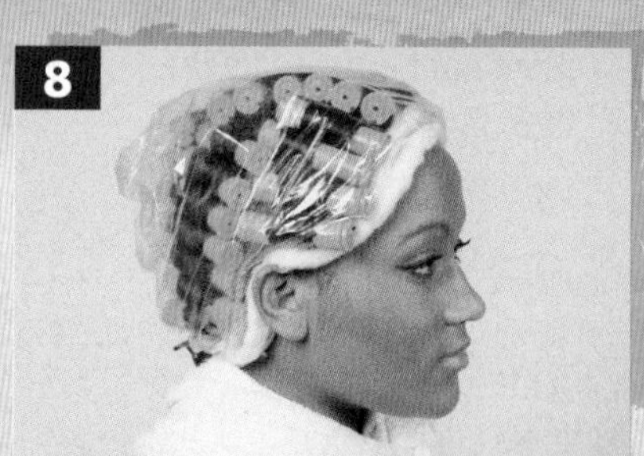
8

8 If a plastic cap is used, punch a few holes in the cap and cover all the hair completely. Do not allow the plastic cap to touch the client's skin. Check cotton and towels. If they are saturated with solution, replace them.

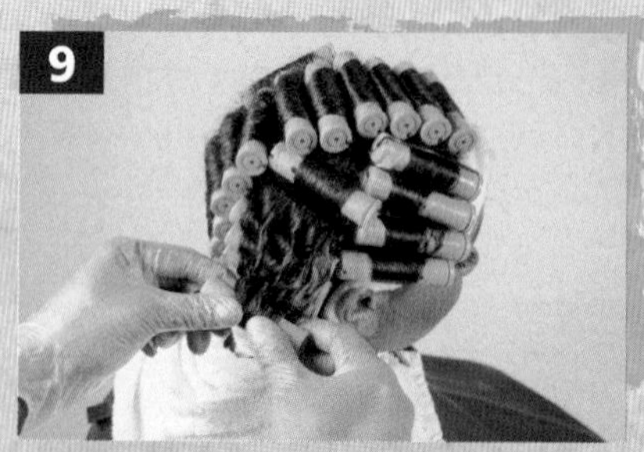
9

9 Process according to manufacturer's directions. Processing time will vary according to the strength of the product, the hair type and condition, and desired results. Processing usually takes less than twenty minutes at room temperature. Check for proper curl development.

10 When processing is completed, rinse the hair thoroughly, for at least five minutes. Then towel-blot the hair on each rod to remove excess moisture. Option: Apply pre-neutralizing conditioner according to the manufacturer's directions.

11 Apply the neutralizer slowly and carefully to the hair on each rod. Avoid splashing and dripping. Make sure each rod is completely saturated. Distribute remaining neutralizer. Set a timer and neutralize according to the manufacturer's directions.

12 Remove the rods, distribute the remaining neutralizer through the ends of the hair, and rinse thoroughly. Option: Shampoo and condition.

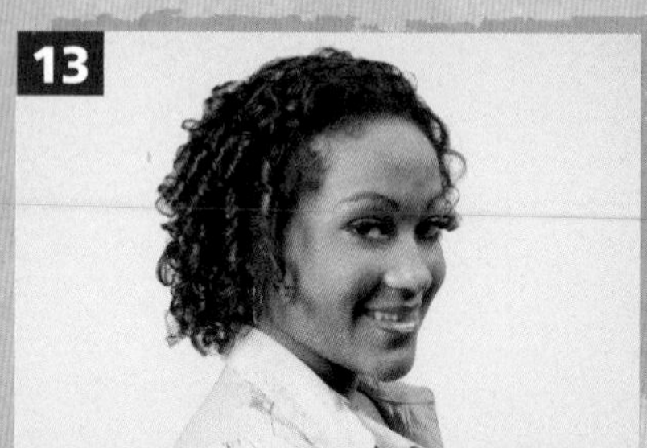
13

13 Style the hair as desired.

Post-Service

- Complete PROCEDURE 15-2 **Post-Service Procedure** SEE PAGE 326

© Milady, a part of Cengage Learning. Photography by Yanik Chauvin.

Review Questions

1. Name the structures of and purpose of each layer of the hair.
2. What are the chemical actions that take place during permanent waving?
3. What is the difference between an alkaline wave and a true acid wave?
4. Why do permanent waves need to be neutralized?
5. How do thio relaxers straighten the hair?
6. How do hydroxide relaxers straighten the hair?
7. What is curl re-forming and what is it best used for?

Chapter Glossary

acid-balanced waves	Permanent waves that have a 7.0 or neutral pH; because of their higher pH, they process at room temperature, do not require the added heat of a hair dryer, process more quickly, and produce firmer curls than true acid waves.
alkaline waves	Also known as *cold waves*; have a pH between 9.0 and 9.6, use ammonium thioglycolate (ATG) as the reducing agent, and process at room temperature without the addition of heat.
amino acids	Compounds made up of carbon, oxygen, hydrogen, nitrogen, and sulfur.
ammonia-free waves	Perms that use an ingredient that does not evaporate as readily as ammonia, so there is very little odor associated with their use.
ammonium thioglycolate (ATG)	Active ingredient or reducing agent in alkaline permanents.
base control	Position of the tool in relation to its base section, determined by the angle at which the hair is wrapped.
base cream	Also known as *protective base cream*; oily cream used to protect the skin and scalp during hair relaxing.
base direction	Angle at which the rod is positioned on the head (horizontally, vertically, or diagonally); also, the directional pattern in which the hair is wrapped.
base placement	Refers to the position of the rod in relation to its base section; base placement is determined by the angle at which the hair is wrapped.
base relaxers	Relaxers that require the application of protective base cream to the entire scalp prior to the application of the relaxer.
base sections	Subsections of panels into which hair is divided for perm wrapping; one rod is normally placed on each base section.
basic permanent wrap	Also known as *straight set wrap*; perm wrapping pattern in which all the rods within a panel move in the same direction and are positioned on equal-sized bases; all the base sections are horizontal, and are the same length and width as the perm rod.
bookend wrap	Perm wrap in which one end paper is folded in half over the hair ends like an envelope.
bricklay permanent wrap	Perm wrap similar to actual technique of bricklaying; base sections are offset from each other row by row, to prevent noticeable splits and to blend the flow of the hair.

Chapter Glossary

chemical hair relaxing	A process or service that rearranges the structure of curly hair into a straighter or smoother form.
chemical texture services	Hair services that cause a chemical change that alters the natural wave pattern of the hair.
concave rods	Perm rods that have a smaller diameter in the center that increases to a larger diameter on the ends.
croquignole perm wrap	Perms in which the hair strands are wrapped from the ends to the scalp in overlapping concentric layers.
curvature permanent wrap	Perm wrap in which partings and bases radiate throughout the panels to follow the curvature of the head.
double flat wrap	Perm wrap in which one end paper is placed under and another is placed over the strand of hair being wrapped.
double-rod wrap	Also known as *piggyback wrap*; a wrap technique whereby extra-long hair is wrapped on one rod from the scalp to midway down the hair shaft, and another rod is used to wrap the remaining hair strand in the same direction.
end papers	Also known as *end wraps*; absorbent papers used to control the ends of the hair when wrapping and winding hair on perm rods.
endothermic waves	Perm activated by an outside heat source, usually a conventional hood-type hair dryer.
exothermic waves	Create an exothermic chemical reaction that heats up the waving solution and speeds up processing.
glyceryl monothioglycolate (GMTG)	Main active ingredient in true acid and acid-balanced waving lotions.
half off-base placement	Base control in which the hair is wrapped at an angle of 90 degrees or perpendicular to its base section, and the rod is positioned half off its base section.
hydroxide neutralization	An acid-alkali neutralization reaction that neutralizes (deactivates) the alkaline residues left in the hair by a hydroxide relaxer and lowers the pH of the hair and scalp; hydroxide relaxer neutralization does not involve oxidation or rebuild disulfide bonds.
hydroxide relaxers	Very strong alkalis with a pH over 13; the hydroxide ion is the active ingredient in all hydroxide relaxers.
keratin proteins	Long, coiled polypeptide chains.
lanthionization	Process by which hydroxide relaxers permanently straighten hair; they remove a sulfur atom from a disulfide bond and convert it into a lanthionine bond.
loop rod	Also known as *circle rod;* tool that is usually about 12-inches long with a uniform diameter along the entire length of the rod.
low-pH waves	Perms that use sulfates, sulfites, and bisulfites as an alternative to ammonium thioglycolate; they have a low pH.

Chapter Glossary

metal hydroxide relaxers	Ionic compounds formed by a metal (sodium, potassium, or lithium) which is combined with oxygen and hydrogen.
no-base relaxers	Relaxers that do not require application of a protective base cream.
normalizing lotions	Conditioners with an acidic pH that restore the hair's natural pH after a hydroxide relaxer and prior to shampooing.
off-base placement	Base control in which the hair is wrapped at 45 degrees below the center of the base section, so the rod is positioned completely off its base.
on-base placement	Base control in which the hair is wrapped at a 45-degree angle beyond perpendicular to its base section, and the rod is positioned on its base.
peptide bonds	Also known as *end bonds*; chemical bonds that join amino acids together, end to end in long chains, to form polypeptide chains.
permanent waving	A two-step process whereby the hair undergoes a physical change caused by wrapping the hair on perm rods, and then the hair undergoes a chemical change caused by the application of permanent waving solution and neutralizer.
polypeptide chains	Long chains of amino acids joined together by peptide bonds.
single flat wrap	Perm wrap that is similar to double flat wrap but uses only one end paper, placed over the top of the strand of hair being wrapped.
soft bender rods	Tool about 12-inches long with a uniform diameter along the entire length.
soft curl permanent	Combination of a thio relaxer and a thio permanent that is wrapped on large rods to make existing curl larger and looser.
spiral perm wrap	Hair is wrapped at an angle other than perpendicular to the length of the rod, which causes the hair to spiral along the length of the rod, similar to the stripes on a candy cane.
straight rods	Perm rods that are equal in diameter along their entire length or curling area.
thio neutralization	Stops the action of a permanent wave solution and rebuilds the hair in its new curly form.
thio relaxers	Use the same ammonium thioglycolate (ATG) that is used in permanent waving, but at a higher concentration and a higher pH (above 10).
thio-free waves	Perm that uses an ingredient other than ATG as the primary reducing agent, such as cysteamine or mercaptamine.
true acid waves	Have a pH between 4.5 and 7.0 and require heat to process; they process more slowly than alkaline waves, and do not usually produce as firm a curl as alkaline waves.
viscosity	The measurement of the thickness or thinness of a liquid that affects how the fluid flows.
weave technique	Wrapping technique that uses zigzag partings to divide base areas.

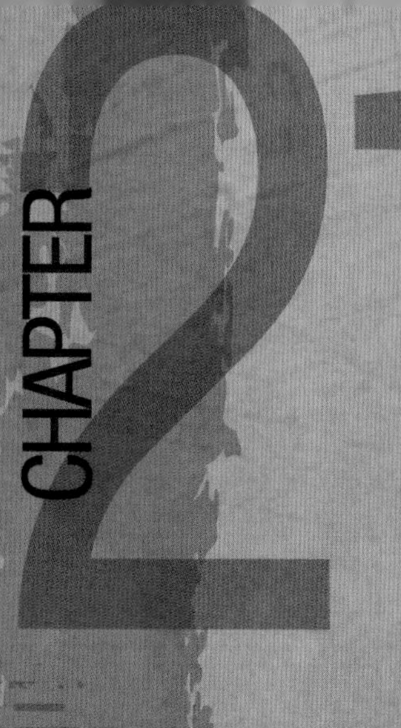

CHAPTER 21 Haircoloring

Chapter Outline

Why Study Haircoloring?

Why People Color Their Hair

Hair Facts

Identifying Natural Hair Color and Tone

Types of Haircolor

Consultation

Haircolor Formulation

Haircolor Applications

Using Lighteners

Using Toners

Special Effects Haircoloring

Special Challenges in Haircolor/ Corrective Solutions

Haircoloring Safety Precautions

Procedures

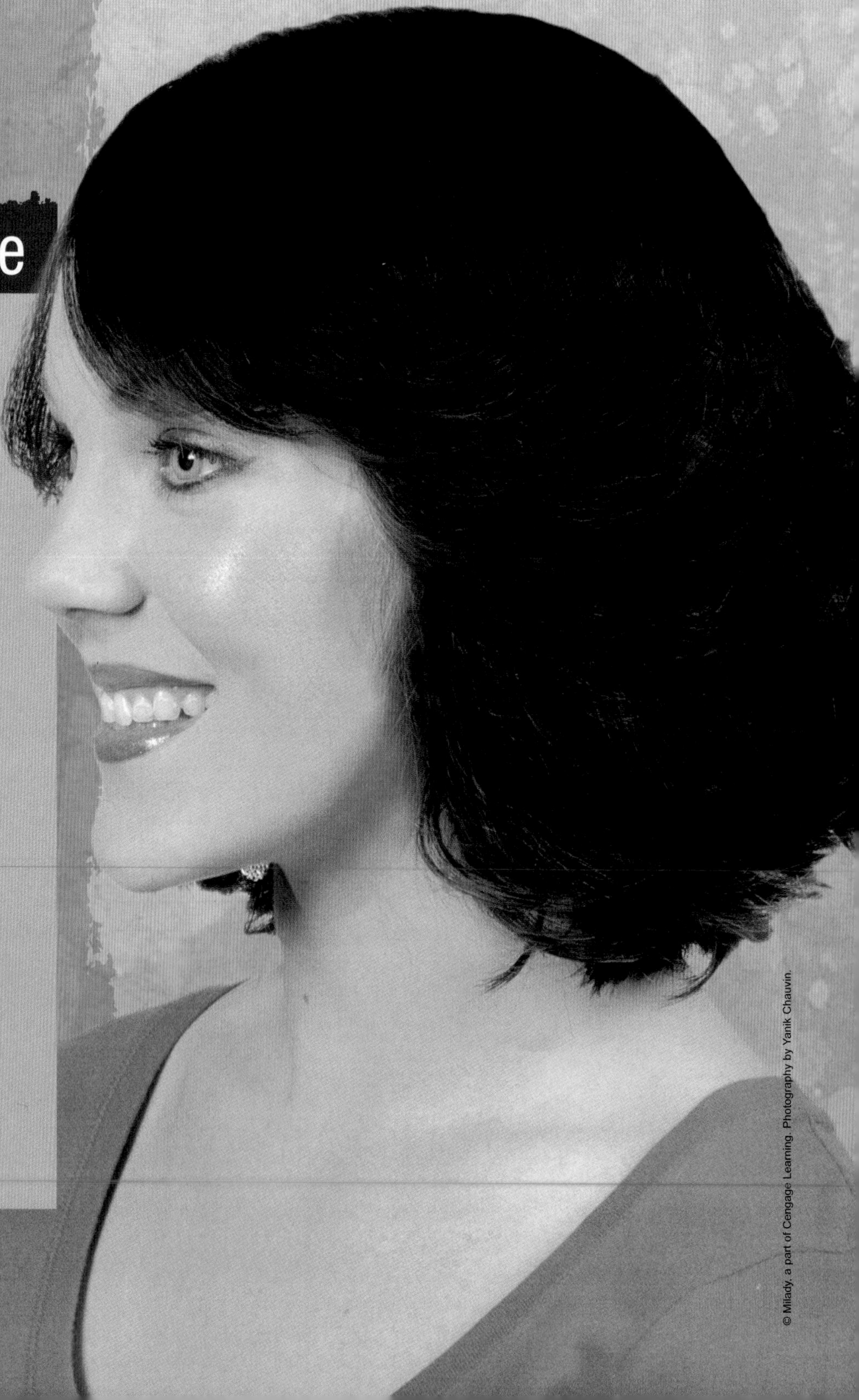

© Milady, a part of Cengage Learning. Photography by Yanik Chauvin.

Learning Objectives

After completing this chapter, you will be able to:

- ✓ **LO1** List the reasons why people color their hair.
- ✓ **LO2** Explain how the hair's porosity affects haircolor.
- ✓ **LO3** Understand the types of melanin found in hair.
- ✓ **LO4** Define and identify levels and their role in formulating haircolor.
- ✓ **LO5** Identify primary, secondary, and tertiary colors.
- ✓ **LO6** Know what roles tone and intensity play in haircolor.
- ✓ **LO7** List and describe the categories of haircolor.
- ✓ **LO8** Explain the role of hydrogen peroxide in a haircolor formula.
- ✓ **LO9** Explain the action of hair lighteners.
- ✓ **LO10** List the four key questions to ask when formulating a haircolor.
- ✓ **LO11** Understand why a patch test is useful in haircoloring.
- ✓ **LO12** Define what a preliminary strand test is and why it is used.
- ✓ **LO13** List and describe the procedure for a virgin single-process color service.
- ✓ **LO14** Understand the two processes involved in double-process haircoloring.
- ✓ **LO15** Describe the various forms of hair lightener.
- ✓ **LO16** Understand the purpose and use of toners.
- ✓ **LO17** Name and describe the three most commonly used methods for highlighting.
- ✓ **LO18** Know how to properly cover gray hair.
- ✓ **LO19** Know the rules of color correction.
- ✓ **LO20** Know the safety precautions to follow during the haircolor process.

Key Terms

Page number indicates where in the chapter the term is used.

activators (boosters, protinators, accelerators)
pg. 650

aniline derivatives
pg. 638

baliage (free-form technique)
pg. 654

base color
pg. 633

cap technique
pg. 653

color fillers
pg. 660

complementary colors
pg. 635

conditioner fillers
pg. 659

contributing pigment (undertone)
pg. 631

demipermanent haircolor (no-lift deposit-only color)
pg. 637

developers (oxidizing agents, catalysts)
pg. 639

double-process application (two-step coloring)
pg. 640

Key Terms

Page number indicates where in the chapter the term is used.

fillers
pg. 659

foil technique
pg. 654

glaze
pg. 649

hair color
pg. 630

hair lightening (bleaching, decolorizing)
pg. 649

haircolor
pg. 630

haircolor glaze
pg. 638

highlighting
pg. 653

highlighting shampoo
pg. 655

hydrogen peroxide developer
pg. 639

intensity
pg. 635

law of color
pg. 633

level
pg. 632

level system
pg. 632

lighteners
pg. 640

line of demarcation
pg. 649

metallic haircolors (gradual haircolors)
pg. 639

mixed melanin
pg. 631

natural haircolors (vegetable haircolors)
pg. 639

new growth
pg. 652

off-the-scalp lighteners (quick lighteners)
pg. 650

on-the-scalp lighteners
pg. 650

patch test (predisposition test)
pg. 647

permanent haircolors
pg. 638

prelightening
pg. 649

presoftening
pg. 658

primary colors
pg. 634

resistant
pg. 631

reverse highlighting (lowlighting)
pg. 653

secondary color
pg. 634

semipermanent haircolor
pg. 637

single-process haircoloring
pg. 648

slicing
pg. 654

soap cap
pg. 638

special effects haircoloring
pg. 653

strand test
pg. 647

temporary haircolor
pg. 637

tertiary color
pg. 634

tone (hue)
pg. 635

toners
pg. 641

virgin application
pg. 648

volume
pg. 639

weaving
pg. 654

One of the most creative, challenging, and popular salon services is haircoloring. It also has the potential for being one of the most lucrative areas in which a stylist can choose to work. You only have to look around while you are dining at a restaurant or standing in line to see a movie to know this is true. Nearly all adults and many teens now color their hair. You will probably find that most of your clients, at some time or another, will want to enhance their hair color, change their hair color, or cover gray. Clients who have their hair colored usually visit the salon every four to twelve weeks. These are the kind of regulars you want in your client base (**Figure 21–1**).

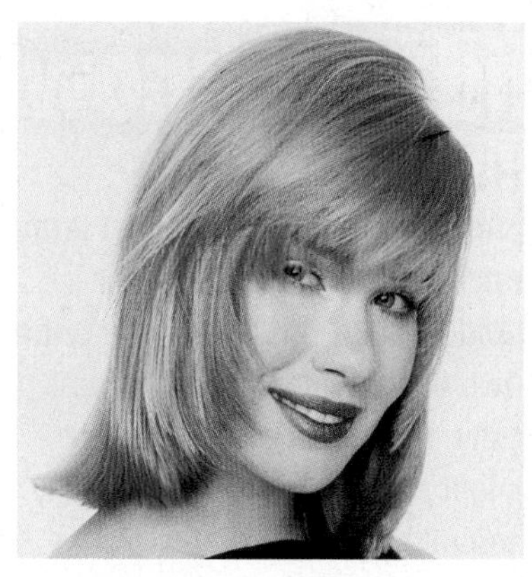

Photo used with the permission of the authors, Martin Gannon and Richard Thompson, as featured in their book, Mahogany: Steps to Cutting, Colouring and Finishing Hair. © Martin Gannon and Richard Thompson.

▲ Figure 21–1
Haircoloring is a popular salon service.

WHY STUDY HAIRCOLORING?

Cosmetologists should study and have a thorough understanding of haircoloring because:

- Haircolor services provide stylists and clients with an opportunity for creative expression and artistry.
- Clients increasingly ask for and require excellent haircoloring services to cover gray, to enhance their haircuts and to camouflage face-shape imperfections.
- Haircolor products employ strong chemical ingredients to accomplish services, so being aware of what these chemicals are and how they work will enable you to safely provide color services for your clients.

Why People Color Their Hair

It is important to have an understanding of what motivates people to color their hair. This information will help you determine which products and haircolor services are appropriate for your client. A few common reasons clients color their hair include the following:

- Cover up or blend gray (unpigmented) hair
- Enhance an existing haircolor
- Create a fashion statement or statement of self-expression
- Correct unwanted tones in hair caused by environmental exposure such as sun or chlorine
- Accentuate a particular haircut

Many people experiment with haircoloring. When a client turns to you for advice and service, you need to have a thorough understanding of the hair structure and how haircoloring products affect it. As a trained professional, you will learn which shades of color are most flattering on your clients and which products and techniques will achieve the desired look. ☑ **LO1**

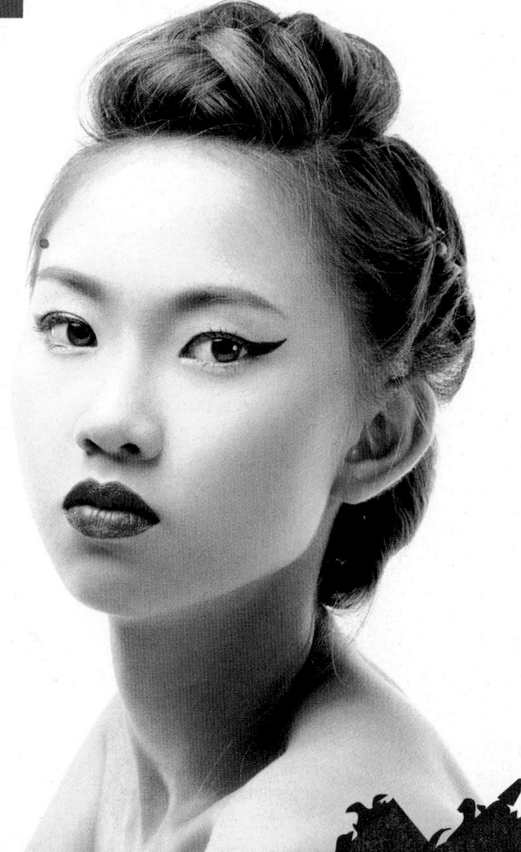

© Nabi Lukic, 2010; used under license from iStockphoto.com.

did you know?

Haircolor (one word) is a professional, industry-coined term referring to artificial haircolor products and services. **Hair color** (two words) refers to the natural color of hair. For example, you might say of a client, "Mrs. Bailey's natural hair color is brown."

Hair Facts

The structure of the client's hair and the desired results determine wwhich haircolor to use. The hair structure affects the quality and ultimate success of the haircolor service. Some haircolor products may cause a dramatic change in the structure of the hair, while others cause relatively little change. Knowing how products affect the hair will allow you to make the best choices for your client.

Hair Structure

In this section, the structure of hair is quickly reviewed. For an in-depth discussion, see Chapter 11, Properties of the Hair and Scalp.

Hair is composed of the following three major components (**Figure 21–2**):

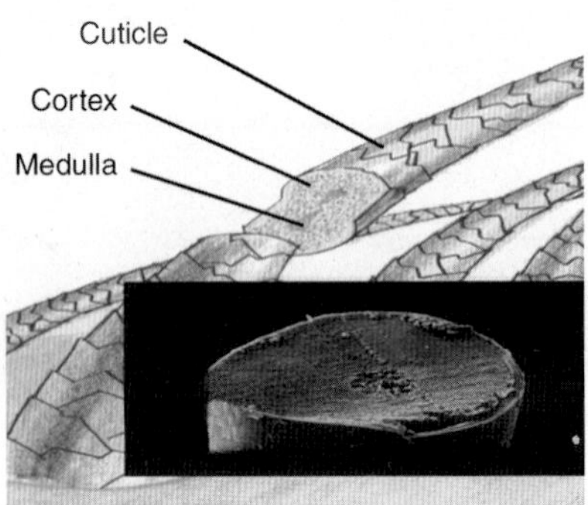

▲ **Figure 21–2**
A cross-section of the hair shaft.

- The cuticle which is the outermost layer of the hair. It protects the interior cortex layer and contributes up to 20 percent of the overall strength of the hair.
- The cortex which is the middle layer and gives the hair the majority of its strength and elasticity. A healthy cortex contributes about 80 percent to the overall strength of the hair. It contains the natural pigment called melanin that determines hair color. Melanin granules are scattered between the cortex cells like chips in a chocolate chip cookie.
- The medulla which is the innermost layer of the hair. It is sometimes absent from the hair and does not play a role in the haircoloring process.

Texture

Hair texture is the diameter of an individual hair strand. Large-, medium-, and small-diameter hair strands translate into coarse, medium, and fine hair textures, respectively. Melanin is distributed differently according to texture. The melanin granules in fine hair are grouped more tightly, so the hair takes color faster and can look darker. Medium-textured hair has an average reaction to haircolor. Coarse-textured hair has a larger diameter and loosely grouped melanin granules, so it can take longer to process (**Figure 21–3**).

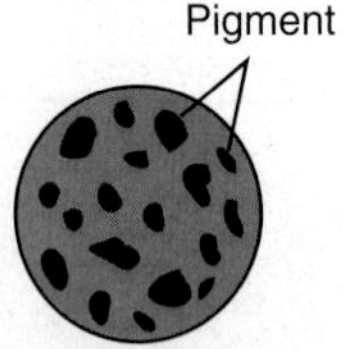

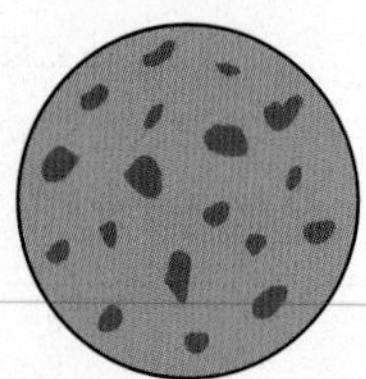

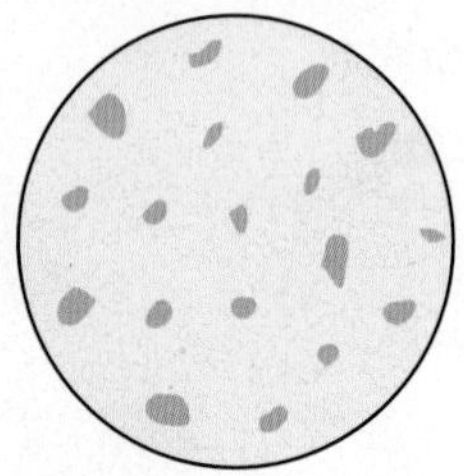

▲ **Figure 21–3**
Melanin distribution according to hair texture.

© Milady, a part of Cengage Learning.

Density

Another aspect of hair that plays a role in haircoloring is density. Hair density, the number of hairs per square inch, can range from thin to thick. Density must be taken into account when applying haircolor, to ensure proper coverage.

Porosity

Porosity is the hair's ability to absorb moisture. Porous hair accepts haircolor faster, and haircolor application on porous hair can result in a cooler tone than applications on less porous hair. Degrees of porosity are described below.

- **Low porosity.** The cuticle is tight. The hair is **resistant**, which means it is difficult for moisture or chemicals to penetrate. Thus, it requires a longer processing time.
- **Average porosity.** The cuticle is slightly raised. The hair is normal and processes in an average amount of time.
- **High porosity.** The cuticle is lifted. The hair is overly porous and takes color quickly; color also tends to fade quickly. Permed, colored, chemically relaxed, and straightened hair will have a high degree of porosity.

Test for porosity:

- Take a several strands of hair from four different areas of the head: the front hairline, the temple, the crown, and the nape.
- Hold the strands securely with one hand and slide the thumb and forefinger of the other hand from the ends to the scalp.
- If the hair feels smooth and the cuticle is compact, dense, and hard, it has low porosity. If you can feel a slight roughness, it has average porosity. If the hair feels very rough, dry, or breaks, it has high porosity.
- Observe hair wet and dry to see porosity.
- Extremely porous hair rejects warmth when color is applied and can process more quickly, which results in deeper color. ✓ **LO2**

Identifying Natural Hair Color and Tone

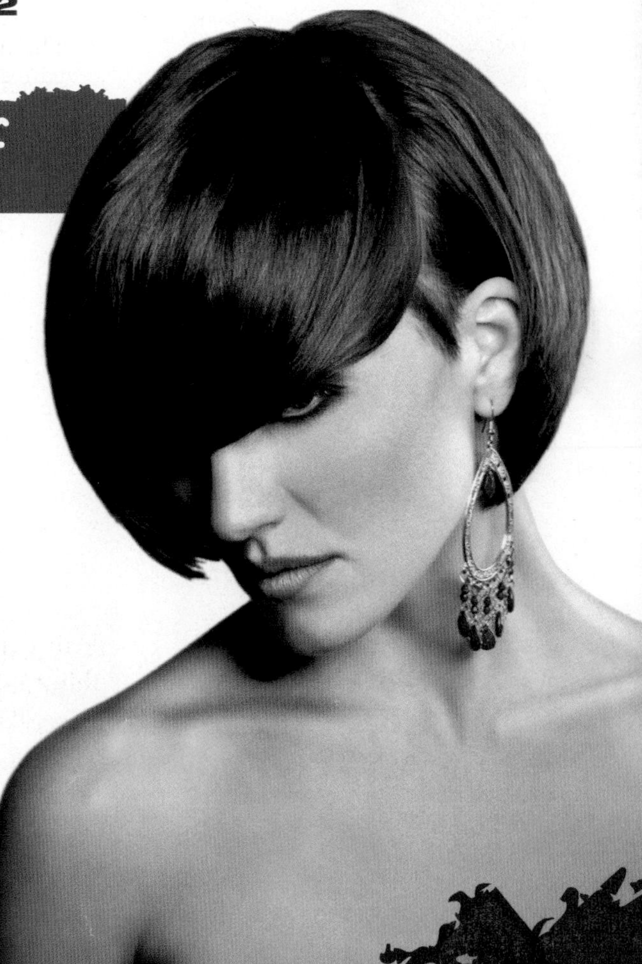

© Puhhha, 2010; used under license from Shutterstock.com.

Learning to identify a client's natural hair color is the most important step in becoming a good colorist. Natural hair color ranges from black to dark brown to red, and from dark blond to light blond. Hair color is unique to each individual; no two people have exactly the same color. There are three types of melanin in the cortex:

- **Eumelanin** is the melanin that lends black and brown colors to hair.
- **Pheomelanin** is the melanin that gives blond and red colors to hair.
- **Mixed melanin** is a combination of natural hair color that contains both pheomelanin and eumelanin. ✓ **LO3**

Contributing pigment, also known as **undertone**, is the varying degrees of warmth exposed during a permanent color or lightening process. Generally, when you lighten natural hair color, the darker the natural level, the more intense the contributing pigment. This must be taken into consideration before the haircolor selection is made. Haircoloring modifies this pigment to create new pigment.

The Level System

Level is the unit of measurement used to identify the lightness or darkness of a color. Level is the saturation, density, or concentration of color. The level of color answers the following question: How much color?

The **level system** is a system that colorists use to determine the lightness or darkness of a hair color (**Figure 21–4**). Haircolor levels are arranged on a scale of 1 to 10, with 1 being the darkest and 10 the lightest. Although the names for the color levels may vary among manufacturers, the important thing is being able to identify the degrees of lightness to darkness (depth) in each level.

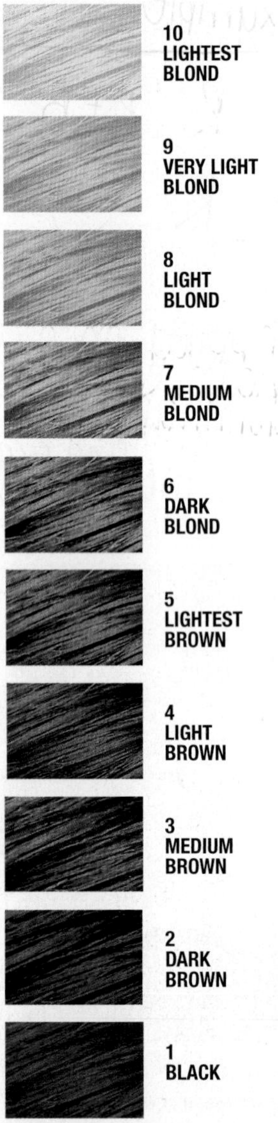

10 LIGHTEST BLOND
9 VERY LIGHT BLOND
8 LIGHT BLOND
7 MEDIUM BLOND
6 DARK BLOND
5 LIGHTEST BROWN
4 LIGHT BROWN
3 MEDIUM BROWN
2 DARK BROWN
1 BLACK

Courtesy of P&G Salon Professional. Clariol Professional.

▲ Figure 21–4
Natural hair color levels.

Identifying Natural Level

Identifying natural level is the first step in performing a haircolor service. Your most valuable tool is the color wheel. Haircolor swatch books provide a visual representation as well (**Figure 21–5**).

To determine the natural level, perform the following four steps:

1. Take a ½-inch square section in the crown area and hold it up from the scalp, allowing light to pass through (**Figure 21–6**).
2. Using the natural level-finder swatches provided by the manufacturer, select a swatch that you think matches the section of hair and place it against the hair. Remember, you are trying to determine depth level (darkness or lightness). Do not part or hold the hair flat against the scalp; that will give you an incorrect reading, as the hair will appear darker (**Figure 21–7**).

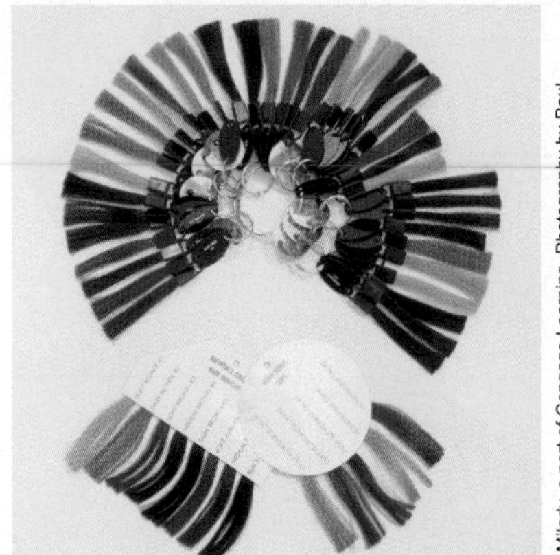

© Milady, a part of Cengage Learning. Photography by Paul Castle, Castle Photography.

▲ Figure 21–5
Manufacturers' swatches are a useful tool.

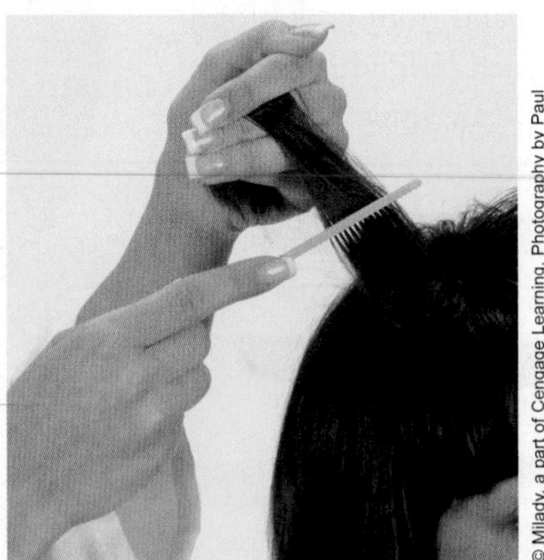

© Milady, a part of Cengage Learning. Photography by Paul Castle, Castle Photography.

▲ Figure 21–6
Take a ½-inch square section in the crown.

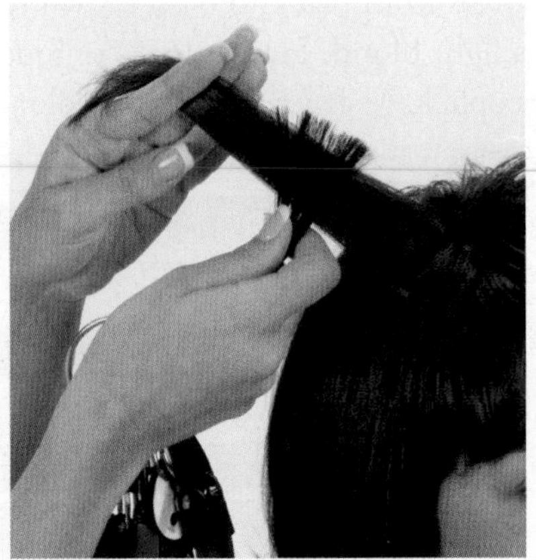

© Milady, a part of Cengage Learning. Photography by Paul Castle, Castle Photography.

▲ Figure 21–7
Hold the color swatch against the hair strand.

3. Move the swatch from the scalp area along the hair strand.

4. Determine the natural-hair color level. ☑ **LO4**

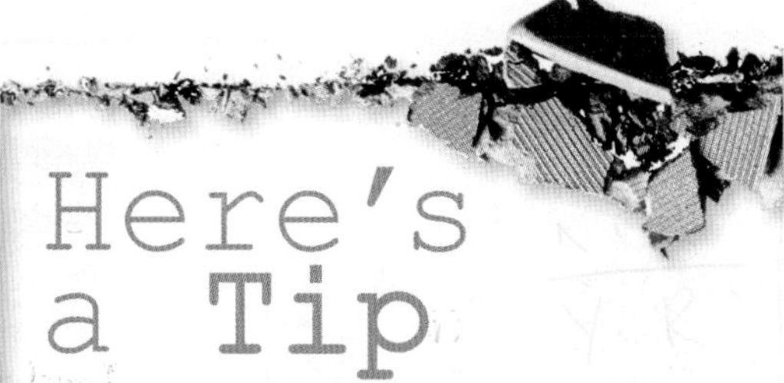

Here's a Tip

Available light is critical in analyzing hair color. Use natural light, walking outside with a client to make your analysis, if possible. Artificial light affects your perception of color. This is especially true of fluorescent light, which can distort color drastically.

Gray Hair

Gray hair is hair that has lost its pigment and is normally associated with aging. Even though the loss of pigment increases as a person ages, few people ever become completely gray haired (**Figure 21–8**). Most retain a certain percentage of pigmented hair (**Table 21-1**). The gray can be solid or blended throughout the head as in salt-and-pepper hair. Gray hair requires special attention in formulating haircolor. This will be discussed later in the chapter.

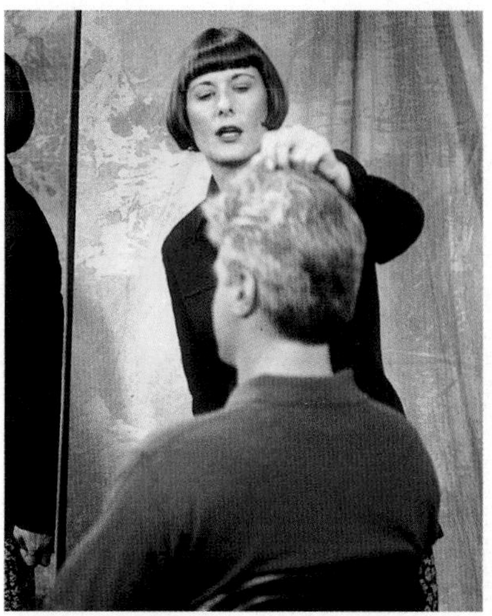

▲ **Figure 21–8**
Many people choose to cover or blend gray hair.

Color Theory

Color is described as a property of objects that depends on the light they reflect and is perceived (by the human eye) as red, green, blue, or other shades. Thus, colors (the light reflected by objects that is perceivable) by definition are in the visible spectrum of light. (See Chapter 13, Basics of Electricity.) Before you attempt to apply haircoloring products, it is important to have a general understanding of color theory. A **base color** is the predominant tone of a color. Once you have a better understanding of color theory, you will see how each haircolor manufacturer associates base colors with color lines.

The Law of Color

The **law of color** is a system for understanding color relationships. When combining colors, you will always get the same result from the same combination. Equal parts of red and blue mixed together always make violet. Equal parts of blue and yellow always make green. Equal parts of red and yellow always make orange. The color wheels in **Figures 21–9** through **21–11** will help you understand colors.

DETERMINING THE PERCENTAGE OF GRAY HAIR

PERCENTAGE OF GRAY HAIR	CHARACTERISTICS
30%	More pigmented than gray hair
50%	Even mixture of gray and pigmented hair
70 to 90%	More gray than pigmented; most of remaining pigment is located in the back of the head
100%	Virtually no pigmented hair; tends to look white

© Milady, a part of Cengage Learning.

Table 21–1 Determining the Percentage of Gray Hair.

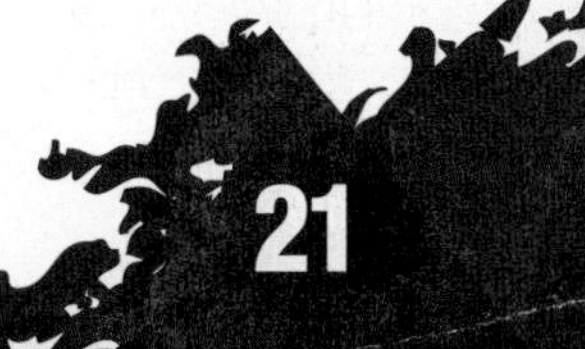

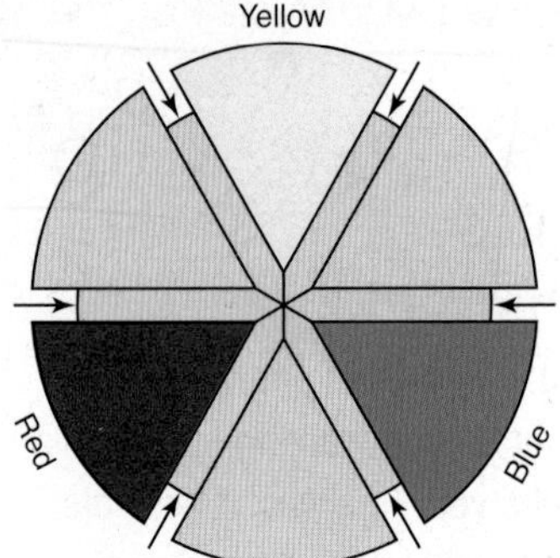

▲ **Figure 21–9**
Primary colors.

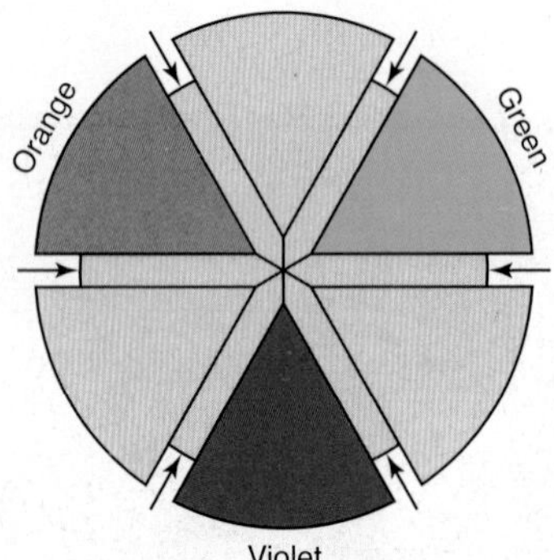

▲ **Figure 21–10**
Secondary colors.

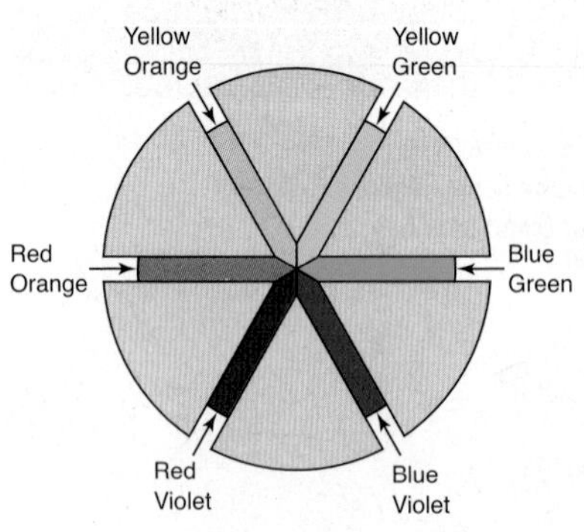

▲ **Figure 21–11**
Tertiary colors.

Primary Colors

Primary colors are pure or fundamental colors (red, yellow, and blue) that cannot be created by combining other colors. All colors are created from these three primaries. Colors with a predominance of blue are cool colors, whereas colors with a predominance of red and/or yellow are warm colors (**Figure 21–9**).

Blue is the strongest of the primary colors and is the only cool primary color. In addition to coolness, blue can also bring depth or darkness to any color.

Red is the medium primary color. Adding red to blue-based colors will make them appear lighter; adding red to yellow colors will cause them to appear darker.

Yellow is the weakest of the primary colors. When you add yellow to other colors, the resulting color will look lighter and brighter.

When all three primary colors are present in equal proportions, the resulting color is brown. It is helpful to think of hair color in terms of different combinations of primary colors. Natural brown, for example, has the primary colors in the following proportions: blue-B, red-RR, and yellow-YYY. Black and white can't be made by mixing colors together. They get excluded from basic color theory. White can be used to lighten a color. Black can be used to deepen a color.

Secondary Colors

A **secondary color** is a color obtained by mixing equal parts of two primary colors. The secondary colors are green, orange, and violet. Green is an equal combination of blue and yellow. Orange is an equal combination of red and yellow. Violet is an equal combination of blue and red (**Figure 21–10**).

Tertiary Colors

A **tertiary color** is an intermediate color achieved by mixing a secondary color and its neighboring primary color on the color wheel in equal amounts. The tertiary colors include blue-green, blue-violet, red-violet, red-orange, yellow-orange, and yellow-green. Natural-looking haircolor is made up of a combination of primary colors, secondary colors, and tertiary colors (**Figure 21–11**). ✔ **LO5**

© Milady, a part of Cengage Learning.

ACTivity

Using primary-colored modeling clay—red, blue, and yellow—create secondary and tertiary colors. You will see that if you mix red clay with yellow clay in equal proportions, you will get orange. If you mix red clay with the orange clay, what is the result? What happens if you change the proportion of each color? The combinations are endless (Figure 21–12).

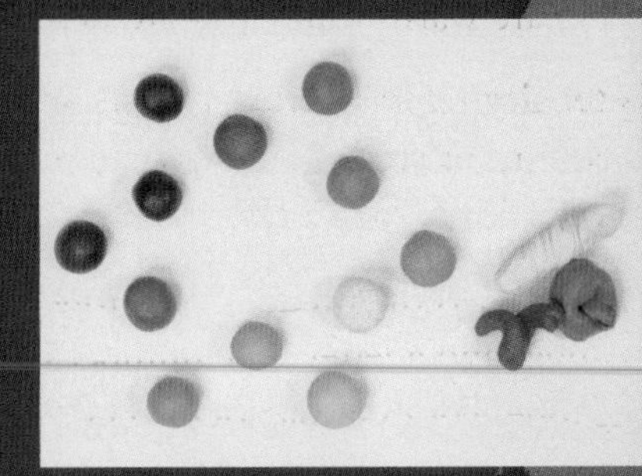

▶ **Figure 21–12**
Creating the color wheel with clay.

ACTivity

Use a plain sugar cookie to represent the color wheel. Use a dollop of vanilla frosting on a dish, along with red, blue, and yellow food coloring. Mix a small amount of frosting with each primary color. Place it on the (cookie) color wheel. Then mix the two primary colors together to make the secondary color. Continue until the color wheel is completed.

Complementary Colors

Complementary colors are primary and secondary colors positioned directly opposite each other on the color wheel. Complementary colors include blue and orange, red and green, and yellow and violet.

Complementary colors neutralize each other (**Figure 21–13**). When formulating haircolor, you will find that it is often your goal to emphasize or distract from skin tones or eye color. You may also want to neutralize or refine unwanted tones in the hair. Understanding complementary colors will help you choose the correct tone to accomplish these goals.

Here is an easy reference guide for color correction:

- When hair is green…use red to balance.
- When hair is red…use green to balance.
- When hair is blue…use orange to balance.
- When hair is orange…use blue to balance.
- When hair is yellow…use violet to balance.
- When hair is violet…use yellow to balance.

Tone or Hue of Color

The **tone**, also known as **hue**, is the balance of color. The tone or hue answers the question of which color to use based on the client's desired results. These tones can be described as warm, cool, or neutral.

Warm tones can look lighter than their actual level. These tones are golden, orange, red, and yellow. Some haircolors use words such as auburn, amber, copper, strawberry, and bronze, which may be a better way to discuss and describe haircolor with the client. Cool tones can look deeper than their actual level. These tones are blue, green, and violet. Some describe cool tones as smoky or ash to the client. Natural tones are warm tones and are described as sandy or tan.

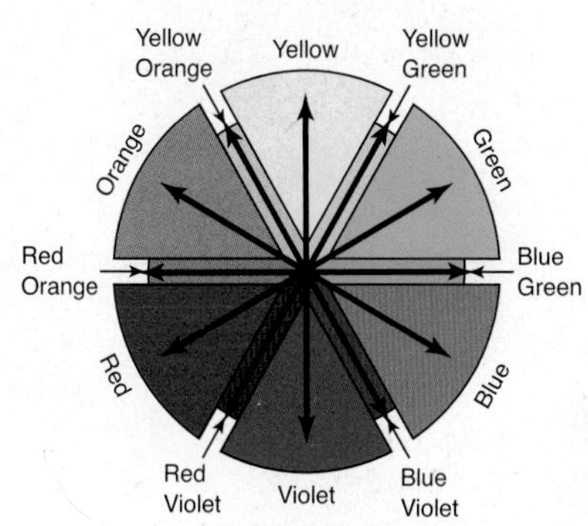

▲ **Figure 21–13 Complementary colors neutralize each other.**

Intensity refers to the strength of a color. It can be described as soft, medium, or strong. Color intensifiers are tones that can be added to a haircolor formula to intensify the result. ☑ **LO6**

Base color is the predominant tone of a color. Each color is identified by a number and a letter. The number indicates the level and the letter indicates the tone. For example: 6G is Level 6-Dark Blond with a G-Gold Base.

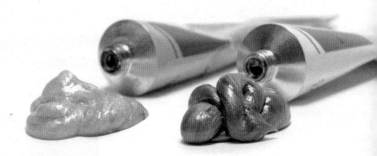

© Milady, a part of Cengage Learning.

When you begin selecting a formula, you must have a good idea of what tones the client likes and dislikes.

Select warm base colors to create brighter colors such as red and gold tones. Select cooler base colors to keep the color result more ash, revealing less gold in the hair. Add a neutral base color to formulate haircolor that will soften and balance colors. Neutral base colors are often used to cover gray hair.

Types of Haircolor

Haircoloring products generally fall into two categories: nonoxidative and oxidative. The classifications of nonoxidative haircolor are temporary and semipermanent (traditional). The classifications of oxidative haircolor are demipermanent (deposit only) and permanent (lift and deposit) (**Table 21–2**). All these products, except temporary color, require a patch test.

Lighteners, metallic haircolors, and natural colors are also discussed in this chapter. Each of these categories has a unique chemical composition that, in turn, affects the final color result and how long it will last.

All permanent haircolor products and lighteners contain both a developer, or oxidizing agent, and an alkalizing ingredient. (See Chapter 12, Basics of Chemistry.) The roles of the alkalizing ingredient—ammonia or an ammonia substitute—are as follows:

REVIEW OF HAIRCOLOR CATEGORIES AND THEIR USES

CLASSIFICATIONS	USES
Temporary color	Creates fun, bold results and easily shampoos from the hair. Neutralizes yellow hair.
Semipermanent color	Introduces a client to haircolor services. Adds subtle color results. Tones prelightened hair.
Demipermanent color	Blends gray hair. Enhances natural color. Tones prelightened hair. Refreshes faded color. Filler in color correction.
Permanent haircolor	Changes existing haircolor. Covers gray. Creates bright or natural-looking haircolor changes.

© Milady, a part of Cengage Learning.

Table 21–2 Review of Haircolor Categories and Their Uses.

© MartiniDry, 2010; used under license from Shutterstock.com.

- Raise the cuticle of the hair so that the haircolor can penetrate into the cortex.
- Increase the penetration of dye within the hair.
- Trigger the lightening action of peroxide.

When the haircolor containing the alkalizing ingredient is combined with the developer (usually hydrogen peroxide), the peroxide becomes alkaline and decomposes, or breaks up. Lightening occurs when the alkaline peroxide breaks up or decolorizes the melanin.

Temporary Haircolor

For those who wish to neutralize yellow hair or unwanted tones, **temporary haircolor**, a nonpermanent color whose large pigment molecules prevent penetration of the cuticle layer, allowing only a coating action that may be removed by shampooing, is a good choice (**Figure 21–14**). Temporary haircolors are nonoxidation colors that make only a physical change, not a chemical change, in the hair shaft, and no patch test is required.

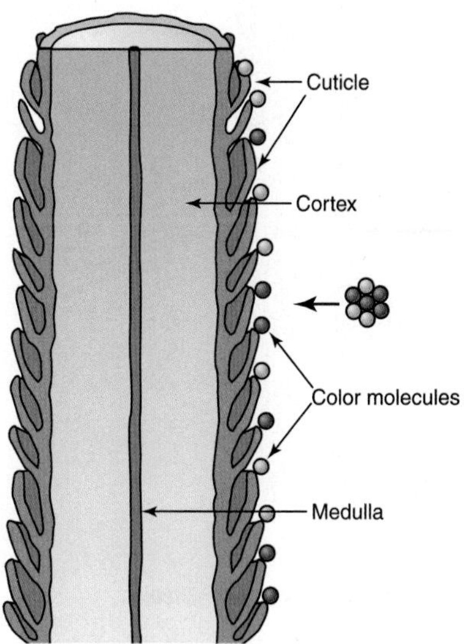

▲ Figure 21–14
Action of temporary haircolor.

Temporary haircolors are available in the following variety of colors and products:

- Color rinses applied weekly to shampooed hair to add color; the hair is styled dry.
- Colored mousses and gels used for slight color and for dramatic effects.
- Hair mascara used for dramatic effects.
- Spray-on haircolor that is easy to apply; used for special effects.
- Color-enhancing shampoos used to brighten, impart slight color, and eliminate unwanted tones.

Semipermanent Haircolor

Traditional **semipermanent haircolor** is a no-lift deposit-only nonoxidation haircolor that is not mixed with peroxide and is formulated to last through several shampoos, depending on the hair's porosity. The pigment molecules are small enough to partially penetrate the hair shaft and stain the cuticle layer, but they are small enough to diffuse out of the hair during shampooing, thus fading with each shampoo. Traditional semipermanent haircolor only lasts four to six weeks, depending on how frequently the hair is shampooed. Semipermanent haircolor is a nonoxidation haircolor. It is not mixed with peroxide, and it only deposits color. It does not lighten the hair, so it does not require maintenance of new growth. Although it is considered gentler than permanent haircolor, it contains some of the same dyes and requires a patch test twenty-four to forty-eight hours before application (**Figure 21–15**). Traditional semipermanent colors are used right out of the bottle.

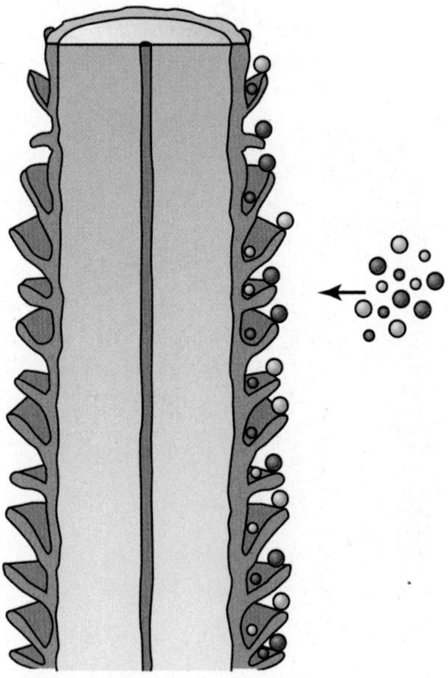

▲ Figure 21–15
Action of semipermanent haircolor.

Demipermanent haircolor, also known as **no-lift deposit-only color**, is formulated to deposit but not lighten color. These products

© Milady, a part of Cengage Learning.

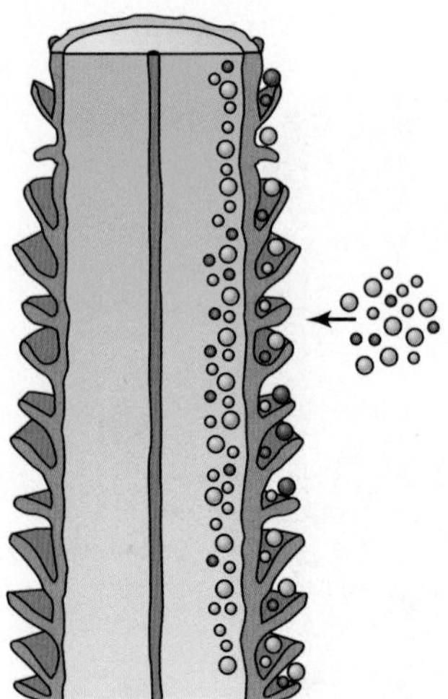

▲ **Figure 21–16**
Action of demipermanent haircolor.

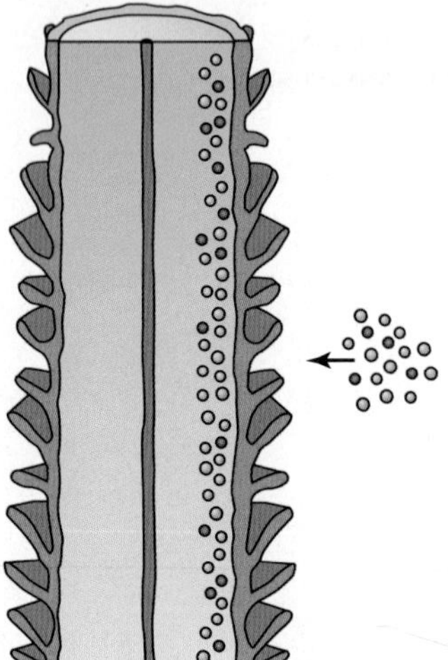

▲ **Figure 21–17**
Action of permanent haircolor.

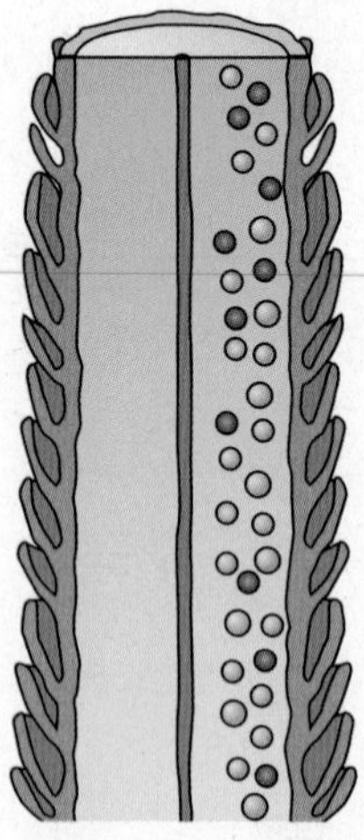

▲ **Figure 21–18**
Permanent haircolor molecules inside the cortex.

are able to deposit without lifting because they are usually less alkaline than permanent colors and are mixed with a low-volume developer. Decolorization requires a high pH and a high concentration of peroxide.

Many demipermanent colors use alkalizing agents other than ammonia, and oxidizing agents other than hydrogen peroxide. It is important to note that these products are not necessarily any less damaging because of the type of alkalizing agent or oxidizer that is used. If they are milder, it is because the concentration of these active ingredients is lower. A **haircolor glaze** is a common way to describe a haircolor service that adds shine and color to the hair. The word *glaze* is a cosmetic word used to describe the services listed below that can be achieved by using a deposit-only or no-lift color.

Demipermanent haircolors are ideal for the following objectives:

- Introducing a client to a color service (because these products create a change in tone without lightening the natural hair color)
- Blending or covering gray
- Refreshing faded permanent color on the midshaft and ends
- Making color corrections and restoring natural color

By their very nature, demipermanent haircolors deepen or create a change in tone on the natural hair color (**Figure 21–16**). In recent years, demipermanent haircolors have been used exclusively on the middle of the hair shaft to the ends after permanent color has been applied to the new growth or scalp area. This method of application refreshes the previously colored hair.

Demipermanent haircolor is available as a gel, cream, or liquid. It requires a patch test twenty-four to forty-eight hours before application.

Permanent Haircolor

Permanent haircolors lighten and deposit color at the same time and in a single process because they are more alkaline than demipermanent colors and are usually mixed with a higher-volume developer.

Permanent haircolor is used to match, lighten, and cover gray hair. Permanent haircolor products require a patch test twenty-four to forty-eight hours before application.

Permanent haircolors contain uncolored dye precursors, which are very small and can easily penetrate into the hair shaft. These dye precursors, called **aniline derivatives**, contain small, uncolored dyes that combine with hydrogen peroxide to form larger, permanent dye molecules within the cortex. These molecules are trapped within the cortex of the hair and cannot be easily shampooed out (**Figures 21–17** and **21–18**). Permanent haircolors can also lighten (make a permanent change in) the natural hair color, which is why these products are considered permanent.

A technique called a **soap cap** is a combination of equal parts of a prepared permanent color mixture and shampoo used during the last

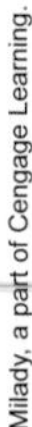
© Milady, a part of Cengage Learning.

five minutes of a haircolor service and worked through the hair to refresh the ends.

Permanent haircoloring products are regarded as the best products for covering gray hair. They remove natural pigment from the hair through lightening, while at the same time adding artificial color to the hair. The action of removing and adding color at the same time, which blends gray and non-gray hair uniformly, results in a natural-looking color.

Natural and Metallic Haircolors

Haircolors that are not generally used in the salon, but which you should still be familiar with, are natural or vegetable haircolors and metallic haircolors. Metallic haircolors is also referred to as gradual colors. Repeated use of these types of color can create a buildup on the hair causing a grayish or green cast.

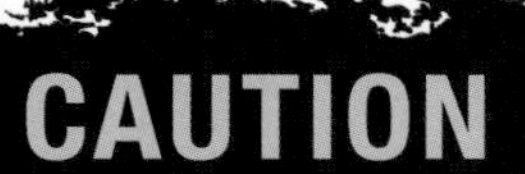

CAUTION

Do not use oxidizing haircolor or haircolor with peroxide on hair that has been treated with metallic hair dye. If you do, the hair will swell and smoke, appearing to be boiling from the inside out.

Natural Haircolors

Natural haircolors, also known as **vegetable haircolors**, such as henna, are colors obtained from the leaves or bark of plants. They do not lighten natural hair color. The color result tends to be weak, and the process tends to be lengthy and messy. Also, shade ranges are limited. For instance, henna is usually available only in clear, black, chestnut, and auburn tones. Finally, when a client who has used natural haircolor comes to the salon for chemical haircoloring services, she may be distressed to find out that many of these chemical products cannot be applied over natural haircolors.

Metallic Haircolor

Metallic haircolors, also known as **gradual haircolors**, are haircolors containing metal salts that change hair color gradually by progressive buildup and exposure to air, creating a dull, metallic appearance. These products require daily application and historically have been marketed to men. The main problems are unnatural-looking colors and a limited range of available colors. ☑ **LO7**

Hydrogen Peroxide Developers

A **hydrogen peroxide developer** is an oxidizing agent that, when mixed with an oxidation haircolor, supplies the necessary oxygen gas to develop the color molecules and create a change in natural hair color. **Developers**, also known as **oxidizing agents** or **catalysts**, have a pH between 2.5 and 4.5. Although there are a number of developers on the market, hydrogen peroxide (H_2O_2) is the one most commonly used in haircolor. Keep in mind, there are different forms of peroxide. There are clear liquids that make it easy to apply the product from an applicator bottle. There are cream forms that are used to make a thicker creamy consistency, sometimes for bowl and brush application. Some manufacturers provide dedicated developers that are used with their own specific haircolor products.

Volume measures the concentration and strength of hydrogen peroxide. The lower the volume, the less lift achieved; the higher the volume, the

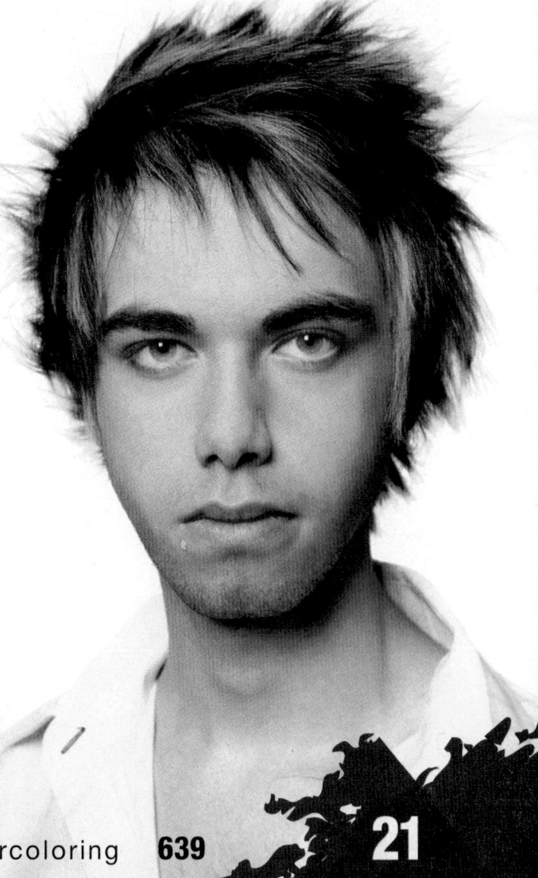

© Jamie Evans, 2010; used under license from iStockphoto.com.

HYDROGEN PEROXIDE VOLUME AND USES	
VOLUME	**WHEN TO USE**
10-Volume	Used when less lift is desired, to enhance a client's natural hair color.
20-Volume	Standard volume; used to achieve most results with permanent haircolor and used for complete gray coverage.
30-Volume	Used for additional lift with permanent haircolor.
40-Volume	Used with most high-lift colors; provides maximum lift in a one-step color service.

Table 21–3 Hydrogen Peroxide Volume and Uses.

greater the lifting action (**Table 21–3**). The majority of permanent haircolor products use 10-, 20-, 30-, or 40-volume hydrogen peroxide for proper lift and color development (**Figure 21–19**). Store peroxide in a cool, dark, dry place.

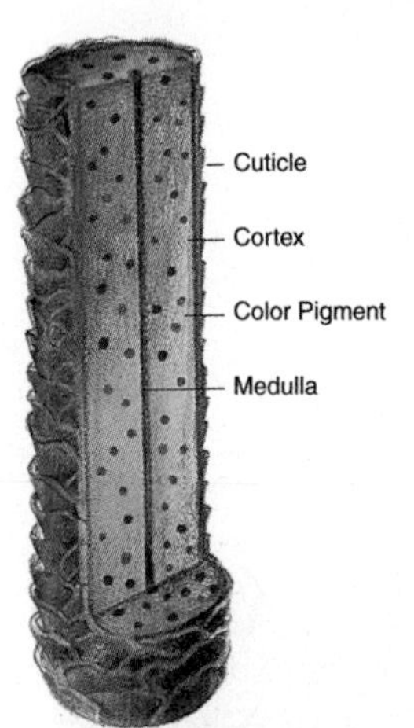

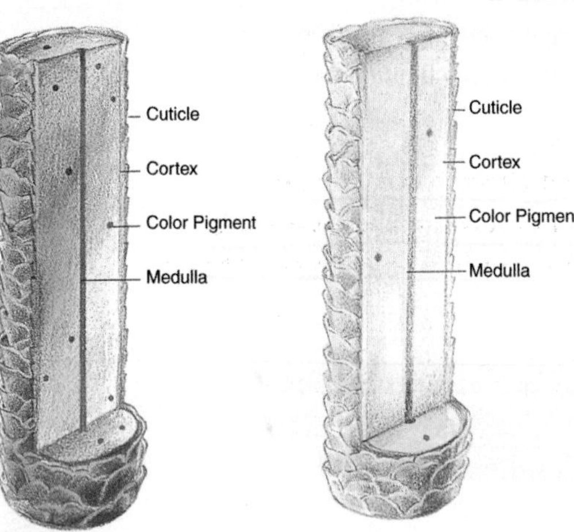

▲ **Figure 21–19 Haircolor lighteners diffuse pigment.**

© Milady, a part of Cengage Learning.

Volume

Use 10-volume peroxide when less lightening is desired. Use 20-volume peroxide with permanent haircolor, as well as for complete gray coverage. For additional lift, use 30-volume peroxide, and to provide maximum lift in a one-step color service, use 40-volume peroxide. ☑ **LO8**

Lighteners

Lighteners are chemical compounds that lighten hair by dispersing, dissolving, and decolorizing the natural hair pigment. As soon as hydrogen peroxide is mixed into the lightener formula, it begins to release oxygen. This is known as oxidation, a process by which oxygen is released, and it occurs within the cortex of the hair shaft. To achieve a very light, pale blond, it is recommended that you use a **double-process application**, also known as **two-step coloring**, which is a coloring technique requiring two separate procedures in which the hair is prelightened before the depositing color is applied. This service includes using a lightener. These products are designed to process up to ninety minutes on the scalp to achieve desired lift. Once the hair is properly decolorized, the second step is to add soft tone back to the hair, called the toning process. There are products called toners designed in a very light shade palette to add tone to the decolorized hair. Demipermanent colors in a light level, such as a Level 8 (Light Blond) to Level 10 (Lightest Blond), are also used to tone hair.

Hair lighteners are used to create a light blond shade that is not achievable with permanent haircolor alone, as well as to accomplish the following objectives:

- Lighten the hair prior to application of a final color
- Lighten hair to a particular shade
- Brighten and lighten an existing shade
- Lighten only certain parts of the hair
- Lighten dark natural or color-treated levels ☑ LO9

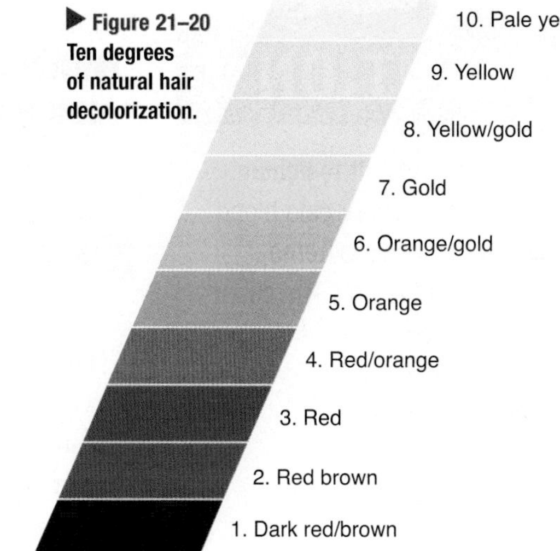

▶ **Figure 21–20** **Ten degrees of natural hair decolorization.**

© Milady, a part of Cengage Learning.

The Decolorizing Process

The hair goes through different stages of color as it lightens. The amount of change depends on the amount of pigment in the hair, the strength of the lightening product, and the length of time that the product is processed. During the process of decolorizing, natural hair can go through as many as 10 stages (**Figure 21–20**).

Decolorizing the hair's natural melanin pigment allows the colorist to create the exact degree of contributing pigment needed for the final result. Contributing pigment is the varying degree of warmth exposed during the lightening process. First, the hair is decolorized to the appropriate level. Then the new color is applied to deposit the desired color. The natural pigment that remains in the hair contributes to the artificial color that is added. Lightening the hair to the correct stage is essential to a beautiful, controlled, final haircoloring result (**Figure 21–21**).

Toners are traditional semipermanent, demipermanent, and permanent haircolor products that are used primarily on prelightened hair to achieve pale and delicate colors. Toners can also be used after dimensional haircolor services. After a highlight service is completed using a lightener, you can tone the hair to create a softer shade of blond. Once the lightener is rinsed, simply towel dry and apply the desired shade of toner over the prelightened hair. This will take up to five minutes for the result.

Not all hair will go through all 10 degrees of decolorization. Each natural hair color starts the decolorization process at a different stage. Remember, the goal is to create the correct degree of contributing pigment as the foundation for the final haircolor.

Hair cannot be safely lifted past the pale yellow stage with lightener. The extreme diffusion of color necessary to give hair a white appearance causes excessive damage to the hair. The result is that when wet, the hair feels mushy and will stretch without returning to its original length. When dry, the hair is harsh and brittle. Such hair often suffers breakage and will not accept a toner properly. However, this does not mean that

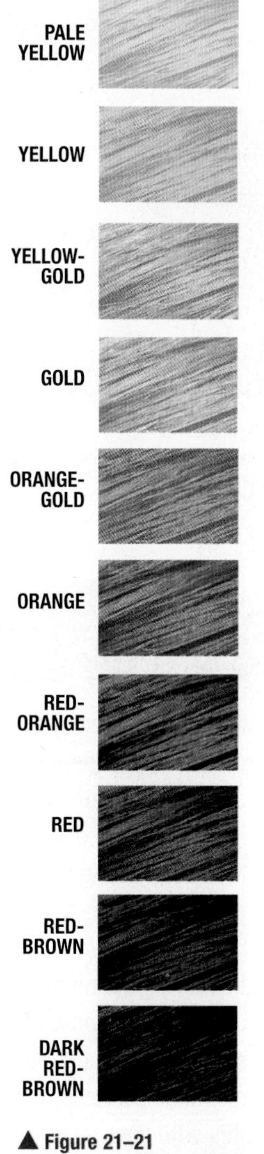

▲ **Figure 21–21** **Level/Contributing pigment.**

Courtesy of P&G Salon Professional. Clariol Professional.

CAUTION

It is often difficult to lighten dark hair to a very pale blond without causing extreme damage to the hair. The client should be alerted to this danger before you proceed with the service.

© Milady, a part of Cengage Learning. Photography by Paul Castle, Castle Photography.

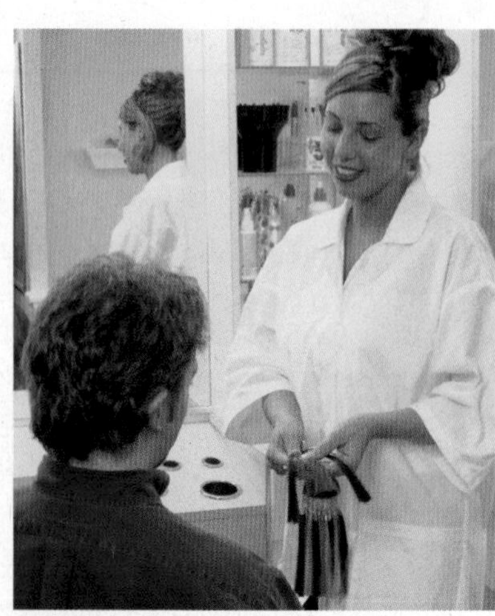

▲ **Figure 21–22**
A client consultation should precede every haircolor service.

CAUTION

Medications can affect hair color. In the consultation, determine whether the client is taking any medications. Medical treatments for conditions such as diabetes, high blood pressure, and thyroid problems may all affect the outcome of color services and most other chemical services. Discuss this with your instructor for more information.

only those born with blond hair can be white-blonds. The baby-blond look can be achieved by lightening to pale yellow and neutralizing the unwanted undertone (contributing pigment) with a toner.

Consultation

A haircolor consultation is the most critical part of the color service (**Figure 21–22**). The consultation is the first important step in establishing a relationship with your client. During the consultation, your client will communicate what he or she is looking for in a haircolor service. You will listen carefully, taking in all the information so that you can make an appropriate haircolor recommendation. Allowing sufficient time for the consultation is the single most reliable way to help ensure a client's satisfaction.

See Chapter 4, Communicating for Success, to review and begin the consultation process. In addition, incorporate the following steps when conducting a haircolor consultation:

1. Book fifteen minutes extra for the consultation. Introduce yourself to the client and welcome him or her to the salon. Offer a beverage. During this time with a new client, make sure there are no interruptions.
2. Have the client fill out a service record card. This allows you to compile a hair history and to note the type of color service the client is looking for. Pay attention to the client's skin and eye color, the condition and length of the client's hair, and the amount of gray in the client's hair.
3. Begin the consultation in an area with proper lighting so that you can accurately determine the client's current hair color. If possible, the walls should be white or neutral.
4. Look at the client directly. Do not look at her through the mirror. Ask what she is thinking about doing with her hair color. Ask leading questions. Let her talk. Keep her on track by discussing the recent history of her hair (over the past six months). Your questions might include the following:
   - Are you looking for a temporary or permanent change?
   - Do you want color all over or just a few highlights?
   - Do you see yourself with a more conservative or dramatic type of color?
   - Have you seen so-and-so's (e.g., a TV celebrity) hair? That color would look great on you.
5. Recommend at least two different haircolor options. Show pictures of different ranges of colors, from brunette to blond, red, and highlighted colors. Review the procedure and application technique, cost of the service, and follow-up maintenance. Sometimes several

steps may be necessary to obtain a haircolor result. A client may love a certain haircolor, but may not be able to afford the service. Have a more economical backup solution ready.

6. Be honest and do not promise more than you can deliver. If you are faced with a corrective situation, let the client know what you can accomplish today and how many more visits it will take to achieve the final results that she wants.
7. Gain approval from the client.
8. Start the haircolor service.
9. Follow through during the service by educating and informing the client about home care, products, and rebooking. Let the client know what type of shampoo and conditioner is needed to maintain the color. Let her know how many weeks it will be before she needs to come back for another service.
10. Fill out the client's Haircolor Service Record Card (**Figure 21–23**).

Release Statement

A release statement is used by schools and many salons when providing chemical services. Its purpose is to explain to clients that there is a risk involved in any chemical service and that if the client's hair is in questionable condition, it may not withstand the requested chemical treatment. It also asks that clients provide more information about any prior chemical services that may affect the current color selection and its end result.

To some degree, the release statement is designed to protect the school or salon from responsibility for accidents or damages. A release statement is required for most malpractice insurance. Take note, however, that a release statement is not a legally binding contract and will not clear the cosmetologist of responsibility for what may happen to a client's hair (see **Figure 21–24**, on page 645). If you are unsure about causing excessive damage to the hair, it is wise to decline to perform the service.

FOCUS ON

COMMUNICATION

The language you use when discussing haircolor can have a huge impact on how a client perceives haircolor services. Using positive descriptive language to discuss products and services with your clients is an important part of the communication process, and it helps you sell your services. Here are some guidelines:

- Use descriptive language when discussing haircolor (e.g., *soft, buttery blond*; *rich chocolate brown*; *spicy, coppery red*).
- Use positive mood words to convey the benefits of haircoloring to your client (e.g., *healthy-looking, richer, natural-looking*, and *subtle*).
- Avoid words that can be interpreted negatively such as *bleached, frosted*, and *roots*.

Haircolor Formulation

Haircolor formulation is another important aspect of creating a successful haircolor. There are four basic questions that must always be asked when formulating a haircolor. Refer to the additional Formulation Checklist to cover more details (see **Figure 21–25**, on page 646).

1. What is the natural level and does it include gray hair?
2. What is the client's desired level and tone?
3. Are contributing pigments (undertones) to be revealed?
4. What colors should be mixed to get the desired result? ☑ **LO10**

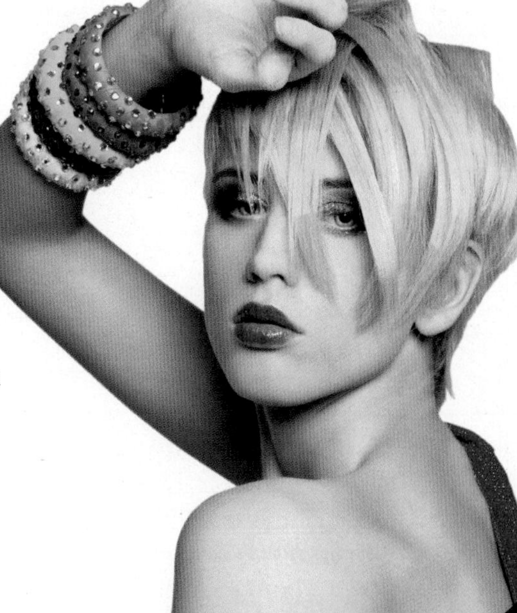

© Ivan Mladenov, 2010; used under license from Shutterstock.com.

HAIRCOLOR SERVICE RECORD CARD

Name ______________________ Tel. ______________________

Address ______________________ City ______________________

Patch Test: ☐ Negative ☐ Positive Date ______________________

Eye Color ______________________ Skin Tone ______________________

DESCRIPTION OF HAIR

Form	**Length**	**Texture**	**Density**	**Porosity**	
☐ straight	☐ short	☐ coarse	☐ low	☐ low	☐ resistant
☐ wavy	☐ medium	☐ medium	☐ medium	☐ average	☐ very resistant
☐ curly	☐ long	☐ fine	☐ high	☐ high	☐ perm. waved

Natural hair color ______________________

Level (1-10) Tone (Warm, Cool, etc.) Intensity (Mild, Medium, Strong)

Scalp Condition

☐ normal ☐ dry ☐ oily ☐ sensitive

Condition

☐ normal ☐ dry ☐ oily ☐ faded ☐ streaked (uneven)

% unpigmented ______________ Distribution of unpigmented ______________

Previously lightened with ______________ for ______________ (time)

Previously tinted with ______________ for ______________ (time)

☐ original hair sample enclosed ☐ original hair sample not enclosed

Desired hair color ______________________

Level (1-10) Tone (Warm, Cool, etc.) Intensity (Mild, Medium, Strong)

CORRECTIVE TREATMENTS

Color filler used ______________ Conditioning treatments with ______________

HAIR TINTING PROCESS

whole head ______________ retouch inches (cm) ______________ shade desired ______________

formula: (color/lightener) ______________ application technique ______________

Results: ☐ good ☐ poor ☐ too light ☐ too dark ☐ streaked

Comments: ______________________

____

____

____

____

Date	**Operator**	**Price**	**Date**	**Operator**	**Price**

© Milady, a part of Cengage Learning.

▲ **Figure 21–23**
Haircolor service record card.

RELEASE FORM

I, the undersigned, ______________________________
(name)

residing at ______________________________
(street, address)

____
(city, state and zip)

about to receive services in the Clinical Department of

____

and having been advised that the services shall be performed by either students, graduate students, and/or instructors of the school, in consideration of the nominal charge for such services, hereby release the school, its students, graduate students, instructors, agents, representatives, and/or employees, from any and all claims arising out of and in any way connected with the performance of these services.

The Proprietor Is Not Responsible for Personal Property

Signed ______________________________

Date ______________________________

Witnessed ______________________________

THIS RELEASE FORM MUST BE SIGNED BY THE PARENT OR GUARDIAN IF THE CLIENT BEING SERVED IS UNDER 18 YEARS OF AGE.

© Milady, a part of Cengage Learning.

◀ **Figure 21–24**
Release form.

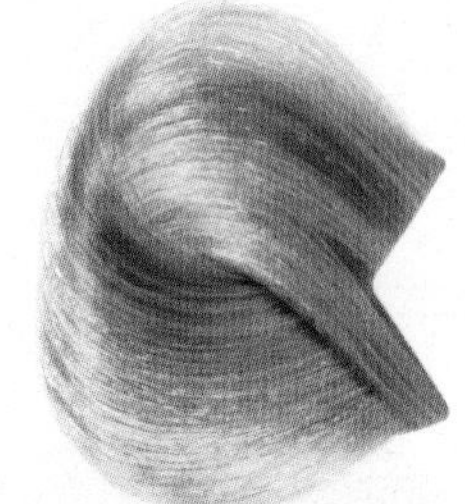
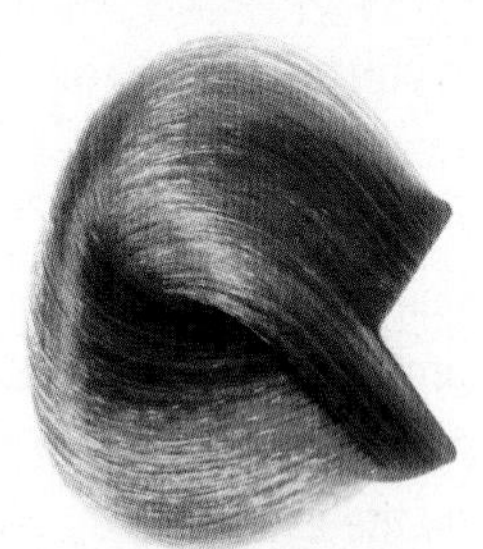
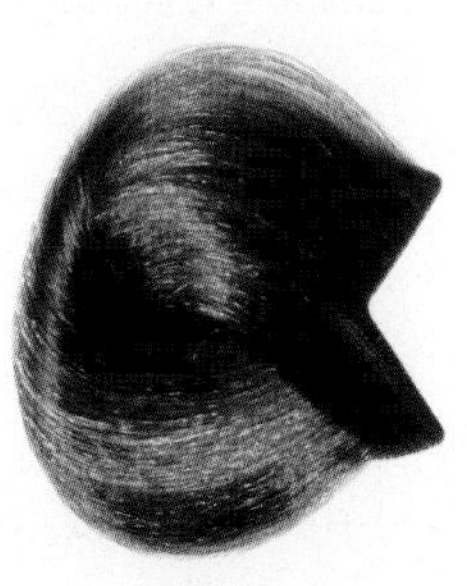
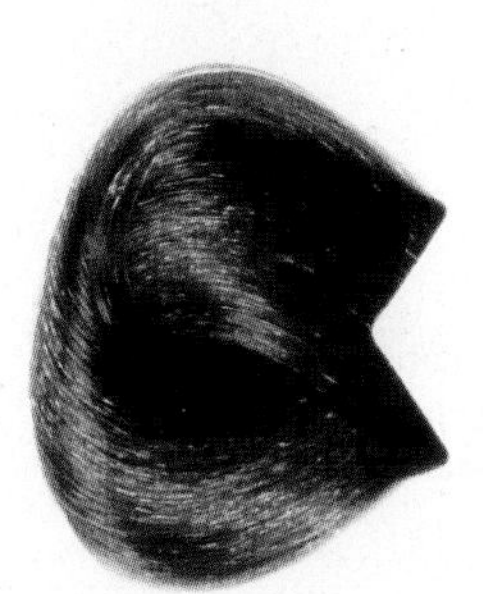
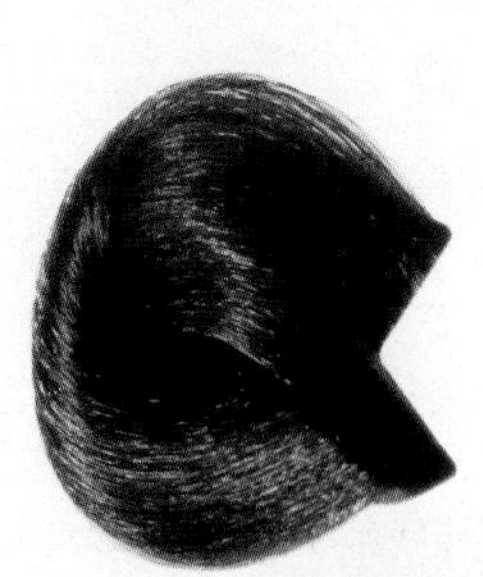

© Ivanova Inga, 2010; used under license from Shutterstock.com.

The combination of the shade selected and the volume of hydrogen peroxide determines the deposit and lifting ability of a haircolor. Always remember to formulate with both lift and deposit in mind in order to achieve the proper balance for the desired end result. A higher-lifting formula, however, may not have enough deposit to cancel the warmth of a client's natural contributing pigment. The volume of hydrogen peroxide mixed with the haircolor product will also influence the lift and deposit.

Mixing Permanent Colors

Your method of mixing permanent colors is determined by the type of application you are using. Permanent color is applied by either the applicator

▶ **Figure 21–25**
Formulation checklist.

FORMULATION CHECKLIST

Be sure to do a complete analysis of the hair to include:

Level and Tone - scalp area, mid-shaft, ends ____________________

Percentage of gray ____________________

Texture and Porosity ____________________

Basic overall condition of the hair ____________________

Color Selection ____________________

What type of product will be used to create end result ____________________

Do you need to lighten or deposit color ____________________

How many levels of lift are required ____________________

What volume of developer will be used ____________________

What undertones are present ____________________

What tone do you want to see ____________________

What tones do you not want to see ____________________

What are the mixing proportions ____________________

Decide on the application method ____________________

How long will the color process ____________________

© Milady, a part of Cengage Learning.

CAUTION

A patch test must be given twenty-four to forty-eight hours before coloring the hair with an aniline derivative product. Aniline derivative haircolors must never be used on the eyelashes or eyebrows. To do so may cause blindness.

bottle or bowl-and-brush method (always follow the manufacturer's directions) (**Figure 21–26**).

- **Applicator bottle.** Be sure that the applicator bottle is large enough to hold both the color and developer, with enough air space to shake the bottle until the mixture is thoroughly mixed. For a 1:1 ratio, pour 1 ounce of the color into the bottle, add 1 ounce of developer, put the top on the bottle, and shake gently. For a 1:2 ratio, pour 1 ounce of the color into the bottle, add 2 ounces of developer, and mix. The latter ratio is for most permanent high-lift blond colors (**Figure 21–27**).

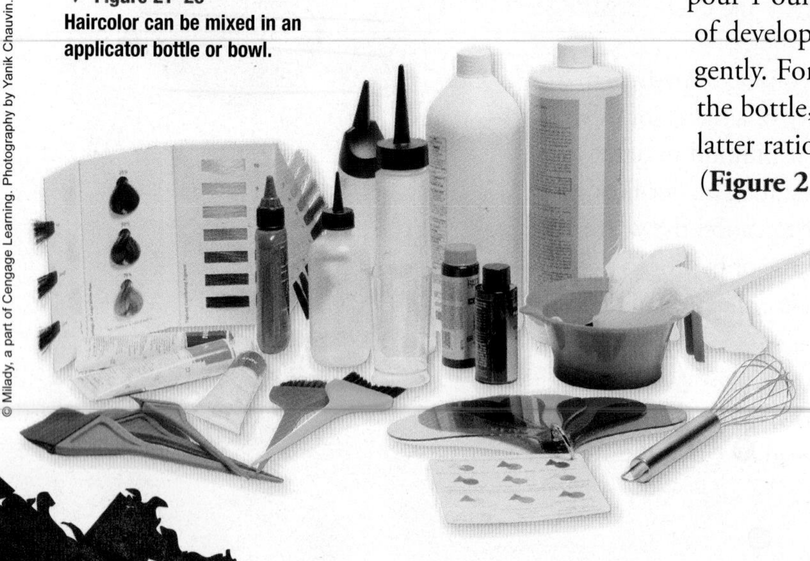

▼ **Figure 21–26**
Haircolor can be mixed in an applicator bottle or bowl.

© Milady, a part of Cengage Learning. Photography by Yanik Chauvin.

- **Brush and bowl.** Use a nonmetallic mixing bowl. Measure and add the developer into the bowl. Add the color or colors you have selected in the appropriate proportions. Using an applicator brush, stir the mixture until it is blended (**Figure 21–28**).

Patch Test

When working with haircolor, you must determine whether your clients have any allergies or sensitivities to the mixture. To identify an allergy in a client, the U.S. Food, Drug, and Cosmetic Act requires that a patch test be given twenty-four to forty-eight hours prior to each application of an aniline haircolor. A **patch test**, also known as **predisposition test**, is a test for identifying a possible allergy in a client. The color used for the patch test must be the same as the color that will be used for the haircolor service (i.e., if a person is having her or his hair colored with 5BR by a particular manufacturer, use the 5BR shade in the patch test). Procedure 21–1 for patch tests should be closely followed.

A negative skin test will show no sign of inflammation and indicates that the color may be safely applied. A positive result will show redness and a slight rash or welt. A client with these symptoms is allergic, and under no circumstances should she receive a haircolor service with the haircolor tested. ☑ **LO11**

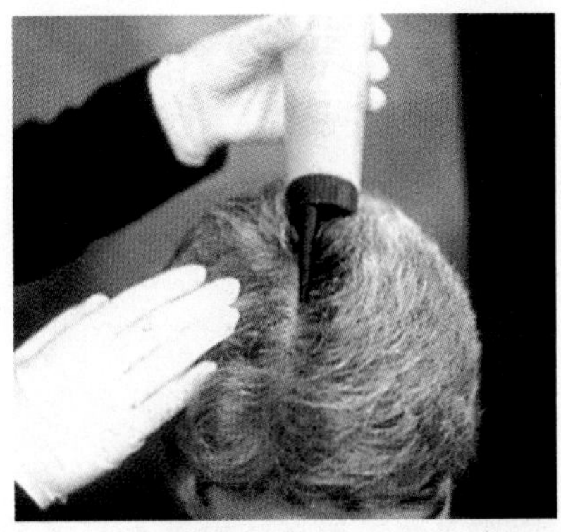
▲ **Figure 21–27**
Applicator bottle.

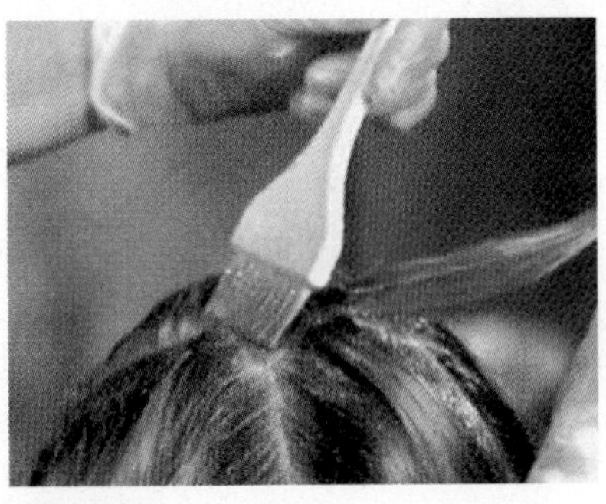
▲ **Figure 21–28**
Application brush and bowl.

PROCEDURE 21-1 Performing a Patch Test SEE PAGE 664

Haircolor Applications

To ensure successful results when performing haircoloring services, the colorist must follow a prescribed procedure. A clearly defined system makes for the greatest efficiency, and the safest and most satisfactory results. Without such a plan, the work will take longer, results will be uneven, and mistakes may be made.

Preliminary Strand Test

Once you have created a color formula for your client, try it out first on a small strand of hair. This preliminary **strand test** determines how the hair will react to the color formula and how long the formula should be left on the hair. The strand test is performed after the client is prepared for the coloring service. ☑ **LO12**

PROCEDURE 21-2 Preliminary Strand Test SEE PAGE 665

Temporary Colors

There are many methods of applying a temporary color, depending on the product used. Your instructor will help you interpret each manufacturer's directions. One method of applying temporary haircolor is outlined in Procedure 21–3. You may apply colored gels, mousses, foams, or sprays at your workstation after your client has been shampooed. Always use and apply these color products according to the manufacturer's directions.

CAUTION

Colorist dermatitis involves the same types of negative reactions to products as those a client may experience. Since a colorist's hands are in contact with chemical solutions repeatedly during an average day, it is important to take proper precautions. Protect yourself from adverse reactions by wearing gloves until the haircolor product is completely removed from the client's hair.

© Milady, a part of Cengage Learning. Photography by Paul Castle, Castle Photography.

PROCEDURE 21-3 Temporary Haircolor Application SEE PAGE 667

Semipermanent Haircolors

Because semipermanent colors do not contain the oxidizers necessary to lift, they only deposit color and do not lighten color. When selecting a semipermanent color, remember that color applied on top of existing color always creates a deeper color and alters the tone.

The porosity of the hair will determine how well these products saturate the hair. Because they are deposit-only, traditional semipermanent colors can build up on the hair ends with repeated applications. A strand test will help determine the formula and processing time before the service.

PROCEDURE 21-4 Semipermanent Haircolor Application SEE PAGE 669

Demipermanent Haircolor

Demipermanent haircolor is a great way to introduce clients to a color service and to enhance their natural hair color in one easy step.

The application procedure for demipermanent haircolor is similar to that of a traditional semipermanent color, since neither process alters the hair's natural melanin or produces lift. Follow the manufacturer's guidelines for application and processing time for the product you have selected.

Gray hair presents special challenges when formulating demipermanent haircolor. Because there is no lift, the resulting depth of color when covering gray hair may appear too harsh unless you allow for some brightness and warmth in your formulation. Selecting a shade that is one level lighter than the natural color is recommended, so that the gray hair looks somewhat highlighted against the natural color. This will deliver a more natural-looking result.

Hair that has previously received a color service will have a greater degree of porosity, which must also be taken into consideration when formulating and applying a demipermanent haircolor.

Single-Process Permanent Color

Single-process haircoloring lightens and deposits color in a single application. Examples of single-process coloring are virgin color applications and color retouch applications. A **virgin application** refers to the first time the hair is colored. Prelightening or presoftening is not required with these applications. ✔ **LO13**

PROCEDURE 21-5 Single-Process Color on Virgin Hair SEE PAGE 671

FOCUS ON

TICKET UPGRADING

Getting your clients interested in haircoloring can be done in indirect as well as direct ways, such as the following:

- **Wear color in your hair.** As a professional hairstylist, you should be an example of what those services can do.
- **Display haircolor-related materials at your workstation.** These could be swatches, pictures of great haircoloring you clip out of magazines, and so forth.
- **Suggest haircolor to every client.** Remember that every client is a potential haircolor client.

Single-Process Color Retouch

As the hair grows, you will need to apply haircolor to the new growth to keep it looking attractive and to avoid a two-toned effect, this is called a retouch.

The procedure provided for applying color to new growth and to refresh faded ends also includes the application of a **glaze**, a nonammonia color that adds shine and tone to the hair. For both applications, follow the same preparation steps as for the virgin single-process procedure, including a consultation and patch test.

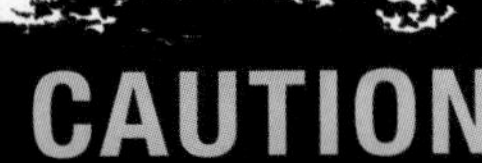

CAUTION

Do not perform any haircoloring service if the client has abrasions or inflammations on the scalp. Do not brush the hair before a haircolor service.

PROCEDURE 21-6 Permanent Single-Process Retouch with a Glaze SEE PAGE 673

Steps for applying color to new growth and faded ends:

1. Apply color to the new growth only, being careful not to overlap on previously colored hair. Overlapping can cause breakage and a **line of demarcation**, which is the visible line separating colored hair from new growth.
2. Process color according to your analysis and strand test results.
3. To refresh faded ends, formulate a demipermanent haircolor for the ends to match the new growth. Work the color through to the ends. Then shampoo and condition. Remember that the same color formula used with different volumes of peroxide will produce different results.

Double-Process Haircolor

First, let us discuss the process of **hair lightening**, also known as **bleaching** or **decolorizing**, which is a chemical process involving the diffusion of the natural hair color pigment or artificial haircolor from the hair.

If the client asks for a dramatically lighter color, the hair has to be prelightened first. Also, to achieve pale or cool colors, it is sometimes more efficient to use a double-process application. By first decolorizing the hair with a lightener and then using a separate product to deposit the desired tone, you will have more control over the coloring process.

Double-process high-lift coloring, also known as *two-step blonding*, is a technique to create light-blond hair in two steps. The hair is prelightened first and then toned. **Prelightening** is the first step of double-process haircoloring, used to lift or lighten the natural pigment before the application of toner.

Because the lightening action and the deposit of color are independent of each other, a wider range of haircolor is possible.

You may find that the contributing pigment of the hair can help you in a double-process color application. By prelightening the hair to the desired color, you can create a perfect foundation for longer-lasting red colors that avoid muddiness and stay true to tone.

The prelightener is applied in the same manner as a regular hair lightening treatment (see the following section). Once the prelightening has reached the desired shade, the hair is lightly shampooed, acidified, and towel dried. After a strand test has been taken, the color is then applied in the usual manner.

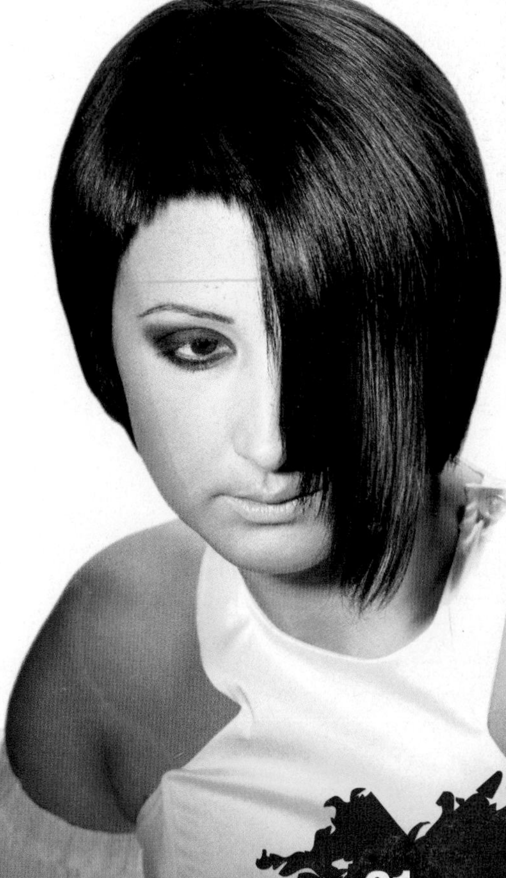

© Ivanchenko, 2010; used under license from iStockphoto.com.

CAUTION

Most powdered lighteners are used exclusively for off-the-scalp applications and special effects, such as foil-wrapped highlighting, highlighting with plastic caps, and hair painting. However, some new powder lighteners can be used directly on the scalp. Refer to manufacturer's directions for best results.

Using an applicator brush, stir the lightener until it is thoroughly mixed. A creamy consistency provides the best control during application. ✓ **LO14**

PROCEDURE 21-7 **Lightening Virgin Hair** **SEE PAGE 675**

Using Lighteners

Colorists can choose from three forms of lighteners: oil, cream, and powder. Oil and cream lighteners are considered **on-the-scalp lighteners**, which are lighteners that can be used directly on the scalp by mixing the lightener with activators. New technology has created powder lighteners that can also be used directly on the scalp. Each type has its unique chemical characteristics and formulation procedures. Refer to the manufacturer's directions for best results.

On-the-Scalp Lighteners

Cream, oil, and some powder lighteners are used on-the-scalp because they are easy to apply. Oil lighteners are the mildest type, appropriate when only one or two levels of lift are desired. Because they are so mild, they are also used professionally to lighten dark facial and body hair.

Cream lighteners are strong enough for high-lift blonding, but gentle enough to be used on the scalp. They have the following features and benefits:

- Conditioning agents give some protection to the hair and scalp.
- Thickeners give more control during application.
- Because cream lighteners do not run or drip, overlapping is prevented during retouching services. Cream lighteners may be mixed with activators in the form of dry crystals.

Activators, also known as **boosters**, **protinators**, or **accelerators**, are powdered persulfate salts added to haircolor to increase its lightening ability. Activators are used in powdered off-the-scalp hair lighteners. They are also added to hydrogen peroxide to increase its lifting power. The more activators you use, the lighter the hair will be. Up to three activators can be used for on-the-scalp applications, and up to four for off-the-scalp applications. Activators increase scalp irritation.

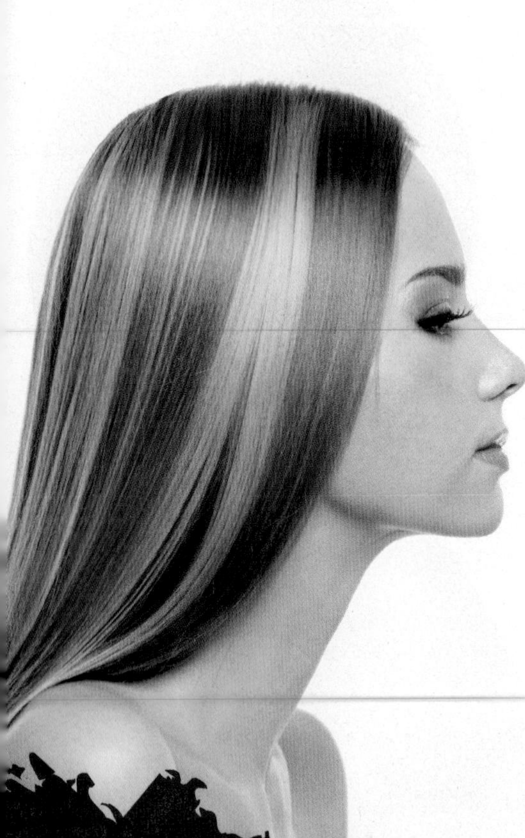

© Valua Vitaly, 2010; used under license from Shutterstock.com.

Powdered Off-the-Scalp Lighteners

Off-the-scalp lighteners, also known as **quick lighteners**, are powdered lighteners that cannot be used directly on the scalp. Powdered lighteners are strong, fast-acting lighteners in powdered form. Some powders are designed for on-scalp, double-process blonding. There are other powders that are specifically designed for off-scalp use.

Powdered off-the-scalp lighteners contain persulfate salts for quicker and stronger lightening. They may dry out more quickly than other types of lighteners, but they do not run or drip. Most powder lighteners expand and spread out as processing continues. **LO15**

© Milady, a part of Cengage Learning.

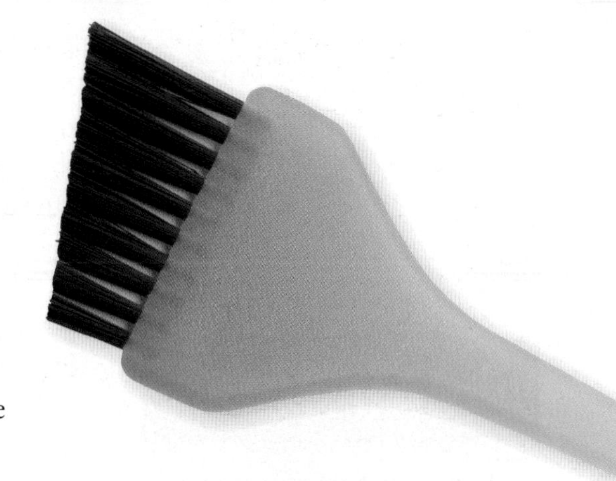

Time Factors

Processing time for lightening is affected by the factors listed below:

- The darker the natural hair color, the more melanin it has. The more melanin it has, the longer it takes to lighten the color.
- The amount of time needed to lighten the natural color is also influenced by the hair's porosity. Porous hair of the same color level will lighten faster than hair that is nonporous, because the lightening agent can enter the cortex more rapidly.
- Tone influences the length of time necessary to lighten the natural hair color. The greater the percentage of red reflected in the natural color, the more difficult it is to achieve the delicate shades of a pale blond. Ash blonds are especially difficult to achieve because the melanin must be diffused sufficiently to alter both the level and tone of the hair.
- The strength of the lightening product affects the speed and amount of lightening. Stronger lighteners produce pale shades in the fastest time.
- Heat leads to faster lightening. But the stages of lightening must be carefully observed to avoid excessive lift. Excess lift could diffuse so much natural pigment that the toner may not produce the desired color. When this occurs, the toner may absorb too much color or *grab*, giving the hair an unwanted ashy, cool tone.

CAUTION

When heat is used with hair lighteners, it softens the hair and makes it more fragile. Excessive heat increases the rate of the reaction and swells the hair. Excessive heat can lift and crack the cuticle and break bonds within the cortex. Therefore, extreme caution must always be exercised when using heat.

Preliminary Strand Test

Perform a preliminary strand test prior to lightening in order to determine the processing time, the condition of the hair after lightening, and the end results. Watch the strand carefully for its reaction to the lightening mixture, especially noting any discoloration or breakage. Reconditioning may be required prior to toning. If the color and condition are good, you can proceed with the lightening service. Carefully record all data on the client's service record card and file it for future use.

If the test shows that the hair is not light enough, increase the strength of the mixture and/or increase the processing time. If the hair strand is too light, decrease the strength of the mixture and/or decrease the processing time.

A patch test must be taken twenty-four to forty-eight hours prior to each application of a toner containing aniline derivatives.

Lightener Retouch

New growth is the part of the hair shaft between the scalp and the hair that has been previously colored. New growth will become obvious as the hair grows. When performing a retouch, always lighten the new growth first. The procedure for a lightener retouch is the same as that for lightening a virgin head of hair, except that the mixture is applied only to the new growth. A cream lightener is generally used for a lightener retouch because it is less irritating to the scalp and its consistency helps prevent overlapping of previously lightened hair. Overlapping can cause severe breakage and lines of demarcation.

Always consult the client's service record card for information about which lightener formulas have been used in the past, timing, and other matters.

CAUTION

In all procedures requiring the use of a towel to check for lightening level, make sure that the towel is damp. Blot—do not rub—the strand. Rubbing could cause a roughening of the cuticle, giving a false reading for the entire process.

Using Toners

Toners are used primarily on prelightened hair to achieve pale, delicate colors. They require a double-process application. The first process is the application of the lightener; the second process is the application of the toner. No-lift demipermanent haircolors are often used as toners.

The contributing pigment is the color that remains in the hair after lightening. It is essential that you achieve the correct foundation in order to create the right color and degree of porosity required for proper toner development.

Toner manufacturers usually provide literature that indicates the contributing pigment necessary to achieve the color you desire. As a general rule, the paler the color you are seeking, the lighter the contributing pigment needs to be. It is important to follow the literature closely and to understand that overlightened hair will grab the color of the toner. Underlightened hair, on the other hand, will appear to have more red, yellow, or orange than the intended color.

It is not advisable to prelighten past the pale-yellow stage. This will create overly porous hair that will not have enough natural pigment left to create the desired effect. Refer to the law of color to select a toner that will neutralize or complement the prelightened hair and produce the desired color. ✓ **LO16**

Toner Application

Administer a patch test for allergies or other sensitivities twenty-four to forty-eight hours before each toner application. Proceed with the application only if the patch test results are negative and the hair is in good condition.

Your speed and accuracy are both important factors in the application and will determine, to a large extent, whether you get good color results. The procedure for applying low- or non-peroxide toners may vary. Check with your instructor for directions.

PROCEDURE 21-8 Toner Application SEE PAGE 677

Special Effects Haircoloring

Special effects haircoloring refers to any technique that involves partial lightening or coloring. Coloring for special effects can be thought of as a pure fashion technique. It is a versatile and exciting haircoloring service.

One way you can create special effects is by strategically placing light and dark colors in the hair. **Highlighting** involves coloring some of the hair strands lighter than the natural color to add a variety of lighter shades and the illusion of depth. Subtle highlights do not contrast strongly with the natural color. Light colors cause the light area to advance toward the eye, to appear larger, and to make details more visible.

Reverse highlighting, also known as **lowlighting**, is the technique of coloring strands of hair darker than the natural color. Contrasting dark areas recede, appear smaller, and make detail less visible.

As you begin to expand your knowledge of haircoloring and lightening and to develop your technical ability, you will become more creative. Your instructor will help you master the basic techniques, but the rest is up to you.

▼ Figure 21–29
Lightening tools.

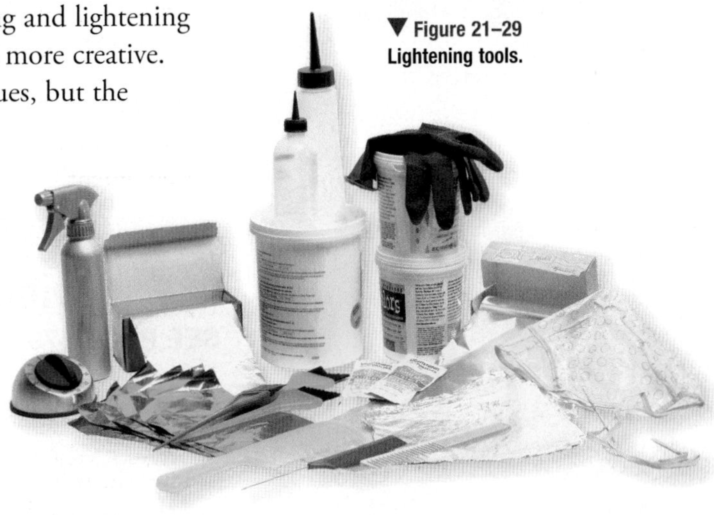

The possibilities are limited only by your imagination and your ability to create a finished style that meets the needs of your clients (**Figure 21–29**).

There are several methods for achieving highlights. The three most frequently used techniques follow:

- Cap technique
- Foil technique
- Baliage or free-form technique

Cap Technique

The **cap technique** involves pulling clean, dry strands of hair through a perforated cap with a thin plastic or metal hook, and then combing them to remove tangles (**Figure 21–30**). The number of strands pulled through determines the amount of hair that will be highlighted or lowlighted. When only a small number of strands are pulled through, the result will be a subtle look. A more noticeable effect is achieved if many strands are pulled through, and the effect is even more dramatic if larger strands of hair are pulled through.

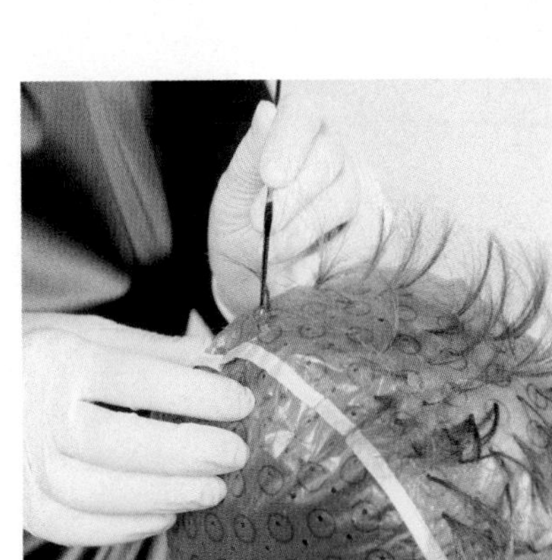

▲ Figure 21–30
Pull strands through holes in cap.

For highlighting, the hair is usually lightened with a powdered off-the-scalp lightener or a high-lift color, beginning in the area that is most

© Milady, a part of Cengage Learning. Photography by Yanik Chauvin.

resistant. The lightener is covered for processing (**Figure 21–31**). Once processed, the lightener is removed by a thorough rinse and a shampoo. After towel blotting and conditioning (if necessary), the lightened hair can be toned, if desired (**Figure 21–32**).

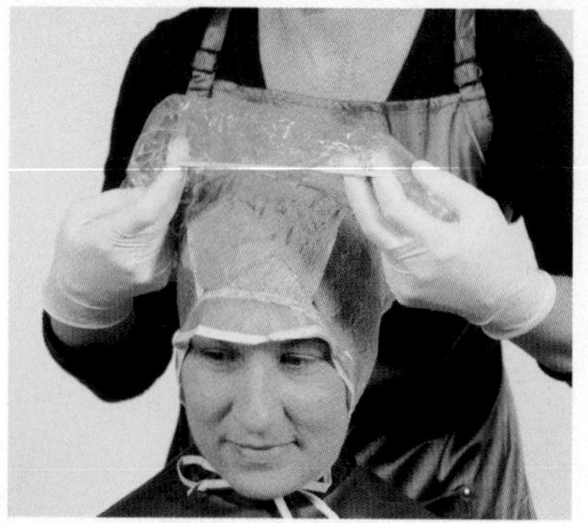

▲ Figure 21–31
Cover loosely with plastic cap.

Foil Technique

The **foil technique** involves coloring selected strands of hair by slicing or weaving out sections, placing them on foil or plastic wrap, applying lightener or permanent haircolor, and then sealing them in the foil or plastic wrap for processing. You can also apply permanent haircolor to the strands to create softer, more natural-looking highlights.

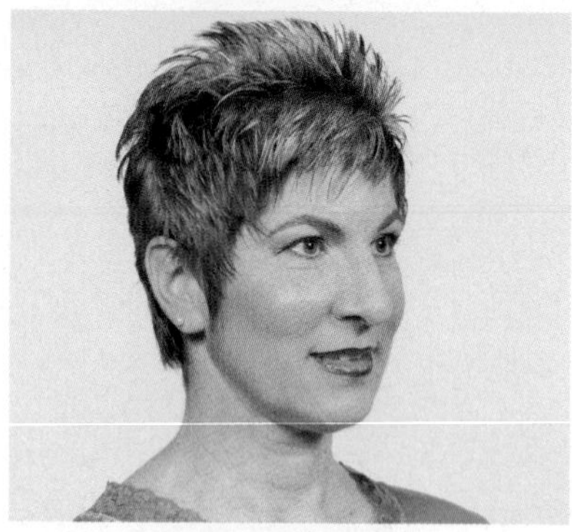

▲ Figure 21–32
Cap technique finished look.

Placing foil in the hair is an art. It takes practice and discipline. To make it easier, start by working to create clean section blocks on the head. Once you have perfected this, you will fully understand the difference between a slice parting and a weave parting. **Slicing** involves taking a narrow, ⅛-inch (0.3 centimeters) section of hair by making a straight part at the scalp, positioning the hair over the foil, and applying lightener or color (**Figure 21–33**). In **weaving**, selected strands are picked up from a narrow section of hair with a zigzag motion of the comb, and lightener or color is applied only to these strands (**Figure 21–34**).

There are many patterns in which foil can be placed in the hair. There are face-frame, half-head, three-quarter head, and full-head foiling patterns that produce different highlights in different portions of the head.

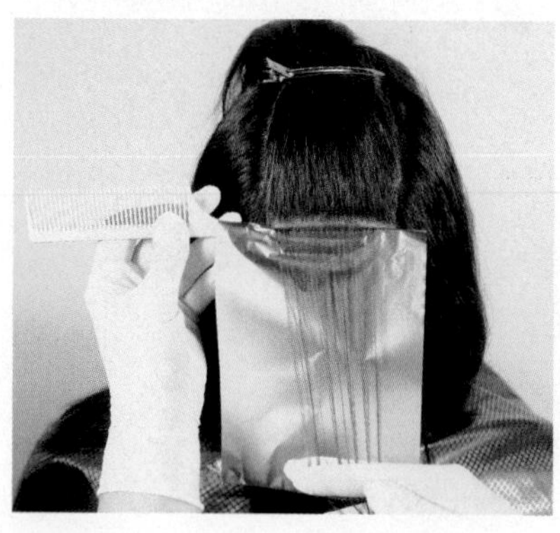

▲ Figure 21–33
Slicing.

PROCEDURE 21-9 Special Effects Haircoloring with Foil (Full Head)

SEE PAGE 679

Baliage Technique

The **baliage** (sometimes spelled balyage), also known as **free-form technique**, involves the painting of a lightener (usually powdered off-the-scalp lightener) directly onto clean, styled hair (**Figure 21–35**). The lightener is applied with an applicator brush or a tail comb from scalp to ends around the head. The effects are extremely subtle and are used to draw attention to the surface of the hair (**Figure 21–36**). ✓ **LO17**

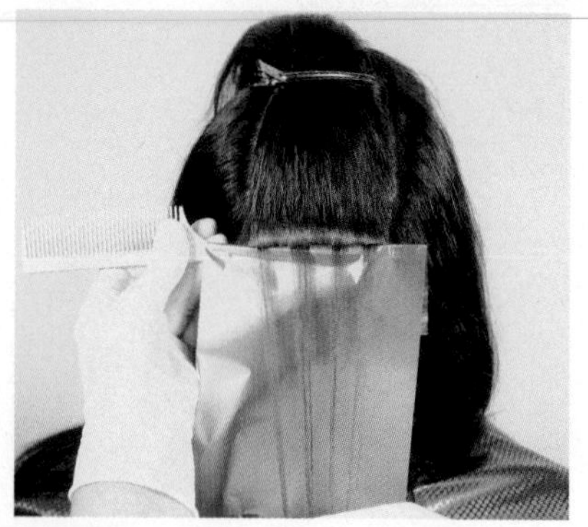

▲ Figure 21–34
Weaving.

Toning Highlighted and Dimensionally Colored Hair

When the hair is decolorized to the desired level during a highlighting service, the use of a toner may not be necessary. However, the use of a pale soft blond with cool or warm tones does create a finished appearance to the overall color result.

When using a toner on highlighted hair, it is important to consider not only the varying degrees of porosity in the hair, but also the

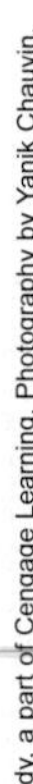

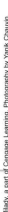

© Milady, a part of Cengage Learning. Photography by Yanik Chauvin.

difference in pigmentation from strand to strand that was created by the lightening process. Although an oxidative toner will add color to the highlighted strands, it might also cause a slight amount of lift to the natural or pigmented hair. Perform a strand test to ensure best results.

To avoid affecting the untreated hair, choose from the following options:

- A nonoxidative toner, which contains no ammonia, requires no developer (thus producing no lift of the natural hair color) and is gentle on the scalp and hair.
- Semipermanent color may be used to deposit color without lift. Select a color that is delicate enough to avoid overpowering the prelightened hair. Always check the manufacturer's color chart to make sure that the combination of your chosen toner and the contributing pigment will produce the desired color results.
- A demipermanent haircolor may also be used to deposit color. It will not cause additional lightening and lasts longer than temporary or traditional semipermanent colors.

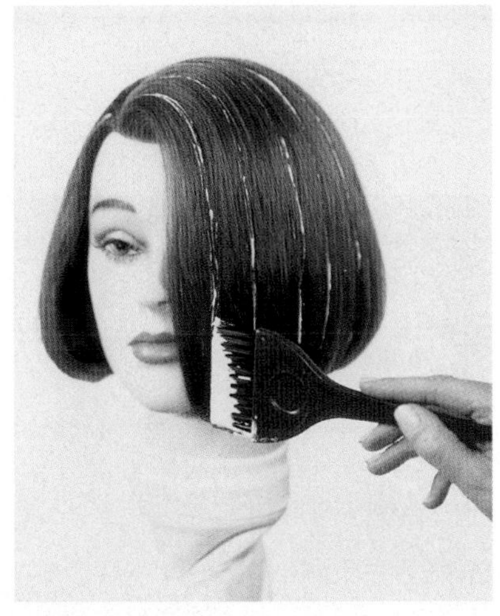

▲ Figure 21–35
Baliage technique.

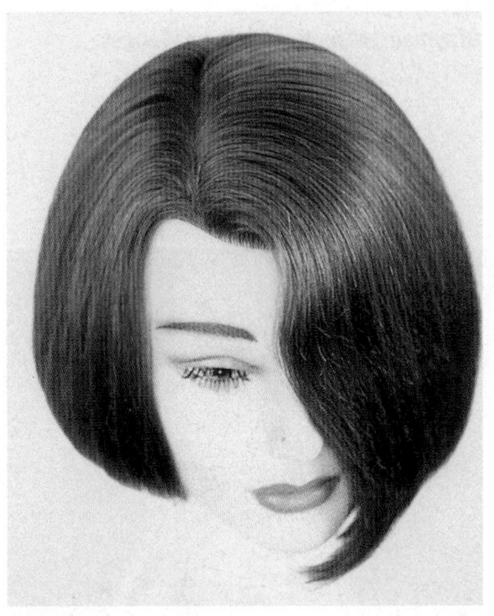

▲ Figure 21–36
Finished hair.

Highlighting Shampoos

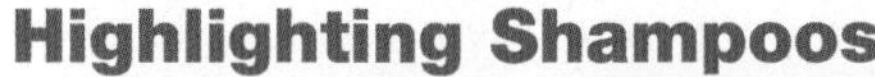

Highlighting shampoo colors are prepared by combining permanent haircolor, hydrogen peroxide, and shampoo. They are used when a slight change in hair shade is desired, or when the client's hair processes very rapidly. This process highlights the hair's natural color in a single application. No patch test is required. Follow the manufacturer's directions.

Special Challenges in Haircolor/Corrective Solutions

Each haircoloring service is unique and can present unique challenges. To give each haircoloring service a good start, the colorist must allow enough time for a complete client consultation and analysis of the client's hair. Strand tests must be performed to ensure satisfactory final results. But even the most skilled colorist will occasionally have a problem that can't be predicted. This may be due to the particular structure or condition of the client's hair. The good news is that most haircoloring problems can be resolved or corrected as long as the colorist remains calm.

Gray Hair: Challenges and Solutions

Gray hair is caused by the reduction of pigment in the cortical layer. Gray, white, and salt-and-pepper hair all have characteristics that present unique coloring challenges. For instance, gray hair can turn orange if the lightener used is not processed long enough. A great many salon

© Milady, a part of Cengage Learning.

coloring services, however, will successfully cover or enhance gray hair if performed correctly (**Figures 21–37** and **21–38**).

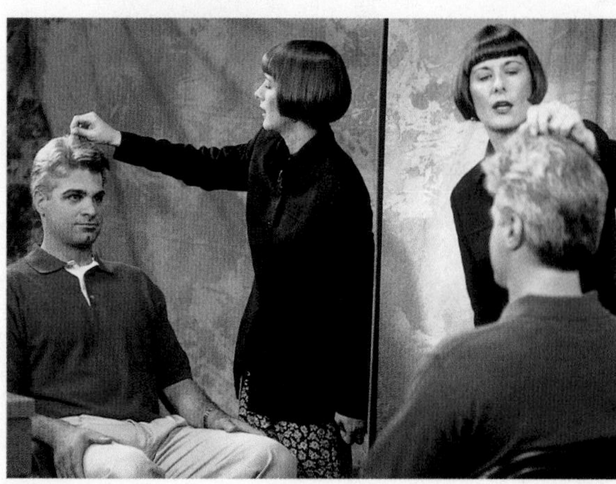

▲ **Figure 21–37**
Gray hair presents certain challenges.

Yellowed Hair

A problem that can occur with gray hair is that it can develop a yellow cast which can be caused by a variety of factors:

- Smoking
- Medication
- Sun exposure
- Hair sprays and styling aids

Lightener and haircolor removers help remove yellow discoloration. Undesired yellow can often be overpowered by the artificial pigments deposited by violet-based colors of an equal or darker level than the yellow.

Formulating for Gray Hair

Gray hair accepts the level of the color applied. However, Level 8 or lighter colors may not give complete coverage because of the low concentration of dye found in these lighter colors. Formulations from Level 7 and darker will provide better coverage, and can be used to create pastel and blond tones if desired.

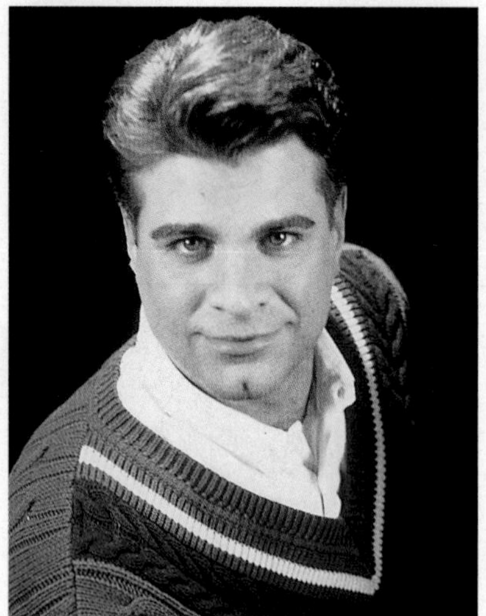

▲ **Figure 21–38**
Many haircolor options cover gray successfully.

For those clients who are 80 to 100 percent gray, a haircolor within the blond range is generally more flattering than a darker shade. This lighter level of artificial color may be selected to give a warm or cool finished color, depending on the client's skin tone, eye color, and personal preference.

One factor to consider when coloring low percentages of gray or salt-and-pepper hair to a darker level is that color on color will always make a darker color. The addition of dark artificial pigment to the natural pigment results in a color that the eye perceives as darker. For this reason, when attempting to cover the unpigmented hair on a salt-and-pepper head, formulate one to two levels lighter than the natural level to ensure a natural result.

For the purposes of a strand test, a manufacturer's product color chart can be used in conjunction with **Tables 21–4** and **21–5** to select a color within the proper level.

The gray hair formulation tables provide general guidelines, but there are other considerations to take into account, such as the following:

- Client's personality
- Personal preferences
- Amount of gray hair and its location on the head

You will note that in the tables there are no colors given in the formulations, only the levels of haircoloring and various techniques. Also note that the table does not consider the location of the gray hair. The

© Milady, a part of Cengage Learning.

SEMIPERMANENT/DEMIPERMANENT COLOR FORMULATION FOR GRAY HAIR

PERCENTAGE OF GRAY HAIR	SEMIPERMANENT/ DEMIPERMANENT COLOR FORMULATION FOR GRAY HAIR
90-100%	desired level
70-90%	equal parts desired and one level lighter
50-70%	one level lighter than desired level
30-50%	equal parts one and two levels lighter
10-30%	two levels lighter than desired level

© Milady, a part of Cengage Learning.

Table 21–4 Semipermanent/Demipermanent Color Formulation for Gray Hair.

PERMANENT COLOR FORMULATION FOR GRAY HAIR

PERCENTAGE OF GRAY HAIR	PERMANENT COLOR FORMULATION FOR GRAY HAIR
90-100%	desired level
70-90%	two parts desired level and one part lighter level
50-70%	equal parts desired and lighter level
30-50%	two parts lighter level and one part desired level
10-30%	one level lighter

© Milady, a part of Cengage Learning.

Table 21–5 Permanent Color Formulation for Gray Hair.

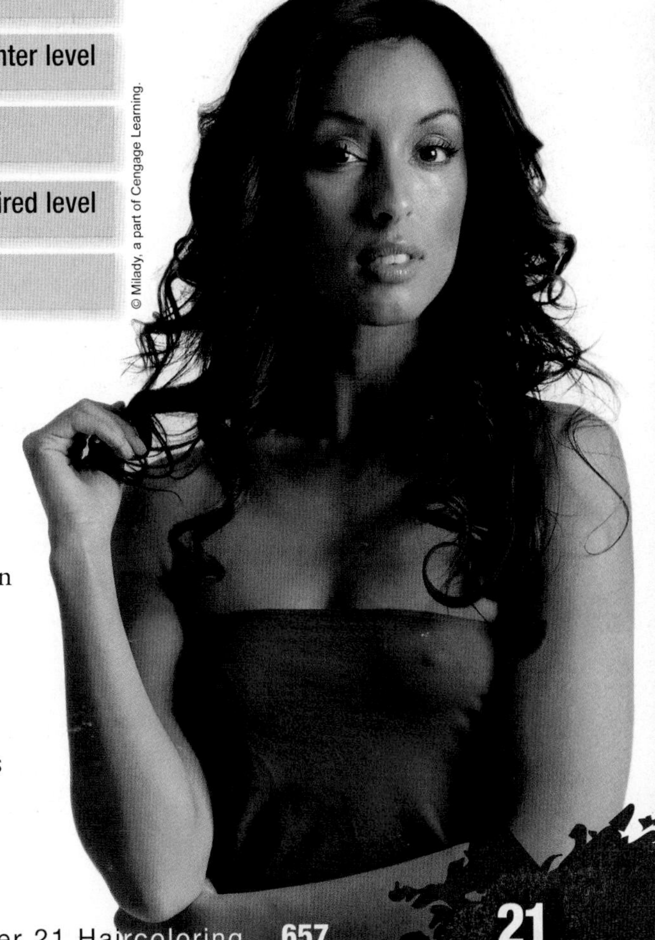

© ABY, 2010; used under license from Shutterstock.com.

percentage assumes that the gray hair is equally distributed throughout the entire head. If, for instance, the majority of gray hair is located in the front section of the head, that section would be considered to have more gray hair, with the back portion containing less gray hair. In that instance, you would have to determine what formulation would best suit the client. The gray hair around the face is what the client sees, so it may be wise to formulate based on the percentage of gray hair the client actually sees. The section of hair that surrounds the face is what influences the client's self-image.

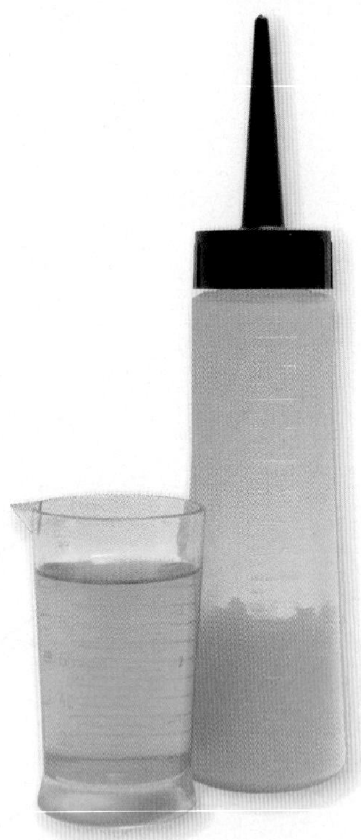

Tips for Achieving Gray Coverage

- Formulate at a Level 7 medium-blond and deeper for best gray coverage.
- Use 20-volume developer.
- Process color for a full forty-five minutes.
- Add neutral tones to the formula.
- If 25 percent gray is present, use 25 percent neutral or natural tones in formula.
- If 50 percent gray is present, use 50 percent neutral or natural tones in formula.
- If 75 percent gray is present, use 75 percent neutral or natural tones in formula.

High-lift blond colors are not designed for gray coverage. To create a very light result, formulate at a Level 7 for the base color and add some highlights over the color to create a balanced blond on blond result. ☑ **LO18**

© Milady, a part of Cengage Learning.

Presoftening

Occasionally, gray hair is so resistant that even when formulation, application, and time are correct, you will find that the coverage is not satisfactory. In such cases, presoftening becomes necessary. **Presoftening** is the process of treating gray or very resistant hair to allow for better penetration of color. Presoftening raises the cuticle layer of the resistant hair to allow for better penetration of color. A presoftener acts like a stain to the hair. It is applied, processed, and removed. Then the haircolor is applied.

Apply the presoftening formula to the resistant areas and allow it to stay on the hair for fifteen minutes. Refer to manufacturer's directions. While presoftening the resistant areas, you may mix the final formula and start to apply it to the rest of the head.

Once the resistant hair has been presoftened, blot the presoftener color off with a towel and apply the final color formula directly over it. Process per the manufacturer's instructions.

FOCUS ON

BUILDING YOUR CLIENT BASE

To build your haircolor clientele:

- Be as knowledgeable about haircolor as you can be. Maintain your skills through continuous education.
- Be honest when recommending color options to your client. That means including information on maintenance, costs, and other issues.
- Keep up to date with celebrity hair trends because your clients will be asking for them.
- Maintain a positive and excited attitude about your work and convey your confidence and enthusiasm to your client.

Rules for Effective Color Correction

Sometimes the color may not turn out as expected. Although this can seem disastrous for your client and for you, it does not need to be. Problems can always be corrected. Keep the following guidelines in mind:

- Do not panic. Remain calm.
- Determine the nature of the problem.
- Determine what caused the problem.
- Develop a solution.

- Always take one step at a time.
- Never guarantee an exact result.
- Always strand test for accuracy. ✔ **LO19**

Damaged Hair

Blowdrying, flat irons, wind, harsh shampoos, and chemical services all take their toll on the condition of the hair. Coating compounds such as hair sprays, styling agents, and some conditioners can block/interfere with color penetration. Hair is considered damaged when it has one or more of the following characteristics:

- Rough texture
- Overporous condition
- Brittle and dry to the touch
- Susceptible to breakage
- No elasticity
- Becomes spongy and matted when wet
- Color fades too quickly or grabs too dark

Any of these hair conditions will create problems during a haircoloring, lightening, permanent waving, or hair relaxing treatment. Therefore, damaged hair should receive reconditioning treatments both before and after the application of these chemical services. Tips for dealing with damaged hair appear below.

- Use a penetrating conditioner that can deposit protein, oils, and moisture-rich ingredients.
- Complete each chemical service by normalizing the pH with an acidic finishing rinse. This will restore the ability of the cuticle to protect the hair.
- Postpone any further chemical service until the hair is reconditioned.
- Schedule the client for between-service conditioning.
- Recommend retail home-care products that will help prepare the hair for the next service.

Fillers

Fillers are used to equalize porosity. Some fillers are ready to use as they come from the manufacturer. Others are a mixture of haircolor and conditioner that your instructor can help you prepare. There are two types of fillers: conditioner fillers and color fillers.

Conditioner fillers are used to recondition damaged, overly porous hair and equalize porosity so that the hair accepts the color evenly from strand to strand and from scalp to ends. They can be applied in a separate procedure or immediately prior to the color application.

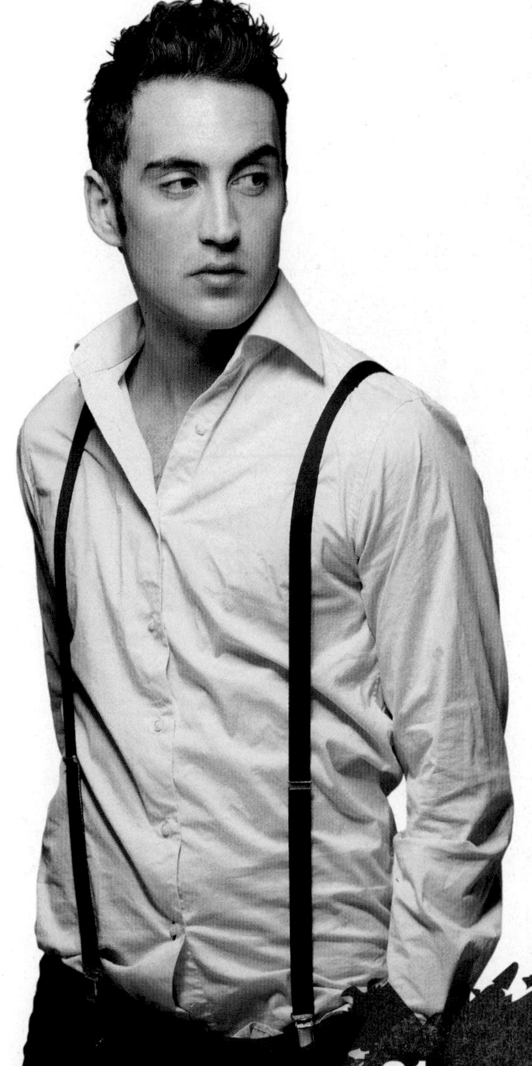

© Andreas Gradin, 2010; used under license from Shutterstock.com.

Color fillers equalize porosity and deposit color in one application to provide a uniform contributing pigment on prelightened hair. Color fillers are used on overly porous, prelightened hair to equalize porosity and provide a uniform contributing pigment that complements the desired finished color. Demipermanent haircolor products are commonly used as color fillers.

Color fillers accomplish the following goals:

- Deposit color to faded ends and hair shaft.
- Help prepare hair to hold a final color by replacing missing building blocks.
- Prevent streaking and dull appearance.
- Prevent off-color results.
- Produce more uniform, natural-looking color.
- Produce uniform color when coloring prelightened hair back to its natural color.

Selecting the Correct Color Filler

All three primary colors must be present to produce a haircolor that looks natural. To correct an unwanted haircolor, always use the primary or secondary color that is missing in the hair. That color is called the complementary color. Remember, complementary colors are directly opposite each other on the color wheel.

Yellow blond hair can be corrected to a natural blond by adding the two missing primary colors, red and blue—in other words, by adding the secondary color violet. Violet cancels yellow. Orange blond hair can be corrected to a natural blond by adding the missing primary color, blue. Blue cancels orange. Adding blue color to yellow hair would make the hair green. Remember that a primary color always cancels a secondary color and a secondary color always cancels a primary color.

Color fillers may be applied directly from their containers to damaged hair prior to coloring. They may also be added to the haircolor and applied to damaged ends.

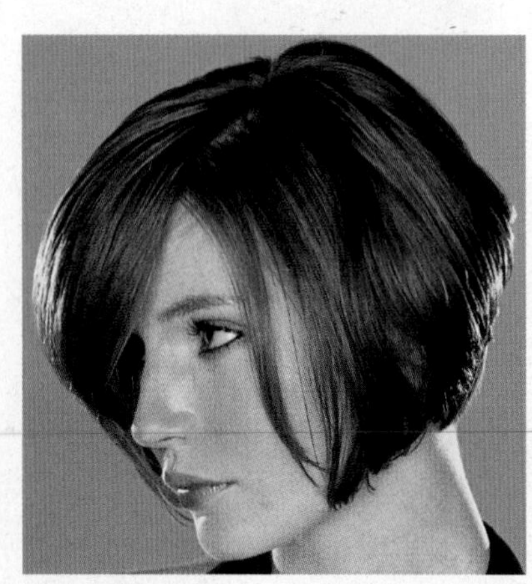

Photo used with the permission of the authors, Martin Gannon and Richard Thompson, as featured in their book, Mahogany: Steps to Cutting, Colouring and Finishing Hair. © Martin Gannon and Richard Thompson.

▲ **Figure 21–39 Vibrant red hair.**

Haircolor Tips for Redheads

Red haircolor is exciting and fun, but fading is a common problem with color-treated red hair (**Figure 21–39**). A daily shampoo and blowdry, an occasional permanent wave, and/or a few days in the pool or at the beach cause the artificial pigment in red hair to oxidize and fade. It is important to recommend the proper products to maintain the finished haircolor. Tips are summarized below.

- To create warm coppery reds, use a red-orange base color (RO, RG).
- To create hot fiery reds, use red-violet or true red colors (R, RR, RV).
- After the hair has been colored with a permanent color, always use a demipermanent color to refresh the shaft and ends.

- If gray hair is present, always add ½ ounce to 1 ounce of a neutral color to the desired red.
- To brighten haircolor, refresh reds with a soap cap of equal parts shampoo and the remaining color formula before rinsing, or mix a demipermanent color and apply it to the ends.

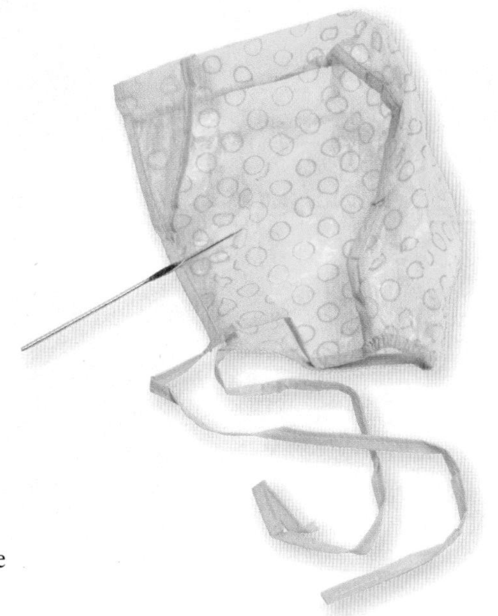

© Milady, a part of Cengage Learning. Photography by Paul Castle, Castle Photography.

Haircolor Tips for Brunettes

- To avoid orange or brassy tones when lifting brown hair with permanent color, always use a cool blue base.
- To avoid unwanted brassy tones, do not lighten more than two levels above the natural color.
- Add 1 ounce of a natural color to cover gray in brunette hair.
- Natural highlights in brunette hair should be deep or caramel colored. Blond highlights have too much contrast with brunette hair. Blond highlights do not look natural and require frequent service.

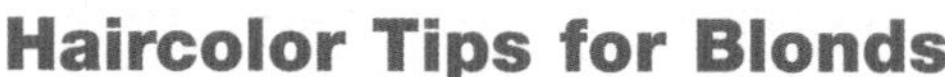

Haircolor Tips for Blonds

Blond haircolor is popular, profitable, and fun. From single-process blond to highlighting, the possibilities are endless. As you work with blond hair, keep the following tips in mind:

- When lightening brown hair to blond, remember that there may be underlying unwanted warm tones.
- When covering gray hair with a blond color, use a Level 7 or darker for the best coverage.
- Double-process blonding is the best way to obtain pale blond results.
- If high-lift blonds that lift only 5 levels are used on Levels 4 and below, the result may be a color that is too warm or brassy.
- If highlights become too blond or all one color, lowlights or deeper strands can be foiled into the hair to create a more natural color. A great lowlight formula using a demipermanent color is 1½ ounces 8N with ½ ounce of 6G. You can also add all-over warmth to the end result with a glaze of 10RO applied all over the hair for five minutes. This will add a sunshine look to the hair.

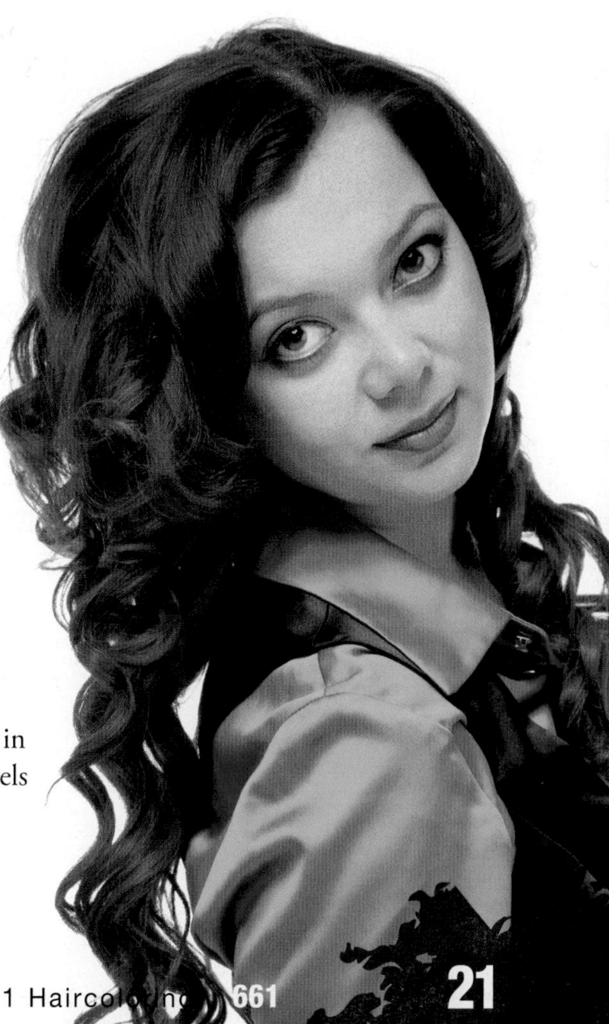

© Beerkoff, 2010; used under license from Shutterstock.com.

Common Haircolor Solutions

Refresh Faded Color

If the hair appears dull and faded, mix a demipermanent haircolor in the same tonal family as the haircolor formula. Stay within two levels of your formula. Apply all over and process up to ten minutes.

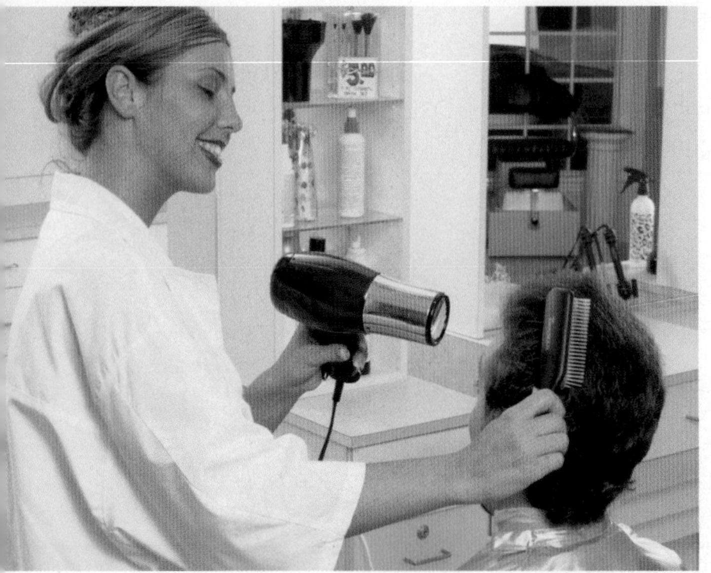

© Milady, a part of Cengage Learning. Photography by Paul Castle, Castle Photography.

Green Cast

If the hair has a buildup of minerals from well water or chlorine, you may want to purify the hair with a product designed to remove the mineral buildup. You can apply a demipermanent color to neutralize any unwanted color that remains in the hair.

Overall Haircolor Is Too Light

This is a result of incorrect formulation. To correct, apply a demipermanent color that is one to two levels darker than the previous formula.

Overall Color Is Too Dark

Determine how much of the color needs to be removed. Use a haircolor remover in cases where the hair is too dark because of buildup or formulation. Apply haircolor remover to the areas that need to be lightened. Process for ten minutes and check development. These removers are designed to remove artificial pigment from the hair. Once you have achieved the desired color, rinse and shampoo.

Restoring Blond to Natural Haircolor

Restoring a client's blond hair back to its natural darker color can be tricky. Even if the client says that she wants to go back to her natural color, she may not like it. She is used to seeing light hair and going too dark could be disastrous. A few tips on how to restore the client's natural color are listed below.

Tips for Restoring Blond Hair to Natural Color

1. If you have a starting regrowth level that is Level 6 dark blond and deeper, soften the new growth with a Level 6 violet base permanent color with 20 volume. Apply to the scalp area, process for twenty minutes, and rinse. Towel dry. If the starting regrowth level is Level 7 medium blond and lighter, soften the regrowth with a Level 8 light blond-violet base permanent color with 20 volume. Apply to the scalp area, process for twenty minutes, and rinse. Towel dry.
2. Next, apply a demipermanent glaze with 1 ounce of a Level 8 light neutral blond and 1 ounce of a Level 9 very light blond red-orange. Apply to all the lightened hair. Do not apply to the scalp area. Process for twenty minutes. Rinse and towel dry. This will turn the hair a very light reddish-gold. Do Not Panic!
3. Finally, mix the final deposit-only glaze. If you formulated with Level 6 dark blond-violet at the base, use 1½ ounces Level 6 dark neutral blond with ½ ounce Level 4 light brown gold base.

If you formulated with Level 8 light violet blond at the base, use 1½ ounces Level 8 light neutral blond with ½ ounce Level 6 dark golden blond. Apply the chosen formula starting on the pieces that were overlightened from the beginning. Work the color through all over. Process up to twenty minutes, checking it every five minutes.

Reevaluate the haircolor at the client's next visit, and determine what is needed to make the color deeper. Apply a separate color to the scalp area and on the remainder of the hair strand for the best results.

Haircoloring Safety Precautions

- Perform a patch test twenty-four to forty-eight hours prior to each application of aniline-derivative haircolor. Apply haircolor only if the patch test is negative.
- Do not apply haircolor if abrasions are present on the scalp.
- Do not apply haircolor if a metallic or compound haircolor is present.
- Do not brush the hair prior to applying color.
- Always read and follow the manufacturer's directions.
- Use cleaned and disinfected applicator bottles, brushes, combs, and towels.
- Protect your client's clothing with proper draping.
- Perform a strand test for color, breakage, and/or discoloration.
- Use an applicator bottle or bowl (glass or plastic) for mixing the haircolor.
- Do not mix haircolor until you are ready to use it; discard leftover haircolor.
- Wear gloves to protect your hands.
- Do not permit the color to come in contact with the client's eyes.
- Do not overlap during a haircolor retouch.
- Use a mild shampoo. An alkaline or harsh shampoo will strip color.
- Always wash hands before and after serving a client. ☑ **LO20**

CAUTION

Sometimes hair is so damaged and overly porous that there may be insufficient structure left within the cortex for the artificial pigment to attach to. Hair that looks gun-metal gray is a real danger sign. Hair that is this porous is very fragile and may be close to the breaking point.

FOCUS ON

RETAILING

Your color client needs to use high-quality salon products at home to help prevent their haircolor from fading. Using the right products increases the longevity of the haircolor, preserves the natural integrity (health) of the hair, and makes your client more likely to return to you for more services. Recommending the right professional products increases your client's satisfaction and your income.

PROCEDURE 21-1

Performing a Patch Test

Implements and Materials

You will need all of the following implements, materials, and supplies:

- **Cotton swab**
- **Developer**
- **Glass or plastic mixing bowl**
- **Haircolor product**
- **Mild soap**
- **Towel**

Preparation

- Perform PROCEDURE 15-1 **Pre-Service Procedure** SEE PAGE 323

Procedure

1 Select a test area, behind the ear or on the inside of the elbow are good choices.

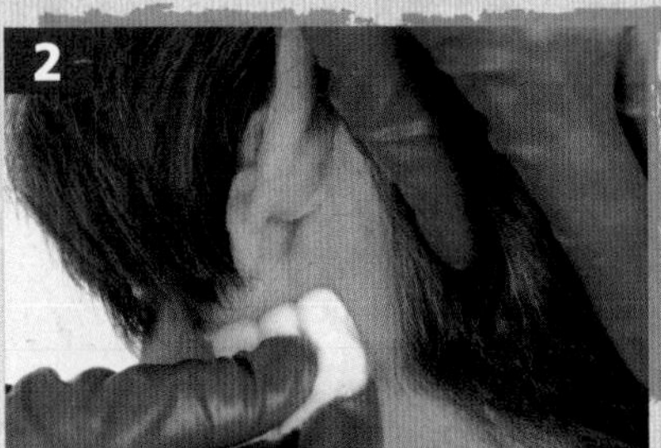

2 Using a mild soap, clean and dry an area about the size of a quarter.

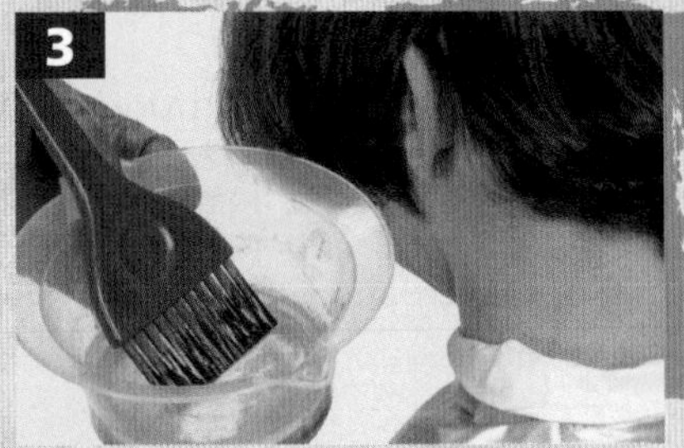

3 Mix a small amount of product according to the manufacturer's directions.

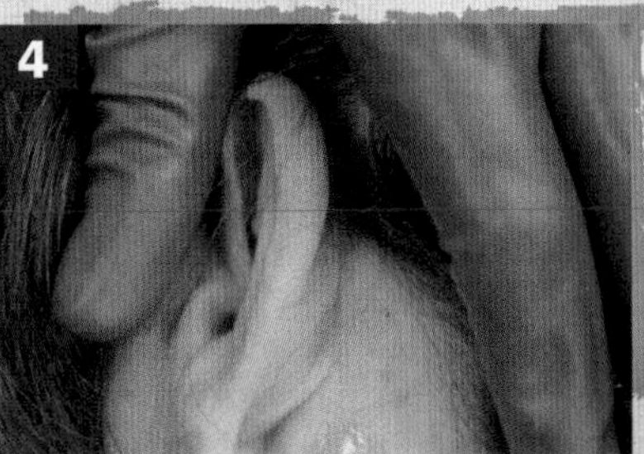

4 Apply a small amount of the haircolor mixture to the test area with a sterile cotton swab.

5 Leave the mixture undisturbed for twenty-four to forty-eight hours.

6 Examine the test area. If there are no signs of redness or irritation, the test result is negative, and you can proceed with the color service.

7 Record the results on the service record card.

Post Service

- Complete PROCEDURE 15-2 **Post-Service Procedure** SEE PAGE 326

© Milady, a part of Cengage Learning. Photography by Paul Castle, Castle Photography.

PROCEDURE 21-2

Preliminary Strand Test

Implements and Materials

You will need all of the following implements, materials, and supplies:

- **Applicator bottle**
- **Chemical cape**
- **Color brushes**
- **Developer**
- **Glass or plastic mixing bowl**
- **Protective gloves**
- **Selected haircolor**
- **Service record card**
- **Shampoo**
- **Sheet of foil or plastic wrap**
- **Spray bottle containing water**
- **Towels**

Preparation

- Perform PROCEDURE 15-1 **Pre-Service Procedure** **SEE PAGE 323**

Procedure

1 Perform a scalp and hair analysis.

2 Drape client to protect skin and clothing.

3 Part off a ½-inch (1.25 centimeters) square section of hair in the lower crown. Using plastic clips, fasten other hair out of the way.

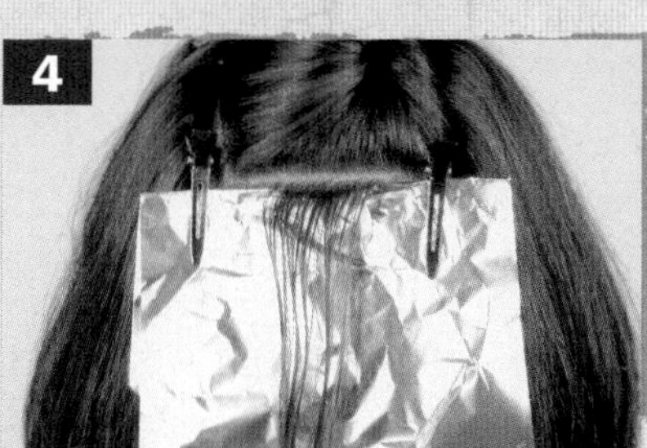

4 Place the hair strand over the foil or plastic wrap and apply the color mixture.

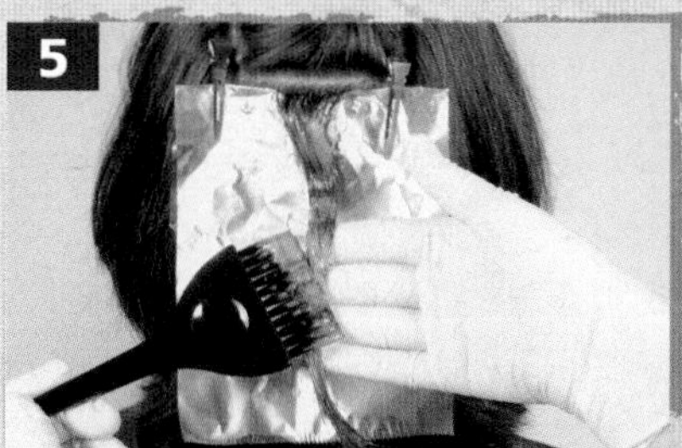

5 Follow the application method for the color you will be using to apply the color mixture.

© Milady, a part of Cengage Learning. Photography by Yanik Chauvin.

Preliminary Strand Test continued

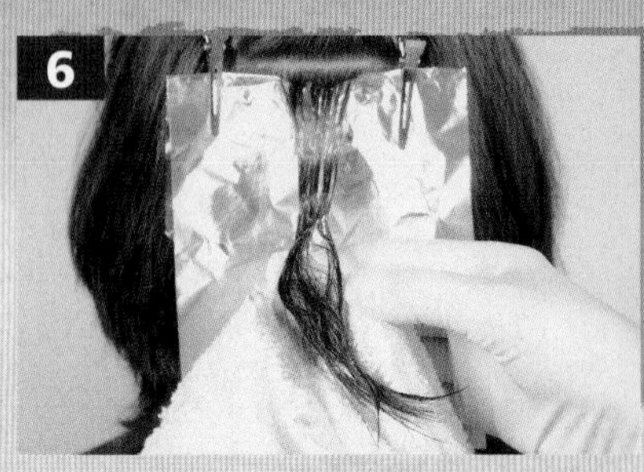

6 Check the development at five-minute intervals until the desired color has been achieved. Note the timing on the service record card.

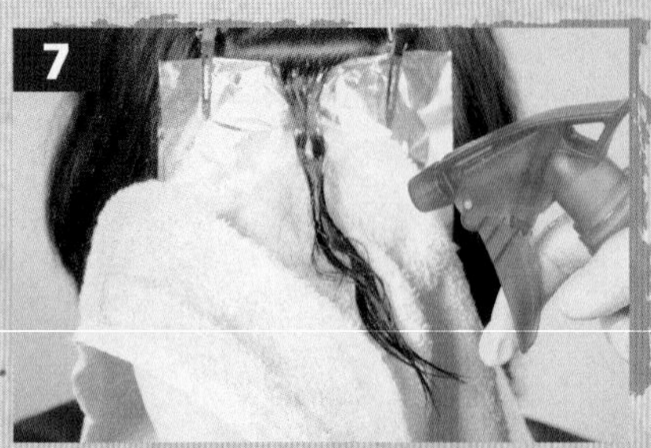

7 When satisfactory color has developed, remove the protective foil or plastic wrap. Place a towel under the strand, mist it thoroughly with water, add shampoo, and massage through. Rinse by spraying with water. Dry the hair strand with the towel and observe the results.

8 Adjust the formula, timing, or application method as necessary and proceed with the color service.

Post Service

- Complete PROCEDURE 15-2 **Post-Service Procedure** SEE PAGE 326

© Milady, a part of Cengage Learning. Photography by Yanik Chauvin.

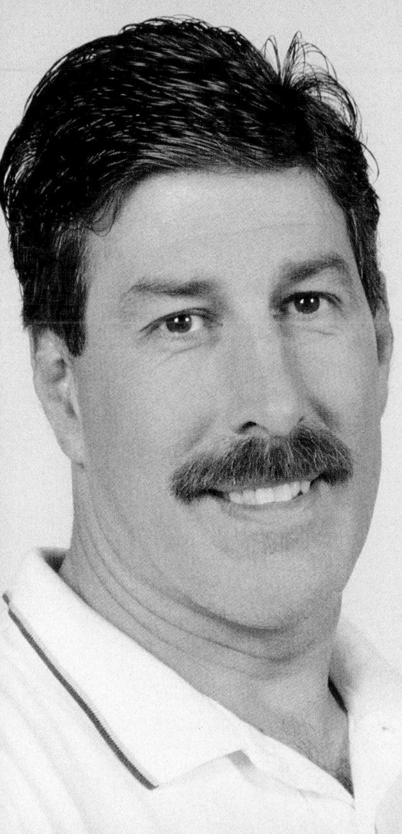

PROCEDURE 21-3

Temporary Haircolor Application

Implements and Materials

You will need all of the following implements, materials, and supplies:

- **Applicator bottle (optional)**
- **Comb**
- **Protective gloves**
- **Service record card**
- **Shampoo**
- **Shampoo cape**
- **Temporary haircolor product**
- **Timer**
- **Towels**

© Milady, a part of Cengage Learning. Photography by Yanik Chauvin.

Preparation

- Perform PROCEDURE 15-1 **Pre-Service Procedure** **SEE PAGE 323**

Procedure

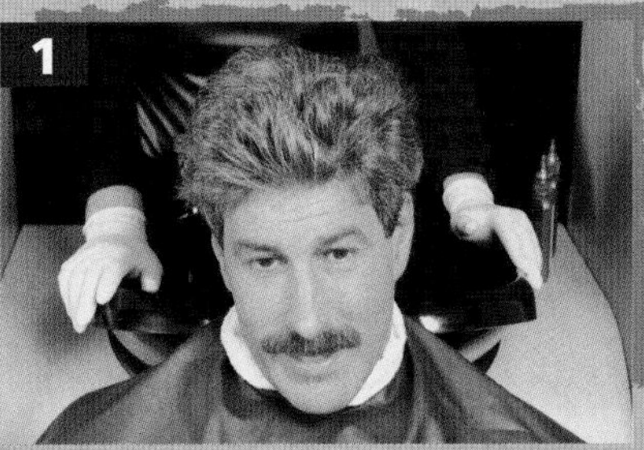

1 Drape the client for a haircoloring service. Slide a towel down from the back of the client's head and place lengthwise across the client's shoulders. Cross the ends of the towel beneath the chin and place the cape over the towel. Fasten the cape in the back. Fold the towel over the top of the cape and secure in front.

2 Shampoo and towel dry the hair.

3 Make sure the client is comfortably reclined at the shampoo bowl.

4 Put on gloves.

PROCEDURE 21-3 Temporary Haircolor Application continued

5 Put the color into an applicator bottle as directed by your instructor or use it directly from its bottle. Shake the bottle gently.

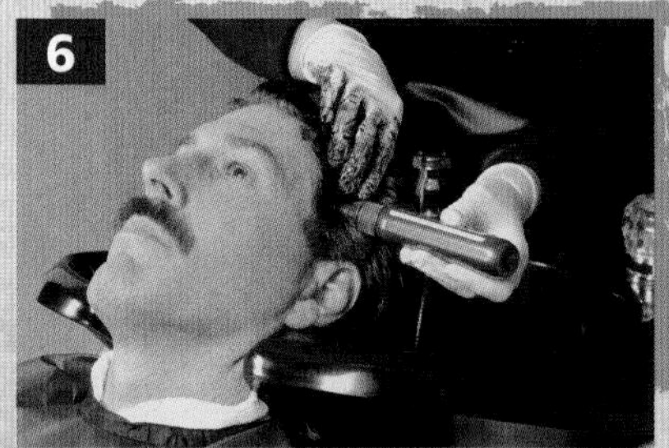

6 Apply the color and work around the entire head.

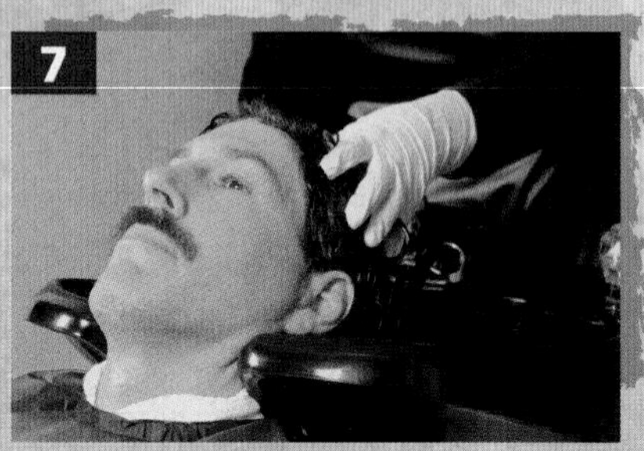

7 Blend the color with your gloved hands or comb it through the hair, applying more color as necessary.

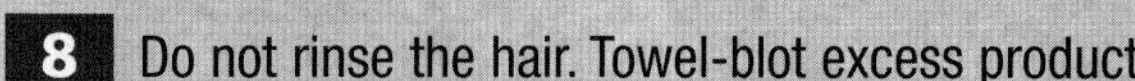

8 Do not rinse the hair. Towel-blot excess product.

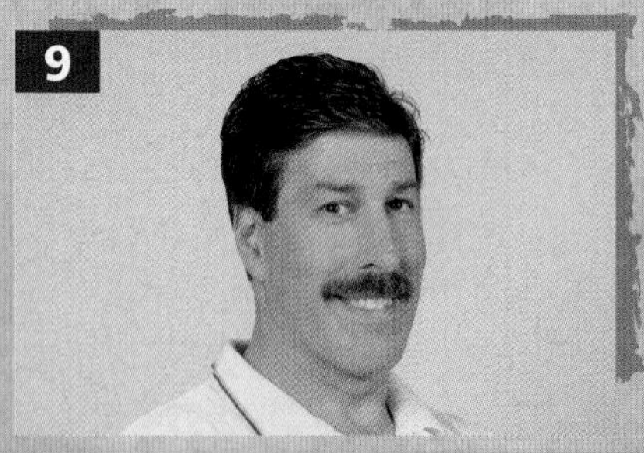

9 Proceed with styling and finish.

Post Service

- Complete PROCEDURE 15-2 Post-Service Procedure SEE PAGE 326

© Milady, a part of Cengage Learning. Photography by Yanik Chauvin.

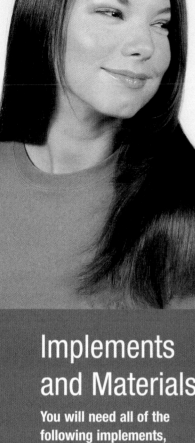

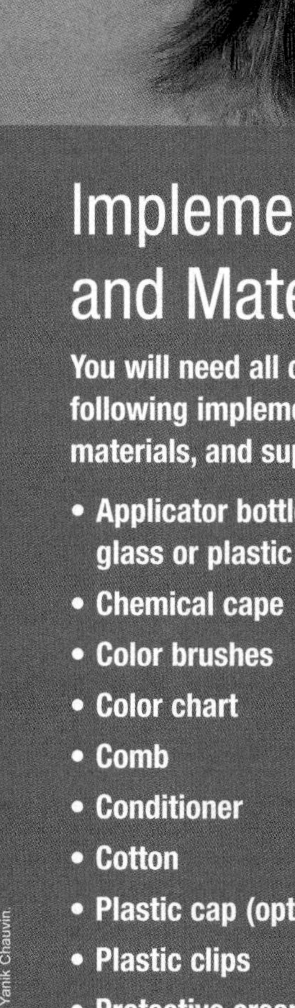

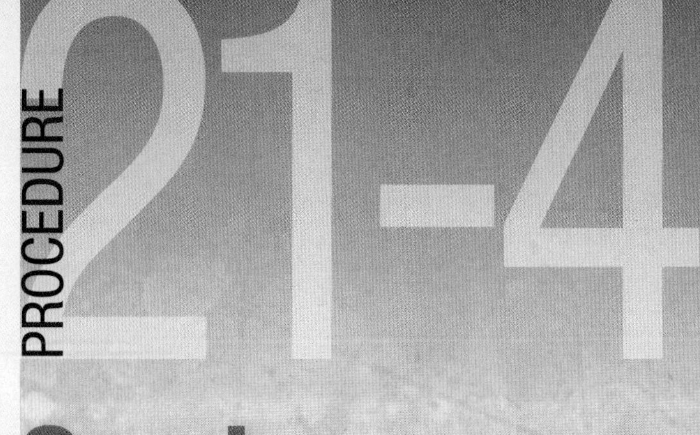

PROCEDURE 21-4

Semipermanent Haircolor Application

Implements and Materials

You will need all of the following implements, materials, and supplies:

- Applicator bottle or glass or plastic bowl
- Chemical cape
- Color brushes
- Color chart
- Comb
- Conditioner
- Cotton
- Plastic cap (optional)
- Plastic clips
- Protective cream
- Protective gloves
- Selected color
- Service record card
- Shampoo
- Timer
- Towels

© Milady, a part of Cengage Learning. Photography by Yanik Chauvin.

Preparation

- Perform PROCEDURE 15-1 Pre-Service Procedure SEE PAGE 323

Procedure

1 Shampoo the client's hair with mild shampoo, and towel dry.

2 Put on gloves.

3 Part the hair into four sections—from ear to ear and from front center of forehead to center nape—and apply protective cream around the hairline and over the ears.

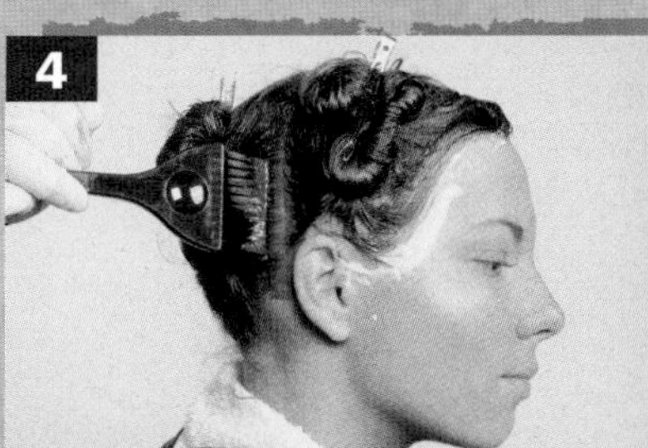

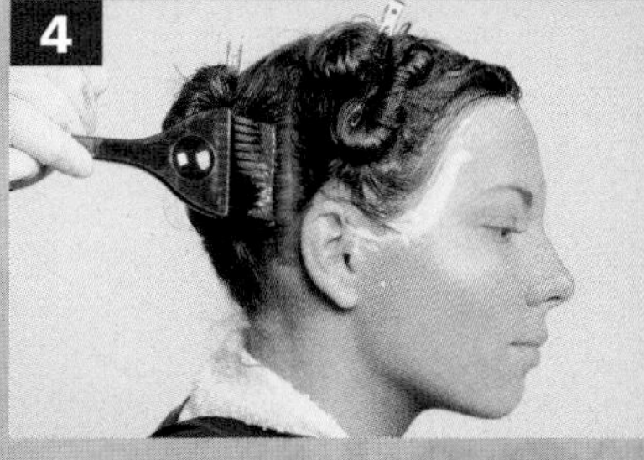

4

4 Outline the partings with color product.

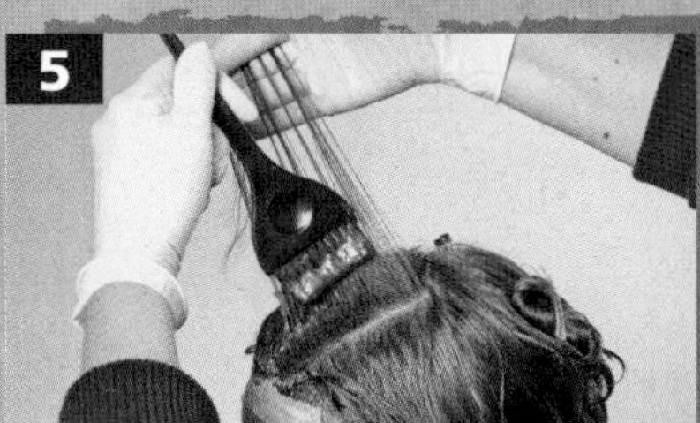

5

5 Take ½-inch partings, and apply the color to the new growth or scalp area in all four sections.

PROCEDURE 21-4

Semipermanent Haircolor Application continued

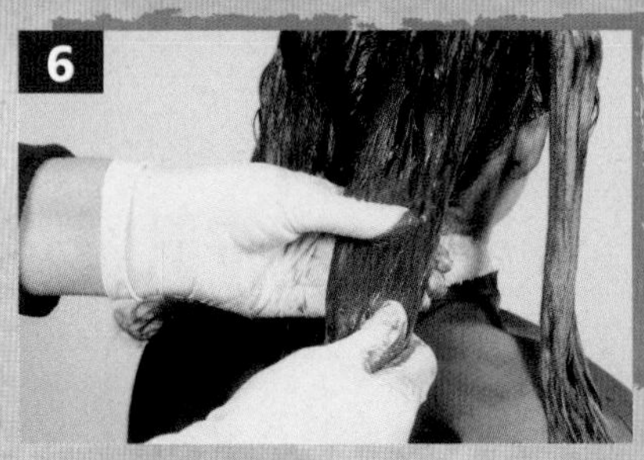

6 After all four sections are completed, work the color through the rest of the hair shaft to the ends until the hair is fully saturated.

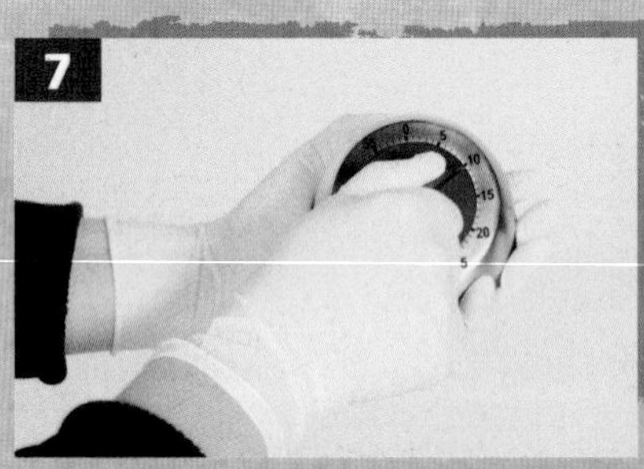

7 Set timer to process. Follow the manufacturer's directions. Some colors require the use of a plastic cap.

8 When processing is complete, massage color into a lather and rinse thoroughly with warm water.

9 Remove any stains from around the hairline with shampoo or stain remover.

10 Shampoo the hair. Condition as needed.

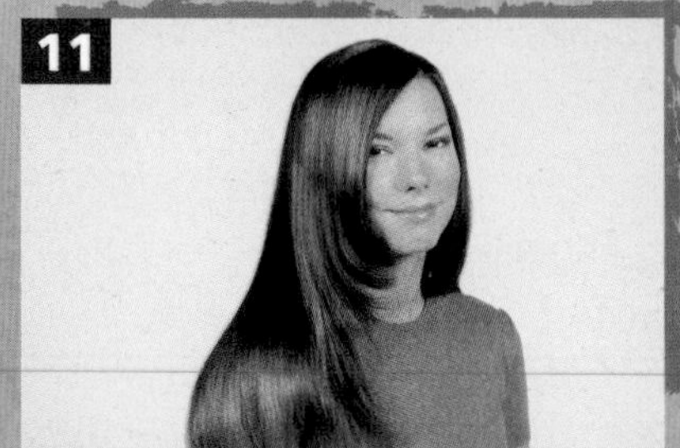

11 Finished look.

Post Service

- Complete PROCEDURE 15-2 Post-Service Procedure SEE PAGE 326

© Milady, a part of Cengage Learning. Photography by Yanik Chauvin.

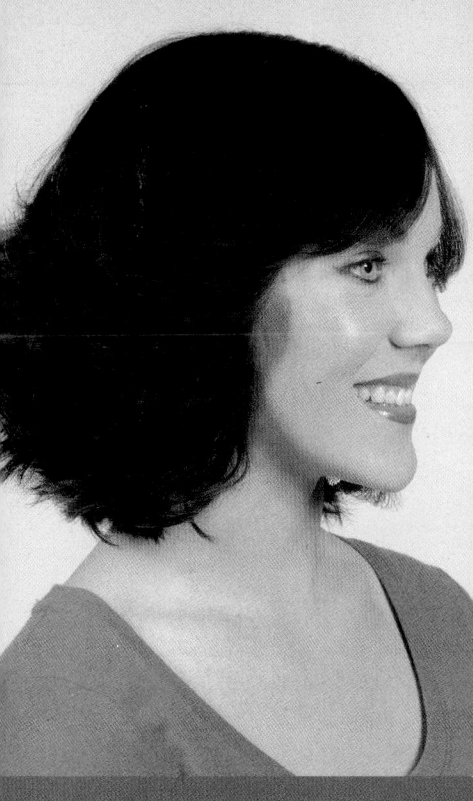

PROCEDURE 21-5

Single-Process Color on Virgin Hair

Implements and Materials

You will need all of the following implements, materials, and supplies:

- **Applicator bottle or glass or plastic mixing bowl**
- **Color brushes**
- **Color chart**
- **Comb**
- **Conditioner**
- **Cotton**
- **Hydrogen peroxide developer**
- **Plastic cap (optional)**
- **Plastic clips**
- **Protective cream**
- **Protective gloves**
- **Selected permanent color**
- **Service record card**
- **Shampoo**
- **Timer**
- **Towels**
- **Waterproof cape**

© Milady, a part of Cengage Learning. Photography by Yanik Chauvin.

Note: The colorist in the photographs completed this application using her left hand. The procedure is exactly the same for right-handed or left-handed application.

Preparation

- Perform PROCEDURE 15-1 **Pre-Service Procedure** **SEE PAGE 323**

Procedure

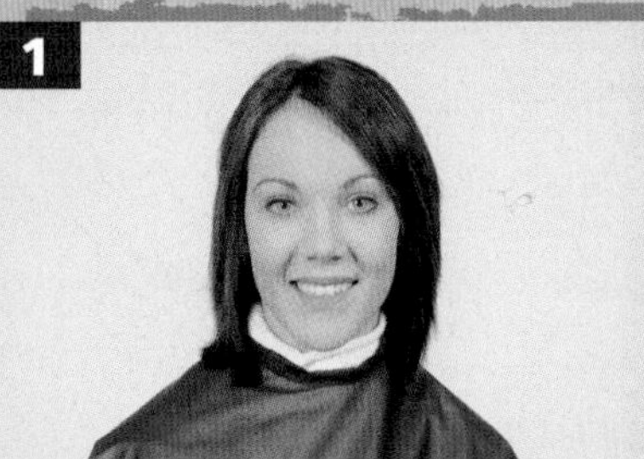

1 Drape the client for a haircolor service.

2 Put on gloves.

3 Part dry hair into four sections.

4 Apply protective cream to the hairline and ears.

5 Prepare the color formula for either bottle or brush application.

PROCEDURE 21-5

Single-Process Color on Virgin Hair continued

Service Tip

The hair at the scalp processes faster due to body heat. For this reason, the color is applied to the mid-strand before being applied to the scalp area. Your strand test will determine the application procedure and timing for even color development.

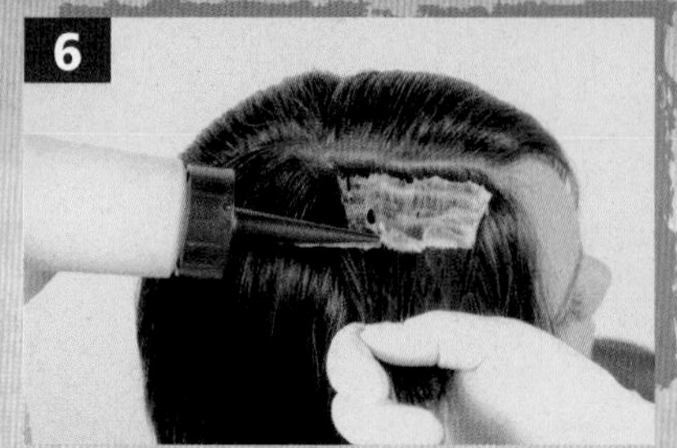

6 Begin in the section where the color change will be greatest or where the hair is most resistant, usually the hairline and temple areas. Part off a ¼-inch (0.6 centimeters) subsection with the applicator.

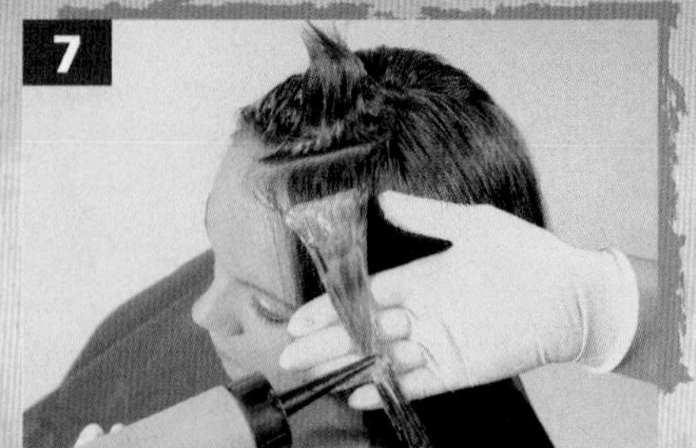

7 Lift the subsection and apply color to the mid-strand area. Stay at least ½ inch (1.25 centimeters) from the scalp, and do not apply to the porous ends.

8 Process according to the strand test results. Check for color development by removing color as described in the strand test procedure.

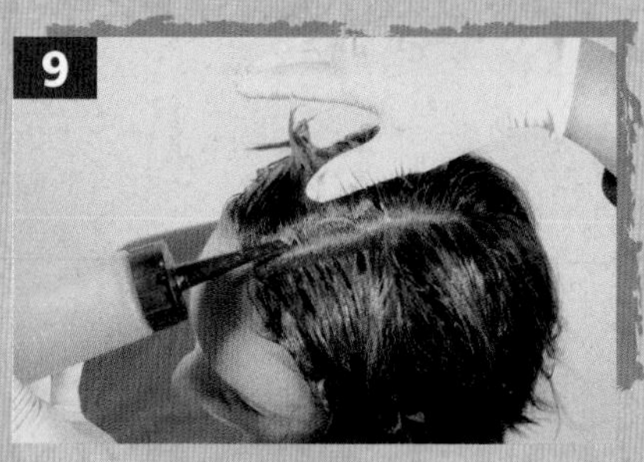

9 Apply color to the hair at the scalp.

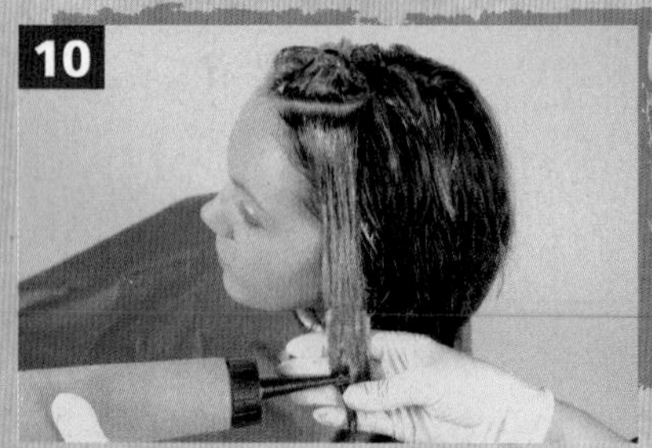

10 Work the color through the ends of the hair.

11 Massage color into a lather and rinse thoroughly with warm water.

12 Remove any stains around the hairline with shampoo or stain remover. Use a towel to gently remove stains.

13 Shampoo the hair. Condition as needed.

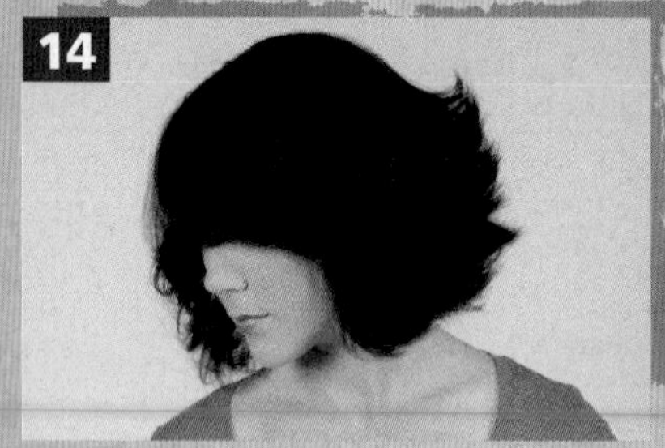

14 Finished look.

Post Service

- Complete PROCEDURE 15-2 Post-Service Procedure SEE PAGE 326

© Milady, a part of Cengage Learning. Photography by Yanik Chauvin.

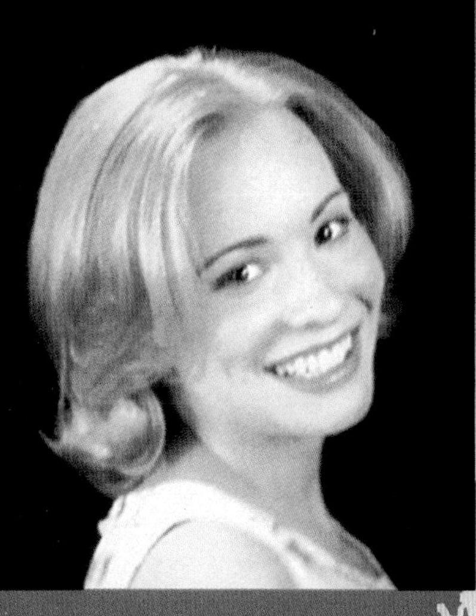

PROCEDURE 21-6

Permanent Single-Process Retouch with a Glaze

Implements and Materials

You will need all of the following implements, materials, and supplies:

- **Applicator bottle or glass or plastic mixing bowl**
- **Color brushes**
- **Color chart**
- **Chemical cape**
- **Comb**
- **Conditioner**
- **Cotton**
- **Developer**
- **Plastic cap (optional)**
- **Plastic clips**
- **Protective cream**
- **Protective gloves**
- **Selected permanent color**
- **Service record card**
- **Shampoo**
- **Timer**
- **Towels**

© Milady, a part of Cengage Learning. Photography by Paul Castle, Castle Photography.

Preparation

- Perform PROCEDURE 15-1 **Pre-Service Procedure** **SEE PAGE 323**

Procedure

1 Drape the client for a haircolor service.

2 Put on gloves.

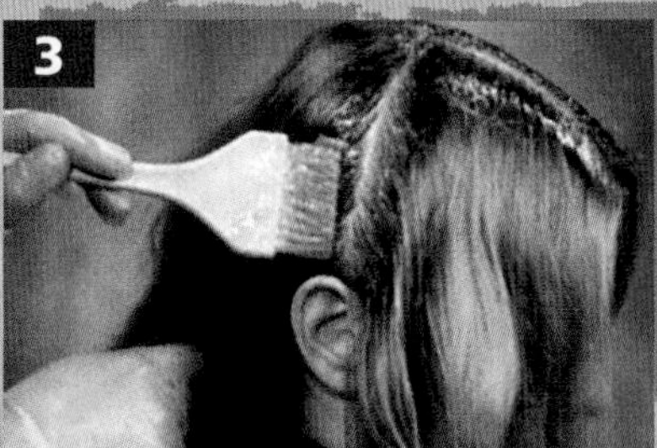

3 Part dry hair into four sections.

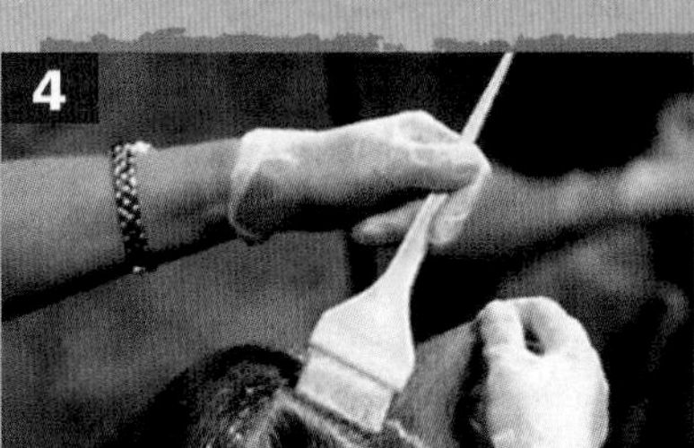

4 Apply the color to the new growth area using ¼-inch partings.

PROCEDURE 21-6

Permanent Single-Process Retouch with a Glaze continued

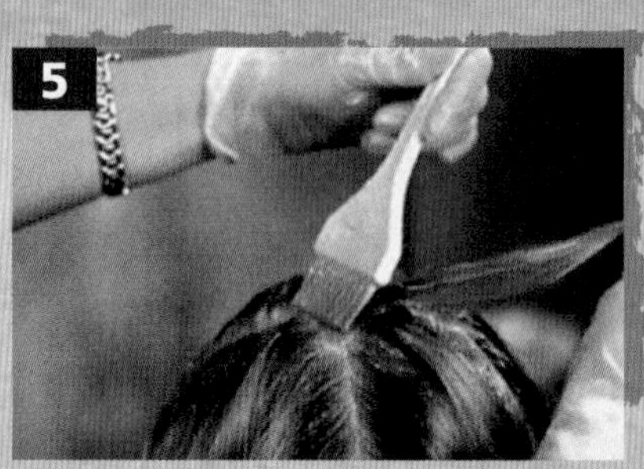
5

5 Complete all four sides and set timer for forty-five minutes or whatever the manufacturer's directions indicate.

6 Prepare a no-lift deposit-only glaze formula to apply to the mid-strand and ends.

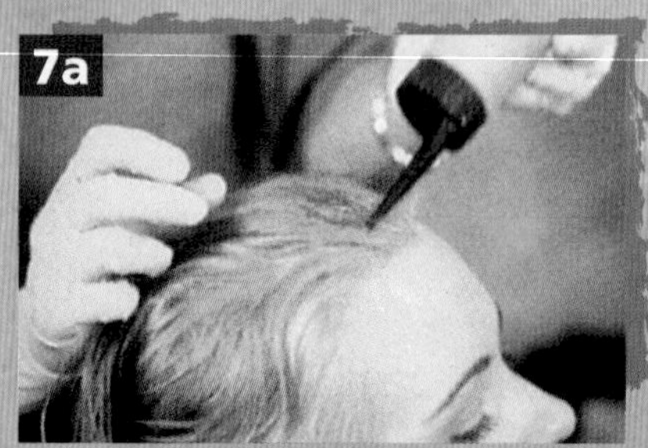
7a

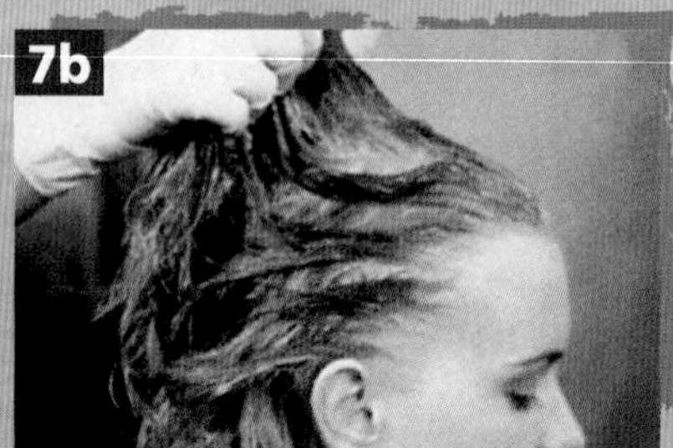
7b

7 Apply the demipermanent glaze and work through the hair.

8 Check haircolor results before rinsing.

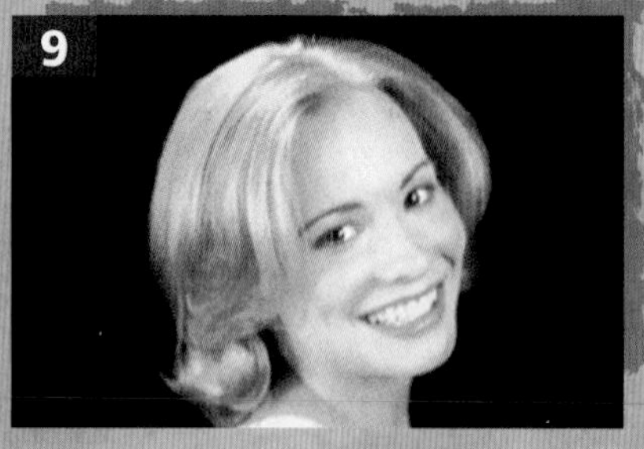
9

9 Finished look.

© Milady, a part of Cengage Learning. Photography by Paul Castle, Castle Photography.

Post Service

- Complete PROCEDURE 15-2 Post-Service Procedure SEE PAGE 326

PROCEDURE 21-7

Lightening Virgin Hair

Implements and Materials

You will need all of the following implements, materials, and supplies:

- **Applicator bottle or glass or plastic mixing bowl**
- **Chemical cape**
- **Color brushes**
- **Comb**
- **Conditioner**
- **Cotton**
- **Hydrogen peroxide developer**
- **Lightener**
- **Plastic clips**
- **Protective cream**
- **Protective gloves**
- **Service record card**
- **Shampoo**
- **Timer**
- **Towels**

Note: The colorist in the photographs completed this application using her left hand. The procedure is exactly the same for right-handed or left-handed application.

Preparation

- Perform PROCEDURE 15-1 Pre-Service Procedure SEE PAGE 323

Procedure

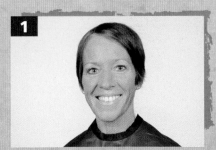

1 Drape the client for a haircolor service.

2 Put on gloves.

3 Part the hair into four sections.

4 Apply a protective cream around the hairline and over the ears.

5 Prepare the lightening formula and use it immediately.

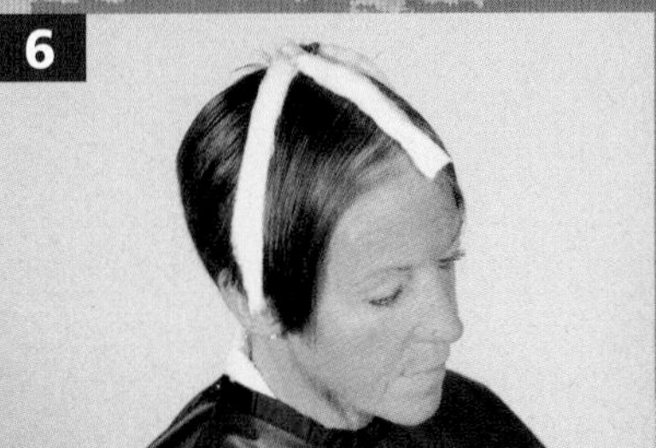

6 Place cotton around and through all four sections to protect the scalp so the lightener does not contact the scalp.

© Milady, a part of Cengage Learning. Photography by Yanik Chauvin.

Lightening Virgin Hair continued

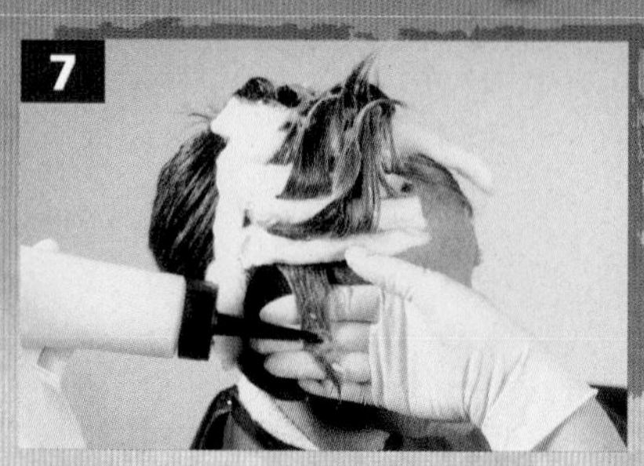

7 Apply the lightener ½-inch away from the scalp, working the lightener through the mid-strand and up to the porous ends.

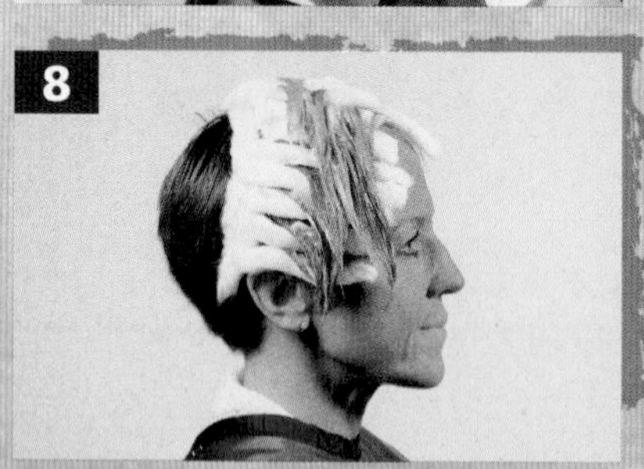

8 Place strips of cotton at the scalp area along the partings to prevent the lightener from touching the base of the hair, and complete all four sections in this manner.

9 Continue to apply the lightener. Double check the application, adding more lightener if necessary. Do not comb the lightener through the hair. Keep the lightener moist during development by reapplying if the mixture dries on the hair.

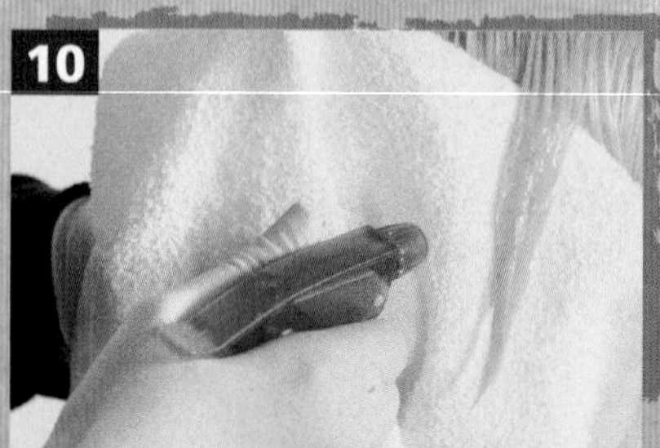

10 Check for lightening action about fifteen minutes before the time indicated by the preliminary strand test. Spray a hair strand with a water bottle and remove the lightener with a damp towel. Examine the strand. If the strand is not light enough, reapply the mixture and continue testing frequently until the desired level is reached.

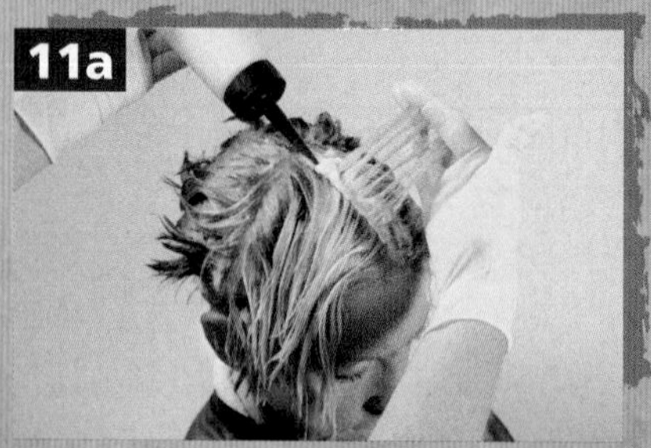

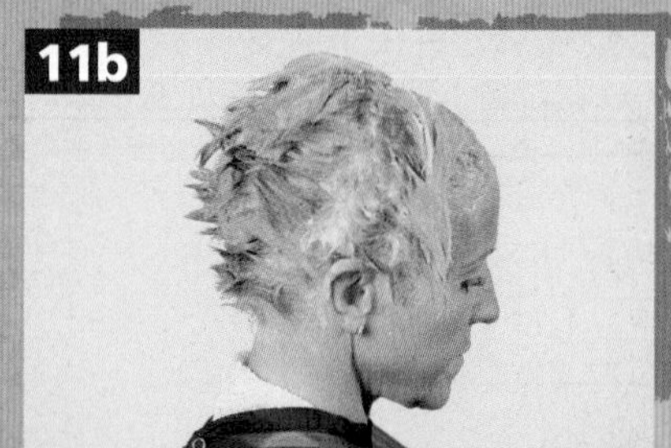

11 Remove the cotton from the scalp area. Apply the lightener to the hair near the scalp with ½-inch (0.3 centimeters) partings. Apply lightener to the porous ends and process until the entire hair strand has reached the desired stage.

12 Rinse the hair thoroughly with warm water. Shampoo gently and condition as needed, keeping your hands under the hair to avoid tangling.

13 Neutralize the alkalinity of the hair with an acidic conditioner. Recondition if necessary.

14 Towel dry the hair, or dry it completely under a cool dryer if required by the manufacturer.

15 Examine the scalp for any abrasions. Analyze the condition of the hair.

16 Proceed with a toner application if desired. (See Procedure 21–8, Toner Application.)

17 If no toner is needed, dry and style the hair.

Post Service

- Complete PROCEDURE 15-2 **Post-Service Procedure** SEE PAGE 326

© Milady, a part of Cengage Learning. Photography by Yanik Chauvin.

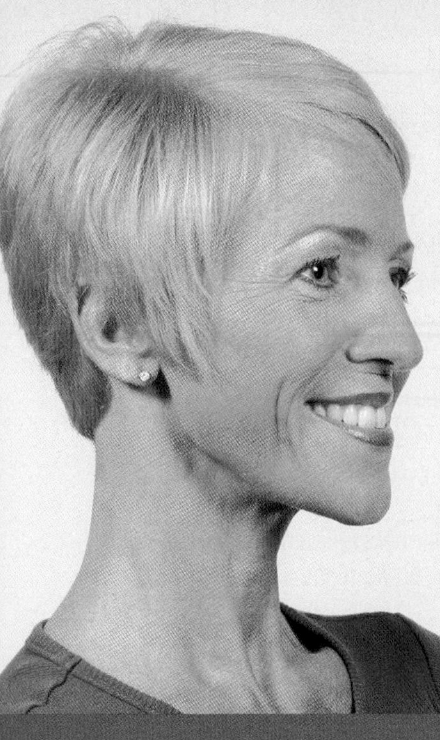

PROCEDURE 21-8

Toner Application

Note: The colorist in the photographs completed this application using her left hand. The procedure is exactly the same for right-handed or left-handed application.

Implements and Materials

You will need all of the following implements, materials, and supplies:

- **Applicator bottle**
- **Chemical cape**
- **Conditioner**
- **Cotton**
- **Glass or plastic mixing bowl**
- **Haircolor brushes**
- **Hydrogen peroxide developer**
- **Protective cream**
- **Protective gloves**
- **Plastic clips**
- **Selected toner**
- **Service record card**
- **Shampoo**
- **Tail comb**
- **Timer**
- **Towels**

© Milady, a part of Cengage Learning. Photography by Yanik Chauvin.

Preparation

- Perform PROCEDURE 15-1 **Pre-Service Procedure** **SEE PAGE 323**

Procedure

1 Prelighten the hair to the desired stage of decolorization.

2 Shampoo the hair lightly, rinse, and towel dry. Condition as necessary.

3 Put on gloves.

4 Select the desired toner shade.

5 Apply protective cream around the hairline and over the ears.

6 Take a strand test and record the results on the client's service record card.

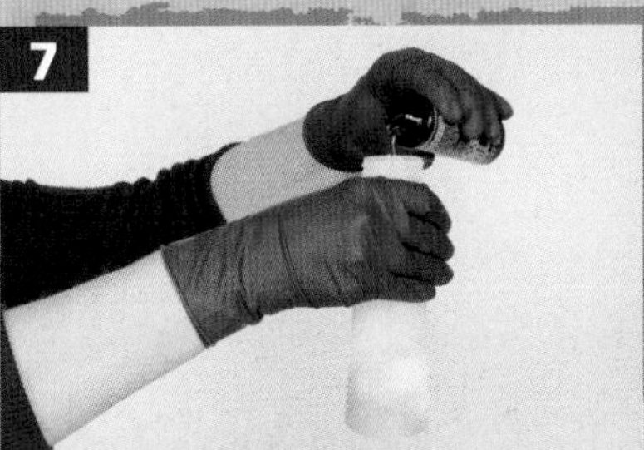

7 If using a toner with developer, mix the toner and the developer in a nonmetallic bowl or bottle, following the manufacturer's directions.

8 Part the hair into four equal sections, using the end of the tail comb or applicator brush. Avoid scratching the scalp.

Toner Application continued

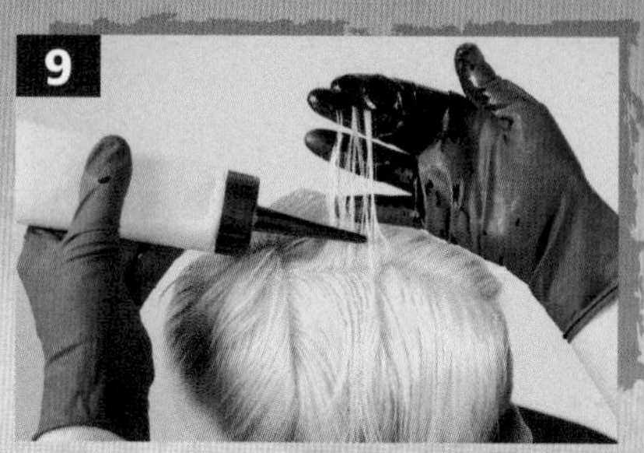

9

9 At the crown of one of the back sections, part off ¼-inch (0.6 centimeters) partings and apply the toner from the scalp up to, but not including, the porous ends.

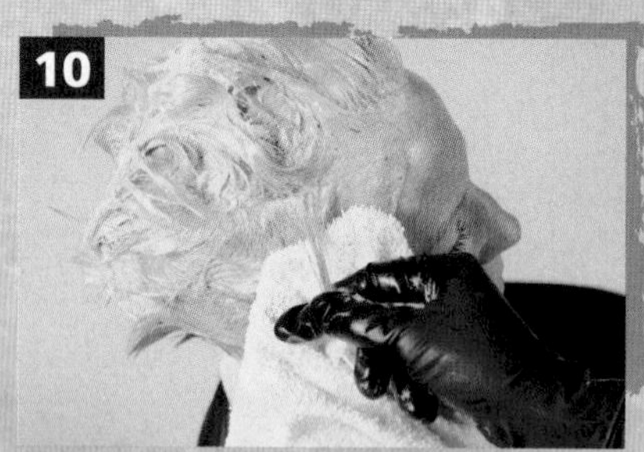

10

10 Take a strand test. If it indicates proper color development, gently work the toner through the ends of the hair, using an applicator brush or your fingers.

11 If necessary for coverage, apply additional toner to the hair and distribute evenly. Leave the hair loose or cover with a plastic cap if required.

12 Time the procedure according to your strand test. Check frequently until the desired color has been reached evenly throughout the entire hair shaft and ends.

13 Remove the toner by wetting the hair and massaging the toner into a lather.

14 Rinse with warm water, shampoo gently, and thoroughly rinse again.

15 Apply an acidic conditioner to close the cuticle, lower the pH, and help prevent fading.

16 Remove any stains from the skin, hairline, and neck.

17 Style as desired. Use caution to avoid stretching the hair.

Service Tip

Do not apply the toner through to the porous ends of the hair until the end of the procedure, and then only do so if you are planning to change the tone or are correcting significant fading. Applying toner through these areas will only make the ends even more porous and more susceptible to continued fading.

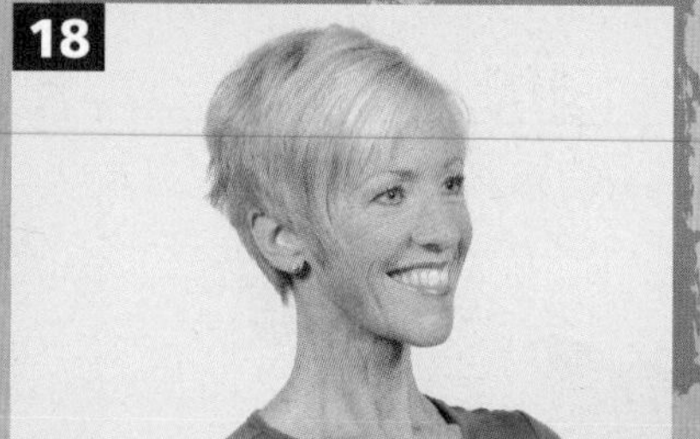

18

18 Finished look.

Post Service

- Complete PROCEDURE 15-2 Post-Service Procedure SEE PAGE 326

© Milady, a part of Cengage Learning. Photography by Yanik Chauvin.

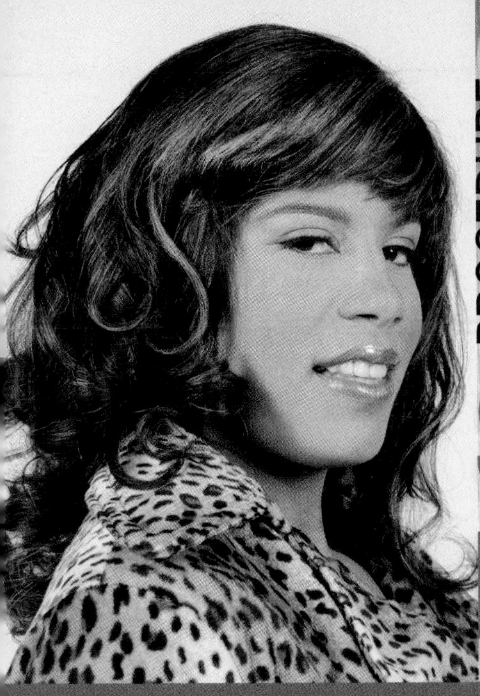

PROCEDURE 21-9 Special Effects Haircoloring with Foil (Full Head)

Implements and Materials

You will need all of the following implements, materials, and supplies:

- Applicator bottle
- Conditioner
- Chemical cape
- Foil
- Glass or plastic mixing bowl
- Gloves
- Haircolor brushes
- Lightener
- Plastic clips
- Service record card
- Shampoo
- Tail comb
- Timer
- Towels

© Milady, a part of Cengage Learning. Photography by Yanik Chauvin.

Note: The colorist in the photographs completed this application using her left hand. The procedure is exactly the same for right-handed or left-handed application.

Preparation

- Perform PROCEDURE 15-1 Pre-Service Procedure SEE PAGE 323

Procedure

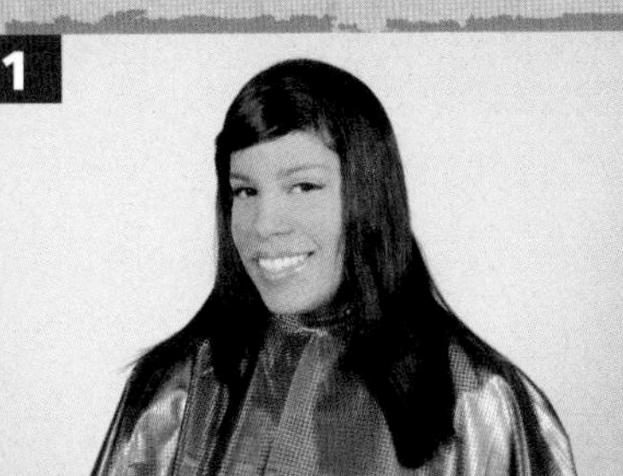

1 Drape the client for a haircolor service.

2 Part the hair into four sections.

3 Apply a protective cream around the hairline and over the ears.

4 Put on protective gloves.

5 Prepare the lightening formula, and use it immediately.

6 Place cotton around and through all four sections to protect the scalp so the lightener does not contact the scalp.

PROCEDURE 21-9

Special Effects Haircoloring with Foil (Full Head) continued

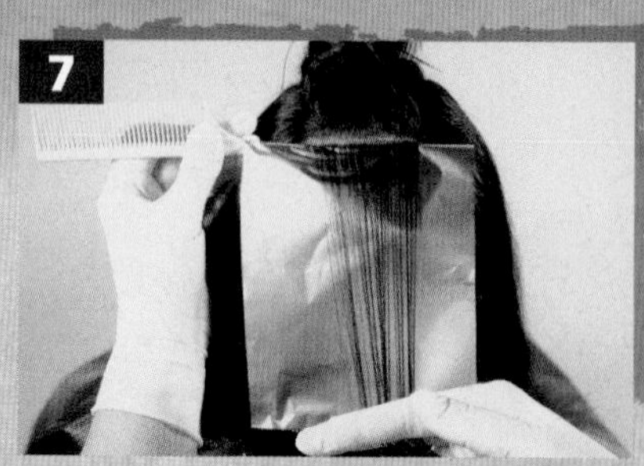

7 With a tail comb, take a slice of hair at the lower crown area of the head and place a piece of foil under the slice of hair.

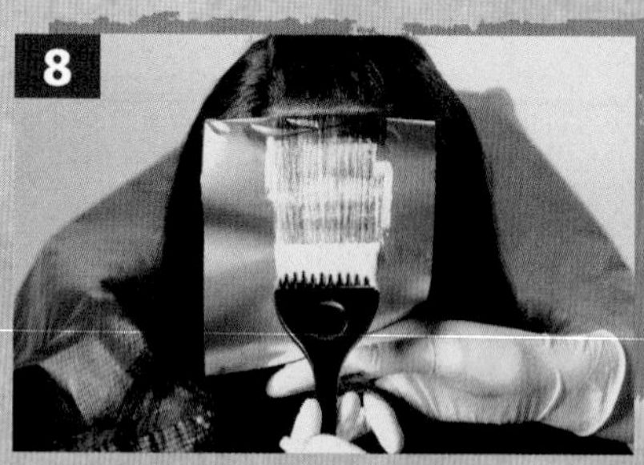

8 Holding the hair taut, brush on the lightener, from the upper edge of the foil to the hair ends.

9 Fold the foil in half until the ends meet.

10 Fold the foil in half again, using the comb to crease it.

11 Clip the foil upward.

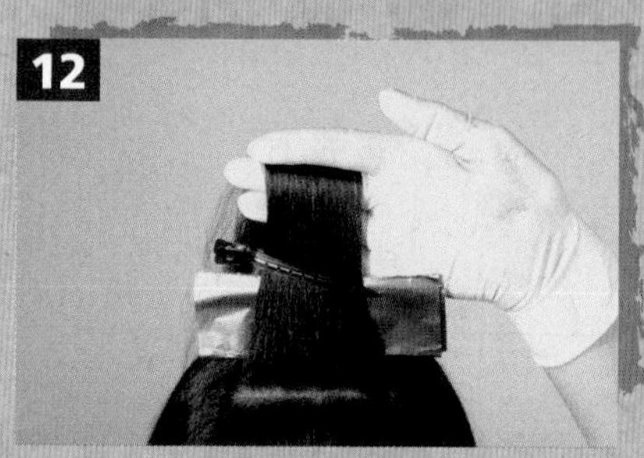

12 Take a ¾-inch (1.8 centimeters) subsection in between foils. Clip this hair up and out of the way. Note the contrast in size between the foiled and unfoiled subsections.

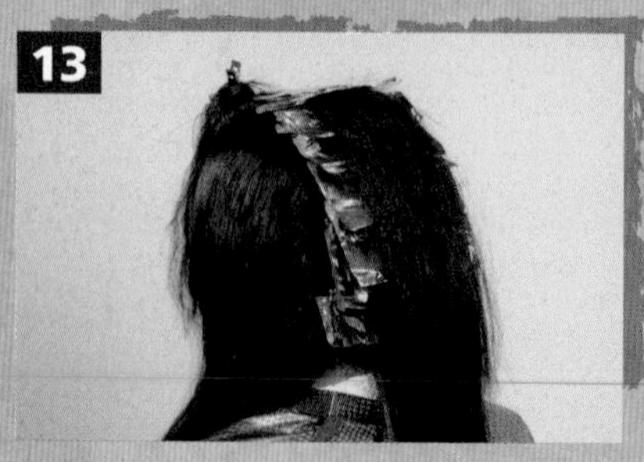

13 Continue working down the back center of the head until the section is complete.

14 Once the section is complete, release the clipped-up foils.

15 Work around the head to the side area; divide it into two smaller sections.

16 Work down the side, bring fine slices of hair into the foil, and apply lightener to the hair. Clip up the foil.

17 Move to the other side of the head and complete the matching sections.

18 Move to the top of the head. Take a fine slice of hair off the top of a large section, place it on the foil, and apply lightener.

© Milady, a part of Cengage Learning. Photography by Yanik Chauvin.

19 Part a larger section and then take a fine slice from the top of this section. Apply lightener.

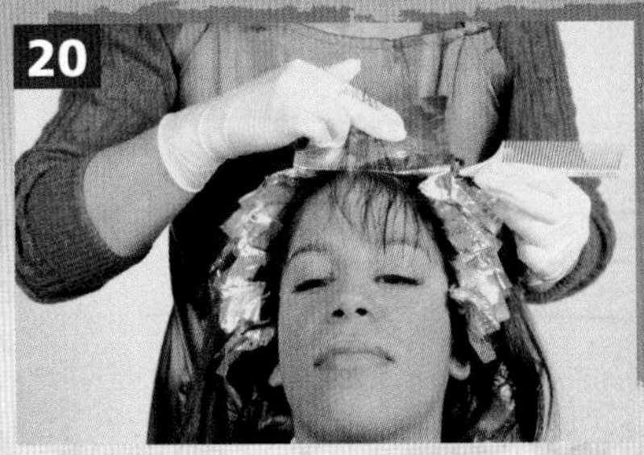

20 Continue toward the front until the last foil is placed.

21 Allow the lightener to process according to the strand test. Check the foils for the desired lightness.

22 Remove the foils one at a time at the shampoo area. Rinse the hair immediately to prevent the color from affecting the untreated hair.

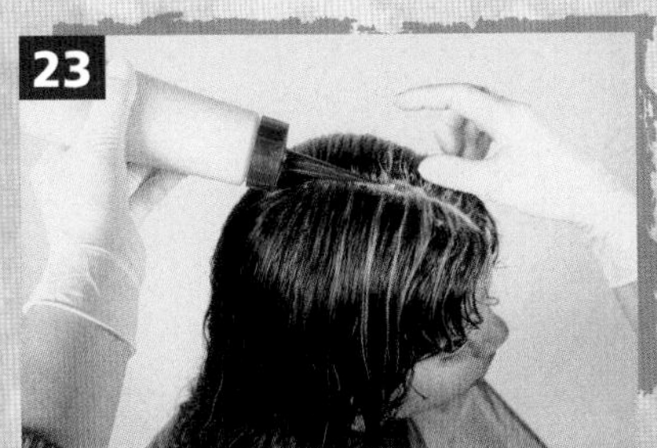

23 Apply a haircolor glaze to the hair, from scalp to ends. A haircolor glaze is an optional service added on to a highlighting to add shine to the finished result.

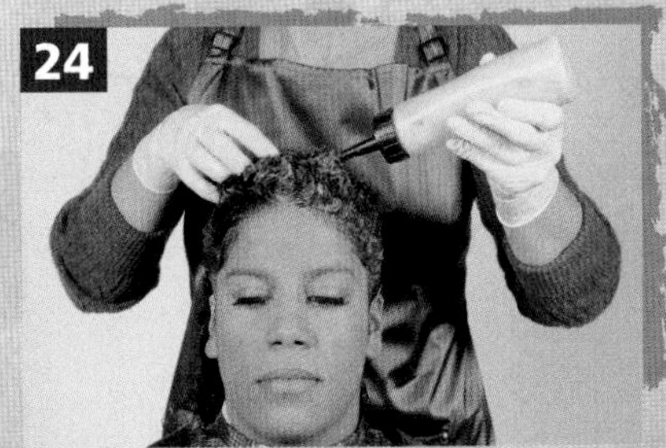

24 Work the glaze into the hair to make sure it is completely saturated and process per the manufacturer's directions.

25 Rinse the hair, shampoo, condition, and style the hair as desired.

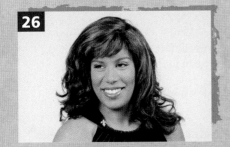

26 Finished look.

© Milady, a part of Cengage Learning. Photography by Yanik Chauvin.

Post Service

- Complete PROCEDURE 15-2 **Post-Service Procedure** **SEE PAGE 326**

Review Questions

1. Why do people color their hair?
2. How does the hair's porosity affect haircolor?
3. How many types of melanin are found in hair? Describe each.
4. What are levels? What does the level system help you to determine when formulating haircolor?
5. Name the primary, secondary, and tertiary colors.
6. What is the role of tone and intensity in haircolor?
7. What are the categories of haircolor? Briefly describe each one.
8. How does hydrogen peroxide developer work in a haircolor formula?
9. What are the four key questions to ask when formulating a haircolor?
10. Why is a patch test useful in haircoloring?
11. What is a preliminary strand test and why is it used?
12. Explain the action of hair lighteners.
13. What is the procedure for a virgin single-process color service?
14. What are the two processes involved in double-process haircoloring?
15. Name and describe the various forms of hair lightener.
16. What is the purpose of toner? When is it used?
17. What are the three most commonly used methods for highlighting? Describe each.
18. List seven tips for achieving gray coverage.
19. List the rules of color correction.
20. List five safety precautions to follow during the haircolor process.

Chapter Glossary

activators	Also known as *boosters*, *protinators*, or *accelerators*; powdered persulfate salts added to haircolor to increase its lightening ability.
aniline derivatives	Contain small, uncolored dyes that combine with hydrogen peroxide to form larger, permanent dye molecules within the cortex.
baliage	Also known as *free-form technique*; painting a lightener (usually a powdered off-the-scalp lightener) directly onto clean, styled hair.
base color	Predominant tone of a color.
cap technique	Lightening technique that involves pulling clean, dry strands of hair through a perforated cap with a thin plastic or metal hook, and then combing them to remove tangles.
color fillers	Equalize porosity and deposit color in one application to provide a uniform contributing pigment on prelightened hair.
complementary colors	A primary and secondary color positioned directly opposite each other on the color wheel.
conditioner fillers	Used to recondition damaged, overly porous hair and equalize porosity so that the hair accepts the color evenly from strand to strand and scalp to ends.
contributing pigment	Also known as *undertone*; the varying degrees of warmth exposed during a permanent color or lightening process.
demipermanent haircolor	Also known as *no-lift deposit-only color*; formulated to deposit but not lift (lighten) natural hair color.

Chapter Glossary

developers	Also known as *oxidizing agents* or *catalysts*; when mixed with an oxidation haircolor, supplies the necessary oxygen gas to develop color molecules and create a change in hair color.
double-process application	Also known as *two-step coloring*; a coloring technique requiring two separate procedures in which the hair is prelightened before the depositing color is applied to the hair.
fillers	Used to equalize porosity.
foil technique	Highlighting technique that involves coloring selected strands of hair by slicing or weaving out sections, placing them on foil or plastic wrap, applying lightener or permanent haircolor, and then sealing them in the foil or plastic wrap.
glaze	A nonammonia color that adds shine and tone to the hair.
hair color	The natural color of hair.
hair lightening	Also known as *bleaching* or *decolorizing*; chemical process involving the diffusion of the natural hair color pigment or artificial haircolor from the hair.
haircolor	Professional, salon industry term referring to artificial haircolor products and services.
haircolor glaze	Common way to describe a haircolor service that adds shine and color to the hair.
highlighting	Coloring some of the hair strands lighter than the natural color to add a variety of lighter shades and the illusion of depth.
highlighting shampoo	Colors prepared by combining permanent haircolor, hydrogen peroxide, and shampoo.
hydrogen peroxide developer	Oxidizing agent that, when mixed with an oxidation haircolor, supplies the necessary oxygen gas to develop the color molecules and create a change in natural hair color.
intensity	The strength of a color.
law of color	System for understanding color relationships.
level	The unit of measurement used to identify the lightness or darkness of a color.
level system	System that colorists use to determine the lightness or darkness of a hair color.
lighteners	Chemical compounds that lighten hair by dispersing, dissolving, and decolorizing the natural hair pigment.
line of demarcation	Visible line separating colored hair from new growth.
metallic haircolors	Also known as *gradual haircolors*; haircolors containing metal salts that change hair color gradually by progressive buildup and exposure to air creating a dull, metallic appearance.
mixed melanin	Combination of natural hair color that contains both pheomelanin and eumelanin.
natural haircolors	Also known as *vegetable haircolors*; colors, such as henna, obtained from the leaves or bark of plants.
new growth	Part of the hair shaft between the scalp and the hair that has been previously colored.
off-the-scalp lighteners	Also known as *quick lighteners*; powdered lighteners that cannot be used directly on the scalp.
on-the-scalp lighteners	Lighteners that can be used directly on the scalp by mixing the lightener with activators.

Chapter Glossary

patch test	Also known as a *predisposition test*; test required by the Federal Food, Drug, and Cosmetic Act for identifying a possible allergy in a client.
permanent haircolors	Lighten and deposit color at the same time and in a single process because they are more alkaline than no-lift deposit-only colors and are usually mixed with a higher-volume developer.
prelightening	First step of double-process haircoloring, used to lift or lighten the natural pigment before the application of toner.
presoftening	Process of treating gray or very resistant hair to allow for better penetration of color.
primary colors	Pure or fundamental colors (red, yellow, and blue) that cannot be created by combining other colors.
resistant	Hair type that is difficult for moisture or chemicals to penetrate, and thus requires a longer processing time.
reverse highlighting	Also known as *lowlighting*; technique of coloring strands of hair darker than the natural color.
secondary color	Color obtained by mixing equal parts of two primary colors.
semipermanent haircolor	No-lift deposit-only nonoxidation haircolor that is not mixed with peroxide and is formulated to last through several shampoos.
single-process haircoloring	Process that lightens and deposits color in the hair in a single application.
slicing	Coloring technique that involves taking a narrow, ⅛-inch (0.3 centimeters) section of hair by making a straight part at the scalp, positioning the hair over the foil, and applying lightener or color.
soap cap	Combination of equal parts of a prepared permanent color mixture and shampoo used the last five minutes and worked through the hair to refresh the ends.
special effects haircoloring	Any technique that involves partial lightening or coloring.
strand test	Determines how the hair will react to the color formula and how long the formula should be left on the hair.
temporary haircolor	Nonpermanent color whose large pigment molecules prevent penetration of the cuticle layer, allowing only a coating action that may be removed by shampooing.
tertiary color	Intermediate color achieved by mixing a secondary color and its neighboring primary color on the color wheel in equal amounts.
tone	Also known as *hue*; the balance of color.
toners	Semipermanent, demipermanent, and permanent haircolor products that are used primarily on prelightened hair to achieve pale and delicate colors.
virgin application	First time the hair is colored.
volume	Measures the concentration and strength of hydrogen peroxide.
weaving	Coloring technique in which selected strands are picked up from a narrow section of hair with a zigzag motion of the comb, and lightener or color is applied only to these strands.

PART 4 SKIN CARE

Chapters

© IKO, 2010; used under license from Shutterstock.com.

CHAPTER 22

Hair Removal

Chapter Outline

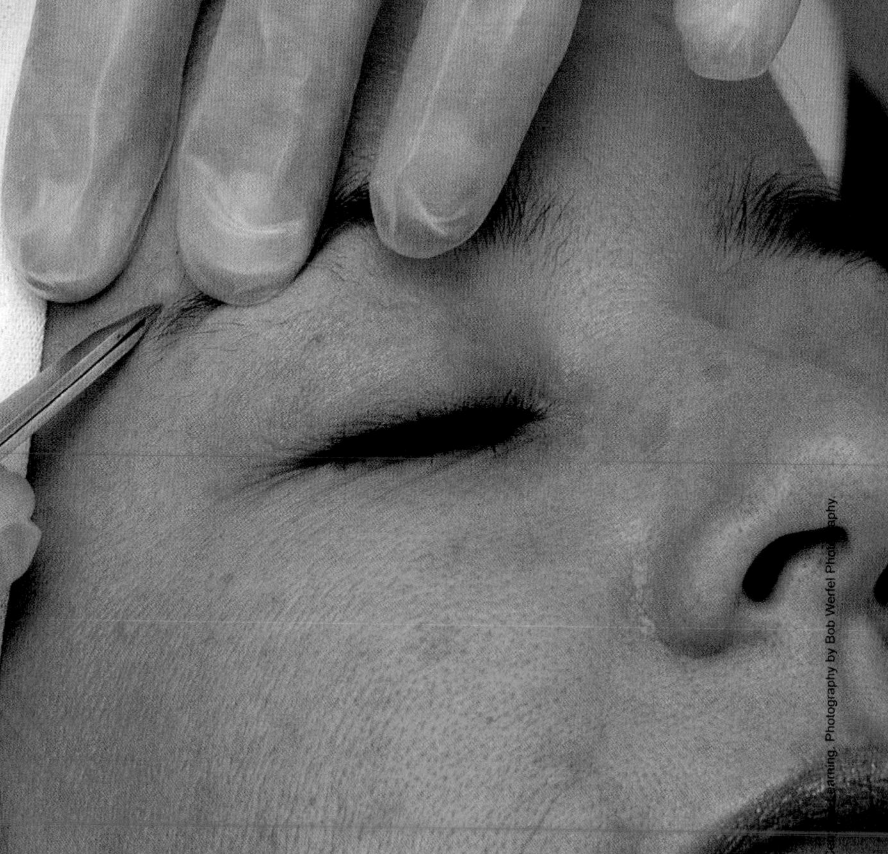

© Milady, a part of Cengage Learning. Photography by Bob Werfel Photography.

Learning Objectives

After completing this chapter, you will be able to:

- ✓ **LO1** Describe the elements of a client consultation for hair removal.
- ✓ **LO2** Name the conditions that contraindicate hair removal in the salon.
- ✓ **LO3** Identify and describe three methods of permanent hair removal.
- ✓ **LO4** Demonstrate the techniques involved in temporary hair removal.

Key Terms

Page number indicates where in the chapter the term is used.

Brazilian bikini waxing
pg. 688

depilatory
pg. 693

electrolysis
pg. 692

epilator
pg. 694

health screening form
pg. 689

hirsuties (hypertrichosis)
pg. 688

hirsutism
pg. 688

laser hair removal
pg. 692

photoepilation (Intense Pulsed Light)
pg. 692

sugaring
pg. 695

threading
pg. 695

tweezing
pg. 693

One of the fastest growing services in the salon and spa businesses is hair removal. Once restricted to an occasional lip or brow service, a growing number of clients want to have their entire face, arms, and legs bare of hair.

Bikini hair removal has also evolved into its own art form, with different designs becoming sought-after services by many clients. **Brazilian bikini waxing,** a waxing technique that requires the removal of all the hair from the front and the back of the bikini area, is a popular style of waxing. The method was named for the completely hairless look required when wearing a Brazilian style bikini. Brazilian bikini waxing requires more specific training than offered in this book. Ask your instructor about advanced courses in Brazilian bikini waxing.

Many men are now frequently requesting hair removal services. It has become a fashion trend for men to have hairless legs, arms, and even chests. Men who participate in sports such as cycling, swimming, body building, and soccer often remove hair from the legs and arms, and occasionally the entire body. The nape of the neck, chest, and back are the most frequent removal requests for men.

The most common form of hair removal in salons and spas is waxing, but with the popularity of these services on the rise, many different methods are now coming into play.

Hirsuties (hur-SOO-shee-eez), also known as **hypertrichosis** (hy-pur-trih-KOH-sis), refers to the growth of an unusual amount of hair on parts of the body normally bearing only downy hair, such as the faces of women and the backs of men. **Hirsutism (HUR-suh-tiz-um)** is an excessive growth or cover of hair, especially in women. Clients with an overabundance of hair are certainly the best candidates for hair removal, although many clients with even just a few unwanted hairs on their arms or legs are now requesting these services.

Facial and body hair removal has become increasingly popular as evolving technology makes it easier to perform with more effective results. All of the various approaches to hair removal fall into two major categories: permanent and temporary. Salon techniques are generally limited to temporary methods.

Why Study Hair Removal?

Cosmetologists should study and have a thorough understanding of hair removal because:

- Removing unwanted hair is a primary concern for many clients, and being able to advise them on the various types of hair removal will enhance your ability to satisfy your clients.
- Offering clients hair removal services that meet their needs and can be scheduled while they are already in the salon can be a valuable extra service you can offer.

© Luba V Nel, 2010; used under license from Shutterstock.com.

- Learning the proper hair removal techniques and performing them safely makes you an even more important part of a client's beauty regimen.

Client Consultation

Before performing any hair removal service, a consultation is always necessary. Ask the client to complete a health screening form. Similar to an intake form, a **health screening form** is frequently used in skin care services and is a questionnaire that discloses all medications, both topical (applied to the skin) and oral (taken by mouth), along with any known skin disorders or allergies that might affect treatment (**Figure 22–1**). Allergies or sensitivities must be noted, highlighted, and documented on the service record card—the client's permanent progress record of services received, and products purchased or used. Keep in mind that many changes can occur between client visits. Since a client's last visit, he or she may have been prescribed medications such as antidepressants, hormones, cortisone, medicine for blood pressure or diabetes, or topical prescriptions such as Retin-A®, Renova®, and hydroquinone. A client using any one of these prescriptions may not be a candidate for hair removal. See **Figure 22–2** for a sample health screening form.

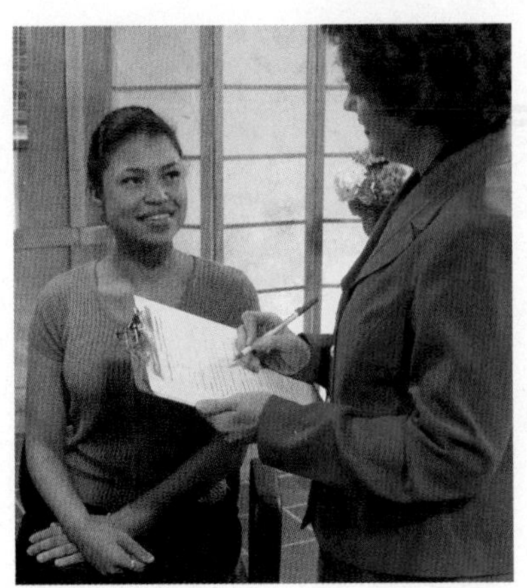

© Milady, a part of Cengage Learning. Photography by Larry Hamill.

▲ **Figure 22–1**
Filling out a service record card.

▼ **Figure 22–2**
Health Screening Form.

HEALTH SCREENING FORM

Date ____________
Name ______________________________ Sex __________
Address ____
City ______________________________ State __________ Zip __________

1. Have you been seen by a dermatologist? Yes_____ No_____ If yes, for what reason? ____________ ____
2. Please list all medications that you take regularly. Include hormones, vitamins, and other similar supplements: ____
3. Do you take steroid drugs or prednisone? Yes _____ No _____
4. Have you ever used Accutane® (isotretinoin)? Yes _____ No _____ If yes, when did you stop taking Accutane® (isotretinoin)? ________
5. Do you use or have you recently used Retin-A®, Renova®, Tazorac®, Differin®, Azelex®, or any other medical peeling agent? Yes_____ No_____ If yes, for how long? __________
6. Do you have any allergies? Are you allergic to any medications? Yes_____ No_____
   If yes, please list allergies: ____
7. Are you pregnant or lactating? Yes_____ No_____
8. Have you had any of the following procedures?
   Laser resurfacing: Yes_____ Date_____ No_____
   Light chemical peel: Yes_____ Date____ No_____
   Medium/heavy chemical peel: Yes_____ Date_____ No_____
   Any microdermabrasion? Yes_____ Date_____ No_____
9. Do you ever experience tightness or flaking of your skin? Yes____ No_____
10. Do you frequent tanning booths? Yes_____ No_____
11. Do you have a history of fever blisters or cold sores? Yes_____ No_____

© Milady, a part of Cengage Learning.

Many of these medications cause changes in the skin that can cause epidermal skin to lift during waxing treatment. In other words, the epidermal skin can peel off along with the wax and the hair.

© Ra 2 Studio, 2010; used under license from Shutterstock.com.

Clients who have autoimmune diseases such as lupus can have reactions to the inflammation caused by waxing, electrolysis, or other hair removal methods.

Clients with conditions such as rosacea or eczema can experience severe inflammation, because these skin conditions are likely to already be inflamed before treatment.

It is imperative that every client fill out a release form for the hair removal service you are going to provide. This should be completed prior to every service. It serves as a reminder to the client to really think about any topical or oral medication they might have started since their last visit. See **Figure 22–3** for a sample release form.

☑ LO1

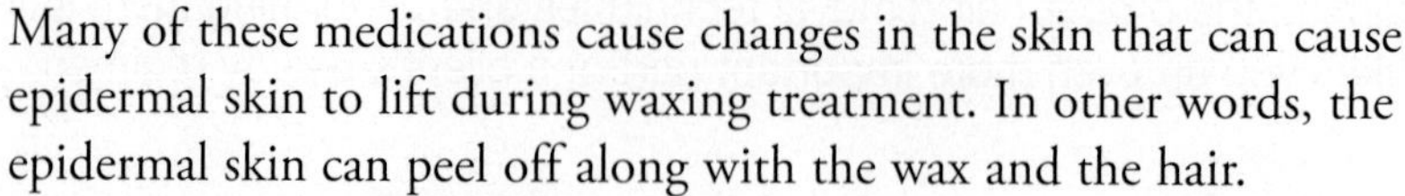

Contraindications for Hair Removal

One of the main purposes of a client consultation is to determine the presence of any contraindications for hair removal. Some medical conditions and medications may cause thinning of the skin or make the skin more vulnerable to injury. Waxing clients with these conditions could cause unnecessary inflammation or severe injuries to the skin. Clients should not have any waxing or

▼ **Figure 22–3**
Sample release form.

RELEASE FORM FOR HAIR REMOVAL

I,______________________________, am_____ am not_____ presently using:

_____ Retin-A, or any other topical prescription medication

_____ Accutane: (isotretinoin)

_____ any alphahydroxy-based products

_____ any medications such as cortisone, blood thinners, or diabetic medication

_____ I understand that if I begin using any of the above products and do not inform my esthetician/cosmetologist prior to hair removal, I am accepting full responsibility for any skin reactions.

_____ The hair removal process has been thoroughly explained to me, and I have had an opportunity to ask questions and receive satisfactory answers.

Client's Signature______________________________ Date______________

Technician's Signature______________________________ Date______________

© Milady, a part of Cengage Learning.

hair removal performed anywhere on the body if one or more of the following is the case, without first obtaining written permission from their physician:

- Client is using or has used isotretinoin (Accutane) in the last six months.
- Client is taking blood-thinning medications.
- Client is taking drugs for autoimmune diseases, including lupus.
- Client is taking predisone or steroids.
- Client has psoriasis, eczema, or other chronic skin diseases.
- Client has a sunburn.
- Client has pustules or papules in area to be waxed.
- Client has recently had cosmetic or reconstructive surgery within the previous three months.
- Client has recently had a laser skin treatment on the body.
- Client has severe varicose leg veins.
- Client has any other questionable medical condition.

Facial waxing should not be performed on clients with any of the following conditions, without first obtaining permission from their physician:

- Client has rosacea or very sensitive skin.
- Client has a history of fever blisters or cold sores. (Waxing can cause a flare-up of this condition without medical pretreatment.)
- Client has had a recent chemical peel using glycolic, alpha hydroxy, or salicylic acid, or other acid-based products.
- Client has recently had microdermabrasion.
- Client uses any exfoliating topical medication, including Retin-A®, Renova®, Tazorac®, Differin®, Azelex®, or other medical peeling agent.
- Client has recently had laser skin treatment or surgical peel.
- Client uses hydroquinone for skin lightening. ☑ **LO2**

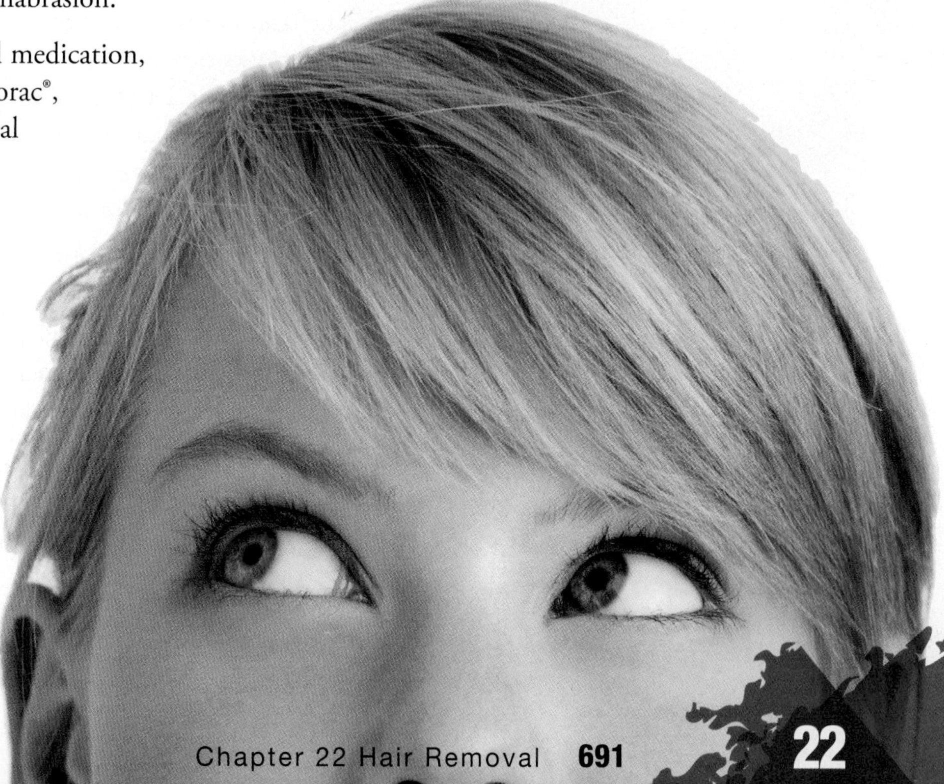

© Yuri Arcurs, 2010; used under license from Shutterstock.com.

Permanent Hair Removal

Although permanent hair removal services are not often offered in salons, it is useful to know the options that exist. Permanent hair removal methods include electrolysis, photoepilation (light-based hair removal), and laser hair removal.

Electrolysis

Electrolysis is the removal of hair by means of an electric current that destroys the growth cells of the hair. The current is applied with a very fine, needle-shaped electrode that is inserted into each hair follicle. This technique must only be performed by a licensed electrologist.

Photoepilation

Photoepilation, also known as **Intense Pulsed Light** (IPL), uses intense light to destroy the growth cells of the hair follicles. This treatment has minimal side effects, requires no needles, and thus minimizes the risk of infection. Clinical studies have shown that photoepilation can provide 50 to 60 percent clearance of hair in twelve weeks. This method can be administered in some salons by cosmetologists and estheticians, depending on state law. Manufacturers of photoepilation equipment generally provide the special training necessary for administering this procedure.

Laser Hair Removal

Lasers are another method for the rapid removal of unwanted hair. In **laser hair removal,** a laser beam is pulsed on the skin, impairing hair growth. It is most effective when used on follicles that are in the growth or anagen phase.

The laser method was discovered by chance when it was noted that birthmarks treated with certain types of lasers became permanently devoid of hair. Lasers are not for everyone; an absolute requirement is that one's hair must be darker than the surrounding skin. Coarse, dark hair responds best to laser treatment. For some clients, this method produces permanent hair removal. For other clients, laser hair removal treatments simply slow down regrowth.

In certain states, cosmetologists or estheticians are allowed to perform laser hair removal under a doctor's supervision. This method requires specialized training, most commonly offered by laser equipment manufacturers.

Laws regarding photoepilation and laser hair removal services vary by state, so be sure to check with your regulatory agency for guidelines. ☑ **LO3**

© Maksim Toome, 2010; used under license from Shutterstock.com.

Temporary Hair Removal

Temporary methods of hair removal, some of which may be offered in the salon or spa, are discussed below.

Shaving

The most common form of temporary hair removal, particularly of men's facial hair, is shaving. The targeted area should be softened by applying a warm, moist towel, and then applying a shaving cream or lotion that has excellent lubrication qualities and calms the skin. An electric clipper may also be used, particularly to remove unwanted hair at the nape of the neck. The application of a preshaving lotion helps to reduce any irritation. An electric trimmer can also make short work of unwanted hair at the nape of the neck.

did you know?

Contrary to popular belief, shaving does not cause the hair to grow thicker or stronger. It only seems that way because the razor blunts the hair ends and makes them feel stiff.

Tweezing

Tweezing is using tweezers to remove hairs, commonly used to shape the eyebrows, and can also be used to remove undesirable hairs from around the mouth and chin. Eyebrow arching is often done as part of a professional makeup service. Correctly shaped eyebrows have a strong, positive impact on the overall attractiveness of the face. The natural arch of the eyebrow follows the orbital bone, or the curved line of the eye socket, but hair can grow both above and below the natural line. These hairs should be removed to give a clean and attractive appearance.

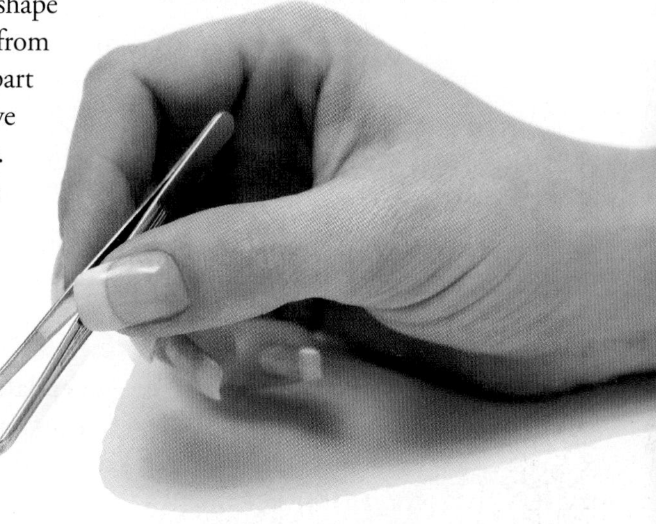

© Marc Dietrich, 2010; used under license from Shutterstock.com.

PROCEDURE 22-3 Eyebrow Tweezing SEE PAGE 701

Depilatories

A **depilatory** is a substance, usually a caustic alkali preparation, used for the temporary removal of superfluous hair by dissolving it at the skin's surface. It contains detergents to strip the sebum from the hair and adhesives to hold the chemicals to the hair shaft for the five to ten minutes necessary to remove the hair. During the application time, the hair expands and the disulfide bonds break. Finally, such chemicals as sodium hydroxide, potassium hydroxide, thioglycolic acid, or calcium thioglycolate destroy the disulfide bonds. These chemicals turn the hair into a soft, jelly-like mass that can be scraped from the skin. Although depilatories are not commonly used in salons, you should be familiar with them in the event that your clients have used them.

Depilatories can be inflammatory to skin, and should not be used on sensitive skin types or on clients who have contraindications for waxing. It is a good idea to patch test any depilatory on your client's skin prior to treatment the first time. Select a hairless part of the arm, apply a small

BODY AREA	APPROPRIATE HAIR REMOVAL PROCEDURES		
	WAXING	TWEEZING	DEPILATORIES
FACE/UPPER LIPS/EYEBROWS	X	X	
UNDERARMS	X		
ARMS	X		X
BIKINI LINE	X	X	
BACK/SHOULDERS	X	X (after waxing or sugaring)	X
LEGS	X		X
TOPS OF FEET/TOES	X		X

© Milady, a part of Cengage Learning.

Table 22–1 Appropriate Hair Removal Procedures.

amount according to the manufacturer's directions, and leave it on the skin for seven to ten minutes. If there are no signs of redness, swelling, or rash, the depilatory can probably be used safely over a larger area of the skin. Follow the manufacturer's directions for application.

For an easy reference guide for which type of hair removal procedure is appropriate for various areas of the body, refer to **Table 22–1**.

FOCUS ON

CLIENT CONSULTATION – EYEBROW DESIGN

As with any procedure, always perform a client consultation prior to tweezing or waxing the eyebrows. Determine the client's wishes for final eyebrow shape. If you remove too much hair, it will generally grow back, but regrowth may take several months. You will also end up with an unhappy client who is not likely to return for your services. Conducting a thorough consultation beforehand will help you avoid such mistakes.

Epilators

An **epilator** removes the hair from the bottom of the follicle. Wax is a commonly used epilator, applied in either hot or cold form as recommended by the manufacturer. Both products are made primarily of resins and beeswax. Cold wax is somewhat thicker and does not require fabric strips for removal. Because waxing removes the hair from the bottom of the follicle, the hair takes longer to grow back. The time between waxings is generally four to six weeks.

Wax may be applied to various parts of the face and body, such as the eyebrows, cheeks, chin, upper lip, arms, and legs. On male clients, wax may be used to remove hair on the back and nape of the neck. The hair should be at least ¼-inch (0.6 centimeters) long for waxing to be effective. Hair shorter than ¼ inch may not adhere to the wax. If hair is more than ½-inch long, it should be trimmed before waxing.

Be aware that removing vellus (lanugo) hair may cause the skin to temporarily feel less soft. When waxing is done properly, the hair will not feel like beard stubble as it grows out.

Before beginning a wax treatment, be sure that the client completes a health screening form, and have the client sign a release form. Wear disposable gloves to prevent contact with bloodborne pathogens.

Safety Precautions for Hot and Cold Waxing

- To prevent burns, always test the temperature of the heated wax before applying to the client's skin. Use a professional wax heater for warming wax. Never heat wax in a microwave or on a stove top. Wax can become overheated and burn the client's skin.
- Use caution so that the wax does not come in contact with the eyes.
- Do not apply wax over warts, moles, abrasions, or irritated or inflamed skin. Do not remove hair protruding from a mole, because the wax could cause trauma to the mole.
- The skin under the arms is sometimes very sensitive. If so, use cold wax.
- Redness and swelling sometimes occur after waxing sensitive skin. Apply an aloe gel and cool compresses to calm and soothe the skin.

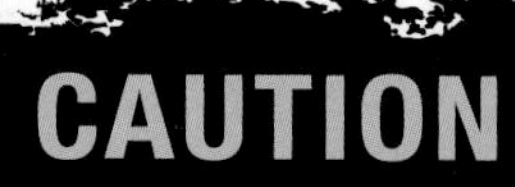

Beeswax can sometimes cause allergic reactions. Always give a small patch test of the product to be used prior to the service.

PROCEDURE 22-4 Eyebrow Waxing SEE PAGE 703

PROCEDURE 22-5 Body Waxing SEE PAGE 705

Threading

Threading is a temporary hair removal method whereby cotton thread is twisted and rolled along the surface of the skin, entwining the hair in the thread and lifting it from the follicle. The technique is still practiced in many Eastern cultures today. Threading has become increasingly popular in the United States as an alternative to other methods. It requires specialized training.

Sugaring

Sugaring is another temporary hair removal method that involves the use of a thick, sugar-based paste and is especially appropriate for more sensitive skin types. Sugaring is becoming more popular and produces the same results as hot or cold wax. One advantage with sugaring is the hair can be removed even if it is only ⅛-inch long.

Removing the residue from the skin is simple, as it dissolves with warm water. ☑ **LO4**

FYI

Threading, sugaring, and specialty waxing, such as Brazilian waxing, are advanced techniques that require additional training and experience. Check with your instructor about advanced training that is often available at trade shows and seminars, as well as through videos.

© Luba V Nel, 2010; used under license from Shutterstock.com.

PROCEDURE 22-1

Pre-Service Procedure

A. Preparing the Facial Room

Check your room supply of linens (towels and sheets) and replenish as needed.

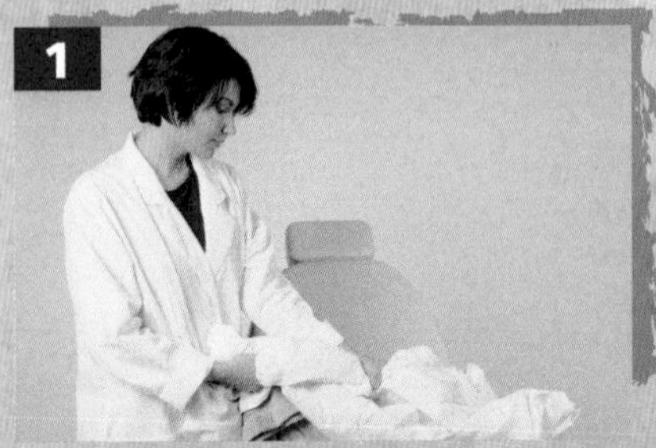

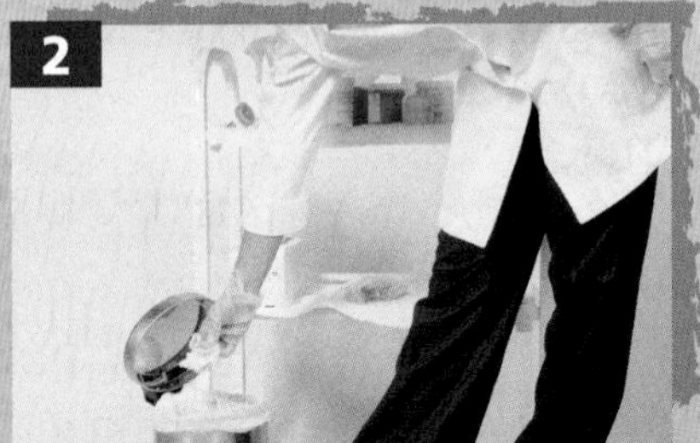

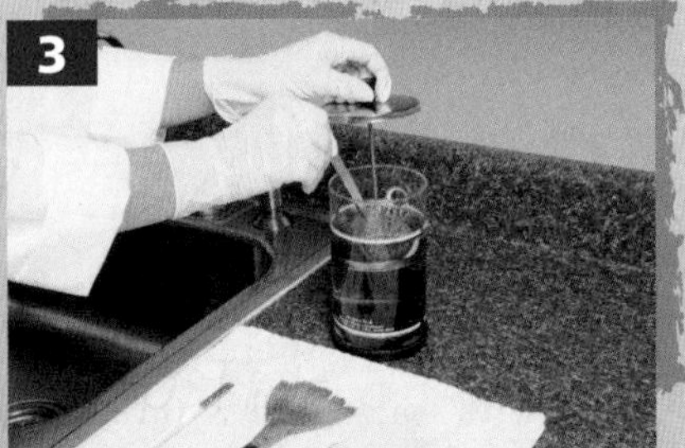

1 Change the bed or treatment chair linens.

2 Throw away any disposables used during the previous service.

3 Clean and disinfect any used brushes or implements, such as mask brushes, comedo extractors, tweezers, machine attachments, and electrodes.

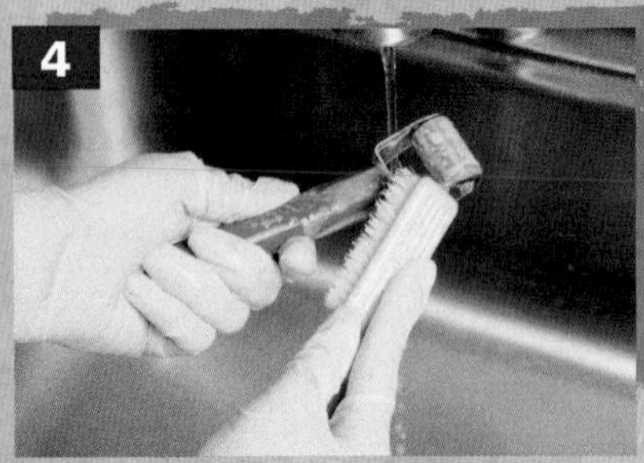

4 Clean and disinfect any machine parts used during the previous service.

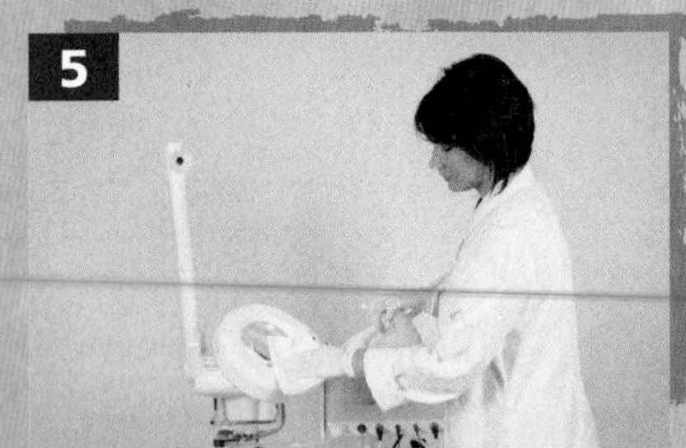

5 Clean and disinfect counters and magnifying lamp or lens.

6 Check water level on vaporizer as needed.

© Milady, a part of Cengage Learning. Photography by Yanik Chauvin.

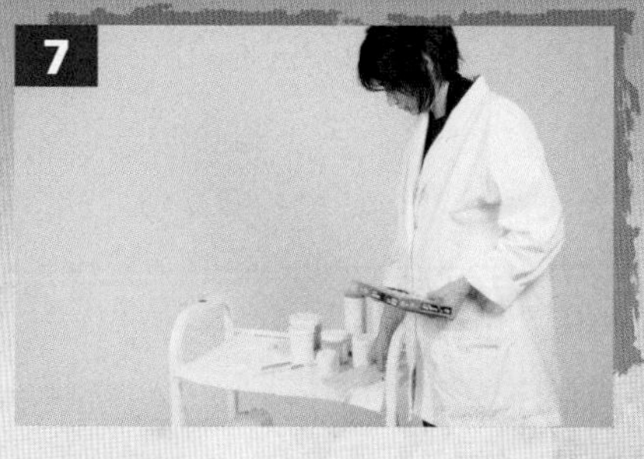

7 Replace any disposable implements you may need, such as gloves, sheet cotton, gauze squares, sponges for cleansing and makeup, disposable makeup applicators (mascara wands, lip brushes, other brushes), spatulas and tongue-depressor wax applicators, cotton swabs, facial tissue, and wax strips.

8 Prepare to greet your next client.

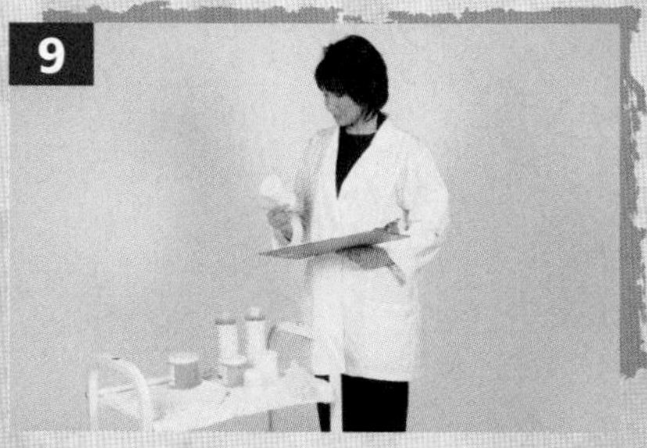

9 Review your client schedule for the day and decide which products you are likely to need for each service. Make sure you have enough of all the products you will be using that day. You may have to retrieve additional product from the dispensary. This is also a good time to refresh your mind about each repeat client you will be seeing that day and his or her individual concerns.

10 Your room should be ready to go from the previous night's thorough cleaning and disinfecting. (See "At the End of the Day" in Procedure 22–2, Post-Service Procedure.)

B. Preparing for the Client

11 Retrieve the client's intake form or service record card and review it. If the appointment is for a new client, let the receptionist know that the client will need an intake form.

12 Organize yourself by taking care of your personal needs before the client arrives—use the restroom, get a drink of water, return a personal call—so that when your client arrives, you can place your full attention on her needs.

13 Turn off cell phone, pager, or PDA. Be sure that you eliminate anything that can distract you from your client while she is in the salon.

14 Take a moment to clear your head of all your personal concerns and issues. Take a couple of deep breaths and remind yourself that you are committed to providing your clients with fantastic service and your full attention.

15 Wash your hands following Procedure 5–3, Proper Hand Washing, before going to greet your client.

Service Tip

Before servicing a client, take a moment to sit on your bed or facial chair and take a good look around. Based on what you see, hear, and feel, ask yourself this question: What kind of an experience will my client have while she is here?

Answering the following questions will enable you to provide your client with a positive experience:

- Is my room clean and organized or cluttered and messy?
- Will the music and the temperature be comfortable for the client?
- Am I wearing too much perfume/cologne? Am I carrying an unpleasant food or tobacco odor? Is my breath pleasant smelling?
- When I look at myself in the mirror, do I see the professional I want to be? Does my personal grooming—my hair, makeup, and clothing—look professional?
- Do I look as if I am happy and enjoying my work?
- Is there some problem bothering me today that is affecting my ability to concentrate on the needs of my client?

Remember the old adage: You only get one chance to make a good first impression. Stack the odds in your favor!

© Milady, a part of Cengage Learning. Photography by Yanik Chauvin.

Pre-Service Procedure continued

C. Greet Client

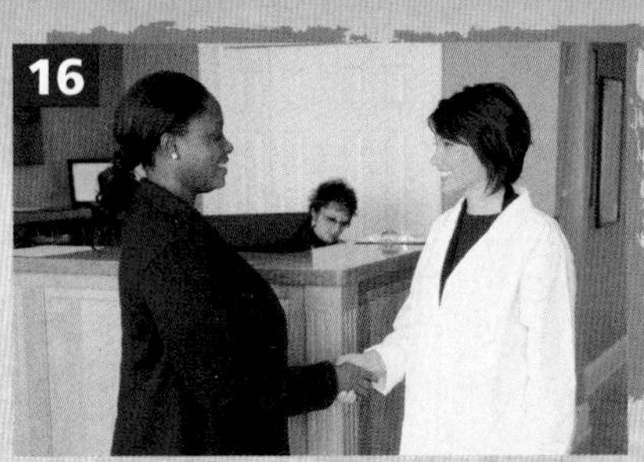
16

16 Greet your client in the reception area with a warm smile and in a professional manner. Introduce yourself if you've never met, and shake hands. The handshake is the first acceptance by the client of your touch, so be sure your handshake is firm and sincere. If the client is new, ask her for the intake form she filled out in the reception area.

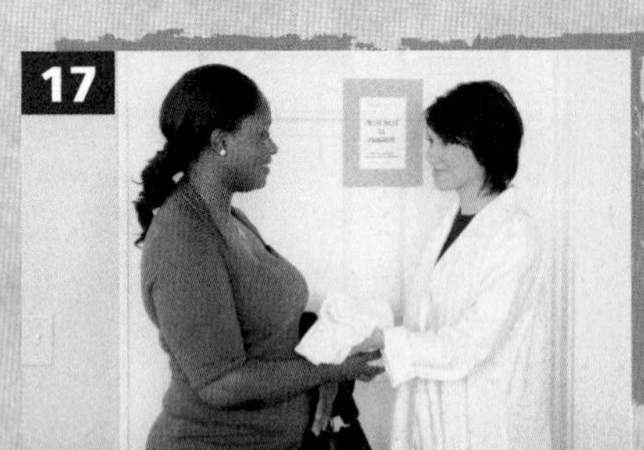
17

17 Escort the client to the changing area for her to change into a smock or robe. Make sure you tell her where to securely place her personal items. If you do not have a changing room or lockers, she will need to change in the treatment room.

18 Ask the client to remove all jewelry and put it in a safe place, because you do not want to stop the service for her to remove the jewelry later.

19 Invite her to take a seat in the treatment chair or to lie down on the treatment table.

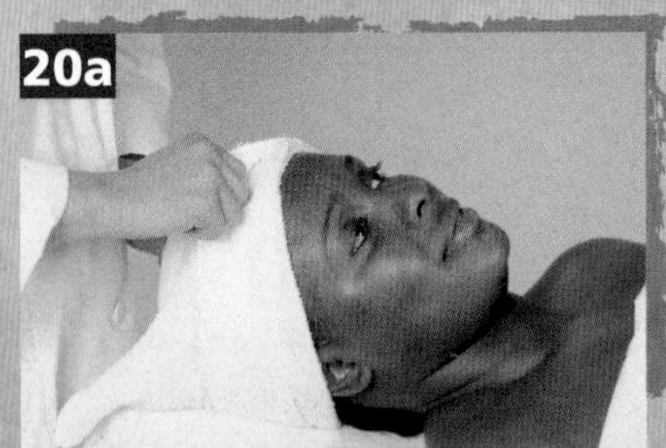
20a

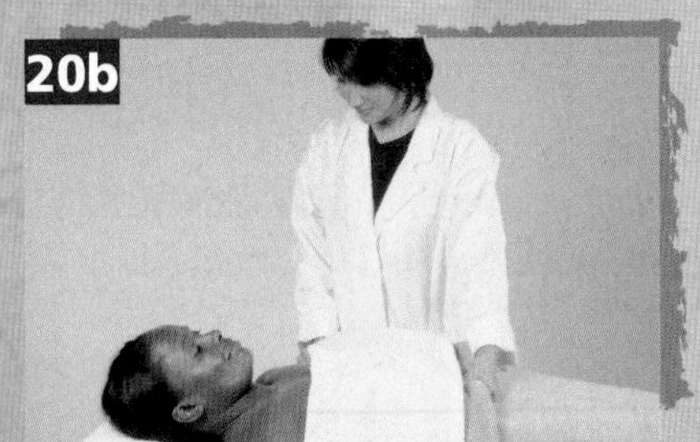
20b

20 Drape the client properly and either place her hair in a protective cap or use a headband and towels to drape her hair properly. Give her a blanket and make sure she is comfortable before beginning the service. Remember, the client is not just a waxing or another service, but a person you want to build a relationship with. By first showing clients respect, you will begin to gain their trust in you as a professional. Openness, honesty, and sincerity are always the most successful approach in winning clients' trust, respect, and, ultimately, their loyalty.

21 Perform a consultation before beginning the service. If you are servicing a returning client, ask how her skin has been since her last treatment. If the client is new, discuss the information on the intake form, and ask any questions you have regarding her skin or any conditions listed on the form. Determine a course of action for the treatment, and briefly explain your plan to the client.

© Milady, a part of Cengage Learning. Photography by Yanik Chauvin.

PROCEDURE 22-2

Post-Service Procedure

A. Advise Clients and Promote Products

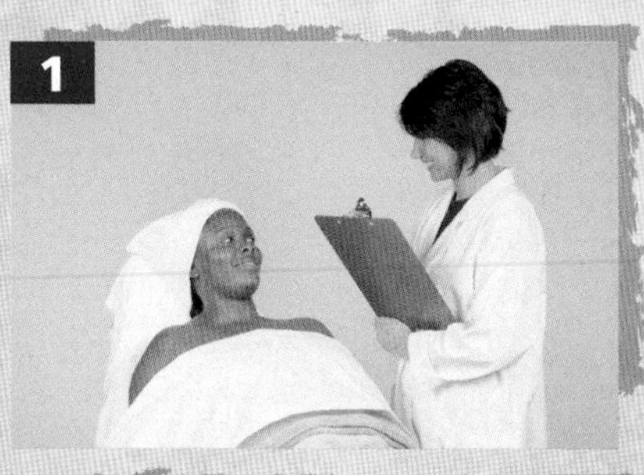

1

1 Before your client leaves your treatment area, ask her how she feels and if she enjoyed the service. Explain the conditions of her skin and your ideas about how to improve them. Be sure to ask if she has any questions or anything else she wishes to discuss. Be receptive and listen. Never be defensive. Determine a plan for future visits. Give the client ideas to think over for the next visit.

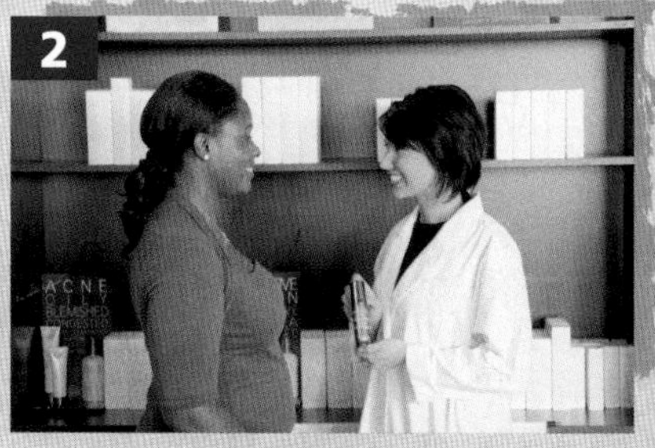

2

2 Advise client about proper home care and explain how the recommended professional products will help to improve any skin conditions that are present. This is the time to discuss your retail product recommendations. Explain that these products are important and explain how to use them.

B. Schedule Next Appointment and Thank Client

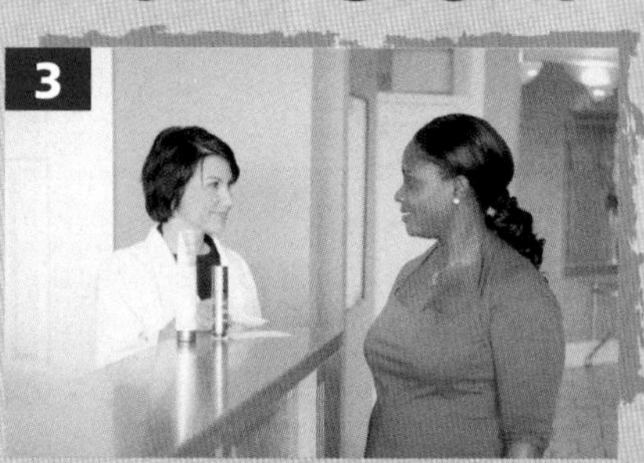

3

3 Escort the client to the reception desk and write up a service ticket for the client that includes the service provided, the recommended home care, and the next visit/service that needs to be scheduled. Place all recommended professional retail home-care products on the counter for the client. Review the service ticket and the product recommendations with your client.

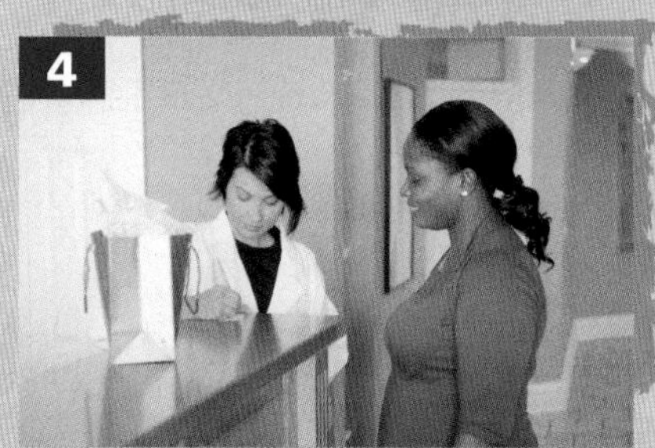

4

4 After the client has paid for her service and take-home products, ask if you can schedule her next appointment. Set up the date, time, and type of service for this next appointment, write the information on your business card, and give the card to the client.

© Milady, a part of Cengage Learning. Photography by Yanik Chauvin.

Post-Service Procedure continued

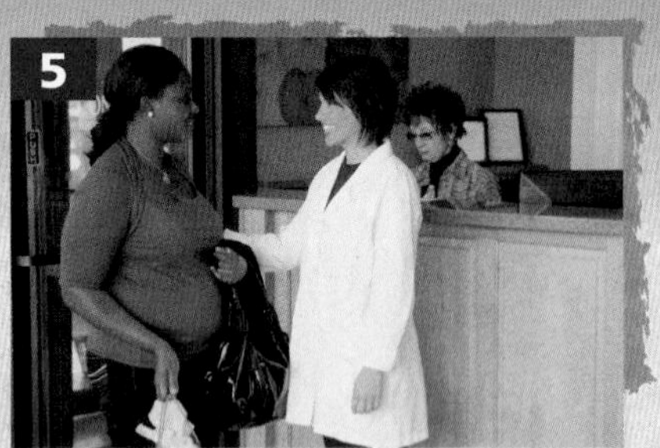

5 Thank the client for the opportunity to work with her. Express an interest in working with her in the future. Invite her to contact you should she have any questions or concerns about the service provided. If the client seems apprehensive, offer to call her in a day or two in order to check in with her about any issues she may have. Genuinely wish her well, shake her hand, and wish her a great day.

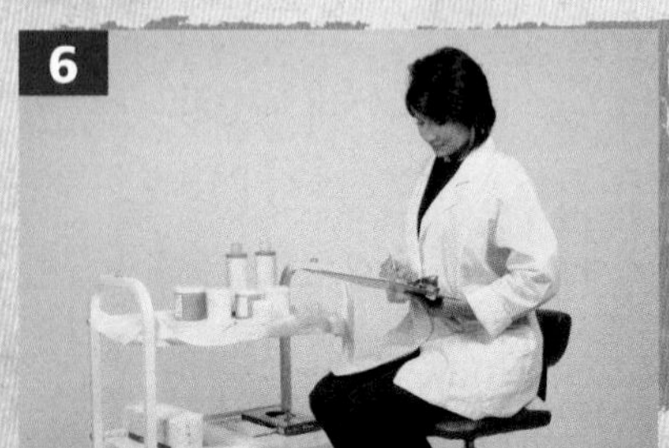

6 Be sure to record service information, observations, and product recommendations on the service record card, and be sure you return it to the proper place for filing.

At the End of the Day

1 Put on a fresh pair of gloves to protect yourself from contact with soiled linens and implements.

2 Remove all dirty laundry from the hamper. Spray the hamper with a disinfectant aerosol spray or wipe it down with disinfectant. Mildew grows easily in hampers.

3 Remove all dirty spatulas, used brushes, and other utensils. Most of these should have been removed between clients during the day.

4 Thoroughly clean and disinfect all multiuse tools and implements.

5 Clean then disinfect all counters, the facial chair, machines, and other furniture with disinfectant. The magnifying lamp should be cleaned and disinfected on both sides in the same manner.

6 Replenish the room with fresh linens, spatulas, utensils, and other supplies, so it is ready for the next day.

7 Change disinfection solution.

8 Maintain vaporizer as necessary.

9 Check the room for dirt, smudges, or dust on the walls, on the baseboards, in corners, or on air vents. Vacuum and mop the room with a disinfectant.

10 Spray the air in the room with a disinfectant aerosol spray.

11 Replenish any empty jars. If you are reusing jars for dispensing creams from a bulk container, always use up the entire content of the small jar and thoroughly clean and disinfect the jar before replenishing. Never add cream to a partially used jar. Rinse the empty jar well with hot water and then disinfect, rinsing thoroughly. Allow the jar to dry before refilling.

© Milady, a part of Cengage Learning. Photography by Yanik Chauvin.

PROCEDURE 22-3

Eyebrow Tweezing

Implements and Materials

You will need all of the following implements, materials, and supplies:

- **Antiseptic lotion**
- **Cotton balls**
- **Disposable gloves**
- **Emollient cream**
- **Eyebrow brush**
- **Gentle eye makeup remover**
- **Soothing toner**
- **Towels**
- **Tweezers**

© Milady, a part of Cengage Learning. Photography by Paul Castle, Castle Photography.

Preparation

- Perform PROCEDURE 22-1 **Pre-Service Procedure** **SEE PAGE 696**

Procedure

1 Cleanse the eyelid area with cotton balls moistened with gentle eye makeup remover.

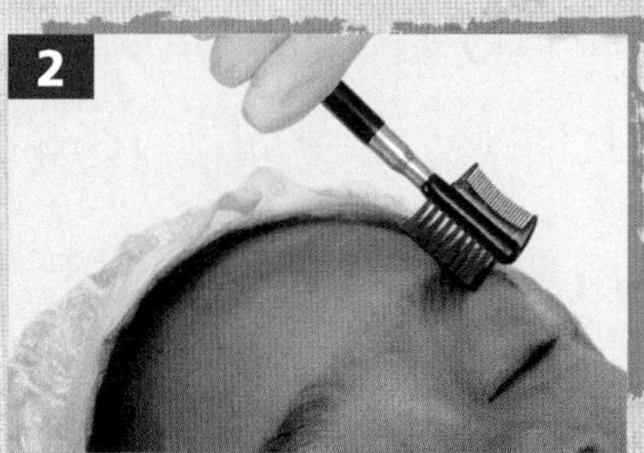

2 Brush the eyebrows with a small brush to remove any powder or scaliness.

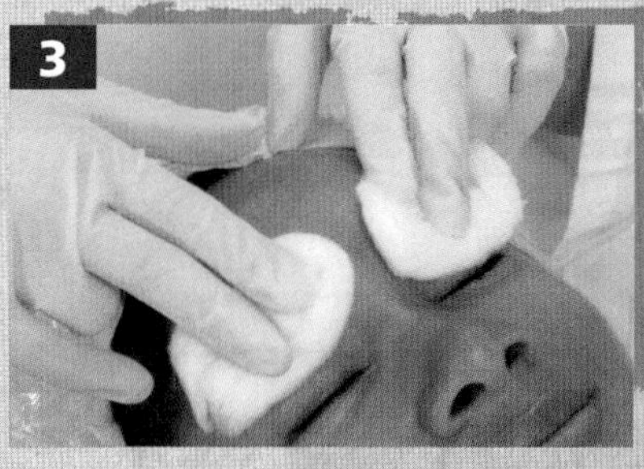

3 Soften brows. Saturate two pledgets (tufts) of cotton, or a towel with warm water, and place over the brows. Allow them to remain on the brows one to two minutes to soften and relax the eyebrow tissue. You may soften the brows and surrounding skin by rubbing a small amount of emollient cream into them.

4 Apply a mild toner on a cotton ball prior to tweezing.

Eyebrow Tweezing continued

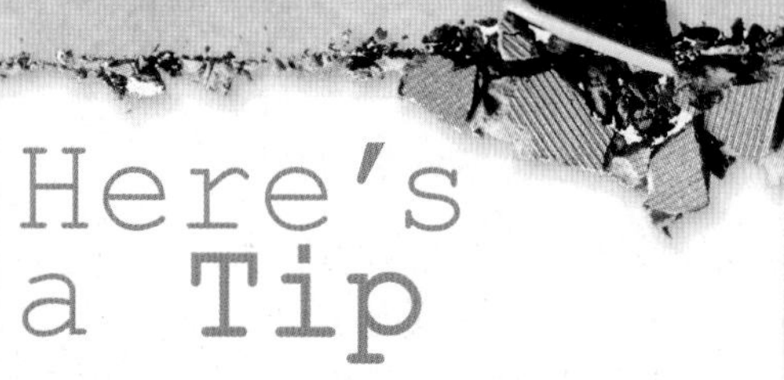
5

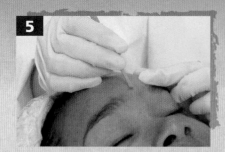

5 Remove the hairs between the brows. When tweezing, stretch the skin taut with the index finger and thumb (or index and middle fingers) of your nondominant hand. Grasp each hair individually with tweezers and pull with a quick motion, always in the direction of growth. Tweeze between the brows and above the brow line first, because the area under the brow line is much more sensitive.

6 Sponge the tweezed area frequently with cotton moistened with an antiseptic lotion to avoid infection.

Here's a Tip

To determine the best shape for the brow, hold the base of a comb or spatula against the corner of the nose, with the other end of the comb or spatula extending straight upward toward the eyebrow. This is where the brow should begin. Hold the comb or spatula so it extends from the corner of the nose to the outside corner of the eye and then across the eyebrow. This is where the brow should end.

The high point of the arch of the brow should be near the outside corner of the iris, if the client is looking straight ahead.

Just like a good haircut, the arch and shape of the eyebrows should be well blended and flow in a natural line. Remove the excess brow hair in an even fashion to avoid sharp angles or obvious thinner areas in the brow line. If the client has an uneven brow line, encourage her to allow the eyebrows in the thin area to grow back, so that you can help her achieve a smoother, well-blended, and more natural-looking line.

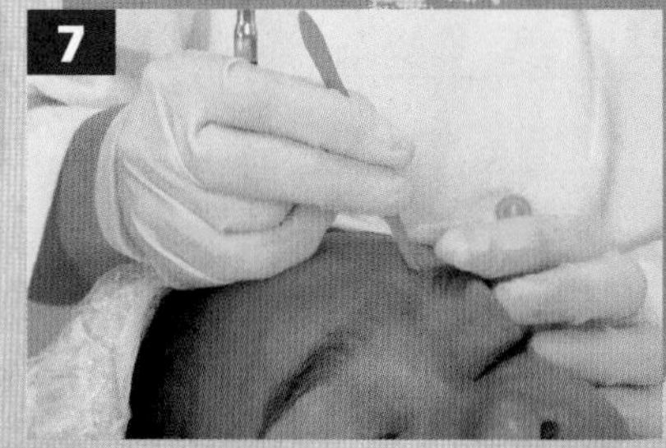
7

7 Brush the hair downward. Remove excessive hairs from above the eyebrow line, being careful to not create a hard line with top of the brow. Shape the upper section of one eyebrow, and then shape the other. Frequently sponge the area with toner.

8 Brush the hairs upward. Remove hairs from under the eyebrow line. Shape the lower section of one eyebrow, and then shape the other. Sponge the area with toner. Optional: Apply emollient cream and massage the brows. Remove cream with cool, wet cotton pads.

9 After tweezing is completed, sponge the eyebrows and surrounding skin with a toner to soothe the skin.

10 Brush the eyebrow hair to its normal position.

Post-Service

- Complete PROCEDURE 22-2 Post-Service Procedure SEE PAGE 699

© Milady, a part of Cengage Learning. Photography by Paul Castle, Castle Photography.

PROCEDURE 22-4

Eyebrow Waxing

Implements and Materials

You will need all of the following implements, materials, and supplies:

- **Disposable gloves**
- **Fabric strips for hair removal**
- **Facial chair**
- **Hair cap or headband**
- **Mild skin cleanser**
- **Roll of disposable paper**
- **Single or double wax heater**
- **Small disposable spatula or small wooden applicators**
- **Soothing emollient or antiseptic lotion**
- **Towels for draping**
- **Wax**
- **Wax remover**

© Milady, a part of Cengage Learning. Photography by Paul Castle, Castle Photography.

Preparation

- Perform PROCEDURE 22-1 **Pre-Service Procedure** **SEE PAGE 696**

Procedure

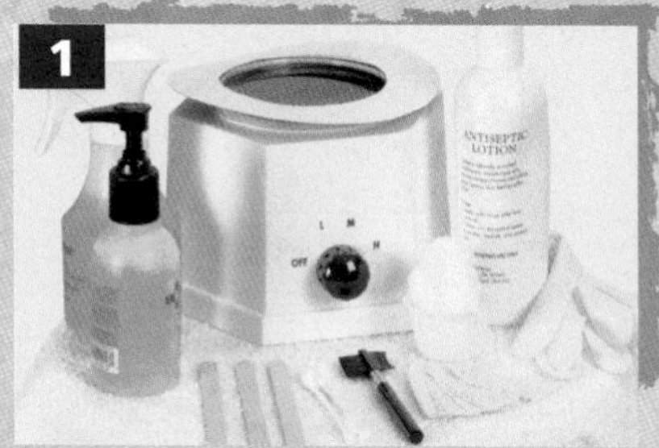

1 Melt the wax in the heater. The length of time it takes to melt the wax depends on how full the wax holder is—fifteen to twenty-five minutes if it is full, and ten minutes if it is one-quarter to one-half full. Be sure it is not too hot or too thin. The hotter the wax is, the thinner the wax becomes. Thin wax is more likely to drip and may cause accidents. Wax should have the thickness of caramel sauce. It should not be runny.

2 Lay a clean towel over the top of the facial chair, and then a layer of disposable paper.

3 Place a hair cap or headband on the client's head to keep hair out of her face.

4 Put on disposable gloves.

5 Remove the client's makeup, cleanse the area thoroughly with a mild cleanser, and dry.

Eyebrow Waxing continued

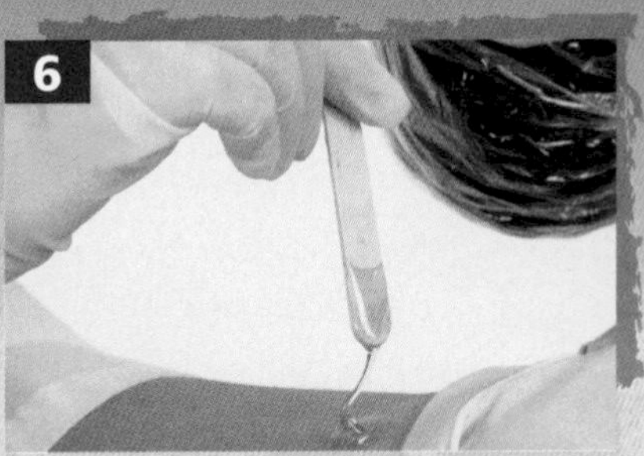

6 Test the temperature and consistency of the heated wax by applying a small drop on your inner wrist. It should be warm but not hot, and it should drip smoothly off the spatula.

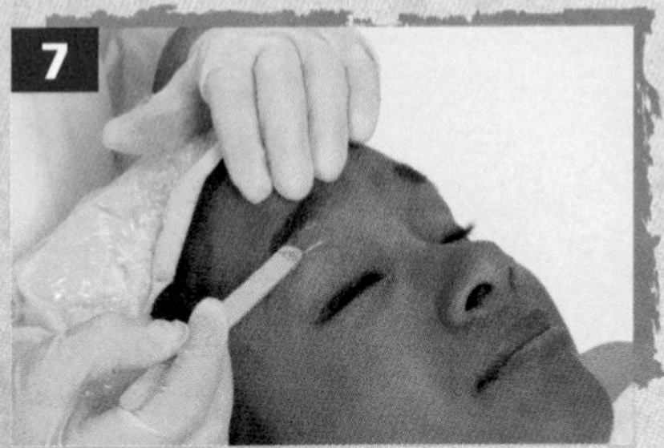

7 With the spatula or wooden applicator, spread a thin coat of the warm wax evenly over the area to be treated, going in the same direction as the hair growth. Be sure not to put the spatula in the wax more than once. No double dips!

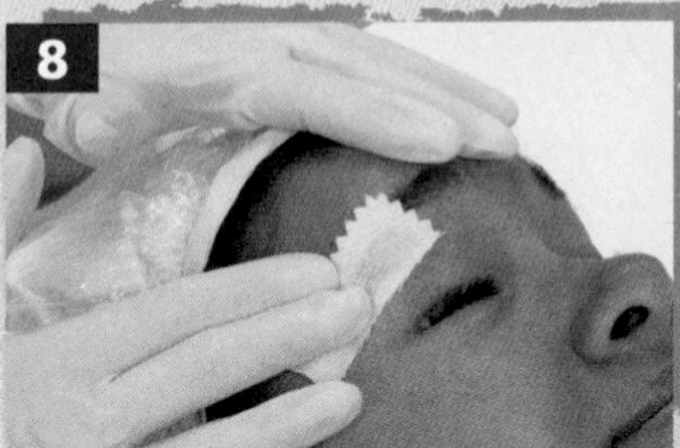

8 Apply a fabric strip over the waxed area. Press gently in the direction of hair growth, running your finger over the surface of the fabric three to five times, always in the direction of the hair growth.

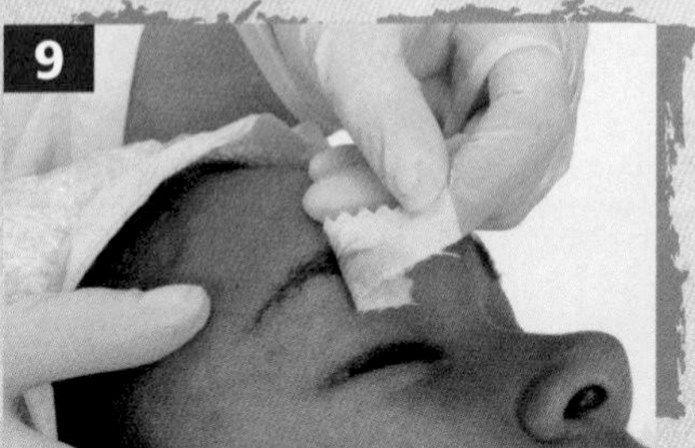

9 Gently applying pressure to hold the skin taut with one hand, quickly remove the fabric strip and the wax that sticks to it by pulling it in the direction opposite the hair growth. Do not pull straight up on the strip.

10 Lightly massage the treated area.

11 Remove any remaining wax residue from the skin with a gentle wax remover.

12 Repeat procedure on the area around the other eyebrow.

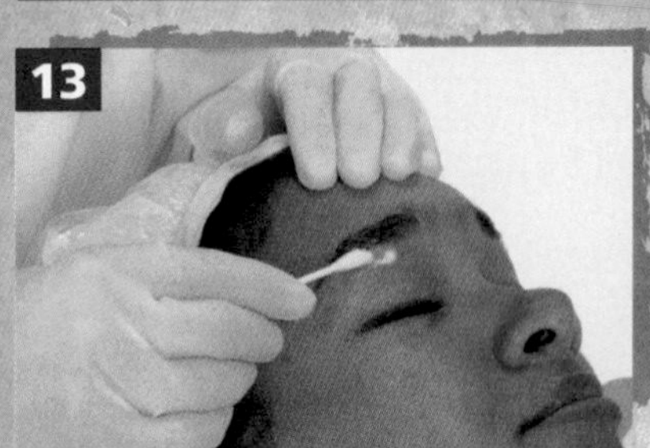

13 Cleanse the skin with a mild emollient cleanser and apply an emollient or antiseptic lotion.

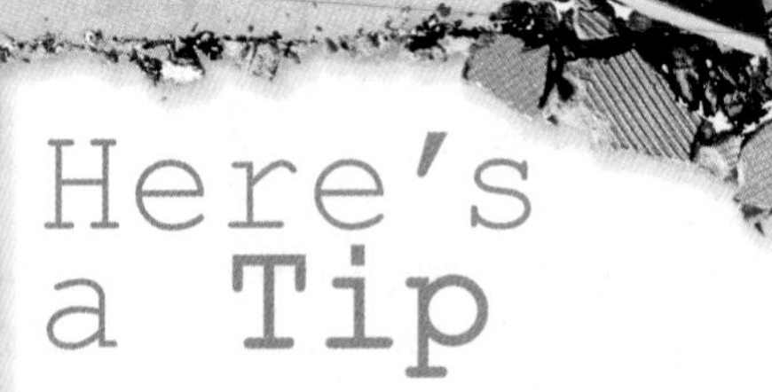

Here's a Tip

Be sure not to use an excessive amount of wax, as it will spread when the fabric is pressed and may spread to hair you do not wish to remove.

Post-Service

- Complete PROCEDURE 22-2 **Post-Service Procedure** SEE PAGE 699

© Milady, a part of Cengage Learning. Photography by Paul Castle, Castle Photography.

PROCEDURE 22-5

Body Waxing

Implements and Materials

You will need all of the following implements, materials, and supplies:

- **Disposable gloves**
- **Fabric strips for hair removal**
- **Facial chair**
- **Mild skin cleanser**
- **Dusting powder**
- **Roll of disposable paper**
- **Single or double wax heater**
- **Small disposable spatula or small wooden applicators**
- **Soothing emollient or antiseptic lotion**
- **Towels for draping**
- **Wax**
- **Wax remover**

© Milady, a part of Cengage Learning. Photography by Paul Castle, Castle Photography.

Preparation

- Perform PROCEDURE 22-1 **Pre-Service Procedure** **SEE PAGE 696**

Procedure

1 Melt the wax in the heater.

2 Drape the treatment bed with disposable paper or a bed sheet with paper over the top.

3 If bikini waxing, offer the client disposable panties or a small clean towel.

4 If waxing the underarms, have the client remove her bra and put on a terry wrap. Offer a terry wrap when waxing the legs as well.

5 Assist the client onto the treatment bed and drape with towels.

6 Thoroughly cleanse the area to be waxed with a mild cleanser and dry.

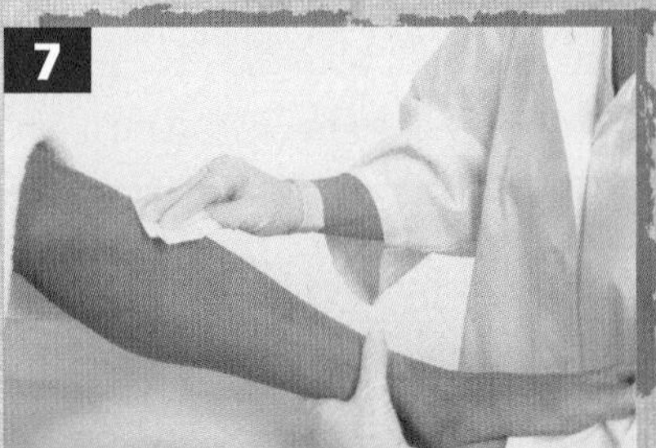

7 Apply a light covering of dusting powder.

Service Tip

Never leave the wax heater on overnight. Doing so presents a fire hazard and can damage the wax. Wax should be covered with a lid when not warm or heating.

Body Waxing continued

8 Test the temperature and consistency of the heated wax by applying a small drop to your inner wrist.

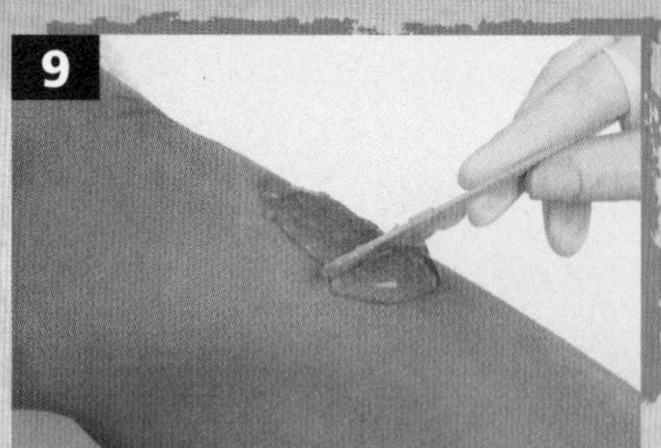
9

9 Using a disposable spatula, spread a thin coat of the warm wax evenly over the skin surface in the same direction as the hair growth. Be sure not to put the spatula in the wax more than once. If the wax strings and lands in an area you do not wish to treat, remove it with lotion designed to dissolve and remove wax.

Service Tip

When waxing sensitive areas, such as underarms or bikini lines, be sure the wax is not too hot. Trim the hair with scissors if it is more than ½-inch (1.25 centimeters) long.

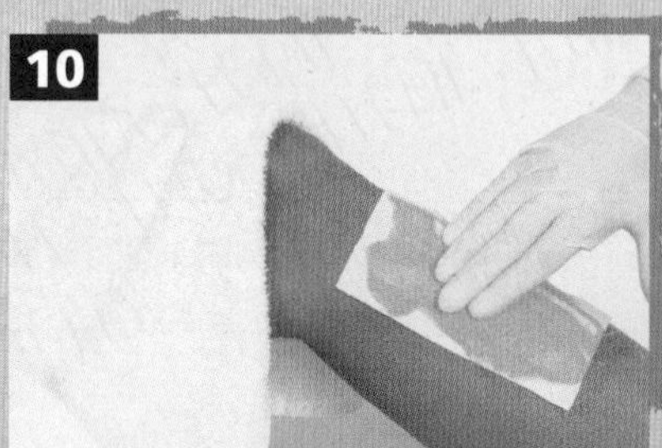
10

10 Apply a fabric strip in the same direction as the hair growth. Press gently, running your hand over the surface of the fabric three to five times.

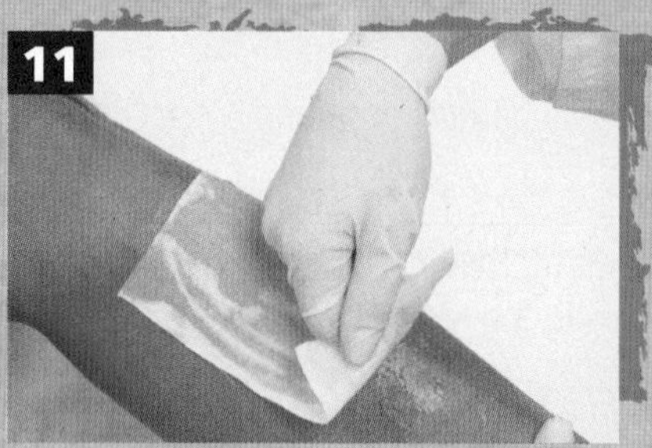
11

11 Gently apply pressure to hold the skin taut with one hand and quickly remove the adhering wax in the opposite direction of the hair growth. Do not pull the fabric strip straight upwards.

12 Apply gentle pressure and lightly massage the treated area.

13 Repeat, using a fresh fabric strip every time.

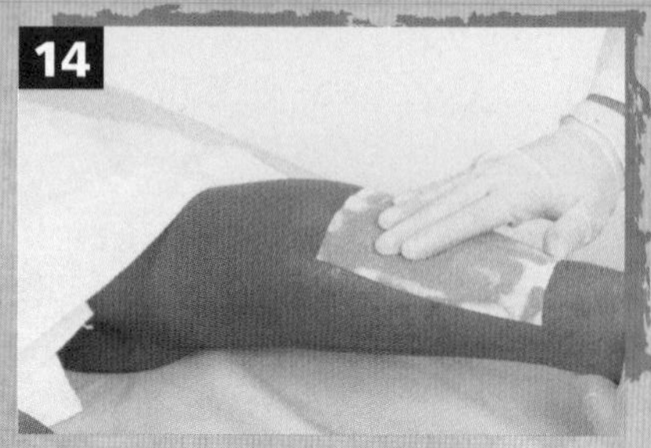
14

14 If waxing the legs, have the client turn over, and repeat the procedure on the backs of her legs.

15 Remove any remaining residue of powder from the skin.

16 Cleanse the area with a mild emollient cleanser and apply an emollient or antiseptic lotion.

17 Undrape the client and escort her to the dressing room.

Post-Service

- Complete PROCEDURE 22-2 **Post-Service Procedure** SEE PAGE 699

© Milady, a part of Cengage Learning. Photography by Paul Castle, Castle Photography.

Review Questions

1. What information should be entered on the health screening form during the consultation?
2. What conditions, treatments, and medications contraindicate hair removal in the salon?
3. What are the two major types of hair removal? Give examples of each.
4. Define electrolysis, photoepilation, and laser removal.
5. Which hair removal techniques should not be performed in the salon without special training?
6. What is the difference between a depilatory and an epilator?
7. Why must a patch test be given before waxing?
8. List safety precautions that must be followed for hot and cold waxing.
9. Define threading and sugaring.

Chapter Glossary

Brazilian bikini waxing	A waxing technique that requires the removal of all the hair from the front and the back of the bikini area.
depilatory	Substance, usually a caustic alkali preparation, used for the temporary removal of superfluous hair by dissolving it at the skin surface level.
electrolysis	Removal of hair by means of an electric current that destroys the root of the hair.
epilator	Substance used to remove hair by pulling it out of the follicle.
health screening form	A questionnaire that discloses all medications, both topical (applied to the skin) and oral (taken by mouth), along with any known skin disorders or allergies that might affect treatment.
hirsuties	Also known as *hypertrichosis*; growth of an unusual amount of hair on parts of the body normally bearing only downy hair, such as the faces of women or the backs of men.
hirsutism	Condition pertaining to an excessive growth or cover of hair, especially in women.
laser hair removal	Permanent hair removal treatment in which a laser beam is pulsed on the skin, impairing the hair growth.
photoepilation	Also known as *Intense Pulsed Light*; permanent hair removal treatment that uses intense light to destroy the growth cells of the hair follicles.
sugaring	Temporary hair removal method that involves the use of a thick, sugar-based paste.
threading	Temporary hair removal method that involves twisting and rolling cotton thread along the surface of the skin, entwining the hair in the thread, and lifting it from the follicle.
tweezing	Using tweezers to remove hairs.

CHAPTER 23

Facials

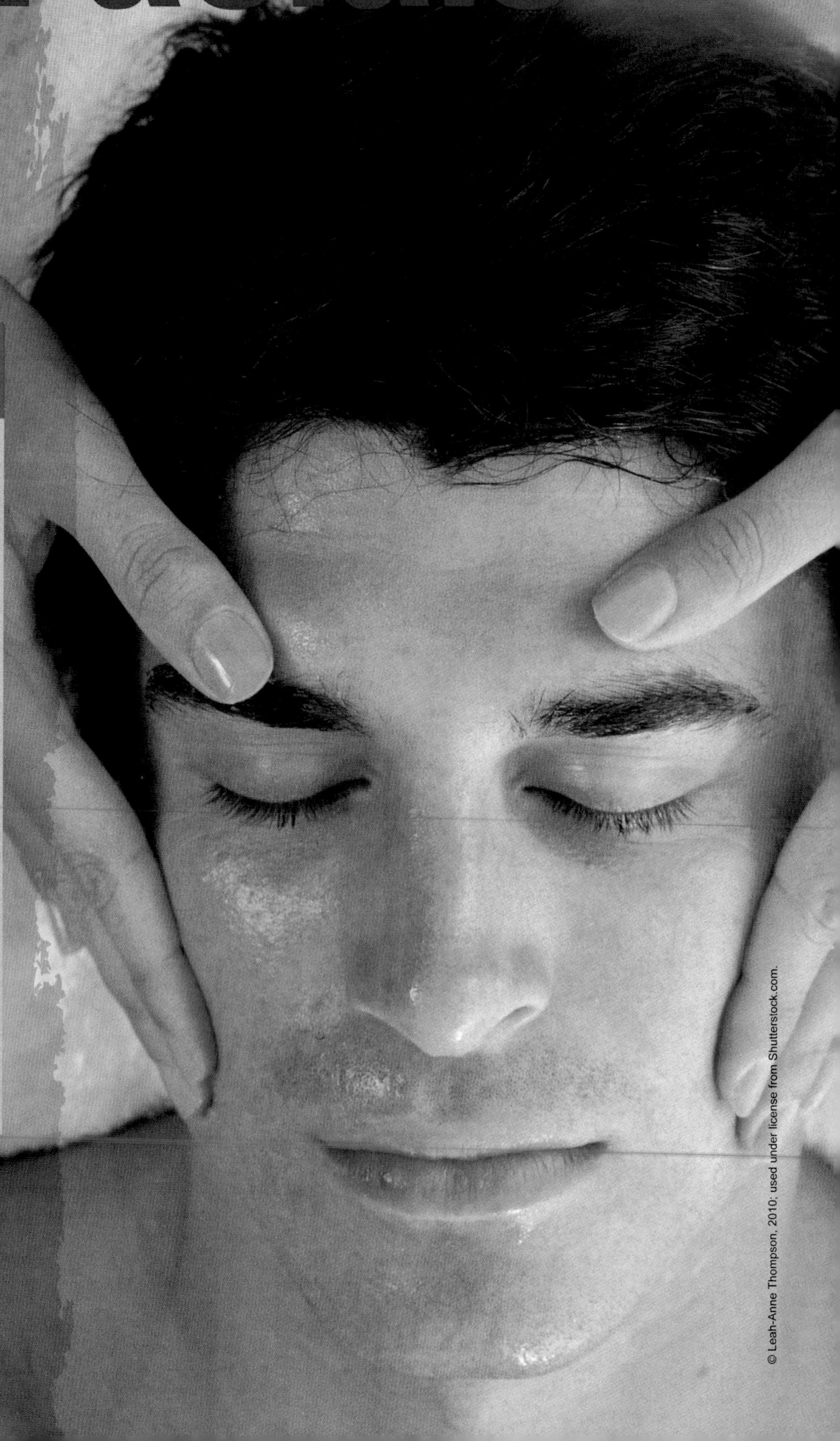

Chapter Outline

Why Study Facials?

Skin Analysis and Consultation

Determining Skin Type

Skin Care Products

Client Consultation

Facial Massage

Facial Equipment

Electrotherapy and Light Therapy

Facial Treatments

Aromatherapy

Procedures

© Leah-Anne Thompson, 2010; used under license from Shutterstock.com.

Learning Objectives

After completing this chapter, you will be able to:

- ✓ **LO1** Explain the importance of skin analysis and client consultation.
- ✓ **LO2** Understand contraindications and the use of a health screening form to safely perform facial treatments.
- ✓ **LO3** List and describe various skin types and conditions.
- ✓ **LO4** Describe different types of products used in facial treatments.
- ✓ **LO5** Perform a client consultation.
- ✓ **LO6** Identify the various types of massage movements and their physiological effects.
- ✓ **LO7** Describe the basic types of electrical equipment used in facial treatments.
- ✓ **LO8** Identify the basic concepts of electrotherapy and light therapy techniques.

Key Terms

Page number indicates where in the chapter the term is used.

alipidic
pg. 716

ampoules
pg. 721

aromatherapy
pg. 740

brushing machine
pg. 733

chemical exfoliants
pg. 719

chucking
pg. 727

clay-based masks
pg. 722

cleansing milks
pg. 718

contraindication
pg. 711

couperose
pg. 718

cream masks
pg. 722

effleurage
pg. 726

electrotherapy
pg. 734

emollients
pg. 721

enzyme peels (keratolytic enzymes, protein-dissolving agents)
pg. 720

exfoliants
pg. 719

exfoliation
pg. 719

foaming cleansers
pg. 719

friction
pg. 727

fulling
pg. 727

gommages (roll-off masks)
pg. 719

hacking
pg. 728

humectants (hydrators, water-binding agents)
pg. 721

masks (masques)
pg. 722

massage
pg. 725

massage creams
pg. 721

mechanical exfoliants
pg. 719

microdermabrasion
pg. 737

microdermabrasion scrubs
pg. 719

modelage masks
pg. 723

moisturizers
pg. 721

motor point
pg. 729

open comedones (blackheads)
pg. 717

ostium
pg. 717

paraffin wax masks
pg. 722

pétrissage
pg. 727

rolling
pg. 727

serums
pg. 721

steamer
pg. 733

tapotement (percussion)
pg. 727

toners (fresheners, astringents)
pg. 719

treatment cream
pg. 728

vibration
pg. 722

wringing
pg. 727

Good skin care can make a big difference in the way skin looks and in the way a client feels about his or her appearance. Besides being very relaxing, facial treatments can offer many improvements to the appearance of the skin (**Figure 23–1**).

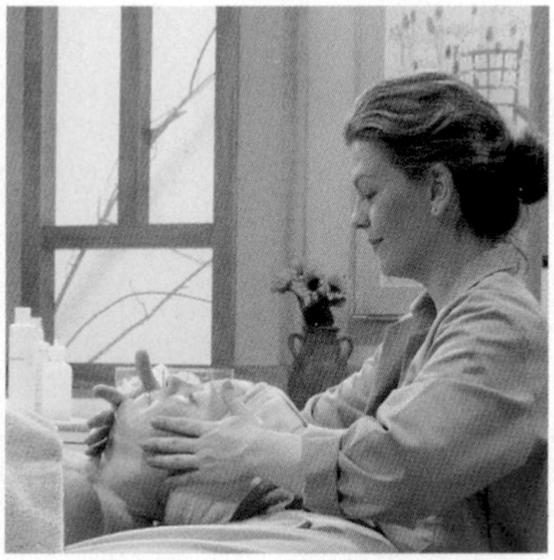

Proper skin care can make oily skin look cleaner and healthier, dry skin look and feel more moist and supple, and aging skin look smoother, firmer, and less wrinkled. A combination of good salon facial treatments and effective, individualized home care will show visible results.

© Milady, a part of Cengage Learning. Photography by Larry Hamill.

▲ **Figure 23–1**
A facial is a soothing, pleasurable experience for the client.

WHY STUDY FACIALS?

Cosmetologists should study and have a thorough understanding of facials because:

- Providing skin care services to clients is extremely rewarding, helps busy clients to relax, improves their appearance, and helps clients feel better about themselves.
- Knowing the basics of skin analysis and basic information about skin care products will enable you to offer your clients advice when they ask you for it.
- Although you will not treat a skin disease, you must be able to recognize adverse skin conditions and refer clients to seek medical advice from a physician.
- Learning the basic techniques of facials and facial massage will give you a good overview of, and an ability to perform, these foundational services.
- You may enjoy this category of services and may consider specializing in skin care services. This study will create a perfect basis for making that decision.

FOCUS ON

SHARPENING YOUR PERSONAL SKILLS

The importance of following hygiene and infection control guidelines when performing facials cannot be overemphasized. As often as possible, perform your cleaning and disinfection procedures in the presence of your clients. When they see you doing this, they will feel more confident in you as a professional.

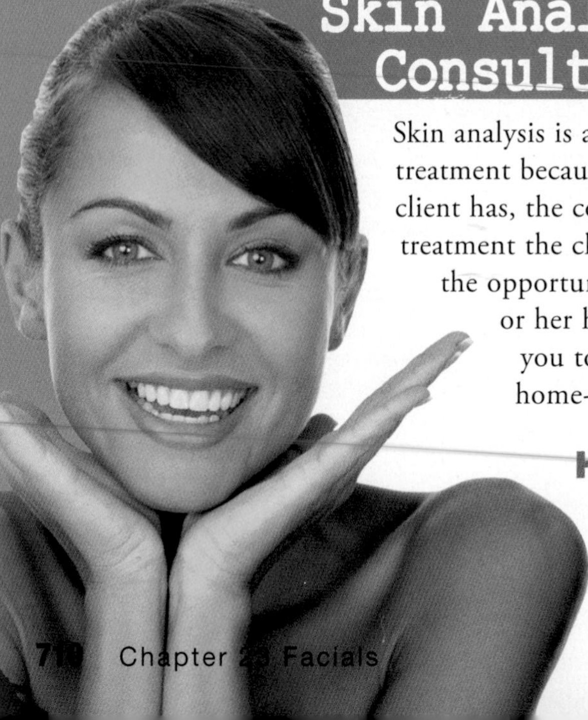

Skin Analysis and Consultation

Skin analysis is a very important part of the facial treatment because it determines what type of skin the client has, the condition of the skin, and what type of treatment the client's skin needs. Consultation allows you the opportunity to ask the client questions about his or her health and skin care history, and it allows you to advise the client about appropriate home-care products and treatments. ☑ **LO1**

Health Screening Form

Before beginning the analysis, you must have the client fill out a health screening

© Dash, 2010; used under license from Shutterstock.com.

form (**Figure 23–2**). Similar to the form used for waxing, the main purpose of the health screening form is to determine whether the client has any contraindications that might prohibit certain skin treatments.

A **contraindication** (kahn-trah-in-dih-KAY-shun) is a condition that requires avoiding certain treatments, procedures or products to prevent

Department of Skin Care

Health Screening Form

Client History

Name____

Address____

City________________State________ Zip Code____________

Home phone______________ Work Phone__________________

Occupation__________Referred by__________Date of Birth________

Is this your first facial treatment? YES___ NO___

Have you ever used:

Retin-A®? YES___ NO___

Accutane®: (isotretinoin)? YES___ NO___

Are you using glycolic or alphahydroxy acids? YES___ NO___

Do you smoke? YES___ NO___

Are you pregnant? YES___ NO___

Do you have acne or frequent blemishes? YES___ NO___

Are you nursing? YES___ NO___

Taking birth control pills? YES___ NO___ If so, how long?______________

Have you had skin cancer? YES___ NO___

Do you experience stress? YES___ NO___ If so, how often?______________

Do you wear contact lenses? YES___ NO___

Are you under a physician's care? YES___ NO___

Physician's Name______________________

Do you have any allergies to cosmetics, foods, or drugs? YES___ NO___

Please list____

Are you presently on any medications - oral or topical-dermatological? YES___ NO___

Please list____

◀ **Figure 23–2**
Health Screening Form.

© Milady, a part of Cengage Learning.

What products do you use presently?______________________________

Please circle: Soap Cleansing Milk Toner Daily Sunscreen Creams

Other____

Please circle if you are affected by or have any of the following:

Have had hysterectomy	Pacemaker/Cardiac Problems	Immune Disorders
Depression or Anxiety	Herpes	Urinary or Kidney Problems
Seborrhea/Psoriasis/Eczema	Chronic Headaches	Hepatitis
Asthma	Fever Blisters	Lupus
High Blood Pressure	Metal Bone Pins or Plates	Epilepsy
Taking Depression/ Mood Altering Medications	Sinus Problems	Other Skin Diseases

Please explain above problems or list any significant others:

____

____

I understand that the services offered are not a substitute for medical care, and any information provided by the therapist is for educational purposes only and not diagnostically prescriptive in nature. I understand that the information herein is to aid the technician in giving better service and is completely confidential.

SALON POLICIES

1. Professional consultation is required before initial dispensing of products.
2. Our active discount rate is only effective for clients visiting every 4 weeks.
3. We do not give cash refunds.

I fully understand and agree to the above salon policies.

______________________________ ______________

Client Signature Date

© Milady, a part of Cengage Learning.

▲ **Figure 23–2 Health Screening Form (continued).**

undesirable side effects. For example, if the client is allergic to fragrance, using a fragranced product would be contraindicated. If a client is using a prescription drug, such as Retin-A® or Tazorac® (both topical drugs that cause skin exfoliation), using other exfoliants in the facial treatment is contraindicated because to do so may injure the skin by causing excessive peeling and inflammation.

Isotretinoin (Accutane), an oral medication for cystic acne, causes thinning of the skin all over the body. Waxing, stimulating treatments, or exfoliation procedures should never be performed on the skin of someone using isotretinoin or someone who has used the drug in the last six months. Because isotretinoin is an oral drug, it stays in the body for several months after the client stops taking it.

The main contraindications to look for are summarized below and in **Table 23–1**:

- Use of isotretinoin or any skin-thinning or exfoliating drug, including Retin-A®, Renova®, Tazorac®, Differin®, and so on: Avoid waxing, exfoliation and/or peeling treatments, and stimulating treatments.
- Pregnancy: Avoid all electrical treatments and any other questionable treatments without a physician's written permission. Some pregnant clients also experience sensitivities from waxing.
- Metal bone pins or plates in the body: Avoid all electrical treatment.
- Pacemakers or heart irregularities: Avoid all electrical treatment.
- Allergies: Strictly avoid any allergic substances listed on the intake form. Clients with multiple allergies should always use nonfragranced products designed for sensitive skin. Food allergies should also be noted, because many skin care products now contain naturally derived food-based extracts such as soy, nut oils, and other ingredients.
- Seizures or epilepsy: Avoid all electrical and light treatments.
- Use of oral steroids such as prednisone: Avoid any stimulating or exfoliating treatment or waxing. Steroids can cause thinning of the skin which could result in blistering or injury.
- Autoimmune diseases such as lupus: Avoid any harsh or stimulating treatments.
- Diabetes: Be aware that many diabetics heal very slowly. If you have questions, you should get approval from the client's physician before treatment. The primary services that need approval are waxing, electrolysis, or any treatment for the feet.
- Blood thinners: No extraction or waxing. To do so may cause bleeding or bruising.

Clients who have obvious skin abnormalities, such as open sores, fever blisters (herpes simplex), or other abnormal-looking signs should be referred to a physician for treatment. They can be rescheduled after they obtain written approval of facial services.

Should you ever have any questions regarding a client's treatment and his or her health conditions, always check with the client's doctor first! Remember one simple rule: When in doubt, don't perform the service.

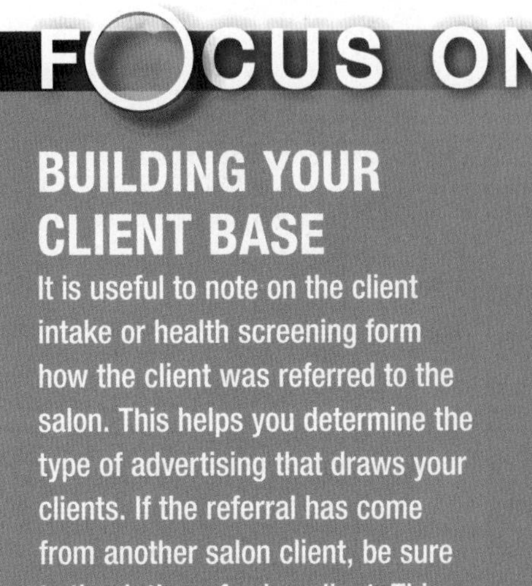

CAUTION

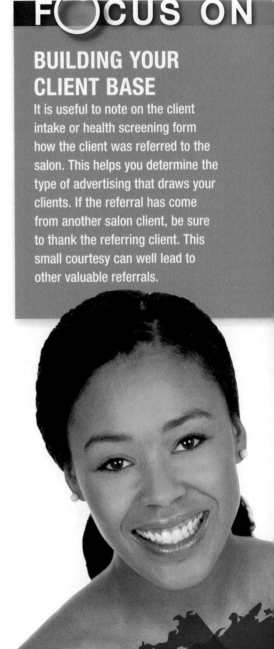

As a cosmetology student, you should receive hands-on training from your instructor before attempting any of the procedures discussed in this chapter.

FOCUS ON

BUILDING YOUR CLIENT BASE

It is useful to note on the client intake or health screening form how the client was referred to the salon. This helps you determine the type of advertising that draws your clients. If the referral has come from another salon client, be sure to thank the referring client. This small courtesy can well lead to other valuable referrals.

© Kurhan, 2010; used under license from Shutterstock.com.

CONTRAINDICATIONS	CONTRAINDICATIONS GRID	
	WHAT TO AVOID	**WHY?**
ISOTRETINOIN (Accutane)	• all waxing anywhere on the body • any peeling agent or drying agent, including alpha hydroxy acids (AHAs) scrubs, microdermabrasion and brushing machines	skin can blister or peel off
EXFOLIATING DRUGS INCLUDING RETIN-A®(TRETINOIN) RENOVA®, TAZORAC®, DIFFERIN®	• all waxing on the area where the drug is used • any peeling agent or drying agent, including AHAs, scrubs, microdermabrasion, and brushing machines	skin can blister or peel off
PREGNANCY	• electrical treatments • any questionable treatment without a physician's written permission • possible sensitivities from waxing	unknown; general safety precaution
METAL BONE PINS OR PLATES IN THE BODY	• electrical treatments	electricity can possibly affect metal
HEART CONDITIONS/ PACEMAKER	• electrical treatments	electricity can possibly affect rhythms and pacemakers
KNOWN ALLERGIES	• avoid known allergens, fragrances	allergic reaction can occur
SEIZURES OR EPILEPSY	• electrical or light treatments	could trigger seizure reaction
USE OF ORAL STEROIDS SUCH AS PREDNISONE	• any stimulating or exfoliating treatment • waxing	steroids can cause thinning of the skin which could result in blistering or injury
AUTOIMMUNE DISEASES SUCH AS LUPUS	• harsh or stimulating treatments without specific physician permission	unpredictable reactions in some cases
DIABETES	• general caution advised (many diabetics heal very slowly; obtain physician approval if you are unsure)	none specific
BLOOD THINNERS	• extraction without physician permission • facial or body waxing without physician permission	may cause bleeding or bruising
SENSITIVE, REDNESS-PRONE SKIN	• heat • harsh scrubs • mechanical treatment • stimulating massage	can aggravate redness
OPEN SORES, HERPES SIMPLEX (COLD SORES)	• avoid all treatments until clear with doctor	can spread or flare; infectious disease
RECENT FACIAL SURGERY OR LASER TREATMENT.	• treat with physician's permission only	treat with physician's permission only

© Milady, a part of Cengage Learning.

Table 23–1 Contraindications Grid.

When the client completes the health screening form, you can obtain important information such as the following:

- Client's name, address, and phone number(s)
- Client's occupation
- Medical conditions that might affect treatment
- All medications being used, including topical drugs for the skin
- Current home skin-care program and salon skin-care history
- Information regarding how the client heard about you and your services

CAUTION

Cosmetologists do not treat skin diseases. However, as a professional, you must be able to recognize the presence of various skin ailments in order to suggest that the client seek medical advice from a physician.

Treatment Records

You should record and highlight with a colored pen any important observations or contraindications in the client's treatment record. File the health screening forms in a secure filing cabinet because the client may have revealed information that is private. The client-treatment record should include the client's name, address, and phone numbers. It should also have spaces to allow for recording the results of the analysis, each treatment performed on the client's skin, your observations on each visit, any home-care products purchased by the client, and the date of each treatment or product purchase. Recording product purchases will help you find products when a client wants to re-purchase but has forgotten the product name. ✔ **LO2**

Analysis Procedure

After carefully reading the client's health screening form and discussing your questions with the client, have the client change into a smock and sit in the facial chair. The client's hair should be covered, and any jewelry should be removed by the client and put away in a safe place. Jewelry can get in the way or become soiled or damaged during treatment.

Cosmetologists should avoid wearing jewelry on the hands or arms while administering facial treatments because rings and bracelets may accidentally injure the client or be damaged.

Recline the client in the chair and drape the client using a hair cap, headband, or towels. After washing your hands thoroughly, warm some cleansing milk in your hands and apply the cleanser to the face in upward circular movements. When cleansing the eye area, use a special cleanser made for eye makeup removal. Apply a small amount to the eye areas, being careful not to use so much that it gets in the eyes. Gently remove the cleanser with warm damp facial sponges or cotton pads. Remember to remove the cleanser using upward and outward movements. When working around the eyes, move outward on the upper lid, and inward on the lower lid.

After thoroughly cleansing the face, apply a cotton eye pad to the client's eyes to avoid exposure to the extreme brightness of the magnifying lamp.

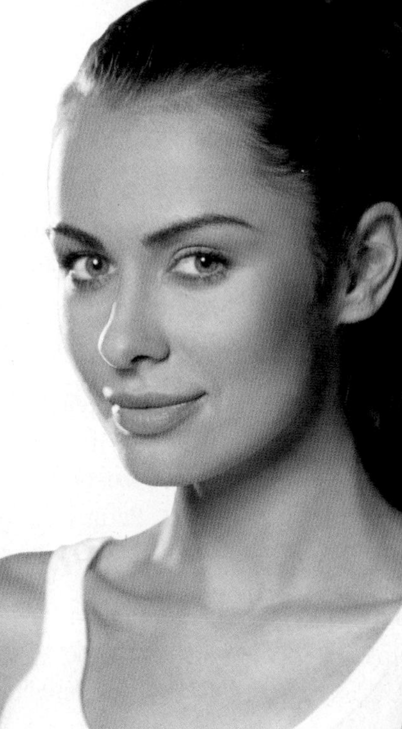

© Dash, 2010; used under license from Shutterstock.com.

Determining Skin Type

Look through the magnifying lamp at the client's skin. Skin type is determined by how oily or dry the skin is. Skin type is hereditary and cannot be permanently changed with treatments, although the skin may look considerably better after treatment. Skin conditions are characteristics associated with a particular skin type (**Table 23–2**).

The first thing you should look for is the presence or absence of visible pores (follicles). The amount of sebum produced by the sebaceous glands determines the size of the pores and is hereditary. Obvious pores indicate oily skin areas, and lack of visible pores indicates dry skin.

Skin Types

The term **alipidic** (al-ah-PIDD-ic) means lack of lipids, and describes skin that does not produce enough sebum, indicated by absence of visible pores. Alipidic skin, also known as *dry skin*, becomes dehydrated because it does not produce enough sebum to prevent the evaporation of cell moisture. Dehydration indicates a lack of moisture in the skin. Dehydrated skin may be flaky or dry looking, with small, fine lines

SKIN	SIGNS AND CONDITIONS ASSOCIATED WITH SKIN TYPES	
	SIGNS OF SKIN TYPE	CONDITIONS ASSOCIATED WITH SKIN TYPE
OILY	Obvious, large pores.	Open and closed comedones, clogged pores. Shiny, thick appearance. Yellowish color. Orange peel texture.
DRY	Pores very small or not visible.	Tight, poreless-looking skin. May be dehydrated with fine lines and wrinkles, dry and rough to the touch.
NORMAL	Even pore distribution throughout the skin. Very soft smooth surface. Lack of wrinkles.	Normal skin is actually very unusual. Most clients have combination skin.
COMBINATION DRY	Obvious pores down center of face. Pores not visible or becoming smaller toward the outer edges of the face.	May have clogged pores in the nose, chin, and center of the forehead. Dry, poreless toward outside edges of the face.
COMBINATION OILY	Wider distribution of obvious or large pores down the center of the face extending to the outer cheeks. Pores become smaller toward edges of the face.	Comedones, clogged pores, or obvious pores in the center of the face.
ACNE	Very large pores in all areas. Acne is considered a skin type because it is hereditary.	Presence of numerous open and closed comedones, clogged pores, and red papules and pustules (pimples).

© Milady, a part of Cengage Learning.

Table 23–2 Signs and Conditions Associated with Skin Types.

and wrinkles. It may look like it has a piece of cellophane on top of it. Dehydrated skin also may feel itchy or tight. Dehydration can occur on almost any skin type. The key to truly alipidic skin is the absence of visible pores.

Oily skin that produces too much sebum will have large pores, and the skin may appear shiny or greasy. Pores may be clogged from dead cells building up in the hair follicle, or may contain **open comedones** (KAHM-uh-dohnz), also known as **blackheads**, which are follicles impacted with solidified sebum and dead cell buildup.

Closed comedones are hair follicles impacted with solidified sebum and dead cell buildup that appear as small bumps just underneath the skin's surface.

The difference between open and closed comedones is the size of the follicle opening, called the **ostium** (AH-stee-um). An open comedo has a large ostium, and a closed comedo has a small one.

CAUTION

Severe or unresponsive cases of acne should be referred to a dermatologist for treatment. If you are ever unsure about treating a client who has acne, always refer that client to a dermatologist!

Acne

The presence of pimples in oily areas indicates acne. Acne is considered a skin type because the tendency to develop acne is hereditary. Acne is a disorder in which the hair follicles become clogged, resulting in infection of the follicle with redness and inflammation. Acne bacteria are anaerobic, which means they cannot survive in the presence of oxygen. When follicles are blocked with solidified sebum and dead-cell buildup, oxygen cannot readily get to the bottom of the follicle where acne bacteria live. Acne bacteria survive from breaking down sebum into fatty acids, which is their only food source. A blocked follicle is an ideal environment for acne bacteria. When acne bacteria flourish from the lack of oxygen and access to a food source such as a blocked follicle filled with sebum, they multiply quickly, eventually causing a break in the follicle wall. This rupture allows blood to come into the follicle causing redness. Acne papules are red pimples that do not have a pus head. Pimples with a pus head are called pustules. Pus is a fluid inside a pustule, largely made up of dead white blood cells that tried to fight the infection.

Analysis of Skin Conditions

Conditions of the skin are generally treatable. They are generally not hereditary, but they may be associated with a particular skin type.

Dehydration is indicated by flaky areas or skin that wrinkles easily on the surface. Very gently pinching the surface of dehydrated skin will result in the visible formation of many fine lines. This is an indication of dehydration. Dehydrated skin can be caused from lack of care, improper or over-drying skin care products, sun exposure, and other causes. Dehydrated skin is treated by using hydrators that help to bind water to the skin surface. These hydrating products should be chosen based on skin type. Hydrators for alipidic skin are generally heavier in

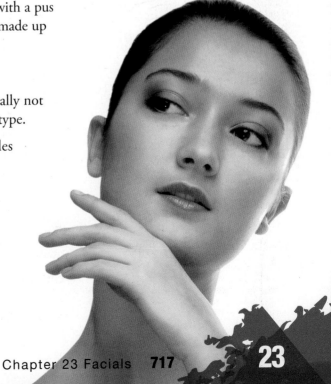

© Yuganov Konstantin, 2010; used under license from Shutterstock.com.

texture. Hydrators for oilier skin are lighter weight. Proper hydration of the skin can result in smoother-looking and softer skin.

Most types of hyperpigmentation, or dark blotches of color, are caused by sun exposure or hormone imbalances. Clients who have spent a lot of time in the sun will often have hyperpigmentation. Hyperpigmentation is treated with mild exfoliation and home care products that discourage pigmentation. Daily use of sunscreen and avoidance of sun exposure are very important for this skin type.

Sensitive skin has a thin, red-pink look. Skin will turn red easily, and is easily inflamed by some skin care products. You should avoid strong products or cleansers, fragranced products, and strong exfoliants when treating sensitive skin. Rosacea is a chronic hereditary disorder that can be indicated by constant or frequent facial blushing.

A person with rosacea often has dilated capillaries, telangiectasis (tel-an-jee-EK-tuh-sus), which are distended or dilated surface blood vessels, and **couperose** (KOO-per-ohs), which are areas of skin with distended capillaries and diffuse redness.

Rosacea is considered a medical disorder and should be diagnosed by a dermatologist. You should treat a client who has rosacea with very gentle products and treatments, avoiding any treatment that releases heat or stimulates the skin.

Aging skin has loss of elasticity, and the skin tends to sag in areas around the eyes and jawline. Wrinkles may be apparent in areas of normal facial expression. Treatments that hydrate and exfoliate improve the appearance of aging skin.

Sun-damaged skin is skin that has been chronically and frequently exposed to sun over the client's lifetime. Sun-damaged skin will have many areas of hyperpigmentation, lots of wrinkled areas including areas not in the normal facial expression, and sagging skin from damage to the elastic fibers. The skin looks older than it should for the age of the client. It is often confused with aging skin. ☑ LO3

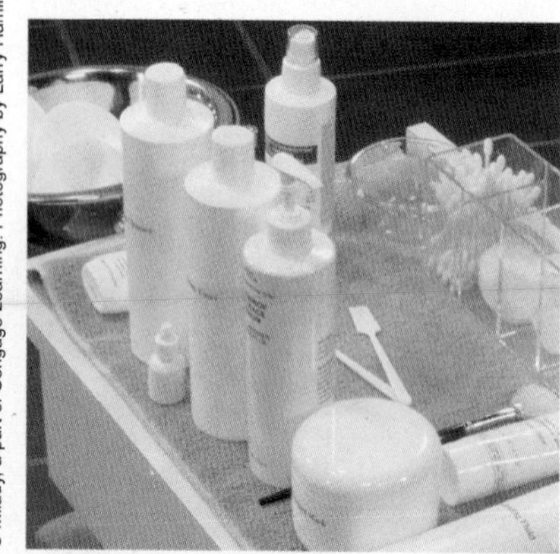
© Milady, a part of Cengage Learning. Photography by Larry Hamill.

▲ **Figure 23–3**
There is a wide variety of skin care products for every skin type.

Skin Care Products

There are many, many types of skin care products available for salon use and for the client's home care. Most skin care products are designed for specific skin types or conditions. Major categories of skin care products are described below (**Figure 23–3**).

Cleansers are designed to clean the surface of the skin and to remove makeup. There are basically two types of cleansers: cleansing milks and foaming cleansers.

Cleansing milks are non-foaming lotion cleansers designed to cleanse dry and sensitive skin types and to remove makeup. They can be applied with the hands or an implement, but they must be removed with a dampened facial sponge, soft cloth, or cotton pad. Ingredients are sometimes added to cleansing milks to make them more specific to a given skin type.

Foaming cleansers are cleansers containing surfactants (detergents) which cause the product to foam and rinse off easily. These products are generally for combination or oilier skin types, although there are some rinse-off cleansers for dry and sensitive skin. Clients love using these products because they may be used quickly and easily in the shower. They have varying amounts of detergent ingredients to treat specific levels of oiliness. Foaming cleansers, like cleansing milks, may have special ingredients to make them more specific for certain skin types. Some have antibacterial ingredients for acne-prone skin.

Toners, also known as **fresheners** or **astringents**, are lotions that help rebalance the pH and remove remnants of cleanser from the skin. They may also contain ingredients that help to hydrate or soothe, and they may sometimes contain an exfoliating ingredient to help remove dead cells. Fresheners and astringents are usually stronger products, often with higher alcohol content, and are used to treat oilier skin types. Toning products are applied with cotton pads after cleansing. Some alcohol-free toners can be sprayed onto the face.

Exfoliants (ex-FO-lee-yahnts) are products that help bring about **exfoliation** (eks-foh-lee-AY-shun), the removal of excess dead cells from the skin surface. Removing dead cells from the surface of the skin allows the skin to look smoother and clearer.

Exfoliants help clear the skin of clogged pores and can improve the appearance of wrinkles, aging, and hyperpigmentation. Cosmetology professionals may use products that remove dead surface cells from the stratum corneum. Deeper, surgical-level peels must only be administered by dermatologists and plastic surgeons.

Exfoliation may be accomplished by using mechanical exfoliants or chemical exfoliants. **Mechanical exfoliants** are products used to physically remove dead cell buildup. **Gommages** (go-mah-jez), also known as **roll-off masks**, are peeling creams that are rubbed off of the skin, and **microdermabrasion scrubs,** scrubs that contain aluminum oxide crystals, along with other granular scrubs, are examples of mechanical exfoliants.

Microdermabrasion can also be used as a machine treatment, which is briefly discussed later in this chapter (**Figure 23–4**). Skin-brushing machines are another example of mechanical exfoliation (**Figures 23–5** and **23–6**).

Chemical exfoliants are products that contain chemicals that either loosen or dissolve dead cell buildup. They are either used for a short time (although some may be worn as a day or night treatment) or combined in a moisturizer. Popular exfoliating chemicals are alpha hydroxy acids (AHAs) (AL-fah hy-DRAHKS-ee AS-uds); these are gentle, naturally

CAUTION

It is important to note that the cosmetology professional's domain is the hair and superficial epidermis. Cosmetology professionals must not perform treatments that remove cells beyond the stratum corneum of the epidermis.

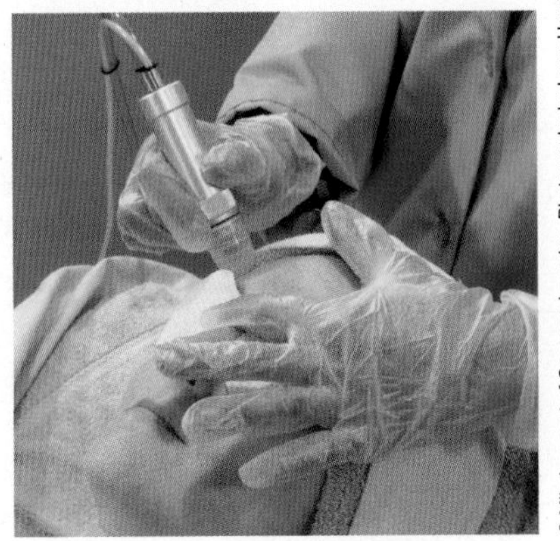

© Milady, a part of Cengage Learning. Photography by Larry Hamill.

▲ Figure 23–4 Microdermabrasion treatment.

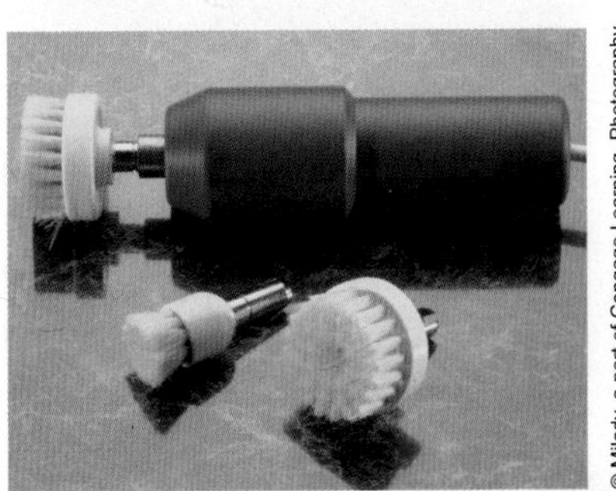

© Milady, a part of Cengage Learning. Photography by Larry Hamill.

▲ Figure 23–5 Skin-brushing machine.

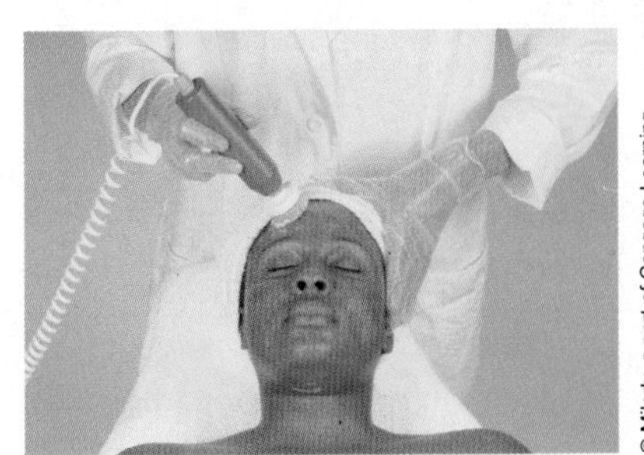

© Milady, a part of Cengage Learning. Photography by Yanik Chauvin.

▲ Figure 23–6 Using a skin-brushing machine during a facial treatment.

CAUTION

Certain skin conditions can be easily inflamed by mechanical exfoliation. Also, certain medications may thin the skin, making it more susceptible to inflammation, bruising, or blistering. Do not use brushing machines, scrubs, or any harsh mechanical peeling techniques on the following skin types and conditions:

- Skin with many visible capillaries
- Thin skin that reddens easily
- Older skin that is thin and bruises easily or the skin of persons using blood thinning medications
- Skin being medically treated with tretinoin (retinoic acid or Retin-A®), isotretinoin, azelaic acid, adapalene (Differin®), AHA, or salicylic acid (found in many common skin products)
- Acne-prone skin with inflamed papules and pustules

occurring acids that remove dead skin cells by dissolving the bonds and intercellular cement between cells. As dead cells are removed from the surface over time, wrinkles appear less deep, skin discolorations may fade, clogged pores are loosened and reduced, new clogged pores are prevented, and skin is smoother and more hydrated. These acids encourage cell renewal, resulting in firmer and healthier-looking skin.

Salon AHA exfoliants, also known as *peels*, contain larger concentrations of AHA, usually around 20 to 30 percent. They should never be used unless the client has been using 10 percent AHA products at home for at least two weeks prior to the higher concentration salon treatment and using a daily facial sunscreen product.

Enzyme peels (EN-zym PEELS), also known as **keratolytic** (kair-uh-tuh-LIT-ik) **enzymes** or **protein-dissolving agents**, are a type of chemical exfoliant that works by dissolving keratin protein in the surface cells of the skin. Usually, enzyme products are made using plant-extracted enzymes from papaya (resulting in an enzyme known as papain, pronounced pa-PAIN) or pineapple (resulting in an enzyme known as bromelain, pronounced bro-ma-LAIN), or they are made from an enzyme derived from beef by-products (resulting in an enzyme known as pancreatin, pronounced pan-cree-at-tin). Enzymes sometimes are blended into scrubs or wearable products, but they are most often designed for use in the salon.

There are two basic types of keratolytic enzyme peels. The first are cream-type enzyme peels (gommage) that usually contain papain. They are applied to the skin and allowed to dry for a few minutes. They form a crust, which is then rolled off the skin (**Figure 23–7**).

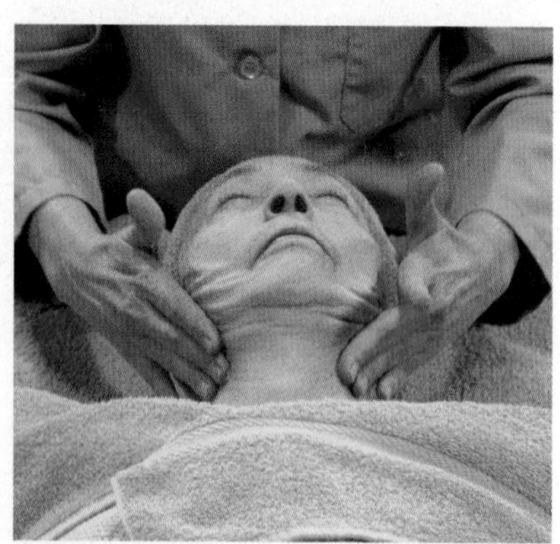

© Milady, a part of Cengage Learning. Photography by Larry Hamill.

▲ **Figure 23–7**
Rolling a gommage mask off the face.

The second and most popular type of enzyme peel is a powder that is mixed with water in the treatment room and applied to the face. This type of enzyme treatment does not dry the skin and can even be used during a steam treatment.

Proper exfoliation may improve the appearance of the skin in the following ways:

- Reduces clogged pores and skin oiliness
- Promotes skin smoothness
- Increases moisture content and hydration
- Reduces hyperpigmentation
- Decreases uneven skin color
- Eliminates or softens wrinkles and fine lines
- Increases elasticity

In addition, proper exfoliation speeds up cell turnover and allows for better penetration of treatment creams and serums. Makeup applies more evenly on exfoliated skin.

CAUTION

You should always receive hands-on training from your instructor before attempting chemical exfoliation treatments!

Moisturizers

Moisturizers are products that help increase the moisture content of the skin surface. Moisturizers help diminish the appearance of fine lines and wrinkles. They are basically mixtures of **humectants** (hyoo-MEKK-tents), also known as **hydrators** or **water-binding agents**, which are ingredients that attract water and **emollients** (ee-MAHL-yunts), which are oily or fatty ingredients that prevent moisture from leaving the skin.

Moisturizers for oily skin are most often in lotion form and generally contain smaller amounts of emollient. Oilier skin does not need as much emollient because oily skin produces more than adequate amounts of protective sebum.

Moisturizers for dry skin are often in the form of a heavier cream, and they contain more emollients, which are needed by alipidic skin.

All moisturizers may have other ingredients that perform additional functions. These ingredients may include soothing agents for sensitive skin, AHAs or peptides for aging skin, or sunscreens.

> **CAUTION**
>
> Over-exfoliation of the skin can result in ultrasensitive and inflamed skin. Never use an exfoliant more often than recommended by the manufacturer. Combining more than one type of exfoliation may lead to irritation. Always carefully advise your client on the proper use of a home care exfoliant, including the need for the use of a daily sunscreen with an SPF of at least 15.

© Marek H., 2010; used under license from Shutterstock.com.

Sunscreens and Day Protection Products

Shielding the skin from sun exposure is probably the most important habit to benefit the skin. Cumulative sun exposure causes the majority of skin cancers and prematurely ages the skin.

Most sun exposure over a lifetime is from casual sun exposure. Therefore, every client should be instructed to use a daily sunscreen. Look for daily moisturizers that contain broad-spectrum sunscreens, which protect against both UVA and UVB light. A sun protection factor (SPF) rating of 15 or higher is considered to be adequate strength for daily use. SPF measures how long someone can be exposed to the sun without burning. For example, if someone normally burns in an hour, an SPF-2 sunscreen allows the person to stay in the sun two times as long without burning. Sunscreens with higher SPF's are appropriate for extended outdoor exposure and for sun-sensitive individuals.

Sunscreens are available in lotion, fluid, and cream forms. Lotions are suitable for combination skin, fluids for oily skin, and creams for dry skin.

Night treatments are usually more intensive products designed for use at night to treat specific skin problems. These products are generally heavier than day-use products, and they theoretically contain higher levels of conditioning ingredients.

Serums (SEH-rums) are concentrated products that generally contain higher concentrations of ingredients designed to penetrate the skin and treat various skin conditions (**Figure 23–8**). They are typically used at home, and they are applied under a moisturizer or sunscreen. **Ampoules** (am-pyools) are individual doses of serum, sealed in small vials.

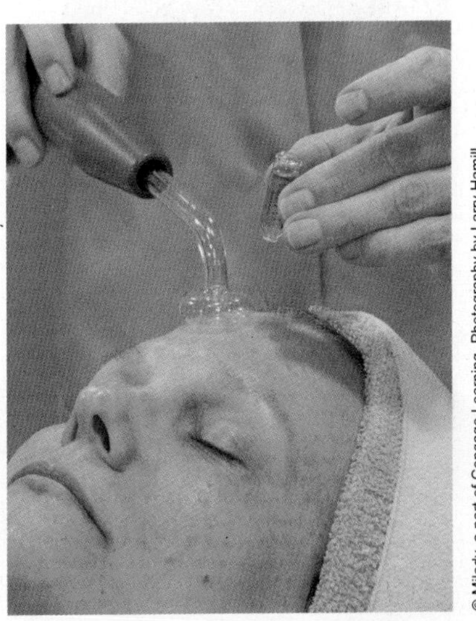

© Milady, a part of Cengage Learning. Photography by Larry Hamill.

▲ **Figure 23–8**
Skin treatment in an ampoule.

Massage creams are lubricants used to make the skin slippery during massage. They often contain oils or petrolatum. If a massage cream is used during a facial treatment, it must be thoroughly removed before any other product can penetrate the skin.

There is a trend toward using treatment products that penetrate the skin during massage. For example, treatment products may be used to increase skin hydration or to soothe redness-prone skin. One of the biggest benefits of massage is that it increases product absorption which, in turn, increases the conditioning effect of treatment products.

did you know?

A valuable ingredient in moisturizers, particularly in day creams, is sunscreen. Not only does sunscreen guard against premature aging of the skin, but also, when used consistently, it is one of the best ways to help prevent skin cancer.

© maryo, 2010; used under license from Shutterstock.com.

Masks

Masks, also known as **masques**, are concentrated treatment products often composed of mineral clays, moisturizing agents, skin softeners, aromatherapy oils, botanical extracts and other beneficial ingredients to cleanse, exfoliate, tighten, tone, hydrate, and nourish the skin.

Clay-based masks are oil-absorbing cleansing masks that have an exfoliating effect and an astringent effect on oily and combination skin, making large pores temporarily appear smaller. They may have additional beneficial ingredients for soothing, or they may include antibacterial ingredients like sulfur, which is helpful for acne-prone skin.

Cream masks are masks often containing oils and emollients as well as humectants, and they have a strong moisturizing effect. They do not dry on the skin like clay masks do, and they are often used to moisturize dry skin.

Gel masks can be used for sensitive or dehydrated skin, and they do not dry hard. They often contain hydrators and soothing ingredients, thus helping to plump surface cells with moisture, making the skin look more supple and more hydrated.

Alginate (al-gin-ate) masks are often seaweed based. They come in a powder form and are mixed with water or, sometime, serums. After mixing, they are quickly applied to the face. They dry to form a rubberized texture. A **treatment cream**, which is a specialty product designed to facilitate change in the skin's appearance, or a serum is generally applied under alginate masks. The alginate mask forms a seal that encourages the skin's absorption of the serum or treatment cream underneath. Alginate masks are generally used only in the salon.

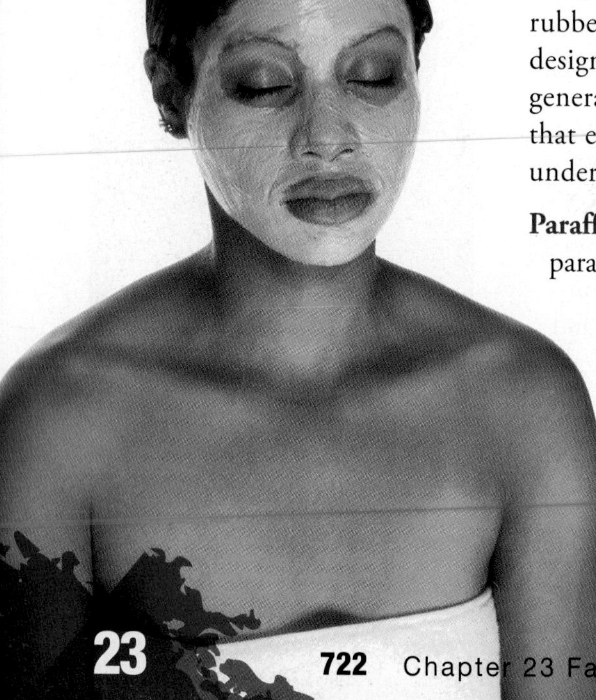

Paraffin wax masks are specially prepared facial masks containing paraffin and other beneficial ingredients. They are melted at a little more than body temperature before application. The paraffin quickly cools to a lukewarm temperature and hardens to a candle-like consistency. Paraffin masks are applied over a treatment cream to allow the cream's ingredients to penetrate more deeply into the surface layers of the skin. Eye pads and gauze are used in a paraffin mask application because facial hair could stick to the wax if it is not covered, making the mask difficult and painful to remove.

© Lev Olkha, 2010; used under license from Shutterstock.com.

Modelage (mod-a-LAHJ) **masks** contain special crystals of gypsum, a plaster-like ingredient (**Figure 23–9**). As with paraffin masks, modelage masks are used with a treatment cream. Modelage masks are mixed with cold water immediately before application and applied about ¼-inch thick. After application, the modelage mask hardens. The chemical reaction that occurs when the plaster and the crystals mix with water produces a gradual increase in temperature that reaches approximately 105 degrees Fahrenheit. As the mask is left on the skin, the temperature gradually cools, until it has cooled down completely. The setting time for modelage masks is approximately twenty minutes. Modelage masks sometimes vary in mixing technique or timing. Always follow the manufacturer's instructions for the product you are using.

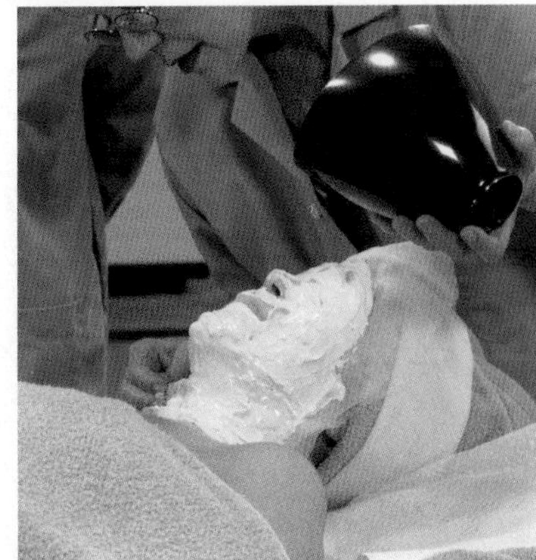

▲ Figure 23–9
Modelage mask.

The heat generated by a modelage mask increases blood circulation and is very beneficial for dry, mature skin or for skin that looks dull and lifeless. This type of mask is not recommended for use on sensitive skin, skin with capillary problems, oily skin, or skin with blemishes. Modelage masks can become quite heavy on the face and should not be applied to the lower neck. These masks should never be used on clients who suffer from claustrophobia, which is a fear of being closed in or confined.

The Use of Gauze for Mask Application

Gauze is a thin, open-meshed fabric of loosely woven cotton (**Figure 23–10**). Masks that have a tendency to run can be applied over a layer of gauze. The gauze holds the mask on the face, while allowing the ingredients to seep through to benefit the skin (**Figure 23–11**). Cheesecloth is sometimes used as well. In some cases, it is necessary to apply a second layer of gauze over the mask to keep the ingredients from sliding off. Gauze is also used to keep paraffin and gypsum/plaster masks from sticking to the skin and the tiny hairs on the skin.

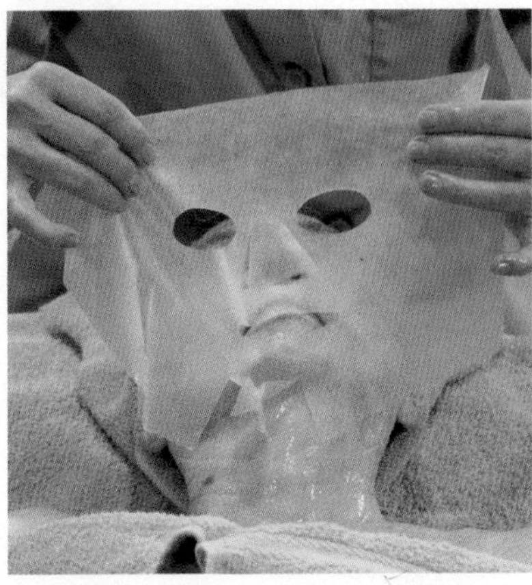

▲ Figure 23–10
Placing gauze on the client's face.

To prepare gauze, cut a piece large enough to cover the entire face and neck. Cut out spaces for the eyes, nose, and mouth. Although the client could breathe through the gauze, the cut-out spaces will make breathing more comfortable for the client. ☑ **LO4**

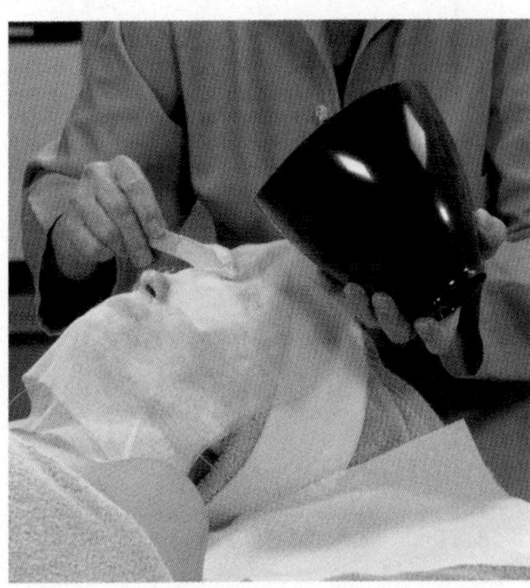

▲ Figure 23–11
Applying a mask over the gauze.

Client Consultation

The salon should designate a quiet area for facial treatments. Not only does the relaxing nature of a facial call for a quiet spot, but also the area needs to be quiet enough that you can conduct a thorough consultation with your client. All facial treatments should begin with a consultation.

Record-Keeping

During the consultation, keep the health screening form and the client intake form at hand so that you can write down all necessary

© Milady, a part of Cengage Learning. Photography by Larry Hamill.

information (**Figure 23–12**). The client intake form should contain the following information:

- Client's name, home address, and home telephone number
- Client's occupation
- Client's date of birth (useful so that you can determine if any signs of aging are premature)
- Client's medical history and current medications, including whether the client is under the care of a physician or dermatologist
- Contraindications—such as a pacemaker, metal implants, pregnancy, diabetes, epilepsy, allergies, high blood pressure—that call for alternative methods of treatment
- Information as to whether the client has had facials before and, if so, what kind of treatments were performed
- Information on any skin care products the client is currently using
- Notation of how the client was referred to the salon
- Observations on the client's skin type, skin condition, and any abnormalities of the skin

Fill out the client intake form to record the date and type of service and/or treatment being performed, the products that are being used, and products purchased by the client for home care. Be sure to

▼ **Figure 23–12**
Client intake form (front).

INTAKE FORM				
Name________________			Date of Consultation ________	
Address________________			D.O.B. ________	
City________	State______	Zip______	Occupation ________	
Tel. (Home)________	(Business)________		Ref. by ________	
Contraindications				
Medical History				
Current Medication				
Previous treatments				
Home Care Products used				
SKIN TYPE	Oily	Normal	Dry (alipidic)	Combination
SKIN CONDITION	Clogged pores	Sensitive	Dehydrated	Mature
Skin Abnormalities				
Remarks				

© Milady, a part of Cengage Learning.

FACIAL RECORD			
Date	Type of treatment	By	Products purchased
2/14	Cleansing, Peel- Relaxing Massage	Mary	Moisturizer with sunscreen
3/16	Cleansing, Peel Modelage Mask	Mary	Cleanser, Toner
4/5	Cleansing, Peel High Frequency indirect	Mary	Moisturizer, Foundation #7
4/26	Cleansing, Peel Massage Alginate Mask	John	
5/13	Cleansing, Peel Iontophoresis Paraffin Mask Skin is showing marked improvement.	Mary	Night cream for dry skin Lipstick #43
6/1	Cleansing, Peel Relaxing Massage	Mary	Eye contour mask

© Milady, a part of Cengage Learning.

▲ **Figure 23–13**
Client intake form (back).

note specific products the client purchases so that you can help her repurchase if she forgets product names (**Figure 23–13**).

As part of the consultation, do not hesitate to recommend services and products that will be beneficial to the client (**Figure 23–14**). Since the client has taken the initiative to come into the salon, they will feel disappointed if you neglect to recommend salon treatments and products, as well as proper home-care products for the skin. Also, if you do not recommend professional products, your client may go elsewhere for advice, such as a department store or drugstore. She might not get the kind of product you would have advised, and you and the salon will not get the retail income.

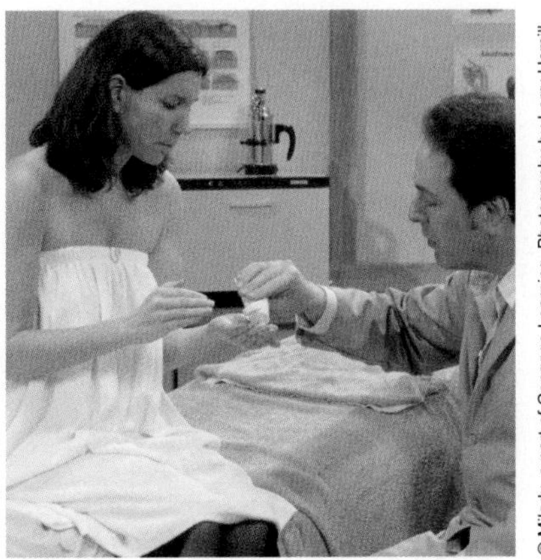

© Milady, a part of Cengage Learning. Photography by Larry Hamill.

▲ **Figure 23–14**
Recommend skin care products to the client.

Make it clear to your client that if they wish to achieve the best results from a treatment, they must follow a proven routine of skin care at home with products that reinforce the salon treatments. Be careful, however, not to make the client feel that the sole purpose of the consultation is to sell products. Review appropriate and discreet retailing techniques with your instructor to make sure you achieve the right tone with your client.

Classification of Skin Types

During the first consultation and before every subsequent facial treatment, it is important to perform a thorough analysis of the client's skin. This analysis should take place prior to cleansing. If the skin is oily, it will often look shiny or greasy. If the skin is dry, it may look flaky. **Table 23–2** lists brief descriptions of basic skin types. ☑ **LO5**

Facial Massage

* summarize!

Massage is the manual or mechanical manipulation of the body by rubbing, gently pinching, kneading, tapping, and other movements to increase metabolism and circulation, to promote absorption, and to relieve pain. Cosmetologists massage their clients to help keep the facial skin healthy and the facial muscles firm.

FOCUS ON

BUILDING YOUR CLIENT BASE

Send your clients a birthday card. This form of advertisement is not expensive, and it is always greatly appreciated. Ask for your clients' e-mail addresses for this purpose and for other kinds of communications. E-mail is now the preferred mode of communication for many people. In fact, many clients now prefer to book appointments using e-mail.

To master massage techniques, you must have a basic knowledge of anatomy and physiology, as well as considerable practice in performing the various movements. It is important that you use a firm, sure touch when giving a massage. To do this, you must develop flexible hands, a quiet temperament, and self-control.

Keep your hands soft by using creams, oils, and lotions. File and shape your nails to avoid scratching your client's skin. Your wrists and fingers should be flexible, and your palms should be firm and warm. Cream or oil should be applied to your hands to permit smoother and gentler hand movements and to prevent drag or damage to the client's skin.

Basic Massage Manipulations

All massage treatments combine one or more basic movements or manipulations. Each manipulation is applied to the superficial muscles in a certain way to achieve a certain end. The impact of a massage treatment depends on the amount of pressure, the direction of movement, and the duration of each type of manipulation involved.

The direction of movement is always from the insertion of the muscle toward its origin. The insertion is the portion of the muscle at the more movable attachment (where it is attached to another muscle or to a movable bone or joint). The origin is the portion of the muscle at the fixed attachment (to an immovable section of the skeleton). Massaging a muscle in the wrong direction could result in a loss of resiliency and sagging of the skin and muscles.

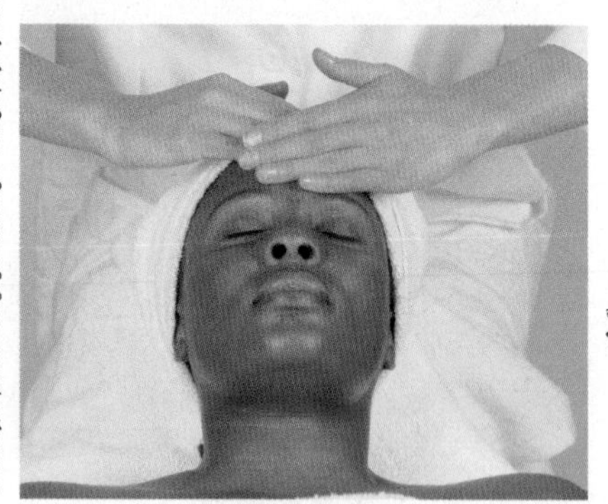

© Milady, a part of Cengage Learning. Photography by Yanik Chauvin.

▲ **Figure 23–15**
Digital effleurage on the forehead.

Effleurage

Effleurage (EF-loo-rahzh) is a light, continuous stroking movement applied in a slow, rhythmic manner with the fingers (digital effleurage) or the palms (palmar effleurage). No pressure is used. The palms work the large surfaces, and the cushions of the fingertips work the small surfaces, such as those around the eyes (**Figure 23–15**). Effleurage is frequently used on the forehead, face, scalp, back, shoulder, neck, chest, arms, and hands for its soothing and relaxing effects. Every massage should begin and end with effleurage.

When performing effleurage, hold your whole hand loosely, and keep your wrist and fingers flexible. Curve your fingers slightly to conform to the shape of the area being massaged, with just the cushions of the fingertips touching the skin. Do not use the ends of the fingertips. They are pointier than the cushions, and will cause the effleurage to be less smooth. Also, the free edges of your fingernails may scratch the client's skin.

FYI

As a cosmetologist, your services are limited to certain areas of the body: the scalp, face, neck, and shoulders; the upper chest; the hands and arms; and the feet and lower legs. Therapeutic massage—including deep muscle massage, deep tissue massage, and lymph drainage—should only be performed by therapists specialized in working on various kinds of tissues. Therapeutic massage requires special training and, in many cases, licensure.

Pétrissage

Pétrissage (PEH-treh-sahj) is a kneading movement performed by lifting, squeezing, and pressing the tissue with a light, firm pressure. Pétrissage offers deeper stimulation to the muscles, nerves, and skin glands, and improves circulation. These kneading movements are usually limited to the back, shoulders, and arms.

Although typically used on larger surface areas such as the arms and shoulders, digital kneading can also be used on the cheeks with light pinching movements (**Figure 23–16**). The pressure should be light but firm. When grasping and releasing the fleshy parts, the movements must be rhythmic and never jerky.

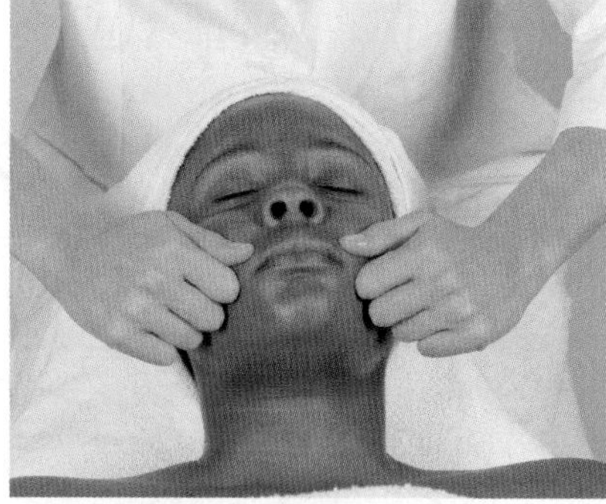

▲ **Figure 23–16**
Pétrissage.

Fulling is a form of pétrissage in which the tissue is grasped, gently lifted, and spread out; this technique is used mainly for massaging the arms. With the fingers of both hands grasping the arm, apply a kneading movement across the flesh, with light pressure on the underside of the client's forearm and between the shoulder and elbow.

Friction

Friction (FRIK-shun) is a deep rubbing movement in which you apply pressure on the skin with your fingers or palm while moving it over an underlying structure. Friction has been known to have a significant benefit on the circulation and glandular activity of the skin. Circular friction movements are typically used on the scalp, arms, and hands. Light circular friction is used on the face and neck (**Figure 23–17**).

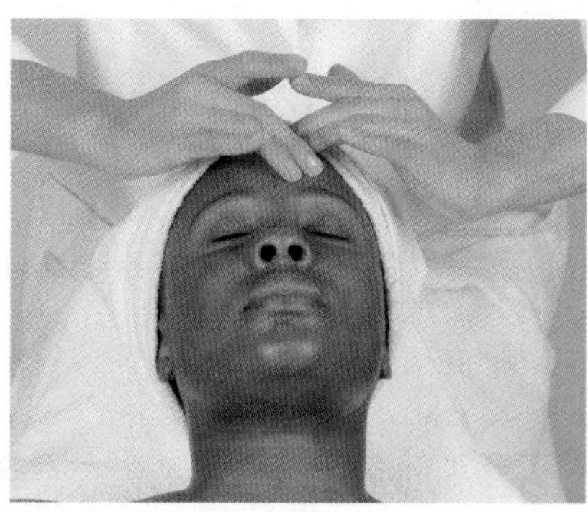

▲ **Figure 23–17**
Friction.

Chucking, rolling, and wringing are variations of friction and are used mainly to massage the arms and legs, as follows:

- **Chucking** is grasping the flesh firmly in one hand and moving the hand up and down along the bone while the other hand keeps the arm or leg in a steady position.
- **Rolling** is pressing and twisting the tissues with a fast back-and-forth movement.
- **Wringing** is a vigorous movement in which the hands, placed a little distance apart on both sides of the client's arm or leg and working downward, apply a twisting motion against the bones in the opposite direction.

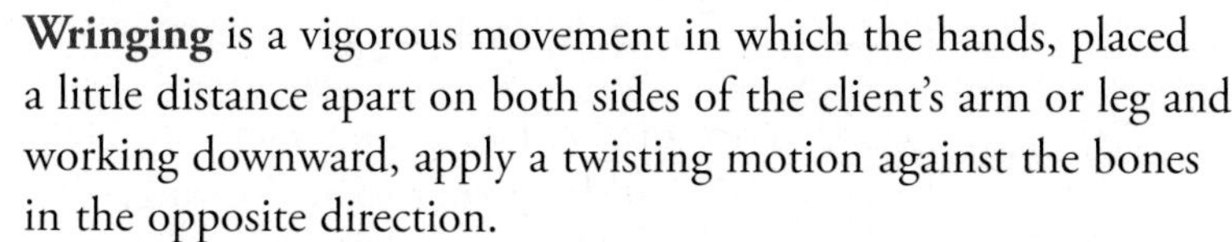

Tapotement

Tapotement (tah-POH-te-ment), also known as **percussion** (pur-KUSH-un), consists of short quick tapping, slapping, and hacking movements. This form of massage is the most stimulating and should be applied with care and discretion. Tapotement movements tone the muscles and impart a healthy glow to the area being massaged.

© Milady, a part of Cengage Learning. Photography by Yanik Chauvin.

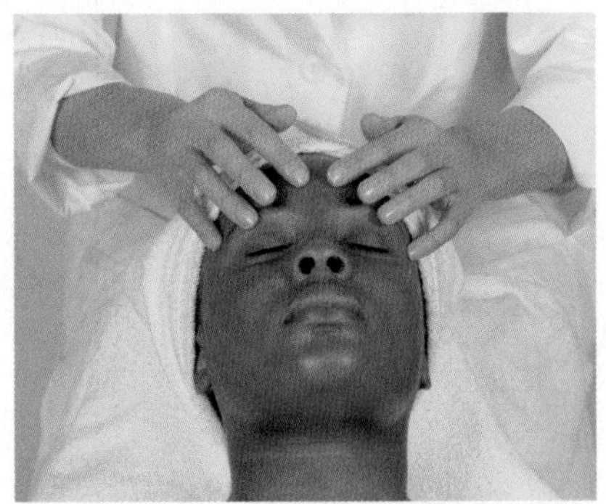

▲ Figure 23–18
Tapotement.

In facial massage, use only light digital tapping. Bring the fingertips down against the skin in rapid succession. Your fingers must be flexible enough to create an even force over the area being massaged (**Figure 23–18**).

In slapping movements, keeping your wrists flexible allows your palms to come in contact with the skin in light, firm, and rapid slapping movements. One hand follows the other. With each slapping stroke, lift the flesh slightly.

Hacking is a chopping movement performed with the edges of the hands. Both the wrists and hands move alternately in fast, light, firm, and flexible motions against the skin. Hacking and slapping movements are used only to massage the back, shoulders, and arms.

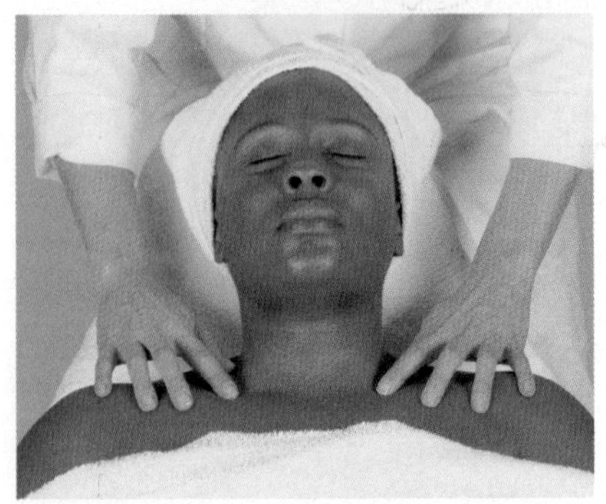

▲ Figure 23–19
Vibration on the top of the shoulders.

Vibration

Vibration (vy-BRAY-shun) is a rapid shaking of the body part while the balls of the fingertips are pressed firmly on the point of application. The movement is accomplished by rapid muscular contractions in your arms. It is a highly relaxing movement, and should be applied at the end of the massage (**Figure 23–19**). Deep vibration in combination with other classical massage movements can also be produced by the use of a mechanical vibrator to stimulate blood circulation and increase muscle tone.

Physiological Effects of Massage

To obtain proper results from a scalp or facial massage, you must have a thorough knowledge of the structures involved, including

FYI

Before performing a service that includes a facial massage, consult the client's intake or health screening form. During the consultation acknowledge and discuss any medical condition that may contraindicate a facial massage. Ask the client if he or she has discussed massage with a physician. If the client has not already sought a physician's advice as to whether or not a facial massage is advisable, encourage him or her to do so before you perform the service.

Many clients who have high blood pressure (hypertension), diabetes, or circulatory conditions may still have facial massage without concern, especially if their condition is being treated and carefully looked after by a physician. Facial massage is, however, contraindicated for clients with severe, uncontrolled hypertension. Also, clients with acne should not be massaged in any area that has breakouts.

If your client expresses a concern about having a facial massage and has a medical condition, advise him or her to speak with a physician before having the service.

If your client has sensitive or redness-prone skin, avoid using vigorous or strong massage techniques.

Do not talk to your client during the massage except to ask once whether your touch should be more or less firm. Talking eliminates the relaxation therapy of the massage.

When making decisions about whether to perform a facial massage on a person who has a medical condition, be conservative. When in doubt, don't include massage as part of your service.

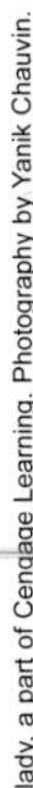
© Milady, a part of Cengage Learning. Photography by Yanik Chauvin.

muscles, nerves, connective tissues, and blood vessels. Every muscle has a **motor point**, which is a point on the skin that covers the muscle where pressure or stimulation will cause contraction of that muscle. Some examples are illustrated in **Figures 23–20** and **23–21**. In order to obtain the maximum benefits from a facial massage, you must consider the motor points that affect the underlying muscles of the face and neck. The location of motor points varies among individuals due to differences in body structure. However, a few manipulations on the proper motor points will relax the client early in the massage treatment.

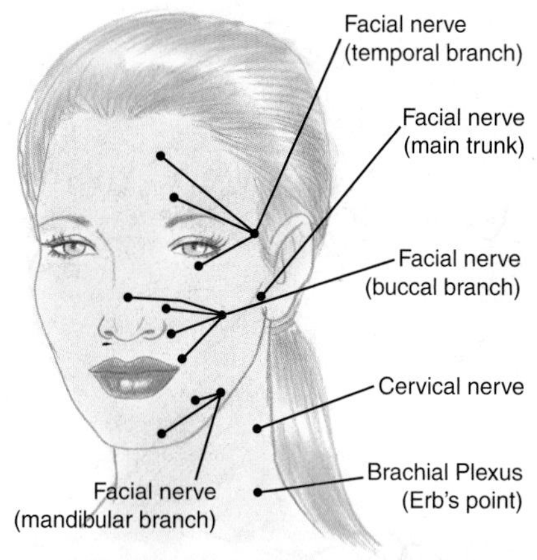

▲ **Figure 23–20**
Motor nerve points of the face.

Relaxation is achieved through light but firm, slow, rhythmic movements, or very slow, light hand vibrations over the motor points for a short time. Another technique is to pause briefly over the motor points, using light pressure.

Skillfully applied massage directly or indirectly influences the structures and functions of the body. The immediate effects of massage are first noticed on the skin. The area being massaged shows increased circulation, secretion, nutrition, and excretion. The following benefits may be obtained by proper facial and scalp massage:

- Skin and all structures are nourished
- Skin becomes softer and more pliable
- Circulation of blood is increased
- Activity of skin glands is stimulated
- Muscle fibers are stimulated and strengthened
- Nerves are soothed and rested
- Pain is sometimes relieved

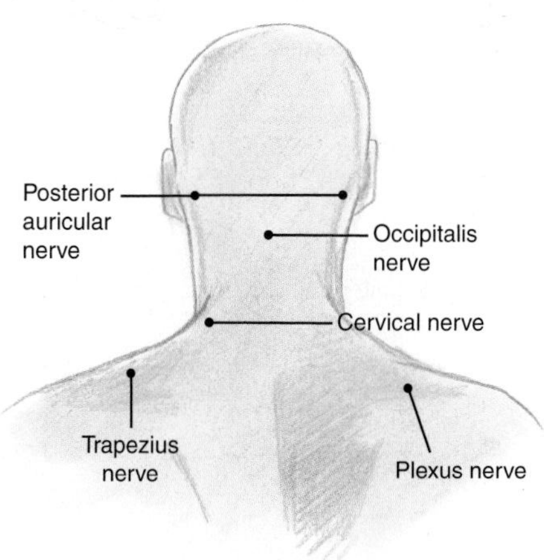

▲ **Figure 23–21**
Motor nerve points of the neck.

The recommended frequency of facial or scalp massage depends on the condition of the skin or scalp, the age of the client, and the condition being treated. As a general rule, normal skin or scalp can be kept in excellent condition with the help of a weekly massage, accompanied by proper home care.

Facial Manipulations

Because an overview of basic massage/manipulation techniques and guidelines is now complete, the best manipulations to use on the face can be discussed in more depth. When performing facial manipulations, keep in mind that an even tempo, or rhythm, is relaxing. Do not remove your hands from the client's face once you have started the manipulations.

Should it become necessary to remove your hands, feather them off, and then gently replace them with feather-like movements. Remember that massage movements are generally directed from the muscle's insertion toward its origin, in order to avoid damage to muscle tissues.

© Milady, a part of Cengage Learning.

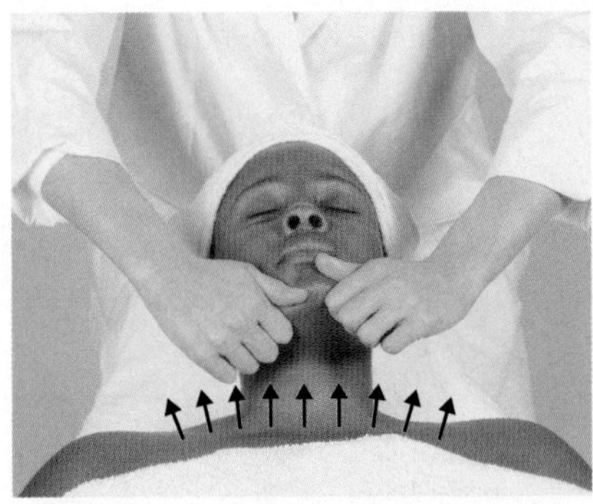

▲ **Figure 23–22**
Chin movement.

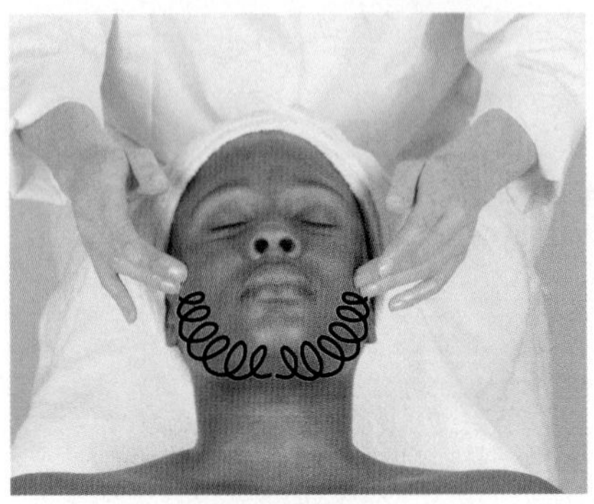

▲ **Figure 23–23**
Circular movement of lower cheeks.

The following photographs show the different movements that may be used on the various parts of the face, chest, and back. Each instructor may have developed her own routine, however. For example, some instructors and practitioners prefer to start massage manipulations at the chin, while others prefer to start at the forehead. Both are correct. Be guided by your instructor.

Chin movement. Lift the chin, using a slight pressure (**Figure 23–22**).

Lower cheeks. Using a circular movement, rotate from chin to ears (**Figure 23–23**).

Mouth, nose, and cheek movements. Follow the diagram (**Figure 23–24**).

Linear movement over the forehead. Slide fingers to the temples and then stroke up to hairline, gradually moving your hands across the forehead to the right eyebrow (**Figures 23–25a** and **b**).

Circular movement over the forehead. Starting at the eyebrow line, work across the middle of the forehead and then toward the hairline (**Figure 23–26**).

Crisscross movement. Start at one side of forehead and work back (**Figure 23–27**).

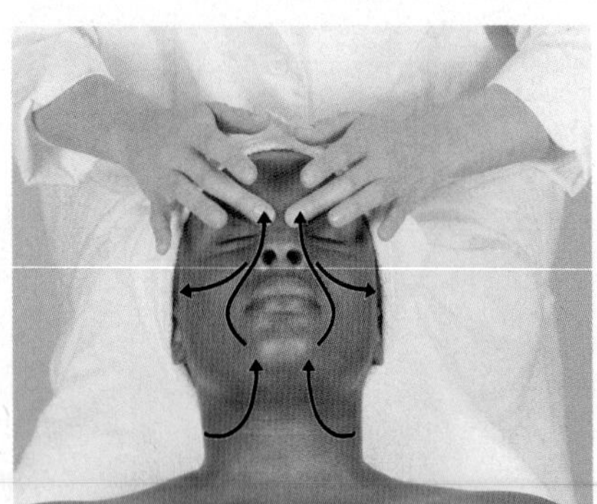

▲ **Figure 23–24**
Mouth, nose, and cheek movements.

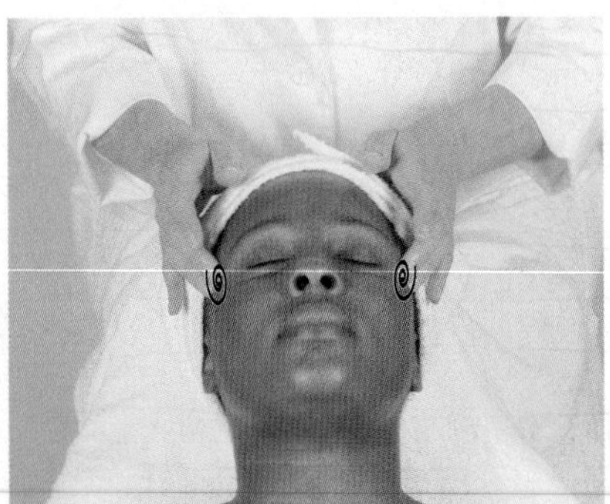

▲ **Figure 23–25a and b**
Light circular movement over the temples continuing with linear movement over forehead.

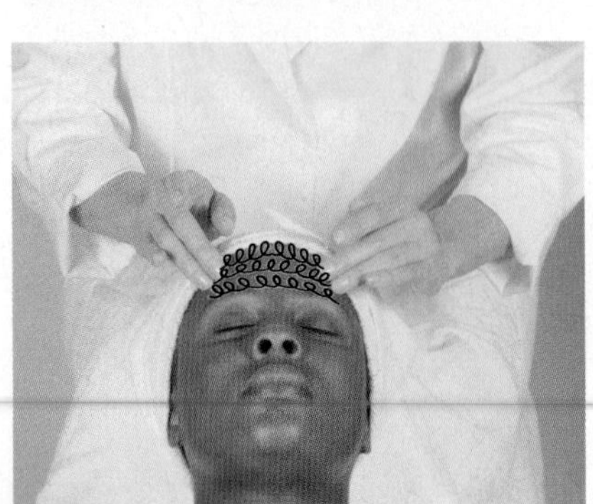

▲ **Figure 23–26**
Circular movement over forehead.

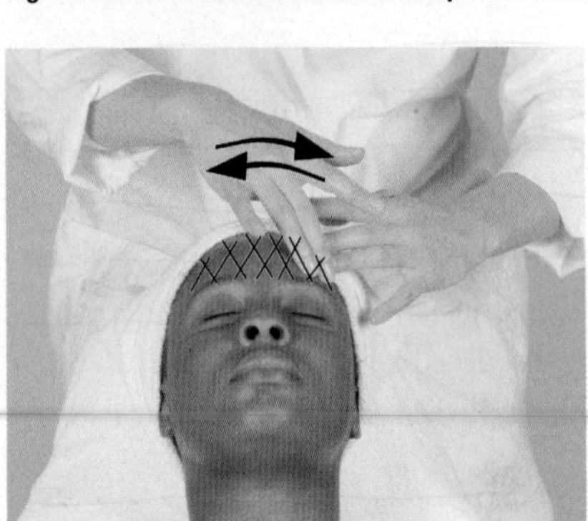

▲ **Figure 23–27**
Crisscross movement.

© Milady, a part of Cengage Learning. Photography by Yanik Chauvin.

Stroking (headache) movement. Slide your fingers toward the center of the forehead and then draw your fingers, with slight pressure, toward the temples and rotate (**Figure 23–28**).

Brow and eye movement. Place your middle fingers at the inner corners of the eyes and your index fingers over the brows. Slide them toward the outer corners of the eyes, under the eyes, and then back to the inner corners (**Figure 23–29**).

Nose and upper cheek movement. Slide your fingers down the nose. Apply a rotary movement across the cheeks to the temples and rotate gently. Slide your fingers under the eyes and then back to the bridge of the nose (**Figure 23–30**).

Mouth and nose movement. Apply a circular movement from the corners of the mouth up to the sides of the nose. Slide your fingers over the brows and then down to the corners of the mouth up to the sides of nose. Follow by sliding your fingers over the brows and down to the corners of the mouth again (**Figure 23–31**).

Lip and chin movement. From the center of the upper lip, draw your fingers around the mouth, going under the lower lip and chin (**Figure 23–32**).

Optional movement. Hold the head with your left hand, and draw the fingers of your right hand from under the lower lip and around mouth, moving to the center of the upper lip (**Figure 23–33**).

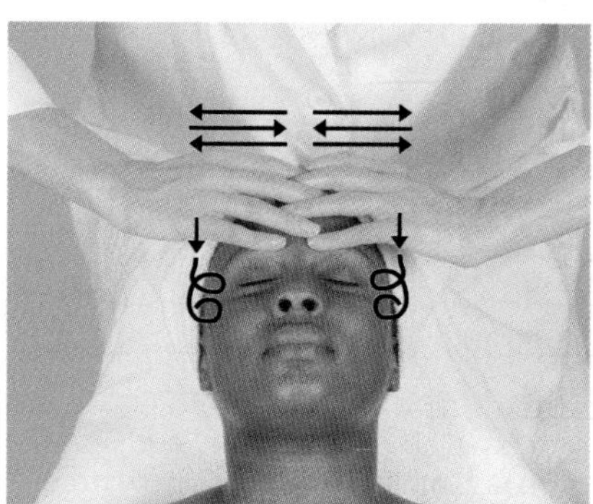

▲ Figure 23–28
Stroking (headache) movement.

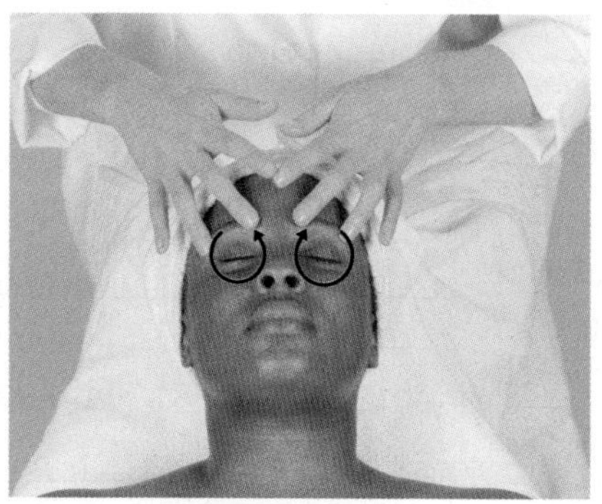

▲ Figure 23–29
Brow and eye movement.

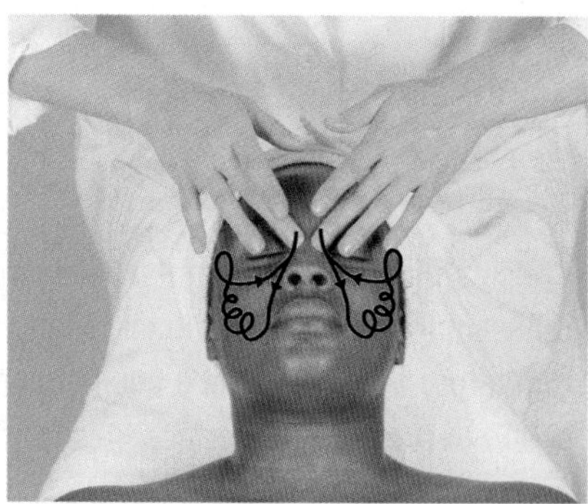

▲ Figure 23–30
Nose and upper cheek movement.

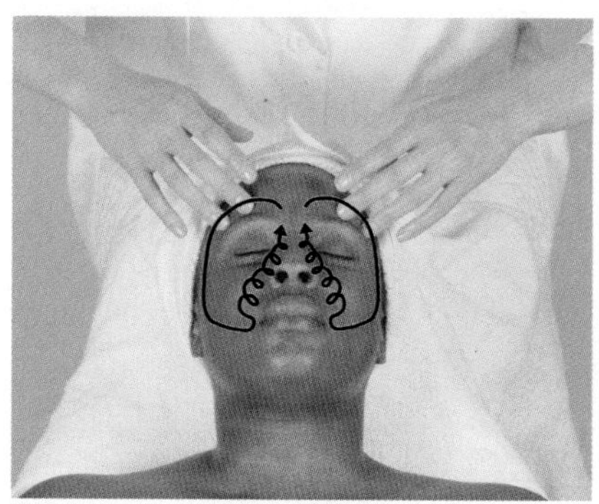

▲ Figure 23–31
Mouth and nose movement.

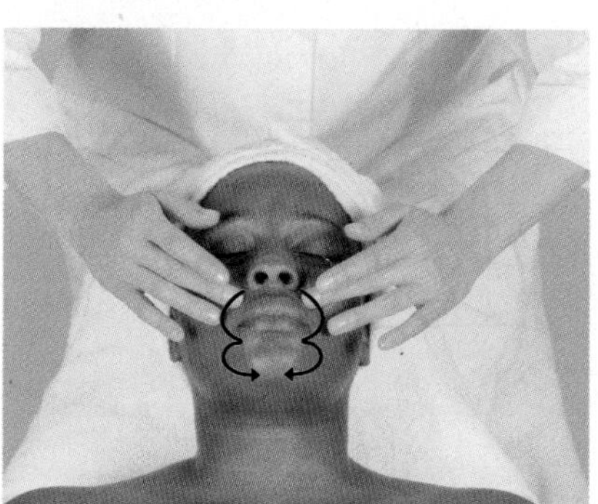

▲ Figure 23–32
Lip and chin movement.

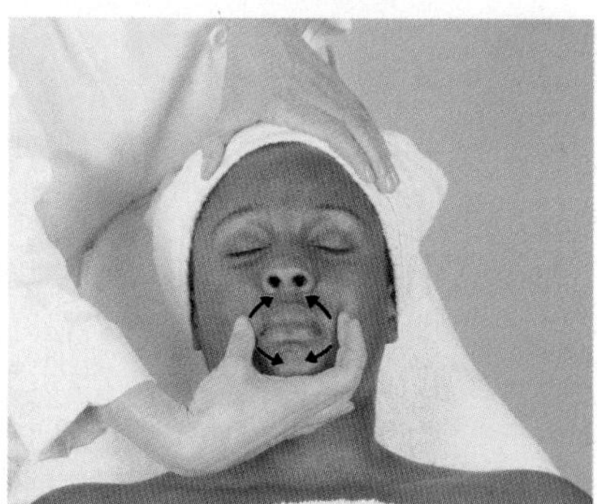

▲ Figure 23–33
Optional movement.

© Milady, a part of Cengage Learning. Photography by Yanik Chauvin.

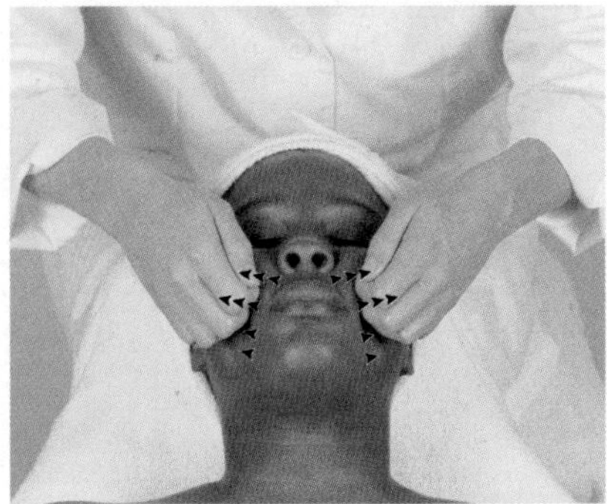

▲ **Figure 23–34**
Lifting movement of cheeks.

Lifting movement of the cheeks. Proceed from the mouth to the ears, and then from the nose to the top part of the ears (**Figure 23–34**).

Rotary movement of the cheeks. Massage from the chin to the ear lobes, from the mouth to the middle of the ears, and from the nose to the top of the ears (**Figure 23–35**).

Light tapping movement. Work from the chin to the earlobe, from the mouth to the ear, from the nose to the top of the ear, and then across the forehead. Repeat on the other side (**Figure 23–36**).

Stroking movement of the neck. Apply light upward strokes over the front of the neck. Use heavier pressure on the sides of neck in downward strokes (**Figure 23–37**).

Circular movement over the neck and chest. Starting at the back of the ears, apply a circular movement down the side of the neck, over the shoulders, and across the chest (**Figure 23–38**).

Massaging male skin is not all that different from massaging female skin. However, it needs more attention in the areas of the face where there is hair growth. For your male clients, use downward movements in the beard area. Massaging against hair growth causes great discomfort. Pressure-point massage in the beard area is much appreciated by male clients.

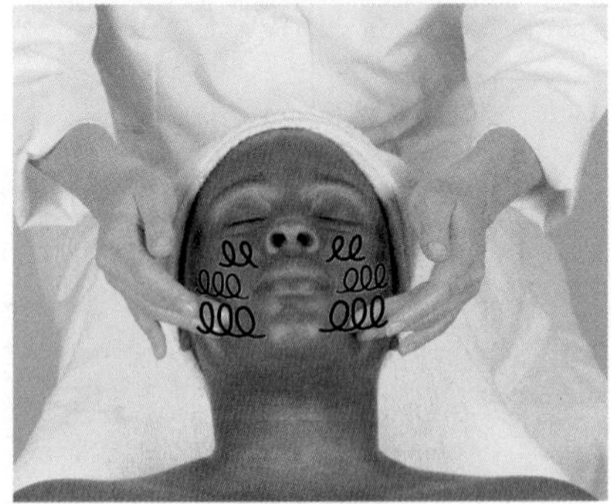

▲ **Figure 23–35**
Rotary movement of cheeks.

Chest, Back, and Neck Manipulations (Optional)

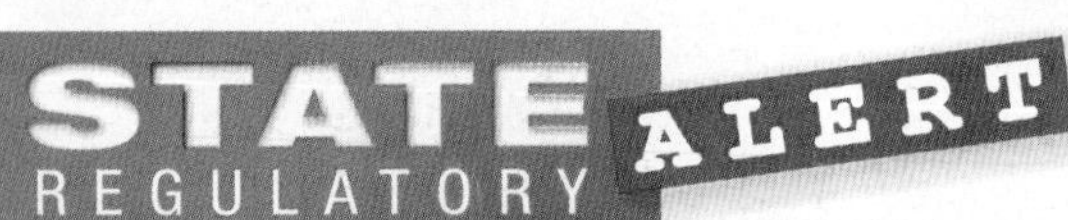

Check with your state regulatory agency before massaging the chest and back. Many state regulatory agencies limit a cosmetologists scope of practice to the face, neck, arms, legs, and shoulders.

Some instructors prefer to treat these areas first before starting the regular facial. Apply cleanser, and remove it with a tissue or a warm, moist towel. Then apply massage cream and perform the following manipulations:

Chest and back movement. Use a rotary movement across the upper chest and shoulders. Then slide your fingers to the base of the neck and rotate three times.

Shoulders and back movement. Rotate the shoulders three times. Glide your fingers to the spine and then to the base of

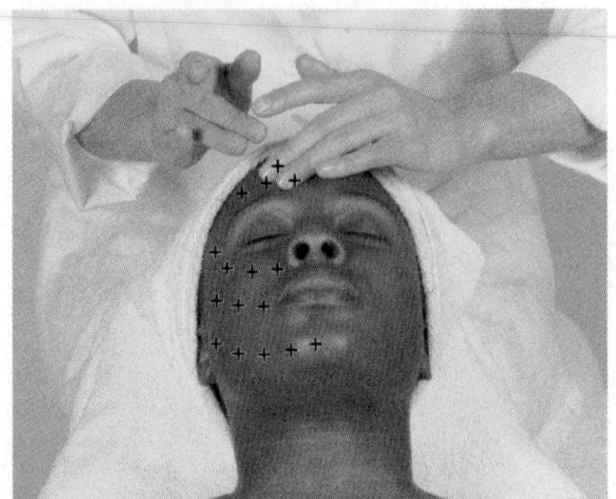

▲ **Figure 23–36**
Light tapping movement.

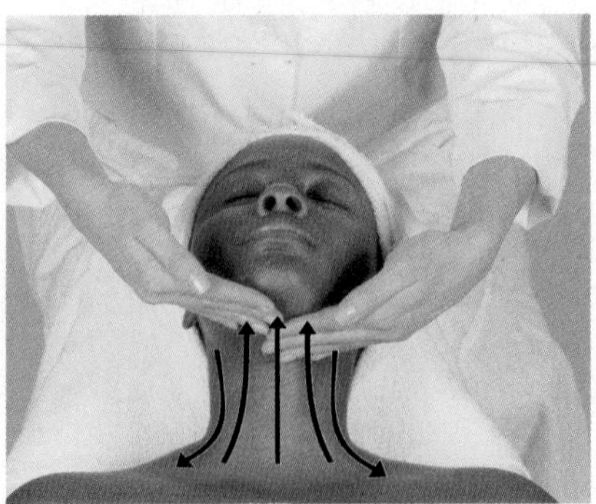

▲ **Figure 23–37**
Stroking movement of neck.

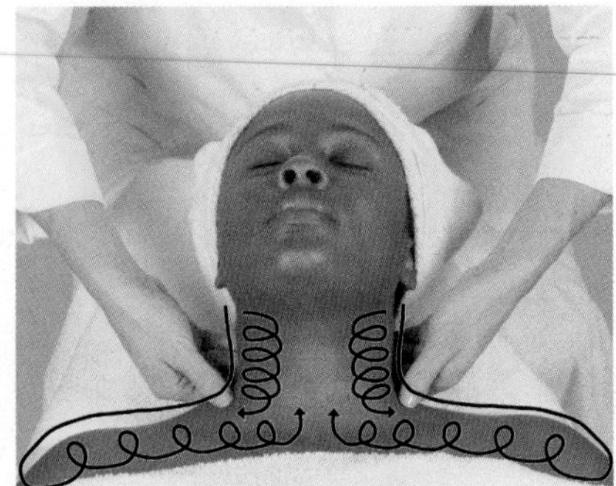

▲ **Figure 23–38**
Circular movement over neck and chest.

© Milady, a part of Cengage Learning. Photography by Yanik Chauvin.

the neck. Apply circular movement up to the back of the ear, and then slide your fingers to the front of the earlobe. Rotate three times.

Back massage. To stimulate and relax the client, use your thumbs and bent index fingers to grasp the tissue at the back of the neck. Rotate six times. Repeat over the shoulders. Remove cream with tissues or a warm, moist towel. Dust the back lightly with talcum powder and smooth.
☑ **LO6**

> **CAUTION**
>
> Information regarding facial equipment in this chapter is intended as an overview. You should receive hands-on experience from your instructor before using any facial equipment! Machine models differ; as a result, precautions vary as well. Consult with your instructor and the specific machine manual for safe operation. In some states, use of certain equipment may not be permissible for cosmetologists. Again, check with your instructor to find out what is allowed in your state.

Facial Equipment

There are many types of facial equipment that can enhance your abilities to perform an outstanding facial treatment. These machines help to increase the efficacy of your products, increase product penetration, and provide for a more complete and relaxing treatment.

We have already mentioned magnifying lamps, which are necessary for both analysis of the skin and procedures such as extraction of comedones and tweezing of excess facial hair.

A facial **steamer** heats and produces a stream of warm steam that can be focused on the client's face or other areas of skin. Steaming the skin helps to soften the tissues, making it more accepting of moisturizers and other treatment products. Steam also helps to relax and soften follicle accumulations such as comedones and clogged follicles, making them easier to extract (**Figure 23–39**).

Most steamers work by having a heating coil that boils water. The steam from the boiling water flows through a pipe that can be focused on the area to be treated, normally the face. Only distilled water should be used in most steamers to avoid mineral buildup in the machine. Steam is usually administered at the beginning of the facial treatment. Most clients enjoy steam, but precautions should be taken with clients who have asthma or other breathing disorders.

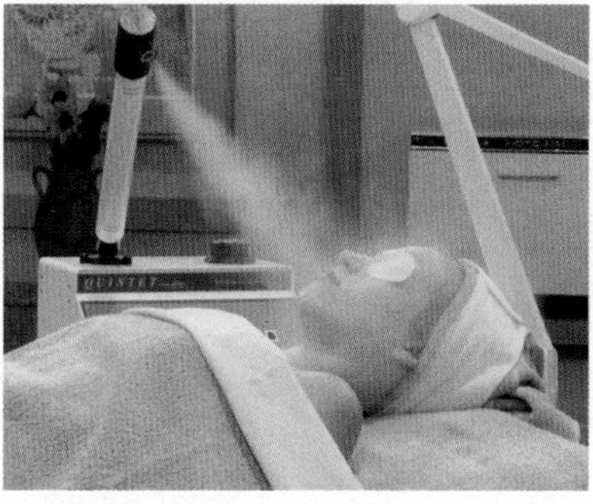

© Milady, a part of Cengage Learning. Photography by Larry Hamill.

▲ **Figure 23–39**
Facial steamer being used during a facial treatment.

* steamer must be 14 inches away from client.

It is strongly recommended that a professional steamer be used, but if one is not available, a warm steamed towel may be gently wrapped around the face, leaving the nose exposed so the client can breathe comfortably. The towel should be comfortably warm, but not hot. Do not use steamed towels on clients who have sensitive skin, redness-prone skin, rosacea, or claustrophobia.

A **brushing machine** is a rotating electric appliance with interchangeable brushes that can be attached to the rotating head. Brushes of various sizes as well as textures are common. Larger and stiffer brushes are used for back treatment, and smaller and softer brushes are used for the face.

Brushing is a form of mechanical exfoliation, and it is usually administered after or during steam. A fairly thick layer of cleanser or moisturizer should be applied to the face before using the brushing machine.

This applied product provides a buffer for the brushes so that they do not scratch the face, which they might do if the face were completely dry.

Brushing helps remove dead cells from the skin surface, making the skin look smoother and more even in coloration. It also helps to stimulate blood circulation.

Brushing should never be used on clients using keratolytic drugs such as Retin-A®, Differin®, Tazorac®, or other drugs that thin or exfoliate the skin. Clients who have rosacea, sensitive skin, pustular acne, or other forms of skin inflammation or reddening should not have brushing administered. Never use a brushing machine at the same time as another exfoliation technique, such as an AHA treatment or microdermabrasion.

Brushes must be thoroughly cleaned and disinfected between clients.

The skin suction and cold spray machine is used to increase circulation, and to jet-spray lotions and toners onto the skin. Skin suction should only be used on nonsensitive and noninflamed skin.

Spray can be used on almost any skin type. Spray is often used to hydrate the skin and to help clean off mask treatments. ☑ LO7

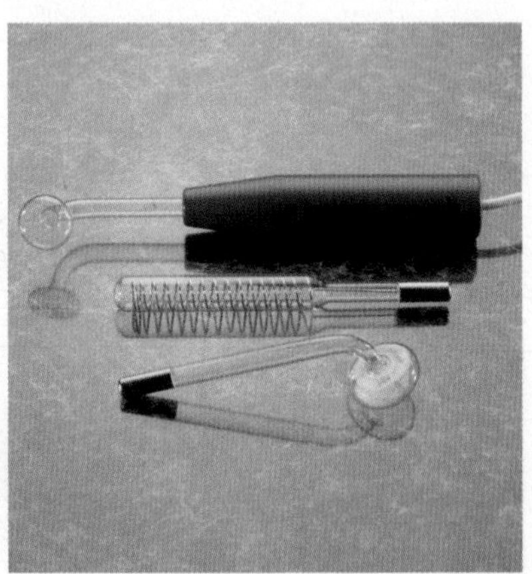

▲ Figure 23–40
Various electrodes.

Electrotherapy and Light Therapy

Galvanic and high-frequency treatment are types of **electrotherapy** (ee-LECK-tro-ther-ah-pee), which is the use of electrical currents to treat the skin.

There are several contraindications for electrotherapy. Electrotherapy should never be administered on heart patients, clients with pacemakers, clients with metal implants, pregnant clients, clients with epilepsy or seizure disorders, clients who are afraid of electric current, or clients with open or broken skin. Furthermore, if you ever have any doubts about whether the client can have electrotherapy safely, request that the client get approval from her physician before receiving this therapy.

An electrode is an applicator for directing the electric current from the machine to the client's skin (**Figure 23–40**). High-frequency machines have only one electrode. Galvanic machines have two positive electrodes called an anode (AN-ohd), which has a red plug and cord, and a negative electrode called a cathode (KATH-ohd), which has a black plug and cord (**Figure 23–41**).

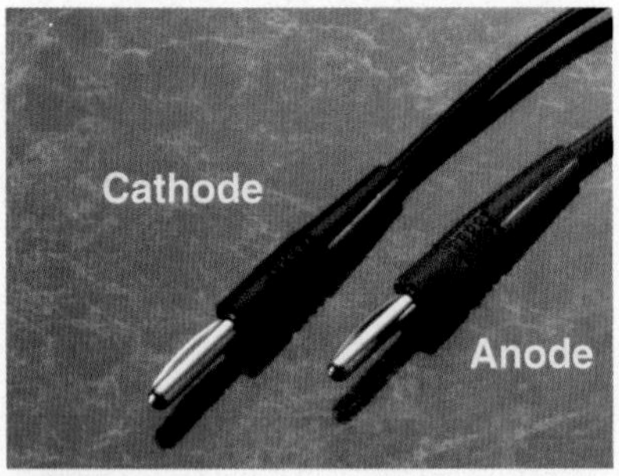

▲ Figure 23–41
Cathode and anode.

© Milady, a part of Cengage Learning. Photography by Larry Hamill.

Galvanic current accomplishes two basic tasks. Desincrustation (des-in-cruh-STAY-shun) is the process of softening and emulsifying hardened sebum stuck in the hair follicles. Desincrustation is very helpful when treating oily areas with multiple comedones and most acne-prone skin. Desincrustation products are alkaline fluids or gels that act as solvents for the solidified sebum. These products make extraction of the impactions and comedones much easier. When the negative pole is applied to the face over a desincrustation product, the current forces the product deeper into the follicle. The current also produces a chemical reaction that helps to loosen the impacted sebum (**Figure 23–42**).

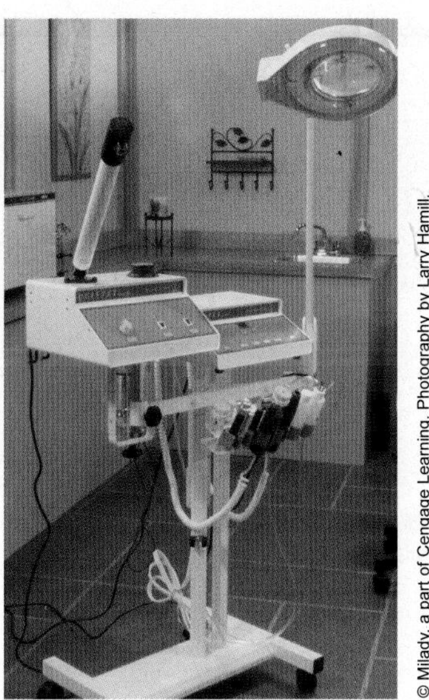
© Milady, a part of Cengage Learning. Photography by Larry Hamill.

▲ **Figure 23–42**
Five-in-one machine, including galvanic electrodes.

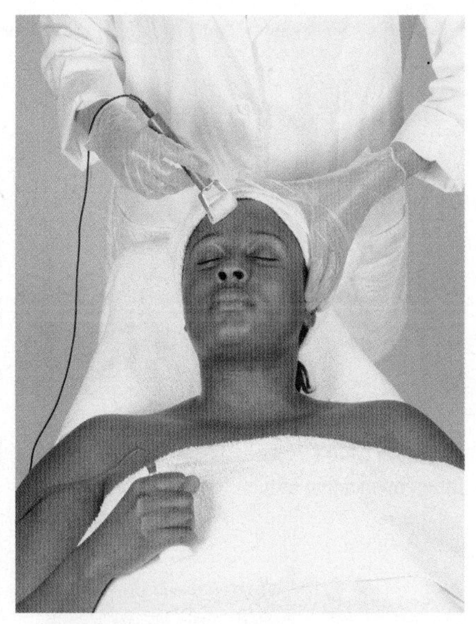
© Milady, a part of Cengage Learning. Photography by Yanik Chauvin.

▲ **Figure 23–43**
Client holding passive electrode.

Both electrodes are wrapped in wet cotton. The active electrode is the one that should be applied to the skin. The active electrode—in the case of desincrustation, the negative electrode—is applied to the oily areas of the face for three to five minutes. The positive electrode (in this case, the inactive electrode) is held by the client in her right hand or attached to a pad that is placed in contact with the client's right shoulder (**Figure 23–43**). After the desincrustation process has taken place, sebum deposits can easily be extracted with gentle pressure.

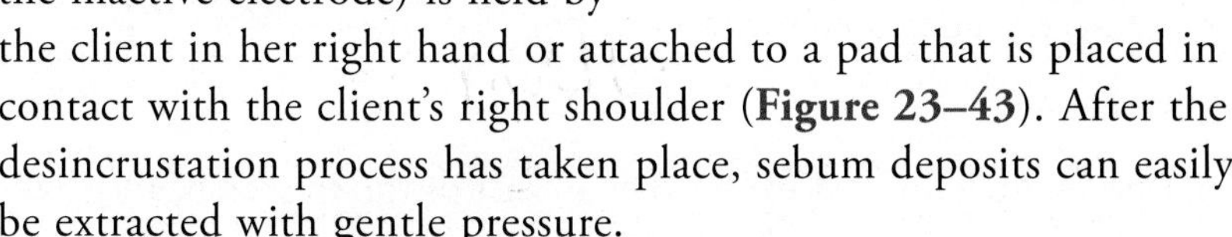

Iontophoresis (eye-ahn-toh-foh-REE-sus) is the process of using galvanic current to enable water-soluble products that contain ions to penetrate the skin. Products suitable for iontophoresis will be labeled as such by manufacturers. When the negative current is applied to the face, products with negative ions are able to penetrate the skin, and when the positive current is applied to the face, products with positive ions are able to penetrate the skin. Many ampoules and serums are prepared for iontophoresis.

Again, you must receive thorough hands-on instruction from your teacher before attempting this procedure.

CAUTION

Do not use the galvanic current on clients who have:

- **metal implants, a pacemaker, or any heart condition.**
- **epilepsy.**
- **pregnancy.**
- **high blood pressure, fever, or any infection.**
- **insufficient nerve sensibility.**
- **open or broken skin (wounds, new scars), including pustular acne.**
- **fear of electrical current.**

Microcurrent

Microcurrent (MY-kroh-KUR-ent) is a type of galvanic treatment using a very low level of electrical current; it has many applications in skin care and is best known for helping to tone the skin, producing a lifting effect for aging skin that lacks elasticity.

High-Frequency Current

High-frequency current, discovered by Nikolas Tesla, can be used to stimulate blood flow and help products penetrate. It works by warming tissues, which allows better absorption of moisturizers and other treatment products. High-frequency current can also be applied after extraction or during treatments for acne-prone skin because it has a germicidal effect.

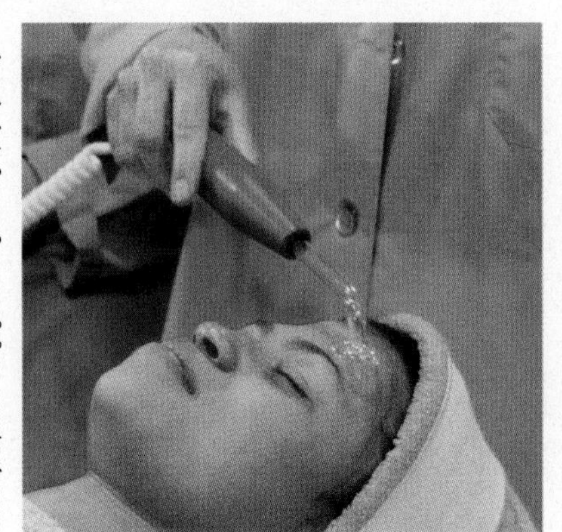

© Milady, a part of Cengage Learning. Photography by Larry Hamill.

▲ **Figure 23–44**
Direct application of high frequency.

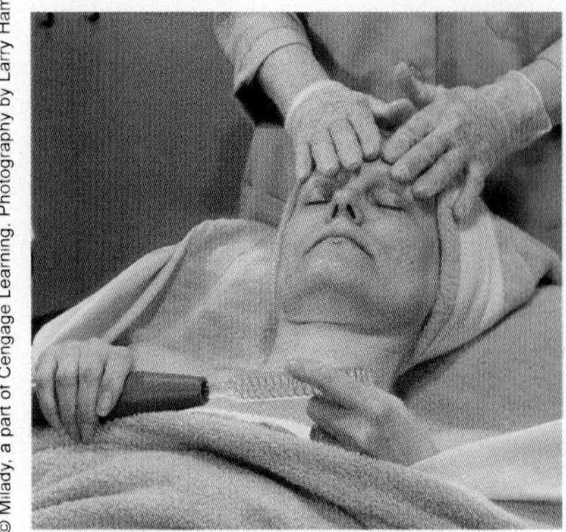

© Milady, a part of Cengage Learning. Photography by Larry Hamill.

▲ **Figure 23–45**
Indirect appplication of high frequency.

Electrodes for the high-frequency machine are made of glass and contain various types of gas, such as neon, which light up as a color when current is flowing through the electrode. Unlike the galvanic machine, high-frequency treatments require the use of only one electrode. There are several different types of electrodes used with high frequency. The most common is shaped like a mushroom, and it is referred to as a *mushroom electrode* (**Figure 23–44**).

CAUTION

Place the passive electrode on the right side of the client's body only (never on the left side) to avoid current flow through the heart.

High frequency can be applied directly to the skin in a technique known as *direct application*. Another application method, known as *indirect massage* or *Viennese massage*, involves the client holding the electrode during treatment, creating an electrical stimulating massage (**Figure 23–45**).

High frequency is applied to the skin as part of the treatment phase of the facial treatment. Again, because machines vary, you should check with your instructor and the manufacturer's manual for instructions for the specific machine you are using.

Light Therapy

Using light exposure to treat conditions of the skin is known as light therapy. There are several different types of light therapy utilizing various types of light. Traditionally, infrared lamps have been used to heat the skin and increase blood flow. Infrared lights have also been used for hair and scalp treatments.

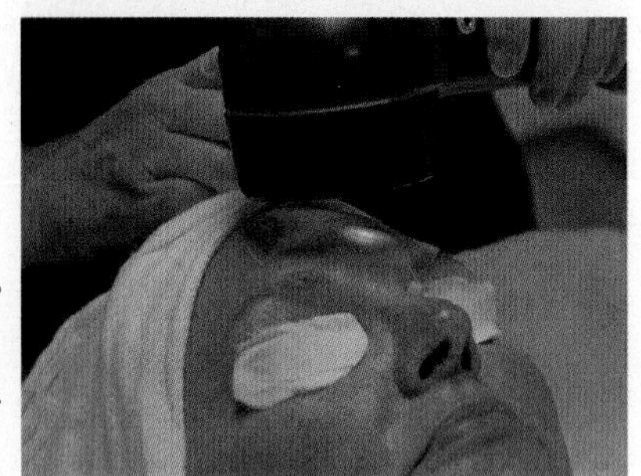

Courtesy of Revitalight.

▲ **Figure 23–46 Light therapy using a LED machine.**

One type of light therapy is called light-emitting diode (LED) treatment (**Figure 23–46**). This treatment uses concentrated light that flashes very rapidly. LEDs were originally developed to help with wound healing. In cosmetology, LED machines are used cosmetically to minimize redness, warm lower-level tissues, stimulate blood flow, and improve skin smoothness. They are applied to improve acne-prone skin. The type and color of the light varies according to treatment objective. Red lights are used to treat aging and redness, and blue light is used for acne-prone skin.

CAUTION

The contraindications for galvanic current also apply to both indirect and direct high-frequency current. Furthermore, in order to prevent burns during the treatment, the client should avoid any contact with metal—such as chair arms, stools, jewelry, and metal bobby pins.

LEDs are a very safe treatment for most clients, but their use should be avoided on clients who have seizure disorders. Flashing lights have been known to trigger seizures in persons with seizure disorders. Any clients with questionable health conditions should receive written approval from a physician before having an LED treatment.

Microdermabrasion

Microdermabrasion (MY-kroh-dur-muh-BRAY-zhun) is a type of mechanical exfoliation that involves shooting aluminum oxide or other crystals at the skin with a hand-held device that exfoliates dead cells. Microdermabrasion uses a closed vacuum to shoot crystals onto the skin, bumping off cell buildup that is then vacuumed up by suction. Microdermabrasion is a popular treatment because it produces fast, visible results. It is used primarily to treat surface wrinkles and aging skin. Performance of safe and effective microdermabrasion treatments requires extensive training. ☑ **LO8**

CAUTION

The client's eyes always should be protected during any light ray treatment. Use cotton pads saturated with alcohol-free freshener or distilled water. The eye pads protect the eyes from the glare of the reflecting rays.

Facial Treatments

A professional facial is one of the most enjoyable and relaxing services available to the salon client. Clients who have experienced this very restful, yet stimulating experience do not hesitate to return for more. When clients receive them on a regular basis, the client's skin tone, texture, and appearance are noticeably improved.

Facial treatments fall into one of the following categories:

- **Preservative.** Maintains the health of the facial skin by cleansing correctly, increasing circulation, relaxing the nerves, and activating the skin glands and metabolism through massage.
- **Corrective.** Correct certain facial skin conditions, such as dryness, oiliness, comedones, aging lines, and minor conditions of acne.

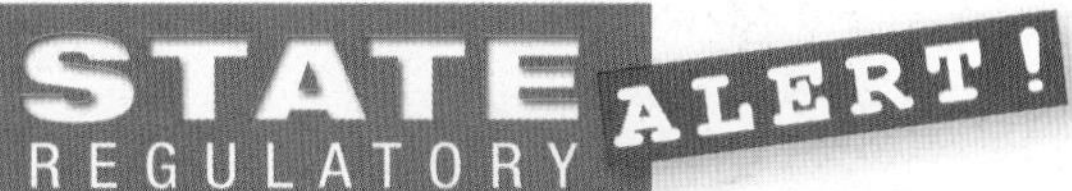

Always check with your state regulatory agency to determine which electrical machines are approved for use in your state.

As with other forms of massage, facial treatments help to increase circulation, activate glandular activity, relax the nerves, maintain muscle tone, and strengthen weak muscle tissues.

Guidelines for Facial Treatments

Your facial treatments are bound to be successful and to inspire return visits if you follow the simple guidelines summarized below:

- Help the client to relax by speaking in a quiet and professional manner.
- Explain the benefits of the products and service, and answer any questions the client may have.
- Provide a quiet atmosphere, and work quietly and efficiently.
- Maintain neat, clean conditions in the facial work area, with an orderly arrangement of supplies.
- Follow systematic procedures.
- If your hands are cold, warm them before touching the client's face.

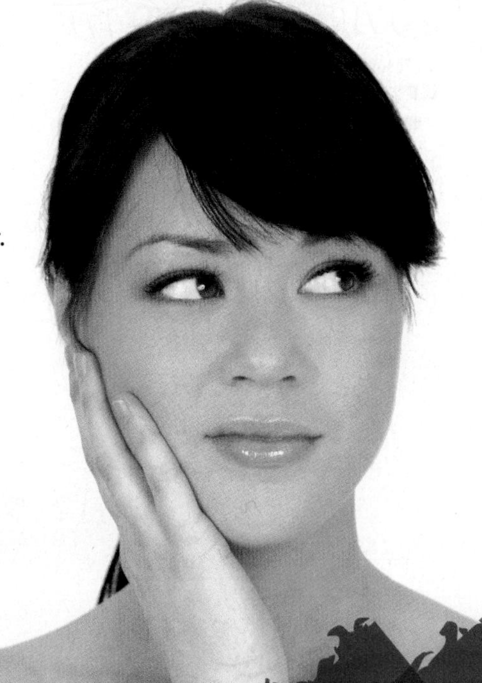

© Phase4Photography, 2010; used under license from Shutterstock.com.

- Keep your nails smooth and short to prevent scratching the client's skin.

Another guideline you must always follow is to perform an analysis of your client's skin. After the client is draped and lying on the facial table (also called a facial bed), you should inspect the skin to determine the following:

- Is the skin dry, normal, or oily?
- Are there fine lines or creases?
- Are comedones or acne present?
- Are dilated capillaries visible?
- Is skin texture smooth or rough?
- Is skin color even?

FYI

To safely and effectively perform advanced skin care treatments—such as microcurrent, microdermabrasion, and LED light—cosmetologists require advanced, specialized training.

The results of your analysis will determine the products to use for the treatment, what areas of the face need special attention, how much pressure to use when massaging, and what equipment should be used.

Basic Facial Application

The steps for performing a basic facial are listed in Procedure 23–1. Some procedures may vary, however, so be guided by your instructor.

The procedure lists the basic implements and materials you will need to perform the basic facial, but you can add other items, such an alternative head covering, if you wish. There are several types of head coverings on the market. Some are a turban design; others are designed with elastic, like a shower cap. They are generally made of either cloth or paper towels. For the paper towel procedure, be guided by your instructor.

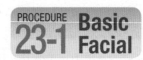

SEE PAGE 741

Special Problems

There are a number of special problems that must be considered when you are performing a facial. These include dry skin, oily skin and blackheads, and acne.

Dry skin is caused by an insufficient flow of sebum (oil) from the sebaceous glands. The facial for dry skin helps correct this condition. Although it can

© Valua Vitaly, 2010; used under license from Shutterstock.com.

be given with or without an electrical current, the use of electrical current provides better results.

PROCEDURE 23-2 Facial For Dry Skin SEE PAGE 746

Oily skin is often characterized by comedones, which are caused by hardened masses of sebum formed in the ducts of the sebaceous glands.

PROCEDURE 23-3 Facial for Oily Skin with Open Comedones SEE PAGE 748

Special Notes for Acne-Prone Skin

Minor problem skin and oily skin should respond well to facial treatments. Unresponsive or severe cases of acne need medical treatment, and clients with such conditions should be referred to a dermatologist.

If a client is under medical care, the role of the cosmetologist is to work under the advisement of the client's physician, following the physician's instructions for the type and frequency of facial treatments. Cosmetologists can help these clients with extraction treatments, assist them in choosing proper home-care products and makeup, and help them to understand how to coordinate medications with a home skin care program.

There are numerous topical prescription medications that can make the skin more sensitive and more reactive to skin care products. Always check with the client's dermatologist if you are performing treatments to clients who are under dermatological care.

Because skin with acne contains infectious matter, you must wear protective gloves and use disposable materials such as cotton cleansing pads when working with clients who have acne.

PROCEDURE 23-4 Facial for Acne-Prone and Problem Skin SEE PAGE 751

Consultation and Home Care

Home care is probably the most important factor in a successful skin care program. The key word here is *program.* Clients' participation is essential to achieve results. A program consists of a long-range plan involving home care, salon treatments, and client education.

Every new client should receive a thorough consultation regarding proper home care for his or her skin conditions.

FOCUS ON

SHARPENING YOUR PERSONAL SKILLS

If a client seems dissatisfied with a facial treatment, check to see if you have been guilty of any of the following:

- Offensive breath or body odor
- Rough, cold hands or ragged nails that may have scratched the client's skin
- Allowing cream or other substances to get into the client's eyes, mouth, nostrils, or hairline
- Towels that were too hot or too cold
- Talking too much
- Manipulating the skin roughly or in the wrong direction
- Being disorganized and interrupting the facial to get supplies

After the first treatment, block out about thirty minutes to explain proper home care for the client.

After the treatment is finished, have the client sit up in the facial chair, or invite the client to move to a well-lighted consultation area. A mirror should be provided for the client, so that he or she can see conditions you will be discussing.

Explain, in simple terms, the client's skin conditions, informing the client of how you propose to treat the conditions. Inform the client about how often treatments should be administered in the salon, and very specifically explain what the client should be doing at home.

You should organize the products you want the client to purchase and use. Explain the use of each one at a time, in the order of use. Make sure to have written instructions for the client to take home.

It is very important to provide clients with products that you believe in and that produce results. Retailing products for clients to use at home is very important for success in the treatment of skin conditions and success in your business.

CAUTION

Aromatherapy is sometimes used as a healing modality by natural healers who have received extensive training in the properties and uses of essential oils and their aromatherapy benefits. Cosmetologists should never attempt to perform healing treatments with aromatherapy.

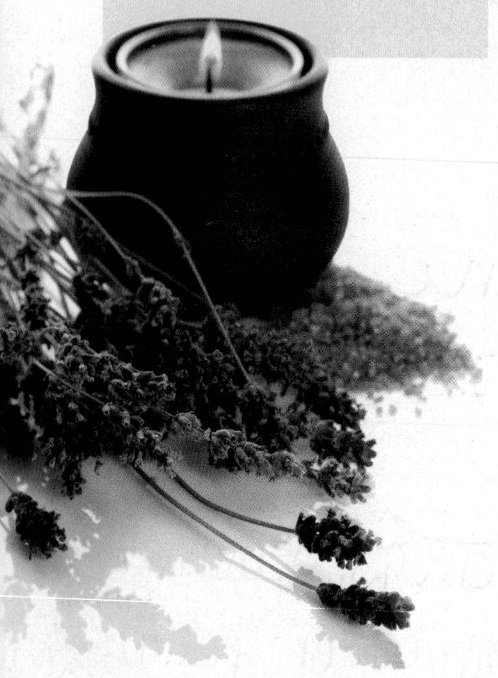

Aromatherapy

The use of essential oils such as lemon verbena, lavender, and rose is a frequent practice in facial skin care. Many essential oils are also used for **aromatherapy**, the therapeutic use of plant aromas for beauty and health treatment. Aromatherapy is thought to benefit and enhance a person's physical, emotional, mental, and spiritual well-being. Using various oils and oil blends for specific benefits is believed to create positive effects on the body, mind, and spirit (**Figure 23–47**).

© Subbotina Anna, 2010; used under license from Shutterstock.com.

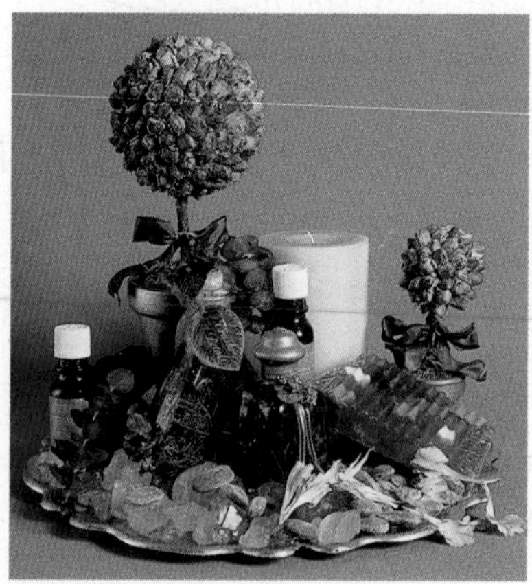

Courtesy of Michael Dzaman.

▲ **Figure 23–47**
Some ingredients for aromatherapy.

Essential oils can be used in a variety of ways. Lighting a cinnamon candle in the winter can give the salon a cozy feeling and cheer up both clients and service providers. You can use a spray bottle to diffuse well-diluted essential oils in the treatment room or on the sheets. You can create your own aromatherapy massage oil by adding a few drops of essential oil to a massage oil, cream, or lotion. Always be careful to use essential oils lightly because they can sometimes be overpowering.

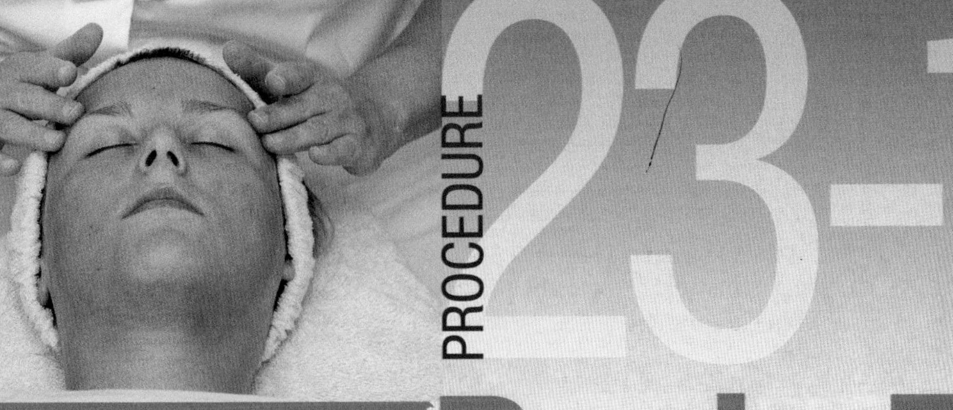

© Milady, a part of Cengage Learning. Photography by Rob Werfel.

PROCEDURE 23-1

Basic Facial

Implements and Materials

You will need all of the following implements, materials, and supplies:

- Antiseptic lotion
- Clean sheet or other covering (blanket if necessary)
- Cleansers and makeup removers
- Cotton (roll)
- Cotton pads
- Cotton swabs and pledgets
- Facial steamer (optional)
- Facial table or chair
- Gauze
- Headband or head covering
- Magnifying lamp
- Masks
- Massage cream or lubricating oil
- Moisturizers
- Bobby pins/safety pins
- Facial gown
- Spatulas
- Sponges
- Sun-protection products
- Tissues
- Toner
- Tonic lotions
- Towels
- Trash can
- Trolley for products and implements

Optional Items:

- Infrared lamp
- Other electrical equipment
- Specialty or intensive care products

Preparation

- Perform PROCEDURE 22-1 **Pre-Service Procedure** SEE PAGE 696

Procedure

1 Ask the client to remove any jewelry such as a necklace or earrings. Store the client's jewelry in a safe place. Clients may wish to keep their handbags nearby during the facial.

2 Show the client to the dressing room and offer assistance if needed.

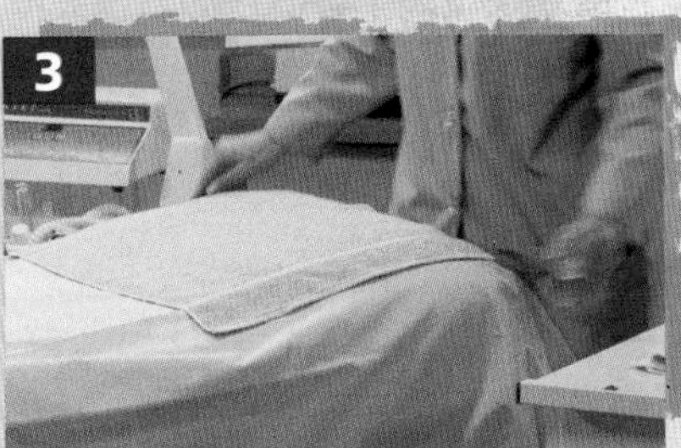

3 Place a clean towel across the back of the facial table to prevent the client's bare shoulders from coming into contact with the bed.

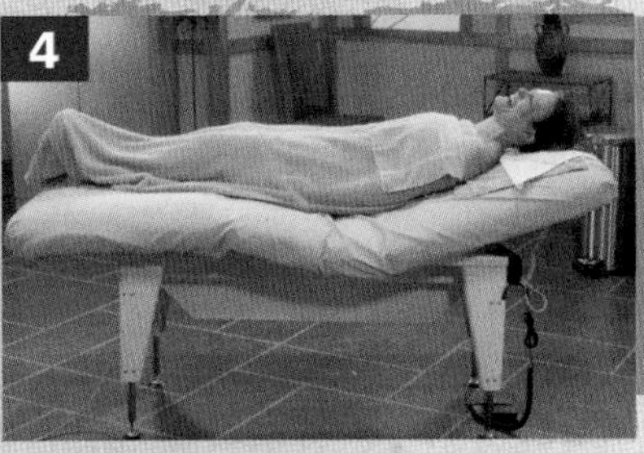

4 If necessary, help your client get onto the facial bed. Place a towel across the client's chest, and place a coverlet or sheet over the client's body, folding the top edge of the towel over it. Remove the client's shoes, and tuck the coverlet around her feet. Some salons provide disposable slippers that can be worn to and from the dressing room.

© Milady, a part of Cengage Learning. Photography by Larry Hamill.
© Milady, a part of Cengage Learning. Photography by Larry Hamill.

Basic Facial continued

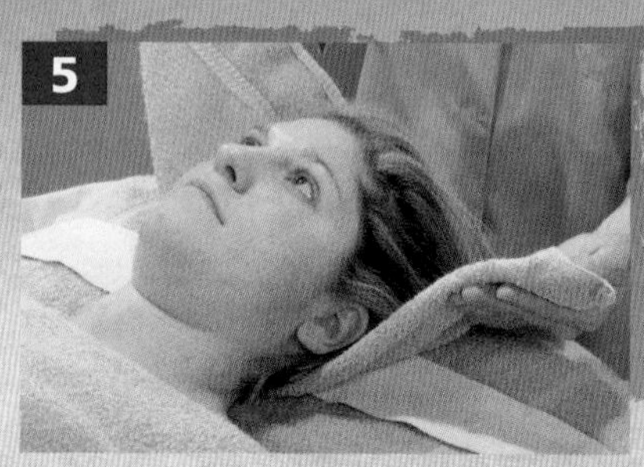

5 Fasten a headband lined with tissue, a towel, or other head covering around the client's head to protect their hair. To drape the head with a towel, follow these steps:

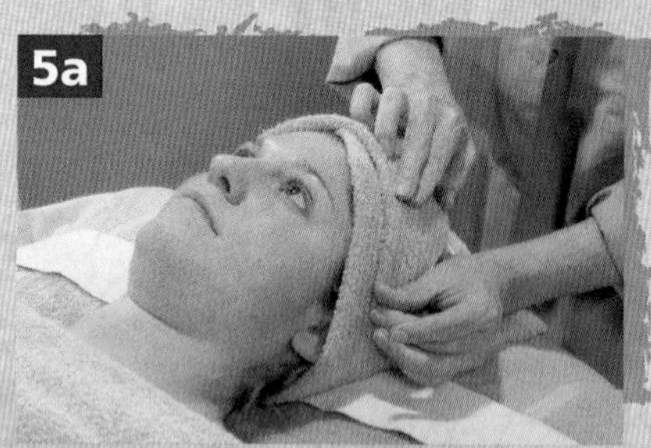

5a Fold the towel diagonally from one of the top corners to the opposite lower corner, and place it over the headrest with the fold facing down. Place the towel on the headrest before the client enters the facial area.

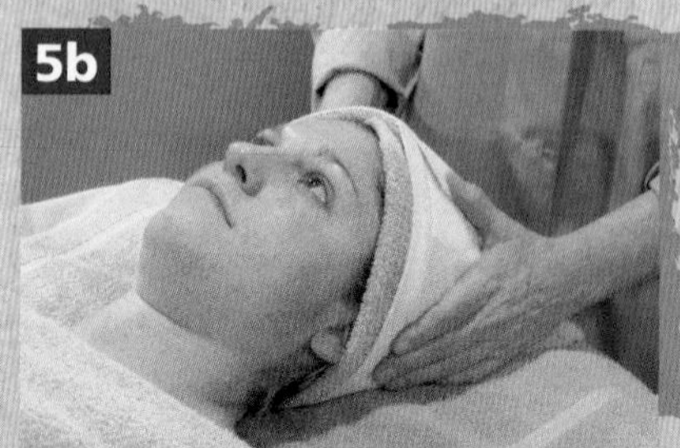

5b When the client is in a reclined position, the back of the head should rest on the towel so that the sides of the towel can be brought up to the center of the forehead to cover the hairline.

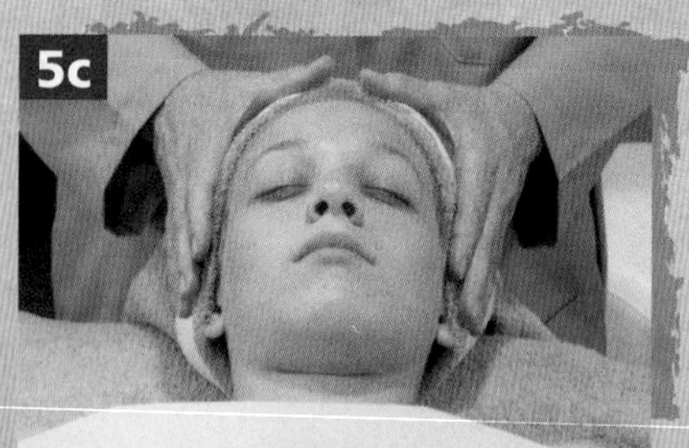

5c Use a headband with a Velcro closure or a pin to hold the towel in place. Make sure that all strands of hair are tucked under the towel, that the earlobes are not bent, and that the towel is not wrapped too tightly.

6 Remove lingerie straps from a female client's shoulders. Alternative method: If client is given a strapless gown to wear, tuck the straps into the top of the gown.

7 If your client wears makeup, use the following steps to remove it. If your client has no makeup, proceed to step 8.

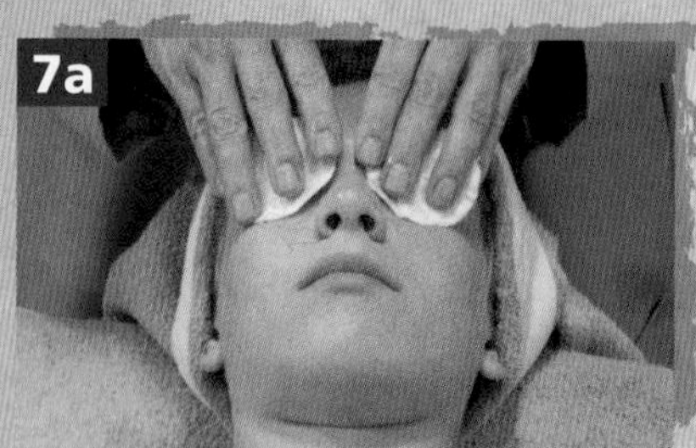

7a Apply a pea-sized amount of eye makeup remover to each of two damp cotton pads and place them on the client's closed eyes. Leave them in place for one minute.

© Milady, a part of Cengage Learning. Photography by Larry Hamill.

13 Apply a moisturizing lotion, cream, or massage product designed for dry skin.

14 Massage the skin with manipulations.

15 If massage cream is used, remove with damp cotton pads, soft sponges, or a warm, moist, soft towel.

16 If you are not using electrotherapy, proceed to step 18.

17 Electrotherapy Option 1, Galvanic Treatment: Apply ionized specialized serum, gel, or lotion. Apply galvanic current as directed by the manufacturer or your instructor. Electrotherapy Option 2, High-frequency Indirect Current Treatment: Use high-frequency machine as directed by the manufacturer or your instructor. Have the client hold the electrode in his or her hand. Perform manipulations, using the indirect method of high frequency, for seven to ten minutes. Do not lift your hands from the client's face. Turn off high-frequency machine.

18 Apply additional moisturizing or specialty product for dry skin with slow massage movements.

19 Starting at the neck and using a soft mask brush, apply a soft-setting cream or hydrating gel mask. Make sure you remove the mask from its container with a clean spatula. Mask should be applied from the center outward.

20 Apply cold cotton eye pads. Allow the mask to process for seven to ten minutes. Make sure client is comfortable and warm.

21 Remove the mask with warm, wet cotton pads, sponges, or warm, moist, soft towels.

22 Apply toner for dry skin with cotton pads.

23 Apply moisturizer or sunscreen designed for dry skin.

24 When the service is completed, remove the head covering and show the client to the dressing room, offering assistance if needed.

Service Tip

For dry skin, avoid using lotions with drying alcohols, such as isopropyl alcohol or SD alcohol.

Post-Service

- Complete PROCEDURE 22-2 **Post-Service Procedure** **SEE PAGE 699**

PROCEDURE 23-3

Facial for Oily Skin with Open Comedones (Blackheads)

Implements and Materials

In addition to the items needed for the Basic Facial, you will also need:

- **Desincrustation gel or lotion**
- **Galvanic or high-frequency machine, depending on treatment**
- **Gloves**
- **Serum, mask, and toner for oily skin**

Preparation

- Perform PROCEDURE 22-1 **Pre-Service Procedure** **SEE PAGE 696**

Procedure

1 Ask the client to remove any jewelry and store it in a safe place.

2 Show the client to the dressing room and offer assistance if needed.

3 Place a clean towel across the back of the facial table to prevent the client's bare shoulders from coming into contact with the bed.

4 If necessary, help your client get onto the facial bed. Place a towel across the client's chest, and place a coverlet or sheet over the client's body, folding the top edge of the towel over it. Remove the client's shoes or slippers and tuck the coverlet around her feet. Some salons provide disposable slippers that can be worn to and from the dressing room.

5 Fasten head covering.

6 Remove lingerie straps.

7 Remove client's makeup.

8 Apply cleanser designed for oily skin, gently massage to apply, and then remove with damp cotton pads, soft sponges, or a warm, moist, soft towel.

9 Remove residue with a damp cotton pad or a soft sponge. Do not tone at this time.

10 Focus steam on the face and allow steaming for five minutes.

11 During or after steaming, apply a mild granular exfoliating product designed for oily or combination skin. Gently massage with light circular movements. Remove with damp cotton pads, soft sponges, or a warm, moist, soft towel.

12 Apply a desincrustation lotion or gel to any area with clogged pores. Negative galvanic current may be applied over this lotion, depending on the manufacturer's instructions. The lotion should generally remain on the skin for five to eight minutes, again, depending on the manufacturer's instructions. Remove the preparation with damp cotton pads, soft sponges, or a warm, moist, soft towel.

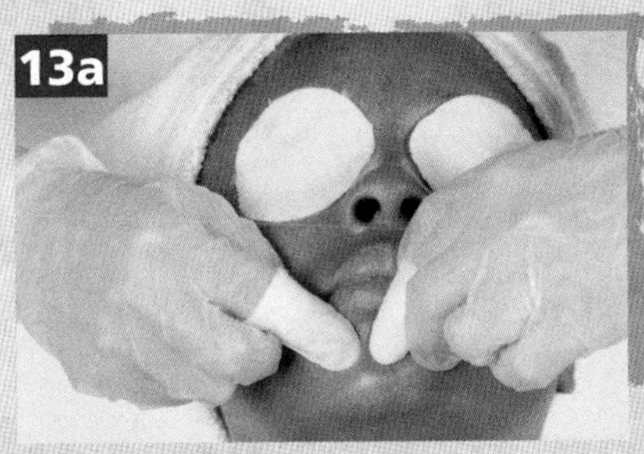

13a Apply latex gloves prior to performing extractions. Apply damp cotton pads to the client's eyes to avoid exposure to the glaring light from the magnifying lamp. Cover your fingertips with cotton, and (using the magnifying lamp) gently pressing out open comedones. Place your middle fingers on either side of the comedone or clogged pore, stretching the skin. Push your fingers down to reach underneath the follicle, and then gently squeeze. Apply the same technique to all sides of the follicle. As an alternative, you may use the same techniques using cotton swabs.

13b Do not extract for more than five minutes for the entire face. Never squeeze with bare fingers or fingernails! If galvanic desincrustation was performed prior to extraction, apply positive galvanic current to the face after extractions are complete. This will help to re-establish the proper pH of the skin surface.

© Milady, a part of Cengage Learning. Photography by Yanik Chauvin.

PROCEDURE 23-3

Facial for Oily Skin with Open Comedones (Blackheads) continued

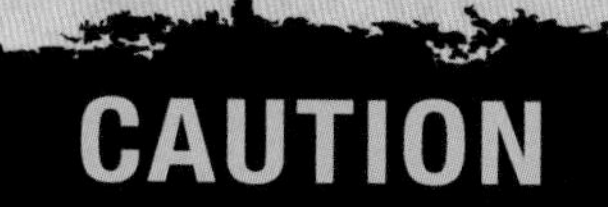

CAUTION

You must receive hands-on instruction to properly perform extraction of clogged pores and comedones. Do not attempt this procedure without first obtaining instruction!

Service Tip

Some people are allergic to latex or rubber. Check with your client to determine whether such an allergy exists and, if so, make a note on the client card. Then proceed, using vinyl gloves. Latex is also used in some facial sponges, so be sure to use cotton pads on clients with latex allergies.

Service Tip

When treating acne-prone skin, disposable gloves should be worn throughout the treatment.

14 After extraction is complete, apply an astringent lotion, a toner for oily skin, or a specialized serum designed to be used following extraction. Allow the skin to dry.

15 Unfold gauze across the face and apply direct high frequency using the mushroom-shaped electrode, according to the machine manufacturer's directions.

16 Extremely oily or clogged skin should not be massaged. If the skin is very clogged, proceed to step 17. If skin is not extremely clogged, apply a hydration fluid or massage fluid designed for oily and combination skin, and perform massage manipulations.

17 Using a mask brush, apply a clay-based mask to all oily areas. To dry areas, such as the eye and neck areas, you may choose to apply a gel mask for dehydrated skin. Allow the mask to process for about ten minutes. Do not allow the mask to overdry so that it cracks.

18 Remove the mask with damp cotton pads, soft sponges, or a warm, moist, soft towel.

19 Apply toner for oily skin with cotton pads.

20 Apply moisturizer or sunscreen designed for oily or combination skin.

21 When the service is completed, remove the head covering and show the client to the dressing room, offering assistance if needed.

Post-Service

- Complete PROCEDURE 22-2 **Post-Service Procedure** SEE PAGE 699

PROCEDURE 23-4

Facial for Acne-Prone and Problem Skin

Implements and Materials

In addition to the items needed for the Basic Facial, you will also need:

- **Antibacterial clay or sulfur mask**
- **Desincrustation gel or lotion**
- **Galvanic or high-frequency machine, depending on treatment**
- **Gloves**
- **Specialized fluids, serums, and toners for acne-prone skin**

Preparation

- Perform PROCEDURE 22-1 **Pre-Service Procedure** **SEE PAGE 696**

Procedure

1 Ask the client to remove any jewelry and store it in a safe place.

2 Show the client to the dressing room and offer assistance if needed.

3 Place a clean towel across the back of the facial table to prevent the client's bare shoulders from coming into contact with the bed.

4 If necessary, help your client get onto the facial bed. Place a towel across the client's chest, and place a coverlet or sheet over the client's body, folding the top edge of the towel over it. Remove the client's shoes or slippers, and tuck the coverlet around her feet.

5 Fasten head covering.

6 Remove lingerie straps.

7 Remove client's makeup.

8 Apply cleanser designed for oily/acne-prone skin, gently massage to apply, and then remove with damp cotton pads, soft sponges, or a warm, moist soft towel.

9 Remove residue with damp cotton pad or soft sponge. Do not tone at this time.

10 Focus steam on the face and allow steaming for five minutes.

PROCEDURE 23-4

Facial for Acne-Prone and Problem Skin continued

11 Apply a desincrustation lotion or gel to any area with pimples or clogged pores. Negative galvanic current may be applied over this lotion, depending on the manufacturer's instructions. The lotion should generally remain on the skin for five to eight minutes, again, depending on the manufacturer's instructions. Remove the preparation with damp cotton pads, soft sponges, or a warm, moist, soft towel.

12 Extract comedones.

13 After extraction is complete, apply an astringent lotion, a toner for oily skin, or a specialized serum designed for use following extraction. Allow the skin to dry. Unfold gauze across the face and apply direct high-frequency using the mushroom-shaped electrode, as directed by the machine manufacturer and your instructor.

14 If galvanic desincrustation was performed prior to extraction, apply positive galvanic current to the face after extractions are complete. This will help to re-establish the proper pH of the skin surface.

15 Acne-prone skin should not be massaged.

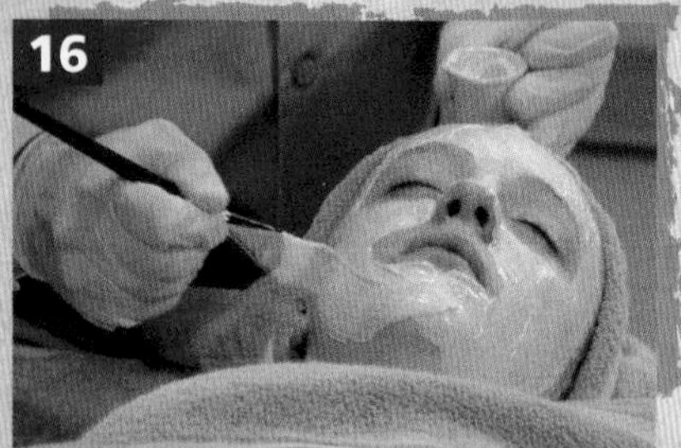

16 Using a mask brush, apply an antibacterial or sulfur-based mask to all oily and acne-prone areas. To dry skin, such as the eye and neck areas, you may choose to apply a gel mask for dehydrated skin. Allow the mask to process for about ten minutes. Do not allow the mask to overdry so that it cracks.

17 Remove the mask with damp cotton pads, soft sponges, or a warm, moist, soft towel.

18 Apply toner for oily skin with cotton pads.

19 Apply specialized lotion or sunscreen designed for oily or acne-prone skin.

20 When the service is completed, remove the head covering and show the client to the dressing room, offering assistance if needed.

Post-Service

- Complete PROCEDURE 22-2 **Post-Service Procedure** SEE PAGE 699

© Milady, a part of Cengage Learning. Photography by Larry Hamill.

Review Questions

1. Explain skin analysis techniques. Why is skin analysis important?
2. What is a contraindication? List five examples.
3. Why is it important to have every client complete a health screening form?
4. Describe the differences between alipidic and oily skin.
5. What is the difference between skin type and skin condition?
6. Name and explain the different categories of skin care products.
7. What are the steps to completing a client consultation?
8. Why is massage used during a facial?
9. Name and briefly describe the five categories of massage manipulations.
10. Name and describe two types of electrical machines used in facial treatments and why these machines add value to a facial.
11. Who is not a good candidate for electrical current treatment? Why?
12. How can aromatherapy be used in the basic facial?

Chapter Glossary

alipidic	Literally means "lack of lipids." Describes skin that does not produce enough sebum, indicated by absence of visible pores.
ampoules	Individual doses of serum, sealed in small vials.
aromatherapy	The therapeutic use of plant aromas for beauty and health treatment.
brushing machine	A rotating electric appliance with interchangeable brushes that can be attached to the rotating head.
chemical exfoliants	Products that contain chemicals that either loosen or dissolve dead cell buildup.
chucking	Massage movement accomplished by grasping the flesh firmly in one hand and moving the hand up and down along the bone while the other hand keeps the arm or leg in a steady position.
clay-based masks	Oil-absorbing cleansing masks that have an exfoliating effect and an astringent effect on oily and combination skin, making large pores temporarily appear smaller.
cleansing milks	Non-foaming lotion cleansers designed to cleanse dry and sensitive skin types and to remove makeup.
contraindication	Condition that requires avoiding certain treatments, procedures, or products to prevent undesirable side effects.
couperose	Distended capillaries caused by weakening of the capillary walls.
cream masks	Masks often containing oils and emollients as well as humectants; have a strong moisturizing effect.

Chapter Glossary

effleurage	Light, continuous stroking movement applied with the fingers (digital) or the palms (palmar) in a slow, rhythmic manner.
electrotherapy	The use of electrical currents to treat the skin.
emollients	Oil or fatty ingredients that prevent moisture from leaving the skin.
enzyme peels	Also known as *keratolytic enzymes* or *protein-dissolving agents*; a type of chemical exfoliant that works by dissolving keratin protein in the surface cells of the skin.
exfoliants	Products that help bring about exfoliation.
exfoliation	The removal of excess dead cells from the skin surface.
foaming cleansers	Cleansers containing surfactants (detergents) which cause the product to foam and rinse off easily.
friction	Deep rubbing movement requiring pressure on the skin with the fingers or palm while moving them over an underlying structure.
fulling	Form of pétrissage in which the tissue is grasped, gently lifted, and spread out; used mainly for massaging the arms.
gommages	Also known as *roll-off masks*; peeling creams that are rubbed off of the skin.
hacking	Chopping movement performed with the edges of the hands in massage.
humectants	Also known as *hydrators* or *water-binding agents*; ingredients that attract water.
masks	Also known as *masques*; concentrated treatment products often composed of mineral clays, moisturizing agents, skin softeners, aromatherapy oils, botanical extracts and other beneficial ingredients to cleanse, exfoliate, tighten, tone, hydrate, and nourish the skin.
massage	Manual or mechanical manipulation of the body by rubbing, gently pinching, kneading, tapping, and other movements to increase metabolism and circulation, promote absorption, and relieve pain.
massage creams	Lubricants used to make the skin slippery during massage.
mechanical exfoliants	Methods used to physically remove dead cell buildup.
microdermabrasion	Mechanical exfoliation that involves shooting aluminum oxide or other crystals at the skin with a hand-held device that exfoliates dead cells.
microdermabrasion scrubs	Scrubs that contains aluminum oxide crystals.
modelage masks	Facial masks containing special crystals of gypsum, a plaster-like ingredient.
moisturizers	Products that help increase the moisture content of the skin surface.

Chapter Glossary

motor point	Point on the skin over the muscle where pressure or stimulation will cause contraction of that muscle.
open comedones	Also known as *blackheads*; follicles impacted with solidified sebum and dead cell buildup.
ostium	Follicle opening.
paraffin wax masks	Specially prepared facial masks containing paraffin and other beneficial ingredients; typically used with treatment cream.
pétrissage	Kneading movement performed by lifting, squeezing, and pressing the tissue with a light, firm pressure.
rolling	Massage movement in which the tissues are pressed and twisted using a fast back-and-forth movement.
serums	Concentrated products that generally contain higher concentrations of ingredients designed to penetrate and treat various skin conditions.
steamer	A facial machine that heats and produces a stream of warm steam that can be focused on the client's face or other areas of skin.
tapotement	Also known as *percussion*; movements consisting of short quick tapping, slapping, and hacking movements.
toners	Also known as *fresheners* or *astringents*; lotions that help rebalance the pH and remove remnants of cleanser from the skin.
treatment cream	A specialty product designed to facilitate change in the skin's appearance.
vibration	In massage, the rapid shaking of the body part while the balls of the fingertips are pressed firmly on the point of application.
wringing	Vigorous movement in which the hands, placed a little distance apart on both sides of the client's arm or leg, working downward apply a twisting motion against the bones in the opposite direction.

CHAPTER 24 Facial Makeup

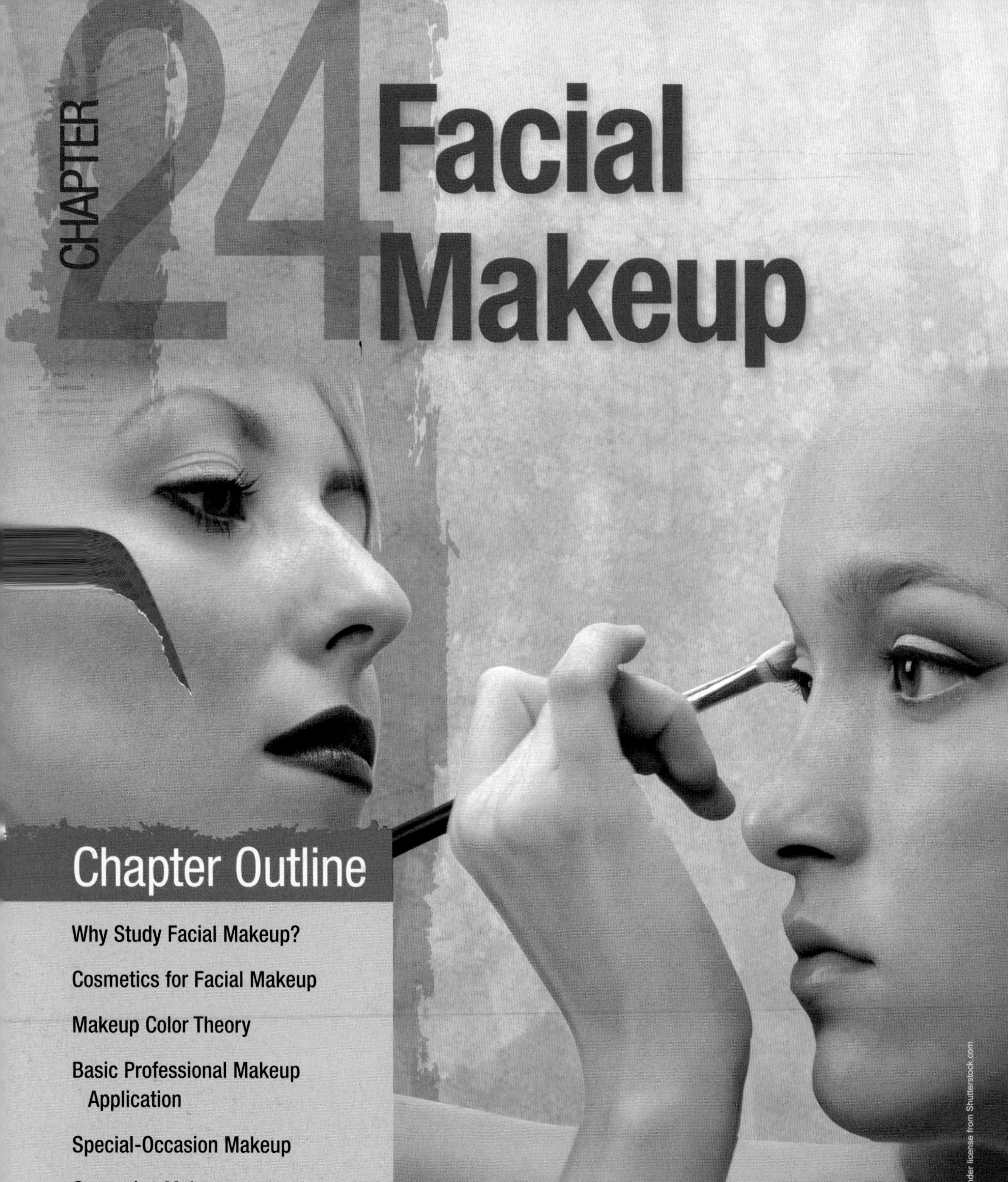

© Brian Chase, 2010; used under license from Shutterstock.com.

Chapter Outline

Why Study Facial Makeup?

Cosmetics for Facial Makeup

Makeup Color Theory

Basic Professional Makeup Application

Special-Occasion Makeup

Corrective Makeup

Artificial Eyelashes

Procedures

Learning Objectives

After completing this chapter, you will be able to:

- ✓ **LO1** Describe the various types of cosmetics and their uses.
- ✓ **LO2** Demonstrate an understanding of cosmetic color theory.
- ✓ **LO3** Perform a consultation for the basic makeup procedure for any occasion.
- ✓ **LO4** Understand the use of special-occasion makeup.
- ✓ **LO5** Identify different facial types and demonstrate procedures for basic corrective makeup.
- ✓ **LO6** Demonstrate the application and removal of artificial lashes.

Key Terms

Page number indicates where in the chapter the term is used.

band lashes (strip lashes)
pg. 783

cake makeup (pancake makeup)
pg. 765

cheek color (blush, rouge)
pg. 761

color primer
pg. 758

concealers
pg. 760

cool colors
pg. 768

eye makeup removers
pg. 765

eye shadows
pg. 762

eye tabbing
pg. 783

eyebrow pencils (eyebrow shadows)
pg. 764

eyelash adhesive
pg. 783

eyeliner
pg. 763

face powder
pg. 760

foundation (base makeup)
pg. 758

greasepaint
pg. 765

individual lashes
pg. 783

line of demarcation
pg. 759

lip color (lipstick, lip gloss)
pg. 761

lip liner
pg. 762

mascara
pg. 764

matte
pg. 759

warm colors
pg. 768

Make up Kit
- pigment powder
- brow pencil
- foundation
- cheek color
- lip color

Makeup is a very interesting part of cosmetology and can produce dramatic and immediate changes in clients' appearance. Most clients prefer a natural look that simply covers or focuses attention away from facial flaws and accents good facial features (**Figure 24–1**). Application of makeup can vary greatly among clients, and the needs of each client can be very different.

WHY STUDY FACIAL MAKEUP?

Cosmetologists should study and have a thorough understanding of facial makeup because:

- Clients will rely on you to advise them on tips and techniques that will help them look their best.
- You will want to use basic makeup techniques to enhance the hair and chemical services you provide for clients, offering them a total look that is harmonious and balanced.
- You will need to understand the various categories of facial makeup products available so that you know when and on whom they should be used (**Figure 24–2**).
- You will also learn about highlighting and contouring and will use these methods to help clients accent attractive features, hide not-so-attractive features, and change the appearance of their face shape.

Cosmetics for Facial Makeup

Foundation

Foundation, also known as **base makeup**, is a tinted cosmetic used to cover or even out the coloring of the skin. It can be used to conceal dark spots, blemishes, and other imperfections. Foundation is usually the first cosmetic used during makeup application (**Figure 24–3**). Foundation comes in liquid, stick, and cream forms. One of the newest trends, mineral powder makeup, is a powder form of foundation.

Occasionally, a special type of foundation product may be applied to the face. A **color primer** is applied to the skin before foundation to cancel out and help disguise skin discoloration. Color primers are available in a variety of colors: green, lavender, amber, and sometimes other colors. For example, green primer helps disguise redness in the skin color, lavender is used to reduce a sallow (yellowish) skin appearance, and amber primer helps cover dark purplish colors like bruising and dark eye circles.

Foundation Chemistry

Most liquid and cream forms of makeup contain a base mixture of water and oil spreading agents that contain

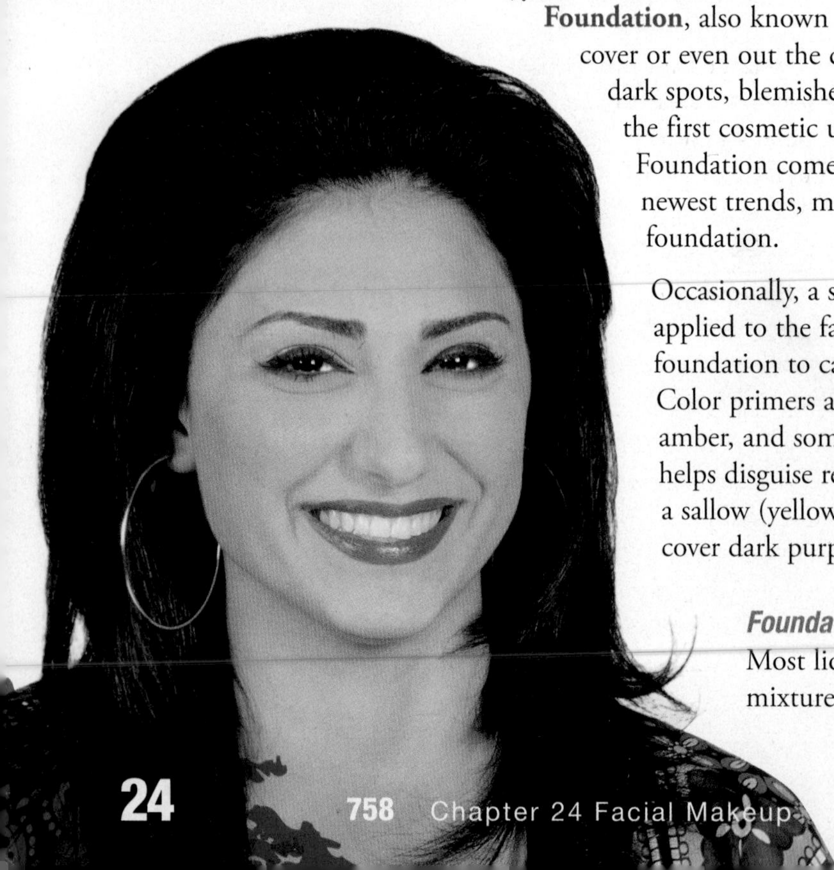

▼ **Figure 24–1**
Enhancing a client's natural beauty.

© Milady, a part of Cengage Learning. Photography by Yanik Chauvin.

a significant amount of talc and various color agents called *pigments*. Pigments can be naturally derived minerals or color agents called *lakes*.

Liquid foundations, also known as *water-based foundations*, are mostly water but often contain an emollient such as mineral oil or a silicone such as cyclomethicone. Some liquid foundations contain alcohols or other drying agents to help the product dry quickly on the skin. The mixture of water and oil helps in applying the makeup color agents evenly and keeps the colors suspended evenly throughout the product. Water-based foundation is most often used for lighter coverage needs and for oily to combination skin types. Water-based foundations dry quickly and produce a **matte** finish, meaning they dry to become nonshiny.

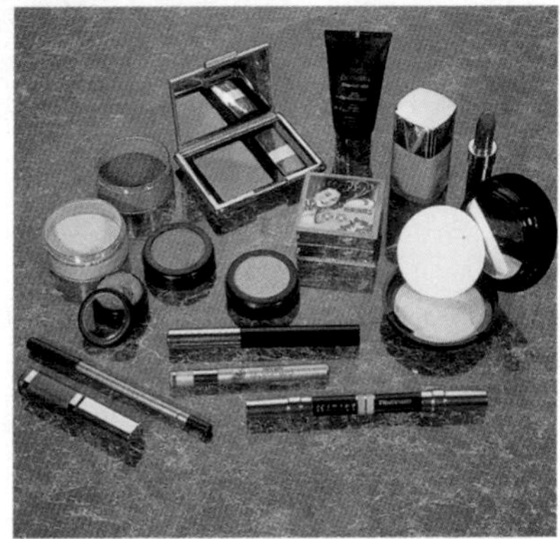

▲ **Figure 24–2**
A wide variety of cosmetics is available to you and your client.

Some foundations are marketed as oil-free. These are usually intended for oilier skin types, but some of these products contain oil substitutes that can actually make them as oily as a foundation containing oil. Be sure to read the label carefully and to check with the manufacturer to make sure it has been tested for oily and acne-prone skin.

Cream foundation, also known as *oil-based foundation*, is a considerably thicker product and is often sold in a jar or a tin. It may or may not contain water. The thicker the product, the less likely it is to contain water. Cream foundations provide heavier coverage and are usually intended for dry skin types. They tend to produce a shinier appearance than water-based products.

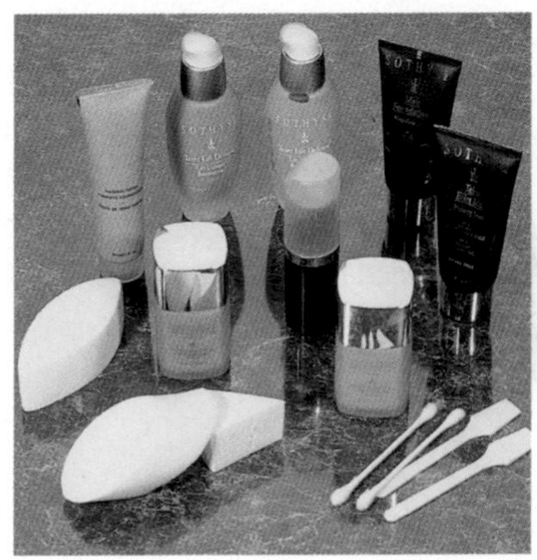

▲ **Figure 24–3**
Foundations.

Using a cream foundation on oily or acneic skin may cause more clogged pores to form. Cosmetic products that cause the formation of clogged pores or comedones are called *comedogenic*, which means that they produce comedones.

All types of foundation can contain sunscreen ingredients.

Using Foundation

Choosing the correct color of foundation is extremely important in making makeup look natural. The foundation should be as close to the client's natural skin coloring as possible. To choose the correct foundation color, have the client sit in a well-lit area. Apply a small amount of the foundation product to the jawline. It is important that the color chosen matches the skin on both the face and neck. If the color of the foundation is too light, it will look dull and chalky. If the color is too dark, it will look muddy or splotchy.

Makeup should be blended onto the skin with a disposable makeup sponge. After choosing the correct color, remove some makeup from the container with a clean spatula. The foundation product may be placed in or on a small disposable palette or plastic cup to avoid contamination of the product container. Using the sponge, blend out the foundation across the skin with short strokes. The product should match the color of the skin very closely. A **line of demarcation** is an obvious line where foundation starts or stops. These are very unattractive. When the correct color of foundation is used and blended well with the natural skin color, lines of demarcation are not visible.

FYI

Some cosmetics companies market a colorless, silicone-based product they call a *primer* or a *skin primer*. These products are used after cleansing and moisturizing the skin or as a moisturizer. Skin primers are applied (before any type of colored foundation is applied) to fill in fine lines, gaps, or other uneven surfaces of the skin, providing a smoother skin surface on which to apply traditional makeup.

© Milady, a part of Cengage Learning. Photography by Larry Hamill.

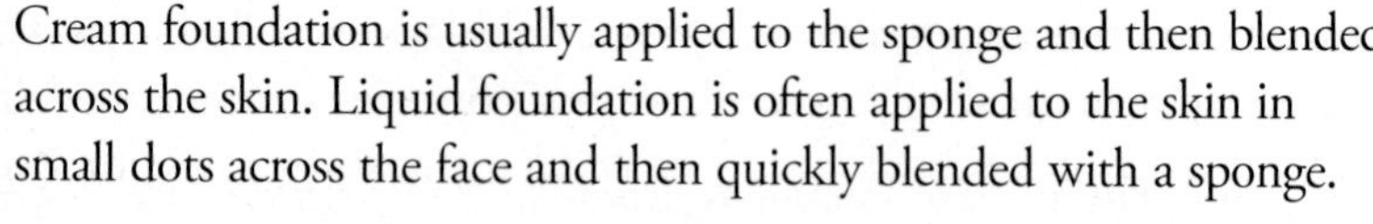

Here's a Tip

A concealer may be worn alone, without foundation, if chosen and blended correctly. Be sure to use it sparingly and soften the edges so that the complexion looks like clear, even skin rather than a heavy makeup application.

Use a clean spatula to remove some of the product, and place it on a palette or a tissue. Using a sponge, dip the sponge into the product and gently apply by patting the sponge over the area that needs concealer. Concealer can also be applied directly to the area by using a disposable cotton swab and then blended by gently tapping with a makeup sponge.

Cream foundation is usually applied to the sponge and then blended across the skin. Liquid foundation is often applied to the skin in small dots across the face and then quickly blended with a sponge.

Mineral powder foundation is applied with a large fluffy brush called a Kabuki brush. Mineral powder contains a lot of pigment for coverage. The pigments stick to the skin, providing natural-looking coverage.

Concealers

Concealers are a thick, heavy type of foundation used to hide dark eye circles, dark splotches, and other imperfections. They contain more talc or pigment for heavier coverage. They are also available in a wide range of colors and should match the skin color very closely. If the color is not matched perfectly, the concealer may draw attention to the area instead of hiding it! Concealers are packaged in tins, jars, or tubes with wands.

Some concealer products contain ingredients to add moisture or control oil, and some concealers actually contain anti-acne ingredients to be used on acne blemishes.

Face Powders

Face powder is a cosmetic powder, sometimes tinted or scented, that is used to add a matte or nonshiny finish to the face. It helps to absorb excess oil and minimizes the shine of oily skin. It is used to set the foundation, making it easier to apply other powder, such as blush (**Figure 24–4**).

Face powder comes in two forms: loose and pressed. Pressed powder is blended with binding agents to keep it in a caked form in the tin. Loose powder does not contain as much binder and comes in a jar.

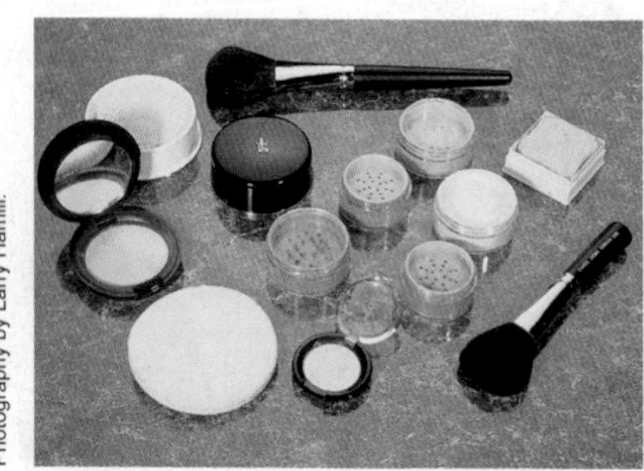

© Milady, a part of Cengage Learning. Photography by Larry Hamill.

▲ **Figure 24–4**
Commonly used forms of face powder.

Both powders are usually a mixture of talc or cornstarch with color pigments added. Some powders that do not contain much color are called *translucent*. They are intended not to add color when applied over a foundation. Pressing agents or binders such as zinc stearate are added to press the foundation and to help it adhere to the skin. If a colored powder is used, it should match the natural skin tone.

Applying Powder

Loose powder is applied with a large powder brush. Remove some loose powder from the container and place it in a disposable cup or tissue. Dip the brush in the powder and fluff it across the face. Make sure all areas of the face are covered, and remove any excess powder. You can also use a disposable cotton ball to apply loose powder.

Powder can also be used to brush out hard edges from blush or eye shadow application. Powder should never look caked, streaked, or blotchy after application.

Pressed powder in compacts is marketed primarily for touch-ups because it can easily be carried in a purse. These products normally come with a powder-puff applicator, which should never be used in the salon because they cannot be easily cleaned and then disinfected.

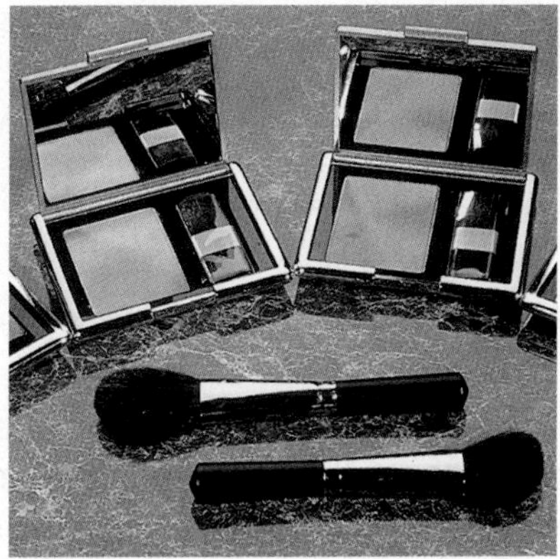

▲ Figure 24–5
Cheek colors.

Cheek Color

Cheek color, also known as **blush** or **rouge**, is used primarily to add a natural-looking glow to the cheeks, but it can also be used to add a little extra color to the face. Cheek color comes in powder, gel, and cream forms (**Figure 24–5**).

Makeup artists have traditionally used cream forms of cheek color; however, powder blushes are easier to use and are much more popular. Cream blush is used immediately after the foundation to blend color into the foundation. Powder blush is used after both the foundation and powder have been applied.

Using Powder Blush

After foundation and face powder have been applied, take a clean or disposable blush brush and stroke the pressed blush once. Do not re-stroke the brush! As an alternative, a disposable cotton puff can be used.

Look carefully at your client's face and notice the natural hollow of the cheek, just under the cheekbone. Apply the blush with short strokes to the area just under the cheekbone and to the area where natural color would normally appear. The application should look soft and natural. It should look as if it fades into the foundation. It is better to apply too little blush than too much. You can always add more if necessary.

Never apply blush in a circle on the apple of the cheek, beyond the corner of the eye, or inward between the cheekbone and the nose.

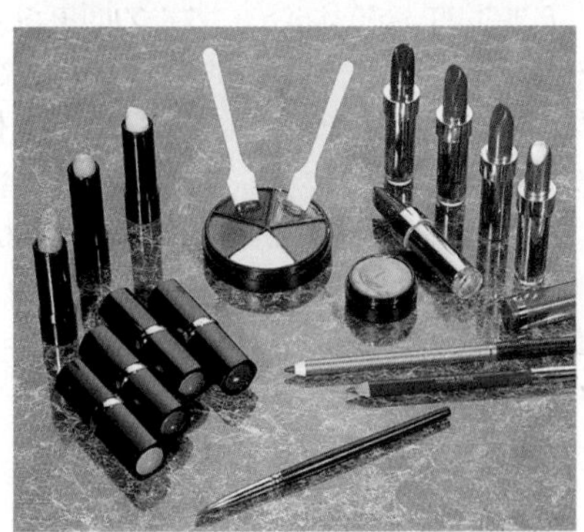

▲ Figure 24–6
Lip colors.

Lip Color

Lip color, also known as **lipstick** or **lip gloss**, is a paste-like cosmetic used to change or enhance the color of the lips. Lip color usually comes in a metal or plastic tube and is available in a wide variety of colors (**Figure 24–6**). Some lip color products contain conditioners to moisturize the lips or sunscreen to protect against sun exposure.

Lip color is available in many forms, including creams, glosses, pencils, gels, and sticks. These products are a mixture of oils, waxes, and color dyes.

Properly selecting lipstick color takes some talent, and an understanding of color theory. The lip color must blend (not match) with the client's hair and eye color and other makeup used.

Current fashion also dictates both lipstick color and application methods. Fashion trends have called for light or dark lip color, shiny versus matte applications, and various application styles.

FOCUS ON

RETAILING

Retailing cosmetics is a great way to increase your income. Most salons will pay you a 5 to 10 percent commission on every product you retail. If you focus on retailing to every client, this amount will add up quickly. It is not unusual for a cosmetologist who is retailing makeup on a daily basis to pay for a long weekend vacation or even make a car payment or two each year using these rewards. And you will be helping your clients by giving them professional advice and allowing them to shop for makeup while receiving other salon services. If you don't take advantage of this opportunity, the department store down the street surely will!

© Milady, a part of Cengage Learning. Photography by Larry Hamill.

FOCUS ON

RETAILING

Lip colors present a huge opportunity for retail. Think of how many lipsticks you own. Most women own several lipsticks, glosses, and pencils. Some carry more than five at a time in their purses. Suggest a few colors to a client in a variety of finishes. Lip color is a simple way to change a look, and it provides a great way for your client to give herself a treat and brighten her day.

Lip color must never be applied directly from the container unless it belongs to the client. Lip color must be removed from the container or applied with a one-application disposable lip brush, which must never be reused! It can also be removed from the container with a spatula and placed on a palette, and then it can be applied more freely.

After placing the lip color on the brush, begin by applying at the outer corners and work toward the middle. Repeat on the opposite side. Connect the center peaks using rounded strokes, following the natural lip line. Repeat on the bottom lip.

Properly applied lipstick should be even and symmetrical on both sides of the mouth. **Lip liner** is a colored pencil used to outline the lips and to keep the lipstick from bleeding into small lines around the mouth. Lip liners are available as thin pencils, thick pencils, and automatic roll-up pencils. Lip liner is usually applied before the lip color to define the shape of the lip. Choose a color that coordinates with the chosen lipstick. The liner color should not be dramatically different from the natural lip shade or the shade of the lipstick.

Before application, sharpen the pencil, and after use, clean the pencil. Remember to clean and then disinfect your sharpener also!

Beginning at the outer corner of the upper lip and working toward the middle, color the natural lip line. Repeat on the opposite side. Connect the center peaks with rounded strokes, following the natural lip line. Outline the lower lip from the outer corners in and then apply liner on the lips, staying within the outline.

Eye Shadow

Eye shadows are cosmetics applied on the eyelids to accentuate or contour them. They are available in almost every color of the rainbow, from warm to cool, neutral to bright, and light to dark. Some powder eye shadows are designed to be used wet or dry. They also come in a variety of finishes, including metallic, matte, frost, shimmer, or dewy.

Eye shadow is available in stick, cream, pressed powder, and dry powder form, and it usually comes with an applicator (**Figure 24–7**).

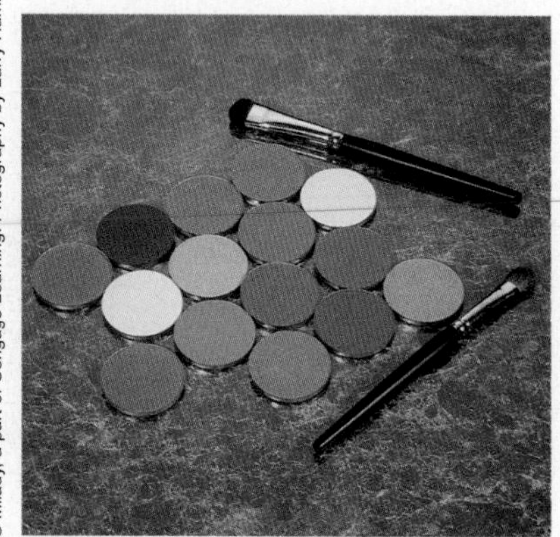

© Milady, a part of Cengage Learning. Photography by Larry Hamill.

▲ **Figure 24–7**
Eye shadows.

Using Eye Shadow

When applied to the lids, eye color or shadow makes the eyes appear brighter and more expressive. Matching eye shadow to eye color creates a flat field of color and should generally be avoided. Using color other than the actual eye color (i.e., a contrasting or complementary color) can enhance the eyes. Using both light and dark colors can also bring attention to the eyes.

Generally, a darker shade of eye color makes the natural color of the iris appear lighter, while a lighter shade makes the iris appear deeper. The only set rules for eye makeup colors are that the chosen colors should enhance the client's eyes, and that the chosen colors should be more subtle for daytime wear. If desired, eye makeup color may match or coordinate with the client's clothing color.

Eye shadow colors are generally referred to as highlight, base, and contour colors. A highlight color is lighter than the client's skin tone and may have any finish. Popular finish choices for highlight colors include matte or iridescent (shiny). As the name suggests, highlight colors highlight a specific area, such as the brow bone. Remember that a lighter color will make an area appear larger.

A base color is generally a medium tone that is close to the client's skin tone. It is available in a variety of finishes. Base color is generally used to even skin tone on the eye and to help cover redness and skin discolorations on the eyelid. The base color is often applied all over the lid and brow bone, from lash to brow, before other colors are applied, thus providing a smooth surface for the blending of other colors. If the base color is to be used this way, a matte finish is generally preferred.

A contour color is a color, in any finish, that is deeper and darker than the client's skin tone. It is applied to minimize a specific area, to create contour in a crease, or to define the eyelash line.

To apply eye shadow, remove the product from its container with a spatula, and then use a fresh applicator or clean brush. Unless you are doing corrective makeup, apply the color close to the lashes on the upper eyelid, sweeping the color slightly upward and outward. Blend to achieve the desired effect. More than one color may be used if a particular effect is desired.

FOCUS ON

RETAILING

One of the biggest challenges that women face when purchasing cosmetics is finding the correct colors and finishes. When you start to use specific and "colorful" language, you will see a great improvement in your selling technique. Consider persuasive phrases such as the following:

- "This cocoa shadow will really make your green eyes look beautiful."
- "You have a great smile. This new peach lipstick will show it off."
- "What a great dress. This silver eyeliner would look fabulous with it."

© Milady, a part of Cengage Learning.

Eyeliners

Eyeliner is a cosmetic used to outline and emphasize the eyes. It is available in a variety of colors, in pencil, liquid, pressed (cake), or felt-tip pen form.

With eyeliner you can create a line on the eyelid close to the lashes to make the eyes appear larger and the lashes appear fuller (**Figure 24–8**).

Eyeliner pencils consist of a wax (paraffin) or hardened oil base (petrolatum) with a variety of additives to create color. Eyeliner pencils are available in both soft and hard form for use on the eyebrow as well as the upper and lower eyelid.

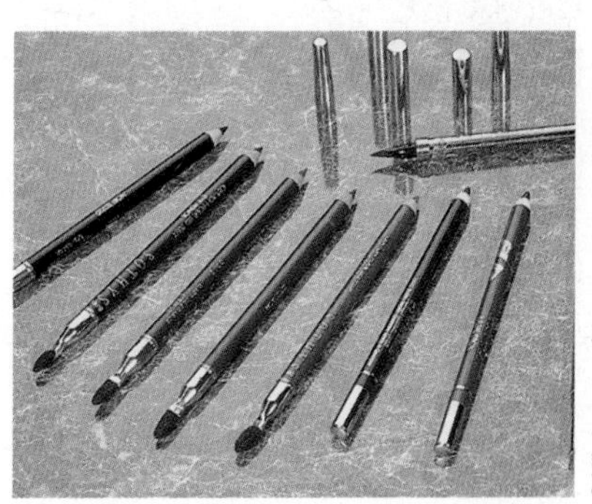
© Milady, a part of Cengage Learning. Photography by Larry Hamill.

▲ **Figure 24–8**
Eyeliners.

Using Eyeliners

Most clients prefer eyeliner that is the same color as the lashes or the same color as the mascara for a more natural look. More dramatic colors may be chosen depending on seasonal color trends.

Be extremely cautious when applying eyeliner. You must have a steady hand and be sure that your client remains still. Sharpening the eyeliner pencil and wiping it with a clean tissue before each use removes sections of the pencil that have touched previous clients. Also, remember to

Here's a Tip

Eye shadow in pressed powder form may be applied to the eyes with an eyeliner brush to create a softer lined effect. Whether using shadow or pencil liner, it may be helpful to pull the skin taut, from right below the eyebrow up, to ensure smooth application.

CAUTION

According to the American Medical Association, eye pencils should not be used to color the inner rim of the eyes because this can lead to infection of the tear duct, causing tearing, blurring of vision, and permanent pigmentation of the mucous membrane lining the inside of the eye.

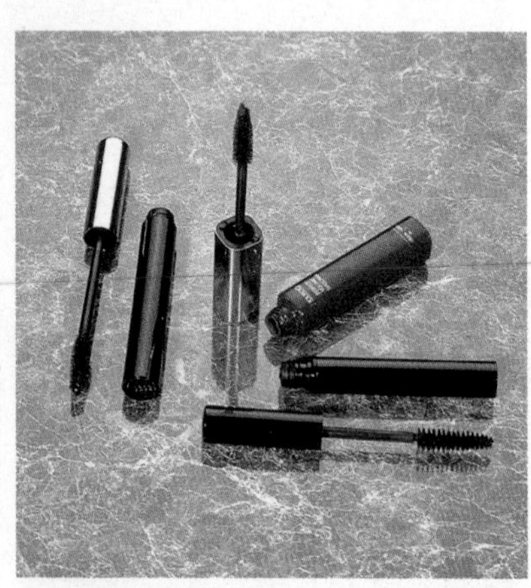
© Milady, a part of Cengage Learning. Photography by Larry Hamill.

▲ Figure 24–9
Mascara products.

clean the sharpener before each use. Apply to the desired area with short strokes and gentle pressure; the most common placement is close to the lash line. For powder shadow liner application, scrape a small amount onto a tissue and apply to the eyes with a disposable applicator or clean brush. If desired, wet the brush before the application for a more dramatic look.

Eyebrow Color

Eyebrow pencils, also known as **eyebrow shadows**, are used to add color and shape to the eyebrows, usually after tweezing or waxing. They can be used to darken the eyebrows, correct their shape, or fill in sparse areas. Brow powders are similar to pressed eye shadows and are applied to the brows with a brush. Brow powders cling to eyebrow hairs, making the brows appear darker and fuller.

The chemistry of eyebrow pencils is similar to that of eyeliner pencils. The chemical ingredients in eyebrow shadows are also similar to those in eye shadows.

Using Eyebrow Color

Sharpen the eyebrow pencil and wipe with clean tissue before each use. Clean the sharpener before each use. For powder shadow application, scrape a small amount onto a tissue and use a disposable applicator or clean brush to apply shadow to brows. Avoid harsh contrasts between hair and eyebrow color, such as pale blond or silver hair with black eyebrows.

Mascara

Mascara is a cosmetic preparation used to darken, define, and thicken the eyelashes. It is available in liquid, cake, and cream form and in a variety of shades and tints (**Figure 24–9**). Mascara brushes can be straight or curved, with fine or thick bristles. The most popular mascara colors are shades of brown and black, which enhance the natural lashes by making them appear thicker and longer.

Mascara is available in tube and wand applicators. Both are polymer products that include water, wax, thickeners, film formers, and preservatives. The pigments in mascara must be inert (unable to combine with other elements) and usually are carbon black, carmine, ultramarine, chromium oxide, and iron oxides. Some wand mascaras contain rayon or nylon fibers to lengthen and thicken the hair fibers.

Using Mascara

Mascara may be used on all the lashes, from the inner to outer corners. Using a disposable wand, dip into a clean tube of mascara and apply from close to the base of the lashes out toward the tips, making sure your client is comfortable throughout the application. Dispose of the wand. Never double dip!

If you are using an eyelash curler, you must curl the lashes before applying mascara. If lashes are curled after mascara, they may be broken or pulled out. Use extreme caution whenever using an eyelash curler.

The easiest way to learn how to use this tool is by first observing its use. Ask your instructor to demonstrate before attempting to use an eyelash curler on someone else.

Other Cosmetics

Eye makeup removers are special preparations for removing eye makeup. Most eye makeup products are water resistant, so wash-off cleansers are generally not very effective for removal. Eye makeup removers are either oil-based or water-based. Oil-based removers are generally mineral oil with a small amount of fragrance added. Water-based removers are comprised of a water solution to which other solvents have been added.

Greasepaint is a heavy makeup used for theatrical purposes. **Cake makeup**, also known as **pancake makeup**, is a heavy-coverage makeup pressed into a compact and applied to the face with a moistened cosmetic sponge. Cake makeup is often used for theatrical purposes. Its most common use outside the theater is to cover scars and pigmentation defects.

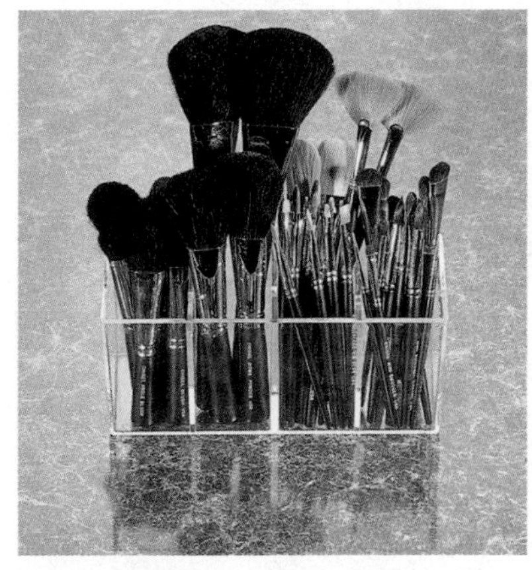

© Milady, a part of Cengage Learning. Photography by Larry Hamill.

▲ Figure 24–10
Makeup brushes.

Makeup Brushes and Other Tools

Makeup brushes come in a variety of shapes and sizes (**Figure 24–10**). They may be made of synthetic or animal hair with wooden or metal handles. Commonly used makeup brushes and implements are listed below:

- **Powder brush.** Large, soft brush used to apply powder and for blending edges of color.
- **Blush brush.** Smaller, more tapered version of the powder brush, excellent for applying powder cheek color.
- **Concealer brush.** Usually narrow and firm with a flat edge, used to apply concealer around the eyes or over blemishes.
- **Lip brush.** Similar to the concealer brush, with a more tapered edge; may be used to apply concealer or lip color.
- **Eye shadow brushes.** Available in a variety of sizes, from small to large, and in finishes from soft to firm. The softer and larger the brush, the more diffused and blended the shadow will be. A firm brush is better for depositing dense color than for blending it.
- **Eyeliner brush.** Fine, tapered, firm bristles; used to apply liquid liner or shadow to the eyes.
- **Angle brush.** Firm, thin bristles; angled for ease of application of shadow to the eyebrows or shadow liner to the eyes.
- **Lash and brow brush.** Comb-like brush used to remove excess mascara on lashes or to comb brows into place.
- **Tweezers.** Available in metal or plastic; used to remove excess facial hair.

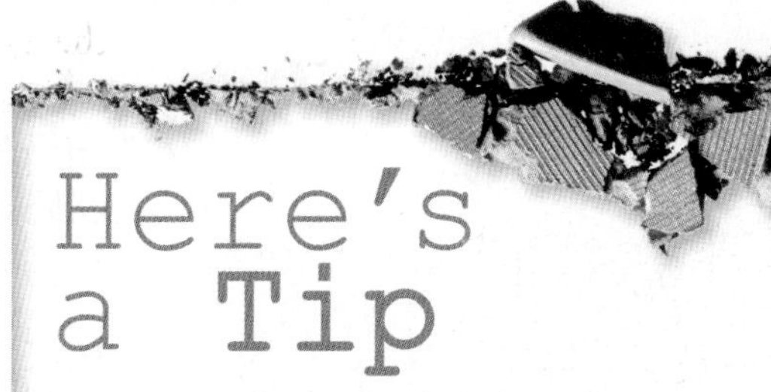

Here's a Tip

Apply mascara carefully. The most common injury with mascara application is poking the eye with the applicator. Practice applying mascara repeatedly until you feel confident enough to apply it on clients.

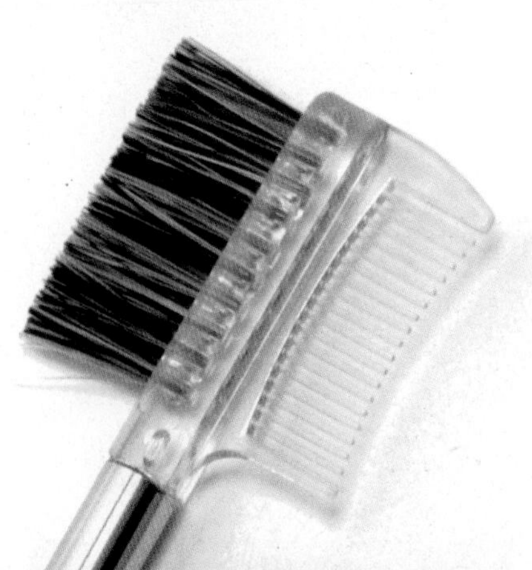

- **Eyelash curler.** Metal or plastic device used to give lift and upward curl to the upper lashes.
- **Pencil sharpener.** Used before each application of eye or lip liner pencil to ensure hygienic application.

Caring for Makeup Brushes

If you invest in high-quality makeup brushes, you will have them for years. Take good care of your brushes by cleaning them gently.

A commercial cleaning solution can be used for quick cleaning of makeup brushes. Spray-on instant sanitizers contain a high level of alcohol and are not recommended because they will dry brushes over time. A gentle shampoo or brush solvent should be used to truly clean the brushes. These products will not hurt brushes and may actually help them last longer. One cautionary note: the brush should always be put into running or still water with the ferrule (the metal ring that keeps bristles and handle together) pointing downward. If the brush is pointed up, the water may remove the glue that keeps the bristles in place. Rinse brushes thoroughly after cleansing. Because they will dry in the shape they are left in, reshape the wet bristles and lay the brushes flat to dry.

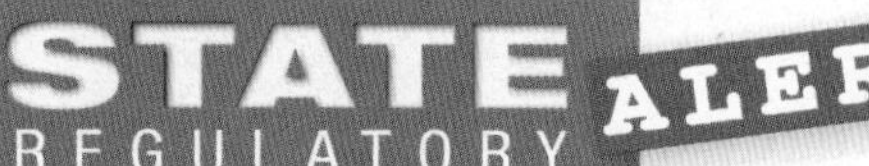

Regulations for cleaning brushes vary from state to state, so check with your regulatory agency.

© Milady, a part of Cengage Learning.

Disposable Implements

Disposable implements include the following items:

- **Sponges.** Available in a variety of sizes and shapes, including wedges and circles, and work well to apply and blend foundation, cream or powder blush, powder, or concealer.
- **Powder or cotton puffs.** May be made of velour or cotton and are used to apply and blend powder, powder foundation, or powder blush.
- **Mascara wands.** Usually plastic and used to apply mascara on a client; generally disposable, so as to ensure proper hygiene.
- **Spatulas.** Wooden or plastic, with a wide, flat base; used to remove makeup such as lipstick, foundation, concealer, powder, blush, and shadow from their containers.
- **Disposable lip brushes.** May be plastic or some other synthetic; used to hygienically apply lip color.
- **Sponge-tipped shadow applicators.** Used to apply shadow and lip color or to blend eyeliner; may be used to remove unwanted makeup from eyes or lips.
- **Cotton swabs.** May be used to apply shadow, blend eyeliner, or remove unwanted makeup from the eyes or lips.
- **Cotton pads or puffs.** May be used with astringents or makeup removers; also used to apply powder products, such as powder blush.

✓ **LO1**

Makeup Color Theory

A strong understanding of how color works is vital to effective makeup application. Everyone sees color a little differently, and it may take a while to learn to see color naturally and easily.

The following guide will help refresh your memory of color theory of primary, secondary, and tertiary colors, as well as warm, cool, and complementary colors.

Primary colors are fundamental colors that cannot be obtained from a mixture. The primary colors are yellow, red, and blue (**Figure 24–11**).

Secondary colors are obtained by mixing equal parts of two primary colors. Yellow mixed with red makes orange. Red mixed with blue makes violet. Yellow mixed with blue makes green (**Figure 24–12**).

Tertiary colors are formed by mixing equal amounts of a secondary color and its neighboring primary color on the color wheel. These colors are named by primary color first and secondary color second. For example, when we mix blue (a primary color) with an equal amount of violet (a neighboring secondary color), we call the resulting color blue-violet (**Figure 24–13**).

Primary and secondary colors directly opposite each other on the color wheel are called *complementary colors*. When mixed, these colors cancel each other out to create a neutral brown or gray color. When complementary colors are placed next to each other, each color makes the other look brighter because of the intense contrast. For example, if you place blue next to orange, the blue seems bluer and the orange seems brighter. Try this with markers or colored paper to compare. The concept of complementary colors is useful when determining color choice. For example, the use of complementary colors will emphasize eye color, making the eyes appear brighter (**Figure 24–14**).

Warm and Cool Colors

Knowing the difference between warm and cool colors is essential to your success as a makeup artist. This is the basis of all color selection, and understanding the difference will enable you to properly enhance your client's coloring.

As you look at the color wheel, think of it as a tool in determining color choice. There are three main factors to consider when choosing colors for a client: skin color, eye color, and hair color.

© Milady, a part of Cengage Learning.

PRIMARY COLORS

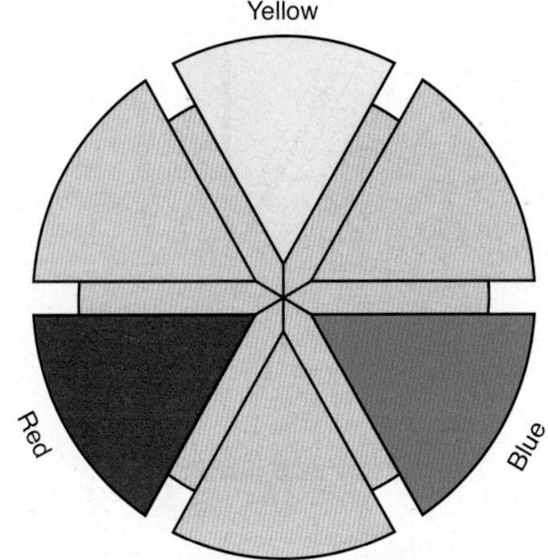

▲ **Figure 24–11**
Primary colors.

SECONDARY COLORS

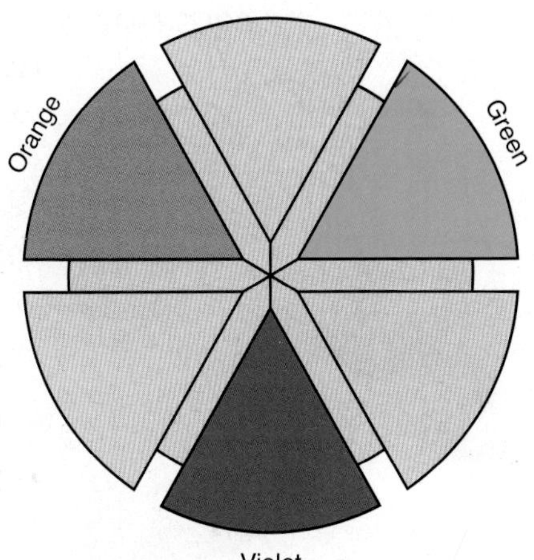

▲ **Figure 24–12**
Secondary colors.

TERTIARY COLORS

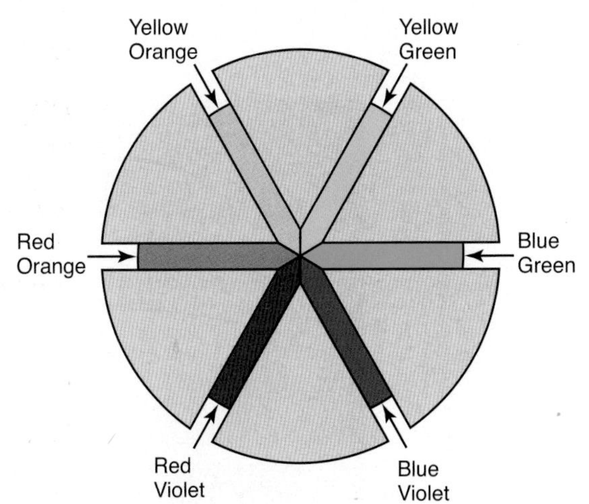

▲ **Figure 24–13**
Tertiary colors.

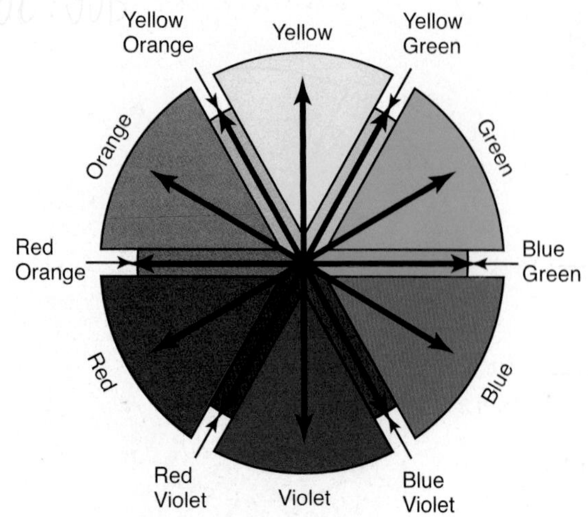

▲ **Figure 24–14**
Complementary colors.

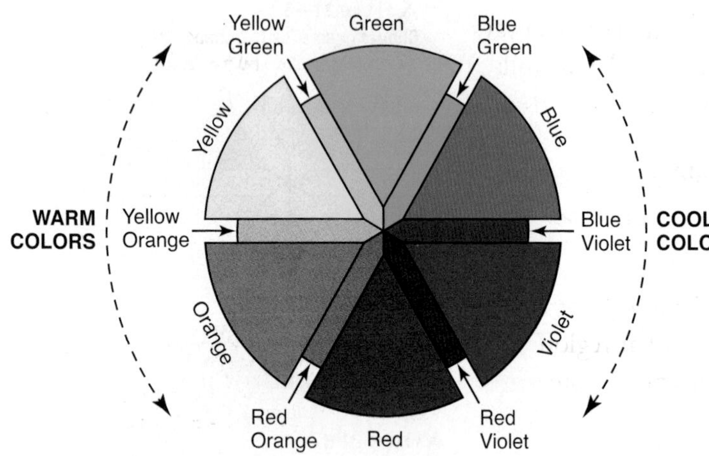

▲ **Figure 24–15**
Warm and cool colors.

Determining Skin Color

When determining skin color, you must first decide if the skin is light, medium, or dark. Then determine whether the tone of the skin is warm or cool (use **Table 24–1** as a guide). You may not see skin colors truly in the beginning. Give yourself time and practice to develop your eye.

Warm colors are the range from yellow and gold through the oranges, red-oranges, most reds, and even some yellow-greens. **Cool colors** suggest coolness and are dominated by blues, greens, violets, and blue-reds (**Figure 24–15**). You will notice that reds can be both warm and cool. If the red is orange-based, it is warm. If it is blue-based, it is cool. Green is similar: if a green contains more gold, it is warm; if it contains more blue, it is cool.

You may hear people refer to a color as having a lot of blue in it. For example: "This lipstick has a blue base" or "That blush is very blue." This does not mean that the color is truly blue. Rather, it means that when the pigments were mixed to create that cosmetic, blue color pigment was added to the formulation. What you are seeing might look primarily violet or magenta.

Selecting Makeup Colors

Now that we have defined warms and cools, it is time to learn a system that will help you feel more comfortable when choosing colors for your clients. Keep in mind that this is simply one way of choosing colors. The art of makeup application allows for more than one way to achieve the result you want.

A neutral skin tone contains equal elements of warm and cool, no matter how light or dark

SKIN COLORS	SKIN COLORS AND TONES	
	WARM	COOL
LIGHT SKIN	yellow, gold, pale peach	pink or slightly ruddy (reddish); florid undertones
MEDIUM SKIN	yellow, yellow-orange, red	olive (yellow-green)
DARK SKIN	red, orange-brown, red-brown	dark olive, blue, blue-black, ebony

Table 24–1 **Skin Colors and Tones.**

© Milady, a part of Cengage Learning.

the skin is. Remember to always match your foundation color to the color of the skin, or use the corrective techniques discussed later in this chapter.

Once you have determined if the skin is light, medium, or dark, you may choose eye, cheek, and lip colors to match the skin color in level, or try contrast for more impact. Most skin tones and levels can wear a surprisingly wide range of eye, cheek, and lip colors.

- If skin color is light, you may use light colors for a soft, natural look. Medium to dark colors will create a more dramatic look.
- If skin color is medium, medium tones will create an understated look. Light or dark tones will provide more contrast and will appear bolder.
- If skin color is dark, dark tones will be most subtle. Medium to medium-light or bright tones will be striking and vivid (**Figure 24–16**).

Be cautious when choosing tones lighter than the skin. If the color is too light, it will turn gray or chalky on the skin. Look for translucent, shimmery colors if you are choosing these tones for use on dark skin.

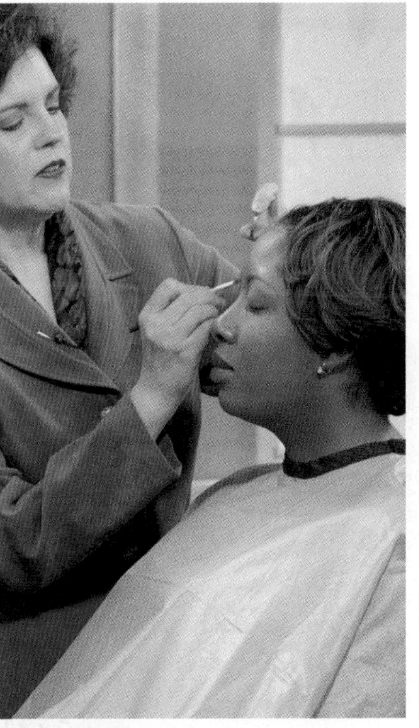

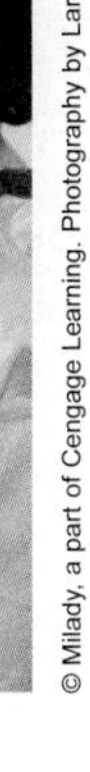

© Milady, a part of Cengage Learning. Photography by Larry Hamill.

▲ **Figure 24–16**
Choose cosmetics to enhance your client's skin color and hair color.

Complementary Colors for Eyes

As you begin recommending eye, cheek, and lip colors, neutrals will always be your safest choice. They contain elements of warm and cool and work well on any skin tone, eye color, or hair color. They come in variations of brown or gray. For instance, they may have a warm or cool base with brown tones. Or you might choose a plum-brown, which would be considered a cool neutral. An orange-brown would be considered a warm neutral. Charcoal gray is a cool neutral, as is blue-gray.

Contrary to popular belief, matching eye color with shadow color is not the best way to enhance this area because it creates a flat region of color. By contrasting eye color with complementary colors, you emphasize the color most effectively.

The following is a procedure for eye color selection. You may refer back to the color wheel for additional help in determining complementary colors.

Reviewing Color Selection Steps

1. Determine skin level: light, medium, or dark.
2. Determine skin undertone: warm, cool, or neutral.
3. Determine eye color: blue, green, brown, and so forth.
4. Determine complementary colors.
5. Determine hair color: warm or cool.
6. Choose eye makeup colors based on complementary or contrasting colors.
7. Coordinate cheek and lip colors within the same color family: warm, cool, or neutral.
8. Apply makeup.

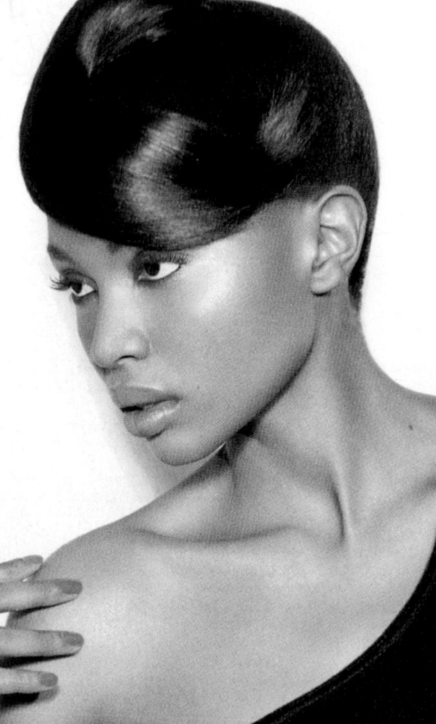

© Iconogenic, 2010; used under license from iStockphoto.com.

The best thing about choosing colors is the unlimited number of choices you have. Try one or all methods of choosing color. Complementary color choices for eye colors are summarized below:

- **Complementary colors for blue eyes.** Orange is the complementary color to blue. Because orange contains yellow and red, shadows with any of these colors in them will make eyes look bluer. Common choices include gold, warm orange-browns like peach and copper, red-browns like mauves and plum, and neutrals like taupe or camel.
- **Complementary colors for green eyes.** Red is the complementary color to green. Because red shadows tend to make the eyes look tired or bloodshot, pure red tones are not recommended. Instead, use brown-based reds or other color options next to red on the color wheel. These include red-orange, red-violet, and violet. Popular choices are coppers, rusts, pinks, plums, mauves, and purples.
- **Complementary colors for brown eyes.** Brown eyes are neutral and can wear any color. Recommended choices include contrasting colors such as greens, blues, grays, and silvers.

© Kin Shing Chan, 2010; used under license from iStockphoto.com.

Adding Cheek and Lip Color

After you have chosen eye makeup, use the color wheel to determine whether your choices are warm or cool, and then coordinate cheek and lip makeup in the same color family as the eye makeup. For example, if your client has green eyes, you might recommend a plum eye color shade, which is cool. Now you should stay with cool colors for the cheeks and lips in order to coordinate with the eye makeup. You may also choose neutrals, as these contain both warm and cool elements and coordinate with any makeup colors.

Hair Color and Eye Color

Hair color needs to be taken into account when determining eye makeup color. For example, if a woman has blue eyes, your instinct might be to select orange-based eye makeup as the complementary choice. But if she has cool blue-black hair, the orange will not be flattering. In this case, you would choose cool colors to coordinate with the hair color. Red-violets (plums) would be a more flattering choice. Look at orange on the color wheel: it is

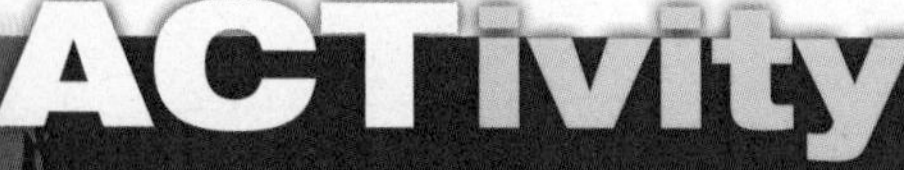

Apply makeup to a partner, using color theory to choose and coordinate makeup colors. Have fun and experiment. Keep track of which colors enhance her appearance and coordinate with her wardrobe and which ones do not. And remember, while a haircut or haircolor may represent a big commitment, makeup does not. If you do not like it, you can simply wash it off and try again!

HAIR COLORS	DETERMINING HAIR COLOR TONES	
	WARM	COOL
BLOND HAIR	yellow, orange	white-blond, ash
RED HAIR	gold, copper, orange, red	red-violet, violet
BROWN HAIR	yellow, gold, orange	ash
DARK BROWN/ BLACK HAIR	copper, red	violet, blue

© Milady, a part of Cengage Learning.

Table 24–2 Determining Hair Color Tones.

warm. Go around the wheel toward the cool end. Red-violets are the closest to orange on the color wheel while still remaining cool. As stated earlier, there is a range of colors to choose from for any client. Use **Table 24–2** as a general guide. ☑ **LO2**

Basic Professional Makeup Application

Client Consultation

The first step in the makeup process, as with all other services that take place in the salon, is the client consultation. This is where you ask the client the questions that will bring out her wishes and concerns. Listen closely and try not to impose your own opinions too much. Your role is to listen to what your client is saying, and only then make recommendations based on your knowledge. If she chooses not to act on your recommendations, do not take it personally. In time, perhaps she will.

Consultation Area

The area that you use for consultations must be clean and tidy. No one wants to see a messy makeup area or dirty brushes lying about. Clean and then disinfect your multiuse brushes after each use, and tidy your makeup area daily. Placing a fresh towel across the work area will help prevent messes and make for easy clean up. Place your brushes on this towel before beginning your makeup work. Also, keep a portfolio in the consultation area that includes photographs of your own work, or pictures from magazines. The client can go through your portfolio to find styles and colors that appeal to her.

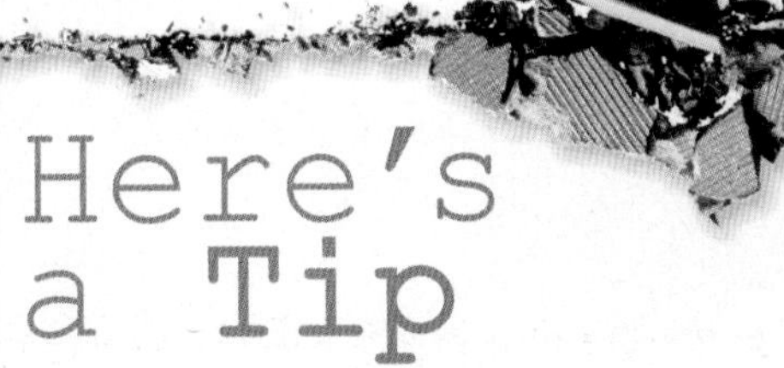

Here's a Tip

Mixing warm and cool colors on a face is not recommended. The colors will compete with each other and will result in an unbalanced appearance. Staying within the color ranges you have chosen will ensure a balanced, beautiful look.

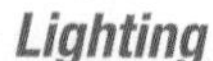

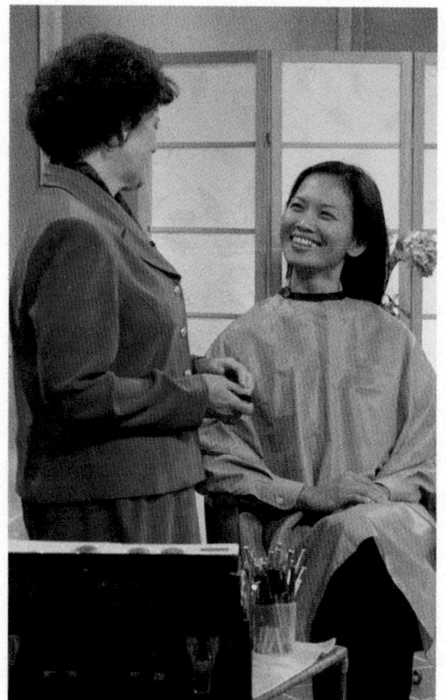

▲ **Figure 24–17**
Client consultation.

Lighting

Adequate and flattering lighting is essential for both the consultation and the application portions of the makeup process. Be sure your client's face is evenly lit without dark shadows. Natural light is the best choice, but if it is necessary to use artificial light, the light should be a combination of incandescent light (warm bulb light) and fluorescent light (cool industrial tube light). If you must choose between the two, incandescent light will be more flattering.

Make sure that the light always shines directly and evenly on the face. And remember, good lighting makes a client look good, and clients who look good are more likely to purchase the products you recommend. When this happens, everyone comes out a winner.

Makeup Consultation

A makeup service should always begin with a warm introduction to your client. Visually assess her to understand her personal style. This will give you cues as you continue your consultation (**Figure 24–17**).

Engaging the client in conversation will help you to determine her needs. Gather whatever information you can about her skin condition, how much or how little makeup she wears daily versus special occasion makeup, the amount of time she spends applying makeup, colors she likes or dislikes, and any makeup issues that are troubling for her.

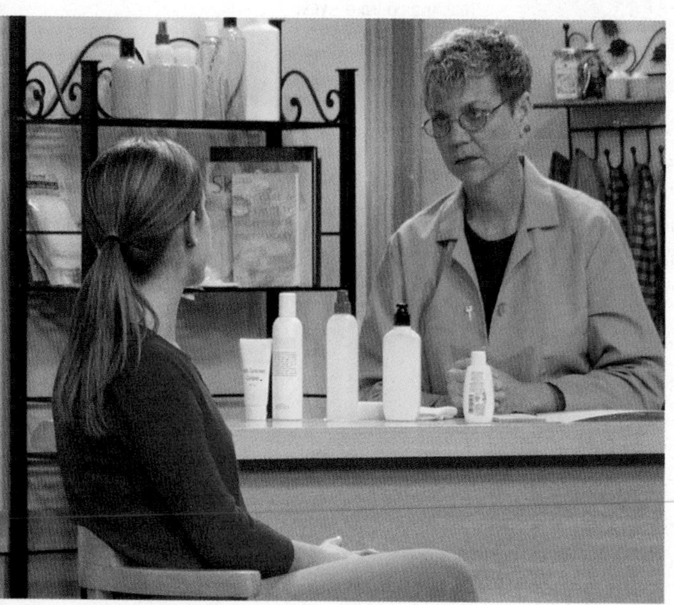

▲ **Figure 24–18**
Retailing cosmetic products.

Record this information on a client consultation card. Also, write down your recommendations so that you may refer back to them at the end of the makeup application. Reviewing and restating your written advice with the client at the end of the service will also help you sell retail products (**Figure 24–18**). Completing an instruction sheet for your client to take home will help her remember the techniques she has been taught, and it will remind her of color and product names that she may wish to purchase at a later time. Escort your client to the reception area where you can assist her in gathering the products that you have recommended. Ask her if she has any other questions and, if so, give clear answers. If possible, set up a time for her next appointment. Then give her a business card with your name on it and shake her hand as you turn her over to the receptionist for checkout. ✓ **LO3**

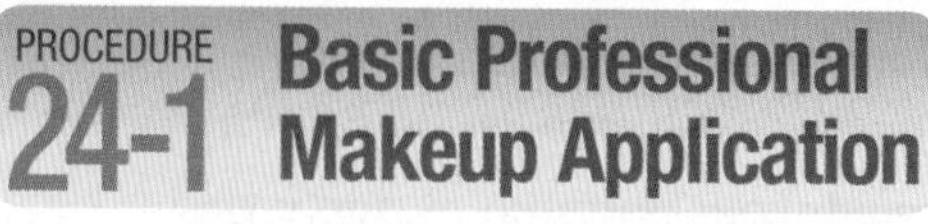

PROCEDURE **24-1** **Basic Professional Makeup Application** SEE PAGE 784

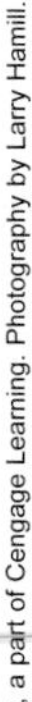

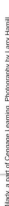

© Milady, a part of Cengage Learning. Photography by Larry Hamill.

Special-Occasion Makeup

When a client asks for makeup for a special occasion, the time is right to work your magic. Special occasions often come with special conditions.

For instance, many special occasions are evening events, when lighting is subdued. That means more definition is required for the eyes, cheeks, and lips. You may also add drama by applying false lashes and using shimmery colors on the eyes, lips, cheeks, or complexion. If the special occasion will include a lot of photographs—such as a wedding—matte colors are recommended because shimmer may reflect light too much. Follow the Basic Professional Makeup Procedure 24-1, but consider the pointers discussed in the following subsections.

Special-Occasion Makeup for Eyes

Option 1: Striking Contour Eyes

1. Apply the base color from the lashes to the brow with a shadow brush or applicator.
2. Apply medium tone on the lid, blending from lash line to crease with the shadow brush or applicator.
3. Apply medium to deep color in the crease, blending up toward the eyebrow, but ending below it.
4. Apply highlight shadow under the brow bone with the shadow brush or applicator.
5. Apply eyeliner on the upper lash line from the outside corner in, tapering as you reach the inner corner. Blend with the small brush or applicator.
6. Apply shadow in the same color as the liner, directly over the liner. This will give longevity and intensity to the liner. Repeat on the bottom lash line, if desired.
7. Apply mascara with a disposable wand (**Figure 24–19**).

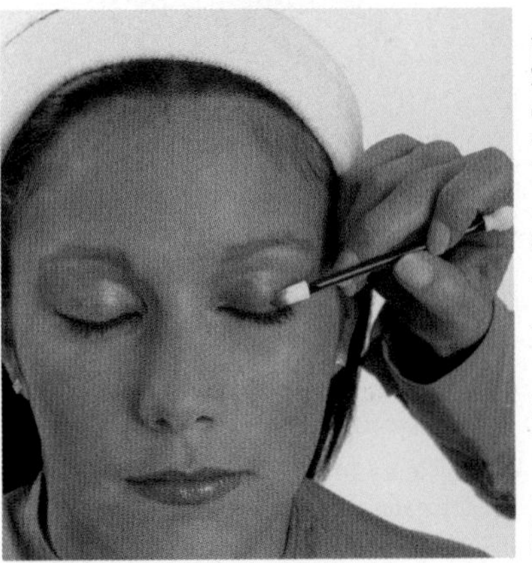

© Milady, a part of Cengage Learning. Photography by Paul Castle.

▲ **Figure 24–19**
Striking contour eyes.

Option 2: Dramatic Smoky Eyes

1. Encircle the eye with dark gray, dark brown, or black eyeliner.
2. Smudge with a small shadow brush or disposable applicator.
3. Using the shadow brush or applicator, apply dark shadow from the upper lash line to the crease, softening and blending as you approach the crease. The shadow should be dark from outer to inner corner. You may choose shimmering or matte finish eye shadows.
4. Repeat on the lower lash line, carefully blending any hard edges.
5. If desired, add a highlight color in a shimmering or matte finish to the upper brow area with the shadow brush or applicator.

ACTivity

Using a model (or yourself) and two different color applications, divide the face in half. Try different foundations, colors, and intensity on each side. This will give you a visual example of how makeup will work on a face. Actually applying makeup is the best way to learn how to use it.

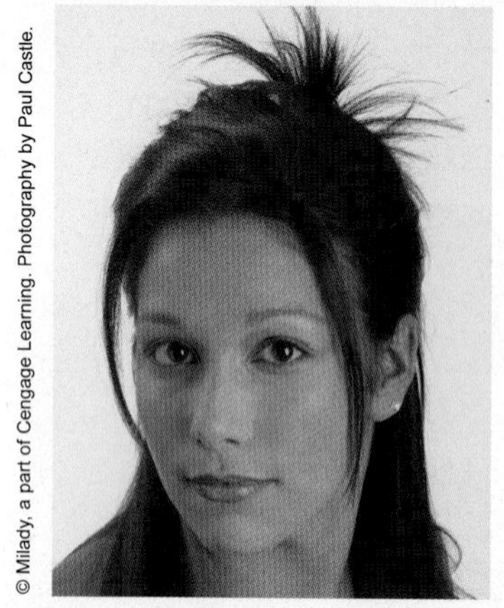

© Milady, a part of Cengage Learning. Photography by Paul Castle.

▲ **Figure 24–20**
Dramatic smoky eyes.

6. Apply mascara with a disposable wand.
7. Add individual or band lashes if desired (**Figure 24–20**).

Special-Occasion Makeup for Cheeks

Refer to the Corrective Makeup section for techniques you can use to remedy less attractive aspects of the cheeks. You can also try one of the following steps:

- Use a darker blush color under the cheekbones to add definition. Apply with a blush brush or applicator and blend carefully. Add a brighter, lighter cheek color to the apples of the cheeks and blend.
- Use a cheek color with shimmer or glitter over the cheekbones for highlight. You may use cream or powder colors.

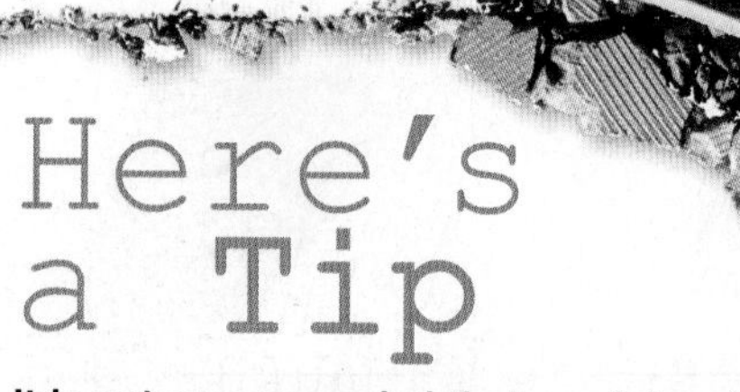

Here's a Tip

It is not recommended that you intensify every feature because this will tend to look overdone and garish. For example, you can intensify the eyes and lips, or the cheeks and lips, but not the eyes, cheeks, and lips.

Special-Occasion Makeup for Lips

Most clients prefer brighter or darker colors for special occasions. You may use shimmer colors or matte colors, if desired.

1. Apply liner color to the lips. Fill in the lip line with pencil and blot.
2. Add similar color in lipstick over the entire mouth with a lip brush or applicator.
3. Apply gloss to the center of the lips with a lip brush or applicator.

☑ **LO4**

Corrective Makeup

All faces are interesting in their own special ways, but few are perfect. When you analyze a client's face, you might see that the nose, cheeks, lips, or jawline are not the same on both sides, or that one eye might be larger than the other, or that the eyebrows might not match. In fact, these tiny imperfections can make the face more interesting if treated artfully. In any case, facial makeup can create the illusion of better balance and proportion when so desired.

Facial features can be accented with proper highlighting, subdued with correct shadowing or shading, and balanced with the proper hairstyle. A basic rule for the application of makeup is that highlighting emphasizes a feature, while shadowing minimizes it. A highlight is produced when a cosmetic, usually foundation that is lighter than the original foundation, is used on a particular part of the face. A shadow is formed when the foundation is darker than the original foundation. The use of shadows (dark colors and shades) minimizes prominent features so they are less noticeable.

Before you undertake any kind of corrective makeup application, you should have a clear sense of how to analyze face shapes.

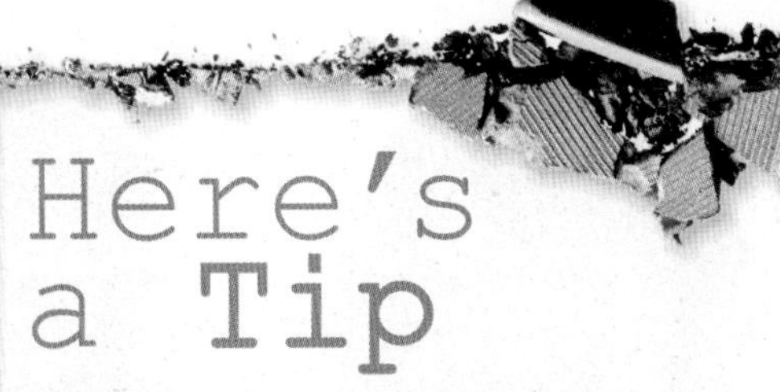

Here's a Tip

When working with older clients who may have wrinkles or sun-damaged skin, be very careful choosing eye shadows and other color products. Shimmering, glitter, or frosted colors can look very bad on dry or mature skin. Stick to muted, softer colors when working with mature clients.

Analyzing Features and Face Shape

The basic rule of makeup application is to emphasize the client's attractive features, while minimizing features that are less appealing. Learning to see the face and its features as a whole and determining the best makeup for an individual takes practice. While the oval face with well-proportioned features has long been considered the ideal, other face shapes are just as attractive in their own way. The goal of effective makeup application is to enhance the client's individuality, not to remake her image according to some ideal standard.

Oval-Shaped Face

The artistically ideal proportions and features of the oval face are the standard to which you will refer when learning the techniques of corrective makeup application. The face is divided into three equal horizontal sections.

The first third is measured from the hairline to the top of the eyebrows. The second third is measured from the top of the eyebrows to the end of the nose. The last third is measured from the end of the nose to the bottom of the chin.

The ideal oval face is approximately three-fourths as wide as it is long. The distance between the eyes is the width of one eye (**Figures 24–21** and **24–22**).

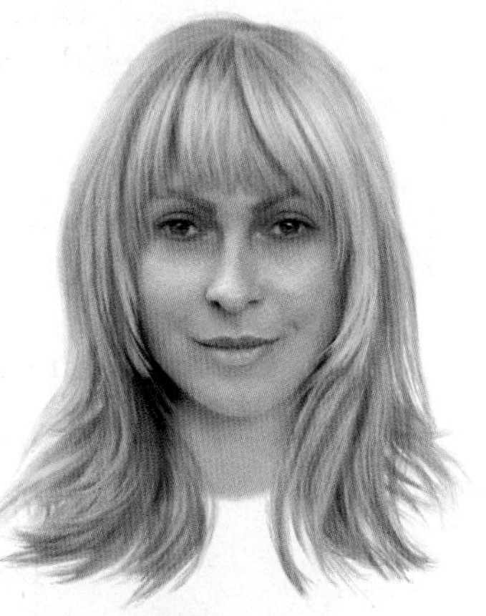

▲ Figure 24–21
Oval face.

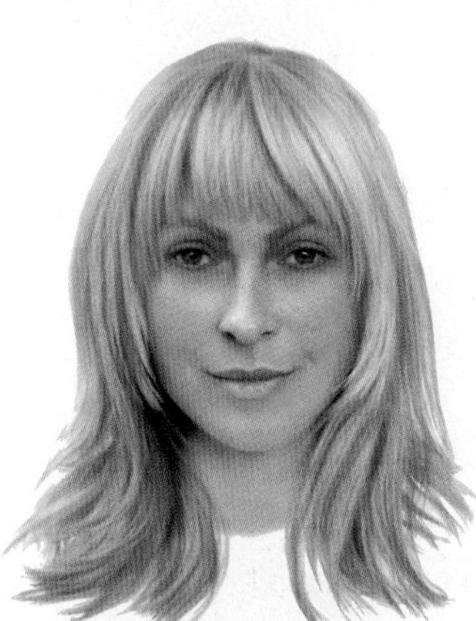

▲ Figure 24–22
Oval face with makeup.

Round Face

The round face is usually broader in proportion to its length than the oval face. It has a rounded chin and hairline. Corrective makeup can be applied to slenderize and lengthen the face (**Figures 24–23** and **24–24**).

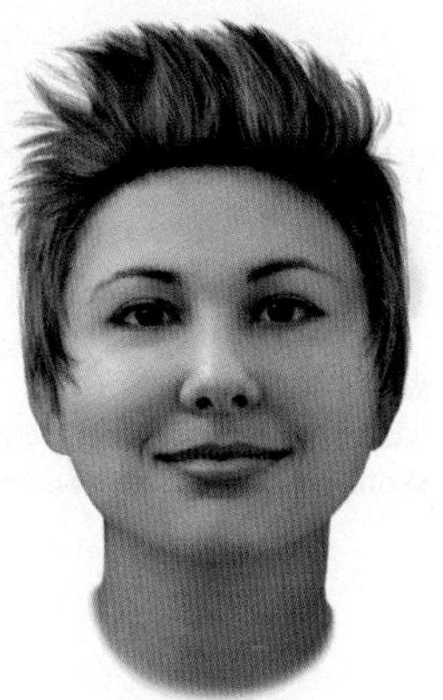

▲ Figure 24–23
Round face.

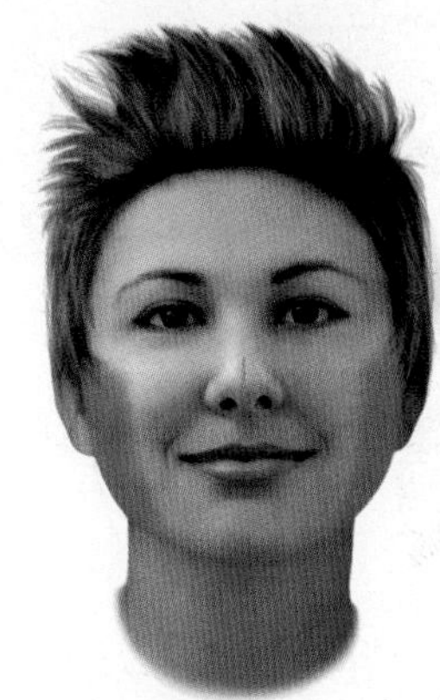

▲ Figure 24–24
Placement of corrective makeup for a round face shape.

© Milady, a part of Cengage Learning.

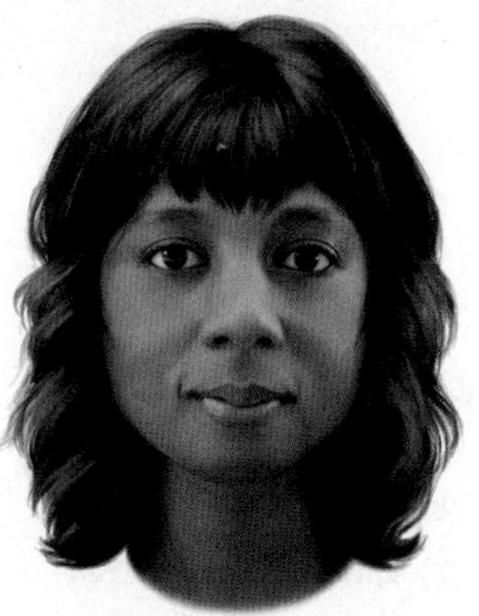

▲ Figure 24–25
Square face.

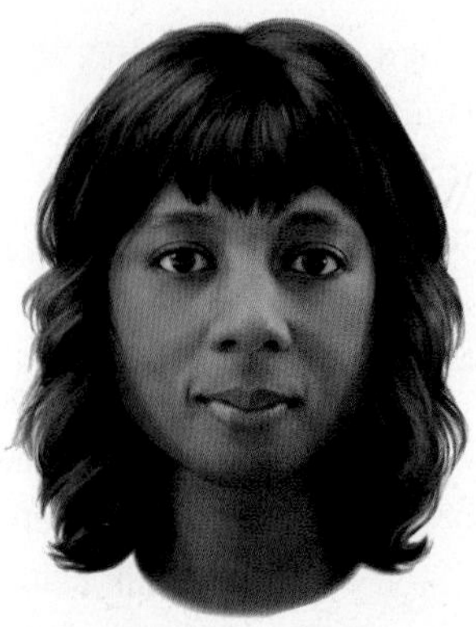

▲ Figure 24–26
Placement of corrective makeup for a square face shape.

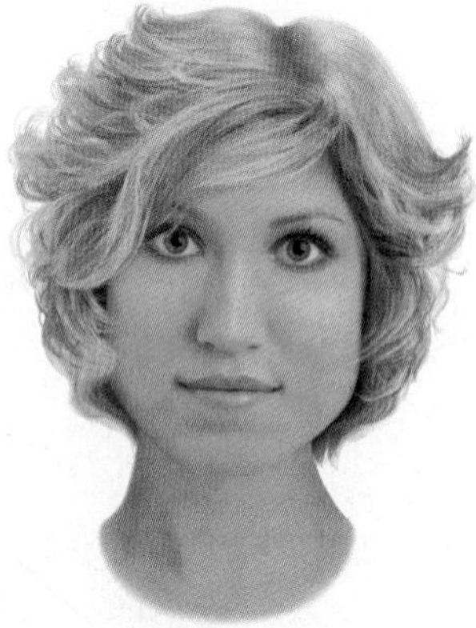

Square-Shaped Face

The square face is composed of comparatively straight lines with a wide forehead and square jawline. Corrective makeup can be applied to offset the squareness and soften the hard lines around the face (**Figures 24–25** and **24–26**).

Triangular (Pear-Shaped) Face

A jaw that is wider than the forehead characterizes the pear-shaped face. Corrective makeup can be applied to create width at the forehead, slenderize the jawline, and add length to the face (**Figures 24–27** and **24–28**).

Inverted Triangle (Heart-Shaped) Face

The inverted triangle or heart-shaped face has a wide forehead and narrow, pointed chin. Corrective makeup can be applied to minimize the width of the forehead and increase the width of the jawline (**Figures 24–29** and **24–30**).

▲ Figure 24–27
Triangular face.

▲ Figure 24–28
Placement of corrective makeup for a triangular face shape.

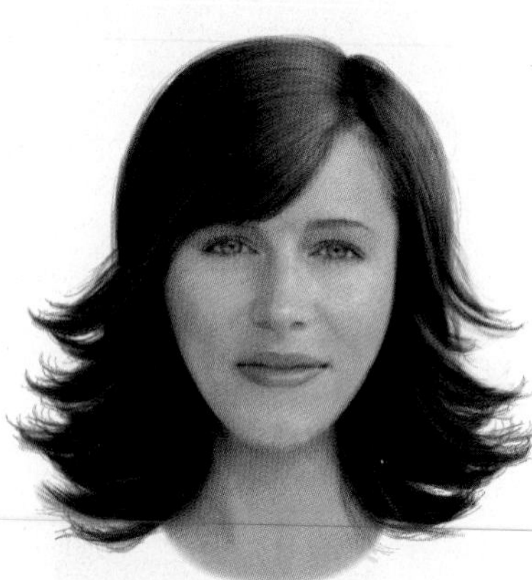

▲ Figure 24–29
Inverted triangle-shaped face.

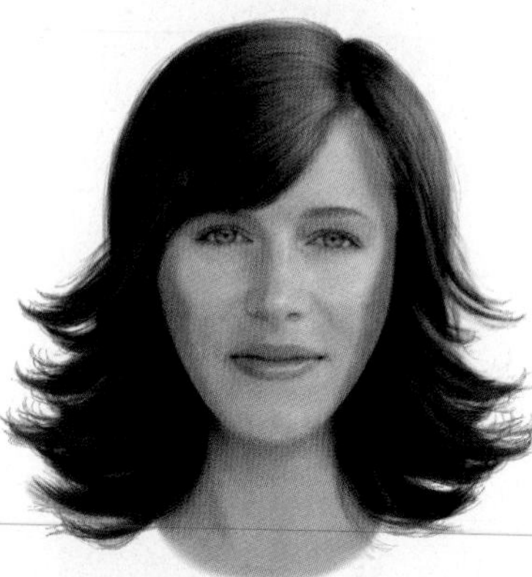

▲ Figure 24–30
Placement of corrective makeup for an inverted triangle-shaped face.

FYI

Corrective makeup can be very effective if applied properly. However, a less-experienced cosmetologist should proceed with caution because improper application, insufficient blending, or the wrong choice of colors can make the face look dirty and artificial.

The illustrations within this chapter are designed to show where contouring or highlighting should be applied to create the illusion of altering the facial shape or emphasizing or minimizing a facial feature. The color in the illustrations is obvious to show exactly where the products should be applied. The actual application should be very well blended and the colors used for shading should only be slightly different than the foundation color.

Corrective makeup techniques using foundation and shading must be very subtle or they will look unnatural and muddy.

© Milady, a part of Cengage Learning.

Diamond-Shaped Face

This face has a narrow forehead. The greatest width is across the cheekbones. Corrective makeup can be applied to reduce the width across the cheekbone line (**Figures 24–31** and **24–32**).

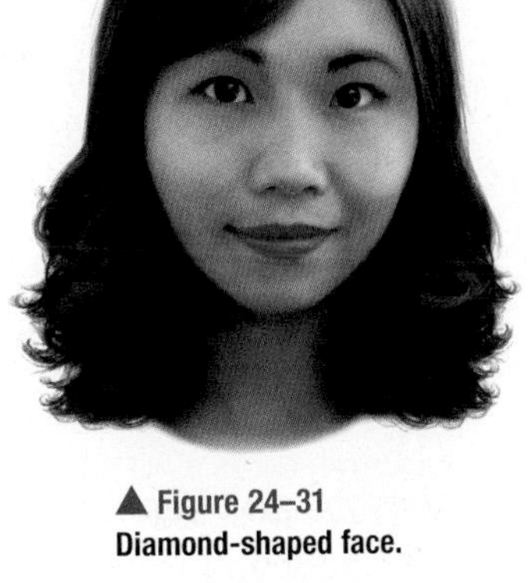

▲ Figure 24–31
Diamond-shaped face.

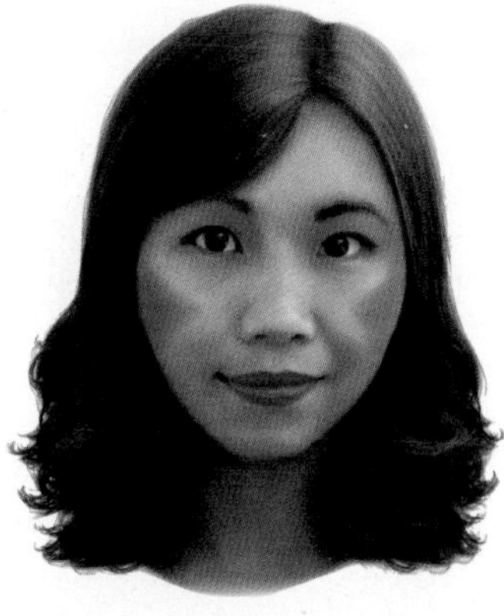

▲ Figure 24–32
Placement of corrective makeup for a diamond-shaped face.

Oblong Face

This face has greater length in proportion to its width than the square or round face. It is long and narrow. Corrective makeup can be applied to create the illusion of width across the cheekbone line, making the face appear shorter (**Figures 24–33** and **24–34**).

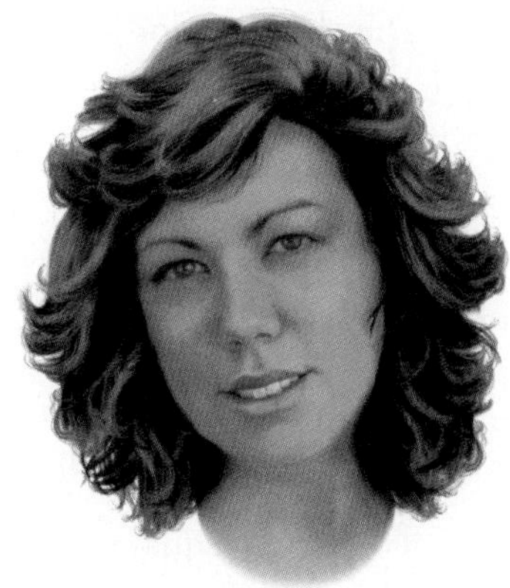

▲ Figure 24–33
Oblong face.

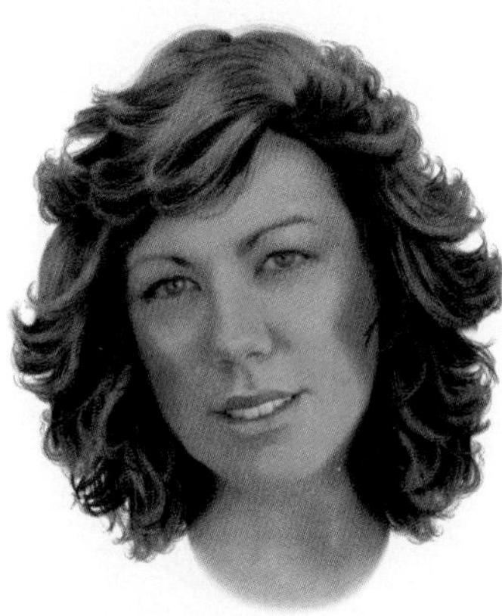

▲ Figure 24–34
Placement of corrective makeup for an oblong face shape.

Forehead Area

For a low forehead, the application of a lighter foundation lends a broader appearance between the brows and hairline. For a protruding forehead, applying a darker foundation over the prominent area gives an illusion of fullness to the rest of the face and minimizes the bulging forehead. A suitable hairstyle also goes a long way toward drawing attention away from the forehead (**Figure 24–35**).

Nose and Chin Areas

For a large or protruding nose, apply a darker foundation on the nose and a lighter foundation on the cheeks at the sides of the nose. This will create fullness in the cheeks and will make the nose appear smaller. Avoid placing cheek color close to the nose.

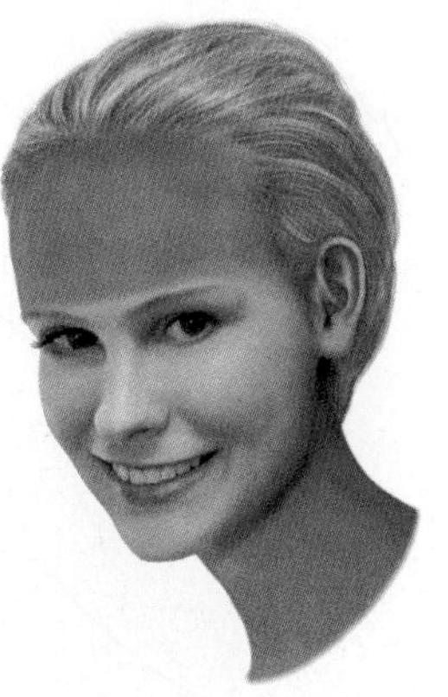

▲ Figure 24–35
Placement of corrective makeup for a protruding forehead.

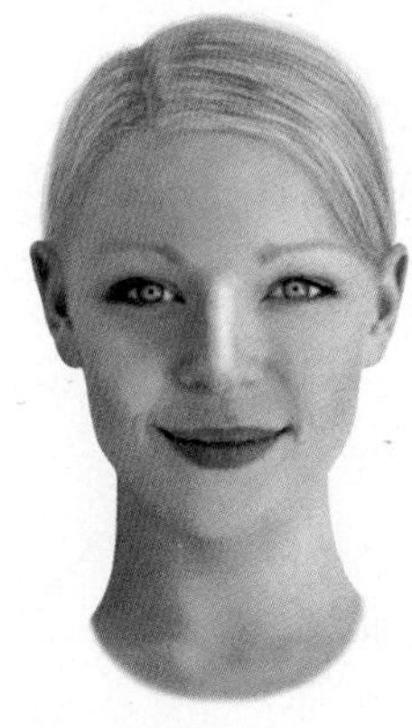

▲ Figure 24–36
Placement of corrective makeup for a short flat nose.

© Milady, a part of Cengage Learning.

For a short and flat nose, apply a lighter foundation down the center of the nose, ending at the tip. This will make the nose appear longer and larger.

If the nostrils are wide, apply a darker foundation to both sides of the nostrils (**Figure 24–36**).

For a broad nose, use a darker foundation on the sides of the nose and nostrils. Avoid carrying this dark tone into the laugh lines because it will

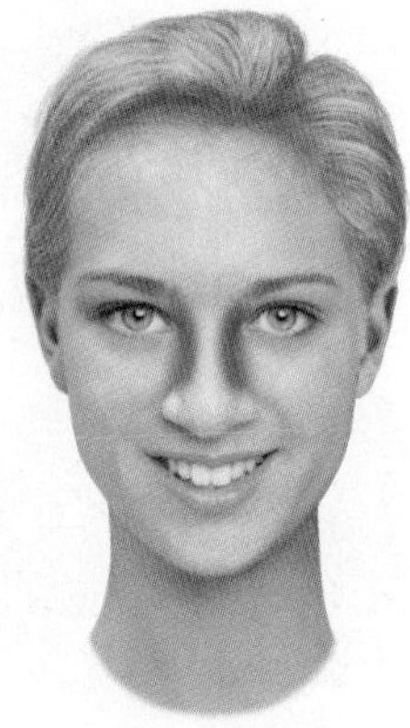

▲ Figure 24–37
Placement of corrective makeup for a broad nose.

accentuate them. The foundation must be carefully blended to avoid visible lines (**Figure 24–37**).

For a protruding chin and receding nose, shadow the chin with a darker foundation and highlight the nose with a lighter foundation. For a receding chin, highlight the chin by using a lighter foundation than the one used on the face.

For a sagging double chin, use a darker foundation on the sagging portion, and use a natural skin tone foundation on the face (**Figure 24–38**).

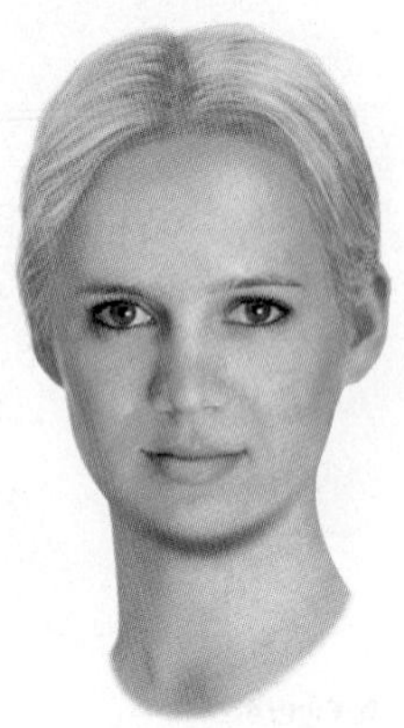

▲ Figure 24–38
Placement of corrective makeup for a double chin.

Jawline and Neck Area

The neck and jaw are just as important as the eyes, cheeks, and lips. When applying makeup, blend the foundation onto the neck so that the client's color is consistent from face to neck. Always set with a translucent powder to avoid transfer onto the client's clothing.

To correct a broad jawline, apply a darker shade of foundation over the heavy area of the jaw, starting at the temples. This will minimize the lower part of the face and create an illusion of width in the upper part of the face (**Figure 24–39**).

To correct a narrow jawline, highlight by using a lighter foundation shade (**Figure 24–40**).

For round, square, or triangular face shapes, apply a darker shade of foundation over the prominent part of the jawline. By creating a shadow over this area, the prominent part of the jaw will appear softer and more oval.

For a small face and a short, thick neck, use a darker foundation on the neck than the one used on the face. This will make the neck appear thinner.

For a long, thin neck, apply a lighter shade of foundation on the neck than the one used on the face. This will create fullness and counteract the long, thin appearance of the neck (**Figure 24–41**).

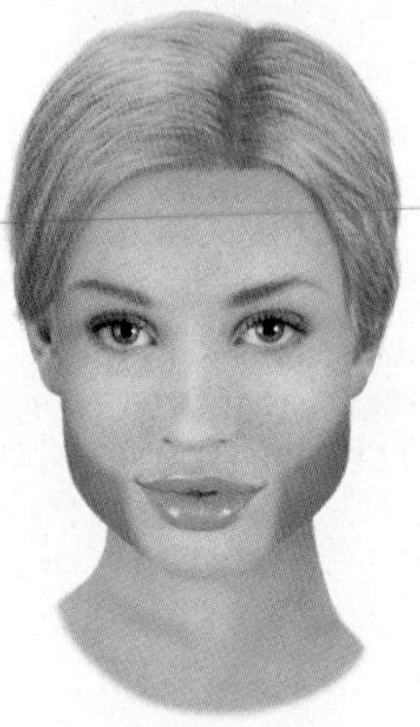

▲ Figure 24–39
Placement of corrective makeup for a broad jawline.

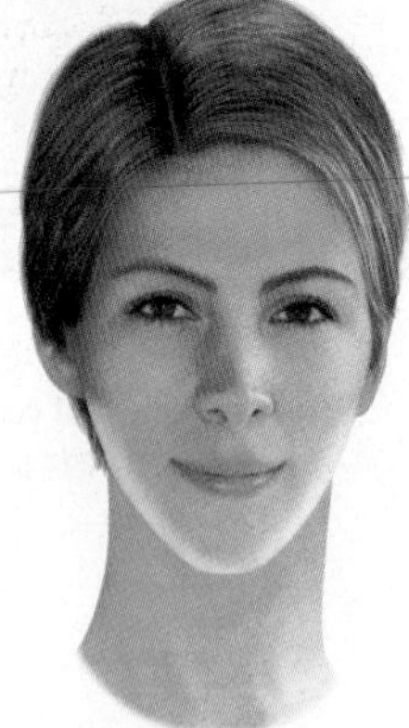

▲ Figure 24–40
Placement of corrective makeup for a narrow jawline.

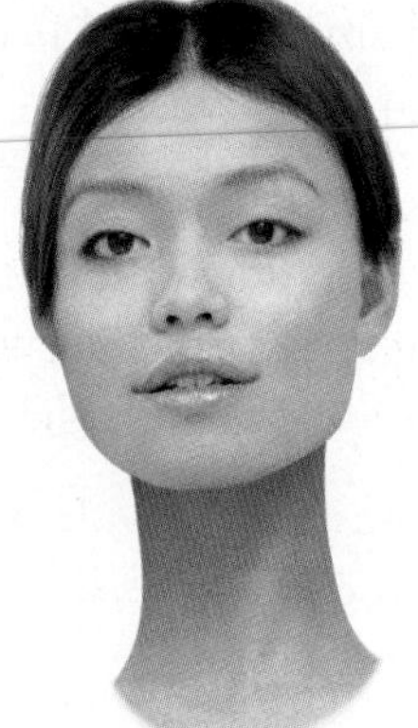

▲ Figure 24–41
Placement of corrective makeup for a long, thin neck.

© Milady, a part of Cengage Learning.

Corrective Makeup for the Eyes

The eyes are very important in balancing facial features. The proper application of eye colors and shadow can create the illusion of the eyes being larger or smaller, and will enhance the overall attractiveness of the face.

Round eyes. This type of feature can be lengthened by extending the shadow beyond the outer corner of the eyes (**Figures 24–42** and **24–43**).

Close-set eyes. The eyes are closer together than the length of one eye. For eyes that are close together, lightly apply shadow up from the outer edge of the eyes (**Figures 24–44** and **24–45**).

Protruding or bulging eyes. This can be minimized by blending the shadow carefully over the prominent part of the upper lid, carrying it lightly toward the eyebrow. Use a medium to deep shadow color (**Figures 24–46** and **24–47**).

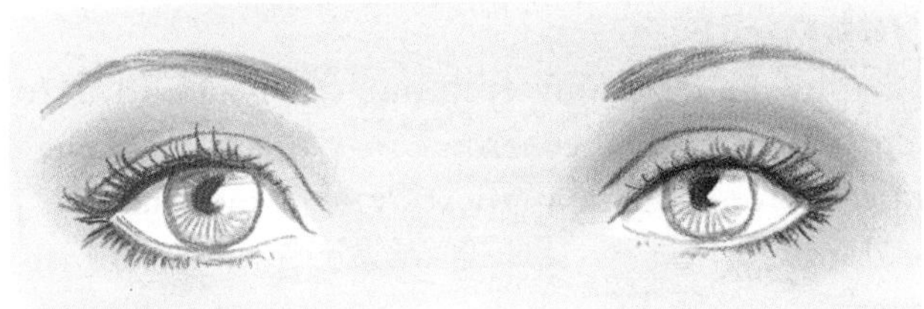

▲ **Figure 24–42**
Round eyes.

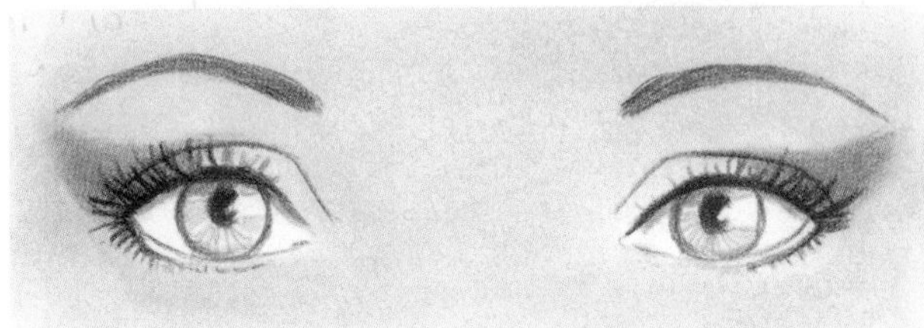

▲ **Figure 24–43**
Placement of corrective makeup for round eyes.

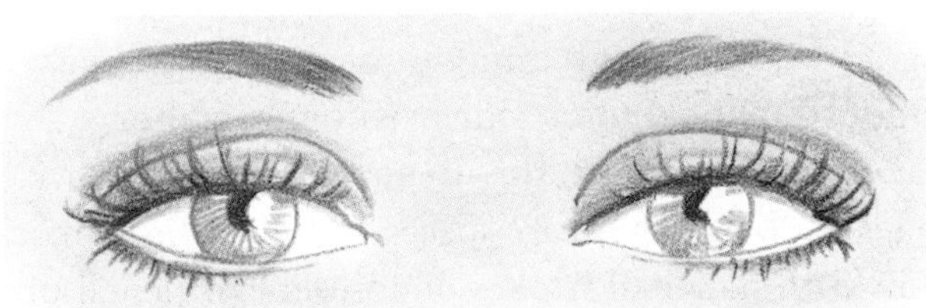

▲ **Figure 24–44**
Close-set eyes.

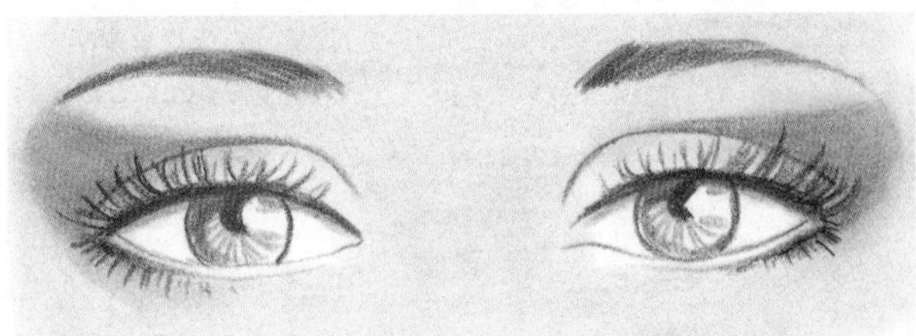

▲ **Figure 24–45**
Placement of corrective makeup for close-set eyes.

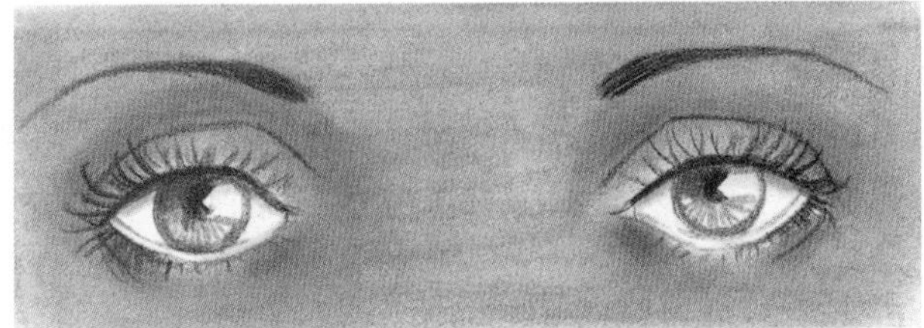

▲ **Figure 24–46**
Protruding eyes.

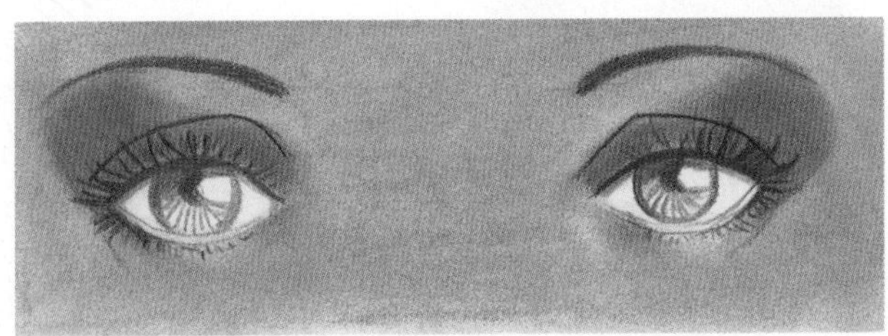

▲ **Figure 24–47**
Placement of corrective makeup for protruding eyes.

© Milady, a part of Cengage Learning.

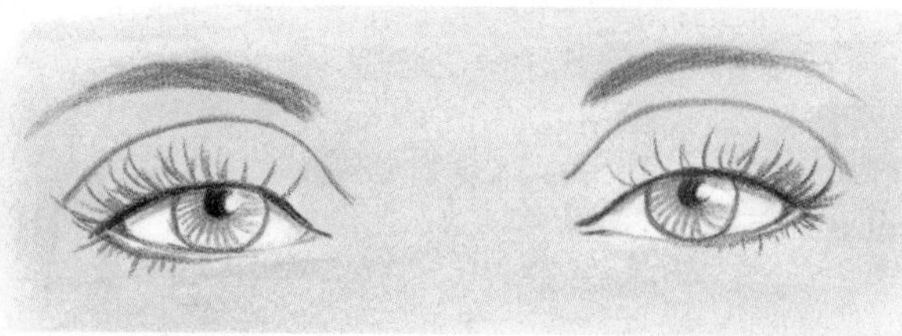

▲ **Figure 24–48**
Heavy-lidded eyes.

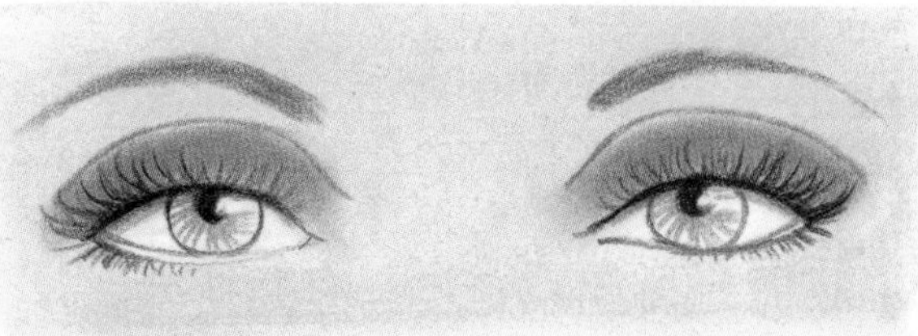

▲ **Figure 24–49**
Placement of corrective makeup for heavy-lidded eyes.

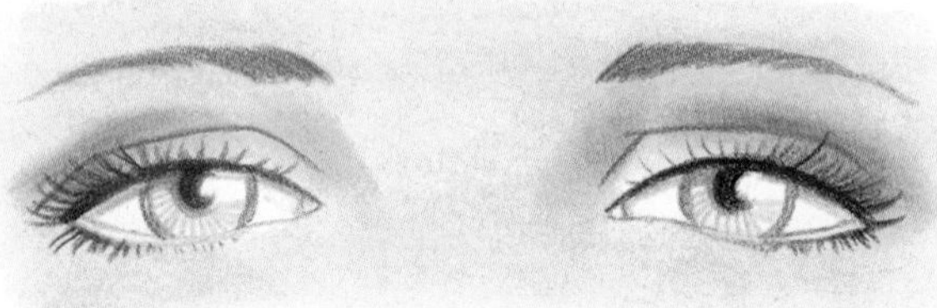

▲ **Figure 24–50**
Deep-set eyes.

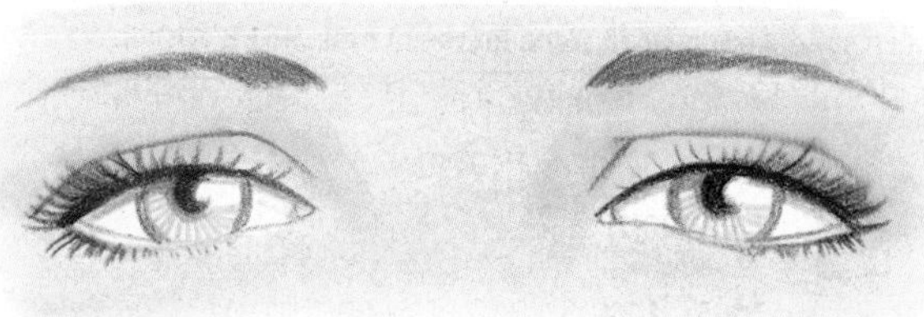

▲ **Figure 24–51**
Placement of corrective makeup for deep-set eyes.

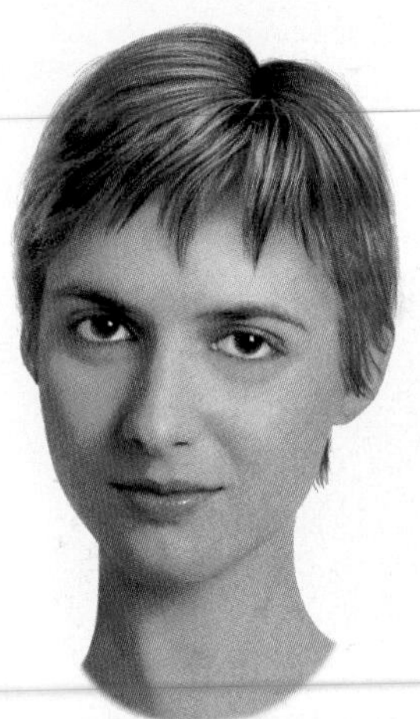

▲ **Figure 24–52**
Dark circles under eyes.

Heavy-lidded eyes. Shadow evenly and lightly across the lid from the edge of the eyelash line to the small crease in the eye socket (**Figures 24–48** and **24–49**).

Small eyes. To make small eyes appear larger, extend the shadow slightly above, beyond, and below the eyes.

Wide-set eyes. Apply the shadow on the upper inner side of the eyelid, toward the nose, and blend carefully.

Deep-set eyes. Use bright, light, reflective colors. Use the lightest color in the crease, and a light-to-medium color sparingly on the lid and brow bone (**Figures 24–50** and **24–51**).

Dark circles under eyes. Apply concealer over the dark area, blending and smoothing it into the surrounding area. Set lightly with translucent powder (**Figure 24–52**).

Eyebrows

Reshaping and defining eyebrows can be an art unto itself. Well-groomed eyebrows are part of a complete and effective makeup application. The eyebrow is the frame for the eye. Overgrown eyebrows can cast a shadow on the brow bone or between the two eyebrows. Over-tweezed eyebrows can make the face look puffy or protruding, or may give the eyes a surprised look.

When a client wants to correct eyebrow shape, begin by removing all unnecessary hairs and then demonstrate how to use the eyebrow pencil or shadow to fill in until the natural hairs have grown in again. When there are spaces in the eyebrow hair, they can be filled in with hair-like strokes of an eyebrow pencil or shadow, applied with an angled brush. Use an eyebrow brush to soften the pencil or shadow marks.

The ideal eyebrow shape can be drawn in three lines (**Figure 24–53**). The first line is vertical, from the inner corner of the eye upward. This is where the eyebrow should begin. The second line is drawn at an angle from the outer corner of the nose to the outer corner of the eye. This is where the eyebrow should end. The third line is vertical, from the outer circle of the iris of the eye upward. The client should be looking straight ahead as you determine this line. This is where the highest part of the arch would ideally be. Of course, not everyone's eyebrows fit exactly within these measurements, so use them only as guidelines.

When the arch is too high, remove the superfluous hair from the top of the brow and fill in the lower part with eyebrow pencil or

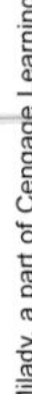
© Milady, a part of Cengage Learning.

shadow. Build up the shape by layering color lightly until the desired effect is achieved.

Adjustments to eyebrow shape can also be used to correct other facial shortcomings listed below:

- **Low forehead.** A low arch gives more height to a very low forehead.
- **Wide-set eyes.** The eyes can be made to appear closer together by extending the eyebrow lines to the inside corners of the eyes. However, care must be taken to avoid giving the client a frowning look.
- **Close-set eyes.** To make the eyes appear farther apart, widen the distance between the eyebrows and slightly extend them outward.
- **Round face.** Arch the brows high to make the face appear narrower. Start on a line directly above the inside corner of the eye and extend to the end of the cheekbone.
- **Long face.** Making the eyebrows almost straight can create the illusion of a shorter face. Do not extend the eyebrow lines farther than the outside corners of the eyes.
- **Square face.** The face will appear more oval if there is a high arch on the ends of the eyebrows. Begin the lines directly above the corners of the eyes and extend them outward.

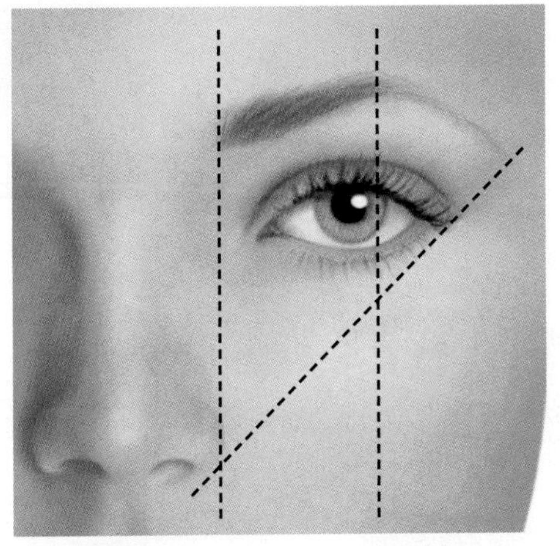

© Milady, a part of Cengage Learning.

▲ **Figure 24–53**
Ideal eyebrow shape.

Here's a Tip

Brow thickness or thinness is sometimes dictated by fashion trends, but today it is more a matter of personal taste and style. Thicker brows are often seen as more natural looking. Keeping thicker brows clean of stray brows is a good grooming technique.

Most thicknesses of eyebrows are accepted in contemporary fashion.

Eyelash Enhancers

There are now treatments available to enhance the eyelashes. Cosmetic lash enhancers are lash lengtheners that contain fibers to make lashes look longer and fuller. Some of these are built into mascaras and some are available as a separate product. Another similar type of product uses a clear polymer to make lashes look thicker.

A prescription drug has now been approved for enhancing lash growth and thickness. Latisse® contains an active drug ingredient called bimatoprost. The drug is applied to the base of the lashes. Most patients using Latisse® see a difference in their lash growth, fullness, and darkness after two to four months of regular use. Latisse® is only available through physicians.

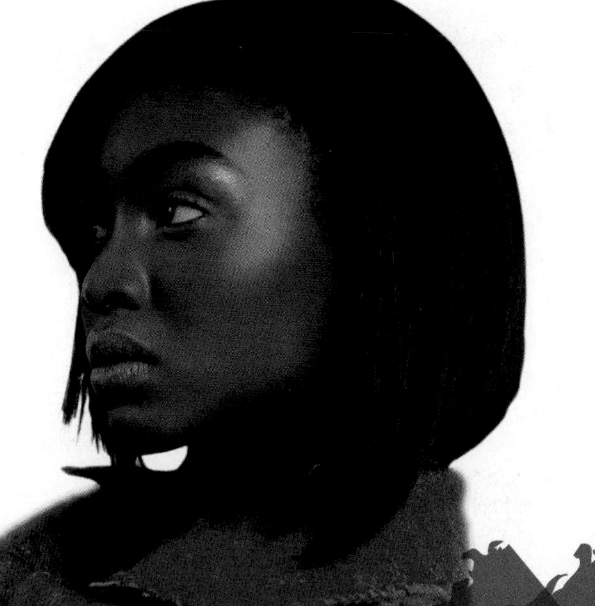

© Iconogenic, 2010; used under license from iStockphoto.com.

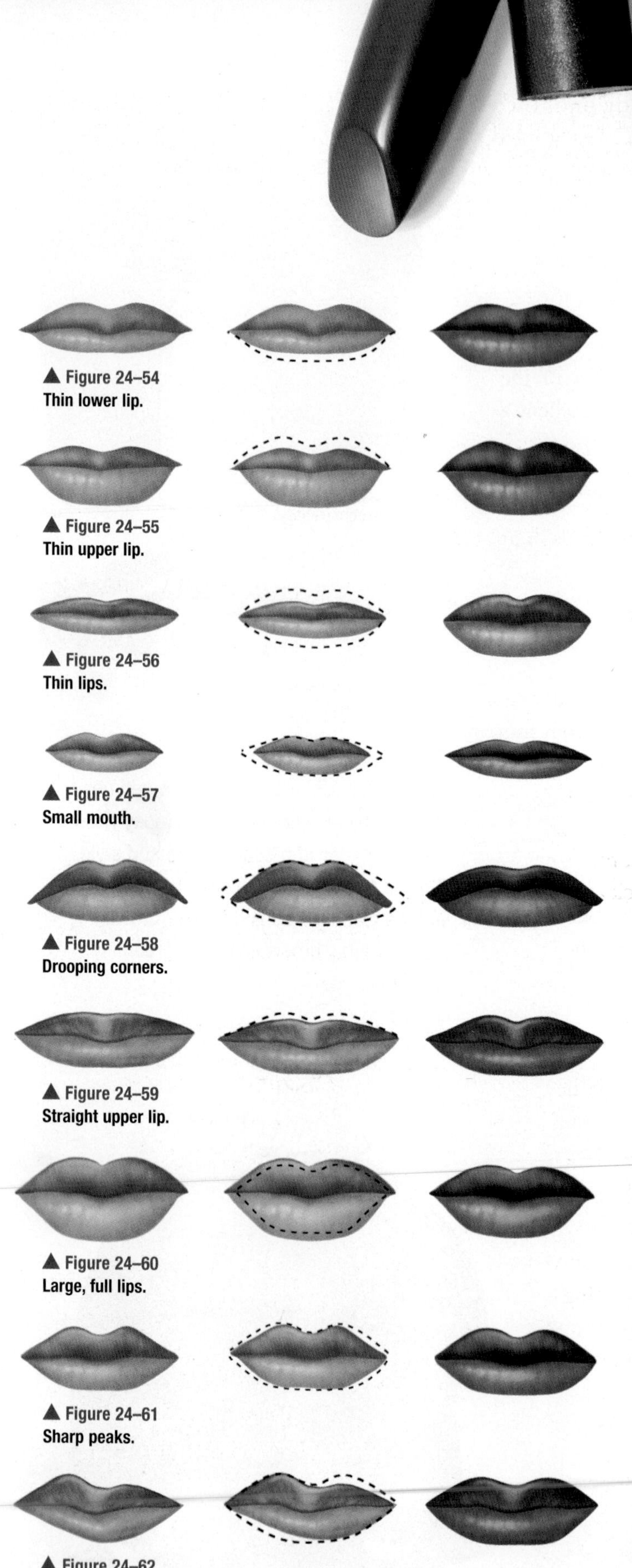

▲ Figure 24–54
Thin lower lip.

▲ Figure 24–55
Thin upper lip.

▲ Figure 24–56
Thin lips.

▲ Figure 24–57
Small mouth.

▲ Figure 24–58
Drooping corners.

▲ Figure 24–59
Straight upper lip.

▲ Figure 24–60
Large, full lips.

▲ Figure 24–61
Sharp peaks.

▲ Figure 24–62
Uneven lips.

© PLAINVIEW, 2010; used under license from iStockphoto.com.

The Lips

Lips are usually proportioned so that the curves or peaks of the upper lip fall directly in line with the nostrils. In some cases, one side of the lips may differ from the other. Lips can be very full, very thin, or uneven. **Figures 24–54** to **24–62** show various lip lines and how lip color can be used to create the illusion of better proportions.

Skin Tones

For whatever reason, some clients may wish to alter their skin tone. In terms of corrective makeup, you will be dealing with two basic skin tones.

For ruddy skin (skin that is red, wind-burned, or affected by rosacea), apply a yellow or green foundation to affected areas, blending carefully. You may then apply a light layer of foundation with a yellow base over the entire complexion. Set it with translucent or yellow-based powder. Avoid red or pink blushes.

For sallow skin (skin that has a yellowish hue), apply a pink-based foundation on the affected areas and blend carefully into the jaw and neck. Set with translucent powder. Avoid yellow-based colors for eyes, cheeks, and lips.

Wrinkles

Age lines and wrinkles due to dry skin can be minimized with a skin primer and foundation. Apply the skin primer evenly and then apply the foundation sparingly and evenly, in a light, outward, circular motion over the entire surface of the face. Care should be taken to remove any foundation that collects in lines and wrinkles of the face. ☑ **LO5**

© Milady, a part of Cengage Learning.

Artificial Eyelashes

The use of artificial eyelashes has grown enormously, mainly because the technology has improved dramatically and fashion has become more reliant on these accessories. Clients with sparse lashes and those who wish to enhance their eyes for special occasions are most likely to request this service. The objective is to make the client's own lashes look fuller, longer, and more attractive without appearing unnatural.

Two types of artificial eyelashes are commonly used. **Band lashes**, also known as **strip lashes**, are eyelash hairs on a strip that are applied with adhesive to the natural lash line. **Individual lashes** are separate artificial eyelashes that are applied to the eyelids one at a time. **Eyelash adhesive** is used to make artificial eyelashes adhere, or stick, to the natural lash line.

CAUTION

Some clients may be allergic to a particular eyelash adhesive. When in doubt, give the client an allergy test before applying the lashes. This test may be done in one of two ways:

- Put a drop of the adhesive behind one ear.
- Attach a single individual eyelash to each eyelid.

In either case, if there is no reaction over the next twenty-four hours, it is probably safe to proceed with the application.

Applying Band Lashes

Band lashes (sometimes referred to as *strip lashes*) are available in a variety of sizes, textures, and colors. They can be made from human hair, certain animal hair such as mink, or synthetic fibers. Synthetic fiber eyelashes are made with a permanent curl and do not react to changes in weather conditions. Artificial eyelashes are available in natural colors ranging from light to dark brown and black or light to dark auburn, as well as bright, trendy colors. Black and dark brown are the most popular choices.

PROCEDURE 24-2 Band Lash Application SEE PAGE 787

CAUTION

Remind the client to take special care with artificial lashes when swimming, bathing, or cleansing the face. Water or cleansing products will loosen artificial lashes.

Removing Band Eyelashes

You may use commercial preparations, such as pads saturated with special lotions, to remove band eyelashes. The lash base may also be softened by applying a face cloth or cotton pad saturated with warm water and a gentle facial cleanser. Hold the cloth over the eyes for a few seconds to soften the adhesive. Starting from the outer corner, remove the lashes carefully to avoid pulling out the client's own lashes. Use cotton-tipped swabs to remove any makeup and adhesive remaining on the eyelid.

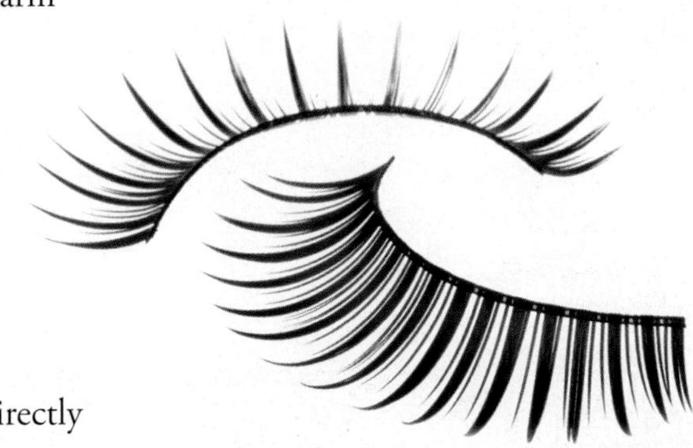

© Shariff Che'Lah, 2010; used under license from iStockphoto.com.

Individual Lashes

Individual lash application, also known as **eye tabbing**, is a procedure in which individual synthetic eyelashes are attached directly to a client's own lashes at their base. Follow the manufacturer's instructions for attaching individual lashes. ☑ **LO6**

PROCEDURE 24-1

Basic Professional Makeup Application

Implements and Materials

You will need all of the following implements, materials, and supplies:

- Assorted makeup brushes (for eye shadow, eyeliner, lip color, concealer, blush, and powder; flat or slanted brush for brows or eyeliner)
- Astringent for oilier skin
- Cheek colors
- Cleansers
- Concealers
- Cotton pads or puffs
- Cotton swabs
- Disposable lip brushes
- Eye shadows
- Eyelash curler
- Eyeliner pencils
- Face powders
- Foundations
- Headband or hair clip
- Lip colors
- Lip liners
- Makeup cape
- Mascara
- Mascara wands
- Moisturizers
- Pencil sharpener
- Shadow applicators
- Small makeup palette
- Spatulas
- Sponge wedges
- Tissues
- Toner for drier skin
- Towels and draping sheets, if desired

Preparation

- Perform PROCEDURE 22-1 **Pre-Service Procedure** SEE PAGE 696

Procedure

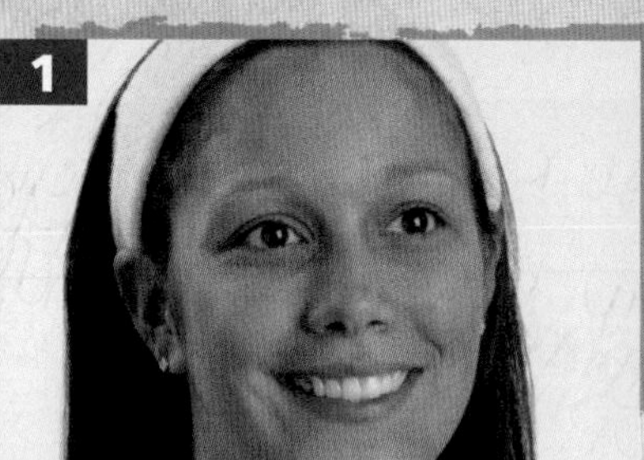

1

© Milady, a part of Cengage Learning. Photography by Paul Castle.

1 Drape the client and use a headband or hair clip to keep her hair out of her face.

2 Cleanse the face and remove cleanser.

3 Apply astringent lotion or toner.

4 Apply moisturizer that is appropriate for the skin type.

5 Before a facial makeup, groom eyebrows, if needed, by removing any stray hairs, tweezing the hair in the same direction in which it grows. For a full eyebrow maintenance or eyebrow arching (tweezing) see Chapter 22, Hair Removal.

Service Tip

Skin varies in color and tone from person to person, regardless of ethnic background. When applying makeup, always remember to analyze the skin and choose makeup that will enhance the client's skin, eyes, and hair color, as well as her features.

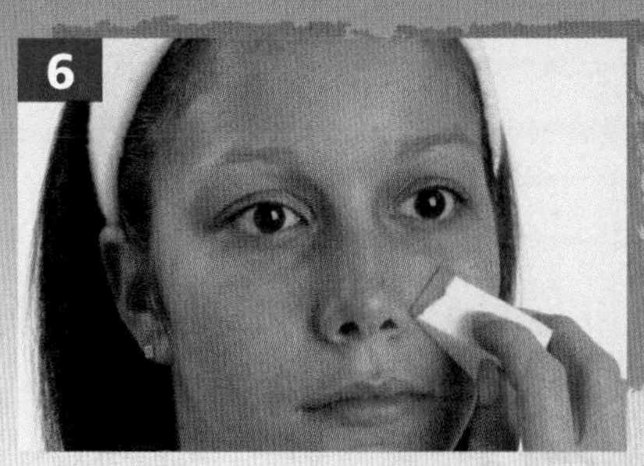

6 Select the proper foundation type for the client's skin type and needs. Test the selected foundation color by blending a small amount of the foundation on the client's jawline. When you are satisfied with your choice, place a small amount of the foundation on a palette, and use a cosmetic sponge to apply it sparingly and evenly over the entire face and around the neckline. Starting at the center of the face, blend with outward and downward motions. Blend near the hairline, and remove excess foundation with a cosmetic sponge or cotton pledget.

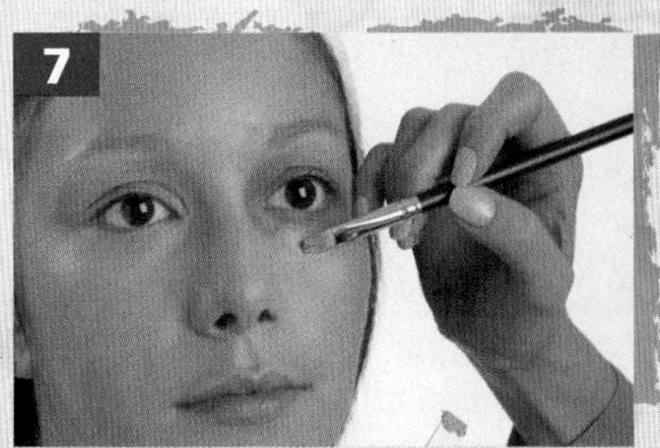

7 Select the appropriate type and color of concealer and scrape a small amount onto a spatula. Using a brush or soft sponge, apply the concealer lightly where needed (under the eyes, over blemishes, over red or dark-colored splotches). Blend in using a cosmetic sponge with a patting motion. If a powder foundation is being used, the concealer must be applied before the foundation. Your instructor may prefer a different method that is also correct.

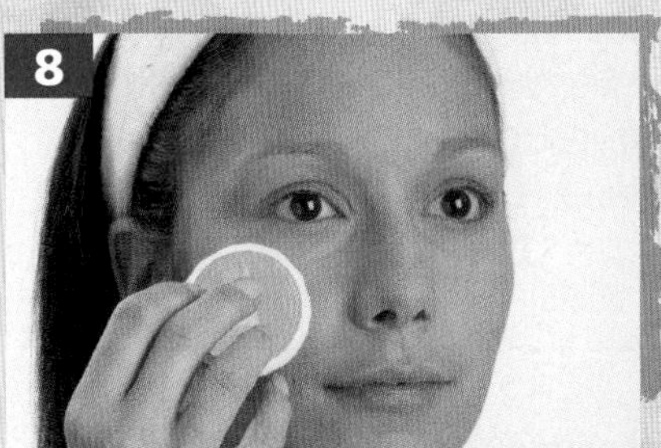

8 Apply face powder with a disposable puff or cosmetic sponge, pressing it over the face and whisking off the excess with a puff or powder brush. As an alternative, a powder brush may be dipped once in loose powder, gently tapped on a facial tissue to remove excess, and gently brushed across the face. A moistened cosmetic sponge may be pressed over the finished makeup to give the face a matte look.

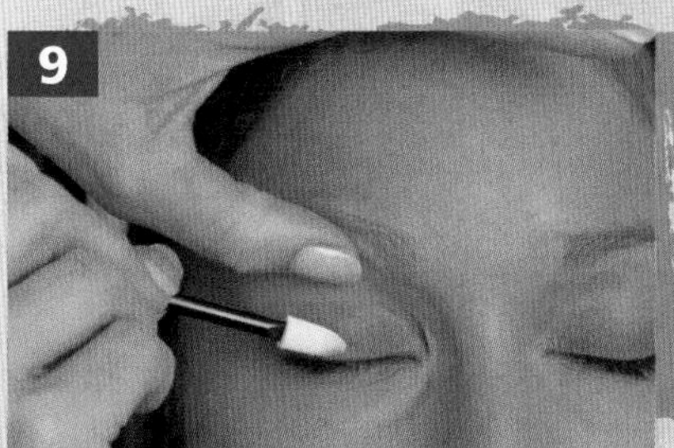

9 Select a complementary eye color in a medium tone. Beginning at the lash line or crease, apply lightly and blend outward with a brush or disposable applicator.

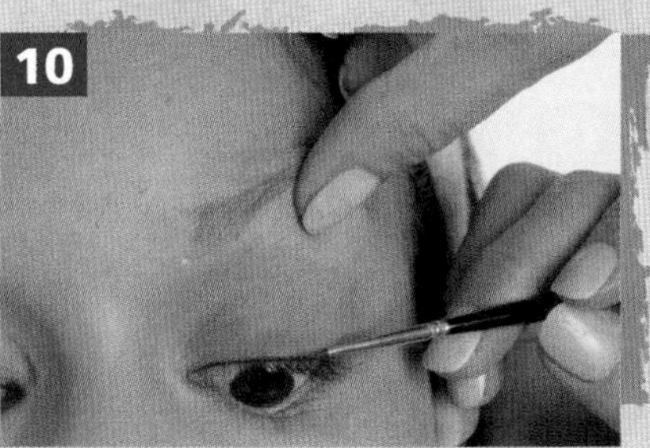

10 Select eyeliner pencil, pressed liner, or liquid liner in a color to harmonize with the mascara you will be applying. Pull the eyelid taut as the client looks down, and draw a very fine line along the entire lid. You may apply to the top and/or bottom lash line. If eyeliner pencil is used, the point should be fine, and care should be taken to avoid injury or discomfort. Be sure to trim the pencil before each use.

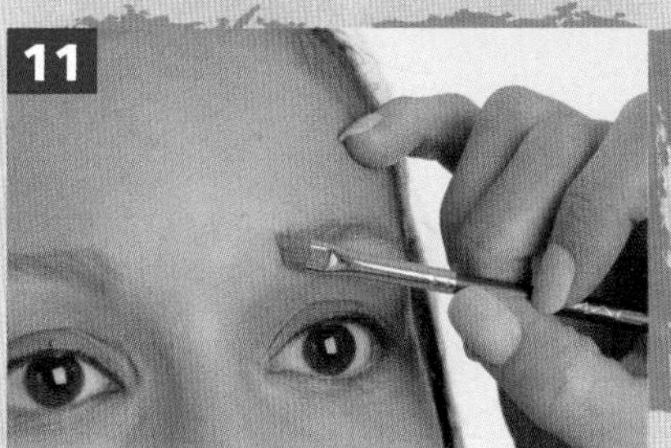

11 Brush the eyebrows into place with light feathery strokes, and either apply color with a fine-pointed pencil or fill in with a brush and shadow. Excess color can be removed with a cotton-tipped swab.

© Milady, a part of Cengage Learning. Photography by Paul Castle.

PROCEDURE 24-1

Basic Professional Makeup Application continued

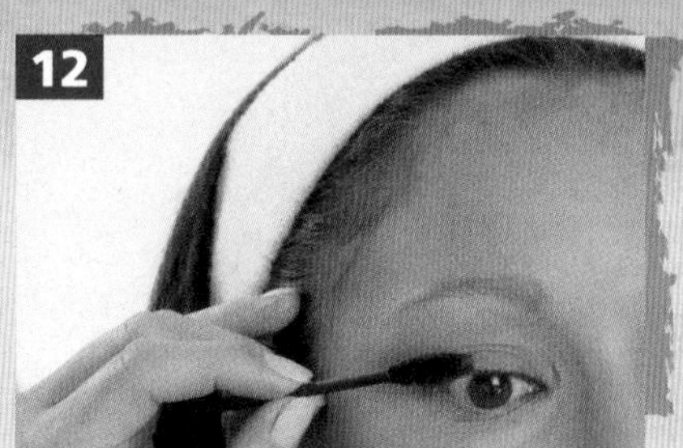

12 Apply mascara to the top and underside of the upper lashes with careful, gentle strokes until the desired effect is achieved. Use a fresh brush or applicator to separate the lashes. Mascara may be applied to the lower lashes if desired, but the effect should be subtle.

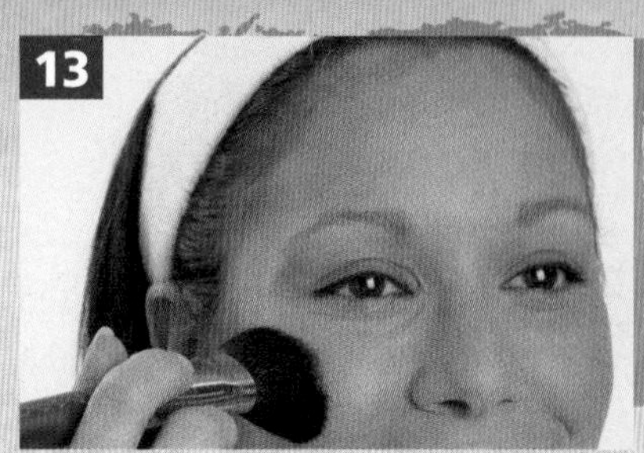

13 Have the client smile to raise her cheeks. Then apply powder cheek color, blending outward and upward toward the temples. Liquid or cream cheek color is applied with a clean applicator before powder and sometimes on bare skin.

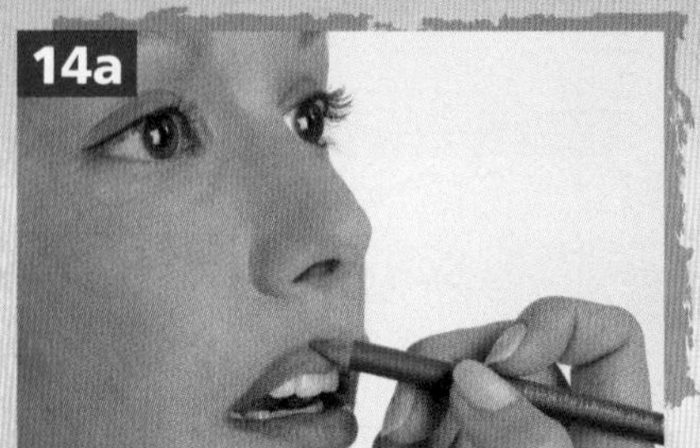

14a Use a freshly sharpened pencil to apply lip liner. Line the lips by beginning at the outer corner of the upper lip and working toward the middle. Repeat on the opposite side. Connect the center peaks using rounded strokes, following the natural line of the lip.

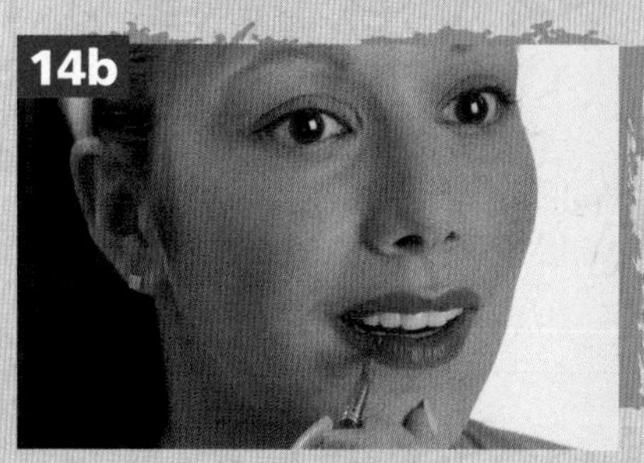

14b Outline the lower lip from the outer corners in. Then apply liner on the lips, staying within the outline. For reasons of hygiene, lip color must not be applied directly from the container unless it belongs to the client. Use a spatula to carefully scrape some of the lip color from the container, and take it from the spatula with a lip brush. Rest your ring finger on the client's chin to steady your hand. Ask the client to relax her lips and part them slightly. Brush on the lip color. Then ask the client to smile slightly so that you can smooth the lip color into any small crevices. Blot the lips with tissue to remove excess product and to set the lip color. Powdering is not recommended because a moist look is more desirable for lips.

CAUTION

When applying mascara, remember to use a disposable mascara wand and dip it into a clean tube of mascara. Then dispose of the wand. Never double dip.

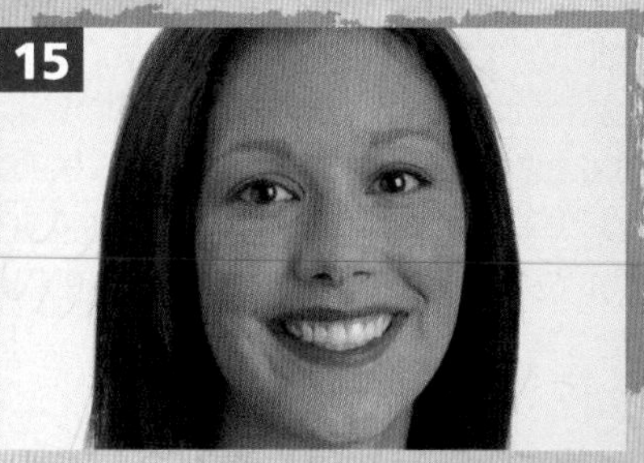

15 Finished makeup application.

Post-Service

- Complete PROCEDURE 22-2 **Post-Service Procedure** SEE PAGE 699

© Milady, a part of Cengage Learning. Photography by Paul Castle.

PROCEDURE 24-2

Band Lash Application

Implements and Materials

You will need all of the following implements, materials, and supplies:

- Adhesive tray
- Adjustable light (gooseneck lamp)
- Cotton pads
- Cotton swabs
- Eye makeup remover
- Eyelash brushes
- Eyelash curler
- Eyelash remover
- Eyelid and eyelash cleanser
- Hand mirror
- Headband or hair clip
- Lash adhesive
- Makeup cape
- Makeup chair
- Manicure scissors
- Pencil sharpener
- Trays of artificial eyelashes
- Tweezers

Preparation

- Perform PROCEDURE 22-1 Pre-Service Procedure SEE PAGE 696

Procedure

1 Properly drape the client to protect her clothing and have her use a hairline strip, headband, or turban during the procedure.

2 If the client wears contact lenses, they must be removed before starting the procedure.

3 If the client has not already done so, remove all eye makeup so that the lash adhesive will adhere properly. Work carefully and gently. Follow the manufacturer's instructions carefully.

4 Brush the client's eyelashes to make sure they are clean and free of foreign matter, such as mascara particles. If the client's lashes are straight, they can be curled with an eyelash curler before you apply the artificial lashes.

5 Carefully remove the eyelash band from the package.

6 Start with the upper lash. If the eyelash band is too long to fit the curve of the upper eyelid, trim the outside edge. Use your fingers to bend the lash into a horseshoe shape to make it more flexible so that it fits the contour of the eyelid.

Band Lash Application continued

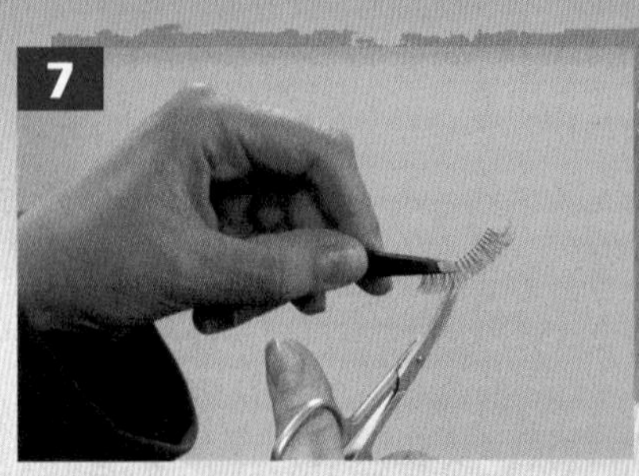

7 Feather the lash by nipping into it with the points of your scissors. This creates a more natural look.

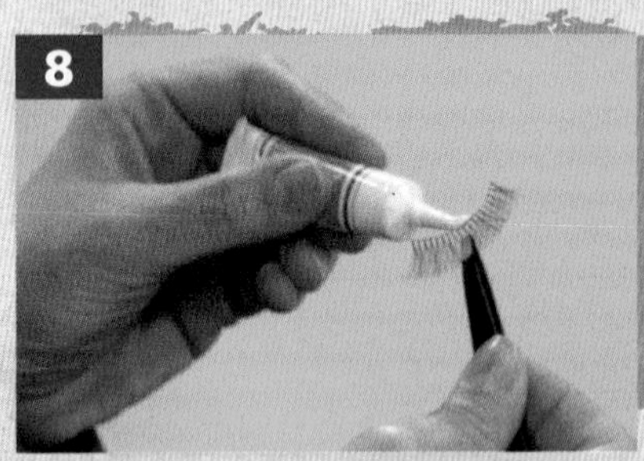

8 Apply a thin strip of lash adhesive to the base of the lash and allow a few seconds for it to set.

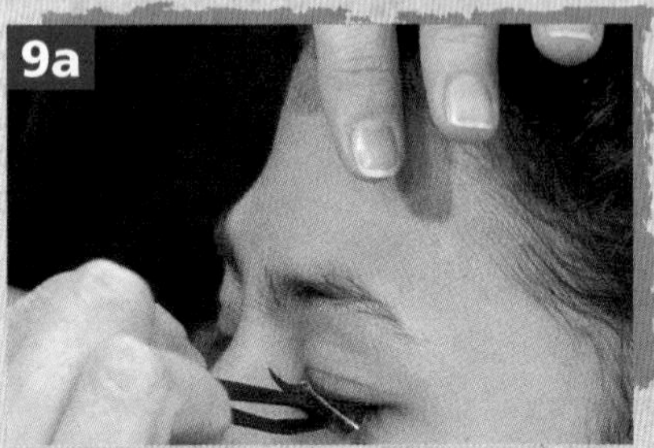

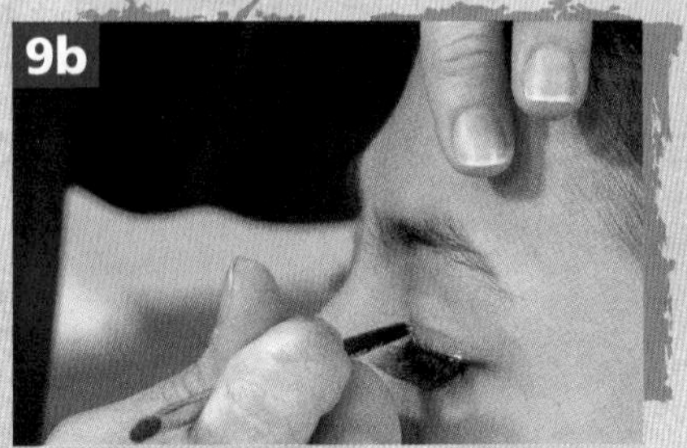

9 Start with the shorter part of the lash and place it on the inner corner of the eye toward the nose. Position the rest of the artificial lash as close to the client's own lash as possible. Use the rounded end of a lash liner brush or tweezers to press the lash on. Be very careful and gentle when applying the lashes. If eyeliner is to be used, the line is usually drawn on the eyelid before the lash is applied, and is retouched when the artificial lash is in place.

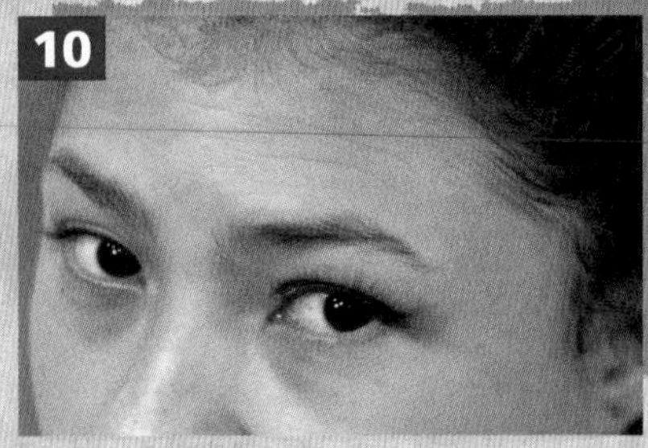

10 Lower lash application is optional because it tends to look less natural. Trim the lash as necessary and apply adhesive in the same way you did for the upper lash. Place the lash on top of the client's lower lash. Place the shorter lash toward the center of the eye and the longer lash toward the outer part of the lid.

Post-Service

- Complete PROCEDURE 22-2 Post-Service Procedure SEE PAGE 699

© Milady, a part of Cengage Learning. Photography by Larry Hamill.

Review Questions

1. List eight types of facial cosmetics and how they are used.
2. Name the primary, secondary, and complementary colors.
3. List the cosmetics used in a basic makeup procedure in the order in which they are applied.
4. What is the purpose of special-occasion makeup?
5. What basic principle is all corrective makeup founded on?
6. Name and describe the two types of artificial eyelashes.

Chapter Glossary

band lashes	Also known as *strip lashes*; eyelash hairs on a strip that are applied with adhesive to the natural lash line.
cake makeup	Also known as *pancake makeup*; a heavy-coverage makeup pressed into a compact and applied to the face with a moistened cosmetic sponge.
cheek color	Also known as *blush* or *rouge*; used primarily to add a natural looking glow to the cheeks.
color primer	Applied to the skin before foundation to cancel out and help disguise skin discoloration.
concealers	Thick, heavy types of foundation used to hide dark eye circles, dark splotches, and other imperfections.
cool colors	Colors that suggest coolness and are dominated by blues, greens, violets, and blue-reds.
eye makeup removers	Special preparations for removing eye makeup.
eye shadows	Cosmetics applied on the eyelids to accentuate or contour.
eye tabbing	Procedure in which individual synthetic eyelashes are attached directly to a client's own lashes at their base.
eyebrow pencils	Also known as *eyebrow shadows*; pencils used to add color and shape to the eyebrows.
eyelash adhesive	Product used to make artificial eyelashes adhere, or stick, to the natural lash line.
eyeliner	Cosmetic used to outline and emphasize the eyes.
face powder	Cosmetic powder, sometimes tinted and scented, that is used to add a matte or nonshiny finish to the face.
foundation	Also known as *base makeup*; a tinted cosmetic used to cover or even out the coloring of the skin.
greasepaint	Heavy makeup used for theatrical purposes.

Chapter Glossary

individual lashes	Separate artificial eyelashes that are applied to the eyelids one at a time.
line of demarcation	An obvious line where foundation starts or stops.
lip color	Also known as *lipstick* or *lip gloss*; a paste-like cosmetic used to change or enhance the color of the lips.
lip liner	Colored pencil used to outline the lips and to help keep lip color from bleeding into the small lines around the mouth.
mascara	Cosmetic preparation used to darken, define, and thicken the eyelashes.
matte	Nonshiny.
warm colors	Range of colors from yellow and gold through oranges, red-oranges, most reds, and even some yellow-greens.

PART 5

NAIL CARE

Chapters

© Crolique, 2010; used under license from Shutterstock.com.

CHAPTER 25

Manicuring

Chapter Outline

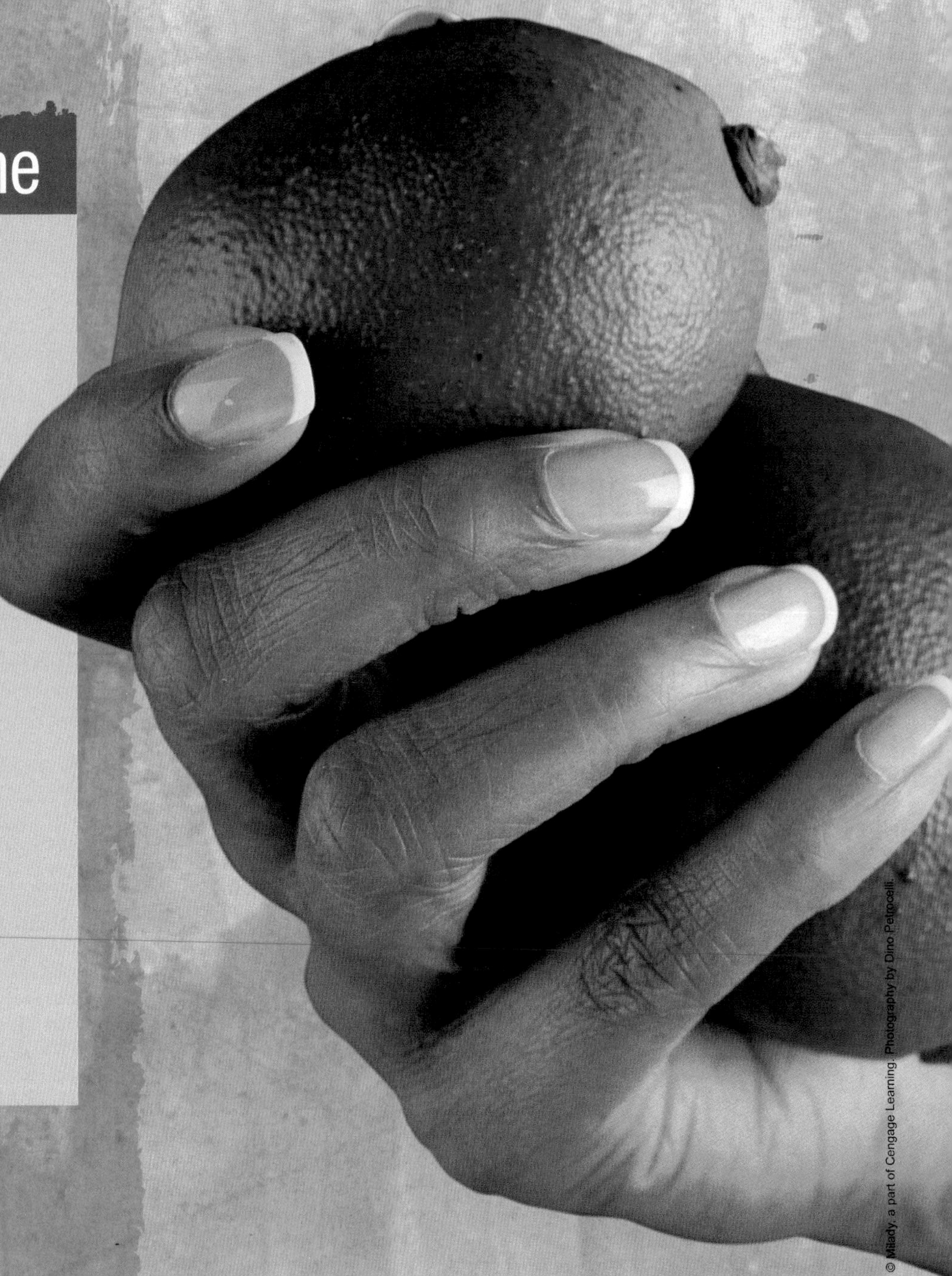

© Milady, a part of Cengage Learning. Photography by Dino Petrocelli.

Learning Objectives

After completing this chapter, you will be able to:

- ✓ **LO1** Identify the four types of nail implements and/or tools required to perform a manicure.
- ✓ **LO2** Explain the difference between reusable and disposable implements.
- ✓ **LO3** Describe the importance of hand washing in nail services.
- ✓ **LO4** Explain why a consultation is necessary each time a client has a service in the salon.
- ✓ **LO5** Name the five basic nail shapes for women.
- ✓ **LO6** Name the most popular nail shape for men.
- ✓ **LO7** List the types of massage movements most appropriate for a hand and arm massage.
- ✓ **LO8** Explain the difference between a basic manicure and a spa manicure.
- ✓ **LO9** Describe how aromatherapy is used in manicuring services.
- ✓ **LO10** Explain the use and benefits of paraffin wax in manicuring.
- ✓ **LO11** Name the correct cleaning and disinfection procedure for nail implements and tools.
- ✓ **LO12** Describe a proper setup for the manicuring table.
- ✓ **LO13** List the steps in the post-service procedure.
- ✓ **LO14** List the steps taken if there is an exposure incident in the salon.
- ✓ **LO15** List the steps in the basic manicure.
- ✓ **LO16** Describe the proper technique for the application of nail polish.
- ✓ **LO17** Describe the procedure for a paraffin wax hand treatment before a manicure.

Key Terms

Page number indicates where in the chapter the term is used.

dimethyl urea hardeners pg. 806

disposable implements (single-use implements) pg. 799

essential oils pg. 814

fine-grit abrasives pg. 802

implements pg. 798

lower-grit abrasives pg. 801

medium-grit abrasives pg. 802

metal pusher pg. 799

microtrauma pg. 799

nail clippers pg. 800

nail creams pg. 804

nail oils pg. 804

nipper pg. 799

oval nail pg. 809

paraffin pg. 798

pointed nail pg. 809

protein hardeners pg. 805

reusable implements (multiuse implements) pg. 798

round nail pg. 809

Scope of Practice pg. 794

service sets pg. 796

square nail pg. 809

squoval nail pg. 809

wooden pusher pg. 800

Once you have learned the fundamental techniques in this chapter, you will be officially on your way to providing clients with a professional manicure. Manicure and pedicure services are currently the fastest-growing services on salon and spa menus.

During your studies you will also learn about regulations when performing these services within your state. These regulations are very important to cosmetologists. They map out what is called your **Scope of Practice** (SOP), the list of services that you are legally allowed to perform in your specialty in your state; the SOP may or may not also state those services you cannot legally perform. Your instructor will provide important guidelines to ensure that you adhere closely to the SOP in your state. Know that if you perform services outside these regulations concerning allowable services, you may lose your license. Also, if damages to a client occur while performing an illegal service, you are fully liable.

WHY STUDY MANICURING?

Cosmetologists should study and have a thorough understanding of manicuring because:

- You will be able to offer your clients a service that they want and enjoy.
- As a professional you should be able to easily recognize manicuring tools and know how they are used.
- You will be able to perform a manicure safely and correctly.

Nail Technology Tools

As a professional cosmetologist, you must learn to work with the tools required for nail services and know all safety, cleaning, and disinfection procedures as defined in your state's regulations.

The four types of nail technology tools that you will incorporate into your services include:

- Equipment
- Implements
- Materials
- Professional cosmetic nail products

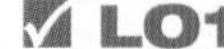
LO1

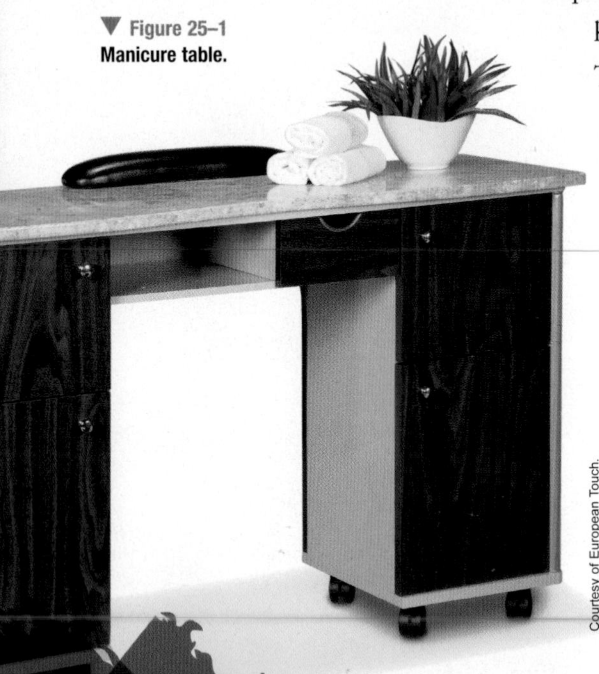
▼ Figure 25–1
Manicure table.

Courtesy of European Touch.

Equipment

Equipment includes all permanent tools that are not implements that are used to perform nail services.

Manicure Table

A standard manicuring table usually includes one or more drawers and shelves (with or without doors) for storing properly cleaned and disinfected implements and professional products

(Figure 25–1). The table can vary in length, but it is usually 36-inches to 48-inches long. The width is normally 16 inches to 21 inches. You must clean and disinfect the surface of the table between clients, so it must be kept clear of clutter and made of something hard and impenetrable, such as Formica or glass.

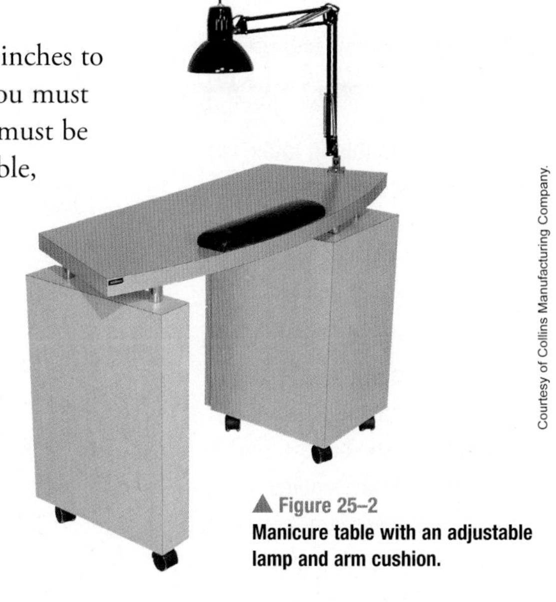

Courtesy of Collins Manufacturing Company.

▲ Figure 25–2
Manicure table with an adjustable lamp and arm cushion.

Adjustable Lamp

An adjustable lamp is attached to the table and should use a 40- to 60-watt incandescent bulb or a fluorescent bulb (Figure 25–2). Fluorescent bulbs are very popular because they emit a cooler light. Most people prefer true-color fluorescent bulb lamps because they show the skin and polishes in their actual color. Fluorescent lights also do not heat up objects underneath the lamp as do high-watt incandescent bulbs. Higher temperatures caused by an incandescent bulb can increase the curing speed of some nail enhancement products.

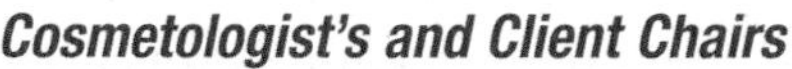

Cosmetologist's and Client Chairs

The cosmetologist's chair should be selected for ergonomics, comfort, durability, resistance to staining, and ease of cleaning. The most appropriate chair has wheels to allow the technician maneuverability and hydraulics to allow adjustment up and down (Figure 25–3).

The client's chair must be durable and comfortable. For the comfort of clients, select a chair that has no or low arms on the sides, so that it can be moved closer to the table. This will allow the client's arms to rest on the nail table and prevent the client and cosmetologist from needing to stretch forward. The chair should also have a supportive back so the client can sit comfortably and relax during the service.

> **CAUTION**
>
> Do not touch or allow your client too close to the light source. Light bulbs, especially incandescent ones, can become very hot while in use, and the possibility of a serious burn is very real.

Gloves

Gloves are Personal Protective Equipment (PPE), worn to protect the cosmetologist from exposure to microbes during services. The Occupational Safety and Health Act (OSHA) defines PPE as "specialized clothing or equipment worn by an employee for protection against a hazard." The hazards in this situation are bloodborne pathogens (BBPs), pathogenic microorganisms that are present in human blood and other body fluids that can cause disease in humans. These pathogens include, but are not limited to, hepatitis B virus (HBV) and human immunodeficiency syndrome (HIV).

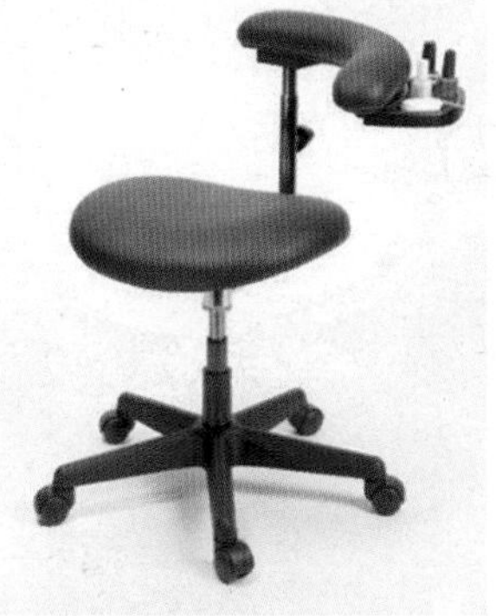

Courtesy of European Touch.

▲ Figure 25–3
Technician chair with wheels for maneuverability and hydraulics for height.

Currently, differences of opinion exist in the nail industry concerning whether gloves must be worn by service providers. Many people say gloves should be worn throughout every service because occasionally cosmetologists are exposed to blood. Other people believe gloves need to be worn only when there is exposure to blood, meaning a large amount of blood.

The rulings from OSHA's Universal Precautions standard, which was implemented in 1993 as an addition to the OSHA Act of 1970, provided

did you know?

Gloves are available in latex, vinyl, and nitrile materials. Know that some clients are allergic to latex, and that latex gloves often shred into pieces when used to apply soak lotions. Vinyl gloves do not protect the wearer from many microbes. For these reasons, many technicians believe nitrile gloves are the best choice for nail services. They come in boxes of 100 and are available at beauty and medical supply stores.

the answer as per federal standards. Universal Precautions include gloves, masks, and eyewear. The Universal Precautions standard within OSHA reads: "Universal Precautions shall be observed to prevent occupational exposure to blood or other potentially infectious materials. Occupational exposure includes any reasonably anticipated skin, eye, mucous membrane, or potential contact with blood or other potentially infectious materials that may result from the performance of an employee's duties."

OSHA does not mention "exposure to a large amount of blood."

PROCEDURE 25-4 **Handling an Exposure Incident During a Manicure** SEE PAGE 824

Remove gloves by inverting the cuffs and pulling the gloves off inside out. The glove taken off first is held in the hand with a glove still on it, and then the glove taken off last is pulled over the first glove. Then they are disposed of together. If a single client receives both a manicure and a pedicure, a new set of gloves must be worn for each service. In addition, when two services are being performed together, the technician must perform hand washing after removing each set of gloves and before putting on a new set. Many cosmetologists use antimicrobial gel cleanser when cleaning the hands between sets of gloves during the same appointment.

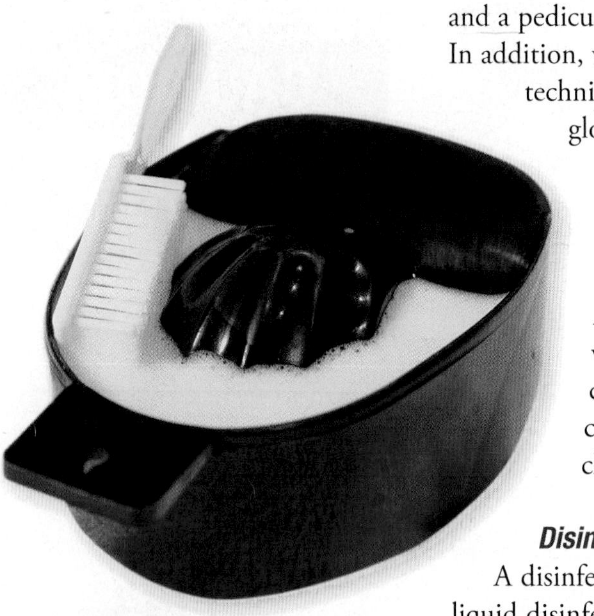

Finger Bowls

A finger bowl is used for soaking the client's fingers in warm water to soften the skin and cuticle. Finger bowls can be made of plastic, metal, glass, or even an attractive ceramic. They should be durable and easy to thoroughly clean and disinfect after use on each client (**Figure 25–4**).

© Milady, a part of Cengage Learning. Photography by Dino Petrocelli.

▲ Figure 25–4
Soak nail tips to soften.

Disinfection Container

A disinfection container must be large enough to hold sufficient liquid disinfectant solution to completely immerse several **service sets,** sets of all the tools that will be used in a service. Containers that do not allow the entire implement, including handles, to be submerged are not acceptable for use in professional salons.

Disinfection containers come in a number of shapes, sizes, and materials, and they must have a lid to keep the disinfectant solution from becoming contaminated when not in use. Most containers are equipped with a tray, and lifting the tray by its handle allows the technician to remove the implements from the solution without contaminating the solution or the implements. After the implements are removed from the disinfectant container, they must be rinsed and air- or towel-dried in accordance with the manufacturer's instructions and state regulations.

Disinfectants must never be allowed to come in contact with the skin. If your disinfectant container does not have a lift tray or basket, always remove the implements with tongs or tweezers and always wear gloves (**Figure 25–5**). It is important to wear gloves when removing and rinsing implements because gloves prevent your fingers from coming into contact with disinfectant solution, which can be irritating to the skin.

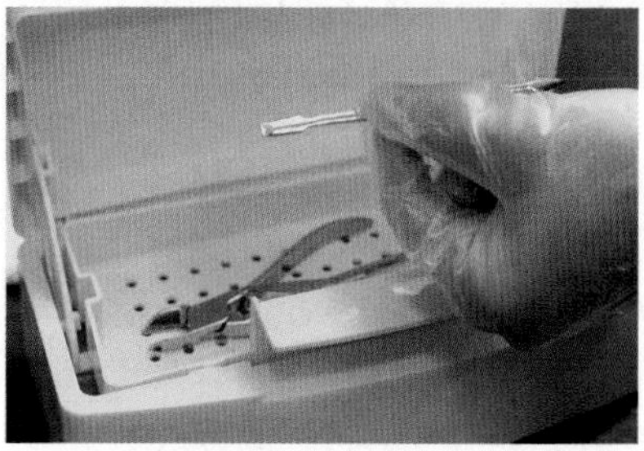

▲ **Figure 25–5**
Disinfection container with removable tray.

All containers must be kept closed when not in use to prevent contamination and/or evaporation.

Client's Arm Cushion

An 8- to 12-inch cushion that can be cleaned with soap and water and that is specifically made for cushioning the client's arm is an option when performing nail services. It must be covered with a fresh, clean towel for each client. A clean towel that is folded or rolled to cushion-size may also be used instead of a commercially purchased cushion.

Service Cushion (Optional)

A foam cushion, higher in the middle and lower on the ends, can be placed between the client and the cosmetologist during a manicure; it is believed to provide more comfort during the service for both parties (**Figure 25–6**). It must be fully covered by a fresh, clean towel throughout each service.

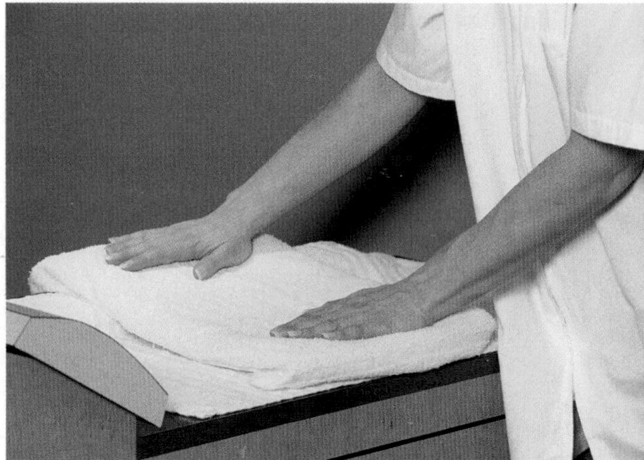

▲ **Figure 25–6**
Service cushion on nail table.

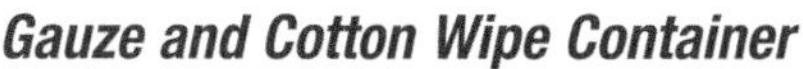

Gauze and Cotton Wipe Container

This container holds absorbent cotton, lint-free wipes, or gauze squares for use during the services. This container must have a lid to protect the contents from dust and contaminants.

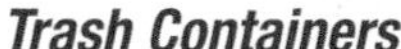

Trash Containers

A metal trash container with a self-closing lid that is operated by a foot pedal should be located next to your workstation (**Figure 25–7**). The trash container should be lined with a disposable trash bag and closed when not in use. It must be emptied at the end of each work day before you leave, and it must be washed and disinfected often. A trash container with a self-closing lid is one of the best ways to prevent excessive odors and vapors in the salon.

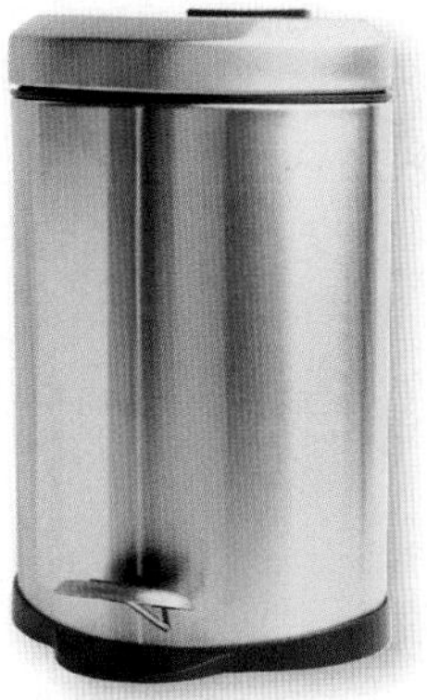

▲ **Figure 25–7**
Metal trash can with self-closing lid.

Supply Tray (Optional)

This sturdy tray holds cosmetics such as polishes, polish removers, and creams. It should be sturdy and easy to clean. Many technicians put every product they need for a service on these trays and then lift the specific service tray on and off a shelf in their station in one efficient movement. This allows the tabletop to be clear and easy to disinfect after each service. This tray should also be cleaned and disinfected between clients.

© Milady, a part of Cengage Learning. Photography by Dino Petrocelli.

did you know?

Implements must be properly prepared or prepped with a thorough cleansing before being placed in the disinfectant solution. Implements must be scrubbed with warm water, liquid soap and a scrub brush, then rinsed and patted dry before placing in the disinfectant liquid (Figure 25–8). Dirty or improperly prepared implements will not be disinfected in the solution.

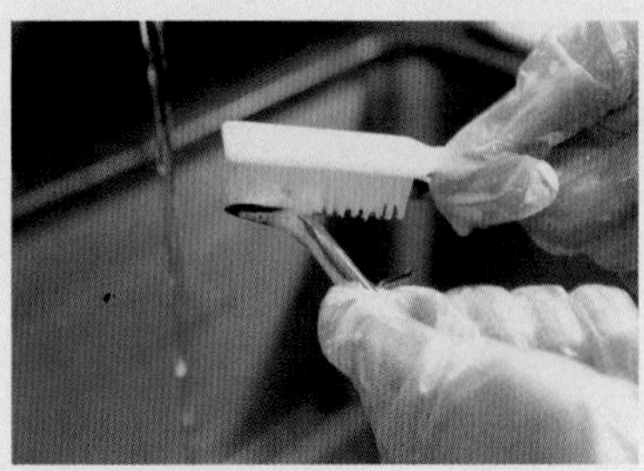

© Milady, a part of Cengage Learning. Photography by Dino Petrocelli.

▲ Figure 25–8
Scrub implements to prepare for disinfection.

Ultraviolet or Electric Nail Polish Dryer (Optional)

A nail polish dryer is designed to shorten the time necessary for the client's nail polish to dry. Electric dryers have heaters and fans that blow warm air onto the nail plates to speed evaporation of solvents from nail polishes, allowing them to harden more quickly. Nail polish dryers that use a light bulb also create warmth to speed drying and work in the same fashion as electric dryers but without fans. Ultraviolet polish dryers are designed to cure polishes that contain an ingredient sensitive to the UVA wavelength of the bulb in the dryer; exposure to this wavelength triggers curing (drying) of the polish.

Electric Hand/Foot Mitts (Optional)

These heated mitts, which are available for both hands and feet, are designed to add a special service to a manicure or pedicure. A manicure that includes heated mitts usually costs more, or their use can be an add-on to a lower-cost service. After the massage during a pedicure, conditioning lotion or even a mask is applied to the feet, which are then placed in a plastic cover and inserted into the foot mitts. The warmth aids in penetration of the conditioning ingredients, adds to the comfort of the service, and provides ultimate relaxation for the client.

Terry Cloth Mitts (Optional)

These washable mitts are placed over a client's hands or feet after a penetrating conditioning product and a cover have been applied. These mitts are routinely used over paraffin to hold in the heat.

Paraffin Bath (Optional)

A paraffin tub has an automatic thermostat that will maintain the paraffin at the ideal temperature for application to the hands and feet. **Paraffin**, a petroleum by-product that has excellent sealing properties (barrier qualities) to hold moisture in the skin, can be added to manicures and pedicures for an extra charge (**Figure 25–9**). Although paraffin from the bath can be applied in many ways, the traditional method is to dip the hands and feet into the paraffin in the bath. The paraffin coating covers the skin, holding the skin's natural moisture in the epidermal layers and thus promoting moisturization of the skin and deeper penetration of other products that have been used on the skin prior to the paraffin. After basic equipment, this bath is often the first purchase for many salons and spas. Check the regulations in your state concerning the use of paraffin in salons.

▼ Figure 25–9
Paraffin bath.

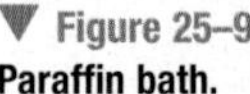

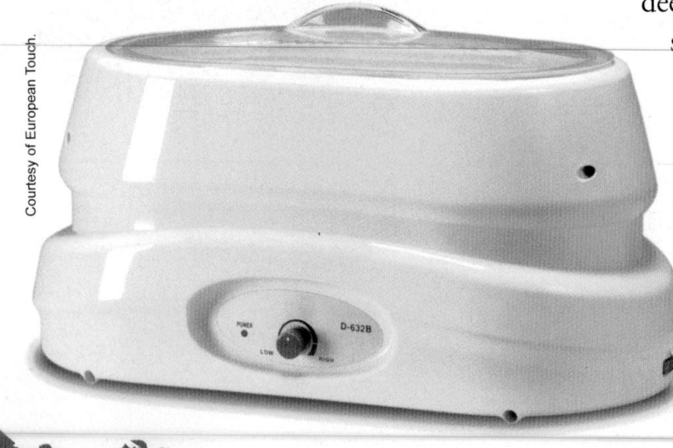

Courtesy of European Touch.

Implements

Implements are tools used to perform your services and are either reusable or disposable. **Reusable implements**, also known as **multiuse implements**, are generally stainless steel because they must be properly cleaned and disinfected after use on one client and prior to use on another. Less expensive nickel-plated metal implements will corrode during disinfection. **Disposable implements**, also known as **single-use implements**, cannot be reused because they cannot be cleaned and disinfected; therefore, they must be thrown away after a single use. It is recommended that cosmetologists have several clean and disinfected service sets of implements available for use at all times. ✓ LO2

did you know?

Many cosmetologists separate their clean, disinfected reusable implements into service sets. These sets can be wrapped in a clean towel and stored in a clean place, or they can be inserted into a sterile pouch before being autoclaved. Open the implements in front of your clients at the start of each service so clients can see that the set has been disinfected prior to their arrival.

Reusable Implements

Metal Pusher

The **metal pusher** (often incorrectly called a cuticle pusher) is designed to gently scrape cuticle tissue from the natural nail plate. It is not to be used to push back the eponychium. Metal pushers must be stainless steel and used carefully to prevent damaging the natural nail and the nail matrix. Improper use on the nail can cause grooving and possible nail growth problems if the nail matrix is accidentally damaged. Improper or careless use of the metal pusher can cause microscopic trauma or injury to the tissues. These injuries are known as **microtrauma**—tiny, often unseen openings in the skin, which can allow microbes to enter the skin, leading to infection.

If you have rough or sharp edges on your metal pusher, use an abrasive to smooth or remove them. This prevents digging into the nail plate or damaging the protective barriers created by the eponychium and cuticle.

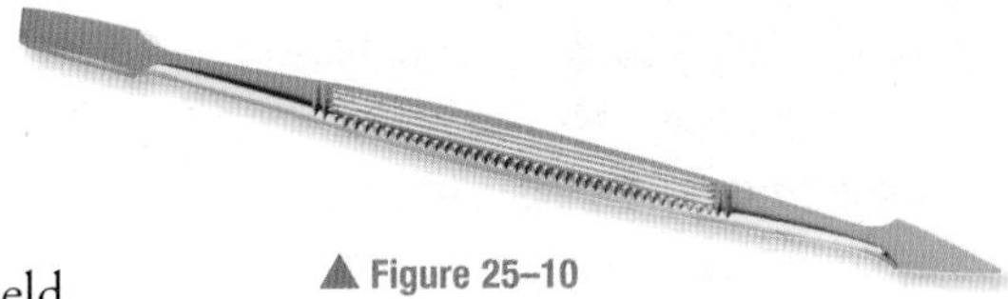

Hold the metal pusher the way you hold a pencil with the flat end held at a 20- to 30-degree angle from the nail plate. The spoon end is used to carefully loosen and push back the dead cuticle tissue on the nail plate (**Figure 25–10**).

▲ Figure 25–10
Metal pusher.

Nippers

A **nipper** is a stainless-steel implement used to carefully trim away dead skin around the nails. It is never used to cut, rip, or tear live tissue because the live nail fold tissue is important to ward off microbes and prevent infection around the nail plate. Nippers must be cleaned and disinfected before use on every client, taking special care to open the hinges for thorough cleaning and disinfecting. Always maintain a sharp edge on your nippers to prevent accidental ripping and tearing into the live tissue.

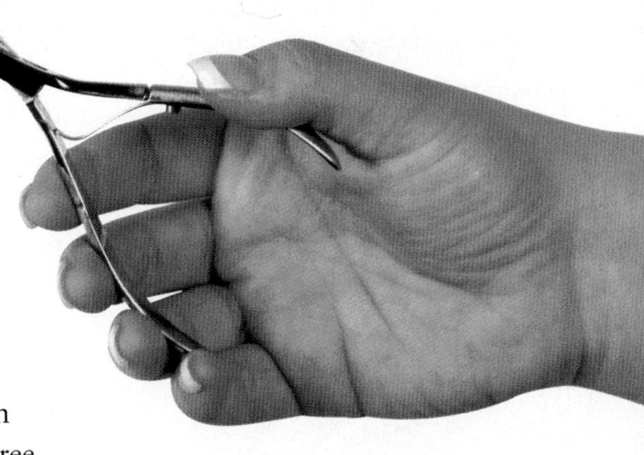

It is important that you learn the correct use of nail nippers while in school. To use nippers, hold your thumb around one handle and three fingers around the other, with the blades facing the nail plate. Your index finger is placed on the box joint to help control the blade and guide it properly (**Figure 25–11**).

▲ Figure 25–11
Nippers.

© Milady, a part of Cengage Learning. Photography by Dino Petrocelli.

Tweezers

Tweezers are multi-task implements for lifting small bits of debris from the nail plate, retrieving and placing nail art, removing implements from disinfectant solutions, and much more (**Figure 25–12**). They must be properly cleaned and disinfected before use on every client because they may come in contact with a client's skin or nails. They must be stainless steel to allow disinfection after use.

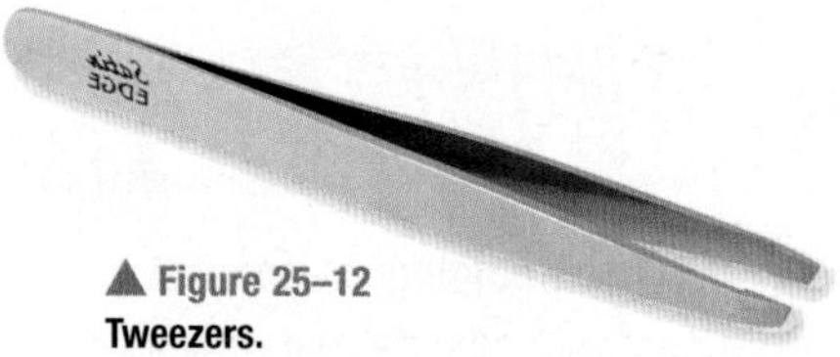

▲ Figure 25–12
Tweezers.

Nail Clippers

Nail clippers shorten the free edge quickly and efficiently. If your client's nails are too long, clipping them will save filing time. Clip the nails from each side to prevent stress damage to the sides of the nail plates and then file to shape the nails. Nail clippers must be properly cleaned and then disinfected before each use on every client. These implements must be stainless steel to be disinfected.

did you know?

A cosmetologist practicing nail procedures full- or part-time will need at least three sets of quality, stainless-steel implements in order to always have a completely clean and disinfected set ready for use on each client. One set is in the disinfectant, one is being used, and another is ready for use. By always having a set of implements ready, you will ensure that clients will not have to wait for the disinfection process. When the current client is finished, the implements in the disinfectant are removed, rinsed and dried, or placed to air-dry. The implements just used are prepared for disinfection, and the set that is prepped and ready is used on the next client. Remember, it takes approximately twenty minutes to properly clean and then disinfect implements after each use.

Disposable Implements

Brushes and Applicators

Any brush or applicator that comes into contact with a client's nails or skin during a manicure or pedicure must be properly cleaned and disinfected before use on another client. If implements cannot be properly cleaned and disinfected according to your state's regulations, they must be disposed of after a single use. Check with the manufacturer if you are unsure whether a brush or applicator can be properly cleaned and disinfected.

Wooden Pusher

The **wooden pusher** is used to remove cuticle tissue from the nail plate, to clean under the free edge of the nail, or to apply products. Hold the stick as you would a pencil with the tip at a 20- to 30-degree angle from the nail plate while pushing the cuticle free (**Figure 25–13**). It is a single-use implement and not intended for reuse or disinfection. Apply nail products by completely wrapping the end of the stick with a small piece of cotton and placing or dipping the cotton tip into the product. If the cotton tip is dipped into product, enough must be retrieved for the entire application. If more product is needed, the cotton on your wooden pusher must be changed to prevent contamination of the product. Using products that have spout lids can shorten time in the application. The spout must not touch the cotton tip, nail plate, or the skin.

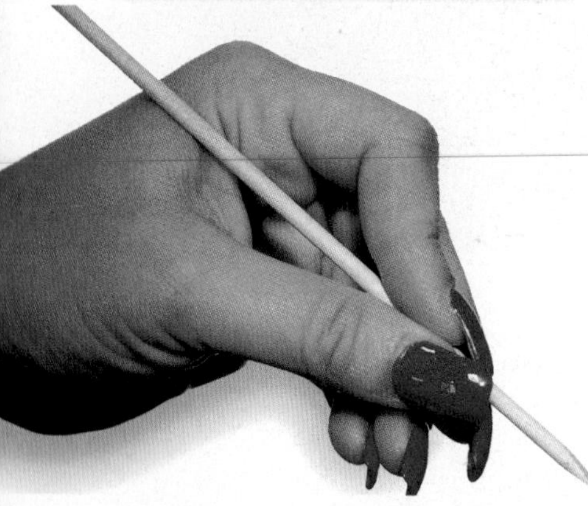

▲ Figure 25–13
Wooden pusher.

Nail Brush

This plastic implement is used in many ways during nail services (**Figure 25–14**). Clients use a nail brush when they arrive at the salon and perform the hand washing procedure. Technicians use a nail brush for hand washing between clients. Nail brushes are also used during the manicure to remove debris from the nail plate. Finally—and very importantly—nail brushes are used to scrub the implements clean before disinfection.

© Milady, a part of Cengage Learning. Photography by Dino Petrocelli.

Application Brush

Application brushes can be used to apply nail oils, nail polish, or nail treatments to client's nails. It is recommended that you purchase inexpensive, readily available packages of disposable application brushes to apply products that can support bacterial growth.

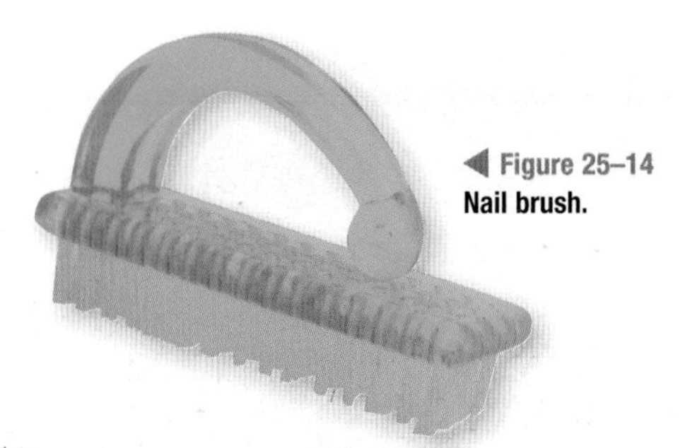

Figure 25–14
Nail brush.

Dip enough product from the container for your entire application using the application brush, or pour enough product for the full application into a clean dappen dish and dip the application brush into this dish throughout the application. Again, these brushes must be disposed of after use on one client.

An exception to this single-use rule is made for brushes used in products that are not capable of harboring or supporting the growth of pathogenic microbes, such as alcohol, nail polish, monomers and polymers, UV gels, nail primers, dehydrators, bleaches, and so forth. Since these products cannot harbor or support pathogen growth, the brushes do not need to be cleaned and disinfected between each use unless the brush touches a contaminated nail immediately before moving to another nail. Since cosmetologists can only work on healthy nails, contaminated nails should not be an issue. However, a brush is considered contaminated if it is used to apply penetrating nail oil to the nail plate and then placed back into the product, because the products themselves can become contaminated with bacteria and support the growth of pathogens. For this reason, disposable application brushes or droppers should be used to apply oils to the nail plate or surrounding skin.

did you know?

It is the salon's choice as to whether nail brushes are reused or disposed of after a single use. To prevent cross-contamination, nail brushes must be clean and fresh for each client. They must be disinfected between services, thrown away after use, or sent home with the client. Many salons find a resource for inexpensive nail brushes so the brushes can be disposed of or sent home with the client. This eliminates the time and effort needed for disinfection, and it eliminates the need for a larger disinfection container and the counter space it would occupy. It also saves the increased cost of disinfection solution for the brush-disinfection process.

Materials

Materials and supplies used during a manicure are designed to be single-use and must be replaced for each client. These items are not considered reusable.

Figure 25–15
Typical abrasive nail file.

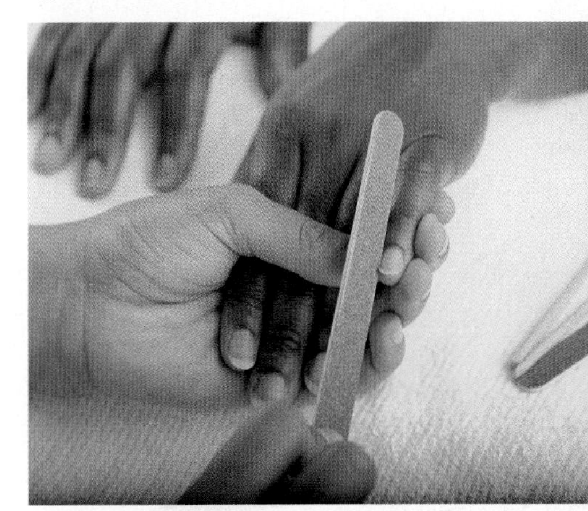

Abrasive Nail Files and Buffers

Abrasive nail files (**Figure 25–15**) and buffers (**Figure 25–16**) are generally single-use only, and they are available in many different types and grits. For example, they come with firm, rigid supporting cores or with padded and very flexible cores. Grits range from less than 180 to over 240 per centimeter. A rule of thumb is the lower the grit, the larger the abrasive particles on the file and the more aggressive its action. Therefore, **lower-grit abrasives** (less than 180 grit) are aggressive and will quickly reduce the thickness of any surface. Lower-grit files also produce deeper and more visible scratches on the surface than do higher-grit. Therefore, lower-grit files must be used with greater care and generally are not used on natural nails since they can cause damage.

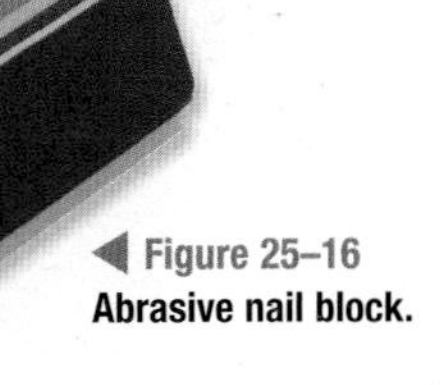

Figure 25–16
Abrasive nail block.

© Milady, a part of Cengage Learning. Photography by Dino Petrocelli.

CAUTION

Abrasives or other implements cannot be stored in a plastic bag or other sealed containers because airtight conditions create the perfect environment for pathogens to grow and multiply before the next use. Always clean, disinfect, and store implements in a clean, unsealed container that allows air to circulate, or roll implements in a towel as a service set (Figure 25–17).

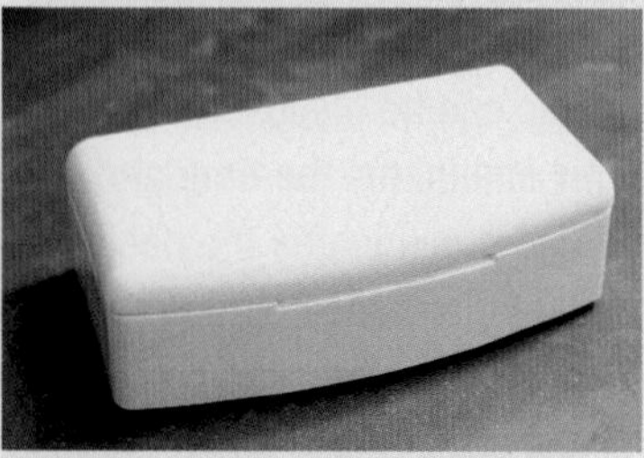

© Milady, a part of Cengage Learning. Photography by Dino Petrocelli.

▲ Figure 25–17
Store disinfected implements in a covered container.

You must prep or edge your abrasive files before using them on a client to prevent harm to the client from the sharp edges of the files. These files are stamped from a large sheet of prepared materials, leaving very sharp edges, and these sharp edges are not removed before the files are shipped. You are responsible for removing this damaging edge from every new file.

To prepare a file for use, rub another (clean, unused) file across the edge to remove that sharp edge; this action is referred to as *file prepping*. Many cosmetologists prepare all their new files and then store them in a clean container. If this edge is not removed on new boards, you may put that client at risk for cuts. Check the corners of buffers also because they may also require prepping.

Medium-grit abrasives (180 to 240 grit) are used to smooth and refine surfaces, and the 180 grit is used to shorten and shape natural nails. **Fine-grit abrasives** are in the category of 240 and higher grits. They are designed for buffing, polishing, and removing very fine scratches.

Abrasive boards and buffers typically have one, two, or three different grit surfaces depending on type, use, and style. Some abrasive boards and buffers can be cleaned and disinfected. Check with the manufacturer to see if the abrasive of your choice can be disinfected. All abrasives must be cleaned and disinfected before reuse on another client. Check with your instructor as to whether your state allows abrasive boards and buffers to be disinfected within the SOP. Abrasives that cannot survive the cleaning and disinfection process without being damaged are considered disposable and must be discarded after a single use.

Two-Way or Three-Way Buffer

The two- or three-way buffer abrasive technology replaces the chamois and creates a beautiful shine on nails (Figure 25–18). The buffer is shaped like a two-sided nail file, long and narrow, with one or two additional grit abrasives and a final shine surface. Begin with the lowest grit abrasive surface in the smoothing task, move to the larger grit, and then finish with the shining surface (usually no grit). The result is a glossy shine on the nails. This buffer is generally used on natural nails and in the final steps of the two-color application of monomer liquid and polymer powder nails, such as the French manicure look, for nails that will be worn with sheer or clear polish only. Most two- or three-way buffers are single-use only and must be thrown away after each use. The salon or technician must find an inexpensive source for purchasing them or a reusable one if regulations in the state allow the use of these buffers.

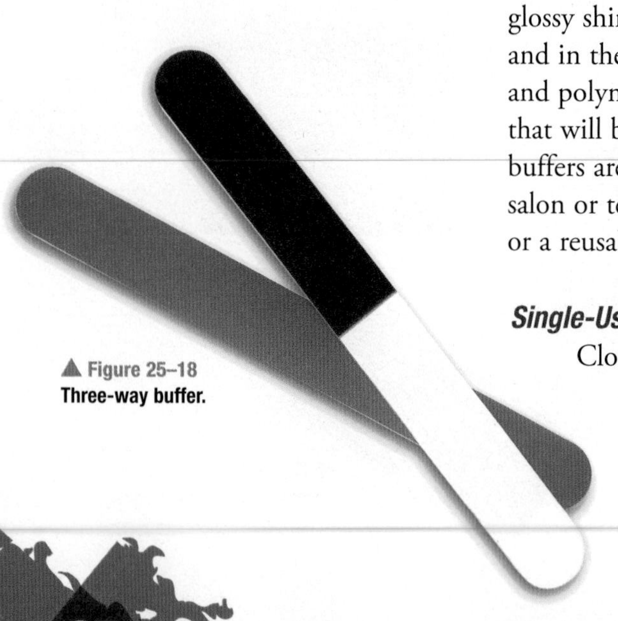

▲ Figure 25–18
Three-way buffer.

Courtesy of purespadirect.com.

Single-Use or Terry Cloth Towels

Cloth towels must be laundered between clients, and paper towels must be thrown away after each use. A fresh, clean terry cloth towel or a new disposable paper towel is used by the client after washing his or her hands. The best terry cloth towels for use in a personal service are white so they can be bleached during their washing between uses. Other clean towels are used to cover any surfaces that can become contaminated during each manicure, including the work area. If spills occur on the table, different terry cloth or disposable towels must be used to wipe them from the surface.

Gauze, Cotton Balls, or Plastic-Backed Pads

Lint-free, plastic-backed, fiber or cotton pads are often used to remove nail polish. Plastic backing protects nail professionals' fingertips from overexposure to drying solvents and other chemicals (**Figure 25–19**).

Gauze squares or cotton balls are also popular for removal of nail polish because they are inexpensive and perfectly designed for this and other application tasks. Gauze squares (2" x 2" or 4" x 4") have many uses in manicure services, from product removal to application. All these materials must be stored in a manner to prevent dust and debris from contaminating them.

STATE REGULATORY ALERT

Reusing implements without properly cleaning and disinfecting them is against the law in every state. The inappropriate and illegal use of implements puts clients, cosmetologists, and the salon at risk of infection and can also put the technician and salon at risk for legal liability, as well as license suspension.

Plastic or Metal Spatulas

A disposable plastic or reusable metal spatula must be used for removing products from their respective containers to prevent contamination of the products and the spread of disease. If a spatula comes into contact with your or the client's skin, it must be properly cleaned and disinfected before being used again, or it must be replaced. Also, never use the same spatula to remove dissimilar products from different containers because the chemistry of the products may be altered.

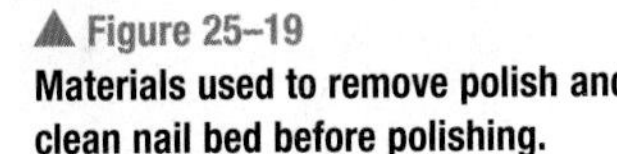

▲ Figure 25–19
Materials used to remove polish and clean nail bed before polishing.

© Milady, a part of Cengage Learning. Photography by Dino Petrocelli.

Professional Cosmetic Products

As a professional, you need to know how to properly use each nail product, what ingredients it contains, and what it does during use. You must also know how to properly store products and remove them from their containers in a hygienic manner. This section provides basic information regarding several professional cosmetic nail products. For more detailed information on products and ingredients see *Nail Structure & Product Chemistry*, Second Edition, by Douglas D. Schoon, published by Milady, a part of Cengage Learning and *Milady's Skin Care and Cosmetic Ingredients Dictionary*, 3rd Edition, by Natalia Michalun and M. Varinia Michalun, also published by Milady, a part of Cengage Learning.

did you know?

The Centers for Disease Control (CDC) states that it does not matter whether the soap/cleanser used in a salon is antibacterial or not; it still removes microbes and debris. However, many clients feel more secure if an antibacterial soap is used at the wash station.

Soap

Soap is used to clean the cosmetologist's and client's hands before a service begins. It acts as an infection control tool during the pre-service hand washing procedure by mechanically removing microbes and debris. Soap is known to remove over 90 percent of pathogenic microbes from the hands, when hand washing is performed properly.

Liquid soaps (**Figure 25–20**) are recommended and preferred because bar soaps harbor bacteria and can become a breeding ground for pathogenic (disease-producing) bacteria.

Polish Remover

Removers are used to dissolve and remove nail polish. There are two types of polish removers available: acetone and non-acetone. Acetone remover works more quickly and is a better solvent than non-acetone removers.

Non-acetone removers will not dissolve enhancement products as quickly as acetone, so they are preferred when removing nail polish from nail enhancements such as wraps. Both acetone and non-acetone polish removers can be used safely. As with all products, read and follow the manufacturer's instructions for use.

Nail Creams, Lotions, and Oils

These products are designed to soften dry skin around the nail plate and to increase the flexibility of natural nails. They are especially effective on nails that appear to be brittle or dry, and they are the number one nail product that should be sold to manicure and pedicure clients. **Nail creams** are barrier products because they contain ingredients designed to seal the surface of the skin and hold in the subdermal moisture in the skin. **Nail oils** are designed to absorb into the nail plate to increase flexibility and into the surrounding skin to soften and moisturize. Typically, oils and lotions can penetrate the nail plate or skin and will have longer-lasting effects than creams, but all three products can be highly effective and useful for clients, especially as daily-use home-care products.

▼ Figure 25–20
Use pump bottles of soap at hand washing stations. Do not use bar soaps because bar soaps harbor bacteria.

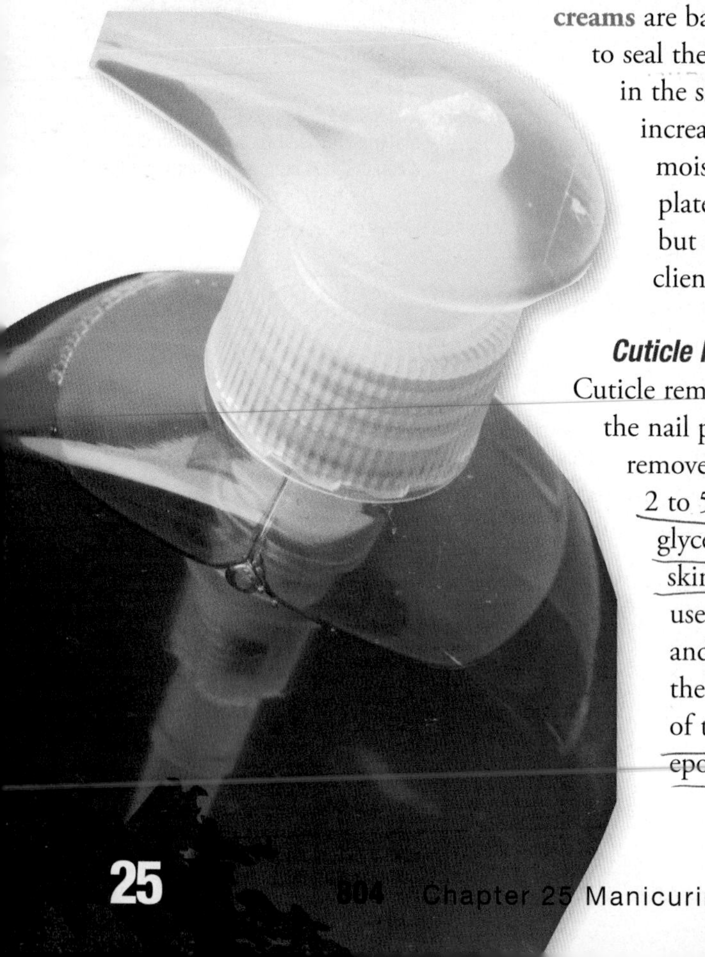

Cuticle Removers

Cuticle removers are designed to loosen and dissolve dead tissue on the nail plate so that this tissue can be more easily and thoroughly removed from the nail plate. These products typically contain 2 to 5 percent sodium or potassium hydroxide, with added glycerin or other moisturizing ingredients to counteract the skin-drying effects of the remover. These products must be used in strict accordance with the manufacturer's directions, and skin contact must be avoided where possible to counter the effects of the alkaline ingredients. Excessive exposure of the eponychium to cuticle removers can cause skin and eponychium dryness, leading to hangnails.

© Milady, a part of Cengage Learning. Photography by Dino Petrocelli.

Nail Bleach

These products are designed to apply to the nail plate and under the free edge of natural nails to remove yellow surface discoloration or stains (e.g., tobacco stains). Usually, nail bleaches contain hydrogen peroxide or some other keratin-bleaching agent. Always use these products exactly as directed by the manufacturer to avoid damaging the natural nail plate or surrounding skin. Because nail bleaches can be corrosive to soft tissue, take care to limit skin contact.

Colored Polish, Enamel, Lacquer, or Varnish

Colored coatings applied to the natural nail plate are known as *polish, enamel, lacquer,* or *varnish.* These are all marketing terms used to describe the same types of products containing similar ingredients. There are no real differences in the products.

Polish is a generic term describing any type of solvent-based colored film applied to the nail plate for the purpose of adding color or special visual effects (e.g., sparkles). Polish is usually applied in two coats over a base coat and then followed by a top coat (**Figure 25–21**).

did you know?

Never shake your polish bottles. Shaking will cause air bubbles to form and make the polish application rough and appear irregular. Instead, gently roll the polish bottles between your palms to thoroughly mix.

Base Coat

The base coat creates a colorless layer on the natural nail and nail enhancement that improves adhesion of polish. It also prevents polish from imparting a yellowish staining or other discoloration to the natural nail plate. Some nail plates are especially susceptible to stains from red or dark colors, so the base coat step is important. Base coats are also important to use on nail enhancements under colored polish to prevent surface staining. Base coats usually rely on adhesives, which aid in retaining polish for a longer time. Like nail polishes, base coats contain solvents designed to evaporate. After evaporation, a sticky, adhesion-promoting film is left behind on the surface of the nail plate to increase adhesion of the colored coating.

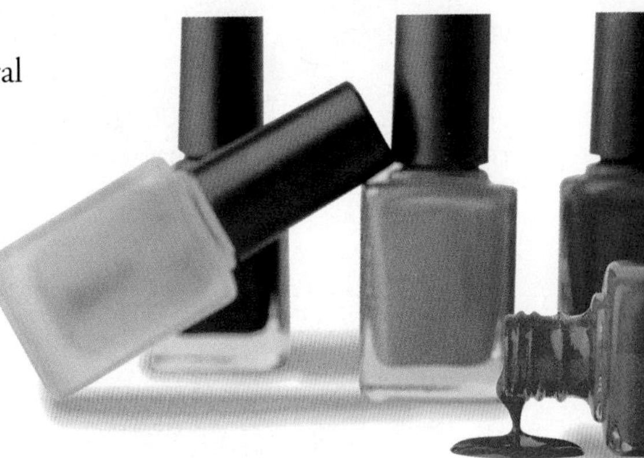

▲ **Figure 25–21**
Polish, top coat, and base coat for manicure.

© Milady, a part of Cengage Learning. Photography by Dino Petrocelli.

Nail Hardener

Nail hardeners are used to improve the surface hardness or durability of weak or thin nail plates. If used properly, some nail hardeners can also prevent splitting or peeling of the nail plate. Hardeners can be applied before the base coat or after as a top coat, according to the manufacturer's directions.

There are several basic types of nail hardeners:

Protein hardeners are a combination of clear polish and protein, such as collagen. These provide a clear, hard coating on the surface of the nail but do not change or affect the natural nail plate itself. Protein (collagen) has very large molecules that cannot be absorbed into the nail plate.

Other types of nail hardeners contain reinforcing fibers such as nylon that also cannot be absorbed into the nail plate. Therefore, the protection they provide comes from the coating itself. They are not therapeutic. These products can be used on any natural nail.

did you know?

Products sold to clients for their use at home are called retail products and are packaged for that purpose. In the beauty industry they are considered home-care products, not retail products, because they are sold under professional recommendation and the client is given instruction on how to use them before taking them home. Home-care products, by law, must have usage directions and cautions listed on the bottles or boxes or have written instructions in the box. Professional products (usually bulk sizes) do not have this labeling requirement.

The ingredient in hardeners that was believed, in the past, to be formaldehyde is actually methylene glycol, an ingredient that creates bridges or cross-links between the keratin strands that make up the natural nail, making the plate stiffer and more resistant to bending and breaking. Methylene glycol is also nonirritating to the skin.

These products are useful for thin and weak nail plates, but should never be applied to nails that are already very hard, rigid, and/or brittle. Methylene glycol hardeners can make brittle nails become so rigid that they may split and shatter. If signs of excessive brittleness or splitting, discoloration of the nail bed, or other signs of adverse nail and skin reactions occur, discontinue use. These products should be used as instructed by the manufacturer until the client's nails reach the desired goal, and then use should be discontinued until the product is needed again. Clients are generally instructed to apply the product daily over nail polish as a top coat, or under nail polish as a base coat when the polish is removed and reapplied. Clients must be instructed to follow manufacturer instructions.

Dimethyl urea hardeners (DY-meth-il yoo-REE-uh **hard**-dn-ers) use dimethyl urea (DMU) to add cross-links to the natural nail plate; DMU does not cause adverse skin reactions. These hardeners do not work as quickly as hardeners containing methylene glycol, but they will not over harden nails as those with methylene glycol can with overuse.

© Milady, a part of Cengage Learning.

Top Coat

Top coats are applied over colored polish to prevent chipping and to add a shine to the finished nail. These products contain ingredients that create hard, shiny films after the solvent has evaporated. Typically the main ingredients are methacrylic or cellulose-type film formers.

Nail polish drying accelerators are designed to be used over a top coat to hasten the drying of nail polishes. They are typically applied with a dropper, a brush or are sprayed onto the surface of the polish. They promote rapid drying by pulling solvents from the nail polish, causing the colored film to form more quickly. These products can dramatically shorten drying time and will reduce the risk of the client smudging the recent polish application.

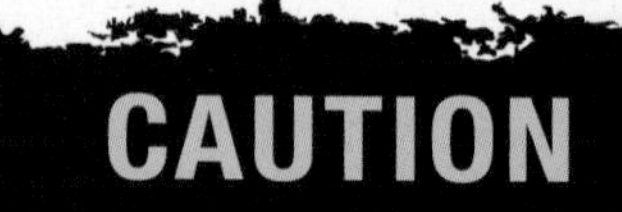

CAUTION

All base coats, top coats, nail polishes, and hardeners are highly flammable.

Hand Creams and Lotions

Hand creams and lotions add a finishing touch to a manicure. Since they soften and smooth the hands, they make the skin and finished manicure look as beautiful as possible. Hand creams are generally designed to be barriers on the skin which help the skin retain moisture, or they contain penetrating ingredients to soften the skin or repair damage. A hand cream's purpose is to make the skin on the hands less prone to becoming dry or cracked. Lotion is generally more penetrating than creams and may treat lower levels of the epidermis. A treatment lotion can be used with warming mitts or paraffin dips to enhance penetration of the ingredients into the skin.

Nail Conditioners

Nail conditioners contain ingredients to reduce brittleness of the nail. They should be applied as directed by the manufacturer. This treatment is especially useful when applied at night before bedtime. Nail conditioners can be oils, lotions, or creams.

Sunscreens

These lotions contain ingredients that protect the skin from damage by the Ultra Violet light (UVA) from the sun. UVA is known to cause age spots (hyperpigmentation) on the backs of the hands and damage to the DNA of skin cells. Overexposure to the sun is known as a major cause of aging and skin cancer. Encourage your clients to purchase and use sunscreen on all their exposed skin.

CAUTION

Material Safety Data Sheets (MSDSs) contain information, compiled by the manufacturer, about product safety, including the names of hazardous ingredients, safe handling and use procedures, precautions to reduce the risk of accidental harm or overexposure, and flammability warnings. Salons must have MSDSs on file for every professional product, easily accessible for reference by employees; MSDSs are not required for retail products. The manufacturer or distributor from which you order a professional product is required by law to provide you with the appropriate MSDS.

The Basic Manicure

The basic manicure is the foundation of all nail technology services, and it is vital that you know and recognize all of the components necessary for making the basic manicure service successful. The information you learn for the basic manicure will serve as your foundation for all of the other nail services you will perform in your career.

Work to get your basic manicure procedure to forty-five minutes at the most, including polishing, before you leave school. This will make you more hirable and more successful in your career. Practice until you can perform the skills automatically, without considering what is next in the protocol, and you will portray the confidence and professional aura that clients prefer in their cosmetologist (and that salon owners prefer in their employees).

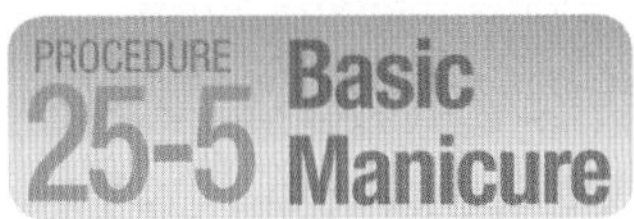

SEE PAGE 826

Hand Washing

To prevent the spread of communicable disease, it is imperative to wash your hands before and after each client—and to have your clients wash their hands before they sit down at your cleaned and disinfected manicure table. The practice of hand washing before any procedure should be so well taught to your regular clients that they go directly to the washing station before coming to your station.

Nail brushes, which are an integral part of the hand washing procedure, should be in a well-known storage place so clients can retrieve one easily and quickly. Mark the clean nail brush container

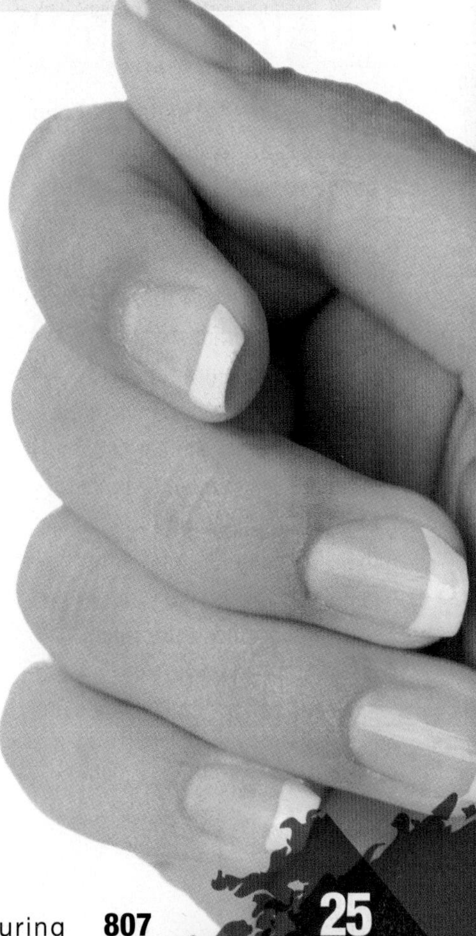

© Tania Zbrodko, 2010; used under license from Shutterstock.com.

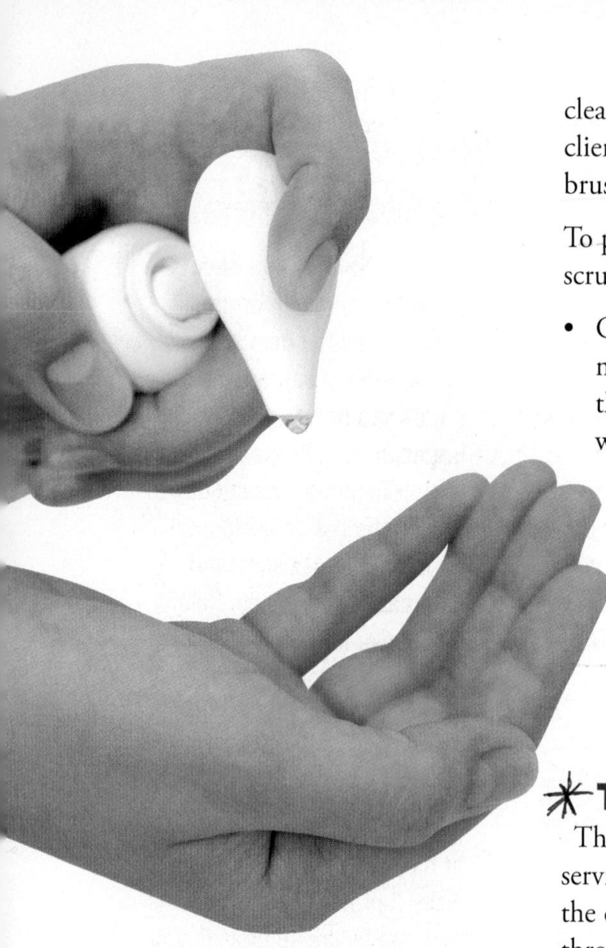

clearly, so the client will know where to retrieve the fresh brush. The client can bring the brush to the table or leave it in a marked dirty-brush container.

To prevent cross-contamination, each client must have a clean brush for scrubbing her hands. There are two choices for providing clean brushes:

- Clean and disinfect your brushes after each client. Many salons clean nail brushes at the end of the day, disinfect them, rinse and dry them, and then place them in a container labeled "Clean Brushes" with convenient access by your clients.
- Purchase them in bulk and give them to clients or throw them away after each service. Clients bring them to the chair for use during their manicure after they wash.

© Stocknadia, 2010; used under license from Shutterstock.com.

PROCEDURE 25-3 **Proper Hand Washing** SEE PAGE 823 ☑ LO3

The Manicure Consultation

The consultation with the client before the manicure, or any other service, is an opportunity for getting to know one another and for the cosmetologist to understand a client's expectations. Do not rush through the consultation—it is an important part of the service!

If the client is new to the salon, he or she should already have filled out the information on the intake form in the waiting room. Use this information to perform the client consultation. Look at the forms closely for important responses from the client, and then record your observations after the service.

Always check the client's nails and skin to make sure that they are healthy and that the service you are providing is appropriate. Next, discuss the shape, color, and length of nails that your client prefers. You must be careful not to diagnose a disease or disorder in any way. All information should then be recorded on the client service form. If there are no health issues observed, continue with the service.

Keep the following considerations in mind: shape of the hands, length of fingers, and shape of the eponychium area. Generally, it is recommended that the shape of the nail's free edge should enhance the overall shape of the fingertips, fingers, and hands of the client. You also need to think about your client's lifestyle; such things as hobbies, recreational activities, and type of work can determine the best nail shape and length. ☑ LO4

did you know?

Although the CDC states that hand sanitizers are appropriate for use, they also note that hand sanitizers are only for use when water is not available for hand washing. It is very important to remember that these products cannot, and do not, replace proper hand washing. Proper hand washing is a vital part of the service, and it cannot be skipped or ignored. Clients must also properly wash their hands before and after the service, and you must properly wash your hands after each customer. Resort to using a hand sanitizer only when it is absolutely necessary!

Basic Nail Shapes for Women

During the consultation, you should discuss the final shape your client wants for her nails, and of course you should do your best to please her. Table 25–1 details the five basic shapes that women most often prefer. ☑ LO5

BASIC NAIL SHAPES	
SHAPE	**DEFINITION**
SQUARE	The **square nail** is completely straight across the free edge with no rounding at the outside edges.
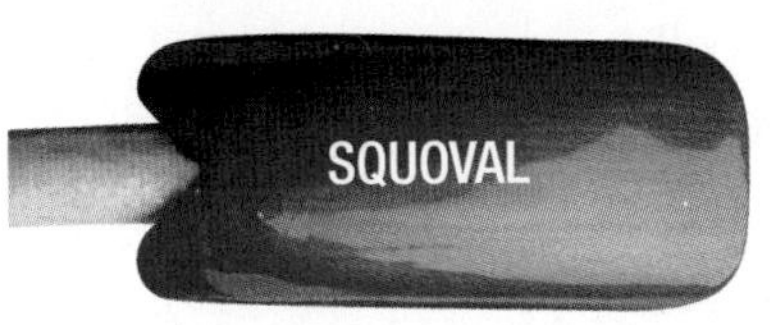	The **squoval nail** has a square free edge that is rounded off at the corner edges. If the nail extends only slightly past the fingertip, this shape will be sturdy because there is no square edge to break off, and any pressure on the tip will be reflected directly back to the nail plate, its strongest area. Clients who work with their hands—nurses, computer technicians, landscapers or office workers—will need shorter, squoval nails.
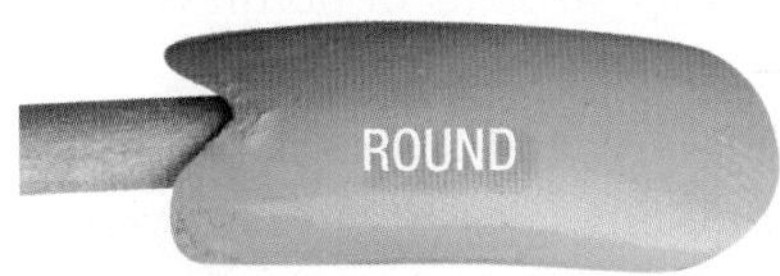	The **round nail** should be slightly tapered and usually should extend just a bit past the fingertip.
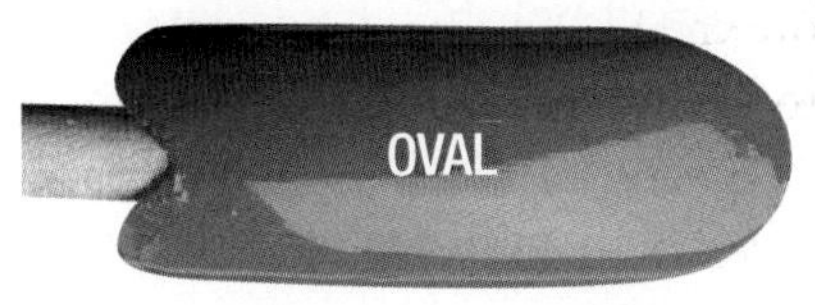	The **oval nail** is a conservative nail shape that is thought to be attractive on most women's hands. It is similar to a squoval nail with even more rounded corners. Professional clients who have their hands on display (e.g., businesspeople, teachers, or salespeople) may want longer oval nails.
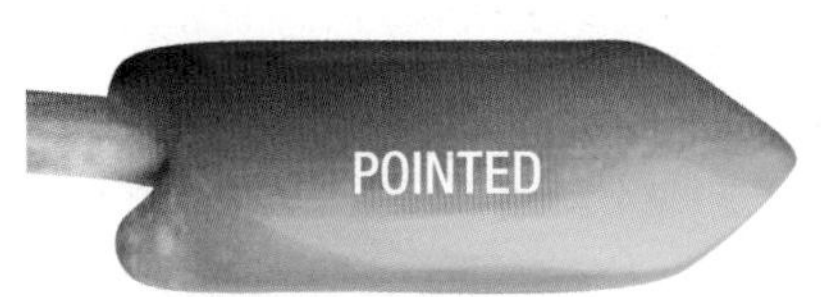	The **pointed nail** is suited to thin hands with long fingers and narrow nail beds. The nail is tapered and longer than usual to emphasize and enhance the slender appearance of the hand. Know, however, that this nail shape may be weaker, may break more easily, and is more difficult to maintain than other nail shapes. Rarely are natural nails successful with this nail shape, so they are usually enhancements. They are for fashion-conscious people who do not need the strongest, most durable shape of nail enhancements.

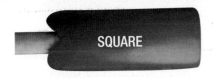

Photos courtesy of European Touch.

© Milady, a part of Cengage Learning.

Table 25–1 Basic Nail Shapes.

Choosing a Nail Color

Polishing is very important for the satisfaction of your clients and for the success of the service, and it may help determine whether clients return to you. Polishing is the last step in a perfect manicure, and it gives your clients a constant visual reminder between visits of the quality of your work. When your clients look at nails that are polished perfectly, they will admire your work and will likely return. If the polish is not applied perfectly, they will have a constant reminder for a week or more of a less-than-perfect manicure and may not return.

Many clients will ask for help in choosing a polish color, or they will ask, "Do you like this color?" When asked for help, suggest a shade that complements the client's skin tone by placing the hand on a white towel under your true-color light, then holding the potential polish colors over

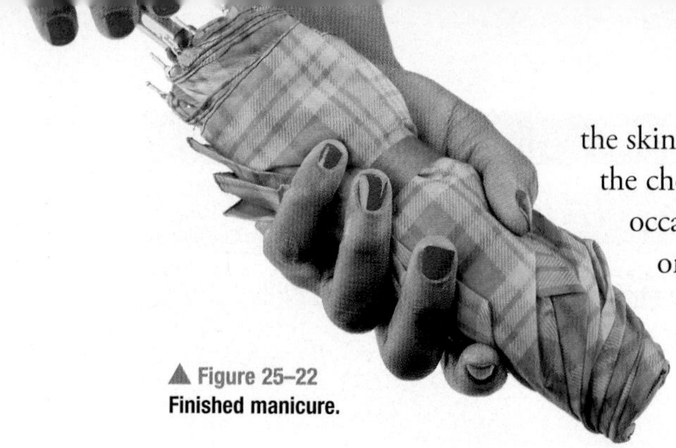

▲ Figure 25–22
Finished manicure.

© Milady, a part of Cengage Learning. Photography by Dino Petrocelli.

the skin on the top of the hand. It is best to allow the client to make the choices to ensure their satisfaction. If the manicure is for a special occasion, you might suggest the client pick a color that matches or coordinates with the clothing they will be wearing, or that represents the holiday, the event, or the season. Some clients will request nail art or other nail fashion enhancements that are popular at the time. Generally, darker shades are appropriate for fall and winter and lighter shades are better for spring and summer; however, this is no longer a hard-and-fast fashion rule. Always have a wide variety of nail polish colors available and the appropriate colors for the French manicure polish techniques.

did you know?

When applying an iridescent or frosted polish, you must make sure the strokes are parallel to the sidewalls of the nail to avoid shadow lines in the polish.

Applying Polish

The most successful nail polish application is achieved by using four coats. The first, the base coat, is followed by two coats of polish color and one application of top coat to give a protective seal. Applying multiple layers of polish improves the longevity and durability of the overall application (**Figure 25–22**). By building layer upon layer, you will improve adhesion and staying power.

The application techniques are the same for all polishes, base coats, and top coats. Apply thin, even coats to create maximum smoothness and minimum drying time. When you have completed the polish application, the nail should look smooth, evenly polished, and shiny.

PROCEDURE 25-7 Polishing the Nails SEE PAGE 835

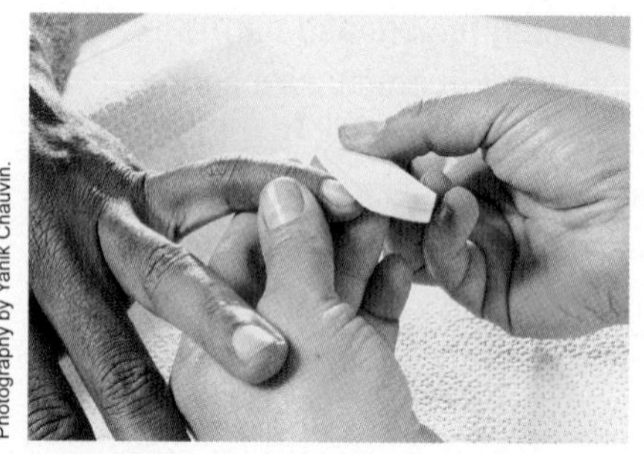

© Milady, a part of Cengage Learning. Photography by Yanik Chauvin.

▲ Figure 25–23
Buffing a male client's nails.

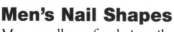

A Man's Manicure Service

Because men are becoming more and more interested in their grooming regimens, many are seeking services for hands and fingernails. A man's manicure is executed using the same procedures as described previously for the basic manicure, though you omit the colored polish and buff the nails with a high-shine buffer (**Figure 25–23**).

Most men tend to go longer between services and will need a little more work than women on their nails and skin. For male clients, a citrus- or spice-scented hand cream is recommended, rather than a flowery scent.

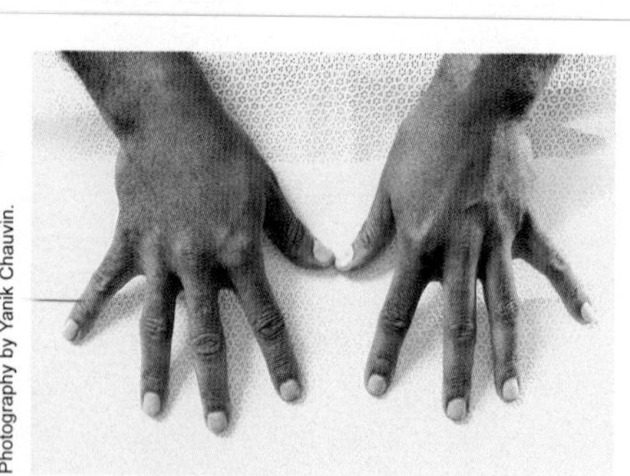

© Milady, a part of Cengage Learning. Photography by Yanik Chauvin.

▲ Figure 25–24
Round nails—the nails most men choose.

Men's Nail Shapes

Men usually prefer their nails shorter than women do. Round nails are the most common choice for male clients because of their natural appearance. Some men, however, prefer their nails really short, with only a small amount of free edge that is shaped according to the base of the nail plate (**Figure 25–24**). ☑ LO6

Men's Massage

Most men enjoy the massage portion of the manicure and want a longer one! Usually men will want a firmer effleurage than women, but this does not mean a deep, sports-type massage—since you are not trained to perform that massage. It just means firmer finger movements on the palm and longer, firmer slides in your effleurage movements (**Figure 25–25**).

Most times, unless the hands are in very poor shape, you can give men a longer massage since polish time is not a factor.

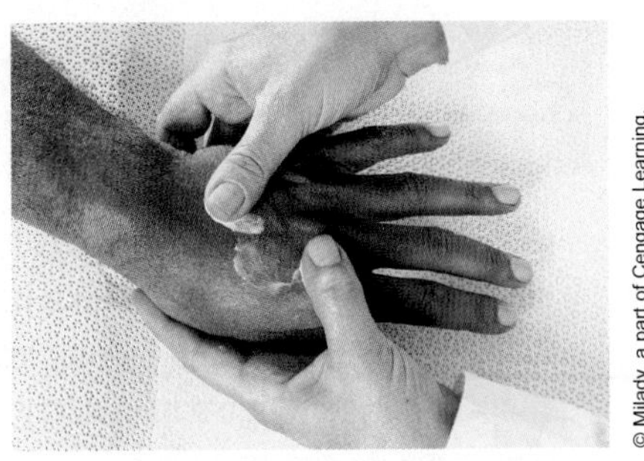
© Milady, a part of Cengage Learning. Photography by Yanik Chauvin.

▲ **Figure 25–25**
Beginning a massage.

Men's Basic Color: Clear

Men usually prefer buffed nails, clear gloss, or a dull, clear satin coating. This satin-coating nail polish finish is designed especially to help men protect their nails without having nails that appear too polished or feminine (**Figure 25–26**). Although a man may rarely want a shiny top coat or colored nail polish on his nails, you should always discuss his preferences during the client consultation.

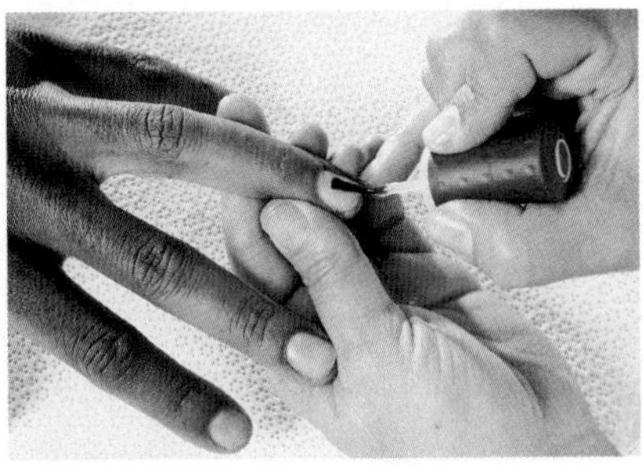
© Milady, a part of Cengage Learning. Photography by Yanik Chauvin.

▲ **Figure 25–26**
Most men prefer buffed nails, clear gloss, or a dull, clear coat.

You must prepare the nails for polish (remove oils and debris) carefully because peeling or chipping gloss is very annoying to men. Use a base coat under clear to encourage staying power; clear without a base tends to peel. Apply a thin base coat and then one thin coat of clear and a quick-drying top coat or just one coat of base and a satin clear.

Always ask for the next appointment and suggest having a pedicure with the manicure. Most men enjoy pedicures!

Marketing to Men

Since most men are new to professional nail care, include on your service menu and your website a brief written description of what is included in the service and a rundown of the benefits. To target men, you may also want to distribute flyers at local athletic gyms and stores, or other places where men gather. Gift certificates sold to your female clients for their boyfriends and husbands are great marketing tools.

To make men feel more at home in your chair, have men's magazines on hand and be careful that your decor is unisex. Staying open later or opening earlier on chosen days makes it easier for your male clients to schedule appointments. Many salons and spas also have a weekly or biweekly men's night, with no women allowed, so male clients can come in without being among women.

Massage

Massage is the manipulation of the soft tissues of the body. It is an ancient therapeutic treatment to promote circulation of the blood and lymph, relaxation of the muscles, and relief from pain. It also has many other benefits. A hand and arm massage, a manicuring specialty, is a service that can be offered with all types of manicures. It is included in all spa manicures, and can be performed on most clients.

STATE REGULATORY ALERT

In a few states, your cosmetology license does not permit you to perform a hand or foot massage. Be guided by your instructor concerning your state's mandatory requirements and procedures for massage during nail services.

A massage is one of the client's highest priorities during the manicure, and often it is the most memorable part of the manicure. Most clients look forward to the soothing and relaxing effects. The massage manipulations should be executed with rhythmic, long, and smooth movements, and you should always have one hand on the client's arm or hand during the procedure.

Hand and arm massages are optional during a basic manicure, but it is to the advantage of the cosmetologist to incorporate this special, relaxing segment of a manicure because it is many clients' favorite part of the service.

General Movements

Massage is a series of movements performed on the human body that, in combination, produce relaxation or treatment.

The following movements are usually combined to complete a massage:

- Effleurage (EF-loo-rahzh) is a succession of strokes in which the hands glide over an area of the body with varying degrees of pressure or contact.
- Pétrissage (PEH-treh-sahz) or kneading is lifting, squeezing, and pressing the tissue.
- Tapotement (tah-POT-ment) is a rapid tapping or striking motion of the hands against the skin.
- Vibration is a continuous trembling or shaking movement applied by the hand without leaving contact with the skin.
- Friction incorporates various strokes that manipulate or press one layer of tissue over another.

The pressure and manipulation of the tissues and muscles vary with each type of movement. Keep in mind that pétrissage and friction are used by massage therapists for therapeutic purposes, and these movements can be painful, even dangerous, when performed by someone without the proper training. The purpose of massage in manicuring is the inducement of relaxation. For that reason, effleurage is the movement that should be perfected, varied, and expertly used. In the traditional manicure, the massage is performed after the basic manicure procedures, right before the polish application. After performing a massage, it is essential that the nail plate be thoroughly cleansed to ensure that it is free from any residue such as oil, cream, wax, or lotion. You can use alcohol or nail polish remover to cleanse the nail plate. ✓ LO7

© Alfred Wekelo, 2010; used under license from Shutterstock.com.

PROCEDURE 25-6 Hand and Arm Massage SEE PAGE 831

Spa Manicures

Spa manicures are fast becoming much-requested and desired salon services, but they require more advanced techniques than basic manicures. Nail professionals who advance their education and knowledge of spa manicures and their specialized techniques will not only make their clients happy, but also may find that these manicures are very lucrative.

© Milady, a part of Cengage Learning.

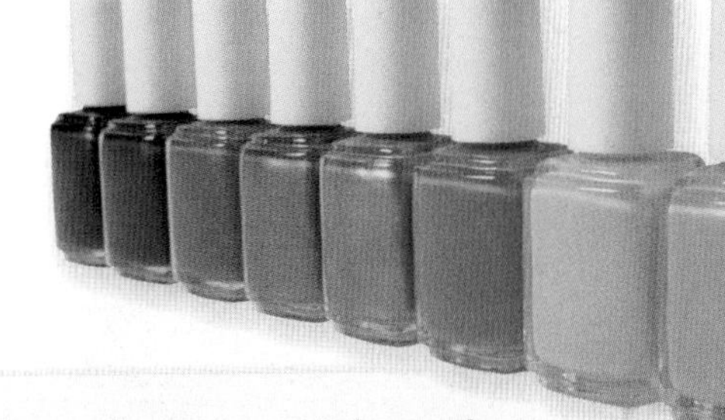

Spa manicures require extensive knowledge not only of nail care, but of skin care as well. Many spa manicures are exceptionally pampering, while others target specific results through the use of advanced skin care–based methods. Most spa manicures include a relaxing massage, and all spa manicures include some form of exfoliation for not only polishing and smoothing the skin, but also for enhancing penetration of professional products.

Spa manicures designed for relaxation may have unique and distinctive names that describe the treatment. For example, "The Rose Garden Rejuvenation Manicure" may incorporate the use of products containing rose oils and may use rose petals for ambiance.

The results-oriented spa manicures, sometimes known as "treatment manicures," often have names that closely represent their purpose. "The Anti-Aging Manicure" may incorporate the use of an alpha hydroxy acid–based product for exfoliation and skin rejuvenation. "The Scrub Manicure" will probably exfoliate callused skin. Many spa manicures have more imaginative names, such as "Spot-Be-Gone," for a manicure designed to lighten age spots. Treatment manicures require further training to produce safe and obvious results. To learn about this and other specialty manicures, see *Spa Manicuring for Salons and Spas* by Janet McCormick, published by Milady, a part of Cengage Learning.

FYI

Some clients may ask for products that are chemical-free. The truth is that no products are or can be chemical-free—even air and water contain chemicals!

When faced with clients who feel strongly about their beliefs and knowledge—whether their information is correct or not—know your product line and its claims, and offer clients the information so they can make informed decisions.

Many clients now base their cosmetic and service decisions on lifestyle choices, such as preferring all-natural products. These clients will seek out spa manicures that meet their needs, and they may ask about the ingredients in the products you are using. In order to know how to answer these questions, you must know whether your product lines make all-natural claims.

The reality is, despite what the product marketing implies, few all-natural products are commercially available and virtually none are chemical-free.

One natural alternative is to mix your own products from fresh ingredients. If you choose to create your own fresh products, you may want to make a small batch for each procedure or per day, because they can spoil very quickly and may require refrigeration in the salon.

did you know?

A newly developed dry manicure eliminates the soak, using lotion and heated mitts to soften the skin and cuticles.

Additional techniques that may be incorporated into a spa manicure consist of aromatic paraffin dips, hand masks, and warm moist-towel applications. When performing any advanced procedures that include oils or cosmetics, always check with your client regarding aroma preferences and allergies. ☑ LO8

Theme Manicures

Many salons and spas have developed services around themes. The entire service contains products—from lotions to oils to masks—that support the theme the salon has chosen, and some salons even serve clients themed refreshments during the service (**Figure 25–27**).

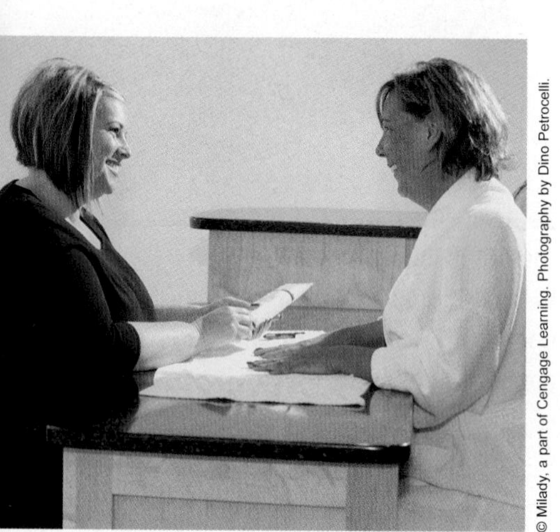

© Milady, a part of Cengage Learning. Photography by Dino Petrocelli.

▲ Figure 25–27
Relaxed client during a spa manicure.

Examples might include the "Chocolate Wonder Manicure and Pedicure" or the "Pumpkin Fall Festival Manicure and Pedicure." The names and themes of these kinds of services are limited only by your imagination. Let yours go wild and have fun developing these well-received manicures and pedicures. Clients love them!

Aromatherapy

In the 1870s, Professor René Maurice Gattefossé, a French scientist, discovered the therapeutic use of essential oils, which are inhaled or applied to the skin. These oils are used in manicures, pedicures, and massages to induce such reactions as relaxation or invigoration, or to simply create a pleasant fragrance during the service. Many clients enjoy the various aromas, so when it is appropriate, incorporate aromatherapy into your nail services.

The practice of aromatherapy involves the use of highly concentrated, nonoily, **essential oils** that are extracted using various forms of distillation from seeds, bark, roots, leaves, wood, and/or resin of plants. Each part of these resources produces a different aroma. For instance, the needles, resin, and wood of a Scotch pine tree all yield a different aroma and, therefore, a different response from the target person. The use of essential oils is limited only by the knowledge of the person controlling their application.

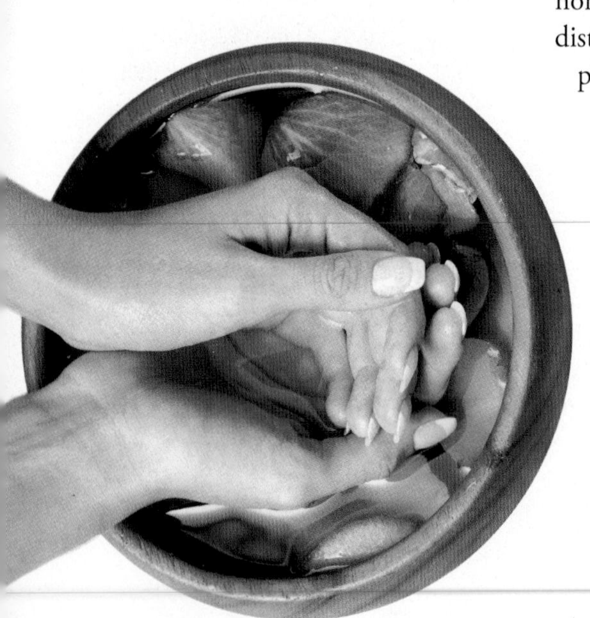

© Niderlander, 2010; used under license from Shutterstock.com.

Performing aromatherapy requires study and expert use of the knowledge gained. The oils are very powerful and can produce actual changes in the client. In some countries, the oils are considered medicines and are only prescribed by physicians. Therefore, unless a cosmetologist is prepared to study these oils in-depth, he or she should use blended oils, those that are already mixed and tested, and apply them only as directed. ☑ LO9

Paraffin Wax Treatments

Paraffin wax treatments are designed to trap moisture in the skin while the heat causes skin pores to open. Besides opening the pores, heat from the warm paraffin increases blood circulation. This is considered to be a luxurious add-on service and can be safely performed on most clients (**Figure 25–28**). Be sure to examine the client's intake form during the client consultation to identify any contraindications to wax or the heat involved in the service and to discuss any additional precautions that should be taken for clients with health factors or risks, such as diabetes or poor circulation.

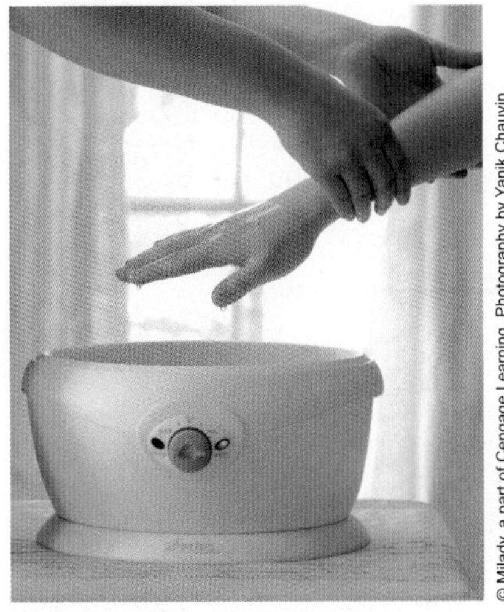
© Milady, a part of Cengage Learning. Photography by Yanik Chauvin.

▲ **Figure 25–28**
Paraffin treatment is a luxury service, as well as a treatment for dry skin.

Paraffin is a petroleum by-product that has excellent sealing properties (barrier qualities) to hold moisture in the skin. Special heating units melt solid wax into a gel-like liquid and maintain it at a temperature generally between 125 and 130 degrees Fahrenheit. When using this treatment, only use the equipment that is designed specifically for this use. Never try to heat the wax in anything other than the proper equipment. This can be very dangerous and may result in painful skin burns or a fire.

If proper procedures are followed, paraffin will not adversely affect nail enhancements or natural nails. A paraffin wax treatment may be offered before a manicure, during a manicure, or as a stand-alone service. Be guided by your instructor and your state regulations, because some states require the service to be performed before the manicure.

PROCEDURE 25-8 **Paraffin Wax Treatment** SEE PAGE 837 ✔ LO10

did you know?

Blended oils are usually mixed to target a particular response from the client, such as relaxation or increased energy. These oils are safe and easy to use by persons who have not studied aromatherapy in-depth and are usually added to such products as massage lotion, body lotion, and masks. These aromas and products are designed to provide maximized results and greater enjoyment for clients.

Before a Manicure

Performing the paraffin wax treatment before beginning a manicure has advantages:

- It allows the client to have her nails polished immediately at the end of the manicure service.
- It is a way to pre-soften rough or callused skin.

Read and follow all operating instructions that come with your paraffin heating unit. Generally, you should avoid giving paraffin treatments to anyone who has impaired circulation or skin irritations such as cuts, burns, rashes, warts, or eczema. Senior citizens and chronically ill clients may be more sensitive to heat because of medications or thinning of the skin. In these cases, ask the clients to bring their physician's permission prior to having a paraffin treatment.

A patch test for heat tolerance can be performed on all clients the first time they have the service. Place a small patch of wax on the client's skin to see if the temperatures can be tolerated.

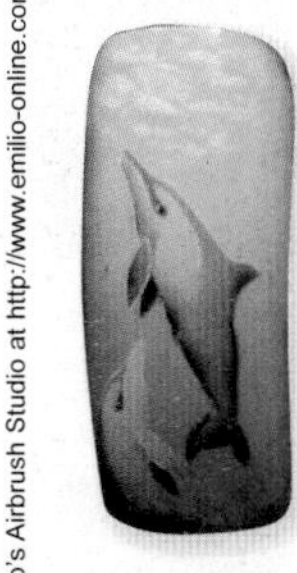
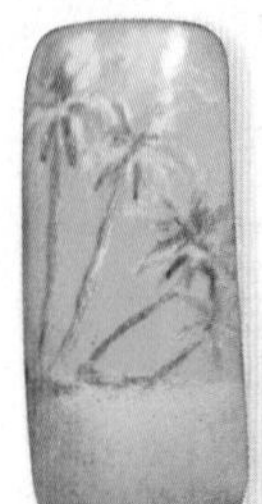
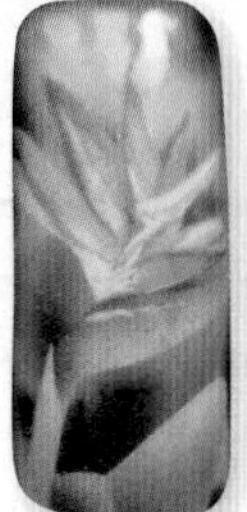
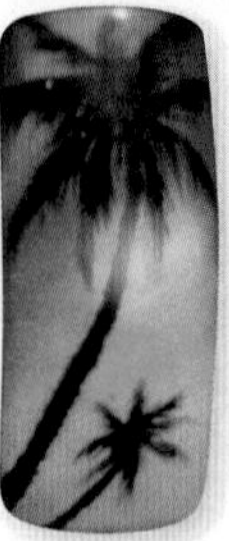

Courtesy of Emilio's Airbrush Studio at http://www.emilio-online.com.

▲ Figure 25–29
Airbrush nail art.

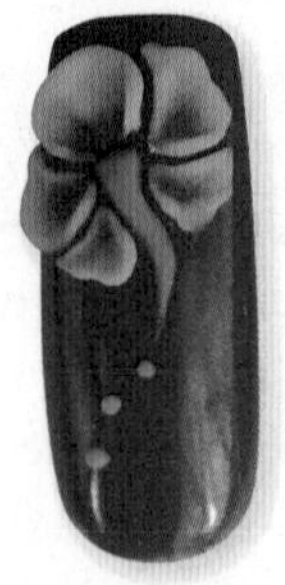
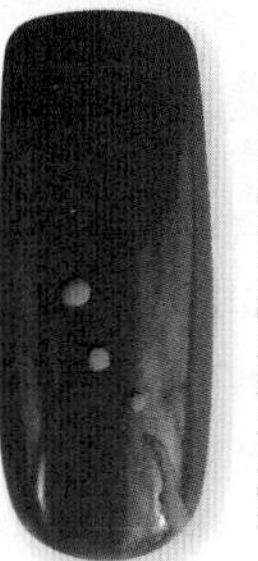

Nail Art by Alisha Rimando Botero.

▲ Figure 25–30
3-D nail art.

During A Manicure

Many salons and spas have developed manicures that include specialized and additional treatments, such as masks and paraffin wax that are performed after the massage and before polishing.

Stand-Alone Service

Many clients enjoy a paraffin treatment. This service can be on the menu with its own price, because clients like the way a paraffin treatment makes their skin feel. The heat provides pain relief for those with arthritis. When the temperature is cold outside, many clients remember the warm feeling the paraffin provides and will book an appointment or drop in for a dip.

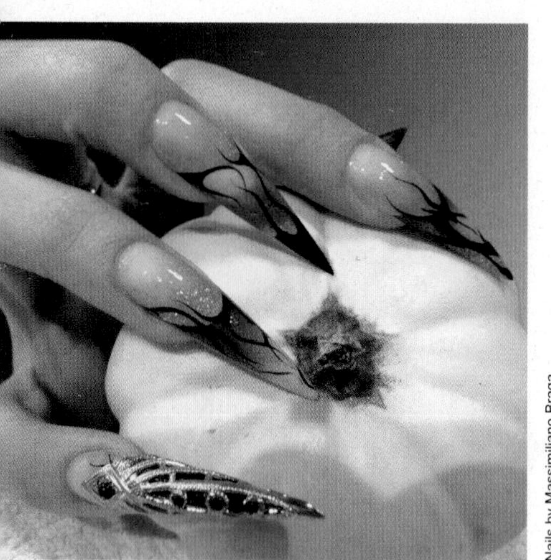

Nails by Massimiliano Braga.

▲ Figure 25–31
Complex nail art.

Nail Art

Many clients love the application of artistic designs on their nails (nail art). The techniques are fun to apply and are only limited by your imagination. Nail art techniques include free-hand designs, airbrush (**Figure 25–29**), glue-on, and even 3-D (**Figure 25–30**). They range from simple to complex (**Figure 25–31**) and from portrait to modern design.

Only the Beginning

During your time in school it is important that you learn the basic procedures of nail technology, as well as the importance of proper cleaning, disinfection, and other skills necessary for ensuring client safety and enjoyment during nail procedures.

Advanced techniques in manicuring may be learned from your instructor or by attending advanced nail care seminars, reading trade magazines, and attending beauty shows. Advanced skill and information books are available from Milady, a part of Cengage Learning. *Spa Manicuring for Salons and Spas* by Janet McCormick will enhance your knowledge of manicures and pedicures.

Business Tip

It is important that you never stop learning about new innovations and continue to seek out information about your industry. Things change, and the wise cosmetologist studies and changes along with the world of cosmetology to remain on the cutting edge.

PROCEDURE 25-1

Pre-Service Procedure

A. Cleaning and Disinfecting

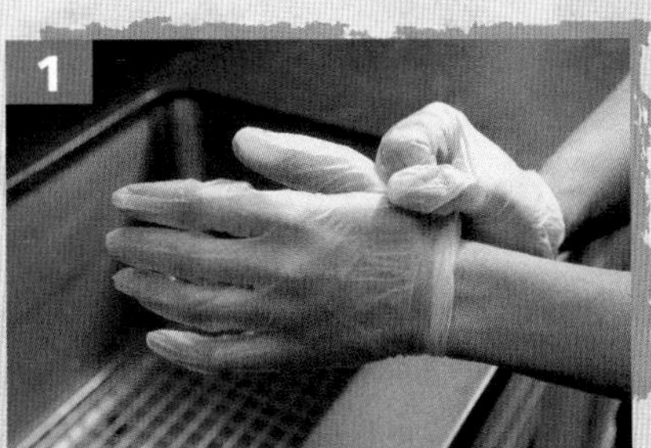

1 It is important to wear gloves while performing this pre-service to prevent possible contamination of the implements by your hands and to protect your hands from the powerful chemicals in the disinfectant solution.

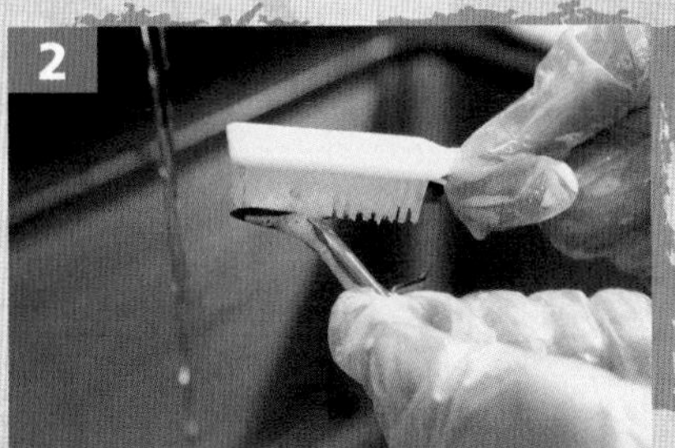

2 Rinse all implements with warm running water, and then thoroughly wash them with soap, a nail brush, and warm water. Brush grooved items, if necessary, and open hinged implements to scrub the area.

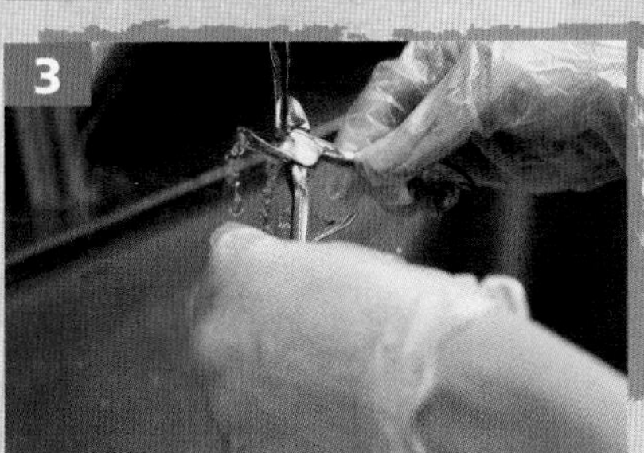

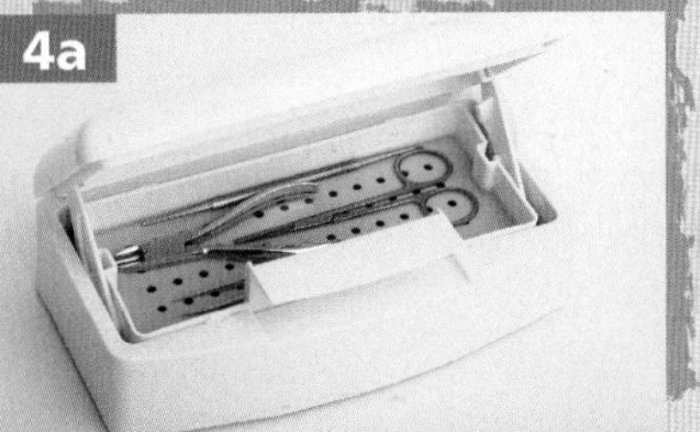

4b

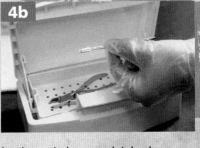

3 Rinse away all traces of soap with warm running water. The presence of soap in most disinfectants can cause them to become inactive. Soap is most easily rinsed off in warm water. Hotter water will not work any better. Dry implements thoroughly with a clean or disposable towel, or allow them to air-dry on a clean towel. Your implements are now properly cleaned and ready to be disinfected.

4 It is extremely important that your implements be completely clean before you place them in the disinfectant solution. If they are not, your disinfectant may become contaminated and rendered ineffective. Immerse cleansed implements in an appropriate disinfection container holding an EPA-registered disinfectant for the required time (usually ten minutes). Remember to open hinged implements before immersing them in the disinfectant solution. If the disinfectant solution is visibly dirty, the solution has been contaminated and must be replaced immediately. Make sure to avoid skin contact with all disinfectants by using tongs or by wearing disposable gloves.

© Milady, a part of Cengage Learning. Photography by Dino Petrocelli.

5 Remove implements, avoiding skin contact, and rinse and dry tools thoroughly.

6 Store disinfected implements in a clean, dry container until needed.

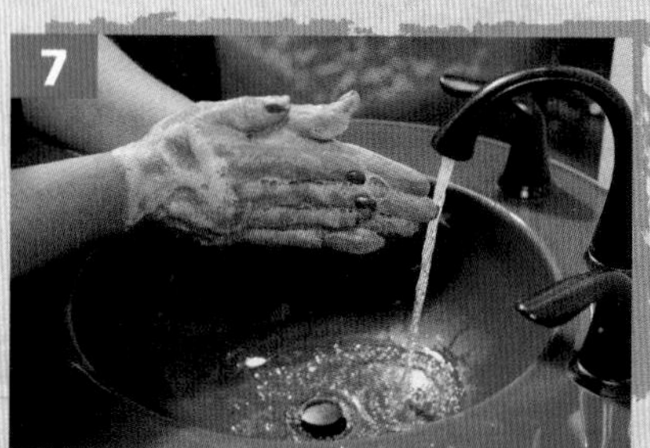

7 Remove gloves and thoroughly wash your hands with liquid soap, rinse, and dry with a clean fabric or disposable towel. ✓ LO11

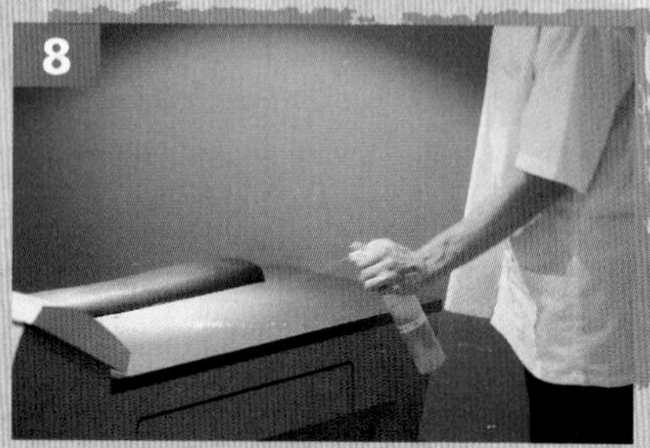

8 Clean and then disinfect manicure table and drawer with an appropriate EPA-approved disinfectant.

B. Basic Table Setup

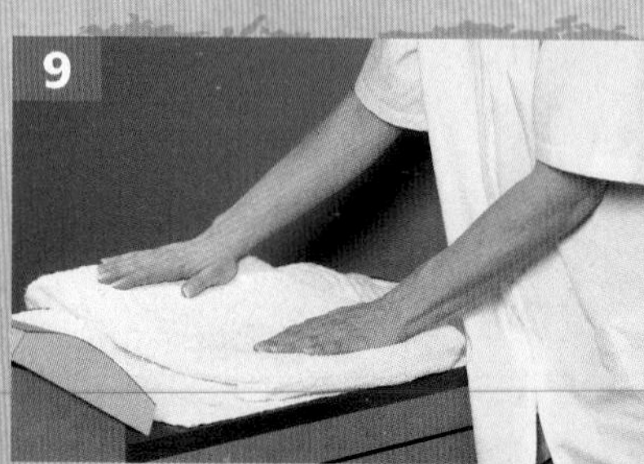

9 Wrap your client's arm cushion, if used, with a clean terry cloth or disposable towel. Place the cushion in the middle of the table so that one end of the towel extends toward the client and the other end extends toward you.

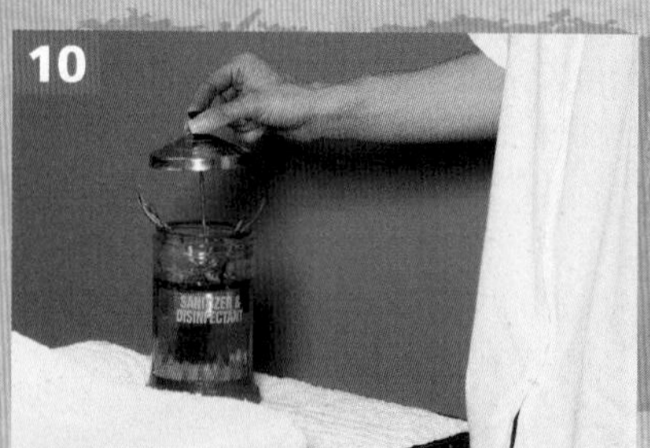

10 Ensure that your disinfection container is filled with clean disinfectant solution at least twenty minutes before your first service of the day. Use any disinfectant solution approved by your state board regulations, but make sure that you use it exactly as directed by the manufacturer. Also make sure that you change the disinfectant every day or according to the manufacturer's instructions. Completely immerse cleaned, reusable implements into the disinfection container for the required time.

© Milady, a part of Cengage Learning. Photography by Dino Petrocelli.

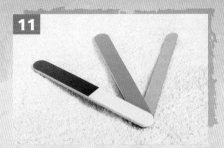

11 Place the abrasives and buffers of your choice on the table to your right (if left-handed, place on the left).

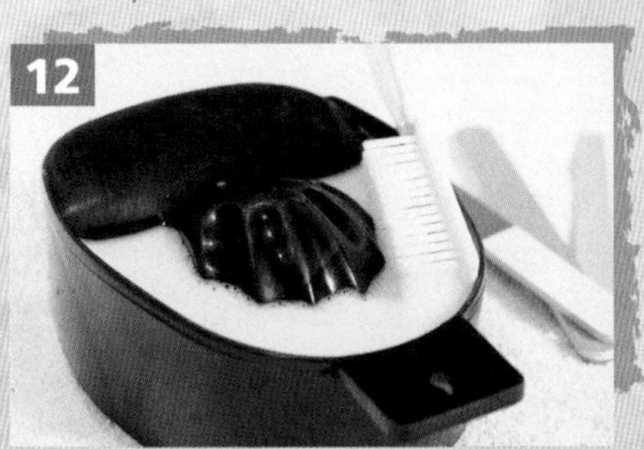

12 Place the finger bowl filled with warm water and the manicure brush in the middle of the table, toward the client. The finger bowl should not be moved from one side to the other side of the manicure table. It should stay where you place it for the duration of the manicure.

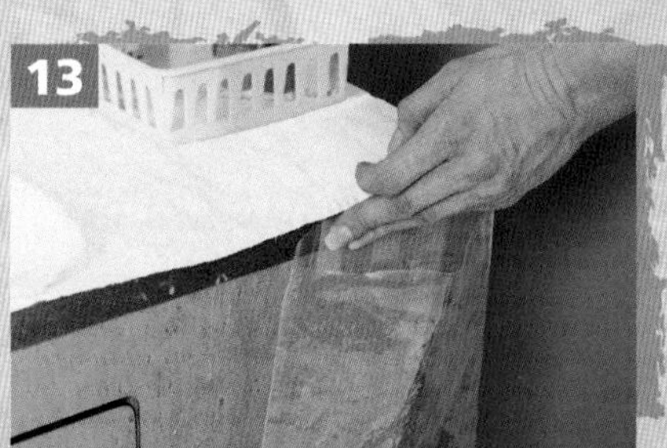

13 If a metal trash receptacle with a self-closing lid is not available, tape or clip a plastic bag that can be closed securely to the right side of the table (if left-handed, tape to the left side). This is used for depositing used materials during your manicure. These bags must be emptied after each client departs to prevent product vapors from escaping into the salon air.

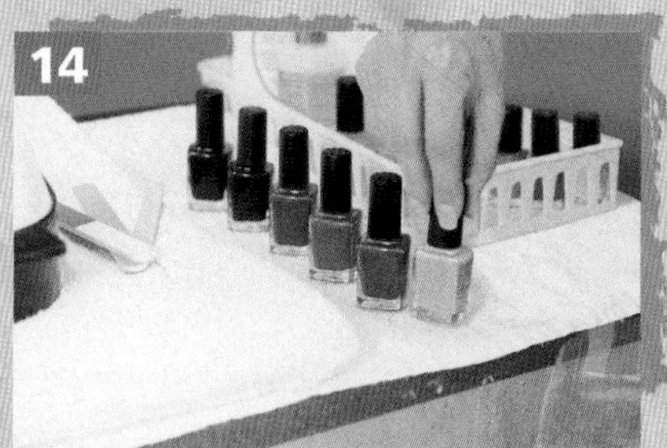

14 Place polishes to the left (if left-handed, place on the right).

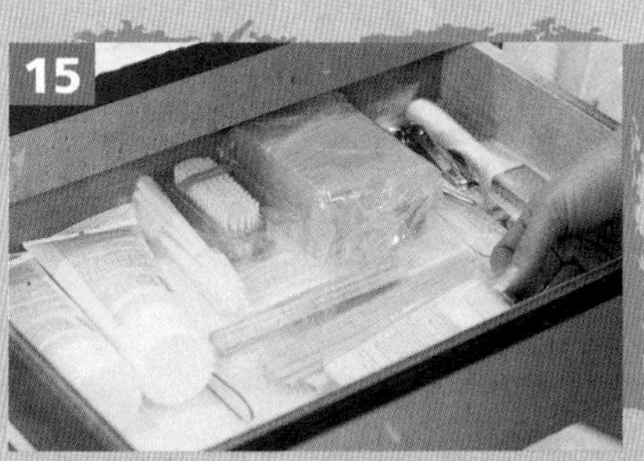

15 The drawer can be used to store the following items for immediate use: extra cotton or cotton balls in their original container or in a fresh plastic bag, abrasives, buffers, nail polish dryer, and other supplies. Never place used materials in your drawer. Only completely cleaned and disinfected implements stored in a sealed container (to protect them from dust and recontamination) and extra materials or professional products should be placed in the drawer. Your drawer should always be organized and clean. ✓ LO12

© Milady, a part of Cengage Learning. Photography by Dino Petrocelli.

Pre-Service Procedure continued

C. Greet Client

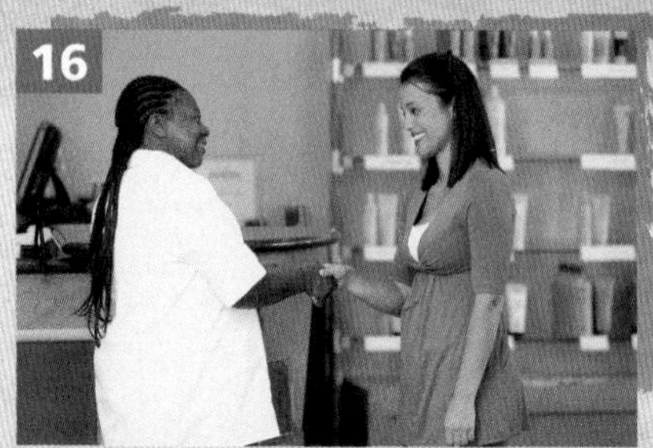
16

16 Greet your client with a smile, introduce yourself if you've never met, and shake hands. If the client is new, ask her for the consultation card she filled out in the reception area.

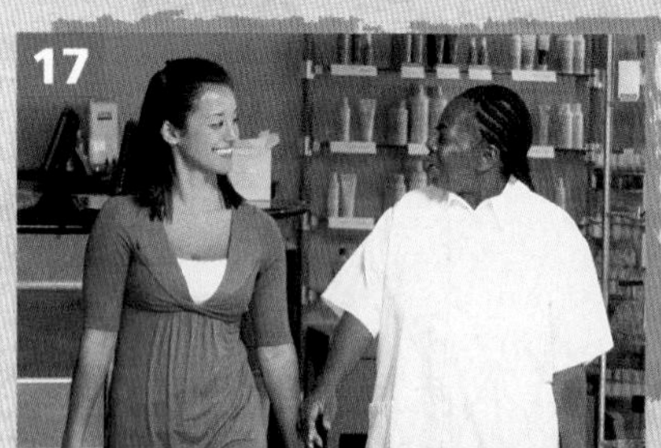
17

17 Escort your client to the hand washing area and demonstrate the hand washing procedure for them on your own hands. Once you have completed the demonstration, hand your client a fresh nail brush and ask her to wash her hands.

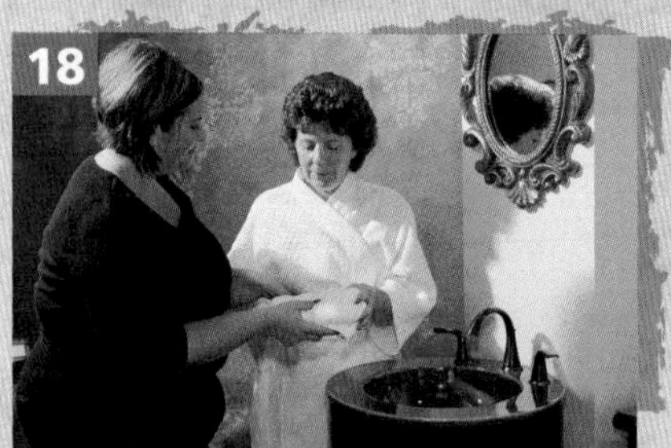
18

18 Be sure that your towels look clean and are not worn. A towel with stains or holes will affect how your client feels about her service. A dirty towel can cause a client either to not come back or to report your salon to the state board.

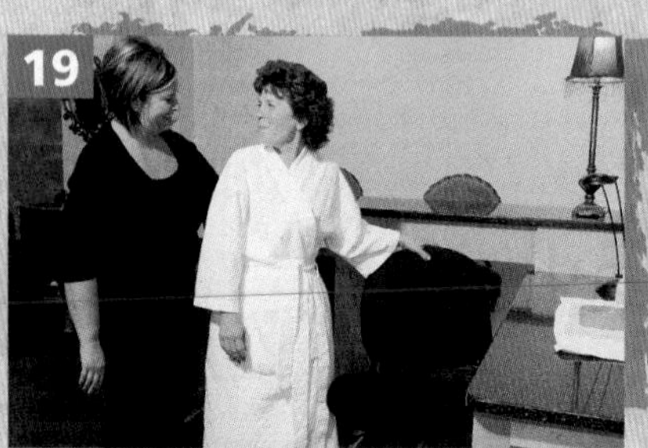
19

19 Show your client to your work table, and make sure they are comfortable before beginning the service.

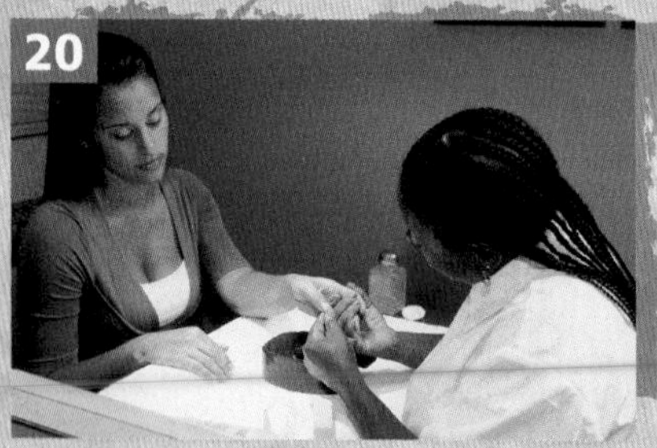
20

20 Discuss the information on the consultation card, and determine a course of action for the service.

© Milady, a part of Cengage Learning. Photography by Dino Petrocelli.

PROCEDURE 25-2

Post-Service Procedure

A. Advise Clients and Promote Products

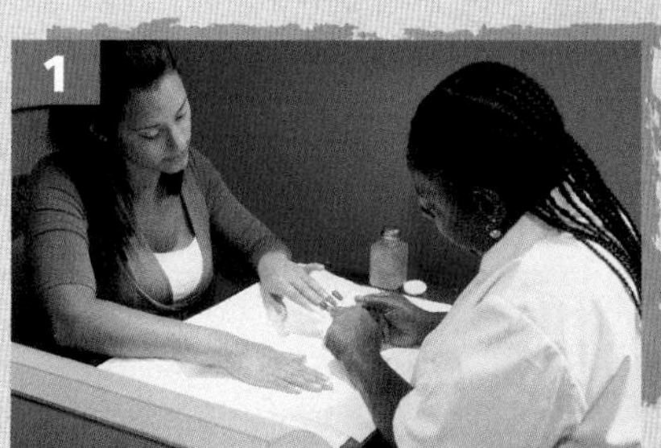

1 Proper home care will ensure that the client's nails look beautiful until he or she returns for another service (in seven to ten days).

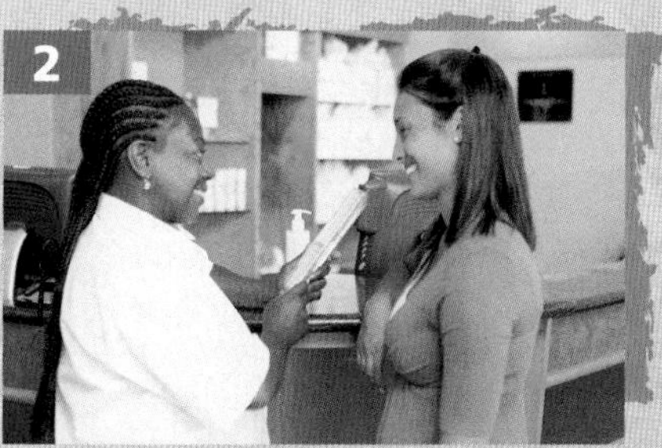

2 Depending on the service provided, there may be a number of retail products that you should recommend for the client to take home. This is the time to do so. Explain why they are important and how to use them.

© Milady, a part of Cengage Learning. Photography by Dino Petrocelli.

B. Schedule Next Appointment and Thank Client

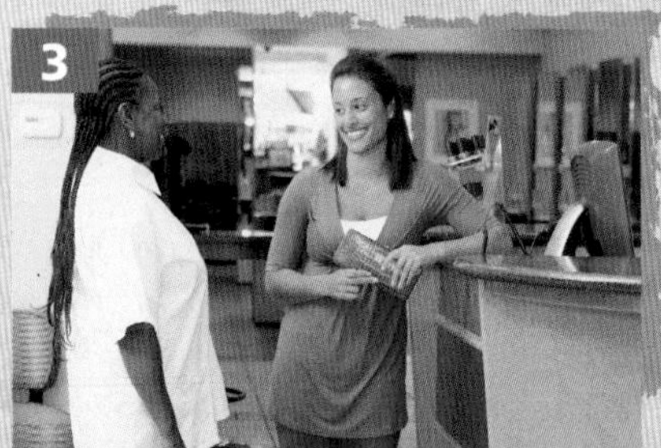

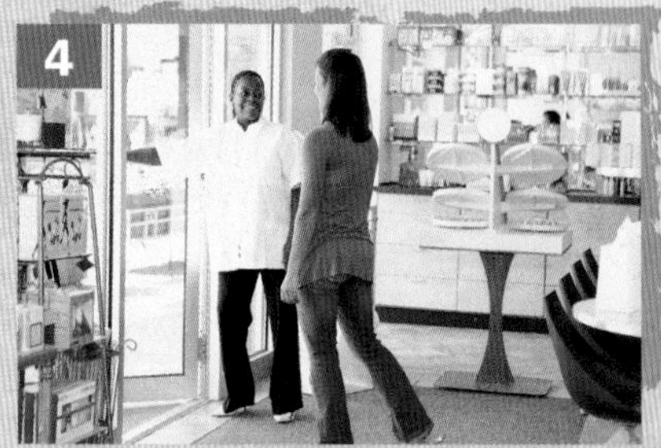

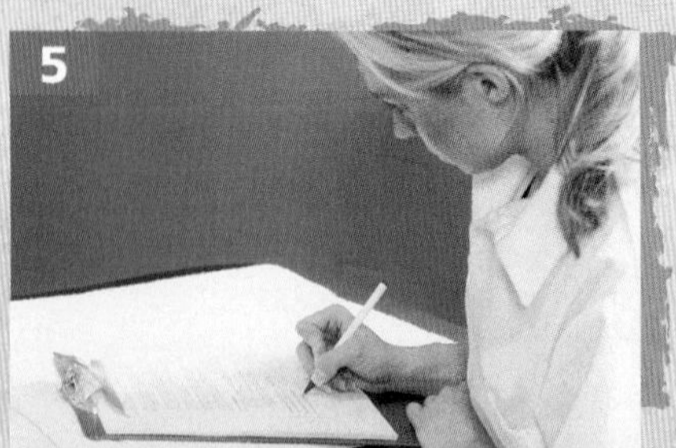

3 Escort the client to the front desk to schedule the next appointment and to collect payment for the service. Set up the date, time, and services. Then write the information on an appointment card and give it to the client.

4 Before the client leaves the salon and you return to your station, be sure to thank her for her business.

5 Record on the client consultation card all service information, products used, observations, and retail recommendations. Then, file the form in the appropriate place.

C. Prepare Work Area and Implements for Next Client

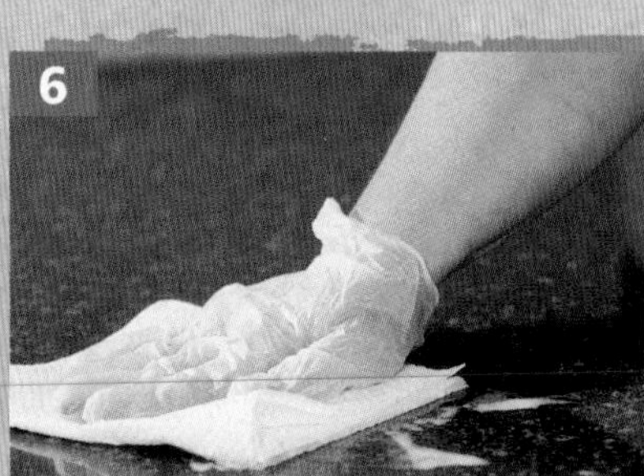

6 Remove your products and tools. Then clean and disinfect your work area and properly dispose of all used materials.

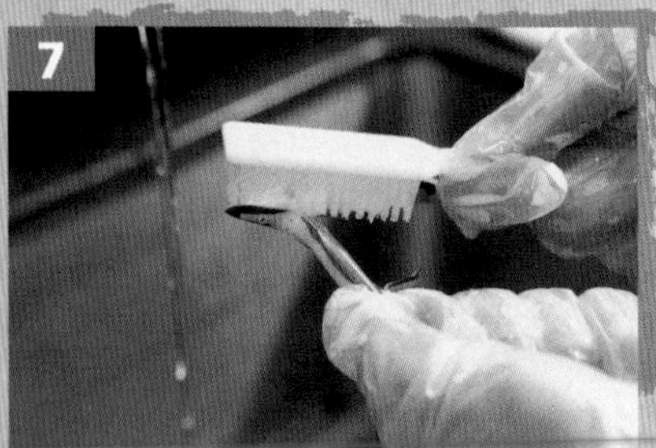

7 Follow steps for disinfecting implements in the pre-service procedure. Reset work area with disinfected tools. ✓ LO13

© Milady, a part of Cengage Learning. Photography by Dino Petrocelli.

PROCEDURE 25-3

Proper Hand Washing

Hand washing is one of the most important procedures in your infection control efforts and is required in every state before beginning any service.

1 Escort the client to the wash station. Before beginning any service, explain the salon or spa's hand washing policy and why it is performed.

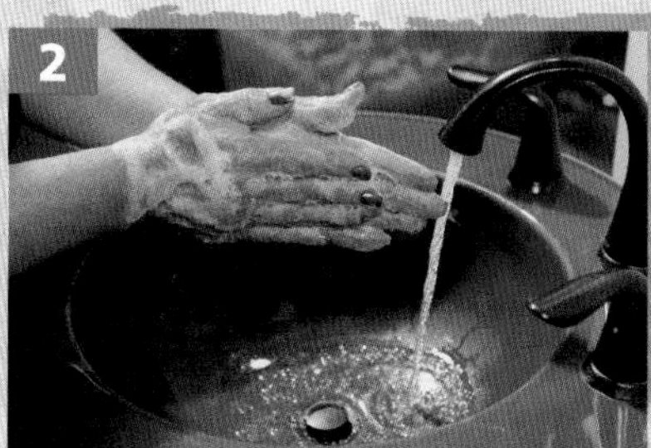

2 Turn the warm water on, wet your hands, and pump soap from a pump container onto the palm of your hand. Rub your hands together, all over and vigorously, until a lather forms. Continue in this manner for about twenty seconds and rinse.

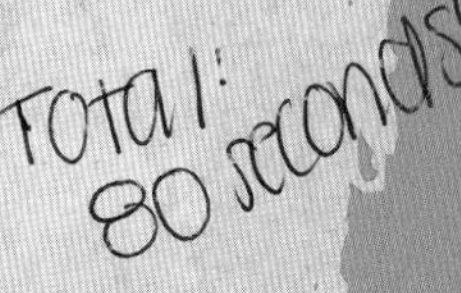

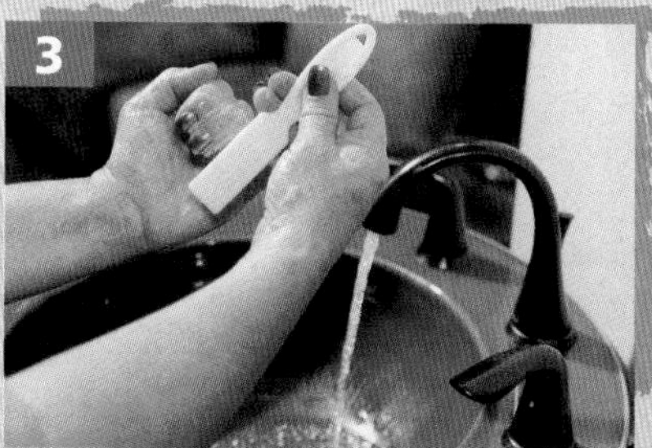

3 Choose a clean nail brush, wet it, pump soap on it, and brush your nails horizontally back and forth under the free edges. Change the direction of the brush to vertical and move the brush up and down along the nail folds of the fingernails. The process for brushing both hands should take about sixty seconds to finish. Rinse hands in running water.

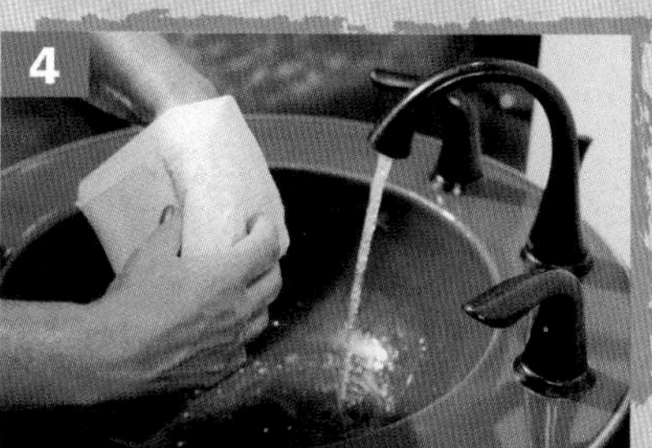

4 After your demonstration, give the client a clean nail brush and instruct her to wash her hands as well.

5 Hand the client a clean towel for drying hands, and inform the client what to do with the towel, or dry the client's hands using a clean cloth or paper towel according to the salon policies for hand drying.

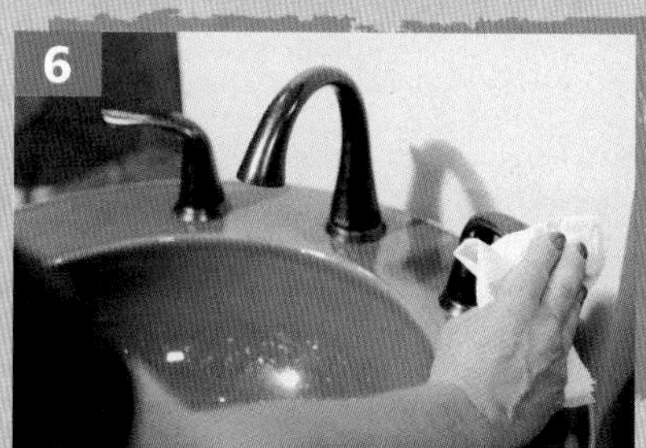

6 After drying, turn off the water with the towel and then dispose of the towel.

7 Escort the client to the table while explaining that hand washing should be performed before every service.

© Milady, a part of Cengage Learning. Photography by Dino Petrocelli.

PROCEDURE 25-4

Handling an Exposure Incident During a Manicure

Should you accidentally cut a client, calmly take the following steps:

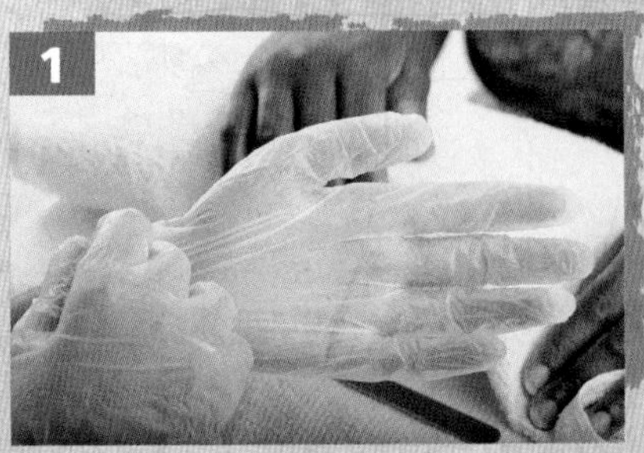

1 Immediately put on gloves unless you already have them on and inform your client of what has occurred. Apologize and proceed.

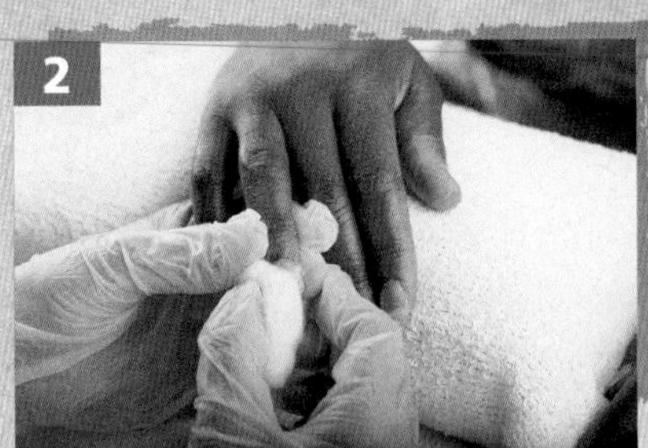

2 Apply slight pressure to the area with cotton to stop the bleeding and then clean with an antiseptic.

© Milady, a part of Cengage Learning. Photography by Dino Petrocelli.

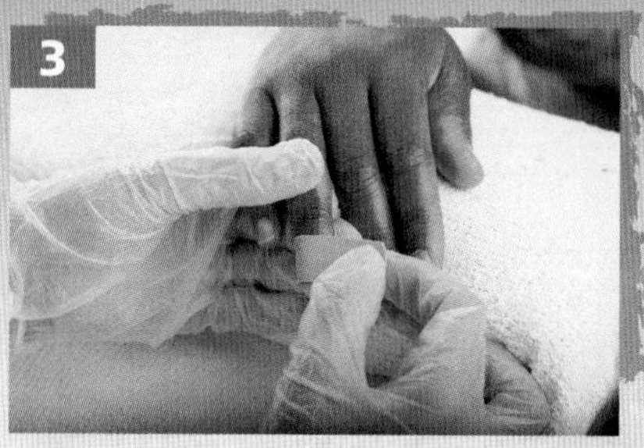

3 Apply an adhesive bandage to completely cover the wound.

Service Tip

Always remember to use the Universal Precautions established by the Occupational Safety and Health Administration (OSHA) when handling items exposed to blood or body fluids. (See Chapter 5, Infection Control: Principles and Practices.) Be guided by your instructor for your state's mandatory requirements and procedures for disinfecting any implements that have come into contact with blood or body fluids.

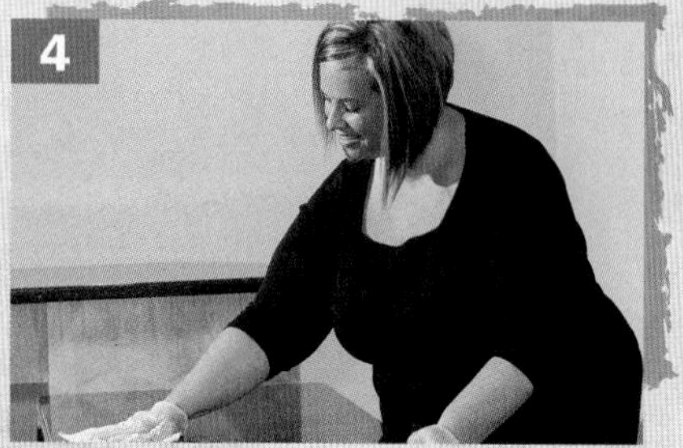

4 Clean and disinfect the workstation, as necessary.

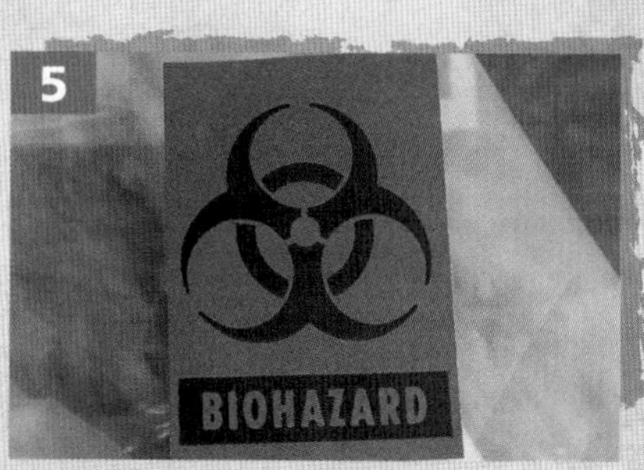

5 Discard all disposable contaminated objects such as wipes or cotton balls by double-bagging (placing the waste in a plastic bag and then in a trash bag). Use a biohazard sticker (red or orange), or a container for contaminated waste. Deposit sharp disposables in a sharps box.

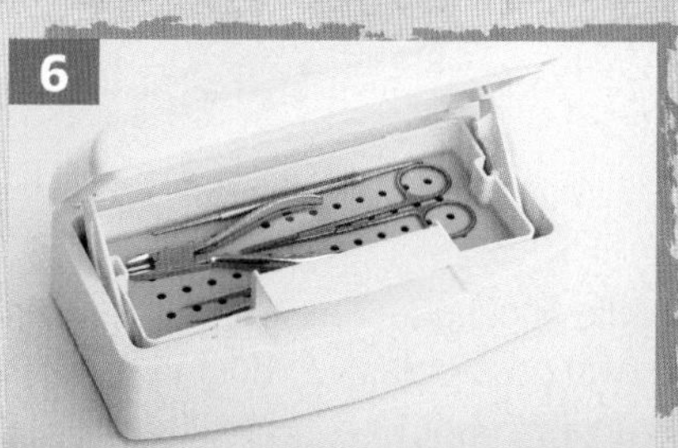

6 Remember, before removing your gloves, all tools and implements that have come into contact with blood or body fluids must be thoroughly cleaned and then completely immersed in an EPA-registered hospital disinfectant solution for ten minutes. Because blood can carry pathogens, you should never touch an open sore or wound with your bare hands.

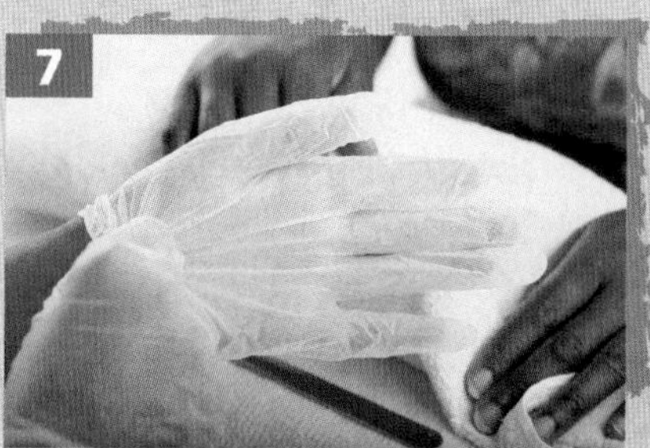

7 Remove gloves and wash your hands with soap and warm water before returning to the service. ✓ LO14

© Milady, a part of Cengage Learning. Photography by Dino Petrocelli.

PROCEDURE 25-5

Performing a Basic Manicure

Implements and Materials

You will need all of the following implements, materials, and supplies on your manicuring table:

- Abrasive nail files and buffers
- Base coat
- Client's arm cushion
- Colored polish, enamel, lacquer, or varnish
- Cuticle removers
- Disposable or terry cloth towels
- Electric hand/foot mitts (optional)
- Finger bowl
- Gauze and cotton wipe container
- Hand creams and lotions
- Nail bleach
- Nail creams, lotions, and penetrating nail oils
- Nail hardener
- Nail polish dryers
- Polish remover
- Service cushion
- Supply tray (optional)
- Terry cloth mitts (optional)
- Top coat
- Trash containers
- Ultraviolet or electric nail polish dryer (optional)
- Wooden pusher

Preparation

- Perform PROCEDURE 25-1 Pre-Service Procedure SEE PAGE 817

Procedure

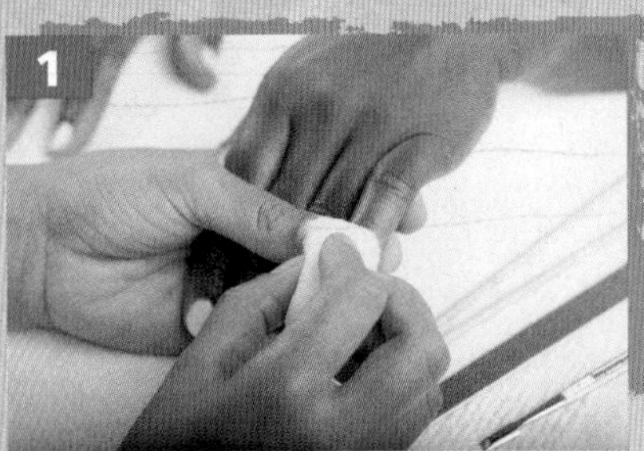

1 Begin with your client's left hand, little finger. Saturate cotton ball, gauze pad, or plastic-backed cotton pad with polish remover. Hold the saturated cotton on each nail while you silently count to 10. The old polish will now come off easily from the nail plate with a stroking motion, moving toward the free edge. Use a confident, firm touch while removing the polish. Continue until all traces of polish are gone.

Complete removal of the polish from the previous manicure is important to client satisfaction. It may be necessary to wrap cotton around the tip of a wooden pusher and use it to clean polish away from the nail fold area. After removal, look closely at the nails to check for abnormalities that could have been hidden by the polish.

© Milady, a part of Cengage Learning. Photography by Dino Petrocelli.

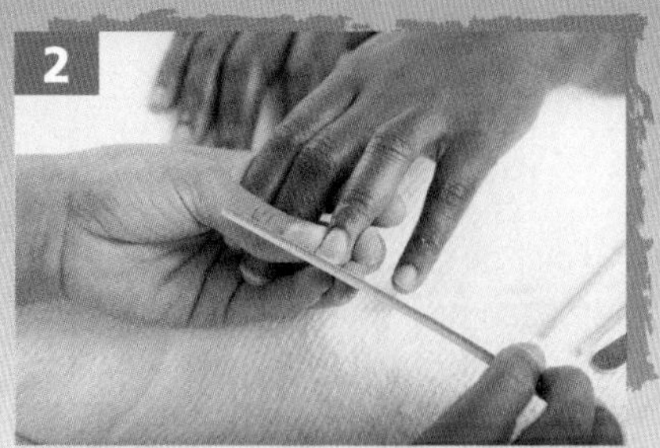

2 Using your abrasive board, shape the nails as you and the client have agreed. Start with the left hand, little finger, holding it between your thumb and index finger. Do not use less than a medium-grit (180) abrasive file to shape the natural nail. File from one side to the center of the free edge, then from the other side to the center of the free edge. Never use a sawing back and forth motion when filing the natural nail, as this can disrupt the nail plate layers and cause splitting and peeling. To lessen the chance of developing ingrown nails, do not file into the corners of the nails. File each hand from the little fingernail to the thumb.

CAUTION

Always file the nails in a manicure before they are soaked, as water will absorb into the nail plate, making it softer and more easily damaged during filing.

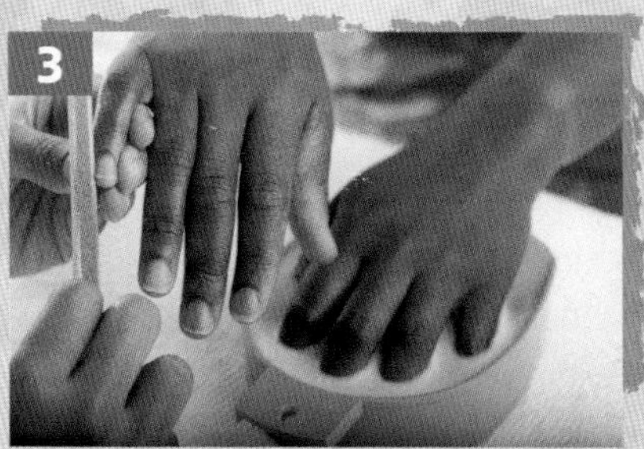

3 After filing the nails on the left hand, and before moving on to the right hand, place the fingertips of the left hand in the finger bowl to soak and soften the eponychium (living skin on the posterior and sides of the nail) and cuticle (dead tissue adhered to the nail plate) while you file the nails on the right hand. When finished with filing of the right hand, remove the left hand from the soak and place the fingertips of the right hand in the finger bowl.

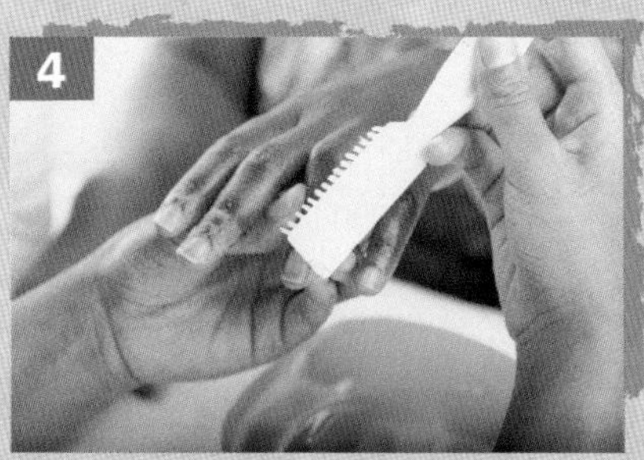

4 Brushing the nails with a nail brush removes service debris from the nail surface. After filing the nails on the right hand, remove the left hand from the soak, holding it above the finger bowl, brush the fingers with your wet nail brush to remove any debris from the fingertips. Use downward strokes, starting at the first knuckle and brushing toward the free edge.

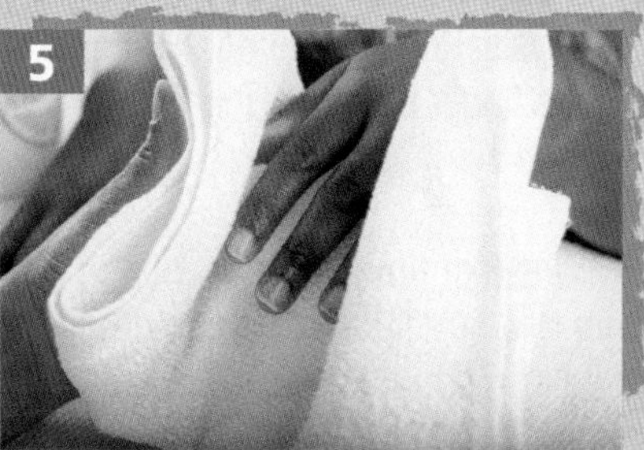

5 Dry the hand with a towel designated as this client's service towel. As you dry, gently push back the eponychium with the towel. Now place the right hand in the soak.

Service Tip

If the nails need to be shortened more than the depth of routine filing, they can be cut with nail clippers, clipping from the sides toward the center of the nails to prevent stress to the sides and possible splitting. This clipping will save time during the filing process. File the free edge after using the nail clipper to perfect the shape.

© Milady, a part of Cengage Learning. Photography by Dino Petrocelli.

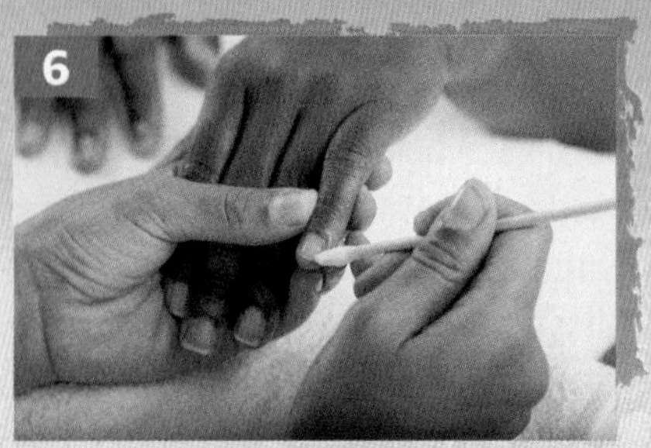

6 Use a cotton-tipped wooden or metal pusher or cotton swab to carefully apply cuticle remover to the cuticle on each nail plate of the left hand. Do not apply this type of product on living skin as it can cause dryness or irritation. Spread evenly on the nail plate. Cuticle removers soften skin by dissolving skin cells, so they are inappropriate for contact with the living skin of the eponychium. Typically, these products have a high pH (caustic) and are irritating to the skin.

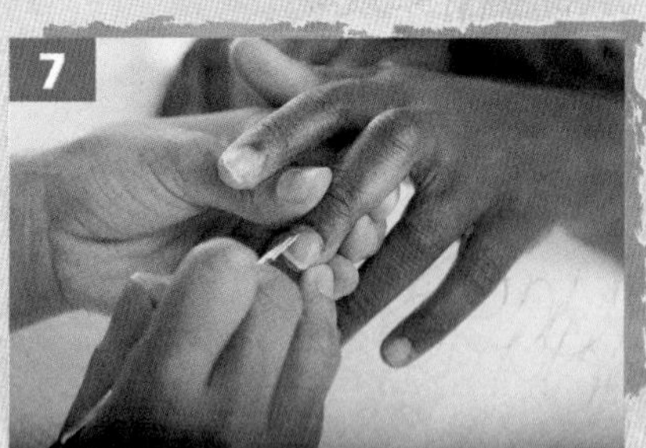

7 After you allow the product to set on the nail for the manufacturer's recommended length of time, the cuticle will be easily removed from the nail plate. Use your wooden pusher or the inside curve of a metal pusher to gently push and lift cuticle tissue off each nail plate of the left hand.

Service Tip

To stabilize the hand that is holding the pusher, balance your pinky finger on the hand that is holding the clients finger. This will allow you to have total control while working with the implement (**Figure 25–32**).

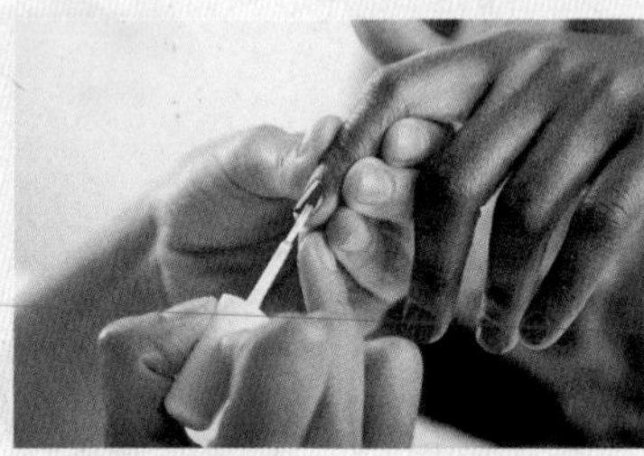

▲ **Figure 25–32**
Correct hold.

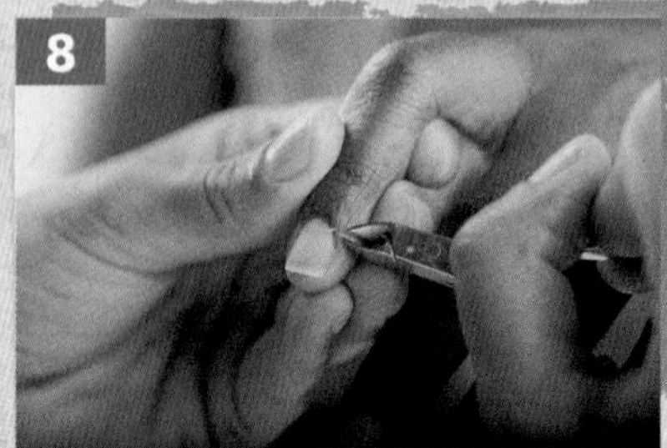

8 Use sharp nippers to remove any loosely hanging tags of dead skin (hangnails). Never rip or tear the cuticle tags or the living skin, since this may lead to infection.

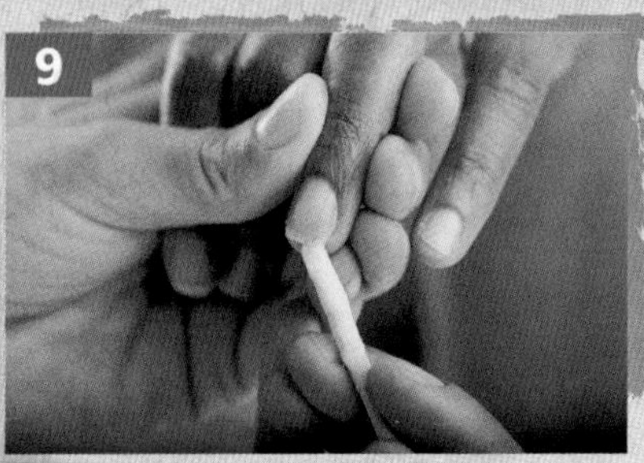

9 Carefully clean under the free edge using a cotton swab or cotton-tipped wooden pusher. Take care to be gentle, as cleaning too aggressively in this area can break the hyponychium seal under the free edge and cause onycholysis. Remove the right hand from the finger bowl, dry the finger bowl, and set it aside.

10 Brush the left hand over the finger bowl one last time to remove bits of debris and traces of cuticle remover. (During this time, the client can be sent to the sink to wash the nail plate with a nail brush.) It is important that all traces of cuticle remover are washed from the skin because remnants can lead to dryness and/or irritation. Instruct the client to rest the left hand on the table towel.

11 Repeat steps 5 through 10 on the right hand.

© Milady, a part of Cengage Learning. Photography by Dino Petrocelli.

12 If the client's nails are yellow, you can bleach them with a nail bleach designed specifically for this purpose. Apply the bleaching agent to the yellowed nail with a cotton-tipped wooden pusher. Be careful not to apply bleach on your client's skin because it may cause irritation. Wear gloves while bleaching the nails.

Repeat the application if the nails are extremely yellow. You may need to bleach certain clients' nails several times during several services because all of the yellow stain or discoloration may not fade after a single service. If this is true, inform the client so he or she will not be disappointed in your work; suggest a series of treatments to address the problem. Surface stains are removed more easily than those that travel deep into the nail plate. In fact, yellow discoloration that penetrates deep into the nail plate will never be completely removed by nail bleaches. However, the yellowing can be improved. These products work best for surface stains (e.g., tobacco). Inform the client if his or her nails have deep staining that cannot be completely removed.

STATE REGULATORY ALERT

State regulations do not permit cosmetologists to cut or nip living skin.

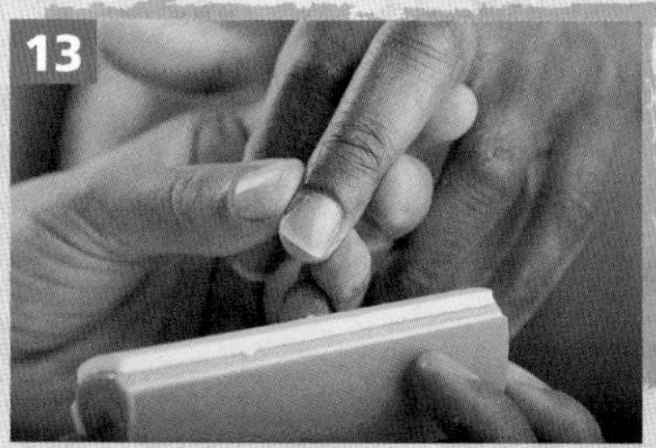

13 Use a three-way or four-way buffer to smooth out surface scratches and give the natural nail a brilliant shine.

14 Use a cotton-tipped wooden pusher, a cotton swab, or an eyedropper to apply nail oil to each nail plate. Start with the little finger, left hand, and massage oil into the nail plate and surrounding skin using a circular motion.

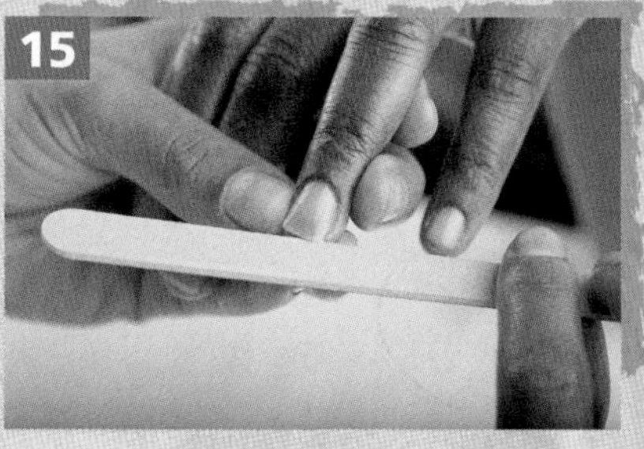

15 To remove any rough edges on the free edges, bevel the underside of the free edge. Hold a medium-grit abrasive board at a 45-degree angle to the underside of the nail and file with an upward stroke. This removes any rough edges or cuticle particles. A fine-grit abrasive board or buffer may be preferable for weak nails.

16 Apply massage lotion or oil and follow hand and arm massage procedure.

CAUTION

When buffing the nail plate, applying excessive pressure or buffing too long can generate excessive and painful heat on the nail bed. This can lead to onycholysis and possible infection. If your client is feeling heat or burning, lighten the pressure, lower the speed of the buffing, and buff fewer times between raising the buffer from the surface.

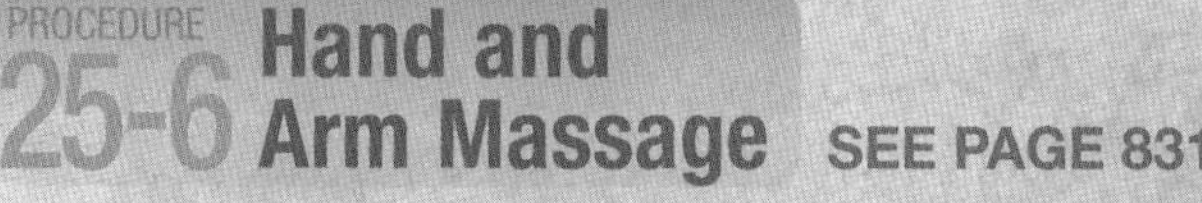

SEE PAGE 831

© Milady, a part of Cengage Learning. Photography by Dino Petrocelli.

Performing a Basic Manicure continued

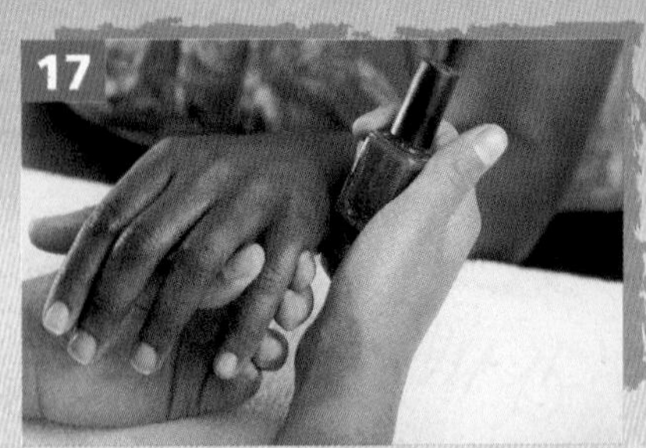

17 After the massage, you must remove all traces of lotion or oil from the nail plate before polishing, or the polish will not adhere well. Use a small piece of cotton saturated with alcohol or polish remover as though you were removing a stubborn, red nail polish. Do not forget to clean under the free edge of the nail plate to remove any remaining massage lotion. The cleaner you get the nail plate, the better the polish will adhere.

18 Most clients will have their polish already chosen before or during the consultation. If not, ask them to choose a color.

19 Always apply a base coat to keep polish from staining the nails and to help colored polish adhere to the nail plate. Nail strengthener/hardener is an option you may recommend for a treatment if the client's nail plates are thin and weak. Apply this before the base coat if the client requests this treatment.

PROCEDURE 25-7 **Polishing the Nails** SEE PAGE 835

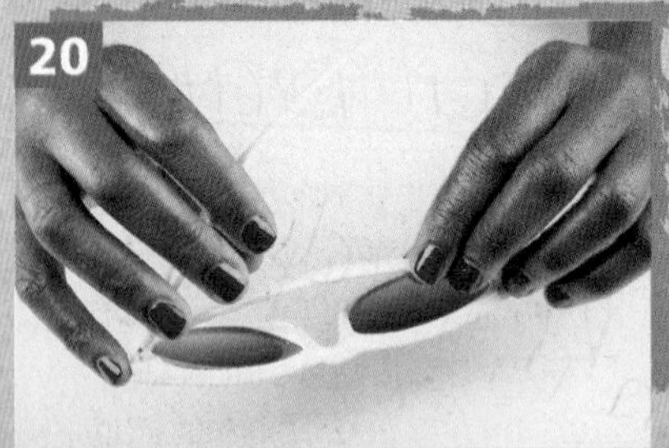

20 You've performed a beautiful, finished manicure.

Post-Service

- Complete PROCEDURE 25-2 **Post-Service Procedure** SEE PAGE 821 ✓ LO15

© Milady, a part of Cengage Learning. Photography by Dino Petrocelli.

PROCEDURE 25-6

Hand and Arm Massage

Implements and Materials

In addition to the basic materials on your manicuring table, you will need the following supplies for the hand and arm massage:

- **Massage lotion, oil, or cream**

Service Tip

Before performing a hand and arm massage, make sure that you are sitting in a comfortable position and are not stretching or leaning forward toward your customer. Your posture should be correct and relaxed, and your feet should be parallel and flat on the floor. Sitting or working in an uncomfortable or strained position can cause back, neck, and shoulder injuries.

Preparation

- Complete PROCEDURE 25-5 **Basic Manicure** **SEE PAGE 826**

Procedure

1 Apply the massage lotion, oil, or cream and distribute to the client's arm. Enough should be applied to allow movement across the skin without resistance (skin drag). Skin drag is not comfortable for the client.

2 The following joint movements are usually performed at the start of the massage to relax the client.

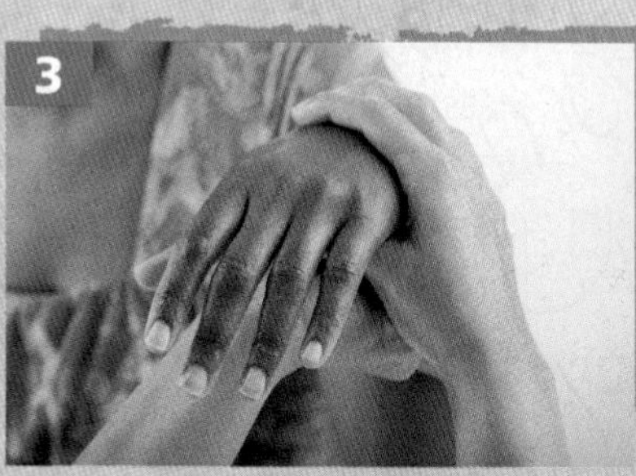

3 At the beginning of the hand massage, place the client's elbow on a cushion covered with a clean towel or a rolled towel. With one hand, brace the client's arm in the wrist area with your nondominant hand. With your other hand, hold the client's wrist and bend it back and forth slowly and gently but with a firm touch, five to ten times, until you feel that the client has relaxed.

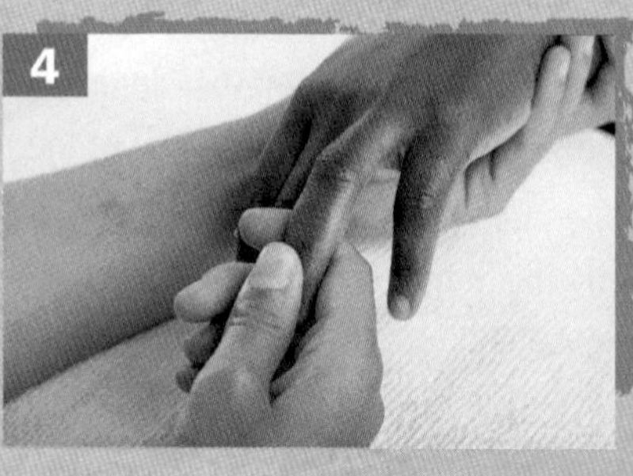

4 Lower the client's arm, brace the arm at the wrist with the left hand, and with your right hand (or dominant hand) start with the little finger, holding it at the base of the nail. Gently rotate fingers to form circles. Work toward the thumb, about three to five times on each finger.

© Milady, a part of Cengage Learning. Photography by Dino Petrocelli.

5

5 Place the client's elbow on the cushion or towel near the center of the table and your elbows on the table at the sides of the client's elbow. With your thumbs in the client's palm, rotate them in a circular movement in opposite directions. The circular movements should start from the bottom, center of the hand and move out, up, and across the underside of the fingers, then back down to the bottom, center, in a smooth pattern of altering movements of each thumb over the palm. This pattern becomes rhythmic and relaxing. You can feel the client's hands relax as you perform these movements.

Service Tip

Be sure to hold the client's hand or arm loosely without too much restraint during the massage. A firm but gentle, slow, and rhythmic movement in a predictable routine is the key to a relaxing massage. Moving quickly sends the message to the client that you are hurrying to get the massage over and do not care about providing a good service.

6a Hold the client's hand gently at the wrist with your nondominant hand and place the palm of your other hand on the back of the client's hand just behind the fingers. Press lightly and move towards the wrist, lift slightly, and move back to the original position and perform the movement. Perform the movement three to five times gently with the palm wrapped warmly around the back of the hand. It is important that enough massage cream, lotion, or oil is on the surface to reduce drag on the skin. Effleurage movements must be smooth and gentle, even predictable, to induce relaxation. After performing the relaxation movements, move to the following effleurage movements.

FYI

Before performing a service that includes a hand and/or arm massage, consult the client's consultation card or intake form. During the consultation acknowledge and discuss any medical condition your client listed that may be contraindicated for a massage. If they have not discussed massage with their physician, encourage them to do so before performing the service.

Many clients who have high blood pressure (hypertension), diabetes, or circulatory conditions may still have hand and/or arm massage without concern, especially if their condition is being treated by a physician. Hand and/or arm massage is, however, contraindicated for clients with severe, uncontrolled hypertension. Avoid using vigorous or strong massage techniques on clients who have arthritis. Do not talk to your client during the massage except to ask once whether your touch should be more or less firm. Talking disturbs the relaxation therapy of the massage.

When making decisions about whether to perform a massage on a person who has a medical condition, be conservative. When in doubt, don't include massage as part of your service.

© Milady, a part of Cengage Learning. Photography by Dino Petrocelli.

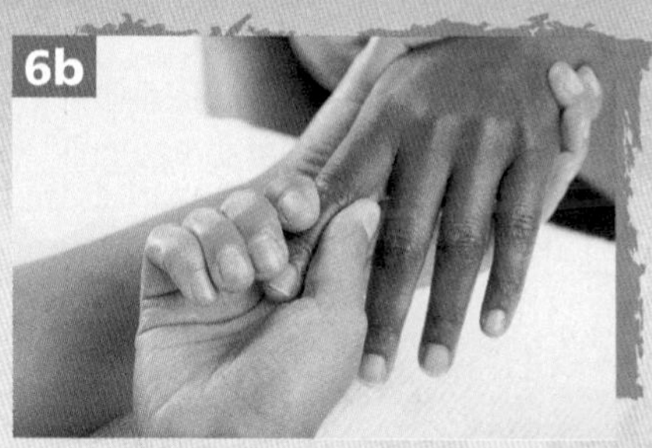

6b Perform the transition movement and then move to the fingers. Now, holding the hand with your nondominant hand, move to the finger tip. Hold each finger with your palm down and the thumb on one side of the finger, the inside of the knuckle of the index finger holding the other side. Gently move the finger back, sliding slowly towards the hand, then turn your hand over completely, moving the thumb to the other side of the finger, your palm up. Then return to the tip, gently pulling the finger. Turn the hand over, back to the original position, and push towards the back of the finger again. Repeat three to five times, then at the fingertip, move the thumb to under the fingertip, the arch of the index finger over the top of the nail plate, and gently squeeze and pull off the finger. Now, move to the next finger. Perform this movement on all fingers the same number of times, moving from small fingers to thumbs. This concludes the hand massage usually performed in the basic manicure, though the last movement of the arm massage is also performed at the end of this massage. It is not if the massage is continuing with an arm massage. Then, it is performed at the end of the arm massage.

7a Now holding the wrist firmly but gently, glide your hand up the arm from wrist to elbow with your palm and fingers on the skin; be certain enough lotion is on the skin to allow a smooth glide of the hand. Cup your movement fingers around the arm, moving up with slight pressure on the skin with your fingers, thumb, and palm to induce relaxation, then move back to the wrist area with a lighter pressure on the skin. Perform this gliding several times. When finishing a movement each time at the top of the arm, rotate the hand to the underside of the arm while pulling the hand back towards you.

7b Now move to the underarm and perform the same movement. When performing the movement on the underarm, press forward, then at the end release the pressure, gently rotate the hand to the top of the arm, and pull it lightly back toward the hand.

Service Tip

If more cream, oil, or lotion is needed during the massage, always leave one hand on the client's hand or arm and retrieve more product with the other. Having your product in a pump container facilitates this important massage technique.

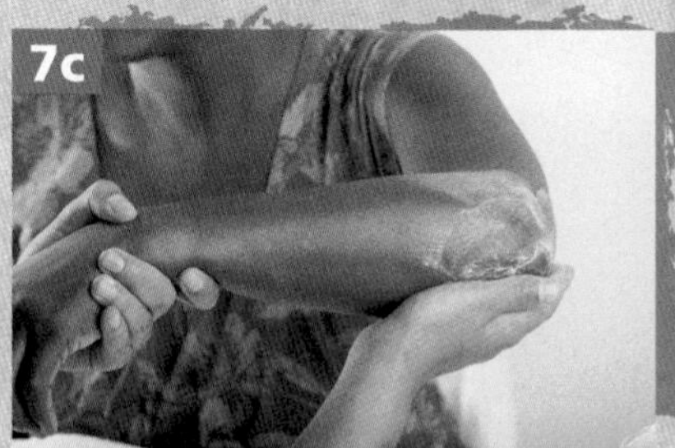

7c Apply lotion on the palm of one of your hands, then apply to the elbow while holding the arm bent and up gently with the other (cupping the elbow). Glide the palm of the hand over and around the elbow to allow moisturization. Take care to be very gentle. Perform the movement for ten to twenty seconds, gently and slowly. Take care not to hit the nerve in the elbow that often is referred to as "the funny bone" as it can be very painful to the client.

© Milady, a part of Cengage Learning. Photography by Dino Petrocelli.

Hand and Arm Massage continued

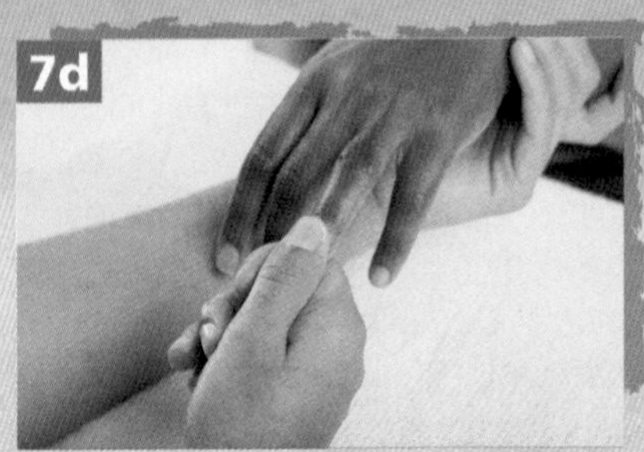

7d Last, holding the hand with your nondominant hand, move to the finger tip, and with your thumb on top and pointer finger below, gently grab and pull the finger down to the tips.

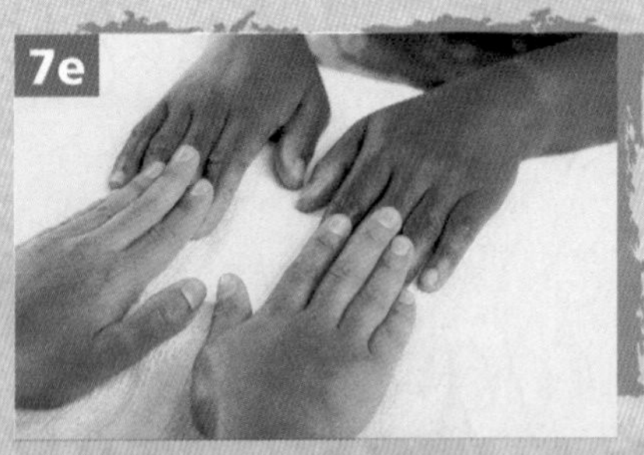

7e After the finger pulls are performed, lay both of the client's hands palms down on the table, cover them with your own hands, palms down on them, and gently press them. Then, as your hands lay on the client's hands, gently, with a light-as-a-feather touch, pull your fingers from the back of the client's hands down the fingers and off the tips of the fingers. Perform two to three times. The client learns quickly this final movement, called "feathering off," is the end of the massage.

Service Tip

Perform the movements several times slowly and rhythmically on each hand or arm and repeat because this is relaxing to the client. Perform the full massage on one arm—palm, back of hand, arm—repeating the gliding movements on each arm several times with transition movements in between. Now, move to the other hand/arm, starting over in the routine you have developed.

CAUTION

Take care not to press or move with pressure over the bones of the arms as this can be quite painful.

© Milady, a part of Cengage Learning. Photography by Dino Petrocelli.

PROCEDURE 25-7

Polishing the Nails

Implements and Materials

In addition to the basic materials on your manicuring table, you will need the following supplies:

- **Base coat**
- **Colored nail polish**
- **Top coat**

Preparation

- Complete PROCEDURE 25-5 **Basic Manicure** SEE PAGE 826

Procedure

1 Be certain the client's nail plates are clean of oil and other debris. Before applying polish, ask your client to put on any jewelry and outerwear she may have taken off before the service and ask her to get car keys ready to avoid smudges to the freshly applied polish. Have the client pay for services also, to avoid smudging the polish later.

2 Polish the client's dominant hand first, apply base coat to cover the entire nail plate of all nails, making sure to use a thin coat. Begin with the pinky finger and work toward the thumb. Once completed, place the client's hand in a nail dryer while you polish the other hand. This will give the most-used, key-holding hand a head start in drying and reduce the likelihood of smudging.

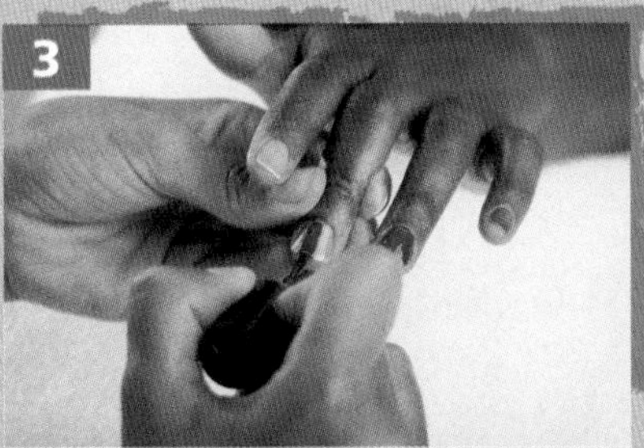

3 When applying nail polish, remove the brush from the bottle and wipe the side of the brush away from you on the inside of the lip of the bottle to remove excess polish. You should have a bead of polish on the end of the other side of the brush large enough to apply one layer to the entire nail plate without having to re-dip the brush (unless the nail plate is unusually long or large). Hold the brush at approximately a 30- to 35-degree angle.

© Milady, a part of Cengage Learning. Photography by Dino Petrocelli.

Polishing the Nails continued

Place the tip of the brush on the nail ⅛ inch away from the cuticle area in the center of the nail. Lightly press the brush onto the nail plate, producing a slight fanning of the brush and then push it toward the eponychium to produce a rounded posterior edge to the polish. Leave a small, rounded area of unpolished nail at the back of the nail. Pull the brush toward the free edge of the nail, down the center.

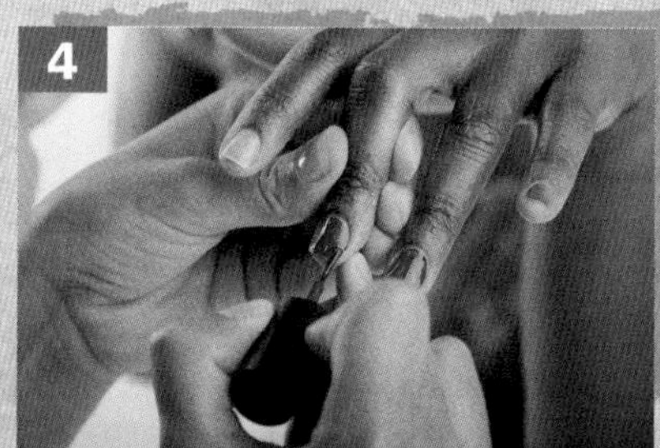

4 Move to each side of the nail and pull in even strokes toward the nail tip.

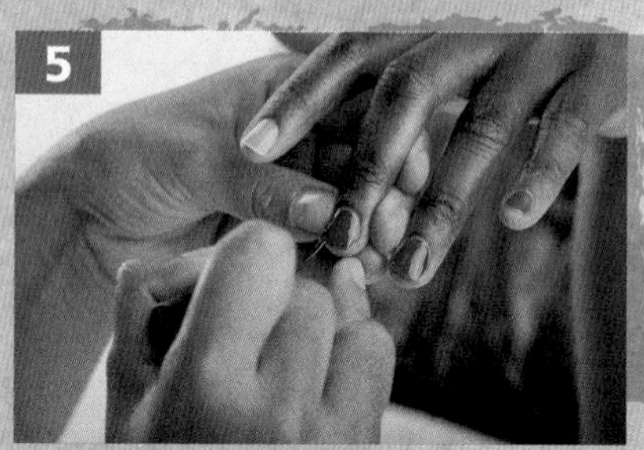

5 After finishing the first coat of each nail, move the brush back and forth on the very end of the free edge, barely touching, to apply color to the edge. Use the same technique for every nail while applying the first coat of color.

6 When you return to apply the second coat, do not fan the brush and do not reapply to the tip. Just start at the base of the polish curve and move toward the free edge.

7 Apply an ample coat of top coat to prevent chipping and to give nails a glossy, finished appearance. Be sure to coat the free edge of the nail with top coat as well.

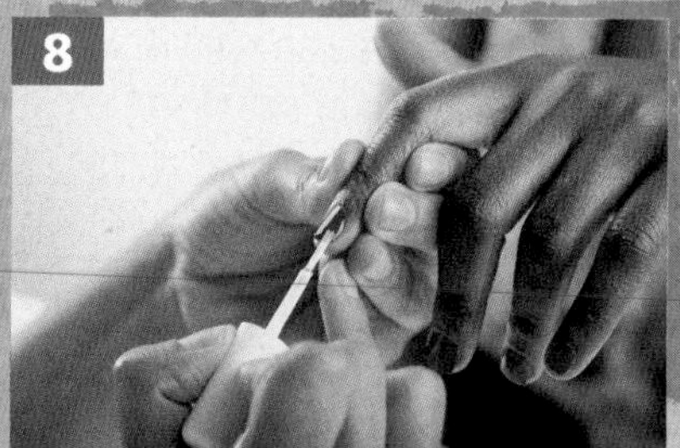

8 If you use a polish-drying top coat product, apply according to the manufacturer's instructions. After the application, ask the client to be seated at a separate table with her hands under a nail dryer or seat her comfortably away from your table. The drying time should be about ten minutes.

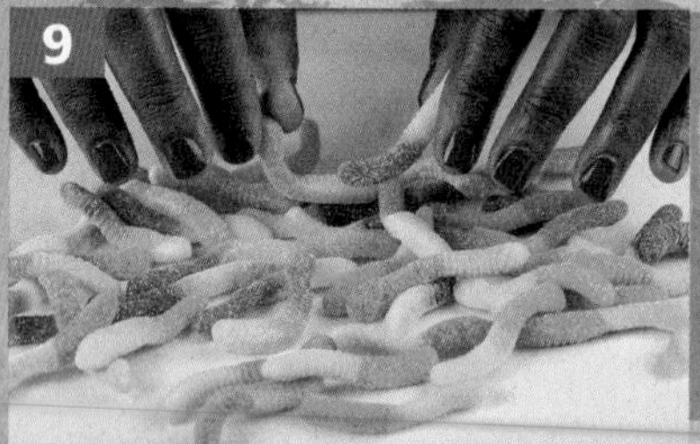

9 Beautifully polished nails. ✓ LO16

© Milady, a part of Cengage Learning. Photography by Dino Petrocelli.

PROCEDURE 25-8

Paraffin Wax Treatment

Implements and Materials

In addition to the basic materials on your manicuring table, you will need the following supplies:

- Moisturizing lotion or penetrating oil
- Paraffin bath and heating unit
- Plastic wrap
- Plastic, terry cloth, or warming (electric) mitts

Preparation

- Perform PROCEDURE 25-1 Pre-Service Procedure SEE PAGE 817
- Perform PROCEDURE 25-3 Proper Hand Washing SEE PAGE 823

Performing a Paraffin Wax Treatment before a Manicure

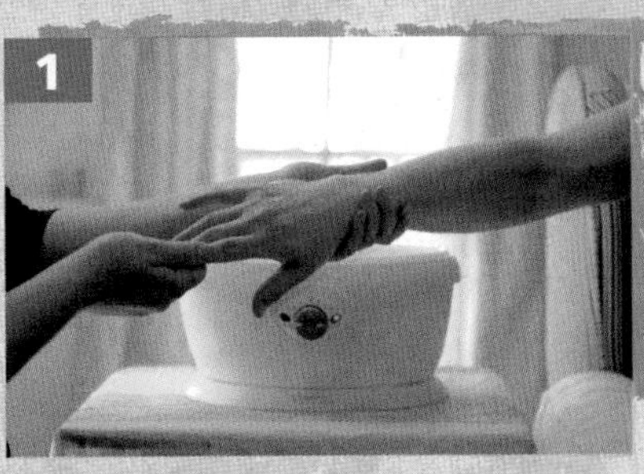

1 Check the hands carefully for open wounds, diseases, or disorders. It is not appropriate to apply heat to clients with abnormal skin conditions. If it is safe to perform the procedure, ensure the client's hands are clean and continue with the service.

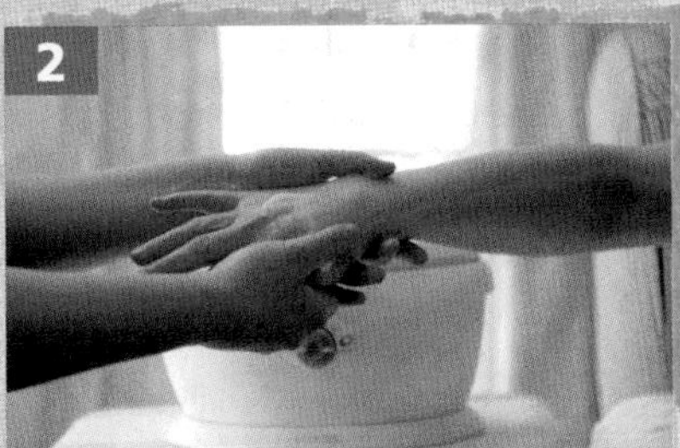

2 Apply moisturizing lotion or penetrating oil to client's hands and gently massage into the skin.

3 Test the temperature of the wax.

© Milady, a part of Cengage Learning. Photography by Yanik Chauvin.

PROCEDURE 25-8 Paraffin Wax Treatment continued

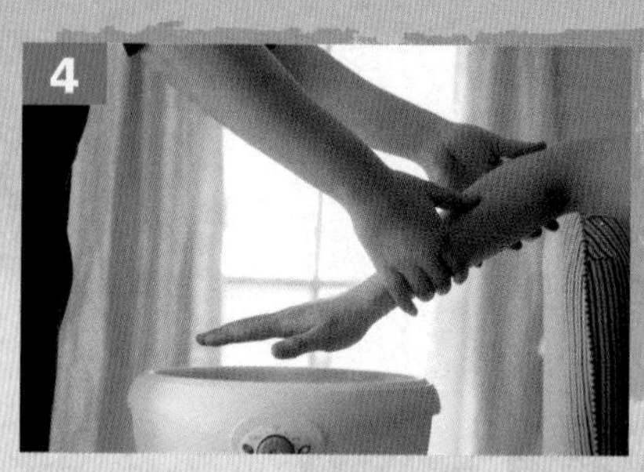

4 Prepare the client's hand for dipping into the paraffin by placing the palm facing down with the wrist slightly bent and the fingers straight and slightly apart.

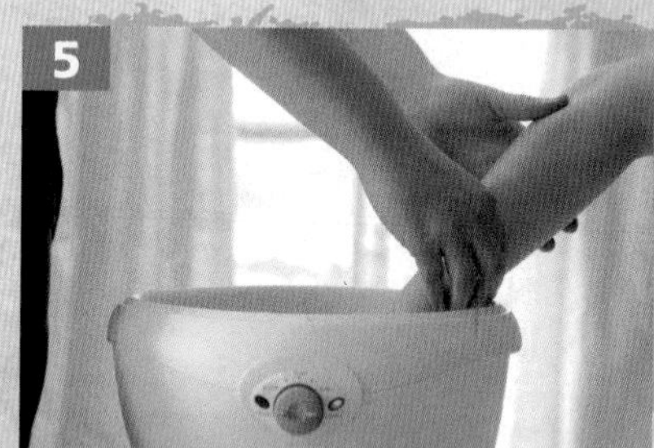

5 Dip the first hand into the wax up to the wrist for about three seconds. Remove. Allow the wax to solidify some before dipping again.

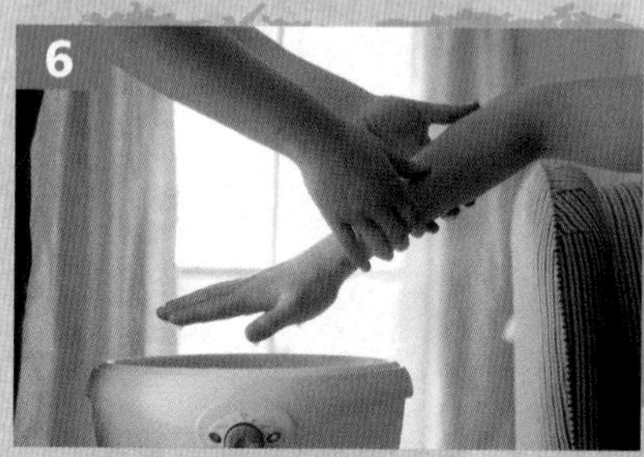

6 Repeat the dip process three to five times on each hand to coat the skin.

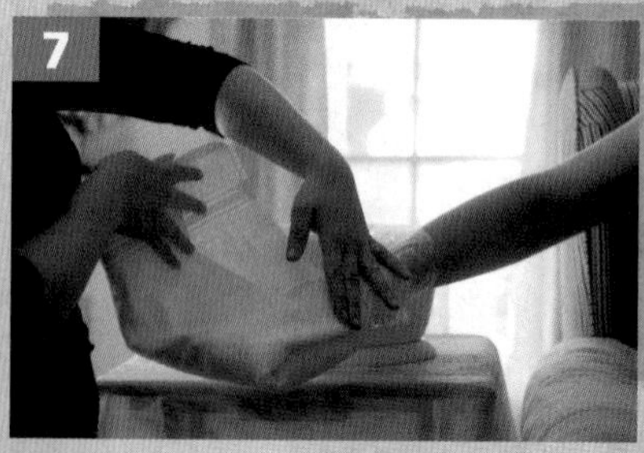

7 Wrap the hands in plastic wrap or insert into plastic mitts designed for this purpose. Then put them into terry cloth or warming (electric) mitts. Allow the paraffin to remain on the hands for approximately five to ten minutes.

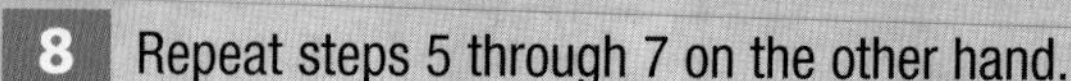

8 Repeat steps 5 through 7 on the other hand.

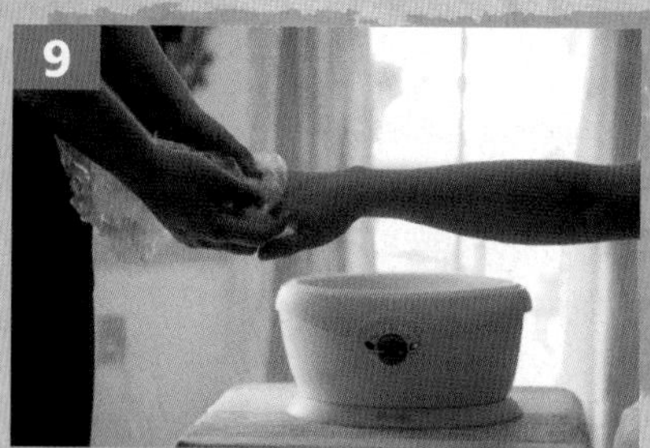

9 To remove the paraffin, turn the plastic cover under at the wrist and peel away at the wrist. The wax will easily come off as you gently pull the cover down the hand to the fingertips. The paraffin removed from the hands will collect in the plastic cover.

© Milady, a part of Cengage Learning. Photography by Yanik Chauvin.

10 Properly dispose of the used paraffin.

11 Begin the manicuring procedure. For many clients who opt to have a paraffin wax treatment before the manicure, soaking is not necessary because the paraffin treatment has already softened the skin sufficiently. ✓ **LO17**

Performing a Paraffin Wax Treatment During a Manicure

1 Perform the basic manicure up to the completion of the massage.

2 Apply a hydrating lotion on one hand and briefly rub it into the hand.

3 Apply the paraffin with your method of choice.

4 Cover the hand with a plastic bag or wrap, then a terry cloth or heated mitt.

5 Repeat steps 1 through 4 on the other hand. Allow the client to relax for five to ten minutes.

6 Remove the paraffin mitt and rub in the remaining lotion.

7 Remove any remaining oils or lotions from the nail plate. Use alcohol or polish remover on a cotton-tipped wooden stick or a cotton ball. Do not allow the alcohol or polish remover on the skin, or the benefits of the treatment will be lessened by the drying effects of these solvents.

8 Polish or clear coat nails, according to client's request.

Performing a Paraffin Wax Treatment as a Stand-Alone Service

- For applying paraffin wax as a stand-alone service, the client must wash her hands. Then you can follow the same steps for Performing a Paraffin Wax Treatment Before a Manicure.

- Complete  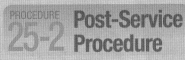

SEE PAGE 821

STATE REGULATORY ALERT

Once paraffin wax is used on a client it becomes contaminated and therefore should never be reused!

Service Tip

If a client is uncomfortable about dipping her hands into the wax bath, there are other ways to apply the wax that will allow it to perform well. Consider the methods below:

- Place about a half cup of paraffin in a plastic bag and insert the client's hand. Then move the wax around the hand, covering the surface.
- Wrap the hands with paraffin-soaked cheesecloth or paper towels. Begin by dipping the cloth into the paraffin bath and allowing the excess paraffin to drip off in the bath. Then, press each piece around the hands until completely covered. Cover the wrap with plastic mitts or plastic wrap.
- Spray paraffin on the hands; then place them in plastic mitts or plastic wrap.
- Purchase one-time-use commercial gloves that heat and have paraffin in them. Merely insert the hands, and the paraffin will heat to become a paraffin mitt.

Review Questions

1. Name the four types of nail implements and/or tools required to perform a manicure.
2. What is the difference between reusable and disposable implements?
3. Why is it important for both the cosmetologist and the client to wash their hands before nail services?
4. Is a consultation necessary each time a client has a service in the salon? Why?
5. Name the basic nail shapes for women.
6. What is the most popular nail shape for men?
7. Which massage movements are most appropriate for a hand and arm massage? Why?
8. What is the difference between a basic manicure and a spa manicure?
9. How is aromatherapy used in manicuring services?
10. Explain the use and benefits of paraffin wax treatments in manicuring.
11. List the correct steps for cleaning and disinfecting nail implements and tools.
12. What is on the manicuring table when it is properly set up?
13. What are the steps in the post-service procedure?
14. What is an exposure incident? If an exposure incident occurs, what steps should be taken?
15. List the steps in the basic manicure.
16. How is nail polish applied properly?
17. What is the procedure for a paraffin wax hand treatment before a manicure?

Chapter Glossary

dimethyl urea hardeners	A hardener that adds cross-links to the natural nail plate. Unlike hardeners containing formaldehyde, DMU does not cause adverse skin reactions.
disposable implements	Also known as *single-use implements*; implements that cannot be reused and must be thrown away after a single use.
essential oils	Oils extracted using various forms of distillation from the seeds, bark, roots, leaves, wood, and/or resin of plants.
fine-grit abrasives	240 grit and higher abrasives designed for buffing, polishing, and removing very fine scratches.
implements	Tools used to perform nail services. Implements can be reusable or disposable.
lower-grit abrasives	Boards and buffers less than 180 grit that quickly reduce the thickness of any surface.
medium-grit abrasives	180 to 240 grit abrasives that are used to smooth and refine surfaces and shorten natural nails.
metal pusher	A reusable implement, made of stainless steel; used to push back the eponychium but can also be used to gently scrape cuticle tissue from the natural nail plate.

Chapter Glossary

microtrauma	The act of causing tiny unseen openings in the skin that can allow entry by pathogenic microbes.
nail clippers	A reusable implement used to shorten the nail plate quickly and efficiently.
nail creams	Barrier products that contain ingredients designed to seal the surface and hold subdermal moisture in the skin.
nail oils	Products designed to absorb into the nail plate to increase flexibility and into the surrounding skin to soften.
nipper	A stainless-steel implement used to carefully trim away dead skin around the nails.
oval nail	A conservative nail shape that is thought to be attractive on most women's hands. It is similar to a squoval nail with even more rounded corners.
paraffin	A petroleum by-product that has excellent sealing properties (barrier qualities) to hold moisture in the skin.
pointed nail	Nail shape suited to thin hands with long fingers and narrow nail beds. The nail is tapered and longer than usual to emphasize and enhance the slender appearance of the hand.
protein hardeners	A combination of clear polish and protein, such as collagen.
reusable implements	Also known as *multiuse implements*; implements that are generally stainless steel because they must be properly cleaned and disinfected between clients.
round nail	A slightly tapered nail shape; it usually extends just a bit past the fingertip.
Scope of Practice	The list of services that you are legally allowed to perform in your specialty in your state.
service sets	Sets of all the tools that will be used in a service.
square nail	A nail shape completely straight across the free edge with no rounding at the outside edges.
squoval nail	A nail shape with a square free edge that is rounded off at the corner edges.
wooden pusher	A wooden stick used to remove cuticle tissue from the nail plate (by gently pushing), to clean under the free edge of the nail, or to apply products.

CHAPTER 26

Pedicuring

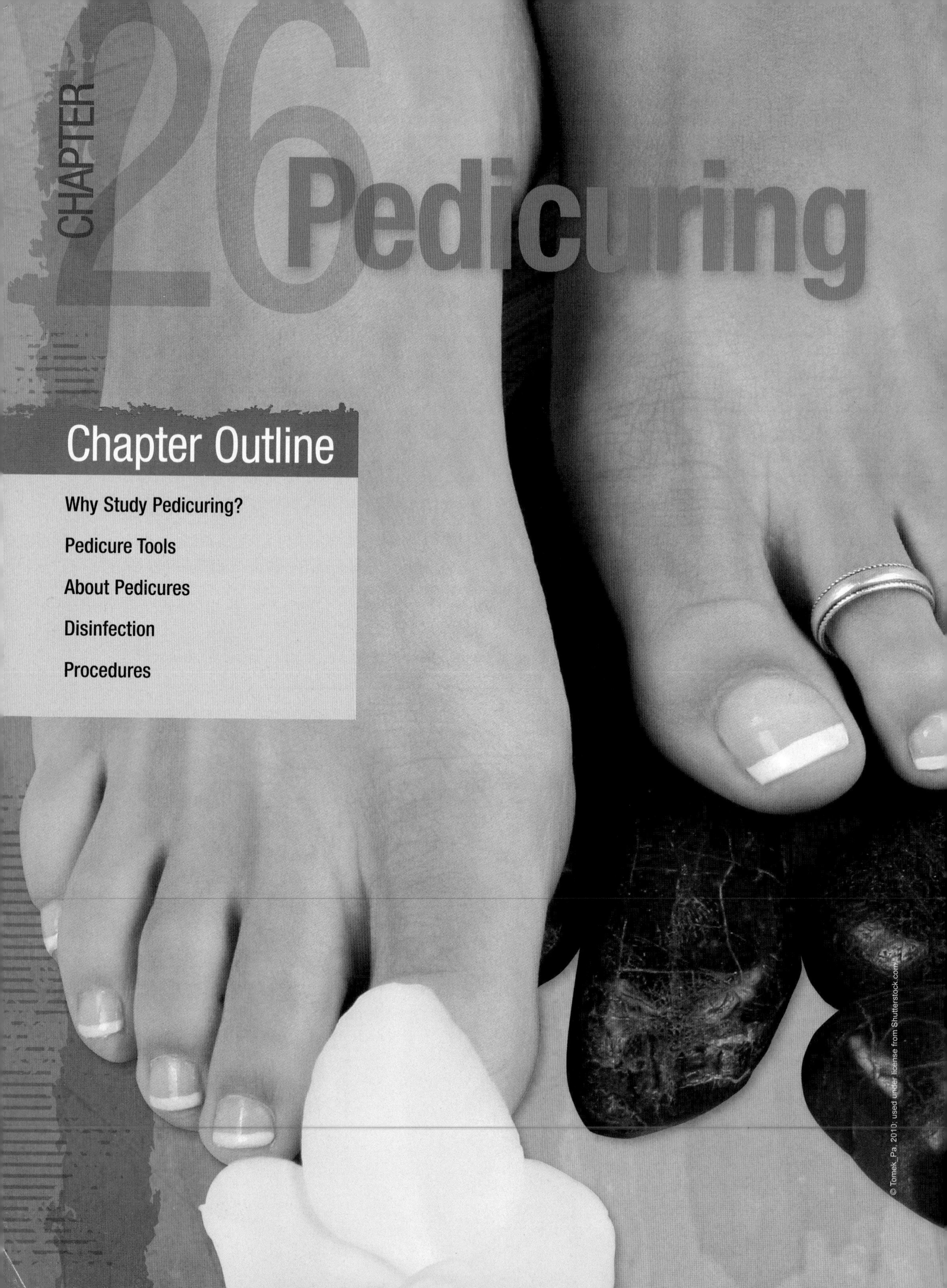

© Tomek_Pa, 2010; used under license from Shutterstock.com

Chapter Outline

Learning Objectives

After completing this chapter, you will be able to:

- ✓ **LO1** Identify and explain the equipment used when performing pedicures.
- ✓ **LO2** Identify and explain three materials used when performing pedicures.
- ✓ **LO3** Describe a callus softener and how it is best used.
- ✓ **LO4** Explain the differences between a basic and a spa pedicure.
- ✓ **LO5** Describe reflexology and its use in pedicuring.
- ✓ **LO6** Know why consistent cleaning and disinfection of pedicure baths must be performed.
- ✓ **LO7** Know and describe the steps involved in the proper cleaning and disinfecting of whirlpool foot spas and air-jet basins.
- ✓ **LO8** Demonstrate the proper procedures for a basic pedicure.
- ✓ **LO9** Demonstrate a foot and leg massage.

Key Terms

Page number indicates where in the chapter the term is used.

callus softeners
pg. 851

curette
pg. 848

exfoliating scrubs
pg. 850

foot file (paddle)
pg. 849

foot soaks
pg. 850

nail rasp
pg. 848

pedicure
pg. 844

reflexology
pg. 858

toe separators
pg. 849

toenail clippers
pg. 847

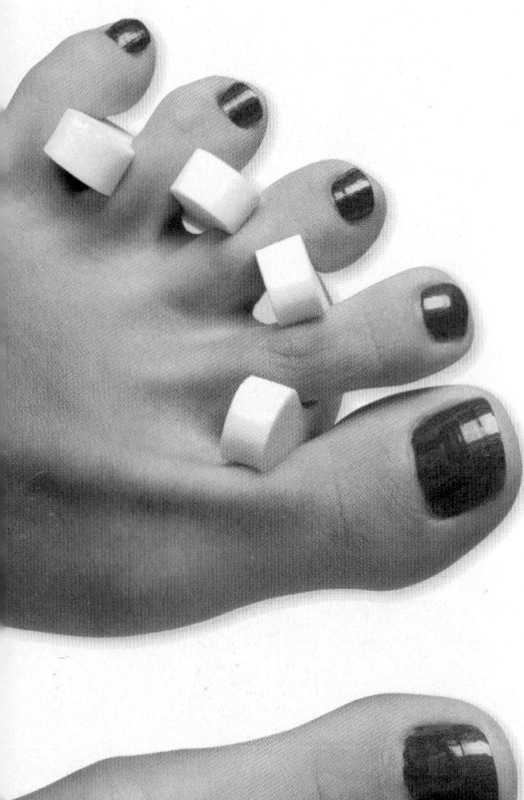

A **pedicure** is a cosmetic service performed on the feet by a licensed cosmetologist or nail technician. Pedicures can include exfoliating the skin, reducing calluses and trimming, shaping, and polishing the toenails. Often pedicures include a foot massage as well. Though pedicures have been performed as foot care since ancient times and in the beauty industry for decades, they were relatively rare even as recently as the late 1980s.

In the 1990s, with the development of the spa industry and new pampering equipment, techniques, and products, pedicures exploded onto service menus and became the fastest-growing service in the industry. Currently pedicures are a regular ritual in many clients' personal-care regimen. Pedicures are now considered a standard service performed in salons by cosmetologists.

The information in this chapter will provide you with the skills you need to perform beautification and routine care on your clients' feet, toes, and toenails. Pedicures are now a basic part of good foot care and hygiene and are particularly important for clients who are joggers, dancers, and cosmetologists—or for anyone who spends a lot of time standing on his or her feet.

Pedicures are not merely manicures on the feet. While they are a similar basic service, they require additional precautions, a specific skill set, and more knowledge of chronic illnesses, disorders, and diseases. Pedicures can cause more damage to clients than manicures. For all of these reasons, experts recommend that you become proficient in performing manicures before learning how to perform pedicures.

Pedicures create client loyalty, produce considerable income, and can be important preventive health services for many clients. In short, pedicure services offer something for everyone. Once your clients experience the comfort, relaxation, and value of a great pedicure they will return for more. For these reasons, you would be wise to perfect your pedicure skills while in school.

© Kirill Zdorov, 2010; used under license from iStockphoto.com.

WHY STUDY PEDICURING?

Cosmetologists should study and have a thorough understanding of pedicuring because:

- It will enable you to add this very desirable service to your service offerings.
- It is important to differentiate between the various pedicure tools and to know how they are properly used.
- It will allow you to perform a pedicure safely and correctly.

Pedicure Tools

In order to perform pedicures safely, you must learn to work with the tools required for this service and to incorporate all safety, cleaning, and disinfection procedures as written in your state's regulations. Pedicures include the standard manicure tools plus a few that are specific to the pedicure service. As with manicures, the four types of nail technology tools that you will incorporate into your services include:

- Equipment
- Implements
- Materials
- Pedicure products

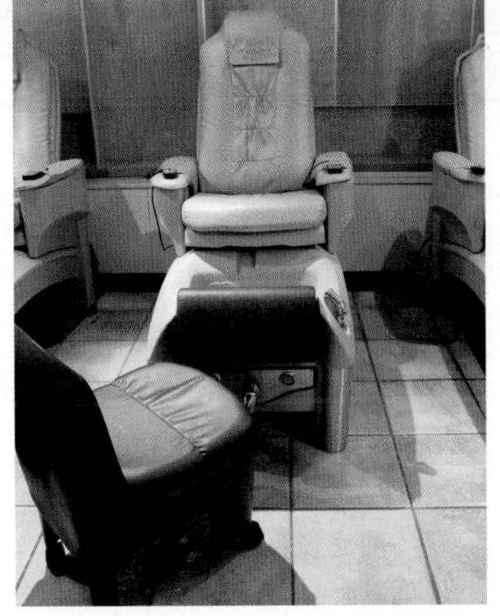
© Milady, a part of Cengage Learning. Photography by Dino Petrocelli.

▲ **Figure 26–1**
Comfortable chair and pedicure chair.

Equipment

Equipment includes all permanent tools, excluding implements, that are used to perform nail services. Some permanent equipment for performing pedicures is different from that used for manicures.

Pedicure Station

Pedicure stations include a comfortable chair with an armrest and footrest for the client and an ergonomic chair for the cosmetologist. Designs vary according to several factors, such as the amount of available space, the availability of water in the salon, and cost (**Figure 26–1**, **Figure 26–2**, and **Figure 26–3**).

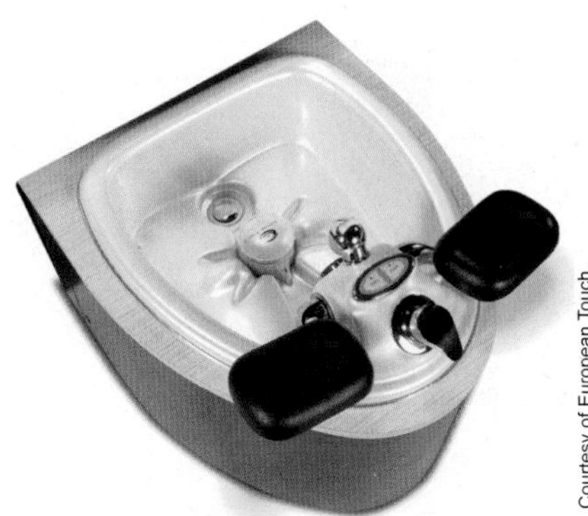
Courtesy of European Touch.

▲ **Figure 26–2**
Sturdy pedicure center with removable foot bath and adjustable footrest.

Pedicure Stool and Footrest

Compared with manicures, pedicures make maintaining healthy posture more challenging for the service provider. The cosmetologist's pedicuring stool is usually low to make it more comfortable and ergonomically correct for the pedicurist to work on the client's feet. Some stools come with a built-in footrest for the client, making it easier for the stylist to reach the client's feet. Alternately, a separate footrest can be used. Your chair must be comfortable and allow ergonomically correct positioning (**Figure 26–4** and **Figure 26–5**).

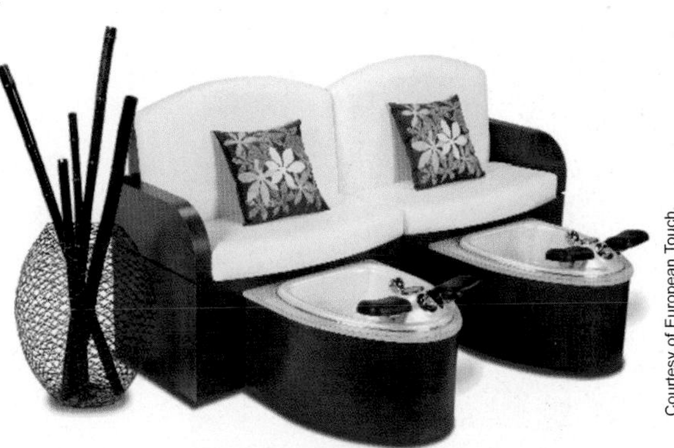
Courtesy of European Touch.

▲ **Figure 26–3**
Fully plumbed station comes with many options.

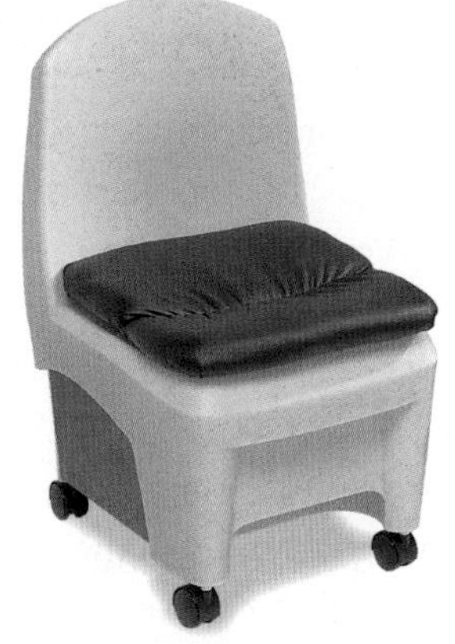
Courtesy of European Touch.

▲ **Figure 26–4**
Low pedicure chair with back support.

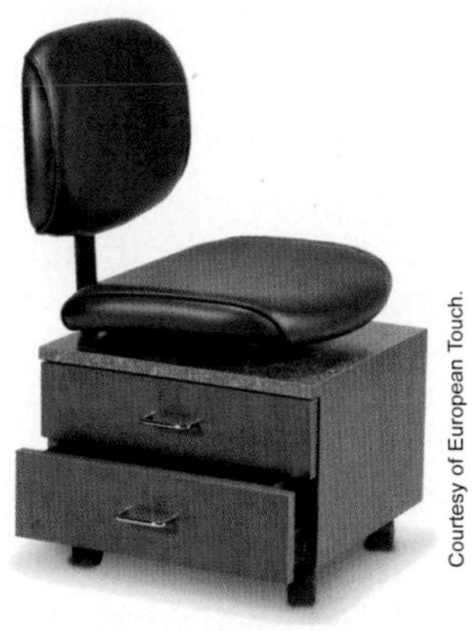
Courtesy of European Touch.

▲ **Figure 26–5**
Pedicure chair with drawers and back support.

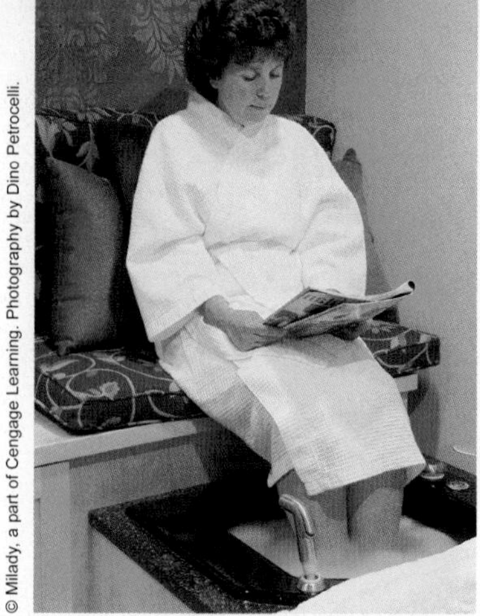

© Milady, a part of Cengage Learning. Photography by Dino Petrocelli.

▲ Figure 26–6
Self-contained foot bath with hose.

Pedicure Foot Bath

Pedicure foot baths vary in design from the basic stainless steel basin to an automatic whirlpool that warms and massages the client's feet. The soak bath is filled with comfortably warm water and a product to soak the client's feet. The bath must be large enough to completely immerse both of the client's feet comfortably.

Basin soak baths can be large stainless steel bowls or beautiful ceramic ones. Small transportable baths can be purchased from retail stores, beauty supply stores, or industry manufacturers. They must be manually filled and emptied for each client's service (**Figure 26–6**).

A step above the portable water baths is the more customized pedicure unit, which has a removable foot bath and the technician's stool built in. Ergonomically, these units are better for the cosmetologist than sitting on the floor to perform the service. A portable pedicure unit includes a place for the foot bath and a storage area for supplies.

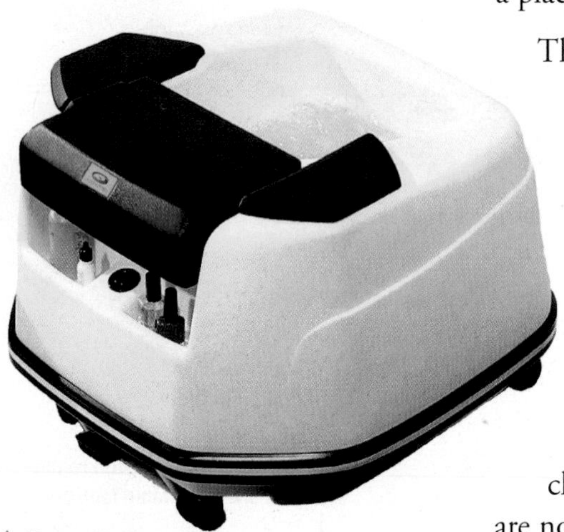

© Courtesy of European Touch.

▲ Figure 26–7
Typical portable foot bath, usually with a whirlpool fan.

The next step up in cost and ease of use is the portable foot basin with built-in whirlpool-action (**Figure 26–7**). These baths add an extra touch to the service by gently massaging the feet with the action of the whirlpool. The bath is filled from the sink through attachable hoses. After the service, the bath is drained by pumping the water back into the sink through the attached hoses. They have built-in footrests, and the surrounding cabinet has areas for storage of pedicure supplies.

The ultimate pedicure foot bath is the fully plumbed pedicure chair, sometimes referred to as a throne-design chair. These units are not portable. They are permanently plumbed to both hot and cold water, as well as to a drain. Most units have a built-in massage feature in the chair and a warmer which adds to the relaxation of the client. Recently, many throne-type chairs with a self-cleaning and disinfection cycle have become available.

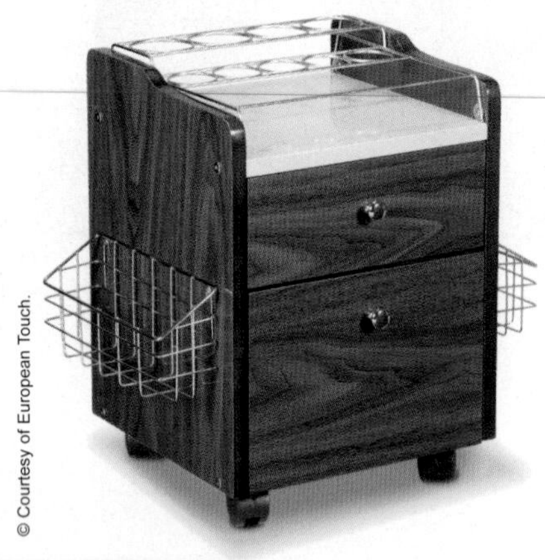

© Courtesy of European Touch.

▲ Figure 26–8
Pedicure cart with drawers.

Pedicure Carts

Pedicure carts are designed to keep supplies organized. There are many different designs available that include a hard surface for placement of your implements and in-service supplies, as well as drawers and shelves for storage of implements, supplies, and pedicure products. Some units include a space for storage of the foot bath. Most take up very little space, and they make it much easier to keep the pedicure area organized (**Figure 26–8**).

Electric Foot Mitts (Optional)

These heated mitts, shaped for the feet but similar to electric manicure mitts, are designed to add a special touch to a more-than-basic pedicure. Pedicures that include the use of heated mitts are a higher-cost service, or their use can be an add-on to a lower-cost service. After a foot massage, a conditioning lotion or a mask is applied to the feet, and then they are placed in a plastic wrap or cover. Last, the feet are placed inside the warm electric foot mitts.

The warmth provided by the mitts helps the conditioning agents of the mask penetrate more effectively, adds to the comfort of the service, and provides ultimate client relaxation.

Terry Cloth Mitts (Optional)

These washable mitts (available for both hands and feet) are placed on a client's feet after a penetrating conditioning product and a cover have been applied. Terry cloth mitts are routinely used over paraffin and a cover because they hold in the heat provided by the warmed paraffin to encourage the product's conditioning of the feet or hands.

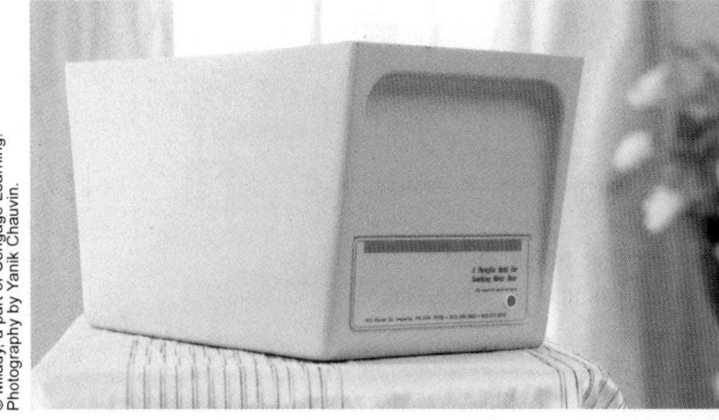
© Milady, a part of Cengage Learning. Photography by Yanik Chauvin.

▲ Figure 26–9
Paraffin foot bath.

Paraffin Bath (Optional)

As discussed in Chapter 25, Manicuring, paraffin is an especially wonderful treatment in a pedicure (Figure 26–9).

Although many clients, salon and spa owners, and cosmetologists prefer other paraffin application methods, the traditional method is to dip and re-dip the hands and feet three to four times into the larger paraffin bath. The paraffin coating covers the skin, sealing the surface of the skin which promotes deeper penetration of previously applied lotions and masks, creating optimum benefits and results from the products. The paraffin bath also stimulates circulation, and the deep heat helps to reduce inflammation and promote circulation to affected joints. Some unique health precautions must be considered for pedicure clients who are chronically ill. Do not provide the paraffin wax treatment to clients with lesions or abrasions, impaired foot or leg circulation, loss of feeling in their feet or legs, or other diabetes-related problems. The skin of elderly clients may be thinner and more sensitive to heat, so a pre-service wax-patch test must be performed to ensure the client will be comfortable having the treatment. ✔ LO1

Implements

The implements mentioned in Chapter 25, Manicuring, are used in pedicures also. There are, however, implements that are specific for use in pedicures. Following is a list of these pedicure-specific implements.

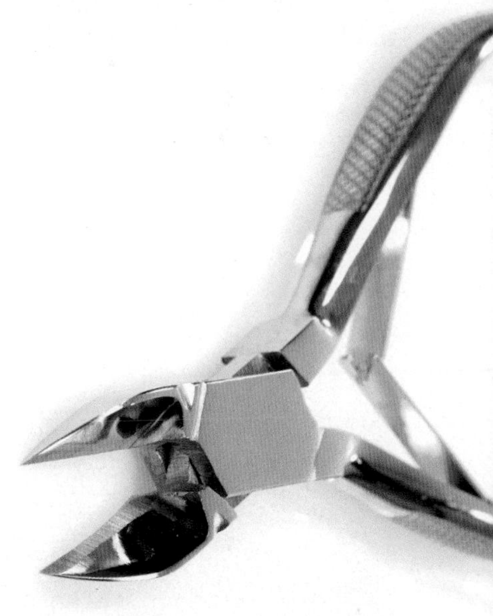
© Peter Zijlstra, 2010; used under license from Shutterstock.com.

Toenail Clippers

Toenail clippers are larger than fingernail clippers, with curved or straight jaws specifically designed for cutting toenails. When performing a pedicure, use only professional toenail clippers. The best clippers for toenails have jaws that are straight and come to a point. Those with blunt points are difficult to use in the small corners of highly curved nail plates. For your client's safety, only use high-quality implements made specifically for performing professional pedicures. They will last longer and make cutting toenails easier for you and safer for your clients.

Curette

A **curette** is a small, scoop-shaped implement used for more efficient removal of debris from the nail folds, eponychium, and hyponychium areas. Curettes are ideal for use around the edges of the big toe nail (**Figure 26–10**). A double-ended curette, which has a 0.06 inch (1.5 mm) diameter on one end and a 0.1 inch (2.5 mm) diameter on the other, is recommended. Some are made with a small hole, making the curette easier to clean after it has been used.

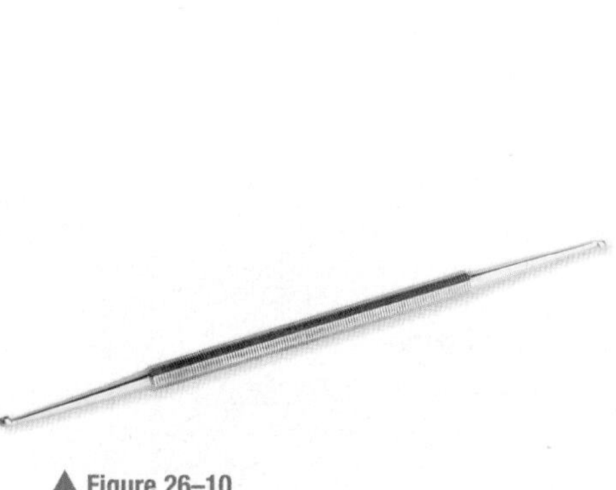

▲ Figure 26–10
Double-ended curette.

Curettes require gentle and careful maneuvers to prevent damage to the skin in the nail folds. Never use curettes to cut out tissue or debris that is adhering to living tissues. Cosmetologists must never use curettes with sharp edges because doing so can result in serious injury. Only those with dull or rounded edges are safe and appropriate for use by cosmetologists.

Nail Rasp

A **nail rasp** is a metal implement with a grooved edge used for filing and smoothing the edges of the nail plate. Ask your instructor to demonstrate its use for you, since it is designed to file in one direction. This implement has a filing surface of about ⅛-inch (3.2 mm) wide and about ¾-inch (19 mm) long attached to a straight or angled metal handle (**Figure 26–11**). The angled file is recommended because it is easier to control under the free edge of the nail.

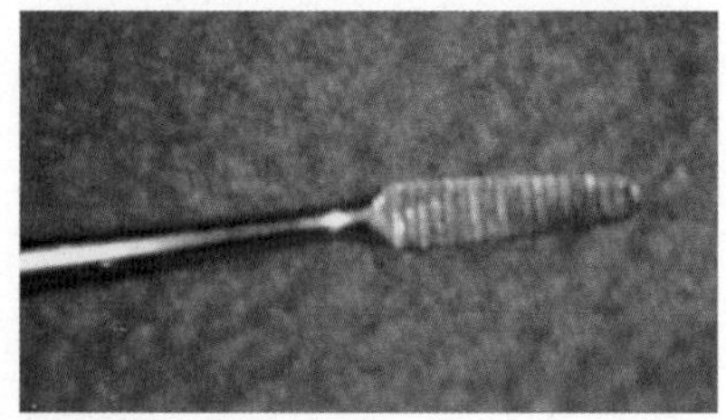

▲ Figure 26–11
Nail rasp.

The file is placed under the nail, angling from the center of the nail out past the side free edge, and then gently pulled toward the center to file free edges that might grow into the tissues, potentially causing an ingrown nail. The filing process may be repeated to make sure there are no rough edges remaining along the free edge. As you become proficient in the use of a nail rasp you will find it to be an invaluable and time-saving implement. Properly used, the nail rasp will add the professional finishing touch required in the care of the toenails. Take special care with this tool and never use it on the top of the nail or past the hyponychium area of the side of the free edge because it can damage the skin and cause infections. Never use it on nails that are already ingrown; refer clients with ingrown toenails to a podiatrist.

Pedicure Nail File

For toenails, a medium grit file will work best for shaping, and a fine grit file will work best for finishing and sealing the edges. Some cosmetologists use a metal file on toenails (**Figure 26–12**). Check with your instructor to find out whether a metal file is legal in your state. Metal files must be either cleaned and then disinfected, or cleaned and then sterilized after each use and before reuse.

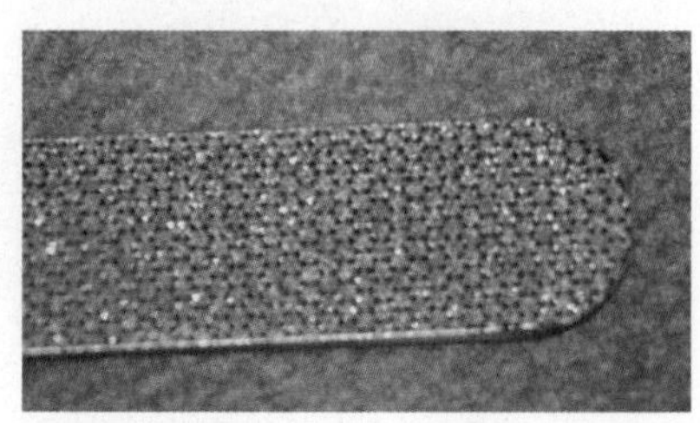

▲ Figure 26–12
Metal abrasive file.

© Milady, a part of Cengage Learning. Photography by Michael Dzaman.

Foot File

A **foot file**, also known as **paddle**, is a large, abrasive file used to smooth and reduce thicker areas of callus (**Figure 26–13**). Foot files come in many different grits and shapes. They must be properly cleaned and disinfected between each use or disposed of after a single use if they cannot be disinfected.

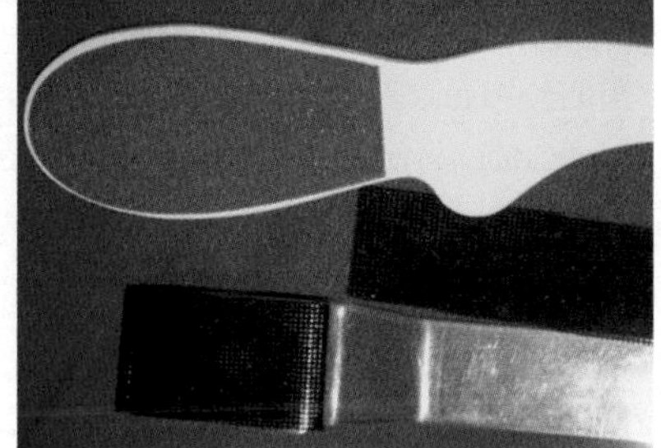

▲ Figure 26–13
Foot files for reducing calluses.

In general, if an abrasive file cannot survive proper cleaning and disinfection procedures without being rendered unusable, it must be considered single-use and be thrown away or given to the client for home use.

Many reasonably priced foot paddles are available for purchase in bulk for single use in pedicures. Foot paddles with disposable and replaceable abrasive surfaces are also available. The handles of these files must be cleaned and disinfected before reuse. Check with your instructor to find out whether these are legal for use in your state.

Nipper

A nipper is an implement used in manicures and pedicures to trim tags of dead skin. Because of the many precautions in performing pedicures, cosmetologists must take great care to avoid cutting, tearing, or ripping living tissue with this implement. Do not use nippers on the feet of clients who have diabetes because the risk of infection, amputation, and even death from accidental injury is great. Also, avoid using nippers on clients with psoriasis since injury to the toenail unit can create new psoriasis lesions where the damage occurs.

Materials

All materials mentioned in Chapter 25, Manicuring, are also used in pedicuring. In addition, a few unique materials are used in this service.

Toe Separators

Toe separators are made of foam rubber or cotton and are used to keep toes apart while polishing the nails. Toe separators are important for performing a quality pedicure (**Figure 26–14**). Since toe separators cannot be cleaned and disinfected, a new set must be used on each client and then thrown away or given to the client for at-home use.

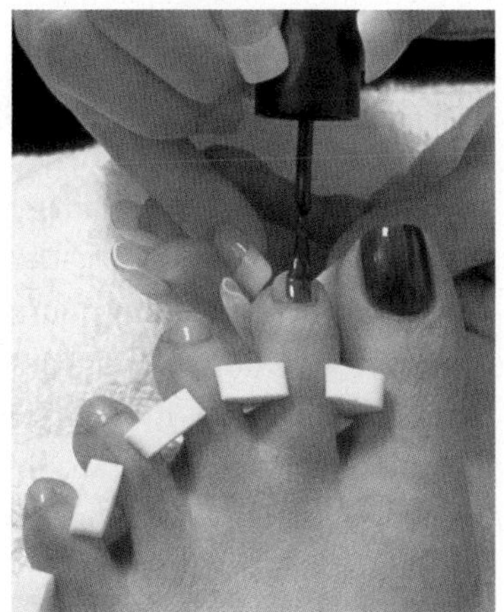

▲ Figure 26–14
Toe separators.

© Milady, a part of Cengage Learning. Photography by Michael Dzaman.

CAUTION

It is illegal for cosmetologists to cut or dramatically reduce calluses on clients unless the cosmetologist is working as an assistant under the direct supervision of a physician or podiatrist. Cutting falls under the category of medical treatment and is not a cosmetic service. For cosmetologists in most states, cutting is considered outside the scope of practice and will be determined so in lawsuits. The service technician may have to explain this truth to some clients who are accustomed to these illegal activities in other salons. Simply say, "I'm sorry, but cutting is a medical treatment and we are not allowed to use blades for that reason. We have excellent products and procedures to reduce calluses without dangerously cutting your skin."

CAUTION

It is especially dangerous to cut into and damage the skin on the feet of immuno-suppressed clients because the healing of their wounds is a slow, sometimes impossible, process. Do not trim cuticles, use metal pushers, or use sharp implements on clients who have any chronic illness. Even a break in the skin that is so tiny it cannot be seen can cause infection, amputation, and even death.

CAUTION

No additive that is added to the water during a pedicure soak kills pathogens and replaces your obligation to clean and disinfect the equipment and implements after the pedicure. Any chemical that is strong enough to adequately kill pathogens is not safe for contact with skin. Disinfectants must never be placed in the foot bath with your client's feet. They can be harmful to the skin.

Pedicure Slippers

Single-use paper or foam slippers are provided for those clients who have not worn open-toed shoes and want to avoid smudging their newly applied toenail polish. They are specially designed not to touch the nails while being worn.

Gloves

Cosmetologists must wear gloves while performing pedicures because repeated exposure to pedicure water can cause extreme dryness and cracking on the hands. Gloves also protect cosmetologists from exposure to pathogens that may be present on the feet or in the water. A new set of gloves is worn for each pedicure and then thrown away. If the client or cosmetologist is allergic to latex, nitrile gloves should be worn. (See Chapter 25, Manicuring, for more information.) ✓ LO2

Professional Pedicure Products

Products for pedicure services include the products discussed in Chapter 25, Manicuring, plus others that are unique to pedicuring. These new product types are:

- Soaks
- Scrubs
- Masks
- Pedicure lotions and creams
- Callus softeners

Foot Soaks

Foot soaks are products containing gentle soaps, moisturizers, and other additives that are used in the pedicure bath to cleanse and soften the skin. A good foot soak product is gentle but effective and thoroughly cleans and deodorizes the feet. It is better to use professionally formulated products because they are designed to properly cleanse without being overly harsh to the skin. Other ingredients may include moisturizing oils with aromatherapy qualities. The soak sets the stage for the rest of the pedicure, so be sure to use a high-quality product to start your pedicure service on a good note.

did you know?

Avoid excessively abrasive scrubs since they may leave tiny, invisible scratches on clients' skin that can be portals of entry for pathogenic microorganisms. Portals of entry are openings in the skin caused by damage during a professional service.

Exfoliating Scrubs

These gritty lotions are massaged on the foot and leg to remove dry, flaky skin and reduce calluses. They leave the skin feeling smoother and moisturized. **Exfoliating scrubs** are usually water-based lotions that contain an abrasive as the exfoliating agent. Sea sand, ground apricot kernels, pumice, quartz crystals, jojoba beads, and polypropylene beads are all exfoliating agents that may be found in pedicure scrubs. Scrubs also contain moisturizers which help to condition the skin. Cosmetologists must wear gloves when using these products as repeated use will irritate the skin on the hands.

Masks

Masks are concentrated treatment products often composed of mineral clays, moisturizing agents, skin softeners, aromatherapy oils, extracts, and other beneficial ingredients to cleanse, exfoliate, tighten, tone, hydrate, and nourish the skin. They are highly valued by clients. Masks are applied to the skin and left in place for five to ten minutes to allow penetration of beneficial ingredients. Menthol, mint, cucumber, and other ingredients are very popular in foot-care masks.

Foot Lotions or Creams

Lotions and creams are important to condition and moisturize the skin of the legs and feet, to soften calluses, and to provide slip for massage. They are also formulated as home-care products for maintenance of the service and improvement of the skin. Cosmetologists who work in a podiatry or medical office will be introduced to treatment-level lotions and creams that are associated with the improvement of medical conditions of the feet. Whether you work in a salon, spa, or medical office, get to know your product line well in order to recommend products to aid the client in maintaining the pedicure benefits.

Callus Softeners

Professional strength **callus softeners** are products designed to soften and smooth thickened tissue (calluses). They are applied directly to the client's heels and over pressure-point calluses. They are left on for a short period of time, according to the manufacturer's directions. After the product softens the callus, it is more easily reduced and smoothed with files or paddles. ✓ LO3

CAUTION

Cuticle removers and callus softeners are potentially hazardous to the eyes. For that reason, safety glasses should be worn whenever using or pouring them. Be sure to wear gloves during their use. Used improperly, these products may cause severe irritation to the cosmetologist's eyes, hands, and skin. Used correctly, they are safe and effective.

About Pedicures

Pedicures have become a part of the American lifestyle to the extent that many people get pedicures more often than they have their hair cut. These clients are as choosy about their pedicure as they are about other salon services. As with most beauty procedures, a pedicure is a service that must be practiced and perfected. You must continually search for education and new ideas to keep up with the changes.

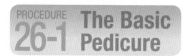

SEE PAGE 863

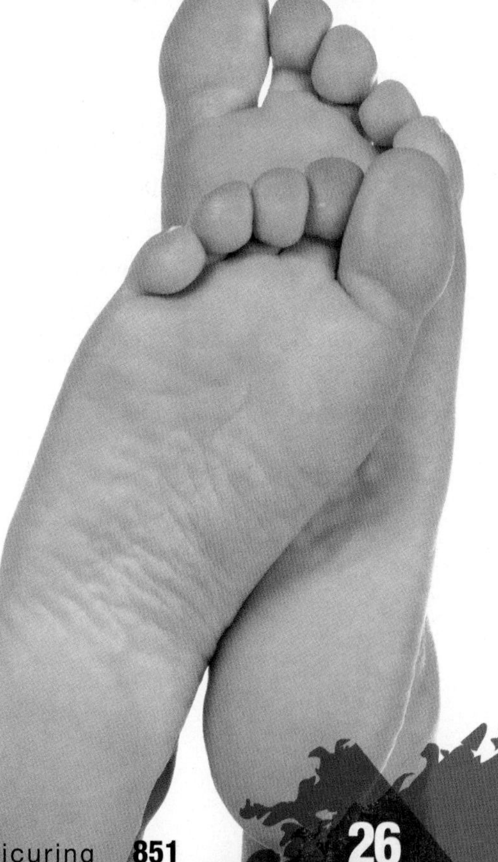

Choosing Pedicure Products

Many pedicure products are available, but the most synergistic ones (those designed to work well together) are developed systems or lines.

© newphotoservice, 2010; used under license from Shutterstock.com.

did you know?

Podiatrists and physicians know that at-risk patients are having, or are interested in having, pedicures. Knowing that these patients are extremely susceptible to infection and that they have poor healing capabilities, many doctors are hiring or referring patients to specially trained pedicure professionals.

These licensed professionals have taken advanced education to learn to perform safe pedicures on at-risk patients. If you are interested in a specialty in nail technology, you might consider becoming an Advanced Nail Technician (ANT). An ANT is a salon-based nail technician who has completed advanced training in how to work safely on at-risk patients. Podiatrists and physicians refer their patients to ANTs for pedicures, feeling confident that the patients will be safe from harm and infection.

Another specialty, the Medical Nail Technician (MNT), may be available for cosmetologists who wish to work in medical offices and who have taken extensive training. These new specialties take nail care to a whole new level and expand professional possibilities for cosmetologists interested in specializing in nail care.

After licensing is achieved, certification courses are usually considered continuing education. They are not licenses.

These products provide the fastest and easiest way to develop an optimal pedicure service. They are available from many manufacturers of professional nail and foot products. Before choosing any one line, check out a variety of product lines, compare them, and then decide for yourself which line is best for your clients.

Always check the quality of the company's educational support and its commitment to the cosmetologists using its products. Find other cosmetologists who use the products and discuss the quality of the company's customer service and its shipping competence, and listen closely to their experiences. Look at your research and make the decision based on which company best meets your and your clients' needs.

When using a manufacturer's product line, follow its recommendations and suggested procedures, because these methods have been tested and found to enhance the effectiveness of the product line.

Service Menu

Tailor your foot-care menu of services to meet the lifestyle and requests of your clientele. For example, younger clients will probably love nail art, while the older clients are more likely to enjoy paraffin wax treatments.

Shorter services are great menu expanders. Not all clients will want or need a full pedicure. Some clients may only want or need a professional nail trimming. Others may want a pampering massage appointment between their full pedicure services to relieve tension and stress. Some may only want a polish change. List these additional services on your menu with your full pedicures to provide options for your clients.

Interaction During the Service

During the procedure, discuss with your client the products that are needed to maintain the pedicure between salon visits. However, only talk to clients who wish to have a discussion. Clients who want to drift off should be allowed the peace and tranquility they are seeking. If this is the case, discuss your product recommendations during polishing or when closing the service. Remember to keep your conversations professional; never discuss personal issues.

Pedicure clients are often in the salon to relax and be pampered. Offer them refreshment and suggest they sit back and relax. Then smile and start the service. There should be no distractions, such as phone calls, others talking with the service provider, and so on, for you or the client during the pedicure. In addition to the foot care provided during a pedicure, clients purchase this service because of the relaxation it provides. Distractions prevent this from happening.

To grow your clientele, you must encourage your clients to schedule regular, monthly pedicures. The accepted time between pedicure appointments is generally four weeks because of the slow growth of the toenails. Mention that their feet are in constant use and need routine maintenance. Remind them that proper foot care, through pedicuring, improves both personal appearance and basic foot comfort.

FYI

When you are performing a pedicure, the foot should be grasped between the thumb and fingers at the mid-tarsal area. The thumb is on the bottom of the foot, while the fingers are wrapped around the dorsal side of the foot. This positioning accomplishes two things:

- It locks the foot into place, allowing the cosmetologist control of its movements.
- A gentle though firm grip has a calming effect on the client and overcomes apprehension in those who dislike their feet being touched.

Never hold the foot lightly or loosely as it can cause a ticklish sensation in many people. Most clients will accept and tolerate a firm, comfortable grip on the foot even if they are ticklish.

Scheduling

When scheduling a client for a pedicure over the telephone, warn female clients not to shave their legs within the forty-eight hours before the pedicure. Why? Shaving the legs increases the presence of tiny microscopic abrasions, and shaving within forty-eight hours before a pedicure may allow portals of entry for pathogenic microbes, increasing the risk of stinging, irritation, or infection. This is an important infection control policy.

To help uphold the policy, post a tasteful sign with the same message in the pedicure area, and place it on your service menu and Web site where your pedicures are listed. Then, before you place your client's feet in the pedicure soak, ask her when she last shaved her legs—if it was within the last forty-eight hours, reschedule the appointment. It is the responsible thing to do. Additionally, when clients are scheduling a pedicure appointment, suggest they wear open-toed shoes or sandals so that polish will not be ruined following the service. Many spas provide single-use pedicure slippers for those who forget to wear open-toed sandals, but a reminder during scheduling is usually appreciated. After all, the appearance of their polish is a priority to most pedicure clients.

© Gubcio, 2010; used under license from iStockphoto.com.

It is important to schedule appointments for the proper length of time, and it is important for the technicians to stay on time. Clients dislike waiting, so you should learn the time that it takes to perform individual steps (toenail shortening, cuticle removal, massage, callus reduction) as assigned on the service menu. Then, practice to meet those times. Knowing where you should be in a service at a specific time also helps you start your next client on time. For example, you must be polishing forty-five to fifty minutes after beginning a one-hour pedicure in order to be on time.

The basic pedicure in most salons does not include a leg massage; a spa pedicure usually does. Pedicures that include leg massages are longer, more upscale and more expensive services. Therefore, they require and deserve additional time. The basic pedicure may be forty-five-minutes, but the spa pedicure, with an added mask and leg massage—perhaps even a paraffin wax service—will be much longer, possibly even half an

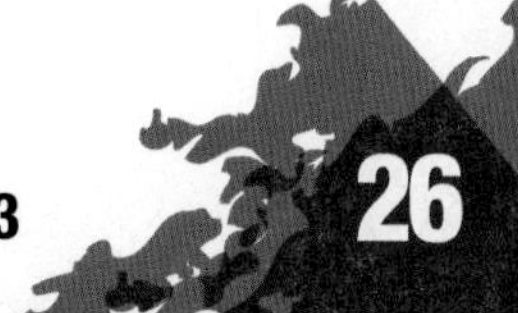

hour longer, depending upon the additional services and how luxurious they might be. Do not cram too much into a pedicure or the experience will not be relaxing for your client or enjoyable for you as a service provider. Rushing through a pedicure may even cause you backaches.

If you time your services appropriately, clients will believe they are receiving better services. As a result, they will be willing to pay what you deserve to receive.

Sometimes when a client books a standard pedicure, his or her feet will be in bad condition requiring more time than was scheduled. When you are completing the client consultation and evaluating the client's feet, you will know quite quickly if this is the case. You must tell this client that you will do the best you can in the time allotted, but he or she must schedule another pedicure very soon in order to get the feet into a condition the client will enjoy. Since clients generally know when they have problem feet, they probably will not be surprised at the need for another appointment and further work. Do not work beyond your scheduled time.

By sticking to the appointment time allotted, you will not only be preserving your schedule, you will also be protecting the client. If the client's feet are in bad shape and you work as long as is necessary to get them in optimal condition in only one service, they may become irritated or painful. The best option is to sell the client home-care products to improve the condition of the feet and schedule another service within one or two weeks.

Series Pedicures

Some improvements in the feet require more than one appointment, this is referred to as a *series*. A situation that may require a series of appointments is callus reduction. When a client comes in with heavy calluses never use a blade. Not only are blades dangerous and a potential cause of infection, but their use is against the law in most states. Using a blade also stimulates heavier growth of calluses as the skin attempts to grow back quickly to protect the damaged skin.

To reduce calluses during a pedicure and to maintain their reduction, perform a safe amount of exfoliation with a scrub. Apply the new, more effective callus reduction products on them and use the foot paddle to remove a safe amount of callus. Explain to the client the negatives regarding rushed removal of calluses. Explain that weekly callus reduction appointments for four to six weeks will lower the calluses and that after that series, the client can receive maintenance pedicures less frequently, about once a month.

© Artbox, 2010; used under license from Shutterstock.com.

© Magdalena Bujak, 2010; used under license from Shutterstock.com.

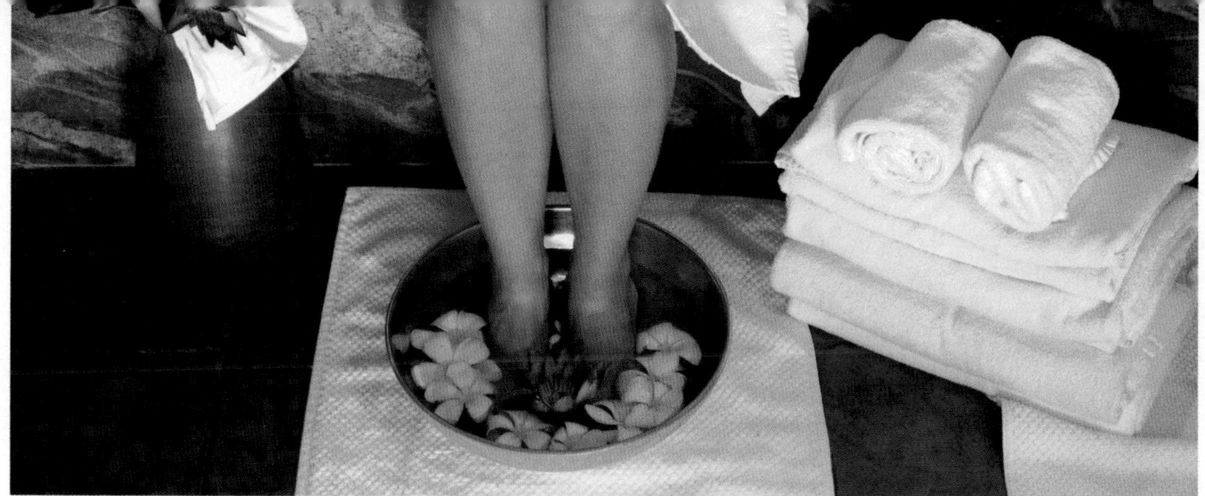

During the series appointments, a full pedicure is not performed between the monthly pedicures; the callus reduction appointment is merely a weekly soak, application of the reduction product for a set time (usually five minutes), reasonable callus reduction, and application of a lotion. It takes about half an hour and should be a less expensive service than an entire pedicure.

At the four-week appointment, a full pedicure is performed with treatments following again. Some clients will require more than the six weeks for a callus reduction series, and this should be explained when the series is suggested. The client can also be sold a glycolic or lactic acid hand and body lotion to use on the feet every other day, and daily use of a lotion containing DMU (Dimethyl urea hardners) should be recommended to soften and prevent the scaly condition from returning. A foot paddle can also be sold to the client for use after showers between treatment appointments. Gloves must be worn during these services.

Another condition that can require weekly treatment is scaly feet. First, however, the client must be sent to a podiatrist to define whether the scaly condition is caused by a fungus. If no fungus is present, the client can return weekly for three to six weeks for a foot exfoliation treatment that includes scrubs and a callus reduction treatment, such as a mask. Remember that masks should be applied all over the feet for one to three minutes, but no longer. These treatments are designed so that the client will have beautiful feet when the series is finished. Home-care products must be recommended to maintain the improved condition.

did you know?

Most salons will have a protocol to follow when finishing services. Follow them closely for two reasons. First, a routine keeps things moving in the salon, and second, clients get used to the closing protocol and know what to expect. If your salon does not have a post-service protocol, or if you work alone, establish one. Clients are more comfortable with a familiar routine.

Spa Pedicure

The pedicure described in Procedure 26–1, The Basic Pedicure, is the basis for all other pedicure services. For example, in the basic pedicure, the massage is performed on the foot only, while in the upgrade to a spa pedicure, the massage is performed on the foot and the lower leg (to the knee).

Another spa pedicure upgrade is the use of a mask on the foot and/or leg. The mask is applied, covered, and allowed to set while the client relaxes and the mask's effectiveness increases. A further upgrade would be the incorporation of special products such as aromatherapy lotions, oils, paraffin, and other specialty products. LO4

Business Tip

You should charge extra for add-on services such as paraffin wax treatments and nail art. Services have dollar value—especially when you consider the time, product expense, skill level, and equipment used. Always be up front about additional service costs, and if a client decides to indulge in one, charge for it.

Elderly Clients

Older people need regular, year-round foot care even more than younger people. Many elderly people cannot reach their feet, cannot see them, or cannot squeeze the nail clippers to trim their own nails. They need continual help in their foot-care maintenance, especially since it can become a health issue. The cosmetologist who offers pedicure services for this segment of the population will be doing these individuals a great service and will find plenty of willing clients in need of their services.

Many of these clients have health issues that require exceptionally gentle care. Never cut their tissues or push back the eponychium as even a microscopic opening, or microtrauma, can be fatal for these clients. Discuss health issues with them; do not perform pedicures on diabetics or on people with circulatory diseases without their physician's permission. Seek training in how to work with these clients, so you will know how to work safely on them.

Pedicure Pricing

Most salons and spas will probably have a price list for services before you join the staff, but you may at some time find yourself in a position to price your own services. In this case, determine the price of your basic pedicure first, and then set your prices for more upscale and luxurious pedicures by increasing the base price of the pedicure according to the value of the added treatments, products, and extra time.

Another great way to upgrade your pedicure service and price is through nail art. Many clients enjoy adding a little something special to their normal pedicure polish, especially if their work prohibits them from wearing polish or art on their hands. It is easy to get your clients addicted to toenail art by giving the first example at no cost. Once they have it and their friends compliment them, they will want it every time, and you will quickly see an increase in revenue with your existing clientele (**Figure 26–15**). Toenail art is especially popular in sandal season and for formal occasions when women often wear open footwear.

Many salons and spas have found that manicure and pedicure packages are well received by their clients and work well for the staff. Manicures and pedicures together are like salt and pepper—although they are different, they go well together.

▼ **Figure 26–15**
Gel toe art.

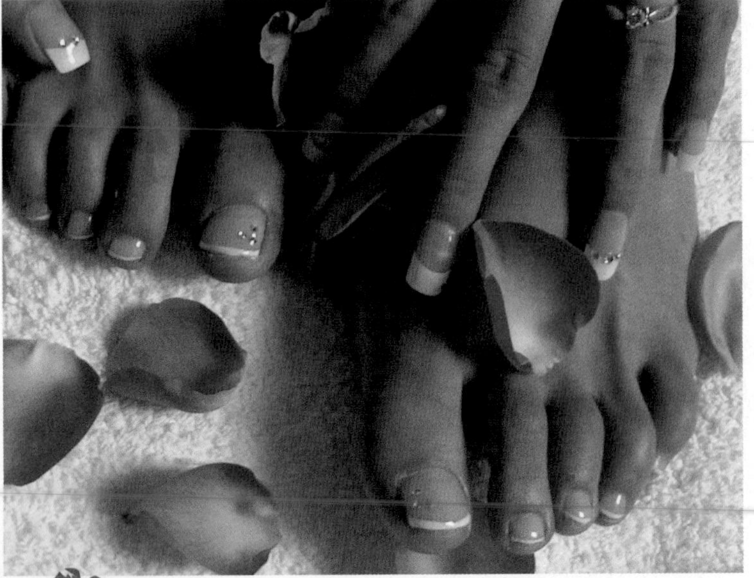

© Courtesy of Noble Nails by Louise Callaway.

One great way to sell these packages is to develop theme services for holidays and special events, such as Christmas, Valentine's Day, Mother's Day, prom, weddings, and birthday packages; market them, and you will see your clientele grow.

Pedicure Massage

According to post-visit client salon surveys, massage is the most enjoyed aspect of any nail service. Because this is especially true for pedicures, you should spend time developing a technique that you will enjoy giving and that your clients will enjoy receiving.

The definition of massage, according to the Merriam-Webster Dictionary, is "a method of manipulation of the body by rubbing, pinching, kneading, tapping." General body massage sometimes has a therapeutic purpose and sometimes focuses on relaxation. However, massage given during manicures and pedicures definitely focuses on relaxation.

The art of massage has a rich and long history. There are many types of massage, and individuals usually develop their own special styles and techniques. No matter what techniques you use, perfect them so foot and leg massage becomes second nature to you. During this part of the pedicure, be keenly aware of your client's health, meet any precautionary requirements, and offer a massage that relaxes the client but is not harmful to him or her.

The foot and leg massage is similar to the hand and arm massage that follows a manicure. The massage technique that is used most is effleurage. This technique is even more important for pedicures than manicures because many clients have circulatory issues that may prevent you from using other massage techniques. During consultation, you must ask clients questions concerning their health. If clients have a circulatory disease, high blood pressure, or other chronic diseases that affect their legs or feet, you must get permission from their physician before providing a full spa pedicure massage.

Most of us enjoy being touched, and the art of massage takes a pedicure to a higher level. Many people think foot massage is more special than

© VladGavriloff, 2010; used under license from Shutterstock.com.

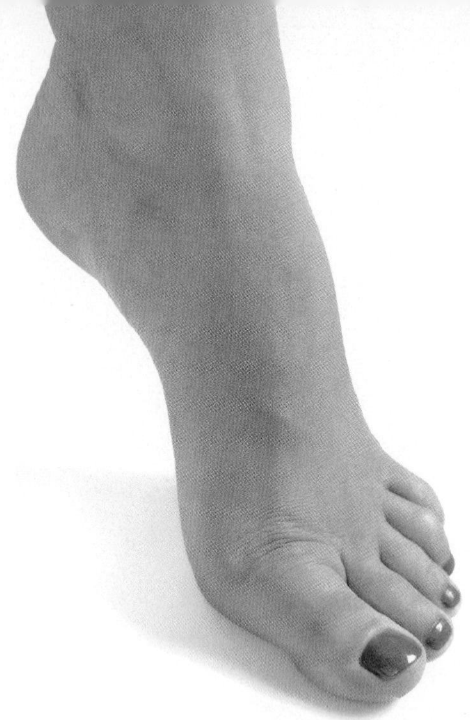

massage on any other part of the body. Foot massage induces a high degree of relaxation and stimulates blood flow. Be aware of the areas of the feet and legs where the client most enjoys massage, and put a greater emphasis in these areas.

Every cosmetologist has his or her own massage style and technique. No matter what you define as yours, perfect it so that it becomes second nature to you.

© Smart-foto, 2010; used under license from Shutterstock.com.

PROCEDURE 26-2 Foot and Leg Massage SEE PAGE 867

Reflexology

Reflexology is a unique method of applying pressure with thumb and index fingers to the hands and feet, and it has demonstrated health benefits. This specialty massage often employs many of the principles of acupressure and acupuncture, and it is considered a science by many technicians.

Reflexology is based on the principle that areas (reflexes) in the feet and hands correspond to all the organs, glands, and parts of the body. Reflexology practitioners believe that stimulating (pressing) these reflexes or points can transmit positive energy and increase blood flow to the specified areas.

Professional, hands-on training is essential in reflexology for two reasons:

- The specific touch used in reflexology can be learned only through hands-on training. Clients who have received a reflexology treatment from a certified expert recognize the appropriate touch and respond negatively to people who attempt reflexology but cannot deliver the same treatment because of minimal or no training.
- An untrained cosmetologist may not be able to produce results for the client, so the client will not be happy about the extra cost and time taken by the service.

If a salon wishes to offer reflexology services, the staff who will perform the services must receive authentic training and certification in the art of reflexology. ✓ LO5

Ergonomics

Pedicures can pose a threat to the health and well-being of cosmetologists who perform them. If technicians are careless about protecting themselves through proper ergonomics, they can develop serious and painful back conditions.

Pay attention to your body's positioning and make sure you are working ergonomically. Always sit in a comfortable position, relaxed and unstrained, to reduce the risk of injury to your back, shoulders, arms, wrists, and hands. For example, avoid leaning forward or stretching to reach your client's feet. Take a minute to stretch before and after each pedicure to keep your body limber, in-line, and more resistant to injury.

Although it is important to give your client the best possible service, it is also important to keep yourself healthy during the process and to avoid injuries caused by strain or repeated motion.

Disinfection

Disinfection of the pedicure bath has been discussed and sensationalized in the media—and for good reason. There are specific criteria and steps that must be followed exactly to ensure proper disinfection and infection control. Improper, rushed, or careless cleaning of the pedicure bath may lead to health and safety concerns for salon clients. The salon and the individual technician bear the responsibility for ensuring that proper disinfection occurs and that proper procedures are followed.

The following cleaning and disinfecting procedures are recommended for all types of pedicure equipment by the Nail Manufacturer's Council (NMC), a group of nail-care company representatives, and the International Nail Technicians Association (INTO), a group of professional nail technicians:

- whirlpool units
- pipeless and all non-whirlpool basins
- bowls
- air-jet basins
- sinks
- tubs

In addition, salons must always use an EPA-registered hospital disinfectant that the label claims is a broad spectrum bactericide, virucide, and fungicide. For accountability purposes, most states require salons to record the time and date of each disinfecting procedure in a pedicure or a disinfection log.

Salon teams should incorporate the disinfection procedures discussed in Chapter 5, Infection Control: Principles and Practices, as well as those on the following pages, into their regular cleaning and disinfecting schedules. These procedures should be displayed in employee areas. Always check your state regulations concerning the required disinfection protocol. ✓ LO6

WEB RESOURCES

For more information concerning disinfection and other important topics pertaining to nails, go to http://www.probeauty.org/research. This site contains many informational brochures, relevant to manicuring and pedicuring. The brochures which are published in several languages, including Vietnamese and Spanish, are written by the leading scientists and technical experts in the industry, and are reviewed by other industry leaders before being published.

Disinfection of Whirlpool Foot Spas and Air-Jet Basins

After Every Client:

1. Drain all water from the basin.
2. Scrub all visible residue from the inside walls of the basin with a brush and liquid soap and water. Use a clean and disinfected brush with a handle. Brushes must be cleaned and disinfected after each use.
3. Rinse the basin with clean water.

4. Refill the basin with clean water and circulate the correct amount (according to the mixing instructions on the label) of the EPA-registered hospital disinfectant through the basin for ten minutes.
5. Drain, rinse, and wipe the basin dry with a clean paper towel.

At the End of Every Day:

1. Remove the screen and any other removable parts. (A screwdriver may be necessary.)
2. Clean the screen and other removable parts and the area behind these with a brush and liquid soap and water to remove all visible residues. Replace the properly cleaned screen and other removable parts.
3. Fill the basin with warm water and chelating detergent (a detergent designed for use in hard water), and circulate the chelating detergent through the system for five to ten minutes (following the manufacturer's instructions). If excessive foaming occurs, discontinue circulation and let soak for the remainder of the time, as instructed.
4. Drain the soapy solution and rinse the basin.
5. Refill the basin with clean water and circulate the correct amount (according to the mixing instructions on the label) of the EPA-registered hospital disinfectant through the basin for ten minutes.
6. Drain, rinse, and wipe the basin dry with a clean paper towel.
7. Allow the basin to dry completely.

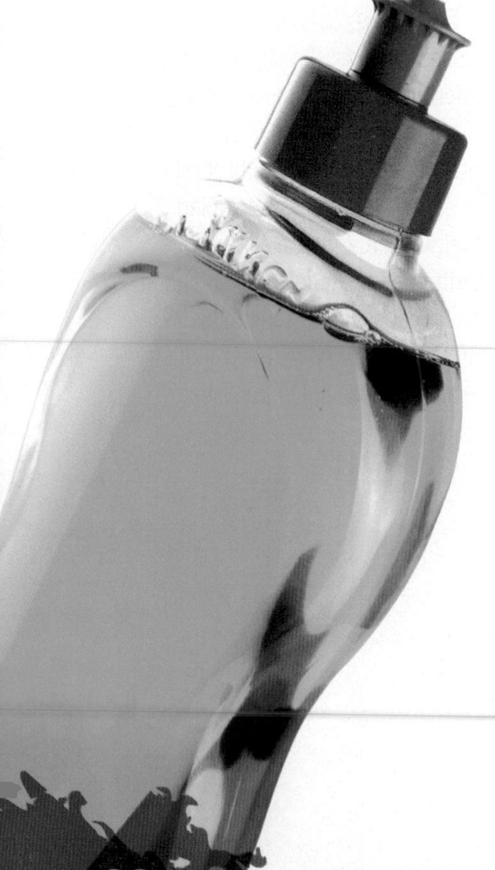

At Least Once Each Week:

1. Drain all water from the basin.
2. Remove the screen and any other removable parts. (A screwdriver may be necessary.)
3. Clean the screen and other removable parts and the area behind these with a brush and liquid soap and water to remove all visible residues. Replace the properly cleaned screen and other removable parts.
4. Scrub all visible residue from the inside walls of the basin with a brush and liquid soap and water. Use a clean and disinfected brush with a handle. Brushes must be cleaned and disinfected after each use.
5. Fill the basin with clean water and circulate the correct amount (according to the mixing instructions on the label) of the EPA-registered hospital disinfectant through the basin.

© Gregory Gerber, 2010; used under license from Shutterstock.com.

6. Do not drain the disinfectant solution. Instead, turn the unit off and leave the disinfecting solution in the unit overnight.
7. In the morning, drain and rinse.
8. Refill the basin with clean water and flush the system.

LO7

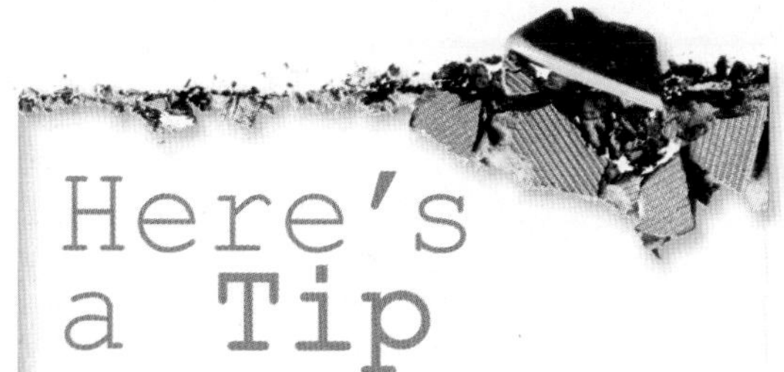

Here's a Tip

Think that you don't have ten minutes between pedicures to disinfect? Try this: before reaching for the massage lotion, clean the basin or foot spa and fill with water and disinfectant solution. Or, if the client is receiving a foot mask, use the mask time to clean the tub, refill it with water, and put in the disinfectant. The disinfectant can remain in the basin while you complete the pedicure, meeting the time requirement for disinfection. This minimizes the procedure time, keeps you on schedule, and allows the client to see you disinfect the tub, which will give them confidence that you consistently provide safe services.

Disinfection of Pipeless Foot Spas

This process is for units with footplates, impellers, impeller assemblies, and propellers.

After Every Client:

1. Drain all water from the basin.
2. Remove impeller, footplate, and any other removable components according to the manufacturer's instructions.
3. Thoroughly scrub impeller, footplate, and/or other components and the areas behind each with a liquid soap and a clean, disinfected brush to remove all visible residues. Then reinsert impeller, footplate, and/or other components.
4. Refill the basin with water and circulate the correct amount (according to the mixing instructions on the label) of the EPA-registered hospital disinfectant through the basin for ten minutes.
5. Drain, rinse, and wipe the basin dry with a clean paper towel.

At the End of Every Day:

1. Fill the basin with warm water and chelating detergent, and circulate the chelating detergent through the system for five to ten minutes (following manufacturer's instructions). If excessive foaming occurs, discontinue circulation and let soak for the remainder of the ten minutes.
2. Drain the soapy solution and rinse the basin.
3. Refill the basin with clean water and circulate the correct amount (according to the mixing instructions on the label) of the EPA-registered hospital disinfectant through the basin for ten minutes.
4. Drain, rinse, and wipe the basin dry with a clean paper towel.

At Least Once Each Week:

1. Drain all water from the basin.
2. Remove impeller, footplate, and any other removable components according to the manufacturer's instructions.
3. Thoroughly scrub impeller, footplate, and/or other components and the areas behind each with a liquid soap and a clean, disinfected brush to remove all visible residues, and then reinsert impeller, footplate, and/or other components.

4. Refill the basin with water and circulate the correct amount (according to the mixing instructions on the label) of the EPA-registered hospital disinfectant through the basin for ten minutes.
5. Do not drain the disinfectant solution. Instead, turn the unit off and leave the disinfecting solution in the unit overnight.
6. In the morning, drain and rinse.
7. Refill the basin with clean water and flush the system.

Disinfection of Non-Whirlpool Foot Basins or Tubs

This includes basins, tubs, foot baths, sinks, and bowls—all nonelectrical equipment that holds water for a client's feet during a pedicure service.

After Every Client:

1. Drain all water from the foot basin or tub.
2. Clean all inside surfaces of the foot basin or tub with a clean, disinfected brush and liquid soap and water to remove all visible residues.
3. Rinse the basin or tub with clean water.
4. Refill the basin with clean water and the correct amount (according to the mixing instructions on the label) of the EPA-registered hospital disinfectant. Leave this disinfecting solution in the basin for ten minutes.
5. Drain, rinse, and wipe the basin dry with a clean paper towel.

At the End of Every Day:

1. Drain all water from the foot basin or tub.
2. Clean all inside surfaces of the foot basin or tub with a brush and liquid soap and water to remove all visible residues.
3. Fill the basin or tub with water and the correct amount (according to the mixing instructions on the label) of the EPA-registered hospital disinfectant. Leave this disinfecting solution in the basin for ten minutes.
4. Drain, rinse, and wipe the basin dry with a clean paper towel.

© Al Rubinetsky, 2010; used under license from Shutterstock.com.

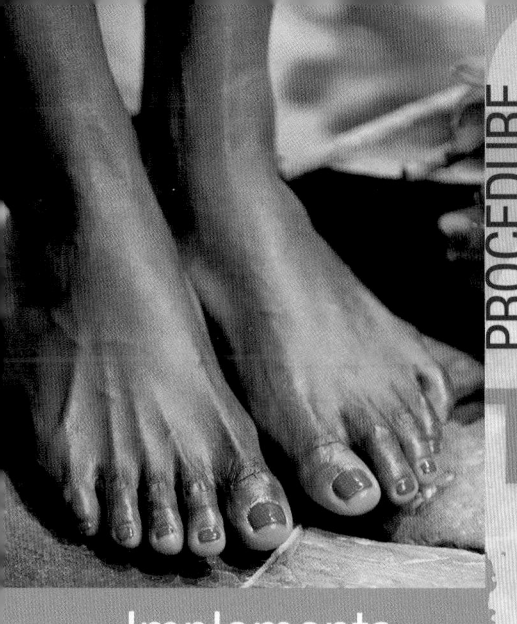

PROCEDURE 26-1 The Basic Pedicure

Implements and Materials

In addition to the basic materials on your manicuring table, you will need the following supplies for the basic pedicure:

- **Callus softeners**
- **Curettes**
- **Electric foot mitts (optional)**
- **Exfoliant**
- **Foot lotions or creams**
- **Foot paddle**
- **Foot soak**
- **Gloves**
- **Nail rasp**
- **Nippers**
- **Paraffin bath (optional)**
- **Pedicure basin or foot bath**
- **Pedicure nail files**
- **Pedicure slippers**
- **Terry cloth mitts (optional)**
- **Toe separators**
- **Toenail clippers**

© Milady, a part of Cengage Learning. Photography by Dino Petrocelli.

Preparation

- Perform PROCEDURE 25-1 **Pre-Service Procedure** SEE PAGE 817

Procedure

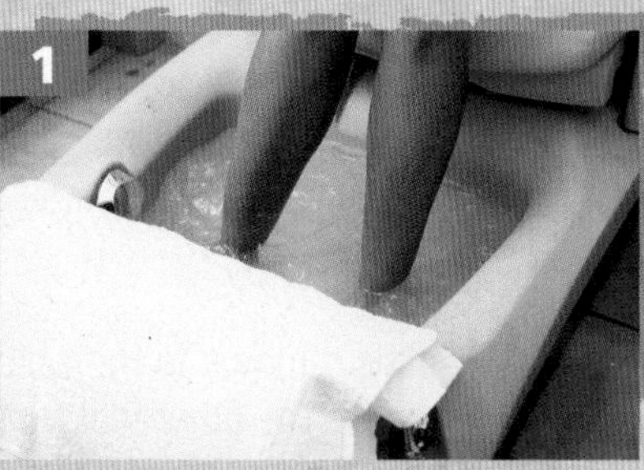

1 Put on a pair of clean gloves and check the temperature of the pedicure bath for safety. Place the client's feet in the bath, and make sure she is comfortable with the water temperature. Allow the feet to soak for five minutes to soften and clean the feet before beginning the pedicure.

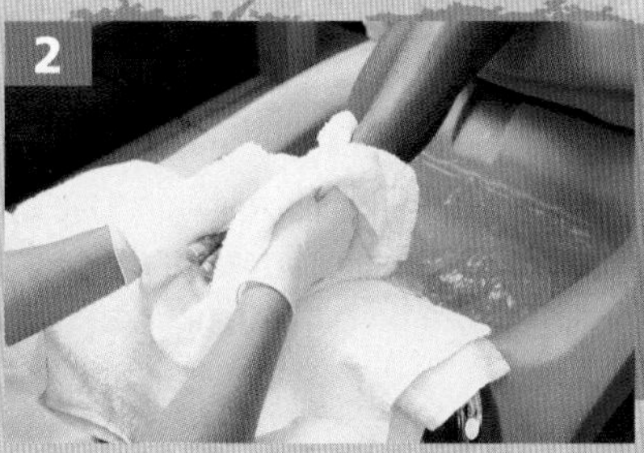

2 Lift one of the client's feet from the bath. Wrap the first towel around the foot and dry it thoroughly. Make sure you dry between the toes. Place the foot on the footrest or on a towel you have placed on your lap.

3 First, remove polish from the little toe and move across the foot toward the big toe. Complete polish removal is important to a quality pedicure finish.

Service Tip

Work on the foot on the client's nondominant side first. (The dominant side of the body is determined by the side of the client's writing hand.) The foot on the client's dominant side usually needs more soaking and attention. It needs to soak those few extra minutes while you are working on the other foot.

The Basic Pedicure continued

CAUTION

Take care not to clip the nails too short and not to break the seal of the hyponychium, an important protection of the toenail unit from infection.

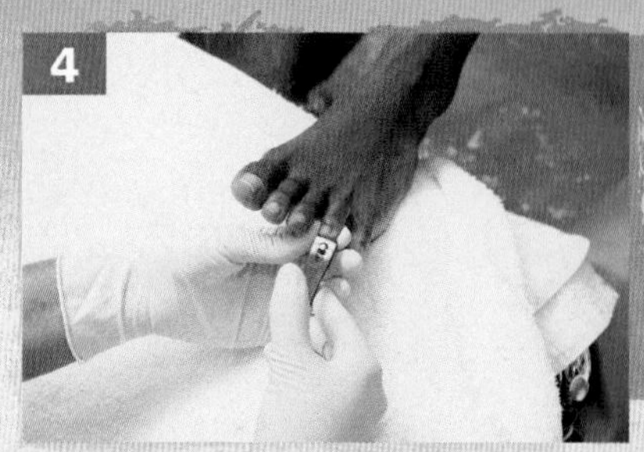

4 Carefully clip the toenails of the first foot straight across and even with the end of the toes. The big toenail is usually the most challenging to trim. Do not leave any rough edges or "hooks" that might create an opportunity for infections.

5 Carefully use the foot rasp, if needed. The rasp is narrow and will only file the nail in one direction. It can be used to remove, smooth, and round off any sharp points on the free edges that might eventually cause infection. Do not probe with the rasp or point the tip toward the hyponychium. Gently draw it along the side free edge that you have just trimmed. Small, short strokes with the file will accomplish the task.

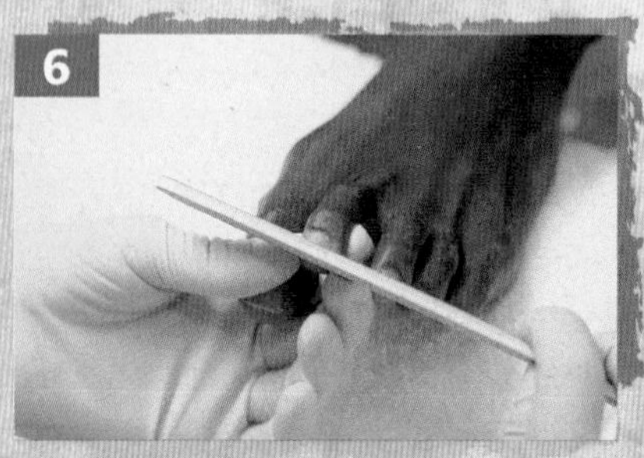

6 Carefully file the nails of the first foot with an appropriate single-use and prepped abrasive file. File them straight across, rounding them slightly at the corners. Smooth rough edges with the fine side of an abrasive file.

7 Apply callus remover to the calluses, wrap the foot in a towel, and lay it aside. Remove the other foot from the water and perform steps 2 through 7 on that foot.

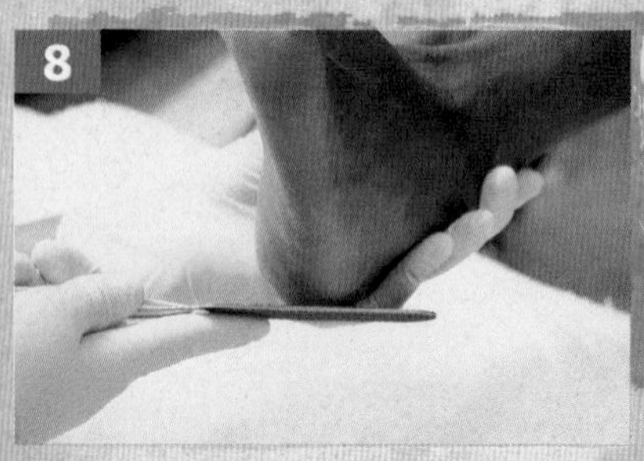

8 Remove the first foot from the towel wrap; use a wooden pusher to gently remove any lose, dead tissue. Next, exfoliate the foot with a scrub to remove the dry or scaly skin. Use extra pressure on the heels and other areas where more calluses and dry skin build up. Next, use a foot file to smooth and reduce the thicker areas of calluses.

9 Place the first foot in the foot bath and rinse off the cuticle softener and callus remover completely. Then, lift the foot to above the water and brush the nails with a nail brush. Remove the foot and dry thoroughly.

10 Repeat steps 8 and 9 on the other foot.

Service Tip

Toe separators can be used to hold the toes apart while filing or applying cuticle remover. Always use new separators for every client.

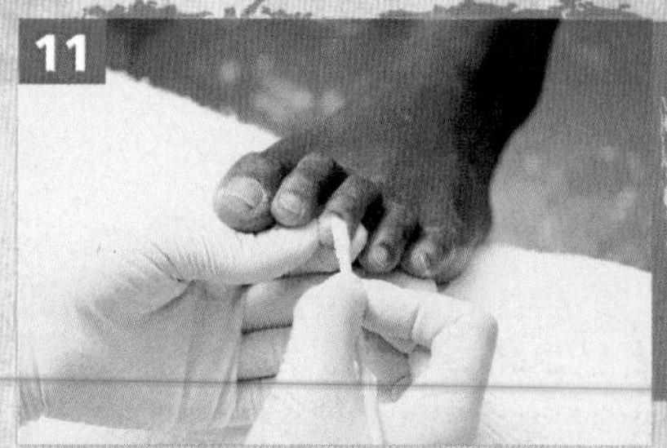

11 Use the single-use cotton-tipped wooden pusher or product dispenser to apply cuticle remover to the second foot. Begin with the little toe and work toward the big toe.

© Milady, a part of Cengage Learning. Photography by Dino Petrocelli.

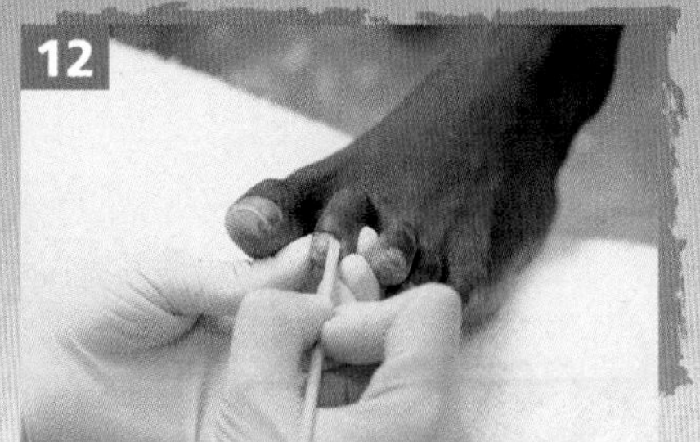

12 Carefully remove the cuticle tissue from the nail plate using a wooden or metal pusher, staying away from the eponychium and taking care not to break the seal between the nail plate and eponychium. Use a nipper to carefully remove any loose tags of dead skin, but don't cut, rip, or tear living skin, since this may lead to serious infections.

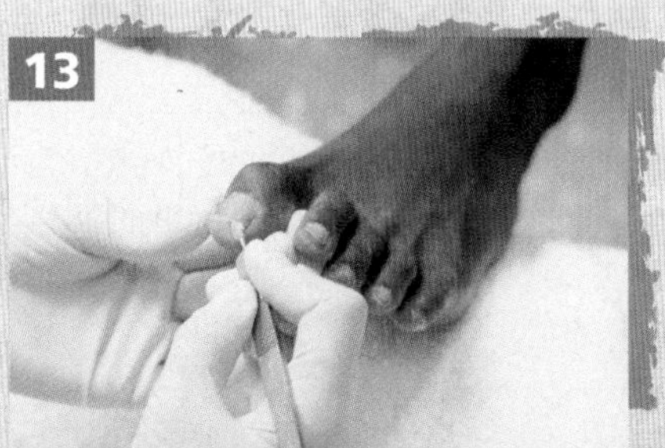

13 Next, if necessary, the curette is used on the first foot to gently push the soft tissue folds away from the walls of the lateral nail plate. This allows you to visually inspect the nail plate and the surrounding tissue. If there is extra buildup of debris between the nail plate and surrounding tissue, it should be gently removed with the curette. To use this implement, place the rounded side of the spoon toward the sidewall of living skin. A gentle scooping motion is then used along the nail plate to remove any loose debris. Take care not to overdo it. Do not use this implement to dig into the soft tissues along the nail fold as injury may occur. If the tissue is inflamed (i.e., ingrown toenail), the client must be referred to a qualified medical doctor or podiatrist.

14 Dip your client's first foot into the foot bath. With the foot over the foot bath, again brush it with the nail brush to remove bits of debris. Dry the foot thoroughly. Wrap it in a towel and perform steps 11 to 13 on the other foot. When finished, wrap that foot in the foot towel and set it aside while performing the coming steps on the first foot.

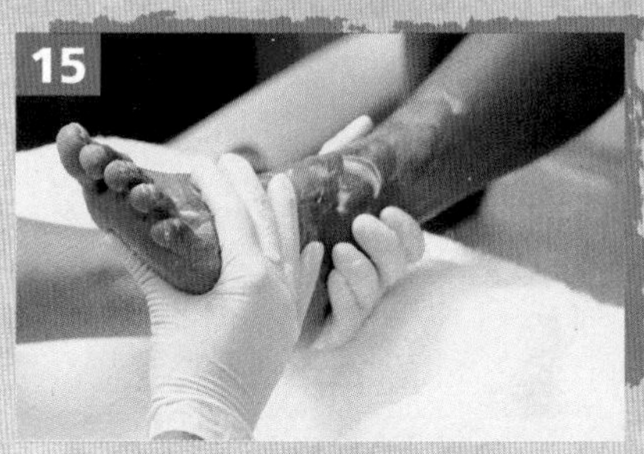

15 Apply lotion, cream, or oil to the first foot for skin conditioning and massage. Use a firm touch to avoid tickling your client's feet.

© Milady, a part of Cengage Learning. Photography by Dino Petrocelli.

CAUTION

Remember that calluses protect the underlying skin from irritation and are there for a purpose. For example, joggers, waitresses, cosmetologists, nurses, teachers, and others are on their feet many hours a day. Calluses protect their feet in stress areas. Remove only enough to make the client comfortable. Calluses should be softened and smoothed, not excessively thinned or removed. Never use a blade on calluses as it is illegal and can cause debilitating infections. Educate your client about callus formation and the protective function calluses provide. Also discuss products for home use to help soften and condition callused areas between salon appointments.

CAUTION

When performing a pedicure, do not push back the eponychium with a metal pusher. Compared with the hands, feet are more susceptible to infections, and pushing back the eponychium (or cutting it) can dramatically increase the risk of serious infections on feet. This tool is designed to remove the tissue that may adhere to the surface of the nail plate, not for pushing back the eponychium. This is especially important for clients with diabetes, psoriasis, and other chronic illnesses.

The Basic Pedicure continued

Service Tip

More expensive pedicures with luxury touches such as masks, paraffin, and mitts should include exfoliation and massage of the legs. The top of the knee may be included, but the underside of the knee is not included. Exfoliate the leg after the foot is exfoliated, but before the use of the foot file, and then apply a lotion to maintain the softness until the massage.

16 Perform a foot massage on the first foot. Then re-wrap the foot and place it on the towel on the floor.

PROCEDURE 26-2 **Foot and Leg Massage** SEE PAGE 867

17 Massage the second foot.

18 Remove traces of lotion, cream, or oil from the nails of both feet with polish remover.

19 Ask the client to put on the sandals he or she will wear home or provide single-use pedicure slippers. Insert the toe separators, if possible. Apply base coat to the nails on both feet, then two coats of color, and finally a topcoat. Apply polish drying product (optional) to prevent smudging of the polish.

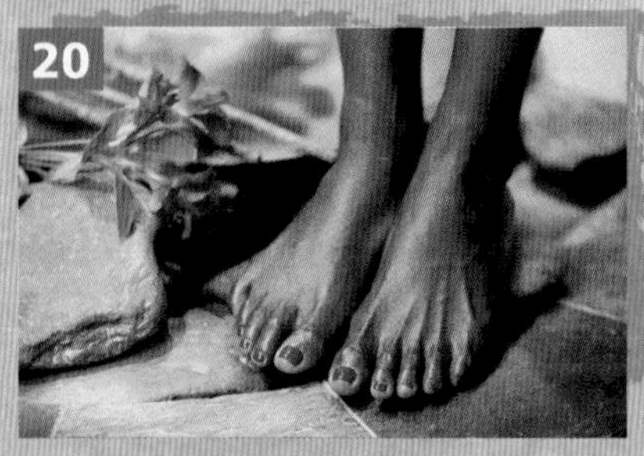

20 Finished look.

21 You may want to escort the client to a drying area and offer him or her refreshment. ✓ LO8

Post-Service

- Complete PROCEDURE 25-2 **Post-Service Procedure** SEE PAGE 821

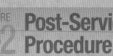

Business Tip

It is very easy to create a specialty pedicure by adding masks, paraffin treatments, or other special applications after the massage and before polishing.

© Milady, a part of Cengage Learning. Photography by Dino Petrocelli.

PROCEDURE 26-2

Foot and Leg Massage

Implements and Materials

In addition to the basic materials on your manicuring table, you will need the following for the massage:

- **Massage oil or lotion**

These techniques and illustrations provide instruction for massage on the feet and legs. A massage for a basic pedicure will include only the foot, while a spa pedicure will also include the leg massage, up to and including the front of the knee.

Foot Massage

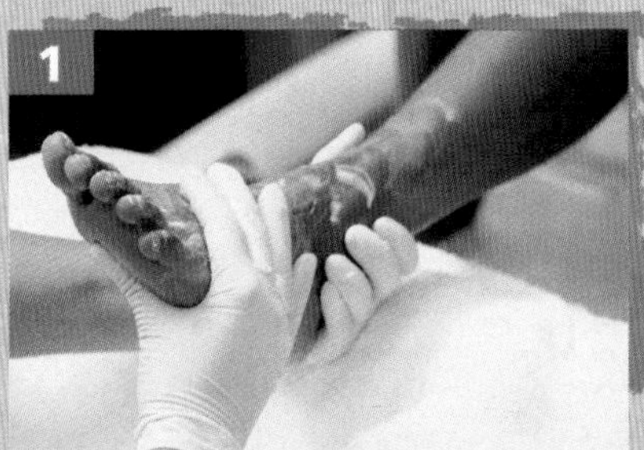

1 Rest the client's heel on a footrest or stool and suggest that your client relax. Grasp the leg gently just above the ankle and use your other hand to hold the foot just beneath the toes; rotate the entire foot in a circular motion.

2 Hold the foot and move the other hand to the dorsal surface of the foot. Place the base of your palm of that hand on top of the foot behind the toes. (Contact is made only with your palm; your fingers do not touch the client's skin and should be lifted away.) Slide up to the ankle area with gentle pressure. Repeat three to five times in the middle, then on the sides of the dorsal surface of the foot. Ever so slightly lift the palm each time to return to the initial position of the slide after reaching the ankle.

© Milady, a part of Cengage Learning. Photography by Dino Petrocelli.

Foot and Leg Massage continued

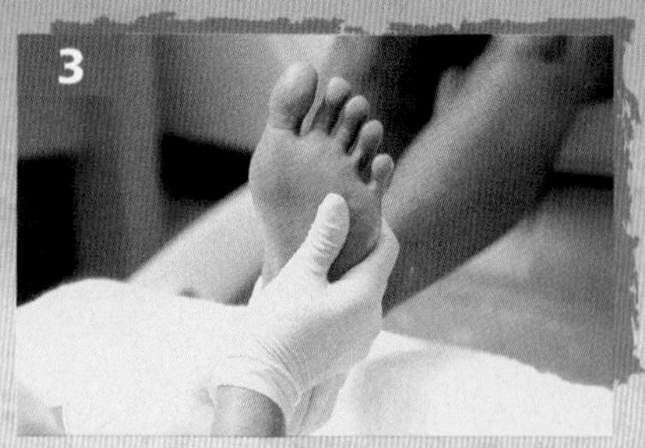

3 Keep one hand in contact with the foot. Slide the other hand and place the thumb on the plantar surface of the foot with the fingers gently holding the dorsal side of the foot. Now, slide the other hand to the same position on the foot, opposite side. Move one thumb in a firm circular movement, moving from one side of the foot, across, above the heel, up the medial side (center side) of the foot to below the toes, across the ball of and back down the other side of the foot (distal side) to the original position. Now, move the thumb of the other hand across and up the outside of the foot, then down to its original position. The base of the thumbs through to the pad of the fingers should be in contact with the skin throughout the movement. Your nails must not touch the client's skin.

4 Alternate the movements of the thumbs in a smooth, firm motion. Repeat several times. This is a very relaxing movement.

5 Perform the same thumb movement on the surface of the heels, rotating your thumbs in opposite directions. Repeat three to five times.

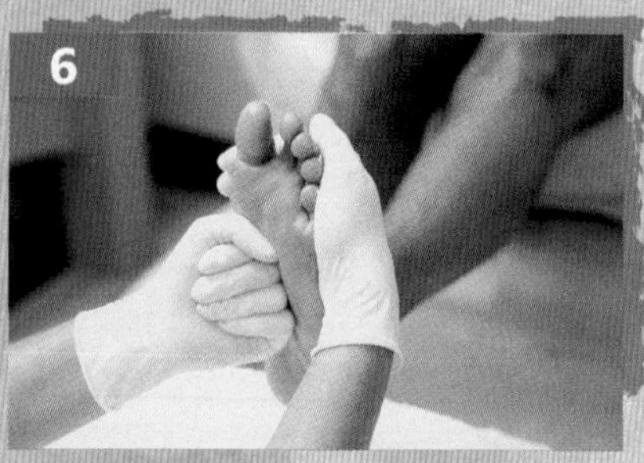

6 Place your one hand on top of the foot, cupping it, and make a fist with your other hand. The hand on top of the foot will press the foot toward you while your other hand twists into the instep of the foot. This helps stimulate blood flow and provides relaxation. Repeat three to five times. This is a friction movement. The bottom of the foot is the only place a friction movement is performed in pedicure services.

Service Tip

Always apply enough lotion or oil to the foot to allow sufficient slide and no skin drag. If there is a need to apply more lotion, stay in contact with the guest by leaving one hand on the foot or leg, while the other hand reaches for a pump of the lotion or oil bottle. Place your thumb over the pump, then press down to deposit more product onto the fingers below the pump. Distribute the lotion and return to the massage.

Business Tip

The basic pedicure does not include the leg massage, only the foot massage, for two reasons: time and money. Most salons schedule less time for the basic pedicure, allowing less time for massage. Second, higher-cost specialty pedicures must be greatly enhanced to be perceived as worth the higher price. The leg massage is one special addition.

© Milady, a part of Cengage Learning. Photography by Dino Petrocelli.

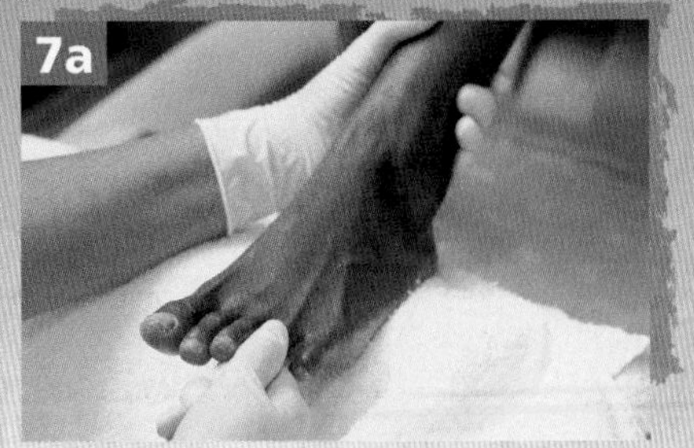

7a Start with the little toe, placing the thumb on the top of the toe and arching the index finger underneath the toe. (Your palm is facing up.) Push the fingers and thumb in that position back to the base of the toe, then rotate the thumb and finger in a circular, effleurage movement until the index finger is arched over the top of the toe, and the thumb is underneath. Pull the toe with index finger and thumb outward, away from the foot.

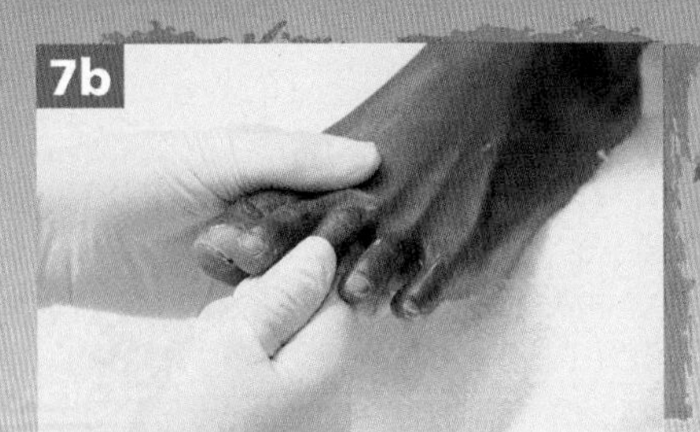

7b Hold the tip of the toe, starting with the little toe, and make a figure eight with each toe. Repeat three to five times on each toe and then move to the next. After the last movement on each toe, gently squeeze the tip of each once, and then move on to the next toe. You must have sufficient lotion for this to be comfortable and relaxing.

Service Tip

The most enjoyable massage is a rhythmic, slow slide with the fingers and palm connecting to the client as much as possible. Maintain a touch connection with the client throughout the massage, sliding the hands from one location to the next in a smooth transition.

---

8 Now, return your hands to the position described in step 4, and repeat steps 3 and 4.

9 Repeat all movements on each foot as many times as you wish, adding other movements that you like to perform, and then move to the other leg/foot.

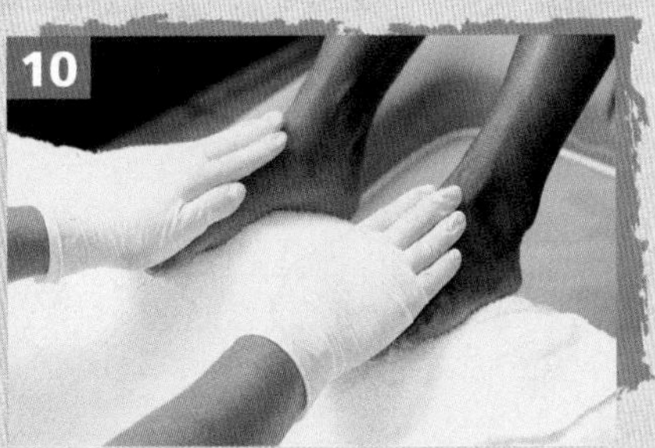

10 Every massage, whether pedicure or body massage, must end. Feathering is a technique used at the end of a massage to provide a signal for experienced clients that the massage is ending, and to provide a gentle release from the client. At the end of the last movement in the pedicure massage, create a smooth transition by gently placing both of the client's feet onto the footrest, or on another stable surface, and move your palms to the top of the feet with your fingers toward the leg. Press your entire hands three times slowly onto the feet. (This should not be a hard press, just a firm push.) Maintain each press for one to two seconds. After the last press, lift your palms slightly, but maintain contact with the feet with your fingertips. Now, gently pull your hand toward the tips of the toes with a feather-light touch of your fingertips. (Do not allow your fingernails to touch the skin.) Pull completely off the end of the toes. Perform the final feather-off movement only once, and then allow the client to relax a minute or two before moving to the next step of the pedicure.

© Milady, a part of Cengage Learning. Photography by Dino Petrocelli.

11 Once the massage of both feet is completed, you may move on in the pedicure procedure. If you are performing a luxury pedicure, do not perform the feather off movement; slide your hands to the leg and move on to the leg massage after step 9.

Leg Massage

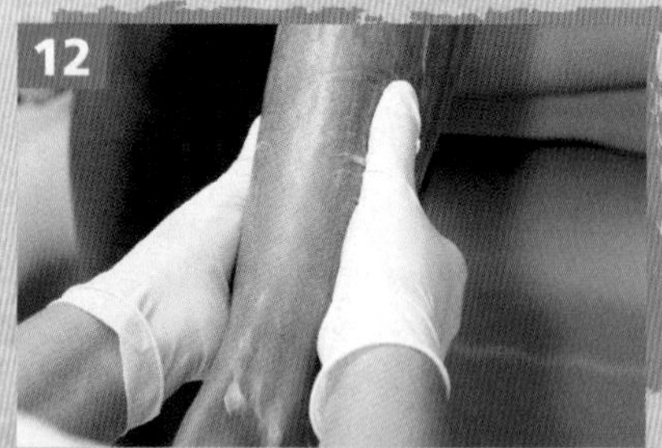

12 Place the foot on the footrest or stabilize it on your lap. Then, gently grasp the client's leg from behind the ankle with one hand. Perform effleurage movements from the ankle to below the knee on the front of the leg with the other hand. Move up the leg and then lightly return to the original location. Perform five to seven repetitions, then move to the sides of the leg and perform an additional five to seven repetitions.

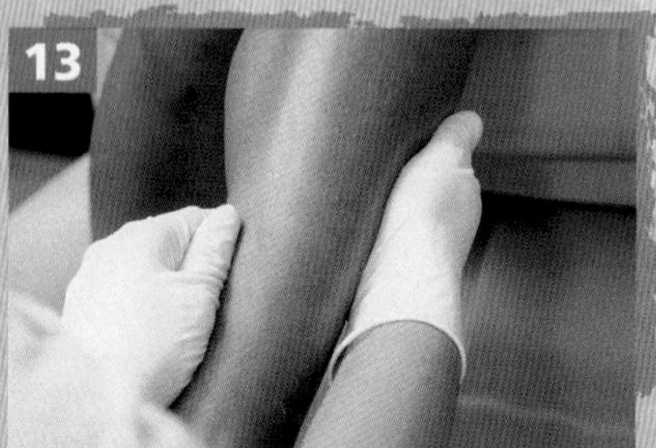

13 Slide to the back of the leg and perform effleurage movements up the back of the leg. Stroke up the leg, then, with less pressure, return to the original location; perform five to seven times. ✓ LO9

14 Once the massage of both legs is completed, you may move on in the pedicure procedure.

© Milady, a part of Cengage Learning. Photography by Dino Petrocelli.

Service Tip

Before performing a service that includes a foot and/or leg massage, consult the client's consultation or intake form. During the consultation, acknowledge and discuss any medical condition your client listed that may be contraindicated for a foot and/or leg massage. Ask the client if they have discussed massage with their physician and if they have not already done so, encourage them to seek their physician's advice as to whether or not a foot and/or leg massage is advisable before performing the service.

Many clients that have high blood pressure (hypertension), diabetes, or circulatory conditions may still have foot and/or leg massage without concern, especially if their condition is being treated and carefully looked after by a physician. Foot and/or leg massage is, however, contraindicated for clients with severe, uncontrolled hypertension. For clients who have circulatory problems such as varicose veins, massaging the foot and/or leg may be harmful because it increases circulation. Ask for written permission from the client's physician before performing this massage.

If your client expresses a concern about having a foot and/or leg massage and has a medical condition, have the client get a note from their physician before performing this part of the service.

If your client has sensitive or redness-prone skin, avoid using vigorous or strong massage techniques. This is especially important for clients who have arthritis. Do not talk to your client during the massage except to ask once whether your touch should be more or less firm. Talking eliminates the relaxation therapy of the massage.

When making decisions about whether to perform a foot and/or leg massage on a person who has a medical condition, be conservative. When in doubt, don't include massage as part of your service.

Review Questions

1. Name five pieces of equipment unique to pedicures.
2. Name three specialty materials used when performing pedicures.
3. What is a callus softener and how is it used?
4. What is the difference between a basic pedicure and a spa pedicure?
5. What is reflexology and how is it used in pedicuring?
6. Why is consistent cleaning and disinfection of pedicure baths so important?
7. What are the steps involved in the proper cleaning and disinfecting of whirlpool foot spas and air-jet basins after each client?
8. List and describe the proper procedures for a basic pedicure.
9. List and explain the procedure for a foot and leg massage.

Chapter Glossary

callus softeners	Products designed to soften and smooth thickened tissue (calluses).
curette	A small, scoop-shaped implement used for more efficient removal of debris from the nail folds, eponychium, and hyponychium areas.
exfoliating scrubs	Water-based lotions that contain a mild, gritty-like abrasive and moisturizers to help in removing dry, flaky skin and reduce calluses.
foot file	Also known as *paddle*; large, abrasive file used to smooth and reduce thicker areas of callus.
foot soaks	Products containing gentle soaps, moisturizers, and other additives that are used in a pedicure bath to cleanse and soften the skin.
nail rasp	A metal implement with a grooved edge that is used for filing and smoothing the edges of the nail plate.
pedicure	A cosmetic service performed on the feet by a licensed cosmetologist or nail technician; can include exfoliating the skin, callus reduction, as well as trimming, shaping, and polishing toenails. Often includes foot massage.
reflexology	A unique method of applying pressure with thumb and index fingers to the hands and feet, and it has demonstrated health benefits.
toe separators	Foam rubber or cotton disposable materials used to keep toes apart while polishing the nails. A new set must be used on each client.
toenail clippers	Professional implements that are larger than fingernail clippers and have a curved or straight jaw, specifically designed for cutting toenails.

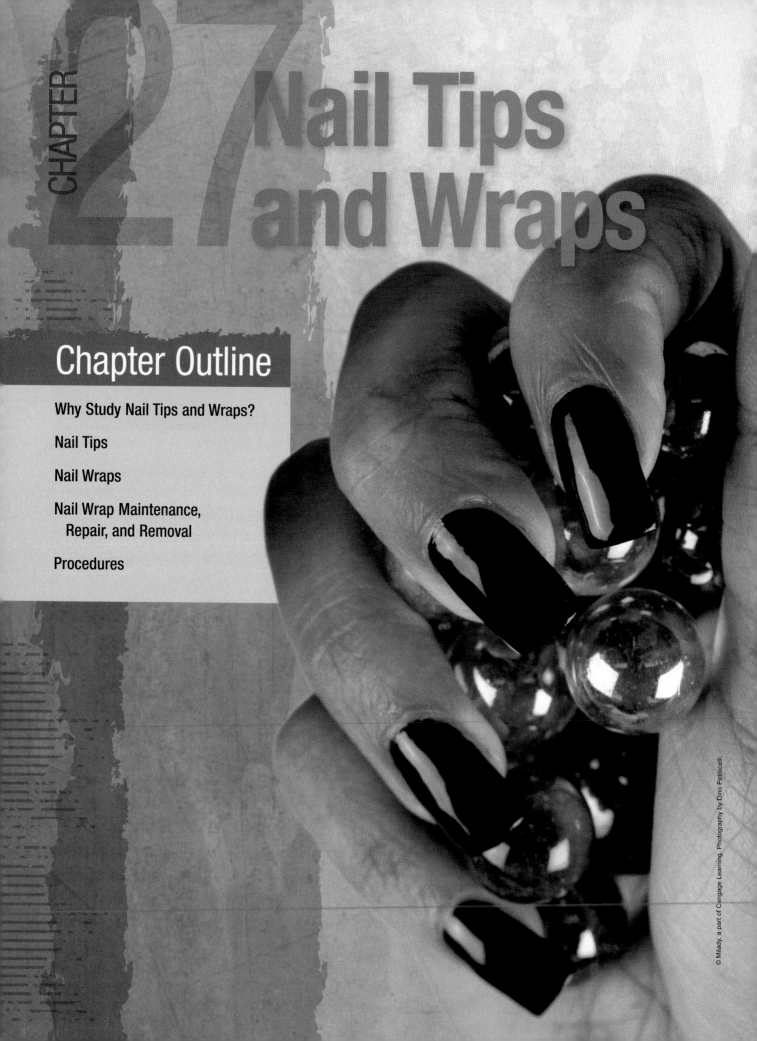

CHAPTER 27

Nail Tips and Wraps

Chapter Outline

© Milady, a part of Cengage Learning. Photography by Dino Petrocelli.

Learning Objectives

After completing this chapter, you will be able to:

✓ **LO1** Identify the supplies, in addition to your basic manicuring table, that you need for nail tip application.

✓ **LO2** Name and describe the types of nail tips available and why it is important to properly fit them for your client.

✓ **LO3** List the types of fabrics used in nail wraps and explain the benefits of using each.

✓ **LO4** Demonstrate the stop, rock, and hold method of applying nail tips.

✓ **LO5** Demonstrate the Nail Tip Application Procedure.

✓ **LO6** Demonstrate the Nail Tip Removal Procedure.

✓ **LO7** Demonstrate the Nail Wrap Application Procedure.

✓ **LO8** Describe the main difference between performing the Two-Week Fabric Wrap Maintenance and the Four-Week Fabric Wrap Maintenance.

✓ **LO9** Demonstrate how to remove fabric wraps and what to avoid.

Key Terms

Page number indicates where the term is used in the chapter.

acrylonitrile butadiene styrene (ABS)
pg. 874

cyanoacrylate
pg. 876

fabric wrap
pg. 876

fiberglass wraps
pg. 876

linen wraps
pg. 876

maintenance
pg. 877

nail dehydrator
pg. 874

nail tip adhesive
pg. 875

nail tips
pg. 874

nail wrap
pg. 876

nail wrap resin
pg. 876

overlay
pg. 874

paper wraps
pg. 876

position stop
pg. 875

repair patch
pg. 878

silk wraps
pg. 876

stress strip
pg. 878

tip cutter
pg. 874

wrap resin accelerator (activator)
pg. 876

One of the most popular services that a cosmetologist can offer clients is the opportunity to wear beautiful nails in an almost endless variety of lengths and strengths.

Regardless of whether a client is interested in wearing long, medium, or short nails, she may decide to have nail tips applied over her natural nails for strength and durability. Once a tip is applied, she will have an opportunity to choose from a variety of products that can be layered over the natural nail and the tip to further secure the strength of the nail and its beauty.

Why Study Nail Tips and Wraps?

Cosmetologists should study and have a thorough understanding of nail tips and wraps because:

- Offering nail extension and wrap services expands your service offerings and enables clients to have a "one stop shop" experience in your salon.
- Learning the proper technique for applying and removing nail tips will aid in helping your client keep her natural nails in the best possible health and condition.
- Understanding the types and uses of nail wraps will enable you to determine the appropriate wrap for your client's specific needs.
- Learning how to safely and correctly apply, maintain, and remove nail tips and wraps will ensure your clients' happiness and loyalty.

Nail Tips

Nail tips are plastic, pre-molded nails shaped from a tough polymer made from **acrylonitrile butadiene styrene** (ak-ruh-loh-NAHY-tril byoo-tuh-DAHY-een STAHY-reen), also known as **ABS**, plastic. They are adhered to the natural nail to add extra length and to serve as a support for nail enhancement products. Tips are combined with an **overlay**, a layer of any kind of nail enhancement product that is applied over the natural nail and tip application for added strength. Nail tips that do not have the reinforcement provided by the overlay are not long-wearing and can break easily.

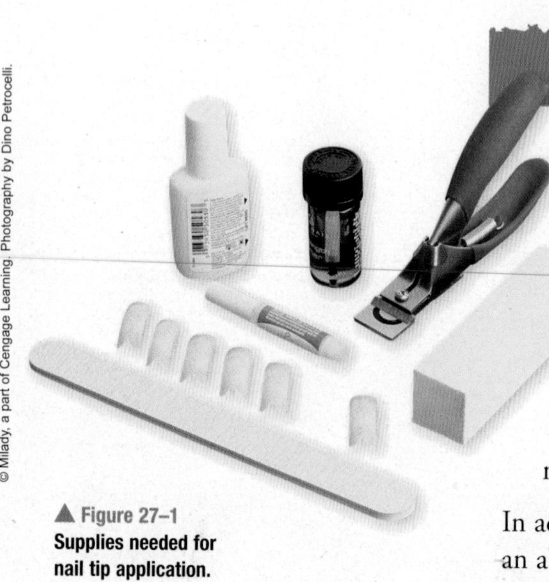

▲ **Figure 27–1 Supplies needed for nail tip application.**

© Milady, a part of Cengage Learning. Photography by Dino Petrocelli.

In addition to the basic materials on your manicuring table, you will need an abrasive board; buffer block; tip adhesive; **tip cutter**, an implement similar to a nail clipper, designed for use on nail tips; **nail dehydrator**, a substance used to remove surface moisture and tiny amounts of oil left on the natural nail plate; and a variety of nail tips for the nail tip application (Figure 27–1). ☑ **LO1**

Many nail tips have a shallow depression called a "well" that serves as the point of contact with the nail plate. The **position stop,** the point where the free edge of the natural nail meets the tip, is where the tip is adhered to the nail. There are various types of nail tips including: partial well, full well, and well-less (no well at all) (**Figure 27–2**).

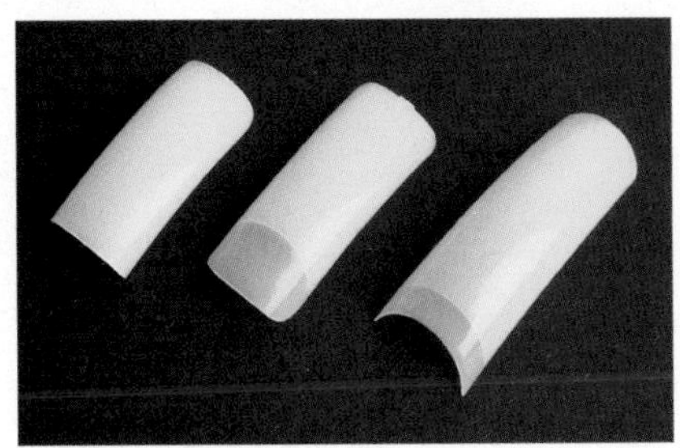

© Milady, a part of Cengage Learning. Photography by Dino Petrocelli.

▲ Figure 27–2
Nail tips that are well-less, partial well, and full well.

Nail tips are available in many sizes, colors, and shapes, making it easy to fit each client with precisely the right size and shape tip. Tips can be purchased in large containers of 100 to 500 pieces, as well as in various individual refill sizes. With such a wide assortment, it is easy to fit each client correctly. Make sure when fitting tips to your client that the tips you choose exactly cover the nail plate from sidewall to sidewall. Do not make the mistake of using a tip that is narrower than the nail plate. This can cause the tip to crack at the sides or split down the middle.

FYI

Do not use fingernail or toenail clippers to cut tips. Cutting the tip with these clippers will weaken the tip and cause it to crack. Instead use a tip cutter.

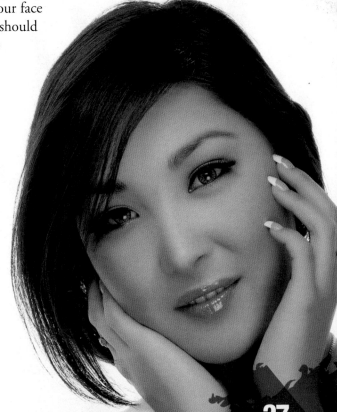

Rather than attempting to force a too-small tip onto the nail, it is better to use a slightly larger tip and use an abrasive board to tailor the tip before you apply it. You can also trim and bevel the well area before applying the tip to the nail, which can save you blending time. Nail tips that are pre-beveled require much less filing on the natural nail after application. This also lessens the potential for damage to the natural nail. ☑ LO2

The bonding agent used to secure the nail tip to the natural nail is called **nail tip adhesive**. Adhesives can be purchased in either tubes or brush-on containers and are available in several different forms, depending on the thicknesses of the adhesive. For instance, gel adhesives, sometimes referred to as *resin*, are the thickest adhesives and require more time to dry than fast-setting, thinner adhesives that dry in about five seconds.

Nail adhesives usually come in either a tube with a pointed applicator tip, a one-drop applicator, or as a brush-on. Use care when opening adhesive containers—always point the opening away from your face and away from your client. Cosmetologists and their clients should always wear eye protection when using and handling nail tip adhesives. Even the smallest amount of adhesive in the eyes can be very dangerous and may cause serious injury.

Once the nail tips are applied, the contact area will need to be reduced with an abrasive, so that the tip blends in with the natural nail. With a perfect tip application, there should be no visible line where the natural nail stops and the tip begins.

PROCEDURE 27-1 **Nail Tip Application** SEE PAGE 879

PROCEDURE 27-2 **Nail Tip Removal** SEE PAGE 882

© Anton Zabielskyi, 2010; used under license from Shutterstock.com.

Nail Wraps

Any method of securing a layer of fabric or paper on and around the nail tip to ensure its strength and durability is called a **nail wrap**. Nail wraps are one type of overlay that can be used over nail tips. Nail wraps are also used to repair or strengthen natural nails or to create nail extensions.

Nail wrap resin is used to coat and secure fabric wraps to the natural nail and nail tip. Wrap resins are made from **cyanoacrylate**, a specialized acrylic monomer that has excellent adhesion to the natural nail plate and polymerizes in seconds.

Fabric wrap is a nail wrap made of silk, linen, or fiberglass. Fabric wraps are the most popular type of nail wrap because of their durability. Fabric wraps are cut to cover the surface of the natural nail and the nail tip and are laid onto a layer of wrap resin to build and strengthen the enhancement. Fabric wraps may be purchased in swatches, rolls, or in packages of pre-cut pieces, some with and some without adhesive backing.

The wrap material is the heart of a nail wrap system and gives this system its unique properties. Nail wraps can be used as an overlay to strengthen natural nails or to strengthen a nail tip application.

Silk wraps are made from a thin natural material with a tight weave that becomes transparent when wrap resin is applied. A silk wrap is lightweight and has a smooth appearance when applied to the nail.

Linen wraps are made from a closely woven, heavy material. It is much thicker and bulkier than other types of wrap fabrics. Nail adhesives do not penetrate linen as easily as silk or fiberglass. Because it is opaque, even after wrap resin is applied, a colored polish must be used to cover it completely. Linen is used because it is considered to be the strongest wrap fabric.

Fiberglass wraps are made from a very thin synthetic mesh with a loose weave. The loose weave makes it easy to use and allows the wrap resin to penetrate, which improves adhesion. Even though fiberglass is not as strong as linen or silk, it can create a durable nail enhancement.

Paper wraps are temporary nail wraps made of very thin paper. Some clients and cosmetologists prefer to use a paper wrap. Paper was one of the very first materials used to create wraps. They are quite simple to use, but they do not have the strength and durability of fabric wraps. For this reason, paper wraps are considered a temporary service and need to be completely replaced each time your client comes in for maintenance. ✓ LO3

A **wrap resin accelerator**, also known as **activator**, acts as the dryer that speeds up the hardening process of the wrap resin or adhesive overlay. Activators come in several different forms: brush-on bottle, pump spray-on, and aerosol. Activator will dissipate in about two

© Milady, a part of Cengage Learning.

minutes after being applied; during this time, do not apply additional wrap resin or you may find that the activator on the nail causes the wrap resin to harden on the brush, tip of the bottle, or extender. Activator also does not need to be applied after every layer of adhesive; this is an optional step; activator can be used as needed.

In addition to your chosen wrap material, you will need wrap resin and resin accelerator, nail buffer and file, small scissors, plastic, and tweezers to perform a nail wrap overlay (**Figure 27–3**).

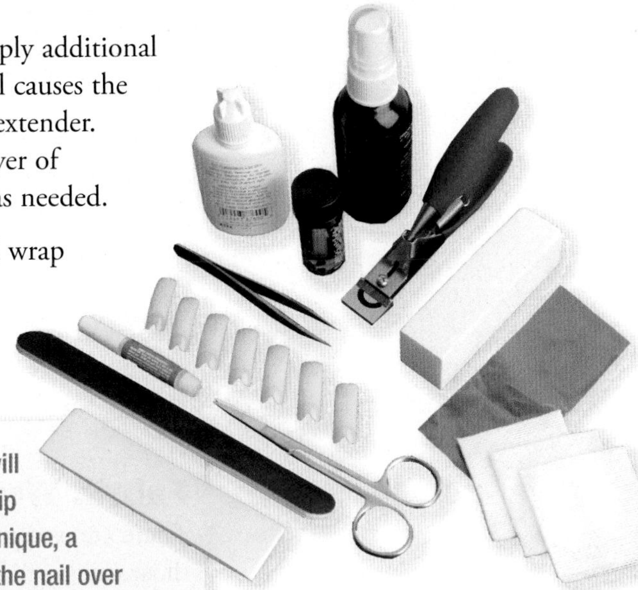

© Milady, a part of Cengage Learning. Photography by Dino Petrocelli.

▲ **Figure 27–3 Supplies needed for nail wrap application.**

FYI

To further strengthen a fabric wrap, some clients will enjoy a method cosmetologists like to use called Dip Powder and Adhesive Enhancements. For this technique, a fine polymer powder is sprinkled or spooned onto the nail over a completed fabric wrap. Several layers of the dip powder can be applied. Any style of adhesive or resin can be used for this procedure. Usually, an activator is used to ensure drying. Many clients who normally cannot wear monomer liquid and polymer powder nail enhancements on their nails because of skin sensitivity or allergy enjoy this service for the additional strength and wearability it provides.

PROCEDURE 27-3 Nail Wrap Application SEE PAGE 884

Nail Wrap Maintenance, Repair, and Removal

Fabric wraps need regular maintenance to keep them looking fresh. In this section, you will learn how to maintain fabric wraps after two weeks and after four weeks. You also will learn how to repair cracks and to remove nail wraps when necessary.

Nail Wrap Maintenance

Nail wraps must have consistent **maintenance** after the initial application.

Maintenance is the term used for when a nail enhancement needs to be serviced after two or more weeks from the initial application of the nail enhancement product. The maintenance service actually accomplishes two goals: it allows the cosmetologist to apply the enhancement product onto the new growth of nail, commonly referred to as a *fill* or a *backfill*. Maintenance also allows the

FYI

You may have heard about, or even tried using, a method of nail enhancement called *No Light Gels*. These were once used professionally but now are popular as do-it-yourself kits. They are available for purchase in grocery and drug stores. If you should encounter a client who has used No Light Gels, you should know that the product consistency is thicker than a wrap resin and made from the same cyanoacrylate. No Light Gels employ a thick adhesive that many companies and marketers mistakenly call a gel.

No Light Gels actually have the same chemical composition as wrap systems with wrap resin and can be used with a spray-on activator to harden or cure the adhesive.

cosmetologist to structurally correct the nail to ensure its strength, shape and durability; this is commonly referred to as a *rebalance*.

Wrap maintenance can be done with either additional wrap resin, as in the Two-Week Fabric Maintenance or with fabric and resin, as in the Four-Week Fabric Maintenance. The maintenance is necessary for the nail's beauty and durability.

PROCEDURE 27-4 **Two-Week Fabric Wrap Maintenance** SEE PAGE 887

Fabric Wrap Repair

There are circumstances when nail wraps will need to be repaired. In those cases, small pieces of fabric can be used to strengthen a weak point in the nail or to repair a break in the nail.

A **stress strip** is a strip of fabric cut to ⅛-inch in length and applied to the weak point of the nail during the Four-Week Fabric Wrap Maintenance in order to repair or strengthen a weak point in a nail enhancement.

A **repair patch** is a piece of fabric cut to completely cover a crack or break in the nail. Use the Four-Week Fabric Wrap Maintenance Procedure to apply the repair patch.

PROCEDURE 27-5 **Four-Week Fabric Wrap Maintenance** SEE PAGE 889

Fabric Wrap Removal

There may be times when a client would like to have their nail wraps removed. When this occurs it is important to remove the wraps as carefully as possible so as not to damage the nail plate. Nail wraps are removed by immersing the entire enhancement into a small glass bowl filled with acetone. Wait for the nail wrap to melt away and then gently and carefully slide the softened wrap material away from the nail with a wooden pusher. Always suggest a manicure after removal of an enhancement to re-hydrate the natural nail and cuticle.

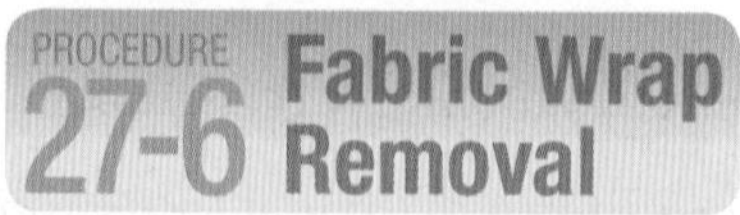

SEE PAGE 892

Business Tip

Host Nail Fashion Nights

Whoever coined the phrase, "Seeing is believing," must have known that people are more likely to purchase something familiar. To acquaint customers firsthand with the latest manicure looks, try hosting a nail fashion night. For a $10.00 to $16.00 admission fee, you can showcase the latest nail looks by giving each attendee a manicure—using the season's most popular fashion colors and hottest new products, of course. To top off the evening, offer each client a nail care fashion kit that includes trial-size products and a gift certificate for 10 to 15 percent off the next nail care purchase or service. Spending an entire night focused on the products creates a buzz about them and shows clients how to use them. The sample size gets them hooked and the gift certificate gives them an incentive to return to you.

PROCEDURE 27-1

Nail Tip Application

Implements and Materials

In addition to the basic materials on your manicuring table, you will need the following supplies for the Nail Tip Application procedure:

- **Abrasive boards**
- **Buffer block**
- **Nail dehydrator**
- **Nail tip adhesive**
- **Nail tips**
- **Tip cutter**

© Milady, a part of Cengage Learning. Photography by Dino Petrocelli.

Preparation

- Perform PROCEDURE 25-1 **Pre-Service Procedure** SEE PAGE 817

Procedure

1 Clean the nails and remove existing polish.

2 Gently push back the eponychium, using a wooden stick, pusher, or other suitable implement.

3 Carefully and gently remove the cuticle tissue from the nail plate, using a wooden stick, pusher, or other suitable implement.

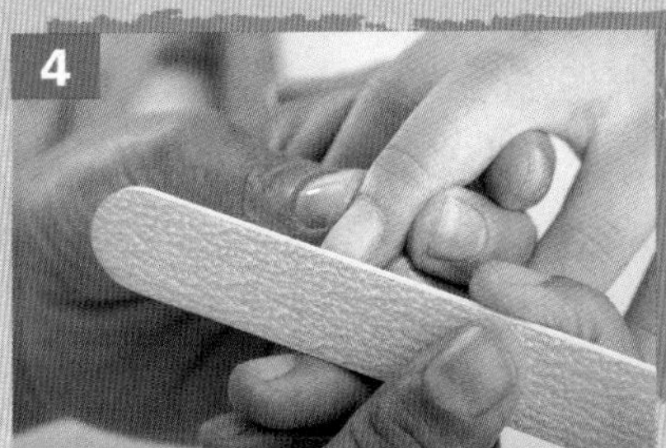

4 Buff very lightly over the nail plate with a medium-fine abrasive (240 grit or higher) to remove the shine caused by natural oil and contaminants on the surface of the nail plate. Do not use a coarse abrasive, and be careful to avoid applying excessive pressure. The goal is to remove only the shine and as little nail plate thickness as possible. Remove the dust with a clean, dry nailbrush by stroking from the cuticle area toward the free edge.

Nail Tip Application continued

CAUTION

If you accidentally touch or contaminate the freshly prepped natural nail, you must clean it again and reapply nail dehydrator.

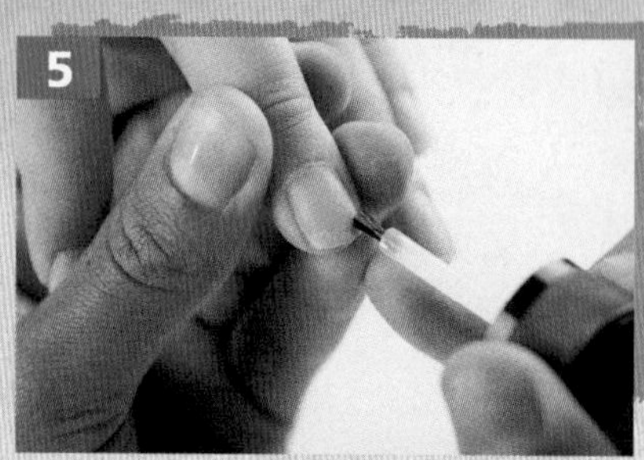

5 Apply nail dehydrator to remove surface moisture and tiny amounts of oil left on the natural nail plate. Be careful not to touch the natural nail with your fingers as any deposit of oils from your fingers could cause lifting of the overlay after it is applied.

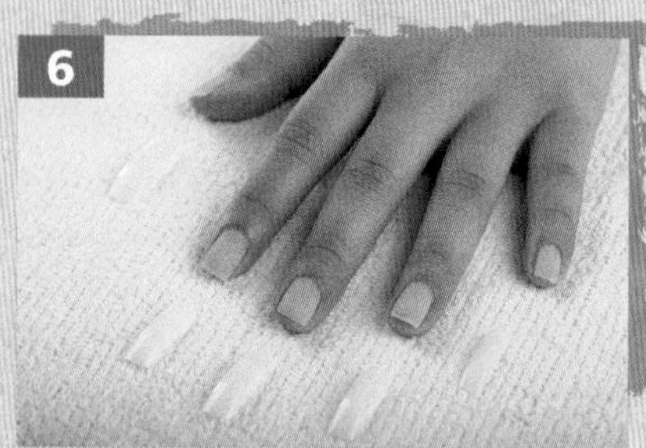

6 Take time to ensure that you are choosing properly sized tips for your client's nail plate before beginning to adhere them to the natural nail. Make sure that the tips you choose exactly cover the nail plate from sidewall to sidewall. Put all of the pre-tailored and pre-sized tips on a towel, in the order of finger position.

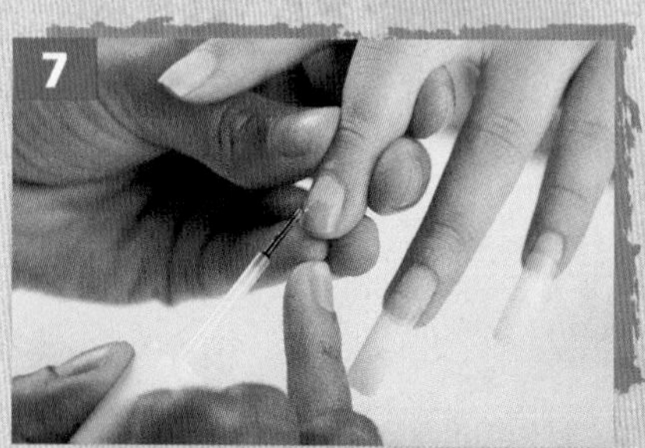

7 Place enough adhesive on the nail plate to cover the area where the tip will be placed, or apply the adhesive to the well of the tip. Do not apply too much: Less is more when it comes to nail tip adhesives! Do not let adhesive run onto the skin. Apply adhesive from the middle of the nail plate to the free edge. You also can use a thin brush-on adhesive and cover the entire nail, then press the tip into it.

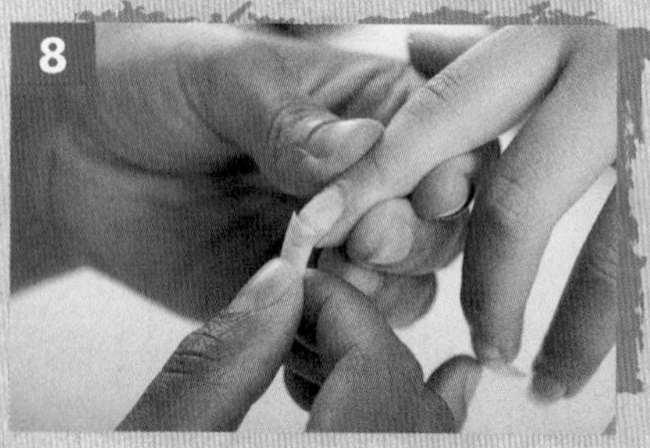

8 Slide the tips onto the client's natural nail and stop, rock, and hold when applying tips. Find the *stop* against the free edge at a 45-degree angle. Rock the tip on slowly. Hold the tip in place for five to ten seconds until the adhesive has dried. You may also apply the adhesive to the well area of the tip. This will ensure that there are fewer air bubbles trapped in the adhesive. This technique also works on well-less tips, followed by positioning on the nail plate and holding it in place for five to ten seconds until the adhesive hardens. ✓ LO4

Service Tip

Consider using a well-less tip that requires no blending with the natural nail. Buff the surface of the nail tip gently once it is applied for better overlay adhesion.

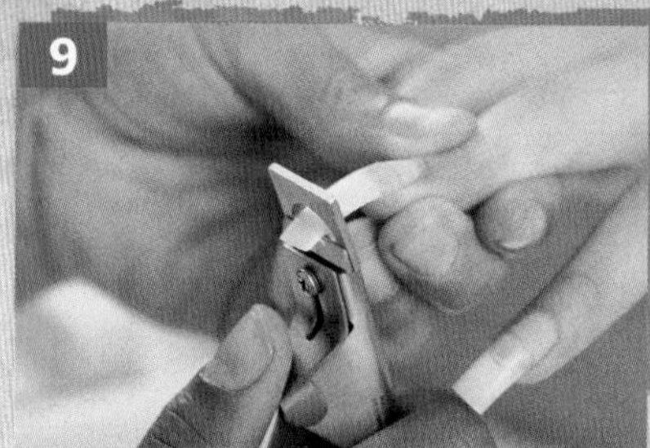

9 Trim the nail tip to desired length using a tip cutter.

© Milady, a part of Cengage Learning. Photography by Dino Petrocelli.

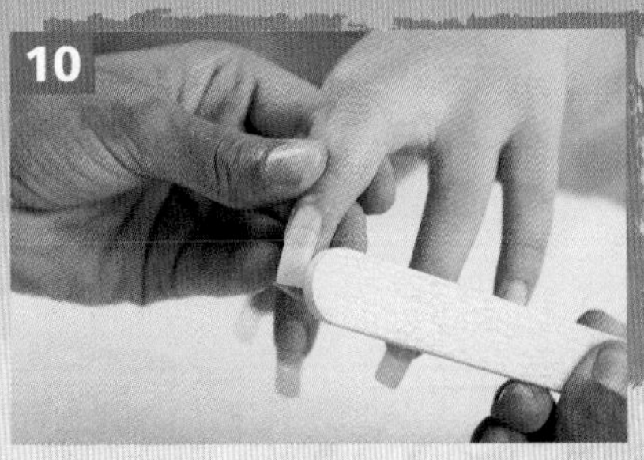

10 If you applied tips with a well, you will still need additional blending to make them match with the surface of the natural nail plate. Take great care because this step can cause damage to the natural nail plate, if done improperly. Using a medium- to fine-grit file or buffing block file (180 grit or higher), carefully smooth the contact area down until it is flush with the natural nail. Make sure to keep your buffer (or board) flat to the nail as you blend the tip. Never hold the file at an angle because the edge of abrasive may gouge the nail plate and damage it. After you finish blending, remove the shine from the rest of the tip.

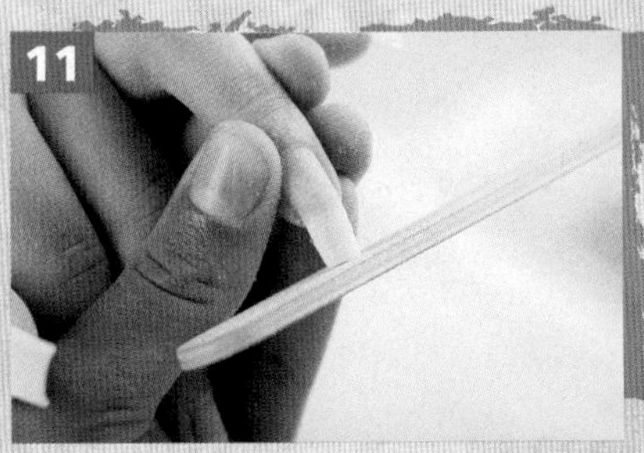

11 Use an abrasive to shape the new, longer nail.

12 Your nail tip application process is now complete. Although your client's tips blend with natural nails, tips should not be worn without an additional nail overlay such as wraps because tips will not be strong enough to wear alone.

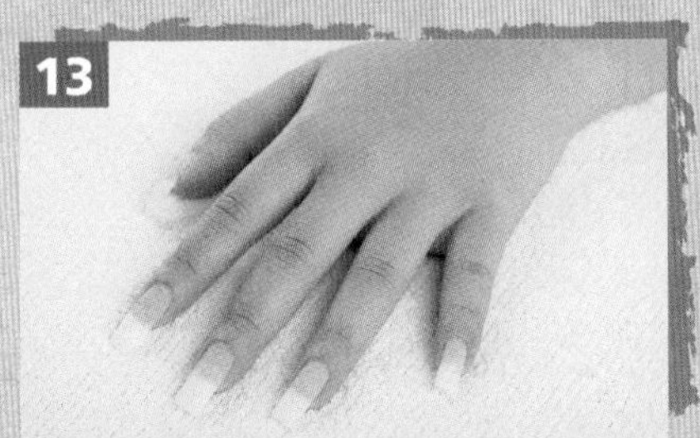

13 Finished look.

Service Tip

During the nail tip application procedure, discuss products such as polish, top coat, and hand lotion or cream that will help your client maintain the beauty and durability of her nails between salon visits.

Service Tip

When applying a tip that has a well, be sure that the well butts up to the natural nail when adhering it to the nail.

Post-Service

- Complete 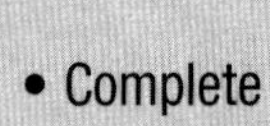 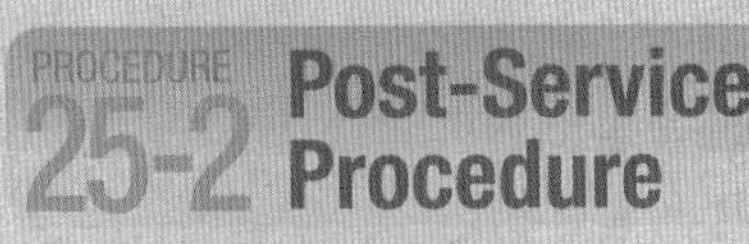 PROCEDURE 25-2 **Post-Service Procedure** SEE PAGE 821 ✓ LO5

© Milady, a part of Cengage Learning. Photography by Dino Petrocelli.

PROCEDURE 27-2

Nail Tip Removal

Implements and Materials

In addition to the basic materials on your manicuring table, you will need the following supplies for the Nail Tip Removal procedure:

- **Buffer block**
- **Small glass bowl**
- **Tip remover solution or acetone**

Preparation

- Perform PROCEDURE 25-1 **Pre-Service Procedure** **SEE PAGE 817**

Procedure

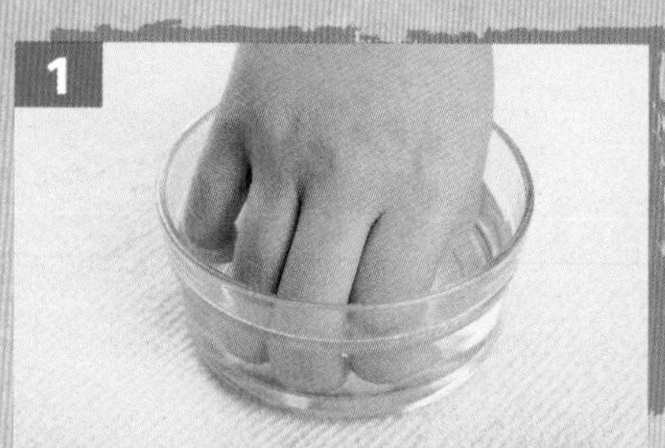

1 Place enough acetone in a small glass bowl to cover nails. Soak for a few minutes.

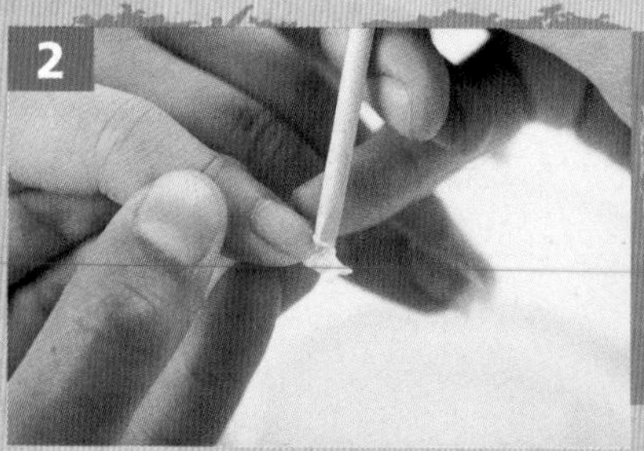

2 Use a pusher to slide off the softened nail tip. Be careful not to pry the nail tip off because you can damage the nail unit. If the nail tip is still too adhered to the nail, have the client soak that nail again for a few more minutes until the entire nail tip is easily removed.

© Milady, a part of Cengage Learning. Photography by Dino Petrocelli.

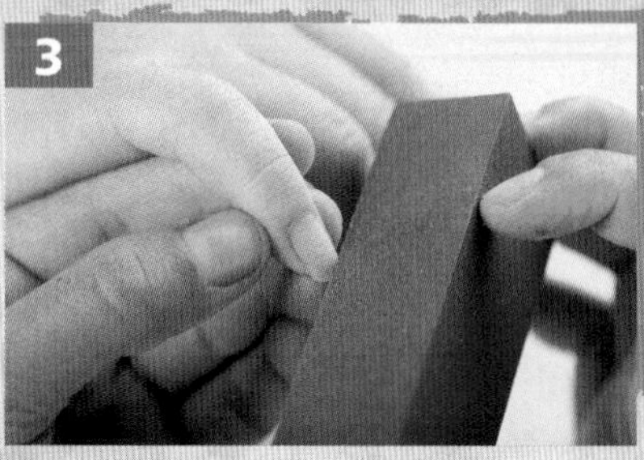

3 Gently buff the natural nail with a fine buffer to remove any adhesive residue.

4 Reapply the nail tip if the client desires, as directed in Procedure 27–1. If not, proceed with the desired service.

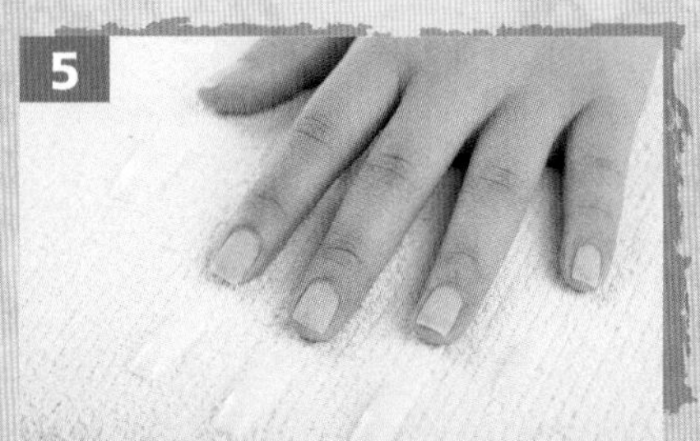

5 Finished look.

CAUTION

Never nip off the nail tip! This may lead to damage of the nail plate by pulling off layers of the natural nail and can break the seal of the remainder of the enhancement.

Post-Service

• Complete 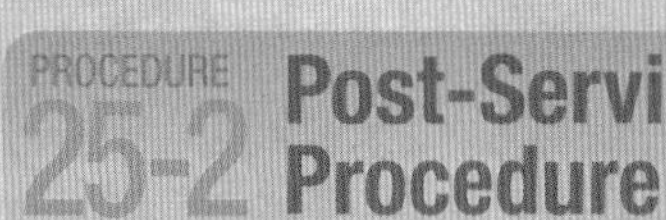

SEE PAGE 821 ✓ LO6

© Milady, a part of Cengage Learning. Photography by Dino Petrocelli.

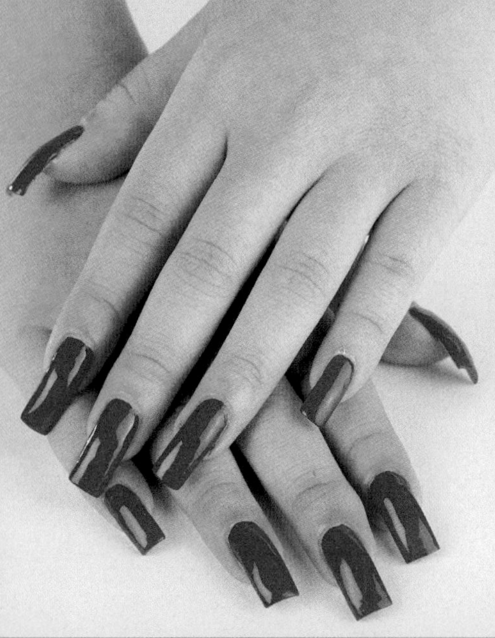

PROCEDURE 27-3

Nail Wrap Application

Implements and Materials

- In addition to the basic materials on your manicuring table, you will need the following supplies for the Nail Wrap Application procedure:
- Adhesive-backed fabric
- Nail buffer
- Nail dehydrator
- Small piece of plastic
- Small scissors
- Tweezers (optional)
- Wrap resin
- Wrap resin accelerator

Preparation

- Perform PROCEDURE 25-1 **Pre-Service Procedure** SEE PAGE 817

Procedure

1 Remove existing polish.

2 Push back the eponychium and remove the cuticle.

3 Lightly buff the nail plate with a medium-fine abrasive (240 grit) to remove shine caused by the oil found on the natural nail plate. Do not use a coarse file, and be careful not to apply pressure. Remove only the oily shine and avoid removing layers from the natural nail plate. Nail wraps can be performed over natural nails or over a set of nail tips. If you are using nail tips, you should use your abrasive to shape the free edges of the natural nails to match the shape of the nail tip to the stop point. Remove the dust with a clean, dry, disinfected nail brush.

4 Spray or wipe a nail dehydrator onto the nail plate. The dehydrator will remove moisture from the surface and will help improve adhesion. Wiping the dehydrator with a plastic-backed cotton pad on the nail plate has the added benefit of removing any remaining natural oil and helps ensure superior adhesion, even on clients with oily skin.

5 Apply nail tips, if desired.

© Milady, a part of Cengage Learning. Photography by Dino Petrocelli.

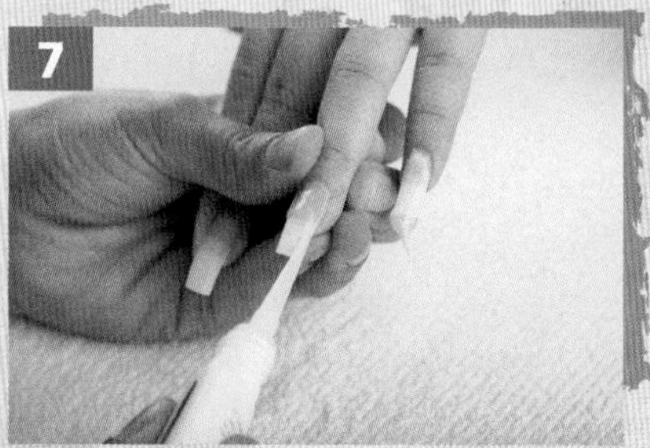

6 Before removing the backing on the fabric, cut it to the approximate width and shape of the nail plate or nail tip.

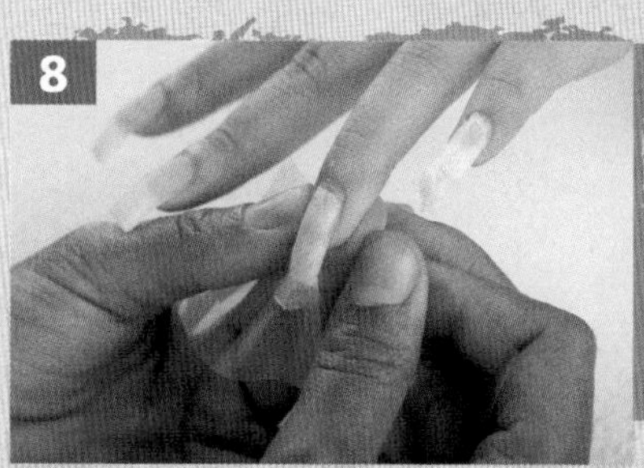

7 Apply a layer of wrap resin over the entire surface of the nail and tip. Remember to keep the nail adhesive off the skin. Besides potentially damaging your client's skin, this could cause the wrap to lift or separate from the nail plate. Begin with the pinky finger of the left hand and apply the wrap resin to all 10 fingers. Once completed return to the first finger and apply fabric wrap.

Service Tip

Using a 6" x 4" piece of flexible plastic sheet—a sandwich baggie works great—to press fabric onto the nail plate will prevent the transfer of oil and debris from your fingers. Wrap resin will not easily penetrate fibers that are contaminated with oil, and those strands become visible in the clear coating. Thus, it is best not to touch them more than you must. Changing to an unused portion of the plastic for each finger is necessary.

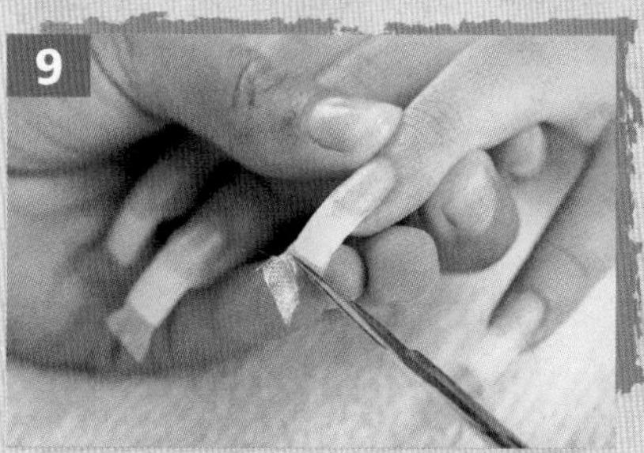

8 Remove the backing from the fabric, being careful to keep the dust and oils on your fingers from contaminating the adhesive side of the fabric, as this could prevent the fabric from adhering to the nail. Gently fit fabric over the nail plate covering the entire nail (you may also use a pair of tweezers to apply the fabric if desired), keeping it $\frac{1}{16}$-inch away from the sidewall and eponychium. Use a small piece of thick plastic to press the fabric onto the nail and to smooth it out.

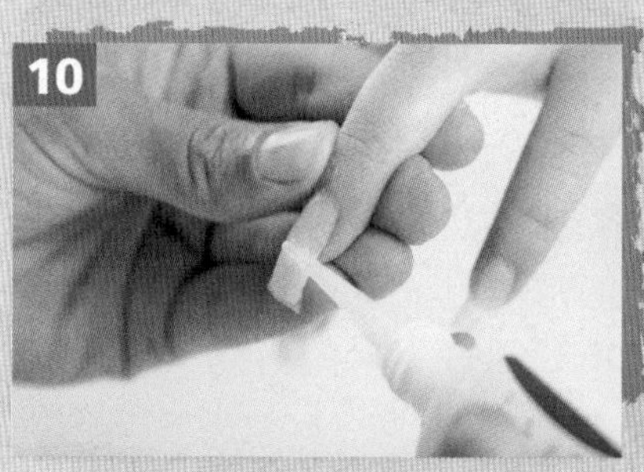

9 Once the fabric is secure on the nail, use small scissors to trim fabric $\frac{1}{16}$-inch away from sidewalls and the free edge. Trimming fabric slightly smaller than the nail plate prevents fabric from lifting and separating from the nail plate.

10 Draw a thin coat of wrap resin down the center of the nail using the extender tip or brush. Do not touch the skin. The wrap resin will penetrate the fabric and adhere to the nail surface. Use the plastic again to make sure that the wrap resin is evenly distributed and that there are no bubbles or areas of bare fabric. Once saturated with wrap resin, the wrap fabric or paper will be almost invisible. (Linen wrap fabric will remain visible because it is quite thick.)

© Milady, a part of Cengage Learning. Photography by Dino Petrocelli.

PROCEDURE 27-3 Nail Wrap Application continued

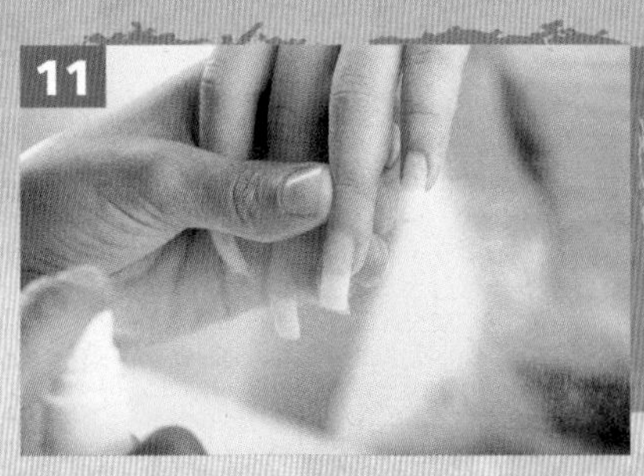
11

11 Wrap resin accelerator is a product specially designed to help any cyanoacrylate glue or wrap resin dry more quickly. Spray, brush, or drop on a wrap resin accelerator that is specifically designed to work with the product you are using. Use accelerator according to manufacturer's instructions. Keep the wrap resin accelerator off skin to prevent overexposure to the product.

12 Apply and spread a second coat of wrap resin and seal free edge to prevent lifting and tip separation.

13 Apply a second coat of wrap resin accelerator.

14 Use medium-fine abrasive (240 grit) to shape and refine the wrap nail.

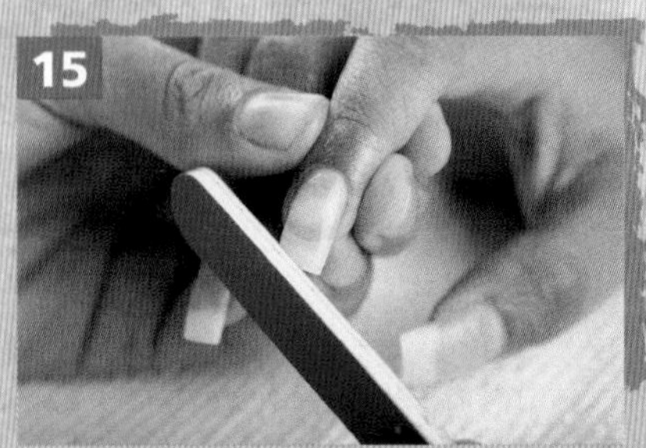
15

15 Apply nail oil and buff to a high shine with a fine (350 grit or higher) buffer. Use the buffer to smooth out rough areas in the fabric. Do not buff excessively or for too long. Overbuffing can wear through the wrap and weaken it.

16 Apply hand lotion and massage the hand and arm.

17 Remove traces of oil. Use a small piece of cotton ball or plastic-backed pad and non-acetone polish remover to eliminate traces of oil from the nail so that the polish will adhere.

18 Polish the nails.

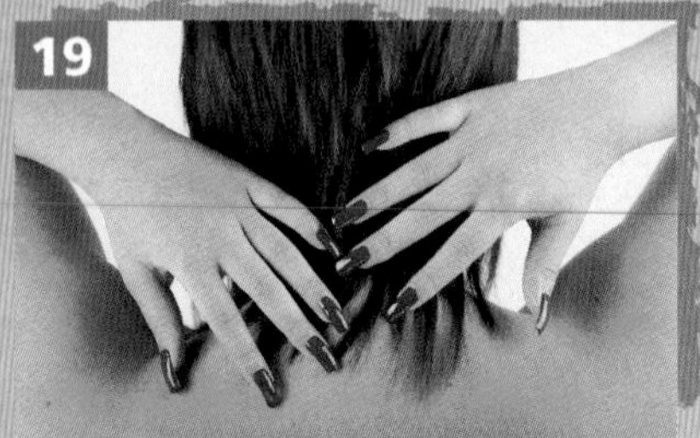
19

19 Finished look.

Post-Service

- Complete 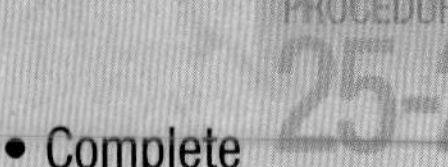 PROCEDURE 25-2 **Post-Service Procedure** SEE PAGE 821 ✓ LO7

© Milady, a part of Cengage Learning. Photography by Dino Petrocelli.

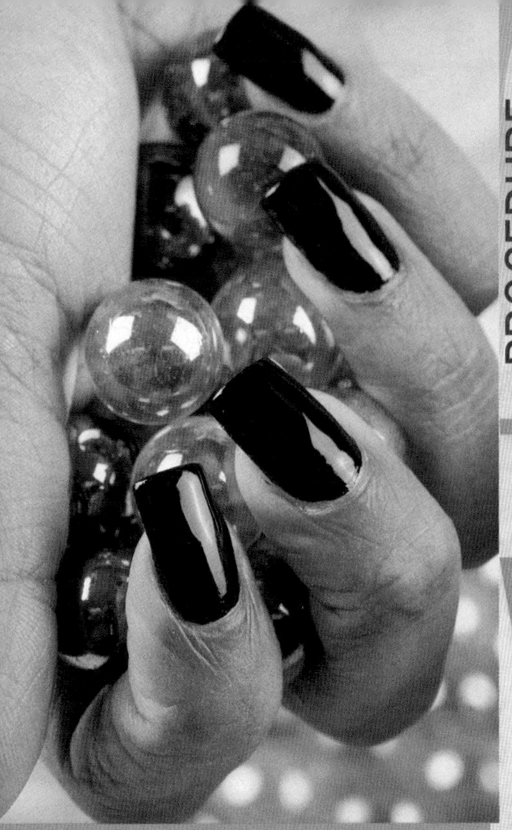

PROCEDURE 27-4

Two-Week Fabric Wrap Maintenance

Implements and Materials

In addition to the basic materials on your manicuring table, you will need the following supplies for the Two-Week Fabric Wrap Maintenance procedure:

- **Abrasive buffer or file**
- **Nail dehydrator**
- **Wrap resin**
- **Wrap resin accelerator**

Preparation

- Perform PROCEDURE 25-1 **Pre-Service Procedure** SEE PAGE 817

Procedure

1 Use a non-acetone polish remover to remove existing nail polish and to avoid damaging nail wraps. Acetone will break down the wrap resin too quickly.

2 Clean the natural nails.

3 Push back the eponychium.

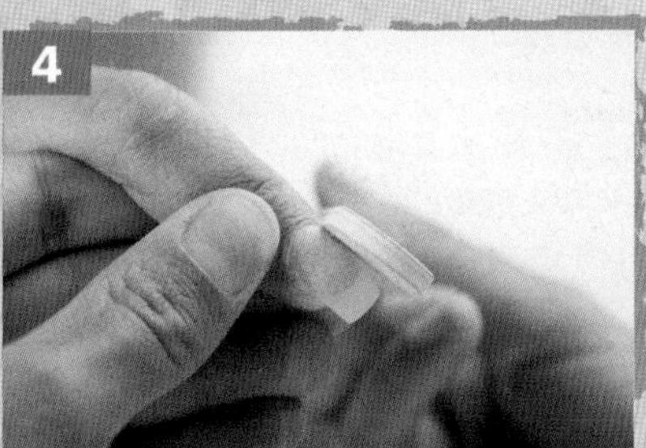

4 Lightly buff the surface of the exposed nail plate to remove oily shine.

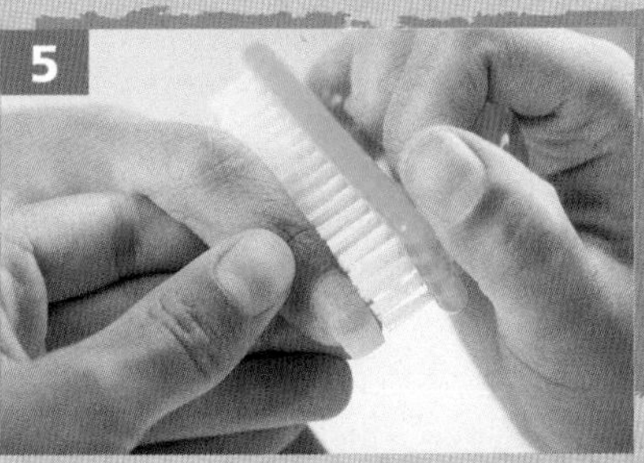

5 Remove the dust with a clean, dry nylon nail brush and apply nail dehydrator to nails with a cotton-tipped wooden pusher, cotton pad with a plastic backing, brush, or spray. Begin with the little finger on the left hand and work toward the thumb. Repeat on the right hand.

© Milady, a part of Cengage Learning. Photography by Dino Petrocelli.

Two-Week Fabric Wrap Maintenance continued

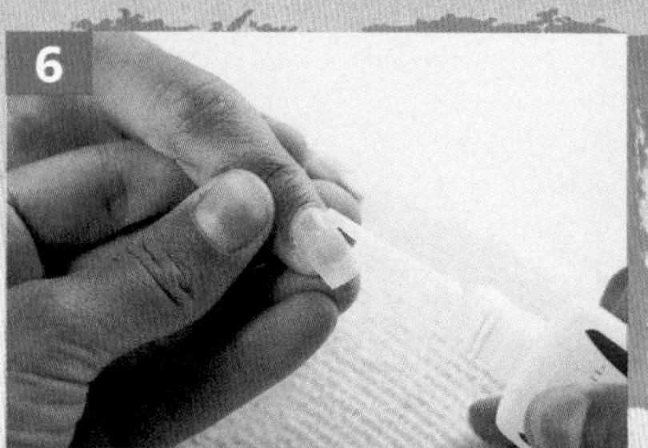

6 Apply a small amount of nail wrap resin to the area of new nail growth. Spread the wrap resin, taking care to avoid touching the skin.

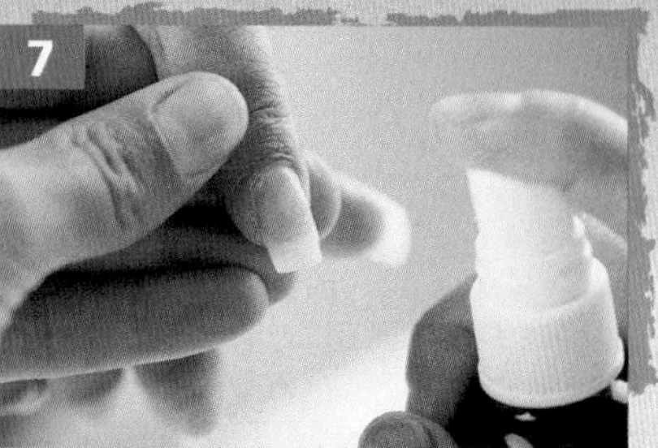

7 Spray, brush, or drop on a wrap resin accelerator that is specifically designed to work with the product you are using. Follow the manufacturer's instructions. Keep the wrap resin accelerator off skin to prevent overexposure to the product.

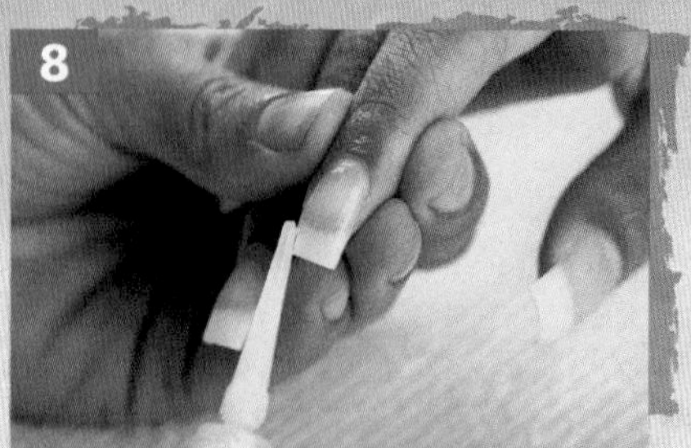

8 Apply a second coat of wrap resin to the entire nail plate to strengthen and reseal the nail wrap.

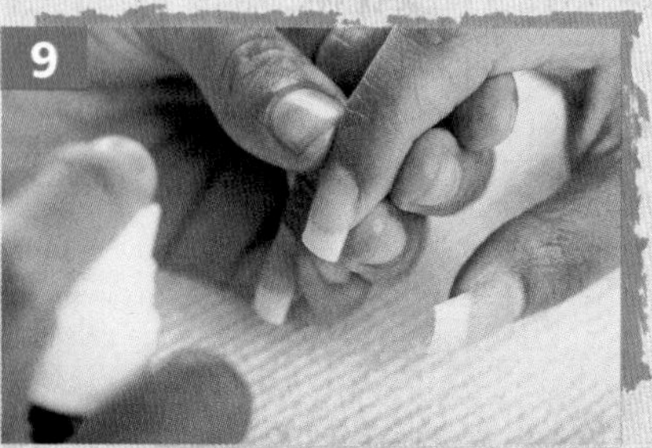

9 Apply a second coat of wrap resin accelerator.

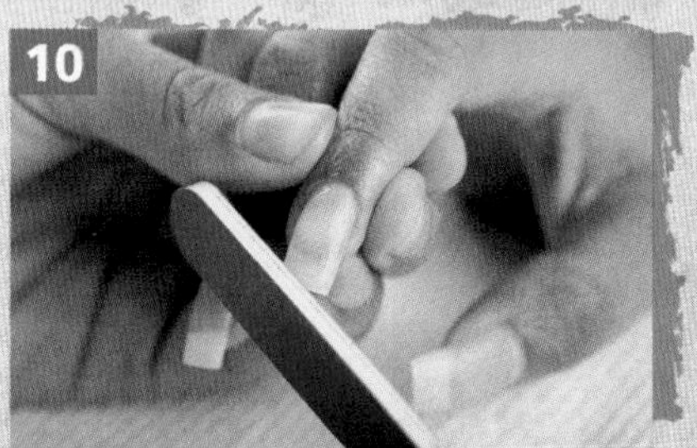

10 Use a medium-fine abrasive over the surface of the nail wrap to remove any high spots and/or other imperfections.

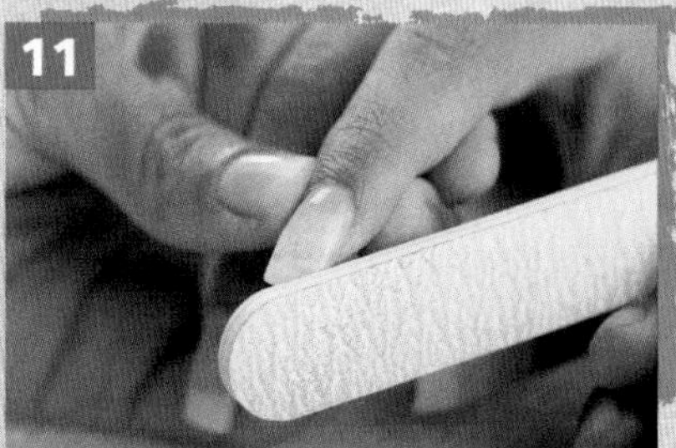

11 Apply nail oil and buff to a high shine with the fine buffer (350 grit or higher).

12 Apply hand lotion and massage the hand and arm.

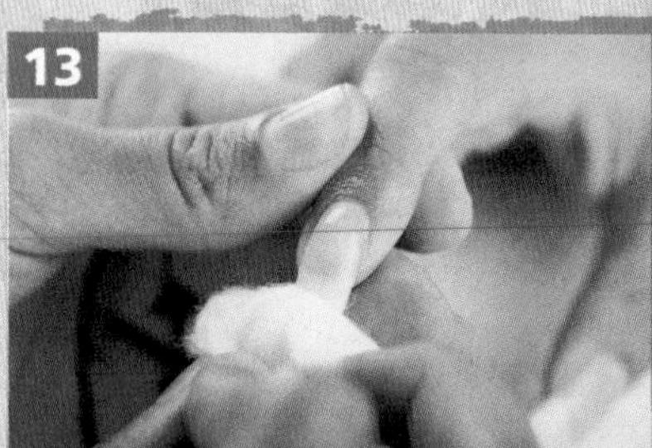

13 Remove traces of oil. Use a small piece of cotton ball or plastic-backed pad and non-acetone polish remover to eliminate traces of oil from the nail so that the polish will adhere.

14 Polish the nails.

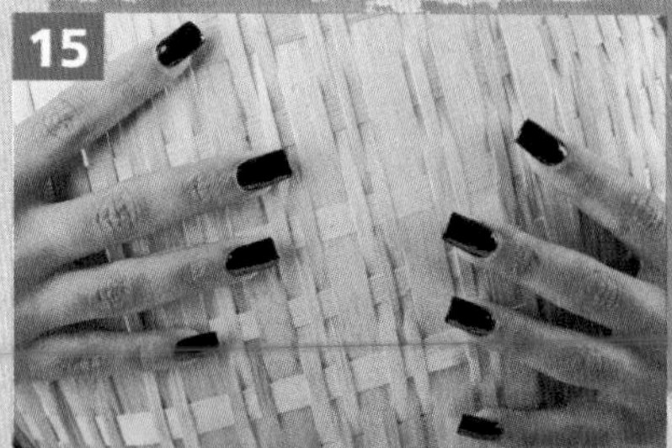

15 Finished look.

Post-Service

- Complete PROCEDURE 25-2 **Post-Service Procedure** SEE PAGE 821

© Milady, a part of Cengage Learning. Photography by Dino Petrocelli.

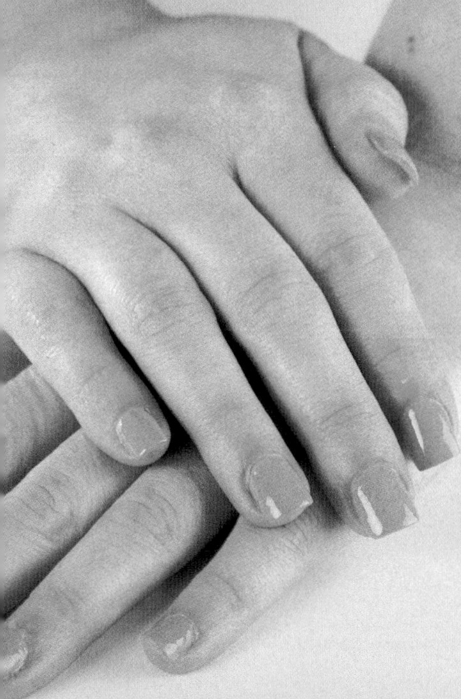

PROCEDURE 27-5

Four-Week Fabric Wrap Maintenance

Implements and Materials

In addition to the basic materials on your manicuring table, you will need the following supplies for the Four-Week Fabric Wrap Maintenance procedure:

- **Abrasive buffer or file**
- **Adhesive-backed fabric**
- **Nail dehydrator**
- **Small piece of plastic**
- **Small scissors**
- **Tweezers (optional)**
- **Wrap resin**
- **Wrap resin accelerator**

© Milady, a part of Cengage Learning. Photography by Dino Petrocelli.

Preparation

- Perform 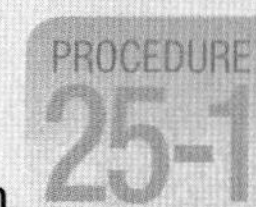 PROCEDURE 25-1 **Pre-Service Procedure** **SEE PAGE 817**

Procedure

1 Use a non-acetone polish remover to remove existing nail polish and to avoid damaging nail wraps. Acetone will break down the wrap resin too quickly.

2 Clean the natural nails.

3 Push back the eponychium.

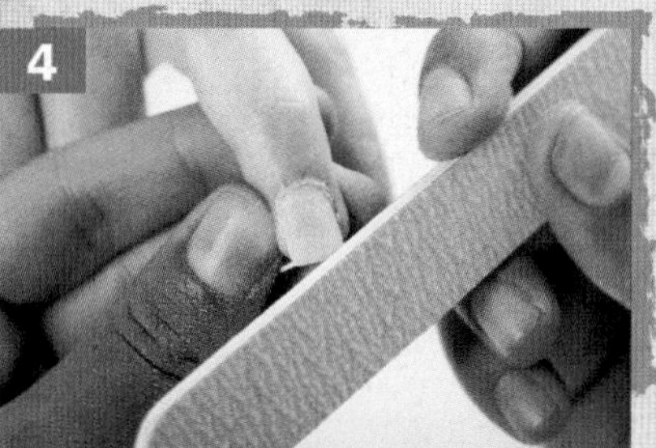

4 Lightly buff the nail plates with a medium-fine (240 grit) abrasive to remove the shine created by natural oils and to remove any small pieces of fabric that may have lifted since the last service. Buff the end of the wrap until smooth, without scratching or damaging the natural nail plate. Carefully refine the nail until there is no obvious line of demarcation between new growth and fabric wrap. Avoid damaging the natural nail with the abrasive.

PROCEDURE 27-5

Four-Week Fabric Wrap Maintenance continued

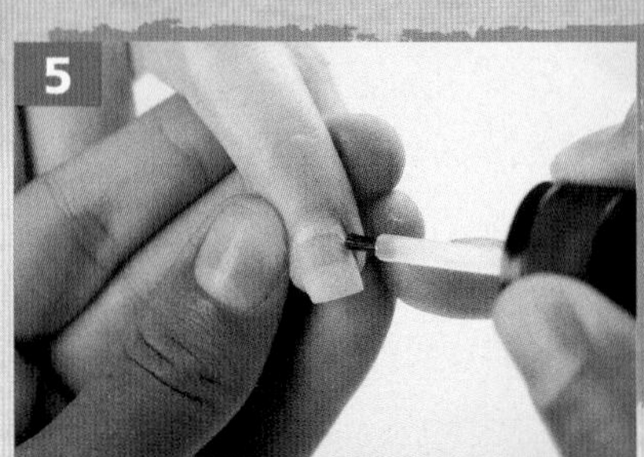

5 Remove the dust with a clean, dry nylon nail brush and apply nail dehydrator to nails with a cotton-tipped wooden pusher, cotton pad with a plastic backing, brush, or spray. Begin with the little finger on the left hand and work toward the thumb. Repeat on the right hand.

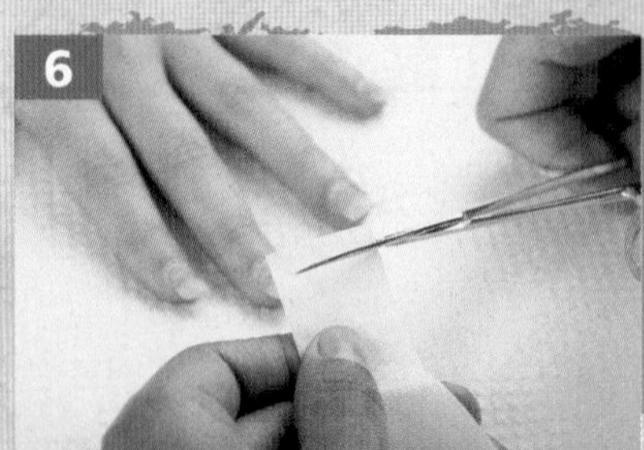

6 Cut a piece of fabric large enough to cover the new growth area and to slightly overlap the old wrap fabric.

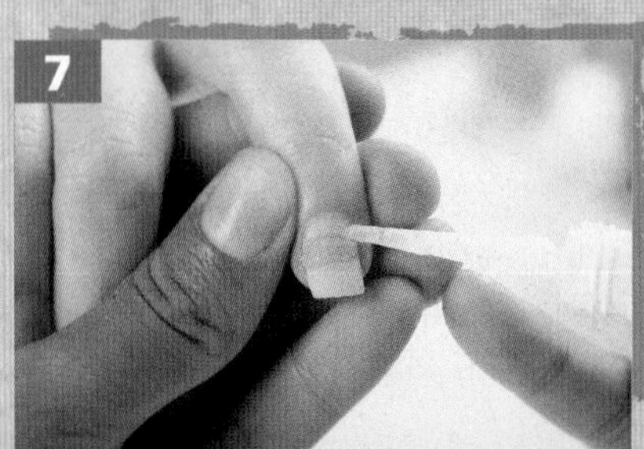

7 Apply a small amount of wrap resin to the fill area and spread throughout the new growth area. Be careful to avoid touching the skin.

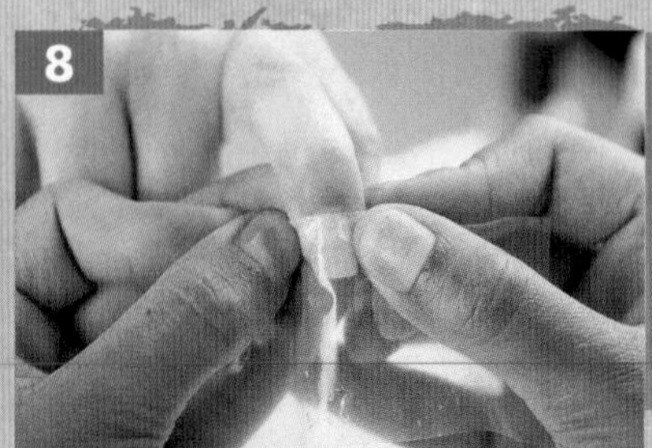

8 Gently fit the fabric over the new growth area and smooth.

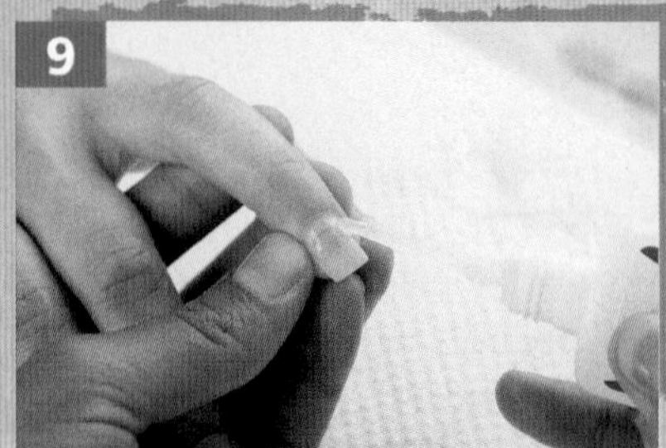

9 Apply another small amount of wrap resin, again avoiding the skin.

© Milady, a part of Cengage Learning. Photography by Dino Petrocelli.

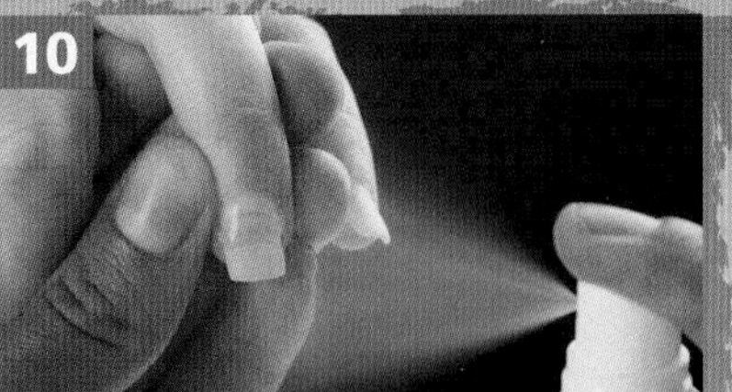

10 Spray, brush, or drop on the wrap resin accelerator to dry the wrap resin more quickly. Follow the manufacturer's instructions.

11 Apply a second coat of wrap resin to the regrowth area.

12 Apply a second coat of wrap resin accelerator.

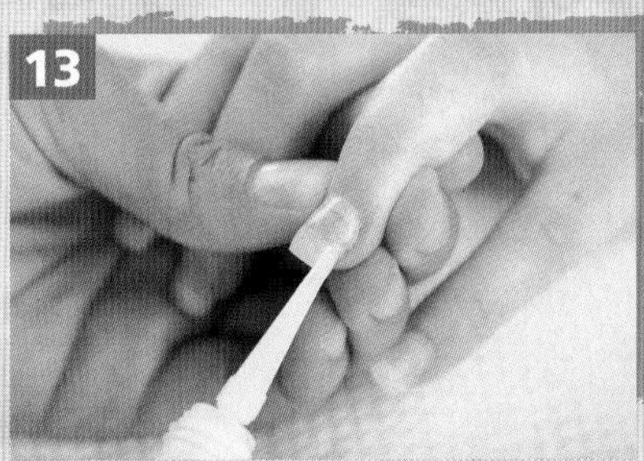

13 Apply a thin coat of nail wrap resin to the entire nail to strengthen and seal wrap.

14 Apply the wrap resin accelerator.

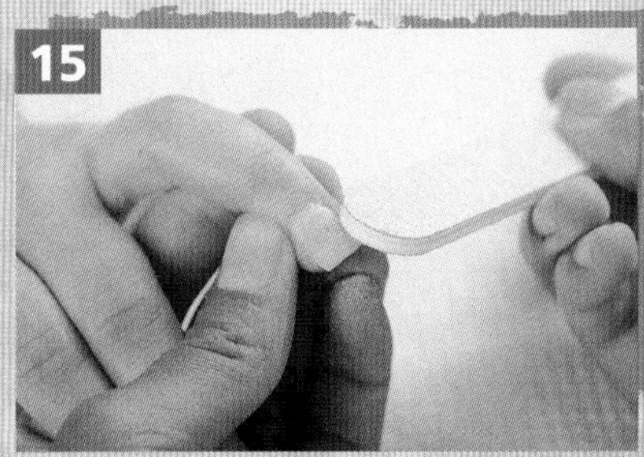

15 Use a medium-fine abrasive (240 grit) over the surface of the nail to remove any high spots or other imperfections. Carefully avoid the skin around the cuticle and sidewalls so that you do not cause cuts or damage.

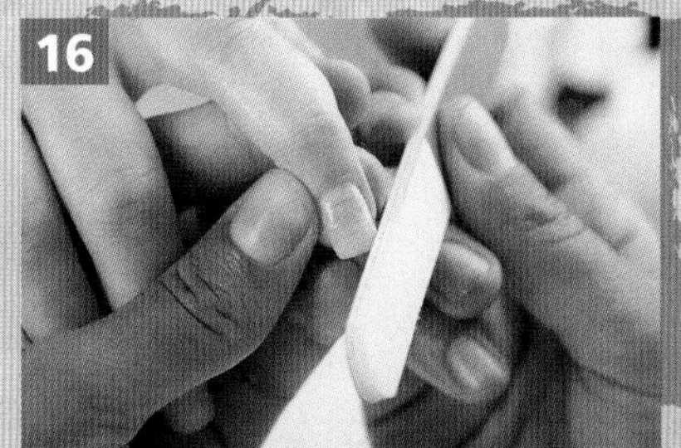

16 Apply nail oil and buff to a high shine with a buffer.

17 Apply hand lotion and massage the hand and arm.

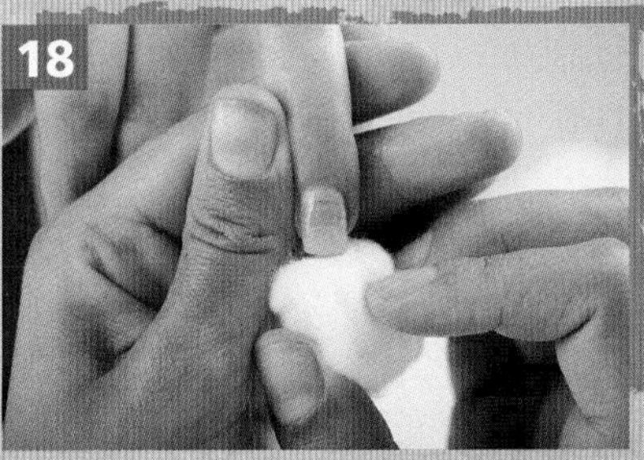

18 Use a small piece of cotton ball or plastic-backed pad and non-acetone polish remover to eliminate traces of oil from the nail so that the polish will adhere.

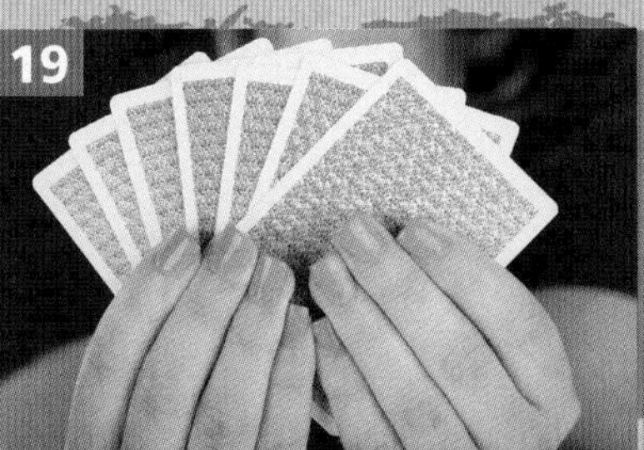

19 Finished look.

© Milady, a part of Cengage Learning. Photography by Dino Petrocelli.

Post-Service

• Complete

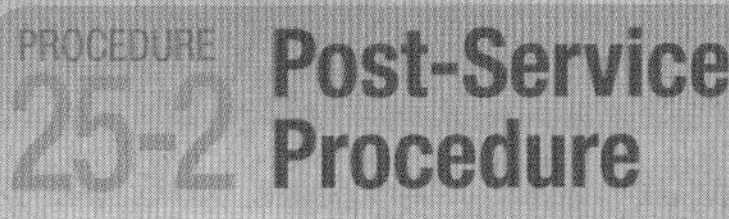

SEE PAGE 821 ✓ LO8

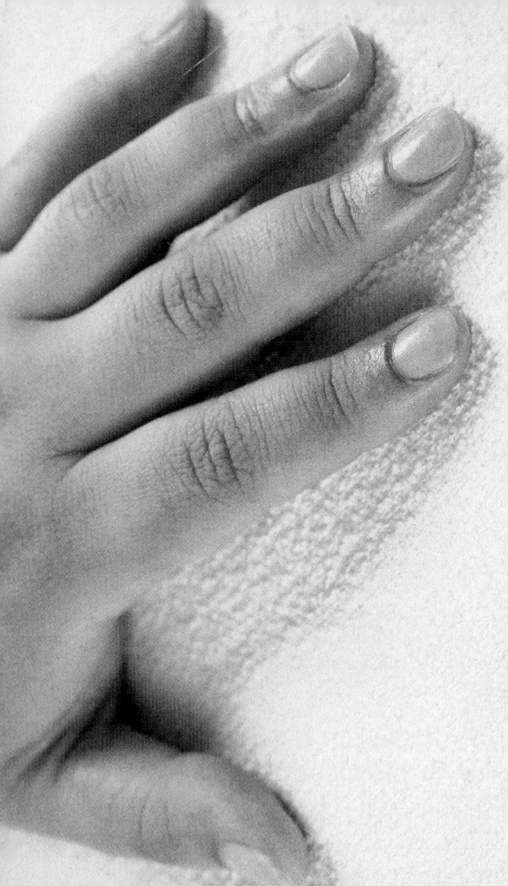

PROCEDURE 27-6

Fabric Wrap Removal

Implements and Materials

In addition to the basic materials on your manicuring table, you will need the following supplies for the Fabric Wrap Removal procedure:

- **Acetone**
- **Small glass bowl**

Preparation

- Perform PROCEDURE 25-1 **Pre-Service Procedure** SEE PAGE 817

Procedure

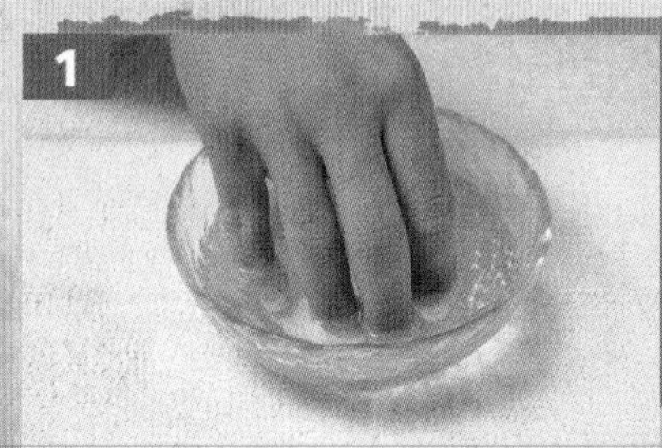

1 Put enough acetone in a small glass bowl to cover the nail wrap. Immerse the client's fingertips in the bowl, making sure that the wraps are covered. Soak for a few minutes. The acetone should be approximately ½-inch above the nail wraps.

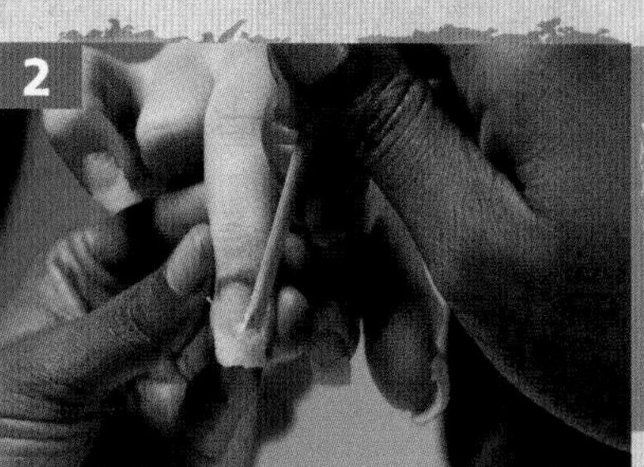

2 Use a pusher to slide softened wraps away from the nail plate.

© Milady, a part of Cengage Learning. Photography by Yanik Chauvin.

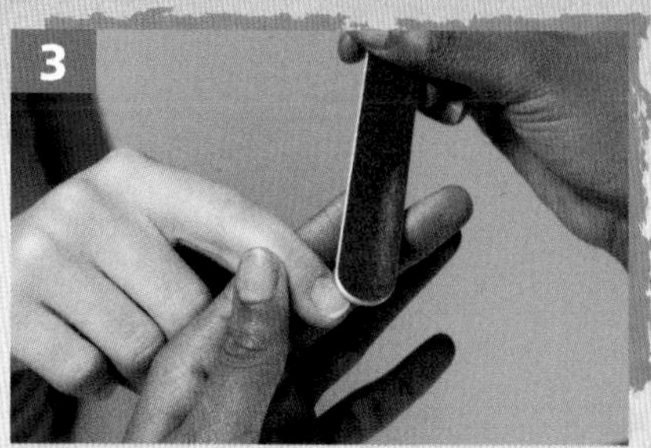

3 Gently buff natural nails with a fine buffer (240 grit) to remove the wrap resin.

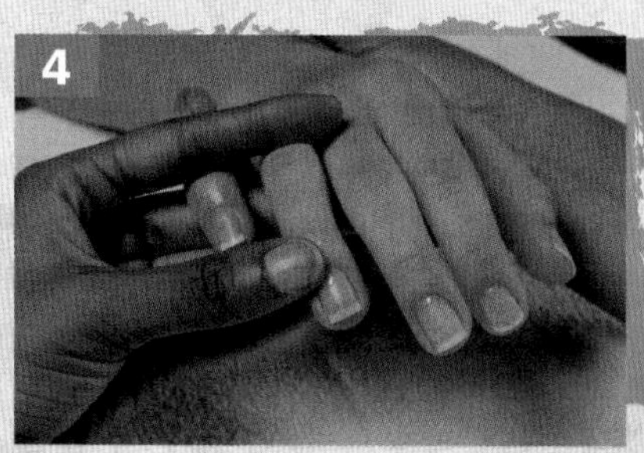

4 Condition the skin surrounding the nail plate with nail oils or lotions designed for this purpose.

5 Proceed to the desired service.

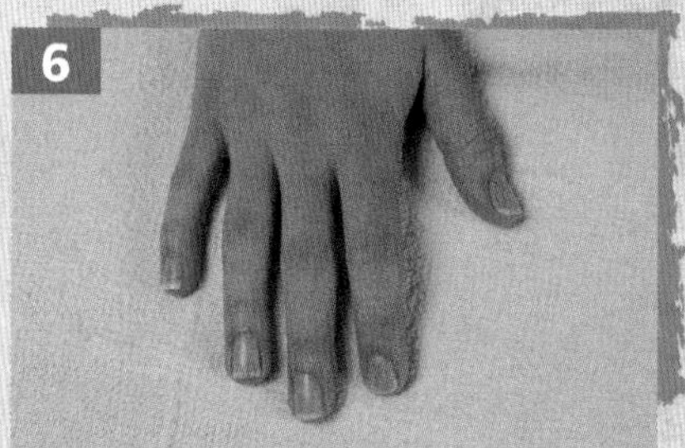

6 Finished look.

Post-Service

- Complete PROCEDURE 25-2 **Post-Service Procedure** SEE PAGE 821 ✓ LO9

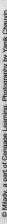

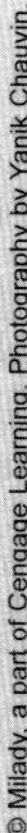
© Milady, a part of Cengage Learning. Photography by Yanik Chauvin.

Review Questions

1. What are the supplies, in addition to your basic manicuring table, that you need for nail tip application?
2. What are the types of nail tips available and why is it important to properly fit them for your client?
3. What types of fabrics are used in nail wraps?
4. What are the benefits of using each of these types of fabric wraps?
5. Describe the stop, rock, and hold method of applying nail tips.
6. Describe the Nail Tip Application Procedure.
7. Describe the Nail Tip Removal Procedure.
8. Describe the Nail Wrap Application Procedure.
9. What is the main difference between performing the Two-Week Fabric Wrap Maintenance and the Four-Week Fabric Wrap Maintenance?
10. Describe how to remove fabric wraps and what to avoid.

Chapter Glossary

acrylonitrile butadiene styrene	Also known as *ABS*; a common thermoplastic used to make light, rigid, molded nail tips.
cyanoacrylate	A specialized acrylic monomer that has excellent adhesion to the natural nail plate and polymerizes in seconds.
fabric wrap	Nail wrap made of silk, linen, or fiberglass.
fiberglass wraps	Made from a very thin synthetic mesh with a loose weave.
linen wraps	Made from a closely woven, heavy material.
maintenance	Term used for when a nail enhancement needs to be serviced after two or more weeks from the initial application of the nail enhancement product.
nail dehydrator	A substance used to remove surface moisture and tiny amounts of oil left on the natural nail plate.
nail tip adhesive	The bonding agent used to secure the nail tip to the natural nail.
nail tips	Plastic, pre-molded nails shaped from a tough polymer made from ABS plastic.
nail wrap	A method of securing a layer of fabric or paper on and around the nail tip to ensure its strength and durability.
nail wrap resin	Used to coat and secure fabric wraps to the natural nail and nail tip.
overlay	A layer of any kind of nail enhancement product that is applied over the natural nail or nail and tip application for added strength.

Chapter Glossary

paper wraps	Temporary nail wraps made of very thin paper.
position stop	The point where the free edge of the natural nail meets the tip.
repair patch	Piece of fabric cut to completely cover a crack or break in the nail.
silk wraps	Made from a thin natural material with a tight weave that becomes transparent when wrap resin is applied.
stress strip	Strip of fabric cut to ⅛-inch in length and applied to the weak point of the nail during the Four-Week Fabric Wrap Maintenance to repair or strengthen a weak point in a nail enhancement.
tip cutter	Implement similar to a nail clipper, designed especially for use on nail tips.
wrap resin accelerator	Also known as *activator*; acts as the dryer that speeds up the hardening process of the wrap resin or adhesive overlay.

CHAPTER 28

Monomer Liquid and Polymer Powder Nail Enhancements

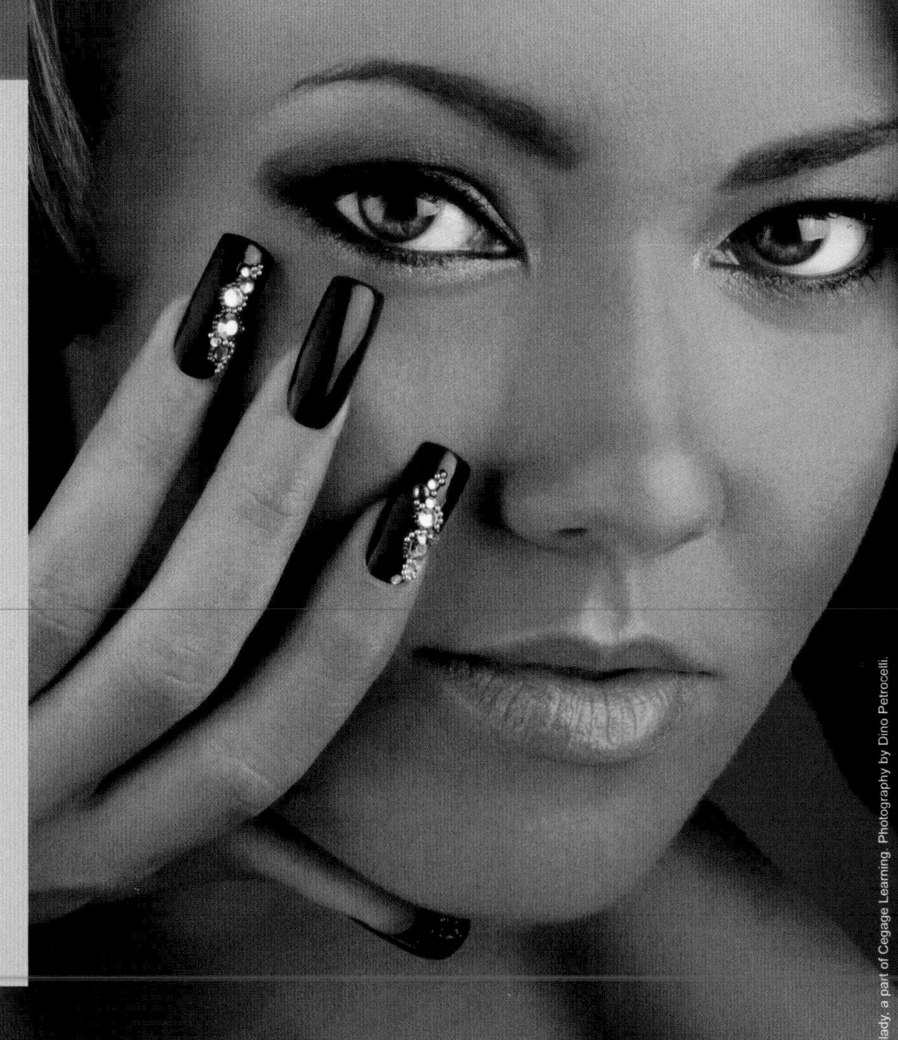

© Milady, a part of Cegage Learning. Photography by Dino Petrocelli.

Chapter Outline

Learning Objectives

After completing this chapter, you will be able to:

- ✓ **LO1** Explain monomer liquid and polymer powder nail enhancement chemistry and how it works.
- ✓ **LO2** Describe the apex, stress area, and sidewall, and tell where each is located on the nail enhancement.
- ✓ **LO3** Demonstrate the proper procedures for applying one-color monomer liquid and polymer powder nail enhancements over tips and on natural nails.
- ✓ **LO4** Demonstrate the proper procedures for applying two-color monomer liquid and polymer powder nail enhancements using forms over nail tips and on natural nails.
- ✓ **LO5** Describe how to perform a one-color maintenance service on nail enhancements using monomer liquid and polymer powder.
- ✓ **LO6** Demonstrate how to perform crack repair procedures.
- ✓ **LO7** Implement the proper procedure for removing monomer liquid and polymer powder nail enhancements.

Key Terms

Page number indicates where in the chapter the term is used.

apex (arch)
pg. 905

chain reaction (polymerization reaction)
pg. 900

initiators
pg. 900

monomer
pg. 898

monomer liquid
pg. 898

monomer liquid and polymer powder nail enhancements (sculptured nails)
pg. 898

nail extension underside
pg. 905

odorless monomer liquid and polymer powder products
pg. 906

polymer
pg. 898

polymerization (curing, hardening)
pg. 899

polymer powder
pg. 898

stress area
pg. 905

Publisher's Note: Nail enhancements based on mixing together liquids and powders are commonly referred to as *acrylic* (a-KRYL-yk) nails. It might surprise you to discover the real definition of *acrylic*, since for many years this word has actually been used incorrectly by the nail enhancement industry. The term *acrylic* actually refers to an entire family of thousands of different substances, all of which share important, closely related features. Acrylics are used to make a wide range of products, including contact lenses, cements for mending broken bones, Plexiglas windows, and even makeup and other cosmetics. Surprisingly, all nail enhancement products are based almost entirely on ingredients that come from the acrylic family. For example, the ingredients in two-part monomer liquid and polymer powder enhancement systems belong to a branch of the acrylic family called methacrylates. In other words, acrylic is a very general term for a large group of ingredients. Monomer liquid and polymer powder nail enhancement products are based on methacrylates (METH-ah-cry-latz). You can see some similarity in the spelling of the terms, which indicates that they are from the same chemical family or group. To be as accurate and specific as possible, this book refers to the two-part monomer liquid and polymer powder enhancement system as monomer liquid and polymer powder. However, please keep in mind that other industry literature, product marketing, and the like may continue to use the word *acrylic*.

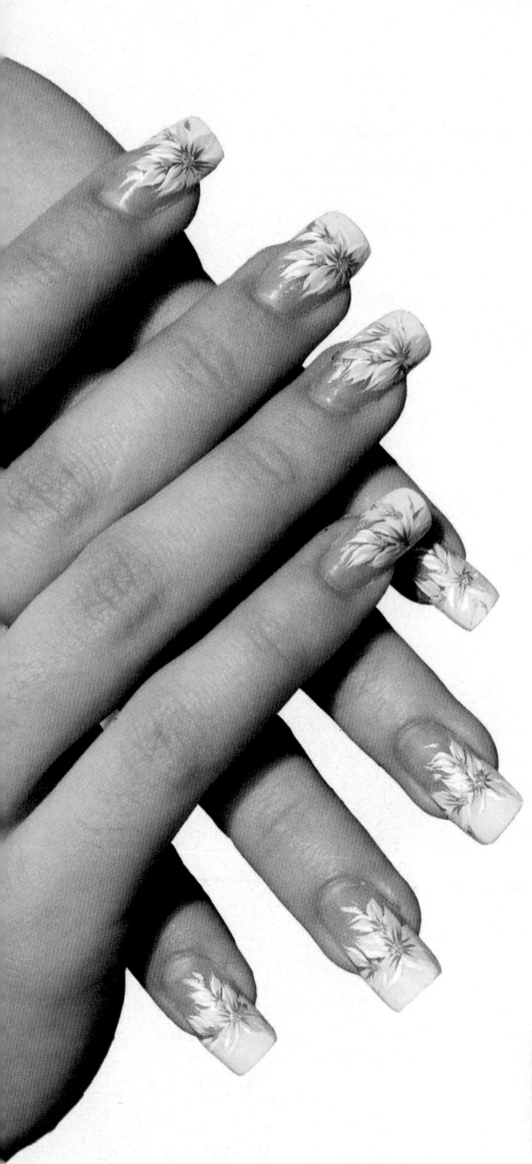

© Pakhnyushcha 2010; used under license from Shutterstock.com.

Today's monomer liquids and polymer powders come in many colors, including variations of basic pink, white, clear, and natural. These colors can be used alone or blended to create everything from customized shades of pink to match or enhance the color of your client's nail beds, to bold primaries or pastels that can be used to create a wide range of designs and patterns. With these powders, you can create unique colors or designs that can be locked permanently in the nail enhancement. They offer a wonderful way to customize your services or to express your artistry and creativity.

WHY STUDY MONOMER LIQUID AND POLYMER POWDER NAIL ENHANCEMENTS?

Cosmetologists should study and have a thorough understanding of monomer liquid and polymer powder nail enhancements because:

- Monomer liquid and polymer powder nail enhancements are popular services that will be frequently requested, and clients will expect expert service.
- Monomer liquid and polymer powder nail enhancements are lucrative services. Clients who desire them are committed to their upkeep, so if you earn clients' trust and respect, you will build a loyal clientele.
- Knowing how to properly work with the enhancement material and understanding its chemical makeup will allow you to perform the service safely for you and for your client.

Monomer Liquid and Polymer Powder Nail Enhancements

Monomer liquid and polymer powder nail enhancements, also known as **sculptured nails**, are created by combining **monomer** (MON-oh-mehr) **liquid**, a chemical liquid mixed with **polymer** (POL-i-mehr) **powder**, a powder in white, clear, pink, and many other colors, to form the nail enhancement. Thus the reason for the terms *liquid* and *powder* is obvious.

Mono means one and *mer* stands for units, so a **monomer** is one unit called a molecule. *Poly* means many, so **polymer** means a substance formed by combining many small molecules (monomers) into very long chain-like structures. This is important to remember, since you will hear these terms many times throughout your career.

Monomer liquid and polymer powder products can be applied in three basic ways:

1. On the natural nail as a protective overlay

2. Over a nail tip

3. On a form to create a nail extension

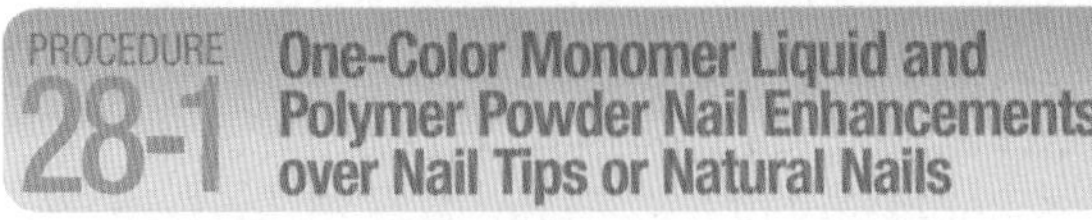

PROCEDURE
28-1
One-Color Monomer Liquid and Polymer Powder Nail Enhancements over Nail Tips or Natural Nails

SEE PAGE 908

A natural hair and pointed, round, or oval application brush is the best brush to use for applying these products. The brush is immersed in the monomer liquid. The natural hair bristles absorb and hold the monomer liquid like a reseroir. The tip of the brush is then touched to the surface of the dry polymer powder, and as the monomer liquid absorbs the polymer powder, a small bead of product forms. This small bead is then carefully placed on the nail surface and molded into shape with the brush.

The monomer liquid portion is usually one of three versions of monomer liquid used in the beauty industry: ethyl methacrylate, methyl methacrylate, or odorless monomer liquid. All three often contain other monomers that are used as customizing additives. The industry standards are the ethyl methacrylate monomer liquid (EMA) and the odorless monomer liquid. Methyl methacrylate (MMA) is not recommended for use on nails and is not legal according to the state board rules in some states.

It may seem strange that polymer powder is also made mostly from ethyl methacrylate monomer liquid. The polymer powder is made using **polymerization** (POL-i-mehr-eh-za-shun), also known as **curing** or **hardening**, a chemical reaction that creates polymers. In this process, trillions of monomers are linked together to create long chains. These long chains create the tiny round beads of polymer powder used to create certain types of nail enhancements.

During the production of polymer powder, the powder forms into tiny round beads of slightly varying sizes. The beads are then poured through a series of special screens that sort the beads by size. The ones that are the right size are separated and then mixed with other special additives and colorants. The final mixture is packaged and sold as polymer powder. It is a surprisingly high-tech process that requires very specific manufacturing equipment, lots of quality control, and scientific know-how to do it right.

Special additives are blended into both the liquid and the powder. These additives ensure complete set or cure, maximum durability, color stability, and shelf life, among other attributes. It is these custom additives that make products work and behave differently. The polymer powders are usually blended with pigments and colorants to create a wide range of shades, including pinks, whites, and milky translucent shades, as well as reds, blues, greens, purples, yellows, oranges, browns, and even jet black.

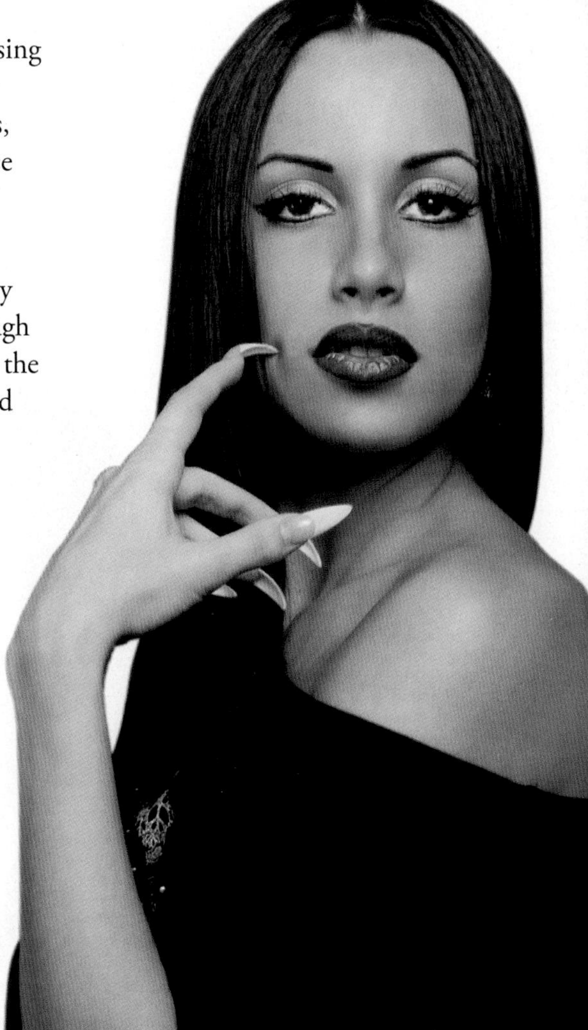

© Konstantynov 2010; used under license from Shutterstock.com.

When liquid is picked up by a brush and mixed with the powder, the bead that forms on the end of the brush quickly begins to harden. It is then put into place with other beads and shaped into place as they harden. In order for this process to begin, the monomers and polymers require special additives called catalysts (KAT-a-lists), substances that speed up chemical reactions between monomer liquid and polymer powder. Catalysts are added to the monomer liquid and used to control the set or curing time. In other words, when the monomer liquid and polymer powder are combined, the catalyst (in the liquid) helps control the set-up or hardening time. How? The catalyst energizes and activates the initiators.

The **initiators** start a chain reaction that leads to the creation of very long polymer chains. It is actually the initiators found in the powder that, when activated, will spring into action and start causing monomer molecules to permanently link together into long polymer chains. This is another example of the polymerization process discussed above, except this time it is actually occurring on the fingernail. The polymerization process begins when the liquid in the brush picks up powder from the container and forms a bead. Creating polymers can be thought of as a **chain reaction**, also known as **polymerization reaction**, a process that joins together monomers to create very long polymer chains, much like many dominos when set on their edges and lined up—tap the first domino, and it hits the next, and so on. This is how polymers form. Once the monomers join together to create a polymer, they do not detach from each other easily.

The initiator that is added to the polymer powder is called benzoyl peroxide (BPO). It is the same ingredient used in over-the-counter acne medicine, except that it has a different purpose in nail enhancement products. BPO is used to start the chain reaction that leads to curing (hardening) of the nail enhancement. There is much less BPO in nail powders than in acne treatments. Diverse nail enhancement products often use different amounts of BPO, since the polymer powders are designed to work specifically with a certain monomer liquid. Some monomer liquids require more BPO to properly cure than others. This is why it is very important to use the polymer powder that was designed for the monomer liquid that you are using. Using the wrong powder can create nail enhancements that are not properly cured and may lead to service breakdown or could increase the risk of your clients developing a skin irritation or sensitivity.

There are many monomer liquid and polymer powder systems available, and you might have to try several in order to find the product that fits best for you and your clients. ☑ **LO1**

To learn more about how products work and how to troubleshoot problems, see *Nail Structure & Product Chemistry*, Second Edition, by Douglas D. Schoon, published by Milady, a part of Cengage Learning.

© Katrina Brown 2010; used under license from Shutterstock.com.

Monomer Liquid and Polymer Powder Nail Enhancement Supplies

Just as every type of nail enhancement service requires specific tools, implements, equipment, and supplies, so do monomer liquid and polymer powder nail enhancements. **Figure 28–1** shows examples of those products and supplies.

© Milady, a part of Cengage Learning. Photography by Dino Petrocelli.

▲ **Figure 28–1**
Supplies needed for monomer liquid and polymer powder nail enhancement applications.

Monomer Liquid

The monomer liquid will be combined with polymer powder to form the sculptured nail. The amount of monomer liquid and polymer powder used to create a bead is called the *mix ratio*. A bead mix ratio can be best described as dry, medium, or wet. If equal amounts of liquid and powder are used to create the bead, it is called a *dry bead*. If twice as much liquid as powder is used to create the bead, it is called a *wet bead*. Halfway between these two is a *medium bead*, which contains one-and-a-half times more liquid than powder. In general, medium beads are the ideal mix ratio for working with monomer liquids and polymer powders.

The mix ratio typically ensures proper set and maximum durability of the nail enhancement. This mixture functions in a similar way as other, more familiar, mixtures. For example, if too much flour is added to cookie batter, the cookies will be dry and crumbly; if too little flour is added, the cookies will be soft and gooey. The same holds true for monomer liquids and polymer powders. If too much powder is picked up in the bead, the enhancement will cure incorrectly and may be brittle or discolored. If too little powder is used, the nail enhancement can become weak, and clients will be at greater risk of developing skin irritation and sensitivity.

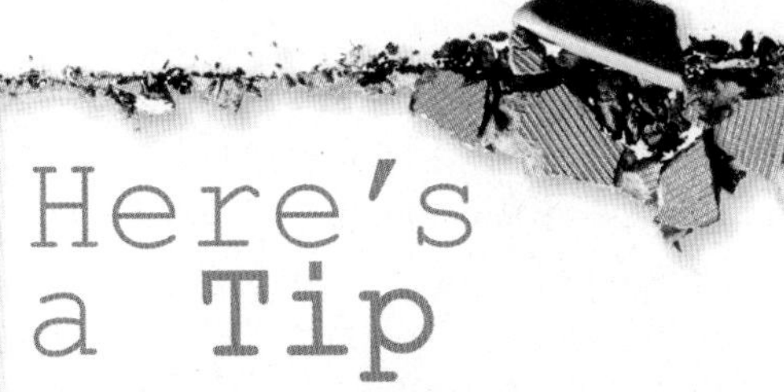

Monomer Liquid Bead Mix Ratio Guidelines

1 part monomer liquid + 1 part polymer powder = dry bead

1½ parts monomer liquid + 1 part polymer powder = medium bead

2 parts monomer liquid + 1 part polymer powder = wet bead

Polymer Powder

Polymer powder is available in white, clear, natural, pink, and many other colors. The color(s) you choose will depend on the nail enhancement method you are using.

Nail Dehydrator

Nail dehydrators remove surface moisture and tiny amounts of oil left on the natural nail plate, both of which can block adhesion. Nail dehydrator should be applied liberally to the natural nail plate only; skin contact should be avoided. This step is a great way to help prevent lifting of the nail enhancement prior to applying primer.

Nail Primer

Many kinds of nail primers are available today. In the past, acid-based nail primer (methacrylic acid) was widely used to help adhere enhancements to the natural nail. Since acid-based nail primer is corrosive to the skin and potentially dangerous to eyes, acid-free and nonacid primers were developed.

FYI

Manufacturer's instructions for using monomer liquid and polymer powder nail enhancement products may differ slightly from the general guidelines presented in this chapter. You should always use products in accordance with the manufacturer's instructions. If you are in doubt about how to use the products, contact the manufacturer.

Acid-free and nonacid primers are the types of primers that are most often used today. They work as well as or better than acid-based nail primers, and have the added advantage of not being corrosive to skin or eyes. All nail primer products must be used with caution, and skin contact must be avoided. Read the manufacturer's instructions and refer to the Material Safety Data Sheet (MSDS) for safe handling recommendations and instructions. Acid-based nail primers must be used with caution and in accordance with the manufacturer's instructions.

For acid-based nail primers: Using a tiny applicator brush, insert the brush tip into the nail primer. Touch the brush tip to the edge of the bottle's neck to release the excess primer back into the bottle. Keeping the brush dry and using a light dotting action, carefully dab the brush tip to the center of the properly prepared natural nail. The acid-based primer will spread out and cover the nail plate. Do not use too much product—it will run onto the skin and cause burns or injury. Be sure to read the label for the manufacturer's suggested application procedures and precautions.

For nonacid and acid-free nail primers: Using the applicator brush, insert brush into the nail primer. Wipe excess product from the brush. Using a slightly damp brush, completely cover the nail plate with the primer. Do not use too much product—it will run onto the skin and cause skin irritation or sensitivity. The brush should hold enough product to treat two or three nails. Be sure the entire nail plate is covered. Before dipping the brush back into the container, gently wipe the brush on a clean table towel so you do not contaminate the bottle with any debris the brush may have picked up. Be sure to read the label for the manufacturer's suggested application procedures and precautions.

FOCUS ON

PROPER HAND WASHING

Always have your clients wash their hands thoroughly with a fingernail brush before any service. Hand sanitizers are an alternative when hand washing is not available, but they do not clean the hands. They cannot remove dirt or debris from hands and underneath the nails. They kill some of the bacteria on skin, but not all of it. Hand sanitizers do give clients peace of mind, though. Clients like to see cosmetologists using hand sanitizers and many clients prefer to use them as well. Keep a high-quality, professional hand sanitizer at your station and offer some to your clients. Let them see you using it, and they will have a greater degree of confidence in the cleanliness of your services. Do not use hand sanitizers in place of hand washing—there is no replacement for proper hand washing.

Abrasives

Select a medium grit (180 to 240) for natural nail preparation and initial shaping. Choose a medium grit for smoothing and a fine buffer (350 grit or higher) for final buffing. A three-way buffer is used to create a high shine on the enhancement when no polish is worn. If you avoid putting the product on too thickly, a 180 grit is usually enough to shape the nail enhancement. Avoid using coarser (lower-grit) abrasives or aggressive techniques on freshly applied enhancement products, because they can damage the freshly created nail enhancement.

Nail Forms

Nail forms are placed under the free edge and used to extend the nail enhancements beyond the fingertip for additional length. Nail forms are often made of paper or Mylar and coated with adhesive backs or are made of preshaped plastic or aluminum. Each of these forms is disposable, except the plastic and aluminum forms, which can be properly cleaned and disinfected.

PROCEDURE 28-2 Two-Color Monomer Liquid and Polymer Powder Nail Enhancements Using Forms SEE PAGE 912

Nail Tips

These are preformed nail extensions made from ABS or tenite acetate plastic and are available in a wide variety of shapes, styles, and colors, including natural, white, and clear.

PROCEDURE 27-1 Nail Tip Application in Chapter 27 SEE PAGE 879

Dappen Dish

The monomer liquid and polymer powder are each poured into a special holder called a *dappen dish*. These dishes must have narrow openings to minimize evaporation of the monomer liquid into the air. Do not use open-mouth jars or other containers with large openings. Those types of containers will dramatically increase evaporation of the liquid and can allow the product to be contaminated with dust and other debris. Dappen dishes must be covered with a tight-fitting lid when not in use.

Each time the brush is dipped into the dappen dish, the remaining monomer liquid is contaminated with small amounts of polymer powder. So never pour the unused portion of monomer liquid back into the original container. Empty the monomer liquid from your dappen dish after the service and wipe it clean with a disposable towel. To avoid skin irritation or sensitivity, do not contact skin with the monomer liquid during this process. Wipe the dish clean with acetone, if necessary, before storing in a dust-free location.

Nailbrush

The best brush for use with these types of procedures is composed of sable hair and is usually an oval or round style application brush. Odorless monomer liquid requires less liquid, and a flat brush holds less liquid.

Synthetic and less expensive brushes do not pick up enough monomer liquid or do not release the liquid properly. Choose the brush shape and size with which you feel the most comfortable. Avoid overly large brushes (sizes 12 to 16), since they can hold excessive amounts of liquid and alter the mix ratio of the powder and liquid.

Having too much monomer liquid on your brush can increase the risk of accidentally touching the client's skin and may increase the risk of developing skin irritation or sensitivities.

Safety Eyewear

Safety eyewear should be used to protect eyes from flying objects or accidental splashes. There are many types and styles. You can get more information by searching the Internet or contacting a local optometrist,

CAUTION

Acid-based nail primers are very effective but can cause serious—and sometimes irreversible—damage to the skin and eyes. Never use acid-based nail primer or any other corrosive material without wearing protective gloves and safety eyewear.

FYI

The best way to dispose of small amounts of monomer liquid is to mix them with small amounts of the powder designed to cure them. (This is safe for amounts ranging from less than a half-ounce of monomer liquid to quarts or gallons.) They should never be disposed of in the trash or down the drain. Tiny amounts left in a dappen dish can be wiped out with a paper towel and disposed of in a metal trash can with a self-closing lid. Be sure to avoid contact with your skin during the process and have the trash disposed of several times during the day so that vapors do not evaporate and escape into the salon air.

who can also help you with both nonprescription and prescription safety eyewear.

Dust Masks

Dust masks are designed to be worn over the nose and mouth to prevent inhalation of excessive amounts of dust. They provide no protection from vapors.

Protective Gloves

Both disposable and multiuse varieties of protective gloves can be purchased. Several types of materials are used to make these gloves. For many salon-related applications, gloves made of nitrile polymer powder work best.

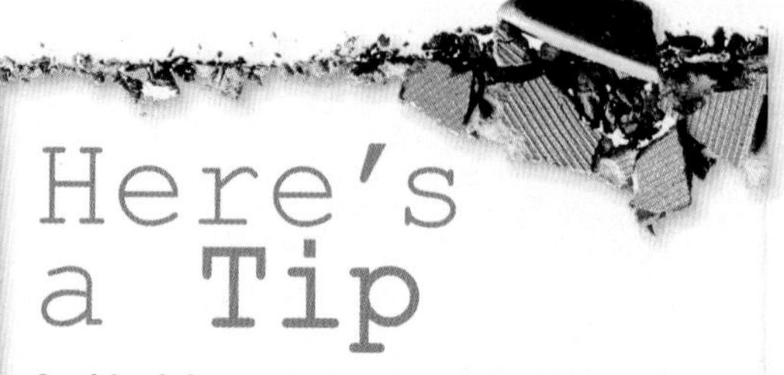

Here's a Tip

Avoid wiping your brush too rapidly or too hard against a table towel. This can press hairs against the sharp edge of the metal ferrule that holds the hairs in place and cut them off.

Storing and Disposing of Monomer Liquid and Polymer Powder Products

Store monomer liquid and polymer powder products in covered containers. Store all primers and liquids separate from each other in a cool, dark area. Do not store products near heat.

After a service, you must discard used materials. Never save used monomer liquid that has been removed from the original container. Use each portion on one client only. To dispose of small amounts of leftover monomer liquid, carefully pour it into a very absorbent paper towel and then place it in a plastic bag. Avoid skin contact with the monomer liquid and never pour it directly into the plastic bag! Should skin contact occur, wash hands with liquid soap and water. After all used materials have been collected, seal them in a plastic bag and discard the bag in a closed waste receptacle. It is important to remove items soiled with enhancement products from your manicuring station after each client. This will help maintain the quality of the air in your salon. Dispose of these items according to local rules and regulations.

Monomer Liquid and Polymer Powder Nail Enhancement Maintenance, Crack Repair, and Removal

Regular maintenance helps prevent nail enhancements from lifting or cracking. If the nail enhancements are not regularly maintained, they have a greater tendency to lift, crack, or break, which increases the risk of the client developing an infection or having other problems.

When a cosmetologist has a client with a piece or section of the monomer liquid and polymer powder enhancement that has broken, lifted, or cracked, it is repaired by filing the area and adding monomer liquid and polymer powder to it. This is called a crack repair.

Proper maintenance must be performed every two to three weeks, depending on how fast the client's nails grow.

If you choose to offer nail enhancement services to your clients, proper maintenance is a critical skill for you to learn. Do not let clients go too long without having a proper maintenance service, or you will have many more repairs to perform when they return. Proper maintenance is both safe and gentle to the nail unit and will not result in injury or damage. In the maintenance service, the nail is thinned down, the apex of the nail is removed, and the entire nail enhancement is reduced in thickness.

PROCEDURE 28-3 One-Color Monomer Liquid and Polymer Powder Maintenance SEE PAGE 916

PROCEDURE 28-4 Crack Repair for Monomer Liquid and Polymer Powder Nail Enhancements SEE PAGE 919

Areas of Concern for Building Properly Structured Nail Enhancements

Nail enhancements should not only look good, but they should also remain strong and healthy while your client is wearing them. Several areas of the nail must be considered when the nail enhancement is being built to accomplish this. Paying particular attention to the following areas of the nail enhancement will help you to create the look your clients' desire and also provide them with the best and longest-lasting nail enhancements.

The **apex**, also known as **arch**, is the area of the nail that has all of the strength. Having strength in the apex allows the base of the nail, sidewalls, and tip to be thin, yet leaves the nail strong enough to resist frequent chipping or breaking. The apex is usually oval shaped and is located in the center of the nail. The high point is visible no matter where you view the nail.

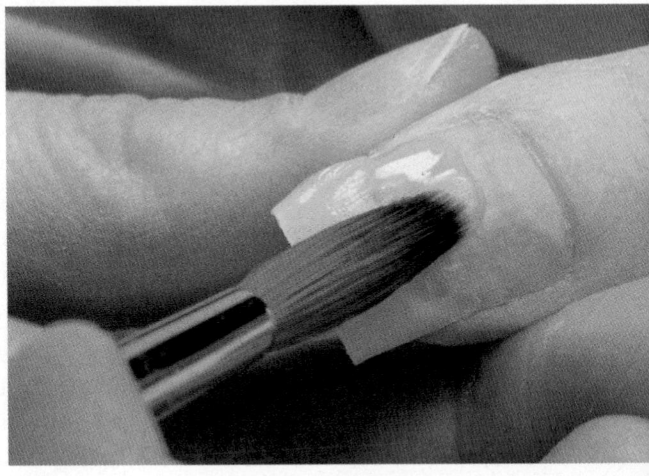

© Christopher Elwell, 2010; used under license from Shutterstock.com.

The **stress area** is where the natural nail grows beyond the finger and becomes the free edge. This area needs strength to support the extension.

The sidewall is the area on the side of the nail plate that grows free of its attachment to the nail fold and where the extension leaves the natural nail.

The **nail extension underside** is the actual underside of the nail extension. The nail extension underside can jut straight out or may dip, depending on the nail style. The nail extension underside should be even, matched on each nail. Undersides should match in length from nail to nail on all fingers. The tip should fit the nail and finger properly, and the underside of the nail extension should be smooth, without any glitches.

The thickness of the nail enhancement should be rather thin if a client is to wear it comfortably while going about her day. The enhancement should graduate seamlessly from the cuticle to the end of the nail extension, so you do not feel an edge. The sidewalls and tip's edge should be credit-card thin.

The C curve of the nail enhancement depends on the C curve of the natural nail. In the salon, a 35 percent C curve is the average. The top surface and bottom side should match perfectly.

To make sure the lengths of the nail extension and enhancements are appropriate and even, be sure to measure the length of the index, middle, and ring fingers; these should be the same length. The thumb and pinkie fingers should also be in proportion and match. ☑ LO2

Monomer Liquid and Polymer Powder Nail Enhancement Removal

There will be circumstances when your client feels that she wants to have her monomer liquid and polymer powder nail enhancements removed. Do not worry. The procedure is simple: You soak the enhancements off of the nail using acetone or the manufacturer's suggested removal solution, remove the enhancement, and complete the service.

PROCEDURE 28-5 Monomer Liquid and Polymer Powder Nail Enhancement Removal SEE PAGE 921

Odorless Monomer Liquid and Polymer Powder Products

Odorless monomer liquid and polymer powder products are nail enhancement products that have little odor. These products do not necessarily have the same chemistry as all other monomer liquid and polymer powder products. Rather than use ethyl acrylic these products rely on monomers that have little odor. Even though these products are called "odorless," they do have a slight odor. Generally, if a monomer liquid does not produce a strong enough odor that others in the salon can detect its presence, it is considered to be an odorless product. Those that create a slight odor in the salon are called "low odor."

In general, odorless products must be used with a dry mix ratio (equal parts liquid and powder in bead). If used too wet, there is the risk of the client developing skin irritation or sensitivity. This mix ratio creates a snowy-appearing bead on your brush. After it is placed on the nail, it will slowly form into a firm glossy bead that will hold its shape until pressed and smoothed with the nailbrush. Wipe your brush frequently to avoid the product sticking to the hairs. Never rewet the brush with monomer liquid. This will change the mix ratio, which can lead to product discoloration, service breakdown, and increased risk of skin irritation and sensitivity.

© Tania Zbrodko, 2010; used under license from Shutterstock.com.

ACTivity

To determine whether you have done the best possible job to ensure a smooth, balanced, and symmetrical nail, and that all nails are consistent, try viewing them from the following perspectives.

Top view. Make sure all the perimeter shapes are consistent.

Left side and right side views. Look at the profile of each nail and make sure your apex is consistently located in the correct place and that the apexes match from nail to nail. Also look at the left side and right side of the nail and make sure the extension's underside matches.

Down the center. Look at the degrees of C curves. Do they match? Is the thinness/thickness of the product consistent and thick enough to withstand wear or are the nails too thin?

From the client's perspective. Turn the client's hand around and fold the fingers toward the palm of the hand so you can view the top surface from the client's perspective. Sometimes you can see lumps and bumps from this view that you couldn't see when looking at them during application.

Line of light. After the nail is smooth and polished, or after a UV gel sealant has been applied, you can follow the line of light that reflects off the surface of the nail to see whether the nail is really smooth. If the nail surface is not smooth, the line of light will not follow perfectly.

Without re-wetting your brush, use the brush to shape and smooth the surface to perfection.

Odorless products harden more slowly and create a tacky layer called the inhibition layer. Once the enhancement has hardened, this layer can be removed with alcohol, acetone, or a manufacturer-recommended product. It is always best to use a plastic-backed cotton pad to avoid skin contact with the inhibition layer, since repeated contact with this layer can lead to skin irritation and sensitivity. The inhibition layer also can be filed away, but avoid skin contact with these freshly filed particles.

Colored Polymer Powder Products

Polymer powders are now available in a wide range of colors that mimic almost every shade available in nail polish. Nail artistry with colored polymer powder is limited only by your imagination. Some professionals use colors to go beyond the traditional pink and white French manicure combinations and offer custom-blended colors to their clients. They maintain recipe cards so that they can reproduce customized nail enhancements that clients cannot get from anyone else. As with all customized techniques, clients are willing to pay a few dollars more for the special service.

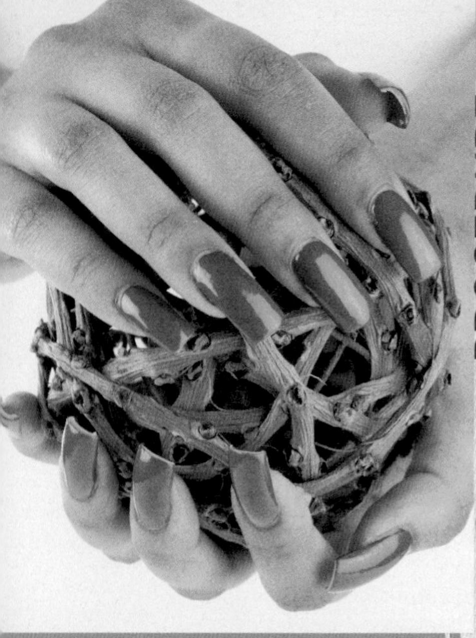

PROCEDURE 28-1

One-Color Monomer Liquid and Polymer Powder Nail Enhancements over Nail Tips or Natural Nails

Implements and Materials

In addition to the basic materials on your manicuring table, you will need the following supplies for the One-Color Monomer Liquid and Polymer Powder Nail Enhancements over Nail Tips or Natural Nails procedure:

- Abrasives
- Application brushes
- Dappen dishes
- Monomer liquid
- Nail dehydrator
- Nail primer
- Polymer powder

Preparation

- Perform PROCEDURE 25-1 Pre-Service Procedure SEE PAGE 817

Procedure

1 Use a pusher to gently push back the eponychium. Then, if needed, apply cuticle remover. Use as directed by the manufacturer, and carefully remove cuticle tissue from the nail plate. Have the client wash and dry their hands again to remove any oils from the cuticle remover.

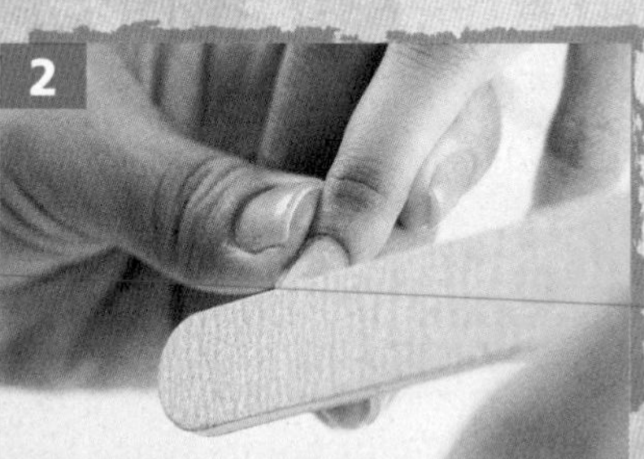

2 Buff (gently) the nail plate with medium-fine abrasive (240 grit) to remove the shine caused by natural oil on the surface of the nail plate. Avoid over-filing of the nail plate. Remove the nail dust with a clean, dry nailbrush, and do not touch the surface of the nails with your fingers as you may deposit oils from your fingertips, degrading the cleanliness of the nail.

3 Apply nail dehydrator to nails. Begin with the little finger on the left hand and work toward the thumb.

4 Apply tips, if your client wants them, as described in Chapter 27, Nail Tips and Wraps. (See Procedure 27–1, Nail Tip Application.) Cut tips to desired length.

© Milady, a part of Cengage Learning. Photography by Dino Petrocelli.

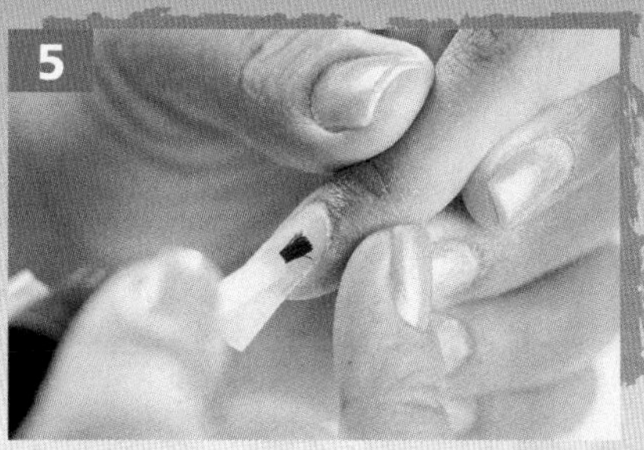

5 Apply nail primer and follow the manufacturer's directions. Allow nail primer to dry thoroughly. Acid-free primer will dry sticky and shiny. Never apply nail enhancement product over wet nail primer. This can cause product discoloration and service breakdown. Avoid overuse of nail primers. Apply primer to the natural nail, but avoid putting it on the nail tips unless instructed by the manufacturer of the nail primer.

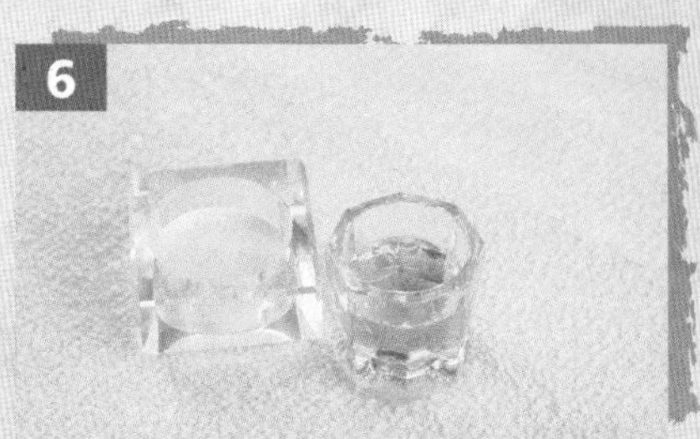

6 Pour monomer liquid and polymer powder into separate dappen dishes.

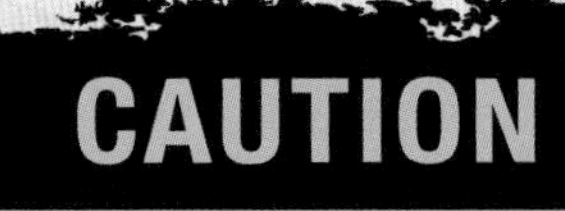

CAUTION

Check your nail primer daily for clarity, to ensure that it does not become contaminated with nail dust and other floating debris, which can dramatically reduce primer effectiveness. Never use nail primers that are visibly contaminated with floating debris. To avoid contamination, wipe the primer brush on a clean, dust-free towel before replacing the brush in the bottle.

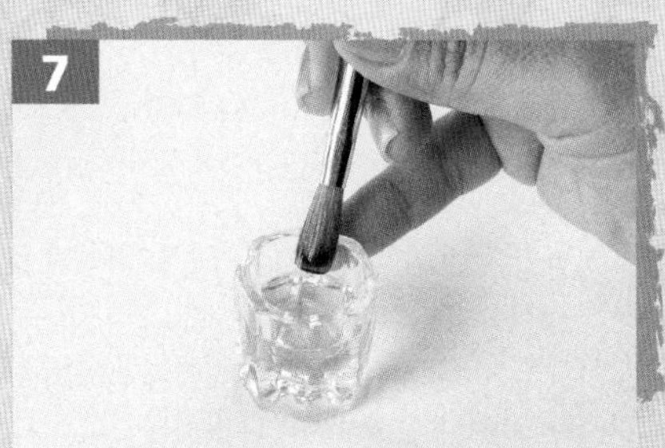

7 Dip brush into the monomer liquid and wipe on the edge of the container to remove the excess.

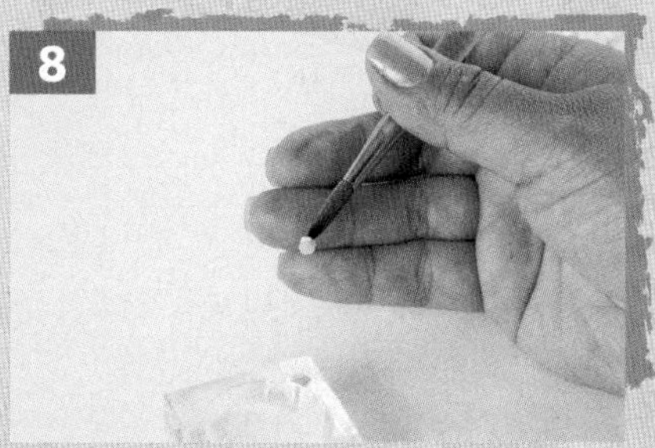

8 Dip the tip of the same brush into the polymer powder and rotate slightly. Pick up a bead of product—with a medium-to-dry consistency, not runny or wet—that is large enough for shaping the entire free-edge extension. If you have trouble using a large bead to shape the edge properly, two smaller beads may be easier.

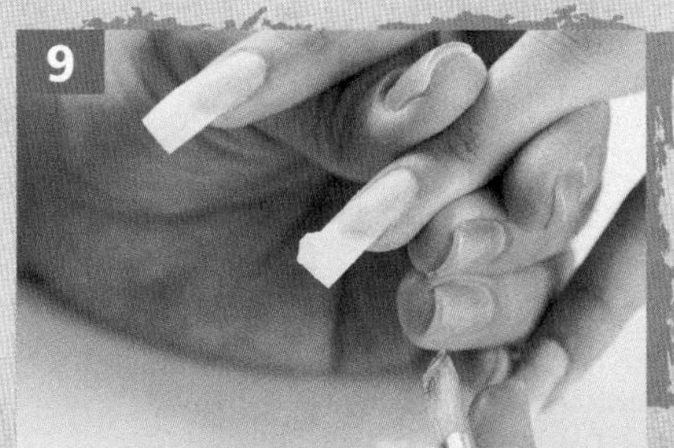

9 Place the pink product bead in the center of the free edge of the tip or natural nail. Immediately wipe your brush on the table towel gently to remove any product left in the bristles and bring brush back to a perfect point.

© Milady, a part of Cengage Learning. Photography by Dino Petrocelli.

PROCEDURE 28-1 One-Color Monomer Liquid and Polymer Powder Nail Enhancements over Nail Tips or Natural Nails continued

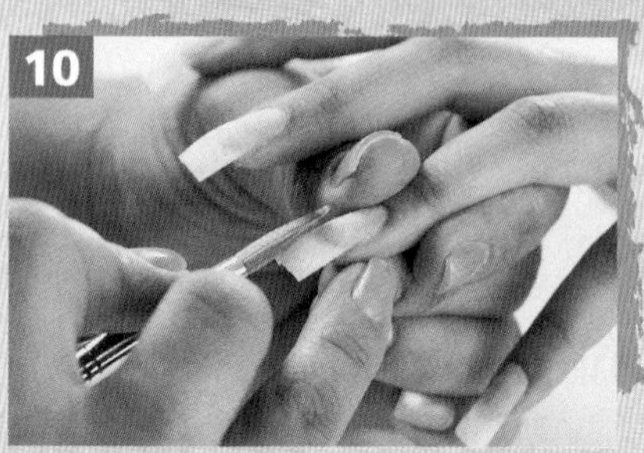

10 Use the middle portion of your sable brush to press and smooth the product to shape the enhancement's free edge. Do not paint the product onto the nail. Pressing and smoothing produces a more natural-looking nail. Keep sidewall lines parallel, and avoid widening the tip beyond the natural width of the nail plate.

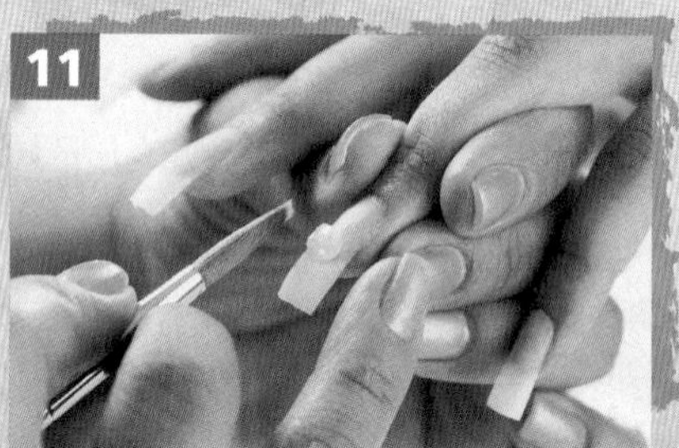

11 Place the second bead—of medium consistency—on the nail plate below the first bead and next to the free-edge line in the center of the nail. Immediately wipe your brush gently on the table towel to remove any product left in the bristles and to bring the brush back to a perfect point.

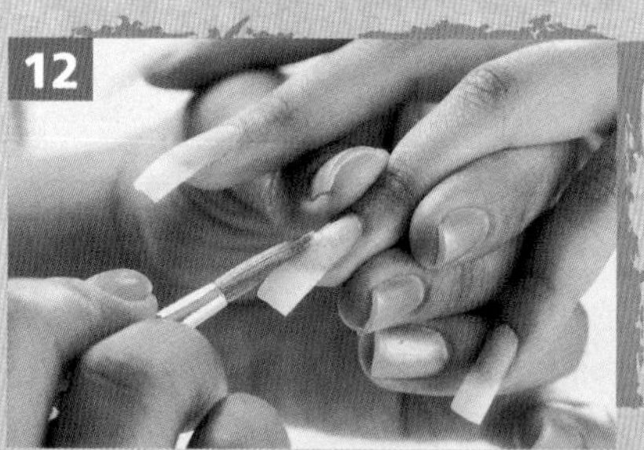

12 Press and smooth the product to sidewalls, making sure that the product is very thin around all edges. Leave a tiny free margin between the product placement and skin. Avoid placing the product too close to the skin, or the product may lift away from the nail plate and may also increase the chance of the client developing a skin irritation or sensitivity. Be sure to use a medium consistency mix that is not too wet.

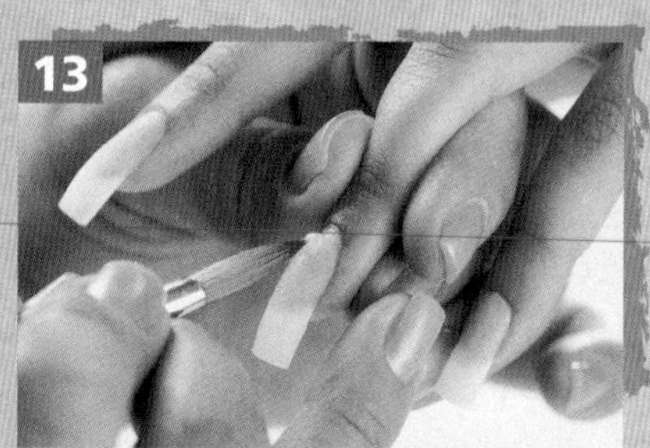

13 Pick up smaller beads of pink polymer powder with your brush and place them at the base of the nail plate, leaving a tiny free margin between the product and the skin. Immediately wipe your brush on the table towel gently to remove any product left in the bristles and to bring the brush back to a perfect point.

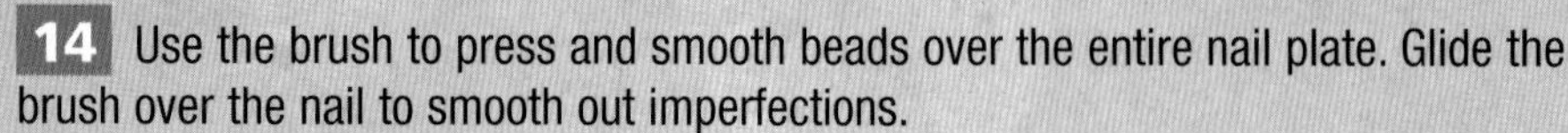

14 Use the brush to press and smooth beads over the entire nail plate. Glide the brush over the nail to smooth out imperfections.

© Milady, a part of Cengage Learning. Photography by Dino Petrocelli.

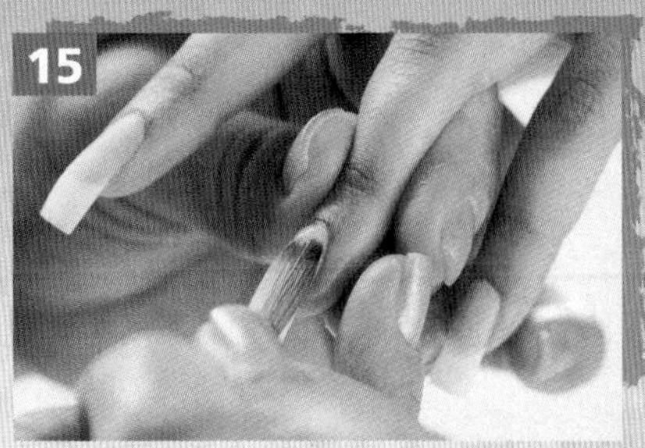

15 Apply more product near eponychium, sidewall, and free edge if needed to complete the application. Be sure that the product in these areas remains thin for a natural-looking nail.

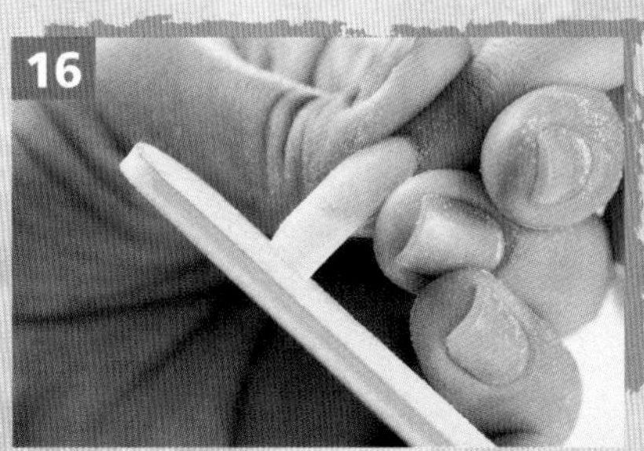

16 Use medium abrasive (180 to 240 grit) to shape the free edge and to remove imperfections. Then refine with medium-fine abrasive (240 grit).

17 Buff the nail enhancement with fine-grit buffer (350 grit or higher) until the entire surface is smooth. If nail polish is to be worn, use a high-shine buffer.

18 Apply and rub nail oil into the surrounding skin and nail enhancement, massaging briefly to speed penetration.

19 Apply hand cream and massage the hand and arm.

20 Ask the client to wash her hands with soap and water at the hand washing station or ask her to use the nailbrush to clean her nails over a finger bowl. Rinse with clean water to remove soap residue that may cause lifting. Dry thoroughly with a clean disposable towel.

21 Polish nail enhancements or apply a gel sealant.

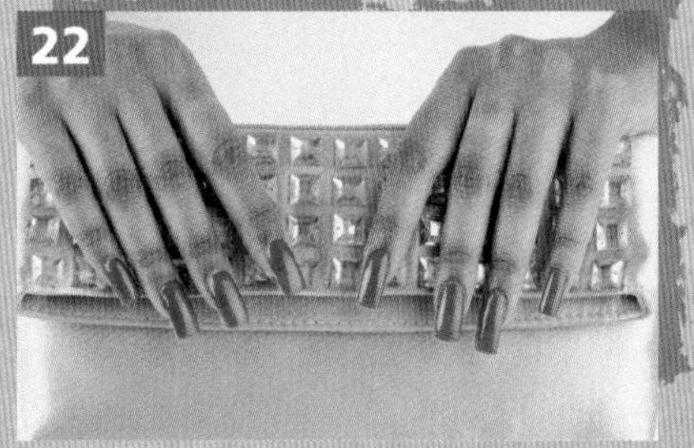

22 Finished look.

© Milady, a part of Cengage Learning. Photography by Dino Petrocelli.

Post-Service

- Complete 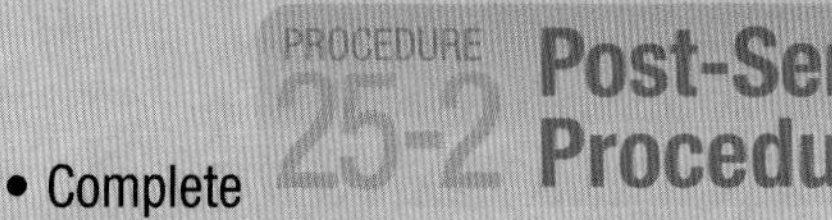 PROCEDURE 25-2 **Post-Service Procedure** SEE PAGE 821 ✓ LO3

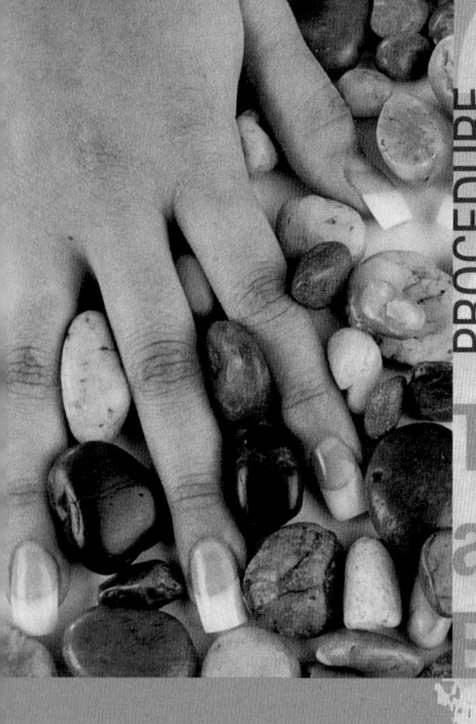

PROCEDURE 28-2

Two-Color Monomer Liquid and Polymer Powder Nail Enhancements Using Forms

Implements and Materials

In addition to the basic materials on your manicuring table, you will need the following supplies for the Two-Color Monomer Liquid and Polymer Powder Nail Enhancements Using Forms procedure:

- **Application brushes**
- **Dappen dishes**
- **Monomer liquid**
- **Nail dehydrator**
- **Nail forms**
- **Nail primer**
- **Polymer powder (pink and white)**

Preparation

- Perform PROCEDURE 25-1 **Pre-Service Procedure** **SEE PAGE 817**

Procedure

1 Clean the nails and remove existing polish or gel sealant.

2 Push back the eponychium and remove the cuticle from the nail plate.

3 Remove oily shine from the natural nail surface with a medium-fine abrasive.

4 Apply nail dehydrator.

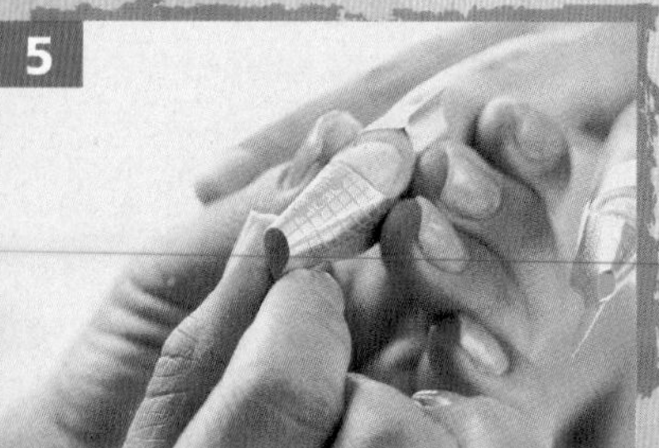
5

5 Position the nail forms. If you are using disposable forms, peel a nail form from its paper backing and, using the thumb and index finger of each of your hands, bend the form into an arch to fit the client's natural nail shape. Slide the form into place and press adhesive backing to the sides of the finger. Check to see that the form is snug under the free edge and level with the natural nail. If you are using multiuse forms, slide the form into place, making sure the free edge is over the form and that it fits snugly. Be careful not to cut into the hyponychium under the free edge. Tighten the form around the finger by squeezing lightly.

© Milady, a part of Cengage Learning. Photography by Dino Petrocelli.

6 Apply nail primer by touching the brush tip to the edge of the bottle's neck to release the excess primer back into the bottle. Using a light dotting action, dab the brush tip to the prepared natural nail only. One end of the primer molecule chemically bonds to the nail protein; the other end of the molecule is a methacrylate, so it can bond to the monomer liquid as it cures. Always follow the manufacturer's directions. Allow the nail primer to dry thoroughly. Acid-free primer will dry to a shiny, sticky surface. Never apply nail enhancement product over wet nail primer, since this can cause product discoloration and service breakdown. Avoid overuse of nail primers.

Service Tip

Do not touch the primed area of the nail with your application brush until you apply enhancement product on the area. The enhancement may become discolored where wet nail primer touches the product. Lifting is another possible result.

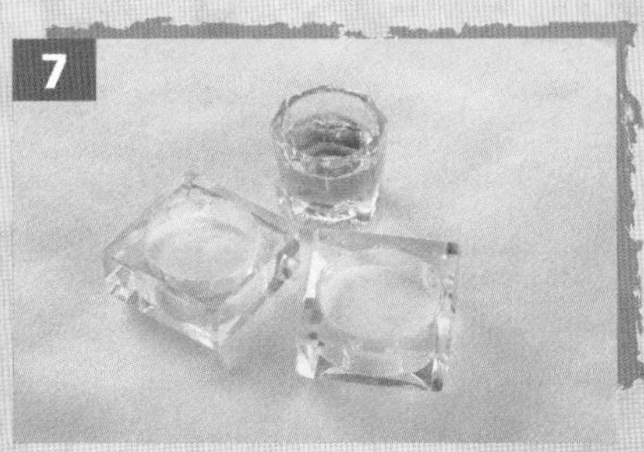

7 Pour monomer liquid and polymer powder into separate dappen dishes. With the two-color method you will need three dappen dishes—one for the white tip powder; one for the clear, natural, or pink powder; and one for the monomer liquid. You can work out of the monomer liquid and polymer powder containers, as well.

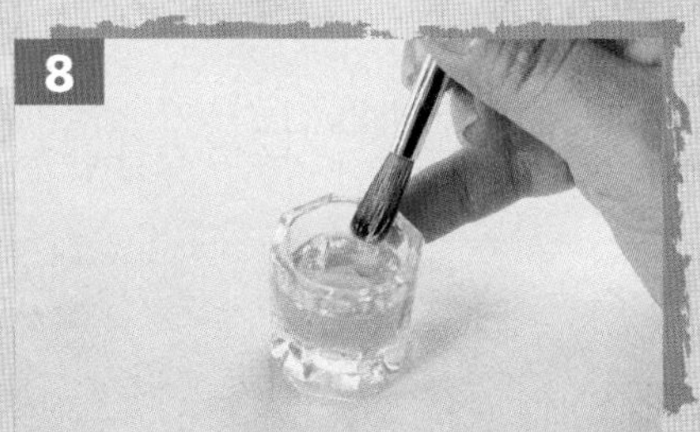

8 Saturate your application brush with monomer liquid and wipe out the liquid completely. Dip the brush in the monomer liquid and wipe on the edge of the container to remove the excess so you can get the liquid you need to pick up the powder.

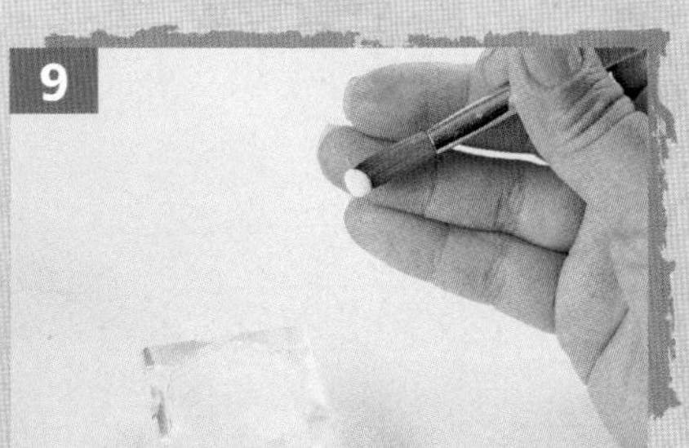

9 Dip the tip of the same brush into the white polymer powder and pick up a bead of product—it should have a dry-to-medium consistency, not runny or wet—that is large enough to cover the entire free-edge extension up to the edge of the smile line. If this is too large a bead to shape properly, using two smaller beads may be easier.

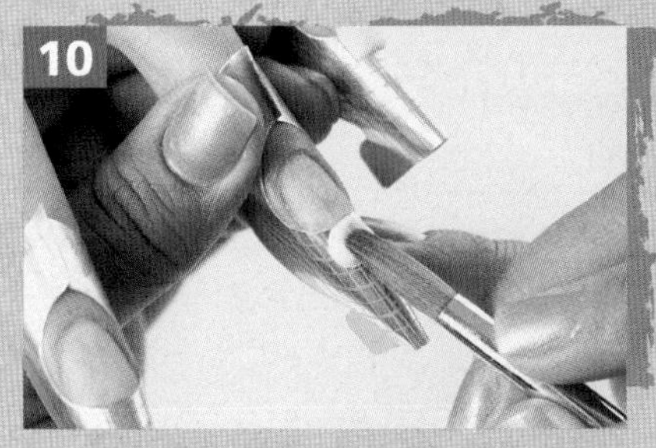

10 Place the white bead in the center of the nail form at the point where the free edge joins the nail form. Wipe your brush gently on a clean or disposable towel—do not use the table towel—to remove any remaining product, and allow your bead to start to self-level and begin setting up. Working with a freshly applied bead of monomer liquid and polymer powder will be sticky; allowing it to set up a bit, will give you a less sticky surface to work with. After the product has set up but still moves, use the tip of your application brush to wipe the smile line so it is crisp.

© Milady, a part of Cengage Learning. Photography by Dino Petrocelli.

PROCEDURE 28-2

Two-Color Monomer Liquid and Polymer Powder Nail Enhancements Using Forms

continued

11 Shape the free edge.

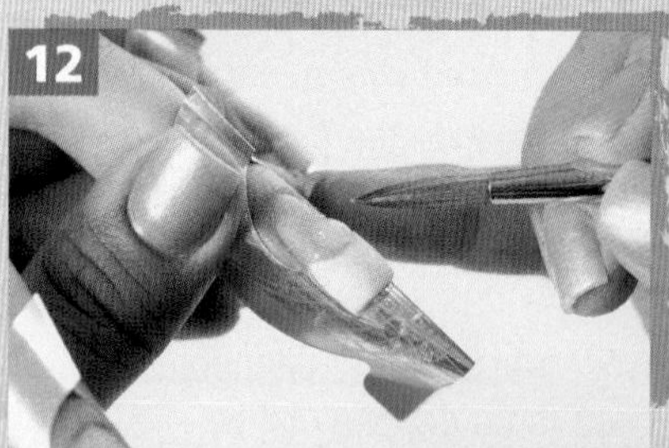

12 Pick up a second bead of white powder, again with a medium consistency, and place it on the natural nail above the last bead, inside the free-edge smile line and in the center of the nail. Wipe your brush gently on a clean or disposable towel—do not use the table towel—to remove any remaining product, and allow your bead to start to self-level and begin setting up.

13 Shape the second bead of white powder.

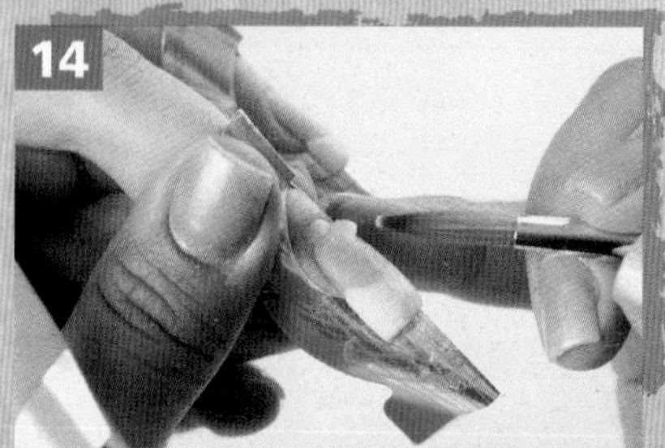

14 Pick up a small bead of pink polymer powder with your brush and place it at the cuticle area of the nail plate, leaving a tiny free margin between it and the skin. Use the brush to press and smooth these beads over the entire nail plate. Glide the brush over the nail to smooth out imperfections. Enhancement product application near eponychium, sidewall, and free edge must be thin for a natural-looking nail.

15 Repeat steps 5 through 14 on remaining nails.

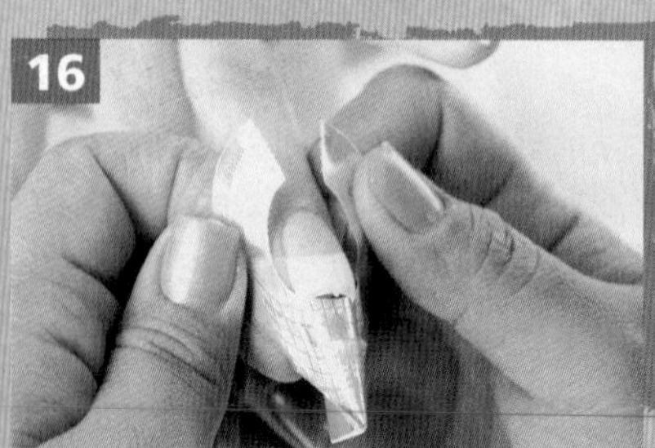

16 When nail enhancements are thoroughly hardened, loosen forms and slide them off. Nail enhancements will harden enough to file and shape after several minutes; they should make a clicking sound when lightly tapped with a brush handle.

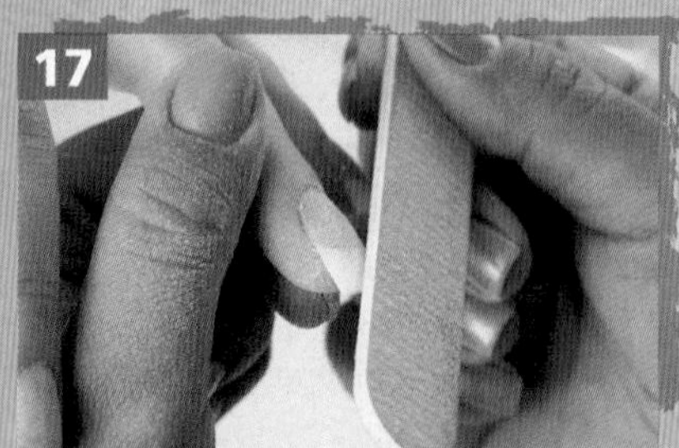

17 Use medium abrasive (180 to 240 grit) to shape the nail and remove imperfections. Begin by shaping the tip's edge on all nails. Be sure to measure the lengths so they are consistent.

© Milady, a part of Cengage Learning. Photography by Dino Petrocelli.

18 File the left side and right side of each nail.

19 File the underside of nail extensions on both sides of each nail.

20 Glide the abrasive over the nail with long sweeping strokes to further shape and perfect the enhancement surface. Thin the product near the base of all nail plates, free edges, and sidewalls.

21 Buff the nail enhancements.

22 Apply nail oil.

23 Apply hand cream and massage the hand and arm.

24 Clean the nail enhancements.

25 Polish the nail with a clear gloss polish or apply a gel sealant.

Service Tip

One of the most common mistakes is applying product too thickly, especially near the base of the nail plate. Avoid this and you will save money and time.

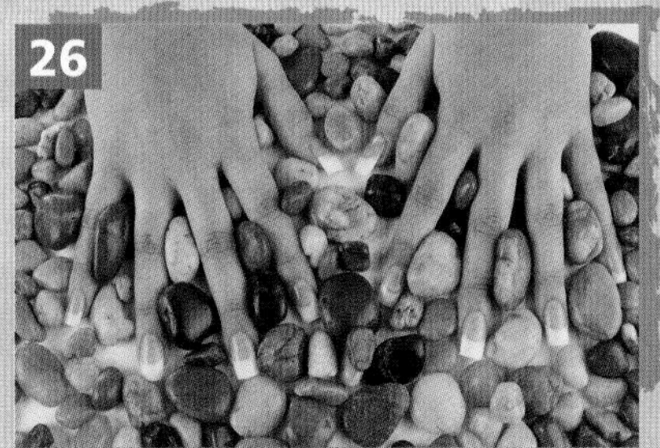

26 Finished look.

Post-Service

- Complete PROCEDURE 25-2 Post-Service Procedure SEE PAGE 821 ✓ LO4

© Milady, a part of Cengage Learning. Photography by Dino Petrocelli.

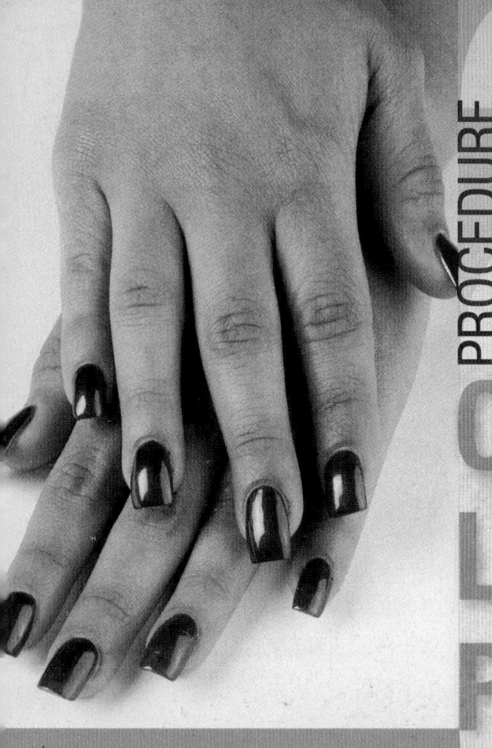

PROCEDURE 28-3

One-Color Monomer Liquid and Polymer Powder Maintenance

Implements and Materials

In addition to the basic materials on your manicuring table, you will need the following supplies for the One-Color Monomer Liquid and Polymer Powder Maintenance procedure:

- Application brushes
- Dappen dishes
- Monomer liquid
- Nail dehydrator
- Nail primer
- Polymer powder

Preparation

- Perform 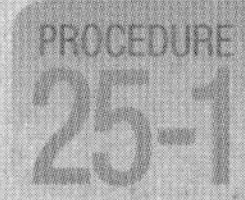 PROCEDURE 25-1 Pre-Service Procedure SEE PAGE 817

Procedure

1 Remove the existing polish or gel sealant.

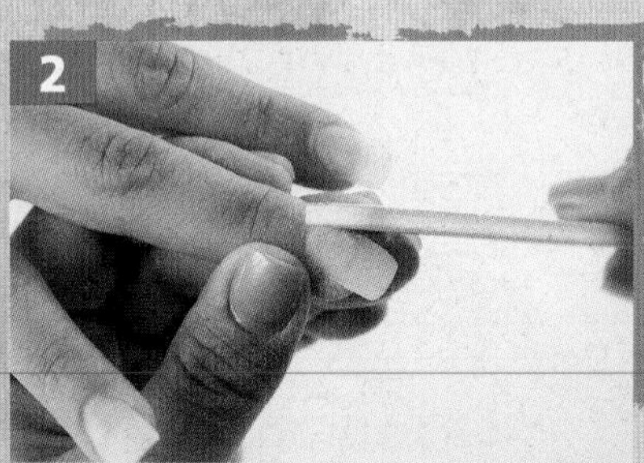

2 Using a medium-coarse abrasive (120 to 180 grit), carefully smooth down the ledge of the existing product until it is flush with the new growth of nail plate. Do not dig into or damage the natural nail plate with your abrasive.

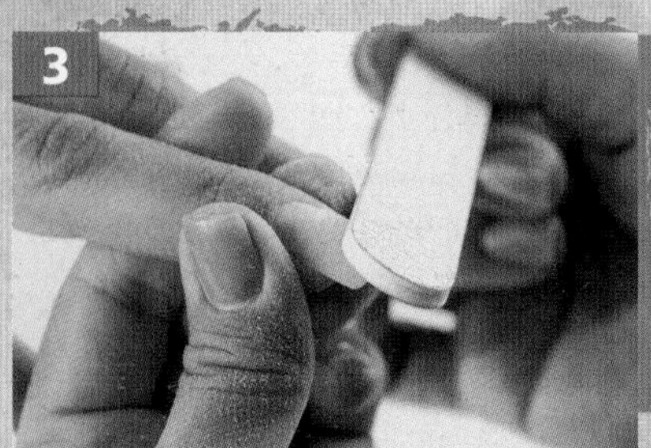

3 Hold the medium abrasive (180 to 240 grit) flat and glide it over the entire nail enhancement to reshape, refine, and thin out the free edge until the white tip appears translucent. Take care not to damage the client's skin with the abrasive.

© Milady, a part of Cengage Learning. Photography by Dino Petrocelli.

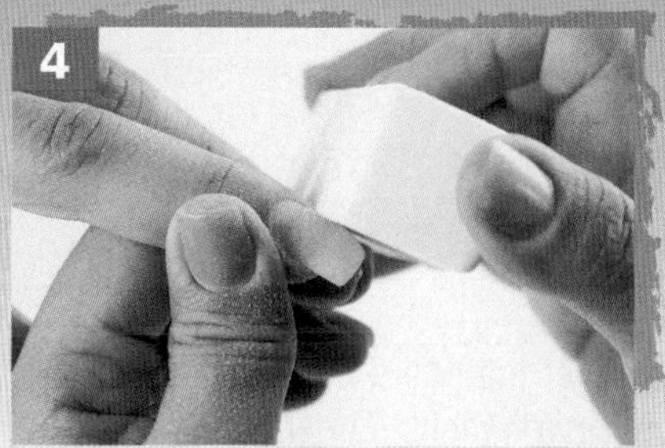

4 Use a fine-grit buffer (350 grit or higher) to buff the product, and smoothly blend it into new growth area without damaging the natural nail plate.

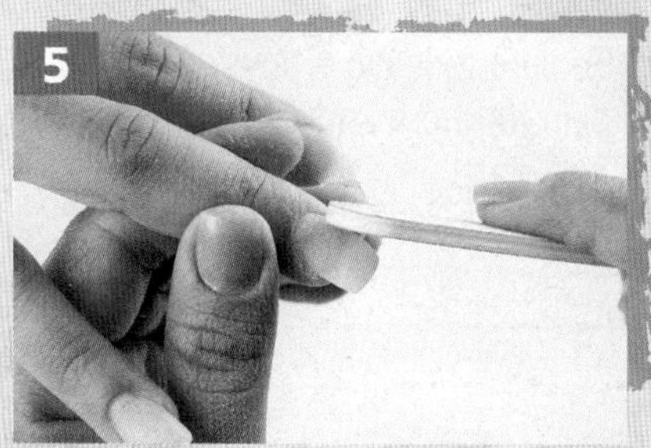

5 Use a medium-abrasive (180 to 240 grit) file to smooth out any areas of product that may be lifting or forming pockets. Do not file into the natural nail plate.

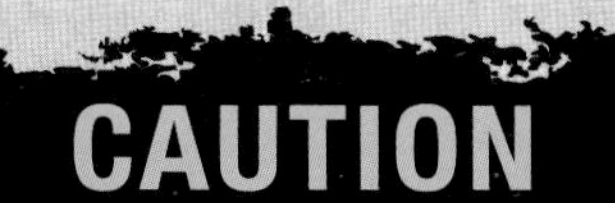

CAUTION

Do not use a nipper to clip away loose nail enhancement product. Nipping may perpetuate the lifting problem and can damage the nail plate. If lifting is excessive, soak off the enhancement and start fresh with a new nail application.

6 Clean the nail enhancements.

7 Remove the oily shine from the natural nail surface.

8 Apply nail dehydrator.

9 Apply nail primer and follow manufacturer's directions. Allow primer to dry thoroughly. Avoid applying nail enhancement product over wet primer, since this can cause product discoloration and service breakdown. Avoid overusing nail primer.

10 Prepare monomer liquid and polymer powder.

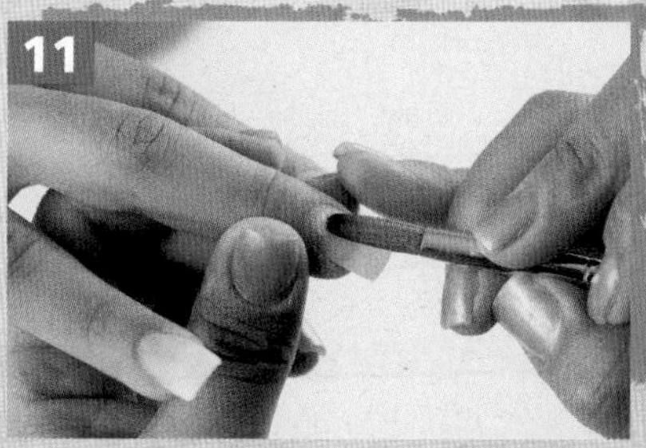

11 Pick up one or more small beads of enhancement product and place at the natural nail area, the regrowth.

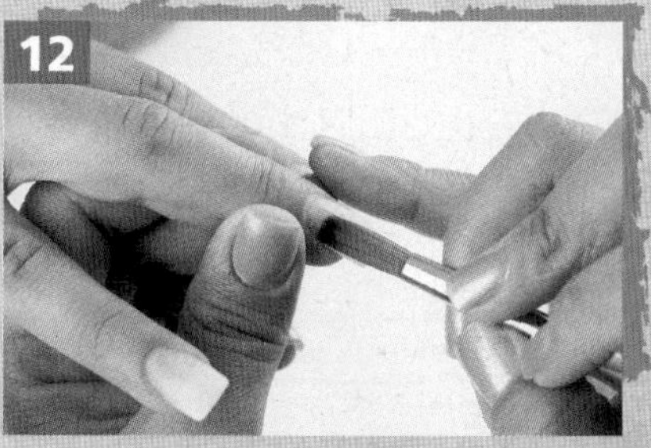

12 Use the brush to smooth these beads over the new growth area. Glide the brush over the nail to smooth out imperfections. Enhancement product application near the eponychium, sidewall areas, and free edge must be extremely thin for a natural-looking nail. Be sure to leave a tiny free margin between the nail enhancement product and skin for more small beads of powder and place them at the center of the nail plate.

13 Pick up one or more small beads of enhancement product and place them at the center or apex of the nail.

© Milady, a part of Cengage Learning. Photography by Dino Petrocelli.

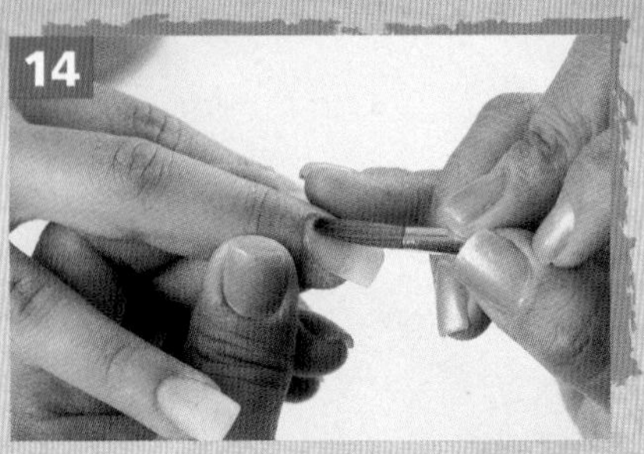

14 Use the brush to smooth these beads over the entire nail enhancement. Glide the brush over the nail to smooth out imperfections. Enhancement product application near the eponychium, sidewall areas, and free edge must be extremely thin for a natural-looking nail. Be sure to leave a tiny free margin between the nail enhancement product and skin for more small beads of powder and place them at the center of the nail plate.

15 Allow the nails to harden. Nails are hard when they make a clicking sound when lightly tapped with a brush handle. Once hardened, shape the nail enhancements with an abrasive board.

16 Buff the nail enhancement.

17 Apply nail oil.

18 Apply hand cream and massage the hand and arm.

19 Clean the nail enhancements.

20 Apply nail polish or gel sealant.

Service Tip

After you have applied the dehydrator and the nail is dry, do not touch the nail plates again with your fingers or allow the client to rest their hands against their face. Touching the prepped nail plate—or getting makeup or moisturizer on it—can deposit oils and cause possible lifting.

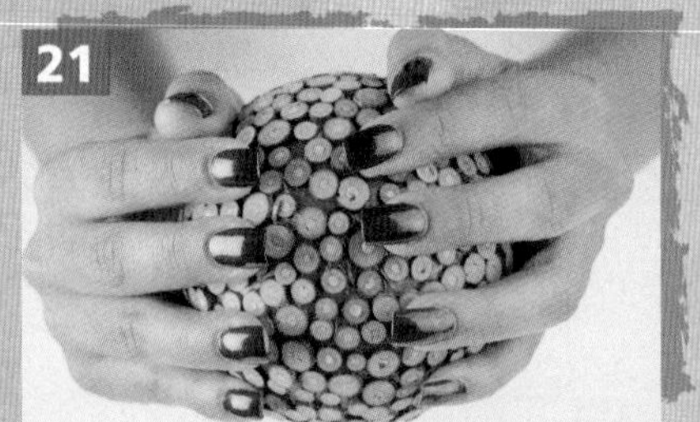

21 Finished look.

Post-Service

- Complete PROCEDURE 25-2 Post-Service Procedure SEE PAGE 821 ✓ LO5

© Milady, a part of Cengage Learning. Photography by Dino Petrocelli.

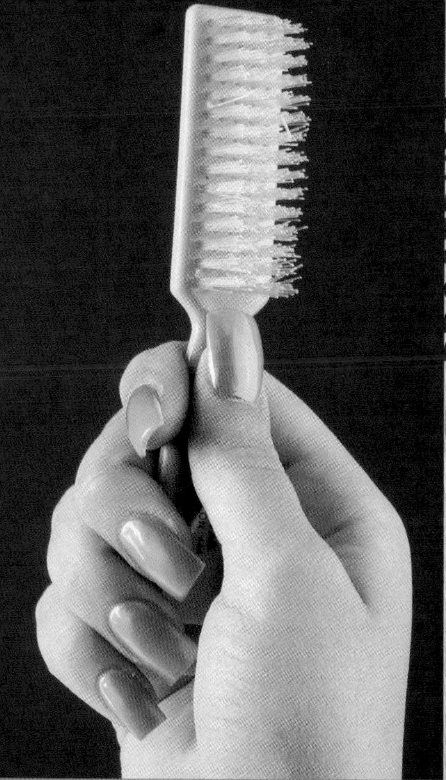

PROCEDURE 28-4

Crack Repair for Monomer Liquid and Polymer Powder Nail Enhancements

Implements and Materials

In addition to the basic materials on your manicuring table, you will need the following supplies for the Crack Repair for Monomer Liquid and Polymer Powder Nail Enhancements procedure:

- **Application brushes**
- **Dappen dishes**
- **Monomer liquid**
- **Nail dehydrator**
- **Nail forms**
- **Nail primer**
- **Polymer powder**

© Milady, a part of Cengage Learning. Photography by Dino Petrocelli.

Preparation

- Perform PROCEDURE 25-1 **Pre-Service Procedure** SEE PAGE 817

Procedure

1 Remove the existing polish or nail sealant.

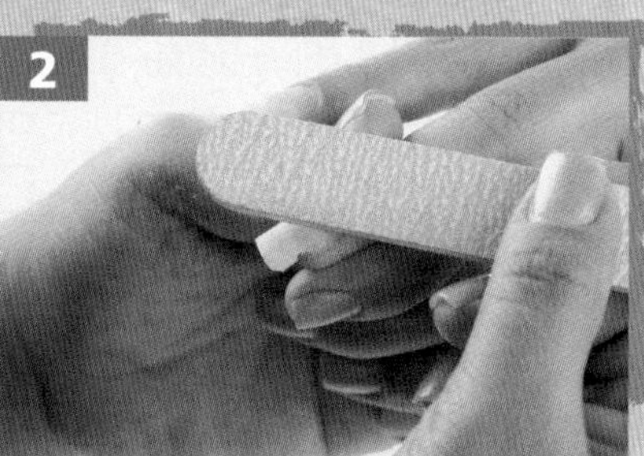

2 File a V shape into the crack or file flush to remove the crack. File more than just the crack for extra protection.

3 Apply nail dehydrator to any exposed natural nail in the crack.

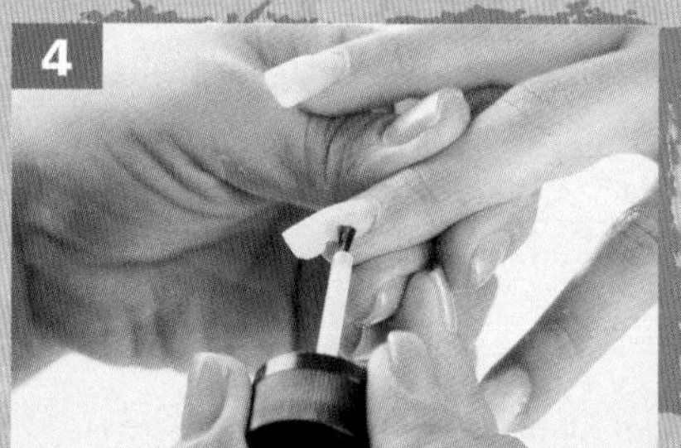

4 Apply nail primer to any exposed natural nail in the crack.

Crack Repair for Monomer Luiquid and Polymer Powder Nail Enhancements continued

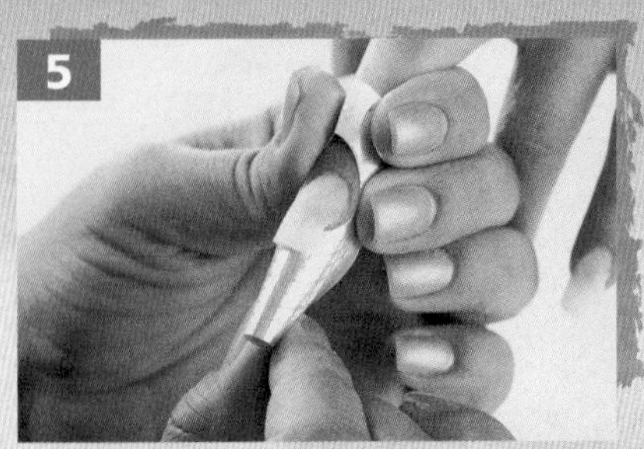

5 If the crack needs support, apply a nail form.

6 Prepare monomer liquid and polymer powder.

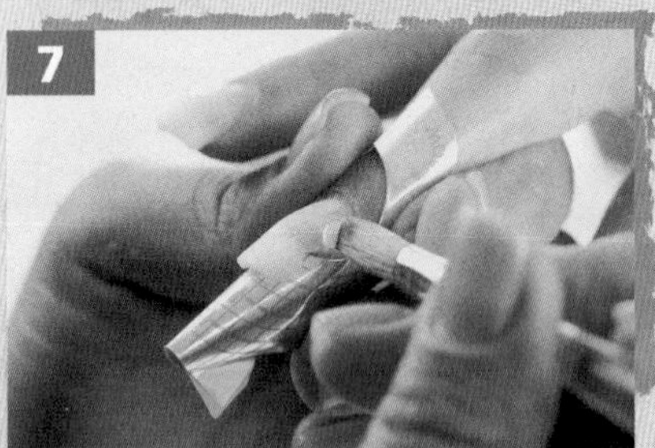

7 Pick up one or more small beads of product, and apply them to the cracked area. If you are using the two-color system, be sure to use the correct color of polymer powder.

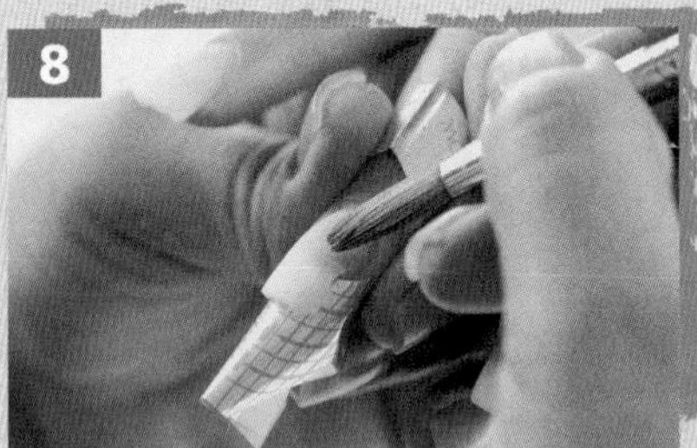

8 Press and smooth the enhancement product to fill the crack. Be careful not to let the product seep under the form.

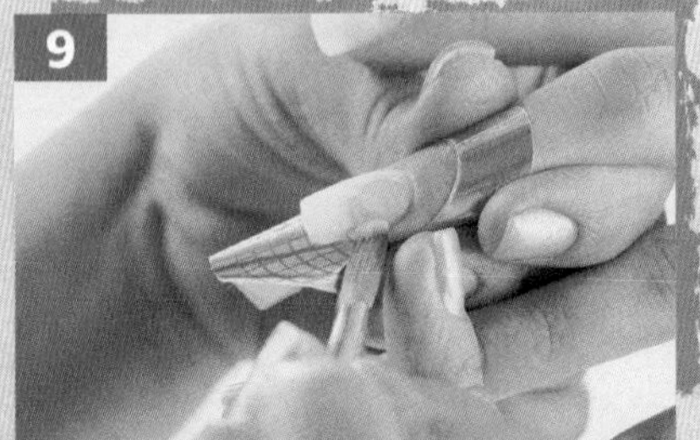

9 Apply additional beads, if needed, to fill in the crack or reinforce the rest of the nail. Shape the enhancement and allow it to harden.

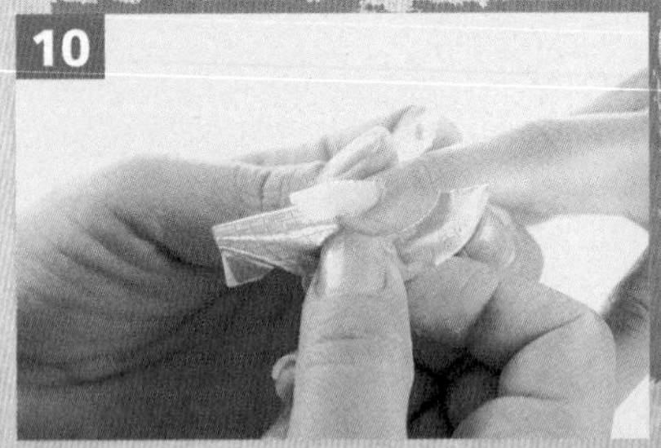

10 Remove the form, if used.

11 Reshape the nail enhancement using a medium abrasive (180 to 240 grit).

12 Use a fine abrasive (350 grit or higher) to buff and smooth the nail. Use a high-shine buffer, if desired.

13 Apply nail oil.

14 Apply hand cream and massage the hand and arm.

15 Clean the nail enhancements.

16 Apply nail polish or gel sealant.

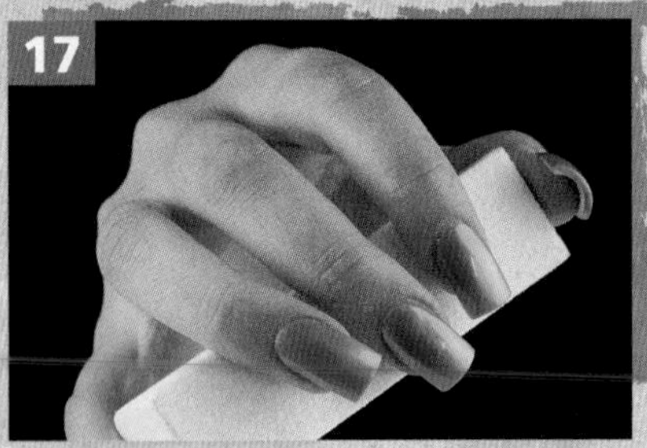

17 Repaired nail.

Post-Service

- Complete PROCEDURE 25-2 Post-Service Procedure SEE PAGE 821 ✓ LO6

© Milady, a part of Cengage Learning. Photography by Dino Petrocelli.

PROCEDURE 28-5

Monomer Liquid and Polymer Powder Nail Enhancement Removal

Implements and Materials

In addition to the basic materials on your manicuring table, you will need the following supplies for the Monomer Liquid and Polymer Powder Nail Enhancement Removal procedure:

- **Acetone**
- **Metal or glass bowl**

Preparation

- Perform 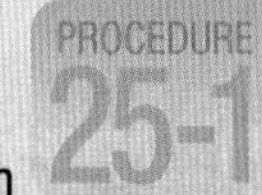

Pre-Service Procedure SEE PAGE 817

Procedure

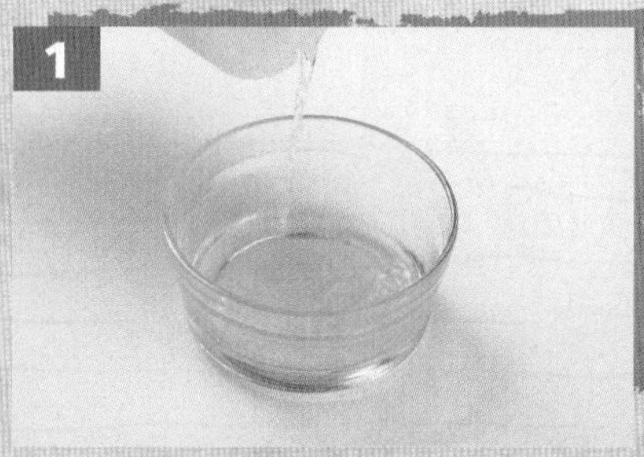

1 Fill the glass bowl with enough acetone or product remover to cover ½ inch higher than client's enhancements. Place the bowl inside another bowl of hot water to heat the acetone safely and speed up the removal procedure.

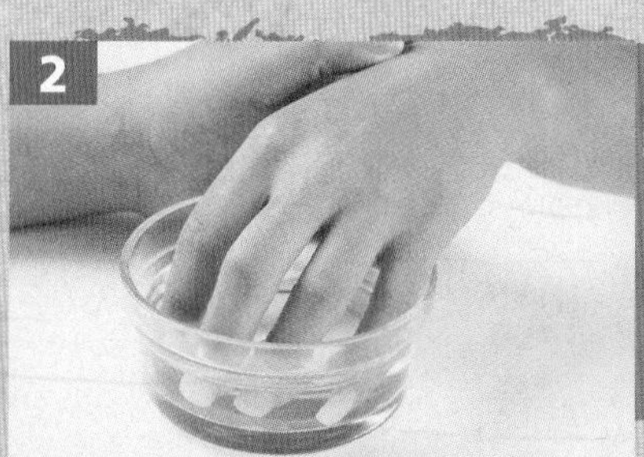

2 Soak the client's nail enhancements for twenty to thirty minutes, or as long as needed to remove the enhancement product. Refer to the manufacturer's directions and precautions for nail enhancement product removal.

© Milady, a part of Cengage Learning. Photography by Dino Petrocelli.

PROCEDURE 28-5

Monomer Liquid and Polymer Powder Nail Enhancement Removal continued

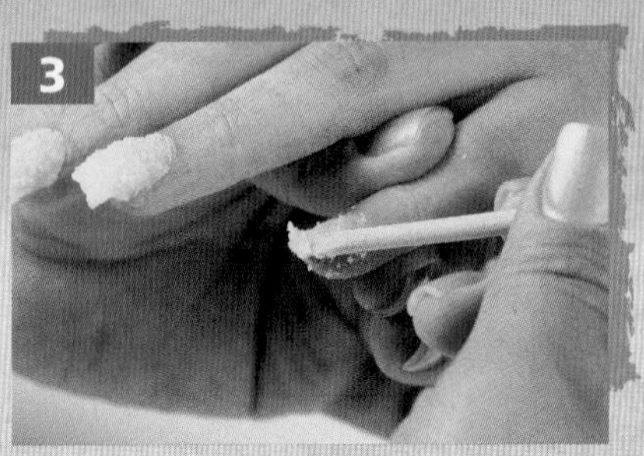

3 Once or twice during the procedure, use a wooden or metal pusher to gently push off the softened enhancement. Repeat until all enhancements have been removed. Do not pry them off with nippers, as this will damage the natural nail plate. Avoid removing enhancements from the acetone or product remover, or they will quickly reharden, making them more difficult to remove. The key is to leave the nails in the acetone until they fall off and leave the natural nail free of product. Use a plastic-backed cotton pad to remove the remaining product.

4 Condition the skin and nails.

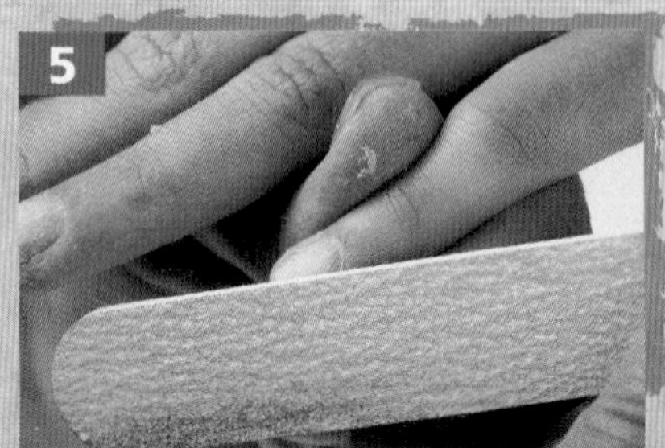

5 Lightly buff the nails to smooth any remaining ridges or residue.

6 Recommend that the client receive a basic manicure.

FYI

Nail plates may appear to be thinner after enhancements have been removed. This is generally because there is more moisture in the natural nail plate, which makes them more flexible. It is not an indication that the nail plates have been weakened by the nail enhancement. This excess flexibility will be lost as the natural nails lose moisture over the next twenty-four hours, and the nail plates will appear to be thicker and more rigid.

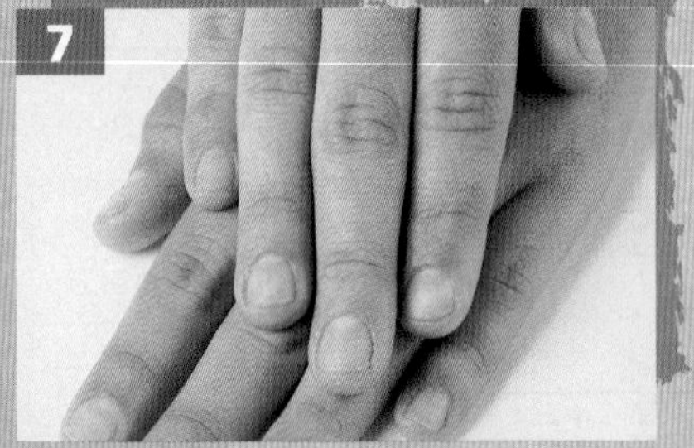

7 Finished look.

Post-Service

- Complete PROCEDURE 25-2 **Post-Service Procedure** SEE PAGE 821 ✓ LO7

© Milady, a part of Cengage Learning. Photography by Dino Petrocelli.

Review Questions

1. What is the chemistry behind monomer liquid and polymer powder nail enhancements and how does it work?
2. What are the definitions of apex, stress area, and sidewall, and where is their location on the nail enhancement?
3. What is the proper procedure for applying one-color monomer liquid and polymer powder nail enhancements over tips and on natural nails?
4. What is the proper procedure for applying two-color monomer liquid and polymer powder nail enhancements using forms?
5. What is the proper procedure for performing a one-color maintenance service on nail enhancements using monomer liquid and polymer powder?
6. How is a crack repair performed?
7. How are monomer liquid and polymer powder removed from the nail?

Chapter Glossary

apex	Also known as *arch*; the area of the nail that has all of the strength.
chain reaction	Also known as *polymerization reaction*; process that joins together monomers to create very long polymer chains.
initiators	Substance that starts the chain reaction that leads to the creation of very long polymer chains.
monomer	One unit called a molecule.
monomer liquid	Chemical liquid mixed with polymer powder to form the sculptured nail enhancement.
monomer liquid and polymer powder nail enhancements	Enhancements created by combining monomer liquid and polymer powder.
nail extension underside	The actual underside of the nail extension.
odorless monomer liquid and polymer powder products	Nail enhancement products that have little odor.
polymer	Substance formed by combining many small molecules (monomers) into very long chain-like structures.
polymerization	Also known as *curing* or *hardening*; chemical reaction that creates polymers.
polymer powder	Powder in white, clear, pink, and many other colors that is combined with monomer liquid to form the nail enhancement.
stress area	Where the natural nail grows beyond the finger and becomes the free edge.

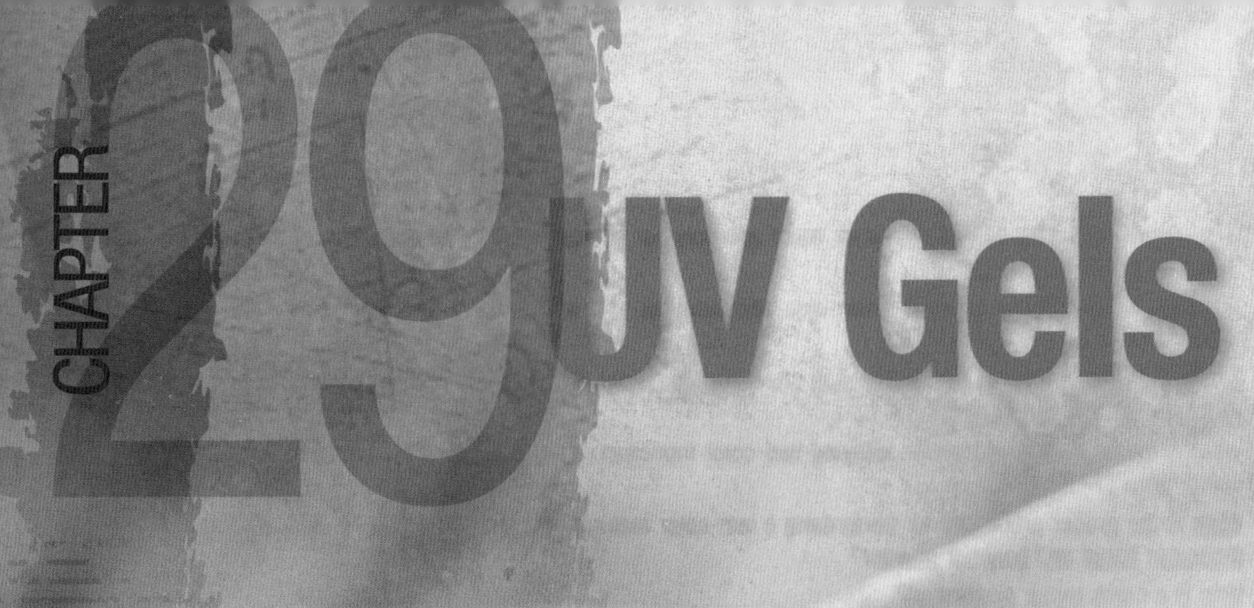

CHAPTER 29 UV Gels

Chapter Outline

Why Study UV Gels?

UV Gels

UV Gel Supplies

When to Use UV Gels

Choosing the Proper UV Gel

UV Light Units and Lamps

UV Gel Polish

UV Gel Maintenance and Removal

Procedures

© Milady, a part of Cengage Learning. Photography by Dino Petrocelli.

Learning Objectives

After completing this chapter, you will be able to:

- ✓ **LO1** Describe the chemistry and main ingredients of UV gels.
- ✓ **LO2** Describe when to use the one-color and two-color methods for applying UV gels.
- ✓ **LO3** Name and describe the types of UV gels used in current systems.
- ✓ **LO4** Identify the supplies needed for UV gel application.
- ✓ **LO5** Determine when to use UV gels.
- ✓ **LO6** Discuss the differences between UV light units and UV lamps.
- ✓ **LO7** Describe how to apply one-color UV gel on tips and natural nails.
- ✓ **LO8** Describe how to apply UV gels over forms.
- ✓ **LO9** Describe how to maintain UV gel nail enhancements.
- ✓ **LO10** Explain how to correctly remove hard UV gels.
- ✓ **LO11** Explain how to correctly remove soft UV gels.

Key Terms

Page number indicates where in the chapter the term is used.

cure
pg. 927

hard UV gels (traditional UV gels)
pg. 934

inhibition layer
pg. 929

oligomer
pg. 926

one-color method
pg. 927

opacity
pg. 929

photoinitiator
pg. 926

pigmented UV gels
pg. 928

soft UV gels (soakable gels)
pg. 934

two-color method
pg. 927

unit wattage
pg. 932

urethane acrylate
pg. 926

urethane methacrylate
pg. 926

UV bonding gels
pg. 928

UV building gels
pg. 928

UV gel
pg. 926

UV gel polish
pg. 928

UV gloss gel (sealing gel, finishing gel, shine gel)
pg. 929

UV lamp (UV light bulb)
pg. 932

UV light unit (UV light)
pg. 932

UV self-leveling gels
pg. 928

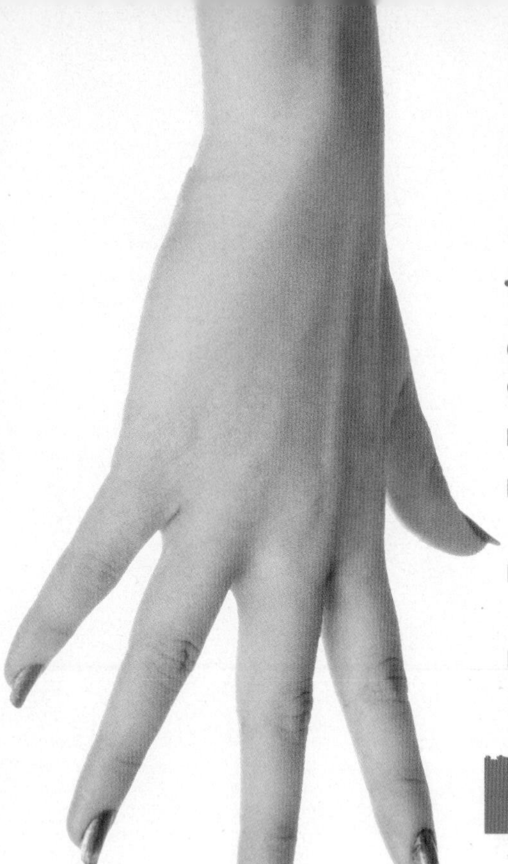

© Valeev, 2010; used under license from Shutterstock.com.

This chapter introduces **UV gel**, a type of nail enhancement product that hardens when exposed to a UV light source. UV gel is an increasingly popular method for nail enhancement services.

WHY STUDY UV GELS?

Cosmetologists should study and have a thorough understanding of UV gels because:

- Clients may be interested in having UV gel services offered to them.
- An understanding of the chemistry of UV gel products will allow you to choose the best system and products to use in your salon.
- An understanding of how UV gel nails are made, applied, and cured will allow you to create a safe and efficient salon service.
- Clients often become loyal and steadfast when they receive excellent UV gel nail services, maintenance, and removal.

UV Gels

Nail enhancements based on UV curing are not traditionally thought of as being methacrylates; however, they are very similar. Like wrap resins, adhesives, monomer liquid, and polymer powder nail enhancements, UV gel enhancements rely on ingredients from the monomer liquid and polymer powder chemical family. Their ingredients are part of a subcategory of this family called acrylates. Wrap resins are called cyanoacrylates, and monomer liquid and polymer powder nail enhancements are from the same category called methacrylates.

Although most UV gels are made from acrylates, new UV gel technologies have been developed that use methacrylates. Like wraps and monomer liquid and polymer powder nail enhancements, UV gels can also contain monomer liquids, but they rely mostly on a related form called an oligomer. The term *mono* means one, and *poly* means many. *Oligo* means few. An **oligomer** (uh-LIG-uh-mer) is a short chain of monomer liquids that is often thick, sticky, and gel-like and that is not long enough to be considered a polymer. These chains are often referred to as prepolymers. Nail enhancement monomer liquids are liquids, while polymers are solids. Oligomers are between solid and liquid.

Traditionally, UV gels rely on a special type of acrylate called a urethane acrylate, while newer UV gel systems use urethane methacrylates by themselves or in combination with urethane acrylates. **Urethane acrylate** (YUR-ah-thane AK-ri-layt) and **urethane methacrylate** (YUR-ah-thane meth-AK-ri-layt) are the main ingredients used to create UV gel nail enhancements. The term *urethane* refers to the type of starting material that is used to create the most common UV gel resins. The chemical family of urethanes is known for high abrasion resistance and durability.

UV gel resins react when exposed to the UV light that is recommended for the gel. A chemical called a **photoinitiator**

(FOH-toh-in-ish-ee-AY-tohr) initiates the polymerization reaction. The key thing to remember here is that it takes the combination of the resin, photoinitiator, and the proper curing lamp to cause the gel to cure. UV gel systems employ a single component resin compound that is cured to a solid material when exposed to a UV light source. UV gels typically do not use a powder that is incorporated into the gel resin. A few UV gels on the market incorporate a powder that is sprinkled into the gel, but the rest of the chapter uses the term *gels* to refer to the more common single component type.

UV gels can be easy to apply, file, and maintain. They also have the advantage of having very little or no odor. Although they typically are not as hard as monomer liquid and polymer powder nail enhancements, UV gels can create beautiful, long-lasting nail enhancements.

The UV gel application process differs from other types of nail enhancements. After the nail plate is properly prepared, each layer of product applied to the natural nail, nail tip, or form requires exposure to UV light to **cure**, which means to harden. The UV light required for curing comes from a special lamp designed to emit the proper type and intensity of UV light. ✓ LO1

There are many types of UV gels. Choosing a favorite and relied-upon UV gel is as important as choosing the monomer liquid and polymer powder system that you prefer. Some cosmetologists favor a UV gel that is thick and will not level by itself. Other cosmetologists like to use UV gels that quickly self-level. It is up to you to find the UV gel that you prefer to use and to learn how to use it well.

The different UV gels can be described as thin-viscosity gels, medium-viscosity gels, thick-viscosity gels, and building or sculpting gels. Remember that viscosity is the measurement of the thickness or thinness of a liquid and that viscosity affects how the fluid flows. Manufacturers have market names for the UV gels, but most UV gels fall under these general categories:

- The **one-color method** is the method whereby one color of UV gel is applied over the entire surface of the nail. This method is used for clients who wish to wear colored polish or UV gel polish over the enhancement.
- The **two-color method** is a method whereby two colors of resin are used to overlay the nail; usually pink and white are used, allowing for a French or American manicure finish in which lacquer is not needed. There are many processes for performing a two-color method over tips or natural nails. The process varies from one UV gel manufacturer to another and can even vary within one manufacturer's product lines. Consult with the UV gel manufacturer about the product you intend to use before you perform a two-color method. ✓ LO2

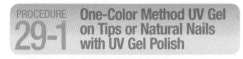

PROCEDURE 29-1 **One-Color Method UV Gel on Tips or Natural Nails with UV Gel Polish** SEE PAGE 935

PROCEDURE 29-2 **Two-Color Method UV Gel on Tips or Natural Nails** SEE PAGE 939

© Milady, a part of Cengage Learning. Photography by Dino Petrocelli.

Types of UV Gels

UV bonding gels are used to increase adhesion to the natural nail plate, similar to a monomer liquid and polymer powder primer. UV bonding gels will vary in consistency and chemical components. The increased adhesion decreases the tendency for enhancements to separate from the natural nail. Some UV bonding gels contain certain chemicals that smell like a monomer liquid and polymer powder primer, while other UV bonding gels do not have a strong odor. UV gel manufacturers are constantly developing new technology in the formulation of UV bonding gels. These technologies could make the use of odiferous chemicals obsolete. Some UV gel manufacturers use air-dry bonding systems. Just because the bonding product may not be cured in an ultraviolet light unit does not make it any less effective than a bonding system that is cured in a UV light unit.

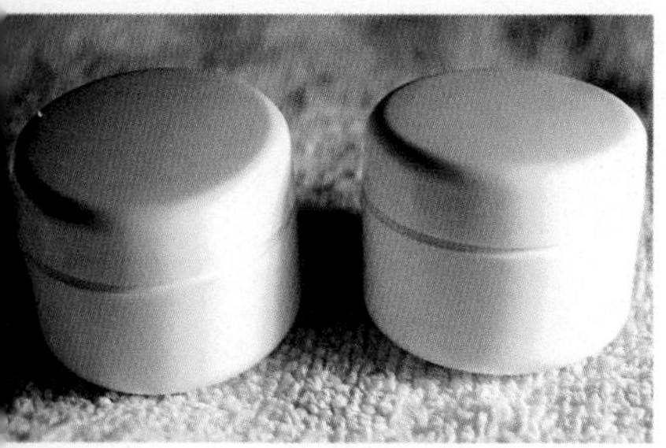

© Katarzyna Krawiec, 2010; used under license from Shutterstock.com.

UV building gels include any thick-viscosity resin that allows the cosmetologist to build an arch and curve to the fingernail. UV building gels can be used with self-leveling UV gels. If done correctly, this combination can reduce the amount of filing and shaping required to contour the enhancement later in the service. Some UV building gels have fiberglass strands compounded into the gel during the manufacturing process. These UV gels typically have hardness and durability properties that closely resemble monomer liquid and polymer powder systems. They are very helpful when repairing a break or crack in a client's enhancement.

UV self-leveling gels are thinner in consistency than building gels, allowing them to settle and level during application. These gels are used to enhance thickness of the overlay while providing a smoother surface. Cosmetologists who are experienced in UV gel application often choose to apply a UV building gel first, and then apply a self-leveling UV gel to reduce filing and contouring.

Pigmented UV gels are building and self-leveling gels that include color pigment. Pigmented building gels are used earlier in the service to create art or a traditional French manicure look using a white-pigmented UV gel. To complete this look, you would use the two-color method, which is similar to a two-color monomer liquid and polymer powder process. Self-leveling pigmented UV gels are used near the final contouring procedure—either before or after filing—because these gels are applied much thinner than the pigmented building gels. Consult the manufacturer's instructions for their use.

UV gel polish is a very thin-viscosity UV gel that is usually pigmented and packaged in a pot or a polish bottle; it is used as an alternative to traditional nail lacquers. UV gel polishes do not dry the same way as nail lacquers; they cure in the UV light unit. When the UV gel polish is finished curing, a gloss gel can be applied over it to create a high lustrous shine. The end result appears lacquered but does not have any solvent odor and will not become smudged the way a traditional nail lacquer might. Another advantage of UV gel polishes is that they do not require any drying time once the service is complete. UV gel polish may be used on natural nails or nail enhancements.

ACTivity

Acquire samples of gels that are on the market by calling a few popular companies. When you receive the gels, place a small amount of gel on a plastic tip that you have adhered to a wooden stick. Study the gel as it moves over the tip. Try applying the gel in a different way (such as brushing a thin layer, then applying a ball of gel in the stress area). Then observe the gel again. Repeat this procedure with all of the samples. The more you know about how the gels work and behave, the easier it will be for you to apply the gels on your client.

UV gloss gel, also known as **sealing gel**, **finishing gel**, or **shine gel**, is used over the finished UV gel application to create a high shine, in much the same way a top coat would be applied over colored nail polish. UV gloss gels do not require buffing and can also be used over a monomer liquid and polymer powder enhancement. There are two types of UV gloss gels: traditional gloss gels that cure with a sticky inhibition layer that requires cleaning, and tack-free gloss gels that cure to a high shine without the inhibition layer. An **inhibition layer** is a tacky surface left on the nail after a UV gel has cured. Choose the gloss gel that is best for you. Traditional UV gloss gels do not discolor after prolonged exposure to UV light, while tack-free gloss gels often discolor. Many UV gel manufacturers are developing tack-free gloss gels that do not discolor upon exposure to UV light. These advancements may make traditional UV gloss gels obsolete, but for now, traditional UV gloss gels still hold the market on non-yellowing performance.

UV gels are available in a wide array of colors. They are available in cream and frosted colors, and some even include glitter! These gels can be mixed together to create a few hundred more colors. UV gels provide the cosmetologist and client with a wide variety of colors and options for expressing their personality and creativity. ☑ LO3

After you have determined how each type of gel behaves on the fingernail, learn how to use the pigmented pink and white gels in the same fashion. Similar to clear gels, pink gels and white gels can be formulated in a variety of viscosities, colors, and degrees of opacity. **Opacity** is the amount of colored pigment concentration in a gel, making it more or less difficult to see through. If a UV gel has a high degree of opacity, the UV gel will be better able to camouflage the nail. If a UV gel has a low degree of opacity, the nail will more clearly show through. There are many different gels on the market, and each of these gels can be combined to give any appearance that you and your client desire.

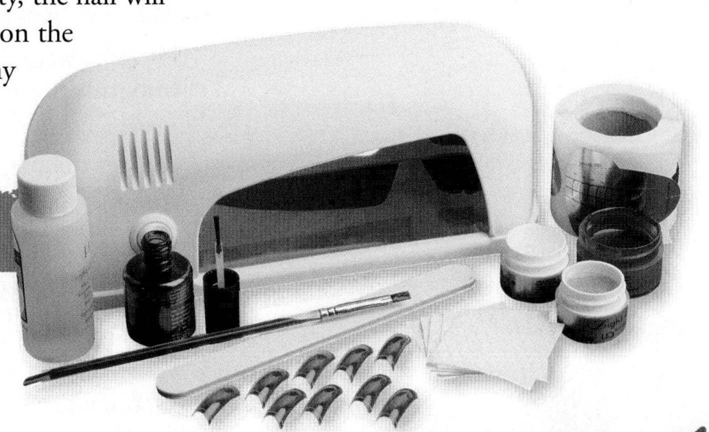

▼ Figure 29–1
Supplies needed for a UV gel service.

© Milady, a part of Cengage Learning. Photography by Dino Petrocelli.

UV Gel Supplies

Just as every type of nail enhancement service requires specific tools, implements, equipment, and supplies, so do UV gel enhancements. Here is a list of those requirements (Figure 29–1). In addition to the supplies in your basic manicuring setup, you will need:

ACTivity

We have discussed how gels require a UV light source to cure properly. Gels will not cure if the light cannot penetrate through the gel. If the gel is pigmented, then the pigment can block the transmission of the UV light into the gel and decrease its curing potential.

Place some gel on a disposable form and spread it using a gel brush. Apply the gel so that you are able to see through it onto the surface of the form. Cure the gel in your UV lamp for the recommended period of time. Clean the surface of the gel to remove the sticky residue—the inhibition layer. Peel the gel from the form and examine the side of the gel that was against the form. If there is a layer of uncured gel, then the gel was applied too thickly. Reapply the gel thinner and repeat the curing and examination process.

- **UV gel light-unit.** Choose a UV gel light-unit designed to produce the correct amount of UV light needed to properly cure the UV gel nail enhancement products you use.
- **Brush.** Choose synthetic brushes with small, flat (or oval) bristles to hold and spread the UV gel.
- **UV gel primer or bonding gel.** Primers and bonding gels are designed specifically to improve adhesion of UV gels to the natural nail plate. Use UV gel primers as instructed by the manufacturer of the product that you are using.
- **UV gel.** This should include pigmented gel(s) for a one-color or two-color service. This will also include a gel that creates a gloss, depending upon the gel system that you choose.
- **Nail tips.** Use nail tips recommended for the UV gel nail enhancement systems.
- **Nail adhesive.** There are many types of nail adhesives for securing preformed nail tips to natural nails. Select a type and size best suited for your work.
- **Nail cleanser or primer.** These products remove surface moisture and tiny amounts of oil left on the natural nail plate, both of which can block adhesion, and help prevent lifting of the nail enhancements.
- **Abrasive files and buffers.** Select a medium abrasive (180 grit) for natural nail preparation. Choose a fine abrasive (240 grit) for smoothing, and a fine buffer (350 grit or higher) for finishing. UV gel manufacturers may have other recommendations for abrasive; please consult the manufacturer's guidelines for more information on the specific system you are using.
- **A cleansing solution.** Cleansing solutions usually contain isopropanol, and they may contain additional solvents. The cleansing solution you choose should be the one recommended by the manufacturer.
- **Lint-free cleansing wipes.** Select an appropriate lint-free wipe. ☑ LO4

When to Use UV Gels

This may seem like a question of personal preference, but it really is a question of logic. The general answer could be, "Anytime!" Gel technology has been able to create some very hard, durable, and tough UV gels. The new UV resin technology allows UV gel manufacturers to create tough, durable, and hard products that will perform as well as many of the monomer liquid and polymer powder systems on the market. The answer also could be, "Never," because there are customers that prefer to wear monomer liquid and polymer powder. It is what they know—they have been wearing these products for years and refuse to change. However, most clients will do what you recommend; if you wear and recommend monomer liquid and polymer powder enhancements, that is what most of your clients will wear. If you wear and recommend UV gels, that will be their preference. You are the professional. As such, you should recommend a system that you have used and that you feel will perform best for the client. There may be a situation when the system you use on your client is not performing as the two of you would like. It may be best to try something else. Maybe using a different gel resin or a changing to monomer liquid and polymer powder would be best. The answer to this question remains in your capable hands. It is also possible to use a monomer liquid and polymer powder system for the fill or full-set and to combine that with a UV gloss gel to create the shine over the enhancement. Pigmented gels, such as UV gel polishes, may also be used over the monomer liquid and polymer powder system, if that is what you prefer. ✔ LO5

PROCEDURE 29-3 UV Gel over Forms SEE PAGE 942

PROCEDURE 29-5 UV Gel over Monomer Liquid and Polymer Powder Nail Enhancements with UV Gel Polish SEE PAGE 948

Choosing the Proper UV Gel

There are many gels to choose from to perform your service. Here are a few guidelines that will help you make the best choice:

- If the client has flat fingernails, more building will need to be done to create an arch and curve. This building will be easiest when done with a thicker UV building gel.
- If the client has fingernails that have an arch and curve, then a self-leveling gel may be the best option. Choose the self-leveling gel that you prefer—either a medium-viscosity or thick-viscosity gel.
- If your client repeatedly returns to the salon with broken enhancements, then a gel that uses fiberglass may be the best product for them.

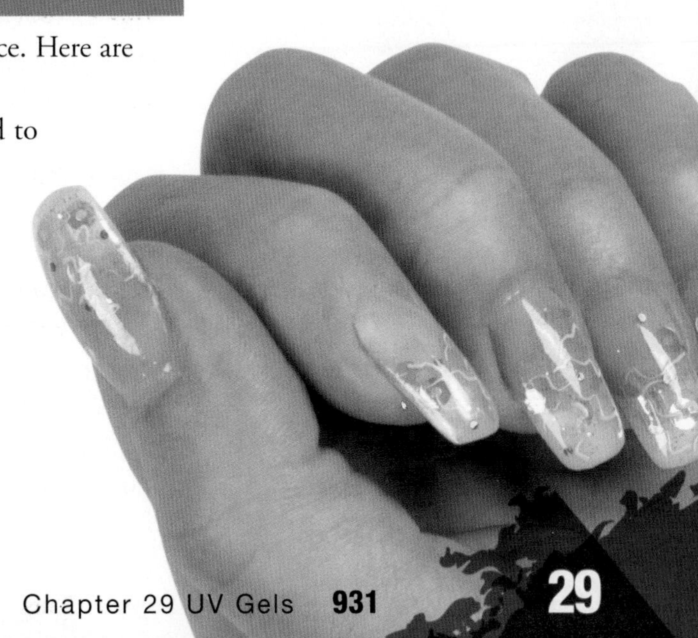

© Mindaugas Makutenas, 2010; used under license from Shutterstock.com.

UV Light Units and Lamps

What is the difference between a UV lamp and a UV light unit?

A **UV lamp**, also known as **UV light bulb**, is a special bulb that emits UV light to cure UV gel nail enhancements. There are a number of different lamps that are used to cure UV gels. There are 4-watt, 6-watt, 7-watt, 8-watt, and 9-watt lamps.

A **UV light unit**, also known as **UV light**, is a specialized electronic device that powers and controls UV lamps to cure UV gel nail enhancements. Light units may look similar at first, but there are differences. The differences include the number of lamps in the unit, the distance the lamps are from the bottom of the unit, and the size of the unit. These factors affect the curing power of the unit.

The names of light units typically indicate the number of lamps inside the light unit multiplied by the wattage of the lamps that are used. Remember that **unit wattage** is the measure of how much electricity the lamp consumes, much like miles per gallon tell you how much gasoline a car requires to drive a certain distance. Miles per gallon will not tell you how fast the car can go, just as wattage does not indicate how much UV light a lamp will produce. For example, if a unit has four lamps in it and each lamp is 9 watts, then the light unit is called a 36-watt light unit. Likewise, if the light unit only has three lamps and each lamp is also 9 watts, then it is called a 27-watt light unit. Wattage does not indicate how much UV light a UV light unit will emit (**Figure 29–2**).

UV gel light-units are designed to produce the correct amount of UV light needed to properly cure UV gel nail enhancement products. UV gels are usually packaged in small opaque pots or squeeze tubes to protect them from UV light. Even though UV light is invisible to the eye, it is found in sunlight and tanning lamps. Also, both true-color and full-spectrum lamps emit a significant amount of UV light. If the UV gel product is exposed to these types of ceiling or table lamps, the product's shelf life may be shortened, causing the product to harden in its container.

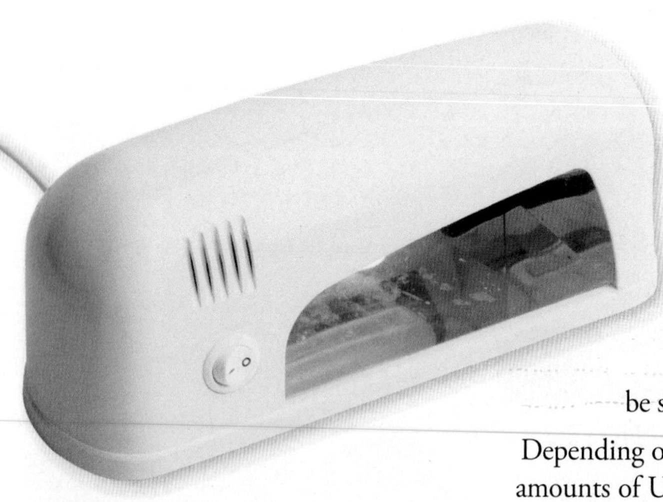

▲ **Figure 29–2**
UV light unit and lamp.

© Milady, a part of Cengage Learning. Photography by Dino Petrocelli.

Depending on their circuitry, different lamps produce greatly differing amounts of UV light. This is referred to as the UV lamp intensity or concentration. The intensity will vary from one light unit to the next and is more important than rating a UV light unit based on the wattage of the lamp or the number of lamps in the unit. For these reasons, it is important to use the UV lamp that was designed for the selected UV gel product. Using the lamp that was specifically designed for the UV gel product will give you a much greater chance of success and fewer problems.

UV lamps will stay blue for years, but after a few months of use they may produce too little UV light to properly cure the enhancement. Typically, UV lamps must be changed two or three times per year, depending on frequency of use. If lamps are not changed regularly, gels may cure inadequately, meaning the oligomers and additional chemicals are not hardened. This can cause service breakdown, skin irritation, and product sensitivity.

The most common UV lamp that is on the market is a 9 watt. Other lamps are 4-watt lamps, 6-watt lamps, 7-watt lamps, and LED (light-emitting diode) lamps. While many of the UV gel systems use the 9-watt lamp, most of the gels can be cured in any manufacturer's 9-watt light unit. A gel that has been specifically designed to cure in a 9-watt light unit may not be able to be cured properly in a 4-watt light unit. The UV gel may become hard when cured in the 4-watt light unit, but it may not become as hard or cure completely. If the gel does not cure completely, it will crack, lift, and separate from the nail. It may not have a high shine, and the client will not be pleased with the service. The result will be similar to a monomer liquid and polymer powder system that has been applied with an incorrect mix ratio between the liquid and the powder.

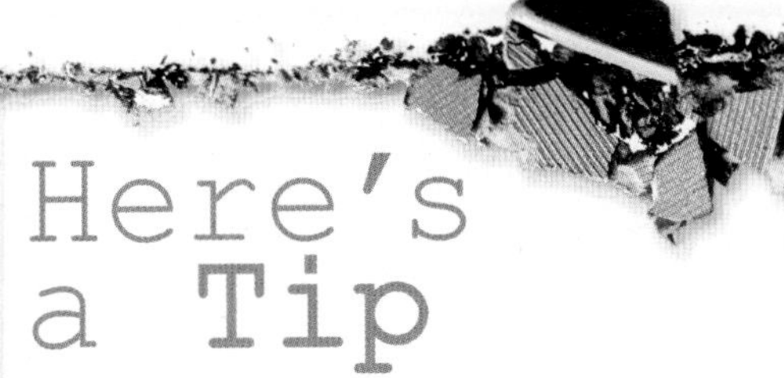

Here's a Tip

The heat from the chemical reaction caused when UV gels cure can make some clients uncomfortable. The heat can be controlled by slowly inserting the hand into the UV lamp. This will help to slow the gel reaction and generate less heat. The heat is a result of the exothermic reaction of the gel as each bond of the polymer is created; the more bonds that are formed when the gel cures, the more heat that is generated. In addition, the more bonds that are created when the gel polymerizes, the stronger the gel will be.

The light unit has as much to do with the proper curing of the UV gel as the lamp! Not all light units are the same. The differences between the structures of the light units will alter the curing potential of the unit. For example, if two light units are similar in every other respect, but light unit A has been constructed with the UV lamps closer to the fingernails than light unit B, light unit A will have more curing potential than B. Thus, the lamps are not going to provide the same results. The light units are both 9 watt and have the same number of lamps, but light unit A is more powerful than light unit B.

Consult with the gel manufacturer to receive more detailed information on which light unit and lamp will properly cure their UV gels. ✓ LO6

UV Gel Polish

UV gel polish has become a popular service to complement gels and all other enhancement services, including natural nails. UV gel polish is a relatively new system that evolved in the year 2000 with the emergence of new chemistries that became available to the beauty industry. The most popular UV gel polishes are highly pigmented, a factor which gives these systems the appearance of a traditional solvent-based nail lacquer. Also, UV gel polishes are available in hundreds of shades, much the same as traditional nail polish, to suit every client.

Wearing UV gel polishes instead of traditional nail lacquers does offer great advantages; however, they are removed differently than traditional nail polish. One advantage of UV gel polishes is that they do not dry—they cure. Cured UV gel polish systems will not imprint or smudge if the client hits her hands while the nail lacquer is still drying. A second advantage is that the UV gel polish does not thicken over time because the solvent does not evaporate. Solvent evaporation makes nail lacquers thicken and dry more slowly after the bottle of nail polish has been opened for a few months. Since the solvent does not evaporate in UV gel polish, a container of such polish will last longer.

To remove a UV gel polish, cosmetologists typically file the polish off, either by hand, using an abrasive, or by using an electric file. However, soakable UV gel polishes are removed by soaking the nails in acetone for five to ten minutes to soften them, allowing the cosmetologist to easily scrape off the polish with a wooden stick.

UV Gel Maintenance and Removal

UV gel enhancements must be maintained regularly, depending on how fast the client's nails grow.

UV Gel Maintenance

Begin the maintenance by using a medium-grit abrasive file (180 grit) to thin and shape the enhancement. Be careful not to damage the natural nail plate with the abrasive when you are performing the fill portion of the UV gel maintenance.

Before filing the nail, be sure to clean the nail with the UV gel manufacturer's recommended cleanser or isopropanol (99 percent or better). This removes oils from the fingernail and results in better adhesion of the gel to the nail plate. It is important to remember that you must file with a lighter touch, because it is usually easier to file UV gel enhancements than monomer liquid and polymer powder enhancements.

Here's a Tip

When you provide enhancement services, ask whether the client would like the enhancements to be easily removable. If the client wants easily removable enhancements, use a soak-off UV gel as the base coat (following the manufacturer's recommendations on the UV gel's application), then perform the remainder of the service. Before the client leaves the salon, arrange a date for her to return to have the UV gels removed.

PROCEDURE 29-4 UV Gel Maintenance SEE PAGE 945

UV Gel Removal

There are two types of gel, and each employs a different removal method.

Hard UV gels, also known as **traditional UV gels**, cannot be removed with a solvent and must be filed off the natural nail to be removed.

Soft UV gels, also known as **soakable gels**, are removed by soaking in acetone. It is important that you read and follow the manufacturer's directions before removing UV gel nails.

PROCEDURE 29-6 UV Gel Removal–Hard Gel SEE PAGE 950

PROCEDURE 29-7 UV Gel Removal–Soft Gel SEE PAGE 951

For more interesting and useful information about UV gel enhancement products, see *Nail Structure & Product Chemistry*, Second Edition, by Douglas D. Schoon, published by Milady, a part of Cengage Learning.

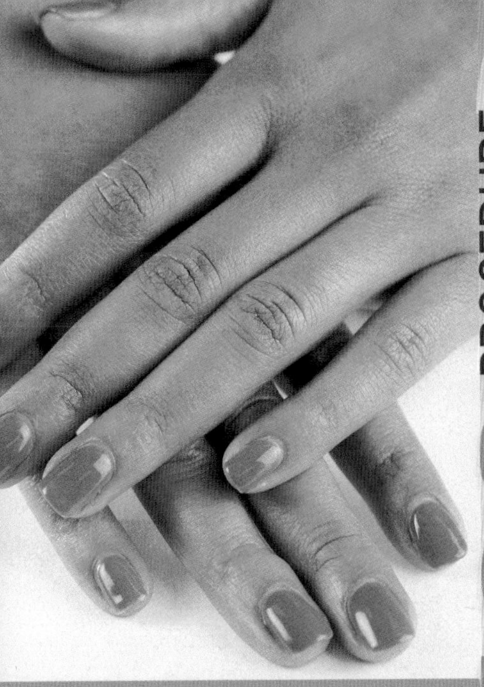

PROCEDURE 29-1

One-Color Method UV Gel on Tips or Natural Nails with UV Gel Polish

Implements and Materials

In addition to the basic materials on your manicuring table, you will need the following supplies:

- **Brush**
- **Cleansing solution**
- **Lint-free cleansing wipes**
- **Nail tips**
- **UV gel for the application**
- **UV gel light-unit**
- **UV gel polish**
- **UV gel primer or bonding gel**

© Milady, a part of Cengage Learning. Photography by Dino Petrocelli.

Preparation

- Perform PROCEDURE 25-1 **Pre-Service Procedure** SEE PAGE 817

Procedure

1 Clean the nails and remove existing polish. Begin with your client's little finger on the right hand and work toward the thumb. Repeat on the left hand. Ask the client to place her nails into a finger bowl with liquid soap. Use a nailbrush to clean the nails over the finger bowl. Thoroughly rinse with clean water to remove soap residues that can cause lifting.

2 Use a cotton-tipped wooden or metal pusher to gently push back the eponychium, then apply cuticle remover to the nail plate. Use as directed by the manufacturer and carefully remove cuticle tissue from the nail plate.

3 Use a solvent-based cleanser per the manufacturer's recommendation. Remove any oils from the fingernail before abrading with a file. This increases the adhesive properties of the gel. Start with the little finger and work toward the thumb.

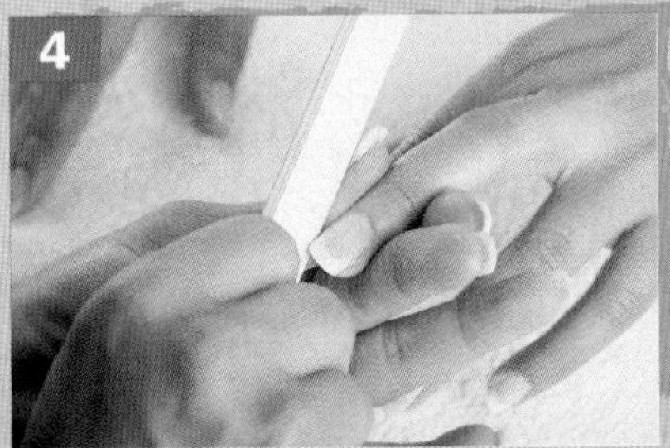

4 Lightly buff the nail plate with a medium (180 grit) abrasive, or the abrasive recommended by the gel manufacturer, to remove the shine on the surface of the nail plate.

One-Color Method UV Gel on Tips or Natural Nails with UV Gel Polish continued

5 Remove the dust from the nail surface per the manufacturer's recommendations.

6 If your client requires nail tips, apply them according to Procedure 27–1, Nail Tip Application, in Chapter 27, Nail Tips and Wraps. Be sure to shorten and shape the tip before the application of the UV gel. During the procedure, the UV gel overlaps the tip's edge to prevent lifting. This seal can be broken during the filing process, allowing the UV gel to peel or lift. Be careful not to break this seal.

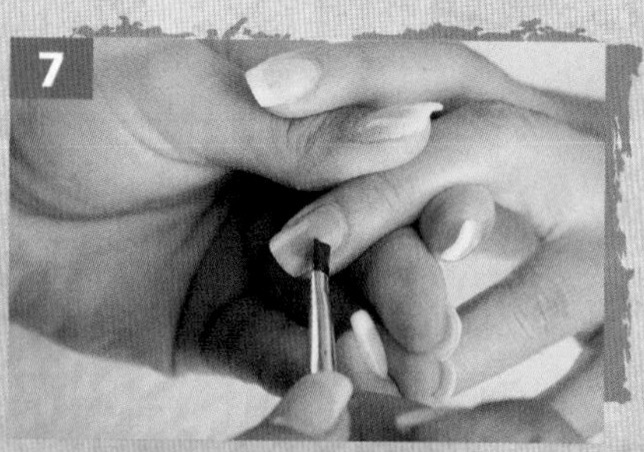

7 Follow the manufacturer's instructions for applying the bonding or priming material. Your success depends on your ability to properly prepare the nail plate for services and apply this bonding material. Using the applicator brush, insert the brush into the nail primer or bonding gel. Wipe off any excess from the brush, and, using a slightly damp brush, ensure that the nail plate is completely covered per the manufacturer's recommendations. Avoid using too much product to prevent running into the skin, which can increase the risks of developing skin irritation or sensitivity to the enhancement system.

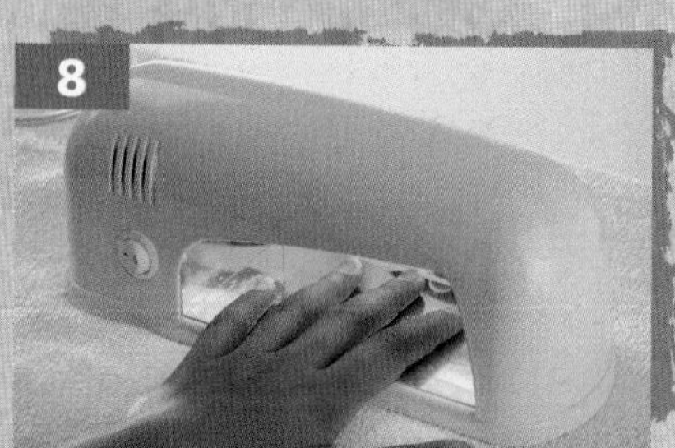

8 Cure the bonding gel according to the manufacturer's directions.

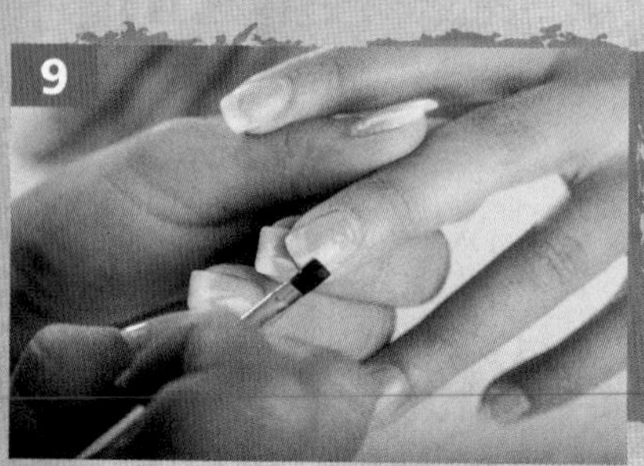

9 Gently brush UV gel onto the fingernail surface, including the free edge. Leave a 3⁄16-inch gap around the cuticle and sidewall area of the fingernail. Keep the UV gel from touching the cuticle, eponychium, or sidewalls. When applying this gel, do not pat the gel as you would monomer liquid and polymer powder material; instead gently brush or float the gel material onto the fingernail. Avoid introducing air into the gel as this will reduce the strength of the cured gel and may lead to bubbles and cracking. Apply to client's right hand from little finger to pointer finger.

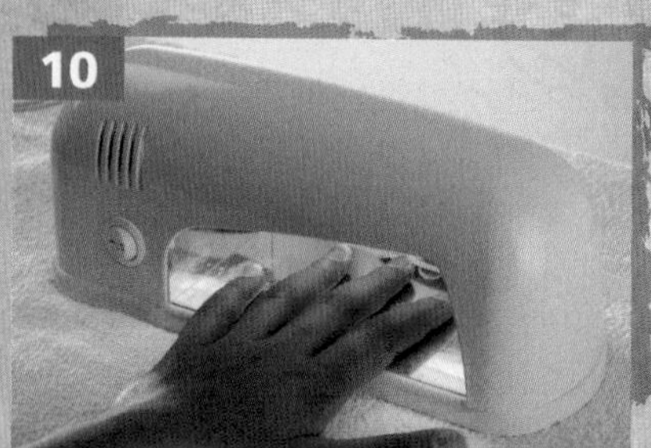

10 Properly position the hand in the UV lamp for the required cure time as indicated by the manufacturer. Always cure each layer of the UV gel for the time required by the manufacturer's instructions. Curing for too little time can result in service breakdown, skin irritation, and/or skin sensitivity. Improper positioning of the hands inside the lamp also can cause improper curing.

© Milady, a part of Cengage Learning. Photography by Dino Petrocelli.

11 Repeat steps 9 and 10 on the left hand, and then repeat the same steps for both thumbs.

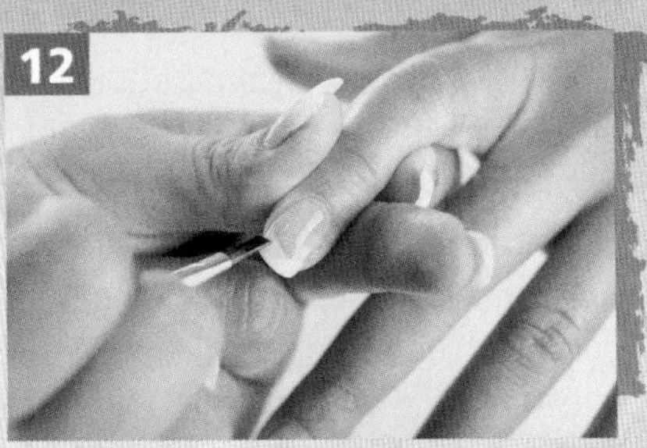

12 Apply a small amount of UV gel to the client's little finger (a self-leveling gel works best at this stage of the application) over the properly cured first layer on the client's right hand. Carefully pull the UV gel across the first layer, and smooth it into place. Avoid patting the brush or pressing too hard because this will introduce air into the gel and decrease its strength. Brush the UV gel over and around the free edge to create a seal. Avoid touching the skin under the free edge to prevent skin irritation and sensitivity. Repeat this application process on the remaining three fingernails.

13 Cure the second UV gel layer (building or self-leveling gel) by properly positioning the hand in the UV lamp for the manufacturer's required cure time.

14 Repeat steps 12 and 13 on the left hand, and then repeat the same steps for both thumbs.

15 Apply another layer of the second UV gel, if needed. Another layer of the second UV gel (building or self-leveling UV gel) will add thickness to the enhancement. Cure for the time required by the manufacturer.

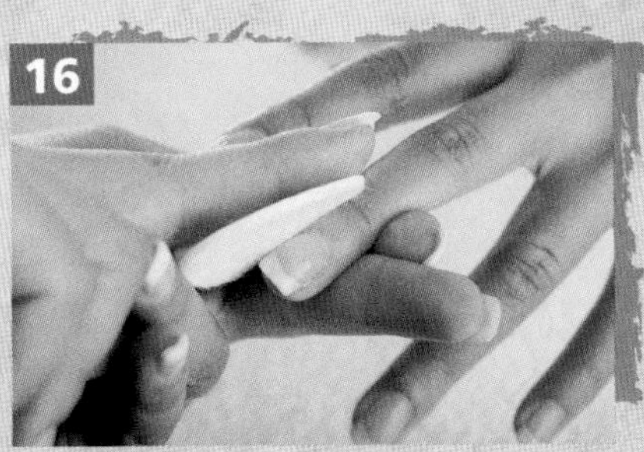

16 Remove the inhibition layer by cleaning with the manufacturer's cleanser on a plastic-backed cotton pad to avoid skin contact. If the cleanser is not available, then alcohol, acetone, or another suitable remover could suffice; confirm with the gel manufacturer. Prolonged or repeated skin contact with the inhibition layer may cause skin irritation or sensitivity.

Service Tip

The procedure recommended for applying and curing UV gel varies from one manufacturer to another. Some systems recommend applying UV gel to the four fingernails on one hand and curing, then repeating this procedure on the other hand before applying and curing UV gel on the thumbnails. Be sure to follow the instructions recommended by the manufacturer of the system that you are using.

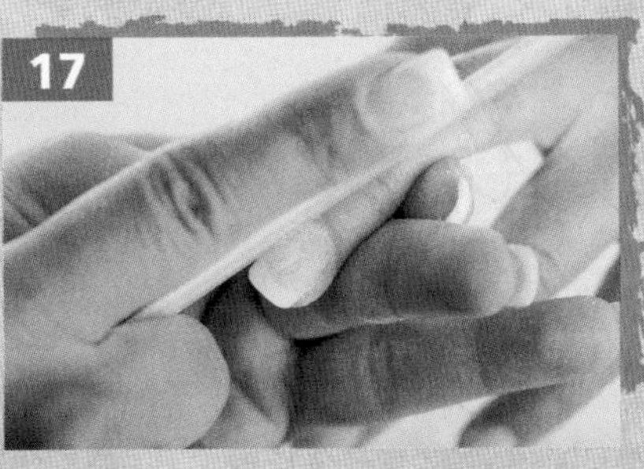

17 Using a medium or fine abrasive (180 or 240 grit), refine the surface contour. File carefully near the sidewalls and eponychium to avoid injuring the client's skin. Bevel down, stroking the file at a 45-degree angle from the top center down to the free edge. Check the free edge thickness and even out imperfections with gentle strokes. Make certain that you avoid excessive filing of the gel on the sidewalls of the enhancements. Excessive filing makes the enhancement too thin, which can result in cracking that begins at the sidewalls.

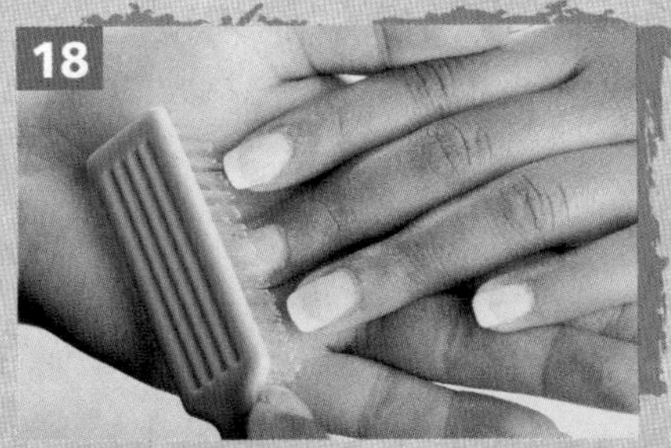

18 Remove dust and filings with a clean and disinfected nylon brush.

19 Remove any oils that may have been deposited on the fingernail during filing. This will decrease potential problems that may cause defects in the final coat of gel.

© Milady, a part of Cengage Learning. Photography by Dino Petrocelli.

One-Color Method UV Gel on Tips or Natural Nails with UV Gel Polish continued

Service Tip

During the procedure, keep the brush and UV gel away from sunlight, UV gel lamps, and full-spectrum table lamps to prevent the gel from hardening. When the service is completed, store your application brush away from all sources of UV light. Do not leave your container of gel open and near a window or UV light unit. If the gel is exposed to these sources of UV light, it will cure and become polymerized in the container.

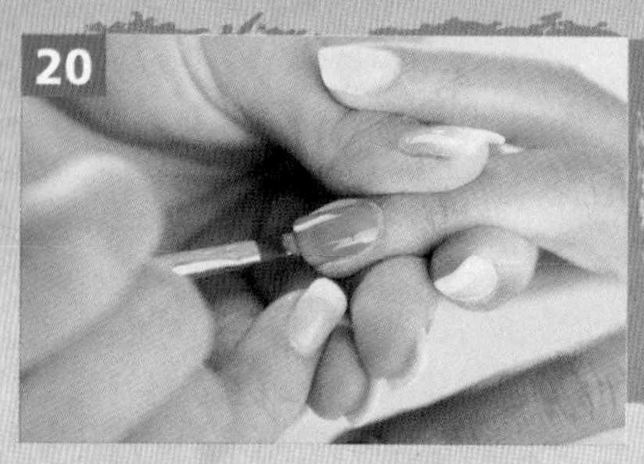

20 Apply the first thin coat of UV gel polish over the entire surface of the enhancement in a brushing technique. Use ample pressure to ensure a smooth finished look to the application. Apply a small amount of the UV gel polish to the free edge of the fingernail to cap the end and create an even and consistent appearance.

21 Place the hand inside the UV light unit in the proper location and cure the first coat of UV gel polish for the recommended period of time.

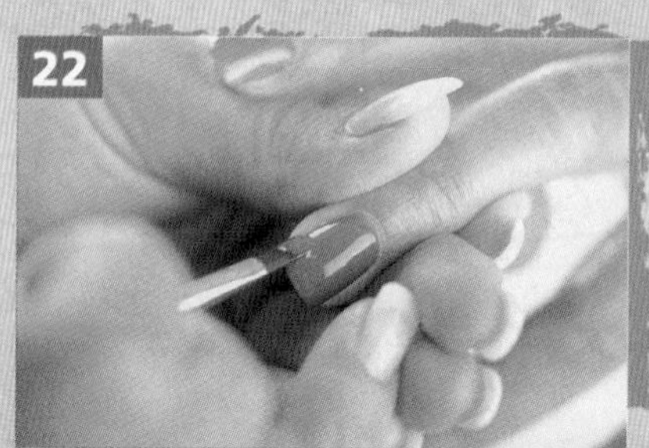

22 Apply a second thin coat of UV gel polish over the entire surface of the enhancement in a brushing technique and apply a small amount of the UV gel polish to the free edge of the fingernail to cap the end and create an even and consistent appearance.

23 Cure second coat of UV gel polish.

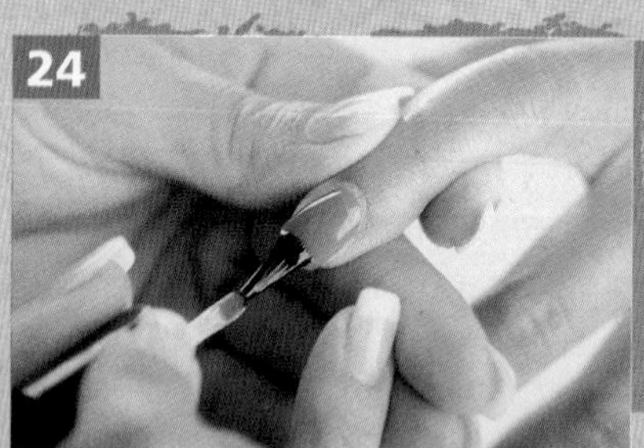

24 Apply gloss UV gel (sealer, gloss, or finisher gel).

25 Cure the gloss gel.

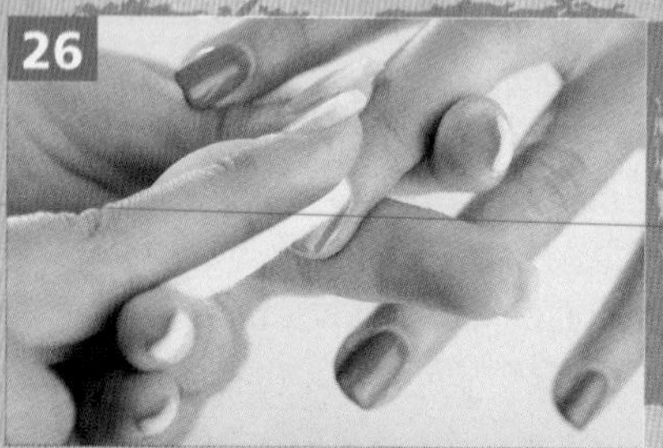

26 Remove the inhibition layer, if required.

27 Apply nail oil.

28 Apply hand lotion and massage the hand and arm.

29 Clean the nail enhancements. Evaluate the work you just completed and make any necessary adjustments.

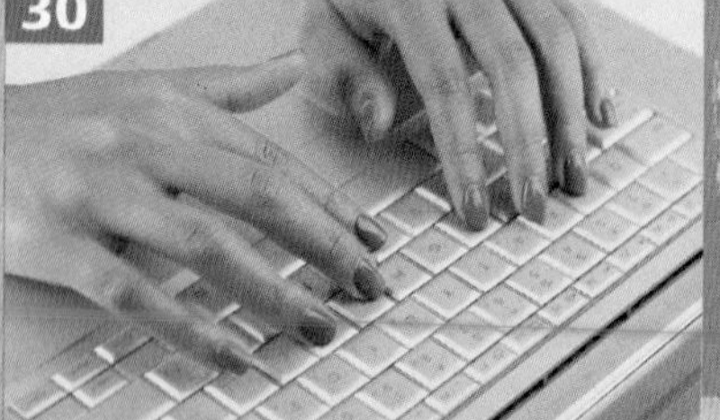

30 Finished look.

Post-Service

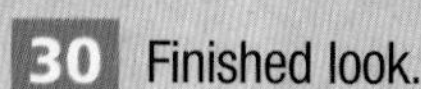

- Complete PROCEDURE 25-2 Post-Service Procedure SEE PAGE 821 ✓ LO7

© Milady, a part of Cengage Learning. Photography by Dino Petrocelli.

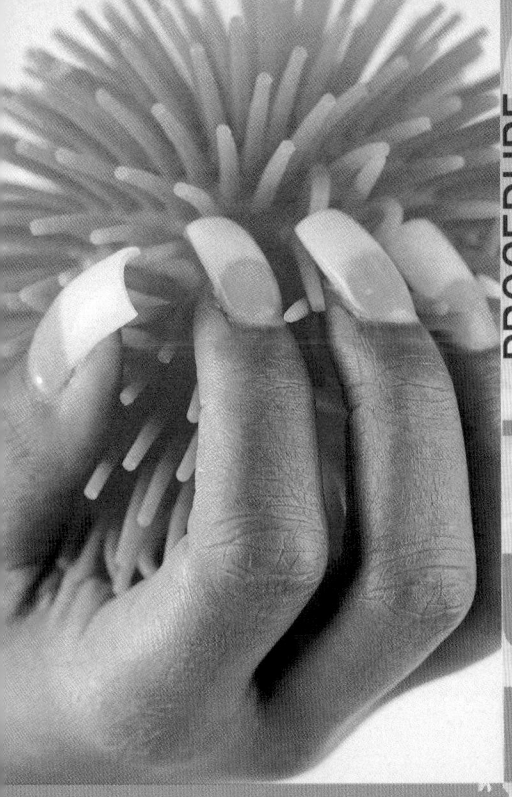

PROCEDURE 29-2

Two-Color Method UV Gel on Tips or Natural Nails

Implements and Materials

In addition to the basic materials on your manicuring table, you will need the following supplies:

- **Brush**
- **Cleansing solution**
- **Lint-free cleansing wipes**
- **Nail tips**
- **Pink UV gel and white UV gel**
- **UV gel light-unit**
- **UV gel primer or bonding gel**

© Milady, a part of Cengage Learning. Photography by Dino Petrocelli.

Preparation

- Perform PROCEDURE 25-1 Pre-Service Procedure SEE PAGE 817

Procedure

1. Clean the nails and remove existing polish.
2. Push back the eponychium and remove the cuticle from the nail plate.
3. Clean and dehydrate the fingernail.
4. Prepare the nails.
5. Remove the dust from the nail surface.
6. Apply nail tips, if desired.
7. Apply primer or bonding gel.
8. Cure bonding resin, if required.

PROCEDURE 29-2

Two-Color Method UV Gel on Tips or Natural Nails continued

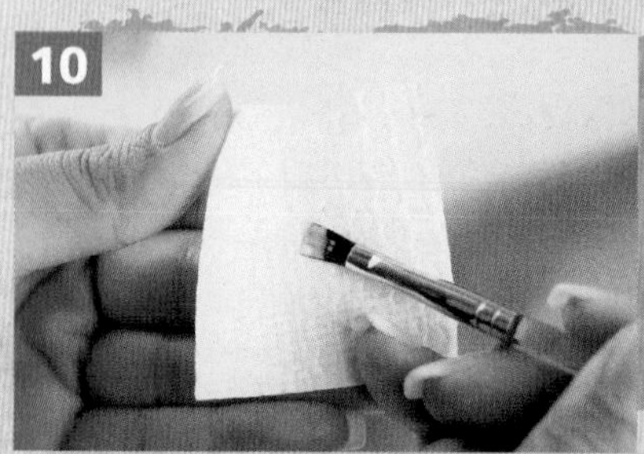
9

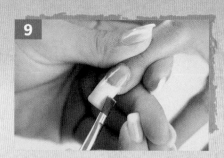

9 Select the desired white gel to create the two-color process. Working from right to left on the hand, apply a coat of the white gel over the tip and along the sidewalls of the fingernail to create the smile line. Be sure to apply this layer of gel thin enough to have the gel cure completely through to the surface of the tip. If the gel does not cure completely through, it will lift from the surface of the tip and fingernail. If there is white UV gel where you do not want it to be, wipe the unwanted gel from the fingernail tip.

10

10 Using a lint-free nail wipe, pinch the bristles of the brush in the nail wipe so that the bristles form a squeegee-like surface. Do not use solvents to clean the bristles.

Service Tip

It is important when using tips with UV gels to size the tip so that the curve of the tip matches the curve of the nail. If the curves do not match and the tip is spread too flat, then the tips could crack lengthwise down the center. So if you find a tip has cracked lengthwise down the center, you know that the curve of your tip was not matched to the curve of the fingernail.

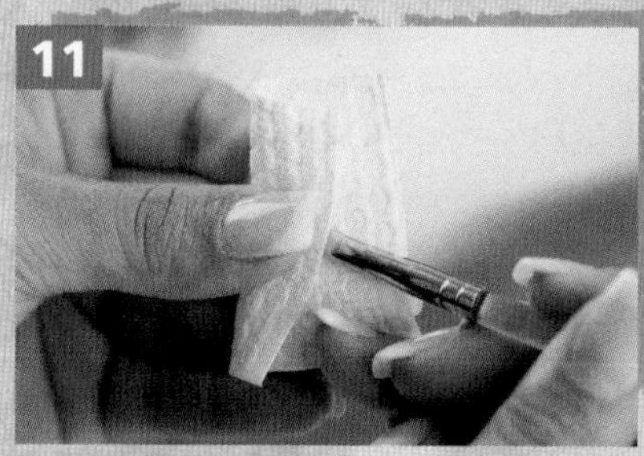
11

11 Using the tip of your clean application brush, wipe away any unwanted gel from the tip to create a crisp smile line. Repeat this process until you have the desired smile line. Make certain that all smile lines are uniform in appearance before curing the gel.

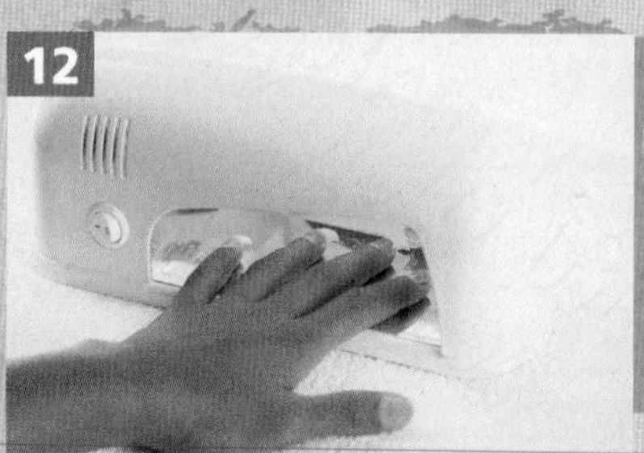
12

12 Cure the white gel in the UV lamp for the recommended time.

13 If the white gel does not have the same brightness on all fingers, repeat steps 9, 10, and 11.

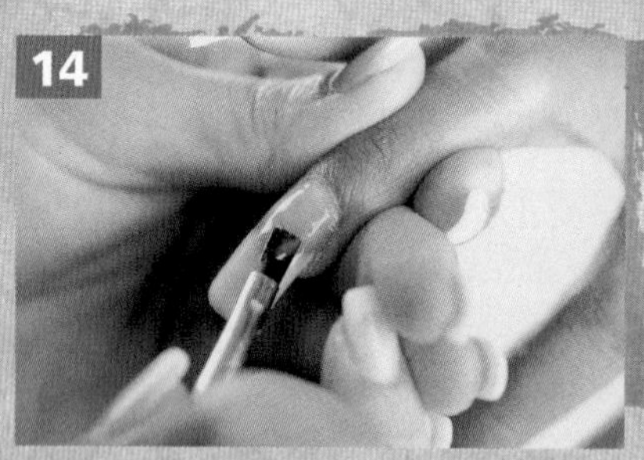
14

14 Gently brush a pink-tinted UV gel onto the fingernail surface, including the free edge. Leave a $^{3}/_{16}$-inch gap around the cuticle and the sidewall area of the fingernail. Keep the UV gel from touching the cuticle, eponychium, or sidewalls. When applying this gel, do not pat the gel as you would a monomer liquid and polymer powder material. Gently brush or float the gel material onto the fingernail. Avoid introducing air into the gel as this will reduce the strength of the cured gel and may lead to cracking. Apply to client's right hand from little finger to pointer finger.

© Milady, a part of Cengage Learning. Photography by Dino Petrocelli.

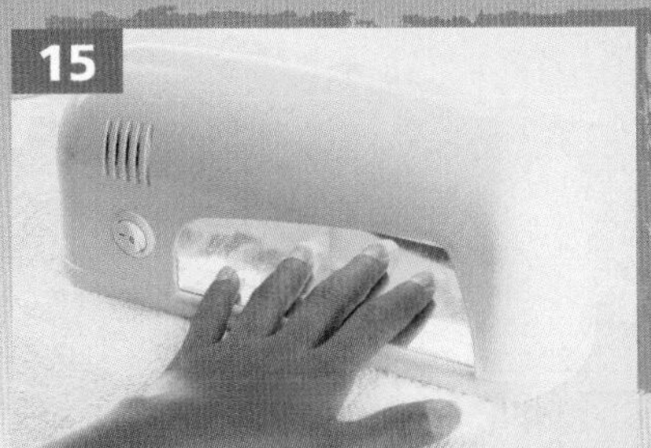

15 Cure the first coat of the UV gel (building gel).

16 Repeat steps 14 and 15 on the left hand, and then repeat the same steps for both thumbs.

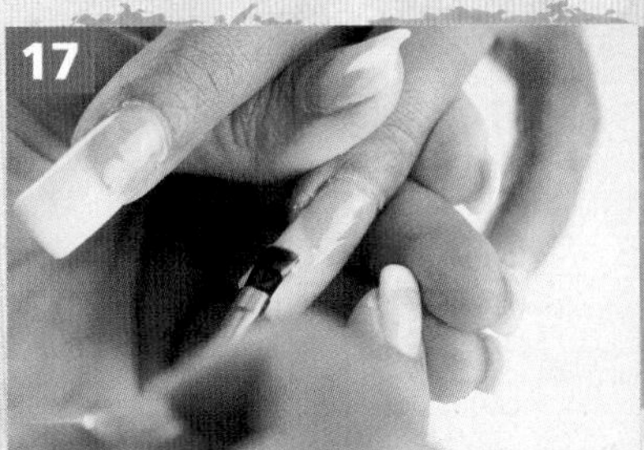

17 Apply a small amount of pink UV gel (a self-leveling gel works best at this stage of the application) over the properly cured first layer. Carefully pull the UV gel across the first layer, and smooth it into place. Avoid patting the brush or pressing too hard as this will introduce air into the gel and decrease its strength. Brush the UV gel over and around the free edge to create a seal. Avoid touching the skin under the free edge to prevent skin irritation and sensitivity. Repeat this application process for the other four nails on the client's right hand from little finger to pointer finger.

18 Cure the second UV gel (building or self-leveling gel).

19 Repeat steps 17 and 18 on the left hand and then repeat the same steps for both thumbs.

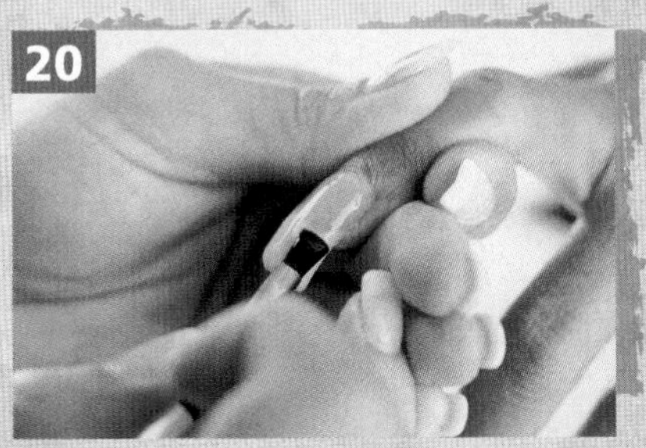

20 Another layer of the second UV gel will add thickness to the enhancement if additional thickness is desired. Cure the nails.

21 Remove the inhibition layer.

22 Check the fingernail contours.

23 Remove dust.

24 Clean the fingernail.

25 Apply the gloss UV gel (sealer, gloss, or finisher gel). Cure the nails.

26 Remove the inhibition layer, if required.

27 Apply nail oil.

28 Apply hand lotion and massage the hand and arm.

29 Clean the nail enhancements. Evaluate the work you just completed and make any necessary adjustments.

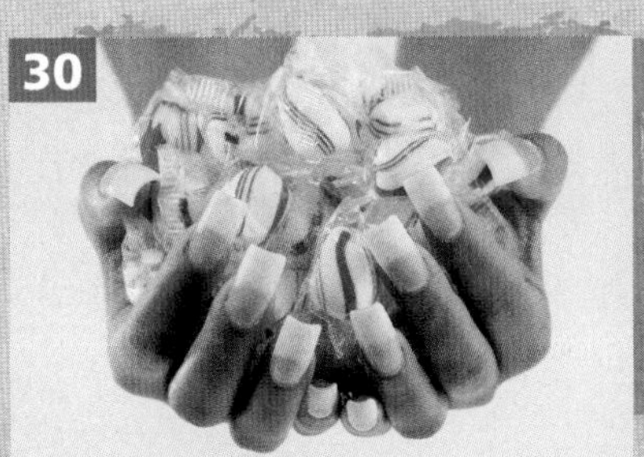

30 Finished look.

Service Tip

It is very common for gel manufacturers to have many colored gels for the two-color method. These pigmented gels can vary in opacity and viscosity. You should follow the manufacturer's recommendations for applying the pigmented gel in a two-color method. Usually, the more opaque gels have thinner viscosities and are applied after the second coat of building gel. The less-opaque pigmented gels are often thicker in viscosity and are applied before the first coat of building gel.

Post-Service

- Complete PROCEDURE 25-2 **Post-Service Procedure** SEE PAGE 821

© Milady, a part of Cengage Learning. Photography by Dino Petrocelli.

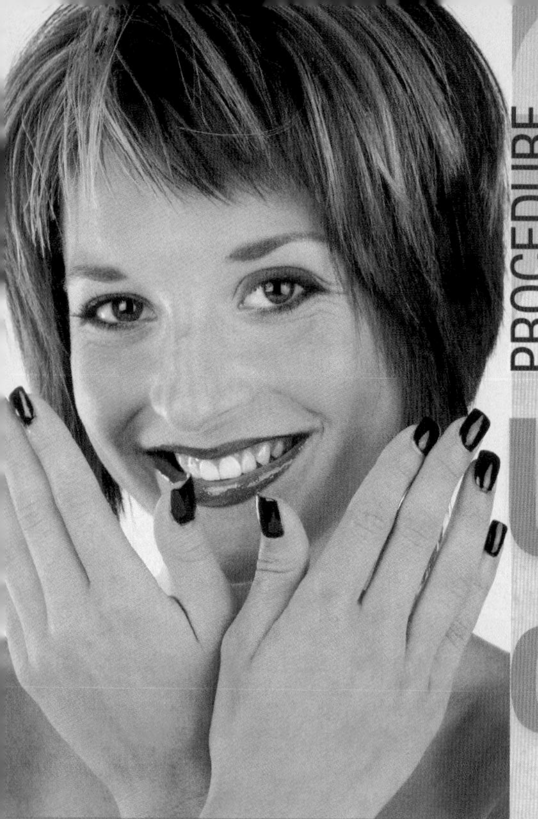

PROCEDURE

29-3 UV Gel over Forms

Implements and Materials

In addition to the basic materials on your manicuring table, you will need the following supplies:

- **Brush**
- **Cleansing solution**
- **Lint-free cleansing wipes**
- **Nail forms**
- **UV gel**
- **UV gel light-unit**
- **UV gel primer or bonding gel**

Preparation

- Perform PROCEDURE 25-1 **Pre-Service Procedure** **SEE PAGE 817**

Procedure

1. Clean the nails and remove existing polish.
2. Push back the eponychium and remove the cuticle from the nail plate.
3. Clean and dehydrate the fingernail.
4. Remove shine from the natural nail surface.
5. Remove the dust from the nail surface.

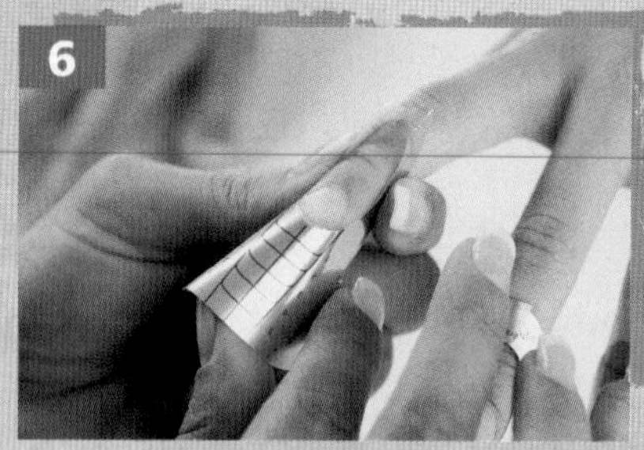

6. Fit forms onto all fingers (as described in Chapter 27, Nail Tips and Wraps). Remember to clean and disinfect multiuse forms, if disposable forms are not used. Clear plastic forms are sometimes used to allow UV light to penetrate from the underside for more complete curing of the free edge.

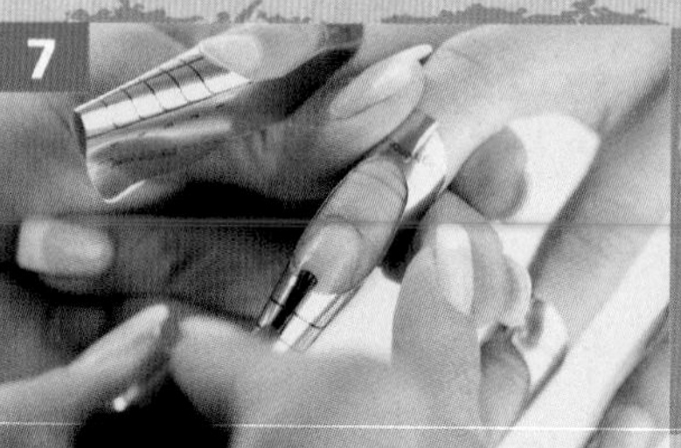

7. Apply the primer or bonding gel.

© Milady, a part of Cengage Learning. Photography by Dino Petrocelli.

8 Cure the bonding gel, if required.

9 Repeat steps 7 and 8 on the left hand and then repeat the same steps for both thumbs.

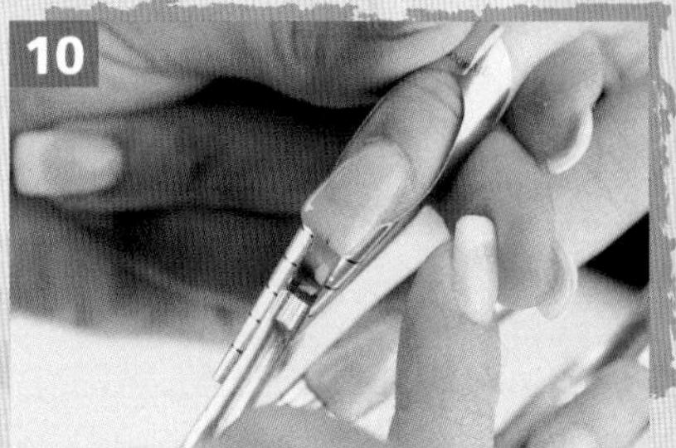

10 Apply the first coat of UV gel (building or self-leveling gel).

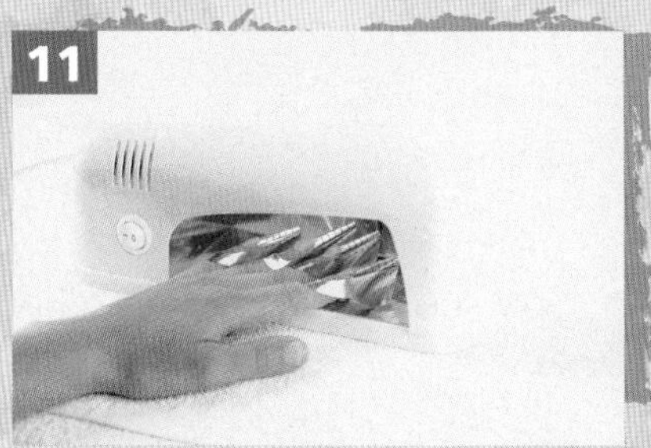

11 Properly position the hand and cure the UV gel for the required time.

12 Apply a second layer of the UV gel (building or self-leveling gel).

13 Properly position the hand and cure the UV gel for the required time.

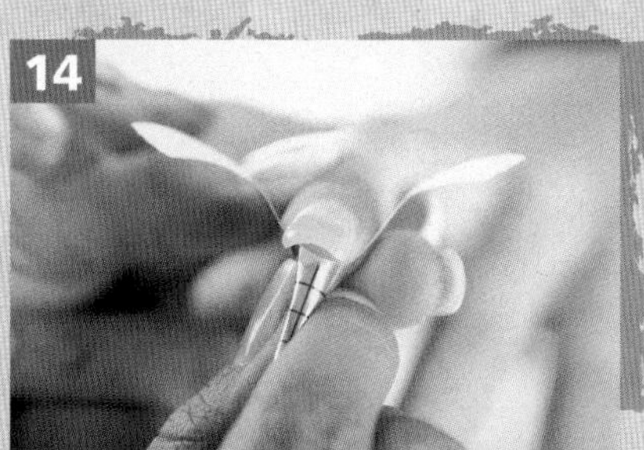

14 Remove nail forms by pinching the form just before the hyponychium of the finger and then gently pulling the form down and away from the finger.

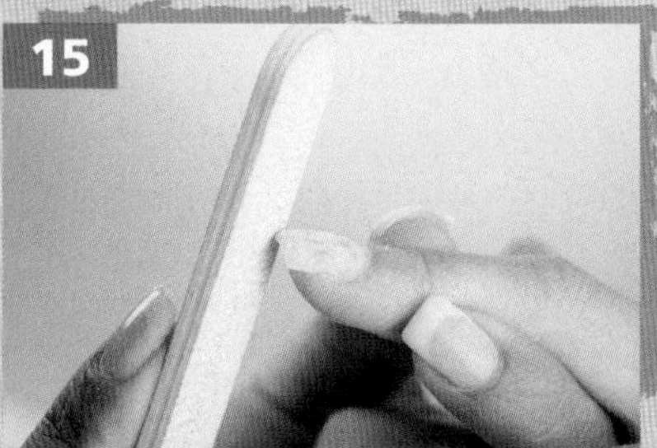

15 Use a medium or fine abrasive (180 or 240 grit) to shape the free edge of the enhancement.

© Milady, a part of Cengage Learning. Photography by Dino Petrocelli.

UV Gel over Forms continued

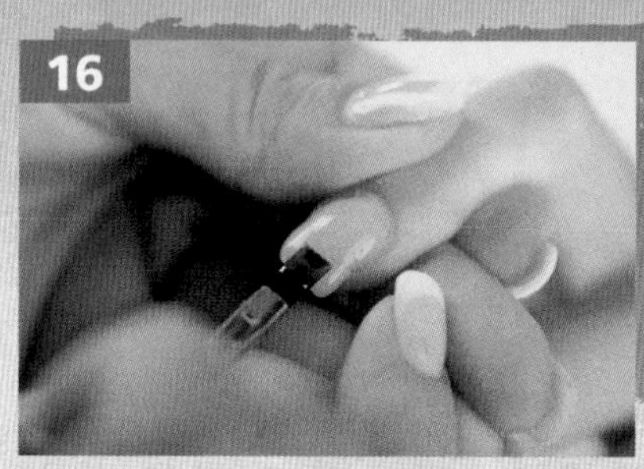
16

16 Apply another layer of UV gel (building or self-leveling gel), if needed, over the entire enhancement.

17 Cure the UV gel (building or self-leveling gel).

18 Remove the inhibition layer.

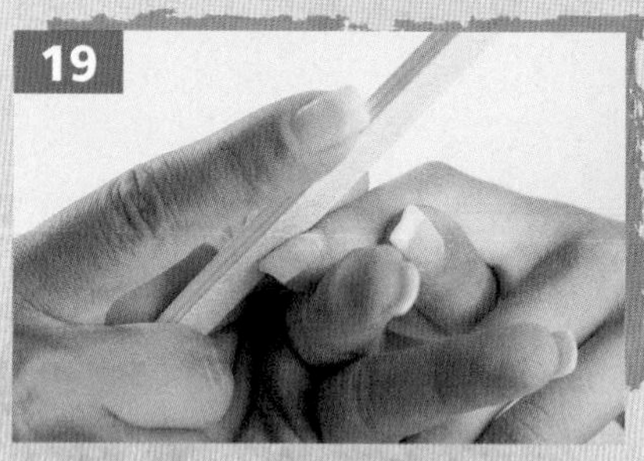
19

19 Using a medium abrasive (180 or 240 grit), refine the surface contour. Be certain to file the enhancement to create an arch and curve into the enhancement in order to optimize the strength of the overlay and create an elegant beauty to the enhancement.

20 Remove the dust.

21 Apply the gloss UV gel (sealer, gloss, or finisher).

22 Cure the UV nail.

23 Remove the inhibition layer, if required.

24 Apply nail oil.

25 Apply hand lotion and massage the hand and arm.

26 Clean the nail enhancements. Evaluate the work you just completed and make any necessary adjustments.

27 Apply nail polish, if desired.

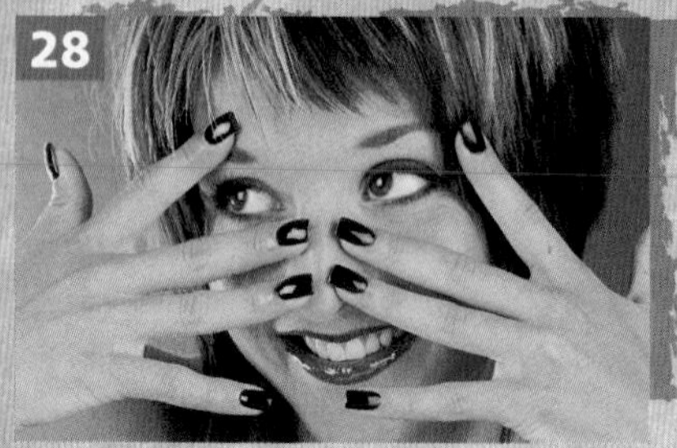
28

28 Finished look.

Post-Service

- Complete PROCEDURE 25-2 Post-Service Procedure SEE PAGE 821 ✓ LO8

© Milady, a part of Cengage Learning. Photography by Dino Petrocelli.

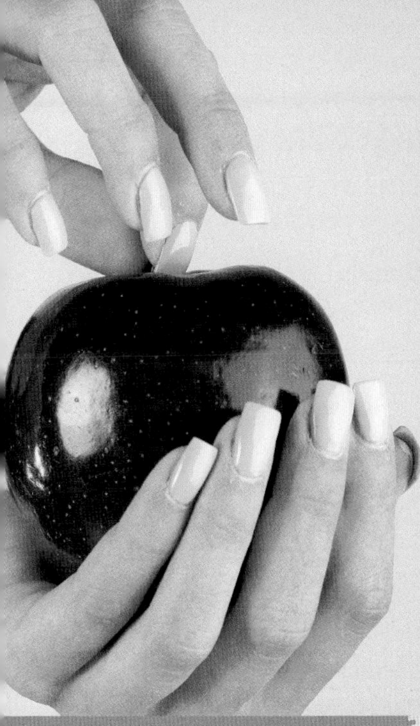

PROCEDURE 29-4

UV Gel Maintenance

Implements and Materials

In addition to the basic materials on your manicuring table, you will need the following supplies:

- **Brush**
- **Cleansing solution**
- **Lint-free cleansing wipes**
- **UV gel**
- **UV gel light-unit**
- **UV gel primer or bonding gel**

© Milady, a part of Cengage Learning. Photography by Dino Petrocelli.

Preparation

- Perform PROCEDURE 25-1 **Pre-Service Procedure** SEE PAGE 817

Procedure

1. Clean the nails and remove existing polish.
2. Push back the eponychium and remove the cuticle from the nail plate.
3. Clean and dehydrate the fingernail.

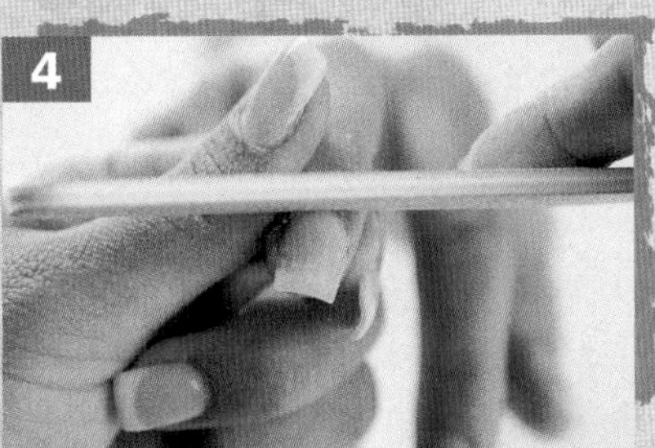

4. Lightly buff the natural nail regrowth with a medium (180 grit) abrasive or the abrasive recommended by the gel manufacturer to remove the shine on the surface of the natural nail plate.

5. Remove the dust from the nail surface.

UV Gel Maintenance continued

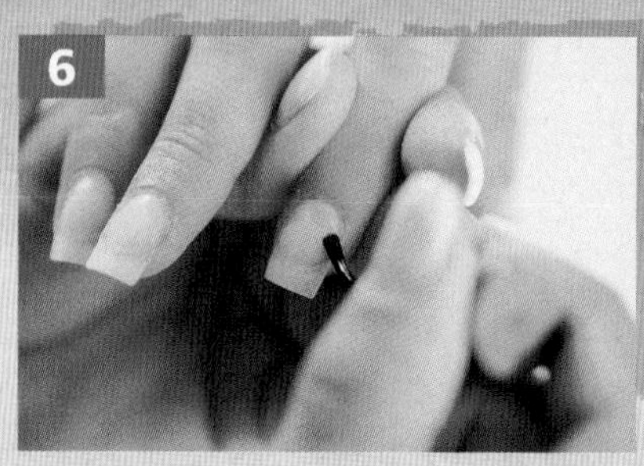

6 Apply primer or bonding gel to the natural nail.

7 Cure the bonding resin.

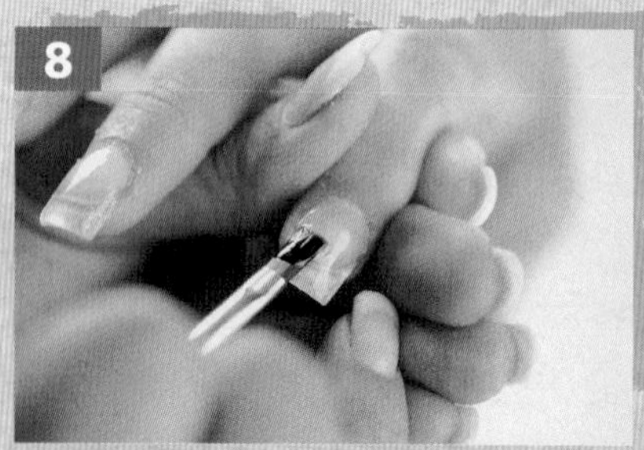

8 Lightly brush the UV gel onto the nail from the natural nail regrowth to the free edge. Keep the UV gel from touching the cuticle, eponychium, or sidewalls. When applying this gel, do not pat the gel as you would a monomer liquid and polymer powder material. Gently brush or float the gel material onto the fingernail. Avoid introducing air into the gel as this will reduce the strength of the cured gel and may lead to cracking. Apply the gel material to the client's right hand from little finger to pointer finger.

9 Cure the first UV gel.

10 Repeat steps 8 and 9 on the other hand. Then repeat the same steps for both thumbs.

11 Cure the UV gel.

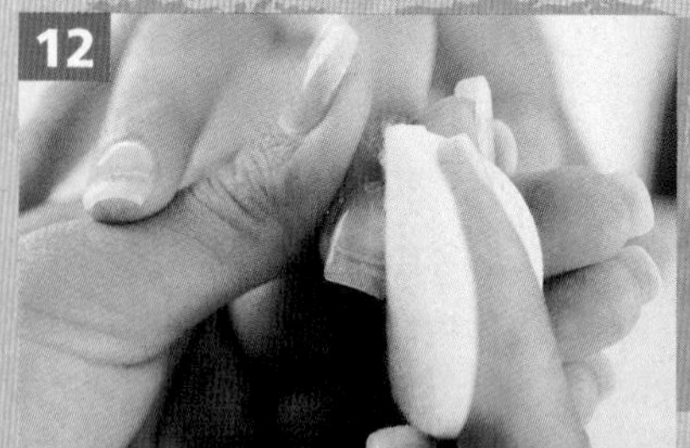

12 Remove the inhibition layer.

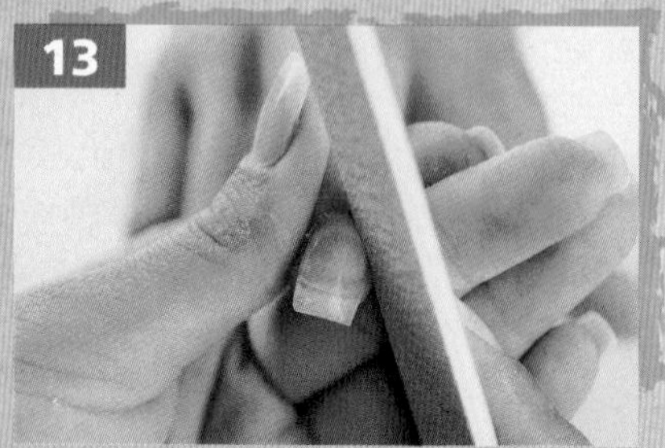

13 UV gel nails can be softer than monomer liquid and polymer powder nail enhancements, so they can file very easily. Using a medium or fine abrasive (180 or 240 grit), refine the surface contour. File carefully near the sidewalls and eponychium to avoid injuring the client's skin. Bevel down, stroking the file at a 45-degree angle from the top center dome to the free edge. Check the free edge thickness and even out imperfections with gentle strokes with the abrasive. Make certain that you avoid excessive filing of the gel on the sidewalls of the enhancements. Excessive filing may lead to the enhancement being too thin, which can result in cracking that begins at the sidewalls of the enhancement.

© Milady, a part of Cengage Learning. Photography by Dino Petrocelli.

14 Remove the dust.

15 Clean the fingernail.

16 Apply the gloss UV gel (sealer, gloss, or finisher gel).

17 Cure the gloss gel.

18 Remove the inhibition layer, if required.

19 Apply the nail oil.

20 Apply hand lotion and massage the hand and arm.

21 Clean the nail enhancements. Evaluate the work you just completed and make any necessary adjustments.

22 Apply nail polish, if desired.

Service Tip

When removing the inhibition layer from the UV gel, avoid cleaning the nail in a manner that would put the gel onto the surface of the skin. Using your nail wipe, start at the top of the fingernail nearest the cuticle and wipe away from the cuticle to the free edge of the fingernail.

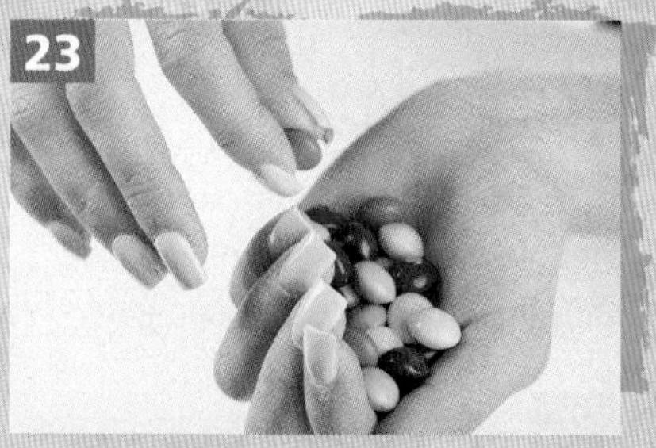

23 Finished look.

Post-Service

- Complete 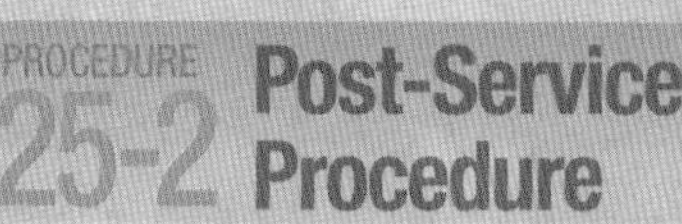 SEE PAGE 821 ✓ LO9

© Milady, a part of Cengage Learning. Photography by Dino Petrocelli.

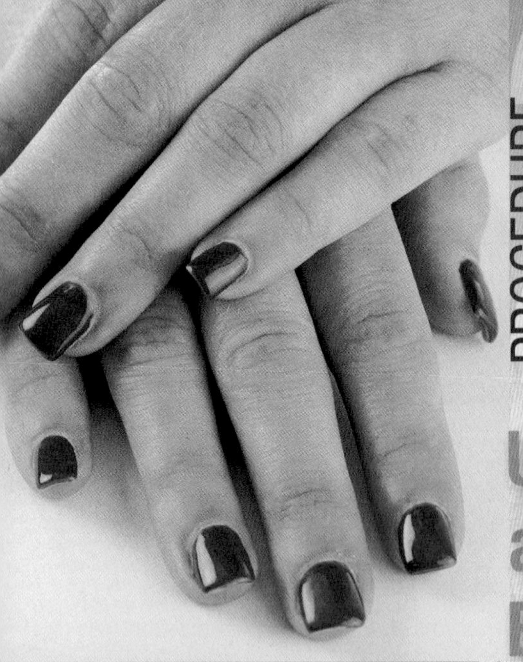

PROCEDURE 29-5

UV Gel over Monomer Liquid and Polymer Powder Nail Enhancements with UV Gel Polish

Implements and Materials

In addition to the basic materials on your manicuring table, you will need the following supplies:

- **Brush**
- **Lint-free cleansing wipes**
- **Nail cleanser**
- **UV gel sealer or top coat**
- **UV gel light-unit**
- **UV gel polish**

Preparation

- Perform PROCEDURE 25-1 **Pre-Service Procedure** SEE PAGE 817

Procedure

1 Perform monomer liquid and polymer powder application described in Chapter 28, Monomer Liquid and Polymer Powder Nail Enhancements.

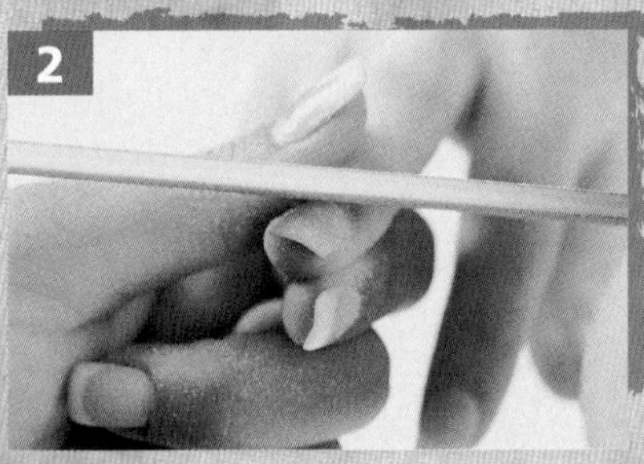

2 After the monomer liquid and polymer powder enhancement has hardened sufficiently to allow it to be filed, contour, smooth, and shape the enhancement. Do not use any oils during this process. Using a buffing or cuticle oil will cause the UV gel to have deformities on its surface and will look undesirable.

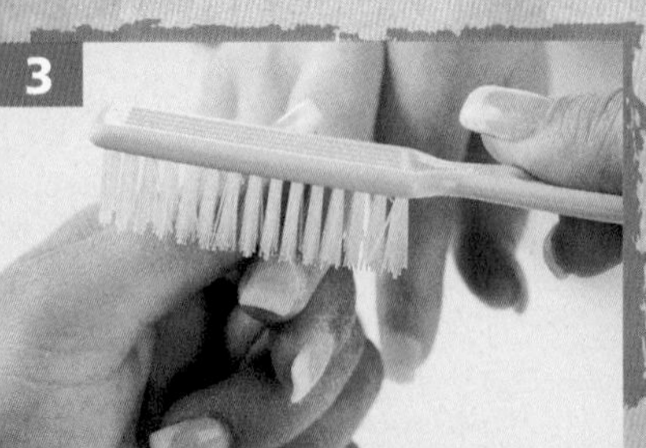

3 Remove dust and filings with a cleaned and disinfected nylon brush.

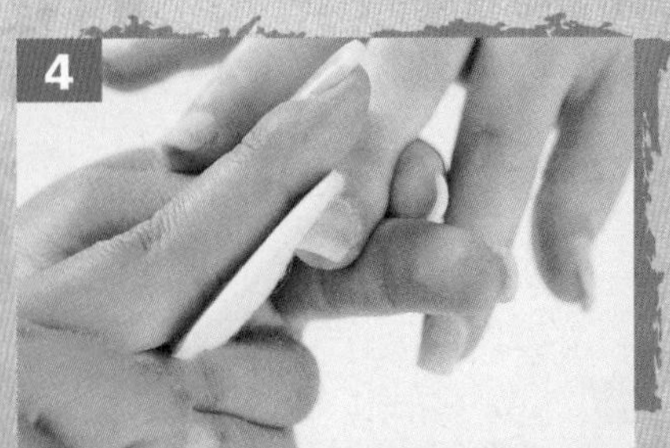

4 Remove any oils that may have been deposited on the fingernail during filing.

© Milady, a part of Cengage Learning. Photography by Dino Petrocelli.

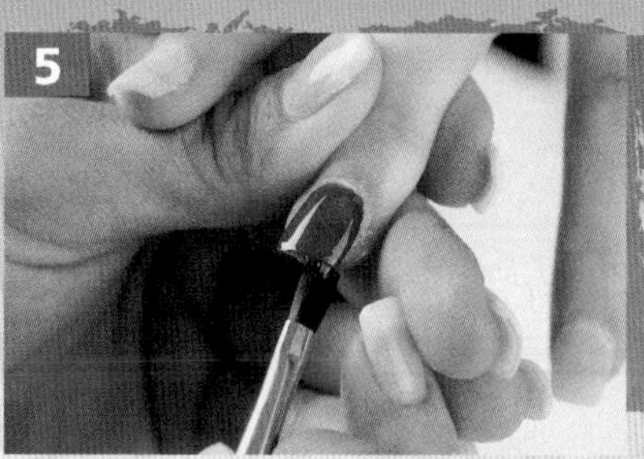

5 Apply a thin coat of UV gel polish over the entire surface of the enhancement in a brushing technique. Use ample pressure to ensure a smooth finished look to the application. Apply a small amount of the UV gel polish to the free edge of the fingernail to cap the end and create an even and consistent appearance.

6 Place the hand inside the UV light unit in the proper location and cure for the recommended period of time.

7 Apply a second thin coat of UV gel polish over the entire surface of the enhancement in a brushing technique. Use ample pressure to ensure a smooth finished look to the application. Apply a small amount of the UV gel polish to the free edge of the fingernail to cap the end and create an even and consistent appearance.

8 Place the hand inside the UV light unit in the proper location and cure for the recommended period of time.

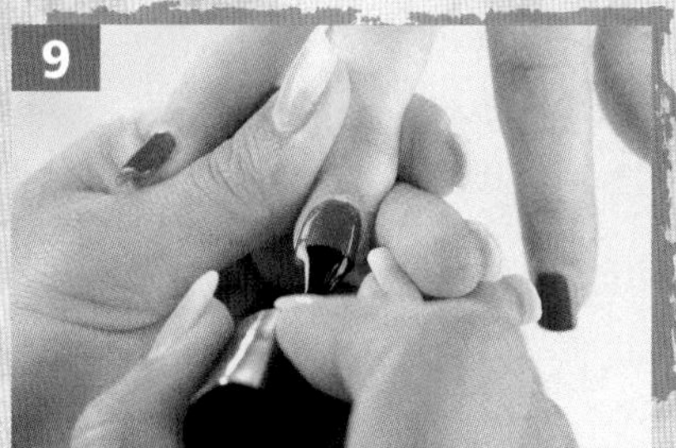

9 Apply a small amount of the third UV gel (sealer or finisher UV gel). Starting from the base of the nail plate, stroke toward the free edge, using polish-style strokes and covering the entire nail surface. Be sure not to contact the skin with the gel and to wrap this final layer under the natural nail's free edge to seal the coating and provide additional protection. Avoid touching the client's skin, as this will cause lifting.

10 Cure the gloss gel.

11 Remove the inhibition layer, if required.

12 Apply nail oil.

13 Apply hand lotion and massage the hand and arm.

14 Clean the nail enhancements. Evaluate the work you just completed and make any necessary adjustments.

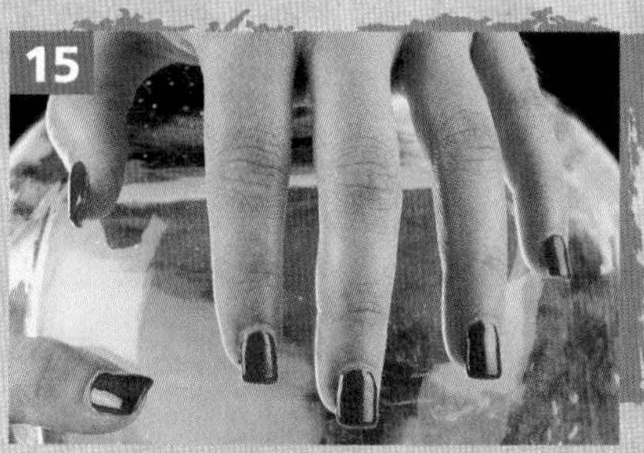

15 Finished look.

© Milady, a part of Cengage Learning. Photography by Dino Petrocelli.

Post-Service

- Complete 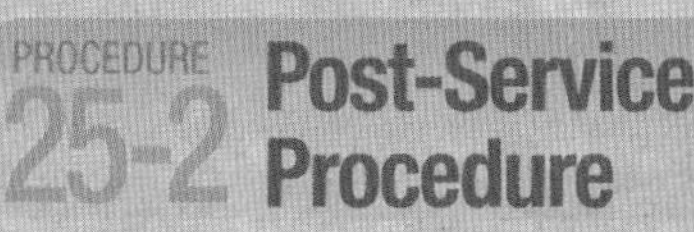

SEE PAGE 821

PROCEDURE 29-6

UV Gel Removal—Hard Gel

Implements and Materials

In addition to the basic materials on your manicuring table, you will need the following supplies:

- **Abrasives**
- **Nail buffer**
- **Polish remover**

Preparation

- Perform PROCEDURE 25-1 **Pre-Service Procedure** SEE PAGE 817

Procedure

1 Remove polish.

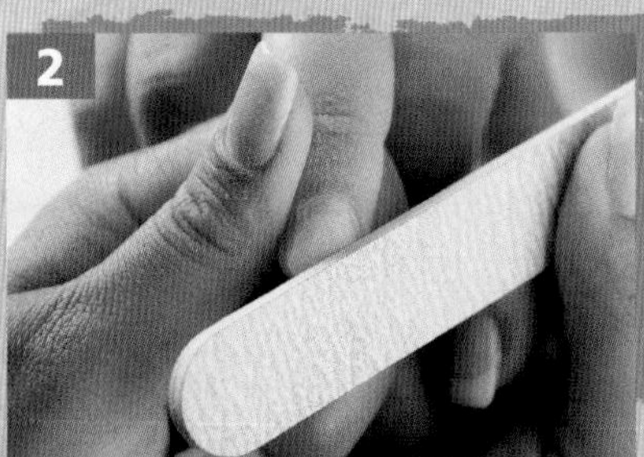

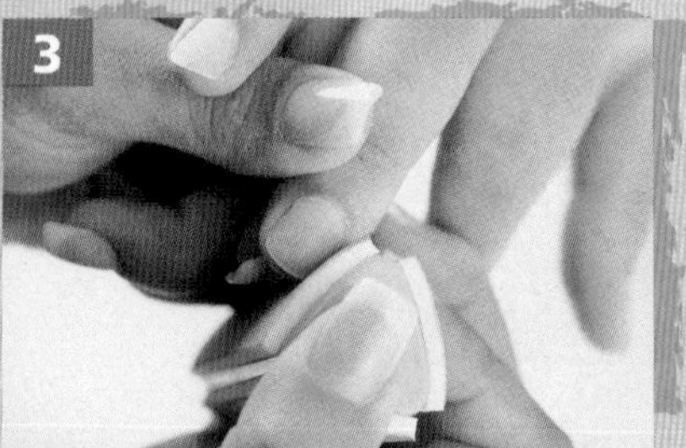

2 Use a medium-grit abrasive (180 grit) to reduce the thickness of the enhancement on the fingernail. Take care not to file into the natural nail.

3 Use a nail buffer (280 grit) to smooth the enhancement for a more natural shine. Talk with the client about how to allow the rest of the enhancements to grow out and off of the fingernails.

4 Suggest that your client have natural nail manicures to ensure that the enhancements grow off correctly. Evaluate the work you just completed and make any necessary adjustments.

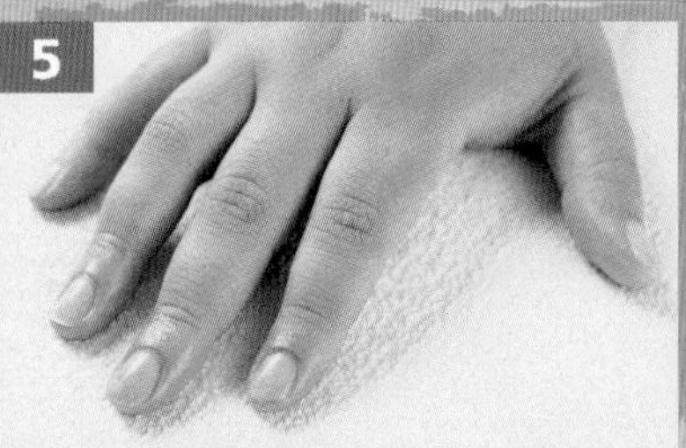

5 Finished look.

Post-Service

- Complete PROCEDURE 25-2 **Post-Service Procedure** SEE PAGE 821 ✓ LO10

© Milady, a part of Cengage Learning. Photography by Dino Petrocelli.

PROCEDURE 29-7

UV Gel Removal—Soft Gel

Implements and Materials

In addition to the basic materials on your manicuring table, you will need the following supplies:

- **Abrasives**
- **Buffer**
- **UV gel remover (as recommended by the gel manufacturer)**

Preparation

- Perform PROCEDURE 25-1 **Pre-Service Procedure** SEE PAGE 817

Procedure

1 Remove polish.

2 File the nail.

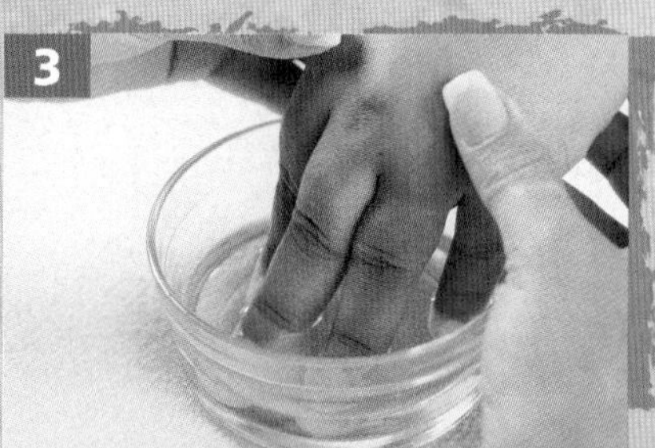

3

3 Deposit the soak-off solution into a finger bowl or other container so that the level of the remover is sufficient to completely immerse the fingernail enhancements in the solution.

4 Soak the client's fingernails in the solution for the manufacturer's recommended period of time.

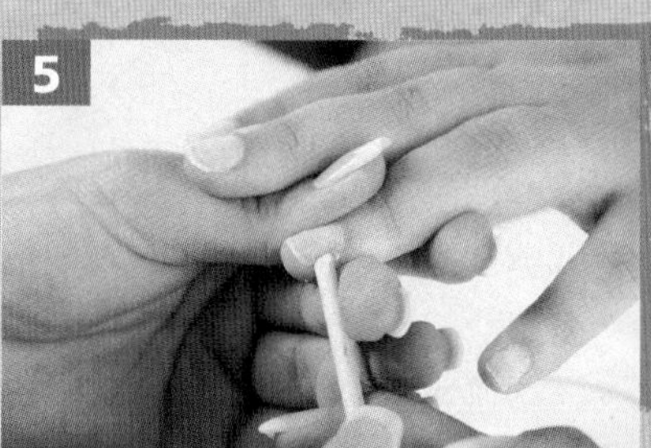

5

5 Use a wooden stick or stainless steel pusher to ease the gel off the fingernail.

© Milady, a part of Cengage Learning. Photography by Dino Petrocelli.

UV Gel Removal-Soft Gel continued

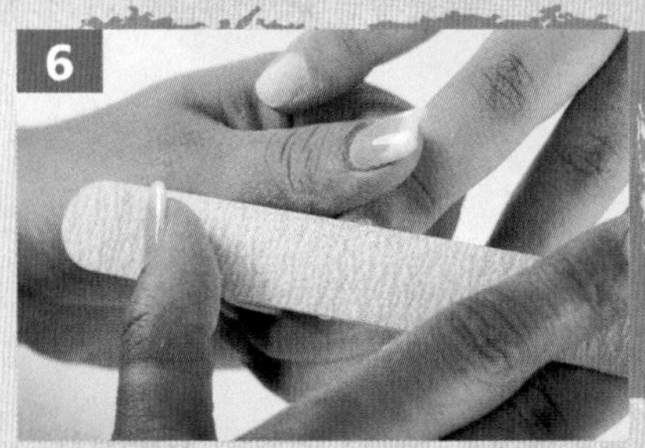

6 Lightly buff the fingernail with a fine-grit buffer (240 or 350 grit) to remove any remaining gel material from the fingernail area. Evaluate the work you just completed and make any necessary adjustments.

7 Suggest natural nail manicures to ensure that the enhancement grows off correctly.

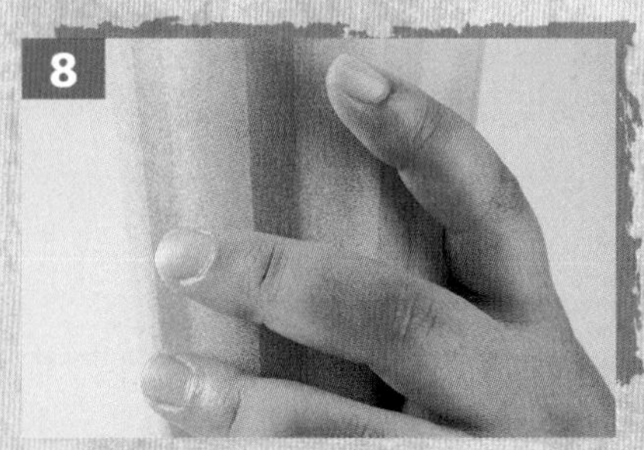

8 Finished look.

Post-Service

- Complete PROCEDURE 25-2 Post-Service Procedure SEE PAGE 821 ✓ LO11

© Milady, a part of Cengage Learning. Photography by Dino Petrocelli.

Review Questions

1. Describe the chemistry and main ingredients of UV gels.
2. When would you use a one-color method of applying UV gels? When would you use a two-color method for applying UV gels?
3. What are the types of UV gels used in current systems?
4. What supplies are needed for UV gel application?
5. When should you use UV gels?
6. When should you use a building gel, a self-leveling gel, or a UV gel that uses fiberglass?
7. What are the differences between UV light units and UV lamps?
8. List the steps to take when applying one-color UV gel on tips or natural nails.
9. Describe how UV gels are applied over forms.
10. Describe how to maintain UV gel nail enhancements.
11. Explain how to correctly remove hard UV gels.
12. Explain how to correctly remove soft UV gels.

Chapter Glossary

cure	To harden.
hard UV gels	Also known as *traditional UV gels*; gels that cannot be removed with a solvent and must be filed off the natural nail.
inhibition layer	The tacky surface left on the nail after a UV gel has cured.
oligomer	Short chain of monomer liquids that is often thick, sticky, and gel-like and that is not long enough to be considered a polymer.
one-color method	When one color of gel, usually clear, is applied over the entire surface of the nail.
opacity	The amount of colored pigment concentration in a gel, making it more or less difficult to see through.
photoinitiator	A chemical that initiates the polymerization reaction.
pigmented UV gels	Any building or self-leveling gel that includes color pigment.
soft UV gels	Also known as *soakable gels*; these gels are removed by soaking in acetone.
two-color method	A method whereby two colors of resin are used to overlay the nail.
unit wattage	The measure of how much electricity the lamp consumes.

Chapter Glossary

urethane acrylate	A main ingredient used to create UV gel nail enhancements.
urethane methacrylate	A main ingredient used to create UV gel nail enhancements.
UV bonding gels	Gels used to increase adhesion to the natural nail plate.
UV building gels	Any thick-viscosity adhesive resin that is used to build an arch and curve to the fingernail.
UV gel	Type of nail enhancement product that hardens when exposed to a UV light.
UV gel polish	A very thin-viscosity UV gel that is usually pigmented and packaged in a pot or a polish bottle and used as an alternative to traditional nail lacquers.
UV gloss gel	Also known as *sealing gel*, *finishing gel*, or *shine gel*; these gels are used over the finished UV gel application to create a high shine.
UV lamp	Also known as *UV light bulb*; special bulb that emits UV light to cure UV gel nail enhancements.
UV light unit	Also known as *UV light*; specialized electronic device that powers and controls UV lamps to cure UV gel nail enhancements.
UV self-leveling gels	Gels that are thinner in consistency than building gels, allowing them to settle and level during application.

PART 6

BUSINESS SKILLS

Chapters

© James Brey, 2010; used under license from iStockphoto.com.

CHAPTER 30

Seeking Employment

Chapter Outline

© zoran… (partially obscured) …photo.com.

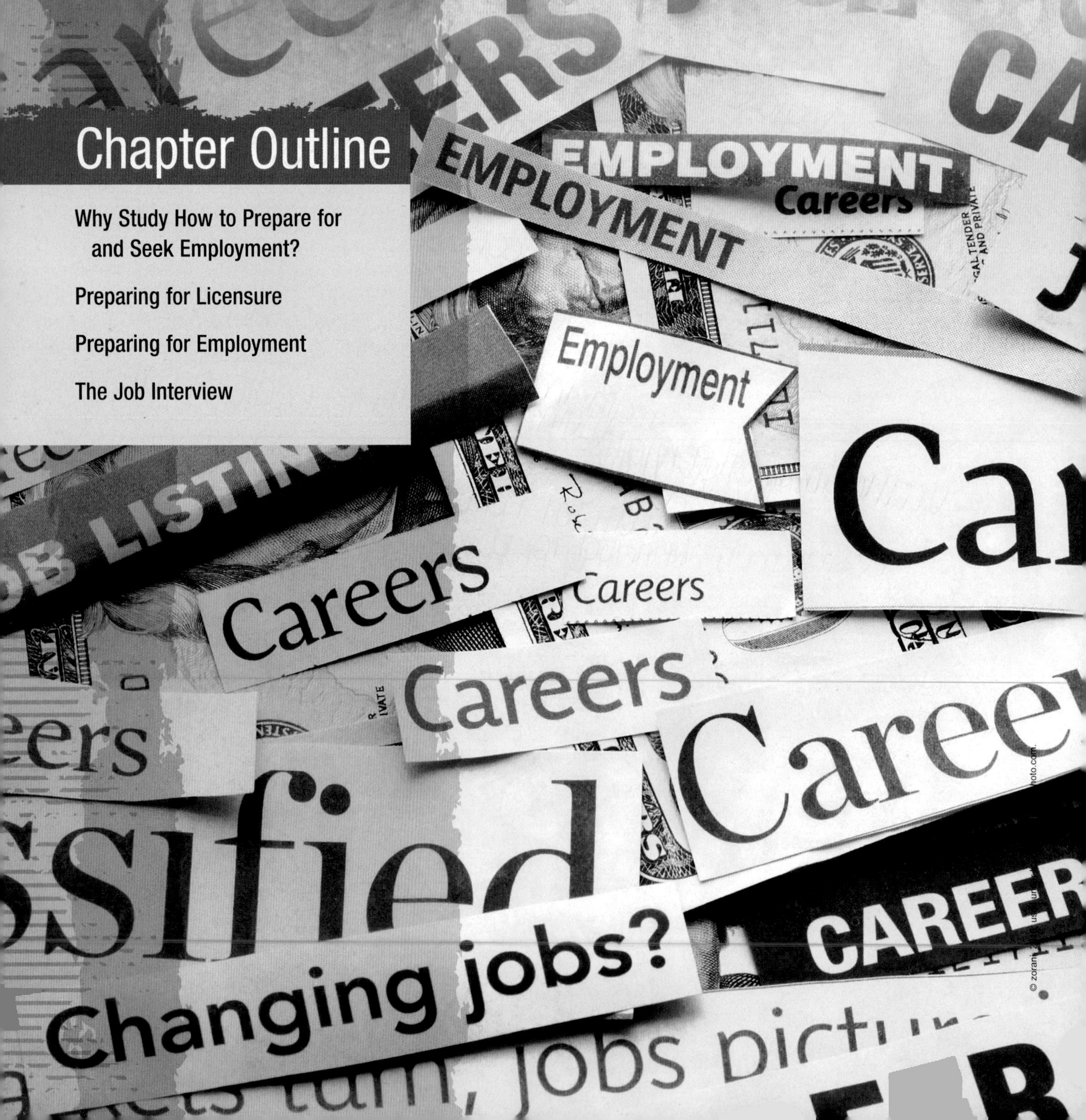

Learning Objectives

After completing this chapter, you will be able to:

✓ **LO1** Understand what is involved in securing the required credentials for cosmetology in your state and know the process for taking and passing your state licensing examination.

✓ **LO2** Start networking and preparing to find a job by using the Inventory of Personal Characteristics and Technical Skills.

✓ **LO3** Describe the different salon business categories.

✓ **LO4** Write a cover letter and resume and prepare an employment portfolio.

✓ **LO5** Know how to explore the job market, research potential employers, and operate within the legal aspects of employment.

Key Terms

Page number indicates where in the chapter the term is used.

deductive reasoning
pg. 960

employment portfolio
pg. 970

resume
pg. 967

stem
pg. 961

test-wise
pg. 959

transferable skills
pg. 969

work ethic
pg. 965

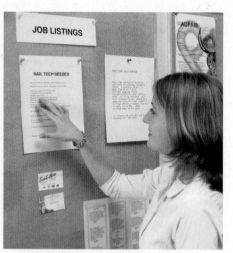

© Milady, a part of Cengage Learning. Photography by Paul Castle, Castle Photography.

▲ Figure 30–1
Job listings are often posted on the school bulletin board.

There are plenty of great jobs out there for energetic, hardworking, talented people. If you look at the top professionals in the cosmetology field, you will find they were not born successful; they achieved success through self-motivation, energy, and persistence. Like you, these stylists began their careers by enrolling in cosmetology school. They were the ones who used their time wisely, planned for the future, went the extra mile, and drew on a reservoir of self-confidence to meet challenges. They owe their success to no one but themselves, because they created it. If you want to enjoy similar success, you must prepare for the opportunities that await you.

No matter what changes occur in the economy, there are often more jobs available for entry-level cosmetology professionals than there are people to fill them. This is a tremendous advantage for you, but you still must thoroughly research the job market in your geographical area before committing to your first job (**Figure 30–1**). If you make the right choice, your career will be on the road to success. If you make the wrong choice, it will not be a tragedy, but it may cause unnecessary delay.

WHY STUDY HOW TO PREPARE FOR AND SEEK EMPLOYMENT?

Cosmetologists should study and have a thorough understanding of how to prepare for and seek employment because:

- You must pass your State Board Exam to be licensed and you must be licensed to be hired; therefore, preparing for licensure and passing your exam is your first step to employment success.
- A successful employment search is a job in itself, and there are many tools that can give you the edge—as well as mistakes that can cost you an interview or a job.
- The ability to pinpoint the right salon for you and target it as a potential employer is vital for your career success.
- Proactively preparing the right materials, such as a great resume, and practicing interviewing will give you the confidence that's needed to secure a job in a salon you love.

Preparing for Licensure

Before you can obtain the career position you are hoping for, you must pass your state licensing examinations (usually a written and a practical exam) and secure the required credentials from your state's licensing board by filling out an application and paying a fee. For details on fees, testing dates, requirements, and more, visit the Web site of your State Board of Cosmetology or your state's department of licensing.

Many factors will affect how well you perform during that licensing examination and on tests in general. They include your physical and psychological state; your memory; your time management skills; and your academic skills, such as reading, writing, note taking, test taking, and general learning.

Of all the factors that will affect your test performance, the most important is your mastery of course content. However, even if you feel that you have truly learned the material, it is still very beneficial to have strong test-taking skills. Being **test-wise** means understanding the strategies for successfully taking tests.

did you know?

If you have a physician-documented disability, such as a learning disability, your state may allow you extra time to take the written exam, or even provide a special examiner. Ask your instructor and check with your state licensing board. Be certain to make any special arrangements well in advance of the test date.

Preparing for the Written Exam

A test-wise student begins to prepare for a test by practicing good study habits and time management. These habits include the following:

- Having a planned, realistic study schedule
- Reading content carefully and becoming an active studier
- Keeping a well-organized notebook
- Developing a detailed vocabulary list
- Taking effective notes during class
- Organizing and reviewing handouts
- Reviewing past quizzes and tests
- Listening carefully in class for cues and clues about what could be expected on the test

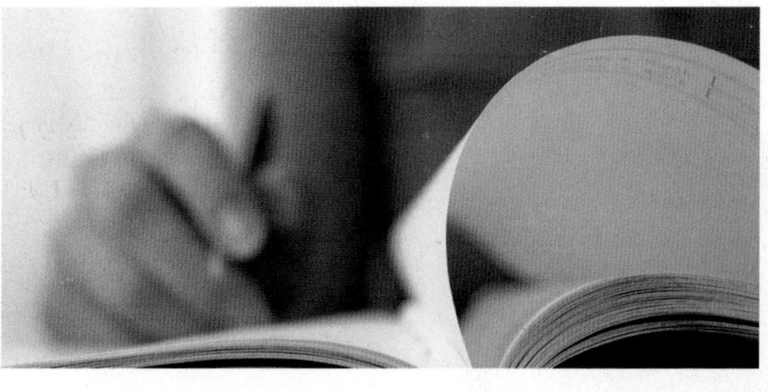

© Petro Feketa, 2010; used under license from Shutterstock.com.

More holistic or "whole you" hints to keep in mind include the following:

- Make yourself mentally ready and develop a positive attitude toward taking the test.
- Get plenty of rest the night before the test.
- Dress comfortably.
- Anticipate some anxiety (feeling concerned about the test results may actually help you do better).
- Avoid cramming the night before an examination.
- Find out if your state uses computers for the written portion of the test. If so, make certain you are comfortable with computerized test taking.

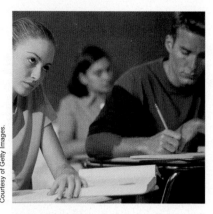
Courtesy of Getty Images.

▲ Figure 30–2
Candidates taking an in-house school exam.

On Test Day

After you have taken all the necessary steps to prepare for your test, there are a number of strategies you can adopt on the day of the exam that may be helpful (**Figure 30–2**):

- Relax and try to slow down physically.
- If possible, review the material lightly the day of the exam.
- Arrive early with a self-confident attitude; be alert, calm, and ready for the challenge.
- Read all written directions and listen carefully to all verbal directions before beginning.
- If there are things you do not understand, do not hesitate to ask the examiner questions.
- Skim the entire test before beginning.
- Budget your time to ensure that you have plenty of opportunity to complete the test; do not spend too much time on any one question.
- Wear a watch so that you can monitor the time.
- Begin work as soon as possible, and mark the answers in the test booklet carefully but quickly.
- Answer the easiest questions first in order to save time for the more difficult ones. Quickly scanning all the questions first may clue you in to the more difficult questions.
- Mark the questions you skip so that you can find them again later.
- Read each question carefully to make sure that you know exactly what the question is asking and that you understand all parts of the question.
- Answer as many questions as possible. For questions that cause uncertainty, guess or estimate.
- Look over the test when you are done to ensure that you have read all questions correctly and that you have answered as many as possible.
- Make changes to answers only if there is a good reason to do so.
- Check the test booklet carefully before turning it in. (For instance, you might have forgotten to put your name on it!)

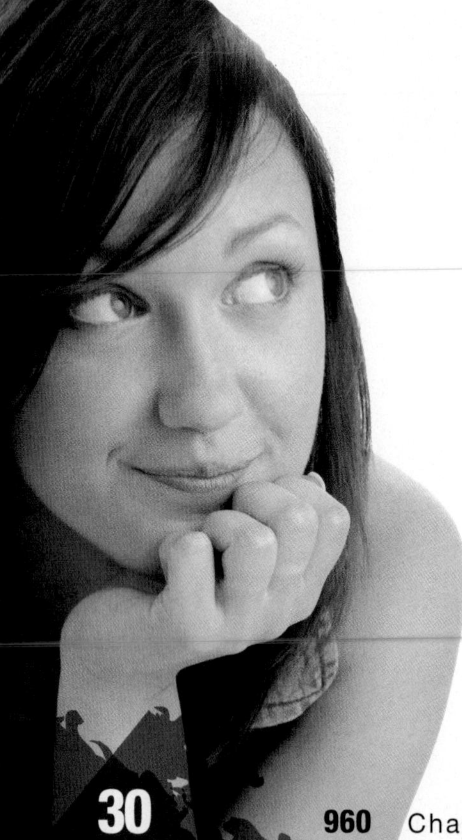

Deductive Reasoning

Deductive reasoning is the process of reaching logical conclusions by employing logical reasoning. Deductive reasoning is a technique that students should learn to use for better test results.

Some strategies associated with deductive reasoning include the following:

- Eliminate options known to be incorrect. The more incorrect answers you can eliminate, the better your chances of identifying the correct answer.

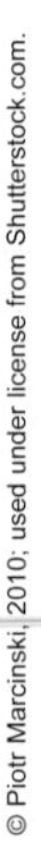
© Piotr Marcinski, 2010; used under license from Shutterstock.com.

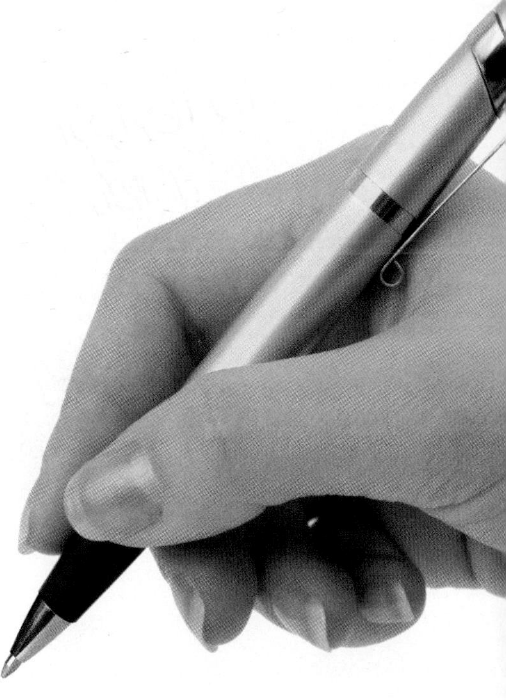

© Tatiana Popova, 2010; used under license from Shutterstock.com.

- Watch for key words or terms. Look for any qualifying conditions or statements. Keep an eye out for phrases and words such as *usually, commonly, in most instances, never,* and *always*.
- Study the **stem**, which is the basic question or problem. It will often provide a clue to the correct answer. Look for a match between the stem and one of the choices.
- Watch for grammatical clues. For instance, if the last word in a stem is *an,* the answer must begin with a vowel rather than a consonant.
- Look at similar or related questions. They may provide clues.
- When answering essay questions, watch for words such as *compare, contrast, discuss, evaluate, analyze, define,* or *describe* and develop your answer accordingly.
- When questions include paragraphs to read and questions to answer, read the questions first. This will help you identify the important information as you read the paragraph.

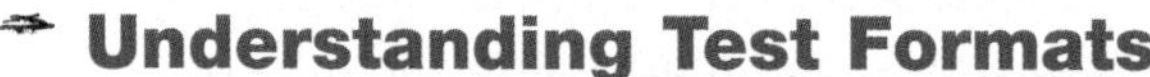

Understanding Test Formats

There are a few additional tips that all test-wise learners should know, especially with respect to the state licensing examination. Keep in mind, of course, that the most important strategy of test taking is to know your material. Beyond that, consider the following tips on the various types of question formats.

True/False

- Watch for qualifying words (*all, most, some, none, always, usually, sometimes, never, little, no, equal, less, good, bad*). Absolutes (*all, none, always, never*) are generally not true.
- For a statement to be true, the *entire* statement must be true.
- Long statements are more likely to be true than short statements. It takes more detail to provide truthful, factual information.

Multiple Choice

- Read the entire question carefully, including all the choices.
- Look for the best answer; more than one choice may be true.
- Eliminate incorrect answers by crossing them out (if taking the test on the test form).
- When two choices are close or similar, one of them is probably right.
- When two choices are identical, both must be wrong.
- When two choices are opposites, one is probably wrong and one is probably correct, depending on the number of other choices.
- "All of the above" and similar responses are often the correct choice.
- Pay special attention to words such as *not, except*, and *but.*

- Guess if you do not know the answer (provided that there is no penalty).
- The answer to one question may be in the stem of another.

Matching

- Read all items in each list before beginning.
- Check off items from the brief response list to eliminate choices.

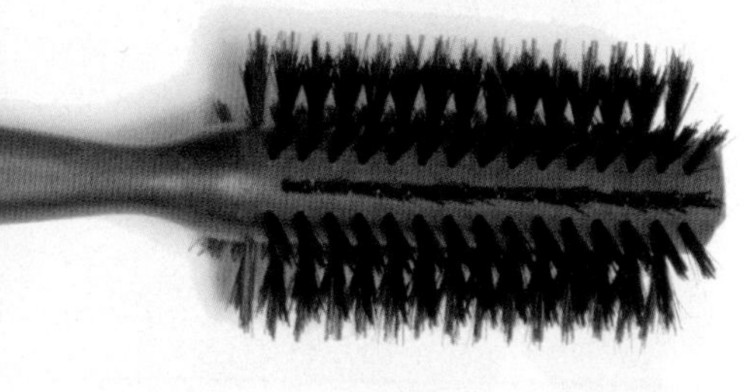

Essays

- Organize your answer according to the cue words in the question.
- Think carefully and outline your answer before you begin writing.
- Make sure that what you write is complete, accurate, relevant to the question, well organized, and clear.

Remember that even though you may understand test formats and effective test-taking strategies, this does not take the place of having a complete understanding of the material on which you are being tested. In order to be successful at taking tests, you must follow the rules of effective studying and be thoroughly knowledgeable of the exam content for both the written and the practical examination.

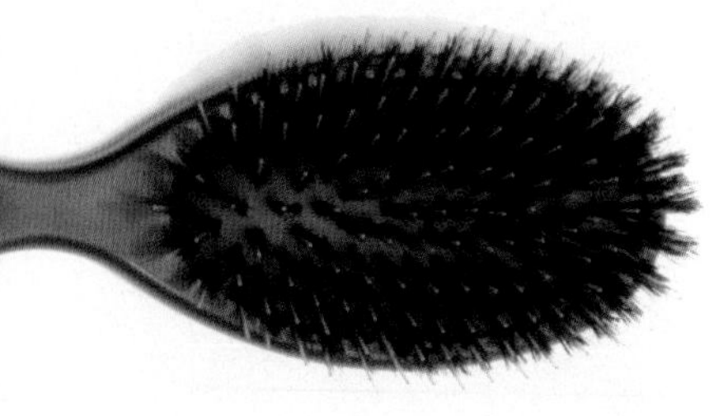

The Practical Exam

In order to be better prepared for the practical portion of the examination, the new graduate should follow these tips:

- Practice the correct skills required in the test as often as you can.
- Participate in mock licensing examinations, including the timing of applicable examination criteria.
- Familiarize yourself with the content contained in the examination bulletins sent by the licensing agency.
- Make a list of equipment and implements you are expected to bring to the examination.
- Make certain that all equipment and implements are clean and in good working order prior to the exam.
- If allowed by the regulatory or licensing agency, observe other practical examinations prior to taking yours.
- If possible, locate the examination site the day before the exam to ensure that you do not get lost on test day. You can also time your drive the day before, just to make sure you are on time for the actual exam.
- As with any exam, listen carefully to the examiner's instructions and follow them explicitly.
- Focus on your own knowledge and do not allow yourself to be concerned with what other test candidates are doing.

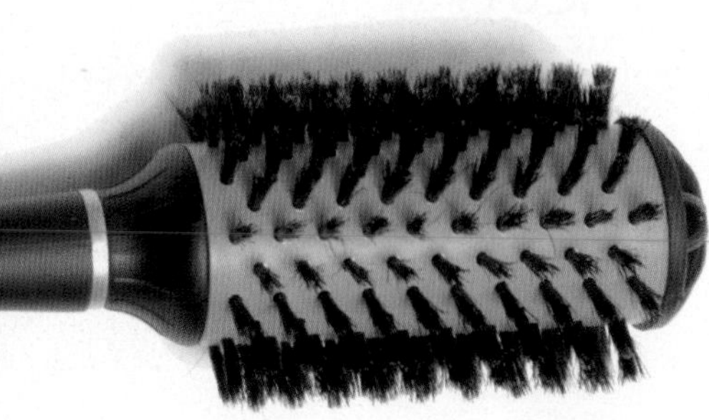

© Milady, a part of Cengage Learning.

- Follow all infection control and safety procedures throughout the entire examination.
- Look the part. Every little bit helps; make certain your appearance is neat, clean, and professional. ✓ LO1

Preparing for Employment

When you chose to enter the field of cosmetology, your primary goal was to find a good job after being licensed. Now you need to reaffirm that goal by reviewing a number of important questions.

- What do you really want out of a career in cosmetology?
- What particular areas within the beauty industry are the most interesting to you?
- What are your strongest practical skills? In what ways do you wish to use these skills?
- What personal qualities will help you have a successful career?

One way that you can answer these questions is to copy and complete the Inventory of Personal Characteristics and Technical Skills (**Figure 30–3**) on the next page. After you have completed this inventory and identified the areas that need further attention, you can determine where to focus the remainder of your training. In addition, you should have a better idea of what type of establishment would best suit you for your eventual employment. ✓ LO2

During your training, you may have the opportunity to network with various industry professionals who are invited to the school as guest speakers. Be prepared to ask them questions about what they like least and most in their current positions. Ask them for any tips they might have that will assist you in your search for the right salon. In addition, be sure to take advantage of your institution's in-house placement assistance program when you begin your employment search (**Figure 30–4**).

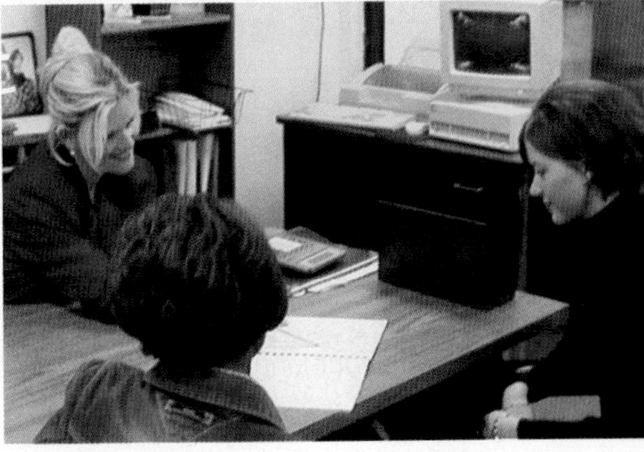

Courtesy of Jerry Kelon Carter, CC's Cosmetology College, Tulsa, OK.

▲ Figure 30–4
Your school advisor can help you find employment.

Your willingness to work hard is a key ingredient to your success. The commitment you make now in terms of time and effort will pay off later in the workplace, where your energy will be appreciated and rewarded. Having enthusiasm for getting the job done can be contagious, and when everyone works hard, everyone benefits. You can begin to develop this enthusiasm by establishing good work habits as a student.

How to Get the Job You Want

There are several key personal characteristics that will not only help you get the position you want, but will also help you keep it. These characteristics include the points listed below:

- **Motivation.** This means having the drive to take the necessary action to achieve a goal. Although motivation can come from external

INVENTORY OF PERSONAL CHARACTERISTICS

PERSONAL CHARACTERISTIC	Exc.	Good	Avg.	Poor	Plan for Improvement
Posture, Deportment, Poise					
Grooming, Personal Hygiene					
Manners, Courtesy					
Communications Skills					
Attitude					
Self-Motivation					
Personal Habits					
Responsibility					
Self-esteem, Self-confidence					
Honesty, Integrity					
Dependability					

INVENTORY OF TECHNICAL SKILLS

TECHNICAL SKILL	Exc.	Good	Avg.	Poor	Plan for Improvement
Hair Shaping/Cutting					
Hairstyling					
Haircoloring					
Texture Services, Perming					
Texture Services, Relaxing					
Manicuring, Pedicuring					
Artificial Nail Extensions					
Skin Care, Facials					
Facial Makeup					
Other					

After analyzing the above responses, would you hire yourself as an employee in your firm? Why or why not?
State your short-term goals that you hope to accomplish in 6 to 12 months:
State your long-term goals that you hope to accomplish in 1 to 5 years:

Ask yourself: Do you want to work in a big city or small town? Are you compatible with a sophisticated, exclusive salon or a trendy salon? Which clientele are you able to communicate with more effectively? Do you want to start out slowly and carefully or do you want to jump in and throw everything into your career from the starting gate? Will you be in this industry throughout your working career or is this just a stopover? Will you only work a 30- or 40- hour week or will you go the extra mile when opportunities are available? How ambitious are you and how many risks are you willing to take?

© Milady, a part of Cengage Learning.

▲ Figure 30–3
Inventory of personal characteristics and technical skills.

ACTivity

For one week, keep a daily record of your performance in the following areas, and ask a few of your fellow students to provide feedback as well.

- Positive attitude
- Punctuality
- Diligent practice of newly learned techniques
- Teamwork
- Professional appearance
- Regular class and clinic attendance
- Interpersonal skills
- Helping others

sources—parental or peer pressure, for instance—the best kind of motivation is internal.

- **Integrity.** When you have integrity, you are committed to a strong code of moral and artistic values. Integrity is the compass that keeps you on course over the long haul of your career.
- **Good technical and communication skills.** While you may be better in either technical skills or communication skills, you must develop both to reach the level of success you desire.
- **Strong work ethic.** In the beauty business, having a strong **work ethic** means taking pride in your work and committing yourself to consistently doing a good job for your clients, employer, and salon team.
- **Enthusiasm.** Try never to lose your eagerness to learn, grow, and expand your skills and knowledge.

A Salon Survey

According to the most recently compiled data as of this printing, there are nearly 370,210 professional salon establishments in the United States alone. These salons employed more than 1,682,641 active cosmetology professionals. (To check for updates, go to http://www.naccas.org.) This year, like every year, thousands of cosmetology school graduates will find their first position in one of the eight basic types of salons described below. As you research salons, focus on the type of salon that you believe will be the best fit for you.

Small Independent Salons

Owned by an individual or two or more partners, this kind of operation makes up the majority of professional salons (**Figure 30–5**). The typical independent salon has 5.1 styling stations, but many salons have up to 40. Usually, the owners are hairstylists who maintain their own clientele while managing the business. There are nearly as many types of independent salons as there are owners. Their image, decor, services, prices, and clientele all reflect

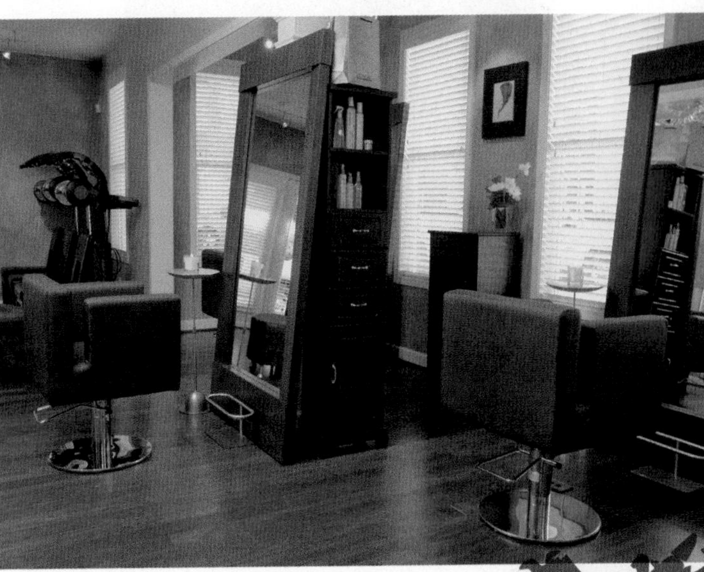

▼ **Figure 30–5**
Perfect 5th, in Mooresville, NC, is an independent salon.

Courtesy of Diane Hughes Photography.

the owner's experience and taste. Depending on the owner's willingness to help a newcomer learn and grow, a beginning stylist can learn a great deal in an independent salon while also earning a good living.

Independent Salon Chains

These are usually chains of five or more salons that are owned by one individual or two or more partners. Independent salon chains range from basic hair salons to full-service salons and day spas. These salons offer everything from low-priced to very high-priced services.

In large high-end salons, stylists can advance to specialized positions in color, nail care, skin care, or other chemical services. Some larger salons also employ education directors and style directors, and stylists are often hired to manage particular locations.

Large National Salon Chains

These companies operate salons throughout the country, and even internationally. They can be budget-priced or value-priced, haircut-only or full service, mid-priced or high-end. Some salon chains operate within department store chains. Management and marketing professionals at the corporate headquarters make all the decisions for each salon, such as size, decor, hours, services, prices, advertising, and profit targets. Many newly licensed cosmetology professionals seek their first jobs in national chain salons because of the secure pay and benefits, additional paid training, management opportunities, and corporate advertising. Also, because the chains are large and widespread, employees have the added advantage of being able to transfer from one location to another.

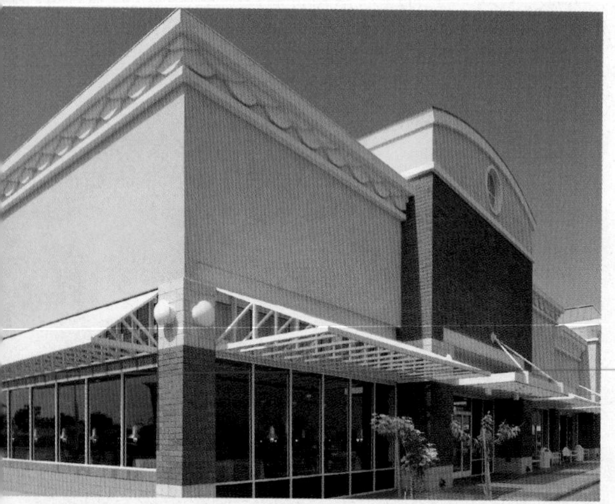

Franchise Salons

Another chain salon organization, the franchise salon has a national name and a consistent image and business formula that is used at every location. Franchises are owned by individuals who pay a fee to use the name; these individuals then receive a business plan and can take advantage of national marketing campaigns. Decisions such as size, location, decor, and prices are determined in advance by the parent company. Franchises are generally not owned by cosmetologists, but by investors who seek a return on their investment.

Franchise salons commonly offer employees the same benefits as corporate-owned chain salons, including on-the-job training, health-care benefits and advancement opportunities.

© Anton Foltin, 2010; used under license from Shutterstock.com.

Basic Value-Priced Operations

Often located in busy, low-rent shopping center strips that are anchored by a nearby supermarket or other large business, value-priced outlets depend on a high volume of walk-in traffic. They hire recent cosmetology graduates and generally pay them by the hour, sometimes adding commission-style bonuses if an individual stylist's sales pass a certain level. Haircuts are usually reasonably priced and stylists are trained to work fast with no frills.

Mid-Priced Full-Service Salons

These salons offer a complete menu of hair, nail, and skin services along with retail products. Successful mid-priced salons promote their most profitable services and typically offer service and retail packages to entice haircut-only clients. They also run strong marketing programs to encourage client returns and referrals. These salons train their professional styling team to be as productive and profitable as possible. If you are inclined to give more time to each client during the consultation, you may like working in a full-service salon. Here you will have the opportunity to build a relationship with clients that may last over time.

High-End Image Salons or Day Spas

This type of business employs well-trained stylists and salon assistants who offer higher-priced services to clients. They also offer luxurious extras such as five-minute head, neck, and shoulder massages as part of the shampoo and luxurious spa manicures and pedicures. Most high-end salons are located in trendy, upscale sections of large cities; others may be located in elegant mansions, high-rent office and retail towers, or luxury hotels and resorts. Clients expect a high level of personal service, and such salons hire professionals whose technical expertise, personal appearance, and communication skills meet their high standards. Medical spas, often owned by physicians, are offshoots of day spas (**Figure 30–6**).

Booth Rental Establishments

Booth renting (also called chair rental) is possibly the least expensive way of owning your own business, but this type of business is regulated by complex laws. For a detailed discussion of booth rental see Chapter 32, The Salon Business. ☑ LO3

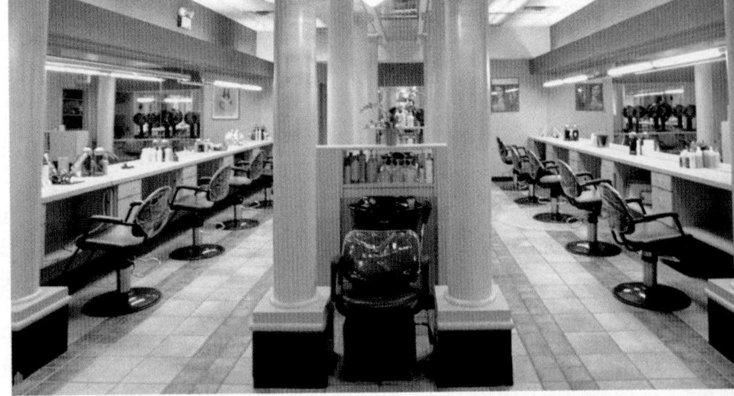

Courtesy of Tom Stock.

▲ Figure 30–6
A high-end salon.

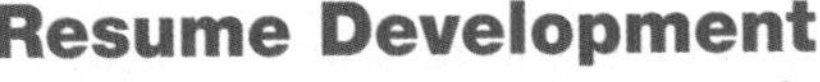

Resume Development

A **resume** is a written summary of a person's education and work experience. It tells potential employers at a glance what your achievements and accomplishments are. If you are a new graduate, you may have little or no work experience, in which case, your resume should focus on skills and accomplishments. Here are some basic guidelines to follow when preparing your professional resume.

- Keep it simple, limit it to one page.
- Print a hard copy from your electronic version, using good-quality paper.
- Include your name, address, phone number, and e-mail address on both the resume and your cover letter.
- List recent, relevant work experience.

- List relevant education and the name of the institution from which you graduated, as well as relevant courses attended.
- List your professional skills and accomplishments.
- Focus on information that is relevant to the position you are seeking.

The average time that a potential employer will spend scanning your resume before deciding whether to grant you an interview is about twenty seconds. That means you must market yourself in such a manner that the reader will want to meet you. If your work experience has been in an unrelated field, show how the position helped you develop transferable skills. Restaurant work, for example, helps employees develop customer-service skills and learn to deal with a wide variety of customers.

As you list former and current positions on your resume, focus on achievements instead of detailing duties and responsibilities. Accomplishment statements enlarge your basic duties and responsibilities. The best way to show concrete accomplishment is to include numbers or percentages whenever possible. As you describe former and current positions on your resume, ask yourself the following questions:

- How many regular clients did I serve?
- How many clients did I serve weekly?
- What was my service ticket average?
- What was my client retention rate?
- What percentage of my client revenue came from retailing?
- What percentage of my client revenue came from color or texture services?

If you cannot express your accomplishment numerically, can you address which problems you solved or other results you achieved? For instance, did your office job help you develop excellent organizational skills?

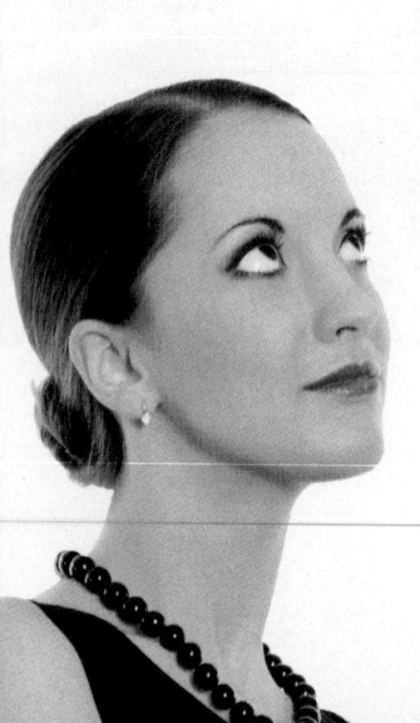

This type of questioning can help you develop accomplishment statements that will interest a potential employer. There is no better time for you to achieve significant accomplishments than while you are in school. Even though your experience may be minimal, you must still present evidence of your skills and accomplishments. This may seem a difficult task at this early stage in your working career, but by closely examining your training and school clinic performance, extracurricular activities, and the full- or part-time jobs you have held, you should be able to create a good, attention-getting resume.

For example, consider the following questions:

- Did you receive any honors during your course of training?
- Were you ever selected "student of the month"?
- Did you receive special recognition for your attendance or academic progress?
- Did you win any cosmetology-related competitions while in school?

© Olga Sapegina, 2010; used under license from Shutterstock.com.

- What was your attendance average while in school?
- Did you work with the student body to organize any fundraisers? What were the results?

Answers to these types of questions may indicate your people skills, personal work habits, and personal commitment to success (**Figure 30–7**).

Since you have not yet completed your training, you still have the opportunity to make some of the examples listed above become a reality before you graduate. Positive developments of this nature while you are still in school can do much to improve your resume.

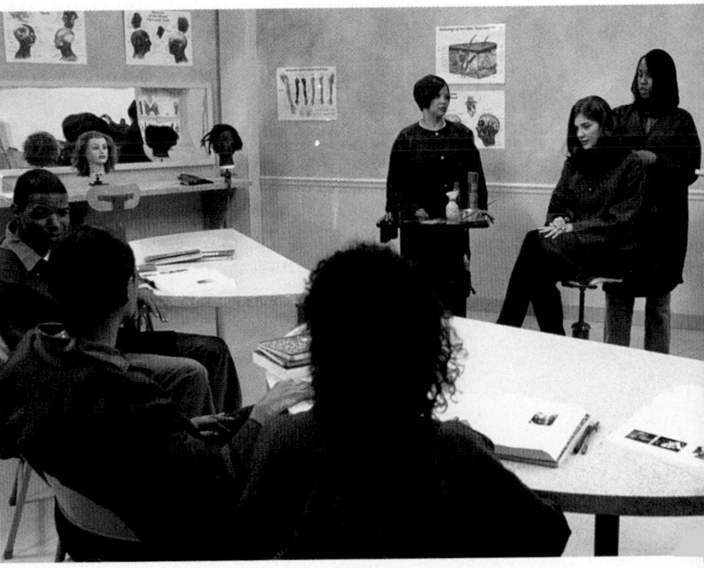

Courtesy of Ed Hille.

▲ Figure 30–7
Excelling in school can help you build a good resume.

The Do's and Don'ts of Resumes

You will save yourself from many problems and a lot of disappointment right from the beginning of your job search if you keep a clear idea in your mind of what to do and what not to do when it comes to creating a resume. Here are some of the do's:

- **Always put your complete contact information on your resume.** If your cell phone is your primary phone, list its number first, and add a backup number.
- **Make it easy to read.** Use concise, clear sentences and avoid overwriting or flowery language.
- **Know your audience.** Use vocabulary and language that will be understood by your potential employer.
- **Keep it short.** One page is preferable.
- **Stress accomplishments.** Emphasize past accomplishments and the skills you used to achieve them.
- **Focus on career goals.** Highlight information that is relevant to your career goals and the position you are seeking.
- **Emphasize transferable skills.** The skills mastered at other jobs that can be put to use in a new position are **transferable skills**.
- **Use action verbs.** Begin accomplishment statements with action verbs such as *achieved, coordinated, developed, increased, maintained,* and *strengthened.*
- **Make it neat.** A poorly structured, badly typed resume does not reflect well on you.
- **Include professional references.** Use only professional references on your resume and make sure you give potential employers the person's title, place of employment, and telephone number.
- **Be realistic.** Remember that you are just starting out in a field that you hope will be a wonderful and fulfilling experience. Be realistic about what employers may offer to beginners.

- **Always include a cover letter.** See **Figure 30-16**, on page 976, for an example of one, which assumes you have targeted and visited salons in advance, as advised in this chapter.
- **Note any skills with new technologies.** Include software programs, web development tools, and computerized salon management systems.

Here are some of the don'ts for resume writing:

- **Avoid salary references.** Don't state your salary history.
- **Avoid information about why you left former positions.**
- **Don't stretch the truth.** Misinformation or untruthful statements usually catch up with you.

If you don't feel comfortable writing your own resume, consider seeking a professional resume writer or a job coach. There may be employment agencies that can help you as well; many online job-search Web sites offer easy-to-use resume templates.

Review **Figure 30–8**, on page 971, which represents an achievement-oriented resume for a recent graduate of a cosmetology course. Remember that you are a total package, not just a resume. With determination, you will find the right position to begin your cosmetology career. Utilize all available resources during your resume development and job search process. For example, there is an abundance of best practice information available on the Internet, or you can communicate with an individual you may already know who has gone through the hiring process and can provide recommendations. Milady also has fantastic resources that can provide you with additional assistance when you begin your job search. One such Milady online resource to help with resume development and overall job search success is Milady's *Beauty & Wellness Career Transitions*.

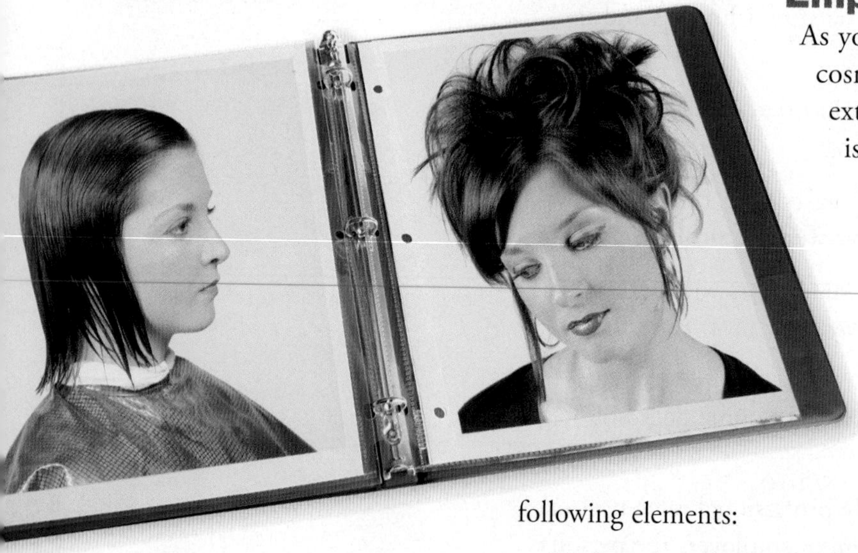

▼ Figure 30–9
Before-and-after photos in an employment portfolio.

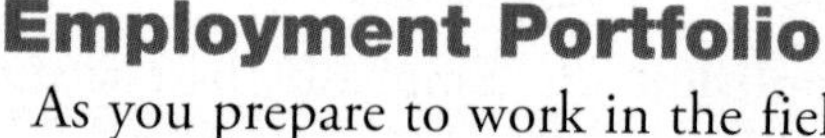

© Milady, a part of Cengage Learning. Photography by Yanik Chauvin.

Employment Portfolio

As you prepare to work in the field of cosmetology, an employment portfolio can be extremely useful. An **employment portfolio** is a collection, usually bound, of photos and documents that reflect your skills, accomplishments, and abilities in your chosen career field (**Figure 30–9**).

While the actual contents of the portfolio will vary from graduate to graduate, there are certain items that have a place in any portfolio.

A powerful portfolio includes the following elements:

- Diplomas, including high school and cosmetology school
- Awards and achievements received while a cosmetology student
- Current resume, focusing on accomplishments

MARY CURL

143 Fern Circle • Anytown, USA 12345 • (123) 555-1234 • Marycurl@gmail.com

Qualifications

- Creative, energetic, and devoted to the cosmetology industry.
- Hold current Arizona license and have strong knowledge of trends.
- Certified image consultant with a history of success.
- An insatiable appetite for industry knowledge, which helped me earn an "A" average throughout my cosmetology training.

Professional Experience

Salon Etc., Spring, 2009

Student Extern: Trained one day weekly for ten weeks in all phases of cosmetology, through state-approved Student Externship Program.

Macy's, Summer, 2008

Retail Sales: Increased the store's retail sales of cosmetics by over 18 percent during part-time employment.

Professional Skills and Achievements

Creative

- Won student contest for best makeover.
- Developed an outstanding digital portfolio of photos, showing cut, color, and style makeovers.

Sales

- Increased chemical services to 30 percent of my clinic volume by graduation.
- Named "Student of the Month" for best attendance, best attitude, highest retail sales, and most clients served.

Client Retention

- Developed and retained a school–clinic client base of over 75 individuals of all ages, both male and female.

Image Consulting

- As a certified Image Consultant, created makeovers for 20 school–clinic clients.
- Advised school–clinic clients on cosmetics and wardrobe, in addition to new cuts and haircolor. All clients were extremely happy with their new looks.

Administration

- Supervised a student "salon team" that developed a business plan for opening a twelve-chair, full-service salon. This project earned an "A" and was recognized for thoroughness, accuracy, and creativity.
- As president of the student council, organized fund-raising activities that funded 19 student trips to a regional hair show.
- Reorganized school facial room for greater efficiency and client comfort.
- Organized the school dispensary, allowing for increased inventory control and the streamlining of clinic operations.

Computers

- Internet savvy with abilities in MS Word, Excel, and PowerPoint.
- Created personal Facebook page, which brought eight new clients into the school clinic.

Education

New Alamo High School, 2008

Milady Career Institute of Cosmetology, August 2009

- Achieved an "A" average in theoretical requirements.
- Achieved "Excellent" ratings in practical requirements.
- Exceeded the number of practical skills required for graduation.

License and Certification

- Licensed as Cosmetologist by the State of Arizona, September, 2009.
- Certified Image Consultant, American Association of Image Consultants, 2009.

References

Available upon request.

© Milady, a part of Cengage Learning.

▲ Figure 30–8

A resume for those with little work experience focuses on achievements.

- Letters of reference from former employers
- Summary of continuing education and/or copies of training certificates
- Statement of membership in industry and other professional organizations
- Statement of relevant civic affiliations and/or community activities
- Before-and-after photographs of services that you have performed on clients or models
- Brief statement about why you have chosen a career in cosmetology
- Any other information that you regard as relevant

Once you have assembled your portfolio, ask yourself whether it accurately portrays you and your career skills. If it does not, identify what needs to be changed. If you are not sure, run it by a neutral party for feedback about how to make it more interesting and accurate. This kind of feedback is also useful when creating a resume. The portfolio, like the resume, should be prepared in a way that projects professionalism.

- For ease of use, you may want to separate sections with tabs.
- If you are technologically savvy, you might want to create a digital portfolio or an online showcase of your work. However, don't expect potential employers to take the extra time to visit a Web site or view a DVD. Bring along a printed copy of everything you want the employer to see.

When you write the statement about why you chose a career in cosmetology, you might include the following elements:

- A statement that explains what you love about your new career
- A description about the importance of teamwork and how you see yourself as a contributing team member
- A description of methods and ideas you would use to increase service and retail revenue (**Figure 30–10**) ✓ **LO4**

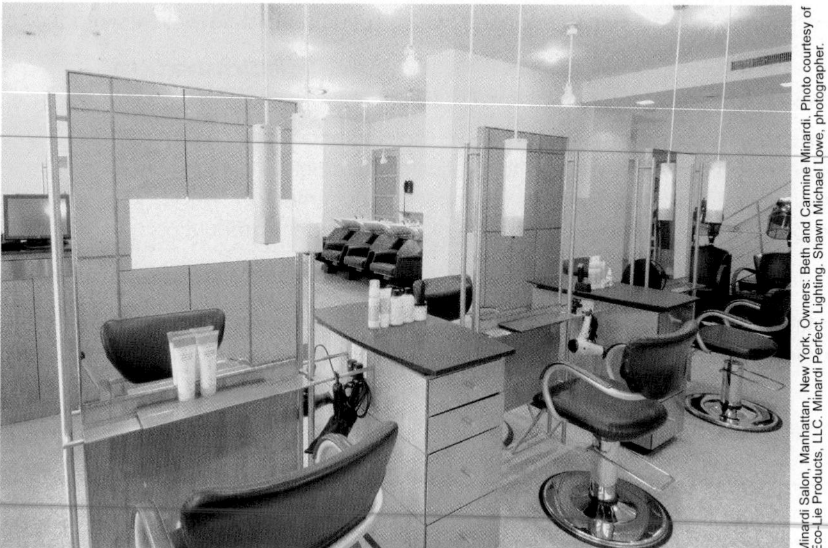

▶ Figure 30–10
Wanna-be colorists should target haircolor specialty salons like Minardi Salon in New York City, which uses Minardi Color Perfect Lighting.

Minardi Salon, Manhattan, New York, Owners: Beth and Carmine Minardi. Photo courtesy of Eco-Lie Products, LLC. Minardi Perfect, Lighting. Shawn Michael Lowe, photographer.

Targeting the Establishment

One of the most important steps in the process of job hunting is narrowing your search. Listed below are some points to keep in mind when targeting potential employers.

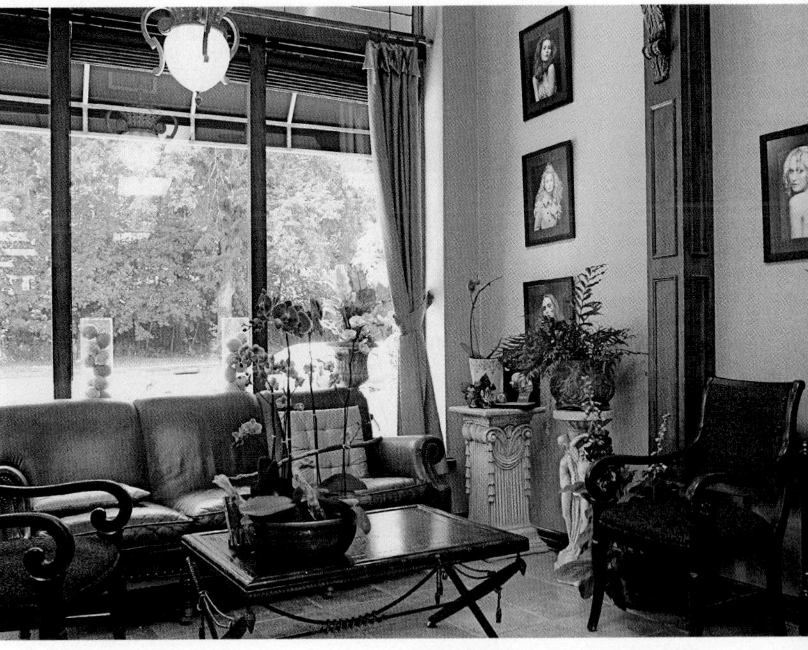

Photo by Michael Watson.

▲ **Figure 30–11**
Independent salons, like Salvatore Minardi in Madison, NJ, reflect the owner's taste, which give you clues as to whether or not you'll fit in.

- Accept that your first job will probably not be your dream job. Few people are so fortunate.
- Do not wait until graduation to begin your search. If you do, you may be tempted to take the first offer you receive, instead of carefully investigating all possibilities before making a decision.
- Locate a salon that serves the type of clients you wish to serve. Finding a good fit with the clients and staff is critical from the outset of your career (**Figure 30–11**).
- Make a list of area salons or spas. The Internet will be your best source for this. If you are considering relocating to another area, go to http://www.anywho.com for a complete listing of businesses in every state, or find top salons in any region or city at http://www.CitySearch.com. You may also want to search at http://www.google.com for your area of interest and city, using key words such as *haircolor salon Portland.*
- Watch for salons that advertise locally, to get a feel for the market each salon is targeting. Then check the salon's Web site or see if it is part of a social network, such as Facebook.
- Check out Web sites and social networking sites for various types of salons. If you contact them, don't waste their time. Get right to the point that you are a student, and ask specific questions about the profession.
- Keep the salon's culture in mind. Do the stylists dress like you? Are the clients in different age groups or just one? Look for the salon that will be best for you and your goals.

Field Research

A great way to find out about potential jobs is to network. Actually get out there, visit salons, and talk to salon owners, managers, educators, and stylists. Whether your first contact is online, in person, or on the phone, sooner or later you'll want to arrange a face-to-face meeting or an exploratory visit to the salon. To set up a salon visit, consider the following:

- If you call, use your best telephone manner; speak with confidence and self-assurance. If you e-mail, be brief, and check spelling and punctuation. Do not text message salon owners or managers, unless they request that you do so.

- Explain that you are preparing to graduate from school in cosmetology, that you are researching the market for potential positions, and that you have a few quick questions.
- If the person is receptive, ask whether the salon is in need of any new stylists, and how many the salon currently employs.
- Ask if you can make an appointment to visit the salon to observe sometime during the next few weeks. If the salon representative is agreeable, be on time! When timing allows, confirm the appointment the day before, via e-mail (**Figure 30–12**).

WEB RESOURCES

To start looking for a cosmetology job, begin at these Web sites:

Industry specific:
http://www.americansalonmag.com
http://www.behindthechair.com
http://www.modernsalon.com
http://www.salonemployment.com
http://www.salongigs.com
http://www.spaandsalonjobs.com
http://www.spawire.com

General:
http://www.careerbuilder.com
http://www.careerfinder.com
http://www.craigslist.org
http://www.jobbank.com
http://www.jobs.net
http://www.monster.com
http://www.snagajob.com

Remember that a rejection is not a negative reflection on you. Many professionals are too busy to make time for this kind of networking. The good news is that you are bound to discover many genuinely kind people who remember what it was like when they started out and who are willing to devote a bit of their time to help others who are beginning their careers.

The Salon Visit

When you visit the salon, take along a checklist to ensure that you observe all the key areas that might ultimately affect your decision making. The checklist will be similar to the one used for field trips that you probably have taken to area salons while in school. Keep the checklist on file for future reference, so that you can make informed comparisons among establishments (**Figure 30–13**).

After your visit, always remember to follow up, thanking the salon representative for his or her time (**Figure 30–14**). Do this even if you did not like the salon and would never consider working there (**Figure 30–15**).

Never burn your bridges. Instead, build a network of contacts who have a favorable opinion of you.

The Job Interview

After you have graduated and completed the first two steps in the process of securing employment—targeting and observing salons—you are ready to pursue employment in earnest. The next step is to contact the establishments that you are most interested in by sending

▶ Figure 30–12
Sample appointment confirmation.

Dear Ms. (or Mr.)________________________

Just a quick reminder that I'll be visiting your salon this Friday, June 12th, at 2:00 PM. I am looking forward to meeting with you, and I am eager to observe your salon and staff at work. If you should need to reach me before that time for any reason, please call me at ______________, e-mail me at ______________, or text me at ______________.

Sincerely,
(Your name)

© Milady, a part of Cengage Learning.

SALON VISIT CHECKLIST

When you visit a salon, observe the following areas and rate them from 1 to 5, with 5 considered being the best.

_____ **SALON IMAGE:** Is the salon's image consistent and appropriate for your interests? Is the image pleasing and inviting? What is the decor and arrangement? If you are not comfortable or if you find it unattractiive, mark the salon off your list of employment possibilities.

_____ **PROFESSIONALISM:** Do the employees present the appropriate professional appearance and behavior? Do they give their clients the appropriate levels of attention and personal service or do they act as if work is their time to socialize?

_____ **MANAGEMENT:** Does the salon show signs of being well managed? Is the phone answered promptly with professional telephone skills? Is the mood of the salon positive? Does everyone appear to work as a team?

_____ **CLIENT SERVICE:** Are clients greeted promptly and warmly when they enter the salon? Are they kept informed of the status of their appointment? Are they offered a magazine or beverage while they wait? Is there a comfortable reception area? Are there changing rooms, attractive smocks?

_____ **PRICES:** Compare price for value. Are clients getting their money's worth? Do they pay the same price in one salon but get better service and attention in another? If possible, take home salon brochures and price lists.

_____ **RETAIL:** Is there a well-stocked retail display offering clients a variety of product lines and a range of prices? Do the stylists and receptionist (if applicable) promote retail sales?

_____ **IN-SALON MARKETING:** Are there posters or promotions throughout the salon? If so, are they professionally made and do they reflect contemporary styles?

_____ **SERVICES:** Make a list of all services offered by each salon and the product lines they carry. This will help you decide what earning potential stylists have in each salon.

SALON NAME: ____

SALON MANAGER: ____

▲ **Figure 30–13**
Salon-visit checklist.

Dear Ms. (or Mr.) ______________________,

I appreciate having had the opportunity to observe your salon/spa in operation last Friday. Thank you for the time you and your staff gave me. I was impressed by the efficient and courteous manner in which your stylists served their clients. The atmosphere was pleasant and the mood was positive. Should you ever have an opening for a professional with my skills and training, I would welcome the opportunity to apply. You can contact me at the address and phone number listed below. I hope we will meet again soon.

Sincerely,

(your name, address, telephone)

◀ **Figure 30–14**
Sample thank-you note.

© Milady, a part of Cengage Learning.

▶ Figure 30–15
Thank-you note to a salon at which you do not expect to seek employment.

Dear Ms. (or Mr.) ____________________,

I appreciate having had the opportunity to observe your salon in operation last Friday. I know how busy you and all your staff are, and want to thank you for the time that you gave me. I hope my presence didn't interfere with the flow of your operations too much. I certainly appreciate the courtesies that were extended to me by you and your staff. I wish you and your salon continued success.

Sincerely,
(your name)

▶ Figure 30–16
Sample resume cover letter.

Your Name
Your Address
Your Phone Number

Ms. (or Mr.) ____________________,
Salon Name
Salon Address

Dear Ms. (or Mr.) ____________________,

We met in August when you allowed me to observe your salon and staff while I was still in cosmetology training. Since that time, I have graduated and have received my license. I have enclosed my resume for your review and consideration.

I would very much appreciate the opportunity to meet with you and discuss either current or future career opportunities at your salon. I was extremely impressed with your staff and business, and I would like to share with you how my skills and training might add to your salon's success.

I will call you next week to discuss a time that is convenient for us to meet. I look forward to meeting with you again soon.

Sincerely,
(your name)

© Milady, a part of Cengage Learning.

them a resume and requesting an interview. Choosing a salon that is the best match to your skills will increase your chances of success.

Many salons have Web sites with special employment areas, others post on salon- or job-related Web sites. Follow instructions exactly for filling out forms or sending resumes. (Some salons don't want attachments, such as letters of recommendation or digital portfolios sent with the resumes.) In rare instances, you may need to send a resume and cover letter (**Figures 30-8** and **30–16**) by traditional snail mail. Comply with the salon's guidelines.

Mark your calendar to remind yourself to make a follow-up contact. A week after submitting your resume is generally sufficient. When you call or e-mail, try to schedule an interview appointment. Keep in mind that some salons may not have openings and may not be granting interviews. When this is the case, send a resume, if you have not already, and ask the salon to keep it on file should an opening arise in the future. Be sure to thank your contacts for their time and consideration.

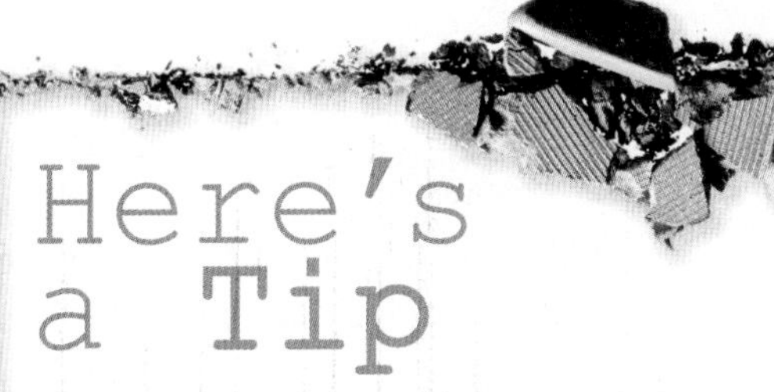

Here's a Tip

When you contact a salon to make an appointment for an interview, you may be told that they are not currently hiring but would be happy to conduct an interview for future reference. Never think that this would be a waste of time.

Take advantage of the opportunity. Not only will it give you valuable interview experience, but it may also provide opportunities that you would otherwise miss.

Interview Preparation

When preparing for an interview, make sure that you have all the necessary information and materials in place (**Figure 30–17**), including the following items:

Identification

- Social Security Number
- Driver's license number
- Names, addresses, and phone numbers of former employers
- Name and phone number of the nearest relative not living with you

▼ Figure 30–17
Preparing for the interview checklist.

PREPARING FOR THE INTERVIEW CHECKLIST
RESUME COMPOSITION 1. Does it present your abilities and what you have accomplished in your jobs and training? 2. Does it make the reader want to ask, "How did you accomplish that?" 3. Does it highlight accomplishments rather than detailing duties and responsibilities? 4. Is it easy to read? Is it short? Does it stress past accomplishments and skills? 5. Does it focus on information that is relevant to your own career goals? 6. Is it complete and professionally prepared?
PORTFOLIO CHECKLIST ——— Diploma, secondary, and post-secondary ——— Awards and achievements while in school ——— Current resume focusing on accomplishments ——— Letters of reference from former employers ——— List of, or certificates from, trade shows attended while in training ——— Statement of professional affiliations (memberships in cosmetology organizations, etc.) ——— Statement of civic affiliations and/or activities ——— Before and after photographs of technical skills services you have performed ——— Any other relevant information Ask: Does my portfolio portray me and my career skills in the manner that I wish to be perceived? If not, what needs to be changed?

© Milady, a part of Cengage Learning.

Interview Wardrobe

Your appearance is crucial, especially since you are applying for a position in the image and beauty industry (**Figure 30–18**). It is recommended that you obtain one or two interview outfits. You may be requested to return for a second interview, hence the need for the second outfit. Consider the following points:

- Is the outfit appropriate for the position?
- Is it both fashionable and flattering, and similar to what the salon's current stylists wear? (If you haven't visited the salon, walk by or check out its Web site to gauge its style culture so that you can dress accordingly.)
- Are your accessories both fashionable and functional (for example, not noisy or so large that they would interfere with performing services)?
- Are your nails well groomed?
- Is your hairstyle current? Does it flatter your face and your overall style?
- Is your makeup current? Does it flatter your face and your overall style?
- (For men:) Are you clean shaven? If not, is your beard properly trimmed?
- Is your perfume or cologne subtle (or nonexistent)?
- Are you carrying either a handbag or a briefcase, but not both?

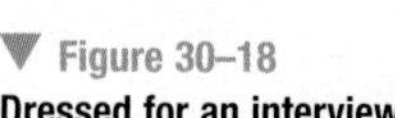

▼ Figure 30–18
Dressed for an interview.

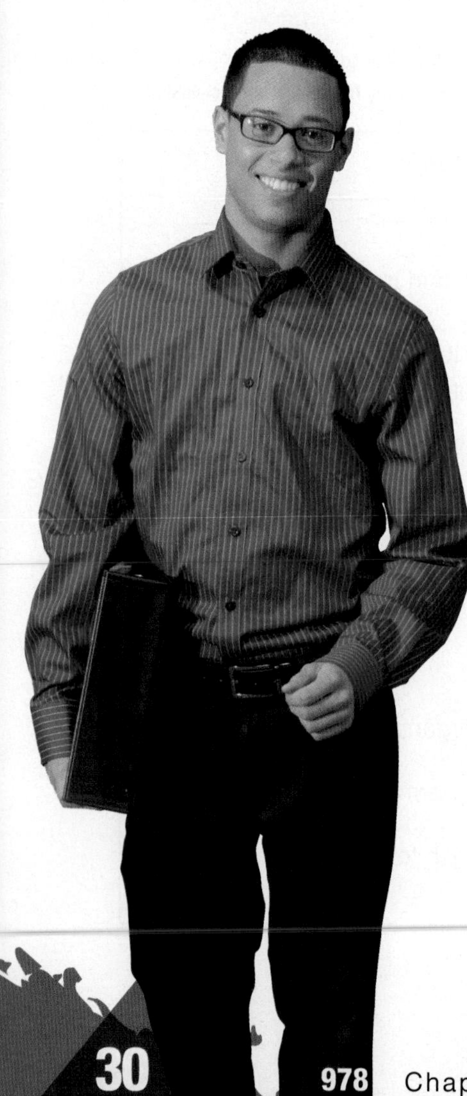

© Milady, a part of Cengage Learning. Photography by Yanik Chauvin.

Supporting Materials

- **Resume.** Even if you have already sent a resume, take another copy with you.
- **Facts and figures.** Have ready a list of names and dates of former employment, education, and references.
- **Employment portfolio.** Even if you have just two photos in your portfolio and they are pictures of haircolor and styles you did for friends, bring them along.

Review and Prepare for Anticipated Interview Questions

Certain questions are typically asked during an interview. Being familiar with these questions will allow you to reflect on your answers ahead of time. You might even consider role-playing an interview situation with friends, family, or fellow students. Typical questions include the following:

- Why do you want to work here?
- What did you like best about your training?
- Are you punctual and regular in attendance?
- Will your school director or instructor confirm this?
- What skills do you feel are your strongest?
- In which areas do you consider yourself to be less strong?
- Are you a team player? Please explain.

- Do you consider yourself flexible? Please explain.
- What are your career goals?
- What days and hours are you available for work?
- Are there any obstacles that would prevent you from keeping your commitment to full-time employment? Please explain.
- What assets do you believe that you would bring to this salon and this position?
- What computer skills do you have?
- How would you handle a problem client?
- How do you feel about retailing?
- Would you be willing to attend our company's training program?
- Would you please describe ways that you provide excellent customer service?
- What consultation questions might you ask a client?
- Are you prepared to train for a year before you have your own clients?

FYI

It can be difficult for new graduates to afford the two or three outfits necessary to project a confident and professional image when going out into the workplace. Fortunately, several nonprofit organizations have been formed to address this need. These organizations receive donations of clean, beautiful clothes in good repair from individuals and manufacturers. These are then passed along to women who need them. For more information, visit Wardrobe for Opportunity at http://www.wardrobe.org and Dress for Success at http://www.dressforsuccess.org.

Be Prepared to Perform a Service

Some salons require applicants to perform a service in their chosen discipline as part of the interview, and many of these salons require you bring your own model. Be sure to confirm whether this is a requirement. If it is, make sure that your model is appropriately dressed and properly prepared for the experience and that you bring the necessary supplies, products, and tools to demonstrate your skills.

The Interview

On the day of the interview, try to make sure that nothing occurs that will keep you from completing the interview successfully. You should practice the following behaviors in connection with the interview itself:

- Always be on time or, better yet, early. If you are unsure of the location, find it the day before, so there will be no reason for delays.
- Turn off your cell phone! Do not arrive with ear buds or a hands-free cell phone device in your ear.
- Project a warm, friendly smile. Smiling is the universal language.
- Walk, sit, and stand with good posture.
- Be polite and courteous.
- Do not sit until you are asked to do so or until it is obvious that you are expected to do so.
- Never smoke or chew gum, even if one or the other is offered to you.
- Do not come to an interview with a cup of coffee, a soft drink, snacks, or anything else to eat or drink.

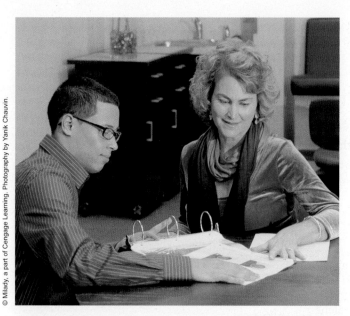
© Milady, a part of Cengage Learning. Photography by Yanik Chauvin.

▲ Figure 30–19
Interview in progress.

- Never lean on or touch the interviewer's desk. Some people do not like their personal space broached without an invitation.
- Try to project a positive first impression by appearing as confident and relaxed as you can be (**Figure 30–19**).
- Speak clearly. The interviewer must be able to hear and understand you.
- Answer questions honestly. Think about the question and answer carefully. Do not speak before you are ready, and not for more than two minutes at a time.
- Never criticize former employers.
- Always remember to thank the interviewer at the end of the interview.

Another critical part of the interview comes when you are invited to ask the interviewer questions of your own. You should think about those questions ahead of time and bring a list if necessary. Doing so will show that you are organized and prepared. Some questions that you might consider include the following:

- What are you looking for in a stylist?
- Is there a job description? May I review it?
- Is there a salon manual? May I review it?
- How does the salon promote itself?
- How long do stylists typically work here?
- Are employees encouraged to grow in skills and responsibility? How so?
- Does the salon offer continuing education opportunities?
- What does your training program involve?
- Is there room for advancement? If so, what are the requirements for promotion?
- What key benefits does the salon offer, such as advanced training and medical insurance?
- What outside and community activities is the salon involved in?
- What is the form of compensation?
- When will the position be filled?
- May I contact you in a week regarding your decision?

Do not feel that you have to ask all of your questions. The point is to create as much of a dialogue as possible. Be aware of the interviewer's reactions and make note of when you have asked enough questions.

By obtaining the answers to at least some of your questions, you can compare the information you have gathered about other salons and choose the one that offers the best package of income and career development.

Remember to follow up the interview with a thank-you note or e-mail. It should simply thank the interviewer for the time he or she spent with you. Close with a positive statement that you want the job (if you do). If the interviewer's decision comes down to two or three possibilities, the one expressing the most desire may be offered the position. Also, if the interviewer suggests that you call to learn about the employment decision, then by all means do so.

Legal Aspects of the Employment Interview

Over the years, a number of legal issues have arisen about questions that may or may not be included in an employment application or interview, including ones that involve race/ethnicity, religion, and national origin. Generally, there should be no questions in any of these categories. Additional categories of appropriate and inappropriate questions are listed below:

- **Age or date of birth.** It is permissible to ask the age if the applicant is younger than 18. Otherwise, age should not be relevant in most hiring decisions; therefore, date-of-birth questions prior to employment are improper.
- **Disabilities or physical traits.** The Americans with Disabilities Act prohibits general inquiries about health problems, disabilities, and medical conditions.
- **Drug use or smoking.** Questions regarding drug or tobacco use are permitted. In fact, the employer may obtain the applicant's agreement to be bound by the employer's drug and smoking policies and to submit to drug testing.
- **Citizenship.** Employers are not allowed to discriminate because an applicant is not a U.S. citizen. However, employers can request to see a Green Card or work permit.

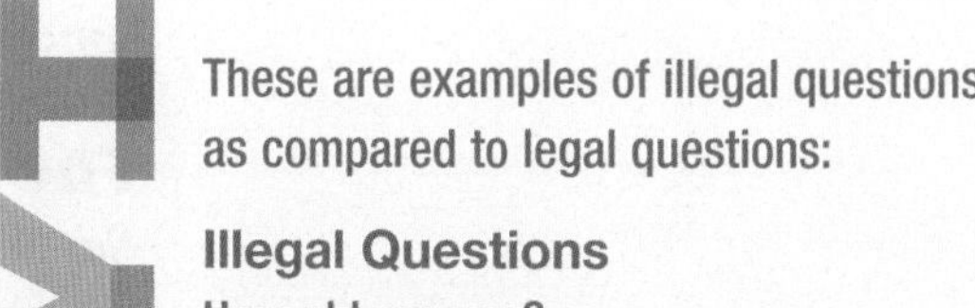

These are examples of illegal questions as compared to legal questions:

Illegal Questions
How old are you?
Please describe your medical history.
Are you a U.S. citizen?
What is your native language?

Legal Questions
Are you over the age of 18?
Are you physically able to perform this job?
Are you authorized to work in the United States?
In which languages are you fluent?

It is important to recognize that not all potential employers will understand that they may be asking improper or illegal questions. If you are asked such questions, you might politely respond that you believe the question is irrelevant to the position you are seeking, and that you would like to focus on your qualities and skills that are suited to the job and the mission of the establishment.

Employee Contracts

Employers can legally require you to sign contracts as a condition of employment. In the salon business, the most common ones are noncompete and confidentiality agreements. Salon owners often invest a great deal in training, and they don't want you taking all that education to a competing salon across the street once your apprenticeship or initial training is complete. Noncompete agreements address this issue, prohibiting you from seeking

ACTivity

Find a partner among your fellow students and role-play the employment interview. Each of you can take turns as the applicant and the employer. After each session, conduct a brief discussion regarding how it went; that is, what worked and what didn't work. Discuss how your performance could be improved. Bear in mind that a role-playing activity will never predict exactly what will occur in a real interview. However, the process will help prepare you for the interview and boost your confidence.

employment within a given time period and geographic area after you leave employment with them. Often, noncompete agreements also forbid employees from gathering and keeping client records, including client phone numbers. A contract cannot interfere with your right to work, and as a result, these contracts must be very specific and are sometimes controversial. If you are presented with any contract, take it home, read it, and make certain you completely understand it. If you do not completely understand any part of it, consult with a labor-law attorney before signing it. ☑ LO5

The Employment Application

Any time that you are applying for any position, you will be required to complete an application, even if your resume already contains much of the requested information. Your resume and the list you have prepared prior to the interview will assist you in completing the application quickly and accurately.

Doing It Right

You are ready to set out on your exciting new career as a professional cosmetologist. The right way to proceed is by learning important study and test-taking skills early and applying them consistently.

Think ahead to your employment opportunities and use your time in school to develop a record of interesting, noteworthy activities that will make your resume more exciting. When you compile a history that shows how you have achieved your goals, your confidence will grow.

Always take one step at a time. Be sure to take the helpful preliminary steps that we have discussed when preparing for employment.

Develop a dynamic portfolio. Keep your materials, information, and questions organized in order to ensure a high-impact interview.

Once you are employed, take the necessary steps to learn all that you can about your new position and the establishment you will be serving. Read all you can about the industry. Attend trade shows and take advantage of as much continuing education as you can manage. Become an active participant in efforts to make the cosmetology industry even better. See Chapter 31, On the Job, to learn some great strategies for ensuring your career success.

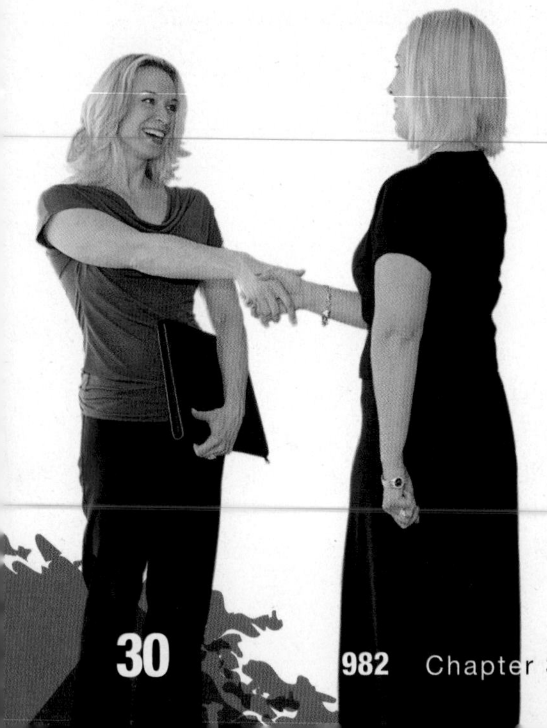

© Milady, a part of Cengage Learning.

Review Questions

1. What habits and characteristics does a test-wise student have?
2. What is deductive reasoning?
3. What are the four most common testing formats?
4. List and describe the different types of salon businesses available to cosmetologists.
5. What is a resume?
6. What is an employment portfolio?
7. List the items that should be included in your employment portfolio.
8. What are some questions that you should never be asked when interviewing for a job?

Chapter Glossary

deductive reasoning	The process of reaching logical conclusions by employing logical reasoning.
employment portfolio	A collection, usually bound, of photos and documents that reflect your skills, accomplishments, and abilities in your chosen career field.
resume	Written summary of a person's education and work experience.
stem	The basic question or problem.
test-wise	Understanding the strategies for successful test taking.
transferable skills	Skills mastered at other jobs that can be put to use in a new position.
work ethic	Taking pride in your work and committing yourself to consistently doing a good job for your clients, employer, and salon team.

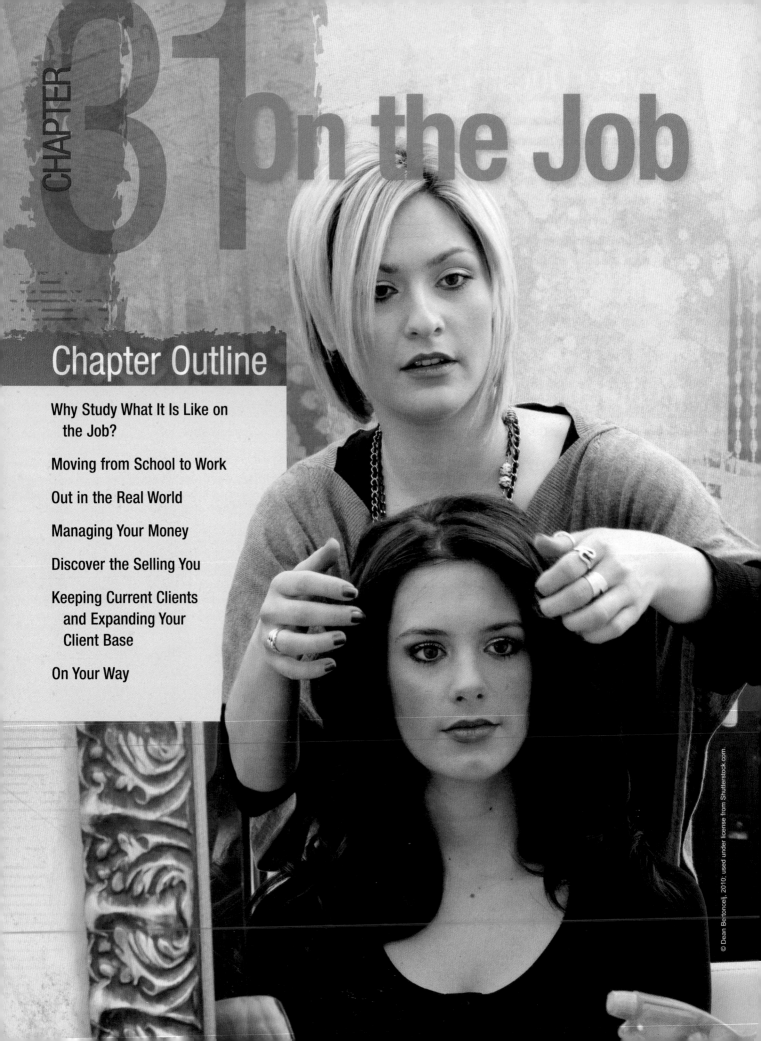

CHAPTER 31

On the Job

Chapter Outline

- Why Study What It Is Like on the Job?
- Moving from School to Work
- Out in the Real World
- Managing Your Money
- Discover the Selling You
- Keeping Current Clients and Expanding Your Client Base
- On Your Way

© Dean Bertoncelj, 2010; used under license from Shutterstock.com.

Learning Objectives

After completing this chapter, you will be able to:

- ✓ **LO1** Describe what is expected of a new employee and what this means in terms of your everyday behavior.
- ✓ **LO2** List the habits of a good salon team player.
- ✓ **LO3** Describe three different ways in which salon professionals are compensated.
- ✓ **LO4** Explain the principles of selling products and services in the salon.
- ✓ **LO5** List the most effective ways to build a client base.

Key Terms

Page number indicates where in the chapter the term is used.

client base
pg. 996

commission
pg. 991

job description
pg. 989

retailing
pg. 996

ticket upgrading (upselling services)
pg. 996

Congratulations! You have worked hard in cosmetology school, passed your state's licensing exam, and been offered your first job in the field. Now, more than ever, you need to prioritize your goals and commit to personal rules of conduct and behavior. These goals and rules should guide you throughout your career. If you let them do so, you can expect to always have work, and to enjoy all the freedom that your chosen profession can offer (**Figure 31–1**).

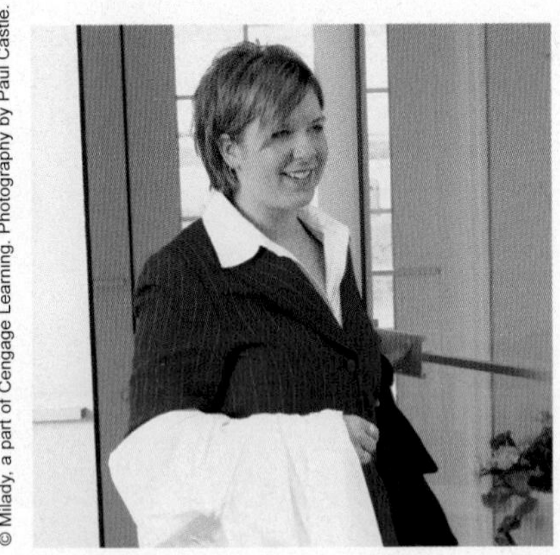
© Milady, a part of Cengage Learning. Photography by Paul Castle.

▲ Figure 31–1
Getting off to a good start.

WHY STUDY WHAT IT IS LIKE ON THE JOB?

Cosmetologists should study and have a thorough understanding of what it is like on the job because:

- Working in a salon requires each staff member to belong to and work as a team member of the salon. Learning to do so is an important aspect of being successful in the salon environment.
- There are a variety of ways that a salon may compensate employees. Being familiar with each way and knowing how they work will help you to determine if the compensation system at a particular salon can work for you and what to expect from it.
- Once you are are working as a salon professional, you will have financial obligations and responsibilities, so learning the basics of financial management while you are building your clientele and business is invaluable.
- As you build your clientele and settle into your professional life, there will be opportunities for you to use a variety of techniques for increasing your income, such as retailing and upselling services. Knowing and using these techniques will help you to promote yourself, build a loyal client base, and create a sound financial future for yourself.

Moving from School to Work

Making the transition from school to work can be difficult. While you may be thrilled to have a job, working for a paycheck brings with it a number of duties and responsibilities that you may not have considered.

Cosmetology school is a forgiving environment. You are given the chance to do a certain procedure over and over again until you get it right. Making and fixing mistakes is an accepted part of the process, and your instructors and mentors are there to help you. Schedules can be adjusted if necessary, and you are given some leeway in the matter of juggling your personal life with the demands of your schooling.

When you become a salon employee, however, you will be expected to put the needs of the salon and its clients ahead of your own.

This means that you must be on time for every scheduled shift and be prepared to perform whatever services or functions are required of you, regardless of what is happening in your personal life. For example, if someone comes to you with tickets for a concert on a day when you are scheduled to work, you cannot just take the day off. To do so would definitely inconvenience your clients, who might even decide not to return to the salon. It could also burden your coworkers, who might feel resentful if they are asked to take on your appointments. ☑ LO1

Out in the Real World

Many cosmetology graduates believe they should be rewarded with a high-paying job, performing only the kinds of services they wish to do, as soon as they graduate from school. It does not work out that way for most people. In a job, you may be asked to do work or perform services that are not your first choice. The good news is that when you are really working in the trenches, you are learning every moment, and there is no substitute for that kind of experience.

What is important is to determine which type of position is right for you by being honest with yourself as you evaluate your skills. If you need help and direction in sorting out the issues around the various workplaces you are considering, ask your instructor for advice. If you chose a salon carefully, based on its culture and the type of salon and benefits you prefer (as discussed in Chapter 30, Seeking Employment), you'll be off to a great start.

FYI

Network with mentors, cosmetology professionals, educators, and classmates; ask questions, take advice, listen, and consider all your options! By doing this, you will open yourself to knowledge, resources, and terrific beauty industry information.

Thriving in a Service Profession

The first reality to remember when you are in a service business is that your career revolves around serving your clients. There will always be some people who do not treat others with respect; however, the majority of people you encounter will truly appreciate the work you do for them. They will look forward to seeing you, and they will show their appreciation for your hard work with their loyalty.

Here are some points that will help guide you as you meet your clients' needs.

- **Put others first.** You will have to quickly get used to putting your own feelings or desires aside, and putting the needs of the salon and the client first. This means doing what is expected of you, unless you are physically unable to do so.
- **Be true to your word.** Choose your words carefully and honestly. Be someone who can be counted on to tell the truth and to do what you say you will do.

- **Be punctual.** Scheduling is central to the salon business. Getting to work on time shows respect not only for your clients, but also for your coworkers who will have to handle your clients if you are late.
- **Be a problem solver.** No job or situation comes without its share of problems. Be someone who recognizes problems promptly and finds ways to resolve them constructively.
- **Be a lifelong learner.** Valued employees continue to learn throughout their careers. Thinking that you are done learning once you are out of school is immature and limiting. Your career might go in all kinds of interesting directions, depending on what new things you learn. This applies to every aspect of your life. Besides learning new technical skills, you should continue gaining more insight into your own behavior and better ways to deal with people, problems, and issues.

Salon Teamwork

Working in a salon requires that you practice and perfect your people skills. A salon is very much a team environment. To become a good team player, you should do your best to practice the following workplace principles.

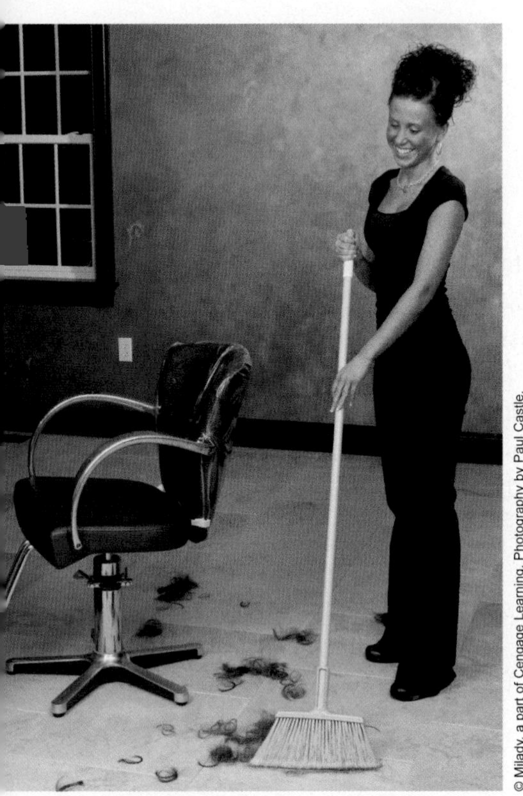
© Milady, a part of Cengage Learning. Photography by Paul Castle.

▲ Figure 31–2
Pitch in wherever you're needed.

- **Strive to help.** Be concerned not only with your own success, but also with the success of others. Be willing to help a teammate by staying a little later or coming in a little earlier.
- **Pitch in.** Be willing to help with whatever needs to be done in the salon—from folding towels to making appointments—when you are not busy servicing clients (**Figure 31–2**).
- **Share your knowledge.** Be willing to share what you know. This will make you a respected member of any team. At the same time, be willing to learn from your coworkers by listening to their perspectives and techniques.
- **Remain positive.** Resist the temptation to give in to maliciousness and gossip.
- **Become a relationship builder.** Just as there are different kinds of people in the world, there are different types of relationships within the salon world. You do not have to be someone's best friend in order to build a good working relationship with that person.
- **Be willing to resolve conflicts.** The most difficult part of being in a relationship is when conflict arises. A real teammate is someone who knows that conflict and tension are bad for the people who are in it, those who are around it, and the salon as a whole. Nevertheless, conflict is a natural part of life. If you can work constructively toward resolving conflict, you will always be a valued member of the team. If you do have a conflict, discuss it with the individual, not with others in the salon.
- **Be willing to be subordinate.** No one starts at the top. Keep in mind that beginners almost always start out lower down in the pecking order.

- **Be sincerely loyal.** Loyalty is vital to the workings of a salon. Salon professionals need to be loyal to the salon and its management. Management needs to be loyal to the staff and clients. Ideally, clients will be loyal to the employee and the salon. As you work on all the team-building characteristics, you will start to feel a strong sense of loyalty to your salon (**Figure 31–3**). LO2

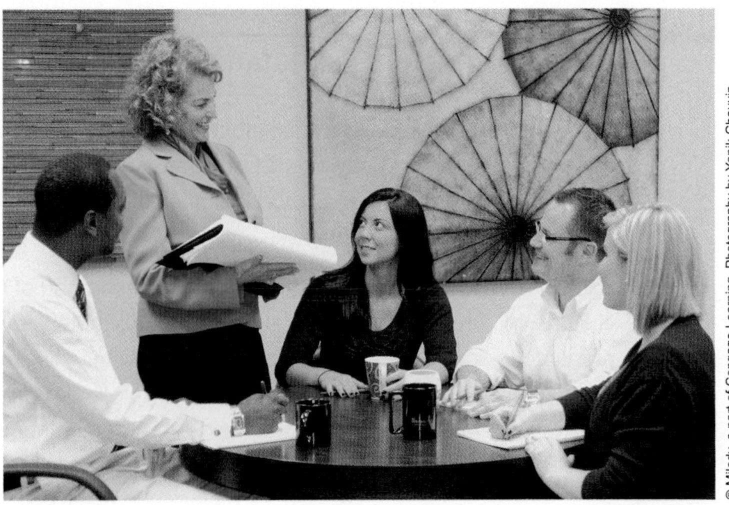

© Milady, a part of Cengage Learning. Photography by Yanik Chauvin.

▲ Figure 31–3
Staff meetings are essential for building a loyal team.

The Job Description

When you take a job, you will be expected to behave appropriately, perform services asked of you, and conduct your business professionally. In order to do this to the best of your abilities, you should be given a **job description**, a document that outlines all the duties and responsibilities of a particular position in a salon or spa. Many salons have a preprinted job description available. If you find yourself at a salon that does not use job descriptions, you may want to write one for yourself. You can then present this to your salon manager for review, to ensure that you both have a good understanding of what is expected of you.

Once you have your job description, be sure you understand it. While reading it over, make notes and jot down questions you want to ask your manager. When you assume your new position, you are agreeing to do everything as it is written down in the job description. If you are unclear about something or need more information, it is your responsibility to ask.

Remember, you will be expected to fulfill all of the functions listed in the job description. How well you fulfill these duties will influence your future at the salon, as well as your financial rewards.

In crafting a job description, the best salons cover all the bases. They outline not only the employee's duties and responsibilities, but also the attitudes that they expect their employees to have and the opportunities that are available to them. **Figure 31–4**, on page 990, shows some highlights from a well-written job description. This is just one example. Like the salons that generate them, job descriptions come in all sizes and shapes, and they feature a variety of requirements, benefits, and incentives.

FOCUS ON

BEING A GOOD TEAMMATE

While each individual may be concerned with getting ahead and being successful, a good teammate knows that no one can be successful alone. You will be truly successful if your entire salon is successful!

Compensation Plans

When you assess a job offer, your first concern will probably be the compensation, or what you will actually get paid for your work. Compensation varies from one salon to another. There are, however, three common methods of compensation that you are most likely to encounter: salary, commission, and salary plus commission.

Job Description: Assistant

Every assistant must have a cosmetology license, as well as the determination to learn and grow on the job. As an assistant you must be willing to cooperate with coworkers in a team environment, which is most conducive to learning and having a good morale among all employees. You must display a friendly yet professional attitude toward coworkers and clients alike.

Excellent time management is essential to the operation of a successful salon. An assistant should be aware of clients who are early and late or stylists who are running ahead or behind in their schedule. You should be prepared to assist in these situations, and to change your routine if necessary. Keep the receptionist and stylists informed about clients who have entered the salon. Be prepared to stay up to an hour late when necessary. Always keep in mind that everyone needs to work together to get the job done.

The responsibilities of an assistant include:

1. Greeting clients by offering them a beverage, hanging up coats, and informing the receptionist and stylist that they have arrived.
2. Shampooing and conditioning clients.
3. Assisting stylists on the styling floor.
4. Assisting stylists in services that require extra help, such as dimensional coloring.
5. Cleaning stations and mirrors, including handheld mirrors.
6. Keeping the styling stations and back bars well stocked with appropriate products.
7. Notifying the salon manager about items and supplies that need to be reordered.
8. Making sure the shampoo sink and drain are always clean and free of hair.
9. Keeping the makeup display neat and clean.
10. Keeping the retail area neat and well stocked.
11. Keeping the bathroom and dressing room neat, clean, and stocked.
12. Performing housekeeping duties such as: emptying trash receptacles, cleaning haircolor from the floor, keeping the lunch room and dispensary neat and clean, helping with laundry, dusting shelves, and maintaining sanitary bathrooms.
13. Making fresh coffee when necessary.
14. Training new assistants.

Continuing Education

Your position as assistant is the first step toward becoming a successful stylist. In the beginning, your training will focus on the duties of an assistant. Once you have mastered those, your training will focus on the skills you will need as a stylist. As part of your continuing education in the salon, you will be required to:

- Attend all salon classes.
- Attend our special Sunday Seminars.
- Acquire all professional tools necessary for training at six weeks (shears, brushes, combs, clips, etc.).

Advancement

Upon successful completion of all required classes and seminars, and your demonstration of the necessary skills and attitudes, you will have the opportunity to advance to the position of Junior Stylist. This advancement will always depend upon your perfomance as an assistant, as well as the approval of management. Remember: how quickly you achieve your goals in this salon is up to you!

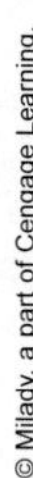
© Milady, a part of Cengage Learning.

▲ Figure 31–4
An example of a job description.

Salary

Being paid an hourly rate is usually the best way for a new salon professional to start out because new professionals rarely have an established clientele. An hourly rate is generally offered to a new cosmetologist, and it is usually based on the minimum wage. Some salons offer an hourly wage that is slightly higher than the minimum wage to encourage new cosmetologists to take the job and stick with it. In this situation, if you earn $10 per hour and you work forty hours, you will be paid $400 that week. If you work more hours, you will get more pay. If you work fewer hours, you will get less pay. Regular taxes will be taken out of your earnings.

Remember, if you are offered a set salary in lieu of an hourly rate, that salary must be at least equal to the minimum wage for the number of hours you work. You are entitled to overtime pay if you work more than forty hours per week. The only exception would be if you were in an official salon management position.

Commission

A **commission** is a percentage of the revenue that the salon takes in from services performed by a particular cosmetologist. Commission is usually offered once an employee has built up a loyal clientele. A commission payment structure is very different from an hourly wage, because any money you are paid is a direct result of the total amount of service dollars you generate for the salon. Commissions are paid based on percentages of your total service dollars, and can range anywhere from 25 to 60 percent, depending on your length of time at the salon, your performance level, and the benefits that are part of your employment package.

Suppose, for example, that at the end of the week when you add up all the services you have performed, your total is $1,000. If you are at the 50 percent commission level, then you would be paid $500 (before taxes). Keep in mind that until you have at least two years of servicing clients under your belt, you may not be able to make a living on straight commission compensation. Additionally, many states do not allow straight commission payments unless they average out to at least minimum wage.

Salary Plus Commission

A salary-plus-commission structure is another common way to be compensated in the salon business. It basically means that you receive both a salary and a commission. This kind of structure is often used to motivate employees to perform more services, thereby increasing their productivity. For example, imagine that you earn an hourly wage that is equal to $300 per week, and you perform about $600 worth of services every week. Your salon manager may offer you an additional 25 percent commission on any services you perform over your usual $600 per week. Or perhaps you receive a straight hourly wage, but

WEB RESOURCES

Most salons require you to take a certain amount of continuing education, even after you've been on the job for years. That's a good thing! The more you learn, the more you'll earn, and salon compensation studies prove it.

Online continuing education is not only travel free and affordable, it also opens up a universe of global ideas and can be taken on your own time. These Web sites will get you started:

- http://www.milady.cengage.com Online courses in salon management, personal and professional development, infection control, and much more.
- http://www.hairdesignertv.com Video lessons from Vivienne Mackinder.
- http://www.prohairstylist.com.au Education and trends from Australia.
- http://www.myhairdressers.com Advanced cutting videos from the UK.
- http://www.modernsalon.com Advanced education and business information.
- http://www.howtocuthair.com Barbering videos.

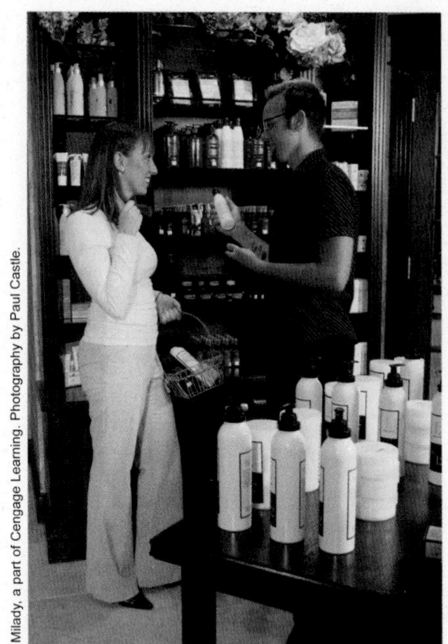

© Milady, a part of Cengage Learning. Photography by Paul Castle.

▲ Figure 31–5
Commissions on retail sales boost income.

you can receive as much as a 15 percent commission on all the retail products you sell. Sometimes, salons call this structure salary plus bonus. With this structure, your salary is actually based on an average of what you would have made if you were paid commission, but you also get a bonus on anything over and above. You can see how this kind of structure quickly leads to significantly increased compensation (**Figure 31–5**). ✓ **LO3**

Tips

When you receive satisfactory service at a hotel or restaurant, you are likely to leave your server a tip. It has become customary for salon clients to acknowledge beauty professionals in this way, too. Some salons have a tipping policy; others have a no-tipping policy. This is determined by what the salon feels is appropriate for its clientele.

The usual amount to tip is 15 percent of the total service ticket. For example, if a customer spends $50, then the tip might be 15 percent of that, or $7.50. Tips are income in addition to your regular compensation and must be tracked and reported on your income tax return. Reporting tips will be beneficial to you if you wish to take out a mortgage or another type of loan and want your income to appear as strong as it really is.

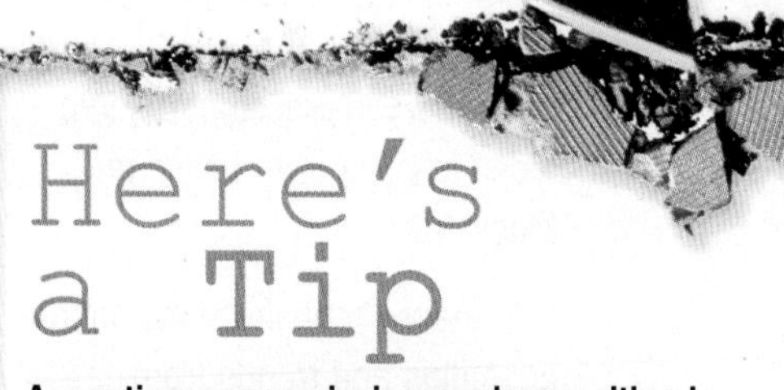

Here's a Tip

Accepting a commission-paying position in a salon can have its positives and negatives for new cosmetologists. If you think you have enough clients to work on commission and can make enough of a paycheck to pay your expenses, then go ahead and give it a try—it could be a great way to work into better commission scales or even booth renting. (Only Pennsylvania forbids booth renting by law, but other states may regulate licensing differently; always check.)

If you don't think you can make enough money being paid solely on a commission basis, then take a job in a salon that is willing to pay you an hourly wage until you build your client base. After you have honed your technical skills and built a solid client base, you can consider working on commission.

As you can see, there are a number of ways to structure compensation for a salon professional. You will probably have the opportunity to try each of these methods at different points in your career. When deciding whether a certain compensation method is right for you, it is important to be aware of what your monthly expenses are and to have a personal financial budget in place. Budget issues are addressed later in this chapter.

Employee Evaluation

The best way to keep tabs on your progress is to ask for feedback from your salon manager and key coworkers. Most likely, your salon will have a structure in place for evaluation purposes. Commonly, evaluations are scheduled ninety days after hiring, and then once a year after that. But you should feel free to ask for help and feedback any time you need it. This feedback can help you improve your technical abilities, as well as your customer-service skills.

Ask a senior stylist to sit in on one of your client consultations and to make note of areas where you can improve. Ask your manager to observe your technical skills and to point out ways you can perform your work more quickly and more efficiently. Have a trusted coworker watch and evaluate your skills when it comes to selling retail products. All of these evaluations will benefit your learning process enormously.

Find a Role Model

One of the best ways to improve your performance is to model your behavior after someone who is having the kind of success that you wish to have. Watch other stylists in your salon. You will easily be able to identify who is really good and who is just coasting along. Focus on the skills of the ones who are really good. What do they do? How do they treat their clients? How do they treat the salon staff and manager? How do they book their appointments? How do they handle their continuing education? What process do they use when formulating color or selecting a product? What is their attitude toward their work? How do they handle a crisis or conflict?

Go to these professionals for advice. Ask for a few minutes of their time, but be willing to wait for it, because it may not be easy to find time to talk during a busy salon workday. If you are having a problem, explain your situation, and ask if the mentor can help you see things differently. Be prepared to listen and not argue your points. Remember that you asked for help, even when what your coworker is saying is not what you want to hear. Thank him for his help, and reflect on the advice you have been given.

A little help and direction from skilled, experienced coworkers will go a long way toward helping you achieve your goals.

did you know?

Beauty pros can increase their chances of building a solid and loyal clientele more quickly if they:

- Live in a large city or choose areas within their cities that have a large number of potential clients.
- Select a location where the competition for clients is less saturated.
- Have advanced training, skills, and certifications.
- Have and use their artistic abilities.
- Employ marketing and publicity strategies.
- Concentrate on an unusual niche within the beauty business (teens, for example).

Managing Your Money

Although a career in the beauty industry is very artistic and creative, it is also a career that requires financial understanding and planning. Too many cosmetology professionals live for the moment and do not plan for the future. They may end up feeling cheated out of the benefits that their friends and family in other careers are enjoying.

In a corporate structure, the human resources department of the corporation handles a great deal of the employees' financial planning for them. For example, health and dental insurance, retirement accounts, savings accounts, and many other items may be automatically deducted and paid out of the employees' salary. Most beauty professionals, however, must research and plan for all of those expenses on their own. This may seem difficult, but in fact it is a small price to pay for the kind of freedom, financial reward, and job satisfaction that a career in cosmetology can offer. And the good news is that managing money is something everyone can learn to do.

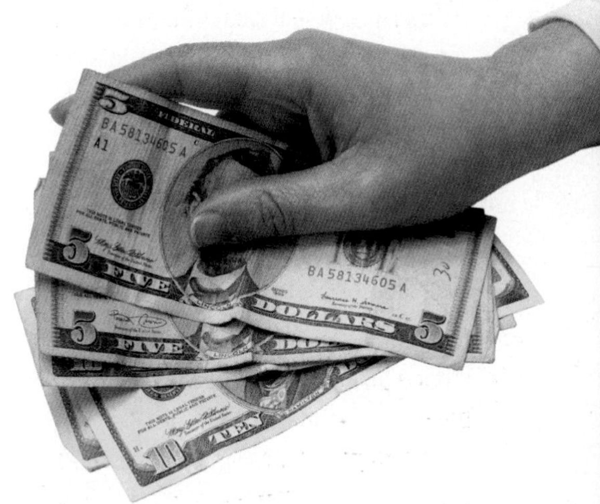

© Rafa Irusta, 2010; used under license from Shutterstock.com.

Meeting Financial Responsibilities

In addition to making money, responsible adults are also concerned with paying back their debts. Throughout your life and your career, you will undoubtedly incur debt in the form of car loans, home mortgages, or

FOCUS ON

SALON TECHNOLOGY

Various surveys show the salon industry is slow to adapt to computerization and new technologies. Nearly one in three or about 33 percent of salons are computerized and have Internet access. However, larger and more upscale salons are far more likely to be computerized and to have Internet and e-mail access. About 22 percent of owners and managers have ordered products online.

The increasing number of computerized salons could be advantageous for technology savvy students. You may be able to master salon software programs more easily than other stylists. These programs now handle cash flow management, inventory tracking, payroll automation, client appointment books, performance evaluation tracking, and more. Just remember, these client records are usually considered the salon's property. Additionally, cost-effective, online continuing education is increasingly popular.

If you are accustomed to working with technology, you may be able to help a salon set up e-mail access, a Web site, social networking pages, and more. With many clients enjoying the freedom of online booking and text-message appointment reminders and with salons benefiting from e-mail or even electronic marketing programs, the more you understand technology, the better. Today, hair care manufacturers even have special educational programs you can access on your mobile phone and social networking pages, where you can swap haircolor formulas or ask for instant help.

student loans. While it is easy for some people to merely ignore their responsibility in repaying these loans, it is extremely irresponsible and immature to accept a loan and then shrug off the debt. Not paying back your loans is called defaulting, and it can have serious consequences regarding your personal and professional credit. The best way to meet all of your financial responsibilities is to know precisely what you owe and what you earn so that you can make informed decisions about where your money goes.

Personal Budget

It is amazing how many people work hard and earn very good salaries but never take the time to create a personal budget. Many people are afraid of the word *budget*, because they think that it will be too restrictive on their spending or that they will have to be mathematical geniuses in order to work with a budget. Thankfully, neither of these fears is rooted in reality.

Personal budgets range from being extremely simple to extremely complex. The right one for you depends on your needs. At the beginning of your career, a simple budget should be sufficient. To get started, take a look at the worksheet in **Figure 31–6** on page 995. It lists the standard monthly expenses that most people have to budget. It also includes school loan repayment, savings, and payments into an individual retirement account (IRA).

Keeping track of where your money goes is one step toward making sure that you always have enough. It also helps you to plan ahead and save for bigger expenses such as a vacation, your own home, or even your own business. All in all, sticking to a budget is a good practice to follow faithfully for the rest of your life.

Giving Yourself a Raise

Once you have taken some time to create, use, and work with your personal budget, you may want to look at ways in which you can have more money left over after paying bills. You might automatically jump to the most obvious sources, such as asking your employer for a raise, or asking for a higher percentage of commission. While these tactics are certainly valid, you will also want to think about other ways to increase your income. Here are a few tips:

- **Spending less money.** Although it may be difficult to reduce your spending, it is certainly one way to increase the amount of money that is left over at the end of the month. These dollars can be used to invest or save or pay down debt.
- **Working more hours.** If possible, choose times when the salon is busiest, which are the most convenient for clients. Come early and stay late to accommodate clients' booking needs. Saturday is a peak workday in most salons.

Personal Budget Worksheet

A. Expenses

1.	My monthly rent (or share of the rent) is	$________
2.	My monthly car payment is	________
3.	My monthly car insurance payment is	________
4.	My monthly auto fuel/upkeep expenses are	________
5.	My monthly electric bill is	________
6.	My monthly gas bill is	________
7.	My monthly health insurance payment is	________
8.	My monthly entertainment expense is	________
9.	My monthly bank fees are	________
10.	My monthly grocery expense is	________
11.	My monthly dry cleaning expense is	________
12.	My monthly personal grooming expense is	________
13.	My monthly prescription/medical expense is	________
14.	My monthly telephone bill is	________
15.	My monthly student loan payment is	________
16.	My IRA payment is	________
17.	My savings account deposit is	________
18.	Other expenses:	________
	TOTAL EXPENSES	$________

B. Income

1.	My monthly take-home pay is	________
2.	My monthly income from tips is	________
3.	Other income:	________
	TOTAL INCOME	$________

C. Balance

Total Income (B)	________
Minus Total Expenses (A)	________
BALANCE	$________

© Milady, a part of Cengage Learning.

▲ Figure 31–6
A budget worksheet.

- **Increasing service prices.** It will probably take some time before you are in a position to increase your service prices. For one thing, to do so, you need a loyal **client base**, customers who are loyal to a particular cosmetologist, which in this instance is you. Also, you must have fully mastered all the services that you are performing. But if you have a loyal client base and service mastery, there is nothing wrong with increasing your prices every year or two, as long as you do so by a reasonable amount. Do a little research to determine what your competitors are charging for similar services, and increase your fees accordingly.
- **Retailing more.** Most salons pay a commission on every product you recommend and sell to your clients. If you sell more products, you make more money!

Seek Professional Advice

Just as you will want your clients to seek out your advice and services for their hair care needs, sometimes it is important for you to seek out the advice of experts, especially when it comes to your finances. You can research and interview financial planners who will be able to give you advice on reducing your credit card debt, on how to invest your money, and on retirement options. You can speak to the officers at your local bank, who may be able to suggest bank accounts that offer you greater returns or flexibility with your money, depending on what you need.

When seeking out advice from other professionals, be sure not to take anyone's advice without carefully considering whether the advice makes sense for your particular situation and needs. Before you buy into anything, be an informed consumer about other people's goods and services.

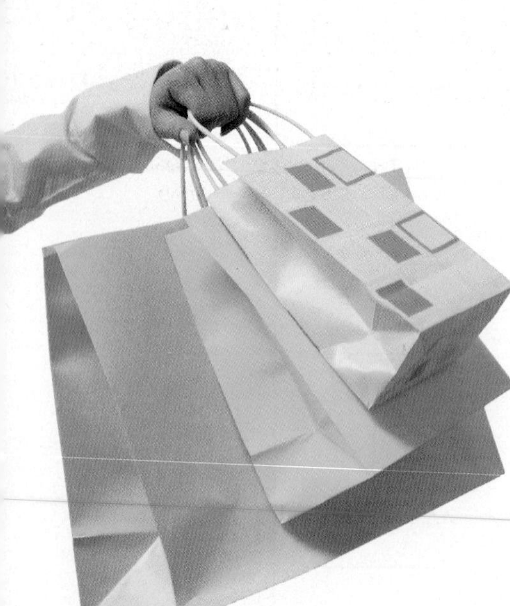

© Stephen Coburn, 2010; used under license from Shutterstock.com.

- How do your expenses compare to your income?
- What is your balance after all your expenses are paid?
- Were there any surprises for you in this exercise?
- Do you think that keeping a budget is a good way to manage money?
- Do you know of any other methods people use to manage money?

Discover the Selling You

Another area that touches on the issue of you and money is selling. As a salon professional, you will have enormous opportunities to sell retail products and upgrade service tickets. **Ticket upgrading**, also known as **upselling services**, is the practice of recommending and selling additional services to your clients. These services may be performed by you or other professionals licensed in a different field (**Figure 31–7**). **Retailing** is the act of recommending and selling products to your clients for at-home use. These two activities can make all the difference

ACTivity

Go through the budget worksheet and fill in the amounts that apply to your current living and financial situation. If you are unsure of the amount of an expense, put in the amount you have averaged over the past three months, or give it your best guess. You may need to have three or four months of employment history in order to complete the income item, but fill in what you can. If the balance is a minus number, start listing ways you can decrease expenses or increase income.

in your economic picture. The following dialogue is an example of ticket upgrading. In this scene, Judy, the stylist, suggests an additional service to Ms. King, her client, who has just had her hair styled for a wedding she will be attending that evening.

Read the script yourself and change the words to make them fit your personality. Then try it the next time you feel that an additional service could help one of your clients.

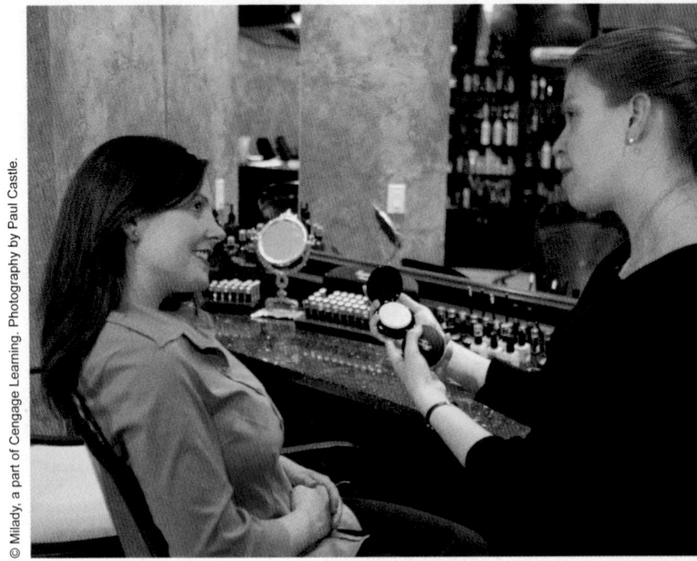
© Milady, a part of Cengage Learning. Photography by Paul Castle.

▲ **Figure 31–7**
This client may wish for a makeup service as well as hairstyling.

Judy: I'm really glad you like your new hairstyle. It will be perfect with the dress you described. Don't you just love formal weddings?

Ms. King: I don't know. To tell you the truth, I don't get dressed up all that often, and putting the look together was harder than I thought it would be.

Judy: Yes, I know what you mean. Are you all set with your makeup for tonight, Ms. King? It would be a shame to have a beautiful new dress and gorgeous hair, and then have to worry about your makeup.

Ms. King: Well, actually, I was sort of wondering about that. I'm wearing this long blue dress and I'm not really sure what the best look is for the occasion. Got any ideas?

Judy: Well, as you know, my specialty is hair care, but we have an excellent makeup artist right here on staff, and she is available for a consultation. You might want to make an appointment with her, and she can do your makeup for you. I don't know if you've ever had a professional do it before, but it's a real treat, and it only costs $25. Plus they throw in a small lipstick to take with you. Shall I get her for you?

Ms. King: Definitely. That sounds terrific!

Judy: You know, since this is such an important occasion, you may want to consider having Marie, one of our nail techs, manicure your nails as well. That will ensure that your total look is the best it can be.

Ms. King: I think that's a great idea. Thanks for the suggestion!

Principles of Selling

Some salon professionals shy away from sales. They think that it is being pushy. A close look at how selling works can set your mind at ease. Not only can you become very good at selling once you understand the principles behind it, but you can also feel good about providing your clients with a valuable service.

▼ Figure 31–8
When you have multiple retail displays, everyone who comes into the salon has the potential to be a retail client.

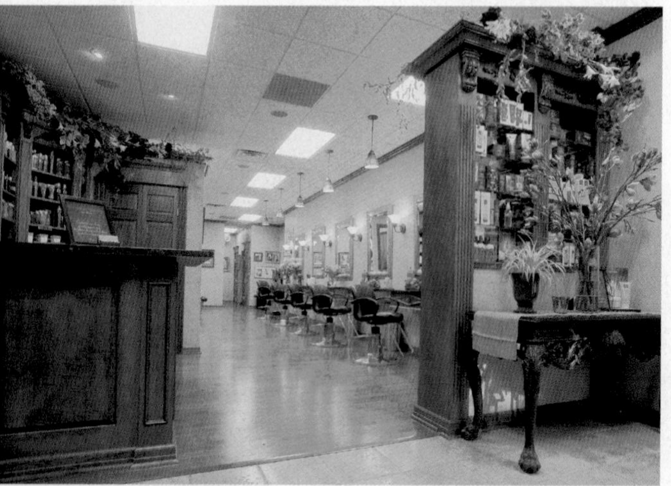

Photography by Michael Watson for Salvatore Minardi Salon, Madison, NJ.

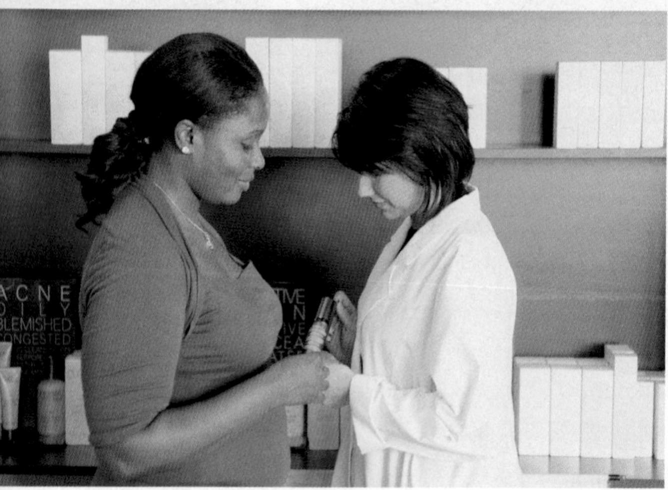

© Milady, a part of Cengage Learning. Photography by Yanik Chauvin.

▲ Figure 31–9
Demonstrate a product's benefits.

To be successful in sales, you need ambition, determination, and a pleasing personality. The first step in selling is to sell yourself. Clients must like and trust you before they will purchase beauty services, cosmetics, skin or nail care items, shampoos and conditioners, or other merchandise.

Remember, every client who enters the salon is a potential purchaser of additional services or merchandise. Recognizing the client's needs and preferences lays the foundation for successful selling (**Figure 31–8**).

To become a proficient salesperson, you must be able to apply the following principles of selling salon products and services:

- Be familiar with the features and benefits of the various services and products that you are trying to sell, and recommend only those that the client really needs. You should try and test all the products in the salon yourself.
- Adapt your approach and technique to meet the needs and personality of each client. Some clients may prefer a soft sell that involves informing them about the product, without stressing that they purchase it. Others are comfortable with a hard-sell approach that focuses emphatically on why a client should buy the product.
- Be self-confident when recommending products for sale. You become confident by knowing about the products you are selling and by believing that they are as good as you say.
- Generate interest and desire in the customer by asking questions that determine a need.
- Never misrepresent your services or products. Making unrealistic claims will only lead to your client's disappointment, making it unlikely that you will ever again make a sale to that client.
- Do not underestimate the client's intelligence or her knowledge of her own beauty regimen or particular needs.
- To sell a product or service, deliver your sales talk in a relaxed, friendly manner. If possible, demonstrate use of the product (**Figure 31–9**).

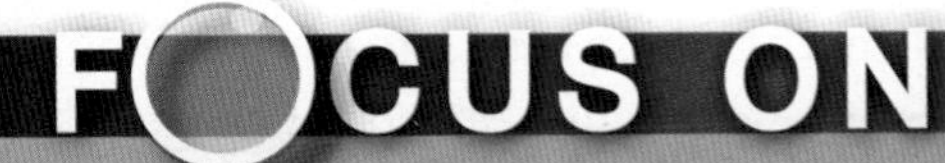

OVERCOMING OBJECTIONS

Making sales won't always be easy. Sometimes, a client is stuck on a haircolor that isn't flattering. Other times, she may not feel convinced a product is any better than a drugstore brand or she may have a genuine price objection.

To overcome an objection, reword the objection in a way that addresses the client's need. For instance, let's say you recommend a shampoo based on the fact that your client has dry hair and she just had it colored. In response, she says she already has a shampoo for color-treated hair.

First, acknowledge what she said. Then reword her objection that she already has the right shampoo in a different way, which gets her thinking. For example:

"Yes, it's good to use a shampoo for color-treated hair. I did notice that your hair is still dry, even before I colored it. This shampoo not only protects your color from fading, it will definitely moisturize it more, which is what adds the shine you told me you wanted. I can leave it at the front desk, so you can think about it."

If the objection is a price objection, base your reaction on the client's. For strong objections, acknowledge the price and offer a free sample, if you can. If the objection is moderate, acknowledge it and reiterate the product's benefits.

"It is a little more expensive, but if you really want your color to last and your hair to be silky and shiny, this is the best product I've ever found. We used it on you at the back bar today. See what you think, and let me know."

Always state things in terms of the client's benefit, based on the information you gathered during the consultation.

- Recognize the right psychological moment to close any sale. Once the client has offered to buy, quit selling. Do not oversell; simply praise the client for making the purchase and assure her that she will be happy with it. ✓ **LO4**

The Psychology of Selling

Most people have reasons for doing what they do, and when you are selling something, it is your job to figure out the reasons that will motivate a person to buy. When dealing with salon clients, you will find that their motives for buying salon products vary widely. Some may be concerned with issues of vanity. (They want to look better.) Some are seeking personal satisfaction. (They want to feel better about themselves.) Others need to solve a problem that is bothersome. (They want to spend less time maintaining their hair.)

Sometimes, a client may inquire about a product or service but still be undecided or doubtful. In this type of situation, you can help the client by offering honest and sincere advice. When you explain a salon service to a client, address the results and benefits of that service. Always keep in mind that the best interests of the client should be your first consideration. You will need to know exactly what your client's needs are, and you need to have a clear idea as to how those needs can be fulfilled. Refer to the sample dialogues in this section—one involves ticket upgrading, and the other involves retailing, both of which demonstrate effective selling techniques.

Here are a few tips on how to get the conversation started on retailing products:

- Ask all your clients what products they are using for home maintenance of their hair, skin, and nails.
- Discuss the products you are using, as you use them. For instance, tell the client why you are using the particular mousse or spray gel and what it will do for her. Also explain how she should use the product at home.

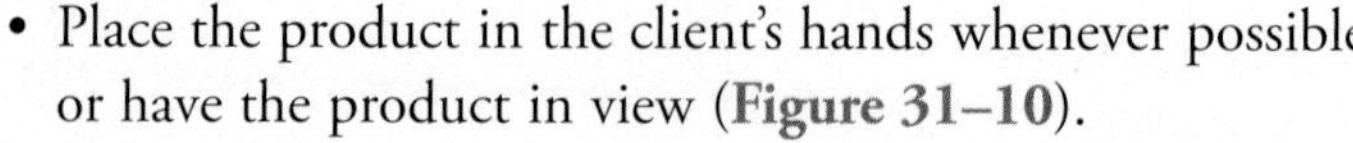

- Place the product in the client's hands whenever possible or have the product in view (**Figure 31–10**).
- Advise the client about how the recommended service will provide personal benefit (more manageable hairstyling or longer-lasting haircolor, for instance).
- Keep retail areas clean, well lit, and appealing.
- Inform clients of any promotions and sales that are going on in the salon.
- Be informed about the merits of using a professional product, as opposed to generic store brands.
- If you have time, offer a quick styling lesson. If your client has difficulty home styling, she'll appreciate your guidance. After demonstrating, watch as the client mimics the recommended styling technique, so you can guide her.

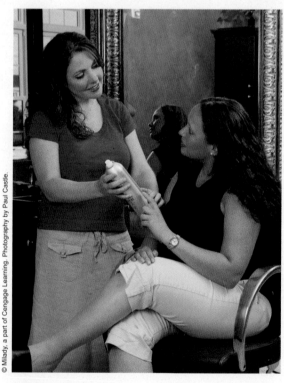

© Milady, a part of Cengage Learning. Photography by Paul Castle.

▲ Figure 31–10
Place the product in the client's hands.

While you realize that retailing products is a service to your clients, you may not be sure how to go about it. Imagine the following scenes and see how Lisa highlights the benefits and features of a product to her client, Ms. Steiner. Notice that price is not necessarily the most important factor.

Scenario 1: Meet a Need

Ms. Steiner: I just love my new haircolor. When should I have it redone? I hope it stays this red.

Lisa: You should come back in six weeks for a retouch. By then, you'll have had time to think about those highlights I suggested. I'm also going to suggest you use this shampoo and conditioner to keep your color vibrant between now and your next visit.

ACTivity

Pick a partner from class and role-play the dynamics of a sales situation. Take turns being the customer and the stylist. Evaluate each other on how you did, with suggestions about where you can improve. Then try this exercise with someone else because no two customers are the same.

Ms. Steiner: Is that what you used on me today? It smelled great.

Lisa: I love that scent, too. Also, the shampoo is a really great moisturizing shampoo that will keep your hair from drying out, in addition to protecting the color. The conditioner adds shine and seals the cuticle. The next time I see you, your hair should be almost as vibrant as it is now.

Ms. Steiner: Great!

Keeping Current Clients and Expanding Your Client Base

Once you have mastered the basics of good service, take a look at some marketing techniques that will expand your client base, the customers that keep coming back to you for services.

The following are only a few suggestions; there are many others that may work for you. The best way to decide which techniques are most effective is to try several!

- **Birthday cards.** Ask clients for their birthday information (just the month and day, not the year) on the client consultation card, and then use it as a tool to get them into the salon again. About one month prior to the client's birthday, send a card with a special offer. Make it valid only for the month of their birthday.
- **Provide consistently good service.** It seems basic enough, but it is amazing how many professionals work hard to get clients, and lose them because they rush through a service, leaving clients feeling dissatisfied. Providing good-quality service must always be your first concern.
- **Be reliable.** Always be courteous, thoughtful, and professional. Be at the salon when you say you will be there, and do not keep clients waiting. (See Chapter 4, Communicating for Success, for tips on how to handle the unavoidable times when you are running late.) Give your clients the hair length and style they ask for, not something else. Recommend a retail product only when you have tried it yourself and know what it can and cannot do.

- **Be respectful.** When you treat others with respect, you become worthy of respect yourself. Being respectful means that you do not gossip or make fun of anyone or anything related to the salon. Negative energy brings everyone down, especially you.
- **Be positive.** Become one of those people who always sees the glass as half full. Look for the positive in every situation. No one enjoys being around a person who is always unhappy.

▼ Figure 31–11
Referral cards help build your client base.

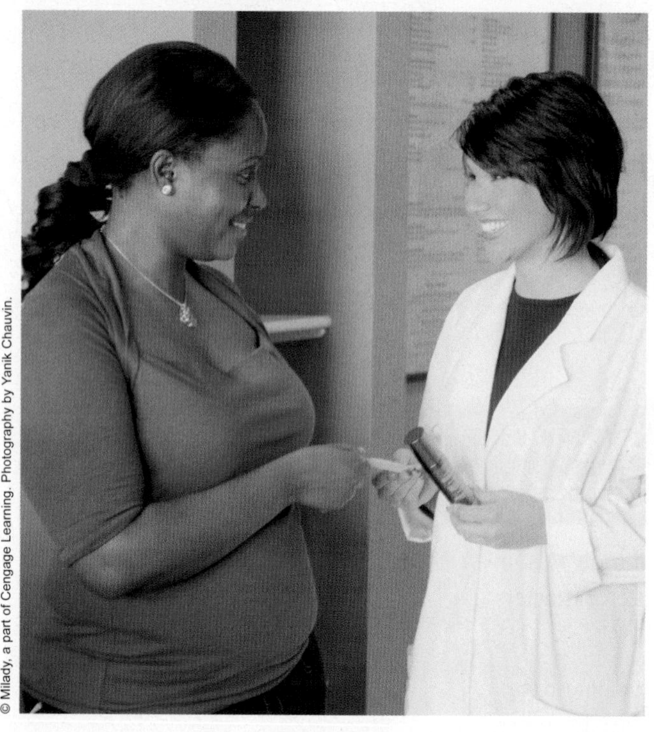

© Milady, a part of Cengage Learning. Photography by Yanik Chauvin.

- **Be professional.** Sometimes, a client may try to make your relationship more personal than it ought to be. It is in your best interest, and your client's best interest, not to cross that line. Remember that your job is to be the client's beauty advisor, not a psychiatrist, a marriage counselor, or a buddy.
- **Business card referrals.** Make up a special business card with your information on it, but leave room for a client to put her name on it as well. If your client is clearly pleased with your work, give her several cards. Ask her to put her name on them and to refer her friends and associates to you. For every card you receive from a new customer with her name on it, give her 10 percent off her next salon service, or a complimentary added service to her next appointment. This gives the client lots of motivation to recommend you to others, which in turn helps build up your clientele (**Figure 31–11**).
- **Local business referrals.** Another terrific way to build business is to work with local businesses to get referrals. Look for clothing stores, florists, gift shops, and other small businesses near your salon. Offer to have a card swap and commit to referring your clients to them when they are in the market for goods or services that your neighbors can provide, if they will do the same for you. This is a great way to build a feeling of community among local vendors and to reach new clients you may not be able to otherwise.
- **Public speaking.** Make yourself available for public speaking at local women's groups, the PTA, organizations for young men and women, and anywhere else that will put you in front of people in your community who are all potential clients. Put together a short program (twenty to thirty minutes) in which, for example, you might discuss professional appearance with emphasis in your chosen field and other grooming tips for people looking for jobs or who are already employed. ☑ LO5

FOCUS ON RETAILING

For quick reference, keep these five points in mind when selling:

1. Establish rapport with the client.
2. Determine the client's needs.
3. Recommend products/services based on these needs.
4. Emphasize benefits.
5. Close the sale.

Rebooking Clients

The best time to think about getting your client back into the salon is while they are still in your salon. It may seem a little difficult to assure your client that you are concerned with their satisfaction on this visit while you are talking about their next visit, but the two go together. The best way to encourage your client to book another appointment before she leaves is to simply talk with her, ask questions, and listen carefully to her answers.

During the time that you are working on a client's hair, for instance, talk about the condition of their hair, their hairstyling habits at home, and the benefits of regular or special salon maintenance. You might raise these issues in a number of ways.

Scenario 2: Color Client

"Mrs. Rivera, when I cut your hair today, I noticed that you need a color retouch. Shall I book a retouch for your next visit?"

Scenario 3: Haircutting Client

"Your son is getting married next month? How wonderful. Have you thought about having a clear glazing so your hair will be bright and shiny and will look as beautiful as the rest of you in that new dress you told me about? I can set up an appointment for the day before the wedding."

Again, you will want to listen carefully to what your clients tell you during their visit, because they will often give the careful listener many good clues as to what is happening in their lives. That will open the door to a discussion about their next appointment.

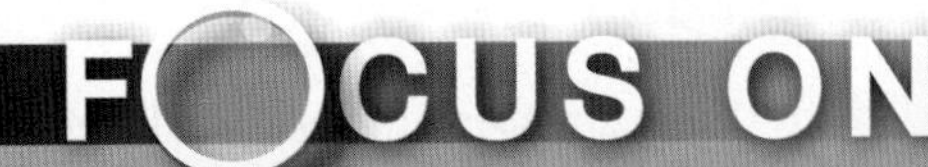

THE GOAL

Always remember that success does not just come to you; you make it happen. How? By being a team player, having a positive attitude, and keeping a real sense of commitment to your work foremost in your mind.

FOCUS ON

BUILDING YOUR EFFICIENCY

Some professionals believe that the more time they spend with their clients performing services, the better the service will be. Not so! Your client should be in the salon only as long as is necessary for you to adequately complete a service.

Be aware of how much time it takes you to perform your various services and then schedule accordingly. As you become more and more experienced, you should see a reduction in the amount of time it takes you to perform these services. That means clients wait less, and you can increase the number of services you perform each day. The increase in services naturally increases your income.

Here's a Tip

There are plenty of books and Web articles that give great strategies for building a client base and keeping those clients coming back to you. Look into these and make a list of the suggestions that seem like a good fit for you, your client base, and your salon. Then, choose one strategy to try every two to three months, and see how well it worked for you. If it helped you to accomplish your goal of getting and keeping new clients, then put a star next to it and save the idea to use again when the time is right!

On Your Way

Your first job in the beauty industry will most likely be the most difficult. Getting started in this business means spending some time on a steep learning curve. Be patient with yourself as you transition from the "school you" to the "professional you." Always remember that in your work life, as in everything else you do, practice makes perfect. You will not know everything you need to know right at the start, but be confident in the fact that you are graduating from cosmetology school with a solid knowledge base. Make use of the many generous and experienced professionals you will encounter, and let them teach you the tricks of the trade. Make the commitment to perfecting your technical and customer service skills.

Above all, always be willing to learn. If you let the concepts that you have learned in this book be your guide, you will enjoy your life and reap the amazing benefits of a career in cosmetology (**Figure 31–12**).

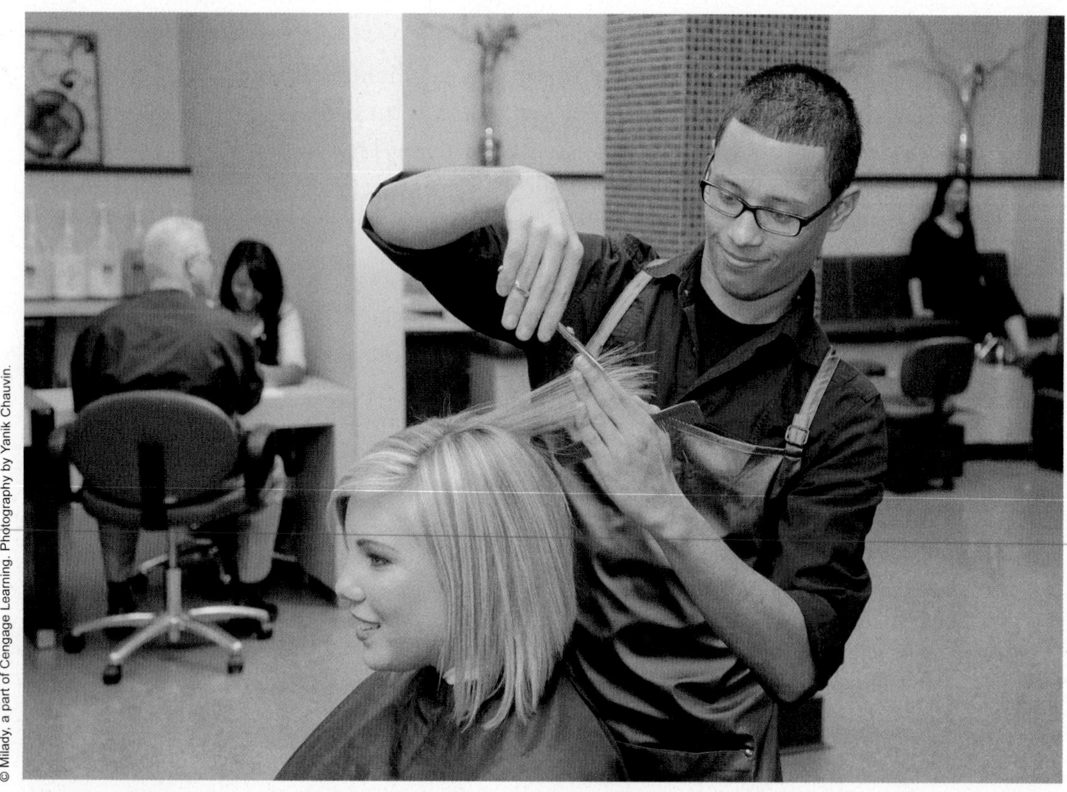

© Milady, a part of Cengage Learning. Photography by Yanik Chauvin.

▲ **Figure 31–12**
Make career satisfaction your goal.

Review Questions

1. What is expected of a new salon employee and what are two things you must do every day?
2. What are six habits of a good team player?
3. What are the three most common methods of salon compensation you are likely to encounter?
4. What are five principles of selling salon products and services? (Explain them.)
5. What are six ways you can work to expand your client base?

Chapter Glossary

client base	Customers who are loyal to a particular cosmetologist.
commission	A percentage of the revenue that the salon takes in from services performed by a particular cosmetologist, usually offered to that cosmetologist once the individual has built up a loyal clientele.
job description	Document that outlines all the duties and responsibilities of a particular position in a salon or spa.
retailing	The act of recommending and selling products to your clients for at-home use.
ticket upgrading	Also known as *upselling services*; the practice of recommending and selling additional services to your clients.

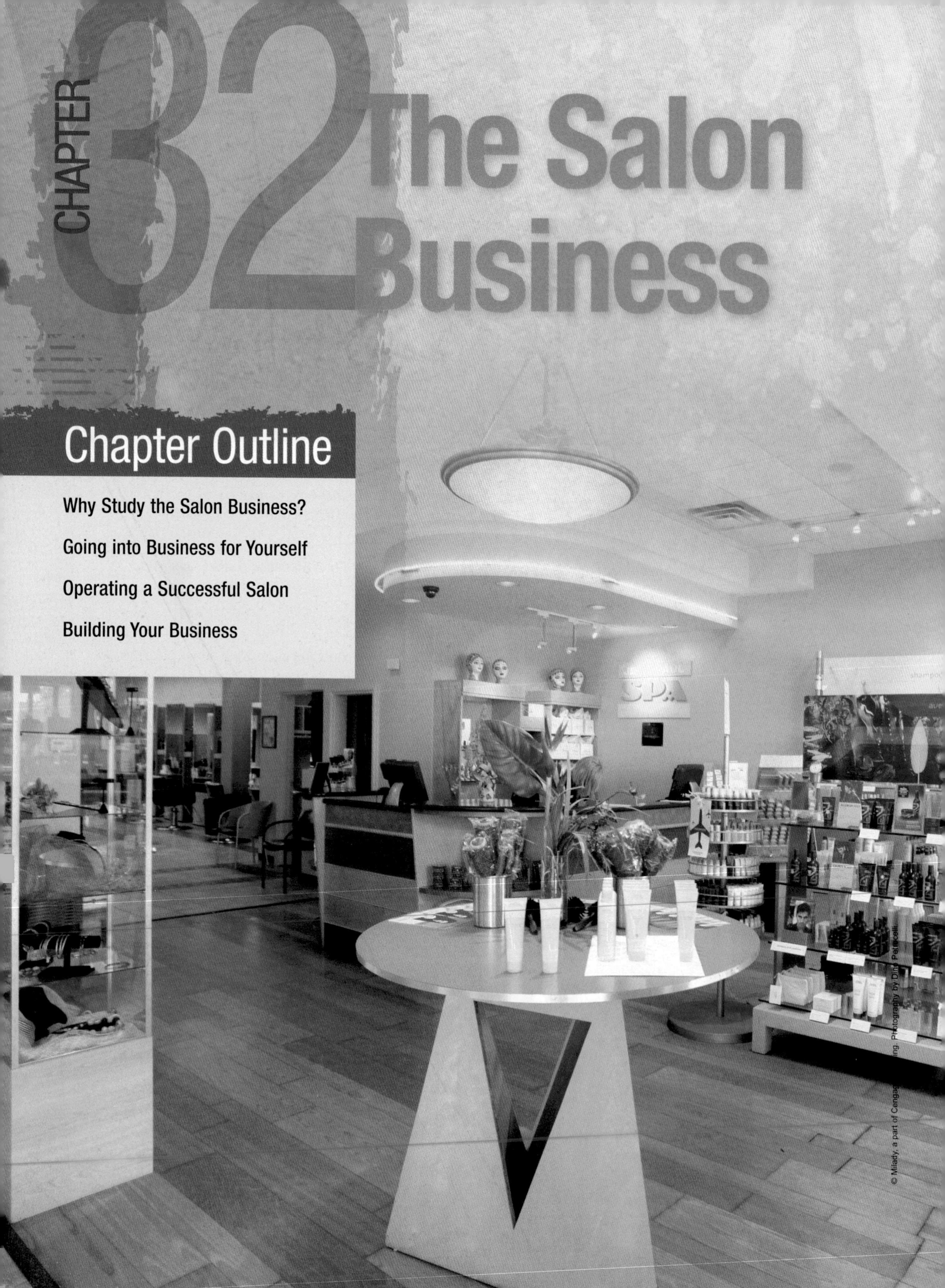

CHAPTER 32 The Salon Business

Chapter Outline

Why Study the Salon Business?

Going into Business for Yourself

Operating a Successful Salon

Building Your Business

© Milady, a part of Cengage Learning. Photography by Dino Petrocelli.

Learning Objectives

After completing this chapter, you will be able to:

- ✓ **LO1** Identify two options for going into business for yourself.
- ✓ **LO2** Understand the responsibilities of a booth renter.
- ✓ **LO3** List the basic factors to be considered when opening a salon.
- ✓ **LO4** Distinguish the types of salon ownership.
- ✓ **LO5** Identify the information that should be included in a business plan.
- ✓ **LO6** Understand the importance of record keeping.
- ✓ **LO7** Recognize the elements of successful salon operations.
- ✓ **LO8** Explain why selling services and products is a vital aspect of a salon's success.

Key Terms

Page number indicates where in the chapter the term is used.

booth rental (chair rental)
pg. 1009

business plan
pg. 1011

business regulations and laws
pg. 1012

capital
pg. 1013

consumption supplies
pg. 1019

corporation
pg. 1013

demographics
pg. 1011

goals
pg. 1010

insurance
pg. 1012

partnership
pg. 1013

personnel
pg. 1021

record keeping
pg. 1012

retail supplies
pg. 1019

salon operation
pg. 1012

salon policies
pg. 1012

sole proprietor
pg. 1013

vision statement
pg. 1010

written agreements
pg. 1011

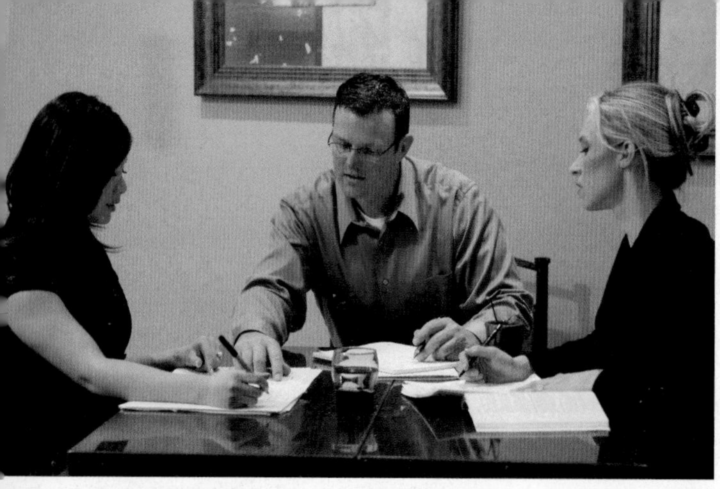

▲ Figure 32–1
Opening your own salon or spa is a big step.

© Milady, a part of Cengage Learning. Photography by Dino Petrocelli.

The better prepared you are to be both a great artist and a successful businessperson, the greater your chances of success (**Figure 32–1**).

Entire books have been written on each of the topics touched on in this chapter, so be prepared to read and research your business idea extensively before making any final decisions about opening a business. The following information is only meant to be a general overview.

WHY STUDY THE SALON BUSINESS?

Cosmetologists should study and have a thorough understanding of the salon business because:

- As you become more proficient in your craft and your ability to manage yourself and others, you may decide to become an independent booth renter or even a salon owner. In fact, most owners are former stylists.
- Even if you spend your entire career as an employee of someone else's salon, you should have a familiarity of the rules of business that affect the salon.
- To become a successful entrepreneur, you will need to attract employees and clients to your business and maintain their loyalty over long periods of time.
- Even if you think you will be involved in the artistic aspect of salons forever, business knowledge will serve you well in managing your career and professional finances, as well as your business practices.

Going into Business for Yourself

If you reach a point in your life when you feel that you are ready to become your own boss, you will have two main options to consider: (1) owning your own salon, or (2) renting a booth in an existing salon.

Both options are extremely serious undertakings that require significant financial investment and a strong line of credit. Salon owners have a very different job than hairdressers. Typically, owners continue to work behind the chair while they manage the business. This is extremely time consuming, and there is no guarantee of profits, which is why salon ownership is definitely not for everyone. Owning your own salon and renting a booth have different pros and cons. ☑ LO1

Booth Rental

Booth rental, also known as **chair rental**, is renting a booth or a station in a salon. This practice is popular in salons all over the United States. Many people see booth rental or renting a station in a salon as a more desirable alternative to owning a salon.

In a booth rental arrangement, a professional generally:

- Rents a station or work space in a salon from the salon owner.
- Is solely responsible for his or her own clientele, supplies, record keeping, and accounting.
- Pays the salon owner a weekly fee for use of the booth.
- Becomes his or her own boss for a very small amount of money.

Booth rental is a desirable situation for many cosmetologists who have large, steady clientele and who do not have to rely on the salon's general clientele to keep busy. Unless you are at least 70 percent booked all the time, however, it may not be advantageous to rent a booth.

did you know?

Currently, booth rental is legal in every state except Pennsylvania, where there is a law prohibiting it. In New Jersey, the state board does not recognize booth rental as an acceptable method of doing business.

Although it may sound like a good option, booth renting has its share of obligations, such as:

- Keeping records for income tax purposes and other legal reasons.
- Paying all taxes, including higher Social Security (double that of an employee).
- Carrying adequate malpractice insurance and health insurance.
- Complying with all IRS obligations for independent contractors. Go to http://www.irs.gov and search for independent contractors.
- Using your own telephone and booking system.
- Collecting all service fees, whether they are paid in cash or via a credit card.
- Creating all professional materials, including business cards and a service menu.
- Purchasing of all supplies, including back-bar and retail supplies and products.
- Tracking and maintaining inventory.
- Managing the purchase of products and supplies.
- Budgeting for advertising or offering incentives to ensure a steady flow of new clients.
- Paying for all continuing education.
- Working in an independent atmosphere where teamwork usually does not exist and where salon standards are interpreted on an individual basis.
- Adhering to state laws and regulations. To date, one state (Pennsylvania) does not allow booth rental at all; others may require that each renter in an establishment hold his or her own establishment license and carry individual liability insurance. Always check with your state regulatory agency.

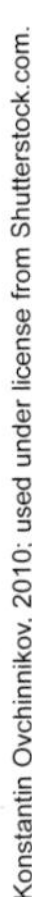
© Konstantin Ovchinnikov, 2010; used under license from Shutterstock.com.

As a booth renter, you will not enjoy the same benefits as an employee of a salon would, such as paid days off or vacation time. Remember, as a booth renter, when you do not work, you do not get paid. Perhaps most importantly, you must continually attract new clients and maintain the ones you have, which means working the hours your clients need you to be available. ✓ LO2

Opening Your Own Salon

Opening your own salon is a huge undertaking—financially, physically, and mentally—because you will face challenges that are complex and unfamiliar to you. Before you can open your doors, you'll need to decide what products to use and carry, what types of marketing and promotions you will employ, the best method and philosophy for running the business, and whom to hire if you need additional staff.

Regardless of the type of salon you hope to open, you should carefully consider basic issues and perform basic tasks, as outlined in the following section.

Create a Vision and Mission Statement for the Business with Goals

A **vision statement** is a long-term picture of what the business is to become and what it will look like when it gets there. A mission statement is a description of the key strategic influences of the business, such as the market it will serve, the kinds of services it will offer, and the quality of those services. **Goals** are a set of benchmarks that, once achieved, help you to realize your mission and your vision. You can set short-term goals and long-term goals for your business.

Create a Business Timeline

While initially you will be concerned with the first two aspects of the timeline, once your business is successful you will need to think about the others as well.

- Year One: It could take a year or more to determine and complete all of the aspects of starting the business.
- Years Two to Five: This time period is for tending to the business, its clientele, and its employees and for growing and expanding the business so that it is profitable.
- Years Five to Ten: This time period, if successfully achieved, can be for adding more locations, expanding the scope of the business (e.g., adding spa services), construction of a larger space, or anything else you or your clients need and want.
- Years Eleven to Twenty: In this time period, you may want to move from being a working cosmetologist into a full-time manager of the overall business and to begin planning for your eventual retirement.

© Yuri Arcurs, 2010; used under license from Shutterstock.com.

- Year Twenty Onward: This may be the perfect time to consider selling your successful business or changing it in some way, such as taking on a junior partner and training him or her to take over the day-to-day operations of the business so you can have time away from the business to explore interests or hobbies.

Determine Business Feasibility

Determining whether or not the business you envision is feasible means addressing certain practical issues. For example, do you have a special skill or talent that can help you set your business apart from other salons in your area? Does the town or area in which you are planning to locate the business offer you the appropriate type of clientele for the products and services you want to offer? Based on what you envision for the business, how much money will you need to open the business? Is this funding available to you?

Choose a Business Name

The name you select for your business explains what it is and can also identify characteristics that set your business apart from competitors in the marketplace. The name you select for your business will also influence how clients and potential clients perceive the business. The name will create a picture of your business in clients' minds, and once that picture exists it can be very difficult to change it if you are not satisfied.

Choose a Location

You will want to base your business location on your primary clientele and their needs. Select a location that has good visibility, high traffic, easy access, sufficient parking, and handicap access (**Figure 32–2**).

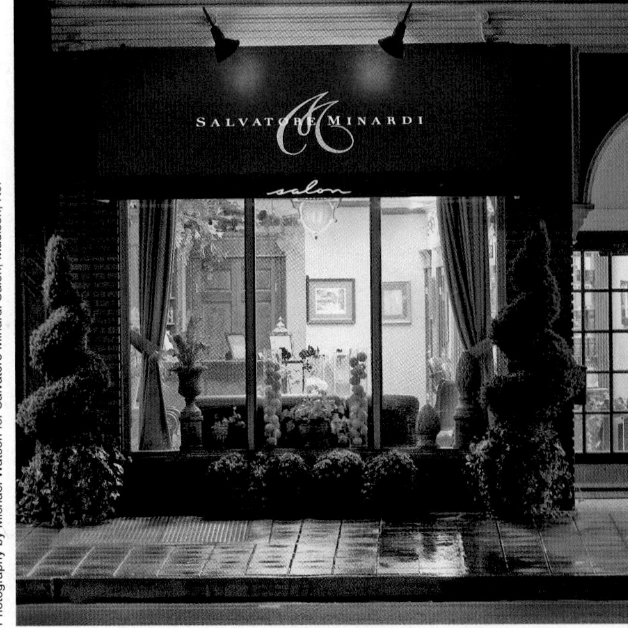

Photography by Michael Watson for Salvatore Minardi Salon, Madison, NJ.

▲ Figure 32–2
Location. Location. Location. Your salon should have good visibility and high pedestrian traffic.

Written Agreements

Many **written agreements** and documents govern the opening of a salon, including leases, vendor contracts, employee contracts, and more. All of these written agreements detail, usually for legal purposes, who does what and what is given in return. You must be able to read and understand them. Additionally, before you open a salon, you must develop a **business plan**, a written description of your business as you see it today and as you foresee it in the next five years (detailed by year). A business plan is more of an agreement with yourself, and it is not legally binding. However, if you wish to obtain financing, it is essential that you have a business plan in place first. The plan should include a general description of the business and the services that it will provide; area **demographics**, which consist of information about a specific population, including data on race, age, income, and educational attainment; expected salaries and cost of related benefits; an operations plan that includes pricing structure and expenses, such as equipment, supplies, repairs, advertising, taxes, and insurance;

and projected income and overhead expenses for up to five years. A certified public accountant (CPA) can be invaluable in helping you gather accurate financial information. The Chamber of Commerce in your proposed area typically has information on area demographics. LO3

did you know?

There are many useful resources for new business owners available online. Try these sites for great information:

- http://www.entrepreneur.com
- http://www.sbaonline.sba.gov
- http://www.score.org
- http://www.sba.gov

Business Regulations and Laws

Business regulations and laws are any and all local, state, and federal regulations and laws that you must comply with when you decide to open your salon or rent a booth. Since the laws vary from state to state and from city to city, it is important that you contact your local authorities regarding business licenses, permits, and other regulations, such as zoning and business inspections. Additionally, you must know and comply with all federal Occupational Safety and Health Administration (OSHA) guidelines, including those requiring that information about the ingredients of cosmetic preparations be available to employees. OSHA requires Material Safety Data Sheets (MSDSs) for this purpose. There are also many federal laws that apply to hiring and firing, payment of benefits, contributions to employee entitlements (e.g., social security and unemployment), and workplace behavior.

Insurance

When you open your business, you will need to purchase **insurance** that guarantees protection against financial loss from malpractice, property liability, fire, burglary and theft, and business interruption. You will need to have disability policies as well. Make sure that your policies cover you for all the monetary demands you will have to meet on your lease.

Salon Operation

Business or **salon operation** refers to the ongoing, recurring processes or activities involved in the running of a business for the purpose of producing income and value.

Record Keeping

Record keeping is the act of maintaining accurate and complete records of all financial activities in your business.

Salon Policies

Salon policies are the rules and regulations adopted by a salon to ensure that all clients and associates are being treated fairly and consistently. Even small salons and booth renters should have salon policies in place.

Types of Salon Ownership

A salon can be owned and operated by an individual, a partnership, or a corporation. Before deciding which type of ownership is most desirable for your situation, research each option thoroughly. There are excellent reference tools available, and you can also consult a small business attorney for advice.

Individual Ownership

If you like to make your own rules and are responsible enough to meet all the duties and obligations of running a business, individual ownership may be the best arrangement for you.

The **sole proprietor** is the individual owner and, most often, the manager of the business who:

- Determines policies and has the last say in decision making.
- Assumes expenses, receives profits, and bears all losses.

Partnership

Partnerships may mean more opportunity for increased investment and growth. They can be magical if the right chemistry exists, or they can be disastrous if you find yourself linked with someone you wish you had known better in the first place. Your partner can incur losses or debts that you may not even be aware of, unless you use a third-party accountant. Trust is just one of the requirements for this arrangement.

In a **partnership** business structure two or more people share ownership, although not necessarily equally.

- One reason for going into a partnership arrangement is to have more **capital** or money to invest in a business; another is to have help running your operation.
- Partners also pool their skills and talents, making it easier to share work, responsibilities, and decision making (**Figure 32–3**).
- Keep in mind that partners must assume one another's liability for debts.

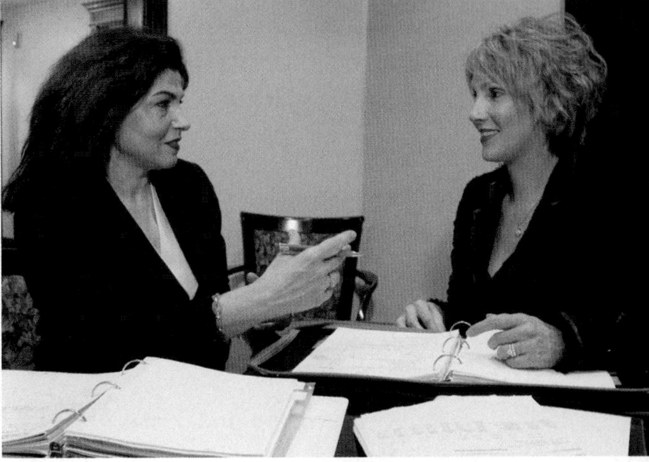

© Milady, a part of Cengage Learning. Photography by Paul Castle.

▲ **Figure 32–3**
Partners share the rewards and the responsibilities.

Corporation

A **corporation** is an ownership structure controlled by one or more stockholders. Incorporating is one of the best ways that a business owner can protect her or his personal assets. Most people choose to incorporate solely for this reason, but there are other advantages as well. For example, the corporate business structure saves you money in taxes, provides greater business flexibility, and makes raising capital easier. It also limits your personal financial liability if your business accrues unmanageable debts or otherwise runs into financial trouble.

Characteristics of corporations are generally as follows:

- Corporations raise capital by issuing stock certificates or shares.
- Stockholders (people or companies that purchase shares) have an ownership interest in the company. The more stock they own, the bigger that interest becomes.
- You can be the sole stockholder (or shareholder), or you can have many stockholders.

- Corporate formalities, such as director and stockholder meetings, are required to maintain a corporate status.
- Income tax is limited to the salary that you draw and not the total profits of the business.
- Corporations cost more to set up and run than a sole proprietorship or partnership. For example, there are the initial formation fees, filing fees, and annual state fees.
- A stockholder of a corporation is required to pay unemployment insurance taxes on his or her salary, whereas a sole proprietor or partner is not.

FYI

When you open your own business, you should consult with an attorney and an accountant before filing any documents to legalize your business. Your attorney will advise you of the legal documents and obligations that you will take on as a business owner, and your accountant can inform you of the ways in which your business may be registered for tax purposes.

Franchise Ownership

A franchise is a form of business organization in which a firm that is already successful (the franchisor) enters into a continuing contractual relationship with other businesses (franchisees) operating under the franchisor's trade name in exchange for a fee. When you operate a franchise salon, you usually operate under the franchisor's guidance and must adhere to a contract with many stipulations. These stipulations ensure that all locations in the franchise are run in a similar manner, look the same way, use the same logos, and sometimes, even train the same way or carry the same retail products.

Franchises offer the advantage of a known name and brand recognition, and the franchisor does most of the marketing for you. Also, many have protected territories, meaning another franchise salon with the same name cannot open up within your fixed geographic area. However, franchise agreements vary widely in what you can and cannot do on your own. Owning a franchise is no guarantee of making a profit, and you should always research the franchise, talk to other owners of the franchise's salons, and have an attorney read the contract and explain anything you do not understand, including your precise obligations and arrangements for paying the franchise fee. In most cases, whether or not you are profitable, you must pay the fee.

Business Plan

Regardless of the type of salon you plan to own, it is imperative to have a thorough and well-researched business plan. Remember, the business plan is a written plan of a business as it is seen in the present and envisioned in the future, and it follows your business throughout the entire process from start-up through many years in the future. Many, many books, classes, DVDs, and Web sites offer much more detailed information than can be provided here, but below is a sampling of the kind of information and material that a business plan should include.

- **Executive Summary.** Summarizes your plan and states your objectives.
- **Vision Statement.** A long-term picture of what the business is to become and what it will look like when it gets there.

- **Mission Statement.** A description of the key strategic influences of the business, such as the market it will serve, the kinds of services it will offer, and the quality of those services.
- **Organizational Plan.** Outlines employees and management levels and also describes how the business will run administratively.
- **Marketing Plan.** Outlines all of the research obtained regarding the clients your business will target and their needs, wants, and habits.
- **Financial Documents.** Includes the projected financial statements, actual (historical) statements, and financial statement analysis.
- **Supporting Documents.** Includes owner's resume, personal financial information, legal contracts, and any other agreements.
- **Salon Policies.** Even small salons and booth renters should have policies that they adhere to. These ensure that all clients and employees are treated fairly and consistently. LO5

Purchasing an Established Salon

Purchasing an existing salon could be an excellent opportunity, but, as with anything else, you have to look at all sides of the picture. If you choose to buy an established salon, seek professional assistance from an accountant and a business lawyer (**Figure 32–4**). You can purchase all the assets of a salon, or some or all of its stock. In general, any agreement to buy an established salon should include the following items:

- A financial audit to determine the actual value of the business once the current owner's bookings are taken out of the equation. Often, the salon owner brings in the bulk of the business income, and it is unlikely you will retain all the former owner's clients without a lot of support and encouragement from that former owner. Any existing financial statements should also be audited.
- Written purchase and sale agreement to avoid any misunderstandings between the contracting parties.
- Complete and signed statement of inventory (goods, fixtures, and the like) indicating the value of each article.
- If there is a transfer of a note, mortgage, lease, or bill of sale, the buyer should initiate an investigation to determine whether there are defaults in the payment of debts.
- Confirmed identity of owner.
- Use of the salon's name and reputation for a definite period of time.
- Disclosure of any and all information regarding the salon's clientele and its purchasing and service habits.

did you know?

Your accountant may suggest that your business become an S Corporation (Small Business Corporation), which is a business elected for S Corporation status through the IRS. This status allows the taxation of the company to be similar to a partnership or sole proprietor as opposed to paying taxes based on a corporate tax structure. Or your accountant may suggest that your business become registered as an LLC (Limited Liability Company), which is a type of business ownership combining several features of corporation and partnership structures. Owners of an LLC also have the liability protection of a corporation. An LLC exists as a separate entity, much like a corporation. Members cannot be held personally liable for debts unless they have signed a personal guarantee. LO4

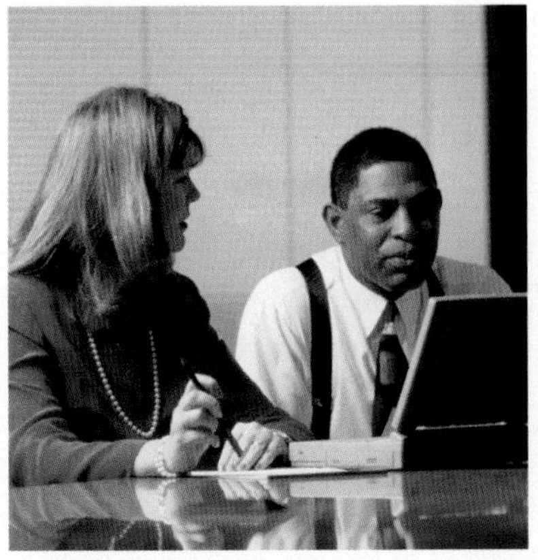

Courtesy of Getty Images.

▲ Figure 32–4
A lawyer specializing in leases and business sales is a good source of professional advice.

ACTivity

Form student groups to plan the practical side of your own salons. Divide into teams. Designate certain tasks to specific team members, or decide if everyone will work on every task as a group. Each group should perform the following tasks:

- Decide on a name for their salon.
- Determine what services will be offered.
- Create fun signage for the salon's exterior.
- Write a vision statement for the salon.
- Write a mission statement for the salon.
- Create an organizational plan and a marketing plan for their salons.

Most students will not be able to develop complex budgets, but if you feel up to it, decide on a specific budget and allocate it to key areas, such as decorating, equipment, supplies and personnel. Ask your instructors to provide feedback about whether your budget is realistic.

- Disclosure of the conditions of the facility. If you are buying the actual building, a full inspection is in order, and many other legalities apply. Be guided by your realtor and attorney.
- Noncompete agreement stating that the seller will not work in or establish a new salon within a specified distance from the present location.
- An employee agreement, either formal or informal, that lets you know if the employees will stay with the business under its new ownership. Existing employee contracts should be transferable.

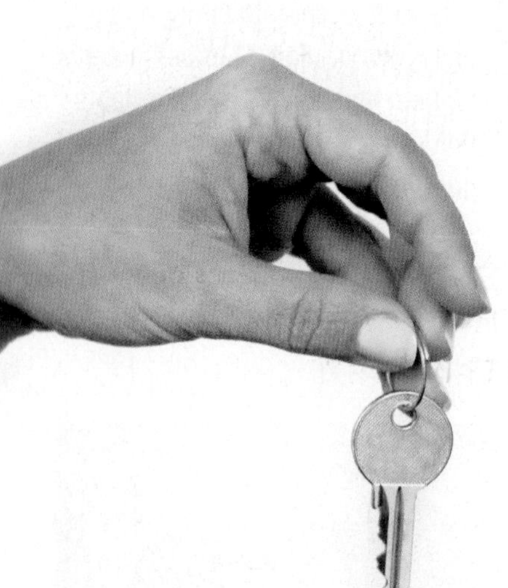

© Tiago Jorge da Silva Estima, 2010; used under license from Shutterstock.com.

Drawing Up a Lease

In most cases, owning your own business does not mean that you own the building that houses your business. When renting or leasing space, you must have an agreement between yourself and the building's owner that has been well thought out and well written. The lease should specify clearly who owns what and who is responsible for which repairs and expenses. You should also secure the following:

- Exemption of fixtures or appliances that might be attached to the salon so that they can be removed without violating the lease.
- Agreement about necessary renovations and repairs, such as painting, plumbing, fixtures, and electrical installation.
- Option from the landlord that allows you to assign the lease to another person. In this way, obligations for the payment of rent are kept separate from the responsibilities of operating the business, should you decide to bring in another person or owner.

Protection Against Fire, Theft, and Lawsuits

- Ensure that your business has adequate locks, fire alarm system, and burglar alarm system.

- Purchase liability, fire, malpractice, and burglary insurance, and do not allow these policies to lapse while you are in business.
- Become thoroughly familiar with all laws governing cosmetology and with the safety and infection control codes of your city and state.
- Keep accurate records of the number of employees, their salaries, lengths of employment, and Social Security numbers as required by various state and federal laws that monitor the social welfare of workers.
- Ignorance of the law is no excuse for violating it. Always check with your regulatory agency if you have any questions about a law or regulation.

▼ Figure 32–5
Coaching a new stylist.

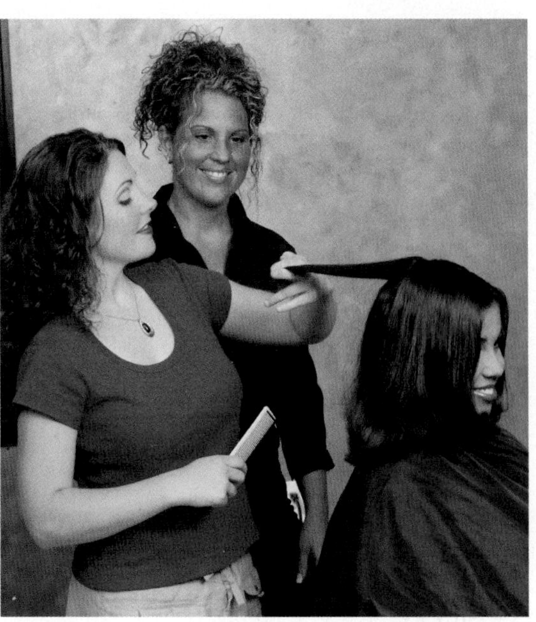

© Milady, a part of Cengage Learning. Photography by Paul Castle.

Business Operations

Whether you are an owner or a manager, there are certain skills that you must develop in order to successfully run a salon. To run a people-oriented business, you need:

- An excellent business sense, aptitude, good judgment, and diplomacy.
- A knowledge of sound business principles.

Because it takes time to develop these skills, you would be wise to establish a circle of contacts—business owners, including some salon owners—who can give you advice along the way. Consider joining a local entrepreneurs' group or your city's Chamber of Commerce in order to extend the reach of your networking.

Smooth business management depends on the following factors:

- Sufficient investment capital
- Efficiency of management
- Good business procedures
- Strong computer skills
- Cooperation between management and employees
- Trained and experienced salon personnel (**Figure 32–5**)
- Excellent customer service delivery
- Proper pricing of services (**Figure 32–6**)

▼ Figure 32–6
Typical salon price list.

STYLES BY DOTTI

Haircuts	
Designer cuts for women	$40
Men's cut	$25
Children's cut	starting at $15
Formal updos	starting at $45
Haircolor Services	
Virgin application, single-process	starting at $40
Color retouch	starting at $35
Double-process	starting at $55
Dimensional highlighting (full head)	$75
Dimensional highlighting (partial head)	$60
Texture Services	
Customized perming*	starting at $80
Spiral perm*	starting at $100

**Includes complimentary home-maintenance product.*

© Milady, a part of Cengage Learning.

Allocation of Money

As a business operator, you must always know where your money is being spent. A good accountant and an accounting system are indispensable. The figures in **Table 32–1** serve as a guideline, but may vary depending on locality.

The Importance of Record Keeping

Good business operations require a simple and efficient record system. Proper business records are necessary to meet the requirements of local, state, and federal laws regarding taxes and employees. Records are of value only if they are correct, concise, and complete. Proper bookkeeping methods include keeping an accurate record of all income and expenses. Income is usually classified as receipts from services and retail sales. Expenses include rent, utilities, insurance, salaries, advertising, equipment, and repairs. Retain check stubs, canceled checks, receipts, and invoices. A professional accountant or a full-charge bookkeeper is recommended to help keep records accurate (**Table 32–1**).

FINANCIAL BENCHMARKS FOR SALONS IN THE UNITED STATES

EXPENSES	PERCENT OF TOTAL GROSS INCOME
SALARIES AND COMMISSIONS (INCLUDING PAYROLL TAXES)	53.5
RENT	13.0
SUPPLIES	5.0
ADVERTISING	3.0
DEPRECIATION	3.0
LAUNDRY	1.0
CLEANING	1.0
LIGHT AND POWER	1.0
REPAIRS	1.5
INSURANCE	0.75
TELEPHONE	0.75
MISCELLANEOUS	1.5
TOTAL EXPENSES	85.0
NET PROFIT	15.0
TOTAL	100.0

Courtesy Kopsa Otte CPAs & Advisors in York, NE, nationally known as the only accounting firm that specializes in salons and spas.

Table 32–1 **Financial Benchmarks for Salons in the United States.**

The term *full-charge bookkeeper* refers to someone who is trained to do everything from recording sales and payroll, to generating a profit-and-loss statement.

Purchase and Inventory Records

The purchase of inventory and supplies should be closely monitored. Purchase records help you maintain a perpetual inventory, which prevents overstocking or a shortage of needed supplies, and they alert you to any incidents of theft. Purchase records also help establish the net worth of the business at the end of the year.

Keep a running inventory of all supplies, and classify them according to their use and retail value. Those to be used in the daily business operation are **consumption supplies** (**Figure 32–7**). Those to be sold to clients are **retail supplies**.

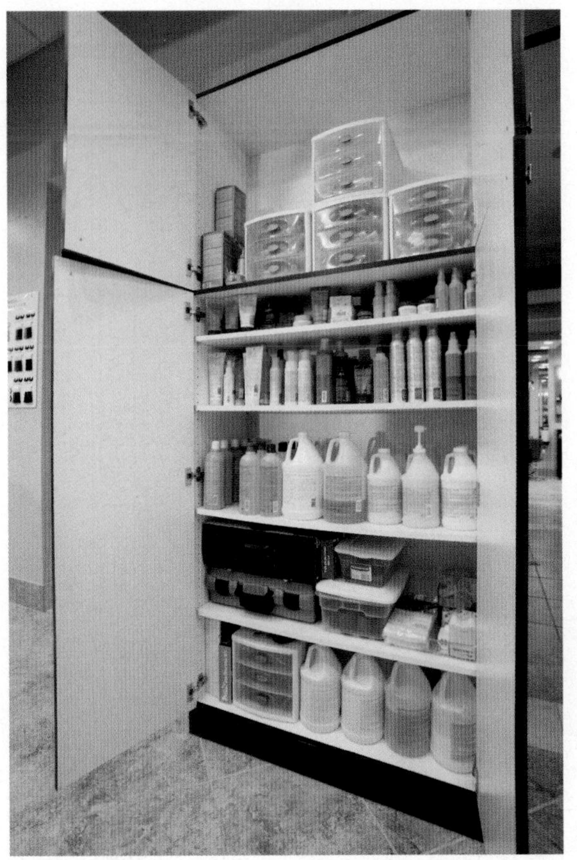

© Milady, a part of Cengage Learning. Photography by Paul Castle.

▲ Figure 32–7
Inventory of consumption supplies.

Service Records

Always keep service records or client cards that describe treatments given and merchandise sold to each client. Using a salon-specific software program for this purpose is highly recommended. All service records should include the name and address of the client, the date of each purchase or service, the amount charged, the products used, and the results obtained. Clients' preferences and tastes should also be noted. For more information on filling out these cards, and for examples of a client record card, see Chapter 4, Communicating for Success. ✓ LO6

Operating a Successful Salon

The only way to guarantee that you will stay in business and have a prosperous salon is to take excellent care of your clients. Clients visiting your salon should feel that they are being well taken care of, and they should always have reason to look forward to their next visit. To accomplish this, your salon must be physically attractive, well organized, smoothly run, and, above all, sparkling clean.

Planning the Salon's Layout

One of the most exciting opportunities ahead of you is planning and constructing the best physical layout for the type of salon you envision. Maximum efficiency should be the primary concern. For example, if you are opening a low-budget salon offering quick service, you will need several stations and a small- to medium-sized reception area because clients will be moving in and out of the salon fairly quickly. Your retail

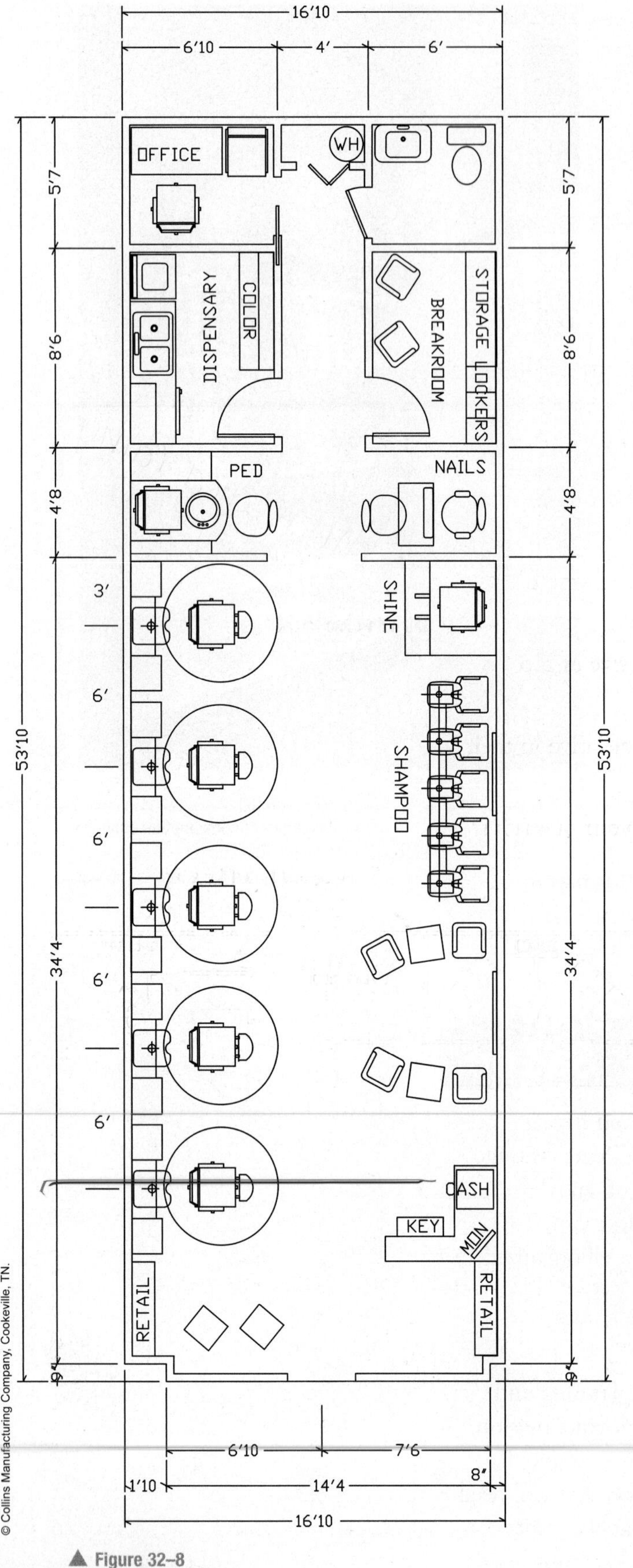

© Collins Manufacturing Company, Cookeville, TN.

▲ **Figure 32–8**
Layout for a typical salon.

area may be on the small side because your clients may not have a lot of disposable income to spend on retail products (**Figure 32–8**).

However, if you are opening a high-end salon or luxurious day spa where clients expect the quality of the service to be matched by the environment, you will want to plan for more room in the waiting area. You may, in fact, choose to have several areas in which clients can lounge between services and enjoy beverages or light snacks. The spa area and quiet rooms should be separated from busy, noisy areas where hair services are performed. Some upscale salons feature small coffee bars that lend an air of sophistication to the environment. Others offer quiet, private areas where clients can pursue business activities, such as phone or laptop work between services. The retail area should be spacious, inviting, and well lit. High-end salons and spas are extremely costly to design, construct, and maintain. Construction alone can be upward of $300 per square foot.

Layout is crucial to the smooth operation of a salon. Once you have decided the type of salon that you wish to run, seek the advice of an architect with plenty of experience in designing salons. For renovations, a professional equipment and furniture supplier will be able to help you (**Figure 32–9**).

Costs to create even a small salon in an existing space can range from $75 to $125 per square foot. Renovating existing space requires familiarity with building codes and the landlord's restrictions before you do anything. All the plumbing should be in the same area, and electrical wiring must be up to code. If they are not, you'll pay thousands extra. Before you begin, get everything in writing from contractors, design firms, equipment manufacturers, and architects. Get more than one quote on everything from cleaning services to salon stations, and negotiate whenever you can (**Figure 32–10**).

Try to estimate how much each area in the salon will earn, so you can use space efficiently. An inviting retail display in your reception area is a good investment; on the other hand, an employee break area produces no income. In addition to start-up costs for creating your salon, you'll need financing for operational expenses. Realistically, you should plan to have several months of expenses available to help get you up and running. It takes most new salons about six months to begin operating at full capacity. ✓ LO7

Personnel

Your **personnel** is your staff or employees. The size of your salon will determine the size of your staff. Large salons and day spas require receptionists, hairstylists, nail technicians, shampoo persons, colorists, massage therapists, estheticians, and hair removal specialists.

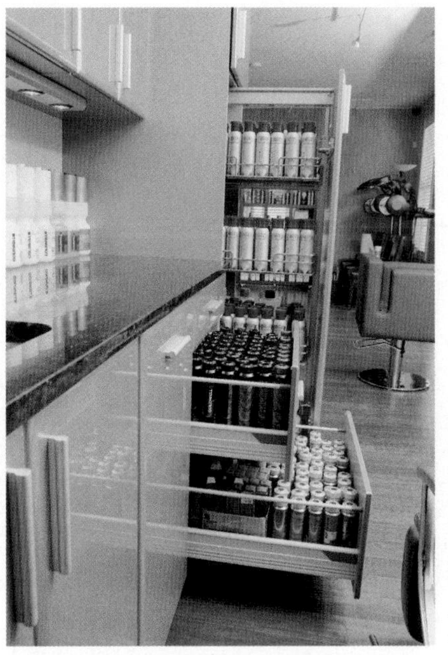

Courtesy of Diane Hughes Photography.

▲ **Figure 32–9**
Salon haircolor dispensary.

Smaller salons have some combination of these personnel who perform more than one type of service. For example, a stylist might also be the colorist and texture specialist. The success of a salon depends on the quality of the work done by the staff.

When interviewing potential employees, consider the following:

- **Level of skill.** What is their educational background? When was the last time they attended an educational event?
- **Personal grooming.** Do they look like professionals you would consult for personal grooming advice?
- **Image as it relates to the salon.** Are they too progressive or too conservative for your environment?
- **Overall attitude.** Are they mostly positive or mostly negative in their responses to your questions?
- **Communication skills.** Are they able to understand your questions? Can you understand their responses?

Making good hiring decisions is crucial. Undoing bad hiring decisions is painful for all involved, and it can be more complicated than one might expect.

▼ **Figure 32–10**
A typical layout for a larger spa/salon.

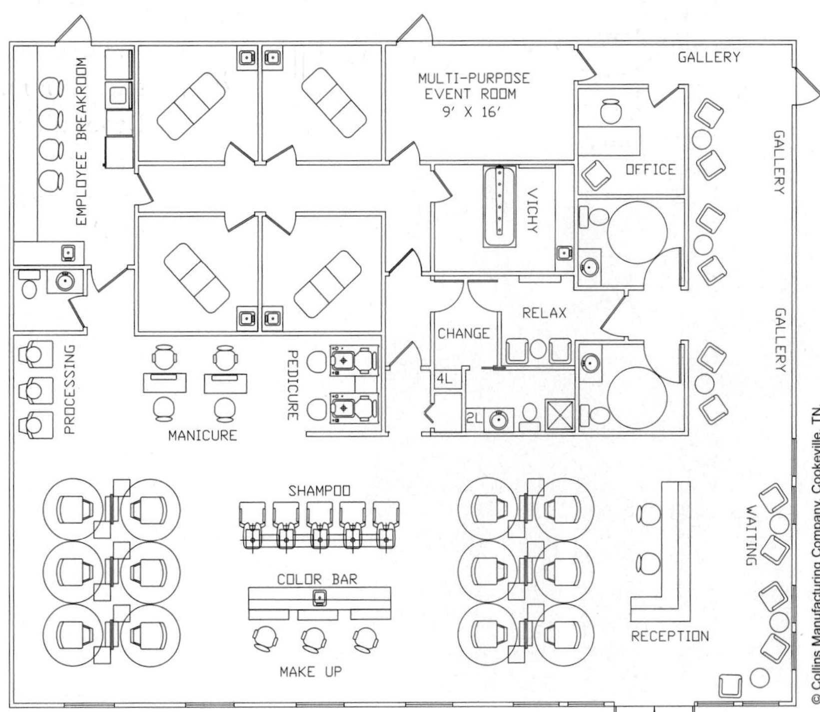

© Collins Manufacturing Company, Cookeville, TN.

Payroll and Employee Benefits

In order to have a successful business, one in which everyone feels appreciated and is happy to work hard to service clients well, you must be willing to share your success with your staff whenever it is financially feasible to do so. You can do this in a number of ways.

- Make it your top priority to meet your payroll obligations. In the allotment of funds, this comes first. It will also be your largest expense.
- Whenever possible, offer hardworking and loyal employees as many benefits as possible. Either

ACTivity

What would your dream salon look like? Try your hand at designing a salon that would attract the kinds of clients you want, offer the services you would like to specialize in, and provide an efficient, comfortable working environment for cosmetology professionals.

Draw pictures, use word pictures, or try a combination of both. Pay attention to practical requirements, but feel free to dream a little, too. Skylights? Fountains? You name it. It's your dream (**Figure 32–11**)!

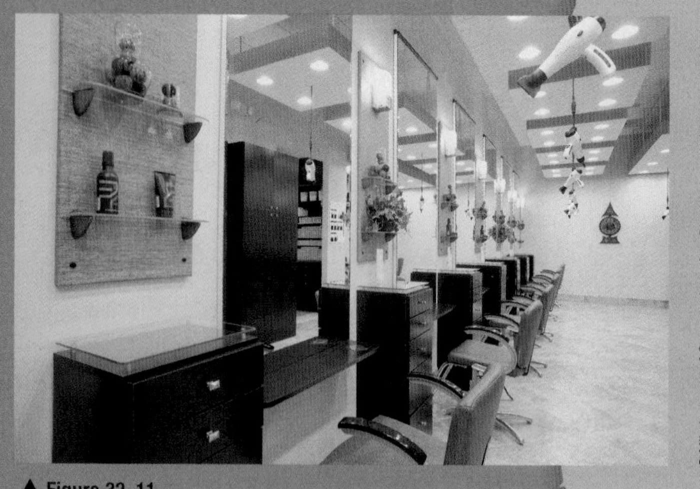

▲ **Figure 32–11**
What does your dream salon look like?

© Milady, a part of Cengage Learning. Photography by Dino Petrocelli.

cover the cost of these benefits or simply make them available to employees, who can decide if they can cover the cost themselves.

- Provide staff members with a schedule of employee evaluations. Make it clear what is expected of them if they are to receive pay increases.
- Create and stay with a tipping policy. It is a good idea both for your employees and your clients to know exactly what is expected.
- Put your entire pay plan in writing.
- Create incentives by giving your staff opportunities to earn more money, prizes, or tickets to educational events and trade shows.
- Create salon policies and stick to them. Everyone in the salon should be governed by the same rules, including you!

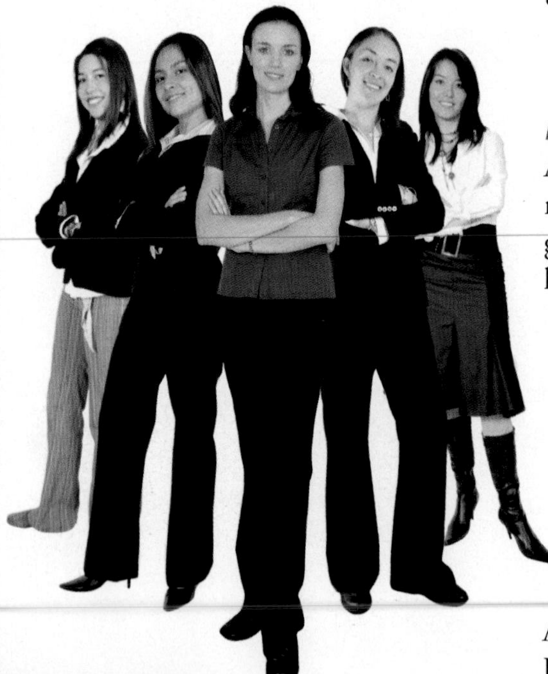

© Andresr, 2010; used under license from Shutterstock.com.

Managing Personnel

As a new salon owner, one of your most difficult tasks will be managing your staff. But this can also be very rewarding. If you are good at managing others, you can make a positive impact on their lives and their ability to earn a living. If managing people does not come naturally, do not despair. People can learn how to manage other people, just as they learn how to drive a car or perform hair services. Keep in mind that managing others is a serious job. Whether it comes naturally to you or not, it takes time to become comfortable with the role.

Human Resources, or HR, is an entire specialty in its own right. It not only covers how you manage employees, it also covers what you can and cannot say when hiring, managing, or firing. All employers must be familiar with various civil rights laws, including Equal Employment Opportunity Commission (EEOC) regulations, and the Americans with Disabilities Act (ADA), which pertains to hiring and firing, as well as business design for accessibility. Every business should have a written personnel policies and a procedures manual, and every employee must read and sign it. The more documented systems you have for managing human resources, the better.

There are many excellent books, both within and outside the professional salon industry, that you can use as resources for learning about managing employees and staff. Spend an afternoon online or at your local bookstore researching the topic and purchasing materials that will educate and inform you. Once you have a broad base of information, you will be able to select a technique or style that best suits your personality and that of your salon.

The Front Desk

Most salon owners believe that the quality and pricing of services are the most important elements of running a successful salon. Certainly these are crucial, but too often the front desk—the operations center—is overlooked. The best salons employ professional receptionists to handle the job of scheduling appointments and greeting clients.

The Reception Area

First impressions count, and since the reception area is the first thing clients see, it needs to be attractive, appealing, and comfortable. This is your salon's nerve center, where your receptionist will sit, where retail merchandise will be on display, and where the phone system is centered.

Make sure that the reception area is stocked with business cards and a prominently displayed price list that shows at a glance what your clients should expect to pay for various services.

The Receptionist

When it comes to staffing, your receptionist is second in importance only to your licensed professionals. A well-trained receptionist is crucial because the receptionist is the first person the client contacts. The receptionist should be pleasant, greet each client with a smile, and address each client by name. Efficient, friendly service fosters goodwill, confidence, and satisfaction.

In addition to filling the crucial role of greeter, the receptionist handles other important functions, including answering the phone, booking appointments, informing professionals that a client has arrived, preparing daily appointment information for the staff, and recommending additional services to clients. The receptionist should have a thorough knowledge of all retail products carried by the salon so that she or he can also serve as a salesperson and information source for clients (**Figure 32–12**).

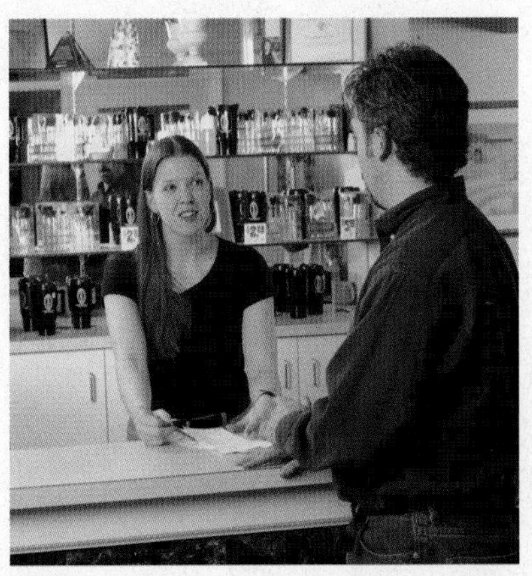

© Milady, a part of Cengage Learning. Photography by Paul Castle.

▲ Figure 32–12
A good receptionist is key to a salon's success.

During slow periods, it is customary for the receptionist to perform certain other duties and activities, such as straightening up the reception area and maintaining inventory and daily reports. The receptionist should also use slow times for making any necessary personal calls or otherwise being away from the front desk.

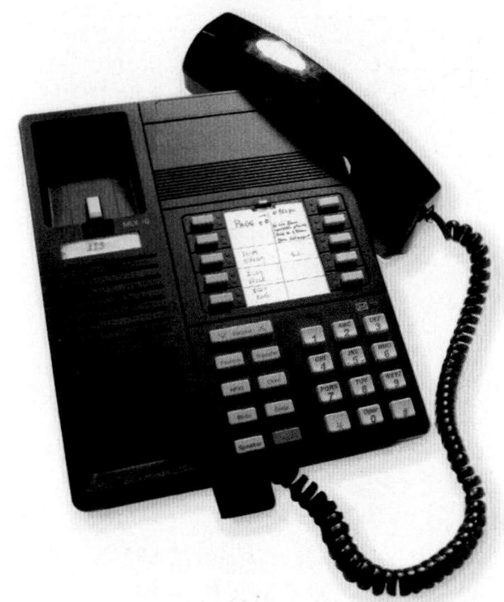

© Donald R. Swartz, 2010; used under license from Shutterstock.com.

Booking Appointments

One of the most important duties the receptionist has is booking appointments. This must be done with care because services are sold in terms of time on the appointment page. Appointments must be scheduled to make the most efficient use of everyone's time. Under ideal circumstances, a client should not have to wait for a service, and a professional should not have to wait for the next client.

Booking appointments is primarily the receptionist's job, but when she is not available, the salon owner or manager or any of the other professionals can help with scheduling. Therefore, it is important for each person in the salon to understand how to book an appointment and how much time is needed for each service. Regardless of who actually makes the appointment, anyone who answers the phone or deals with clients must have a pleasing voice and personality.

In addition, the receptionist must have the following qualities:

- Appearance that conveys your salon's image
- Knowledge of the various services offered
- Unlimited patience with both clients and salon personnel

Appointment Book

The appointment book helps professionals arrange time to suit their clients' needs. It should accurately reflect what is taking place in the salon at any given time. In most salons, the receptionist prepares the appointment schedule for staff members; in smaller salons, each person may prepare his own schedule (**Figure 32–13**).

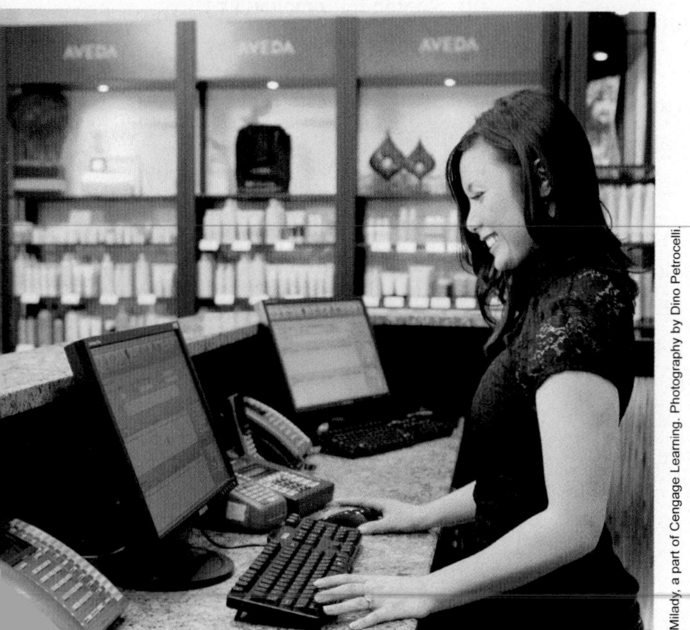

▼ Figure 32–13
Computerized appointment book.

© Milady, a part of Cengage Learning. Photography by Dino Petrocelli.

Increasingly, the appointment book is a computerized book that is easily accessed through the salon's computer system. It may also be an actual hard copy book that is located on the reception desk. Some salons have Web sites with online booking systems, that tie in to salon management software.

Use of the Telephone in the Salon

An important part of the business is handled over the telephone. Good telephone habits and techniques make it possible for the salon owner and employees to increase business and improve relationships with clients and suppliers. With each call, a gracious, appropriate response will help build the salon's reputation.

Good Planning

Because it can be noisy, business calls to clients and suppliers should be made at a quiet time of the day or from a quiet area of the salon.

When using the telephone, you should:

- Have a pleasant telephone voice, speak clearly, and use correct grammar. A smile in your voice counts for a lot.
- Show interest and concern when talking with a client or a supplier.
- Be polite, respectful, and courteous to all, even though some people may test the limits of your patience.
- Be tactful. Do not say anything to irritate the person on the other end of the line.

Incoming Telephone Calls

Incoming phone calls are the lifeline of a salon. Clients usually call ahead for appointments with a preferred stylist, or they might call to cancel or reschedule an appointment. The person answering the phone should have the necessary telephone skills to handle these calls. The following section offers additional guidelines for answering the telephone.

When you answer the phone, say, "Good morning (afternoon or evening), Milady Salon. May I help you?" or "Thank you for calling Milady Salon. This is Jane speaking. How may I help you?" Some salons require that you give your name to the caller. The first words you say tell the caller something about your personality. Let callers know that you are glad to hear from them.

Answer the phone promptly. On a system with more than one line, if a call comes in while you are talking on another line, ask to put the first person on hold, answer the second call, and ask that person to hold while you complete the first call. Take calls in the order in which they are received.

If you do not have the information requested by a caller, either put the caller on hold and get the information, or offer to call the person back with the information as soon as you have it.

Do not talk with a client standing nearby while you are speaking with someone on the phone. You are doing a disservice to both clients.

Booking Appointments by Phone

When booking appointments, take down the client's first and last name, their phone number, and the service booked. Many salons call the client to confirm the appointment one or two days before it is scheduled. Automated systems can send an e-mail or even a text message confirmation.

You should be familiar with all the services and products available in the salon and their costs, as well as which cosmetology professionals perform specific services, such as color correction. Be fair when making

WEB RESOURCES

This chapter provides a general overview of the complex issues involved in salon ownership. There are many resources on the Internet for further study. These can get you started:

Design

- http://www.beautydesign.com

Click on the Design Center to view various salon layouts and to see salon photos of salons from all over the world.

- http://www.collinsmfgco.com

Get an overview of equipment, furniture, and its costs. This site includes a multi-cultural product category.

- http://www.momoy.com

At the search line, enter: salon spa layouts.

Human Resources

- http://www.dol.gov/compliance/guide

The Department of Labor's Web site. Search for: employment law guide.

- http://www.eeoc.gov

Research relevant equal employment opportunity regulations; check out the compliance manual.

- http://hr.blr.com

Human resources—related business and legal reports. Find a forum, dozens of topics, and regulations by state.

Continued next page

WEB RESOURCES

Small Business Ownership and Operation

- http://www.business.com
Advice on business topics from A to Z and business resources for accounting, sales, marketing, technology, and more.

- http://www.isquare.com
The Small Business Advisor.

- http://www.salonbuilder.com
Information on starting a salon.

- http://www.smallbusinessnotes.com
Various business-related articles.

- http://www.strategies.com
The source for salon business growth seminars, training, and coaching.

Salon Software

- http://www.harms-software.com
- http://www.shortcuts.net
- http://www.salonbiz.com
- http://www.salon2k.com
- http://www.salon-software.com

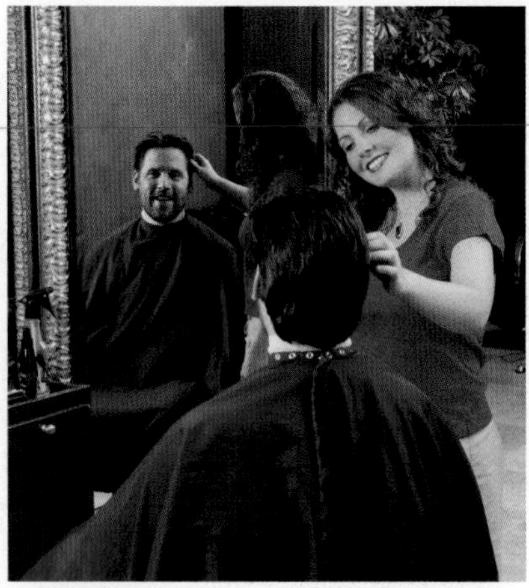

© Milady, a part of Cengage Learning. Photography by Paul Castle.

▲ Figure 32–14
Customer satisfaction is your best advertising.

assignments. Don't schedule six appointments for one professional and only two for another, unless it's necessary because you are working with specialists.

However, if someone calls to ask for an appointment with a particular cosmetology professional on a particular day and time, make every effort to accommodate the client's request. If the professional is not available when the client requests, there are several ways to handle the situation:

- Suggest other times that the professional is available.
- If the client cannot come in at any of those times, suggest another professional.
- If the client is unwilling to try another professional, offer to call the client if there is a cancellation at the desired time.

Handling Complaints by Telephone

Handling complaints, particularly over the phone, is a difficult task. The caller is probably upset and short tempered. Respond with self-control, tact, and courtesy, no matter how trying the circumstances. Only then will the caller feel that she has been treated fairly.

The tone of your voice must be sympathetic and reassuring. Your manner of speaking should convince the caller that you are really concerned about the complaint. Do not interrupt the caller. After hearing the complaint in full, try to resolve the situation quickly and effectively.

Building Your Business

A new salon owner will want to get the business up and running as soon as possible to start earning some revenue and to begin paying off debts. One of the first items the new salon owner should consider is how to advertise the salon. It is important to understand the many aspects of advertising.

Advertising includes all activities that promote the salon favorably, from newspaper ads to radio spots to charity events that the salon participates in, such as fashion shows. In order to create a desire for a service or product, advertising must attract and hold the attention of readers, listeners, or viewers.

A satisfied client is the very best form of advertising because she will refer your salon to friends and family. So make your clients happy (**Figure 32–14**)! Then, develop a referral program in which both the referring client and the new client reap some sort of reward.

If you have some experience developing ads, you may decide to do your own advertising. On the other hand, if you need help, you can hire a small local agency or ask a local newspaper or radio station to help you produce the ad. As a general rule, an advertising budget should not

ACTivity

All the planning in the world can't guarantee success as much as a happy client can. Great customer service and a fabulous customer experience are the most important aspects of salon success. What will your customer service look like? Imagine you are calling or walking into your dream salon. Write down everything about your ideal experience as a customer, from the way you are greeted to the actual service to checkout at the desk when you leave. Include all five senses.

exceed 3 percent of your gross income. Plan well in advance for holidays and special yearly events, such as proms, New Year's Eve, or the wedding season.

Make certain you know what you are paying for. Get everything in writing. No form of advertising can promise that you'll get business. Sometimes, local circulars can work as well as a costly Web site. You must know your clientele, which types of media they use, and what kinds of messages attract them.

Here are some tools you may choose to use to attract customers to the salon:

- Newspaper ads and coupons (**Figure 32–15**)

Spring Specials
at
The Manor Day Spa

Celebrate the coming of spring!
Let us pamper you with one of our new deluxe packages

The Getaway:	Swedish massage, facial, manicure, pedicure, makeup, haircut and styling (includes complimentary lunch)	$200
The Refresher:	deep cleansing facial, makeup, haircut and styling	$100
Body Sensations:	aromatherapy massage, facial, makeup	$75
Tips and Toes:	spa manicure, hot stones pedicure	$55

Feb. 15 through May 15 only

Deep conditioning treatment with every haircolor service!
Call now to reserve an hour, two hours, or a whole day
of relaxation and pampering at the Manor.

Bring in this ad to receive a 5% discount on any service.

The Manor Day Spa, 123 Main Street, Hometown, USA 12345
(300-555-1111)

Open Tuesday - Friday 10-6,
Saturday 10-4

© Milady, a part of Cengage Learning.

Figure 32–15
Newspaper advertisement for services at a salon.

- Direct mail to mailing lists and your current salon client list
- Classified advertising
- E-mail newsletters and discount offers to all clients who have agreed to receive such mailings (Always include an *Unsubscribe* link.)
- Web site offerings, including those on your own Web site, social networking Web sites, and blogs
- Giveaway promotional items or retail packages, such as "Buy a shampoo and conditioner, and get a hairbrush for free."
- Window displays that attract attention and feature the salon and your retail products
- Radio advertising
- Television advertising
- Community outreach by volunteering at women's and men's clubs, church functions, political gatherings, charitable affairs, and on TV and radio talk shows
- Client referrals
- In-salon videos that promote your services and products

Many of these vehicles can help you attract new clients, but the first goal of every business should be to maintain current clients. It takes at least three salon visits for a new client to become a loyal current client. Once you have a loyal client base, it is far less expensive to market to that base. That is why you should follow up every visit to determine the client's satisfaction and why you should personally contact any client who has not been in the salon for more than eight weeks.

▼ Figure 32–16
Selling retail products benefits everyone.

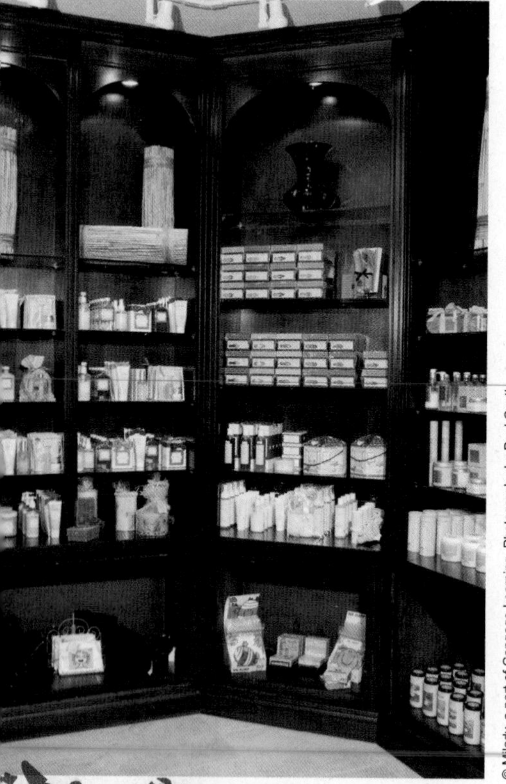

© Milady, a part of Cengage Learning. Photography by Paul Castle.

Selling in the Salon

An important aspect of the salon's financial success revolves around the sale of additional salon services and take-home or maintenance products. Whether you own or manage a large salon with several employees or you are a booth renter with only yourself to worry about, adding services or retail sales to your service ticket means additional revenue.

In general, beauty professionals seem to feel uncomfortable about having to make sales of products or additional services. It is important to work at overcoming this feeling. When professionals are reluctant to sell, it is often because they carry a negative stereotype of salespeople, and they do not want to be seen this way themselves. Helpful and knowledgeable sales professionals make customer care their top priority. These people play a major role in the lives of their customers and are very valuable to clients because they offer good advice. In fact, the successful salon owner, like the successful stylist, makes his or her living by giving complete beauty advice every day (**Figure 32–16**). ✓ **LO8**

Review Questions

1. Name and describe the two most common options for going into business for yourself.
2. What responsibilities does a booth renter assume? What are the disadvantages of booth renting?
3. List at least three of the basic factors that potential salon owners should consider before opening their business.
4. How many types of salon ownership are there? Describe each.
5. List and describe the categories of information that should be included in a business plan.
6. Why is it important to keep good records? What type of records should be kept?
7. List and describe the five elements of a successful salon.
8. Why is selling services and products such a vital aspect of a salon's success?

Chapter Glossary

booth rental	Also known as *chair rental*; renting a booth or station in a salon.
business plan	A written description of your business as you see it today, and as you foresee it in the next five years (detailed by year).
business regulations and laws	Any and all local, state, and federal regulations and laws that you must comply with when you decide to open your salon or rent a booth.
capital	Money needed to invest in a business.
consumption supplies	Supplies used in the daily business operation.
corporation	An ownership structure controlled by one or more stockholders.
demographics	Information about a specific population including data on race, age, income, and educational attainment.
goals	A set of benchmarks that, once achieved, help you to realize your mission and your vision.
insurance	Guarantees protection against financial loss from malpractice, property liability, fire, burglary and theft, and business interruption.
partnership	Business structure in which two or more people share ownership, although not necessarily equally.
personnel	Your staff or employees.

Chapter Glossary

record keeping	Maintaining accurate and complete records of all financial activities in your business.
retail supplies	Supplies sold to clients.
salon operation	The ongoing, recurring processes or activities involved in the running of a business for the purpose of producing income and value.
salon policies	The rules or regulations adopted by a salon to ensure that all clients and associates are being treated fairly and consistently.
sole proprietor	Individual owner and, most often, the manager of a business.
vision statement	A long-term picture of what the business is to become and what it will look like when it gets there.
written agreements	Documents that govern the opening of a salon, including leases, vendor contracts, employee contracts, and more; all of which detail, usually for legal purposes, who does what and what is given in return.

Appendix A: Associations

Accrediting Commission of Career Schools and Colleges (ACCSC)
2101 Wilson Boulevard, Suite 302
Arlington, VA 22201
(703) 247-4212
http://www.accsc.org

Allied Beauty Association (ABA)
145 Traders Boulevard East
Units 26 & 27
Mississauga ON L4Z 3L3
Canada
(905) 568-0158
http://www.abacanada.com

American Association of Cosmetology Schools (AACS)
9927 E. Bell Road, Suite 110
Scottsdale, AZ 85260
(800) 831-1086
http://www.beautyschools.org

American Board of Certified Haircolorists (ABHC)
PO Box 9090
San Pedro, CA 90734
(310) 547-0814
http://www.haircolorist.com

American Health & Beauty Aids Institute (AHBAI)
PO Box 19510
Chicago, IL 60619
(312) 644-6610
http://www.ahbai.org

Barbers International (BI)
2708 Pine Street
Arkadelphia, AR 71924
(870) 230-0777
http://www.barbersinternational.com

Personal Care Products Council (formerly CTFA)
1101 17th Street NW, Suite 300
Washington, DC 20036
(202) 331-1770
http://www.personalcarecouncil.com

Cosmetology Educators Association (CEA)
9927 E. Bell Road, Suite 110
Scottsdale, AZ 85260
(800) 831-1086
http://www.beautyschools.org

Cosmetology Industry Association of British Columbia (CIABC)
899 West 8th Avenue
Vancouver BC V5Z 1E3
Canada
(604) 871-0222
http://www.ciabc.net

The Day Spa Association
310 17th Street
Union City, NJ 07087
(201) 865-2065
http://www.dayspaassociation.com

Independent Cosmetic Manufacturers and Distributors (ICMAD)
1220 W. Northwest Highway
Palatine, IL 60067
(800) 334-2623
http://www.icmad.org

Intercoiffure, America • Canada
7628 Densmore Avenue
Van Nuys, CA 91406
http://www.intercoiffure.us

International Nail Technicians Association
8286 Solutions Center
Chicago, IL 60677-8002
(312) 321-5161
http://www.americasbeautynetwork.com/OURNETWORK/InternationalNailTechniciansAssociation/tabid/139/Default.aspx

International SPA Association (ISPA)
2365 Harrodsburg Road, Suite A325
Lexington, KY 40504
(888) 651-4772
http://www.experienceispa.com

National Association of Barber Boards of America (NABBA)
2703 Pine Street
Arkadelphia, AR 71923
(501) 682-2806
http://www.nationalbarberboards.com

National Accrediting Commission of Cosmetology Arts & Sciences (NACCAS)
4401 Ford Avenue, Suite 1300
Alexandria, VA 22302
(703) 600-7600
http://www.naccas.org

National Beauty Culturists League
25 Logan Circle NW
Washington, DC 20005-3725
(202) 332-2695
http://www.nbcl.org

National Coalition of Estheticians, Manufacturers/Distributors and Associations (NCEA)
484 Spring Avenue
Ridgewood, NJ 07450-4624
(201) 670-4100
http://www.ncea.tv

National Cosmetology Association (NCA)
15825 N 71st Street, Suite 100
Scottsdale, AZ 85254
(866) 871-0656
http://www.ncacares.org

National-Interstate Council of State Boards of Cosmetology (NIC)
7622 Briarwood Circle
Little Rock, AR 72205
(501) 227-8262
http://www.nictesting.org

Professional Beauty Association
15825 N. 71st Street, Suite 100
Scottsdale, AZ 85254
(800) 468-2274
http://www.probeauty.org

Society of Permanent Cosmetic Professionals
69 North Broadway
Des Plaines, IL 60016
(847) 635-1330
http://www.spcp.org

SkillsUSA (Vocational Industrial Clubs of America, Inc.)
14001 SkillsUSA Way
Leesburg, VA 20176
(703) 777-8999
http://www.skillsusa.org

Metric Conversion Tables

U.S. MEASUREMENT–METRIC CONVERSION TABLES

The following tables show standard conversions for commonly used measurements in the 2012 edition of Milady Standard Cosmetology:

Conversion Formula for Inches to Centimeters: (number of) inches x 2.54 = centimeters

LENGTH	
INCHES	**CENTIMETERS**
⅛ inch (.125 inches)	0.317 centimeters
¼ inch (.25 inches)	0.635 centimeters
½ inch (.50 inches)	1.27 centimeters
¾ inch (.75 inches)	1.9 centimeters
1 inch	2.54 centimeters
2 inches	5.1 centimeters
3 inches	7.6 centimeters
6 inches	15.2 centimeters
12 inches	30.5 centimeters

Conversion Formula for U.S. Fluid Ounces to Milliliters:
(amount of) U.S. fluid ounce (fl. oz.) x 29.573 milliliters (ml)
Conversion Formula for U.S. Fluid Ounces to Liters:
(amount of) U.S. fluid ounce (fl. oz.) x .029573 liters (l)

VOLUME (LIQUID)	
U.S. FLUID ONCES	**MILLILITERS/LITERS**
1 fluid ounce (⅛ cup)	29. 57 milliliters/.02957 liters
2 fluid ounces (¼ cup)	59.14 milliliters/.05914 liters
4 fluid ounces (½ cup)	118.29 milliliters/.11829 liters
6 fluid ounces (¾ cup)	177.43 milliliters/.17743 liters
8 fluid ounces (1 cup)	236.58 milliliters/.23658 liters
16 fluid ounces (1 pint)	473.16 milliliters/.47316 liters
32 fluid ounces (1 quart)	946.33 milliliters/.94633 liters
33.81 fluid ounces (1 liter)	1,000 milliliters/1 liter
64 fluid ounces (½ gallon)	1,892.67 milliliters/1.8926 liters
128 fluid ounces (1 gallon)	3,785.34 milliliters/3.78534 liters

Conversion Formula for Degrees Fahrenheit (°F) to Degrees Celsius (°C): °C = (°F-32) x (5/9) ***

TEMPERATURE	
DEGREES FAHRENHEIT (°F)	DEGREES CELSIUS (°C)
32°	0°
40°	4.444°
50°	10°
60°	15.556°
70°	21.111°
80°	26.667°
98.6°	37°
200°	93.333°
300°	148.889°
400°	204.444°

*** If you have a Fahrenheit temperature of 40 degrees and you want to convert it into degrees on the Celsius scale: Using the conversion formula, first subtract 32 from the Fahrenheit temperature of 40 degrees to get 8 as a result. Then multiply 8 by five and divide by nine (8 x 5)/9 to get the converted value of 4.444 degrees Celsius.

Glossary/Index

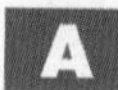

A. *See* Ampere

ABCDE Cancer Checklist, 185

Abductor digiti minimi, muscles that separate the fingers and the toes, 126

Abductor hallucis, muscle that moves the toes and helps maintain balance while walking and standing, 126

Abductors, muscles that draw a body part, such as a finger, arm, or toe, away from the midline of the body or of an extremity, 125

AC. *See* Alternating current

Accelerated hydrogen peroxide (AHP), 85

ACD. *See* Allergic contact dermatitis

Acetone, 804, 934

Acid waves, 573, 576

Acid-alkali neutralization reactions, 258

Acid-balanced shampoo, 588

Acid-balanced waves, permanent waves that have a 7.0 or neutral pH; because of their higher pH, they process at room temperature, do not require the added heat of a hair dryer, process more quickly, and produce firmer curls than true acid waves, 574

Acidic solution, a solution that has a pH below 7.0 (neutral), 257

Acne, also known as *acne vulgaris*; skin disorder characterized by chronic inflammation of the sebaceous glands from retained secretions and Propionibacterium acnes (P. acnes) bacteria, 163

signs and conditions associated with, 716

Acquired immune deficiency syndrome (AIDS), a disease that breaks down the body's immune system. AIDS is caused by the human immunodeficiency virus (HIV), 80

Acquired immunity, immunity that the body develops after overcoming a disease, through inoculation (such as flu vaccinations), or through exposure to natural allergens, such as pollen, cat dander, and ragweed, 82

Acrylonitrile butadiene styrene, also known as *ABS*; a common thermoplastic used to make light, rigid, molded nail tips, 874

Actinic light, 275

Activators, also known as *boosters*, *protinators*, and *accelerators*; powdered persulfate salts added to haircolor to increase its lightening ability, 650

Active electrode, electrode used on the area to be treated, 270

Additives, cleaning, 91

Adductors, muscles that draw a body part, such as a finger, arm, or toe, inward toward the median axis of the body or of an extremity, 125

Adipose tissue, technical term for fat; gives smoothness and contour to the body, 114, 159

Adrenal glands, glands that secrete about 30 steroid hormones and control metabolic processes of the body, including the fight-or-flight response, 139

Advanced Nail Technician (ANT), 858

Advertising, 1027–1028

AHAs. *See* Alpha hydroxy acids

AHP. *See* Accelerated hydrogen peroxide

AIDS. *See* Acquired immune deficiency syndrome

Albinism, congenital hypopigmentation, or absence of melanin pigment of the body, including the skin, hair, and eyes, 183

Alginate masks, 724

Alipidic, literally means "lack of lipids." Describes skin that does not produce enough sebum, indicated by absence of visible pores, 716

Alkaline solution, a solution that has a pH above 7.0 (neutral), 257

acid-alkali neutralization reactions, 258

Alkaline waves, also known as *cold waves*; have a pH between 9.0 and 9.6, use ammonium thioglycolate (ATG) as the reducing agent, and process at room temperature without the addition of heat, 573

Alkalis, also known as *bases*; compounds that react with acids to form salts, 257

Alkanolamines, alkaline substances used to neutralize acids or raise the pH of many hair products, 255

Allergic contact dermatitis (ACD), an allergy to an ingredient or a chemical, usually caused by repeated skin contact with the chemical, 190

Allergy, reaction due to extreme sensitivity to certain foods, chemicals, or other normally harmless substances, 83. *See also* Dimethyl urea hardeners

Alopecia, abnormal hair loss, 230

surgical treatment for, 232

Alopecia areata, autoimmune disorder that causes the affected hair follicles to be mistakenly attacked by a person's own immune system; usually begins with one or more small, round, smooth bald patches on the scalp, 231

Alopecia totalis, total loss of scalp hair, 231

Alopecia universalis, complete loss of body hair, 231

Alpha hydroxy acids (AHAs), acids derived from plants (mostly fruit) that are often used to exfoliate the skin, 257

Alternating current (AC), rapid and interrupted current, flowing first in one direction and then in the opposite direction; produced by mechanical means and changes directions 60 times per second, 265

American Cancer Society, ABCDE Cancer Checklist, 185

Amino acids, units that are joined together end to end like pop beads by strong, chemical peptide bonds (end bonds) to form the polypeptide chains that comprise proteins, 233, 566

in hair, 222–224

Aminomethylpropanol, 576

Ammonia, colorless gas with a pungent odor that is composed of hydrogen and nitrogen, 255

Ammonia-free waves, perms that use an ingredient that does not evaporate as readily as ammonia, so there is very little odor associated with their use, 575

Ammonium thioglycolate (ATG), active ingredient or reducing agent in alkaline permanents, 572

Ampere (A), also known as *amp*; unit that measures the strength of an electric current, 266

Ampoules, individual doses of serum, sealed in small vials, 721

Anabolism, constructive metabolism, the process of building up larger molecules from smaller ones, 114

Anaerobic, cannot survive in the presence of oxygen, 186

Anagen phase, also known as *growth phase*; phase during which new hair is produced, 227

Anaphoresis, process of infusing an alkaline (negative) product into the tissues from the negative pole toward the positive pole, 270

Anatomy, study of human body structure that can be seen with the naked eye and how the body parts are organized and the science of the structure of organisms or of their parts, 112

body systems, 114–115, 116

cells, 113–114

circulatory system, 116, 131–137

digestive system, 116, 138–139

endocrine system, 116, 137–138

excretory system, 116, 139–140

integumentary system, 116, 140–141

lymphatic/immune system, 116, 137

muscular system, 116, 120–126, 138

nervous system, 116, 121, 126–131, 137

organs, 114–120, 127, 139, 140

reproductive system, 116, 141

respiratory system, 116, 120, 140

skeletal system, 115, 116–120

tissues, 112–113

Androgenic alopecia, also known as *androgenetic alopecia*; hair loss characterized by miniaturization of terminal hair that is converted to vellus hair; in men, it is known as male pattern baldness, 230

Angle, space between two lines or surfaces that intersect at a given point, 346. *See also* Specific haircut

Angular artery, supplies blood to the side of the nose, 135

Anhidrosis, deficiency in perspiration, often a result of fever or certain skin diseases, 181

Aniline derivatives, contain small, uncolored dyes that combine with hydrogen peroxide to form larger, permanent dye molecules within the cortex, 638

Anion, an ion with a negative electrical charge, 256

Anode, positive electrode; the anode is usually red and is marked with a *P* or a plus (+) sign, 269

Anorexia, 221

ANS. *See* Autonomic nervous system

ANT. *See* Advanced Nail Technician

Anterior auricular artery, supplies blood to the front part of the ear, 135

Anterior tibial artery, artery that supplies blood to the lower leg muscles and to the muscles and skin on the top of the foot and adjacent sides of the first and second toes. This artery continues to the foot where it becomes the dorsalis pedis artery, 136

Antibiotics, 71

Antidandruff shampoo, 234, 319

Antidandruff treatment, 310, 331

Antiseptics, chemical germicides formulated for use on skin; registered and regulated by the Food and Drug Administration (FDA), 92

Aorta, the largest artery in the body, 133

Apex, highest point on the top of the head, 345; **also known as *arch*; the area of the nail that has all of the strength**, 905

Application brush, 801

Applicator bottle, 646

Appointment book, 1024

Aromatherapy, involves the use of highly concentrated, nonoily, and volatile essential oils to induce such reactions as relaxation and invigoration, or to simply create a pleasant fragrance during a service, 740

manicure with, 814

Arrector pili muscles, small, involuntary muscles in the base of the hair follicle that cause goose flesh, sometimes called *goose bumps*, and papillae, 158

Arteries, thick-walled, muscular, flexible tubes that carry oxygenated blood away from the heart to the arterioles, 131

Arterioles, small arteries that deliver blood to capillaries, 133

Artistry, of hairstyling, 447

Asymmetrical balance, is established when two imaginary halves of a hairstyle have an equal visual weight, but the two halves are positioned unevenly. Opposite sides of the hairstyle are different lengths or have a different volume. Asymmetry can be horizontal or diagonal, 292

Asymptomatic, showing no symptoms or signs of infection, 93

ATG. *See* Ammonium thioglycolate

Atoms, the smallest chemical components (often called particles) of an element; structures that make up the element and have the same properties of the element, 247

Atrium, thin-walled, upper chamber of the heart through which blood is pumped to the ventricles. There is a right atrium and a left atrium, 131

Attentiveness, 48

Auricularis anterior, muscle in front of the ear that draws the ear forward, 121

Auricularis posterior, muscle behind the ear that draws the ear backward, 121

Auricularis superior, muscle above the ear that draws the ear upward, 121

Auriculotemporal nerve, affects the external ear and skin above the temple, up to the top of the skull, 128

Autoclave, 84, 89

Autonomic nervous system (ANS), the part of the nervous system that controls the involuntary muscles; regulates the action of the smooth muscles, glands, blood vessels, heart, and breathing, 126–127. *See also* Specific organs

Avicenna, 6, 11

Axon, the extension of a neuron through which impulses are sent away from the body to other neurons, glands, or muscles, 127

Axon terminal, the extension of a neuron through which impulses are sent away from the body to other neurons, glands, or muscles, 127

B

Bacilli, short rod-shaped bacteria. They are the most common bacteria and produce diseases such as tetanus (lockjaw), typhoid fever, tuberculosis, and diphtheria, 74–75

Back massage, 733

Backbrushing, also known as *ruffing*; technique used to build a soft cushion or to mesh two or more curl patterns together for a uniform and smooth comb out, 429

Backcombing, also called *teasing, ratting, matting,* or *French lacing*; combing small sections of hair from the ends toward the scalp, causing shorter hair to mat at the scalp and form a cushion or base, 429

Bacteria, also known as *microbes* or *germs*; one-celled microorganisms that have both plant and animal characteristics, 74

movement of, 75–76

nail infections, 210

pathogenic, 76–78, 81

Bactericidal, capable of destroying bacteria, 73

Balance, establishing equal or appropriate proportions to create symmetry. In hairstyling, it is the relationship of height to width, 291

Balancing shampoo, shampoo that washes away excess oiliness from hair and scalp, while preventing the hair from drying out, 317

Baliage, also known as *free-form technique*; painting a lightener (usually a powdered off-the-scalp lightener) directly onto clean, styled hair, 654

Band lashes, also known as *strip lashes*; eyelash hairs on a strip that are applied with adhesive to the natural lash line, 783

Bang area, also known as *fringe area*; triangular section that begins at the apex, or high point of the head, and ends at the front corners, 302

cutting of, 372–373

safety around face area, 365

Barber comb, 354, 382

Barber's itch, 80–81

Barber spa, 9

Barrel curls, pin curls with large center openings, fastened to the head in a standing position on a rectangular base, 425

Basal cell carcinoma, most common and least severe type of skin cancer; often characterized by light or pearly nodules, 184

Base, stationary, or nonmoving, foundation of a pin curl (the area closest to the scalp); the panel of hair on which a roller is placed, 422

Base coat, 805

Base color, predominant tone of a color, 633

Base control, position of the tool in relation to its base section, determined by the angle at which the hair is wrapped, 579

Base cream, also known as *protective base cream*; oily cream used to protect the skin and scalp during hair relaxing, 587

Base direction, angle at which the rod is positioned on the head (horizontally, vertically, or diagonally); also, the directional pattern in which the hair is wrapped, 570

Base placement, refers to the position of the rod in relation to its base section; base placement is determined by the angle at which the hair is wrapped, 569

Base relaxers, relaxers that require the application of protective base cream to the entire scalp for the application of the relaxer, 587

Base sections, subsections of panels into which hair is divided for perm wrapping; one rod is normally placed on each base section, 569

Basic haircuts, 366–371

Basic permanent wrap, also known as a *straight set wrap*; perm wrapping pattern in which all the rods within a panel move in the same direction and are positioned on equal-sized bases; all the base sections are horizontal, and are the same length and width as the perm rod, 579

Beard, 303, 383

Beau's lines, visible depressions running across the width of the natural nail plate; usually a result of major illness or injury that has traumatized the body, 207, 211

Bed epithelium, thin layer of tissue that attaches the nail plate and the nail bed, 199

Belly, middle part of a muscle, 120

Benzalkonium chloride, 92

Benzoyl peroxide (BPO), 900

Beveling, technique using diagonal lines by cutting hair ends with a slight increase or decrease in length, 347

Bicep, muscle that produces the contour of the front and inner side of the upper arm; lifts the forearm and flexes the elbow, 124

Binary fission, the division of bacteria cells into two new cells called daughter cells, 76

Bioburden, the number of viable organisms in or on an object or surface or the organic material on a surface or object before decontamination or sterilization, 85

Birthmark, 183

Bitten nails, 208

Blackhead, 163

Bleach, 85, 86, 87

Blending shear, 360

Block, head-shaped form, usually made of canvas-covered cork or Styrofoam, on which the wig is secured for fitting, cleaning, coloring, and styling, 546

Blood, nutritive fluid circulating through the circulatory system (heart and blood vessels) to supply oxygen and nutrients to cells and tissues and to remove carbon dioxide and waste from them, 133

- arteries of head, face, and neck, 134–136
- blood vessels, 133–136
- as connective tissue, 114–115
- properties and functions, 133
- supply to arm and hand, 136
- supply to lower leg and foot, 136–137
- unexpected skin bleeding, 184
- veins of head, face, and neck, 136

Blood thinners, 713

Blood vascular system, consists of the heart, arteries, veins, and capillaries that distribute blood throughout the body, 131

Blood vessels, tube-like structures that include arteries, arterioles, capillaries, venules, and veins, 133

Bloodborne pathogens, disease-causing microorganisms carried in the body by blood or body fluids, such as hepatitis and HIV, 79, 92

Bloodletting, 8

Blowdry styling, technique of drying and styling damp hair in a single operation, 431

- blunt or long-layered, straight to wavy hair into straight style
  - left-handed, 479
  - right-handed, 476
- combs, picks, and brushes, 432–433
- concentrator, 431
- diffuser, 431–432
- of graduated haircuts, 435
- hood dryer *vs.* blowdryer, 431
- long, curly hair in its natural wave pattern, 471
- sectioning clips, 433
- short, curly hair in its natural wave pattern, 469
- short, layered, curly hair to produce smooth, full finish, 465

straight or wavy hair with maximum volume, 472

styling products, 433–434

Blunt haircut, also known as a *one-length haircut*; haircut in which all the hair comes to one hanging level, forming a weight line or area; hair is cut with no elevation or overdirection, 366

with fringe

left-handed, 388

right-handed, 384

Blush, 761, 765

Boar-bristle brush, 510, 550

Body systems, also known as *systems*; groups of body organs acting together to perform one or more functions. The human body is composed of 11 major systems, 114, 116

Body waxing procedure, 705

Bonding, method of attaching hair extensions in which hair wefts or single strands are attached with an adhesive or bonding agent, 556

Bonding UV gels. *See* UV bonding gels

Bonds, chemical, of hair, 224–225

Bookend wrap, perm wrap in which one end paper is folded in half over the hair ends like an envelope, 568

Booth rental, also known as *chair rental*; renting a booth or station in a salon, 1009

BPO. *See* Benzoyl peroxide

Braid-and-sew method, attachment method in which hair extensions are secured to client's own hair by sewing braids or a weft onto an on-the-scalp braid or cornrow, which is sometimes called the track, 554

Braiding

caution about, 514

cornrows, 516, 533

with extensions, 516, 535

facial shapes and, 517

fishtail braid, 515, 524

hair analysis for, 509–510

invisible braid, 514, 515, 526

locks, 518–519

origins, 508–509

overhand technique, 514

preparing textured hair for, 520

rope braid, 514, 522

single braids, 515

with extensions, 530

without extensions, 528

tools for, 510–512

tree braids, 518

underhand technique, 514

visible braid, 514

working with wet *vs.* dry hair, 513–514

Brain, part of the central nervous system contained in the cranium; largest and most complex nerve tissue and controls sensation, muscles, gland activity, and the power to think and feel emotions, 127

Brazilian bikini waxing, a waxing technique that requires the removal of all the hair from the front and the back of the bikini area, 688

Brazilian straightening treatments, 11

Breedlove, Sarah, 7, 10

Bricklay permanent wrap, perm wrap similar to actual technique of bricklaying; base sections are offset from each other row by row, to prevent noticeable splits and to blend the flow of the hair, 580

Bromhidrosis, foul-smelling perspiration, usually noticeable in the armpits or on the feet, that is caused by bacteria, 181

Bruised nails, condition in which a blood clot forms under the nail plate, causing a dark purplish spot. These discolorations are usually due to small injuries to the nail bed, 207, 211

Brush and bowl, haircoloring, 646

Brushing machine, a rotating electric appliance with interchangeable brushes that can be attached to the rotating head, 733

Buccal nerve, affects the muscles of the mouth, 129

Buccinator muscle, affects the muscles of the mouth, 123

Bulla, large blister containing a watery fluid; similar to a vesicle but larger, 178, 179

Business, your own, 1008. *See also* Retailing

advertising, 1027–1028

booth rental, 1009

business operation, 1017

drawing up a lease, 1016

fire, theft, and lawsuit protection, 1016–1017

opening your own salon, 1010

business plan, 1014

regulations and laws, 1012

written agreements, 1011

operating a successful salon
front desk, 1023–1024
personnel, 1021
planning salon layout, 1019–1020
telephone use, 1024–1026
purchasing an established salon, 1015
record keeping, 1018–1019
types of salon ownership, 1012
corporation, 1013
franchise, 1014
individual, 1013
partnership, 1013
Business card, 1002
Business plan, a written description of your business as you see it today, and as you foresee it in the next five years (detailed by year), 1011
Business regulations and laws, any and all local, state, and federal regulations and laws that you must comply with when you decide to open your salon or rent a booth, 1012

C

Cake makeup, also known as *pancake makeup*; a heavy-coverage makeup pressed into a compact and applied to the face with a moistened cosmetic sponge, 765
Calcaneus bone, 119, 120
Callus, thickening of the skin caused by continued, repeated pressure on any part of the skin, especially the hands and feet, 157
cutting of, 849
removal, 79
Callus softeners, products designed to soften and smooth thickened tissue (calluses), 851
Cancer, 178
ABCDE skin cancer checklist, 185
LGFB program, 232
skin, 184–186
Canities, technical term for gray hair; results from the loss of the hair's natural melanin pigment, 232
Cap technique, lightening technique that involves pulling clean, dry strands of hair through a perforated cap with a thin plastic or metal hook, and then combing them to remove tangles, 653
Cap wigs, wigs constructed of elasticized, mesh-fiber bases to which the hair is attached, 544
Capes, cleaning of, 90. *See also* Draping
Capillaries, tiny, thin-walled blood vessels that connect the smaller arteries to the veins. Capillaries bring nutrients to the cells and carry away waste materials, 133
Capital, money needed to invest in a business, 1013
Capless wigs, also known as *caps*; machine-made from human or artificial hair which is woven into rows of wefts. Wefts are sewn to elastic strips in a circular pattern to fit the head shape, 544
Carbohydrates, 164–170
Carbuncle, inflammation of the subcutaneous tissue caused by staphylococci; similar to a furuncle but larger, 236
Carcinogenics, 87. *See also* Cancer
Carcinoma, 178, 184
Cardiac muscle, the involuntary muscle that is the heart. This type of muscle is not found in any other part of the body, 120
Carpus, also known as *wrist*; flexible joint composed of eight small, irregular bones (carpals) held together by ligaments, 119
Carved curls, also known as *sculptured curls*; pin curls sliced from a shaping and formed without lifting the hair from the head, 425
left-handed procedure, 459
right-handed procedure, 457
Carving, haircutting technique done by placing the still blade into the hair and resting it on the scalp, and then moving the shears through the hair while opening and partially closing the shears, 377
Cascade curls, also known as *stand-up curls*; pin curls fastened to the head in a standing position to allow the hair to flow upward and then downward, 425
Cast, method of manufacturing shears; a metal-forming process whereby molten steel is poured into a mold and, once the metal is cooled, takes on the shape of the mold, 355
Catabolism, the phase of metabolism that involves the breaking down of complex compounds within the cells into smaller ones. This process releases energy that has been stored, 114
Catagen phase, the brief transition period between the growth and resting phases of a hair follicle. It signals the end of the growth phase, 228
Catalysts, substances that speed up chemical reactions, 275, 900
Cataphoresis, 270
Cathode, negative electrode; the cathode is usually black and is marked with an *N* or a minus (–) sign, 269,

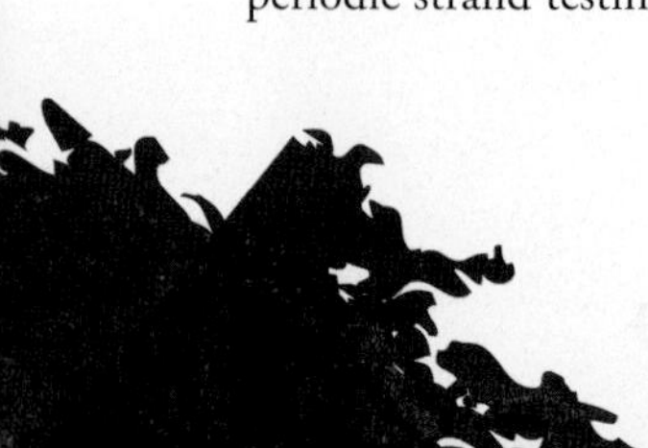

Cyst, closed, abnormally developed sac that contains fluid, pus, semifluid, or morbid matter above or below the skin, 178

Cysteine, an amino acid joined with another cysteine amino acid to create cystine amino acid, 224

Cystine, an amino acid that joins together two peptide strands, 225

Cytoplasm, the protoplasm of a cell, except for the protoplasm in the nucleus, that surrounds the nucleus; the watery fluid that cells need for growth, reproduction, and self-repair, 113

D

Damaged hair, 320, 660

Day spas, salon survey, 965

DC. *See* Direct current

DeCaprio, Noel, 11

Decolorizing process, 641, 649

Decontamination, the removal of blood or other potentially infectious materials on an item's surface and the removal of visible debris or residue such as dust, hair, and skin, 78, 82

Method 1, 82–84

Method 2, 84

Deductive reasoning, the process of reaching logical conclusions by employing logical reasoning, 960

Deep peroneal nerve, also known as *anterior tibial nerve*; extends down the front of the leg, behind the muscles. It supplies impulses to these muscles and also to the muscles and skin on the top of the foot and adjacent sides of the first and second toes, 130

Deep-conditioning treatment, also known as *hair mask* or *conditioning pack*; chemical mixture of concentrated protein and intensive moisturizer, 320

Deionized water, water that has had impurities, such as calcium and magnesium and other metal ions that would make a product unstable, removed, 314

Deltoid, large, triangular muscle covering the shoulder joint that allows the arm to extend outward and to the side of the body, 124

Demipermanent haircolor, also known as *no-lift deposit-only color*; formulated to deposit but not lift (lighten) natural hair color, 637

Demographics, information about a specific population including data on race, age, income, and educational attainment, 1011

Dendrites, tree-like branching of nerve fibers extending from a nerve cell; carry impulses toward the cell and receive impulses from other neurons, 127

Department of Agriculture, U. S. (USDA), 165–170

Department of Labor, U. S., 69

Depilatory, substance usually a caustic alkali preparation, used for the temporary removal of superfluous hair by dissolving it at the skin surface level, 693

Depressor labii inferioris muscle, also known as *quadratus labii inferioris muscle*; muscle surrounding the lower lip; depresses the lower lip and draws it to one side, as in expressing sarcasm, 123

Dermal papillae, small, cone-shaped elevations at the base of the hair follicles that fit into the hair bulb, 159, 221

Dermatitis, inflammatory condition of the skin, 182

contact, 190–191

Dermatologist, physician who specializes in diseases and disorders of the skin, hair, and nails, 156, 178

Dermatology, medical branch of science that deals with the study of skin and its nature, structure, functions, diseases, and treatment, 156, 171

Dermis, also known as *derma*, *corium*, *cutis*, or *true skin*; underlying or inner layer of the skin, 158–159, 162

Design texture, wave patterns that must be taken into consideration when designing a style, 287

Desincrustation, process used to soften and emulsify grease deposits (oil) and blackheads in the hair follicles, 270, 734–735

Developers, also known as *oxidizing agents* or *catalysts*; when mixed with an oxidation haircolor, supplies the necessary oxygen gas to develop color molecules and create a change in hair color, 640–641

Diabetes, 713

Diagnosis, determination of the nature of a disease from its symptoms and/or diagnostic tests. Federal regulations prohibit salon professionals from performing a diagnosis, 78

Diagonal asymmetry, 292

Diagonal lines, lines positioned between horizontal and vertical lines. They are often used to emphasize or minimize facial features, 286

Diaphragm, muscular wall that separates the thorax from the abdominal region and helps control breathing, 140

Dietary guidelines, 165–166

Dietary supplements, 166–167

Diffuser, blowdryer attachment that causes the air to flow more softly and helps to accentuate or keep textural definition, 431

Digestive enzymes, chemicals that change certain types of food into a soluble (capable of being dissolved) form that can be used by the body, 139

Digestive system, also known as *gastrointestinal system*; responsible for breaking down foods into nutrients and wastes; consists of the mouth, stomach, intestines, salivary and gastric glands and other organs, 116, 138–139,

Digital nerve, sensory-motor nerve that, with its branches, supplies impulses to the fingers, 129

Dimethyl urea hardeners, a hardener that adds cross-links to the natural nail plate. Unlike hardeners containing formaldehyde, DMU does not cause adverse skin reactions, 806

Dip Powder and Adhesive Enhancements, 877

Diplococci, spherical bacteria that grown in pairs and cause diseases such as pneumonia, 74

Diplomacy, 31

Direct current (DC), constant, even-flowing current that travels in one direction only and is produced by chemical means, 265

Direct transmission, transmission of blood or body fluids through touching (including shaking hands), kissing, coughing, sneezing, and talking, 75

Directional lines, lines with a definite forward or backward movement, 287

Discolored nails, nails turn a variety of colors; may indicate surface staining, a systemic disorder, or poor blood circulation, 208, 211

Disease, an abnormal condition of all or part of the body, or its systems or organs, that makes the body incapable of carrying on normal function, 70, 78

Disinfectants, chemical products that destroy all bacteria, fungi, and viruses (but not spores) on surfaces, 70–72, 84, 85

- additives, powders, and tablets, 91
- choosing, 85–86
- contraindicated for skin contact, 87–88
- dispensary for, 91
- EPA registration number, 84
- improper mixing of, 84
- labels for, 84, 86, 88
- proper use, 86
- safety tips for, 88
- soaps and detergents, 90
- types, 87
- for work surfaces, 90

Disinfection, the process that eliminates most, but not necessarily all, microorganisms on nonporous surfaces. This process is not effective against bacterial spores, 73

- disinfect *vs.* dispose, 88–89
- electrical tools and implements, 89–90
- foot spas and pedicure equipment, 86, 89, 90
- logbook recording of, 89–90
- manicure implements, 798
- nail infections, 210
- nonelectrical tools and implements, 89, 96
- pedicure procedures, 71, 90, 859–862
- pipe-less foot spas, 99–100
- of towels, linens, and capes, 90

Disinfection container, for manicure service sets, 796

Disposable implements, also known as *single-use implements*; implements that cannot be reused and must be thrown away after a single use, 799

Distribution, where and how hair is moved over the head, 372

Distributor sales consultants (DSCs), 12

Disulfide bond, strong chemical side bond that joins the sulfur atoms of two neighboring cysteine amino acids to create one cystine, which joins together two polypeptide strands like rungs on a ladder, 224, 225

Dorsal nerve, also known as *dorsal cutaneous nerve*; a nerve that extends up from the toes and foot, just under the skin, supplying impulses to toes and foot, as well as the muscles and skin of the leg, where it is becomes the superficial peroneal nerve or the musculocutaneous nerve, 130

Dorsalis pedis artery, artery that supplies blood to the foot, 136

Double flat wrap, perm wrap in which one end paper is placed under and another is placed over the strand of hair being wrapped, 568

Double press, technique of passing a hot curling iron through the hair before performing a hard press, 442

Double-process application, also known as *two-step coloring*; a coloring technique requiring two separate procedures in which the hair is prelightened before the depositing color is applied to the hair, 640

Double-rod wrap, also known as *piggyback wrap*; a wrap technique whereby extra-long hair is wrapped on one rod from the scalp to midway down the hair shaft, and another rod is used to wrap the remaining hair strand in the same direction, 571

Dramatic look, 52

Draping, 320–322

- basic shampoo and conditioning, 333
- chemical service, 334
- cleaning of capes, 90

Dreadlocks, 518–519

Drug abuse, 80, 188

Dry bead, 901

Dry hair, 240, 315
products, 320
and scalp treatment, 309–310, 329
Dry shampoo, also known as *powder shampoo*; shampoo that cleanses the hair without the use of soap and water, 317–318
Dry skin, 782
facial procedure, 746
signs and conditions associated with, 716
DSCs. *See* Distributor sales consultants
Duodenum, 139
Dust mask, 904
Dyschromias, abnormal colorations of the skin that accompany many skin disorders and systemic disorders, 183

Ear hair trimming, 383
Eczema, an inflammatory, uncomfortable, and often chronic disease of the skin, characterized by moderate to severe inflammation, scaling, and sometimes severe itching, 182
Effective communication, the act of sharing information between two people (or main groups of people) so that the information is successfully understood, 49
Efficacy, the ability to produce an effect, 85
disinfectants', 85–86
Effleurage, a succession of strokes made by gliding the hands over an area of the body with varying degrees of pressure or contact, 726
Eggshell nails, noticeably thin, white nail plates that are more flexible than normal, 207, 211
Egyptians, 4–5, 10, 11
Elastin, protein base similar to collagen that forms elastic tissue, 161, 162
Electric current, flow of electricity along a conductor, 264
Electrical equipment, 256, 270, 737
common tools, 271–272
disinfecting of tools and implements, 89–90
safety, 266–269
two-prong and three-prong plugs, 268
Electricity, the movement of particles around an atom that creates pure energy, 264
electrical measurement, 266
types of current, 265
Electrode, also known as *probe*; applicator for directing electric current from an electrotherapy device to the client's skin, 269
Electrolysis, removal of hair by means of an electric current that destroys the root of the hair, 692
Electromagnetic spectrum, also known as *electromagnetic spectrum of radiation*; name given to all of the forms of energy (or radiation) that exist, 272–274
Electrotherapy, the use of electrical currents to treat the skin, 734
Element, the simplest form of chemical matter; an element cannot be broken down into a simpler substance without a loss of identity, 247
Elemental molecule, molecule containing two or more atoms of the same element in definite (fixed) proportions, 248
Elevation, also known as *projection* or *lifting*; angle or degree at which a subsection of hair is held, or lifted, from the head when cutting, 347. *See also* Specific haircut
Eleventh cranial nerve, also known as *accessory nerve*; a motor nerve that controls the motion of the neck and shoulder muscles, 129
Emollients, oil or fatty ingredients that prevent moisture from leaving the skin, 721
Emotions, 32
Emphasis, also known as *focus*; the place in a hairstyle where the eye is drawn first before traveling to the rest of the design, 292
Employee benefits, 1021-1022
Employment
employee contracts, 981
employment portfolio, 970–972
field research, 973
Interests Self-Test, 23
job interview, 974–981
managing your career, 22–23
paths, 9, 12–14
preparing for
getting the job you want, 963–965
salon survey, 965–967
resume, 967–972
cover letter for, 976
in salon management, 13–14
salon visit checklist, 975
targeting potential employers, 973
thank you note, 975, 976, 981

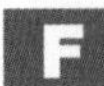

Form, the mass or general outline of a hairstyle. It is three-dimensional and has length, width, and depth, 287

Formal style, 447

Formaldehyde gas, 87

Foundation, also known as *base makeup*; a tinted cosmetic used to cover or even out the coloring of the skin, 758

Four corners, points on the head that signal a change in the shape of the head, from flat to round or vice versa, 345

Fragilitas crinium, technical term for brittle hair, 233

Freckles, 178, 183

Free edge, part of the nail plate that extends over the tip of the finger or toe, 199, 203

Free radicals, unstable molecules that cause biochemical aging, especially wrinkling and sagging of the skin, 188

Free-hand notching, haircutting technique in which pieces of hair are snipped out at random intervals, 377

Free-hand slicing, technique used to release weight from the subsection, allowing the hair to move more freely, 378

French braid, 514

Friction, deep rubbing movement requiring pressure on the skin with the fingers or palm while moving them over an underlying structure, 727

Front desk, operation of, 1023

Frontal artery, supplies blood to the forehead and upper eyelids, 135

Frontal bone, bone that forms the forehead, 117

Frontalis, front (anterior) portion of the epicranius; muscle of the scalp that raises the eyebrows, draws the scalp forward, and causes wrinkles across the forehead, 121, 122

Full-base curls, thermal curls that sit in the center of their base; strong curls with full volume, 440

Fulling, form of pétrissage in which the tissue is grasped, gently lifted, and spread out; used mainly for massaging the arms, 727

Full-stem curl, curl placed completely off the base; allows for the greatest mobility, 423

Fumigants, 87

Fungi, microscopic plant parasites, which include molds, mildews, and yeasts; can produce contagious diseases such as ringworm, 80–81, 235, 242, 243

- malassezia, 234
- nail, 210
- onychomycosis, 215, 217

Fungicidal, capable of destroying fungi, 73

Furuncle, boil; acute, localized bacterial infection of the hair follicle that produces constant pain, 236

Fuse, prevents excessive current from passing through a circuit, 267

Fuse box, 267

Fusion bonding, method of attaching extensions in which extension hair is bonded to the client's own hair with a bonding material that is activated by heat from a special tool, 557

G

Galvani, Luigi, 269

Galvanic current, constant and direct current having a positive and negative pole that produces chemical changes when it passes through the tissues and fluids of the body, 269–270, 736

Game plan, the conscious act of planning your life, instead of just letting things happen, 20

Gas, state of matter, 248, 249

Gastrocnemius, muscle attached to the lower rear surface of the heel and pulls the foot down, 125

Gattefossé, René, 814

Gauze

- manicure squares, 803
- for mask application, 723

Gel, thickened styling preparation that comes in a tube or bottle and creates a strong hold, 433

Gel masks, 722

Gelb, Lawrence, 8, 11

Glands, specialized organs that remove certain elements from the blood to convert them into new compounds, 137. *See also* Specific gland

- over-functioning of, 78, 107

Glasses, hairstyle appropriate for, 302

Glaze, a nonammonia color that adds shine and tone to the hair, 649

Gloves, safety, 96, 795, 850, 904

- avoiding contact dermatitis, 190–191

Glycerin, sweet, colorless, oily substance used as a solvent and as a moisturizer in skin and body creams, 255

Glyceryl monothioglycolate (GMTG), main active ingredient in true acid and acid-balanced waving lotions, 573

GMTG. *See* Glyceryl monothioglycolate

H

Hair cuticle, outermost layer of hair; consisting of a single, overlapping layer of transparent, scale-like cells that look like shingles on a roof, 221–222

Hair density, the number of individual hair strands on 1 square inch (2.5 square centimeters) of scalp, 238

analysis: thin, medium, or thick, 352–353

Hair design

elements of, 285–290

facial structure and hairstyle, 295–303

hair type influencing hairstyle, 293–295

men's facial hair, 303, 383

philosophy of design, 284–285

principles of, 290–293

Hair elasticity, ability of the hair to stretch and return to its original length without breaking, 239

Hair extensions, hair additions that are secured to the base of the client's natural hair in order to add length, volume, texture, or color, 553

blending client's hair with, 554

bonding method, 556

braid-and-sew attachment method, 554–555

fusion bonding method, 557–558

guidelines for, 553–554

linking, 559

materials and implements for, 512–513

retailing, 559–560

tube shrinking, 559

Hair follicle, the tube-like depression or pocket in the skin or scalp that contains the hair root, 220, 221

miniaturization, 230

Hair lightening, also known as *bleaching* or *decolorizing*; chemical process involving the diffusion of the natural hair color pigment or artificial haircolor from the hair, 650

Hair loss

emotional impact of, 229–230

treatments to counter, 231–232

types of abnormal, 230–231

Hair porosity, ability of the hair to absorb moisture, 238–239, 632

Hair pressing, method of temporarily straightening extremely curly or unruly hair by means of a heated iron or comb, 441

conditioning treatments, 443

hair texture and, 442–443

pressing combs, 443–444

pressing oil or cream, 444–445

reminders and hints, 445

safety, 442

scalp condition, 443

service notes, 443

special considerations, 446

types of, 441–442

Hair removal

body areas and appropriate procedures, 693

body waxing procedure, 705

client consultation, 689

contraindications for, 690

depilatory, 693

electrolysis, 692

epilator, 694

eyebrows

tweezing procedure, 701

waxing procedure, 703

Health Screening Form, 689

lasers for, 276, 693

photoepilation, 693

post-service procedure, 699

pre-service procedure, 696

shaving, 693

sugaring, 695

threading, 695

tweezing, 693, 701

Hair root, the part of the hair located below the surface of the epidermis, 220

Hair shaft, the portion of hair that projects above the epidermis, 220

structures of, 221–222

Hair spray, also known as *finishing spray*; a styling product applied in the form of a mist to hold a style in position; available in a variety of holding strengths, 434

Hair stream, hair flowing in the same direction, resulting from follicles sloping in the same direction, 240

Hair structure, 630

Hair texture, thickness, or diameter of the individual hair strand, 237, 239, 294, 631. *See also* Chemical texture services

analysis of, 352–353

coarse, 237, 238

analysis of, 352–353

pacemaker, 714

Helix, spiral shape of a coiled protein created by polypeptide chains that intertwine with each other, 223

Hemoglobin, complex iron protein in red blood cells that binds to oxygen; gives blood color, 134

Hepatitis, a bloodborne virus that causes disease and can damage the liver, 71, 79–80, 86

Herpes simplex, recurring viral infection that often presents as a fever blister or cold sore, 178, 182, 714

Herpes zoster, 178

High heels, 39

High-frequency current, 735–736

Highlighting, coloring some of the hair strands lighter than the natural color to add a variety of lighter shades and the illusion of depth, 653

Highlighting shampoo, colors prepared by combining permanent haircolor, hydrogen peroxide, and shampoo, 655

Hirsuties, also known as *hypertrichosis*; growth of an unusual amount of hair on parts of the body normally bearing only downy hair, such as the faces of women or the backs of men, 688

Hirsutism, condition pertaining to an excessive growth or cover of hair, 688

Histology, also known as *microscopic anatomy*; the study of tiny structures found in living tissues, 112

History, of cosmetology, 4–9

timeline, 10–11

HIV. *See* Human immunodeficiency virus

Hives, 178

Hood dryer, 431, 511

Horizontal finger waving

left-handed, 454

right-handed, 450

Horizontal lines, lines parallel to the floor or horizon; create width in design, 285

Hormones, secretions, such as insulin, adrenaline, and estrogen, that stimulate functional activity or other secretions in the body. Hormones influence the welfare of the entire body, 138

nail growth influenced by, 202

Horny layer, 157

Hospital disinfectants, disinfectants that are effective for cleaning blood and body fluids, 70

Hospital Grade, 70

Hot rollers, 428

HPV. *See* Human papilloma virus

Human immunodeficiency virus (HIV); virus that causes acquired immune deficiency syndrome (AIDS), 79, 80, 86, 795

Human papilloma virus (HPV), also known as *plantar warts*; a virus that can infect the bottom of the foot and resembles small black dots, usually in clustered groups, 79

Human relations, 46–49

Humectants, substances that absorb moisture or promote the retention of moisture, 319; **also known as *hydrators* or *water-binding agents*; ingredients that attract water**, 721

Humerus, uppermost and largest bone in the arm, extending from the elbow to the shoulder, 119

Hydrogen bond, a weak, physical, cross-link side bond that is easily broken by water or heat, 223–224, 225, 256

Hydrogen peroxide developer, oxidizing agent that, when mixed with an oxidation haircolor, supplies the necessary oxygen gas to develop the color molecules and create a change in natural hair color, 639

Hydrogen relaxers, 585–586

Hydrophilic, easily absorbs moisture; in chemistry terms, capable of combining with or attracting water (water-loving), 238

Hydrophobic, naturally resistant to being penetrated by moisture, 238

Hydroxide neutralization, an acid-alkali neutralization reaction that neutralizes (deactivates) the alkaline residues left in the hair by a hydroxide relaxer and lowers the pH of the hair and scalp; hydroxide relaxer neutralization does not involve oxidation or rebuild disulfide bonds, 587

Hydroxide relaxers, very strong alkalis with a pH over 13; the hydroxide ion is the active ingredient in all hydroxide relaxers, 585

procedures, 588–589

retouch, 617

on virgin hair, 614

Hygiene, personal, 37

Hyoid bone, u-shaped bone at the base of the tongue that supports the tongue and its muscles, 118

Hyperhidrosis, excessive sweating, caused by heat or general body weakness, 181

Hyperpigmentation, darker than normal pigmentation, appearing as dark splotches, 183

Hypertrichosis, also known as *hirsuties*; condition of abnormal growth of hair, characterized by the growth of terminal hair in areas of the body that normally grow only vellus hair, 232–233, 688

Hypertrophy, abnormal growth of the skin, 184

Hyponychium, slightly thickened layer of skin that lies between the fingertip and free edge of the natural nail plate, 199, 200, 203

Hypopigmentation, absence of pigment, resulting in light or white splotches, 183

Hypothalamus, 139

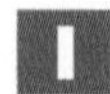

IA. *See* International Alliance of Theatrical Stage Employees, Moving Picture Technicians, Artist and Allied Crafts of the United States and Canada

ICD. *See* **Irritant contact dermatitis**

Image, client's, 52

Immersion, in disinfectant, 86, 96

Immiscible, liquids that are not capable of being mixed together to form stable solutions, 252

Immunity, the ability of the body to destroy and resist infection Immunity against disease can be either natural or acquired and is a sign of good health, 82

Impetigo, contagious bacterial skin infection characterized by weeping lesions, 178, 182

Implements, tools used to perform services. Implements can be reusable or disposable, 798. *See also* Specific implement

manicure, 798–801

Inactive electrode, opposite pole from the active electrode, 270

Indentation, the point where curls of opposite directions meet, forming a recessed area, 428

Indirect transmission, transmission of blood or body fluids through contact with an intermediate contaminated object such as a razor, extractor, nipper, or an environmental surface, 75

Individual lashes, separate artificial eyelashes that are applied to the eyelids one at a time, 783

Infection, the invasion of body tissues by disease-causing or pathogenic bacteria, 71, 75

entrance to body, 81

Infection control, the methods used to eliminate or reduce the transmission of infectious organisms, 72

difference between laws and rules, 72

pathogenic disease, 76–81

principles

of infection, 72–82

of prevention, 82–92

regulations, 69–72

Infectious, caused by or capable of being transmitted by infection, 71

Infectious disease, disease caused by pathogenic (harmful) microorganisms that enter the body. An infectious disease may or may not be spread from one person to another person, 73

Inferior labial artery, supplies blood to the lower lip, 135

Inflammation, a condition in which the body reacts to injury, irritation, or infection; characterized by redness, heat, pain, and swelling, 76, 78

wrist, 118

Influenza, 79

Infraorbital artery, supplies blood to the muscles of the eye, 134

Infraorbital nerve, affects the skin of the lower eyelid, side of the nose, upper lip, and mouth, 128

Infrared light, infrared light has longer wavelengths, penetrates more deeply, has less energy, and produces more heat than visible light; makes up 60 percent of natural sunlight, 275–276

Infratrochlear nerve, affects the membrane and skin of the nose, 128

Inhalation, breathing in through the nose or mouth, 140

Inhibition layer, the tacky surface left on the nail after a UV gel has cured, 929

Initiators, substance that starts the chain reaction that leads to the creation of very long polymer chains, 900

Inorganic chemistry, the study of substances that do not contain the element carbon, but may contain the element hydrogen, 246–247

Insect bite, 178

Insertion, part of the muscle at the more movable attachment to the skeleton, 121

Insurance, guarantees protection against financial loss from malpractice, property liability, fire, burglary and theft, and business interruption, 1009, 1011, 1012, 1017

Integration hairpiece, hairpiece that has openings in the base through which the client's own hair is pulled to blend with the hair (natural or synthetic) of the hairpiece, 551

Integumentary system, the skin and its accessory organs, such as the oil and sweat glands, sensory receptors, hair, and nails; serves as a protective covering and helps regulate the body's temperature, 116, 140–141

Intense pulse light, a medical device that uses multiple colors and wavelengths (broad spectrum) of focused light to treat spider veins, hyperpigmentation, rosacea and redness, wrinkles, enlarged hair follicles and pores, and excessive hair, 277

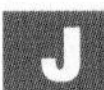

J

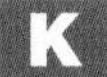

K

Knot also known as *chignon*; a technique used for formal hairstyling that creates the look of a knot or bun, 446, 496

kosmetikos, 4

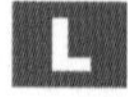

Labels

biohazard, 91, 93

chemical, 247

disinfectant, 84, 86, 88

food nutritional value, 166

UL certification for electric appliances, 267–268

Lacrimal bones, small, thin bones located at the front inner wall of the orbits (eye sockets), 117–118

Lady Godiva, 220

Lanthionine bonds, the bonds created when disulfide bonds are broken by hydroxide chemical hair relaxers after the relaxer is rinsed from the hair, 225

Lanthionization, process by which hydroxide relaxers permanently straighten hair; they remove a sulfur atom from a disulfide bond and convert it into a lanthionine bond, 585

Lanugo hair, 227

Laser, acronym for *light amplification stimulation emission of radiation*; a medical device that uses electromagnetic radiation for hair removal and skin treatments, 276

Laser hair removal, permanent hair removal treatment in which a laser beam is pulsed on the skin, impairing the hair growth, 692

Lateral nail fold, 201

Lateral pterygoid, muscles that coordinate with the masseter, temporalis, and medial pterygoid muscles to open and close the mouth and bring the jaw forward; sometimes referred to as chewing muscles, 122

Latex gloves, 801–802

Latissimus dorsi, large, flat, triangular muscle covering the lower back, 123

Laughing, benefit of, 48

Law of color, system for understanding color relationships, 633

Layered haircut, graduated effect achieved by cutting the hair with elevation or overdirection; the hair is cut at higher elevations, usually 90 degrees or above, which removes weight, 366

Layers, create movement and volume in the hair by releasing weight, 366

Layout planning, 1019–1022

Lease, 1016

Leave-in conditioner, 319

LED. *See* Light-emitting diode

Legal aspects of employment interview, 981

Length guard attachments, 381

Lentigines, technical term for freckles; small yellow-colored to brown-colored spots on skin exposed to sunlight and air, 183

Lesion, mark on the skin; may indicate an injury or damage that changes the structure of tissues or organs, 178–180, 186

Leukoderma, skin disorder characterized by light abnormal patches (hypopigmentation); caused by a burn or congenital disease that destroys the pigment-producing cells, 183, 216

Leukonychia spots, also known as *white spots*; whitish discolorations of the nails, usually caused by injury to the matrix area; not related to the body's health or vitamin deficiencies, 208

Levator anguli oris muscle, also known as *caninus muscle*; muscle that raises the angle of the mouth and draws it inward, 123

Levator labii superioris muscle, also known as *quadratus labii superioris muscle*; muscle surrounding the upper lip; elevates the upper lip and dilates the nostrils, as in expressing distaste, 122, 123

Level, the unit of measurement used to identify the lightness or darkness of a color, 632

Level system, system that colorists use to determine the lightness or darkness of a hair color, 632

LGFB. *See* Look Good . . . Feel Better

Lice infection, 81–82, 235–236

Licensure

preparing for, 958–959

test day, 960–963

Life skills, 18, 24

creative capability, 21–22

ethics, 29–30

goal setting checklist, 25

guidelines, 19–20

Interests Self-Test, 23

managing your, 22–23

motivation and self-management, 21

personality development and attitude, 31–32

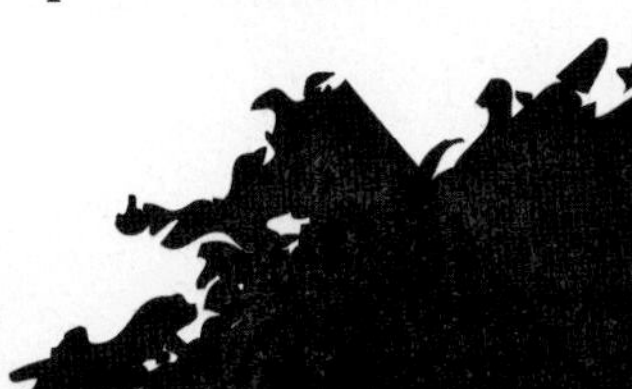

Madam C. J. Walker Hair Culturists Union of America, 7, 10, 11

Maintenance, term for when a nail enhancement needs to be serviced after two or more weeks from the initial application of the nail enhancement product, 877

Makeup. *See* Facial makeup

Makeup and Hairstylists Union, 12

Malassezia, naturally occurring fungus that is present on all human skin, but is responsible for dandruff when it grows out of control, 234

Malignant melanoma, most serious form of skin cancer; often characterized by black or dark brown patches on the skin that may appear uneven in texture, jagged, or raised, 184, 185

Mandible, lower jawbone; largest and strongest bone of the face, 117–118

Mandibular nerve, branch of the fifth cranial nerve that affects the muscles of the chin, lower lip, and external ear, 128, 129

Manicure

- aromatherapy with, 814
- basic, 807
- basic nail shapes, 809
  - men, 810
  - women, 808
- chemical-free products, 813
- equipment and implements, 794–803
- handling exposure incidents, 824
- iridescent or frosted polish, 810
- massage of hands and arms, 811, 831
- man's manicure service, 810
- materials, 801
- nail art, 816
- nail color choice, 809
- nail polishing procedure, 835
- paraffin wax treatment, 815, 837
- procedure
  - post-service, 821
  - pre-service, 817
- professional cosmetic products, 803
- proper hand washing, 823
- service sets, 799
- spa manicures, 813
- theme, 814

Manicure table, 794

- disinfecting of, 90

Marginal mandibular nerve, branch of the seventh cranial nerve that affects the muscles of the chin and lower lip, 129

Mascara, cosmetic preparation used to darken, define, and thicken the eyelashes, 764

Masks, also known as *masques*; concentrated treatment products often composed of mineral clays, moisturizing agents, skin softeners, aromatherapy oils, beneficial extracts, and other beneficial ingredients to cleanse, exfoliate, tighten, tone, hydrate, and nourish the skin, 722

Massage, manual or mechanical manipulation of the body by rubbing, gently pinching, kneading, tapping, and other movements to increase metabolism and circulation, promote absorption, and relieve pain, 725

- back, 733
- facial, 725
- manicure with, 811

Massage creams, lubricants used to make the skin slippery during massage, 721

Masseter, muscles that coordinate with the temporalis, medial pterygoid, and lateral pterygoid muscles to open and close the mouth and bring the jaw forward; sometimes referred to as chewing muscles, 121–122, 135

Matching test format, 962

Material Safety Data Sheet (MSDS), information compiled by the manufacturer about product safety, including the names of hazardous ingredients, safe handling and use procedures, precautions to reduce the risk of accidental harm or overexposure, and flammability warnings, 69, 70, 1012

- for disinfectants, 88
- product manufacturer or distributor provision of, 807
- for sodium hydroxide products, 258

Matrix, area where the nail plate cells are formed; this area is composed of matrix cells that produce the nail plate, 199–200, 203

Matte, nonshiny, 759

Matter, any substance that occupies space and has mass (weight), 247

- atoms, 247
- elements, 247
- molecules, 247–248
- physical and chemical properties, 249–250
- pure substances and physical mixtures, 251–256
- states of, 248–249

Maxillae, bones of the jaw, 117, 118

Maxillary nerve, branch of the fifth cranial nerve that supplies impulses to the upper part of the face, 128

Mayonnaise, 255

Measles, 79

Mechanical exfoliants, methods used to physically remove dead cell buildup, 719

Medial pterygoid, muscles that coordinate with the masseter, temporalis, and lateral pterygoid muscles to open and close the mouth and bring the jaw forward; sometimes referred to as chewing muscles, 122

Median nerve, sensory-motor nerve, smaller than the ulnar and radial nerves that, with its branches, supplies the arm and hand, 130

Medical Nail Technician (MNT), 852

Medicated scalp lotion, conditioner that promotes healing of the scalp, 319

Medicated shampoo, shampoo containing special chemicals or drugs that are very effective in reducing dandruff or relieving other scalp conditions, 317

Medium bead, 901

Medium press, technique that removes 60 to 75 percent of the curl by applying a thermal pressing comb once on each side of the hair, using slightly more pressure than in the soft press, 441

Medium texture hair, 237, 352–353

Medium-grit abrasives, 180 to 240 grit abrasives that are used to smooth and refine surfaces and shorten natural nails, 802

Medulla, innermost layer of the hair, often called the *pith* or *core* of the hair, 221, 222, 565

Melanin, tiny grains of pigment (coloring matter) that are produced by melanocytes and deposited into cells in the stratum germinativum layer of the epidermis and in the papillary layers of the dermis. There are two types of melanin: pheomelanin, which is red to yellow in color, and eumelanin, which is dark brown to black, 158, 160–161, 172, 221, 222

Melanocytes, cells that produce the dark skin pigment called melanin, 158

Melanoma, 186

Melanonychia, darkening of the fingernails or toenails; may be seen as a black band within the nail plate, extending from the base to the free edge, 208, 211

Men

- androgenic alopecia, 230
- basic clipper cut, 383, 413
- facial/ear hair trimming, 383
- hirsuties on back, 688
- manicure service, 810
- marketing to, 811
- mustache trimming, 303, 383
- -only specialty spa, 9, 71
- permanent wave, 582

Mental nerve, affects the skin of the lower lip and chin, 128

Mentalis muscle, muscle that elevates the lower lip and raises and wrinkles the skin of the chin, 123

Mercaptamine/cysteamine, 576

Metabolism, chemical process that takes place in living organisms through which the cells are nourished and carry out their activities, 114, 138, 139

Metacarpus, bones of the palm of the hand; parts of the hand containing five bones between the carpus and phalanges, 119

Metal hydroxide relaxers, ionic compounds formed by a metal (sodium, potassium, or lithium), which is combined with oxygen and hydrogen, 585

Metallic haircolors, also known as *gradual haircolors*; haircolors containing metal salts that change hair color gradually by progressive buildup and exposure to air creating a dull, metallic appearance, 639

Metal pusher, a reusable implement, made of stainless steel; used to push back the eponychium but can also be used to gently scrape cuticle tissue from the natural nail plate, 799

Metatarsal, one of three subdivisions of the foot; long and slender bones, like the metacarpal bones of the hand. The other two subdivisions are the tarsal and phalanges, 119

Methicillin-resistant staphylococcus aureus (MRSA), a type of infectious bacteria that is highly resistant to conventional treatments such as antibiotics, 77

Microcurrent, an extremely low level of electricity that mirrors the body's natural electrical impulses, 270–271, 737

Microdermabrasion, mechanical exfoliation that involves shooting aluminum oxide or other crystals at the skin with a hand-held device that exfoliates dead cells, 737

Microdermabrasion scrubs, scrubs that contains aluminum oxide crystals, 719

Microorganism, any organism of microscopic or submicroscopic size, 74

Microtrauma, the act of causing tiny unseen openings in the skin that can allow entry by pathogenic microbes, 799

Middle Ages, 5–6

Middle temporal artery, supplies blood to the temples, 135

Mildew, a type of fungus that affects plants or grows on inanimate objects, but does not cause human infections in the salon, 80

Milia, benign, keratin-filled cysts that can appear just under the epidermis and have no visible opening, 180

Miliaria rubra, also known as *prickly heat*; an acute inflammatory disorder of the sweat glands, characterized by the eruption of small red vesicles and accompanied by burning, itching skin, 181

Milliampere (mA), one-thousandth (1/1000) of an ampere, 266

Mineral deposits, 317

Minerals, 165–170

Miniaturized hair, 230

Minoxidil, 231

Miscible, liquids that are mutually soluble, meaning that they can be mixed together to form stable solutions, 252

Mission statement, a statement that establishes the values that an individual or institution lives by, as well as future goals, 22, 1010

Mitosis, usual process of cell reproduction of human tissues that occurs when the cell divides into two identical cells called daughter cells, 113

Mitral valve, also known as *bicuspid valve*; the valve between the left atrium and the left ventricle of the heart, 132

Mixed melanin, combination of natural hair color that contains both pheomelanin and eumelanin, 631

MNT. *See* Medical Nail Technician

Modalities, currents used in electrical facial and scalp treatments, 269

Modelage masks, facial masks containing special crystals of gypsum, a plaster-like ingredient, 723

Moisturizer, product formulated to add moisture to dry hair or promote the retention of moisture, 315

Moisturizers, products that help increase the moisture content of the skin surface, 721

Mole, small, brownish spot or blemish on the skin, ranging in color from pale tan to brown or bluish black, 184

Cancer Checklist, 185

removal of hair in, 184

Molecule, a chemical combination of two or more atoms in definite (fixed) proportions, 247–248

Money management, 993–996

Monilethrix, technical term for beaded hair, 233

Monomer, one unit called a molecule, 898

Monomer liquid, chemical liquid mixed with polymer powder to form the sculptured nail enhancement, 898

Monomer liquid and polymer powder nail enhancements, also known as *sculptured nails*; enhancements created by combining monomer liquid and polymer powder, 898

disposal of, 903

removal, 906

storage, 904

Motility, self-movement, 75

Motivation, 21

Motor nerve fibers, fibers of the motor nerves that are distributed to the arrector pili muscles attached to hair follicles. Motor nerves carry impulses from the brain to the muscles, 160

face and neck motor nerve points, 729

Motor nerves, also known as *efferent nerves*; carry impulses from the brain to the muscles or glands, 126, 127, 160

Motor point, point on the skin over the muscle where pressure or stimulation will cause contraction of that muscle, 729

Mousse, styling products, 433

MRSA. *See* Methicillin-resistant staphylococcus aureus

MSDS. *See* Material Safety Data Sheet

Multiple choice test format, 962–963

Multiuse, also known as *reusable*; items that can be cleaned, disinfected, and used on more than one person , even if the item is accidentally exposed to blood or body fluid, 89

Mumps, 79

Muscle tissue, tissue that contracts and moves various parts of the body, 114, 120

Muscular system, body system that covers, shapes, and holds the skeleton system in place; muscular system contracts and moves various parts of the body, 116, 120–126, 138

Mustache, 303, 383

Mycobacterium fortuitum, a microscopic germ that normally exists in tap water in small numbers, 71

Myology, study of the nature, structure, function, and diseases of the muscles, 120

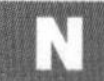

N

NAAF. *See* National Alopecia Areata Foundation

NACCAS. *See* National Accrediting Commission of Cosmetology Arts and Sciences

Nail adhesive, 930

Nail art, 816

Natural nail unit, composed of several major parts of the fingernail including the nail plate, nail bed, matrix, cuticle, eponychium, hyponychium, specialized ligaments, and nail fold. Together, all of these parts form the nail unit, 199

Needle sharing, 80, 82

Nerve tissue, tissue that carries messages to and from the brain and controls and coordinates all body functions, 114

Nerves, whitish cords made up of bundles of nerve fibers held together by connective tissue, through which impulses are transmitted, 112, 114, 116, 127. *See also* Central nervous system

- arm and hand, 130, 141
- circulatory system, 130–131
- head, face, and neck, 128–129
- lower leg and foot, 130
- motor, 126, 127
- sensory, 127
- types of nerves, 127

Nervous system, body system composed of the brain, spinal cord, and nerves; controls and coordinates all other systems of the body and makes them work harmoniously and efficiently, 116, 121, 126, 129, 131, 137

- brain and spinal cord, 127
- divisions of, 126–127
- nerves of arm and hand, 130
- nerves of head, face, and neck, 128–129
- nerves of lower leg and foot, 130

Nessler, Charles, 6, 8, 10

Neurology, scientific study of the structure, function, and pathology of the nervous system, 126

Neuron, also known as a *nerve cell*; primary structural unit of the nervous system, consisting of cell body, nucleus, dendrites, and axon, 114, 126, 127, 128

Nevus, also known as a *birthmark*; small or large malformation of the skin due to abnormal pigmentation or dilated capillaries, 183

New growth, part of the hair shaft between the scalp and the hair that has been previously colored, 652

Nipper, a stainless-steel implement used to carefully trim away dead skin around the nails, 799

Nitrile gloves, 796

No-base relaxers, relaxers that do not require application of a protective base cream, 587

Nodosum, 178

Nodule, a solid bump larger than .4 inches (1 centimeter) that can be easily felt, 178

No-lye relaxers, 586

Non-acetone nail polish remover, 804

Noncomedogenic, product that has been designed and proven not to clog the follicles, 187

Nonconductor, also known as *insulator*; a material that does not transmit electricity, 265

Nonpathogenic, harmless microorganisms that may perform useful functions and are safe to come in contact with since they do not cause disease or harm, 74

Nonporous, an item that is made or constructed of a material that has no pores or openings and cannot absorb liquids, 70. *See also* Porous

Nonstriated muscles, also known as *smooth muscles*; these muscles are involuntary and function automatically, without conscious will, 120

Nonstripping, product that does not remove artificial color from the hair, 317

Normal skin, 199, 200, 203, 716

Normalizing lotions, conditioners with an acidic pH that restore the hair's natural pH after a hydroxide relaxer and for shampooing, 589

No-stem curl, curl placed directly on its base; produces a tight, firm, long-lasting curl and allows minimum mobility, 423

Notching, version of point cutting in which the tips of the scissors are moved toward the hair ends rather than into them; creates a chunkier effect, 377

Nucleus, dense, active protoplasm found in the center of the cell; plays an important part in cell reproduction and metabolism, 113, 120, 127

Nutrition, 164–170, 188, 221

Nylon synthetic, 512–513

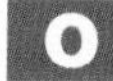

O. *See* **Ohm**

O/W emulsion. *See* Oil-in-water

Occipital artery, supplies blood to the skin and muscles of the scalp and back of the head up to the crown, 135, 136

Occipital bone, hindmost bone of the skull, below the parietal bones; forms the back of the skull above the nape, 117, 345

Occipital ridge, 345

Occipitalis, back of the epicranius; muscle that draws the scalp backward, 121

Occupational disease, illness resulting from conditions associated with employment, such as prolonged and repeated overexposure to certain products or ingredients, 78

contact dermatitis, 190–191

Occupational Safety and Health Act of 1970, 69, 795

Occupational Safety and Health Administration (OSHA), 69–70

business regulations, 1012

gloves *vs.* pathogens, 795

on single-use supplies, 91

Universal Precautions, 92–94, 795

Odorless monomer liquid and polymer powder products, nail enhancement products that have little odor, 906

Off base, the position of a curl or a roller completely off its base for maximum mobility and minimum volume, 427

Off-base curls, thermal curls placed completely off their base, offering only slight lift or volume, 440

Off-base placement, base control in which the hair is wrapped at 45 degrees below the center of the base section, so the rod is positioned completely off its base, 570

Off-the-scalp lighteners, also known as *quick lighteners*; powdered lighteners that cannot be used directly on the scalp, 650

Ohm (O), unit that measures the resistance of an electric current, 266

Oil glands, 141, 163

Oil-in-water (O/W) emulsion, oil droplets emulsified in water, 254

Oily hair, 240, 310, 330

Oily skin, 186, 718

with open comedones, 748

Oligomer, short chain of monomer liquids that is often thick, sticky, and gel-like and that is not long enough to be considered a polymer, 926

-ology, word ending meaning study of, 112

On base, also known as *full base*; position of a curl or roller directly on its base for maximum volume, 427

On-base placement, base control in which the hair is wrapped at a 45-degree angle beyond perpendicular to its base section, and the rod is positioned on its base, 569

One-color method, when one color of gel, usually clear, is applied over the entire surface of the nail, 927

One-length haircut, 366

On-the-scalp lighteners, lighteners that can be used directly on the scalp by mixing the lightener with activators, 650

Onychia, inflammation of the nail matrix, followed by shedding of the natural nail, 212, 213

Onychocryptosis, also know as *ingrown nails*; nail grows into the sides of the tissue around the nail, 213

Onycholysis, lifting of the nail plate from the nail bed without shedding, usually beginning at the free edge and continuing toward the lunula area, 212, 213, 835

Onychomadesis, the separation and falling off of a nail plate from the nail bed; affects fingernails and toenails, 214

Onychomycosis, fungal infection of the natural nail plate, 215, 217

Onychophagy, also known as *bitten nails*; result of a habit of chewing the nail or chewing the hardened skin surrounding the nail plate, 208, 211

Onychorrhexis, split or brittle nails that have a series of lengthwise ridges giving a rough appearance to the surface of the nail plate, 208

Onychosis, any deformity or disease of the natural nails, 213

Onyx, 198

Opacity, the amount of colored pigment concentration in a gel, making it more or less difficult to see through, 929

Open comedones, also known as *blackheads*; follicles impacted with solidified sebum and dead cell buildup, 717

Open-center curls, pin curls that produce even, smooth waves and uniform curls, 423

Ophthalmic nerve, branch of the fifth cranial nerve that supplies impulses to the skin of the forehead, upper eyelids, and interior portion of the scalp, orbit, eyeball, and nasal passage, 128

Orbicularis oculi muscle, ring muscle of the eye socket; enables you to close your eyes, 121, 122

Orbicularis oris muscle, flat band of muscle around the upper and lower lips that compresses, contracts, puckers, and wrinkles the lips, 122, 123

Organic chemistry, the study of substances that contain the element carbon, 246

Organs, structures composed of specialized tissues designed to perform specific functions in plants and animals, 114, 116–120, 127, 139, 140

major, 115

Origin, part of the muscle that does not move; attached to the skeleton and usually part of a skeletal muscle, 120

Os, bone, 115

OSHA. *See* Occupational Safety and Health Administration

Osteology, the study of anatomy, structure, and function of the bones, 115

Ostium, follicle opening, 717

OTC. *See* Over the counter

Oval face type, 296

Oval nail, a conservative nail shape that is thought to be attractive on most women's hands. It is similar to a squoval nail with even more rounded corners, 809

Ovaries, female sexual glands that function in reproduction, as well as determining female sexual characteristics, 138, 139, 141

Over the counter (OTC), 231

Overdirection, combing a section away from its natural falling position, rather than straight out from the head, toward a guideline; used to create increasing lengths in the interior or perimeter, 349

Overhand technique, a technique in which the first side section goes over the middle one, then the other side section goes over the middle strand, 514

Overlay, a layer of any kind of nail enhancement product that is applied over the natural nail or nail and tip application for added strength, 874

Oxidation, a chemical reaction that combines a substance with oxygen to produce an oxide, 250

Oxidation-reduction, also known as *redox;* a chemical reaction in which the oxidizing agent is reduced (by losing oxygen) and the reducing agent is oxidized (by gaining oxygen), 250

Oxidizing agent, substance that releases oxygen, 250

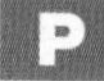

P

Pacemaker, heart, 713

Pain receptor, 164

Palm roll technique, 519

Palm-to-palm, cutting position in which the palms of both hands are facing each other, 365

Pancake makeup, 10

Pancreas, secretes enzyme-producing cells that are responsible for digesting carbohydrates, proteins, and fats. The islet of Langerhans cells within the pancreas control insulin and glucagon production, 138, 139

Papaya, 720

Paper wraps, temporary nail wraps made of very thin paper, 876

Papillary layer, outer layer of the dermis, directly beneath the epidermis, 158–161, 172

Papule, also known as *pimple*; small elevation on the skin that contains no fluid but may develop pus, 163, 178, 179, 186

Paraffin, a petroleum by-product that has excellent sealing properties (barrier qualities) to hold moisture in the skin, 798

Paraffin bath, 798, 847

Paraffin wax masks, specially prepared facial masks containing paraffin and other beneficial ingredients; typically used with treatment cream, 722

Paraffin wax treatment, 820, 837

Parallel lines, repeating lines in a hairstyle; may be straight or curved, 286

Parasites, organisms that grow, feed, and shelter on or in another organism (referred to as the host), while contributing nothing to the survival of that organism Parasites must have a host to survive, 75, 81–82

head and scalp infections, 235–236

Parasitic disease, disease caused by parasites, such as lice and mites, 75, 78

Parathyroid glands, glands that regulate blood calcium and phosphorus levels so that the nervous and muscular systems can function properly, 138, 139

Parietal artery, supplies blood to the side and crown of the head, 135

Parietal bones, bones that form the sides and top of the cranium, 117

Parietal ridge, widest area of the head, usually starting at the temples and ending at the bottom of the crown, 345

Paronychia, bacterial inflammation of the tissues surrounding the nail causing pus, swelling, and redness, usually in the skin fold adjacent to the nail plate, 212, 214, 215

Part/parting, line dividing the hair at the scalp, separating one section of hair from another, creating subsections, 347

Partial perm, 581

Partnership, business structure in which two or more people share ownership, although not necessarily equally, 1013

Small Business Corporation status *vs.* LLC, 1015

Patch test, also known as a *predisposition test*; test required by the Federal Food, Drug, and Cosmetic Act for identifying a possible allergy in a client, 647

Patella, also known as *accessory bone* or *kneecap*; forms the kneecap joint, 119

Pathogenic, harmful microorganisms that can cause disease or infection in humans when they invade the body, 71–73, 74, 76–81

classifications of, 74–75

description of, 74

entrance to body, 81

principles of prevention, 82–92

Pathogenic disease, disease produced by organisms, including bacteria, viruses, fungi, and parasites, 76–81

entrance to body, 81

principles of prevention, 82–92

Payroll and employee benefits, 1018, 1021–1022

Pectoralis major, muscles of the chest that assist the swinging movements of the arm, 124

Pectoralis minor, muscles of the chest that assist the swinging movements of the arm, 124

Pediculosis capitis, infestation of the hair and scalp with head lice, 81–82, 235–236

Pedicure, a cosmetic service performed on the feet by a licensed cosmetologist or nail technician; can include exfoliating the skin, callus reduction, as well as trimming, shaping, and polishing toenails. Often includes foot massage, 844

disinfection procedures for, 71, 90, 859

elderly clients, 856

ergonomics, 858

interaction during service, 852

massage, 857

pricing, 856

professional pedicure products, 851

proper grip on foot, 853

reflexology, 858

scheduling, 853

series pedicures, 854

spa pedicure, 855

tools, 845

Pedicure chair, 845

Pedicure foot bath, 846

Pedicure professionals, 852

Pedicure slippers, 850

Peptide bond, also known as *end bond*; chemical bond that joins amino acids to each other, end to end, to form a polypeptide chain, 223, 566

Perfectionism, an unhealthy compulsion to do things perfectly, 20

Pericardium, double-layered membranous sac enclosing the heart; made of epithelial tissue, 131

Perimeter, outer line of a hairstyle, 348

Periodic strand testing, 587

Peripheral nervous system, system of nerves that connects the peripheral (outer) parts of the body to the central nervous system; it has both sensory and motor nerves, 126

Permanent haircolors, lighten and deposit color at the same time and in a single process because they are more alkaline than no-lift deposit-only colors and are usually mixed with a higher-volume developer, 638

Permanent waving, a two-step process whereby the hair undergoes a physical change caused by wrapping the hair on perm rods, and then the hair undergoes a chemical change caused by the application of permanent waving solution and neutralizer, 567

basic permanent wrap, 595

bricklay permanent wrap, 601

categories, 576

chemistry of, 571

curl re-forming, 620

curvature permanent wrap, 598

double-rod (piggyback) technique, 605

hydroxide relaxer on virgin hair, 614

hydroxide relaxer retouch, 617

for men, 582

partial perm, 581

preliminary test curl procedure, 593

procedures, 593–620

processing, 576–577

reduction reaction, 571–573

safety precautions, 591–592

selecting the right type, 575

spiral wrap technique, 607

thio neutralization: stages one and two, 578–579

thio relaxer on virgin hair, 610

thio relaxer retouch, 612

types of, 572

underprocessed hair, 577

weave technique, 603

Peroneous brevis, muscle that originates on the lower surface of the fibula and bends the foot down and out, 125

Peroneous longus, muscle that covers the outer side of the calf and inverts the foot and turns it outward, 125

Persians, 11

Personal budget, 994

Personal grooming, 38–39

job interview wardrobe, 978, 979

makeup, 39

Personal hygiene, daily maintenance of cleanliness by practicing good healthful habits, 37

Personal Protective Equipment (PPE), 795

Point cutting, haircutting technique in which the tips of the shears are used to cut *points* into the ends of the hair, 376

Pointed nail, suited to thin hands with long fingers and narrow nail beds. The nail is tapered and longer than usual to emphasize and enhance the slender appearance of the hand, 809

Poison oak, 179

Polarity, negative pole or positive pole of an electric current, 269

Polio, 79

Pollution, premature aging and, 188–189

Polymer, substance formed by combining many small molecules (monomers) into very long chain-like structures, 898

Polymer powder, powder in white, clear pink, and many other colors that is combined with monomer liquid to form the nail enhancement, 898

Polymerization, also known as *curing* or *hardening*; a chemical reaction that creates polymers, 899

Polymerization reaction, 900

Polypeptide chain, long chains of amino acids joined together by peptide bonds, 223, 566

Pomade, also known as *wax*; styling products that add considerable weight to the hair by causing strands to join together, showing separation in the hair, 434

Ponytail, wraparound, 551–552

Popliteal artery, artery that supplies blood to the foot; divides into two separate arteries known as the anterior tibial artery and the posterior tibial artery, 136, 137

Porous, made or constructed of a material that has pores or openings. Porous items are absorbent, 89, 632

Port wine stain, skin discoloration, 183

Position stop, the point where the free edge of the natural nail meets the tip, 875

Posterior auricular artery, supplies blood to the scalp, the area behind and above the ear, and the skin behind the ear, 135, 136

Posterior auricular nerve, affects the muscles behind the ear at the base of the skull, 128, 129

Posterior tibial artery, artery that supplies blood to the ankle and the back of the lower leg, 136

Postpartum alopecia, temporary hair loss experienced at the conclusion of a pregnancy, 231

Posture and body position, 40–42, 364–366

- for manicuring, 831
- for shampooing, 311

Potential hydrogen (pH), the abbreviation used for potential hydrogen. pH represents the quantity of hydrogen ions, 256–258

PPE. *See* Personal Protective Equipment

Practical exam, test format, 962

Prednisone, 714

Pregnancy, 202, 714

Prelightening, first step of double-process haircoloring, used to lift or lighten the natural pigment before the application of toner, 649

Preliminary strand test, 665

Preliminary test curl procedure, 593

Presoftening, process of treating gray or very resistant hair to allow for better penetration of color, 658

Pressed hair, 442

- curling iron for, 437
- soft pressing for normal curly hair, 493
- tempering, heating, and cleaning the comb, 444

Pressure receptor, 164

Pricing. *See* Retailing

Prickley heat, 181

Primary colors, pure or fundamental colors (red, yellow, and blue) that cannot be created by combining other colors, 634

Primary lesions, lesions that are a different color than the color of the skin, and/or lesions that are raised above the surface of the skin, 178

Prioritize, to make a list of tasks that needs to be done in the order of most-to-least important, 26

Procerus muscle, covers the bridge of the nose, lowers the eyebrows, and causes wrinkles across the bridge of the nose, 122, 123

Procrastination, putting off until tomorrow what you can do today, 20

Professional image, the impression you project through both your outward appearance and your conduct in the workplace, 38

- beauty and wellness, 37
- ergonomics and your body, 41–42
- personal grooming, 38–39
- personal hygiene, 37
- physical presentation, 40–42
- wardrobe, 94–95
- "you are what you eat," 221

Professional image of, 68–73, 94–95

Profile, outline of the face, head, or figure seen in a side view, 298–299

Pronators, muscles that turn the hand inward so that the palm faces downward, 124, 125

Propionibacterium acnes (P. acnes), technical term for acne bacteria, 163

Proportion, the comparative relation of one thing to another; the harmonious relationship among parts or things, 290

Protection, as skin function, 163

Protein conditioner, product designed to penetrate the cortex and reinforce the hair shaft from within, 319

Protein hardeners, a combination of clear polish and protein, such as collagen, 805

Protein-dissolving agents, 720

Proteins, long, coiled complex polypeptides made of amino acids, 164–170, 223

of hair, 222–224

Protoplasm, colorless jelly-like substance found inside cells in which food elements such as protein, fats, carbohydrates, mineral salts, and water are present, 113

Pseudomonas aeruginosa, one of several common bacteria that can cause nail infection, 210

Psoriasis, skin disease characterized by red patches covered with silver-white scales; usually found on the scalp, elbows, knees, chest, and lower back, 182

light treatment for, 275

nail, 211, 212, 214

Pterygium, nail, 209, 211

Puberty, 227

Pulmonary circulation, sends the blood from the heart to the lungs to be purified, then back to the heart again, 131, 133

Pure substance, a chemical combination of matter in definite (fixed) proportions, 251

Pus, a fluid created by infection, 76, 178

Pustule, raised, inflamed papule with a white or yellow center containing pus in the top of the lesion referred to as the head of the pimple, 163, 178, 179

Pyogenic granuloma, severe inflammation of the nail in which a lump of red tissue grows up from the nail bed to the nail plate, 212, 215

Pyrithione zinc, 234

Q

Quaternary ammonium compounds, also known as *quats*; disinfectants that are very effective when used properly in the salon, 87

R

Rabies, 79

Radial artery, artery, along with numerous branches, that supplies blood to the thumb side of the arm and the back of the hand; supplies the muscles of the skin, hands, fingers, wrist, elbow, and forearm, 136

Radial nerve, sensory-motor nerve that, with its branches, supplies the thumb side of the arm and back of the hand, 130

Radius, smaller bone in the forearm (lower arm) on the same side as the thumb, 119, 125

Rayon synthetic, 512–513

Razor, haircutting, 354, 379

of bang area, 373–374

Method A, 363

Method B, 363

sharps box, 93

texturizing with, 378–379

Razor rotation, texturizing technique similar to razor-over-comb, done with small circular motions, 379

Razor-over-comb, texturizing technique in which the comb and the razor are used on the surface of the hair, 379

RDA. *See* Recommended daily allowance

RDA Chart for Vitamins and Minerals: Natural Sources, Functions, and Deficiency Symptoms, 168–170

Recommended daily allowance (RDA), 166

Record keeping, maintaining accurate and complete records of all financial activities in your business, 1012

Rectifier, apparatus that changes alternating current (AC) to direct current (DC), 265

Red blood cells, blood cells that carry oxygen from the lungs to the body cells and transport carbon dioxide from the cells back to the lungs, 133

Redding, Jheri, 317

Reducing agent, a substance that adds hydrogen to a chemical compound or subtracts oxygen from the compound, 250

Reduction, the process through which oxygen is subtracted from or hydrogen is added to a substance through a chemical reaction, 250

Reduction reaction, a chemical reaction in which oxygen is subtracted from or hydrogen is added to a substance, 250

Reference points, points on the head that mark where the surface of the head changes or the behavior of the hair changes, such as ears, jawline, occipital bone, apex, and so on; used to establish design lines that are proportionate, 344

Reflective listening, listening to the client and then repeating, in your own words, what you think the client is telling you, 55

Reflex, automatic reaction to a stimulus that involves the movement of an impulse from a sensory receptor along the sensory nerve to the spinal cord. A responsive impulse is sent along a motor neuron to a muscle, causing a reaction (for example, the quick removal of the hand from a hot object). Reflexes do not have to be learned; they are automatic, 127

Reflexology, a unique method of applying pressure with thumb and index fingers to the hands and feet, and it has demonstrated health benefits, 858

Repair patch, piece of fabric cut to completely cover a crack or break in the nail, 878

Reproductive system, body system that includes the ovaries, uterine tubes, uterus and vagina in the female and the testes, prostate gland, penis and urethra in the male. This system performs the function of producing offspring and passing on the genetic code from one generation to another, 116

Resistant, hair type that is difficult for moisture or chemicals to penetrate, and thus requires a longer processing time, 631

Respiration, act of breathing; the exchange of carbon dioxide and oxygen in the lungs and within each cell, 140

Respiratory system, body system consisting of the lungs and air passages; enables respiration, supplying the body with oxygen and eliminating carbon dioxide as a waste product, 116, 120, 140

Resume, written summary of a person's education and work experience, 967

cover letter for, 976

Retailing, the act of recommending and selling products to your clients for at-home use, 996

client retention, 318

commissions on, 991–992

cosmetics, 762,

extra cost for add-on services, 856

hair extensions, 560–561

hair product recommendations, 237

lip colors, 763

marketing to men, 811

Nail Fashion Night, 878

nail products, 806

pedicure pricing, 856

principles of selling, 998–999

psychology of selling, 999–1001

sale of products and additional services, 1028

tips for product sales, 996

Retail supplies, supplies sold to clients, 1019

Retention hyperkeratosis, the hereditary tendency for acne-prone skin to retain dead cells in the follicle, forming an obstruction that clogs follicles and exacerbates inflammatory acne lesions such as papules and pustules, 186

Reticular layer, deeper layer of the dermis that supplies the skin with oxygen and nutrients; contains fat cells, blood vessels, sudoriferous (sweat) glands, hair follicles, lymph vessels, arrector pili muscles, sebaceous (oil) glands, and nerve endings, 158, 159, 172

Reusable implements, also known as *multiuse implements*; implements that are generally stainless steel because they must be properly cleaned and disinfected between clients, 798

Reverse highlighting, also known as *lowlighting*; technique of coloring strands of hair darker than the natural color, 653

Revlon, 8, 11

Rhythm, a regular pulsation or recurrent pattern of movement in a design, 292

Ribboning, technique of forcing the hair between the thumb and the back of the comb to create tension, 424

Ribs, twelve pairs of bones forming the wall of the thorax, 118, 140

Ridge curls, pin curls placed immediately behind or below a ridge to form a wave, 425

Ridges, vertical lines running through the length of the natural nail plate that are caused by uneven growth of the nails, usually the result of normal aging, 209, 211

Ringed hair, variety of canities characterized by alternating bands of gray and pigmented hair throughout the length of the hair strand, 232

Ringworm, 77, 78, 80–81, 210, 235

Risorius muscle, muscle of the mouth that draws the corner of the mouth out and back, as in grinning, 123

Rod, round, solid prong of a thermal iron, 436

Role model, 993

Role-playing, for job interview, 982

Roller curls, 425–429

Rolling, massage movement in which the tissues are pressed and twisted using a fast, 727

Romans, 5

Rope braid, braid created with two strands that are twisted around each other, 514

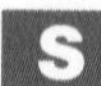

S

Submental artery, supplies blood to the chin and lower lip, 135

Subsections, smaller sections within a larger section of hair, used to maintain control of the hair while cutting, 347

Sudoriferous glands, also known as *sweat glands*; excrete perspiration and detoxify the body by excreting excess salt and unwanted chemicals, 162, 173

Sugaring, temporary hair removal method that involves the use of a thick, sugar-based paste, 695

Sunscreen, 189–190, 721, 807

Superficial peroneal nerve, also known as *musculocutaneous* nerve; extends down the leg, just under the skin, supplying impulses to the muscles and the skin of the leg, as well as to the skin and toes on the top of the foot, where it becomes the dorsal nerve, also known as the dorsal cutaneous nerve, 130

Superficial temporal artery, a continuation of the external carotid nerve artery; supplies blood to the muscles of the front, side, and top of the head, 135

Superior labial artery, supplies blood to the upper lip and region of the nose, 135

Supinator, muscle of the forearm that rotates the radius outward and the palm upward, 125

Supraorbital artery, supplies blood to the upper eyelid and forehead, 134, 135

Supraorbital nerve, affects the skin of the forehead, scalp, eyebrow, and upper eyelid, 128

Supratrochlear nerve, affects the skin between the eyes and upper side of the nose, 129

Sural nerve, supplies impulses to the skin on the outer side and back of the foot and leg, 130

Surfactants, a contraction of *surface active agents*; substances that allow oil and water to mix, or emulsify, 254, 315

Suspensions, unstable physical mixtures of undissolved particles in a liquid, 252

Sweat glands, 138, 141, 162

Sweat pore, 162

Symmetrical balance, two halves of a style; form a mirror image of one another, 291

Synthetic hair, 542

Systemic circulation, also known as *general circulation*; carries the blood from the heart throughout the body and back to the heart, 130, 131

Systemic disease, disease that affects the body as a whole, often due to under-functioning or over-functioning of internal glands or organs. This disease is carried through the blood stream or the lymphatic system, 78

Tactile corpuscles, small epidermal structures with nerve endings that are sensitive to touch and pressure, 159

Tail comb, 354, 511

Talus, also known as *ankle bone*; one of three bones that comprise the ankle joint. The other two bones are the tibia and fibula, 119, 120

Tan, change in pigmentation of skin caused by exposure to the sun or ultraviolet light, 183, 275

skin aging and, 161, 187–188

Taper, haircutting effect in which there is an even blend from very short at the hairline to longer lengths as you move up the head; *to taper* is to narrow progressively at one end, 380

Tapotement, also known as *percussion*; movements consisting of short quick tapping, slapping, and hacking movements, 727

Tarsal, one of three subdivisions of the foot. There are seven bones— talus, calcaneus, navicular, three cuneiform bones, and the cuboid The other two subdivisions are the metatarsal and the phalanges, 119, 120

Teamwork, 988

Telangiectasis, distended or dilated surface blood vessels, 181, 692

Telephone use, 1024–1026

Telogen phase, also known as *resting phase*; the final phase in the hair cycle that lasts until the fully grown hair is shed, 227, 228

Temper, a process used to condition a new brass pressing comb so that it heats evenly, 444

Temporal bones, bones that form the sides of the head in the ear region, 117

Temporal nerve, affects the muscles of the temple, side of the forehead, eyebrow, eyelid, and upper part of the cheek, 128, 129

Temporalis, muscles that coordinate with the masseter, medial pterygoid, and lateral pterygoid muscles to open and close the mouth and bring the jaw forward; sometimes referred to as chewing muscles, 122

Temporary haircolor, nonpermanent color whose large pigment molecules prevent penetration of the cuticle layer, allowing only a coating action that may be removed by shampooing, 637

Tension, amount of pressure applied when combing and holding a section, created by stretching or pulling the section, 364

Terminal hair, long, coarse, pigmented hair found on the scalp, legs, arms, and bodies of males and females, 227, 230

Two-color method, a method whereby two colors of resin are used to overlay the nail, 927

Two-way buffer, 802

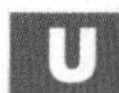

UL. *See* Underwriter's Laboratory

Ulcer, open lesion on the skin or mucous membrane of the body, accompanied by pus and loss of skin depth and possibly weeping fluids or pus, 179, 180

Ulna, inner and larger bone in the forearm (lower arm), attached to the wrist and located on the side of the little finger, 119

Ulnar artery, artery, along with numerous branches, that supplies blood to the muscle of the little-finger side of the arm and palm of the hand, 136

Ulnar nerve, sensory-motor nerve that, with its branches, affects the little-finger side of the arm and palm of the hand, 130

Ultraviolet light (UV light), also known as *cold light* or *actinic light*; invisible light that has a short wavelength (giving it higher energy), is less penetrating than visible light, causes chemical reactions to happen more quickly than visible light, produces less heat than visible light, and kills germs, 89, 161, 167, 272, 274–275

change in skin pigmentation, 183

nail polish dryer, 798

premature aging and, 189

Underhand technique, also known as *plaiting*; a technique in which the left section goes under the middle strand, then the right section goes under the middle strand, 514

Underwriter's Laboratory (UL), 267–268

Uniform layers, hair is elevated to 90 degrees from the scalp and cut at the same length, 370

left-handed, 405

right-handed, 401

Unit wattage, the measure of how much electricity the lamp consumes, 932

Universal Precautions, a set of guidelines published by OSHA that require the employer and the employee to assume that all human blood and body fluids are infectious for bloodborne pathogens, 92–94, 795

Updo, hairstyle in which the hair is arranged up and off the shoulders, 446

braided, and face shapes, 517

Urethane acrylate, a main ingredient used to create UV gel nail enhancements, 926

Urethane methacrylate, a main ingredient used to create UV gel nail enhancements, 926

USDA. *See* Department of Agriculture, U. S.

UV bonding gels, gels used to increase adhesion to the natural nail plate, 928

UV building gels, any thick-viscosity adhesive resin that is used to build an arch and curve to the fingernail, 928

when to use, 931

UV gel, type of nail enhancement product that hardens when exposed to a UV light, 926

maintenance of, 934

removal of, 934

UV gel polish, a very thin-viscosity UV gel that is usually pigmented and packaged in a pot or a polish bottle and used as an alternative to traditional nail lacquers, 928

UV gloss gel, also known as *sealing gel, finishing gel,* or *shine gel*; these gels are used over the finished UV gel application to create a high shine, 929

UV lamp, also known as *UV light bulb*; special bulb that emits UV light to cure UV gel nail enhancements, 932

UV light unit, also known as *UV light*; specialized electronic device that powers and controls UV lamps to cure UV gel nail enhancements, 932

UV self-leveling gels, gels that are thinner in consistency than building gels, allowing them to settle and level during application, 928

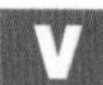

Valves, structures that temporarily close a passage or permit blood flow in only one direction, 131

Veins, thin-walled blood vessels that are less elastic than arteries; veins contain cup-like valves that keep blood flowing in one direction to the heart and prevent blood from flowing backward, 133

Velcro rollers, 428

Vellus hair, also known as *lanugo hair*; short, fine, unpigmented downy hair that appears on the body, with the exception of the palms of the hands and the soles of the feet, 227

Vellus-like hair, 230

Ventricle, a thick-walled, lower chamber of the heart that receives blood pumped from the atrium. There is a right ventricle and a left ventricle, 131–133

Venules, small vessels that connect the capillaries to the veins. They collect blood from the capillaries and drain it into veins, 133

Verruca, also known as *wart*; hypertrophy of the papillae and epidermis, 184

Vertical lines, lines that are straight up and down; create length and height in hair design, 286

Vesicle, small blister or sac containing clear fluid, lying within or just beneath the epidermis, 178, 179

Vibration, in massage, the rapid shaking of the body part while the balls of the fingertips are pressed firmly on the point of application, 728

Victorian Age, 6

Virgin application, first time the hair is colored, 648

Virucidal, capable of destroying viruses, 73

Virus, a parasitic submicroscopic particle that infects and resides in cells of biological organisms. A virus is capable of replication only through taking over the host cell's reproductive function, 79

Viscosity, the measurement of the thickness or thinness of a liquid that affects how the fluid flows, 583

Visible braid, three-strand braid that is created using an underhand technique, 514

Visible spectrum of light, the part of the electromagnetic spectrum that can be seen. Visible light makes up only 35 percent of natural sunlight, 274

Vision statement, a long-term picture of what the business is to become and what it will look like when it gets there, 1010

Vitamins, 164–167

RDA Chart, 168–170

Vitamin A, supports the overall health of the skin; aids in the health, function, and repair of skin cells; has been shown to improve the skin's elasticity and thickness, 166

Vitamin C, an important substance needed for proper repair of the skin and tissues; promotes the production of collagen in the skin's dermal tissues; aids in and promotes the skin's healing process, 167

Vitamin D, enables the body to properly absorb and use calcium, the element needed for proper bone development and maintenance. Vitamin D also promotes rapid healing of the skin, 167 275

Vitamin E, helps protect the skin from the harmful effects of the sun's UV light, 167

Vitiligo, hereditary condition that causes hypopigmented spots and splotches on the skin; may be related to thyroid conditions, 183

VOCs. *See* **Volatile organic compounds**

Volatile alcohols, alcohols that evaporate easily, 255

Volatile organic compounds (VOCs), compounds that contain carbon (organic) and evaporate very easily (volatile), 256

Volt (V), also known as *voltage*; unit that measures the pressure or force that pushes electric current forward through a conductor, 266

Volume, measures the concentration and strength of hydrogen peroxide, 639

Volume-base curls, thermal curls placed very high on their base; provide maximum lift or volume, 439

Volumizer, styling product that adds volume, especially at the base, when wet hair is blown dry, 434

W. *See* **Watt**

W/O emulsion. *See* Water-in-oil

Wall plate, also known as *facial stimulator*; instrument that plugs into an ordinary wall outlet and produces various types of electric currents that are used for facial and scalp treatments, 269

Wardrobe, for job interview, 978, 979

Warm colors, range of colors from yellow and gold through oranges, red-oranges, most reds, and even some yellow-greens, 768

Wart, 178, 184

Water-binding agents, 721

Water-in-oil (W/O) emulsion, water droplets emulsified in oil, 254

Watt (W), unit that measures how much electric energy is being used in one second, 266

Wave pattern, the shape of the hair strands; described as straight, wavy, curly, and extremely curly, 225–227, 288, 352–353

chemically altered, 288–289

Waveform, measurement of the distance between two wavelengths, 273

Wavelength, distance between successive peaks of electromagnetic waves, 273, 276

Waving lotion, type of hair gel that makes the hair pliable enough to keep it in place during the finger-waving procedure, 421

Wavy hair, 287–288

Weave technique, wrapping technique that uses zigzag partings to divide base areas, 580, 603–604

Weaving, interweaving a weft or faux hair with natural hair, 510; **coloring technique in which selected strands are picked up from a narrow section of hair with a zigzag motion of the comb, and lightener or color is applied only to these strands**, 654

Web resources, 974, 991

Wefts, long strips of human or artificial hair with a threaded edge, 544,

Weight line, visual line in the haircut, where the ends of the hair hang together, 366

Wet bead, 901

Wet set with rollers, 428, 461

Wet styling basics, 421

Wheal, itchy, swollen lesion that lasts only a few hours; caused by a blow or scratch, the bite of an insect, urticaria (skin allergy), or the sting of a nettle. Examples include hives and mosquito bites, 178, 179

White blood cells, also known as *white corpuscles* or *leukocytes*; blood cells that perform the function of destroying disease-causing bacteria, 134

White spots, on nails, 208

Whorl, hair that forms in a circular pattern on the crown of the head, 240

Wide-tooth comb, 354, 382

Wig, artificial covering for the head consisting of a network of interwoven hair, 544. *See also* Hair extensions

- basic types, 544–545
- block, 546
- cleaning of, 318, 549
- coloring and hair additions, 549
- curling iron for, 437
- cutting, 546–547
- hairpieces, 550–553
- human *vs.* synthetic hair, 541–542
- Look Good . . . Feel Better Foundation, 232, 541
- methods of construction, 545
- putting on, 546
- quality and cost, 543–544
- special tools, 550
- styling, 547–548
- taking measurements, 545–546
- tips for styling the hairline, 548–549

Willatt, Arnold F., 10

Wooden pusher, a wooden stick used to remove cuticle tissue from the nail plate (by gently pushing), to clean under the free edge of the nail, or to apply products, 800

Work ethic, taking pride in your work and committing yourself to consistently doing a good job for your clients, employer, and salon team, 965

Wraparound ponytail, 552

Wrap resin accelerator, also known as *activator*; acts as the dryer that speeds up the hardening process of the wrap resin or adhesive overlay, 876

Wringing, vigorous movement in which the hands, placed a little distance apart on both sides of the client's arm or leg, working downward apply a twisting motion against the bones in the opposite direction, 727

Wrinkle therapies, 277

Wrist inflammation, 118

Written agreements, documents that govern the opening of a salon, including leases, vendor contracts, employee contracts, and more; all of which detail, usually for legal purposes, who does what and what is given in return, 1011

- drawing up a lease, 1016

Yak, 513, 543

Yarn, as hair adornment, 513

Yellow fever, 79

Yellow nails, 829

Z

Zygomatic bones, also known as *malar bones* or *cheekbones*; bones that form the prominence of the cheeks, 117–118

Zygomatic nerve, affects the muscles of the upper part of the cheek, 129

Zygomaticus major muscles, muscles on both sides of the face that extend from the zygomatic bone to the angle of the mouth. These muscles pull the mouth upward and backward, as when you are laughing or smiling, 123

Zygomaticus minor muscles, muscles on both sides of the face that extend from the zygomatic bone to the upper lips. These muscles pull the upper lip backward, upward, and outward, as when you are smiling, 123